A TEXTBOOK OF

Medicine

Edited by

RUSSELL L. CECIL, M.D., Sc.D.

Professor of Clinical Medicine Emeritus, Cornell University, New York

ROBERT F. LOEB, M.D., Sc.D., D. Hon. Causa., LL.D.

Bard Professor of Medicine, Columbia University, New York

Associate Editors

ALEXANDER B. GUTMAN, M.D., Ph.D.

Professor of Medicine, Columbia University, New York

WALSH McDERMOTT, M.D.

Livingston Farrand Professor of Public Health and Preventive Medicine, Cornell University, New York

HAROLD G. WOLFF, M.D.

Professor of Medicine (Neurology), Cornell University, New York

Ninth Edition, Illustrated

W. B. SAUNDERS COMPANY

Philadelphia, London · *1955*

Preface to the Ninth Edition

Year by year Internal Medicine continues to make rapid advances, and to meet this constant change, textbooks of medicine must progress also. In this, the Ninth Edition, the Editors have tried to reflect the many strides which have taken place in medicine during the past four years. Again we have emphasized the physiologic and biochemical aspects of disease and we still believe that this important part of modern medicine can best be covered by combining physiology and biochemistry with the actual description of the disease rather than by presenting them in a separate section of the book.

The Ninth Edition contains the following articles on subjects which have not been covered in previous editions:

Melanosis .... Dr. Alexander B. Gutman

Carotenemia .... Dr. Franklin M. Hanger

Portal Hypertension .... Dr. Arthur J. Patek

Pulmonary Arteriovenous Fistula .... Dr. Dickinson W. Richards

Cystic Disease of the Lungs .... Dr. Herbert C. Maier

Asbestosis .... Dr. William S. McCann

Acute Nonspecific Pericarditis .... Dr. Johnson McGuire

Senile Heart Disease (Presbycardia) ...... Dr. Hugh Morgan

Introduction to Diseases of the Muscles..... Dr. Joseph L. Lilienthal, Jr.

The Painful Shoulder
    Calcific Tendinitis
    Adhesive Peritendinitis
    Arthritis of the Shoulder
    Shoulder-Hand Syndrome .... Dr. Russell L. Cecil

Hyperostosis Frontalis Interna .... Dr. Walter Bauer

Hemiplegia .... Dr. Louis Hausman

Delirium .... Dr. Desmond Curran

The Dementias .... Dr. William H. Dunn

Nonpurulent Meningitis .... Dr. Chester H. Keefer

Developmental Anomalies of the Cervico-
    medullary Juncture .... Dr. Bronson S. Ray

Petrositis .... Dr. A. Earl Walker

In addition to this new material, the retirement or death of a number of former contributors has necessitated the preparation of fifty-eight new treatises on subjects previously covered. There have been several transpositions of material: Bartonellosis (Carrion's Disease) has been transferred from Rickettsial Diseases to Bacillary Diseases. Hepatolenticular Degeneration, Familial Periodic Paralysis and Phenylpyruvic Oligophrenia have been moved from the section on Nervous Diseases to the section on Inborn Errors of Metabolism. The Dystrophies have been transposed from Diseases of the Nervous System to Diseases of the Muscles.

It is with deepest regret that the Editors must report the death of seven contributors: Drs. William DeWitt Andrus, Francis G. Blake, William H. Dunn, George M. Mackenzie, Wilbur A. Sawyer, James Stevens Simmons and Williard O. Thompson.

The Editors wish to extend their sincere thanks to the distinguished contributors who have written for this Ninth Edition. Their cooperation has been of the greatest aid in editing the new edition. We also wish to express our appreciation to the officers and staff of the W. B. Saunders Company for their constant help and advice. Grateful acknowledgment is due to Mrs. Natalie J. Hoyt, for proofreading, editorial work and the preparation of an exceptionally comprehensive index.

THE EDITORS

June 1955

Contributors

RAYMOND D. ADAMS, M.A., M.D., M.A. (Hon.)
Myelitis; Acute Idiopathic Polyneuritis
Bullard Professor of Neuropathology, Harvard University; Chief of Neurology Service, Massachusetts General Hospital, Boston.

FULLER ALBRIGHT, M.D.
Introduction to Diseases of the Ductless Glands
Associate Professor, Harvard University Medical School; Physician, Massachusetts General Hospital, Boston.

HARRY L. ALEXANDER, M.D.
Contact Dermatitis; Revision of Angioneurotic Edema; Urticaria; Purpura; Erythemas
Emeritus Professor of Clinical Medicine, Washington University Medical School; Associate Physician, Barnes Hospital, St. Louis.

HATTIE E. ALEXANDER, M.D.
Hemophilus Influenzae Infections; Hemophilus Ducreyi Infections
Associate Professor in Pediatrics, College of Physicians and Surgeons, Columbia University; Attending Pediatrician, Babies Hospital and Vanderbilt Clinic, New York.

THOMAS PATTISON ALMY, M.D., F.A.C.P.
Regional Ileitis
Associate Professor of Medicine, Cornell University Medical College; Visiting Physician and Director, Second (Cornell) Medical Division, Bellevue Hospital; Associate Attending Physician, The New York Hospital; Assistant Attending Physician, Memorial Cancer Center; Consultant in Medicine, Manhattan Veterans Administration Hospital, New York.

BERNARD J. ALPERS, M.D., Sc. D. Med.
Diseases of the Motor Tracts
Professor of Neurology, Jefferson Medical College; Neurologist, Jefferson Hospital; Consulting Neurologist, Pennsylvania Hospital, Philadelphia.

AFRÂNIO do AMARAL, M.D., D. Hyg. (Trop. Med.) (Harvard)
Snake Venom Poisoning
Professor, Escola Paulista de Medicina, São Paulo (ret.); Postgraduate Course in Experimental Pathology, Instituto Butantan and University of São Paulo; General Director, Instituto Butantan (incl. Vital Brazil Hospital); Chief, Department of Ophiology and Medical Zoology, Instituto Butantan, São Paulo, Brazil.

J. BURNS AMBERSON, M.D.
Tuberculosis
Professor of Medicine, College of Physicians and Surgeons, Columbia University; Visiting Physician in Charge, Chest Service, Bellevue Hospital, New York.

DANA W. ATCHLEY, M.D.
The Nephroses; Uremia
Professor of Clinical Medicine, College of Physicians and Surgeons, Columbia University; Visiting Physician, Presbyterian Hospital, New York.

GEORGE BAEHR, M.D., F.A.C.P.
Disseminated Lupus Erythematosus
Formerly Clinical Professor of Medicine, Columbia University; Consulting Physician, Mount Sinai Hospital, New York.

A. B. BAKER, M.S., M.D., Ph.D.
Scalenus Anticus Syndrome; Neuromas
Professor of Neurology, University of Minnesota Medical School; Chief of the Neurological Service, University of Minnesota Hospitals, Minneapolis.

JANET S. BALDWIN, M.D., F.A.A.P.
Congenital Heart Disease
Associate Professor of Pediatrics, New York University-Bellevue Medical Center; Chief, Children's and Adolescents' Cardiac Clinic, Bellevue Hospital; Attending Physician and Chief, Children's Cardiac Clinic, Lenox Hill Hospital, New York.

ALVAN L. BARACH, M.D., F.A.C.P.
Motion Sickness
Clinical Professor of Medicine, College of Physicians and Surgeons, Columbia University; Associate Attending Physician, Presbyterian Hospital, New York.

JOHN B. BARNWELL, M.D., Sc.D. (Hon.)
Pleurisy; Pleural Effusion; Pneumothorax; Uncommon Pleural Affections
Formerly Associate Professor of Internal Medicine, University of Michigan Medical School; Director, Tuberculosis Service, U.S. Veterans Administration, Washington, D. C.

DAVID P. BARR, M.D., Sc.D., LL.D.
Atherosclerosis; Xanthomatosis; Diseases of the Thyroid Gland
Professor of Medicine, Cornell University

Medical College; Physician-in-Chief, New York Hospital; Consulting Physician, Bellevue Hospital, New York.

FREDERIC C. BARTTER, M.D.
Diseases of the Parathyroid Gland; Osteoporosis; Fragilitas Ossium; Osteomalacia; Osteitis Fibrosa Cystica Generalisata; Fibrous Dysplasia of Bone; Osteitis Deformans; Leontiasis Ossea; Dyschondroplasia; Achondroplasia; Oxycephaly; Hyperostosis Frontalis Interna; Hypertrophic Osteoarthropathy
Chief, Section on Clinical Endocrinology, Clinic of General Medicine and Experimental Therapeutics, National Heart Institute, National Institutes of Health, Bethesda, Md.

WALTER BAUER, M.D., F.A.C.P.
Osteoporosis; Fragilitas Ossium; Osteomalacia; Osteitis Fibrosa Cystica Generalisata; Fibrous Dysplasia of Bone; Osteitis Deformans; Leontiasis Ossea; Dyschondroplasia; Achondroplasia; Oxycephaly; Hyperostosis Frontalis Interna; Hypertrophic Osteoarthropathy
Jackson Professor of Clinical Medicine, Harvard University Medical School; Chief of Medical Services, Massachusetts General Hospital, Boston.

PAUL B. BEESON, M.D., C.M.
Typhoid Fever; The Leptospiroses
Professor of Medicine and Chairman of the Department of Internal Medicine, Yale University School of Medicine; Physician-in-Chief, University Service, Grace-New Haven Community Hospital, New Haven, Conn.

ROBERT W. BERLINER, M.D.
Dehydration and Fluid Balance: Physiological Principles
Associate Director (In Charge of Research), National Heart Institute, National Institutes of Health, Bethesda, Md.

HERRMAN L. BLUMGART, M.D.
Diseases of the Coronary Arteries
Professor of Medicine, Harvard University Medical School; Physician-in-Chief, Beth Israel Hospital, Boston.

WILLIAM L. BRADFORD, M.D.
Pertussis
Professor of Pediatrics, University of Rochester School of Medicine and Dentistry; Pediatrician-in-Chief, Strong Memorial Hospital and Rochester Municipal Hospital, Rochester, N. Y.

RANDOLPH K. BYERS, M.D.
Lead Poisoning
Assistant Clinical Professor of Pediatrics, Harvard Medical School; Neurologist, Children's Medical Center, Boston.

ANNE C. CARTER, M.D.
Diseases of the Female Gonads
Assistant Professor of Medicine, Cornell University Medical College; Assistant Attending Physician, New York Hospital, New York.

WILLIAM B. CASTLE, M.S. (Hon.), M.D., M.D. (Hon.), S.D. (Hon.), F.A.C.P.
Introduction to Diseases of the Blood; The Anemias; Hemorrhagic Diseases; Polycythemia
Professor of Medicine, Harvard University; Director, Thorndike Memorial Laboratory; Director, Second and Fourth Medical Services, Boston City Hospital, Boston.

RUSSELL L. CECIL, M.D., Sc.D., F.A.C.P.
Miliary Fever; Ainhum; Milk Sickness; Diseases of the Joints
Professor of Clinical Medicine, Emeritus, Cornell University Medical College; Attending Physician, Bellevue Hospital; Consulting Physician, New York Hospital, New York.

F. SARGENT CHEEVER, M.D.
Diphtheria; Bacillary Dysentery
Professor of Microbiology, Graduate School of Public Health, University of Pittsburgh; Lecturer in Bacteriology, School of Medicine, University of Pittsburgh.

CHARLES G. CHILD, 3RD, M.D., F.A.C.S.
Diseases of the Pancreas
Professor of Surgery, Tufts College Medical School; Director, First Surgical Service (Tufts), Boston City Hospital; Consultant in Surgery, New England Center Hospital, Boston.

STANLEY COBB, M.D., D.Sc.
Psychosomatic Medicine
Bullard Professor of Neuropathology, Emeritus, Harvard University; Consultant, Massachusetts General Hospital, Boston.

L. T. COGGESHALL, M.D., F.A.C.P.
Malaria
Rawson Professor of Medicine, Dean of Division of Biological Sciences, Director of University Clinics, University of Chicago.

BRADLEY L. COLEY, M.D., F.A.C.S.
Tumors of Bone
Associate Professor of Clinical Surgery, Cornell University Medical College; Attending Surgeon, Memorial Hospital, New York.

KENDALL B. CORBIN, M.D.
Cervical and Lumbosacral Radiculitis, Including the Syndrome Due to Displacement of an Intervertebral Disk
Professor of Neurology, Mayo Foundation, University of Minnesota Graduate School; Consultant, Section of Neurology, Mayo Clinic, Rochester, Minn.

DESMOND CURRAN, M.D. (Camb.), F.R.C.P. (Lond.), D.P.M.
Delirium
St. George's Hospital Medical School, University of London; Senior Consultant Psychiatrist, St. George's Hospital, London, England.

G. M. DACK, M.D., Ph.D.
Food Poisoning
Professor of Microbiology, University of Chicago.

WORTH B. DANIELS, M.D., F.A.C.P.
Cat Scratch Disease
Clinical Professor of Medicine, Georgetown University School of Medicine; Senior Consultant in Medicine, Veterans Administration Hospital; Attending Physician, Emergency Hospital, Washington, D.C.

MARGARET DANN, M.D., Ph.D., F.A.A.P.
Phenylpyruvic Oligophrenia
Assistant Professor of Pediatrics, Cornell University Medical College; Associate Attending Pediatrician, New York Hospital, New York.

ROBERT C. DARLING, M.D.
Heat Exhaustion, Heat Stroke and Heat Cramps; Decompression Illness; Blast Injury
Professor of Physical Medicine and Rehabilitation, College of Physicians and Surgeons, Columbia University; Director and Attending Physician, Physical Medicine and Rehabilitation Service, Presbyterian Hospital, New York.

MICHAEL E. DeBAKEY, M.D., M.S., F.A.C.S.
Intestinal Obstruction; Intestinal Neoplasms; Affections of the Mesentery
Professor and Chairman, Department of Surgery, Baylor University College of Medicine; Surgeon-in-Chief, Jefferson Davis and Methodist Hospitals, Houston, Texas.

ARTHUR CHRISTIAN DeGRAFF, M.D., F.A.C.P.
Neurocirculatory Asthenia; Carotid Sinus Syncope
Professor of Therapeutics, New York University College of Medicine; Visiting Physician, Bellevue Hospital; Attending Physician, University Hospital, New York University-Bellevue Medical Center; Senior Consultant in Medicine, Bronx Veterans Administration Hospital, New York.

DEREK DENNY-BROWN, A.M. (Lond.), M.D., Ph.D., F.R.C.P.
Hepatolenticular Degeneration; Hereditary Chorea; Familial Spastic Paralysis; Progressive Familial Neuritic Atrophies; Dystonia Musculorum Deformans; Combined System Disease; Paralysis Agitans; Tic and Torticollis
Putnam Professor of Neurology, Harvard University Medical School; Neurologist-in-Chief and Director of Neurological Unit, Boston City Hospital, Boston.

LEWIS DEXTER, M.D., F.A.C.P.
Toxemia of Pregnancy; Vascular Hypertension; Vascular Hypotension
Assistant Professor of Medicine and Tutor in Medicine, Harvard University Medical School; Physician, Peter Bent Brigham Hospital; Consultant in Medicine, Children's Medical Center, Boston.

FRANCIS R. DIEUAIDE, M.D.
Cholera; Plague; Leishmaniasis
Scientific Director, The Life Insurance Medical Research Fund; Clinical Professor of Medicine, Columbia University, New York; Formerly Professor of Medicine and Head of Department of Medicine, Peiping Union Medical College, China.

JOHN H. DINGLE, M.D., Sc.D.
Meningococcal Infections
Professor of Preventive Medicine and Associate Professor of Medicine, School of Medicine, Western Reserve University; Associate Physician, University Hospitals; Senior Consultant in Medicine, Crile Veterans Administration Hospital, Cleveland.

CHARLES AUSTIN DOAN, M.D., F.A.C.P.
Diseases of the Spleen
Dean and Professor of Medicine, Director of Medical Research, Ohio State University College of Medicine; Director, the University Hospitals, Ohio State University.

WILLIAM H. DUNN, M.D.
The Dementias
Late Associate Professor of Clinical Psychiatry, Cornell University Medical College; Late Associate Attending Psychiatrist, New York Hospital, New York.

DAVID P. EARLE, M.D., Med. Sc.D.
Epidemic Hemorrhagic Fever
Professor of Medicine, Northwestern University Medical School, Chicago.

GEORGE LIBMAN ENGEL, M.D.
Syncope
Associate Professor of Psychiatry and Medicine, University of Rochester School of Medicine and Dentistry; Associate Psychiatrist and Associate Physician, Strong Memorial and Rochester Municipal Hospitals, Rochester, N. Y.

JOHN B. ERICH, M.S., D.D.S., M.D., F.A.C.S.
Diseases of the Mouth, Salivary Glands and Pharynx
Associate Professor of Plastic Surgery, Graduate School, University of Minnesota; Head of Department of Plastic Surgery, Mayo Clinic, Rochester, Minn.

ERNEST CARROLL FAUST, M.A., Ph.D.
Sporozoan Infections; Toxoplasmosis; Ciliate Infections; Sarcosporidiosis; The Platyhelminthes; The Nematoda; Trichocephaliasis; Strongyloidiasis; Creeping Eruption; Ascariasis; Visceral Larva Migrans; Enterobiasis; Filariasis; Dracunculosis; Arthropods and Human Disease; Arthropods as Causative Agents of Disease; Arthropods as Mechanical Carriers or Essential Hosts
William Vincent Professor of Tropical Diseases and Hygiene, and Head, Division of Parasitology, Department of Tropical Medicine and

Public Health, Tulane University, New Orleans. Parasitologist, Hutchinson Memorial Clinic; Resident Consultant, Armed Forces Institute of Pathology.

CLEMENT A. FINCH, M.D.
Hemochromatosis
Associate Professor of Medicine, University of Washington School of Medicine; Attending Physician, King County Hospital and Veterans Administration Hospital, Seattle.

MAXWELL FINLAND, M.D.
Klebsiella Infections (Friedländer's Bacillus)
Associate Professor of Medicine, Harvard University Medical School; Chief, Fourth Medical Service, Boston City Hospital; Associate Director, Thorndike Memorial Laboratory, Boston.

LLOYD FLORIO, M.D., D.P.H., F.A.C.P.
Colorado Tick Fever
Professor and Head, Department of Preventive Medicine, University of Colorado School of Medicine; Manager, Health and Hospitals, City of Denver; Consultant, Denver General Hospital, Children's Hospital, Denver.

LEROY D. FOTHERGILL, M.D.
Equine Encephalomyelitis
Camp Detrick, Frederick, Md.

GEORGE DAVIS GAMMON, M.D., F.A.C.P.
Diphtheritic Polyneuritis; Acroparesthesia
Chairman, Department of Neurology, and Professor of Clinical Neurology, University of Pennsylvania; Hospital of the University of Pennsylvania; Neurologist, Children's Hospital; Consultant, Veterans Administration Hospital, Philadelphia.

FRANK GLENN, M.D.
Diseases of the Peritoneum
Lewis Atterbury Stimson Professor of Surgery, Cornell University Medical College; Surgeon-in-Chief, New York Hospital, New York.

IRVING GORDON, M.D.
Acute Infectious Nonbacterial Gastroenteritis
Associate Professor of Medicine and Bacteriology, Albany Medical College; Assistant Director, Division of Laboratories and Research, New York State Department of Health; Associate Attending Physician, Albany Hospital, Albany, N.Y.

WALLACE GRAHAM, M.D., M.R.C.P. (Lond.), F.R.C.P., (Can.)
The Fibrositis Syndrome
Assistant Professor of Medicine, University of Toronto, Faculty of Medicine; Attending Physician, Toronto General Hospital; Consultant and Chief of Arthritis Service, Sunnybrook Veterans Hospital.

ASHTON GRAYBIEL, A.M., M.D., F.A.C.C.
Aviation Medicine
Director of Research, U.S. Naval School of Aviation Medicine, Pensacola, Fla.

ALEXANDER B. GUTMAN, M.A., Ph.D., M.D., F.A.C.P.
Inborn Errors of Metabolism; The Lipomatoses; Amyloidosis; Melanosis and Melanuria
Professor of Medicine, College of Physicians and Surgeons, Columbia University; Director, Department of Medicine, Mount Sinai Hospital, New York.

THOMAS HALE HAM, M.D., F.A.C.P.
Hemoglobinuria and Myohemoglobinuria
Professor of Medicine, School of Medicine, Western Reserve University; Physician, University Hospitals, Cleveland.

FRANKLIN M. HANGER, M.D.
Introduction to Diseases of the Liver; Jaundice
Professor of Medicine, College of Physicians and Surgeons, Columbia University; Attending Physician, Presbyterian Hospital, New York.

KENDRICK HARE, Ph.D., M.D.
Diabetes Insipidus
Professor of Pediatrics and Pharmacology, Medical College of Alabama, Birmingham.

GEORGE T. HARRELL, M.D., F.A.C.P.
Trichinosis
Professor of Medicine and Dean, College of Medicine, University of Florida, Gainesville.

A. McGEHEE HARVEY, M.D., F.A.C.P.
Dermatomyositis; Polyarteritis; Progressive Systemic Sclerosis; Scleredema; Diseases of the Thymus Gland; Myasthenia Gravis
Professor of Medicine, Johns Hopkins University; Physician-in-Chief, Johns Hopkins Hospital, Baltimore.

LOUIS HAUSMAN, M.D.
Hemiplegia
Professor of Clinical Medicine (Neurology), Cornell University Medical College; Clinical Professor of Neuropsychiatry, New York University College of Medicine; Director of the Neurological Service, Second (Cornell) Medical Division, Bellevue Hospital, New York.

JOSEPH H. HAYMAN, JR., M.D.
Non-Parasitic Chyluria; Pneumaturia; Anomalies and Malformations of the Kidneys; Circulatory Disturbances of the Kidneys; Nephroptosis; Hydronephrosis; Bacterial Infections of the Kidney and Urinary Passages; Nephrolithiasis; Cysts of the Kidney; Tumors of the Kidney
Dean and Professor of Medicine, Tufts College Medical School; Senior Physician, New England Center Hospital, Boston.

CLYDE A. HEATLY, M.D., F.A.C.S.
Diseases of the Nose; Diseases of the Larynx
Associate Professor of Surgery in Charge of Otolaryngology, University of Rochester School of Medicine; Otolaryngologist-in-Chief, Strong Memorial and Municipal Hospitals; Consultant, Rochester General, Highland, and Genesee Hospitals, Rochester, N.Y.

PHILIP S. HENCH, M.D., Sc.D., LL.D., F.A.C.P.
Gout and Gouty Arthritis
Professor of Medicine, University of Minnesota (Mayo Foundation); Senior Consultant, Department of Rheumatic Diseases, Mayo Clinic, Rochester, Minn.

THOMAS H. HOLMES, M.D.
Muscle Spasms, Professional Cramp and Backache
Associate Professor of Psychiatry, University of Washington School of Medicine; Attending Physician, King County Hospital; Psychiatric Consultant, Firland Sanatorium; Attending Staff, Veterans Administration Hospital, Seattle; Consultant in Neuropsychiatry, Bremerton Naval Hospital.

FRANK L. HORSFALL, JR., M.D., C.M.
Introduction to Viral Diseases; Influenza; Herpes Simplex; Herpes Zoster; Psittacosis; Encephalitis Lethargica; St. Louis Encephalitis; Postinfection Encephalitis
Member, The Rockefeller Institute for Medical Research; Physician, Hospital of The Rockefeller Institute, New York.

ROBERT J. HUEBNER, M.D.
Coxsackie Viral Infections
Associate Professor of Medicine, Georgetown University School of Medicine; Medical Director, U.S. Public Health Service; Chief, Virus Section, L.I.D., National Microbiological Institute, Bethesda, Md.

THOMAS HARRISON HUNTER, M.D.
Endocarditis
Professor of Medicine and Dean, School of Medicine, University of Virginia, Charlottesville, Va.

HARRIS ISBELL, M.D., F.A.C.P.
Barbiturate Poisoning; Opium Poisoning; Cocaine Poisoning; Chronic Poisoning with Sympathomimetic Amines
Lecturer in Pharmacology, University of Cincinnati Medical School; Director, National Institute of Health Addiction Research Center, U.S. Public Health Service Hospital, Lexington, Ky.

LEON O. JACOBSON, M.D.
Radiation Injury
Professor of Medicine, University of Chicago; Director, Argonne Cancer Research Hospital, University of Chicago.

CHARLES A. JANEWAY, M.D.
Lymphocytic Choriomeningitis; Salmonellosis Other than Typhoid Fever; Infections with the Coliform, Proteus and Pseudomonas Groups of Bacilli
Thomas Morgan Rotch Professor of Pediatrics, Harvard University Medical School; Physician-in-Chief, Infants' and Children's Hospitals; Consultant in Infectious Diseases, Peter Bent Brigham Hospital; Pediatrician, Boston Lying-in Hospital, Boston.

GEORGE A. JERVIS, M.D., Ph.D.
Mental Deficiency
Instructor in Psychiatry, Columbia University; Director of Laboratories, Letchworth Village, New York State Department of Mental Hygiene.

FREDERICK A. JOHANSEN, M.D., F.A.C.P.
Leprosy
Medical Director, U.S. Public Health Service (Ret.); Formerly Medical Officer in Charge, U.S. Public Health Service Hospital (National Leprosarium), Carville, Louisiana; Member, Medical Advisory Board, Leonard Wood Memorial, (American Leprosy Foundation); Member, World Health Organization Expert Advisory Panel on Leprosy.

CHESTER M. JONES, M.D., D.Sc.
Diseases of the Esophagus
Clinical Professor of Medicine, Harvard University School of Medicine; Consulting Visiting Physician, Massachusetts General Hospital, Boston.

ELVIN A. KABAT, Ph.D.
Introduction to Diseases of Allergy
Professor of Microbiology (Assigned to Neurology), College of Physicians and Surgeons, Columbia University, and Neurological Institute, Presbyterian Hospital, New York.

CHESTER S. KEEFER, M.S., M.D., F.A.C.P.
Introduction to Bacterial Diseases; Meningitis
Wade Professor of Medicine, Boston University School of Medicine; Director, Evans Memorial Hospital; Physician-in-Chief, Massachusetts Memorial Hospitals, Boston.

ALLAN T. KENYON, M.D.
Diseases of the Pituitary Gland
Professor of Medicine, University of Chicago.

J. AUSTIN KERR, M.D.
Yellow Fever
Staff Member, Division of Medicine and Public Health, The Rockefeller Foundation, New York.

EDWIN D. KILBOURNE, M.D.
Measles; Rubella
Associate Professor of Medicine and Director of Division of Infectious Disease, Tulane-University of Louisiana School of Medicine; Attending Physician, Charity Hospital; Consultant, Veterans Administration Hospital, New Orleans.

WILLIAM M. M. KIRBY, M.D.
Gonococcal Infections
Associate Professor of Medicine, University of Washington School of Medicine, Seattle.

PAUL KLEMPERER, M.D.
Introduction to Collagen Diseases
Pathologist, Mount Sinai Hospital; Professor of Pathology, College of Physicians and Surgeons, Columbia University, New York.

WALTER O. KLINGMAN, M.D.
Acute Chorea
Professor of Neurology and Psychiatry, School of Medicine, University of Virginia; Chief of Neurology, Department of Neurology and Psychiatry, University of Virginia Hospital, Charlottesville.

YALE KNEELAND, Jr., M.D., F.A.C.P.
Common Upper Respiratory Disease
Associate Professor of Medicine, Columbia University; Attending Physician, Presbyterian Hospital; Clinical Director, Columbia Service, Goldwater Memorial Hospital, New York; Consulting Physician, Sharon (Conn.) Hospital and St. Francis Hospital, Poughkeepsie, N.Y.

HILARY KOPROWSKI, M.D.
Rabies
Assistant Director, Viral and Rickettsial Research, American Cyanamid Company, Pearl River, N.Y.; Member of the Expert Committee on Rabies, World Health Organization, Geneva, Switzerland.

E. CHARLES KUNKLE, M.D. F.A.C.P.
Diseases of Nerve Roots, Plexuses and Nerves; Neuritis
Associate Professor of Medicine (in Charge of Neurology), Duke University School of Medicine; Assistant Physician, Duke Hospital, Durham, N.C.

PAUL H. LAVIETES, M.D.
Acidosis; Alkalosis
Associate Clinical Professor of Medicine, Yale University School of Medicine; Attending Physician, Grace-New Haven Community Hospital, New Haven, Conn.

JOHN S. LAWRENCE, M.D., F.A.C.P.
Infectious Mononucleosis
Professor of Medicine, University of California at Los Angeles; Consultant in Internal Medicine, Wadsworth Veterans Administration Hospital and Harbor County General Hospital; Honorary Consultant, Santa Monica Hospital; Honorary Staff Member, St. John's Hospital, Santa Monica, Cal.

WILLIAM GORDON LENNOX, M.A., M.D., ScD. (Hon.)
Epilepsy
Associate Professor of Neurology (Emeritus), Harvard University; Chief of Seizure Division, Children's Medical Center, Boston.

SAMUEL Z. LEVINE, M.D.
Phenylpyruvic Oligophrenia
Professor of Pediatrics, Cornell University Medical College; Pediatrician-in-Chief, New York Hospital, New York.

THEODORE LIDZ, M.D.
Causalgia
Professor of Psychiatry, Yale University School of Medicine; Psychiatrist-in-Chief, Yale Psychiatric Institute; Psychiatrist-in-Chief, University Services to the Grace-New Haven Community Hospital; Consultant, Veterans Administration Hospital, West Haven, Conn.

JOSEPH L. LILIENTHAL, Jr., M.D.
Enterogenous Cyanosis; Introduction to Diseases of the Muscles
Professor of Environmental Medicine, Associate Professor of Medicine, Johns Hopkins University; Physician, Johns Hopkins Hospital, Baltimore.

ROBERT F. LOEB, M.D., ScD., D. *hon. causa,* LL.D.
Diabetes Mellitus; Spontaneous Hypoglycemia; Nephritis
Bard Professor of Medicine, College of Physicians and Surgeons, Columbia University; Director of Medical Service, Presbyterian Hospital, New York.

JOHN A. LUETSCHER, Jr., M.D.
Urinary Suppression
Associate Professor of Medicine, Stanford University School of Medicine, San Francisco.

CYRIL M. MacBRYDE, M.D., F.A.C.P.
Obesity
Associate Professor of Clinical Medicine, Washington University School of Medicine; Assistant Physician, Barnes Hospital; Director, Metabolism and Endocrine Clinics, Washington University Clinics; Attending Physician, St. Luke's Hospital; Chief, Department of Medicine, St. Joseph Hospital, St. Louis.

GEORGE M. MACKENZIE, M.D.
Late Director, Mary Imogene Bassett Hospital, Cooperstown, N.Y.

JOHN D. MacLENNAN, M.D.
Histotoxic Infections
Assistant Professor of Microbiology, College of Physicians and Surgeons, Columbia University, New York.

HERBERT C. MAIER, M.D., M.S., Med. Sc.D., F.A.C.S.
Abscess of the Lung; Cystic Disease of the Lungs; New Growths in the Lungs
Assistant Clinical Professor of Surgery, Columbia University; Director of Surgery, Lenox Hill Hospital; Visiting Surgeon, Bellevue Hospital; Associate Surgeon, Presbyterian Hospital, New York.

DONALD D. MATSON, M.D., F.A.C.S.
Internal Hydrocephalus; Birth Injuries of the Central Nervous System
Assistant Professor of Surgery, Harvard University Medical School; Neurosurgeon, Children's Medical Center; Senior Associate in Neurosurgery, Peter Bent Brigham Hospital, Boston.

WILLIAM S. McCANN, M.D., D.Sc. (Hon.), LL.D. (Hon.), F.A.C.P.
Pneumonconiosis
Charles A. Dewey Professor of Medicine, University of Rochester School of Medicine; Physician-in-Chief, Strong Memorial and Rochester Municipal Hospitals, University of Rochester Medical Center, Rochester, N.Y.

MACLYN McCARTY, M.D.
Rheumatic Fever
Member, Rockefeller Institute for Medical Research; Physician, Hospital of The Rockefeller Institute, New York.

WILLIAM J. McCONNELL, M.D.
Mountain Sickness; Electric Shock; Carbon Monoxide Poisoning; Carbon Tetrachloride Poisoning; Benzene Poisoning; Chronic Bromide Poisoning; Arsenic Poisoning; Mercury Poisoning; Beryllium Poisoning
Associate Professor, New York University School of Management; Associate Medical Director, Metropolitan Life Insurance Co., New York.

WALSH McDERMOTT, M.D.
Foot-and-Mouth Disease; Syphilis
Livingston Farrand Professor of Public Health and Preventive Medicine, Cornell University Medical College; Attending Physician, New York Hospital-Cornell Medical Center, New York.

JOHNSON McGUIRE, M.S., M.D., F.A.C.P.
Diseases of the Pericardium
Professor of Clinical Medicine, University of Cincinnati College of Medicine; Director, Cardiac Laboratory and Cardiac Clinic; Visiting Physician, Cincinnati General Hospital, Cincinnati, Ohio.

RUSTIN McINTOSH, M.D.
Vitamin C Deficiency
Carpentier Professor of Pediatrics, Columbia University; Director of Pediatric Service, Babies Hospital, Presbyterian Hospital, New York.

GORDON MEIKLEJOHN, M.D., C.M.
Mumps
Professor of Medicine, University of Colorado School of Medicine; Chief of Medical Service, Colorado General Hospital and Denver General Hospital, Denver.

HENRY EDMUND MELENEY, M.D.
Hookworm Disease
Research Professor of Medicine, School of Medicine, Louisiana State University; Visiting Physician, Charity Hospital of Louisiana, New Orleans.

H. HOUSTON MERRITT, M.D.
Affections of the Blood Vessels of the Spinal Cord; Cerebral Hemorrhage; Cerebral Thrombosis; Cerebral Embolus; Management of Cerebral Vascular Accidents; Common Syndromes of Cerebral Vascular Accidents;

Vascular Lesions of the Brain Stem; Pseudobulbar Palsy; Cerebral Venous Lesions; Subdural Hematoma
Professor of Neurology, College of Physicians and Surgeons, Columbia University; Director of Service of Neurology, Neurological Institute, Presbyterian Hospital, New York.

KARL F. MEYER, M.D., Ph.D.
Tularemia; Glanders; Anthrax
Professor of Experimental Pathology, Emeritus, and Director, Emeritus, Hooper Foundation, University of California Medical Center, San Francisco.

WILLIAM S. MIDDLETON, M.D., Sc.D., M.A.C.P., F.R.C.P. (Lond.)
Sarcoidosis
Professor of Medicine and Dean, University of Wisconsin Medical School; Physician, University Hospitals, Madison, Wis.

A. T. MILHORAT, M.D.
Familial Periodic Paralysis; The Dystrophies
Associate Professor of Medicine in Psychiatry, Cornell University Medical College; Attending Physician, New York Hospital, New York.

CARL V. MOORE, M.D., F.A.C.P.
Diseases of the Reticuloendothelial System; The Leukopenic State and Agranulocytosis
Professor of Medicine, Washington University School of Medicine; Associate Physician, Barnes and Allied Hospitals, St. Louis.

HUGH J. MORGAN, M.D., D.Sc. (Hon.), M.A.C.P.
Syphilitic Aortitis and Aneurysm; Diseases of the Myocardium; Arteriosclerosis
Professor of Medicine, Vanderbilt University School of Medicine; Physician-in-Chief, Vanderbilt University Hospital, Nashville, Tenn.

CARL MUSCHENHEIM, M.D., F.A.C.P.
Bronchiectasis; Foreign Bodies in the Bronchi; Diseases of the Mediastinum; Diseases of the Diaphragm
Associate Professor of Clinical Medicine, Cornell University Medical College; Attending Physician, New York Hospital, New York.

ELLIOT V. NEWMAN, M.D.
Renal Physiology and Tests of Renal Function
Professor of Experimental Medicine, Vanderbilt University School of Medicine, Nashville, Tenn.

JOHANNES MAAGAARD NIELSEN, M.D.
Aphasia
Clinical Professor of Medicine (Neurology), University of Southern California; Senior Attending Neurologist (Chairman of Staff), Los Angeles General Hospital; Attending Neurologist, Good Samaritan Hospital, Los Angeles; National Consultant in Aphasia, Area Consultant in Neurology and Psychiatry, Veterans Administration; Senior Consultant in Neurology, Methodist Hospital, Los Angeles.

WALTER LINCOLN PALMER, M.S., M.D., Ph.D.,
F.A.C.P.
*Diseases of the Stomach; Diseases of the Duo-
denum; Visceroptosis; Diarrhea; Constipation; Irritable Colon; Dilatation of the
Colon; Diverticula of the Intestines; Ulcerative Colitis*
Richard T. Crane Professor of Medicine, University of Chicago School of Medicine, Chicago.

ALTON OCHSNER, M.D., D.Sc. (Hon.), F.A.C.S.
*Intestinal Obstruction; Intestinal Neoplasms; Af-
fections of the Mesentery*
William Henderson Professor of Surgery and
Chairman of the Department of Surgery, Tu-
lane-University of Louisiana School of Med-
icine; Director, Section on Surgery, Ochsner
Clinic and Ochsner Foundation Hospital;
Senior Visiting Surgeon and Surgeon-in-Chief,
Tulane Surgical Service at Charity Hospital;
Senior Surgeon, Touro Infirmary; Consultant
in Thoracic Surgery, Veterans Administration
Hospital and Eye, Ear, Nose and Throat Hos-
pital; Attending Specialist in Chest Surgery,
U.S. Public Health Service Hospital; Consult-
ing Surgeon, Illinois Central Hospital, New
Orleans.

ARTHUR J. PATEK, Jr., M.D.
*Circulatory Disturbances of the Liver; Ascites;
Cirrhosis of the Liver; Abscess of the Liver;
Neoplasms of the Liver; Cysts of the Liver;
Fatty Liver*
Associate Clinical Professor of Medicine, Col-
lege of Physicians and Surgeons, Columbia
University; Research Fellow, Goldwater Me-
morial Hospital; Assistant Attending Physician,
Presbyterian Hospital; Medical Consultant, St.
Barnabas Hospital, New York.

JOHN R. PAUL, A.M. (Hon.), M.D., F.A.C.P.
Poliomyelitis
Professor of Preventive Medicine, Yale Uni-
versity School of Medicine; Associate Physi-
cian, Grace-New Haven Community Hospital;
Consultant to the Meriden (Conn.) Hospital.

HENRY PINKERTON, M.D.
Trench Fever; Bartonellosis
Professor of Pathology, St. Louis University
School of Medicine; Pathologist-in-Chief, St.
Mary's Group of Hospitals, St. Louis.

FRED PLUM, M.D.
*Syringomyelia; Facial Hemiatrophy; Hemifacial
Spasm*
Assistant Professor of Medicine (Neurology),
University of Washington School of Medicine;
Attending Neurologist, King County, U.S. Vet-
erans, and Children's Orthopedic Hospitals,
Seattle.

WILLIAM B. PORTER, M.D., F.A.C.P.
Miscellaneous Pathologic Conditions of the Heart
Professor of Medicine and Chairman of the
Department, Medical College of Virginia; Hos-
pital Division, Medical College of Virginia,
Richmond.

CHARLES H. RAMMELKAMP, Jr., M.D.
*Introduction to Staphylococcal Infections; Fu-
runcles and Carbuncles; Staphylococcal
Pneumonia; Osteomyelitis; Staphylococcal
Bacteremia*
Professor of Medicine, Western Reserve University School of Medicine, Cleveland; Director
of Research Laboratories, Cleveland City Hospital; Director, Streptococcal Disease Laboratory, Warren Air Force Base, Wyoming.

LOWELL A. RANTZ, M.D.
Scarlet Fever
Associate Professor of Medicine, Stanford Uni-
versity School of Medicine, San Francisco.

ISIDOR S. RAVDIN, M.D.
Appendicitis
John Rhea Barton Professor of Surgery, Uni-
versity of Pennsylvania; Professor of Surgery,
Graduate School of Medicine, University of
Pennsylvania; Surgeon-in-Chief, Hospital of
the University of Pennsylvania, Philadelphia.

BRONSON S. RAY, M.D., Sc.D. (Hon.), F.A.C.S.
*Tumors of the Spinal Cord and Spinal Canal; De-
velopmental Anomalies of the Cervicomedul-
lary Juncture*
Professor of Clinical Surgery, Cornell University Medical College; Chief, Department of
Neurosurgery, and Attending Surgeon (Neurosurgery), New York Hospital, New York.

THOMAS A. C. RENNIE, M.D.
*Alcoholism; Methyl Alcohol Poisoning; Mari-
huana Intoxication; The Psychoneuroses*
Professor of Psychiatry (Social Psychiatry),
Cornell University Medical College; Attending
Psychiatrist, New York Hospital, New York;
Consultant in Psychiatry, Franklin Delano
Roosevelt Veterans Administration Hospital,
Montrose, N.Y.

DICKINSON W. RICHARDS, M.D., F.A.C.P.
*Bronchitis; Pulmonary Function in Health and
Disease; Circulatory Disturbances in the
Lungs; Pulmonary Atelectasis; Pulmonary
Fibrosis; Radiation Pleuropneumonitis;
Lipoid Pneumonitis; Allergic Pneumonia;
Emphysema*
Lambert Professor of Medicine, College of
Physicians and Surgeons, Columbia University;
Director and Visiting Physician, First (Colum-
bia University) Medical Division, Bellevue
Hospital; Attending Physician, Presbyterian
Hospital, New York.

HARRY M. ROSE, M.D.
*Pneumonia Due to Filterable Agents; Neurotoxic
Infections*
John E. Borne Professor of Medical and Sur-
gical Research, and Executive Officer of the
Department of Microbiology, College of Physi-
cians and Surgeons, Columbia University; At-
tending Microbiologist, Presbyterian Hospital,
New York.

GEORGE A. SCHUMACHER, M.D.
Multiple Sclerosis
Professor of Neurology, University of Vermont College of Medicine; Attending Neurologist, Mary Fletcher Hospital, Bishop DeGoesbriand Hospital, Burlington, Vt.

VIRGIL SCOTT, M.D.
Lymphogranuloma Venereum
Professor of Medicine, American University of Beirut, Beirut, Lebanon; Formerly Associate Professor of Medicine and Preventive Medicine, Washington University Medical School, St. Louis.

WILLIAM B. SHERMAN, M.D., F.A.C.P.
Hay Fever; Asthma
Associate Clinical Professor of Medicine, College of Physicians and Surgeons, Columbia University; Attending Physician, Roosevelt Hospital; Assistant Attending Physician, Presbyterian Hospital, New York.

HOWARD B. SHOOKHOFF, M.D., D.T.M. & H. (Lond.)
Amebiasis
Assistant Professor of Tropical Medicine, Columbia University (School of Public Health of the Faculty of Medicine); Assistant Attending Physician, Presbyterian Hospital; Attending Physician, Tropical Diseases, Beth David Hospital; Consultant, Tropical Medicine, St. Albans Naval Hospital, New York.

EPHRAIM SHORR, M.D.
Diseases of the Female Gonads
Associate Professor of Medicine, Cornell University Medical College; Attending Physician, New York Hospital, New York.

JAMES S. SIMMONS, M.D., Ph.D., D.P.H., Sc.D. (Hon.)
Relapsing Fever
Late Dean and Professor of Public Health, Harvard University School of Public Health, Boston.

DONALD J. SIMONS, M.D.
Narcolepsy
Associate Professor of Clinical Medicine (Neurology), Cornell University Medical College; Associate Attending Physician, New York Hospital; Associate Visiting Neuropsychiatrist, Bellevue Hospital, New York.

CHARLES H. SLOCUMB, M.S., M.D.
Myositis
Professor of Medicine, The Mayo Foundation for Medical Education and Research, Graduate School, University of Minnesota; Consultant in Medicine, Mayo Clinic, St. Mary's Hospital, Rochester, Minn.

JOSEPH E. SMADEL, M.S. (Hon.), M.D.
Rocky Mountain Spotted Fever; Scrub Typhus; Rickettsialpox
Chief, Department of Virus and Rickettsial Diseases, and Director, Communicable Diseases

Division, Army Medical Service Graduate School, Walter Reed Army Medical Center, Washington, D.C.

DAVID T. SMITH, M.D.
The Mycoses
Professor of Bacteriology and Associate Professor of Medicine, Duke University School of Medicine, Durham, N.C.

JOHN C. SNYDER, M.D.
Introduction to Rickettsial Diseases; The Typhus Group; Q Fever
Professor of Microbiology, Harvard University School of Public Health, Boston; Consultant on Virus and Rickettsial Diseases for the Veterans Administration.

HARRY C. SOLOMON, M.D., F.A.P.A.
Syphilis of the Central Nervous System
Professor of Psychiatry, Harvard University Medical School; Medical Director, Boston Psychopathic Hospital, Boston.

TOM D. SPIES, M.D., F.A.C.P.
Hypervitaminosis; Vitamin A Deficiency; Vitamin B Deficiencies; Vitamin E Deficiency; Vitamin K Deficiency; Mixed Deficiency Diseases
Professor and Chairman of Department of Nutrition and Metabolism, Northwestern University Medical School, Chicago; Director, Nutrition Clinic, Hillman Hospital, Birmingham, Alabama.

WESLEY W. SPINK, M.D., Sc.D., F.A.C.P.
Introduction to Streptococcal Infections; Acute Tonsillitis; Peritonsillar Abscess; Erysipelas; Brucellosis
Professor of Medicine, University of Minnesota Medical School, Minneapolis; Staff Physician, University of Minnesota Hospitals; Consulting Physician, Minneapolis General Hospital and Minneapolis Veterans Administration Hospital.

EUGENE A. STEAD, Jr., M.D., F.A.C.P.
Pathologic Physiology of Generalized Circulatory Failure; Cardiac Dilatation and Hypertrophy; The Treatment of Congestive Heart Failure; Circulatory Collapse and Shock
Professor of Medicine, Duke University School of Medicine; Physician-in-Chief and Chairman, Department of Medicine, Duke Hospital, Durham, N.C.

J. MURRAY STEELE, M.D.
Alcaptonuria and Ochronosis
Professor of Medicine, New York University College of Medicine; Director, New York University Research Service, Goldwater Memorial Hospital, New York.

LEWIS D. STEVENSON, M.D.
Malformations of the Brain Meninges and Spinal Cord; Little's Disease; Hereditary Hemiplegia; Hereditary Spinal Ataxia; Hereditary Cerebellar Ataxia
Professor of Clinical Neurology, Cornell Uni-

versity Medical College; Associate Professor of Neuropathology, Cornell University Medical College and New York University College of Medicine; Associate Neuropsychiatrist, Bellevue Hospital; Attending Neurologist, French Hospital, New York; Consulting Neurologist, New York Hospital, Westchester Division, White Plains, N.Y.

HAROLD J. STEWART, M.A., M.D., F.A.C.P.
Cardiac Arrhythmias
Associate Professor of Medicine, Cornell University Medical College; Attending Physician, New York Hospital; Head of Subdepartment of Cardiology of Department of Medicine, New York Hospital-Cornell University Medical Center, New York.

JOSEPH STOKES, JR., M.D., Sc.D.
Varicella; Smallpox; Vaccinia
William H. Bennett Professor of Pediatrics, School of Medicine, University of Pennsylvania; Physician-in-Chief, Children's Hospital of Philadelphia; Chairman, Pediatric Clinic, Hospital of the University of Pennsylvania, Philadelphia.

CYRUS C. STURGIS, M.D.
The Leukemias
Professor of Internal Medicine, Chairman of Department of Internal Medicine, Director of Simpson Memorial Institute for Medical Research, University of Michigan, Ann Arbor.

RAMON M. SUAREZ, M.D., Sc.D. (Hon.), F.A.C.P.
Sprue
Director, Fundación de Investigaciones Clinicas; Internist, Hospital Mimiya, Santurce; Consultant, Veterans Administration, U.S. Army, Presbyterian Hospitals, P.R.

V. P. SYDENSTRICKER, M.A., M.D., M.A.C.P.
Dengue
Professor of Medicine, Medical College of Georgia, Augusta; Physician-in-Chief, University Hospital; Consultant, V.A. Hospital, Augusta; Consultant, Milledgeville State Hospital; Consultant, Battey State Hospital, Rome, Ga.

W. H. TALIAFERRO, Ph.D., Sc.D., LL.D.
Trypanosomiasis
Eliakim H. Moore Distinguished Service Professor of Microbiology and Chairman of the Department of Microbiology, University of Chicago, Chicago.

LEWIS THOMAS, M.D.
Drug Allergy; Serum Sickness
Professor and Chairman, Department of Pathology, New York University-Bellevue Medical Center, New York.

WILLARD OWEN THOMPSON, M.D., F.A.C.P.
Diseases of the Male Gonads
Late Clinical Professor of Medicine, University of Illinois College of Medicine; Attending

Physician, Grant Hospital; Attending Physician, Senior Staff, Henrotin Hospital; Attending Physician, University of Illinois Research and Educational Hospitals, Chicago.

GEORGE W. THORN, M.D.
Diseases of the Adrenal Glands
Hersey Professor of the Theory and Practice of Physic, Harvard University Medical School; Physician-in-Chief, Peter Bent Brigham Hospital, Boston.

WILLIAM S. TILLETT, M.D., Sc.D. (Hon.)
Empyema
Professor of Medicine, New York University College of Medicine; Director and Visiting Physician, Third (N.Y.U.) Medical Division, Bellevue Hospital, New York.

THOMAS B. TURNER, M.D.
Nonsyphilitic Treponematoses; Yaws; Bejel; Pinta; Rat-Bite Fever
Professor of Microbiology, Lecturer in Medicine, Johns Hopkins University, Baltimore.

A. EARL WALKER, M.D., LL.D. (Hon.), F.A.C.S.
Intracranial Tumors; Intracranial Abscesses
Professor of Neurological Surgery, Johns Hopkins University; Neurological Surgeon-in-Charge, Johns Hopkins Hospital, Baltimore.

CECIL J. WATSON, M.D., Ph.D., F.A.C.P.
Porphyria; Diseases of the Gallbladder and Bile Ducts
Professor and Head, Department of Medicine, University of Minnesota; Chief of Medical Service, University of Minnesota Hospital, Minneapolis.

A. ASHLEY WEECH, M.D.
Vitamin D Deficiency
B. K. Rachford Professor of Pediatrics, University of Cincinnati College of Medicine; Medical Director, The Children's Hospital; Director, The Children's Hospital Research Foundation; Director, Pediatric-Contagious Division, Cincinnati General Hospital, Cincinnati, Ohio.

JOHN C. WHITEHORN, M.D.
The Psychoses
Professor of Psychiatry, Johns Hopkins University; Psychiatrist-in-Chief, Johns Hopkins Hospital, Baltimore.

ROBERT W. WILKINS, M.D., F.A.C.P.
General Considerations in Diseases of the Peripheral Vessels. Peripheral Vascular Diseases Due to Organic Arterial Obstruction; Peripheral Vascular Diseases Due to Abnormal Vasoconstriction or Vasodilatation; Peripheral Vascular Diseases Due to Exposure to Cold; Peripheral Vascular Diseases Due to Abnormal Communications between Arteries and Veins; Diseases of the Peripheral Veins; Diseases of the Peripheral Lymphatic Vessels

CONTRIBUTORS

Associate Professor of Medicine, Boston University School of Medicine; Member, Robert Dawson Evans Memorial and Massachusetts Memorial Hospitals; Visiting Physician, Massachusetts Memorial Hospital, Boston.

GEORGE ANTHONY WOLF, Jr., M.D., F.A.C.P.
Spontaneous Subarachnoid Hemorrhage
Dean and Professor of Clinical Medicine, University of Vermont College of Medicine; Attending, Mary Fletcher Hospital; Consulting, Bishop DeGoesbriand Hospital, Burlington, Vt.

HAROLD G. WOLFF, M.D.
Headache
Professor of Medicine (Neurology), Cornell University Medical College; Attending Physician, New York Hospital; Consultant, Neurology, Veterans Administration.

FRANCIS C. WOOD, M.D., F.A.C.P.
Rheumatic Heart Disease; Chronic Valvular Heart Disease
Professor of Medicine and Chairman of the Department, University of Pennsylvania School of Medicine; Chief of Medical Clinic and Director of the Robinette Foundation for the Study of Cardiovascular Disease, Hospital of the University of Pennsylvania, Philadelphia.

JOHN R. WOOD, M.S., M.D., Sc.D. (Hon.),
Colonel, Medical Corps, U.S. Army
War Gases
Commandant, Army Medical Service Graduate School, Walter Reed Army Medical Center, Washington, D.C.

W. BARRY WOOD, Jr., M.D., F.A.C.P.
Pneumococcal Pneumonia; Other Forms of Acute Bacterial Pneumonia
Busch Professor of Medicine, Washington University School of Medicine; Physician-in-Chief, Barnes and Wohl Hospitals, St. Louis.

JOHN B. YOUMANS, M.S., M.D., F.A.C.P.
Introduction to Deficiency Diseases; Undernutrition
Professor of Medicine, Vanderbilt University School of Medicine; Visiting Physician, Vanderbilt University Hospital, Nashville, Tenn.

HARRY F. ZINSSER, Jr., M.D., A.A.C.P.
Rheumatic Heart Disease; Chronic Valvular Heart Disease
Assistant Professor of Medicine, University of Pennsylvania Medical School; Staff Member of Medical Clinic and Member of Robinette Foundation for the Study of Cardiovascular Disease, Hospital of the University of Pennsylvania; Consultant in General Medicine, Veterans Administration Hospital, Philadelphia.

Contents

THE INFECTIOUS DISEASES

CONTENTS

THE MYCOSES

SPIROCHETAL INFECTIONS

DISEASES DUE TO CHEMICAL AGENTS

DEFICIENCY DISEASES

DISEASES OF METABOLISM

DISEASES OF THE DUCTLESS GLANDS

DISEASES OF THE DIGESTIVE SYSTEM

DISEASES OF THE RESPIRATORY SYSTEM

DISEASES OF THE KIDNEYS

DISEASES OF THE SPLEEN AND RETICULOENDOTHELIAL SYSTEM

DISEASES OF THE BLOOD

DISEASES OF THE CARDIOVASCULAR SYSTEM

DISEASES OF THE LOCOMOTOR SYSTEM

DISEASES OF THE NERVOUS SYSTEM

IMPORTANT SYMPTOMS AND SIGNS

DISEASES OF THE MOTOR TRACTS

HEREDITARY, FAMILIAL AND CONGENITAL DISEASES

CONTENTS   xxxiii

The Infectious Diseases

VIRAL DISEASES

INTRODUCTION

Infectious diseases are usually classified according to the kind of infectious agent which induces them. The clinical manifestations of these various diseases differ widely, and the agents which cause them are also dissimilar. The following groups of infectious agents are recognized: protozoa, fungi, bacteria, rickettsiae and viruses. These causal agents have a single property in common: all are capable of multiplication in an appropriate environment. The degree of their structural differention as well as their size decreases from the protozoa to the viruses in the order given; viruses are the smallest of known agents capable of inducing infectious disease. One or another of the pathogenic agents included among the viruses is either known or believed to be the primary cause of each of fifty different infectious diseases of man. These are:

B virus infection	Infectious hepatitis and
Colorado tick fever	serum hepatitis
Common cold	Infectious mononucleosis
Dengue	Infectious polyneuritis
Encephalitis lethargica	Influenza (A, B and C)
Encephalitis, Japanese	Kerato-conjunctivitis
type B	Louping ill
Encephalitis, Murray	Lymphocytic choriomen-
Valley type	ingitis
Encephalitis, Russian	Lymphogranuloma vene-
type	reum
Encephalitis, St. Louis	Measles
type	Molluscum contagiosum
Encephalitis, West Nile	Mumps
type	Newcastle disease
Encephalomyocarditis	Ovine pustular der-
Epidemic pleurodynia	matitis
Equine encephalomyeli-	Pappataci fever
tis, Eastern	Poliomyelitis
Equine encephalomyeli-	Primary atypical pneu-
tis, Venezuelan	monia
Equine encephalomyeli-	Pseudolymphocytic chori-
tis, Western	omeningitis
Equine infectious anemia	Psittacosis
Exanthem subitum	Rabies
Foot-and-mouth disease	Rift Valley fever
Hemorrhagic meningo-	Rubella
encephalitis	Smallpox
Herpes simplex	Trachoma
Herpes zoster	Vaccinia
Inclusion conjunctivitis	Varicella
Infections due to Cox-	Warts
sackie viruses	Yellow fever

The nature of viruses is not yet definitely known, but certain facts appear well established. Viruses are particulate entities, which can be visualized by sufficiently powerful instruments, e.g., the electron microscope. Multiplication of viruses occurs under suitable conditions in the presence of living cells, but in the absence of living cells no virus has as yet shown any evidence of multiplication. Discontinuous variation has been observed with certain ones. Viruses differ widely in size, stability and degree of apparent structural differentiation.

The smallest viruses (with dimensions of 10 to 28 millimicrons)—e.g., those responsible for foot-and-mouth disease and poliomyelitis —are particles only slightly larger than serum globulin molecules and are actually considerably smaller than the hemocyanin molecules of certain animal species. The largest viruses (with dimensions of 225 to 400 millimicrons) —e.g., those of psittacosis and vaccinia—are but little smaller than certain bacteria and are, in fact, larger than pleuropneumonia organisms. Between these two extremes the viruses form an almost unbroken series in regard to their size; at one end the dimensions of viruses overlap those of protein molecules, at the other those of living micro-organisms. Vigorous discussion has centered around the question: Are viruses living or nonliving entities? Viruses have certain properties which are usually attributed to living things, as well as certain others which are usually associated with nonliving things, and there is as yet no satisfactory basis upon which to determine the relative viability or nonviability of these infectious agents. At the present time it is convenient to think of viruses as obligate intracellular parasites of very small size.

The pathologic changes resulting from infections by viruses depend primarily upon alterations in cell metabolism which are induced by the presence of a virus; the nature of such metabolic aberrations is not known. It is known that different viruses affect the same cells in different ways, and it is well established that certain viruses selectively attack different types of cells. Consequently it would be expected that viral diseases might present exceedingly diverse clinical manifestations and that the ultimate pathologic changes would be dissimilar. This is, in fact, the case, as will be evident from a consideration of the foregoing list of widely different infectious diseases, each of which is either known or believed to be induced by a particular virus. The primary pathologic phenomena common to all viral diseases appear to be the following: hyperplasia, hyperplasia accompanied by necrosis, and necrosis. Some viral diseases are characterized by the occurrence of inclusion bodies in affected cells; others do not show these peculiar morphologic elements. The exudative phenomena commonly associated with inflammation occur in varying degrees in most viral diseases, but are thought to be secondary to the changes induced by the virus in cells of the infected tissues.

An enduring immunity develops after many but not all viral diseases (those not followed by persistent immunity are common cold, influenza and herpes simplex). This phenomenon serves additionally to distinguish viral infections from diseases caused by most other infectious agents. The basis for the lasting immunity which follows most viral diseases is not known. It is thought that changes induced as a result of the intimate association between virus and infected cell, or the prolonged, possibly persistent, presence of some viruses in infected hosts, may account for the continuing immunity. It is because of the prolonged active immunity of many viral diseases that specific prophylactic measures have been so effective in protecting against some of them, e.g., smallpox and yellow fever.

At the present time almost no effective specific therapeutic measures have been devised for viral diseases. However, some diseases caused by the largest of known viruses—e.g., the psittacosis-lymphogranuloma venereum group—appear to be favorably influenced by various chemotherapeutic substances. Therapy with specific antiserum apparently is of no value once clinical manifestations of the infection have ensued, since by this time the virus is widely disseminated in the infected tissues and most, if not all, susceptible cells have already been affected. During the incubation period, that is, before wide dissemination of the virus has occurred, specific immune serum appears to be useful as a preventive measure in a few viral diseases, e.g., measles.

FRANK L. HORSFALL, JR.

References

Boycott, A. E.: The Transition from Live to Dead: the Nature of Filtrable Viruses. Proc. Roy. Soc. Med. (Path. Sect.), 22:55, 1928–29.
Burnet, F. M.: Virus as Organism. Cambridge, Harvard University Press, 1945.
Dale, H. H.: The Biological Nature of the Viruses. Nature, 128:599, 1931.
Goodpasture, E. W.: Etiological Problems in the Study of Filterable Virus Diseases. The Harvey Lectures, 25:77, 1929–30.
Rivers, T. M.: Pathologic and Immunologic Problems in the Virus Field. Am. J. M. Sc., 190:435, 1935.
———: Viral and Rickettsial Infections of Man. Philadelphia, J. B. Lippincott Company, 1952.
———, and others: Virus Diseases. Ithaca, N. Y., Cornell University Press, 1943.
Stanley, W. M.: The Isolation and Properties of Tobacco Mosaic and Other Virus Proteins. The Harvey Lectures, 33:170, 1937–38.

COMMON UPPER RESPIRATORY DISEASE

(The Common Cold; Acute Undifferentiated Respiratory Disease; Nonstreptococcal Exudative Pharyngitis)

The term, "common upper respiratory disease," is used to denote a group of infections of the upper respiratory tract, presumably of viral origin, which are world-wide in distribution, and to which the human race is almost universally susceptible. Common respiratory disease is by all odds the most widespread of all infections, and is a leading cause of minor incapacitation and absence from work. It is not an entity, but rather a diagnostic residuum after the exclusion of disease caused by such recognizable agents as the influenza viruses or streptococci.

Extensive studies in the U. S. Army during World War II by the Commission on Acute Respiratory Disease resulted in a certain degree of redefinition and clarification of the components entering into common respiratory disease, and the scheme thus evolved will be followed here. The subject will be presented under three headings: The Common Cold; Acute Undifferentiated Respiratory Disease; and Nonstreptococcal Exudative Pharyngitis.

THE COMMON COLD

(Acute Coryza)

Definition. The common cold is an acute inflammation of the upper respiratory tract which is ordinarily communicable and caused by a filterable virus. Such terms as "acute rhinitis," "pharyngitis" and "laryngitis" have often been used to denote the area chiefly involved.

Etiology. Kruse, in 1914, was the first to adduce evidence of a filterable virus in colds. These observations were considerably extended by Dochez and his co-workers, who repeatedly demonstrated the presence of a filterable agent in acute coryza capable of causing colds when introduced into an anthropoid ape or a susceptible human volunteer, and succeeded in cultivating it in tissue culture medium and the developing chick embryo. These filterable agents were obtained early in the course of the coryzal type of cold, and the experimental disease had a short incubation period of twelve to forty-eight hours. Some observers have been unable to cultivate the cold virus, but in recent years Atlas reported success in a large series of transmission experiments, and actually used a biochemical test to determine growth of the agent in allantoic fluids. Moreover, C. H. Andrewes in England, after a long series of unsuccessful attempts at artificial cultivation, has now reported positive results using embryonal lung as part of the culture medium. There seems little doubt, therefore, that a filterable virus of the common cold exists and presumably is the causative agent in the great majority of cases, notably of the epidemic type. A great deal, however, still remains to be elucidated. It is not known how many different cold viruses there are; there is no precise information as to how long the virus is carried in the respiratory tract, or what the conditions of transmission may be; and little knowledge concerning the immunity to colds is available. Moreover, it cannot be said with certainty that under certain conditions the common respiratory pathogenic bacteria do not initiate colds, although the evidence is against this possibility. Studies of small, isolated communities, such as those conducted by Paul and Freese in Spitzbergen, imply that, in the absence of the virus, the common cold almost wholly disappears. Presumably the residuum of sporadic, noncommunicable colds may be due to bacterial infection.

In spite of extensive investigation for many decades, the exact role of the bacterial inhabitants of the nasopharynx is not clear. Most students agree that a considerable part of the so-called "basal flora" of the upper respiratory tract consists of nonpathogenic and inconsequential agents. In this category would be placed the various Neisserieae, diphtheroids, nonhemolytic streptococci, most of the staphylococci, and so on. On the other hand, hemolytic streptococci, pneumococci and *Hemophilus influenzae* are proved respiratory pathogens, and, when they are recovered in considerable numbers from a patient with a cold, it is tempting to assume that they are playing a role of some sort. Undoubtedly, hemolytic streptococci can initiate exudative pharyngitis without any assistance from a filterable virus, as evidenced by the food- and milk-borne outbreaks of this disease. Perhaps *H. influenzae* can, in unusual circumstances, do the same sort of thing, as in "Woodside throat," which was described in the Australian Army at the outbreak of the last war. On the other hand, any of these organisms may appear in the normal nasopharynx without causing symptoms, and the mere recovery of one of them from a case of coryza may be of little significance. Most authors tend to designate them as "secondary invaders," assuming that the cold virus paves the way for their entry into the mucous membranes. Yet when effective chemotherapeutic agents have been used in large-scale controlled experiments on adults with colds, there is little evidence that suppression of the bacterial component alters the average duration of the disease. Perhaps the best way to define the activity of the bacteria is in relation to the susceptibility of the population under scrutiny. Infants and small children, together with certain remote rural populations (note Burkey's and Smillie's experience in Labrador and Alabama), appear to be much more susceptible to the activity of these bacteria than do adults in urban localities. In all likelihood, secondary infection with pathogenic bacteria in the young age and rural groups does intensify the local inflammation of the mucous membranes and heighten the constitutional reaction as well as prolongs the course. Support for this view is derived from the fact that antibiotics do seem to modify the severity of colds in children, in contrast to the adult experience cited before. Thus it appears that most colds in adults, unless they are accompanied by a purulent complication such as sinusitis or otitis, are probably not much affected by the mere presence of a bacterial pathogen.

In summary, it can be stated that the common cold is due to one or more filterable viruses and that only in highly susceptible persons is there an "etiologic complex," i.e., a bacterium acting in concert with a virus. The bacterial effect may be either the general intensification of symptoms already referred to or a clear-cut complication, such as purulent sinusitis or otitis.

It is to be noted that in the foregoing no reference has been made to chilling and exposure as factors in the etiology of colds. This may be surprising, since the very name of the malady presupposes an important etiologic relationship. Moreover, it is mainly a disease of the colder months of the year, and chilling of the body surface has been shown to cause vasoconstriction in the mucous membranes of the upper respiratory tract. The latter observation lends some physiologic basis to the notion that chilling may reduce local resistance to infection, and thus supports the age-old human belief that one can catch cold as a result of exposure. It would be rash indeed to deny that chilling has any effect on the likelihood of catching cold. It can be stated, however, that chilling in the absence of a primary infecting agent will not cause colds, and that its role is at best a minor auxiliary one in an environment where primary agents are ubiquitous.

Pathologic Anatomy and Physiology. In the presence of a cold there is an inflammation of the mucous membranes of the upper respiratory tract which often begins as a local affair in the throat. The most intense reaction takes place in the nasal passages, turbinates and so forth, where a good deal of secretion, mucoid at first, and then mucopurulent, is produced. The principal pathologic changes are edema, hyperemia and hypersecretion, with comparatively little cellular infiltration. An appreciable amount of epithelial desquamation takes place as the disease progresses. Stained smears of the secretions show considerable numbers of epithelial cells and leukocytes, and the finding of eosinophils suggests that an allergic rhinitis is present.

The effects of this disturbance are local and general. With regard to the former, in addition to the difficulty in breathing and the troublesome secretions, there may be symptoms from blockage of the eustachian tubes or the paranasal sinuses. The general effects, presumably due to "absorption," are relatively minor, particularly in adults.

Epidemiology. The epidemiology of colds can best be understood by remembering that they are highly communicable, notably indoors and in childhood, that the period of active immunity is short, and that for reasons not entirely clear they appear mainly in the colder months of the year.

Many surveys of the incidence of colds have yielded various estimates of their frequency, depending on the age of the group under scrutiny, its geographic location, habitat and modus vivendi. It seems likely that in urban communities in the temperate zone the general population averages about three colds a year. This average number is often greatly exceeded in susceptible persons, particularly children.

When the weekly incidence of common respiratory diseases is charted for large masses of population, there is ordinarily a low rate during the summer, a rise in the autumn, a single high midwinter peak, and a spring decline. When smaller urban groups are studied, however, a different pattern may appear in which not one but three peaks are discernible. The first is in early autumn, and all evidence would indicate that this is a result of the reopening of schools with the massing together of young susceptibles indoors. The winter peak is often associated with an increased incidence of more severe respiratory infections such as pneumonia, and may be accompanied by a wider dissemination of pathogenic bacteria. Finally, there may be a smaller secondary peak in the spring.

As has been stated, most colds appear to be communicable, and transmitted directly by droplet infection. Susceptibility being almost universal, there is no practicable method of limiting the spread of colds under the ordinary conditions of urban life.

Symptoms. The onset of a cold is usually fairly abrupt, and the first symptom is likely to be a sensation of soreness and dryness localized to a small area of the pharynx. Within a few hours a sense of congestion develops in the nasal passages, usually accompanied by sneezing, and shortly thereafter by nasal discharge, which in the early stages is thin and watery. At the end of forty-eight hours the full-blown clinical picture has ordinarily developed; the eyes are suffused, the voice is husky, there is fairly intense congestion of the upper respiratory mucosa with obstructed breathing, nasal discharge is abundant, the sense of smell and taste are diminished, and there is some cough. Unless the patient has a tendency to chronic bronchitis, the cough is usually nonproductive in the early stages; later on there may be some mucoid sputum. Along with these local symptoms there is a variable amount of general malaise. The patient feels lethargic and may complain of some vague aching pains in the back and limbs. Marked malaise and prostration are not features of the common cold in adults, however, and the ordinary case is afebrile throughout.

In children the disease is likely to be more severe, and temperatures of 102° F. or even higher are frequently noted. Malaise is more pronounced, and anorexia is common. Other digestive symptoms are rare.

Once the full symptoms have developed, the common cold runs a variable course. The whole illness may subside rapidly. More commonly, however, there is a period of several days of excessive nasal secretion and cough, with thick, mucopurulent discharge, which then gradually begins to abate. Ordinarily the uncomplicated cold lasts from seven to fourteen days.

Precisely where the common cold ends and complications begin is a matter of definition. Some degree of laryngitis and tracheitis may be part of the primary picture, but clinical signs of tracheobronchitis are properly to be considered as complications, in all likelihood due to secondary bacterial infection. Similarly, it seems probable that there is some inflammation of the paranasal sinuses as part of the uncomplicated cold, yet acute clinical sinusitis (which may occur late in the course of a cold) is a complication. Otitis media is mainly a problem for the pediatrician. It occurs most often in infancy and early childhood, and may appear at any stage of the disease, although most often it is fairly early. It is more common in the winter months and is caused by the common respiratory bacterial pathogens.

Diagnosis. The characteristic appearance of a person with a full-blown cold in the head is too familiar to require further comment. Some mention, however, should be made of the appearance of the throat. Close inspection will usually reveal a slightly shiny and edematous appearance of the mucous membrane, with swelling and redness of the lymphatic aggregations. Postnasal drip may be present, but is not diagnostic. True exudate on the tonsils or pharynx is not part of the picture of the common cold. Such an exudate, together with swelling and tenderness of the upper deep cervical lymph nodes, indicates the presence of so-called "exudative pharyngitis," often caused by infection with hemolytic streptococci. On the whole, however, the adult pharynx, particularly in heavy smokers, may show little or no recognizable deviation from the normal in the course of an acute cold. In children, on the other hand, the normal pharynx is usually paler, and evidences of acute inflammation are thus much easier to detect.

It must be borne in mind that there is a catarrhal stage at the onset of certain specific diseases such as measles, rubella, chickenpox, pertussis and cerebrospinal fever, which may be indistinguishable from the common cold. Moreover, it is now known that infection with the viruses of influenza and atypical pneumonia may take the form of a mild disease simulating acute coryza. These entities (in the absence of pneumonia) can only be differentiated from the common cold by serologic means. A purely allergic rhinitis may mimic the common cold. In this situation the history is most important in differential diagnosis, and the rapid development of symptoms, the lacrimation, sneezing, itching and the pale boggy appearance of the turbinates, are fairly characteristic. An element of allergy may be present in infectious colds. This is particularly true in some of the so-called "cold susceptible" children with a tendency to asthma. In such instances the allergy is presumably directed toward bacterial products.

There are no abnormal laboratory findings in the common cold. If a leukocytosis is present it strongly suggests a bacterial complication.

Finally it may be remarked that, except in infancy, the diagnosis of common cold is usually made by the patient, not the physician. His function is to exclude other conditions, to search for complications and to institute appropriate therapy.

Prophylaxis. The prevention of any communicable disease may be attempted by interrupting the lines of communication or increasing the resistance of the person. In a disease such as typhoid fever both methods are used with success. It is obvious that the common cold falls into a different category.

As the malady is ubiquitous and nonincapacitating, strict isolation is not a practicable measure. Under conditions of urban life, exposure is inevitable. This must not be construed as an argument for total defeatism. When one is dealing with highly susceptible groups, such as nursery schools, every endeavor should be made to exclude children in the acute stages of a cold. Attempts to effect quarantine in the home, and the wearing of masks, are also laudable, albeit usually doomed to failure. Recently the use of germicidal aerosols and ultraviolet light barriers have been extensively studied. It is obvious that these measures have a limited application, but it has been shown that ultraviolet light, if properly applied, seems to prevent cross infection in nurseries. It is costly, however, and only warranted when special, small populations are at risk.

Attempts to increase individual resistance to an infection may be either specific or general. In regard to the first, it may be stated that there is no specific vaccine against the common cold, and vaccination with virus-containing material has, up to the present, been unsuccessful. Indeed, in a disease which leaves so short a period of active immunity in its wake, this is not surprising. Moreover, in experimental transmission of the common cold, it has been shown that there is little resistance to homologous reinoculation after a brief period of time. In a somewhat different category are the so-called "cold vaccines," composed of mixed bacterial antigens, which are supposed to enhance resistance to the secondary invaders. On the whole, these have been disappointing, and most large controlled studies indicate that they are not effective in reducing the incidence of, or invalidism from, colds. In the occasional patient who is highly susceptible to bacterial complications, the vaccines have at times appeared to be of some limited benefit.

The general measures are mainly concerned with nutrition, hygiene, "hardening" procedures and the eradication of focal diseased areas. Here again the record is a disappointing one. There is no statistical evidence in controlled studies that the state of nutrition, the addition of vitamins in excess, the type of clothing worn, exposure to sunlight, fresh air and similar measures have any effect on susceptibility to colds. In regard to the presence of diseased tonsillar and adenoidal tissue there is some difference of opinion. Though the removal of tonsils is generally admitted to influence recurrent severe streptococcal throat infections, its effect on colds is debatable. In all likelihood the presence of adenoid tissue influences the severity of colds in early childhood. On the other hand, surveys of older children indicate that there is little difference in cold susceptibility between those who have undergone tonsillectomy and adenoidectomy and those who have not.

Long-term chemoprophylaxis with small doses of sulfadiazine or oral penicillin will strikingly reduce the incidence of streptococcal infections. There is also evidence that it may reduce the severity of common respiratory disease in highly susceptible infants or children. In adults, on the others hand, such chemoprophylaxis appears to have relatively little effect.

Treatment. Up to the present no specific agent has been developed which is effective against the virus of the common cold. In consequence, therapy is directed at general management, relief of symptoms and the control of complications.

In ideal circumstances it would probably be advisable to treat all sufferers from the common cold with rest and isolation, but in practice this is impossible. Bed rest should, however, be enforced in the more highly susceptible, i.e., infants and young children, and in adults with temperatures over 100° F. or some complicating chronic disease.

Symptomatic relief in the very young can usually be afforded by small doses of acetylsalicylic acid (aspirin). In adults, particularly if cough is troublesome, it is customary to give some codeine as well. This may be administered in the form of codeine cough mixture or in the traditional "grippe capsule." The following prescription has the weight of tradition behind it and is effective:

Codeine sulfate	0.015 gm.
Acetylsalicylic acid	0.3 gm.
Phenacetin	0.12 gm.
Caffeine citrate	0.03 cc.

One of these capsules may be given every three or four hours.

Capsules containing 0.015 gm. each of codeine and papaverine are also popular, and it has been suggested that they may aid in "aborting" a cold. In the writer's experience they do not do so, but are merely symptomatic in their effect.

Local therapy directed toward lessening secretions and improving the nasal airway is not recommended in the early acute stages of a cold. Later on, however, when secretions have thickened, it is often helpful, not only in relieving symptoms, but also in promoting sinus drainage. One per cent ephedrine in saline, used either in an atomizer or in the form of nose drops, is safe and relatively nonirritating. An amphetamine inhaler is convenient for the ambulatory patient. It is important not to use these agents more than once in four hours, and their habitual use in persons with a tendency to chronic nasal inflammations is not recommended.

A few years ago the antihistaminic drugs were introduced as therapy for the common cold, and it was claimed that, if they were employed early enough, the disease could be aborted in a large percentage of cases. This received widespread publicity and in consequence of a tremendous advertising campaign these agents, either by themselves or incorporated with other drugs, have been taken by the public on a huge scale. Subsequent carefully controlled studies have quite failed to substantiate the original claims. The conclusions of the present writer, based on an admittedly small series, were that in perhaps one half of the cases the antihistaminics appeared to exert some benefit on the intensity of the catarrhal symptoms, but that usually the fundamental course of the disease remained unchanged. Fortunately these drugs, in the dosages employed, have been singularly innocuous as far as untoward side effects are concerned. Nevertheless they are not recommended unless there is an allergic element present.

The routine use of sulfonamides or antibiotics in colds is contraindicated. These drugs should be used only with a specific objective in mind, i.e., the control of bacterial secondary infection. In other words, their use should be limited to those cases in which there is a strong likelihood that a complication is developing. Thus, clinical signs of bronchopulmonary infection, or sinusitis or otitis media, are indications for their use. The use of antimicrobial drugs may also be justified in highly susceptible persons who give a history of the regular occurrence of complications with their colds. In such cases penicillin is the safest and most generally desirable agent. A daily intramuscular injection of 1 cc. of a mixture containing 300,000 units of procaine penicillin and 100,000 units of crystalline penicillin is recommended. The suggestion of parenteral rather than oral penicillin is deliberate, for the latter is so much easier to administer that it leads to much more indiscriminate use. It must be borne in mind that as time goes on more and more persons disclose some sensitivity to penicillin, and the drug should not be used without reasonable indications. Obviously, if it is employed the patient's past history in regard to penicillin therapy must be queried. The tetracyclines and chloramphenicol are not recommended for routine use owing to their side effects.

The treatment of subacute and chronic complications of the common cold is outside the scope of this discussion. In adults the treatment of these complications usually falls into the purview of the otolaryngologist. The pediatrician, too, is confronted with a small group of children, often of the "allergic" type, who may be literally incapacitated by recurrent upper respiratory infections. For such cases many expedients have been tried: sulfadiazine or penicillin prophylaxis, injections of stock and autogenous bacterial vaccines, bacterial filtrates and similar procedures. Change of climate is sometimes an essential recourse in the treatment of these recurrent respiratory infections.

ACUTE UNDIFFERENTIATED RESPIRATORY DISEASE

The separation of this condition from the mosaic of common respiratory disease, as has been stated, resulted from the work of the Commission on Acute Respiratory Disease during World War II. In their experimental transmission of colds to human subjects with bacteria-free filtrates, they not only confirmed earlier experiments in regard to the coryzal type with a short incubation period, but also produced another variety with a longer incubation period—four to seven days. A study of this second type showed other clinical differences as well. The symptoms of nasal inflammation were less striking, there was more discomfort in the throat, and in particular the tendency to constitutional symptoms was more marked. Chilliness, headache and malaise were present in about half the cases, and a fever of about 101° F. lasting two or three days was frequently noted. There were no distinguishing physical signs observed in this condition, and laboratory findings were usually normal except for a very occasional slight elevation in the leukocyte count or erythrocyte sedimentation rate.

It must be emphasized that there is no method of differentiating on clinical grounds between infection with this virus and that of the common cold. Moreover, the number of transmission experiments thus far reported is much too small to form the basis of an opinion as to the relative frequency of the two conditions. Infection with the virus of undifferentiated respiratory disease appears to be fairly common, however, under certain circumstances such as military life. Transmission experiments performed by the Commission indicated that infection with this virus is followed by considerable immunity to homologous reinoculation. This is a plausible explanation to the phenomenon of "seasoning" of troops, i.e., the fact that the noneffective rate owing to common respiratory disease is much higher in recruits than in troops during their second year of military service.

If undifferentiated respiratory disease cannot be distinguished clinically from the common cold at one end of the scale, at the other it may mimic influenza. Studies by the Commission during the 1943 epidemic of influenza A showed that in only about half the proved cases were the symptoms "typical" of influenza. The rest of them resembled undifferentiated respiratory disease. Moreover, instances of what they believed to be the latter condition were noted in which the clinical picture was that of "typical" influenza.

Such was the situation with respect to undifferentiated respiratory disease (or "ARD," as it is now often called) as appraised after World War II. Recently, new information of extraordinary interest has appeared on the subject. Hilleman and Werner studied an outbreak of respiratory illness in 1953 at Fort Leonard Wood, and by means of newly discovered tissue culture techniques isolated an agent, presumably a virus. This virus was isolated not only from ARD patients but from patients who, except that they did *not* show cold agglutinins, had an illness identical with primary atypical pneumonia. This agent could be identified by serologic means, the antibody titer in human serum rising sharply during convalescence. Dingle has now retested serums collected a decade ago from his studies at Fort Bragg and from his human transmission experiments, and the results indicate that what the Commission designated "ARD" at that time was due to this newly discovered agent. These observations are, as yet, preliminary, but they would appear to indicate that the virus of "ARD" is quite widespread, and that it may give rise to varying clinical pictures, including that of primary atypical pneumonia. At about the same time as the Hilleman-Werner studies, a closely related virus or viruses was isolated in high incidence from specimens of human adenoidal tissue by Huebner and his associates.

There is no specific treatment for undifferentiated respiratory disease, and the general principles of therapy are the same as those of the common cold.

NONSTREPTOCOCCAL EXUDATIVE PHARYNGITIS

The Commission on Acute Respiratory Disease also drew attention to the entity nonstreptococcal exudative pharyngitis as a result of their studies of hemolytic streptococcal throat infections. Pharyngitis was encountered under endemic rather than epidemic conditions, and formed a relatively small part of the large body of respiratory diseases under scrutiny. The clinical manifestations of the pharyngeal disease were those of acute exudative tonsillitis and pharyngitis familiar to practitioners of medicine, and generally assumed to be caused by beta hemolytic streptococci. When the Commission began to examine such cases bacteriologically, however, a very considerable number were found from which no hemolytic streptococci could be cultivated. The subject was therefore studied further and in brief their conclusions were as follows:

The florid picture of exudative tonsillitis or pharyngitis is ordinarily due to infection with beta hemolytic streptococci. That is to say, a patient with real pain on swallowing, high fever, marked involvement of the upper deep cervical lymph nodes, leukocytosis, and a very inflamed pharynx with exudate, ordinarily shows an abundant growth of beta hemolytic streptococci. Moreover, serologic tests during convalescence, such as the antistreptolysin titer, usually give evidence of antibody response to streptococcal infection. On the other hand, patients with less severe disease, less involvement of the lymph nodes, little or no leukocyte response, but nevertheless showing an exudative pharyngeal reaction, may yield no hemolytic streptococci at all or no antibody response.

Quantitatively speaking, endemic exudative pharyngitis divided itself roughly in this manner: About one quarter of the cases were unquestionably due to hemolytic streptococcal infection, and from another quarter some streptococci could be cultivated, although serologic evidence of infection was lacking. *In one half the cases, however, no proof of streptococcal etiology could be established.* This was the group designated as nonstreptococcal exudative pharyngitis, and the disease was presumed to be due to some unidentified agent, possibly a virus.

Clinically, as has been stated, these cases

in the aggregate differ from those of streptococcal origin. In the individual case, however, mild streptococcal pharyngitis may be indistinguishable from the nonstreptococcal variety. This raises an important point in relation to therapy. There is no specific treatment for nonstreptococcal exudative pharyngitis, and the results of antimicrobial therapy in the mild streptococcal cases are not very striking in terms of immediate clinical change. However, it is becoming increasingly clear that the likelihood of late nonsuppurative complications, such as rheumatic fever, is lessened by early penicillin therapy. Therefore it seems wise to treat all streptococcal pharyngitis with penicillin, and, when facilities for a prompt bacteriologic diagnosis are unavailable, this practice will obviously involve treatment of the nonstreptococcal cases as well.

As has been stated, the whitish or yellowish-white exudate on an inflamed background, seen in these diseases, is fairly characteristic, and distinguishable from the ulcerated lesions of Vincent's pharyngitis, or the tenacious gray membrane of diphtheria. The clinician should never rely too heavily on his visual diagnosis, however, and it is wise practice to submit all exudative cases to routine throat culture for *C. diphtheriae*.

YALE KNEELAND, JR.

References

Andrewes, C. H.: Report to the International Congress of Microbiology. 1953.

Annals of the Pickett-Thomson Research Laboratory: The Common Cold. London, 1932, Vol. VIII. (Complete review of literature.)

Atlas, L. T., and Hottle, G. A.: The Common Cold: Titration of M.R.–1 Virus in Embryonated Eggs. Science, 108:743, 1948.

Commission on Acute Respiratory Diseases: Experimental Transmission of Minor Respiratory Illness to Human Volunteers by Filter-Passing Agents. J. Clin. Investigation, 26:957, 974, 1947.

————: Endemic Exudative Pharyngitis and Tonsillitis. J.A.M.A., 125:1163, 1944.

————: Clinical Patterns of Undifferentiated and Other Respiratory Diseases in Army Recruits. Medicine, 26:441, 1947.

Cooke, B., Atkinson, N., Mawson, J., and Hurst, E. W.: Acute Infection of the Upper Respiratory Tract in South Australia: Note on "Woodside Throat." Med. J. Australia, 1:3, 1941.

Dingle, J. H., et al.: Evidence for Specific Etiology of "Acute Respiratory Disease (ARD)." Tr. A. Am. Physicians, 1954.

Dochez, A. R., Mills, K. C., and Kneeland, Y., Jr.: Studies on the Common Cold. VI. Cultivation of the Virus in Tissue Medium. J. Exper. Med., 63: 559, 1936.

Hilleman, M. R., and Werner, J. H.: Recovery of New Agent from Patients with Acute Respiratory Illness. Proc. Soc. Exper. Biol. & Med., 85:183, 1954.

Kneeland, Y., Jr., and Dawes, C. F.: The Relationship of Pathogenic Bacteria to Upper Respiratory Disease in Infants. J. Exper. Med., 55:735, 1932.

Paul, J. H., and Freese, H. L.: Epidemiological and Bacteriological Study of "Common Cold" in Isolated Arctic Community (Spitzbergen). Am. J. Hyg., 17:517, 1933.

Rowe, W. P., Huebner, R. J., Gilmore, L. K., Parrott, R. H., and Ward, T. G.: Isolation of a Cytopathogenic Agent from Human Adenoids Undergoing Spontaneous Degeneration in Tissue Culture, Proc. Soc. Exper. Biol. & Med., 84:570, 1953.

Shibley, G. S., Hanger, F. M., and Dochez, A. R.: Observations of the Norman Bacterial Flora of Nose and Throat with Variations Occurring during Colds. J. Exp. Med., 43:415, 1926.

INFLUENZA

(La Grippe, Grip, Catarrhal Fever, Epidemic Influenza)

Definition. Influenza is a specific infectious disease of man and is caused by a virus of the influenza group. The disease is an acute, self-limited infection and is characterized by constitutional symptoms, although the infection is restricted to the respiratory tract. It occurs most commonly in epidemics of varied size. Between epidemics, sporadic cases are encountered. Three distinct etiologic types of the disease are known: *influenza A, influenza B* and *influenza C*. Influenza A occurs more commonly than influenza B; influenza C appears to be rare. A distinction between the etiologic types cannot be made on clinical or pathologic grounds. The disease is usually of short duration and is rarely serious. Complications are uncommon but may be severe, particularly if secondary bacterial pneumonia develops. The cause of great pandemics, such as that in 1918–19, has not been established.

History. The disease has been recognized since ancient times. Many widespread epidemics and occasional great pandemics have occurred during the past four centuries. In recent times, extensive pandemics appeared in 1889–92 and 1918–19. The latter affected persons in all areas of the earth and is thought to have led to the death of about 20,000,000 people. Much the most common cause of death was secondary bacterial pneumonia.

Modern knowledge of influenza stems from the discovery by Smith, Andrewes and Laidlaw in 1933 that the disease is caused by a virus. This agent is now designated influenza A virus. In 1936, Smith and Stuart-Harris demonstrated that after passage in experimental animals the virus could still cause influenza in man. Epidemics of varying extent have occurred, frequently during the past twenty years; recently they have appeared almost yearly, but the disease involved has not been commonly associated with complications. In 1940, Francis and Magill independently discovered influenza B virus. This agent is unrelated antigenically to influenza A virus; one does not produce immunity against the other. In 1944, Francis and co-workers showed that after passage in experimental animals influenza B virus could still induce influenza in man. That the two major types of influenza, now designated A and B, are caused by influenza A virus and influenza B virus, respectively, is generally accepted. In 1949, Taylor discovered influenza C virus. This agent is unrelated antigenically to either influenza A or B virus. Relatively few patients with influenza C have been studied as yet and far less is known of this disease than of influenza A or influenza B. In the absence of satisfactory material from patients with the pandemic disease, it has not been possible to determine whether any of the known influenza viruses or some other infectious agent was the primary causal factor.

Etiology. The disease is caused by a virus of the influenza group. These agents are spherically shaped and of medium size, about 100 mμ in diameter. During the acute phase of the disease, the virus is present in the respiratory tract but not in other areas of the body nor in the blood. Sputum, saliva and nasal secretions contain the agent. It can be demonstrated in washings of the nose or throat from the first day of illness to the fifth, occasionally the seventh day. There are three distinct and immunologically unrelated serologic types: *influenza A, influenza B* and *influenza C* virus, respectively. Influenza A and B viruses are infective for ferrets, mice, hamsters and chick embryos. Influenza C virus appears to be infective but less virulent for most of these species, although it has not caused infection in mice. Animals appear not to be infected by these agents in nature and there is no evidence for an interepidemic reservoir for the viruses other than man himself. Usually, the agents are recovered from throat washings of patients by inoculation into the amniotic sac of chick embryos. With the exception of swine influenza virus, which is immunologically related to some strains of influenza A virus, no other virus is known to be serologically related to any of the agents in the influenza group. Progressive variation in antigenic composition, particularly marked with influenza A and B viruses, is more striking than with any other virus infecting man,

and has seriously affected efforts to prevent the disease with vaccines.

Infection or immunization with influenza A virus does not lead to immunity against influenza B or C virus and vice versa. Despite these striking immunologic differences, the agents possess many common properties. One of the most useful is their capacity to cause agglutination of erythrocytes *in vitro,* a reaction which has provided simple techniques for identification and measurement of the viruses or antibodies against them. An increase in antibodies against the type of virus which caused the infection may be demonstrated seven to ten days after the onset of illness; the maximal antibody response is observed two to four weeks after onset. Antibody levels against a soluble antigen of the virus are measured by complement fixation; against the virus itself by hemagglutination inhibition, or by neutralization *in vivo.* Because many persons of school age or older possess antibodies against each of the three types of virus in their serum, measurement of the antibody levels in a single serum specimen is not helpful in reaching an etiologic diagnosis. A comparison of the antibody levels in acute phase and convalescent serum specimens is the most reliable means of establishing the diagnosis and the etiologic type of the disease.

Incidence and Epidemiology. Although occasional sporadic cases occur during interepidemic periods, they do not often lead to many secondary cases among contacts. Influenza appears most commonly in epidemics which may be localized or widely spread. During the past twenty years, epidemics have broken out in some parts of the world almost annually. Localized epidemics may appear nearly at the same time in different areas, even in different countries, or large epidemics may seem to spread from one area or country to another. Pandemic outbreaks have appeared only rarely and have been separated by long intervals of varying duration. It should be emphasized that the nature of the agent responsible for pandemics of the disease has not been established.

Although epidemics tend to appear during winter months, they may occur at any time of the year, even in the summer. Large epidemics show some cyclic tendency; those of influenza A have occurred at about two- to three-year intervals, while those of influenza B have appeared roughly at four- to five-year intervals. Epidemics of influenza A tend to be more extensive than those of influenza B. Occasionally, the two diseases occur in the same epidemic and rarely concurrent infection with the two viruses may develop in the same patient. The attack rate may vary widely in different epidemics, from as low as 1 to 2 per cent to as high as 20 to 30 per cent. Usually, the more crowded the conditions of living, the higher is the attack rate. Under conditions of crowding, epidemics build up rapidly and then quickly "burn out," the whole occupying no more than two to three weeks. In dispersed populations, events are less dramatic and the epidemic may smolder along for two to three months.

Persons of any age or race and of either sex are about equally susceptible. Transmission is probably through infective droplets distributed from the upper respiratory tract which is also the portal of entry for the virus. The existence of persistent carriers of influenza virus has not been demonstrated. It is thought that the viruses are maintained during interepidemic periods by a chain of sporadic infections in man. Infection with the agents is very common and after five years of age most persons possess specific antibodies in their serum. Inapparent or subclinical infections are at least as frequent as is the manifest disease and account in part for the high incidence of antibodies against the viruses in the serum of healthy persons. Neither influenza A nor B leads to persistent immunity; second infections of the same type may develop after six to eight months. Influenza A induces no immunity to influenza B and vice versa. Resistance to infection is directly correlated with the type-specific antibody level in the serum; the higher the titer, the less likely is infection.

Morbid Anatomy. Little is known of the pathologic alterations associated with uncomplicated influenza in man. In the ferret, the virus causes necrosis of the respiratory epithelium of the nasal mucous membrane. There is also an inflammatory reaction in the submucosa. Repair begins on about the fourth day after infection. In man, fatal attacks are commonly complicated by secondary bacterial infection. Many of the pathologic changes seen may be largely attributable to the latter. In such cases, there is tracheal and bronchial inflammation with marked epithelial desquamation and some epithelial necrosis. The interstitial tissues show an inflammatory reaction and there is necrosis of the alveolar walls associated with hemorrhage. Extensive bronchopneumonia or interstitial pneumonia is usually present. In the pandemic disease of 1918–19, Goodpasture described a lesion which appeared to be peculiar to the infection. This consisted of dilated alveolar ducts, with a hyaline membrane covering their walls and those of adjacent alveoli, and was found with great consistency during the pandemic.

Pathologic Physiology and Chemistry. The leukocyte count is commonly within the normal range. Leukopenia, when it occurs, is found early in the disease, usually in patients with high fever and marked symptoms. The differential leukocyte pattern is usually normal, even if leukopenia is present. The erythrocyte sedimentation rate is increased. The urine is usually normal, although slight albuminuria may occur. In the uncomplicated disease, cyanosis is not present, cultures of the blood are sterile and the roentgenogram does not show evidence of pneumonia in the great majority of patients. The evidences of toxicity and the marked prostration so commonly seen may be attributable to toxic properties of the virus itself.

Symptoms. Both influenza A and B lead to an array of clinical pictures which vary widely in severity and duration. Neither of the infections produces signs or symptoms which are pathognomonic. Too little is known as yet about influenza C to permit generalization.

The incubation period of influenza A or B is usually only one or two days, and the onset generally is abrupt. The first and most prominent symptoms are constitutional. In the more typical cases, these are commonly: chilliness or a frank chill, fever, headache, malaise, lassitude, anorexia and muscular pains. Prostration of varying degree is common. Symptoms referable to the respiratory tract usually are not marked, and consist of sneezing, nasal irritation or discharge, fullness or irritation of the nasopharynx, larynx or trachea. Cough is common but usually is not productive. Epistaxis, hoarseness, nausea or substernal pain may develop. In the less typical cases, similar symptoms usually appear but may vary markedly in degree. In some patients, the disease may simulate any of the minor acute respiratory infections. In other patients, the disease may resemble more severe or generalized infections.

Fever is commonly remittent and usually persists for two or three days; the range is one to six days. Generally, the highest temperature is between 101 and 103° F., though in the more severe cases it may reach 105° F. Commonly, the fever is highest on the first or second day of disease. The pulse rate is increased generally in proportion to the fever and may be quite rapid. The respiratory rate is normal or only slightly increased.

Physical signs usually are neither definite nor striking. The face may be flushed and the conjunctivae are sometimes injected. The nasal mucosa may be somewhat injected and swollen. The fauces, soft palate and posterior pharynx may be mildly injected and the lymphoid follicles may be prominent. The physical signs over the chest are usually normal although fine moist rales may be found in the lower lung fields posteriorly. Definite signs of pulmonary consolidation occur only in rare instances and commonly are indicative of secondary bacterial infection. The remainder of the physical examination does not ordinarily reveal abnormal findings attributable to influenza.

Course and Complications. The severity of the infection and the course of the illness vary widely. Usually, patients are not acutely ill for more than three to five days, though some may be miserable for a week or more. The fever tends to come down by lysis and thereafter symptoms gradually disappear. Convalescence is commonly uneventful and may be fairly rapid in previously healthy persons. Patients with marked symptoms may complain of considerable prostration, increased sweating and fatigability for a week or more after fever has disappeared.

The infections which occurred during the pandemic disease of 1918–19 were in general more severe than those which have developed during the two decades since influenza viruses were discovered. In this pandemic, pneumonia appeared in many patients and was the major cause of death. Usually, the first evidence of pneumonia developed two to four days after the onset. In some patients, very severe or fulminating infections occurred and rapidly were fatal. In others, pneumonia did not develop until the acute phase of the initial infection was over. The pneumonia was attributable to bacterial infection in almost every instance and a variety of bacterial species was associated with the infection. Staphylococci, beta hemolytic streptococci, *H. influenzae* and pneumococci were the most frequent invaders. Infection of the pleura and empyema were common complications usually associated with beta

hemolytic streptococci or pneumococci. Occasionally, lung abscess developed following staphylococcal or beta hemolytic streptococcal infection. Bronchiectasis, chronic bronchitis or pulmonary fibrosis sometimes developed.

In striking contrast is the experience of the past two decades with epidemics of influenza of known cause. During this period, previously healthy persons who contracted either influenza A or B, only, rarely developed serious complications. A small number of attacks of influenza have been associated with staphylococcal pneumonia and some with pneumococcal pneumonia, but in the great majority of patients frank pulmonary disease has not occurred.

Diagnosis. During an epidemic of influenza, the diagnosis is usually not difficult because of the fairly typical clinical picture presented by the majority of patients. Common features are: abrupt onset with fever, headache, prostration, muscular pains, cough and nasal symptoms in the absence of markedly abnormal physical signs. During interepidemic periods, sporadic cases, though presenting somewhat similar clinical pictures, are difficult to diagnose without aid from the laboratory.

A number of other infectious diseases may closely resemble influenza. Among these are: the common cold, undifferentiated acute upper respiratory infections, primary atypical pneumonia, paranasal sinusitis, abortive measles, dengue, Rift Valley fever, lymphocytic choriomeningitis and Venezuelan equine encephalomyelitis. In some instances, influenza can be distinguished from these diseases only by laboratory procedures.

Infection with either influenza A or B virus may cause a wide variety of clinical pictures, ranging from very mild to moderately severe illnesses. During epidemics, subclinical or inapparent infections not associated with definite symptoms are common. Influenza A may lead to somewhat more marked symptoms than influenza B but the clinical findings do not distinguish one from the other.

An etiologic diagnosis can be established only by laboratory procedures. The virus may be recovered from the upper respiratory tract during the acute phase of the illness by intra-amniotic inoculation in embryonated chicken eggs. The virus cannot be recovered from the blood, cerebrospinal fluid or feces. A specific antibody response to the infecting virus may be demonstrated with appropriate serum specimens by various immunologic techniques. Complement fixation, virus neutralization and hemagglutination inhibition procedures can all yield satisfactory results. Two specimens of serum are needed from each patient; one should be obtained less than five days after onset, and the other two or three weeks later. Before throat-washings or serum specimens are obtained, the laboratory which is to carry out the tests should be consulted.

Prognosis. In previously healthy children or adults, the prognosis is excellent and an uneventful recovery may be anticipated in the great majority of patients. In undernourished or debilitated persons, those with chronic diseases, or persons of advanced age, the prognosis may not be as good. Such patients appear to be more liable to develop secondary bacterial infections of the respiratory tract and pneumonia may arise. Under these circumstances, the prognosis becomes that usually associated with the particular bacterial infection. Antimicrobial therapy appears to be about as effective in controlling secondary bacterial infection associated with influenza as in similar infections in the absence of the virus disease.

Prophylaxis. During the past fifteen years, vaccines capable of inducing temporarily increased resistance to influenza A and B have been developed and gradually improved. The currently available vaccines contain a number of strains of both viruses which have been inactivated and to some degree purified from the allantoic fluid of infected chick embryos. Subcutaneous or intramuscular injection of such a vaccine usually results in the production of antibodies against the viruses in the vaccine. An increase in the antibody levels of the serum begins about a week after injection of the vaccine and the maximal antibody response is present at about two weeks. Another another month or six weeks, the increased antibody levels gradually decline. To a considerable extent, the degree of increase in resistance to infection with either influenza A or B virus is directly correlated with the serum antibody level.

Vaccination leads in general to reduced susceptibility to infection for some months; estimates range from two to twelve months. Protection is not complete and vaccinated persons can still contract the disease. Available vaccines, although capable of diminishing the likelihood of infection, are effective for a relatively short period. As a consequence, they are most useful when given shortly before an epidemic. Predictions on the occurrence of epidemics are notably unreliable. Influenza virus vaccines possess toxic properties and, if a sufficient quantity is injected, may lead to unpleasant symptoms, especially in children. In addition, they contain some chick embryo material which is antigenic. This may induce sensitization or, in rare instances, lead to serious reactions in persons hypersensitive to egg products.

Treatment. Effective chemotherapy against the virus infection has not yet been developed. Supportive and symptomatic treatment similar to that used in other acute upper respiratory infections provides some relief. During the febrile period, the patient should remain in bed, large quantities of fluid should be taken, and the diet should be liquid or light. Acetylsalicylic acid, 0.3 to 1.0 gm., and codeine, 0.016 to 0.032 gm., are the drugs most commonly employed. Barbiturates may be used to control sleeplessness. Sulfonamide drugs and penicillin, even in large doses, are ineffective. Similarly, the tetracyclines and chloramphenicol do not favorably affect the course of the disease. The injection of influenza virus vaccine after the disease has appeared is not beneficial and may increase symptoms.

Because secondary bacterial infections occur in only a small proportion of patients, it is in general unwise to attempt to prevent their development with antimicrobial drugs. However, when definite bacterial infection does develop, appropriate chemotherapy should be instituted and carried out as it would be in the absence of the virus infection. This is especially important when bacterial pneumonia appears.

FRANK L. HORSFALL, JR.

References

Francis, T., Jr.: A New Type of Virus from Epidemic Influenza. Science, 92:405, 1940
————, Pearson, H. E., Salk, J. E., and Brown, P. N.: Immunity in Human Subjects Artificially Infected with Influenza Virus, Type B. Am. J. Pub. Health, 34:317, 1944.
Horsfall, F. L., Jr.: Influenza, in Rivers, T. M.: Viral and Rickettsial Infections of Man. 2nd ed. Philadelphia, J. B. Lippincott Co., 1952, pp. 392–413.
Magill, T. P.: A Virus from Cases of Influenza-like Upper Respiratory Infection. Proc. Soc. Exper. Biol. & Med., 45:162, 1940.
Opie, E. L., Blake, F. G., Small, J. C., and Rivers,

T. M.: Epidemic Respiratory Disease. St. Louis, C. V. Mosby Co., 1921.

Smith, W., Andrewes, C. H., and Laidlaw, P. P.: A Virus Obtained from Influenza Patients. Lancet, 2:66, 1933.

————, and Stuart-Harris, C. H.: Influenza Infection of Man from the Ferret. Lancet, 2:121, 1936.

Taylor, R. M.: Studies on Survival of Influenza Virus between Epidemics and Antigenic Variants of the Virus. Am. J. Pub. Health, 39:171, 1949.

DENGUE

Definition. Dengue, or "breakbone fever," is an acute, specific febrile disease caused by a filterable virus and transmitted by mosquitoes of the genus *Aedes*. It is characterized by sudden onset with fever and prostration and by intermission of fever on the third or fourth day, in the American type of the disease, with recurrence after eighteen to thirty hours. A rash appears during the period of apyrexia or with the second rise in temperature on the third to fifth day in the disease as seen in this country. The duration is seldom longer than seven days.

History. The first known epidemics of dengue occurred in Egypt and Java in 1779; a year later Philadelphia experienced the severe outbreak described by Rush. It is possible that a disease recorded in Seville during the seventeenth century was dengue. During the past 150 years many widespread epidemics have occurred in the southern United States and in many other areas.

Incidence. Dengue occurs wherever the mosquito *Aedes aegypti* abounds and climatic conditions are suitable for the survival of the virus in this vector. It is endemic in the tropics and mildly so in certain subtropical and even temperate regions. During the past twenty years there have been severe epidemics in the Southeastern and Gulf states of the United States, in Australia, Egypt and Greece. Between epidemics, sporadic cases are occasionally seen.

Mode of Transmission. In 1903, Graham suggested that dengue was transmitted by mosquitoes and suspected *Culex fatigans.* Four years later, Ashburn and Craig, working in the Philippines, demonstrated that the causative agent could be transmitted by blood, that it was filterable and that a mosquito was the vector, though they erroneously implicated *Culex quinquefasciatus.* In 1916, Cleland, Bradley and McDonald in Australia showed that *Aedes aegypti* could transmit the

disease, but that culicine mosquitoes could not be infected. This observation was confirmed by Koizumi and his collaborators and by American investigators in the Philippines. The latter group demonstrated that *Aedes albopictus* could also be infected. It has been rather reliably reported that *Aedes scutellaris* also can be a vector (MacKerris, quoted by Fairley). A mosquito having once ingested the blood of a person with dengue is able to transmit the disease during the remainder of its life, though Blanc and Caminopetros found that the virus became noninfective when mosquitoes known to carry it were kept at temperatures below 20° C. (64.4° F.). This observation probably explains the rapid subsidence of epidemics of dengue with the advent of cool weather.

Period of Infectivity. Though Blanc and Caminopetros were able to transmit dengue with intravenous injections of patients' blood taken during the first five days of illness, Simmons, St. John and Reynolds showed that for mosquitoes to become infected, it was necessary for them to ingest blood during the first forty-eight hours. They also proved that there is then a period of "extrinsic" incubation or presumable multiplication of the virus in the mosquito of at least nine days, usually twelve, before the vector is able to infect by its bite.

Immunity. An attack of dengue produces transient immunity, probably for not longer than five years in most persons, perhaps as long as ten in some. Major epidemics in certain localities have occurred at five-year intervals, affecting from 50 to 60 per cent of the population on each occasion. No protection is afforded by the injection of convalescent serum or blood, nor is filtered infectious plasma or serum rendered avirulent by treatment with immune serum. Second and third attacks are likely to be mild and somewhat atypical.

Etiology. The specific causative factor of dengue is a filterable virus capable of passing Chamberland candles L_2 and L_3. It resists refrigeration for at least fifty-four days and drying for at least ten months. Koizumi was able to transmit the disease by injection of as little as 0.00005 cc. of blood drawn during the first febrile period. Experimental animals do not show fever or symptoms after inoculation, but Blanc and Caminopetros observed that the blood of guinea pigs was infectious for human subjects five days after the injection of virulent blood or serum. They also produced a transient asymptomatic and afebrile carrier state in some nonimmune human subjects. Intensive investigations carried out during World War II showed that there are several strains of the virus which may produce slightly different clinical manifestations. Dengue seen in the Pacific area differs from American dengue in that the period of remission of fever is likely to be absent and the secondary rash may be petechial.

Epidemiology. Noteworthy epidemics of dengue occur when there is a coincidence of free propagation of *Aedes aegypti* with waning immunity of the human population. Such conditions exist when, after a period of five or more years, there is unusual warmth and abundant rainfall during the late summer and early autumn in almost any locality between the parallels 32° 50′ north and 23° 25′ south. *Aedes aegypti* is thoroughly domesticated and able to breed in small amounts of water, so that the innumerable containers present in any center of population offer optimum facilities for oviposition. Since dengue is mildly endemic throughout its distribution and it has been shown that some infected persons remain free from symptoms, an excessive number of mosquitoes soon become infected. An epidemic of dengue spreads with rapidity comparable only to pandemic influenza. In Athens 80 to 90 per cent of the population were ill during the epidemic of 1928–29, and in the 1934 epidemic in Florida at least 30 per cent of the permanent residents of Miami were infected. The epidemiology of dengue is important, since it reflects the potential distribution of yellow fever, *Aedes aegypti* being the vector of the virus of both diseases. Several species of monkeys are susceptible to natural or experimental infection with the virus of dengue. It is suspected that these animals may be a constant reservoir of the disease in the tropics.

Morbid Anatomy. Hemorrhagic or petechial lesions have been described in the central nervous system, endocardium, the various serous membranes, the mucous membranes of the gastrointestinal tract and in the muscles and skin. Nonspecific degenerative changes have been observed in the brain, myocardium, liver and kidneys. The lymph nodes and spleen may be moderately enlarged. The specific lesion, described by Sabin, is a vasculitis involving the small blood vessels; there is endothelial swelling, perivascular edema and infiltration with mononuclear cells. The petechiae are simple hemorrhages without inflammatory reaction. Inclusion bodies have not been demonstrated.

Symptoms and Signs. The incubation period is from four to ten days. The onset is abrupt with severe headache, often localized behind the eyes, pain on moving the eyeballs, lumbar backache and extreme prostration. Occasionally there is rigor, and children may have convulsions. Loss of the sense of taste and complete anorexia are usual, nausea and vomiting frequent and constipation almost constant. The temperature rises in a few hours to 102° to 104° F. and may reach 106° F. Relative bradycardia is the rule, and some patients have heart rates as low as forty. Systolic blood pressure is depressed, often below 100 mm. of mercury, and the pulse may be dicrotic. During the first few hours all the larger joints, particularly those of the knees, hips and vertebrae, become intensely painful, so that motion is almost impossible, though passive movement may be tolerated. A transient, pale pink, macular rash is often seen at the onset. The face is flushed, the conjunctivas and sclerae are much congested, and mild injection of the pharynx is common. Some enlargement of the lymph nodes is present in about three fourths of the cases, the epitrochlear, inguinal and posterior cervical nodes being most frequently palpable. The spleen is not infrequently palpable just below the costal border and is quite soft. Fever and symptoms persist for three, sometimes four, days; there is then rapid defervescence accompanied by profuse sweating and, often, diuresis. Sometimes there is epistaxis or diarrhea. All symptoms are greatly improved during the period of intermission, which is most often of twenty-four hours' duration. There is then a second rapid rise in temperature to 102° to 103° F., all symptoms recur and the characteristic rash appears. This is almost always morbilliform, but varies in distribution. Typically it appears first over the knees, ankles and elbows, which may show periarticular swelling. The entire body except the face may be involved, or there may be a patchy distribution over the trunk and the flexor surfaces of the extremities. The palms and soles may be bright red and often so edematous that flexion of the hands and feet is painful. Some patients have marked pruritus before or with the eruption. The rash and symptoms persist until final defervescence, which occurs with great regularity after two days, on the sixth or seventh

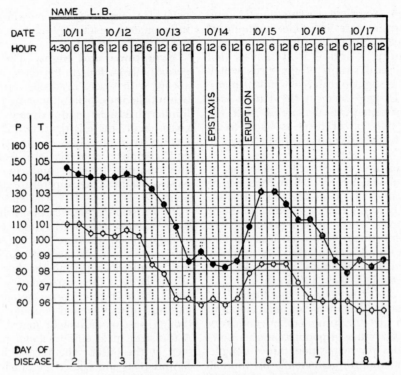

Fig. 1. Temperature chart of a patient with dengue.

day of illness. Desquamation is frequent. Certain cases are atypical in that the second febrile period does not occur. Convalescence is likely to be slow; bradycardia, hypotension and asthenia may persist for weeks.

The blood constantly shows leukopenia due to granulocytopenia. The leukocyte count is usually between 2000 and 6000 per cu. mm. with 20 to 45 per cent of granulocytes. Many of the polymorphonuclear cells show "toxic" or degenerative changes. Vacuolization, pyknosis and fragmentation of nuclei, basophilic granulation and vacuoles in the cytoplasm are common. Coles has described minute, round and oval diplococcoid bodies in the red cells which are demonstrable by prolonged staining with dilute Giemsa stain. Their significance is not established.

The urine is often scanty and concentrated from vomiting and inadequate intake of fluids. Albuminuria and cylindruria are seldom more prominent than could be explained by the presence of the fever.

Complications. Bleeding from the nose, gastrointestinal tract and uterus may occur and seems to have been unusually common in the Greek epidemic. Heart failure and acute renal insufficiency have been observed in patients with arteriosclerosis. The syndrome of neurocirculatory asthenia is a rather frequent sequel to dengue.

Diagnosis. Illness beginning suddenly with headache, muscle and joint pains, nausea and fever during a time when *Aedes* mosquitoes are abundant should suggest dengue. At the onset it may be mistaken for influenza, malaria or measles. In areas where typhus or yellow fever is endemic it may be confused with them. Seen first after the exanthem has appeared, it may suggest scarlet fever. In unvaccinated persons smallpox may be suspected. The course of the illness speedily differentiates influenza and measles; malaria can be excluded by examination of the blood. Yellow fever can be eliminated from consideration by the absence of icterus and albuminuria. Lack of angina, of marked cervical adenitis and of leukocytosis serves to differentiate dengue from scarlet fever, but occasionally smallpox cannot be excluded until the eruption appears.

Prognosis. Death from uncomplicated dengue probably occurs in less than one case in 10,000. In severe epidemics the rate may far exceed this because of prevalence of the disease among the higher age groups with advanced vascular disease of the brain, heart or kidneys.

Prevention. The prevention of dengue is largely a matter of adequate mosquito control. All breeding places must be sought out and destroyed or screened and treated with larvicide. Buildings should be screened and treated with residual DDT spray. Area spraying with DDT by aircraft may be of great value in epidemics. The use of effective mosquito repellents by persons exposed to attack by mosquitoes during work or sleep is advisable. Vaccines for immunization against dengue have been prepared and may prove important in prevention of the disease.

Treatment. This is entirely symptomatic. Pain is often mitigated by codeine, 0.033 gm., and acetylsalicylic acid, 0.3 gm, given as frequently as necessary; codeine, 0.06 gm., or morphine, 0.008 gm., given hypodermically may be required when nausea is severe; atropine should be combined with these. Ice caps to the head, cold sponges or packs and cool rectal irrigations give some relief from fever. Diet should be liquid and fluids forced to tolerance. Fluids must be given parenterally when nausea prevents an adequate intake by mouth. During convalescence the diet should be increased slowly. Rest is essential and should be prolonged for elderly patients.

V. P. SYDENSTRICKER

References

Ashburn, P. M., and Craig, C. E.: Experimental Investigations Regarding the Etiology of Dengue Fever, with a General Consideration of the Disease. Philippine J. Sc., 2:93, 1907.

Cleland, J. B., Bradley, B., and McDonald, W.: On the Transmission of Australian Dengue by the Mosquito, Stegomyia fasciata. M. J. Australia, 2:179, 200, 1916.

Fairley, N. H.: Medicine in Jungle Warfare. Proc. Roy. Soc. Med., 38:195, 1945.

Graham, H.: The Dengue: A Study of Its Pathology and Mode of Propagation. J. Trop. Med., 6:209, 1903.

Griffiths, T. H. D., and Hanson, H.: Significance of Epidemic of Dengue, J.A.M.A., 107:1107, 1936.

Mackie, T. T., Hunter, G. W., III, and Worth, C. B.: Manual of Tropical Medicine. 2nd ed. Philadelphia, W. B. Saunders Company, 1954.

Sabin, A. B., and others: Dengue, in Viral and Rickettsial Diseases of Man. Philadelphia, J. B. Lippincott Company, 1948, p. 445.

Siler, J. F., Hall, M. W., and Hitchens, A. P.: Results Obtained in the Transmission of Dengue Fever. Proc. Soc. Exper. Biol. & Med., 23:197, 1925.

Stewart, F. H.: Dengue; Analysis of Clinical Syndrome at a South Pacific Advance Base. U. S. Nav. M. Bull., 42:1233, 1944.

COLORADO TICK FEVER

Definition and Etiology. Colorado tick fever is a distinct disease entity of viral etiology transmitted by ticks. It is clinically indistinguishable from dengue except for the absence of a rash.

Incidence, Epidemiology and Prevention. The disease is unfortunately named, since it has been reported in all the western states in which the wood tick, *Dermacentor andersoni,* is found. In Colorado, it is by far the most common of the tick-borne diseases, probably outnumbering Rocky Mountain spotted fever 100 to 1. Although it has never been reported on the eastern seaboard, the virus has been isolated from Long Island dog ticks, *Dermacentor variabilis.* Colorado tick fever, therefore, is probably not confined to the west, but, like Rocky Mountain spotted fever, will be found in other parts of the United States.

The disease occurs in the spring and early summer when the ticks are active. Invariably the victim has been in a tick-infested area four to six days prior to onset. In most cases either the patient will have found the feeding tick prior to the illness or a careful search at the time of onset will demonstrate it. The person involved is not aware of the presence of this arthropod, since the bite is painless. Persons who visit in the mountains, particularly if they walk through tall grass and low shrubs, are likely to pick up one or more ticks. The entire body should be thoroughly inspected several times a day, particularly the short hair of the neck, and all ticks removed. The feeding or attached tick is removed with some difficulty, the best method being to apply some irritant such as turpentine, iodine or acetone. Then the tick can be teased out of the skin by inserting a needle between the mouth parts. Should the mouth parts be left in the skin, a small shallow, indolent ulcer is likely to develop.

The virus is transmitted transovarially and consequently the infection is self-perpetuating in the tick. No animal host has as yet been demonstrated. It is easy to infect the hamster or newborn mice with blood from a patient.

No one has ever been reported to have had the disease twice. Several individuals who had had Colorado tick fever were experimentally challenged with virus and remained well. A few persons have had both Colorado tick fever and Rocky Mountain spotted fever at different times.

Morbid Anatomy; Pathologic Physiology. Deaths have never been reported; consequently, nothing is known about pathologic changes in the tissues. Like dengue, however, the disease causes a definite reduction in the leukocyte count. Counts lower than 2000 per cu. mm. are frequently recorded, the low point usually occurring during the second attack. All the leukocytes are reduced in absolute numbers except the monocytes. There is a marked increase in the band forms. Hematologic recovery follows clinical recovery by four to seven days.

Symptoms and Clinical Course. The onset is sudden with chilly sensations and mild photophobia. This is quickly followed by generalized aching, especially in the muscle and tendon insertions around the joints. The other prominent features of this aching consist of headache, deep ocular pain and backache, particularly in the lumbar region. Anorexia and nausea are common. Vomiting occurs in children. The first attack lasts approximately two days, followed by a complete remission of all signs and symptoms for about the same length of time, with the second attack usually lasting somewhat longer than the first. Either episode may be more severe than the other. Although the usual pattern is for each attack and for the remission to last approximately two days each, variations of one to four days do occur. Third attacks have been reported. A single episode lasting five to seven days is likewise possible. While disappearance of symptoms occurs rapidly at the end of the second attack, the patient usually has a period of four to five days of mild lassitude. Figure 2 is typical of most of the cases recognized in the western states.

Diagnosis. The diagnosis is made on the basis of the following criteria: (1) A history of having been bitten by a tick or having been in a tick-infested area four to six days prior to onset. (2) A fever curve and symptoms identical with dengue. The temperature rises rapidly to between 102° to 104° F., and occasionally to 105° F. During the remission it is frequently subnormal. (3) Absence of physical findings other than fever with a corresponding increase in pulse rate, slight erythema of the skin and conjunctival injection. (4) A reduced leukocyte count with an increase in immature forms. (5) Other confirmatory laboratory tests, usually unnecessary in the typical case.

Complement fixation tests during the acute phase and three weeks following recovery may be a useful procedure. The first test should be negative and the second positive. Injection intraperitoneally or intracerebrally into baby mice or baby hamsters of blood serum obtained during any phase of the disease will

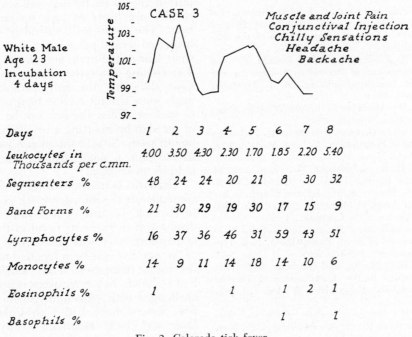

Fig. 2. Colorado tick fever.

cause the death of these animals, while neutralization of the virus with immune serum results in survival.

Care must be exercised not to confuse Colorado tick fever with the much more severe and frequently fatal Rocky Mountain spotted fever, especially since specific treatment is available for the latter. The difference in severity between the two is most helpful, while the rash of Rocky Mountain spotted fever will always differentiate the two. There is no disease in the United States with which typical Colorado tick fever should be confused except dengue. The mode of spread and the frequent presence of a rash in dengue suffice to differentiate them. Colorado tick fever is not a tick-borne dengue, since neither disease gives an immunity to the other, although each confers immunity to itself.

Prognosis. The prognosis is excellent. No complications or sequelae have ever been observed except for a mild stiffness of the neck in an occasional child. Although the virus is found in the cerebrospinal fluid, no increase in pressure or other abnormalities of the fluid have been observed.

Treatment. Treatment is symptomatic. Acetylsalicylic acid in standard doses is usually sufficient to reduce the fever and aching. There is no evidence that any of the available antimicrobial drugs is of value.

LLOYD FLORIO

References

Becker, F. E.: Tick-Borne Infections in Colorado; I. The Diagnosis and Management of Infections Transmitted by the Wood Tick; II. A Survey of the Occurrence of Infections Transmitted by the Wood Tick. Colorado Med., 27:36, 87, 1930.

———, Miller, M. S., and Mugrage, E. R.: Colorado Tick Fever: Isolation of the Virus From Dermacentor andersoni in Nature and a Laboratory Study of the Transmission of the Virus in the Tick. J. Immunol., 64:257, 1950.

———, Miller, M. S., and Mugrage, E. R.: Colorado Tick Fever; Isolations of Virus from Dermacentor variabilis Obtained from Long Island, New York, with Immunologic Comparisons Between Eastern and Western Strains. J. Immunol. 64:265, 1950.

———Miller, M. S., and Mugrage, E. R.: Colorado Tick Fever. Recovery of Virus from Human Cerebrospinal Fluid. J. Infect. Dis., 91:285, 1952.

Florio, L., Stewart, M. O., and Mugrage, E. R.: The Experimental Transmission of Colorado Tick Fever. J. Exper. Med., 80:165, 1944.

———, Stewart, M. O., and Mugrage, E. R.: The Etiology of Colorado Tick Fever. J. Exper., Med. 83:1, 1946.

YELLOW FEVER

Definition. Yellow fever is an acute viral disease characterized by sudden onset, prostration, moderately high fever, a pulse rate slow in relation to temperature and, when severe, by vomiting of altered blood, albuminuria and jaundice. It is endemic in the tropical rain forests of Africa and South America; in the past, summer epidemics have been widespread in the temperate zone. There are two epidemiologic types of the disease. When the virus is transmitted from man to man by the domestic mosquito, *Aedes aegypti,* it is called *urban yellow fever,* but when it occurs in a forest environment and is transmitted to man by some forest mosquito, usually in the absence of *A. aegypti,* it is called *sylvan (or jungle) yellow fever.*

Etiology and Epidemiology. Yellow fever virus is small, about 17 to 25 millimicrons in diameter. In nature the virus is pantropic, in that it has viscerotropic and neurotropic characteristics. Viscerotropism enables the virus to attack the liver, kidneys and heart, while neurotropism permits it to infect cells of the central nervous system. The virus becomes more neurotropic and loses its viscerotropism almost entirely during long-continued brain-to-brain passage through mice. Prolonged passage of the virus in tissue culture has produced an attenuated strain, 17D, suitable for use as vaccine.

Man is universally susceptible to the virus, and the characteristic symptoms and lesions of yellow fever in man are due to its viscerotropism, severe disease being the exception rather than the rule. The rhesus monkey, while no more susceptible to infection by the virus, is much more likely to die of the disease. Albino mice, especially of the Swiss strain, are highly susceptible to the neurotropic element of pantropic strains of the virus, provided they are inoculated by the intracerebral route.

In urban yellow fever, the aegypti mosquito transmits the virus by biting a human host during his initial three-day period of viremia and later biting a susceptible person. An extrinsic incubation period of nine to twelve days must elapse before the mosquito becomes infectious by bite.

In sylvan yellow fever man acquires his infection through the bite of some mosquito other than aegypti. In South America the virus has been isolated from wild-caught mosquitoes of the genus *Haemagogus* and from

Aedes leucocelaenus. In Africa it has been obtained from wild-caught *Aedes simpsoni* and *A. africanus.* The more important of these vectors, *Haemagogus* and *A. africanus,* inhabit chiefly the forest canopy which is also the habitat of the monkeys which are most frequently infected in nature. The exact role of monkeys in the epidemiology of sylvan yellow fever has not been elucidated.

Since 1934 no large epidemics of urban yellow fever have been reported from the Western Hemisphere, and the few small aegypti-transmitted epidemics which have occurred have been secondary to sylvan yellow fever. In Africa, in areas contiguous to the rain forest areas where sylvan yellow fever is endemic, there are still frequent epidemics of urban yellow fever. An important epidemic occurred in Nigeria in 1946. Beginning in 1948 in Panama, an epidemic wave of sylvan yellow fever has been spreading northward through the forests of Central America.

There is no evidence that yellow fever has ever been present in the Orient.

Morbid Anatomy. Yellow fever produces characteristic lesions in the liver of man. There is necrosis and necrobiosis of the parenchymal cells, most evident in the midzones of the lobules, with normal, or much less involved, cells around the central and portal veins. The necrosis is scattered and irregular, rather than massive and uniform. Scattered among the necrotic cells are Councilman bodies, parenchymal cells which have undergone eosinophilic hyaline necrosis. There are also fatty changes in the parenchymal cells. The liver lobules are not collapsed.

Clinical Manifestations. The great majority of attacks of yellow fever are mild, and show few of the classic symptoms. Not infrequently the only symptoms are low fever and headache, both of short duration.

The incubation period is from three to six days. The onset is sudden, often with a chill, and without prodromal symptoms. The first stage of the disease, which lasts about three days, is the *period of infection.* The symptoms are fever, severe headache, backache, pain in the legs and prostration. The face is flushed and the eyes are injected; there is photophobia. The tongue is bright red at the tip and edges. There is no jaundice at the onset of the illness. The temperature rises abruptly to about 104° F., sometimes higher. The pulse may rise to 90 or 100 initially, only to become increasingly slow in relation to the temperature (Faget's sign). The pulse

is full and strong during this stage. Nausea and vomiting are the rule, as are epigastric distress and tenderness. Constipation is to be expected. A progressive leukopenia, sometimes pronounced, has frequently been observed early in the disease. The sudden development of intense albuminuria about the third or fourth day is characteristic.

After a short remission the *period of intoxication* begins about the fourth day. The remission in fever is often indefinite or absent, and it may be accompanied by a deceptive temporary improvement. In this period, lassitude and depression may replace restlessness and agitation. Headache may diminish and jaundice gradually develops. While jaundice is always present in severe cases, it is usually not so marked as the name of the disease would indicate. The gums are swollen and bleed easily, either spontaneously or when pressed; the nose may bleed. There may be petechiae in the skin. Hemorrhages from the stomach, intestine or uterus, or subcutaneously, may be massive. The pulse rate falls progressively and may go below 50 per minute. Even in otherwise mild attacks there may be marked dilatation of the heart and low blood pressure as evidence of myocardial damage. Vomiting may be frequent and distressing, and the vomitus in this stage usually contains altered blood. The amount of albumin in the urine rises, often to 3 to 5 gm. per liter, sometimes much higher. Fatal cases often exhibit hiccup, copious vomiting of altered blood, tarry stools and anuria; coma may last two or three days. Or death may be immediately preceded by a short period of wild delirium. Death occurs most frequently from the sixth to the ninth day.

When there is recovery from a severe case, the temperature is likely to reach normal by the seventh or eighth day. Convalescence begins then and progresses rapidly to complete recovery, with rapid disappearance of the albuminuria. Relapses do not occur, and there are no sequelae. Complications are rare. A life-long immunity follows the attack, whether it be mild or severe.

A peculiarity of yellow fever is the great variation in the degree to which different organs are affected. With much renal involvement there may be no cardiac symptoms, and vice versa. In mild and moderate cases there is little or no albuminuria, jaundice or hemorrhage.

Diagnosis. In a severe febrile illness with "black vomit," intense albuminuria and jaundice, yellow fever must be suspected. Diseases which must be differentiated from severe yellow fever are: infectious and serum hepatitis, "acute yellow atrophy" of the liver, carbon tetrachloride poisoning, other jaundices and even malaria. In mild cases of yellow fever, which have been confused with dengue and influenza, clinical diagnosis is notoriously inaccurate. The necessary laboratory diagnostic procedures are highly specialized. These are two: the isolation of the virus in mice or rhesus monkeys; and yellow fever neutralization tests on paired acute-phase and convalescent serums.

For postmortem diagnosis, specimens of liver and other tissues should be preserved in 10 per cent formalin for histologic examination.

Prognosis. Early in the disease the prognosis should always be guarded, since sudden changes for the worse are not uncommon. If early symptoms are mild, rapid recovery is probable, though some severe cases will end favorably. Hiccup, copious black vomit, melena and anuria require a very grave prognosis.

The over-all average case fatality rate is less than 10 per cent, and rates of less than 5 per cent have been observed in epidemics involving completely susceptible populations. Rates as high as 85 per cent have been observed, but they are most exceptional. Even the often cited 50 per cent rate is false because large numbers of mild cases have been missed.

Treatment. There is no specific treatment. A patient should be moved as little as possible, and should be kept quiet in bed. The severe headache and body aches may require relief with an analgesic. The heart should be watched carefully throughout the illness and into early convalescence.

Water should be given in adequate amounts, parenterally if necessary. Easily assimilated food should be given to the extent which the patient will tolerate. Citrus fruit juices ad lib. are a time-honored prescription, but milk in moderate quantities would appear to be much more useful to a damaged liver. Procaine hydrochloride by mouth should control stubborn vomiting. When vomiting has ceased and the temperature is down, full diet may be given. Full activity should be gradually resumed.

Prevention. If a case of yellow fever is treated in a place in which vector mosquitoes exist, the patient must be kept under a bed net or in a mosquito-proof room during the first four days of his illness.

Vaccination is essential for persons who intend to visit yellow fever endemic areas and for the people resident in such areas. Two strains of living virus have been used extensively for human vaccination. The 17D vaccine is prepared in chick embryos and is given by subcutaneous inoculation. At the Pasteur Institute of Dakar the technique of vaccination by scarification of the skin was developed, using the neurotropic French strain suspended in gum arabic solution. This procedure is used extensively in French West Africa. With either strain an effective immunity to yellow fever is regularly produced. Severe reactions to the Dakar-type of vaccine seem to be more frequent than are reactions to 17D. The advantages of the Dakar method are its simplicity and low cost for large-scale application. Vaccination ordinarily gives protection in a week, and the consequent immunity has been shown to last at least six years. Communities infested with *Aedes aegypti* should protect themselves by exterminating that mosquito, making use of the efficient methods now available. An urban epidemic can best be stopped by mass vaccination of the population combined with a DDT spraying campaign.

J. AUSTIN KERR

References

Elton, N. W.: Progress of Yellow Fever Wave in Central America: Nicaragua and Honduras. Am. J. Pub. Health, 42:1527, 1952.
Strode, G. K.: Yellow Fever. New York, McGraw-Hill Book Co., 1951.
Theiler, M.: In Rivers, T. M.: Viral and Rickettsial Infections of Man. 2nd ed. Philadelphia, J. B. Lippincott Co., 1952, pp. 531–551.
Theiler, M., and Smith, H. H.: The Effect of Prolonged Cultivation in vitro upon the Pathogenicity of Yellow Fever Virus. J. Exper. Med., 65:767, 1937.

MEASLES

(Moribilli, Rubeola)

Definition. Measles is an extremely contagious febrile disease of high morbidity characterized by rash and catarrhal inflammation of the eyes and respiratory tract. It is principally a benign disease of children but may afflict with equal frequency persons of any age not previously attacked by its virus.

History. Although exanthems comparable to measles were described in Arabian writings as early as the tenth century, Sydenham in the seventeenth century was probably the first to distinguish the disease clearly from other infections. The infectious nature of measles was first conclusively demonstrated by Hektoen in 1905 in man-to-man transmission experiments. Convalescent serum was shown to be effective in the prevention of the disease by Nicolle and Conseil in 1918.

Etiology. Measles is caused by a virus of narrow host range which induces manifest disease only in man and monkeys. Although filterable agents from measles patients have been propagated in chick embryos (Rake and Shaffer) and in chick embryo tissue culture (Plotz), the demonstration of measles virus has been definitely dependent upon inoculation of human subjects or monkeys. By this tedious method certain limited information has been garnered concerning distribution within the host of the virus and some of its physical properties. The virus may be passed through Berkefeld N or Seitz EK filters. It may remain infective for four weeks at low temperatures (−35° F. or −72° C.) or for at least 34 hours at room temperature; it may be dried from the frozen state and retain viability for at least fifteen weeks. Virus has been demonstrated in the blood and nasopharyngeal washings of human and simian subjects during the period of prodromal symptomatology and the initial appearance of rash.

Recently Enders and Peebles have announced the recovery and passage in human kidney tissue culture of virus-like agents from the blood and throat washings of patients with typical measles. It appears highly probable that these agents represent isolates of measles virus. Neutralizing and complement fixing antibodies against these agents were demonstrated to appear in serums of convalescent patients. Should this preliminary report receive confirmation, techniques will be available for the first time for the specific laboratory diagnosis of measles.

Incidence and Epidemiology. Measles is a disease of cosmopolitan distribution, endemic in all but isolated populations. It may occur at any time of the year, but most outbreaks are in the late winter and early spring. The disease recurs in epidemic cycles at two- to three-year intervals in most civilized communities which have been studied. This epidemic periodicity is best explained as a result of the introduction of new susceptibles into the population by birth or ingress from other areas. When the proportion of nonimmunes reaches a certain crucial concentration, disease and coincident dissemination of virus may occur to produce an epidemic. It is likely that virus is introduced from sources external to the involved population, probably by incoming susceptibles; there is no solid evidence of subclinical infection or a postinfection carrier state with unmodified measles to suggest local persistence of virus in interepidemic periods. Isolated communities such as the Faeroe Islands (Panum) are infrequently attacked by measles, at which times manifest illness appears in virtually all persons not previously infected. In Greenland, a country not known to have been invaded previously by the disease, a recent epidemic resulted in overt measles in 99.9 per cent of the indigenous population (Christiansen et al.).

Throughout most of the world measles is a disease of children; the blood of most adults possesses neutralizing antibodies against the virus. Morbidity and mortality rates do not appear to be influenced by sex or race. Case fatality rates are highest in children less than five years of age, and are also relatively high in the aged. Congenital infection has occurred.

There is no evidence that the virus may vary in virulence in nature. The oft-cited and notorious virulence of the disease in primitive, isolated or crowded populations may be explained as a corollary of (1) more prevalent infection of feeble and aged adults, (2) poor environmental conditions, (3) inadequate medical care and (4) secondary bacterial infections. Because measles virus *per se* rarely induces fatal disease, it is evident that fatalities attributable to measles may vary in incidence according to the prevalence of bacterial pathogens and the resistance of the population to their presence.

Communicability. Measles is one of the most contagious of infections. Demonstration of virus in nasopharyngeal secretions is in accord with epidemiologic evidence that infection is disseminated and acquired by the respiratory tract. Close physical proximity or direct person-to-person contact is the usual requisite for infection, but third person transfer has occurred.

Immunity. An unmodified attack of measles usually confers lifelong immunity. Able observers have described apparently authentic instances of second or even multiple infections. Definitive proof of recurrent infection with measles virus is lacking, however, because specific, diagnostic laboratory tests are not available. Detailed study of a family subject to recurrent attacks suggests an hereditary defect in the capacity to develop immunity in certain cases. One such patient was found to be capable of antibody formation, and electrophoretic analysis of the serum showed no deficit of gamma globulin (Thamdrup). Temporary immunity may be passively acquired by receipt of convalescent serum or gamma globulin derived from the pooled serums of human adults (see Treatment). Humoral antibody is demonstrable in patients convalescent from gamma globulin-modified measles. The low incidence of measles in early infancy (0 to 6 months) is attributed to transient protection by placentally transferred maternal antibody.

Morbid Anatomy. Pathologic changes in fatal measles usually represent the compound effect of viral and secondary bacterial infection. Bronchopneumonia is almost invariably present; it is most frequently interstitial, but may be lobular with purulent exudate within the alveoli. More representative of the pathology of the uncomplicated viral disease are changes within the tonsillar, nasopharyngeal and appendiceal tissue removed during the prodrome. These changes consist of subepithelial round cell infiltration and the presence of large, multinucleated giant cells (Warthin). The latter are so characteristic that skilled pathologists have predicted the development of rash from their presence in surgical specimens. The lesions clinically apparent as Koplik's spots derive from inflammatory mononuclear cell infiltration of buccal submucous glands and necrosis of focal vesicular lesions of the mucosa. Rash is the result of proliferation of capillary endothelial cells in the corium and the coincident exudation of serum, and occasionally erythrocytes, into the epidermis.

Pathologic Physiology. No consistent or characteristic aberrations in physiology are observed with measles. The transient hemoconcentration and albuminuria found with other febrile diseases may occur. A normal total leukocyte count or leukopenia is observed throughout the febrile period. Initially, the leukopenia is occasioned by a decline in lymphocytes on the first day of fever; subsequently, granulocytopenia ensues as well. The incubation period is characterized by neutrophilia, and convalescence by a relative lymphocytosis. A false positive serologic test for syphilis may be observed.

Hormone-like Effects of Measles Infection. Several striking physiologic effects of measles, although poorly understood, mimic the influence of cortisone or corticotropin. These are: transient suppression of the tuberculin reaction, improvement in eczema and allergic asthma, delay in wound healing, and the induction of remissions in leukemia, Hodgkin's disease and lipoid nephrosis. Whether these effects are directly attributable to the virus or are hormonally mediated is not known.

Symptoms. Following an incubation period which averages eleven days, measles becomes clinically manifest with symptoms of fever, malaise, myalgia and headache. Within hours *ocular symptoms* of photophobia and burning pain are evidenced by conjunctival injection, tearing and exudate is the conjunctival sac. Concomitantly, or soon thereafter, *catarrhal inflammation of the respiratory tract* is manifested by sneezing, coughing and nasal discharge. Less commonly, hoarseness and aphonia may reflect laryngeal involvement. In this prodromal stage of one to four days' duration, petechial lesions of the palate and pharynx or tiny white spots on the buccal mucosa (*Koplik's spots*) may herald the appearance of skin rash. The white lesions described by Koplik characteristically occur lateral to the molar teeth and typically are mounted on red areolae of injected mucosa which may coalesce to form a diffuse red background. Not invariably present, they constitute a valuable, if not em pathognomonic, diagnostic sign. The enanthem may involve other mucous membranes such as the vaginal lining. It may "overlap" the subsequent appearance of the cutaneous rash by one to three days. Rarely, a transient, erythematous exanthem may occur in the prodromal period.

The *rash* of measles follows the prodromal symptoms by two to four days, occasionally as late as seven days. It first appears behind the ears or on the face as a blotchy erythema, spreads downward to cover the trunk, and finally is manifest on the extremities. The hands and feet may escape involvement. Initially, the eruption consists of discrete, reddish-brown macules which blanch with pressure. Subsequently, these lesions become slightly elevated, tend to coalesce and may develop a hemorrhagic, nonblanching component. The rash fades in the order of its appearance, disappearing about five days after onset attended by a fine, powdery desquamation which spares the hands and feet. At its

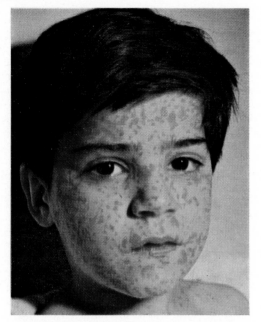

Fig. 3. *a*, Early measles eruption. (Reproduced from Therapeutic Notes, by Courtesy of Park, Davis & Company.)

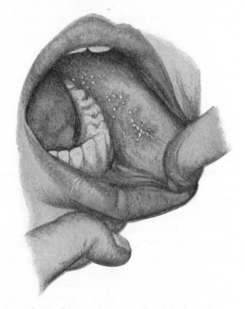

Fig. 3. *b*, Koplik's spots in measles (Hecker, Trumpp, and Abt).

maximum the exanthem usually marks the termination of malaise and fever in the uncomplicated illness.

The *fever* of measles is commonly of the typhoidal, progressively rising type and falls by lysis. It persists for about six days, and frequently reaches 103° F. In the adult,

fever may follow rather than antedate the catarrhal symptoms. Throughout the febrile period productive *cough* and auscultatory evidence of bronchiolitis may be evident. These manifestations may persist after defervescence, and cough is often the last symptom to disappear. It is probable that bronchopulmonary symptomatology is an integral part of the primary virus infection; roentgenographic evidence of pulmonary involvement is frequently seen in the uncomplicated disease in the absence of leukocytosis and obvious bacterial infection.

Complications. It is difficult to distinguish between those complications directly attributable to the virus of measles and those resulting from secondary bacterial infections. The persistence or recurrence of fever and the occurrence of leukocytosis are presumptive evidence of the usual bacterial sequelae of *otitis media* or *bronchopneumonia*. Beta hemolytic streptococci are the most frequent secondary invaders, but pneumococci or influenza bacilli may be implicated. The incidence of bacterial complications is increased by crowding, debility and the prevalence of bacterial pathogens in the population. Bacterially engendered sequelae may be unduly frequent in crowded contagious disease hospitals.

Serious complications directly related to the measles virus are rare. *Laryngitis* of sufficient severity to embarrass respiration has been observed, and may warrant tracheotomy. *Electrocardiographic abnormalities* may be found in as many as 30 per cent of children (Ross), but clinical evidence of cardiac disease is meager in such cases. *Abdominal pain* or *diarrhea* may be related to invasion of lymphoid tissue of the appendix or Peyer's patches. These symptoms may lead to unnecessary surgery before the appearance of the typical rash.

A rare (0.01 to 0.5 per cent) but serious consequence of measles is a demyelinating *encephalomyelitis* which may appear from one to fourteen days after the onset of infection. This complication is associated with a recurrence of fever, and headache, vomiting and stiff neck. Stupor and occasionally convulsions follow. Localizing neurologic symptoms may or may not be present. Death ensues in about 10 per cent of patients; about half of survivors suffer permanent residuals of varying severity (see chapter on Postinfection Encephalitis).

Other late sequelae of measles are thrombocytopenic purpura and exacerbation or activation of preexisting pulmonary tuberculosis.

Measles Modified by Antibody Administration. Attenuation of the natural disease by antibody prophylaxis may result in an illness of lessened severity comparable with the milder infection of the maternally immunized newborn. Fever alone may be observed, but some degree of exanthem is usually apparent. Koplik's spots may not appear. In general, the course is truncated and relatively uncomplicated.

Prognosis. Uncomplicated measles is rarely fatal, and complete recovery from the disease is the rule. Fatalities are almost always the result of secondary streptococcal or pneumococcal pneumonia, occurring principally in children below the age of five who become infected after the dissipation of passive neonatal immunity. Case fatality rates are also high in elderly and tuberculous patients. Cardiac decompensation is a common cause of death in patients over fifty.

The introduction of antimicrobial drugs effective against the usual secondary invaders

A Guide to the Differential Diagnosis of Measles

	CONJUNC-TIVITIS	RHINITIS	SORE THROAT	ENANTHEM	LEUKO-CYTOSIS	SPECIFIC LABORATORY TESTS AVAILABLE
Measles	++	+	0	+	0	0
Rubella	±	±	±	±	0	0
Exanthem subitum	±	±	0	0	0	0
Scarlet fever	±	±	++	0	+	+
Infectious mononucleosis	0	0	+	0	±	+
Drug rash	0	0	0	0	0	0

0 not usually present; no test available
± variable in occurrence; test available
+ present
++ present and severe

Diagnosis. The experienced layman can diagnose typical measles. The querulous, bleary-eyed child, his face blotched and his nose crusted with exudate, presents a characteristic, if miserable, picture as he breathes open-mouthed between paroxysms of sneezing and coughing. The severity of the catarrhal symptoms distinguishes the disease from other eruptive fevers. In the prodromal period the diagnosis should be suggested by (1) fever higher than that of the usual common cold, (2) known measles in the community and (3) Koplik's spots on the buccal mucosa.

Differential diagnosis (see table) includes consideration of rubella, scarlet fever, exanthem subitum, infectious mononucleosis, secondary syphilis and drug eruptions. Of value in excluding these possibilities are: the milder course and pinker rash of rubella, the sore throat and leukocytosis of scarlet fever, and serologic tests for infectious mononucleosis and syphilis. The rash of exanthem subitum does not appear until the termination of fever. Fever, enanthem and catarrh are uncommon with the cutaneous manifestations of drug hypersensitivity.

No specific laboratory tests are available for the diagnosis of measles.

has reduced the case fatality rate of measles sharply in recent years. The incidence of otitis media and pneumonia may be lowered by the prophylactic use of penicillin or a tetracycline early in illness (Karelitz et al.).

Encephalitis occurs as frequently in mild as in severe measles. However, modification of measles by gamma globulin prophylaxis (see below) affords an improved prognosis with reference to the encephalitic complication.

Treatment. There is no specific treatment for the fully developed disease. The administration of convalescent serum or gamma globulin during the period of incubation may prevent or modify the manifestations of illness. The degree of modification obtained is dependent upon the quantity of antibody given and the time of its administration. In children of less than six years, the intramuscular injection of 0.025 cc./lb. of gamma globulin in the first half of the incubation period results in disease of lessened severity. Two to four times this amount will prevent disease in nearly 80 per cent of children. In older children and adults, one and one-half to two times as much globulin is recommended. In young or debilitated children the aim is complete prevention of disease. In children over five, less subject to complications, the goal of prophylaxis is attenuation of the infection sufficient to lessen symptomatology but not the development of effective immunity. However, recent studies indicate that recurrences of measles may follow the gamma globulin-modified disease, in contrast to the solid permanent immunity conferred by the unaltered natural infection.

Symptomatic Therapy. In the absence of complications, bed rest is the essence of treatment in this benign, self-limited disease. Codeine sulfate (0.015 to 0.06 gm.) is useful in the amelioration of headache and myalgia and is effective in the management of cough. Acetylsalicylic acid (0.3 to 0.6 gm.) may be employed for its analgesic and antipyretic actions. Diet should be unrestricted. Bright light is not an ocular hazard, but photophobia may require darkening of the patient's room.

Antimicrobial prophylaxis. The course of uncomplicated measles is not influenced by antimicrobial therapy. In common practice the incidence of serious bacterial infections is not sufficient to justify the routine prophylactic use of antimicrobials. Certain special circumstances may warrant full therapeutic dosage with penicillin or the tetracyclines in anticipation of the potentially fatal sequelae of pneumococcal or beta hemolytic streptococcal infections. These circumstances include treatment of the chronically ill, the very young or the aged, and the treatment of patients under crowded conditions which foster the increase and dissemination of pathogenic bacteria, as may occur in contagious disease hospitals. If careful observation of the patient is possible, rational therapy is based on the prompt recognition and etiologic definition of complications, followed by initiation of the appropriate antimicrobial drug in proper dosage.

Vaccination. No vaccine is available for the production of effective active immunity. A chick embryo vaccine of attenuated living virus failed to protect its recipients from the natural disease, although the vaccine induced a mild form of measles in some subjects (Maris et al.).

EDWIN D. KILBOURNE

References

Christiansen, P. E., et al.: An Epidemic of Measles in Southern Greenland, 1951. Acta med. Scandinav., *144*:313, 430, 450, 1952–53.

Enders, J. F., and Peebles, T. C.: Propagation in Tis-sue Culture of Cytopathogenic Agents from Patients with Measles. Proc. Soc. Exper. Biol. & Med., 86:277, 1954.

Karelitz, S., King, H., Curtis, B., and Weichsel, M.: Use of Aureomycin and Penicillin in the Treatment of Rubeola in the Pre-eruptive and Early Eruptive Phase. Pediatrics, 7:193, 1951.

Koplik, H.: The Diagnosis of the Invasion of Measles from a Study of the Exanthema as It Appears on the Buccal Mucous Membrane. Arch. Pediat., *13*:918, 1896.

Maris, E. P., et al.: Vaccination of Children with Various Chorioallantoic Passages of Measles Virus; a Follow-up Study. Pediatrics, 4:1, 1949.

Panum, P. L.: Observations made during the Epidemic of Measles on the Faröe Islands in the Year 1847. English Translation. Panum on Measles, Delta Omega Society, 1940.

Plotz, H.: Culture "in vitro" du virus de la rougéole. Bull. Acad. de méd., Paris, *119*:598, 1938.

Rake, G., and Shaffer, M. F.: Propagation of the Agent of Measles in the Fertile Hen's Egg. Nature, *144*:672, 1939.

Ross, L. J.: Electrocardiographic Findings in Measles. Am. J. Dis. Child., 83:282, 1952.

Thamdrup, E.: Re-infections with Measles. Acta paediat., *41*:276, 1952.

Warthin, A. S.: Occurrence of Numerous Large Giant Cells in the Tonsils and Pharyngeal Mucosa in the Prodromal Stage of Measles. Arch. Path., *11*:864, 1931.

RUBELLA

(German Measles)

Rubella is an apparently benign but potentially malignant infection of children and young adults. This mild disease, usually manifest only by its pale pink rash and posterior cervical lymphadenitis, is now recognized as an important factor in the genesis of certain fetal abnormalities. Accordingly, recognition and prevention of the disease are matters of far reaching consequence.

Etiology. The causative agent of rubella is considered to be a virus, largely on the basis of its filterability. Study of the virus has been limited by its restricted host range; its presence is demonstrable only by infection of humans (Hiro and Tasaka) or monkeys (Habel). The virus is detectable in both blood and nasopharyngeal washings soon after the rash appears, and may be found in the blood two days before the eruption (Krugman et al.). Nasopharyngeal washings may retain infectivity for as long as two years when stored at −70° C. (Anderson, 1950).

Incidence and Epidemiology. Accurate information on the incidence of rubella is not available. The mildness and brevity of its clinical signs may confound the diagnosis and reporting of many instances of infection. Studies of the experimental disease lend support to prior clinical evidence that infection may occur without rash, and indicate a further diagnostic pitfall. It can be said, however, that the disease is seen on every continent, may occur in epidemic form and has its highest incidence in the early spring. The disease is less frequently acquired in childhood than measles, as is attested by the fact that rubella is more common than measles in young adults. The higher incidence of infection in younger age groups in institutional outbreaks argues against a greater susceptibility of the adult. It is probable that rubella is spread by the respiratory route by close personal contact. The infection is contagious during the period of prodromal symptoms and the first day of rash. Like measles, rubella rarely occurs in the first six months of life, and is uncommon beyond the age of 40.

Immunity is lasting. Authenticated second attacks are rare, and are virtually unprovable because of the nebulous nature of the clinical syndrome. Passive immunity of questionable efficacy may be conferred by the injection of gamma globulin from the serums of patients convalescent from the disease (see Treatment). Rubella has no immunologic relationship to measles.

Morbid Anatomy. Death from uncomplicated rubella is unknown. Histologic changes characteristic of the disease have not been demonstrated. The onset of disease is attended by leukopenia resulting from a decrease in both lymphocytes and neutrophils. After five days absolute lymphocytosis is manifest. The total leukocyte count is normal at the tenth day (Hynes).

Necropsies of fetal and infantile victims of maternal infection have shown a variety of embryonal defects related to developmental arrest involving all three germ layers. Those defects most consistently associated with maternal rubella are microcephaly, cataract, patency of the ductus arteriosus and defects of the interventricular septum. Limited evidence suggests that agenesis of the organ of Corti underlies the deafness observed in affected infants.

Symptoms. Fourteen to twenty-one days after exposure to the infection, the onset of rubella is evidenced by symptoms variable in their occurrence and severity. Cough, sore throat and coryza may initiate the illness, but are often absent; headache, malaise and myalgia may precede the eruption, especially in young adults. Commonly, fever and obvious enlargement of posterior cervical nodes antedate the appearance of the rash. Fever, when present, rarely exceeds 101° F. and seldom persists beyond 48 hours. Injection of the bulbar conjunctivas may be noted. Palpable, tender and occasionally visible lymphadenopathy involves postauricular and suboccipital nodes with sufficient frequency to be an important diagnostic sign. Generalized peripheral lymphadenitis, and, more rarely, splenomegaly, may occur.

The exanthem of rubella is usually apparent within 24 hours of the first symptoms as a faint macular erythema which first involves the face and neck. Characterized by its brevity and evanescence, it spreads rapidly to the trunk and extremities, sometimes leaving one site even as it appears at the next. The pink macules which constitute the rash blanch with pressure and rarely stain the skin. Diffuse erythema on the second day of rash may closely simulate scarlet fever. The eruption has vanished by the third day. Rubella may occur without rash. An enanthem has been described (Forchheimer) which is inconstant in form and occurrence, and lacks the premonitory significance of the Koplik spots of measles. The lesions consist of red macules which usually involve the soft palate.

Complications. Recovery is almost always prompt and uneventful, although relapse occurs with greater frequency than with most virus diseases (5 to 8 per cent). Secondary bacterial infections do not occur. Rare complications are arthralgia, neuritis, gingivitis, thrombocytopenic purpura and increased capillary fragility. Heart block has been described. A meningoencephalitis of short duration may occur one to six days after the appearance of rash. Its incidence is estimated at 1 in 6000 cases (Margolis et al.), and it is fatal in approximately 20 per cent of those afflicted.

Embryopathic Effects. The importance of rubella attaches to the well substantiated observation of Gregg that the occurrence of certain fetal abnormalities may be correlated with a history of maternal infection in the first trimester of pregnancy. Infection of the mother may lead to intrauterine fetal death or stillbirth, or more commonly to delivery of a viable infant of small size. Such infants show retardation in mental and physical development and varying degrees of congenital abnormality. The nature of the congenital defects observed has been related to the time of onset of the maternal infection and time of active proliferation of the primordia of organs subsequently manifesting defects. Clinical manifestations in the infant may range in severity from dental hypoplasia to complete or partial blindness, deafness and acyanotic cardiovascular disease. Blindness is usually related to cataract, deafness is of the inner ear type and patent ductus arteriosus is the most frequently observed cardiovascular abnormality. The latter condition has been related epidemiologically to the occurrence of rubella, in contrast to other congenital cardiac defects.

The true incidence of congenital lesions following rubella is not known; most of the available data are retrospective and hence unreliable. Studies are in progress in England and the United States to answer this important question.

Diagnosis. Rubella may be diagnosed with assurance only during an epidemic. It may be difficult to distinguish from mild or modified measles, infectious mononucleosis or scarlet fever. Distinction from measles may be made on the basis of the pinker, nonstaining rash, the milder course and the lesser catarrh of rubella. Sore throat is a more prominent complaint in scarlet fever; the course of infectious mononucleosis is often more protracted, and splenomegaly is more frequent than in rubella. Definitive diagnosis of scarlet fever and infectious mononucleosis may be made by laboratory means. No specific laboratory test is available for the diagnosis of rubella.

Prognosis. Complete recovery from rubella is almost invariable. The rare deaths attributable to rubella follow the infrequent complication of meningoencephalitis. Infection in pregnancy constitutes a hazard to the fetus but not to the mother.

Treatment. There is no specific treatment for the disease. Few patients suffer discomfort severe enough to warrant symptomatic medication. Headache and myalgia may be controlled by acetylsalicylic acid; bed rest is advisable for the duration of the fever.

Prophylaxis. In contrast to measles, current evidence is conflicting with regard to the prophylaxis of rubella with convalescent serum and gamma globulin. Various lots of gamma globulin appear to vary in prophylactic potency, some being completely ineffective. Trials of convalescent serum gamma globulin have been equally disappointing; prophylactic injection of susceptibles fails to protect them from the experimental disease. In natural epidemics an equivocally significant preventive effect has been noted (Anderson, 1953). *Women exposed to rubella in early pregnancy should receive the benefit of gamma globulin prophylaxis (as recommended for measles) despite its ambiguous status.*

Effective active immunization may be induced only by natural or experimental infection. The experimental infection is contagious (Krugman et al.) and constitutes a potential hazard to pregnant women in the community.

EDWIN D. KILBOURNE

References

Anderson, S. G.: Epidemiological Aspects of Rubella. M. J. Australia, 2:389, 1950.

————, and McLorinan, H.: Convalescent Rubella Gamma Globulin as a Possible Prophylactic against Rubella. M. J. Australia, *1*:182, 1953.

Forchheimer, F.: Enanthem of German Measles. Philadelphia M. J., 2:15, 1898.

Gregg, N. M.: Congenital Cataract Following German Measles in the Mother. Tr. Ophth. Soc. Australia, 3:35, 1941.

Habel, K.: Transmission of Rubella to *Macacus mulatta* Monkeys. Pub. Health Rep., 57:1126, 1942.

Hiro, Y., and Tasaka, S.: Die Röteln sind eine Viruskrankheit. Monatschr. f. Kinderheilk., 76:328, 1938.

Hynes, M.: Leucocyte Count in Rubella. Lancet, 2: 679, 1940.

Krugman, S., Ward, R., Jacobs, K. G., and Lazar, M.: Studies on Rubella Immunization. 1. Demonstration of Rubella without Rash. J.A.M.A., *151*: 285, 1953.

Margolis, F. J., Wilson, J. L., and Top, F. H.: Post-rubella Encephalomyelitis; Report of Cases in Detroit and Review of the Literature. J. Pediat., 23:158, 1943.

HERPES SIMPLEX

(Herpes Febrilis, Symptomatic Herpes, Fever Blisters, Cold Sores)

Definition. Herpes simplex is an acute infectious disease of man characterized by the development, in the skin or mucous membranes, of groups of superficial vesicles containing clear fluid. The infection is transmissible to a number of animal species, particularly the rabbit.

Etiology. Herpes simplex is caused by a

virus. With the exception of herpes zoster, all herpetic eruptions are thought to be induced by the same virus. This agent is of medium size and is 100 to 150 millimicrons in diameter. Löwenstein and Grüter showed that herpes simplex is caused by an infectious agent. There are two types of herpetic disease: *(a) primary* infections in persons without antibodies and *(b) recurrent* infections in persons with antibodies who are believed to be carriers of the virus. The virus is capable of infecting the central nervous system of various experimental animals and humans.

Morbid Anatomy. Hyperplasia of epithelial cells and necrosis and the development of vesicles containing clear fluid are the alterations usually seen in affected tissues. Inflammation in the adjacent corium is associated with these changes. Infected cells often show nuclear inclusion bodies.

Incidence. Herpetic eruptions often develop without evident cause and in the absence of other pathologic conditions. Frequently they occur during the course of various infectious diseases such as pneumonia, cerebrospinal meningitis, malaria, diphtheria, and so forth. In some persons recurrent herpes is seen, and in women it may be associated with menstruation. Injections of foreign proteins, e.g., vaccines or fever therapy, may precipitate an attack of herpes.

Symptoms. Primary infections, common in young children, are associated frequently with vesicular gingivostomatitis and may produce a constitutional reaction with fever, irritability, malaise and local lymphadenopathy. The disease is self-limited, but symptoms may persist for seven to ten days.

Recurrent infections, common in adults, usually are associated with herpetic eruptions which may occur anywhere in the skin or mucous membranes. Common sites are the lips, face, mouth, genitalia, conjunctiva and cornea. The lesions at first cause small painful swellings that rapidly develop into vesicles surrounded by areas of erythema. The vesicles are usually filled with clear, watery fluid, but suppuration may ensue. At times, particularly in the skin of the face, the distribution of lesions is similar to that seen in herpes zoster. Recurrent herpes simplex is usually a mild local lesion; when it is not associated with another infectious disease, general symptoms are rarely encountered.

Prognosis. In the absence of secondary infection the herpetic eruption gradually recedes and disappears. Corneal herpes may cause serious scarring and impairment of vision. One attack does not confer immunity against subsequent infections by the virus.

Treatment. No specific treatment has been developed. Local applications may relieve pain and swelling, but do not shorten the course of the eruption.

FRANK L. HORSFALL, JR.

References

Goodpasture, E. W.: Herpetic Infection with Especial Reference to Involvement of the Nervous System. Medicine, 8:223, 1929.
Grüter, W.: Experimentelle und klinische Untersuchungen über den sog. Herpes Corneae. Klin. Monatsabl. Augenheilk., 65:398, 1920.
Löwenstein, A.: Aetiologische Untersuchungen über den fieberhaften Herpes. Münch. med. Wchnschr., 66:769, 1919.
Scott, T. F. M., and Steigman, A. J.: Acute Infectious Gingivostomatitis. Etiology, Epidemiology and Clinical Picture of a Common Disorder Caused by the Virus of Herpes Simplex. J.A.M.A., 117:999, 1941.
Warren, S. L., Carpenter, C. M., and Boak, R. A.: Symptomatic Herpes, A Sequela of Artificially Induced Fever. Incidence and Clinical Aspects; Recovery of a Virus from Herpetic Vesicles, and Comparison with a Known Strain of Herpes Virus. J. Exper. Med., 71:155, 1940.

HERPES ZOSTER

(Zona, Zoster, Shingles)

Definition. Herpes zoster is an acute infectious disease characterized by inflammation of one or more dorsal root ganglia or extramedullary cranial nerve ganglia, and associated with a painful vesicular eruption in the skin or mucous membranes. The surface lesions are distributed along the course of peripheral sensory nerves arising in the affected ganglia.

History. Bärensprung (1863) showed that the disease was associated with inflammation of the corresponding dorsal root ganglion. Unna (1896) described the histology of the zoster vesicle. Head and Campbell (1900) made a classic study of the neuropathology. Bokay (1909) suggested that zoster and varicella were related etiologically. Lipschütz (1921) described the inclusion bodies seen in affected cells. Teague and Goodpasture (1921) pointed out the similarity between certain lesions of zoster and herpes simplex. Kundratitz (1925) reported successful attempts to transmit the disease to human beings. Numerous workers have failed in attempts to transmit the infection either to animals or to man.

Etiology. Present evidence strongly suggests that herpes zoster is caused by a virus, even though the infectious agent has not been definitely demonstrated by experimental procedures. The most direct indications that the agent is a virus are the presence of intranuclear inclusions in cells of the surface lesion, the reported successes in experimental transmission to man, and the presence of immunity following the disease.

The portal of entry of the infectious agent is unknown. It is not certain how the agent reaches the ganglia it affects. The occurrence of so-called symptomatic herpes zoster, in association with various pathologic processes about the ganglia, e.g., tuberculosis, syphilis or neoplasms, suggests that the agent may either be present commonly in the environment or often latent in human tissues.

Morbid Anatomy. The basic lesion is in the dorsal root or extramedullary cranial nerve ganglia corresponding to the sensory innervation to the areas of herpetic eruption. The lesions consist of severe inflammation and destruction of ganglion cells and fibers. These changes are followed by degeneration in the peripheral sensory nerve, in the posterior nerve root and in the corresponding fibers of the spinal cord.

The cutaneous vesicle is situated in the epithelial layer, and there is marked inflammation of the corium. Acidophilic intranuclear inclusions are found in epithelial cells about the vesicle.

Symptoms. In cases of so-called essential or idiopathic herpes zoster a typical attack rises without any obvious cause. There is a prodromal period, usually of three or four days' duration, during which the patient feels ill, the temperature is elevated and there is more or less pain. At this time a definite diagnosis cannot be made, but suddenly the erythematous and vesicular eruption appears with its characteristic distribution along the course of a sensory nerve, usually of the trunk, occasionally in a trigeminal area. The eruption is frequently preceded or accompanied by enlargement of the regional lymph nodes. There is often an increase in the number of cells in the cerebrospinal fluid.

The febrile period lasts usually from three to five days, and with its subsidence drying and healing of the cutaneous lesions take place. Secondary infection may delay healing and increase the tendency to scarring. Neuralgic pains may persist, especially in elderly people, and rarely there is some local residual paralysis.

Herpes zoster of the face occurs and is often severe. It usually results from involvement of the first branch of the sensory division of the trigeminal nerve and may lead to serious corneal ulceration which requires special care. The other cranial nerves are rarely affected.

Diagnosis. Because of the characteristic sensory nerve distribution of the vesicular eruption, the diagnosis is usually not difficult after the lesions appear. In children and rarely in adults the local eruption may be followed by the appearance of numerous other vesicles apparently unrelated to cutaneous innervation. In cases in which a generalized vesicular exanthem appears there may be a question, especially in children, whether the disease is not, in reality, varicella. There is some clinical and epidemiologic evidence indicating that the viruses of herpes zoster and of chickenpox are related etiologic agents. The histopathology of the cutaneous lesions offers no distinction between the two, for acidophilic intranuclear inclusions occur in the epithelial cells about the vesicles and in the corium of cutaneous lesions of varicella; and these, as well as other elements of the affected skin areas, are similar to those of herpes zoster.

Occasionally the virus of herpes simplex causes a vesicular eruption along the course of a cutaneous nerve, usually limited in extent, and it may involve the supraorbital branch of the ophthalmic nerve. This may closely simulate a mild herpes zoster. In such cases the presence of the virus of herpes simplex can be determined by inoculating vesicular contents into the scarified cornea of a rabbit. The viruses of herpes zoster and of varicella, on the other hand, have never been proved to be transmissible to any species other than man.

Treatment. There is no specific treatment for herpes zoster. Relief of pain and prevention of secondary infection of the surface lesions are the most important considerations. In mild cases salicylates or codeine are sufficient, but in severe cases morphine or Demerol may be required to relieve pain. Locally, antiseptic powders or ointments containing phenol, cocaine and the like may be used. Numerous special remedies have been offered, e.g., paraffin coating, ultraviolet irradiation, x-ray therapy, pituitary extracts, certain antimicrobial drugs, and so on, but there is no convincing evidence that any of these procedures is of value. In so-called symptomatic herpes zoster, treatment should be directed to the cause of the associated condition, i.e., syphilis, tuberculosis, tumor, and so forth.

Postherpetic neuralgia may be prolonged and refractory to treatment. In patients who suffer intractable pain, posterior root section or ganglionectomy may be necessary.

FRANK L. HORSFALL, JR.

References

Bärensprung: Fernere Beiträge zur Kenntniss des Zoster. Ann. d. Char.-Krankenh. zu Berlin, 11: Hft. 96, 2, 1863.
Bokay, J.: Ueber den ätiologischen Zusammenhang der Varizellen mit gewissen Fällen von Herpes zoster. Wien. klin. Wchnschr., 22:1323, 1909.
Head, H., and Campbell, A. W.: The Pathology of Herpes Zoster and Its Bearing on Sensory Localization. Brain, 23:353, 1900.
Kundratitz, K.: Experimentelle Uebertragungen von Herpes Zoster auf Menschen und die Beziehungen von Herpes zoster zu Varicellen. Ztschr. f. Kinderh., 39:379, 1925.
Lipschütz, B.: Untersuchungen über Aetiologie der Krankheiten der Herpes Gruppe (Herpes Zoster, Herpes Genitalis, Herpes Febrilis). Arch. f. Dermat. u. Syph., 136:428, 1921.
Philadelphy, A., and Haslhofer, L.: Varicellen bei Leukämischer Lymphadenose. Arch. f. Dermat. u. Syph., 169:512, 1934.
Teague, O., and Goodpasture, E. W.: Experimental Herpes Zoster. J. Med. Res., 44:185, 1923.
Tyzzer, E. E.: The Histology of the Skin Lesions in Varicella. Philippine J. Sc., 1:349, 1906.

VARICELLA

(Chickenpox)

Varicella is a mild communicable disease of childhood characterized by fever and a vesicular eruption with erythema around the vesicles, and involving the skin over the entire body and the mucous membranes of the mouth and throat.

Etiology and Epidemiology. The causative agent is a virus estimated to be approximately 145 to 250 millimicrons in diameter. It is found in the vesicular fluids in largest amounts from twenty-four to forty-eight hours after appearance of the lesions, and electronmicrographs have recently shown it to be a cuboidal or bricklike body about two

thirds the size of the vaccinia or the smallpox virus. All three of these viruses have a similar cuboidal or bricklike appearance. The virus of herpes zoster also is indistinguishable morphologically from that of varicella, and is quite similar antigenically.

The virus of varicella has been grown successfully in tissue cultures by Weller, but animals other than man do not appear to be susceptible.

Convalescent serums from cases of varicella effectively agglutinate the virus of herpes zoster, and vice versa. Herpes zoster in adults will often initiate an epidemic of varicella in children, and data also appear to indicate that varicella in children will cause zoster in an adult on rare occasions. In varicella of children, posterior root involvement, indistinguishable from zoster, is frequent. Varicella has been produced experimentally in children by intradermal inoculation with zoster vesicular fluid. The relation between zoster and varicella could well be explained on the basis of their antigenic identity—varicella representing the original invasion of the virus and zoster an accelerated reaction of an immune or partially immune person. The former would presumably occur at an early age, the latter in adults or older children who were able to localize the virus.

Varicella epidemics are rarely seen in persons over twenty years of age. The disease strikes both sexes equally. It occurs more frequently in the winter and spring, and the frequency of epidemic recurrence depends upon the density of susceptibles.

A striking characteristic of varicella, in which it resembles measles, is the highly communicable nature of the virus, which appears to spread chiefly by the air-borne route, although direct contact and droplet "hits" from sneezing, coughing or speaking at times must play an important role. The virus apparently enters through the respiratory tract and is spread by the same route during the early catarrhal stages of the disease, when mild inflammatory reactions of the mucous membranes of the nasopharynx are more evident. Spread of the disease also occurs from the vesicles on the skin during the early stages of the eruption, but probably no spread of the virus occurs after the appearance of crusts.

Immunity is usually permanent after a single attack. Transplacental passive immunity may be present in newborn infants, although cases have been recorded in infants within the first two weeks of life. The rarity of exposure of newborn infants to varicella has delayed conclusive evidence on this question.

Morbid Anatomy. The vesicular lesions of varicella and zoster in the skin are identical histologically, showing marked ballooning of the prickle cells, amitotic giant cells and numerous acidophilic intranuclear inclusions. Though in the early stages of the development of lesions some proliferation of the epidermis occurs, the corium remains virtually unaltered. The typical vesicle is the result of disintegration of the multinucleated giant cells and the ballooned prickle cells with the entrance of tissue fluids. The larger vesicles may involve all layers of the skin and result in scarring. In the later stages of the vesicle, acidophilic inclusion bodies may be seen both in the nuclei and in the cytoplasm of the cells. In the few postmortem examinations carried out the same cellular changes and intranuclear inclusions were found in the esophagus, pancreas, liver, renal pelvis, ureters, bladder and adrenal glands.

Incubation. The incubation period usually is fourteen to sixteen days, but in many instances the first symptoms and signs occur as late as twenty-one days from the time of exposure.

Symptoms and Signs. Prodromal symptoms may be severe, particularly in adults, but in childhood they are apt to be mild or absent, with nasopharyngitis, mild fever, headache, malaise and anorexia. Within twenty-four to forty-eight hours crops of papules and later of vesicles begin to appear on the face and trunk, particularly about the shoulders, and usually a few appear on the buccal mucosa or pharynx. The majority of lesions are vesicular. The vesicles are slightly elevated with a surrounding circular erythema or areola, and it is difficult to mistake them for any other lesion, except possibly those of variola. In variola, however, in addition to the severity of the symptoms and the more extensive character of the rash, the vesicles appear almost simultaneously and are usually larger, with a greater tendency to umbilication.

In varicella the appearance of fresh crops of vesicles in the same area of skin over a period of twenty-four to seventy-two hours is characteristic; for this reason, in contrast to variola, the lesions are usually seen in various stages of development, some as small, translucent vesicles, some with slight um-

bilication, as the vesicles dry from the center, and some with dry, firmly attached crusts. Also, in variola, the severe symptoms precede the eruption, while in varicella the symptoms accompany the eruption unless the disease is unusually severe. Severe irritation and itching usually accompany vesiculation in varicella, and for this reason in younger children the larger lesions are rarely permitted to heal "by first intention" unless care is taken to prevent scratching and to relieve the severe itching. Excoriated areas and larger crusts are the inevitable result.

On the buccal mucosa or the pharynx the vesicles early become small ulcer craters with a surrounding erythema and resemble closely the type of ulcer frequently seen in herpetic stomatitis. Two particularly annoying points of attack are the larynx and the conjunctivas. At times vesicles in these structures may be dangerous because of complicating bacterial infections. The genitalia also must be examined daily, since lesions on these areas are often scratched and secondarily infected. Another area frequently overlooked is the scalp, where the matting of hair over scratched and crusted lesions results in severe secondary bacterial infections, with enlarged and tender occipital and posterior cervical lymph nodes.

In the mildest cases, only ten to twenty lesions may appear on the skin, and there may be no fever or only a transient fever of a few hours; in the more severe cases the discrete vesicles will dot the entire body surface and the temperature rises to 103° or 104° F. for several days at the time of the appearance of the rash. The disease in adults may at times be dangerously severe before and during the appearance of the eruption. Rarely, necrosis occurs around the vesicles, resulting, if widespread, in lesions which have been termed "varicella gangrenosa."

Complications. The most severe complications may occur in children who are subject to eczema or staphylococcal infections of the skin. In such children the vesicles rapidly fill with pus and are usually ruptured by scratching, with a resultant spread of infection and ulceration. Such ulceration and crusting are typical of impetigo contagiosa, and many cases of varicella observed first in the late stages would be diagnosed as impetigo were a proper history not available. After the usual case of severe varicella a few small scars or pox marks remain about the face or shoulders even though scratching has been avoided, but in the secondarily infected case with pus and crusting, the pox marks may be large and disfiguring. Hemolytic streptococci, resulting in severe cellulitis and erysipelas, have been less common secondary invaders, but, until the advent of effective antimicrobial therapy, they were the complicating organisms most feared. A small percentage of cases of acute glomerular nephritis are the result of skin infections, and varicella with its complications plays an important role in this group of causative factors. Pneumonia from laryngeal ulceration, abscesses of lymph nodes draining secondarily infected areas, and serious eye infections are other less common complications to be avoided by proper preventive measures.

A rather infrequent but important complication, due probably to the activity of the virus only, is encephalitis, which is similar to that caused by measles and by other communicable diseases. It occurs in the more severe cases of varicella, usually toward the end of the febrile period, but may at times appear one to three weeks after the attack of the disease. It is rarely fatal, and complete recovery usually occurs.

Diagnosis. The appearance of vesicles on the skin, each surrounded by a ring of erythema, and accompanied by a fever, however slight, is the *sine qua non* of varicella. If the disease is seen in this stage of vesiculation, when the crops of eruption in the various stages of translucent vesicles, vesicles with umbilication, and crusting are seen, it cannot readily be mistaken for any other disease. The severe constitutional reaction caused by smallpox, together with uniformity of development of the eruption in all areas of the skin at the same time, serves to separate it from varicella. Smallpox lesions also appear in somewhat larger numbers on the extremities and face and involve the skin more deeply than the lesions of varicella.

Varicella must also be differentiated from impetigo, herpes zoster, urticaria and eruptions resulting from various drugs, such as the sulfonamide group, bromides and others.

Treatment. The treatment must be directed almost entirely toward increasing the patient's comfort and preventing secondary infections. In severe cases with widespread eruption it is difficult to prevent extreme discomfort, and sedatives, such as phenobarbital, should be used in adequate doses. If, despite local treatment, pustular infections, abscesses, erysipelas or impetigo occur, the patient should receive appropriate antimicrobial

therapy. In addition, if the patient is first seen in the later stages and a widespread pustular eruption and crusting are present, extensive application of potassium permanganate solution, 1 to 5000, in wet dressings at regular intervals is very effective. In the uncomplicated case of varicella the crusts should be permitted to loosen slowly and drop off in order to avoid extensive scars, and even in the complicated pustular eruption, for the same reason, the crusts should be handled with considerable care. In children the fingernails should be kept short and the ends of the fingers and the fingernails should be scrubbed carefully with soap and water and alcohol.

Prevention. Quarantine is rarely successful. The prophylactic use of convalescent or pooled adult serum has been also rarely successful, even when used early in the incubation period. However, at times, in hospitals and institutions for children the use of large amounts of convalescent serum in the exposed susceptibles has apparently stopped the spread of the disease. For attempted complete protection, 15 cc. of convalescent serum should be used for a child less than six years of age, and 20 cc. of serum for a child over this age. Mere modification of the disease by serum in childhood is not indicated because of its usually mild nature. The recent work by Weller may well explain the variability in protection afforded by convalescent serum or plasma, inasmuch as neutralization tests have indicated a sharp but quite temporary rise of antibodies very early in convalescence. The time of obtaining such antibodies for passive protection would thus be very important.

Vaccination with vesicular fluid or by other methods has not as yet been successful.

It appears possible to prevent the spread of infection by the air-borne route with the use of ultraviolet irradiation, but except for nurseries such protection would be inadvisable.

JOSEPH STOKES, JR.

References

Johnson, H. N.: Visceral Lesions Associated with Varicella. Arch. Path., 30:292, 1940.
Kundratitz, K.: Experimentelle Uebertragungen von Herpes zoster auf Menschen und die Beziehungen von Herpes zoster zu Varicellem. Ztschr. f. Kinderh., 39:379, 1925.
Rivers, T. M., and Eldridge, L. A., Jr.: Relation of Varicella to Herpes Zoster. I. Statistical Observa-

tions. II. Clinical and Experimental Observations. J. Exper. Med., *49*:899, 907, 1929.

The School Epidemics Committee: Epidemics in Schools. Med. Research Council Special Report Series No. 227, 181, 1938.

Tyzzer, E. E.: The Histology of the Skin Lesions in Varicella. Philippine J. Sci., *1*:349, 1906.

Von Bokay, J.: Ueber den ätiologischen Zusammenhang der Varizellen mit gewissen Fallen von Herpes zoster. Wien. klin. Wchnschr., 22:1323, 1909.

SMALLPOX

(*Variola*)

Definition. Smallpox is an acute communicable disease characterized by severe constitutional symptoms and a single crop of skin lesions all proceeding at the same rate through a macular, papular, vesicular and pustular stage over a period of approximately three to ten days.

History. In addition to certain evidence in the earliest records of China and Egypt suggesting its presence in both Asia and Africa, the disease undoubtedly changed the course of the Roman Empire and later altered the course of history among nations, kings and men of all nationalities throughout Europe and the British Isles, up to the time of Jenner. In the Western Hemisphere the conquest of the natives by the European races may be attributed in no small degree to the devastating effect of the introduction of the virus of smallpox among the Indians by their conquerors. However, the discovery of vaccination by Jenner dramatically altered the role of the virus from that of the conqueror to that of the conquered.

Etiology and Epidemiology. Smallpox is apparently caused by a virus which in size and shape closely resembles the cuboidal or bricklike vaccinia virus. These viruses can readily be grown on the chorioallantois of the embryonated egg and have a diameter of about 200 millimicrons. They are readily stained by certain aniline dyes. The virus of smallpox is found in the vesicular fluid, being slightly larger than the varicella virus. It withstands drying for long periods without refrigeration, which probably accounts for the ease with which it is transmitted. Dry desquamated crusts, dust or bed clothes from a patient's room may remain infective for long periods. The protection against smallpox afforded man by the vaccinia virus was a historic event in preventive medicine. Both *in vitro* and *in vivo* tests have indicated the presence of common antigens and antibodies for both viruses.

Variolation, the practice of using material from active lesions or variola crusts for transmission of the disease with a view to controlling it, marks the first use historically of any active virus in planned transmission. The use of crusts or pustular lesions was later replaced by the use of fluid from early vesicles for scarification of human susceptibles. The resulting disease resembled varioloid (modified smallpox; see below) in that a local lesion occurs at the point of scarification followed in about eleven days by a mild generalized eruption which usually leaves no scars. Variola virus generally produces a mild disease similar to varioloid in anthropoids, and in monkeys it may occur by contact simultaneously with a human epidemic. Other animals are far less susceptible and develop only local lesions, as, for example, the rabbit, in which vaccinia virus multiplies rapidly in contrast to the localized lesions of variola virus.

Transmission of smallpox to susceptibles may occur during all stages of the disease and until the scabs have disappeared.

Occurrence of small outbreaks of the disease even among the carefully vaccinated U.S. Army has demonstrated the need for vaccination in the presence of epidemics of the disease. For example, in 1945 and 1946 the U.S. Army in Korea suffered 121 cases of smallpox with 25 deaths. Revaccination of troops in this area with fresh vaccinia virus completely controlled the outbreaks, which, however, continued among the surrounding natives.

The incidence of smallpox has been greater in the United States, where vaccination is not nationally compulsory, than in countries which require vaccination. In the United States the incidence is particularly high in those states which make little effort to vaccinate children against the disease, but cases have been occurring in every state. In Philadelphia there were 2585 deaths from smallpox in 1872, and as late as 1904 over 200 deaths occurred yearly; with the advent of compulsory vaccination no deaths from smallpox have occurred since 1924.

Smallpox is more frequently fatal in infants and children, and no transplacental immunity appears to be established—a situation similar to that of varicella. Smallpox contracted during pregnancy may involve the fetus, and infants have been born suffering from a typical eruption. Pregnant women suffering from a severe attack of the disease usually abort. Men and women are equally susceptible. Complete natural immunity is extremely rare, but permanent immunity is generally established by a single attack, since there have been only a few reports of second attacks.

There appears to be a greater susceptibility among the colored races, especially the Negro, to the virus of smallpox. Although smallpox generally occurs during the winter months, this is probably due to closer contacts within inclosed spaces in the colder weather. Epidemics have been known to occur during the summer weather. There is a great variation in the severity of epidemics, and fortunately those of recent years have been mild, possibly because of greater emphasis upon cleanliness of the skin with resultant diminished danger of secondarily invading bacteria. The virus itself also appears to vary in virulence, and many mild cases termed *varioloid* may occur. Such mild cases in the majority of instances appear to be a result of previous vaccination. On the other hand, the virus appears at times to gain in virulence as the epidemic progresses.

Morbid Anatomy. The pathologic lesions are almost entirely in the skin and mucous membranes. The lack of a cornified epithelium in the mucous membrane prevents the development of a typical vesicle and pustule, while ulcers with a deep crater and a surrounding red areola are common, similar to those of varicella, but usually more extensive. These ulcers often occur in the buccal and nasopharyngeal mucosa, larynx, trachea, esophagus, vagina, and even in the intestinal mucosa at times. The bladder, ureters and urethra are rarely involved. Secondarily invading streptococci and staphylococci frequently are present and increase the severity of the disease, but the pustular stage of the eruption occurs irrespective of the presence or absence of these organisms. The local skin lesion is a multilocular pock in which the epithelium becomes degenerated and vacuolated with transudation of serum and the formation of a reticulum. As the reticular spaces swell with transudate and later with exudate, their walls rupture to form the typical pustule. This pustule may be only in the epidermis, but frequently extends into the corium. Such lesions contain both the typical cytoplasmic acidophilic inclusions lying close to the cell nucleus and termed the Guarnieri bodies, and also the intranuclear inclusions. A single cell apparently does not include both types of inclusions, i.e., both cytoplasmic and intranuclear. The round or oval Guarnieri body, which is about 10 microns in diameter with an unstained halo around it, is probably a mass of variola virus imbedded in a matrix, while the intranuclear inclusion apparently does not contain virus. The latter is also round or oval, somewhat smaller than the Guarnieri body, is acidophilic, and is separated from the nuclear membrane in histologic preparations by an unstained halo.

Two types of hemorrhage may occur with the lesions: (1) *purpura variolosa,* in which extensive hemorrhages invade the corium, only occurring, however, in the most severe cases soon after the onset of the disease, and usually fatal; and (2) *variola haemorrhagica pustulosa,* in which small localized hemorrhages occur into the pock—a severe form of the disease, but causing fewer fatalities than purpura variolosa.

Aside from the local changes in the cutaneous lesions of smallpox, the general pathologic picture, as far as has been determined, differs little from that resulting from other severely toxic states. The lungs are frequently involved by secondarily invading organisms such as pneumococci and streptococci, resulting in bronchopneumonia which may be hemorrhagic at times. The liver is usually enlarged at the time the pustules develop and may also contain hemorrhagic foci. The spleen is similarly enlarged during the pustular stage and hemorrhages may also occur into the pulp. Because of the marked involvement of the skin of the face, the cervical lymph nodes are also considerably enlarged, chiefly with edema which extends beyond the capsule of the node. The marrow is notable for the absence of polymorphonuclear elements, and hemorrhages frequently occur in the more severe cases. Hemorrhages also may occur into the pelvis of the kidneys and into the ureters, usually beneath the mucous membranes, and severe degenerative changes in the kidneys themselves are often noted.

There is a characteristic proliferation in the hematopoietic system and extensive infiltration, particularly in the liver, kidney, adrenals and testicle of mononuclear basophilic cells, which in areas such as the testicle appear to cause pressure severe enough to produce occasionally localized necrosis.

Symptoms. *Clinical History.* The *period of incubation* lasts usually from eight to twelve days, but may be somewhat shorter or longer. At onset the constitutional symptoms are severe, with marked headache, usually a chill or chilliness, aching of the back and limbs quite similar to that of epidemic influenza, and a mounting fever which may reach a height of 106° or 107° F. In children, convulsions and vomiting or drowsiness, quickly followed by coma, may occur. The patient is usually prostrated, the face is flushed, the pulse is usually full and bounding, and marked restlessness, which at times amounts to delirium, supervenes.

shotty, 2 to 4 mm. in diameter, with an appearance unlike any other exanthematous disease. Widespread tuberculids, all of the same size and symmetrically distributed, could have the same appearance. With the increasing size and tenderness of the papules, *multilocular vesicles* begin to form over the papules on about the sixth day, characteristically umbilicated because of a dry and depressed center. Some vesicles are superficial, while others are deeper and not so readily rec-

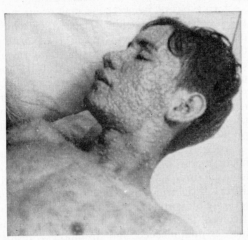

Fig. 4. Smallpox in a young man during the active stage of the disease. Note the even distribution of lesions on the face and trunk. (Courtesy of Drs. Vernon Knight and A. Ruiz-Sanchez.)

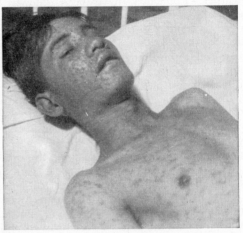

Fig. 5. Same patient as in Figure 4 during convalescence after treatment with intravenous injections of oxytetracycline (Terramycin) for secondary invaders.

Transient rashes resembling scarlet fever or measles may occur during the *prodromal stages* of the disease while the temperature is approaching or when it has reached its highest point. Such rashes occur only during the first two days and are found usually over the lower abdomen and the inner aspects of the thighs. The position of the rash and its lack of elevation serve to distinguish it from measles or scarlet fever. At times such a rash initiates the more severe types of smallpox.

On the third or fourth day, *raised macules* begin to appear over the face. The earlier these macules appear, the more likely is the rash to become confluent. The macules rapidly develop into *papules,* and with this development there is associated an immediate diminution in the severity of symptoms and the fever, the patient becoming considerably more comfortable. Fever and symptoms usually increase later irrespective of multiplication of staphylococci or streptococci in the pustules with their attendant complications. The single crop of papules are firm and

ognized. By approximately the eighth day the vesicle becomes full of cloudy fluid and the typical *pustular rash* is in full bloom. The pustular nature of the lesion apparently is not dependent upon the presence of secondarily invading bacteria, although they are often present and greatly increase the danger of complications. The pustules are slightly larger than the papules, with somewhat greater elevation, and have a characteristic greenish or grayish-yellow color. A small red areola forms about each lesion at the time of vesiculation, a phenomenon which occurs synchronously with the development of an allergic response of the skin to variolous material.

Although the lesions may vary slightly in size, they proceed through each stage of development at the same time and do not appear in crops, as is characteristic of varicella, with which otherwise mild smallpox might be readily confused. Although all the lesions appear at approximately the same time, a small percentage of them do not progress through all the characteristic steps, but remain at times only as papules or with very slight evidence of vesiculation. In such lesions involution occurs frequently in the earlier stage of the disease.

The rash usually appears on the face and about the wrists only slightly in advance of its appearance on the rest of the body, and then rather rapidly involves the rest of the forearms, upper arms, and thorax. The lateral region of the neck from the clavicle to the lower jaw, the inguinal areas and around the eyes usually have very few pocks. The abdomen and legs are often only slightly involved, but in severe cases this may not be true. Such severe cases, in which the rash is widespread and in which the lesions are so closely studded over the skin that they coalesce, are termed *confluent;* whereas in the absence of coalescence the term *discrete* may be used.

Frequently these two forms, confluent and discrete, occur in the same patient, the confluent lesions appearing on the face and about the wrists, while the discrete lesions appear on the thorax, abdomen and legs. In certain confluent lesions the area involved has almost the appearance of a large abscess. On the face these lesions can be particularly distressing, often producing extreme discomfort; edema may close the eyelids and involve the tissues of the neck as well. Edema of the hands and feet often occurs in children. At the height of the pustulation, lesions frequently occur in areas which must be watched closely for secondary infection: the mouth and nasopharynx, the prepuce, the labia and the vagina. Lesions on the palms and plantar surfaces are not apt to develop into vesicles and pustules, but nevertheless form crusts. Marked pitting of the face or arms occurs, as a rule, only in the areas where the lesions are confluent.

With the appearance of pustules in the more severe cases, the temperature, which has fallen with the earlier appearance of the papules, again begins to rise and subsides only when satisfactory crusting has occurred. Staphylococcal and streptococcal invasions of the pustules apparently are not responsible for the secondary febrile reactions, although they may increase them. The pustules and crusts itch severely, and scratching must be prevented. Desquamation may begin at the twelfth to the fourteenth day, and, unlike the branny desquamation of measles and scarlet fever, the desquamating crusts are thick and brownish-yellow in appearance. A dark blue discoloration of the skin occurs in the area from which the crust has separated, but this gradually and completely disappears.

Blood. There is usually a leukopenia together with a relative mononucleosis in the earlier stages of the disease, but later a leukocytosis occurs, particularly during the pustular stage and when secondary complications occur. Anemia usually occurs together with enlargement of both the spleen and the liver. In the two hemorrhagic types of smallpox previously mentioned, considerable depression of the bone marrow and the liver may occur, resulting apparently in alterations in the platelets, fibrinogen and prothrombin. The exact origin of such hemorrhagic phenomena, however, is not entirely clear.

Varioloid. This term is usually applied to smallpox modified by a vaccination which has "taken" successfully within approximately five years. The lesions are of the discrete type, the prodromal symptoms are rarely severe, there is no secondary rise of fever, and the lesions frequently undergo involution with a markedly shortened course.

Abortive Types. Occasionally in recently vaccinated persons early involution of the eruption occurs, even before vesicles are well established, and in rare instances the eruption never develops, a condition which is known as *variola sine eruptione.*

Complications. The common complications of smallpox may be considered as largely due to the secondary invasions of staphylococci and streptococci. Abscesses, septicemia, nephritis, erysipelas, laryngitis and the various lower respiratory infections can usually be traced to these organisms together with, at times, pneumococci. Corneal ulcers and pustules of the eyelids are not uncommon. Rarer, though still important, complications are diarrhea and otitis media in children, and, in adults, hemiplegia, encephalitis, polyneuritis, decubitus ulcers and gangrene.

Diagnosis. Difficulties in diagnosis arise chiefly from the following conditions:

Varioloid with the involution of many of the lesions can be confused at times with varicella. In such cases one must depend upon the appearance of varicella in crops of lesions in all stages of development and also upon the difference in distribution of varicella, which is more plentiful on the trunk.

The *severe hemorrhagic forms* can be confused with septicemia or severe meningococcal infection. Blood cultures should establish the diagnosis.

The *initial rash* which occurs in severe forms may be confused with that of measles or scarlet fever. The short duration of the early evanescent rash of smallpox and the other accompanying symptoms should assist in differentiation.

Pustular syphilids are at times extremely difficult to differentiate from smallpox. In

from lesions of varicella does not produce pocks. Since differentiation from varicella presents clinical difficulties at times, such isolation may be important. The best method of diagnosis, however, is in the microscopic study of smears from the smallpox lesions in which the elementary bodies are readily distinguished.

Prognosis. The prognosis in smallpox depends largely upon the severity of the particular case. In the epidemics of recent years

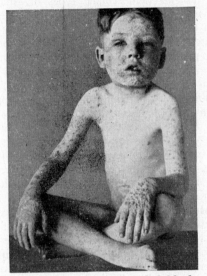

Fig. 6. Smallpox in an unvaccinated child, showing distribution of eruption.

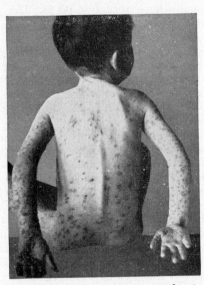

Fig. 7. Same patient as in Figure 6, showing eruption on back and palms.

certain instances one can depend only upon the history and serologic tests for syphilis for differentiation.

The injection intradermally of heat-killed vaccine virus may be used also as a diagnostic test for smallpox after the vesicles have appeared, or the contents of the vesicles may be used in a similar manner. If positive for smallpox, a local reaction occurs at the site of injection within a few hours and reaches its maximum within approximately twenty-four hours. If the patient has been vaccinated previously, this test is not significant. A similar test has utilized rabbits sensitized to cowpox vaccine and the vesicular contents. The vesicular contents have also been used successfully as antigen in a complement fixation test with serum from sensitized rabbits.

The isolation of the virus on the chorioallantois of the embryonated egg also has been quite successful inasmuch as pocks are produced by variola or vaccinia, while material

the mortality has been distinctly lower than in the prevaccination era. The cases accompanied by high fever are more likely to be fatal. Complications, particularly those in the respiratory tract, add to the seriousness of the prognosis.

Prophylaxis. The problem of vaccination is considered properly in the chapter on Vaccinia. Emphasis must be placed upon the fact that vaccination even during the incubation period of the disease may prevent its development. Strict quarantine is essential.

The disease at times is air-borne, as well as transmitted by contact or by direct droplet "hits" from the patient's nasopharyngeal secretions; and means of sterilization of the air, if practicable, must be considered, as well as the prevention of close contacts and of spread by fomites.

Treatment. The principal consideration in the treatment of smallpox is the prevention of secondary infection of the vesicles and

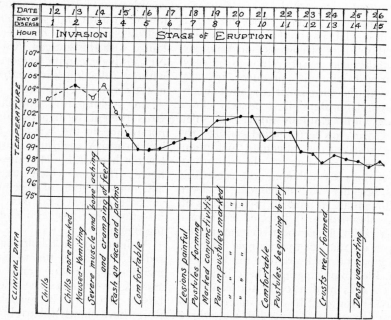

Fig. 8. Typical temperature curve from a case of smallpox, illustrating the secondary rise.

pustules. The secondary elevation of temperature which usually follows the appearance of the vesicles and pustules may depend partially upon the bacterial invasion of the lesions, particularly by staphylococci and streptococci. Treatment therefore should be aimed essentially, as in varicella, toward the prevention of itching and the cleansing of fingers, the skin, and garments or clothing which may come in contact with the lesions. Also scrupulous care must be taken by those caring for the patient. The advent of the sulfonamide drugs and penicillin has assisted greatly in the control of secondary infection of the lesions of smallpox. Swabbing the lesions in wet dressings of potassium permanganate, 1:4000, may prevent serious infection. It is important that crusts should not be removed too quickly, in view of the possible resultant scarring. Bathing the lesions gently with hot water or antipruritic lotions should be done to alleviate the itching.

Dehydration is a frequent severe complication of smallpox and should be avoided by rectal, intravenous or hypodermic fluids, particularly glucose, if vomiting occurs. The possible benefit of convalescent serum has not yet been determined. The isolation period should be at least fourteen days, and longer if the lesions remain in an active stage.

JOSEPH STOKES, JR.

References

American Public Health Association: Smallpox, in The Control of Communicable Diseases. 6th ed. New York, Am. Pub. Health A., 1945, pp. 113–115.

Bulletin of U.S. Army Medical Department: Smallpox in Japan and Korea. Bull. U.S. Army Med. Dept., 6:101, 1946.

Councilman, W. T., Magrath, G. B., and Brinkerhoff, W. R.: The Pathological Anatomy and Histology of Variola. J. Med. Res., 11:12, 1904.

Downie, A. W., and Dumbell, K. R.: Survival of Variola Virus in Dried Exudate and Crusts from Smallpox Patients. Lancet, 1:550, 1947.

Guarnieri, G.: Ricerche sulla patogenesi ed etiologia dell' infezione vaccinica e variolosa. Arch. per le sci. med., 16:403, 1892.

Irons, J. V., Bohls, S. W., Cook, E. B. M., and Murphy, J. N., Jr.: The Chick Membrane as a Differential Culture Medium with Suspected Cases of Smallpox and Varicella. Am. J. Hyg., 33:50, 1941.

Parker, R. F.: Variola and Vaccinia, in Diagnostic Procedures for Virus and Rickettsial Diseases. New York, Am. Pub. Health A., 1948.

VACCINIA

Vaccination, or active immunization against smallpox by means of the virus of cowpox, is the first procedure of this type known to medicine, and its discovery and development by Jenner long before bacteria or viruses had been identified is one of the most dramatic events of medical history. The antigenic, serologic or possible morphologic relationships between the viruses of cowpox and smallpox are not understood as yet, although in view of the proved immunity produced by vaccination with the cowpox virus against smallpox, these relationships must be very close.

Etiology and Epidemiology. Vaccinia, or cowpox virus, has been studied as diligently and has received as adequate definition as any virus. According to the definition of some workers it is cuboidal and, according to others, bricklike, with a diameter of about 236 millimicrons. In purified preparations of the virus obtained from infected epidermal cells of a rabbit, it has been determined by a variety of calculations that a single infective particle apparently will produce the lesion of vaccinia. Electronmicrographs have indicated a spherical area of density in the center of the virus, surrounded by four smaller areas of similar density. Its density lies somewhere between that of bacteria, 1.10, and that of proteins, 1.33. A number of different antigens have been separated from the virus particles as well as cholesterol, phospholipids and neutral fats. No iron is demonstrable, but copper as well as thymonucleic acid, biotin and flavin is present in the virus.

Some of its antigenic relationships to variola virus have already been discussed. When variolation is performed five days after vaccination, only a local lesion results, while at eleven days variolation produces no lesion. Vaccination "takes" during the prodromes of smallpox, but not when performed a few days after the eruption has appeared. Serums obtained from cases of either vaccinia or variola neutralize both viruses. A soluble antigen from the surface of the vaccinia virus has been obtained and purified by Craigie and Wishart. It is termed the LS antigen and is common to both variola and vaccinia viruses, but is unable to produce either immunity or neutralizing antibody. This antigen can be separated into LL and S antigens which, when injected, produce specific antibodies to each antigen. Erythrocytes are agglutinated by both vaccinia and variola viruses, but it is not known whether the LS antigen is associated with this reaction.

Vaccinia virus (not proved for variola virus) contains another antigen, termed NP or nucleo-protein, which constitutes approximately half of the virus particle and contains 6 per cent thymonucleic acid. Precipitin and complement fixation reactions can be obtained with the antigen. Immunity and neutralizing antibodies, however, cannot be obtained with this antigen. Also, by adsorption, NP antibody can be removed from serums without affecting the neutralizing capacity of the serums for the virus.

An agglutinating antibody for vaccinia virus present in hyperimmune serums and not related to the NP and LS antigens has ben termed X agglutinin, but its significance has not been fully determined. Thus the antigenic fraction which produces immunity and neutralization of vaccinia virus has not yet been characterized. For this reason, only infection itself has been effective in producing immunity.

Malnutrition in rabbits has been shown to reduce the size of the vaccinial lesion. Also methionine, choline and estrogenic substances have reduced the susceptibility of rabbits to vaccinia. The available antimicrobial drugs have shown relatively slight inhibiting effects on the vaccinia virus. Storage with glycerol, at 10° C., and by lyophilization have been adequate to maintain viral activity. Ultraviolet light and x-ray radiation inactivate the virus.

Radiation inactivation recently has suggested that the virus has genes distributed through at least half of the particle, which finding would be consistent with the estimated amount and nature of the NP antigen.

The virus of vaccinia has been ordinarily preserved by glycerination of lymph from inoculated calves. More recently it has been grown in tissue cultures by the methods of Rivers and Goodpasture, which have almost entirely eliminated bacterial contamination. These latter preparations can be used intradermally and produce a much milder reaction, with a closed lesion. Although the protection afforded against smallpox is probably as solid as that produced by the more usual material, sufficient experience with its value in the face of an epidemic of smallpox has not been obtained to warrant its widespread use.

Proper Age for Vaccination. In view of the fact that severe reactions, particularly the complication of encephalomyelitis, are less apt to occur when vaccination is performed during the first year, it is best to vaccinate an infant about the fourth to the sixth month. The choice of months, however, should vary according to a number of factors. It is essential that no fixed or invariable order of immunization procedures be followed in infants, since epidemics of communicable diseases, respiratory infections, the convenience of the family and the physician, the weather and other factors should all be considered in such procedures. It is wise to avoid hot weather because of the possibility of a marked febrile reaction, and to avoid vaccination within a certain period following illness, and until the latter half of the first year in premature infants or those who have suffered from nutritional difficulties. The presence of such cutaneous conditions as eczema, impetigo and others should cause postponement of vaccination until the skin is normal, but in chronic eczema or in other cutaneous conditions which are not readily curable, tissue culture virus injected by the intradermal method can often be used successfully with less danger of bacterial contamination.

Choice of Site for Vaccination. The area of choice for both sexes is the skin on the posterior and upper portion of the arm close to the axilla where the scar is not readily visible and where the friction is minimal.

Method of Vaccination. In the development of techniques for vaccination over many years the objective has been to produce a lesion which results in as inconspicuous a scar as possible, but still produces an optimal degree of immunity. Although serologic means of determining such immunity are not available, experience in the presence of epidemics of smallpox and with the results of revaccinations has indicated that the "take" from the recent methods of vaccination, resulting in a small scar, is as highly protective as the "take" with the large scar resulting from the older methods of vaccination. Unfortunately, many physicians still believe that scarification or drilling of a large area of skin and the resultant disfiguring lesion are essential for a solid and more lasting immunity. Even were this true, the danger of secondary infections from the larger lesions and the added discomfort and fever would not justify such a procedure.

The methods recommended at present are of three types: (1) single scratch or incision method; (2) drill method; (3) multiple pressure method. In these methods the objective is to permit the virus to enter the skin in as small an area as possible without sufficient trauma to draw blood. The skin of the selected site should be cleansed thoroughly with sterile cotton and ethyl alcohol,

acetone or ether, care being taken to avoid abrasions which might result in multiple "takes." The site should also be permitted to dry thoroughly after cleansing, in order to avoid inactivation of the virus.

1. *Scratch or Incision Method.* A single scratch, ⅛ to ¼ inch in length, should be made in the skin with a sterile needle or point drawn through the drop of lymph. More than one scratch may be made if the first appears to be insufficient, but cross scratches should never be used. The needle or point should then be placed horizontal with the skin and rubbed gently over the scratched area, after which the drop of lymph should be rubbed off lightly with dry sterile cotton.

2. *Drill Method.* Multiple pricks are made through the drop of lymph with the needle held vertical to the skin surface. The number of pricks should be limited to five or six, and the lymph may then be wiped off with dry sterile cotton.

3. *Multiple Pressure Method.* The needle or point is held at an angle of approximately 45 degrees with the skin surface and is moved up and down rapidly with pressure on the skin sufficient to puncture it lightly six to ten times. Erythema but no blood or serum should be noted after the procedure, and the lymph may be wiped away immediately with sterile cotton, as in the other methods.

In all these methods no dressing should be used, but scrubbing the area with soap and water should probably be avoided for the following twenty-four hours.

Types of Reaction. In general it may be said that the longer the incubation period, the greater is the susceptibility of the vaccinated person and the more severe is the reaction. The small-sized reaction which occurs within the first twenty-four to seventy-two hours and disappears rather rapidly denotes a high type of immunity, whereas the usual "take," with the large reaction, which begins to develop typical signs after five or six days and reaches its height at eight or nine days, is evidence of a highly susceptible person. Between these extremes of reaction and susceptibility there are many intermediate responses and degrees of immunity which follow a characteristic pattern.

In order of degree of immunity which they indicate, the following reactions can be classified, approximately as follows:

1. *Immediate Reaction.* This occurs as a

papule with a light surrounding erythema, usually reaching its height during the first three days after the inoculation and then receding rapidly in size and reactivity. Persons showing this type of reaction often have been previously vaccinated within a relatively short time.

Inactive virus as well as active virus can give an immune reaction, although the former cannot produce immunity. Thus, unless vaccination is performed on a number of persons, some of whom would have primary "takes" or accelerated (vaccinoid) reactions, one may be mistaken concerning the immunizing value of the vaccine material used.

2. *Accelerated Reaction.* In such persons the immunity is less than in the preceding case, the reaction reaches its height in from three to five days, and there is a vesicle rather than a papule, with a marked erythema extending well out from the base of the vesicle. The entire area rarely extends over ½ to ¾ inch in diameter. Slight fever, malaise, chilliness, aching, local tenderness and slight enlargement of the draining lymph nodes frequently occur. By some this type of reaction has been termed "vaccinoid."

3. *Primary Vaccination Reaction or Typical "Take."* In the typical "take" little is noted at the site of inoculation, except for a punctate area of erythema, until the fifth day, when a vesicle appears with a rapidly increasing erythema and induration about it. Usually the vesicle, erythema and induration increase up to the ninth day, when the total area involved ranges approximately from the diameter of a silver half dollar up to the diameter of a grapefruit or even, at times, beyond, in adults. The vesicle itself, if the vaccination is properly performed, rarely exceeds ¼ to ½ inch in diameter, but the area of erythema and induration may not only extend in a wide circular areola, but may reach out toward the draining lymph nodes to involve areas of skin many inches from the central vesicle. In certain instances where primary "takes" have occurred, by mistake, on the tips of the fingers, acute lymphangitis resembling that due to hemolytic streptococci may occur during the height of the reaction and extend well up the arm—apparently the result of the tension produced in such a restricted area. In the larger reactions the draining lymph nodes are swollen and tender. Fever is usually present, in infants at times reaching 104° or 105° F. and remaining at that elevation for several days. Extreme discomfort with chills, aching and localized tenderness is common. Also in such reactions small additional vesicles may occur about the periphery of the indurated area. As a result of the irritation and itching, infants will frequently scratch the vesicle and inoculate themselves elsewhere on the body at the site of open skin lesions or scratch marks. As the reaction subsides, the vesicle, which is typically umbilicated, becomes darker in color, with a deeper central crater, and gradually changes into a hard, black crust which falls off in several weeks. The remaining scar is bluish-red at first and in time becomes a firm white area, characteristically round and irregularly pocked.

Failure to react in one of these manners is not an indication of immunity, as is often incorrectly supposed, but rather an evidence in almost all instances of an inactive virus vaccine. In certain cases the lymph may have been washed off with soap and water, or possibly methyl alcohol or some other improper antiseptic may have been used for preparation of the site of inoculation; but it is probable that in only rare instances does the child fail to react when the virus is active and applied properly, on a dry site.

Care of Reaction. Of primary importance in the care of the lesion resulting from the typical "take" is maintenance of dryness and a free flow of air about the vesicle. For this reason, shields should never be used. In addition, a relatively sterile surface may be maintained on the vesicle and on the entire area about the reaction by sponging them gently with alcohol and cotton at least twice daily, being careful to leave the surface of the vesicle intact. If a serous discharge occurs from the vesicle because of excessive tension or, more commonly, trauma, alcohol and cotton should be used three to four times daily and a loose piece of gauze attached to the clothing over the vesicle or attached to the skin by adhesive tape placed well outside the indurated area. If a discharge sufficient to cause crusting occurs, so that the gauze becomes attached to the vesicle, an antibiotic ointment may be applied to the vesicle at least twice daily, following the usual cleansing with alcohol, and a piece of gauze may be added as further protection for the clothing.

Frequency of Vaccination. Opinions vary as to the required frequency of revaccination, but in general, five to seven years may be considered a proper interval between vaccinations, with the additional provision that vaccination be performed whenever epidemics of smallpox are impending.

Complications and Sequelae. The most dangerous complication of vaccination is that of pyogenic infection, resulting from neglect, dirt, scratching, and other skin infections. Such infection is usually of staphylococcal

veloped by Kempe and given parenterally in 10 cc. amounts every one or two weeks for four to six weeks appeared to be of curative value in a single case in which it was used.

The additional necrosis caused by pyogenic complications is an excellent medium for the growth of tetanus bacilli. Tetanus occurs less frequently now than formerly, but is still an important consideration where dirt and

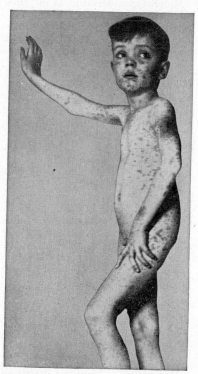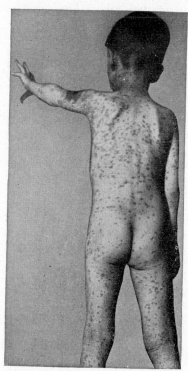

Fig. 9. Hyperallergy, expressed as roseola vaccinosa. Note the marked area of the vaccination lesion on the arm.

origin with cellulitis, but hemolytic streptococci may at times be responsible, and septicemia, erysipelas or scarlet fever may also be seen. Such infections increase the size and severity of the reaction considerably and result finally in a large and disfiguring scar.

Vaccinia gangrenosa or prolonged generalized vaccinia, an almost invariably fatal but rather rare complication, occurs as a slowly spreading gangrenous vaccinial involvement of the skin surrounding the "take" with serpiginous ulceration, edema with gangrene, and satellite "takes" which are incorporated into the slowly spreading swollen and gangrenous slough. This is associated with extreme toxicity, fever, and incapacity of the skin to localize the infection.

Hyperimmune human gamma globulin de-

squalor prevail. Under such conditions the use of tetanus toxoid for immunization should precede vaccination against smallpox. The elimination of shields in the care of the usual "take" has also eliminated much of the danger of tetanus.

Scratching may cause secondary vesicles at distant points, particularly about the genitalia and face, where severe scarring can occur. A generalized vaccinia is seen at times in an infant with eczema or some other generalized skin disease when it has been exposed to another vaccinated member of the household. Umbilicated lesions may extend over most of the body with high fever and extreme toxemia. In such cases lesions of the eye should be handled most carefully because of the danger of corneal perforation. At times generalized urticaria, roseola or purpura is seen when the reaction is at its height.

Postvaccinal Encephalitis. Encephalitis has rarely been reported in the United States, but has been recorded more often in England and Europe. It usually appears about ten days to two weeks after the height of the vaccination reaction, although it may be seen earlier or later. The severity of this complication appears to be entirely unrelated to the severity of the "take." The onset is generally abrupt, with high fever, disorientation, and at times with coma or convulsions. A stiff neck, positive Kernig sign, increase or absence of reflexes, and positive Babinski sign are usually present. Weakness and paralysis of the extraocular muscles are common, as well as paralyses of the face, pharynx and limbs. As a rule the cells are increased in the cerebrospinal fluid, chiefly the lymphocytes, although at first there may be an increase in polymorphonuclear cells. The sugar and chloride of the spinal fluid ordinarily are not greatly altered, but the protein is usually increased, as is also the spinal fluid pressure. The reflex control of the bladder and bowel is often disturbed. The course of the disease is usually extremely stormy with either a rapid progression to death or an equally rapid improvement. The case mortality of this complication ranges from 30 to 40 per cent, and even though rapid improvement occurs, residual mental retardation or spasticity may remain. There is no specific therapy available other than lumbar punctures for relief of cerebrospinal fluid pressure and the proper orthopedic care of any paralyzed or spastic skeletal muscles.

JOSEPH STOKES, JR.

References

Barbero, G., Gray, A., Scott, T. F. McN., and Kempe, C. H.: Vaccinia Gangrenosa Treated with Hyperimmune Vaccinia Gamma Globulin. Pediatrics, to be published.

Blaxall, F. R.: Animal Pock Diseases in a System of Bacteriology in Relation to Medicine. London, His Majesty's Stationery Office, 7:140, 1930.

Craigie, J., and Wishart, F. O.: Studies on the Soluble Precipitable Substances of Vaccinia. I. The Dissociation in Vitro of Soluble Precipitable Substances from Elementary Bodies of Vaccinia. J. Exper. Med., 64:803, 1936.

————, and Wishart, F. O.: Studies on the Soluble Precipitable Substances of Vaccinia. II. The Soluble Precipitable Substances of Dermal Filtrate. J. Exper. Med., 64:819, 1936.

Downie, A. W.: The Immunological Relationship of the Virus of Spontaneous Cowpox to Vaccinia. Brit. J. Exper. Path., 20:158, 1939.

Goodpasture, E. W., Buddingh, G. J., Richardson, L., and Anderson, K.: The Preparation of Anti-Smallpox Vaccine by Culture of the Virus in the Chorio-allantoic Membrane of Chick Embryos, and Its Use in Human Immunization. Am. J. Hyg., 21:319, 1935.

Gordon, M. H.: Studies of the Viruses of Vaccinia and Variola. Med. Res. Council, Special Report Series No. 98, London, His Majesty's Stationery Office, 1925.

Green, R. H., Anderson, T. F., and Smadel, J. E.: Morphological Structure of the Virus of Vaccinia. J. Exper. Med., 75:651, 1942.

Jenner, E.: An Inquiry into the Causes and Effects of the Variolae Vaccinae, a Disease Discovered in Some of Western Counties of England, Particularly Gloucestershire, and Known by the Name of Cow Pox, 1798. Reprinted by Cassell and Company, Ltd., 1896. Available in pamphlet, Vol. 4232. Army Medical Library, Washington, D. C.

Parker, R. F.: Statistical Studies of the Nature of the Infectious Unit of Vaccine Virus. J. Exper. Med., 67:725, 1938.

Rivers, T. M., Ward, S. M., and Baird, R. D.: Amount and Duration of Immunity Induced by Intradermal Inoculation of Cultured Vaccine Virus. J. Exper. Med., 69:857, 1939.

Smadel, J. E., and Hoagland, C. L.: Elementary Bodies of Vaccinia. Bact. Rev., 6:79, 1942.

Tyzzer, E. E.: The Etiology and Pathology of Vaccinia. J. Med. Res., 11:180, 1904.

van Rooyen, C. E., and Rhodes, A. J.: The Variola-Vaccinia Virus, in Virus Diseases of Man. London, Oxford University Press, 1940, pp. 280–353.

MUMPS

(Epidemic Parotitis)

Definition. Mumps is an acute communicable disease caused by a virus, which usually manifests itself by involvement of the salivary glands, but frequently involves other tissues, notably those of the testes and the central nervous system.

History. The clinical and epidemiologic features of mumps were well described long before the etiology was known. Advances in knowledge have been rapid since 1934, when Johnson and Goodpasture isolated the virus by inoculating saliva of patients into the parotid duct of monkeys. Enders and associates developed a complement fixation test which made possible a definite diagnosis and was useful in epidemiologic and immunologic studies. A notable advance was made by Habel, who succeeded in growing the virus in chick embryos. Levens and Enders then adapted the virus to the allantoic sac and demonstrated its hemagglutinating properties. These developments facilitated studies on prophylaxis and immunization which have been carried on by Henle and associates, Habel, and others. Infection of volunteers by Maris provided data on the frequency of subclinical infection and the period of communicability. Kilham showed that the virus was pathogenic for suckling hamsters and mice.

Etiology. Mumps virus is of medium size, with a diameter calculated by various observers to be between 90 and 135 millimicrons. It is readily isolated from the saliva of patients with parotitis and from the cerebrospinal fluid of patients with meningo-encephalitis. In monkeys it causes parotitis. In suckling mice or hamsters it may cause fatal meningo-encephalitis. It grows readily, but slowly, in the yolk sac or amniotic sac of chick embryos and can be adapted to the allantoic sac. After multiple chick embryo passages the virus may become less virulent for man. Erythrocytes of chickens and human are agglutinated by virus suspensions.

Morbid Anatomy. Observations of infected parotid tissue from humans are few. In general, the changes observed resemble those noted in infected monkeys. Serofibrinous exudate in the interstitial tissue, vascular engorgement, and lymphocytic infiltration of the tubules are noted. Necrotic glandular cells and polymorphonuclear cells are found within the lumina. Biopsy specimens from the testis show marked edema, perivascular lymphocytic infiltration, focal hemorrhages, pronounced destruction of germinal epithelium, and plugging of the tubules by epithelial debris, fibrin and polymorphonuclear cells. In most instances the lesions are focal and some areas escape.

Pathologic Physiology. The serum amylase of most patients is elevated during the first few days of illness, apparently because of the acute inflammatory process in the parotid glands rather than an accompanying pancreatitis.

Incubation Period. The incubation period is most frequently between seventeen and twenty-one days. Extremes of from eight to thirty-five days have been reported.

Communicability. The virus has been repeatedly recovered from the saliva during the three days following onset and, on one occasion, as late as the sixth day after onset. Experimental studies show that it may be present for several days before the onset of symptoms and may also be recovered from persons with inapparent infections. It is presumed to enter the host by the oral or respiratory route through the medium of infected droplet or direct contact. Spread to other tissues probably takes place by way of the blood stream. The degree of communicability of

mumps is relatively low. Many persons reaching adult life are susceptible to infection.

Age Incidence. The disease is most frequent between the ages of five and fifteen. All ages may be affected. High attack rates have been noted in all age groups in isolated populations such as the inhabitants of Pacific islands.

Immunity. Immunity is generally of long duration. Second or, even more rarely, third attacks have been reported, but are exceed-

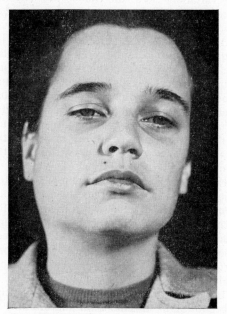

Fig. 10. Mumps. Second day.

ingly uncommon. There is no convincing evidence that the patient with unilateral parotitis is any more likely to experience a second attack than one with a bilateral parotitis. The development of immunity as a result of inapparent infection is a common occurrence.

Clinical Picture. *Parotitis.* Before the appearance of parotid swelling, there may be a prodrome of one or two days' duration during which the patient experiences feverishness, chilliness, malaise, anorexia and headache. In mild cases this is not observed. Swelling of one or both parotid glands then occurs. In the latter event the two glands may be affected at the same time or in sequence. The swelling is accompanied by variable amounts of pain about the angle of the jaw, and by difficulty in moving the jaw.

The swelling in the parotid region fills the area behind, below and anterior to the angle of the jaw, extending up to the zygomatic arch. The lobe of the ear is pushed out and upward. The affected glands feel firm and are moderately or extremely tender. The orifice of Stensen's duct may appear reddened. The temperature is usually between 100° and 103° F., but may rise to higher levels. By the second or third day the swelling has usually reached a maximum and begins to subside. The time required for swelling to disappear completely is subject to considerable variation. As a rule this occurs within a week, but swelling may persist for considerably longer periods.

Accompanying the parotitis or, rather infrequently, in the absence of obvious parotitis, swelling of the submaxillary or sublingual glands may occur. This is more readily determined by palpation than by inspection. Edema of tissues surrounding affected glands is commonly observed and may involve much of the anterior surface of the neck and the area lying over the anterior surface of the manubrium sterni.

Orchitis. Orchitis is an infrequent manifestation of mumps before puberty, but is common in adults. The over-all incidence has been estimated as approximately 20 per cent. Considerable variation in incidence has been reported in different epidemics. A small proportion of patients may have orchitis without evidence of parotitis.

In general, orchitis develops as the parotitis is beginning to subside. Pain and swelling of the affected testis are noted, and the temperature rises, accompanied by chilliness and malaise. The affected testis may enlarge to two or three times its normal size and is painful and exquisitely tender. Epididymitis, hydrocele and scrotal edema may be present. Usually only one gonad is involved, but both may be affected. The swelling and constitutional symptoms progress for two or three days and then subside over a period of a week or more. In certain instances fever drops precipitously rather than by lysis. A considerable amount of atrophy, as determined by palpation, occurs in approximately one half of the patients, but sterility seldom ensues. This may be explained by the fact that, even when there is extensive involvement of both testes, the distribution of the inflammatory reaction is spotty, and certain seminiferous tubules are spared. Psychologic rather than organic factors are presumably responsible for the occasional development of impotence following an attack of mumps orchitis.

Meningo-encephalitis. Wide variations in the incidence of meningo-encephalitis in different epidemics have been reported. In certain series in which the cerebrospinal fluid has been examined routinely, pleocytosis has been found in as many as one half, and signs of meningo-encephalitis in more than one fourth, of the patients. Though signs of central nervous system involvement commonly follow the development of parotitis, they may be observed before or simultaneous with the parotid involvement. Furthermore, it is important to stress the fact that meningo-encephalitis may occur in the absence of any salivary gland involvement.

The temperature is usually markedly elevated in the presence of meningo-encephalitis, and the patient complains of severe headache, photophobia, neck stiffness, nausea and vomiting. Delirium may occur, but in most instances the sensorium remains clear. On physical examination the patient is often drowsy, but can be roused, the neck and back are stiff, and Kernig's sign is present. Lumbar puncture shows an increased cerebrospinal fluid pressure, an increase in cell count, and a slight increase in protein. The cells are predominantly lymphocytes, and the cell count, though variable, tends to be higher than in certain other neurotropic virus diseases. The prognosis is favorable. There is reason to believe that death, when it occurs, results from a chain of events initiated by the mumps infection rather than from a direct effect of the virus. Convalescence may be slow, but sequelae are uncommon.

Other Manifestations. Pancreatitis is suggested by the appearance of epigastric pain, nausea and vomiting. There may be tenderness on deep palpation, and, occasionally, the pancreas is palpable. Determination of the serum amylase is of no value in this situation, however, for elevated serum amylase values occur commonly in apparently uncomplicated mumps. Oophoritis is probably not uncommon, but the diagnosis is difficult to establish with certainty. It should be considered when a patient complains of lower quadrant or low back pain and when a tender, enlarged ovary is felt. Other less common manifestations of mumps include mastitis, in either sex, involvement of lacrimal glands, thyroiditis, deafness, seventh nerve paralysis and optic neuritis. Myocarditis has also been described. Polyneuritis and myelitis occur, but can hardly be considered to be due to a specific effect of the mumps virus, since they have been observed in a wide variety of infectious diseases.

Diagnosis. The clinical diagnosis in a patient with parotitis who has been exposed to mumps is seldom difficult. Occasionally, cervical lymphadenitis, parotitis of bacterial etiology, and salivary calculi must be considered. The diagnosis may be more difficult when only submaxillary or sublingual glands are involved. Meningo-encephalitis without accompanying parotitis must be differentiated from other neurotropic virus diseases, in particular, nonparalytic poliomyelitis. A history of exposure to mumps is often an important clue. When the issue is in doubt, it can now be resolved by serologic tests.

Complement fixation, agglutination inhibition and neutralization tests have been developed for the diagnosis of mumps. In all tests two serum specimens should be tested, for definitive diagnosis rests on the demonstration of a significant increase in antibody titer. The first specimen should be taken as early as possible and the second between ten and twenty-one days after onset.

The total leukocyte count may be low, normal or slightly elevated. A considerable proportion of patients show a lymphocytosis. Because this is not uniform, the blood picture is not of great value in diagnosis.

Prognosis. The outlook is almost invariably favorable. A fatal outcome is stated to occur less than once in a thousand cases.

Prevention. *Tests to Determine Susceptibility.* Intradermal tests and measurement of serum antibodies have been used to determine susceptibility in exposed persons. Both procedures may provide useful information, but neither is infallible.

Passive Immunization. Gamma globulin from normal serum or, preferably, from serum known to contain mumps antibody in high titer may prevent the development of mumps when given within a week of exposure. Convalescent serum may also be effective, but carries the risk of viral hepatitis even when irradiated. Passive immunity is of short duration and the patient remains susceptible to infection later in life, when complications are more likely to occur.

Active Immunization. Some reduction in the incidence of mumps has been shown among persons vaccinated with either inactivated virus preparations or with live virus attenuated by chick embryo passage. The degree of protection obtained has fallen somewhat short of expectations.

Treatment. Patients should be kept at rest in bed. Pain associated with parotitis can usually be relieved by salicylates supplemented, if necessary, by codeine. Application of heat or cold may afford comfort. In orchitis, Demerol (0.05 to 0.1 gm.) or morphine (0.01 to 0.015 gm.) may be necessary. The testes are more comfortable when supported. In extremely severe cases of orchitis surgical incision may be advisable.

Convalescent serum and pooled gamma globulin have been recommended for alleviating the severity of the illness and preventing the development of orchitis. Stilbestrol has been widely used in treating orchitis. Evidence for the effectiveness of all these substances is conflicting. There is limited, but more convincing, evidence that gamma globulin prepared from mumps convalescent serum may reduce the incidence of orchitis.

GORDON MEIKLEJOHN

References

Applebaum, I. L.: Serum Amylase in Mumps. Ann. Int. Med., *21*:35, 1944.

Bashe, W., Jr., Gotlieb, T., Henle, G., and Henle, W.: Studies on the Prevention of Mumps. VI. The Relationship of Neutralizing Antibodies to the Determination of Susceptibility and to the Evaluation of Immunization Procedures. J. Immunol., *71*:76–85, 1953.

Enders, J. F.: Mumps, in Rivers, T. M., Jr.: Viral and Rickettsial Infections of Man. 2nd ed. Philadelphia, J. B. Lippincott Co., 1952, pp. 513–521.

Habel, K.: Cultivation of Mumps Virus in the Developing Chick Embryo and Its Application to Studies of Immunity to Mumps in Man. Pub. Health Rep., *60*:201, 1945.

Johnson, C. D., and Goodpasture, E. W.: An Investigation of the Etiology of Mumps. J. Exper. Med., *59*:1, 1934.

Kilham, L., and Overman, J. R.: Natural Pathogenicity of Mumps Virus for Suckling Hamsters on Intracerebral Inoculation. J. Immunol., *70*:147–151, February, 1953.

Levens, J. H., and Enders, J. F.: The Hemoagglutinative Properties of Amniotic Fluids from Embryonated Eggs Infected with Mumps Virus. Science, *102*:117, 1945.

Maris, E. P., Enders, J. F., Stokes, J., Jr., and Kane, L. W.: Immunity in Mumps. IV. The Correlation of the Presence of Complement-Fixing Antibody and Resistance to Mumps in Human Beings. J. Exper. Med., *84*:323, 1946.

Wesselhoeft, C.: Mumps: Its Glandular and Neurologic Manifestations, in Gordon, J. E., Mueller, J. H., Zinsser, H., and others: Virus and Rickettsial Diseases. Cambridge, Harvard University Press, 1940, pp. 309–344.

PSITTACOSIS

(Ornithosis)

Definition. Psittacosis (ornithosis) is a specific infectious disease endemic among various members of the bird kingdom. The infectious agent is transmissible to man, in whom it usually induces an atypical form of pneumonia. In a strict sense the term *psittacosis* designates the disease in birds of the order Psittaciformes (parrots, parrakeets and the like) and the disease communicated by them to man. The discovery that birds belonging to other orders may be infected similarly and may transmit the infection to man led to the suggestion (Meyer) that all instances of the disease, whether avian or human, be included under the broader term *ornithosis.*

History. Psittacosis in man was a rarely recognized disease until 1929. The disease was described by Jürgensen, 1876, and by Ritter, 1880, who noted the association between it and the presence of ill birds. Morange, 1895, gave the disease its name. The etiologic agent was discovered by Bedson, Western and Simpson, 1930, who showed it to be filterable and present in infected tissues of parrots and human beings. Levinthal, and Coles, as well as Lillie, 1930, independently described "elementary bodies" in infectious material. Krumwiede, McGrath and Oldenbusch, 1930, demonstrated the susceptibility of mice to infection with psittacosis virus. Rivers and Berry, 1930, 1932, induced psittacosis pneumonia in monkeys. Coles, 1940, showed that pigeons were infected with the virus, and Meyer, Eddie and Yanamura, 1942, demonstrated that these birds could cause infections in man.

Etiology. The etiologic agent is usually included among the viruses of the psittacosis-lymphogranuloma group. The agent of psittacosis, one of the largest of known viruses, is filterable and has not been shown to be capable of multiplication in the absence of living cells. Elementary bodies, which are often termed Levinthal-Coles-Lillie bodies, are readily demonstrable in infected tissues of birds, mammals and human beings; many investigators consider them to represent the virus. A number of different strains of the virus are recognized. Infected birds represent the source of infection in the majority of human cases. In man the disease appears to be more severe when acquired from members of the parrot family, but pigeons have been responsible for numerous infections in human beings, and some cases have been attributed to contact with infected canaries, finches, petrels or chickens. Infected birds may or may not appear ill. The virus is present in the nasal discharges and droppings of most infected birds and contaminates their feathers and cages. It is relatively stable, withstands prolonged drying, and enters man via the upper respiratory tract. Both sexes and persons of all ages are susceptible, although children appear to be more resistant than adults. The virus is present in the sputum of patients, and direct transmission from man to man occurs, although it is not common. Extensive epidemics have not occurred. The disease usually occurs in a sporadic manner or affects small groups of persons exposed to a common avian source of infection.

Morbid Anatomy. Infection by viruses of the psittacosis-lymphogranuloma group induces a variety of pathologic alterations. Among infected birds the lungs are seldom altered. The chief abnormalities are seen in the liver and spleen, which are enlarged and show areas of focal necrosis. Similar lesions are seen in infected mice; pnuemonia seldom occurs unless the virus has been given intranasally.

In man, as in monkeys, the chief abnormalities are seen in the lungs. The pneumonic lesions are usually patchy and irregularly distributed. They develop near the hilum and spread toward the pleura, which is only rarely involved. Bronchitis is not striking. There is cellular infiltration of the alveolar walls and spaces; lymphocytes and other mononuclear cells predominate. Bronchioles and small bronchi often show cuffing due to peripheral collections of mononuclear cells. If the lungs become infected secondarily by bacterial microorganisms, the lesions become altered accordingly.

Pathologic Physiology and Chemistry. The leukocyte count is usually within normal limits, although transient leukocytosis or leukopenia may occur, and a relative monocytosis may develop. Albuminuria is seldom marked and may be absent. The erythrocyte sedimentation rate is increased. Cyanosis is seldom a striking feature, probably because the alveolar spaces in the pneumonic lesions are usually not completely filled with exudate.

Symptoms. The incubation period ranges from seven to fifteen days. The symptoms vary widely, as does the severity of the disease. The source of the virus appears to be of some importance; infections derived from birds of the parrot family are often more severe than those contracted from pigeons. The onset may be abrupt or insidious. The initial symptoms are malaise, anorexia, fever, headache and backache. Chills may occur. The cough is usually nonproductive, and may be severe and paroxysmal. The temperature rises fairly rapidly, is usually remittent, and may remain elevated for two or three weeks, after which it falls by lysis. The pulse rate is usually slow in relation to the temperature. The respiratory rate is often normal or only slightly increased. Pleural pain is rarely present. In severe cases a high temperature, restlessness, insomnia and delirium may develop; headache, cough and constipation with abdominal distention may be prominent features; marked increase in both the pulse and respiratory rates may occur and indicates a poor prognosis. Pulmonary consolidation develops in the great majority of patients, but may be difficult to detect by physical examination, particularly during the first week of illness. Usually it begins at the hilum and spreads outward. Despite the absence or paucity of physical signs of consolidation, roentgenograms of the chest usually show evidence of pneumonia early in the course of the disease. The roentgenogram reveals hazy, patchy, irregularly distributed areas of increased density which are seldom lobar in distribution. Pleural fluid rarely is evident, and, when present, is small in amount. Diarrhea, epistaxis and even scattered macules resembling rose spots may occur. Some patients produce large amounts of sputum which may be slightly blood streaked, but is not rusty. Extension and spread of the pneumonic process occurs frequently, and migratory pneumonia has been observed. Relapses occur occasionally. Complications are not frequent, but phlebitis may develop. Convalescence is slow and, after a severe attack, may be prolonged.

Diagnosis. The development of symptoms and signs indicative of an atypical form of pneumonia in a person who has recently had contact with birds should suggest the possibility of psittacosis. A normal respiratory rate, a relatively slow pulse rate, a normal leukocyte count, the absence of classical physical signs of pneumonia, and the presence of consolidation on the roentgenogram are characteristic but not pathognomonic. Without the assistance of laboratory tests the disease rarely can be distinguished from atypical pneumonias of other etiology. Mild cases may be confused with pulmonary tuberculosis or sporadic influenza. Severe cases may resemble typhoid fever. In appropriately equipped laboratories experienced personnel may be able to recover psittacosis virus from the sputum, and thereby establish the diagnosis. The complement fixation reaction with serum and psittacosis antigen is an important diagnostic aid.

Prognosis. The prognosis is influenced by the source of the virus, the age of the patient and the extent of pneumonia. Infections derived from birds of the parrot family are most severe; the case mortality rate is approximately 20 per cent. Infections contracted from other members of the bird kingdom appear to be less severe, and the case mortality rate is lower. In general, the older the patient, the poorer the prognosis; most deaths occur in persons over forty years of age.

Prophylaxis. Psittacosis in man could be eradicated if exposure to infected birds could be eliminated. Birds belonging to the parrot family and pigeons appear to constitute the chief sources of human infections. Patients with the disease may transmit it to those who care for them. The virus is present in the sputum and may be disseminated by coughing.

Treatment. Psittacosis is one of the very few viral diseases for which specific treatment is available. Chemotherapy with modern antimicrobial drugs is effective in the disease in man. Sulfonamides are not of much value, nor is streptomycin. Penicillin, however, in doses of 300,000 to 600,000 units per day, may in some cases be curative. The tetracyclines (Aureomycin or Terramycin) are the drugs of choice and appear to be more effective than chloramphenicol. Doses of 1 gm. of a tetracycline drug by mouth every six to eight hours during the first two days and every twelve hours thereafter should be given for one week. Symptomatic and supportive therapeutic measures should also be used.

FRANK L. HORSFALL, JR.

References

Bedson, S. P., Western, G. T., and Simpson, S. L.: Observations on the Aetiology of Psittacosis. Lancet, 1:235, 345, 1930.

Meyer, K. F.: The Ecology of Psittacosis and Ornithosis. Medicine, 21:175, 1942.

———, and Eddie, B.: The Value of the Complement Fixation Test in the Diagnosis of Psittacosis. J. Infect. Dis., 65:225, 1939.

Peterson, E., Spaulding, O. B., and Wildman, O.: Psittacosis: A Clinical and Roentgenologic Study of Seven Cases with Postmortem Observations in One Case. J.A.M.A., 95:171, 1930.

Rabinowitz, M. A., and Livingston, S. H.: Psittacosis. Report of Five Cases. Arch. Int. Med., 49: 464, 1932.

Rivers, T. M., and Berry, G. P.: Psittacosis. IV. Experimentally Induced Infections in Monkeys. J. Exper. Med., 54:129, 1931.

LYMPHOGRANULOMA VENEREUM

(Lymphopathia Venerea, Climatic Bubo)

Definition. Lymphogranuloma venereum is an infectious disease systemic in nature and varied in manifestations, which pro-

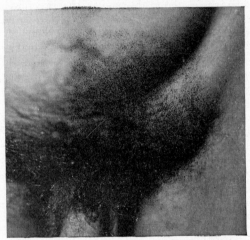

Fig. 11. Lymphogranuloma venereum; unilateral involvement five days after appearance of inguinal adenitis. (Courtesy of Howard and Strauss: New England Journal of Medicine.)

duces specific involvement with acute and chronic inflammation of the lymph channels and nodes of the genitals and rectum. The disease is transmitted by sexual contact. Early manifestations include an evanescent genital lesion followed by subacute regional lymphadenitis progressing to suppuration and sinus formation. General dissemination of the infective agent, constitutional symptoms and, rarely, involvement of distant structures occur. Later, progressive inflammatory disease of the local lymphatics and surrounding tissues leads to lymphedema, ulceration and disfigurement of the genitals, and to proctitis, perianal fistulas and rectal stricture.

Etiology. The causative agents of lymphogranuloma, and of psittacosis, trachoma and certain diseases of birds and animals, are known as the psittacosis-lymphogranuloma group and are tentatively classified inter-

mediate between the viruses and rickettsiae. Common characteristics of the psittacosis-lymphogranuloma group include large particle size, antigenic interrelationships and susceptibility to certain antimicrobial agents. The lymphogranuloma micro-organism is pathogenic for the chick embryo and produces meningo-encephalitis on intracerebral inoculation into mice.

Epidemiology. Although lymphogranuloma venereum was long considered a disease of warm climates, there is ample evidence of its world-wide distribution. As with other venereal diseases, the prevalence of the infection is determined by the promiscuity of the population and is greatest in young adults. Surveys based on intradermal reactions to killed lymphogranuloma agent suggest that inapparent infection and latent disease are frequent in promiscuous persons. Existence of the carrier state has been shown by isolation of the agent from the genitals or rectum of asymptomatic persons of both sexes (Coutts). Accidental infections of laboratory personnel have been described.

Pathogenesis. After a variable incubation period of from three to twenty days, an initial lesion (vesicular, papular or ulcerative) may occur at the site of infection. More commonly, the first evidence of the disease is involvement of the inguinal lymph nodes beginning two weeks to three months after exposure, the primary lesion having been unnoticed or absent.

The inguinal adenitis, unilateral or bilateral, is a subacute diffuse process affecting the entire chain of lymph nodes, and often the femoral group as well, producing the "sign of the groove." Characteristic of the inflammatory reaction is the formation of multiple small abscesses within the nodal parenchyma, subsequently spreading to the surrounding pericapsular tissues and to the overlying skin. The tissues become indurated, matted and fused, the skin reddened and brawny. Pain and tenderness are variable. Ultimately, rupture of abscesses through the skin results in chronically draining sinuses.

The isolation of the micro-organism from peripheral blood by Beeson and co-workers indicates that constitutional symptoms (fever, headache, arthralgia) which commonly accompany early lymphogranuloma are due to systemic invasion. Further evidence of dissemination has been provided by recovery of the agent from involved distant sites (cerebrospinal fluid, supraclavicular lymph node).

In females, the less frequent occurrence of early external manifestations is presumably related to the lymphatic drainage of the site of entry of the agent. On this basis, primary infection of the vulva or introitus results in inguinal involvement; inoculation through mucous membranes of the upper vagina or cervix leads to inflammation of perirectal and pelvic lymphatics. The latter type, which in its early stages may simulate gonococcic disease, has serious long-term implications in the form of proctitis and rectal stricture.

Late manifestations of lymphogranuloma venereum include disfiguring lesions of the external genitals (elephantiasis or, in females, esthiomene) and the anorectal syndrome. In the former, persistence of the infectious process in the skin, subcutaneous tissues and lymphatics of the genitals produces brawny induration and slowly developing enlargement of affected soft tissues over periods of months or years. Finally suppuration, fistula formation and scarring lead to disfigurement and to functional impairment. The anorectal syndrome is initiated early in the disease by proctitis with tenesmus and a bloody or purulent discharge. Later, chronic cicatrizing inflammation of the rectum and perirectal tissues leads to obstipation and to diminished caliber of the stools. At the onset of rectal stricture edema is a contributing factor and, at this stage, the process is amenable to medical treatment. The late fibrous stricture, however, may require colostomy. In addition, there may be involvement of the rectovaginal septum progressing to fistula formation. Perianal fistulas also occur and, because of lymphatic obstruction, dilated perianal lymph channels (lymphorrhoids), resembling hemorrhoids, develop. It is to be emphasized that lymphogranuloma is the commonest cause of benign rectal stricture.

Diagnosis. Isolation and identification of the infective agent of lymphogranuloma are experimental rather than practical procedures. Consequently, the diagnosis must usually be based on clinical grounds combined with indirect laboratory evidence and the exclusion of other diseases. Both early syphilis and chancroid mimic *early* lymphogranuloma. Tuberculosis and lymphoma frequently require diagnostic consideration as may tularemia and plague under appropriate circumstances. Clinical similarities, as well as terminology, cause confusion between lymphogranuloma venereum and granuloma inguinale, a separate disease caused by the Donovan body. *Late* anorectal lymphogranuloma must be differentiated principally from ulcerative colitis and cancer.

To ensure the absence of early syphilis, darkfield examinations of material expressed from genital lesions or aspirated from enlarged inguinal nodes should be performed, as well as follow-up serologic observations. It should be pointed out that false positive serologic tests for syphilis occur in about 20 per cent of patients with lymphogranuloma. The clinical manifestations of chancroid and lymphogranuloma may be indistinguishable.

The *intradermal test,* introduced by Frei, now employs as antigen killed lymphogranuloma agent harvested from yolk sacs of chick embryos (Lygranum). Sensitivity develops in from ten to thirty days after onset of the disease and persists for years in the absence of treatment. Thus, a positive reaction is indicative of either present or past infection. The sensitivity of the test is high, 90 per cent or more of patients with lymphogranuloma giving positive results. Positive reactions are not induced by use of the test material itself, but reactivation of latent lymphogranuloma has been described following this procedure. Cross-reactions with diseases due to other agents of this group may occur.

The *complement fixation test* uses an antigen similar to the skin-testing material. As with the intradermal test, a positive complement fixation reaction (except as noted subsequently) indicates present or previous infection. In Heyman's study all of 27 patients with early lymphogranuloma, proved by isolation of the agent, had complemented fixation titers of 1:40 or more, and most had titers of 1:160 or higher. However, more important than titer was the serologic trend determined by study of acute phase and convalescent serums collected over periods of weeks, frozen, and tested simultaneously. "Cross-reactions" may occur in infections due to other agents of the lymphogranuloma-psittacosis group. Ordinarily these do not constitute a problem because of differing clinical manifestations as well as because of the lower titer of most cross-reacting serums, as in trachoma. In psittacosis, however, high-titered complement fixation reactions with lymphogranuloma antigen may occur.

Hyperglobulinemia. Hyperglobulinemia with elevated total serum proteins and reversal of the albumin-globulin ratio is common. Although the increase in globulin may develop within a few days after the appearance of buboes, several weeks or more may be required. In addition, administration of effective antimicrobial agents may prevent or reverse hyperglobulinemia.

As chancroid may simulate lymphogranuloma with respect to both primary lesion and bubo, diagnostic tests for both diseases should be carried out concurrently. For chancroid, smears and cultures employing appropriate techniques and an intradermal test using killed Ducrey bacilli as antigen have demonstrated value. Inasmuch as the histopathology of each of these two venereal infections is distinctive and frequently diagnostic, biopsy may prove helpful. Biopsy is usually necessary for the diagnosis of either tuberculous lymphadenitis or lymphoma.

Prognosis. Early lymphogranuloma has a variable and unpredictable course. Prompt diagnosis and adequate treatment to terminate infectiousness and to prevent late complications are important. The longer the duration, the slower and less complete is the therapeutic response. The end-stages of late lymphogranuloma, fibrous strictures and scars, are usually resistant to medical treatment.

It has been suggested that there is an increased occurrence of genital and anal cancer in patients with symptomatic late lymphogranuloma. In view of this possibility biopsy should be freely utilized in patients with known or suspected lymphogranuloma.

Treatment. Although penicillin has been demonstrated to be active against experimental lymphogranuloma infections, it has not proved effective clinically in the dosages employed. Both the sulfonamides and the tetracyclines are somewhat effective, but the therapeutic response to either may be incomplete. In the treatment of early lymphogranuloma with sulfonamides, 3 or 4 gm. should be administered daily for three to six weeks depending on clinical response. For disease of long duration treatment may be initiated as above, then the dosage decreased to 2 gm. daily for a prolonged period (several months). With tetracycline therapy (chlortetracycline or oxytetracycline) 500 mg. four times daily is recommended. The individual dose may be reduced later to 250 mg. and continued three to six weeks for early infections and for more prolonged periods for late lymphogranuloma.

Fluctuant buboes respond to repeated aspirations; incision and drainage or the excision of involved structures are unnecessary and may be harmful. With respect to rectal stricture, digital dilatation should accompany administration of antimicrobial agents, and combined treatment should be continued for several months, if possible, before resorting to surgical procedures. Plastic operations on the genitals should likewise be deferred until the effects of antimicrobial therapy have been observed. In spite of longstanding disease, surprising recovery of form and function may occur. Conversely, treatment may not be wholly effective even in early lymphogranuloma.

VIRGIL SCOTT

References

Beeson, P. B., Wall, M. J., and Heyman, A.: Isolation of Virus of Lymphogranuloma Venereum from Blood and Spinal Fluid of a Human Being. Proc. Soc. Exper. Biol. & Med., 62:306, 1946.

Coutts, W. E.: Lymphogranuloma Venereum, A General Review. Bull. World Health Org., 2: 545, 1950.

Greenblatt, R. B.: Management of Chancroid, Granuloma Inguinale and Lymphogranuloma Venereum in General Practice. 2nd ed., United States Public Health Service, Publication No. 255, 1953.

Koteen, H.: Lymphogranuloma Venereum. Medicine, 24:1, 1945.

Wall, M. J., Heyman, A., and Beeson, P. B.: Studies on the Complement Fixation Reaction in Lymphogranuloma Venereum, Am. J. Syph., Gonorr. & Ven. Dis., 31:289, 1947.

FOOT-AND-MOUTH DISEASE

(Aphthous Fever)

Foot-and-mouth disease is a viral infection of animals, chiefly cattle, which occurs in man only with great rarity. Infection, when it does occur in man, presumably results from direct contact with the virus either in the laboratory or from handling the tissues or body fluids of infected animals. The disease in man is characterized by a short incubation period followed by the appearance of a febrile illness with vesicular lesions of palms, soles and the oropharyngeal mucosa. Neurologic involvement has not been reported and the disease is self-limited. There is no treatment of established value; the tetracycline drugs have yielded inconclusive results in the treatment of animals. Prevention of the disease in man has not been extensively studied, for man generally has a high degree of resistance to the infection. An effective vaccine for use in cattle has been developed.

WALSH McDERMOTT

References

British Foot-and-Mouth Disease Research Committee —First, Second, Third, and Fourth Progress Reports. London, His Majesty's Stationery Office, 1927, 1928, 1929, 1931.

Flaum, A.: Foot-and-Mouth Disease in Man. Acta path. et microbiol. Scandinav., 16:197, 1939.

LYMPHOCYTIC CHORIOMENINGITIS

Definition. Lymphocytic choriomeningitis is an acute disease of man characterized by a grippelike systemic illness which is followed in certain instances by an acute aseptic meningitis.

Etiology. The causative agent is a filterable virus of medium size, which is pathogenic for guinea pigs, hamsters and monkeys by various routes of inoculation and for rats and mice by the intracerebral route. It produces inapparent infection with the subsequent development of antibodies in dogs, pigs and rabbits. The virus belongs to the viscerotropic group of filterable agents, producing an interstitial type of pneumonia, areas of round cell infiltration, particularly in the liver, and choriomeningitis. During infection a soluble antigen is produced, to which complement-fixing antibodies develop in convalescence. Neutralizing antibodies to the virus itself are distinct and do not appear until several months after infection.

Incidence. The disease occurs sporadically. Cases have been recognized in various parts of the United States, the British Isles, Europe and Asia. The disease is usually seen in the fall, winter or spring.

Epidemiology. The virus causing the disease is harbored by mice in which the infection is latent and passes from one generation to the next. A number of cases have been traced to direct or indirect contact with these rodents. Dogs develop inapparent infection with this virus, and the ability of certain blood-sucking insects to transmit the disease has been demonstrated experimentally, so that other possible sources of human infection exist. Among laboratory animals this infection is a frequent source of difficulty, because of its high degree of communicability, and the disease has been contracted by a number of laboratory workers. Transmission of infection from one human being to another has not been observed.

Pathology. Few proved fatal cases have been studied. The principal findings have been interstitial bronchopneumonia and lymphocytic infiltration of the choroid plexus and meninges in the acute phases. The meningeal inflammation subsides slowly and may occasionally be followed by thickening, infiltration and scarring of the ventricular walls and subarachnoid space.

Symptoms. The incubation period is short. Within a period of a few days after exposure, fever develops. This is usually irregular and may be accompanied by chills and symptoms of "the grippe": malaise, headache, generalized aches and pains and anorexia. Pharyngitis, cough and signs of pneumonia may occur. During this phase of the disease, which lasts from a few days to two weeks, there is a leukopenia. In some patients complete recovery ensues, while in others, approximately fifteen to twenty days after exposure, and often after a remission of a day or two, the temperature again rises, and the symptoms of meningitis appear: headache, drowsiness, nausea, vomiting, nuchal rigidity, Kernig's sign, bradycardia and changes in the deep tendon reflexes. During this second phase the leukocyte count is usually normal, and lumbar puncture yields fluid under increased pressure, with an increased amount of protein, a normal concentration of glucose, and from 50 to 2500 cells per cubic millimeter, almost all lymphocytes. The meningeal phase of the disease lasts about a week with gradual subsidence of fever and symptoms, but considerably slower disappearance of the changes in the cerebrospinal fluid. Cases exhibiting only the systemic symptoms of the prodromal phase have been diagnosed rarely, but probably occur as often as cases with meningitis. The majority of proved cases have had the syndrome of "aseptic meningitis" (see section on Nonpurulent Meningitis). Several patients have been observed in whom the stage of invasion of the central nervous system was characterized by encephalomyelitic symptoms with both motor and sensory disturbances. Two fatal cases with pharyngitis, pneumonitis, high fever, prostration and leukopenia which gradually changed to a leukocytosis have been described.

Diagnosis. The syndrome of "acute aseptic meningitis," as originally described by

Wallgren, is relatively common. A few instances of this syndrome are actually due to the virus of lymphocytic choriomeningitis. The diagnosis of lymphocytic choriomeningitis should be entertained in those cases in which there has been an exposure to mice, other animals capable of harboring the virus, or blood-sucking insects, and in patients tral nervous system, such as those of herpes simplex, herpes zoster, meningopneumonitis, lymphogranuloma inguinale, poliomyelitis and the various forms of encephalitis. In any case with a lymphocytic reaction in the cerebrospinal fluid such conditions as brain abscess, torulosis, tuberculosis, leptospirosis and syphilis should be excluded.

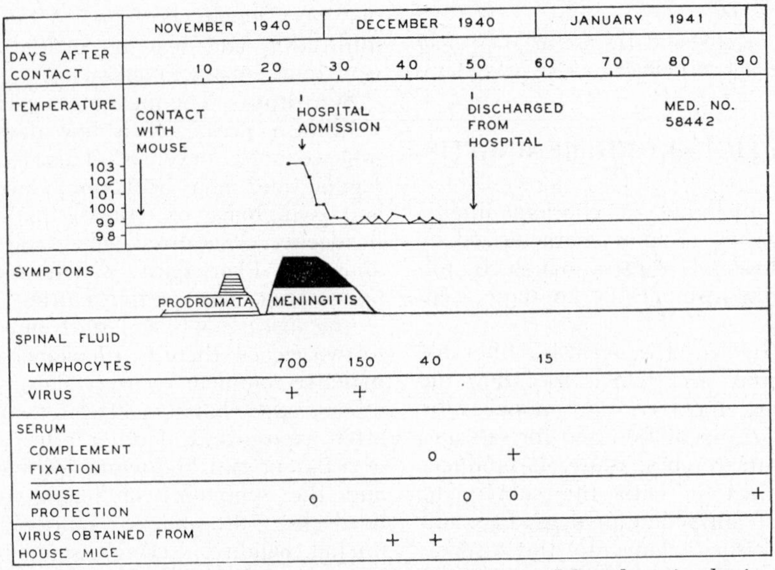

Fig. 12. Course and laboratory findings in a patient with proved lymphocytic choriomeningitis, probably acquired from handling a recently trapped mouse, since the virus of this disease was subsequently obtained from mice trapped in the home. (Reprinted from Medicine, Vol. 21, with permission of the publishers, Williams and Wilkins.)

whose disease has been characterized by a prodromal illness of several days' duration with a latent period before the development of meningitis. The diagnosis is made by isolation of the virus by subcutaneous or intraperitoneal inoculation of guinea pigs with blood taken during the prodromal phase or cerebrospinal fluid obtained during the meningeal phase. Intracerebral inoculation of white mice with infectious material in most instances gives rise to characteristic convulsions and death in six to ten days. The serologic diagnosis depends upon demonstration of the development of complement-fixing antibodies for the soluble antigen (four to six weeks after onset) and of neutralizing antibodies for the virus which appear later (two to three months after onset).

A common cause of acute aseptic meningitis is mumps. It also occurs in infectious mononucleosis and in infections due to many viruses capable of invading the cen-

Prognosis. Most patients with this infection recover completely. Death due to overwhelming infection and sequelae due to fibrosis and scarring of the choroid plexus or meninges have been observed in a few instances.

Prophylaxis. Because the disease is rare, no attempts at immunization have been made. Control of rodents and vermin in the home and in places where laboratory animals are kept should reduce the incidence of the disease. Persons trapping mice should handle animals and traps with care.

Treatment. Treatment of the disease is purely symptomatic.

CHARLES A. JANEWAY

References

Armstrong, C., Wallace, J. J., and Ross, L.: Lymphocytic Choriomeningitis; Gray Mice, *Mus Musculus*, a Reservoir for the Infection. Pub. Health Rep., 55:1222, 1940.

Farmer, T., and Janeway, C. A.: Infections with the Virus of Lymphocytic Choriomeningitis. Medicine, *21*:1, 1942.

Lépine, P., Mollaret, P., and Kreis, K.: Réceptivité de l'Homme au Virus Murin de la Chorioméningite Lymphocytaire. Reproduction Expérimentale de la Méningite Lymphocytaire Bénigne. Compt. rend. Acad. d. Sc., *204*:1846, 1937.

Rivers, T. M., and Scott, T. F. McN.: Meningitis in Man Caused by a Filterable Virus. II. Identification of the Etiological Agent. J. Exper. Med., *63*: 415, 1936.

Scott, T. F. McN., and Rivers, T. M.: Meningitis in Man Caused by a Filterable Virus. I. Two Cases and the Method of Obtaining a Virus from Their Spinal Fluids. J. Exper. Med., *63*:397, 1936.

Smadel, J. E., Green, R. H., Paltauf, R. M., and Gonzales, T. A.: Lymphocytic Choriomeningitis: Two Human Fatalities Following an Unusual Febrile Illness. Proc. Soc. Exper. Biol. & Med., *49*:683, 1942.

Wallgren, A.: Une Nouvelle Maladie Infectieuse du Système Nerveux Central? Acta Pediat., *4:158*, 1925.

RABIES

(Hydrophobia, Lyssa)

Definition. Rabies is an acute infectious disease of the central nervous system to which all warm-blooded animals and man are susceptible. The virus, frequently present in the saliva of an infected host, is usually transmitted by bites or licks. The disease, characterized by a profound dysfunction of the central nervous system, ends almost invariably in death.

History. Rabies was probably the disease to which Homer referred in the Iliad when he write, " κυνα λυσσώζα." Democritus and Aristotle recognize it as a disease of animals, and Celsus described its transmissibility to man. Rabies as a disease of wild animals had been known in Europe as early as the 13th century, and in the 18th century epizootics among domestic animals were recorded in urban centers. It was first reported in the Americas in 1709 by Fray José Gil Ramirez in Mexico, and was described in the Virginia Colony in 1753. Since that time, its presence has been evident throughout the North and South American continents.

The transmission of rabies from the saliva of a rabid dog to a normal dog was first recounted by Zinke in 1809, and in 1879 Galtier described the susceptibility of rabbits to rabies and their use for diagnostic purposes. The modern concept of the disease was developed by Pasteur and his associates (1881). They not only identified the causative agent, but also were able to modify its pathogenicity by serial intracerebral passages in laboratory animals (1884).

Etiology, Host Range and Experimental Infection.

Virus recovered in nature, the so-called *street virus,* is characterized by extremely variable, usually long, incubation periods, and by its ability to invade salivary glands as well as central nervous tissue. The term *fixed virus* is used for strains of rabies which have been adapted to laboratory animals by means of serial intracerebral passages. Fixed virus is characterized by a short incubation period (usually four to six days) and by its apparent inability to multiply in salivary glands. Prolonged cultivation of some strains of rabies virus in the developing chick embryo has resulted in modification to the point of complete loss of pathogenicity for animals injected extraneurally.

In discussing the properties of the virus both the type of virus and the source of infected material have to be considered. In general, it may be said that the virus, having a diameter of 100 to 150 millimicrons, can be filtered through bacteria-retaining porcelain filters. It is filterable, but not readily, through Seitz EK filter pads. Rabies virus is speedily inactivated by sunlight, ultraviolet irradiation, formalin, bichloride of mercury and strong acids. It is relatively resistant to ether and chloroform, and quite resistant to phenol. In aqueous solution, its thermal death point is reached at 56° C. after an exposure of one hour. It survives desiccation from the frozen state, and may be best preserved in dry form.

The host range of rabies is one of the widest in the disease spectrum. All mammals, including bats, are susceptible. The virus is also pathogenic for birds, but to a lesser degree than for mammals. The disease is not transmissible by insects or arthropods. The virus cannot invade the body through intact skin, and is apparently harmless when ingested. However, infection through unabraded mucosa seems possible.

Rabbits, guinea pigs, Swiss albino mice and hamsters are most commonly employed for experimental infection. Hamsters are remarkably susceptible to intramuscular infection with street virus, but intracerebral injection of albino mice is usually employed for diagnostic purposes.

Epidemiology and Epizootiology. Johnson distinguishes two epidemiologic patterns of the disease: the natural, sylvatic type maintained in wildlife, and the urban type which occurs in domestic dogs. The sylvatic type is present in enzootic form in many areas of the world in such wild animals as wolves (Arctic regions of Canada, Eastern Europe, Turkey, Iran), mongooses (South Africa, the Caribbean), bats (Central and South America, and only recently the United States), foxes, coyotes, skunks (United States). In the urban type a number of domestic animals, including cows and cats, may become involved; but the propagation of the virus in dogs is solely responsible for the epizootics, and after the elimination of canine rabies there is no evidence that rabies persists in urban areas.

Epizootics of rabies can occur in any climate during any season of the year. Wars and mass movements of men and animals favor the geographic spread of the disease. Man becomes an accidental host upon exposure to the infected saliva of the biting animal, and although wild animals are often sources of human rabies, dogs are mostly responsible for human infection. The attack rate in man following exposure depends to a certain extent on the location and severity of the inflicted wounds. Head and neck bites lead to a higher incidence of infection than bites on other parts of the body. Although the bites of rabid wolves are apparently very dangerous, an attack rate of 47 per cent was recently observed in 32 persons bitten by the same animal.

Morbid Anatomy. At autopsy, the brain is friable, edematous and congested; the convolutions are broad and flattened. Marked vascular congestion of the white and gray matter may extend to the medulla and the spinal cord. Virus-infected salivary glands are usually soft and swollen. On microscopic examination of the central nervous system, the nonspecific findings consist of hyperemia, perivascular and perineuronal infiltration with mononuclear cells, and marked neuronal degeneration. Mononuclear cell infiltration of periacinal interstitial tissue accompanied by degeneration of acinar cells may be observed in the parotid, sublingual and submaxillary salivary glands.

If proper staining technique is applied, intracytoplasmic inclusion bodies can be demonstrated in the neurons of the majority of rabies cases. These so-called Negri bodies are pathognomonic for rabies encephalitis. In their absence, the lesions cannot be distinguished from those observed in other viral encephalitides.

Incubation. The incubation period varies from ten days to over twelve months. As minor and seemingly insignificant contacts with rabies virus in the saliva of an animal not obviously sick at the time of exposure are sometimes forgotten, claims of extended incubation periods (one to two years) have to be critically evaluated. In dogs, signs of rabies may appear after an incubation period of ten days to several months. In one instance rabies developed in a dog eight and one-half months after artificial exposure by intramuscular inoculation with street virus.

The length of the incubation period is related to the amount of virus introduced at the time of exposure and to the severity of the laceration. The site of the original exposure does not seem to affect the duration of the incubation period.

Clinical Manifestations. *Dogs.* In dogs the prodromal phase of the disease consists of fever, failure to eat, hyperesthesia and very frequently change in the tone of the bark. However, often these signs are so slight that only a trained observer may note them. Altered disposition of the animal is also characteristic. The prodromal period may last from a few hours to several days, and gives way to the excitation phase in which the animal grows unnaturally restless and agitated. General tremor due to stimulation of the muscular system is frequent. In the furious type of the disease, agitation intensifies as the illness progresses. The animal, erratic and aggressive, growls and barks constantly. It will grab viciously at any object or animal encountered. At this stage, an unrestrained animal sometimes leaves home and travels great distances, inflicting damage on other animals and humans along the way. Convulsive seizures are often observed, and the animal may become completely paralyzed. In many cases, however, the excitation phase predominates until the time of death.

In the paralytic type of rabies, the excitation phase may be slight or totally absent, and the disease is characterized only by the paralytic syndrome. Paralysis of the lower jaw, accompanied by excessive salivation, appears as an early symptom, and the animal acts as though choking on a foreign body. Paralysis of the muscles of phonation may lead to loss of the bark. As the disease progresses, paralysis of the posterior extremities sets in, followed by general paralysis and death. The time from the onset of the disease to the death of the animal ranges from one to eleven days. On the other hand dogs may die suddenly without noticeable signs of illness.

Man. In man, the prodromal phase is marked by fever, malaise, nausea and sore throat. Abnormal sensations around the site of infection, such as intermittent pain, tingling or burning, are of diagnostic significance. Extreme stimulation of the general sensory system is manifested by hyperesthesia of the skin to temperature changes and to drafts, and by acute sensitiveness to sound and light. Increased muscular tonus, prompt gag and corneal reflexes, dilation of pupils and increased salivation may be present.

As the disease progresses, spasmodic contractions of the muscles of the mouth, pharynx and larynx on drinking—and later at the mere sight of fluid—are observed in the majority of cases. This dysfunction of deglutition lent the disease its common name, *hydrophobia,* or fear of water. Spasms of respiratory muscles and convulsive seizures leading to opisthotonos may occur. The pulse is very rapid. Periods of irrational and often maniacal behavior are interspersed with those of alertness and responsiveness. Paralysis of the muscles of phonation may lead to hoarseness or loss of voice.

The excitation phase may remain predominant until the time of death. However, in many cases it gives way shortly before death to cessation of muscle spasms, hyporeflexia or areflexia, and to general paralysis of the flaccid type.

In some cases, particularly those in Trinidad resulting from vampire bat infection, the excitation phase is almost totally absent, and the disease is characterized by ascending paralysis without hydrophobia. Without an adequate history of exposure, this type is indistinguishable from other viral encephalitides, and the diagnosis may be overlooked.

Diagnosis. Profound dysfunction of the central nervous system accompanied by impairment in deglutition, following a history of exposure to a bite or lick of an animal, facilitates the clinical diagnosis. Isolation of virus from saliva obtained in the course of the disease and from brain tissue obtained at autopsy, followed by proper identification of the agent by means of neutralization test, will confirm the diagnosis. Syrian hamsters, rabbits, guinea pigs and mice are used for diagnostic purposes. The presence of Negri bodies is pathognomonic, but their absence does not exclude the diagnosis of rabies encephalitis since isolation of the virus may still be accomplished.

Prognosis. Although inapparent infection with street virus may be induced artificially in laboratory animals, and although animals have recovered completely after exhibiting signs of the disease, *there is no proved instance of the recovery of man from rabies.*

Treatment–Prevention. A treatment for rabies does not exist in the strict sense of the word, for there are no therapeutic measures available which would save the life of a person exhibiting symptoms of the disease. A *protective type of treatment* can be used following exposure to the virus and prior to the development of the disease. Particularly in a rabies endemic area and adjacent territory, this protective treatment has to be based on the assumption that every animal inflicting a wound on a human may be rabid, until proved otherwise by clinical observation or by failure to discover the virus in its tissues after death.

Local Treatment of Wounds. All bite wounds, including skin abrasions exposed to licks of animals, should be treated *immediately* by thorough cleansing with soap or detergent solutions. This does not preclude the use of strong mineral acids, such as nitric acid, which may be particularly useful in the treatment of deep puncture wounds where other methods of cleansing are not very effective. In laboratory animals a cationic detergent, Zephiran chloride, applied in a 1 per cent solution to wounds artificially contaminated with the virus, has been found to be more effective in preventing rabies than either nitric acid or 20 per cent soap solution. The detergent does not cause burns, and does not interfere with wound healing.

The local or parenteral application of an antimicrobial drug is of no value as a prophylactic measure, except in combating concomitant bacterial infections.

Indications for Specific Treatment. These are summarized in a table prepared by the Expert Committee on Rabies of the World Health Organization. Emphasis is placed on the condition of the biting animal at the time of the exposure and during the ensuing ten days. It is assumed that the saliva of an animal which is not obviously ill at the time of exposure may be infectious during a maxi-

Indications for Specific Post-Exposure Treatment*

NATURE OF EXPOSURE	CONDITION OF ANIMAL		RECOMMENDED TREATMENT
	At time of exposure	During observation period of 10 days	
I. No lesions Indirect contact only	Rabid	—	None†
II. Licks			
1. Unabraded skin	Rabid	—	None†
2. Abraded skin and abraded or un-abraded mucosa	(a) Healthy	Healthy	None
	(b) Healthy	Clinical signs of rabies or proven rabid	Start vaccine at first signs of rabies in animal
	(c) Signs suggestive of rabies	Healthy	Start vaccine immediately. Stop treatment if animal is normal on 5th day after exposure‡
	(d) Rabid, escaped, killed or unknown	—	Start vaccine immediately
III. Bites			
1. Simple exposure	(a) Healthy	Healthy	None
	(b) Healthy	Clinical signs of rabies or proven rabid	Start vaccine at first signs of rabies in animal
	(c) Signs suggestive of rabies	Healthy	Start vaccine immediately. Stop treatment if animal is normal on 5th day after exposure‡
	(d) Rabid, escaped, killed or unknown; or any bite by wolf, jackal, fox or other wild animal	—	Start vaccine immediately
2. Severe exposure (Multiple; or face, head or neck bites)	(a) Healthy	Healthy	Hyperimmune serum immediately No vaccine as long as animal remains normal
	(b) Healthy	Clinical signs of rabies or proven rabid	As in III, 2, (a), but start vaccine at first sign of rabies
	(c) Signs suggestive of rabies	Healthy	Hyperimmune serum immediately, followed by vaccine. Vaccine may be stopped if animal is normal on 5th day after exposure
	(d) Rabid, escaped, killed or unknown. Any bite by wild animal	—	Hyperimmune serum immediately, followed by vaccine

Hyperimmune serum to be effective must be given within 72 hours of exposure.

These indications apply equally well whether or not the biting animal has been previously vaccinated.

* Prepared by Expert Committee on Rabies of World Health Organization.

† Start vaccine immediately in young children and patients where a reliable history cannot be obtained.

‡ Alternative treatment would be to give hyperimmune serum and not start vaccine as long as animal remained normal.

mum period of five days preceding the appearance of clinical signs of disease.

Passive immunization against rabies by the administration of hyperimmune antiserum is introduced as a standard procedure in view of the overwhelming experimental evidence obtained in favor of such treatment. Because of the existence of various vaccine preparations, no emphasis is placed on the use of any special type of vaccine provided it meets the standard potency requirement.

Administration of antirabies vaccine may give rise to local allergic reactions, and to those of a general neuroparalytic nature. The latter are caused by the presence of nervous tissue in the vaccine, and occur most frequently during a repeated course of protective treatment. No vaccine preparation is at present available which is free from the paralysis-producing factor, and therefore the administration of vaccine should be interrupted if even slight signs of dysfunction of the central or peripheral nervous system are observed. By the same token, antirabies vaccine treatment should not be given unless specifically indicated. (See table.)

Control Measures. The majority of human exposures can be prevented by the use of control methods which will rid an area of enzootics or epizootics of rabies.

The following measures should be applied in an efficiently organized rabies control program conducted by public health authorities: control of the canine population (registration, restraint, elimination of stray dogs), reduction in number of susceptible dogs by mass vaccination, reduction in number of wildlife species which are a reservoir of the virus, and continuous educational campaigns for the general public.

HILARY KOPROWSKI

References

Babes, V.: Traité de la rage. Paris, Librairie J.-B. Baillière et Fils, 1912.

Expert Committee on Rabies. Report on the Second Session. Geneva, World Health Organization Technical Report Series No. 82, 1954.

Gremliza, L.: Rabies: Kasuistik zum Lyssa-Problem. Ztschr. Tropenmed. u. parasitol., 4:382, 1953.

Habel, K.: Seroprophylaxis in Experimental Rabies. Pub. Health Rep., 60:545–560, 1945.

Johnson, H. N.: Rabies. In Rivers, T. M. ed.: Viral and Rickettsial Infections of Man. 2nd ed. Philadelphia, J. B. Lippincott Company, 1952, pp. 267–299.

———, and Sellers, T. F.: Laboratory Techniques in Rabies. Geneva. World Health Organization Monograph Series No. 23, 1954.

Koprowski, H.: Immunization with Modified Living Virus with Particular Reference to Rabies and Hog Cholera. Vet Med., 47:144–150, 1952.

Kraus, R., Gerlach, F. and Schweinburg, F.: Lyssa bei Mensch und Tier. Berlin, Urban and Schwarzenberg, 1926.

Shaughnessy, H. J., and Zichis, J.: Treatment of Wounds Inflicted by Rabid Animals. Bull. World Health Organization, 10:805, 1954.

Webster, L. T.: Rabies. New York, The Macmillan Company, 1942.

POLIOMYELITIS

(*Infantile Paralysis*)

Definition. Poliomyelitis is a common, acute viral disease characterized clinically by a brief, febrile illness with sore throat, headache and vomiting, and often with stiffness of the neck and back. In certain cases a lower neuron paralysis develops in the early days of illness.

History. References to conditions which may have been poliomyelitis date from earliest times, but no descriptions of this disease have been found in medical literature before the end of the eighteenth century. At this time mention of acute paralysis in childhood was made in England by Michael Underwood in his textbook on diseases of children. During the subsequent fifty years there were several descriptions of poliomyelitis, the best being that by the German orthopedist Heine which was published in 1840. During most of the nineteenth century the disease was regarded as a sporadic and ubiquitous affliction of young infants. Its contagious and epidemic character did not receive emphasis until Medin's work appeared in Sweden in 1890. From that time forward the disease ceased to be a curiosity and became a periodic scourge in some countries. The principles of its epidemiology were first reviewed by Medin's pupil, Wickman, who published his monograph in 1908, the same year in which Landsteiner discovered the virus.

Etiology. The virus of poliomyelitis has been commonly isolated from patients acutely ill with this disease, the best sources being intestinal excreta, the oropharynx, occasionally the blood, and, at necropsy, the central nervous system. It is extremely small as viruses go. The virus is labile in some respects, being sensitive to drying, and stable in others, resisting ether and certain other so-called disinfectants. It remains viable at ice-box temperature in aqueous suspensions of feces for months, and in pieces of infected spinal cord for years, when stored in 50 per cent glycerol. As for its resistance to heat, the virus has been inactivated when suspended in water, milk or ice cream at pasteurization temperatures.

With most strains of poliomyelitis virus, primates are the only animals which can be infected, the rhesus monkey (*Macaca mulatta*) being the experimental animal most often used. However, infection of mice has been achieved, particularly with the Lansing (or Type 2) group of strains. A fundamental discovery by Enders and his collaborators has been the demonstration that poliomyelitis virus will grow in tissue culture. As a result of the practical application of this method, the isolation, typing and neutralization of this virus can now be carried out *in vitro*.

Within the poliomyelitis virus family there are three immunologic types, designated as: *Brunhilde* (Type 1); *Lansing* (Type 2); and *Leon* (Type 3). It has been shown repeatedly in the laboratory (particularly in work on feeding chimpanzees) that, although *type-specific immunity* can be induced, an animal can be reinfected with an *heterologous* type of poliomyelitis virus. This is the reason usually given to explain why the same person may contract poliomyelitis more than once. The practical implication is that any proposed poliomyelitis vaccine should probably contain all three types of virus.

Epidemiology and Pathogenesis. Poliomyelitis is an endemic and epidemic disease of world-wide distribution, primarily affecting children, and spread by *contact,* with clinical and inapparent "cases" acting as carriers. Although regarded as a "contact disease" there is still much to be learned as to how this disease is actually transmitted. Some of the present mystery vanishes, however, with the recognition that unlike certain other contact diseases, such as measles, in which the disease passes from one recognized case to another, the spread of poliomyelitis often occurs through the medium of mild cases, many of which are so mild as to escape recognition. Evidence is convincing that during an average epidemic of poliomyelitis those who are ill enough to be diagnosed or become paralyzed represent a small fraction of those who become infected. Nevertheless, the contact theory does not cover the whole story, for it does not explain why cases of poliomyelitis occur at a much higher rate in the summer and early autumn than they do in the winter. There are two possible explanations: either something happens in summer which enormously facilitates the dissemination of the virus throughout a community, or something happens which makes people far more susceptible.

Poliomyelitis virus has been found under natural circumstances, in sewage and on food (contaminated by flies) and in flies and cockroaches during epidemics. An obvious question is whether the patient's immediate or remote environment is not only contaminated but "infectious," serving to spread the disease through the agency of contaminated water, food or insects. However, there is at least no evidence that insects are an *essential* link in the chain, as are mosquitoes in the transmission of malaria or yellow fever.

Children are more susceptible to poliomyelitis than are adults. As in measles, this is an expression of acquired immunity on the part of the adult populations. The age at which this immunity is acquired differs in different places. In the United States, although most of the cases fall within the age group of 4 to 15, many cases occur in young adults.

How the virus of poliomyelitis actually enters the human body is a subject of controversy. It is unlikely, however, that it gains access to the central nervous system directly by way of the nasal mucosa and the olfactory bulbs. It is more likely that it penetrates through the mucosa of the oral cavity, the alimentary tract or, conceivably, the skin. Very early in the disease, or late in the incubation period, the virus has been recovered from the blood stream, but the central nervous system, the oral cavity and the intestinal tract are sites for which it has affinity and where it soon settles.

Prior to, during and after an acute attack, virus can be demonstrated in the oropharynx and in the intestinal tract; in the former site it persists for about a week from onset, and in the latter for about three to six weeks or even longer. This (acute and convalescent) carrier state can be initiated by an attack so mild as to go undiagnosed or even unnoticed. Although usually not more than one person in a family becomes paralyzed at a single time, simultaneous multiple infections within families are common. Evidence suggests, however, that in certain families a high prevalence of the paralytic form of the disease has prevailed through several generations.

As to *predisposing influences,* recent tonsillectomy (performed within three months of onset) is regarded as one. During epidemics this operation has been followed by bulbar poliomyelitis more often than might be expected. Furthermore, such minor procedures as inoculations for diphtheria or pertussis also fall into this category. Severe exertion, or stress or an injury, if sustained on the day or two preceding or following the onset of acute poliomyelitis, tend to make the prognosis less favorable. A theoretical explanation of this is that if the "injury" occurs during the stage of viremia the virus may gain access to the nervous system and spread within it more readily. Therapeutic and prophylactic implications inherent in this situation are discussed later.

Morbid Anatomy. Important lesions occur in the central nervous system, notably in the gray matter of the spinal cord. Hyperplasia of lymph nodes (cervical, axillary and mesenteric) also occurs. Myocarditis has been described in fatal cases.

Classic *neural* lesions are the result of the neuronotropic character of the virus. Ganglion cells in the anterior horns of the spinal cord are characteristically involved, particularly in the cervical and lumbar regions. These lesions pass through stages marked by diffuse chromatolysis, destruction of neurons, neuronophagia and perivascular and interstitial infiltration of round cells. The brain stem is nearly always involved in fatal cases, whereas lesions of the cerebral cortex are re-

of the neck and spine muscles, unlike that seen in meningitis, can be overcome by slight resistance and diminishes or even disappears with the patient in a prone position. Probably this relaxation is explainable in terms of reciprocal innervation and is the result of an inhibition of an exaggerated extensor reflex.

The occurrence of "spasm" in paralytic and nonparalytic muscles has been the subject of extensive discussion. Some investigators consider it to be due to increased myotatic reflex

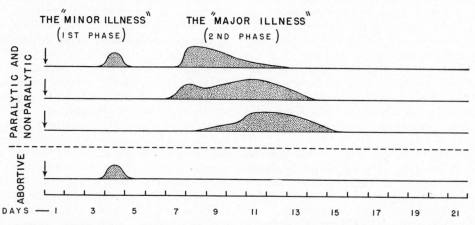

Fig. 13. Diagrams illustrative of various clinical forms which poliomyelitis may assume. The stippled areas indicate periods of fever. Arrows on the left mark the hypothetical time of exposure. The top diagram is more typical of the disease in infancy; the diagram which is third from the top is more typical of the adult form.

stricted to the precentral gyrus (motor area). Rarely have lesions been found in the olfactory bulbs in human cases, an important negative finding.

Pathologic Physiology. Although physical signs attributable to a disturbance within the central nervous system can often be explained on the basis of a *diffuse* inflammatory reaction, in acute poliomyelitis a correlation between direct nerve cell injury and the physical sign should be considered first, before incriminating the accessory influences of edema or other secondary factors. Since muscular function is often regained in previously paretic muscles during convalescence, this would seem to indicate that the changes in certain virus-infected cells are *reversible*. Illustrative of the reversible affections are the transient paresis of the urinary bladder and the intestinal tract.

The stiff neck and back in acute poliomyelitis have been considered in the past to be signs of meningeal reaction, but there is some evidence to the contrary. The rigidity

activity; others, to reflex contraction secondary to pain in hyperirritable muscles.

Incubation Period. Usually stated as about ten days, the incubation period is probably less. It may range from as short as four to as long as thirty-five days. Average figures indicate nine to thirteen days for paralytic cases and four to ten for abortive cases, the difference being that first-phase symptoms may be so slight as to escape notice. Opinions differ as to the best method of dating the onset of the disease. It is the writer's practice to consider the earliest (first-phase or minor illness) symptoms, when present, as marking the onset of the disease.

Symptoms. Common clinical forms which poliomyelitis may assume are illustrated in Figure 13. Recently an improvement in nomenclature has been proposed, calling for the terms, "minor illness" and "major illness," to supplant the terms, "first or systemic phase" and "second or neurologic phase," respectively.

The "Minor Illness." These brief illnesses,

so commonly seen during poliomyelitis epidemics, usually last only 24 hours, and are more frequent in children than adults. They are the critical indications that infection has started and are probably contemporaneous with the period of viremia, but they cannot be diagnosed with certainty by clinical methods. Clinical manifestations include: fever, headache, vomiting, listlessness, sore throat and, rarely, diarrhea. Sore throat is a much more frequent complaint in the *minor* as opposed to the *major* illness, and thus becomes a useful symptom in determining the stage of the disease. The cerebrospinal fluid findings are almost always normal here and the symptoms comparable to those of a variety of mild, acute illnesses. A tentative diagnosis can be made, however, on those patients who have been in close association with a recognizable case of poliomyelitis. For a positive diagnosis, virus isolation or antibody tests are almost essential.

The minor illness in poliomyelitis may be followed by signs of *paralytic* or *nonparalytic* poliomyelitis, or it may represent the entire course of the disease. In the latter event, it is also known as *abortive poliomyelitis.**

The "Major Illness." This term relates to both nonparalytic and paralytic poliomyelitis. It designates that important "complication" of acute poliomyelitis which may occur with or without antecedent symptoms and which indicates that lesions have developed within the central nervous system to an extent sufficient to give rise to neurologic symptoms. The onset may be abrupt or gradual over a period of several days. If the onset is sudden, fever, vomiting and severe headache are again commonly encountered. These early symptoms may be accompanied or followed quickly by spontaneous pain in the extremities—deep pain, hyperesthesia and sometimes paresthesia. Soreness and stiffness of the neck and back and hamstring muscles become promi-

* Definitions of the terms abortive and nonparalytic poliomyelitis are not easily made. In the writer's clinic an *abortive* case is a case of "minor illness," without clinical or laboratory signs of central nervous system involvement. Obviously, an illness of this type can be diagnosed only in epidemic times. The *nonparalytic* case, on the other hand, is an example of the "major illness" in which *residual paralysis* does not occur. Physical signs include stiff neck and/ or positive findings in the cerebrospinal fluid. The criterion for the absence of paralysis is that during and shortly after the course of the disease no weakness of any muscles should be evident on two examinations made at least 24 hours apart.

nent early. Severe lumbar back pain not associated with motion of the spine (in fact relieved by motion) is relatively common in adults with severe infections. Abdominal pain may also occur.

If "major illness" symptoms develop insidiously, as is often the case with adults, there may be no fever at first, or only slight fever, not above 100° F. This gradual onset may be puzzling and responsible for a delay in diagnosis. Such patients appear uncomfortable and restless, rather than sick. They complain of listlessness, intermittent headache, anorexia with occasional vomiting, pains in the extremities and, again, hyperesthesia and paresthesia followed by stiffness of the neck and back, and pain in the back.

During the febrile period, temperatures may range from 100° to 103° F., depending on the age of the patient, and may last three to ten days. The onset of weakness or flaccid paralysis usually occurs while fever is still present, but may appear as the fever begins to fall. Thus, concurrently with an improvement in the general clinical picture, the patient discovers that his limbs will not function properly. Acute retention of urine is not uncommon, particularly when severe paralysis of the lower extremities is present. Constipation or obstipation is also common.

Spinal Paralytic Poliomyelitis. This is the classic form of poliomyelitis in which the presence of flaccid paralysis makes the clinical diagnosis quite definite. Muscles commonly paralyzed, in order of frequency, are those of the legs (by far the most frequent), arms, back, thorax, face, intercostal region and diaphragm.

Respiratory Paralysis. Difficulty in breathing results from several causes which will be considered later.

Other Types of Paralysis. The encephalomyelitic and bulbar forms also represent examples of paralytic poliomyelitis, but actually the disease is seldom limited to any of these anatomic categories.

Encephalitic symptoms occur at any stage, and in some epidemics are very frequent. Symptoms include dizziness, which is not a true vertigo, but rather a lightheadedness, apprehension, yawning, twitching of the limbs and irritability, to be followed by lassitude, drowsiness and even coma. Convulsions are rare.

The *bulbar* form is most serious. It includes those cases in which cranial nerve nuclei are involved. When the tenth (and often the eleventh) cranial nerves are implicated, there is unilateral or bilateral weakness of the soft palate which sags unnaturally in the back of the throat. There may also be weakness of the pharynx and vocal cords. This results in an inability to swallow or to talk clearly, and occasionally in regurgitation of fluid through the nose. Other patients have symptoms and signs indicating involvement of the autonomic centers of the medulla, notably the respiratory center. Respiratory failure may progress with great rapidity.

Diagnosis. Initial symptoms and signs of the acute disease are likely to be nonspecific. Often a preliminary diagnosis is "tonsillitis" or "summer grippe." An important point of differentiation is that signs indicating respiratory tract involvement, other than sore throat, are absent. If the disease progresses, stiffness of the neck, back and hamstring muscles soon becomes prominent. At this stage there is apt to be an increase of cells and protein in the cerebrospinal fluid. These clinical and laboratory findings are again not specific for poliomyelitis, being essentially those of benign, nonpurulent meningitis, which may be due to a variety of agents of viral, bacterial, spirochetal or even protozoan origin. Thus it may not be possible to make a positive diagnosis of *nonparalytic* poliomyelitis without resort to virologic or immunologic tests.

Nevertheless, stiffness of the back is a characteristic sign of poliomyelitis. It is best elicited with the patient sitting up in bed with the knees naturally flexed and asking him to "kiss his knees." If the back is stiff, attempts to do this will cause pain. Another sign is "head drop," demonstrated by having the patient lie on his back, placing one's hands beneath his shoulders and lifting him up from the bed. In the normal person the head follows along in a plane with the body as it is raised, but in poliomyelitis (even in its earliest stages) the head falls back limply in a position of hyperextension. This sign is not specific for poliomyelitis; it occurs in children severely ill with a number of prostrating diseases, including pneumonia and meningitis, but in the obvious absence of such diseases it is useful.

Tightness and soreness of the hamstring muscles and resistance to extension of the leg are common.

The *reflexes* in early stages of the "major illness" may be normal and active. Later, if the onset of paralysis is imminent, there is an irregular shift to hyperactivity, and then sudden (and sometimes transient) shifts to diminished (or absent) reflexes. Usually the appearance of reflex changes precedes the appearance of weakness or paralyses by 12 to 24 hours. Superficial reflexes, i.e., the abdominal, cremasteric and spinal reflexes, are the first to disappear.

Although the periodic but cautious examination for muscle power is part of the daily examination of the patient, ill patients should be spared from exhaustive and exhausting muscle examinations during the acute stage of the disease. Patients in whom there is progressive muscle weakness, however, require frequent observation for evidence of diminished excursions of the intercostals and diaphragm.

A valuable laboratory test is the examination of the *cerebrospinal fluid*. If the (white) cell count is elevated above 8 cells per cu. mm. and the protein is above 35 mg. per 100 ml., the diagnosis in a suspicious case is more likely, but one cannot rely on a negative test to exclude poliomyelitis. Furthermore, there is an element of timing, because during the "minor illness," a normal cerebrospinal fluid is to be expected. One should also recall that these positive findings are those of so-called benign lymphocytic meningitis. The cerebrospinal fluid cell count is likely to be highest during the first week of the "major illness," and although the predominant cell type is usually mononuclear, early in the disease polymorphonuclear forms predominate. Usually the white cell count does not exceed 300 cells per cu. mm. The protein content of the fluid is low and often normal during the first week, but rises later, remaining up through the fourth week and then gradually decreasing to normal. Thus a high and rising protein content may exist after the cell count has returned to normal.

There is no consistent change in the peripheral *blood picture*. As a rule the total leukocyte count is only moderately elevated (10,000 to 16,000 per cu. mm.) with a relative lymphopenia. Rapid erythrocyte sedimentation rates have recently been reported in about half the patients tested. Routine *urinalysis* reveals no abnormalities.

Serologic tests (neutralization and complement fixation tests) which can be done on matched (early and convalescent) blood samples for purposes of clinical diagnosis require a special laboratory. The availability of these tests is likely to increase.

Differential Diagnosis. Paralytic poliomyelitis should be considered whenever flaccid paralysis (particularly paralysis without sensory changes) occurs in the presence of fever and in the absence of traumatic or other types of injury to the cord. It can be confused with the summer, arthropod-borne encephalitides, but serious paralysis of the limbs does not usually occur in these conditions.

Nonparalytic poliomyelitis can be confused with *mumps encephalitis*, particularly when mumps occurs without involvement of the salivary glands, and with *postmeasles encephalitis, meningoencephalitis* (of undetermined type), *lymphocytic choriomeningitis* and *infectious neuronitis* (Guillain-Barré syndrome). Infections by members of the Coxsackie group of viruses may be easily mistaken for poliomyelitis, as may also be the case with leptospirosis.

Rheumatic fever is often diagnosed as poliomyelitis. Other conditions which have been confused are *acute meningitides* (of various types) and *tuberculous meningitis*. In these conditions the diagnosis is likely to become apparent in the course of time. More rarely, *acute osteomyelitis, trichinosis, acute appendicitis, infectious mononucleosis* and *lead poisoning* are mistaken for poliomyelitis.

It is also well to recall that generalized weakness of limbs may occur in the presence of acute fever, as in influenza or acute enteritis.

Prognosis. During the early and acute stage of poliomyelitis, predictions as to eventual outcome are risky. Extreme agitation, restlessness and apprehension in the febrile stages may indicate a poor prognosis, and, if physical exertion has been undertaken in the early days of illness (in the "major illness"), a less favorable result can be expected. The height of fever bears little relationship to the extent of paralysis which may ensue but the duration of high fever may be significant.

The *mortality rate* for any given epidemic will vary according to diagnostic criteria. It may range from 1 to 4 per cent or higher. By far the highest mortality occurs in bulbar cases. The severity of the illness and the case fatality rate increase with the age of the patient.

Paralysis shows a remarkable tendency to improve in this disease but the *extent of recovery* is subject to variables, and primarily to the degree of irreversible change which the virus has inflicted on the infected nerve cells. When all the anterior horn cells which control a given area are irreversibly damaged, a complete and permanent loss of power inevitably occurs.

The rate of recovery of strength in individual muscles or muscle groups follows a fairly definite pattern. By the end of the third month from the onset, a muscle will usually recover approximately 60 per cent of the total strength that it will ever recover under treatment. During the next three months an additional 20 per cent may return. After this the recovery rate becomes increasingly slower, so that by the end of eighteen months of treatment it is more than likely that no further increase in muscle strength can be expected.

Treatment. At present, no specific treatment is available for poliomyelitis. None of the antimicrobial drugs which have been tried has any effect in destroying the virus or controlling its spread within the body. Although it was believed at one time that convalescent serum was valuable, this has proved not to be the case, and even concentrated immune globulin (gamma globulin) has proved ineffective as a therapeutic measure. This is not surprising, as, by the time of onset of the major illness, the patient is usually manufacturing his or her own antibodies.

Mild Cases. It is impossible to determine within the first few hours or days of illness whether a given case will or will not go on to the eventual development of paralysis. But the clinician's responsibility in the management of these early, though potentially severe, cases seems clear. Thus, *during epidemics,* all patients with brief, febrile illnesses of the type described above deserve to be regarded with suspicion, physical activities should be curtailed, and the patient should be kept quiet and in bed under observation preferably at home for at least a week. Seldom do they require special types of therapy, such as drugs, hot packs, orthopedic care or physiotherapy. Potentially, such patients may be infectious and therefore require some degree of isolation.

Paralytic Cases. Hospitalization is advisable for paralytic cases. An isolation hospital is not necessary, for general hospitals can care for poliomyelitis patients, provided isolation precautions can be carried out. Care should be exerted that the trip to the hospital involves a minimum of exertion and trauma. Within a large hospital the management of a patient with acute and advancing paralysis often involves the services of a team, composed of a physician (internist or pediatrician), an orthopedic surgeon, a physiotherapist, and perhaps specially trained nurses.

GENERAL MEASURES. Orthopedists recommend that a hard bed be provided from the beginning. The bed should be fitted with a footboard placed several inches beyond the mattress, allowing room for the heels or toes when the patient lies supine or prone. The footboard also serves to protect the extremities from the pressure of bedclothing and allows proprioceptive reflexes to be stimulated when the feet rest against it. If the legs are weak, the knees should be supported in a slightly flexed position; weak arms should be in external rotation alongside the body but not against it. If the patient is acutely ill or irrational, it will not be possible to keep him in this position, but the sooner it can be achieved the better.

Early in and during the stage of active myelitis (in which fever is usually present) there are four important aspects of general therapy: adequate rest; cautious use of sedation and analgesia; adequate fluids; and proper nursing care.

For all patients whether at home or in the hospital, *early bed rest* is important. As part of the program of rest the patient should be spared from undue fatigue, and from injections which are not essential.

Sedation and other means for the relief of pain are important considerations. Relief may be aided by the intermittent application of hot moist packs. Green and Gucker believe that the value of hot packs has been exaggerated, but their moderate use seems to be helpful, tending to relieve pain and to assist in promoting relaxation of tight muscles. The availability of equipment and personnel often determines the type and methods of applying hot foments. Although numerous types of packs have been advocated, two general types are in current use, the so-called "wrap-around pack," and the "lay-on pack." Woolen cloth is favored material. Both types of pack call for application directly to the skin of the hot wet wool from which the water has been well wrung. This is then covered by two ad-

ditional layers, one of which is of waterproof material and the second is for insulation.

The response to common analgesics and sedatives is not very satisfactory in early stages, but sedatives are often used. Often, if pain is relieved by hot packs, drugs will not be necessary. This is desirable, for the danger of aggravating incipient or actual respiratory difficulty makes it necessary to use sedatives cautiously. Some physicians are convinced, however, that the physical activity of the restless patient represents a danger in precipitating paralysis, and adequate sedation is indicated if there is no obvious respiratory embarrassment.

In recent years several •drugs, including neostigmine and curare, have been advocated for the relaxation of muscle tightness and relief of pain, but they are not recommended. It would seem that none of the drugs is as effective as the more cumbersome method of hot packs.

Fluid should be given freely and, whenever hot packs or hot baths are used, salt tablets should be added to make up for excessive salt loss in perspiration.

Nursing care for the acute disease should follow general principles used in acute infections. The diet should be light. Isolation technique with so-called "typhoid precautions" should be followed for one to three weeks, depending upon local rules. The patients' stools should be disposed of as quickly and safely as possible. The use of chemical disinfectant to "sterilize" the stools is not recommended.

CARE OF PARALYZED LIMBS. Protection of the recently paralyzed limb (rather than fixation) is the objective. The ultimate care of such limbs is essentially an orthopedic problem and consequently will not be discussed here.

Complications. Urinary retention is common in patients with severe involvement of the lower extremities. Before resorting to catheterization, an adequate trial of drug therapy should be given. The parasympatheticomimetic drug, furfuryl trimethylammonium iodide (Furmethide), has proved efficacious if given subcutaneously in adequate dosage. In infants, doses of 1.25 mg. (0.3 to 0.5 cc.) have been used. In children the dose has ranged from 2 to 5 mg., and in adults from 5 to 7 mg. If there is no response, catheterization is indicated, together with prophylactic antimicrobials. In general, urinary retention is a complication that lasts but a few days.

Patients with *bulbar paralysis* require special nursing care. Loss of ability to swallow is the most common cause of respiratory tract obstruction in poliomyelitis patients. Steps involved in treating this condition begin with *postural drainage* to maintain a free airway, with the bed tilted at an angle of 10 to 12 degrees off horizontal. Patients are usually more comfortable in a side-lying than a prone position. When mechanical aspiration is done, a rubber or polyethylene catheter may be passed through the nose into the hypopharynx. The catheter is then connected to an electrically driven suction machine, or water pump; the ideal is to provide gentle intermittent suction. If swallowing is impaired, fluid, salt and nutriment are administered either by hypodermoclysis, intravenously or by proctoclysis. The amount of fluid depends on the age, size and condition of the patient; 3000 cc. or more are recommended daily for adults. Intravenous saline and glucose should be given slowly and in small amounts, not more than 500 cc. at a time.

Respiratory difficulty may reflect at least four types of disturbances. In any given case of poliomyelitis several of them may coexist, but it is important to recognize which are involved. They are: (1) Disturbance of function of the muscles which perform the respiratory movements. (2) Disturbances of the central control of respiration so that damaged neurons do not respond in the normal manner to changes in the CO_2 concentration, pH and O_2 saturation of arterial blood. (3) Obstruction of the airway caused by inability to swallow and by paralysis of intrinsic muscles of the larynx; aspiration of oral secretions may lead to atelectasis of portions of the lung and further loss of respiratory function. (4) Pulmonary edema which may occur when extensive bulbar disease is present. It brings about serious impairment of gas exchange in the lungs.

In estimating the condition of the respiratory muscles, the appearance of the patient is extremely important. With mild degrees of respiratory muscle weakness the patient exhibits anxiety by facial expression, restlessness, irritability, emotional lability and wakefulness. With more weakness of the respiratory muscles, the face becomes flushed, hypoxia and CO_2 retention increase, pallor replaces the florid appearance, there is inability to cough, and respiration becomes rapid and labored with the use of accessory muscles. Certain clinical and laboratory procedures have proved of value in estimating the adequacy of the respiratory muscles. The strength of intercostal muscles is tested by having the patient expand the chest against manual pressure exerted against the lower portion of the rib cage. Intercostal muscles are also tested by restriction of the diaphragmatic excursion by manual force supplied to the upper part of the abdomen. As sniffing is brought about by descent of the diaphragm, ability to carry out this action constitutes a test of diaphragmatic function. The resting small child with normal respiratory muscle function is able to hold its breath for 15 to 20 seconds; the child suffering from respiratory muscle impairment of relatively slight degree falls far short of this. Under certain circumstances a fluoroscopic examination to test diaphragmatic excursion is useful; furthermore, a spirometer may be used to estimate the state of pulmonary ventilation.

RESPIRATORY AIDS. When only a small loss of function of respiratory muscles is present, there is no need for mechanical aid to respiration. However, when respiratory muscles are so impaired that conscious effort is necessary to supplement their action and this compensation does not appear adequate, then mechanical therapy is necessary. One of the factors indicative of respiratory inadequacy is the inability of the patient to obtain sleep. It is a mistake to wait for signs of hypoxia or CO_2 accumulation before using mechanical therapy, for they represent signs of respiratory decompensation. In the use of mechanical aids to respiration the general principle is that the patient's possible needs must be anticipated and unexpected crises should be avoided. Every effort should be made to allay the patient's anxiety, and emphasis should be placed upon the usually successful outcome. The apparatus to be used should be at hand, and obviously members of the medical and nursing staff should be familiar with its operation.

For severe degrees of respiratory muscle weakness, the *tank respirator* is the apparatus of choice. When relatively minor degrees of respiratory muscle weakness exists, the cuirass respirator and the rocking bed may be employed to give rest and sleep. In general, however, both of these machines are of greatest use in the recovery period and in "weaning" patients from the tank respirator period.

In the United States "positive pressure" devices seem to have been less well suited for prolonged use and are probably most valuable as an adjuvant for the tank respirator period. The main use of the *electrophrenic respirator* is in the treatment of respiratory impairment due to injury to the respiratory center.

For initiating the use of the tank respirator, it should be appreciated that since respirator patients no longer control their respiratory rate they often attempt to breathe voluntarily and out of time with the bellows. By persistent instruction the patient is urged to relax and let the respirator "do the work." In general younger children are given a more rapid respiratory *rate* than older children or adults, but the rate should be determined by clinical observation in steering a course between underventilation as opposed to hyperventilation with excessive loss of CO_2 and alkalosis. Of the two, hyperventilation is by far the lesser danger. Rates range from 30 per minute in young children to 18 per minute in the adult. Younger children are subjected to smaller pressure ranges than adults, although some competent and experienced physicians do not follow this practice. For small children, an *intra-tank pressure* starting at 0 and reaching −12 cm. of water at its peak is suggested for the beginning; 0 to −15 for older children, and 0 to −18 for adults may be tried. Some workers employ pressures which range from a positive reading of +3 or +4 to −18. Signs of improvement which indicate successful action of a respirator include improvement or disappearance in the signs of anoxia, such as restlessness, pallor or cyanosis; acceptance of the rhythm of the respirator, and cessation of voluntary respiratory movements with relaxation, so that the patient may fall asleep.

It should be appreciated that when respiratory difficulty is due entirely to weakness of the respiratory muscles, the tank respirator is of great benefit. When improvement is not quickly obtained, complicating factors must be sought. These include: obstruction of the airway, pulmonary atelectasis, pneumonia or pulmonary edema.

Nursing care required by the patient in the tank respirator is of a special type. The patient's skin must be cared for; fluid, mineral and nutritional requirements must be met. Excessive handling of painful extremities should be avoided, although the patient's position should be changed, if possible, every two hours. Physical therapy should be postponed until the patient has become well adjusted to the respirator. Infections of the upper respiratory passages—bronchitis and pneumonia—are serious and must be treated promptly. When pneumonia is present, oxygen therapy is of value. Atelectasis is also a serious complication. Danger of its occurrence may be minimized by frequently changing the patient's position, by obtaining maximum safe pulmonary ventilation, by prevention of aspiration of secretions. When atelectasis of any considerable degree occurs, bronchoscopic drainage is usually necessary. In the event of pulmonary edema, oxygen therapy should be given. When cardiac insufficiency is present, digitalis and other measures to improve cardiac function are indicated. If the difficulty is caused by injury of the medullary respiratory centers, such patients nearly always require mechanical aids to respiration. If the bank respirator fails, here the electrophrenic respirator may be used but certain difficulties in its use limit its value.

Obstruction of the airway resulting from an inability to swallow may induce respiratory difficulties. Not only does it interpose a barrier to the air entering the larynx and trachea, but during inspiration the pooled secretions may be drawn into the trachea and bronchi. The general principle of treatment is to provide a free airway by postural drainage and mechanical aspiration of the secretions in the pharynx. This should be done if possible without trauma. If this fails, *tracheotomy* is performed, providing an airway which cannot be obstructed. A cooperative patient is less likely to require tracheotomy than a panic-striken one. Adults and older children are less likely to need it than very young children. Mechanical respiration is of no value in the treatment of respiratory tract obstruction.

Differing views exist as to the *indications for tracheotomy* and there are no dogmatic rules. It perhaps goes without saying that it should be performed, if possible, by one expert in the technique, and not as a hurried last resort type of procedure.

It is wiser to operate when there is doubt as to the advisability of further watchful waiting even though, occasionally, the subsequent course of the patient may prove that survival without tracheotomy would have followed. A careful, unhurried tracheotomy is neither mutilating nor dangerous.

The particular type of anesthesia selected

depends upon the emotional state of the patient. In exceedingly frightened, panicky adults and in children general anesthesia is desirable. An endotracheal tube is passed and cyclopropane in high oxygen concentration is introduced via the tube. Cyclopropane accords rapid induction and rapid release from anesthesia. Local anesthesia is adequate in the more controlled adult. During local anesthesia artificial respiration is maintained by the anesthesia machine through a pharyngeal airway using 100 per cent oxygen. In either case, artificial respiration with the anesthesia machine through the tracheotomy is continued as the patient is returned from the operating room.

The tracheotomy should be performed as high as possible, i.e., just below the first tracheal ring, so that the tube will be outside the respirator.

For the first 24 to 48 hours after operation the patient is given nothing by mouth. Fluid and electrolyte balance is maintained by intravenous administration. At the end of 48 hours, feedings of a soft diet are carefully given by an attendant, and over the next several days solid foods are slowly introduced.

MANAGEMENT IN RESPIRATOR. Once the tracheotomy is done, a free airway can be maintained by repeated suctioning. In general the patient is placed in the tank respirator postoperatively. If the patient is able to maintain adequate respiration unaided, he may be placed on the respirator bed with the respirator tank open and the bellows not operating. In this situation artificial respiration may be instituted at a moment's notice.

The respirator must be provided with an adjustable collar bar so that the tracheotomy is outside the respirator at all times.

The next most important task is to maintain a clear airway. First, the physician must consider the tube itself. The tracheotomy tube should be changed 48 hours after initial installation and weekly thereafter. Second, there should be ample opportunity for secretions to drain from both sides of the lungs. This is accomplished by placing the patient in the Trendelenburg position every one to two hours for about 20 minutes, and by turning him from side to side every two hours. Intermittently he should be given a period on his back. In the case of severe respiratory involvement the periods of Trendelenburg position may need to be lengthened. Suctioning should be at frequent intervals to keep the airways free from secretions at all times. The immediate postoperative period may require nearly constant suctioning.

"Weaning" from the tank respirator should be instituted as early as possible and started when the patient is afebrile and as soon as he is able to do without the respirator for 30 to 60 seconds. The tank respirator is gradually replaced by a simpler device, i.e., a cuirass respirator or a rocking bed.

Early Convalescent Care. The aim in convalescent care is to restore the maximal functional capacity which is possible within the limits imposed by the actual damage to the nervous system. It should be done with an awareness of the psychologic impact on the patient, which not only the illness but the therapy may have produced. During the period of after-care and rehabilitation, favorable conditions should be provided for the restoration of normal function and the preservation of the limbs in the best condition for late orthopedic operations, if such become necessary. Rehabilitation today calls for more than the care of limbs and should be directed from the start by physicians, orthopedists and technicians.

Prevention. In the early stages of an epidemic it is well to seek the counsel of the local health officer so that a uniform plan may be adopted in which local physicians may join. This includes the adoption of criteria of diagnosis.

Although the *isolation* of patients as usually practiced has not proven to be effective in controlling the spread of the disease, it is reasonable to regard acute poliomyelitis patients as infectious for a period of ten to twenty days following onset. Therefore early recognition, isolation and reporting of cases are all important. The period of isolation of a patient with poliomyelitis ranges from one to three weeks from onset, depending on local rulings. Mention has already been made of techniques to be followed in disposing of feces.

Quarantine of an exposed family or intimate group of contacts, although not of proved value, seems wise, particularly in the form of modified quarantine, which calls for the restriction of familial juvenile contacts for seven to fourteen days.

Vaccination. The large scale trials conducted during the spring of 1954 with the trivalent, formalinized vaccine developed by

Salk indicated that *active immunization* against poliomyelitis is now feasible. Salk recommends that two intramuscular inoculations of 1 cc. apiece be administered two to four weeks apart, and that a third "booster" injection be given no sooner than seven months thereafter.

It is Salk's belief that the first two inoculations accomplish primary vaccination. He feels that the third inoculation may effect full immunization, with a persistence of high antibody levels for years. Untoward reactions to the vaccine seem negligible and its effectiveness in preventing paralytic poliomyelitis in the 1954 trial was about 68% for Type I and in the range of 85–90% for Types II and III.

For *passive immunization* in unvaccinated individuals or in members of groups subjected to heavy exposure, concentrated immune globulin (gamma globulin) may be administered in a dosage of 0.1 cc. per pound of body weight.

Certain measures have been found useful *during epidemics.* These are: (1) the isolation in bed of all children with fever, pending diagnosis; (2) the education in such technique of bedside nursing as will prevent distribution of infectious discharges to others from patients isolated at home; (3) the protection of children as far as practicable against unnecessary contacts with other persons, and the avoidance of unnecessary travel and visiting, especially of children, during the high prevalence of the infection; (4) postponement of elective nose and throat operations, dental extractions or other types of induced trauma, including certain immunization procedures; (5) the avoidance of violent exercise and stress if the person has been intimately exposed to poliomyelitis or feels ill in the slightest degree; (6) finally, as a means of reducing the incidence or degree of paralysis in the mildly or severely ill case, one should avoid so-called *meddlesome* procedures. In this category are multiple physical examinations, exhausting muscle testing and inoculations which are not essential.

JOHN R. PAUL

References

A series of papers by various authors, including Green and Gucker, will be found in A Symposium on Poliomyelitis. Am. J. Med., 6:537–632, 1949. For general information reference is also made to: Poliomyelitis, Papers and Discussions, presented at the Second International Poliomyelitis Conference, Philadelphia, J. B. Lippincott Co., 1952. See also the Third International Poliomyelitis Conference, *Ibid.* (In press).

Enders, J. F., Weller, T. H., and Robbins, F. C.: Cultivation of the Lansing Strain of Poliomyelitis Virus in Cultures of Various Human Embryonic Tissues. Science, 109:85, 1949.

Hammon, W. McD., and others: Evaluation of Red Cross Gamma Globulin as a Prophylactic Agent for Poliomyelitis. J.A.M.A., 156:21, 1954.

Heine, J.: Beobachtungen über Lähmungszustände der unteren Extremitäten und deren Behandlung. Stuttgart, F. H. Köhler, 1840.

Horstmann, D. H., McCollum, R. W. and Mascola, A. D.: Viremia in Human Poliomyelitis. J. Exper. Med., 99:355, 1954.

Langmuir, A.: Evaluation of Gamma Globulin in Prophylaxis of Paralytic Poliomyelitis in 1953. Summary of the Report of the National Advisory Committee for Evaluation of Gamma Globulin. J.A.M.A., 154:1086, 1954.

Russell, W. R.: Poliomyelitis. London, Edward Arnold & Co., 1952.

Management of Poliomyelitis Patients with Respiratory Difficulty, Publication of the National Foundation for Infantile Paralysis (120 Broadway, New York 5, New York).

Salk, Jonas E.: Present Status of the Problem of Vaccination Against Poliomyelitis. Am. J. Pub. Health. 45:285 (Mar.) 1955.

COXSACKIE VIRAL INFECTIONS

(Herpangina and Epidemic Pleurodynia)

The first Coxsackie virus was reported in 1948 by Dalldorf and Sickles, having been obtained from poliomyelitis patients in Coxsackie, New York. By 1953, eighteen apparently similar but immunologically distinct new viruses of man had been described. They are grouped together because of similar physical and chemical properties, and because they produce paralysis and death in newborn mice and hamsters, but little or no overt illness in older mice or other laboratory animals.

Coxsackie viruses produce widespread infections in man, usually but not always during early childhood. Many, perhaps most, of these infections are clinically inapparent, but because the viruses occur abundantly in the oral secretions and stools of children during the summer months, persisting often for weeks in the stools, they have frequently been found in association with serious illnesses prevalent in similar age groups at the same time, particularly poliomyelitis. Most early studies suggested that some of the viruses may be important in the etiology of that disease. Despite many reports seemingly confirming this hypothesis, epidemiologic studies have failed to produce convincing evidence in support of it. Studies designed to test this hypothesis have revealed extremely high prevalence of these agents during the warm months in well children and in children ill with diseases other than poliomyelitis. Thus, the operation of chance and of other demonstrated factors such as rapid spread among exposed persons within household and community groups, and even among patients on hospital poliomyelitis wards, render their frequent occurrence in a series of poliomyelitis patients no more significant or unexpected than in a similar series of well persons or patients suffering from noninfectious diseases.

Evidence of high order suggests, however, that two different groups of Coxsackie viruses are indeed

in sewage and on flies. One strain has been found in mosquitoes.

HERPANGINA
(Vesicular Pharyngitis, Aphthous Pharyngitis)

Definition. Herpangina is a mild specific disease characterized by fever, lassitude, and

Classification of Coxsackie Viruses According to Disease and Some of Their Attributes

DALLDORF'S CLASSIFICATION

	Group A	Group B
Prevalence in man:	Many strains prevalent in children in summer. Endemic and epidemic. Nearly 100% of adults have antibodies to multiple types.	Less prevalent than A's. Prevalent during epidemics of pleurodynia. In certain areas most persons devoid of antibodies.
Mode of transmission:	Person to person most important.	Usually person to person.
Laboratory host range:	Suckling mice, suckling hamsters, chimpanzee, chick embryo (several types) *Tissue culture:* human and mouse tissue.	Same as A's including adult mice (subclinical illness).
Pathology in mice:	*Suckling mice:* generalized myositis only. *Adult mice:* — None.	*Suckling mice:* Pancreatitis, encephalitis, myositis, panniculitis, hepatitis, myocarditis. *Adult mice:* pancreatitis.
Size:*	25–37 mμ	Same.
Resistance to inactivation:	*Resistant to:* Lysol, phenol, ether, alcohol and dyes. *Susceptible to:* Heat, halogens and mercurial germicides.	Same.
Chief disease in man:	*Herpangina:* Types 2, 4, 5, 6, 8, 10 (probably 3 and possibly others).	*Epidemic Pleurodynia:* Types 1 and 3. (Possibly 2 and 4.)
Immunity in man:	Type-specific in neutralization. Group-specific in complement fixation.	Same as A's.
Strains for which specific disease is undetermined ("nonpurulent meningitis"?)	Types 1, 3, 7, 9, 11, 12, 13 and 14.	Types 2 and 4.

* Determined in ultracentrifuge and electron microscope. Ultrafiltration studies give lower figures (15–25 mμ).

responsible for two specific diseases: *herpangina* and *epidemic pleurodynia*. Evidence that certain Coxsackie viruses cause a nonspecific syndrome usually called "nonpurulent meningitis" or "nonparalytic poliomyelitis" is based on simple associations of Coxsackie virus infection with illness. Epidemiologic studies to evaluate the importance of these associations and an adequate definition of this clinical syndrome as a specific entity must still be achieved.

Dalldorf's classification of Coxsackie viruses into groups A and B is modified in the accompanying table in order to present current information about the diseases which they probably cause as well as some of their attributes. Besides their prevalence during the summer months, Coxsackie viruses resemble the poliomyelitis viruses in other respects. They are very small, occurring in comparatively large amounts in oral secretions and in stools; they are resistant to antimicrobial drugs, commonly used germicides and natural conditions unfavorable to the survival of most other viruses. Undoubtedly this accounts to some extent for their widespread occurrence in man and in his environment, particularly

small papular, vesicular and ulcerative lesions on the soft palate and the faucial areas. Although it is one of the most frequent summer illnesses of early childhood, the specific nature of the illness in individual cases is often missed by the clinician, somewhat more often recognized when it occurs in epidemic form in newly established residential areas or in summer camps for children.

History. The disease was first recognized as a specific entity by Zahorsky in 1920. He suggested the name *herpangina* in a report of 80 cases in 1924. Reports of outbreaks of a similar illness in a summer camp and nursery school appeared in 1939 and 1941. The illness was not reported again until 1950 when certain Group A Coxsackie viruses were suggested as etiologic agents. Since 1950, the disease has been recognized with increasing frequency and viral studies have repeatedly confirmed certain Group A viruses as etiologic agents. Reports of the same agents found in association with similar illnesses in other countries leaves little doubt that herpangina is a common occurrence in all parts of the world.

Etiology and Pathology. Six strains of Group A viruses have repeatedly been found causing herpangina (see table). During four years of study at the National Institutes of Health, they have been demonstrated in cases located in Washington, D. C., Southern Maryland, Camp LeJeune, North Carolina, Southern California and Texas. The same viruses have been reported from typical cases in Pennsylvania, New York, West Virginia, Canada, Cuba and Sweden.

All virus types found in herpangina, while immunologically distinct from each other, produce after brief incubation, identical generalized destruction of the skeletal muscles of suckling mice and hamsters—followed promptly by death. No other lesions are observed. Mice over two weeks of age are completely resistant.

The pathology of herpangina in man is obscure. The illness does not result in death; consequently, postmortem tissues are not available. Biopsies of muscle tissue from a typical case revealed neither pathologic changes nor the presence of virus.

Epidemiology. The disease has been found during the summer months in nearly every community in which an effort to find cases has been made. Most illnesses occur in early childhood, and large urban pediatric clinics such as exist in Washington, D. C., and Philadelphia are an abundant source of cases. As many as 10 per cent of children randomly selected from such clinics may be found harboring herpangina strains of virus during July, August and September.

When observed entering a household or a community, herpangina viruses rapidly infect nearly all intimate susceptible contacts including an occasional parent. However, even when under constant surveillance only about 30 per cent of those infected manifest typical faucial lesions. Nevertheless, a variable number of the infected family contacts will present a similar picture of mild febrile illness without the typical throat lesions. As in poliomyelitis and many other viral infections, a large proportion of the infections are not attended by any clinical manifestations.

Although immunity to the infecting strain appears permanent, the frequent presence of other strains in the community provides ample opportunity for a repetition of the typical illness within the same or a subsequent summer. Herpangina has been observed twice within one year in several children, each subsequent episode being caused by a strain different from that found during the initial illness. Most urban adults possess neutralizing antibodies against herpangina viruses, the number of types neutralized increasing with age. Unlike age, differences in sex and race have not been associated with observable differences in attack rates.

Clinical Manifestations. In a typical case the disease begins with a sharp elevation of temperature (102° to 105° F.). In the very young, vomiting may be common and convulsions may occur. The patient complains of headache and frequently of pain and tenderness in the neck, abdomen and extremities. Infants often salivate excessively and refuse food. Older children usually complain only mildly of a sore throat. During the first 24 to 48 hours, the fever reaches its peak and only minute petechiae or papules may be observed on the soft palate and tonsillar pillars, but 12 to 24 hours later, two to six superficial ulcers with grayish bases surrounded by red areolae are observed at these sites. The ulcerations heal within one to five day. Fever seldom lasts longer than three days and by the fourth day the patient is usually asymptomatic. There are no complications and a good immune response is produced. Hematologic and cerebrospinal fluid studies have revealed no characteristic abnormalities.

Diagnosis. In a typical case a clinical diagnosis of herpangina is not difficult if a careful inspection of the pharynx is made, particularly when, as frequently occurs, there are similar cases in the household or the immediate neighborhood. Herpetic stomatitis occurs at all seasons of the year and is characterized by larger, more persistent and more painful ulcers located in the anterior part of the mouth; lesions seldom occur exclusively in the pharynx. When laboratory facilities are available and suitable virus procedures can be carried out, differential diagnosis can be made by recovering either Coxsackie or herpes viruses from the lesions or by demonstrating a specific rise in antibody titer. Unfortunately, few laboratories are at present in a position to perform such studies. Recurrent aphthae and Bednar's aphthae seldom occur in the pharynx and are not usually associated with constitutional symptoms.

Relation to Poliomyelitis. The distribution and spread of herpangina parallels that of poliomyelitis, and simultaneous infection with agents of both diseases is common. In a mixed epidemic, a majority of persons infected with either or both of these agents can be expected not to show pathognomonic signs of specific illness, and when they do show signs of illness characteristic of one agent this fact does not exclude infection with the other; thus a clinical separation of herpangina from nonparalytic or "abortive" poliomyelitis without cerebrospinal fluid abnormalities may on many occasions be extremely difficult if not impossible. Even laboratory efforts to unscramble mixed outbreaks are liable to encounter insurmountable difficulties unless accompanied by exhaustive epidemiologic studies.

Prognosis. The disease tends to run a mild course; it may occasionally seem more severe in an adult. No complications or deaths have been reported. The ability of the physician to recognize this illness and give a hopeful prognosis is much appreciated by parents worried about poliomyelitis, often occurring at the same time in the community.

Treatment. None of the antimicrobial drugs appears to influence the severity or the duration of herpangina. Symptomatic treatment is often efficacious and should be used when indicated.

EPIDEMIC PLEURODYNIA

(*Bornholm Disease, Epidemic Myalgia, Devil's Grip*)

Definition. Epidemic pleurodynia is an acute specific viral disease, characterized by sudden onset of severe paroxysmal pain in the region of the attachment of the diaphragm which is aggravated by respiration and accompanied by intermittent fever, headache, anorexia and malaise. Uncommon, except during localized epidemics, the specific nature of such alarming symptoms occurring abruptly in previously healthy persons often is not recognized.

History. The disease was first described by Daae and Homann in Norway in 1872. Although Finsen observed the disease in Iceland as early as 1856, he did not publish these observations until 1874. In 1888, Dabney described the first outbreak in the United States. Following extensive observations of this disease on the Island of Bornholm, Sylvest in 1933 published a monograph reviewing all previous reports thus stimulating much interest in this disease. Numerous reports of outbreaks in England and the United States followed. Although viral etiology was postulated by many observers, all efforts to demonstrate such an agent failed until 1949, when Curnen, Shaw and Melnick reported a Coxsackie virus, type B-1 (Conn. 5 strain) in a single case. Subsequent reports have confirmed this agent as well as Coxsackie virus B-3 as etiologic agent in epidemic pleurodynia.

Etiology and Pathology. All four Group B Coxsackie viruses have been found in illnesses resembling epidemic pleurodynia. However, only B-1 and B-3 have been confirmed as etiologic agents. Several reports describe Group A viruses in sporadic cases. However, the much greater prevalence of these latter viruses renders the etiologic significance of these occasional isolations from pleurodynia illnesses extremely dubious. Furthermore, etiologic studies of outbreaks have uniformly incriminated Group B viruses as causative agents. The pathology of this disease in man is unknown since a postmortem examination has never been reported. The occurrence of high fever and the demonstration of Coxsackie B type viruses in throat secretions and stools suggest a generalized infection.

In suckling mice, B-1 and B-3 viruses produce lesions in the brain, pancreas, fat tissue and muscles. Following injection with these strains the adult mouse develops a clinically inapparent, immunity-producing infection and at necropsy presents lesions only in the pancreas; these, however, may be extensive often leading to loss of nearly all acinar tissue. There are no available data suggesting that similar lesions occur in man.

Epidemiology. Most reports of epidemic pleurodynia have come from Europe and the United States where outbreaks have been described over wide geographic areas. Strictly a summer and early autumn disease, the illness occurs in all age groups but is most common in children and young adults. Long-lasting immunity against the infecting strain of virus results. Although endemic areas have occasionally been described, pleurodynia is not generally prevalent each summer and most reports deal with sharp outbreaks confined to geographically limited areas. Similarly, Group B Coxsackie viruses are also not generally prevalent in most areas as are the Group A viruses. However, Group B viruses may be extremely prevalent during an epidemic of pleurodynia.

Most evidence suggests person-to-person spread and multiple cases frequently occur in a household. The incubation period appears to be three to five days. Many apparently susceptible household contacts may escape infection but when infection with a Group B virus is demonstrated, it is nearly always associated with a clinically apparent illness. Thus Group B and Group A Coxsackie viruses while similar in many respects differ not only with respect to the illnesses they cause in mice and in man, but also with respect to their basic epidemiologic patterns.

Clinical Manifestations. The disease begins with sudden onset of pain either in the abdomen or chest. Although fever invariably follows in all cases, it is pain in the epigastrium often shifting to the lower part of the anterior thorax on either side which is the most characteristic manifestation of epidemic pleurodynia. The pain is frequently so extreme that the patient seems on the verge of collapse. He is observed breathing rapidly and shallowly, leaning forward and to one side, splinting his chest by holding one arm tightly against it. It is obvious that both movement and respirations aggravate the pains. The physician faced with such a spectacle is moved to promptly administer analgesics or opiates unless a surgical emergency is suggested. In either case, arrangements for hospitalization may be made—then cancelled within the hour because the patient rather suddenly feels well—all negotiations to be reopened a short time later by a recurrence of severe pain. After several such attacks the patient becomes extremely apprehensive of future exacerbations and is usually content to remain in bed for several days. The patient often has difficulty describing his pain accurately, localizing it over the area of the epigastrium and in the region of the attachment of the diaphragm. Very often the patient expresses his difficulty by saying "I can't breathe" or "It hurts to breathe," indicating a feeling of constriction in the chest—a feeling which undoubtedly led to the early American designation, "Devil's grip," for this disease. The pain is described as a dull ache, "like a toothache," occasionally as a "stabbing pain." Children are usually restless, with knees drawn up, their sobbing or crying jerkily interrupted by painful stitches. Convulsions are common in infants during bouts of high fever. Moderate tenderness in the affected area is often accompanied by hyperesthesias, localized muscle swellings and al-

tered reflexes, the latter most often in the abdominal areas.

Fever, a constant finding during the initial attacks, may occasionally exceed 104° F., but usually will fluctuate from 101° to 103° F. The fever is intermittent, recurring usually during exacerbations of pain. Other prominent symptoms are headache, sore throat and malaise. Nausea and vomiting occur during the early stage of illness in young children; however, the severe pain tends to suppress excessive vomiting. Although pleural rubs are occasionally reported, there appears to be no evidence of lung involvement and coughing is conspicuously absent. Hematologic findings are usually within normal limits. *Relapses may occur a few days after apparent recovery* and continue to occur over a period as long as a month.

Complications. Orchitis lasting three to seven days would appear to be the complication most frequently reported, occurring in nearly all large outbreaks. Fibrinous pleuritis is irregularly reported but is not uncommon. Nonpurulent meningitis has been reported as an infrequent complication in some of the larger urban epidemics, particularly when large numbers of cases have been hospitalized and cerebrospinal fluid examinations performed. Since studies capable of excluding the presence of nonparalytic poliomyelitis and lymphocytic choriomeningitis infection are rarely done, the significance of such observations in many instances cannot be determined. However, laboratory infections of man with Group B viruses have resulted in meningitic involvement, thus supporting the hypothesis that pleurodynia viruses may produce similar effects in naturally occurring cases.

Diagnosis. A clinical diagnosis is seldom difficult once the existence of an epidemic is apparent. However, during the early stages of an epidemic or when only sporadic cases are encountered, the occurrence of severe pain in the chest or abdomen may suggest serious medical or surgical emergencies. This impression is often reinforced when the disease occurs in older persons perhaps with a previous history of cardiac disease, or in children when attended by fever, nausea and vomiting. Fortunately, in the former instance, the moderately elevated but otherwise normal pulse plus the shifting character of the pain will suggest the proper diagnosis. In the latter instance the absence of deep-seated tenderness, the presence of superficial hyperesthesias of the skin and the usually early remissions of pain are helpful in differentiating pleurodynia from acute appendicitis. Since herpangina may also be prevalent, and in children may be characterized occasionally by abdominal pain, careful inspection of the pharynx and faucial areas will be helpful in making a correct clinical diagnosis.

A tentative laboratory diagnosis can be made by demonstrating Coxsackie Group B viruses in the stool or throat washing taken during or shortly following the acute illness. A rise in specific neutralizing antibodies against one of the Group B viruses during the illness and convalescent periods provides good evidence for infection concomitantly with the illness. As with the Group A viruses the complement fixation test for antibodies, while apparently group-specific, gives non-specific reactions within the Coxsackie group and is of little use by itself in establishing the identity of the infecting virus. Unfortunately, all currently used tests for Coxsackie viruses are available only for research purposes. Even should they be available in diagnostic laboratories, a laboratory diagnosis cannot be made during the course of a specific illness. All of which means that for the present the physician must rely upon clinical signs and symptoms for the diagnosis of epidemic pleurodynia.

Prognosis and Treatment. Despite its sometimes stormy course, virtually no deaths have been attributed to this disease. There is no specific treatment for the disease or its complications. Modern antimicrobial drugs are ineffective against the Coxsackie viruses. Symptomatic relief from pain and high fever can be usually achieved by analgesics and antipyretics. Opiates are occasionally required to alleviate severe pain. Rest in bed is, of course, mandatory during the period of pain and fever. Too rapid return to normal activity seems associated with more frequent sequelae, particularly orchitis.

ROBERT J. HUEBNER

References

Curnen, E. C., Shaw, E. W., and Melnick, J. L.: Disease Resembling Nonparalytic Poliomyelitis Associated with Virus Pathogenic for Infant Mice. J.A.M.A., 141:894, 1949.
Dalldorf, G., and Sickles, G. M.: Unidentified, Filtrable Agent Isolated from Feces of Children with Paralysis. Science, 108:61, 1948.
Huebner, R. J., Cole, R. M., Beeman, E. A., Bell, J.

A., and Peers, J. H.: Herpangina: Etiological Studies of Specific Infectious Disease. J.A.M.A., 145:628, 1951.
———, Risser, J. A., Bell, J. A., Beeman, E. A., Beigelman, P. M., and Strong, J. C.: Epidemic Pleurodynia in Texas. A Study of 22 Cases. New England J. Med., 248:267, 1953.
Johnsson, T., and Lindahl, J.: Herpangina. A Clinical and Virological Study. Arch. ges. Virusforsch., 5:96, 1943.
Melnick, J. L., Walton, M., and Myers, I. L.: Isolation of a Coxsackie Virus during a Summer Outbreak of Acute Minor Illness. Pub. Health Rep., 68:1167, 1953.
———, and Curnen, E. C.: The Coxsackie Group. In Rivers, T. M. ed.: Viral and Rickettsial Infections of Man. 2nd ed. Philadelphia, J. B. Lippincott Co., 1952.
Sylvest, E.: Epidemic Myalgia: Bornholm Disease. Copenhagen and London, Oxford University Press, 1934.
Weller, T. H., Enders, J. F., Buckingham, M., and Finn, J. J., Jr.: Etiology of Epidemic Pleurodynia: Study of Two Viruses Isolated from Typical Outbreak. J. Immunol., 65:337, 1950.

ENCEPHALITIS LETHARGICA

(Von Economo's Disease, Epidemic Encephalitis, Type A Encephalitis [Japan])

Definition. Encephalitis lethargica is a malady which causes both degenerative and disseminated inflammatory changes in the central nervous system and is characterized by a marked diversity of symptoms in different cases and in successive stages of the same case. It is unfortunate that the name *epidemic encephalitis* has been used to designate this disease; other types of encephalitis occur in epidemic form, and encephalitis lethargica now occurs only sporadically.

History. The disease became known after a pandemic broke out in the winter of 1916–17. Von Economo carefully described the disease at that time and called it "lethargic encephalitis." The first cases were seen in Rumania in 1915. Thereafter epidemics of the illness occurred in many parts of the world. In 1918 it appeared in the United States. After 1926 no further epidemics developed. If the disease still occurs, it is represented only by occasional sporadic cases.

Etiology. The cause of encephalitis lethargica is not known, but there are reasons for thinking that the etiologic agent is a virus. The idea that a streptococcus or a neurotropic strain of herpes simplex virus is the causal agent is not substantiated by experimental facts.

Morbid Anatomy. There may be areas of hyperemia in the meninges. Hyperemia and minute hemorrhages may be present in the basal ganglia, midbrain and pons. Microscopically, the lesions are of two sorts: one degenerative, the other inflammatory and infiltrative. The degenerative process is characterized by destruction of nerve cells, the inflammatory process by perivascular cuffing, scattered patches of glial cell proliferation and lymphocytic infiltration, especially in the gray matter. The lesions are more chronic and productive than those seen in the established viral encephalitides. Demyelination is not a prominent feature. Lesions in the spinal cord are not marked.

Incubation. It is thought that the incubation period is four to fifteen days.

Symptoms. The onset may be sudden or gradual. Almost any type of neurologic syndrome may be simulated by the disease; there is a wide diversity of signs and symptoms. The symptom-complex may be divided into three stages.

In the first stage there are a large number and variety of symptoms in diverse combination and sequence. Most common are either a somnolent-ophthalmoplegic syndrome or an irritative hyperkinetic syndrome, which may be choreiform or myoclonic. Psychic disturbances may occur, with symptoms ranging from mental impairment to those of the major psychoses. Paralyses may develop and simulate poliomyelitis. There is a fulminating type in which the patient may succumb within a few hours. The fever may be slight or severe; many afebrile cases have been noted. Inapparent disease occurs and may lead to the appearance of parkinsonism.

In the second, or pseudopsychoneurotic, stage there are many subjective complaints, often without demonstrable objective findings of organic nervous disease. Headache, insomnia, dizziness, fatigability, irritability and restlessness are common. Such symptoms may persist for months or years, after which the symptoms of the third stage appear. Occasionally the third stage follows almost immediately upon the first.

In the third, or chronic, stage, peculiar motor, vegetative and psychic symptoms make their appearance. The disturbances of motility are like those of the Parkinson syndrome, with or without tremor. Among the more common vegetative disturbances are sialorrhea, dacryorrhea and seborrhea. There may be intellectual and emotional torpor with marked slowing of thought.

Diagnosis. In the absence of an epidemic the diagnosis is difficult and the disease must be differentiated from the numerous encephalitides of established cause. When the disease is epidemic and typical cases are occurring, encephalitis lethargica may be suspected in puzzling cases of fever, somnolence or delirium. There are no laboratory procedures available which are helpful in confirming the diagnosis.

Prognosis. The case mortality rate varied in past epidemics, but may have been as high as 20 to 30 per cent. Among patients who survive, a large number recover rapidly; others are partially disabled for six months to two years; still others are permanently disabled because of the severe symptoms of the third stage.

Treatment. Symptomatic and careful supportive treatment is all that is available. In spite of claims to the contrary, there is no evidence that any of the vaccines or serums used in the treatment of the disease are of value.

FRANK L. HORSFALL, JR.

References

Association for Research in Nervous and Mental Diseases: Acute Epidemic Encephalitis (Lethargic Encephalitis), an Investigation by the Association for Research in Nervous and Mental Diseases, etc. New York, Paul B. Hoeber, Inc., 1921.

von Economo, C.: Encephalitis Lethargica. Its Sequelae and Treatment. Translated and Adapted by K. O. Newman. New York, Oxford Press, 1931.

Jelliffe, S. E.: Psychopathology of Forced Movements and the Oculogyric Crises of Lethargic Encephalitis. New York, Nerv. and Ment. Dis. Pub. Co., 1932.

Matheson Commission, Epidemic Encephalitis: Etiology, Epidemiology, Treatment. Second Report, William Darrach, chairman. New York, Columbia University Press, 1932.

ST. LOUIS ENCEPHALITIS

Definition. St. Louis encephalitis is a viral disease characterized by signs and symptoms referable to the central nervous system and its meninges. It may occur either epidemically or sporadically.

History. In the summer of 1933, in and around St. Louis, more than 1000 cases of encephalitis occurred. Muckenfuss, Armstrong and McCordock, and Webster and Fite demonstrated that the epidemic was caused by a filterable virus previously un-recognized. The malady is now endemic in America, cases having been reported each year since 1933.

Epidemiology. The mode of spread is not definitely established, but certain species of mosquitoes have been shown capable of transmitting the infection. The malady occurs most frequently during the summer and fall months. No age is exempt, but the highest incidence is in persons from fifteen to fifty years of age.

Etiology. The disease is caused by a small virus with dimensions of 20 to 30 milli-microns. The agent has been propagated in media containing viable susceptible cells. Albino mice and rhesus monkeys are susceptible hosts; the former is the one of choice for the demonstration of virus in suspected material and for the performance of neutralization tests used in arriving at a diagnosis.

Incubation. It has been estimated that incubation periods range from four to twenty-one days.

Morbid Anatomy. Edema, vascular congestion and small hemorrhages are evident upon gross examination of the brain and cord. Microscopic examination reveals an infiltration of the meninges with lymphocytes, plasma cells, large mononuclear elements and an occasional polymorphonuclear cell. In the brain and cord are evidences of an acute inflammation, e.g., vascular congestion, small hemorrhages, cellular infiltration, perivascular cuffing, degeneration of nerve cells, neuronophagia and proliferation of glial elements. The focal accumulations of cells around the blood vessels are limited to the Virchow-Robin spaces and for the most part consist of lymphocytes. In many instances there are foci of mononuclear cells bearing no relation to blood vessels; these seem to consist of lymphocytes and glial elements.

Symptoms. The fact that the clinical picture varies tremendously can be explained upon the basis of differences in the severity of the infection and the localization of lesions in the brain and cord. According to Hempel-mann the cases may be placed in three large groups.

Group I. Patients exhibit an abrupt onset without prodromal symptoms. High fever, nausea, vomiting, headache, vertigo, nuchal rigidity, Kernig's sign, lethargy, difficulty with speech, ataxia, mental confusion and tremor of tongue, lips or hands are the most common signs and symptoms. Not all patients are lethargic; paralyses are not common, and when they do occur are usually of the spastic type; involvement of the eye muscles is extremely rare, a state of affairs very different from that met with in lethargic encephalitis. The abdominal reflexes are usually absent, while the deep reflexes tend to be exaggerated instead of diminished. Constipation is common. The pulse is usually proportional to the temperature, but a bradycardia may occur.

The cerebrospinal fluid may be under increased pressure, is free from ordinary bacteria, and contains a normal amount of sugar, an increased amount of globulin, and an increased number of cells consisting chiefly of lymphocytes and other mononuclear elements. The leukocyte count may be normal or show a moderate increase.

As the patient's condition improves, the temperature falls by lysis and in most instances reaches the normal level within seven to ten days; in a few cases, however, the fever persists for four to six weeks.

Group II. In this group a stage of invasion, lasting from one to four days and characterized by headache, general malaise, abdominal pains, chilly sensations, fever, generalized muscular pains, sore throat and a mild conjunctivitis, accompanied by photophobia, precedes the picture of encephalitis, which, after its development, is similar in all respects to that described for Group I.

Group III. The third group consists of mild or abortive cases, exhibiting only headache and fever of undetermined cause, which would be missed in the absence of an epidemic and incorrectly diagnosed without the aid of a lumbar puncture.

Diagnosis. Clinical or pathologic observations may lead to a diagnosis of encephalitis but usually do not serve to distinguish one type of viral encephalitis from another. A specific etiologic diagnosis may be made by laboratory procedures. With specimens of serum taken during the acute phase and during convalescence, neutralization and complement fixation tests may be of great aid in reaching a correct diagnosis.

Prognosis. From 5 to 30 per cent of patients die; the mortality rate is reported to increase directly with age. Those who recover do so quickly as a rule and are not usually bothered by troublesome or disastrous sequelae.

Treatment. Treatment is symptomatic. No antimicrobial drugs have been shown to be of any effectiveness.

FRANK L. HORSFALL, JR.

References

Casals, J., and Palacios, R.: The Complement Fixation Test in the Diagnosis of Virus Infections of the Central Nervous System. J. Exper. Med., 74: 409, 1941.

Hammon, W. McD., and Reeves, W. C.: Recent Advances in the Epidemiology of the Arthropod-Borne Virus Encephalitis. Am. J. Pub. Health, 35: 994, 1945.

Muckenfuss, R. S., Armstrong, C. A., and McCordock, H. A.: Encephalitis: Studies on Experimental Transmission. Pub. Health Rep., 48:1341, 1933.

Neal, J. B.: Encephalitis, a Clinical Study. New York, Grune and Stratton, 1942.

Report on the St. Louis Outbreak of Encephalitis. Pub. Health Bull., No. 214, 1935.

Webster, L. T., and Fite, G. L.: Experimental Studies on Encephalitis. I. Transmission of St. Louis and Kansas City Encephalitis to Mice. II. The Specific Virus Character of the Infectious Agent from Cases of St. Louis and Kansas City Encephalitis, 1933. J. Exper. Med., 61:103, 411, 1935.

POSTINFECTION ENCEPHALITIS

(Acute Demyelinating Encephalitis, Acute Disseminated Encephalitis, Postvaccinal Encephalitis, Postmeasles Encephalitis)

Definition. Postinfection encephalitis is an acute malady of the central nervous system characterized by perivascular demyelination, exhibiting itself as a rule in patients convalescing from infectious diseases, particularly those caused by viruses, or in those who are being vaccinated against virus maladies such as smallpox or rabies. In certain instances the disease manifests itself in the absence of a history of preceding infection.

History. An involvement of the central nervous system may complicate the picture of smallpox and measles. In 1874, Westphal recorded descriptions of pathologic changes observed in the cords of patients who had died with nervous manifestations developing during an attack of smallpox, and, in 1886, Barlow and Penrose gave an account of a similar case that arose during the course of measles. Soon after the initiation of vaccination against rabies it was realized that an occasional patient receiving the injections met with "paralytic accidents" which at times resulted in death. In 1907, Comby described a case with involvement of the central nervous system as a complication of jennerian prophylaxis; this observation was followed by a similar one made by Turnbull in 1912. Although isolated cases of the nature just mentioned had been described from time to time, it was not until the outbreak of postvaccinal encephalitis in England, Holland and other countries in 1922 that attention was focused on them. As the result of extended clinical, pathologic and experimental observations, the tendency at present is to consider this type of nervous accident following in the wake of acute infections as a clinical entity.

Epidemiology. The disease has been shown to occur during the course of and after vaccination against rabies and smallpox, and after measles, German measles, varicella, mumps or influenza; a few cases have been reported in which no history of a preceding infection was obtained. The incidence varies from year to year, being lower now after jennerian prophylaxis than it was in 1922–1925. It is not distributed uniformly throughout the population of a country, nor are the inhabitants of all countries equally affected. No age is exempt; the malady occurs, however, more frequently in children than in infants and adults. There is no evidence that the disease is contagious.

Etiology. The cause of postinfection encephalitis is not known, nor has the malady been transmitted from man to experimental animals. The three most prevalent ideas regarding the etiology are (a) the viruses that cause the primary disease, e.g., smallpox, measles, and so forth, also give rise to the complicating encephalitis; (b) a latent neurotropic virus is activated by the primary disease process; (c) inasmuch as the encephalitis occurs during convalescence from some infectious malady or after vaccination, certain workers have suggested that it is an expression of allergic phenomena. There is no convincing evidence that any of these ideas is correct. It seems unlikely, however, that the direct action of a virus is the cause of the disease, because no virus is known to produce a perivascular demyelination similar to that seen in this disease. Furthermore, Rivers and his co-workers, by means of repeated intramuscular injections of emulsions of fresh normal rabbit brain, have produced a perivascular demyelination in monkeys manifested clinically by ataxia and paralyses. This work has recently been confirmed and expanded.

Incubation. In view of the indecision regarding the etiology of the disease, it may seem inappropriate to speak of an incubation period. Regardless of the cause of the encephalitis, one cannot deny that there is a definite relation between it and the primary infections. In any event, there is a comparative constancy of incubation—that is, of the period which elapses between the onset of the primary disease and the occurrence of the complicating encephalitis. In postvaccinal encephalitis the "incubation" period in most instances lies between the ninth and thirteenth days, the most favored day being the eleventh. In antirabic vaccination the encephalitis, or myelitis, usually comes during the second half of the Pasteur treatment or after it has been completed. In measles the "incubation" period is not constant, but as a general rule the encephalitis follows the appearance of the rash at variable intervals—usually it comes after the defervescence, and at times the patient may have fully recovered from measles.

Morbid Anatomy. Pathologic changes are found in both the white and gray matter of the brain and cord and are characterized by a minimal involvement of nerve cells, and a perivascular infiltration or accumulation of cells accompanied by a destruction of myelin. The perivascular collections of cells are not limited to the Virchow-Robin spaces, and consist largely of altered glial elements undergoing proliferation, many of which become phagocytic and take up large amounts of fat and degenerated myelin. This pathologic picture is decidedly unlike that seen in the encephalitides caused by viruses; on the other hand, in many respects, it is similar to that seen in acute multiple sclerosis and allied conditions.

Symptoms. There are two main types of the disease, the encephalitic and the myelitic; the former is more common in postvaccinal encephalitis, the latter during antirabic vaccination, while both types occur with almost equal frequency after smallpox. Under such conditions it is to be expected that the clinical picture will vary and that the form it takes will depend on whether the brain or cord is predominantly involved.

The onset of the disease, if not abrupt, is rarely insidious and is manifested in the encephalitic cases by pyrexia, headache, vomiting and drowsiness—cardinal symptoms "constantly present in severe, and rarely absent in mild, cases; they may be the only symptoms present even in fatal cases." Photophobia, irritability, delirium, general or local convulsions, trismus, strabismus, incontinence of urine, extensive paralyses (spastic at first and then flaccid) or transient weakness of muscles, incoordination and ataxia are symptoms that may occur. Kernig's sign may be present; the deep and superficial reflexes are variable. In the myelitic cases, symptoms caused by mild or severe involvement of the cord, such as paralyses, anesthesias, paresthesias and disturbances of sphincter control, are observed.

The cerebrospinal fluid may be under increased pressure, is sterile, and may contain an increased number of cells which are usually mononuclear elements; the amount of sugar is within normal limits.

Diagnosis. The clinical picture of postinfection encephalitis is at times not unlike that caused by certain known viruses, for example, St. Louis encephalitis virus. Consequently, it is important to remember that not all cases of encephalitis occurring in the wake of infectious diseases are necessarily postinfection encephalitis. In certain instances they undoubtedly represent other types; for example, some cases of encephalitis following antirabic vaccination are in reality rabies, and some that occur after measles are of the hemorrhagic rather than the demyelinating type. Often it is difficult, and at times impossible, by means of clinical observations alone to differentiate postinfection encephalitis from the other types. In view of this fact, a history of an encephalitis during convalescence from a virus malady usually results in a diagnosis of postinfection encephalitis. As a rule such a diagnosis is correct, but not always. At present a definite diagnosis of postinfection encephalitis can be arrived at only by a careful examination of the brain and cord which should show a characteristic perivascular demyelination.

Prognosis. Ten to 50 per cent of the patients die; the mortality rate is much higher in postvaccinal encephalitis (50 per cent) than it is in postmeasles encephalitis (10 per cent); the rate also varies from years to year in the same type, being considerably lower now in postvaccinal encephalitis than it was in 1922–1925. The patients who recover usually do so completely; sequelae occasionally occur, and seem to be more frequent in cases developing after measles than in those following jennerian prophylaxis.

Treatment. The treatment is symptomatic. Headache may be relieved by repeated lumbar punctures and the intravenous administration of hypertonic glucose solution. Definite evidence is lacking, in spite of claims to the contrary, that convalescent measles serum and the like are of therapeutic value.

FRANK L. HORSFALL, JR.

References

Ferraro, A.: Pathology of Demyelinating Diseases as an Allergic Reaction of the Brain. Arch. Neurol. & Psychiat., 52:443, 1944.

Hurst, E. W.: A Review of Some Recent Observations of Demyelination. Brain, 67:103, 1944.

Jorge, R.: Postvaccinal Encephalitis: Its Association with Vaccination and with Post-Infectious and Acute Disseminated Encephalitis. Lancet, 1:215, 267, 1932.

Mackie, T. T., Hunter, G. W., III, and Worth, C. B.: Manual of Tropical Medicine. 2nd ed. Philadelphia, W. B. Saunders Company, 1954.

Marsden, J. P., and Hurst, E. W.: Acute Perivascular Myelinoclasis ("Acute Disseminated Encephalomyelitis") in Smallpox. Brain, 55: Part 2, 181, 1932.

Perdrau, J. R.: The Histology of Post-Vaccinal Encephalitis. J. Path. & Bact., 31:17, 1928.

Rivers, T. M., and Schwentker, F. F.: Encephalomyelitis Accompanied by Myelin Destruction Experimentally Produced in Monkeys. J. Exper. Med., 61:689, 1935.

Report of the Committee on Vaccination, Ministry of Health, London, 1928.

EQUINE ENCEPHALOMYELITIS

THE DISEASE IN HORSES

Equine encephalomyelitis has undoubtedly been present among horses and mules in this country for many years, but was diagnosed as botulism, forage poisoning and similar illnesses. In 1931 it was proved to be caused by a filterable virus by Meyer, Haring and Howitt during the course of their studies of an epidemic in the San Joaquin Valley in California. Since then our knowledge of its extent, epidemiology, transmission, prevention and so on has accumulated rapidly.

In 1933 an epidemic occurred along the seacoast of Virginia and New Jersey and was shown by Ten Broeck and Merrill to be due to a virus immunologically distinct from that causing the disease in the West. The eastern disease, moreover, is more severe than the western, with a considerably higher mortality rate (about 90 per cent as compared to 25 to 30 per cent). The two diseases are referred to as the eastern and western types of equine encephalomyelitis.

Epidemiology. The first important clue to the mechanism of spread of epidemics was provided by Kelser's experiments, in which he demonstrated that the virus could be transmitted by the mosquito, *Aedes aegypti.* Subsequently, Kelser, as well as other investiga-

tors, showed that other mosquitoes, including *A. sollicitans, A. cantator, A. vexans, A. taeniorhynchus, A. dorsalis, A. nigromaculis* and *A. albopictus,* may transmit the virus. It is of interest that the *Anopheles* mosquitoes fail to transmit the virus. Recent experiments have demonstrated transmission of the virus by *Culex tarsalis.* The mosquito transmission of the virus accounts for the spread of the disease in a particular area; however, it does not explain the sudden appearance of the malady in widely separated areas.

Giltner and Shahan showed that pigeons were susceptible to infection after intracerebral inoculation of the virus and suggested that birds may play a role in the epizootiology of the disease. Other investigators demonstrated that other species of birds were also susceptible. During the course of the 1938 epidemic in Massachusetts, Tyzzer, Sellards and Bennett isolated the virus from pheasants dying in their natural state, and Fothergill and Dingle isolated the virus from a pigeon in similar circumstances. These findings clearly implicate birds in the epidemiology of the disease and explain its spread to widely separated areas. Indeed, it appears likely that the malady is primarily a disease of birds and that man and horses are accidental secondary hosts.

The final link in the chain of epidemiologic circumstances to be accounted for is the mechanism whereby the virus survives from one season to the next. Syverton and Berry showed that the tick, *Dermacentor andersoni,* could be infected by feeding on an infected animal. This insect harbored the virus throughout its life and could pass it on to a succeeding generation through the ova.

Prevention. Shahan and Giltner showed that a vaccine could be prepared by treating an emulsion of infective horse brain with formalin. Although some evidence of protection was obtained with this preparation, the results were not entirely satisfactory. In 1935, Higbie and Howitt showed that the developing chick embryo could be infected with this virus. In 1938, Beard, Finkelstein, Sealy and Wyckoff prepared a vaccine by formalinizing a suspension of infected chick embryo tissue. Such tissues were found to contain a much higher content of virus than infective horse brain. This material has been widely used. Vaccination of horses and mules is achieved by subcutaneous injection, at weekly intervals, of two doses of 10 cc. each of the vaccine of triturated chick embryo tissue treated with 0.4 per cent formalin. Experimental and field studies have shown that this method is very effective. Practical sanitary measures should, of course, be used, such as screening stables and removing horses and mules from pastures after dark.

THE DISEASE IN MAN

Meyer, in 1932, described three cases of encephalitis in persons having contact with sick horses which he suspected might be due to the virus of the equine disease. No proof for this suspicion was obtained, however, by biologic test.

During the summer of 1938 an epidemic of the eastern variety of the disease occurred among horses in southeastern Massachusetts. During this time and in the same area an unexpected number of human cases of encephalitis occurred. These were proved by Fothergill, Dingle, Farber and Connerley and by Webster and Wright to be caused by the equine virus, by isolating the infectious agent from the brain tissue of fatal cases.

There were about 40 human cases in this outbreak with a mortality of 65 per cent. The majority of cases occurred in young children, 70 per cent of them less than ten years of age. During the summer of 1941 more than 3000 cases occurred in the north central states.

Clinical Picture. The onset of the disease was usually sudden, particularly in young children. The temperature rose rapidly to 103° to 105° F. and generally remained at a high level during the course of the disease. In some cases the disease was ushered in by a convulsion. Repeated convulsions occurred during the course of the illness in many patients. Deep coma occurred rapidly and persisted throughout the acute stage. Nuchal rigidity, stiffness of the back and positive Kernig's sign were usually present. Many of the younger patients exhibited a peculiar edema about the face and upper extremities. In some of the older patients the onset was more gradual.

Laboratory Findings. Certain laboratory findings were of importance, particularly during the first few days of illness. A leukocytosis was always present. The cerebrospinal fluid was under increased pressure and contained an increased amount of protein and a normal content of sugar. The cell count varied from 200 to 2000 per cubic millimeter. Of considerable importance was the fact that from 60 to 90 per cent of the cells were polymorphonuclear leukocytes.

In fatal cases death occurred at variable times during the course of the disease, most commonly during the first few days. In the few patients who recovered, the acute phase of the illness terminated by lysis six to ten days after the onset. The majority of the patients who survived were left with severe mental and physical damage.

Diagnosis. It must be emphasized that a diagnosis of encephalitis in man due to the virus of equine encephalomyelitis cannot be made on the basis of the clinical findings. It may be confused with other types of acute infectious encephalitis, such as polioencephalitis and St. Louis encephalitis. An increase in the incidence of encephalitis in man in an area where an epidemic of the disease in horses and mules is in progress should lead one strongly to suspect the equine type of the disease. Virus was not isolated from any of the Massachusetts cases by inoculation of animals with blood or cerebrospinal fluid.

A diagnosis can eventually be established in the majority of cases by certain biologic tests. The most important of these is the isolation of the virus from the brain tissue of acute fatal cases obtained at necropsy. It is advisable to take small portions of brain tissue from various regions in the brain and brain stem. The tissue is emulsified in physiologic salt solution and inoculated intracerebrally into white Swiss mice or guinea pigs. If virus is recovered it can be identified by immunologic tests (protective tests in actively immunized animals or by serum neutralization tests). If it is impossible to inoculate animals immediately, brain tissues can be preserved in the ice box in a mixture of 50 per cent neutral glycerin in buffered Tyrode solution. It is important to preserve such material in a buffered mixture, since the virus is inactivated rapidly by the developing cadaveric acidity. Histologic examination is, of course, of great value in diagnosis.

In cases with a prolonged illness and in convalescent patients a diagnosis may be made by neutralization tests with patients' serum. Neutralizing antibodies appear seven to ten days after the onset of the illness.

Treatment. There is no specific therapy for this disease. Treatment is entirely symptomatic, consisting in the administration of sedatives for the control of convulsions, administration of fluids parenterally and food by gavage during the period of coma.

Prevention of the disease in man, if an epidemic occurs, should consist largely in sanitary measures. Houses and particularly sleeping quarters should be screened against mosquitoes, and children should not be allowed outside after sundown. A vaccine, similar to that for horses, could be developed for use in man. However, the infrequency of the disease in the latter does not justify large-scale vaccination. The vaccination of laboratory personnel is indicated.

LeRoy D. Fothergill

References

Beard, J. W., Finkelstein, H., Sealy, W. C., and Wyckoff, R. W. G.: Immunization against Equine Encephalomyelitis with Chick Embryo Vaccines. Science, 87:490, 1938.

Fothergill, L. D., and Dingle, J. H.: A Fatal Disease of Pigeons Caused by the Virus of the Eastern Variety of Equine Encephalomyelitis. Science, 88: 549, 1938.

———, Dingle, J. H., Farber, S., and Connerley, M. L.: Human Encephalitis Caused by the Virus of the Eastern Variety of Equine Encephalomyelitis. New England J. Med., 219:411, 1928.

Higbie, E., and Howitt, B.: The Behavior of the Virus of Equine Encephalomyelitis on the Chorioallantoic Membrane of the Developing Chick. J. Bact., 29:399, 1935.

Meyer, K. F.: A Summary of Recent Studies on Equine Encephalomyelitis. Ann. Int. Med., 6: 645, 1932–1933.

Shahan, M. S., and Giltner, L. T.: Some Aspects of Infection and Immunity in Equine Encephalomyelitis. J. Am. Vet. M. A., 84:928, 1934.

Syverton, J. T., and Berry, G. P.: An Arthropod Vector for Equine Encephalomyelitis, Western Strain. Science, 84:186, 1936.

Tyzzer, E. E., Sellards, A. W., and Bennett, B. L.: The Occurrence in Nature of "Equine Encephalomyelitis" in the Ring-Necked Pheasant. Science, 88:505, 1938.

Webster, L. T., and Wright, F. H.: Recovery of Eastern Equine Encephalomyelitis Virus from the Brain Tissue of Human Cases in Massachusetts. Science, 88:305, 1938.

INFECTIOUS AND SERUM HEPATITIS

See under Diseases of the Liver.

EPIDEMIC HEMORRHAGIC FEVER

(Manchurian Fever)

Definition. Epidemic hemorrhagic fever is an acute disease of unknown etiology which occurs during the spring and fall in Northeast Asia. It is characterized by fever, prostration, vomiting, proteinuria, hemorrhagic manifestations, shock and renal failure.

History. Beginning in 1951 seasonal outbreaks of a disease previously unknown to Western medicine occurred among the UN troops in Korea. It was soon learned that the Japanese had encountered an identical clinical entity in eastern Manchuria which they named epidemic hemorrhagic fever. This disease was apparently first described in Far Eastern Siberia under the name hemorrhagic nephroso-nephritis by the Russians in the mid-1930's.

Etiology. Russian investigators reproduced the disease in human volunteers by the parenteral injection of serum or urine obtained prior to the fifth day of illness from patients with the naturally occurring disease. They further found that the disease agent was filterable through a Berkefeld filter (grade N), that the incubation period was usually twelve to sixteen days, and that a single attack conferred immunity. Extensive efforts to grow the causative agent on media and tissue cultures were failures, as were efforts to establish the disease in a variety of lower animal hosts.

Epidemiology and Mode of Transmission. Hemorrhagic fever has been limited to Far Eastern Siberia, Northern Manchuria and Korea north of Seoul. Sporadic cases occur throughout the year, but large outbreaks in the late spring and fall account for the majority of attacks. All ages, sexes and races are susceptible. The disease occurs only in rural areas and the majority of cases occur as isolated events, widely separated in time and place, even during large epidemics. Person-to-person transmission does not occur. Inability to isolate the causative agent has precluded definitive demonstration of the mode of transmission of epidemic hemorrhagic fever. However, its epidemiology is reminiscent of that of scrub typhus, and careful studies strongly incriminate one or more species of trombiculid mites which infest certain field rodents.

Morbid Anatomy. A profound, protein-rich retroperitoneal edema is characteristic of early deaths due to shock, but not of deaths in the later stages. Certain viscera are also edematous, although dehydration of most regions is the rule. In practically all autopsies, the kidneys are swollen and exhibit extreme congestion sharply localized to the medulla, while the right atrium appears hemorrhagic and the anterior pituitary exhibits marked congestion or hemorrhagic necrosis. Less often, similar congestion or hemorrhage is noted in the stomach, adrenals, lungs and central nervous system. Histologic preparations reveal that most of the congested or hemorrhagic areas derive their appearance from extremely dilated and con-

Clinical Course and Pathologic Physiology. The clinical and laboratory manifestations of hemorrhagic fever make up a confusing array of problems that occur in rapid sequence with considerable overlapping and variation in severity. However, most patients

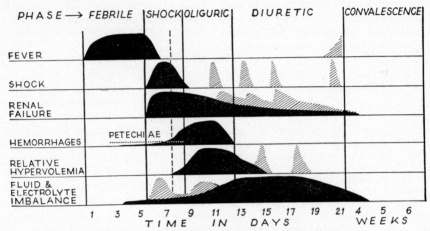

Fig. 14. Hemorrhagic fever; abnormal physiology.

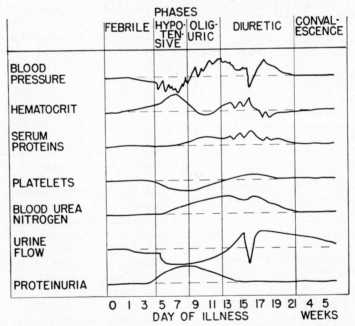

Fig. 15. Severe hemorrhagic fever; course of certain laboratory findings.

gested small blood vessels, especially in the renal medulla. Glomeruli and convoluted tubules are usually normal except for proteinaceous deposits. In addition, petechial hemorrhages may occur in the skin, heart, adrenals and brain. In certain areas there may be mononuclear cell infiltrations and, at times, bland, localized necrosis.

follow a fairly typical course which is conveniently considered in relation to several phases. The course of important clinical and laboratory features of a moderately severe case is shown in Figures 14 and 15. Although all patients exhibit proteinuria and many have petechiae and some degree of hemoconcentration, hypotension and renal failure, consequences such as shock, serious hemorrhages and fluid and electrolyte imbalances occur in no more than 20 per cent.

The febrile phase lasts three to eight days and is characterized by fever, malaise, a flush of the face and neck, injection of the eyes and palate and other nonspecific features. Physiologic evidence suggests widespread arteriolar dysfunction at this time. Towards the end of the febrile phase, petechiae occur, blood platelets decrease, the hematocrit begins to increase and faint traces of protein appear in the urine.

The hypotensive phase develops suddenly during defervescence and generally lasts one to three days. Despite shock, which accounts for a third of all deaths, the extremities may remain warm, and evidence suggests that persistence of arteriolar dysfunction contributes to the hypotension. The dominant feature, however, is a reduction in blood volume due to loss of plasma from the vascular system, as evidenced by a rapid increase in hematocrit to as high as 70 per cent, and to trapping of erythrocytes in dilated capillaries. Heavy proteinuria, oliguria, acute renal failure and hemorrhages of capillary origin associated with thrombocytopenia are prominent clinical features, whether or not hypotension develops. Nausea and vomiting are common while backache and abdominal discomfort result from localized edemas. The leukocytes, which earlier were normal or reduced, now show a leukemoid reaction.

The oliguric phase begins as the hematocrit decreases and the sequestered plasma returns to the vascular system. It usually lasts for three to five days. Deaths in this phase are due to pulmonary edema; electrolyte abnormalities and shock secondary to dehydration or pulmonary complications. This phase is one of increasing renal failure and nitrogen retention, continued vomiting and dehydration. Hyperkalemia is common, but curiously, acidosis is rare. Despite improvement in many of the earlier symptoms, increasing confusion and extreme restlessness are common, as is hypertension. Some patients exhibit a *hypervolemic syndrome* which may respond to phlebotomy. Hemorrhages into the skin, sclerae, gastrointestinal tract, lungs and renal pelvis continue but rarely are large in amount and generally decrease toward the end of the oliguric phase.

The diuretic phase, which may last for days or weeks, usually initiates clinical recovery and rapid improvement in renal function. However, a diuresis of 3 to 8 liters daily represents a real hazard to patients who are already extremely dehydrated and who have had limited caloric intake for seven to ten days. These patients exhibit a brittle fluid volume homeostasis and may fluctuate rapidly between shock on one hand and hypertension and pulmonary edema on the other, depending on the state of the fluid balance. Serious potassium deficiency is not uncommon, while hypernatremia can be troublesome. Deaths in this phase account for a third of the total and are usually due to shock secondary to dehydration and to pulmonary complications. The diuresis characteristic of this phase does not represent mobilization of edema fluid but is the result of residual renal tubular damage.

Convalescence requires three to twelve weeks and is characterized by gradual return of appetite, strength and urinary concentrating ability to normal.

Diagnosis. In the absence of any specific test, the diagnosis must be made on clinical evidence and should be suspected when an acute febrile illness associated with the characteristic flush and petechiae occurs in a subject who has been in an endemic area. The subsequent developments such as hypotension or shock, increased hematocrit, thrombocytopenia, oliguria and renal failure assist in establishing the diagnosis, but 3 to 4 plus proteinuria developing near the time of defervescence is the single most useful diagnostic sign.

Prognosis. The case fatality rate among U.S. Armed Forces, once techniques for prompt diagnosis and early, adequate treatment were developed, has been 5 per cent. No single finding is of great prognostic value in individual patients. However, prolonged high fever, protracted or recurrent shock and persistent hemoconcentration are all ominous features. With rare exceptions, survivors who have not had central nervous system hemorrhages make apparently complete recoveries.

Prevention. Preventive measures are based on the assumption that the disease is transmitted by an arthropod parasite of a rodent. Control of the rodent population and individual measures such as dipping all clothing in miticide solution and use of insect repellents have been used by the Armed Forces in Korea. The effectiveness of such measures has not yet been established, although each outbreak of hemorrhagic fever in Korea has been smaller than the preceding epidemic.

Treatment. Since antimicrobial drugs, convalescent serum, hormones and other agents are entirely ineffective, the management of hemorrhagic fever must be supportive and based on an understanding of its physiologic and biochemical characteristics, and on frequent clinical observations. Adequate sedation with barbiturates or opiates is frequently required for restlessness. Contrary to the practice in other febrile diseases, fluid intake must be limited since any excess will simply leak out of damaged capillaries and increase edema and symptoms. When intravenous fluid is required, it usually should be 5 per cent dextrose in water and must be given very slowly. If shock fails to respond to simple measures such as shock blocks, then concentrated (salt-poor) human serum albumin to restore plasma volume and continuous intravenous infusion of pressor drugs (preferably Arterenol) may be required. Doses of the latter must be based on the response of the shock, blood pressure and hematocrit. Occasionally, large doses of both albumin and pressor drugs are required. Treatment in the olguric phase is that of acute renal failure, with careful control of electrolytes and particular attention paid to hyperkalemia. Phlebotomy may be required for the fully developed hypervolemic syndrome. The chief problem of the diuretic phase is one of careful matching of fluid intake against the brisk urinary output, so as to avoid excessive dehydration and shock on one hand and hypervolemia and pulmonary edema on the other. Electrolyte abnormalities are still a problem, especially potassium deficiency.

DAVID P. EARLE

References

Katz, S., Leedham, C. L., and Kessler, W. H.: Medical Management of Hemorrhagic Fever. J.A.M.A., 150:1363, 1952.

McNinch, J. H., and others: Far East Command Conference on Epidemic Hemorrhagic Fever. Ann. Int. Med., 38:53, 1953.

Steer, A., and Hullinghorst, R. L.: Epidemic Hemorrhagic Fever. 1951 Yearbook of Pathology and Clinical Pathology. Chicago, The Yearbook Publishers, 1952, p. 7.

Symposium on Epidemic Hemorrhagic Fever. Am. J. Med., 16:617, 1954.

INFECTIOUS MONONUCLEOSIS

Definition. Infectious mononucleosis is a disease of unknown etiology and of protean symptomatology occurring principally in the first three decades of life, and characterized typically by lymphadenopathy, lymphocytosis (largely due to abnormal lymphocytes) and an elevated titer of sheep cell agglutinins in the serum.

History. Emil Pfeiffer in 1889 is generally credited with having first called attention to the disease, which he termed "glandular fever." West was the first to report the disease in the United States. The increase in the small mononuclear elements in the blood was reported by Burns in 1909. Between 1909 and 1920 various reports were made of what appear to have been sporadic forms of the disease. In 1920 the term "infectious mononucleosis" was proposed by Sprunt and Evans, who also called attention to the presence of abnormal cells in the blood. Downey and McKinlay made a detailed report of the hematologic findings in 1923. Paul and Bunnell in 1932 were the first to call attention to the presence of sheep cell agglutinins in the serum in this disorder.

Incidence. Infectious mononucleosis is not limited to any one geographic location. It has been reported in America, Europe, Egypt, Australia, China, Japan and elsewhere. It may occur in either the epidemic or the sporadic form, although most reports have dealt with the latter type. The disease may occur at any age, cases having been reported at 7 months and 70 years, but the great preponderance of patients with the disease is found between the ages of 10 and 35. Until recently it has been thought that the incidence in Negroes was low. However, a number of cases of the disease in the Negro have been reported in the past few years. Wechsler and his co-workers found that 49 Negroes, or 8.7 per cent of the total number of patients in a large epidemic, were affected.

Etiology. Infectious mononucleosis presumably represents either a single infection or a common host reaction pattern to several infections, for it may occur as a localized epidemic as well as in the form of sporadic cases. It is generally considered that a virus or filterable agent is responsible for the condition, but as yet no definitive proof of this has been offered. Transfer of the disease to monkeys by means of a filtrate of nasal washings has been reported, but there has been failure to confirm this work. During recent years a wide variety of inoculums have been used in sixty-one individual attempts to transfer the disease to human volunteers. Successful results have been claimed in only two instances. Evans, who is responsible for twenty-one of the experiments in human beings, had negative results as regards transmission of the disease in every instance. He suggested that failure to transmit the disease might be due to extreme lability of the causative organism and/or to low individual susceptibility. Whatever the answer may be, the evidence at the present time does not justify any designation of the causative factor.

Morbid Anatomy. The morbid anatomy of infectious mononucleosis is much more clearly understood than previously as a result of postmortem studies on several patients who succumbed to the disease. Gross changes are limited almost entirely to enlargement of the lymphoid tissue, including the spleen. Other gross features include frequent enlargement of the liver, rare icterus and occasional skin lesions. The histologic lesions tend to be generalized, and closely resemble those of some of the viral diseases. They consist mainly of perivascular aggregates of normal and abnormal lymphocytes. Most of the tissues, with the exception of the bone marrow, have been shown to have these lesions. The lymphocytes are absent in the bone marrow sections, whereas aspirated marrow specimens do contain them as a consequence of admixture with peripheral blood. Recently granulomatous lesions have been demonstrated in the bone marrow. The lymph nodes, which contain large numbers of the abnormal lymphocytes, show varying pictures from follicular hyperplasia to changes simulating those of a malignant lymphoma. Lymphocytic infiltration of the capsule and trabeculae of the spleen occurs regularly. The trabeculae are often dissolved by these infiltrations, resulting in rupture of the spleen in rare instances. Perivascular accumulation of the lymphocytes about the arteries of the trabeculae is to be expected. Moreover, subintimal accumulation of these cells in the veins of the spleen is constantly found. Pneumonic exudate of either the round cell or neutrophilic types may occur. Small myocardial infiltrates are found frequently. In addition, periportal round cell accumulation in the liver and various lesions of the nervous system, in particular meningo-encephalitis, are often encountered.

Symptoms. Infectious mononucleosis is protein in its manifestations; the classic or so-called "typical" case may be described as follows:

A young adult is typically affected, probably five to fifteen days after exposure to the causative organism. Malaise, with or without sore throat, but with fever and lymphatic enlargement—more typically of the posterior cervical nodes, but frequently of all the nodes—characterizes the onset. The fever is of no definite type, but usually is not pronounced. It lasts ordinarily for five to ten days, but variations from absence to persistence for several weeks may occur. The nodes, which are moderate in size (usually not over 3 cm. in diameter), discrete, slightly indurated, nonsuppurative and sometimes slightly tender, generally return to normal size in three to four weeks. Slight splenomegaly occurs in approximately one third of the cases and, ordinarily, recedes at the same time as the lymphadenopathy. The duration of active clinical signs and/or symptoms varies from a few days to a few weeks or more. Leukopenia is common in the first week of the disease, followed by moderate leukocytosis in the second and third weeks. This leukocytosis is due to an increase in the number of lymphocytes, many of which are abnormal. In general, the white blood cell picture returns to normal gradually within three to four weeks. The sheep cell or heterophile agglutination test becomes positive usually within the first two weeks of the illness. The thymol turbidity test is said to be positive in as high a percentage of cases as the sheep cell agglutination test. Some of the other liver function tests have also shown abnormal findings. Serologic tests for syphilis may be positive in 3 to 10 per cent of the cases. No other significant abnormal laboratory findings occur in the usual patient with this disease.

Toxic symptoms, such as headache, malaise, generalized aching, anorexia and so forth, are present in the acute phase in many instances. Also gingivitis and tonsillitis with or without Vincent's organism and/or streptococci occur in an appreciable percentage of the cases.

Some of the many variations which may be found in this disease are worthy of special comment.

Latent Forms. The disease occurs in an appreciable number of persons in the absence of signs or symptoms, the diagnosis being made by means of changes in the white blood cell picture and/or serologic tests.

Cutaneous Eruption. Skin eruptions of one type or another occur frequently. Wechsler and his associates reported dermatologic lesions in 16 per cent of their patients, but the incidence in other reports has varied from 4 to 100 per cent. The most common skin rashes are of the macular and/or maculopapular types. Other types, such as morbilliform, polymorphous, nodular, vesicular, urticarial and hemorrhagic, are found at times.

Abdominal Types. Jaundice with or without hepatomegaly may occur in a small number of patients, being found in 6 per cent (34 cases) of those composing the epidemic studied by Wechsler. Liver biopsies, abnormal liver function tests and autopsy findings have indicated that hepatitis rather than obstruction of the common duct by enlarged lymph nodes is responsible for the jaundice. In very rare instances, the hepatitis may be extreme. It must be emphasized, however, that there is no certain way to distinguish between hepatitis as a complication of mononucleosis, and viral hepatitis. Hence, in the absence of serologic evidence of infectious mononucleosis, it is advisable to manage the illness as if serum or infectious hepatitis were present.

Abdominal pain secondary to enlarged mesenteric nodes is not uncommon. Rarely, appendiceal involvement and rupture of the spleen may occur. Thirteen cases of rupture of the spleen with 5 deaths have been reported.

Cardiac Involvement. Focal myocarditis and electrocardiographic changes, such as abnormal T waves and prolonged P-R intervals, are common. However, clinical symptoms referable to the heart are conspicuously absent.

Pulmonary Involvement. Clinical evidence of pulmonary involvement is rare. Wechsler and his colleagues have reported that 2.5 per cent of their cases showed pulmonary lesions similar to those of atypical pneumonia. Whether the pulmonary changes in these cases were due to infectious mononucleosis or to some secondary complicating infection is not established.

Neurologic Involvement. Symptoms indicative of involvement of the cerebral meninges, the brain, the cranial nerves, the peripheral nerves, the spinal roots and the spinal cord have been reported. Typical cases of the Guillain-Barré syndrome have occurred; in two of these, deaths resulted. Also, cases of encephalomyelitis with a symptomatology suggesting poliomyelitis have been reported. Pleocytosis and changes in the protein content of the cerebrospinal fluid may occur. Seven patients with central nervous system involvement are known to have died as the result of neurologic complications.

Hematologic Abnormalities. Granulocytopenic leukopenia at the onset followed by lymphocytic leukocytosis constitutes the principal abnormality in the blood. In some instances, polymorphonuclear leukocytosis precedes the lymphocytic leukocytosis and the granulocytic leukopenia. The leukopenia is usually supplanted by leukocytosis during the second week of illness, owing to an increase in the number of lymphocytes, many of which are abnormal. Downey's description of the three types of abnormal lymphocytes that may occur still remains one of the best. His *Type I* cell is characterized by heavy-staining, irregular or bean-shaped nuclei, without nucleoli, and with dark blue, foamy cytoplasm. His *Type II* cell is characterized by relatively large amounts of light blue cytoplasm and a relatively normal-appearing eccentrically placed nucleus. His *Type III* cell occurs much less often than either *Type I* or *Type II* and is distinguished by its resemblance to malignant or leukemic cells. The lymphocytosis is of varying degrees and is both relative and absolute. The percentage of lymphocytes varies widely, at times being above 90. Further, the actual percentage of abnormal lymphocytes varies greatly from patient to patient. These abnormal cells are *in no sense specific,* being found in a variety of clinical disorders, particularly some of the viral infections. Epidemic or infectious hepatitis, at times, has a leukocyte picture indistinguishable from that found in infectious mononucleosis. A similar but less marked blood picture may be found at times in a number of acute illnesses of viral origin. Most of the lymphocytes are approximately the size of small or intermediate lymphocytes, but there are usually a few cells much larger and with nuclei showing nucleoli.

In most patients the leukocyte picture is the only blood change of any significance. However, a few cases with anemia and/or thrombocytopenia have been reported. Also, hemolytic anemia may occur rarely. Agranulocytosis has been noted in only one instance. An increased erythrocyte sedimentation rate is found, but, of course, is in no sense specific.

Serologic Findings. The sheep cell or heterophile agglutination test constitutes one of the most important diagnostic procedures in this disease. Paul and Bunnell were the first to call attention to this fact. They assumed that the heterophile antibody of infectious mononucleosis was of the Forssman type, but Bailey and Raffel, and Stuart, showed later that this antibody could be distinguished from that of serum sickness and from that of normal serum. Thus, there may be at least three types of agglutinins for sheep cells in the serum of human beings. The agglutinins associated with serum sickness have been said to be completely adsorbed by either guinea pig kidney or beef erythrocytes; those associated with normal serum to be almost completely adsorbed by guinea pig kidney, but not by beef erythrocytes; and those associated with infectious mononucleosis to be completely adsorbed by beef erythrocytes, but not significantly by guinea pig cells. However, Dempster has called attention recently to the fact that there are distinct exceptions even to these latter assumptions.

There has been considerable argument as to what constitutes a significant titer in infectious mononucleosis. This probably varies from laboratory to laboratory, depending upon the technique used. Paul has suggested the following ranges for titers: 1:10 to 1:40, negative; 1:80 to 1:160, suspicious; above 1:160, positive. A rising titer is the best criterion in the early stages of the disease. The differential adsorption tests are of distinct advantage, particularly when the titer is in the lower ranges. In rare instances, Hodgkin's disease and leukemia may have very high titers which are completely abolished by adsorption with guinea pig kidney. Usually adsorption with guinea pig kidney is satisfactory, but in some instances adsorption by both guinea pig kidney and beef erythrocytes is needed to clarify the diagnosis. The exact incidence of the positive sheep cell agglutination test in infectious mononucleosis is not established. Certainly, all cases do not show the positive test. In Paul's series the test was positive for 20 to 40 per cent of the cases in the first week, for 60 per cent of the cases in the second week, and for considerably fewer in the fourth week. In Dempster's series 66 per cent of the cases of infectious mononucleosis gave positive agglutinin adsorption reactions.

As previously indicated, the serologic tests for syphilis are falsely positive for a small number of these patients, possibly 3 to 10 per cent. Moreover, *cold agglutinins* in significant titer and abnormal liver function tests have been reported.

Prognosis. In general, the prognosis of infectious mononucleosis may be considered good. Most of those affected recover within three to six weeks without sequelae. However, severe complications, such as hepatitis, thrombocytopenia, myocarditis, spontaneous rupture of the spleen, and involvement of the central and/or peripheral nervous system, may occur. Several instances of fatal outcome from rupture of the spleen, involvement of the nervous system and myocarditis have been recorded. In rare instances the spleen and/or lymph nodes may remain enlarged for long periods of time. Neurologic symptoms may persist for varying intervals. Neurologic complications and rupture of the spleen account for most of the deaths (12 out of 16) from this disorder. Recurrences and relapses have been reported, but the author's experience is in conformity with that of Contratto, to the effect that they are generally absent in patients who have actually shown recovery.

Diagnosis. The diagnosis of infectious mononucleosis is not difficult in the typical case with lymphadenopathy, splenomegaly, lymphocytosis and positive sheep cell agglutination. All these findings may be absent in certain stages of the disease, however, and one or more of them may be absent throughout the illness. Streptococcal sore throat, Vincent's angina and diphtheria may be confused with the oropharyngeal lesions. Infectious hepatitis and homologous serum jaundice may be mistaken for this disease, and vice versa, since the leukocyte picture may be identical in these disorders. Typhoid fever and undulant fever may be confused with the disease at times when leukopenia is present. The skin lesions may lead to confusion with typhus fever, rubella, secondary syphilis and scarlet fever. The neurologic involvement may raise the question of a large number of neurologic disorders, such as lymphocytic choriomengitis, encephalitis, Guillain-Barré disease and poliomyelitis. Leukemia, idiopathic thrombocytopenic purpura and infectious lymphocytosis may be simulated at times. Infectious lymphocytosis is differentiated by hyperleukocytosis, negative sheep cell agglutination test and the absence of atypical lymphocytes.

Treatment. There is no specific treatment for infectious mononucleosis. Sulfonamides, penicillin, chloramphenicol and the tetracyclines have been tried without evidence of benefit. Rest is indicated in the presence of acute symptoms. It is probably wise to limit activities considerably in any known case, even when fever and acute symptoms are absent, because of the danger of rupture of the spleen. When jaundice is present, a high carbohydrate and protein diet in addition to limitation of activities is indicated. Palliative measures of various types, depending upon the symptomatology in individual cases, are indicated. In severely ill patients a prompt remission can usually be obtained by the use of corticotropin or cortisone but the advantages and disadvantages of such treatment have not yet been defined.

JOHN SEWARD LAWRENCE

References

Cohn, C., and Lidman, B. I.: Hepatitis without Jaundice in Infectious Mononucleosis. J. Clin. Investigation, 25:145, 1946.

Contratto, A. W.: Infectious Mononucleosis—A Study of One Hundred and Ninety-six Cases. Arch. Int. Med., 73:449, 1944.

Custer, R. P., and Smith, E. B.: The Pathology of Infectious Mononucleosis. Blood, 3:830, 1948.

Dempster, G.: Some Serological Aspects of Infectious Mononucleosis with Special Reference to the Use of Agglutinin Absorption Tests in Diagnosis. Edinburgh Med. J., 53:296, 1946.

Dolgopol, Vera B., and Husson, G. S.: Infectious Mononucleosis with Neurologic Complications—Report of a Fatal Case. Arch. Int. Med., 83:179, 1949.

Downey, H., and McKinlay, C. A.: Acute Lymphadenosis Compared with Acute Lymphatic Leukemia. Arch. Int. Med., 32:83, 1923.

Evans, A.: Experimental Attempts to Transmit Infectious Mononucleosis to Man. Yale J. Biol. & Med., 20:19, 1947.

————: Liver Involvement in Infectious Mononucleosis. J. Clin. Investigation, 27:106, 1948.

Gendel, B. R., and Cottrell, J. E.: Infectious Mononucleosis. Amer. Pract., 2:472, 1948.

Halcrow, J. P. A., Owen, L. M., and Rodger, N. C.: Infectious Mononucleosis with an Account of an Epidemic in an E. M. S. Hospital. Brit. M. J., 2: 443, 1943.

Hovde, Ruth F., and Sundberg, R. Dorothy: Granulomatous Lesions in the Bone Marrow in Infectious Mononucleosis. A Comparison of the Changes in the Bone Marrow in Infectious Mononucleosis with Those in Brucellosis, Tuberculosis, Sarcoidosis and Lymphatic Leukemia. Blood, 5: 209, 1950.

Paul, J. R.: Diagnosis of Virus and Rickettsial Infections. New York, Columbia University Press, 1949, Chap. 10, pp. 108–116.

Templeton, H. F., and Sutherland, R. T.: Exanthem of Acute Mononucleosis. J.A.M.A., 113: 1215, 1939.

Wechsler, H. F., Rosenblum, A. H., and Sills, C. T.: Infectious Mononucleosis—Report of an Epidemic in an Army Post, Ann. Int. Med., 25:113, 236, 1946.

CAT SCRATCH DISEASE*

(Cat Scratch Fever: Sterile Regional Lymphadenitis: Benign Lymphoreticulosis of Inoculation)

Definition. Cat scratch disease is a benign, subacute, regional lymphadenitis which may proceed to sterile suppuration or subside spontaneously. An indolent primary skin lesion at the site of a cat scratch precedes the adenitis.

History. About 1932 Foshay in Cincinnati differentiated the disease from tularemia and Debré in Paris independently recognized it as a specific entity. Hanger and Rose devised a specific intradermal test in 1945.

Incidence. Since its first description by Debré in 1950, hundreds of cases have been recognized throughout the world. It is a common disease and wherever physicians become informed of its manifestations many cases are found.

Epidemiology. Most victims have cat contacts, the majority being scratched and a few bitten. Occasionally inoculation follows the prick of a thorn or splinter. Household epidemics center about the family cat. Suspected cats appear healthy and presumably transmit the disease passively. Children are affected more frequently than adults.

Etiology. The causative agent has not been isolated. The disease has been transmitted to monkeys and one human by intracutaneous inoculation of infected lymph node suspension. "Granular corpuscles" found in cells of nodes are considered by some to be a visible form of the "virus" and by others to be nonspecific. There appears to be a serologic relationship to the lymphogranuloma-psittacosis group of viruses, in that complement fixation tests with Lygranum have been positive in one third of one series of patients so studied.

Pathology. Histologically the lymph nodes have shown reticuloendothelial hyperplasia and later focal granulomas with necrotic centers surrounded by epithelioid cells. Langhans giant cells are common. The process fre-

* Appreciation is expressed to Dr. Frank G. MacMurray for his assistance in the preparation of this chapter.

quently involves the pericapsular connective tissue.

Clinical Manifestations. A few days following a cat scratch or other skin injury about half the patients develop an indolent primary skin lesion. This appears as a persistent, infected, scabbed ulcer or scratch or a papule surmounted by a vesicle or pustule. About one to three weeks later the regional lymph nodes become remarkably enlarged and fever and symptoms of infection usually develop. The nodes may be elastic, movable and virtually insensitive or fixed, red and tender. They may recede spontaneously in weeks to months or suppurate with the development of sterile pus. Lymphangitis does not occur. The epitrochlear-axillary and inguinale-femoral forms are unilateral; the cervical form is frequently bilateral. Enlarged nodes may occur in unusual sites as under the edge of the pectoral or trapezius muscles. Infected thyroglossal cyst may be simulated.

Rarely the eye is the site of inoculation, causing *Parinaud's oculoglandular syndrome* (unilateral conjunctivitis with enlargement of the homolateral preauricular lymph node). Encephalitis occasionally complicates the disease, recovery occurring without residuals. Macular or papular rashes and erythema nodosum are occasionally seen.

Laboratory Findings. *Intradermal Test:* Aspirated pus is diluted 1:5 with isotonic sodium chloride solution and heated to 60° C. for one hour on two consecutive days. When proved sterile, 0.1 cc. is injected intracutaneously. At 48 hours a positive reaction is indicated by a papule 0.5 to 1.0 cm. in diameter or an area of erythema 1 to 6.0 cm. in diameter, or both. A positive reaction is indicative of past or present infection. Negative reactions, however, have been obtained in a few patients who had illnesses clinically and often pathologically suggestive of cat scratch disease.

The leukocyte count is usually normal. The erythrocyte sedimentation rate is often rapid. Cultures of pus or removed nodes are sterile.

Diagnosis. Cat scratch disease may simulate a wide variety of lymph node diseases such as tularemia, infectious mononucleosis, lymphosarcoma, Hodgkin's disease, tuberculous adenitis, pyogenic adenitis, subcutaneous abscesses, lymphogranuloma venereum and both benign and malignant tumors. Appropriate examinations to exclude other diseases and the intradermal test with cat scratch disease antigen will lead to the proper diagnosis. In the presence of a typical clinical history, pathologic findings consistent with this disease and a positive intradermal test, an unequivocal diagnosis can be made. Whenever there is doubt as to the etiology of a lymph node disease, an intradermal test with cat scratch antigen may avoid the necessity of biopsy and release the patient and physician from the fear of some more serious ailment.

Prognosis. This is a benign, self-limited disease which may last from two weeks to two years.

Treatment. Chloramphenicol or the tetracyclines may shorten the course of the disease and prevent suppuration. Suppurative nodes should be aspirated. Excision or drainage may be necessary.

WORTH B. DANIELS

References

Cassady, J. V., and Culbertson, C. S.: Cat Scratch Disease and Parinaud's Oculoglandular Syndrome. A.M.A. Arch. Ophth., 50:68, 1953.

Daniels, W. B., and MacMurray, F. G.: Cat Scratch Disease: Non-bacterial Regional Lymphadenitis. Arch. Int. Med., 88:736, 1951.

———, and MacMurray, F. G.: Cat Scratch Disease: Nonbacterial Regional Lymphadenitis: A Report of 60 Cases. Ann. Int. Med., 37:697, 1952.

———, and MacMurray, F. G.: Cat Scratch Disease. A Report of 160 Cases. J.A.M.A., 154:1247, 1954.

Debré, R., Lamy, M., Jammet, M. L., Costil, L., and Mozziconacci, P.: La maladie des griffes de chat. Bull. et mém. Soc. méd. d. hôp. de Paris, 66:76, 1950.

Mollaret, P., Reilly, J., Bastin, R., and Tournier, P.: La découverte du virus de la lymphoréticulose benigne d'inoculation. I. Caractérisation serologique et immunologique. Presse méd., 59:681, 1951.

———: La découverte du virus de la lymphoréticulose benigne d'inoculation. II. Inoculation expérimentale au singe et colorations. Presse méd., 59:701, 1951.

Winship, T.: Pathologic Changes in So-called Cat-scratch Fever. Am. J. Clin. Path., 23:1012, 1953.

ACUTE INFECTIOUS NONBACTERIAL GASTROENTERITIS

Definition. So-called nonbacterial gastroenteritis or viral enteritis is an acute, self-limited infection. The afebrile type is characterized by watery diarrhea, abdominal cramps, nausea and vomiting. There is also a febrile nondiarrheal type, apparently unrelated to the first. Both are presumed to be due to viruses.

Incidence and Epidemiology. The epidemiologic unit seems to be the family, in which nonbacterial gastroenteritis may rank second only to common respiratory disease as a cause of illness. Both sexes and all ages are affected. The most likely mode of transmission is by the fecal-oral route. The afebrile disease, which is highly communicable, occurs in large epidemics, more frequently in the cold months, and also sporadically. The incubation period ranges from one to five days, averaging three days. The febrile type has an incubation period of one or two days and is less contagious than the afebrile form.

Etiology and Pathology. The causative agents have not been propagated in the laboratory but human volunteers were infected when fed bacteria-free fecal supernates. Volunteers were actively immune to one strain of the afebrile agent for a year, but there may be antigenic variants. The afebrile agent has been passed through ultrafilters. Neither disease causes fatalities. Rarely, however, the afebrile type is a terminal complication in the aged or in patients seriously ill of other diseases. The pathologic findings, consisting of hyperemia and occasional ulceration of the intestines, can be attributed to hypermotility.

Symptoms. The onset of the afebrile disease is often abrupt with profuse watery diarrhea, anorexia, nausea and vomiting, occurring singly or in combination. Usually there are hyperperistaltic abdominal cramps, often preceding a watery stool. Dizziness, mild headache and malaise are frequent complaints. When there is fever, it is low and related to mild or moderate dehydration. The abdomen is relaxed and the colon, distended with gas, may be palpated. Borborygmi are heard and felt. Symptoms and signs referable to the respiratory tract are conspicuously absent, or if present are thought to be adventitious. The blood count and other clinical laboratory values are normal, and the feces seldom contain blood, pus or mucus. The acute illness lasts only a day or so, although stools may be loose for a week.

The gastrointestinal symptomatology of the febrile type resembles that described above with the important difference that there is no watery diarrhea. Some patients are constipated. Abdominal pain tends to be persistent and frequently is intense. It is often accompanied by moderate fever, headache and malaise. Patients recover within two days.

Diagnosis and Treatment. Culture and microscopy of the feces are important in differentiation of nonbacterial gastroenteritis from salmonellosis, shigellosis or amebiasis, particularly in epidemics of the afebrile type. Absence of fever or leukocytosis may be helpful. Food poisoning can often be excluded by the distribution and timing of new cases, which continue to appear in outbreaks for over a week. Treatment is rarely needed, and consists only of fluid replacement. Febrile nonbacterial gastroenteritis can resemble early acute surgical conditions but fails to progress and is soon over.

IRVING GORDON

References

Britten, S. A., Rubenstein, A. D., Raskin, N., and Strassman, G.: Epidemic Diarrhea of Unknown Cause. Report of Outbreaks in Three Massachusetts State Hospitals. New England J. Med., 244: 749, 1951.

Cook, G. T., and Marmion, B. P.: Gastroenteritis of Unknown Aetiology. An Outbreak in a Maternity Unit. Brit. M. J., 2:446, 1947.

Dingle, J. H., and collaborators: A Study of Illness in a Group of Cleveland Families. I. Plan of Study and Certain General Observations. Am. J. Hyg., 58:16, 1953.

Gordon, I., Ingraham, H. S., and Korns, R. F.: Transmission of Epidemic Gastroenteritis to Human Volunteers by Oral Administration of Fecal Filtrates. J. Exper. Med., 86:409, 1947.

Gray, J. D.: Epidemic Nausea and Vomiting. Brit. M. J., 1:209, 1939.

Jordan, W. S., Jr., Gordon, I., and Dorrance, W. R.: A Study of Illness in a Group of Cleveland Families. VII. Transmission of Acute Non-bacterial Gastroenteritis to Volunteers: Evidence for Two Different Etiologic Agents. J. Exper. Med., 98: 461, 1953.

Kojima, S., and collaborators: Studies on the Causative Agent of the Infectious Diarrhoea. Records of the Experiments on Human Volunteers. Japanese Med. J., 1:467, 1948.

Reimann, H. A., Hodges, J. H., and Price, A. H.: Epidemic Diarrhea, Nausea, and Vomiting of Unknown Cause. J.A.M.A., 127:1, 1945.

RICKETTSIAL DISEASES

INTRODUCTION

The rickettsial diseases of man are caused by micro-organisms which are classified as a family (*Rickettsiaceae*) between the bacteria and the viruses because they have characteristics in common with both. These micro-organisms were named "*rickettsiae*" to honor the observation made by Dr. H. T. Ricketts in his studies of Rocky Mountain spotted fever and epidemic typhus fever. In 1910, while investigating the etiology of typhus, Ricketts contracted this disease and died. Several species of rickettsiae are now recognized as pathogenic for man. Their individual characteristics are described in the sections dealing with the various human infections which they induce. In general, the rickettsiae have four common features: (*a*) they are pleomorphic, cocco-bacillary forms, readily visible in the ordinary light microscope (see Fig. 16); (*b*) they multiple only within certain cells of susceptible animals; (*c*) they occur in various arthropods in nature; and (*d*) they cause acute, febrile, self-limited illnesses in man, most of which are accompanied by a skin rash.

The principal rickettsial diseases are divided into groups as indicated in the accompanying table.

The distinctive clinical course typical of each disease has been the primary basis for the classification shown in the table. There are also differences between the usual mode of transmission. The specific immunologic properties of the rickettsiae and their differences biologically as revealed in laboratory studies are more valuable and more reliable in the classification of the rickettsial diseases than either the clinical features or the arthropod vectors. After recovery from any one of the individual diseases shown in the table, the blood serum of man and certain animals has highly specific antibodies in complement fixation or rickettsial agglutination tests. These serologic procedures not only indicate the main group to which a particular disease belongs, but also distinguish between the members of the same group in certain instances.

Before specific serologic techniques with rickettsial antigens were fully developed, the Weil-Felix test was the only simple procedure available for laboratory differentiation of the rickettsial diseases. The Weil-Felix test is described in the section on the diagnosis of typhus fever. The basis of the reaction is believed to be a fortuitous occurrence of a common antigenic component between

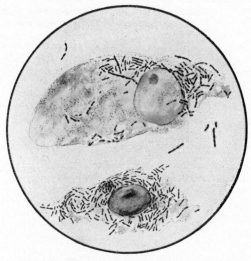

Fig. 16. *Rickettsia prowazeki*. Camera lucida drawing of infected peritoneal cells of x-rayed mouse. (Courtesy, editors, Journal of Experimental Medicine.)

some rickettsiae and certain strains of the bacillus *Proteus vulgaris*. It should be emphasized that there is no etiologic relationship between rickettsial diseases and the strains of *Proteus vulgaris* used in the Weil-Felix test. Although this test is immensely helpful in epidemics of classic typhus and in the investigation of scrub typhus, it has important limitations and no longer serves as a primary criterion in the identification and classification of rickettsial diseases.

The immunity produced by the rickettsial diseases is usually of long duration. The members of one group confer either partial or complete immunity to the other diseases of the same group, but no cross-immunity occurs between the different groups. Unfortunately, there are several instances of fatal infections

Rickettsial Diseases of Man

GROUP	PRINCIPAL DISEASES	SYNONYMS	ETIOLOGIC AGENT	USUAL MODE OF TRANSMISSION TO MAN	USUAL OCCURRENCE
Typhus	Epidemic typhus	Classic, historic, human, European typhus[1]	*Rickettsia prowazeki*	Human body louse[2]	Winter and spring in cold climates over most of world
	Brill-Zinsser disease	Brill's disease, recrudescent typhus	*Rickettsia prowazeki*	Not established[3]	U.S.A., Europe, probably world-wide[3]
	Murine typhus	Endemic typhus, urban or shop typhus of Malaya	*Rickettsia mooseri*[4]	Rat flea[5]	World-wide
Rocky Mountain spotted fever[6]	Rocky Mountain spotted fever	Spotted fever, tick fever, tick typhus, etc.	*Dermacentroxenus rickettsi*[7]	Ticks[8]	North and South America
	Fièvre boutonneuse	Button fever, Mediterranean fever	*Dermacentroxenus conori*[9]	Ticks[10]	Mediterranean countries and North Africa
	South African tick bite fever		*Dermacentroxenus pijperi*	Ticks[11]	South Africa
	Rickettsialpox	Kew Gardens fever	*Rickettsia akari*[12]	Mites[13]	Northeastern U.S.A.[3]
Tsutsugamushi disease	Scrub typhus	Mite-borne typhus, Japanese river fever, tropical typhus, rural typhus, Sumatran mite fever, etc.	*Rickettsia tsutsugamushi (orientalis)*	Mites[14]	Korea, Japan, China, Formosa, India, Burma, Ceylon, Indonesia, the Philippines and Australia
Q fever	Q fever	Nine mile fever, Australian Q fever, Balkan grippe	*Coxiella burneti*[15]	Probably airborne route; occasionally ticks; possibly milk[3]	Australia, U.S.A., Panama, Europe, North Africa (probably world-wide)

[1] Jail fever, war fever, camp fever, *Fleckfieber* (German), *typhus exanthematique* (French), *tifus exantematico* (Spanish), *dermotypho* (Italian).

[2] *Pediculus humanus corporis.*

[3] See text for further explanation.

[4] Bergey's Manual classification: *Rickettsia typhi.*

[5] *Xenopsylla cheopis.*

[6] In addition to the diseases listed, there are others which probably belong in this group, such as North Queensland tick typhus, tick-borne rickettsioses of India and Kenya.

[7] Bergey's Manual classification: *Rickettsia rickettsii.*

[8] *Dermacentor andersoni; D. variabilis; Amblyomma americanum.*

[9] Bergey's Manual classification: *Rickettsia conorii.*

[10] *Rhipicephalus sanguineus.*

[11] *Amblyomma hebraeum; Haemaphysalis leachi.*

[12] In author's opinion, name *Dermacentroxenus akari* would be preferable.

[13] *Allodermanyssus sanguineus.*

[14] *Trombicula akamushi; T. deliensis.*

[15] *Rickettsia diaporica* was the name first used for the American variety of Q fever rickettsiae.

among laboratory workers which emphasize this point; for example, tsutsugamushi disease has taken the lives of persons who had previously experienced epidemic typhus.

The rickettsial diseases include one of the notorious diseases of medical history, epidemic typhus fever, which has been a scourge of mankind for more than four centuries, as well as two "new" diseases not recognized clinically before 1935 (Q fever) and 1946 (rickettsialpox). Some of the rickettsial diseases, such as murine typhus, are world-wide in distribution, others are known only in certain areas, for example, rickettsialpox. It is of considerable interest that micro-organisms indistinguishable in appearance from pathogenic rickettsiae are found as harmless symbionts in many different arthropods. Students of the rickettsiae, particularly Wolbach and Zinsser, have stressed the possible occurrence of rickettsial diseases whenever man, rodents and ectoparasites common to both are closely associated. Indeed, the list of rickettsial diseases in the accompanying table indicates only the principal human rickettsial infections. For example, a disease called North Queensland tick typhus has been reported from Australia (1947) which probably is a member of the Rocky Mountain spotted fever group, but it has not been completely characterized; trench fever, or Wolhynian fever, is reputed to be a rickettsial disease of man, transmitted by the human body louse from man to man, yet its position in respect to the other rickettsiae has not been established.

One final point of general interest in respect to the rickettsial diseases should be mentioned. Recent developments have added enormously to our ability to prevent, to control and to treat these infections. Satisfactory vaccines have been prepared on a large scale against some of the rickettsial diseases. The methods for rapid mass delousing with the insecticide DDT have demonstrated how effectively the once dread epidemics of typhus can be sharply arrested. Finally, several of the new antimicrobial drugs, if used early in the illness, have a dramatic effect on the clinical course of the rickettsial diseases. These advances greatly reduce the severity and the magnitude of the problems associated with the rickettsial diseases.

JOHN C. SNYDER

THE TYPHUS GROUP

Definition. Typhus fever is an acute infectious disease characterized by severe headache, sustained high fever, generalized macular or maculopapular rash, and termination by rapid lysis in approximately two weeks.

Three diseases compose the typhus group: epidemic louse-borne typhus fever, Brill-Zinsser disease, and murine flea-borne typhus fever. Clinically and pathologically, these three illnesses are nearly identical, differences occurring only in the intensity of the symptoms and signs, the severity of the course, and the case fatality rate. Epidemiologically and historically, however, the three members of the typhus group are so different that they are described in separate sections.

EPIDEMIC LOUSE-BORNE TYPHUS FEVER

(*Classic, Historic, Human, European Typhus; Jail Fever; War Fever; Camp Fever; Fleckfieber [German]; Typhus Exanthematique [French]; Tifus Exantematico, Tabardillo [Spanish]; Dermotypho [Italian]*).

History. It is probable that typhus fever has afflicted mankind since ancient times, but the account of Fracastorius in 1546 is the earliest medical record which describes typhus fever with sufficient accuracy to permit its definite identification. The word *typhus* is derived from the Greek *typhos,* meaning smoky or hazy. Although the term had been used by Hippocrates to describe a "confused state of intellect with a tendency to stupor," it was not applied to cases which were clearly typhus fever itself until 1760. Despite the work of Fracastorius, typhoid and typhus fevers were usually regarded as one entity by physicians until 1837, when Gerhard in Philadelphia clearly differentiated the two disorders on the basis of important differences clinically and pathologically. Even today, however, confusion in terminology persists in those parts of Europe where *typhoid* fever is called "typhus abdominalis."

Typhus fever has had a major role in the history of the past four centuries. It followed in the wake of wars, famines and human misfortunes of all kinds. It has often had a more decisive effect on military campaigns than the actual battles themselves, a subject admirably treated by Zinsser in his book *Rats, Lice, and History.* The typhus epidemics in eastern Europe and Russia between 1918 and 1922 are estimated to have caused 30 million cases and at least three million deaths. It is worthy of comment that the ravages of typhus have characteristically been even greater among medical personnel than among the general population. In the 1915 epidemic in Serbia nearly all of the 400 doctors in that country contracted typhus, and 126 died. Thus typhus has established its reputation as one of the major epidemic diseases.

Etiology and Transmission. In 1916, da Rocha Lima showed that typhus was caused by the micro-organism which he named *Rickettsia prowazeki.* This micro-organism has been found in nature only in man and the human louse, *Pediculus humanus.* Several other species can be experimentally infected with *R. prowazeki* — for example, monkeys, guinea pigs, cotton rats, gerbilles, mice, fleas and developing chick embryos. The numerous instances of typhus fever among laboratory investigators working with experimental typhus infection clearly indicate the validity of the conclusions reached by Wolbach, Todd and Palfrey in their classic monograph on the etiology of typhus fever (1922).

The micro-organism is present in the blood of typhus patients during the febrile period, particularly in the first few days of the illness. Human lice feeding on the patients ingest the typhus rickettsiae, which then multiply

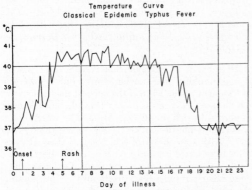

Fig. 17. Temperature curve in a case of classic epidemic typhus. (Courtesy of Dr. T. M. Rivers: Viral and Rickettsial Infections of Man. J. B. Lippincott Company.)

within the lining cells of the intestinal tract of the louse. The cells become greatly distended with masses of *R. prowazeki* and may burst into the lumen of the gut, whereupon the micro-organisms invade other lining cells or pass out of the louse in the feces. After several days the louse gut becomes occluded by the distended, typhus-infected cells, and the louse dies of intestinal obstruction. Chronic infection of lice with typhus rickettsiae has not been demonstrated. The micro-organisms do not pass to new generations via the louse egg.

When the louse feeds, it makes a small puncture in the skin; secretions of the louse introduced during the act of feeding irritate the skin, causing the bitten person to scratch. It is characteristic of the louse that it defecates as it feeds, so that conditions are ideal for the rubbing of typhus rickettsiae into the skin punctures. Two factors explain the movement of typhus-infected lice from the person whose blood has infected them to normal persons: the insects tend to leave a patient who has a high fever if other hosts are available; and if the host dies of typhus, the body becomes cold, and the lice promptly crawl away in search of another host. These

facts probably account for much of the transmission of typhus during epidemics.

Another important way in which transmission may occur is by contact with infected louse feces. The garments of a typhus patient, toward the end of his febrile course and for several days early in his convalescence, are contaminated by large quantities of louse feces containing viable typhus rickettsiae. Agitation of the garments disperses many particles of infected feces into the air of the room, so that they may gain access to the respiratory tract or the conjunctivas of persons thus exposed. It is possible, therefore, to become infected with typhus without being louse-infested at any time.

Morbid Anatomy. The typhus rickettsiae invade the endothelial cells of small arteries, capillaries and venules. The affected cells tend to proliferate, and the injury soon results in thrombus formation with small areas of necrosis and perivascular accumulations of phagocytic cells. The lesions thus produced are sometimes referred to as typhus nodules and are scattered throughout the various organs and tissues, particularly the skin, the brain and the heart muscle.

Bacterial bronchopneumonia is a frequent finding at autopsy in patients who did not receive specific therapy. When penicillin or sulfonamides have been used, an interstitial pneumonitis may be observed which is ascribed to the typhus rickettsiae themselves; when death is delayed to the third week of the disease, a necrotizing, fibrinoid arteritis has been encountered which is similar to that found in numerous clinical conditions, including hypersensitivity, infection or renal disease (McAllister).

Pathologic Physiology and Chemistry. Although epidemic typhus has developed in millions of patients, there have been remarkably few studies of the physiology and chemistry of this illness. The explanation of the paucity of data lies in the association of typhus epidemics and human misery. The disease breaks out under precisely those conditions which make hospitalization, medical care and scientific investigation largely impossible.

Suspensions of living, fully virulent typhus rickettsiae are toxic for white mice, producing death in a few hours. This phenomenon has not been explained biochemically or physiologically. Possibly the toxicity of rickettsiae is responsible for some of the clinical features of the disease. On the other hand, the widespread distribution of lesions in blood vessels can account for many of the manifestations of the illness in man.

It is characteristic of typhus that a severe hypotension may occur, often followed by evidence of renal insufficiency with a drop in urea clearance and a rise in blood urea nitrogen. Oliguria and fixed specific gravity of the urine accompany the other findings. If the patient recovers, a diuresis is often value for ten to fourteen days, subsiding by rapid lysis in three or four days if recovery is to ensue (Fig. 17). Death occurs between the ninth and the eighteenth days in about 20 per cent of patients (for all age groups) during epidemics.

One or more shaking chills may occur at the onset. Unproductive cough may be troublesome. Constipation is more frequent than diarrhea. Other symptoms and signs are

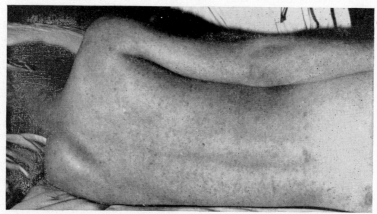

Fig. 18. Rash of epidemic typhus, eleventh day of disease. (Courtesy of U.S.A. Typhus Commission and of Dr. T. M. Rivers: Viral and Rickettsial Infections of Man. J. B. Lippincott Company.)

noted concomitant with improvement in clinical condition.

The plasma volume of several patients measured at various stages of typhus was found to lie within normal limits despite clinical impressions that dehydration was a feature of the clinical course in untreated cases. Usually the hemoglobin and the plasma albumin values fall below normal, and a rise in plasma globulin is observed particularly in the second week of the untreated disease (Yeomans).

When typhus occurs in a previously immunized person or when specific treatment is instituted early in the disease, the abnormal findings described above may be entirely absent.

Symptoms and Clinical Course. *Untreated, Nonimmunized Patients.* The incubation period of typhus is approximately ten days to two weeks. The onset may be preceded by variable prodromal symptoms, such as lassitude, headache and mild anorexia. More often the onset is abrupt with a severe headache and generalized aches and pains over the entire body. The temperature rises in the course of two or three days to 40° C. (104° F.) and usually remains above this sometimes present, but the most constant and characteristic feature in the first week of illness is the severe headache, which resists all attempts to alleviate it with the usual drugs.

Toward the end of the first week the patient may appear to be slightly deaf. His face may be flushed and dusky. His conjunctivas are suffused, and photophobia is usually apparent. The pulse is often somewhat slower than is expected with a fever of 40° C. or more. The blood pressure is below normal. A macular or maculopapular rash usually appears between the fourth and the seventh days (most commonly on the fifth day) on the back and chest, spreading later to the abdomen and the extremities, but sparing the face, palms and soles except in severely ill patients (Fig. 18).

The lesions are 1 to 4 mm. in diameter with somewhat irregular outlines and, when first apparent, are pinkish to reddish in color. At first they fade on light pressure, but later become fixed. The rash lasts about as long as the fever, rarely being visible in convalescence. During the second week the lesions often become dark red or purplish as small hemorrhages occur in the lesions. Frankly purpuric or confluent rashes are observed only in severe cases, which usually end fatally.

During the second week of typhus the pulse becomes more rapid. The patient tends to be stuporous or to have bouts of active delirium followed by profound stupor. This may progress to coma in severely stricken patients. Skin necrosis over the sacrum and other pressure points may occur. Otitis media and bacterial bronchopneumonia are frequent complications. Gangrene of the toes, the fingers, the penis, the scrotum, the ear lobes or the tip of the nose may appear. Parotitis, sometimes bilateral, often develops toward the end of the second week. Pneumonitis may be present and is often found more easily by roentgenographic than by physical examination.

Death from typhus usually occurs after gradual progression from stupor to coma. Less often there may be peripheral vascular collapse with a fall in body temperature and death after a short period of unconsciousness. Rarely, a convulsion may bring an abrupt end to an illness which had not seemed particularly severe.

The reader is referred to Murchison for an excellent and detailed description of the course of epidemic typhus.

Typhus Fever in Previously Immunized Persons. The symptoms and clinical course of epidemic typhus are greatly modified as a consequence of active immunization, which has been widely used in recent years since the development of formalin-treated rickettsial vaccines. "Adequate immunization" is defined in the material on Prevention and Control. The clinical course in "adequately immunized" persons varies from an illness characterized only by a mild headache and slight fever of one or two days' duration to an illness of several days with a rash consisting of a few macules which disappear in a day or two. Complications are rare, and the diagnosis often cannot be established except by laboratory tests. The mortality is close to zero.

Typhus Fever Modified by Specific Treatment. Although clinical experience with the tetracycline drugs (Aureomycin, Terramycin) and chloramphenicol is less extensive in epidemic typhus than in scrub typhus and Rocky Mountain spotted fever, the data at present indicate the probability of entirely similar beneficial results, particularly if treatment is started early in the disease. Thus any one of these drugs may be expected to arrest the clinical course of typhus at whatever stage is present when they are first administered. They should bring about a drop in temperature to normal in thirty-six to seventy-two hours. Clinical recovery depends on the rate of healing of the widespread vascular lesions of typhus, which may take several days, depending upon the extent of their development when therapy was begun.

If the tetracyclines or chloramphenicol are not available, para-aminobenzoic acid may be used in the treatment of typhus. The clinical response to this substance takes three to five days, and beneficial results are to be expected only when scrupulous attention is given to the recommended method of administration (Snyder et al.).

Diagnosis. *Clinical Diagnosis.* Before the characteristic rash appears, it is impossible to assert on clinical grounds alone that a patient is suffering from epidemic typhus. The early stages of several acute infectious diseases closely resemble the first few days of epidemic typhus—for example, smallpox, relapsing fever, malaria, typhoid fever, meningococcal infection, yellow fever, the other rickettsial diseases, and so on. The typhus rash is a distinguishing feature of considerable value; the first lesions appear on the trunk and later spread to the extremities, sparing the face, palms and soles except in severely ill patients. This is helpful in distinguishing between typhus fever and Rocky Mountain spotted fever. The typhus rash, however, is not present in 10 to 15 per cent of cases and may be difficult to recognize in dark-skinned subjects. The clinical diagnosis of epidemic typhus is particularly difficult in children or in persons who have previously received immunization. In such instances a rash may be detected for short intervals only or may be entirely absent, the symptoms are much less severe, and the fever may persist for only a few days.

Laboratory Diagnosis. SPECIFIC SEROLOGIC TESTS. Agglutinins for typhus rickettsiae and complement-fixing antibodies for specific rickettsial antigens appear in the serums of patients beginning about the end of the first week of the illness. The titer rises toward the end of the illness and during the first and second weeks of convalescence, tending to subside slowly thereafter. In some instances persons recovered from typhus still show significant titers in their serums for months or years after an attack of the disease. Sometimes, on the other hand, the specific antibodies may be no longer detectable a few weeks after the illness. The use of killed rickettsial vaccines for active immunization often is followed by the development of specific antibodies which may add slight confusion to the interpretation of complement fixation tests taken during the course of a febrile illness. The most important point in the serologic diagnosis of typhus by specific rickettsial tests is the demonstration of a rise in titer from the early stage of the disease to a later stage. A fourfold change in value is usually considered diagnostic.

The rickettsial antigens prepared from infected yolk sac suspensions must be processed to eliminate a factor ordinarily present in the yolk sac, which results in falsely positive complement fixation tests if the patient has positive serologic tests for syphilis. The antigens currently being prepared in this country are free of this cross-reacting factor. The specific antibodies for the typhus group serve to distinguish it clearly and definitely from the other rickettsial diseases. Any laboratory which is able to perform routine complement fixation tests can purchase rickettsial antigens and perform specific diagnostic tests for the typhus group, although the antigens are relatively more expensive than those for other tests.

WEIL-FELIX TEST. Strains of the bacillus *Proteus vulgaris,* referred to as OX-19, OX-2, and OX-K, have been relied upon in the past for the diagnosis of epidemic typhus. As indicated in the Introduction, the basis of the Weil-Felix reaction with these strains of *P. vulgaris* is an accidental occurrence of an antigenic component common to both Proteus and the rickettsiae. Usually patients suffering from a disease in the typhus group develop agglutinins for Proteus OX-19. The titer rises from a low level to more than 1:160 in most instances. Furthermore, some of the members of the Rocky Mountain spotted fever group likewise agglutinate Proteus OX-19. Thus the test does not distinguish between the two groups. As ordinarily performed, the reaction is carried out in test tubes with either living or killed suspensions of *P. vulgaris* in the smooth, nonmotile form. Slide tests developed by various workers are helpful during epidemics, since the result may be obtained at the bedside in a matter of minutes with reasonable accuracy if suitable controls are performed.

ISOLATION OF RICKETTSIAE FROM THE PATIENT. The laboratory diagnosis of typhus may be made by inoculation of blood from a patient into susceptible species, such as cotton rats, guinea pigs or chick embryos, if facilities are available for the further manipulations required to establish the identity of the micro-organisms thus obtained. The procedure is somewhat complicated and suitable only for specially equipped laboratories. Colonies of human body lice may be used with success in the detection of living rickettsiae in patients. Biopsy of skin lesions might also be of diagnostic help in the hands of an experienced pathologist.

Prognosis. The case fatality rate in epidemic typhus is less than 10 per cent in children. As age increases, the fatality rate rises until, in persons over fifty, it is 60 per cent or more. However, active immunization and the use of specific therapy greatly affect the mortality figures.

In the absence of specific treatment the appearance of renal insufficiency is an early sign that a patient's illness will be severe or fatal. The extent and severity of the typhus rash are roughly indicative of the severity of the disease. Complications such as bronchopneumonia or gangrene of the skin are likewise serious prognostic signs. A fall in systolic blood pressure to values below 80 mm. of mercury for a few hours or longer may cause damage from which the patient may not recover, even though the blood pressure rises after the period of severe hypotension.

When epidemic typhus occurs in persons who have received "adequate immunization," the prognosis is excellent unless the exposure to infection has been overwhelming.

Treatment. The tetracyclines (Aureomycin, Terramycin) and chloramphenicol are highly effective if administered early, in adequate dosage, by mouth. The clinician must decide on the basis of his own preference which of the three he will use. The initial dose for adults is 2 to 3 gm., split into three parts, at hourly intervals. This should be followed by a maintenance dose of 0.5 gm. every six hours until the patient's temperature is normal. The dose may then be cut in half and continued for at least two or three days longer.

If treatment is terminated too soon, the fever and symptoms may recur, but will respond promptly when antimicrobial therapy is resumed.

Para-aminobenzoic acid (PABA) is a simple chemical compound, which, when given in adequate dosage, has a beneficial therapeutic effect on the course of epidemic typhus. It is far more difficult to administer than the three drugs mentioned previously. It is necessary to give large amounts every two hours and to make measurements of the blood concentration at frequent intervals to assure adequate and safe concentration. It is to be recommended only if the tetracyclines or chloramphenicol is not available, and should be given with careful attention to details of administration. The reader is referred to original articles for dosage schedules, precautions, complications and contraindications (Snyder et al.).

Penicillin and streptomycin may have slight activity against typhus rickettsiae, but their use in the clinical course of epidemic typhus should be considered only when secondary infections which respond specifically to penicillin or streptomycin are present. The sulfonamides may have a harmful effect on the course of typhus and should not be given.

Persons who handle typhus cases should be actively immunized. A louse-infested typhus patient on admission to the hospital should be bathed and dusted with DDT. His garments should be sterilized. It is not necessary to shave the patient in order to achieve satisfactory delousing with DDT.

General Supportive Care. Good nursing care is of great importance in the management of a patient with epidemic typhus. A rise in temperature above 105° F. is an indication for prompt administration of cold packs. Barbiturates and morphine are to be avoided if possible. Codeine may be tried for relief of headache, but is likely to be ineffective. It is expected that the use of the new antimicrobial drugs will so alter the clinical picture of typhus that many of the recommendations and precautions in general supportive care of patients will be obviated. The reader is referred to the excellent account by Yeomans for further details in the management of epidemic typhus.

Prevention and Control. The accomplishments in prevention and control of epidemic typhus during World War II constitute a milestone in the history of preventive medicine. Active immunization by means of killed rickettsial vaccines is now possible on a wide scale and has a profound effect on the severity and mortality of the illness. "Adequate immunization" consists in an initial course of two subcutaneous inoculations of 1 cc. each, ten days to two weeks apart, followed by stimulating doses of 0.5 cc. each at intervals of a few months if exposure is expected. The American military forces prefer the Cox-type vaccine, derived from the yolk sac membrane of developing chick embryos. "Adequate immunization" probably reduces the *incidence* of typhus fever among exposed persons; it definitely reduces the mortality close to zero and greatly lessens the severity of the illness.

DDT as a 10 per cent powder effectively delouses large numbers of people quickly if the dust is blown up the sleeves, down the neck, and around the waistband with a hand duster or a power duster. If our knowledge of prevention and control is properly applied, it should be possible to eliminate outbreaks of typhus before they achieve serious proportions.

BRILL-ZINSSER DISEASE
(Brill's Disease; Recrudescent Typhus)

History. Nathan Brill, after observing an epidemic of *typhoid* fever in the Mount Sinai Hospital in New York City, subsequently encountered sporadic cases of an atypical typhoid-like disease in which the Widal tests and blood cultures were negative. In 1910 he reported 255 such cases and called attention to their several common features: The disease usually occurred in immigrants from Russia or Poland; there was no infectiousness (only in one household did a second case occur); headache, fever and malaise were the prominent symptoms; and the most characteristic aspect of the disease was a macular or maculopapular rash beginning on the fifth or sixth day. Clinicians in other large cities of the eastern United States promptly reported cases which were referred to as "Brill's disease." In 1912, Anderson and Goldberger showed by cross-immunity tests in monkeys that Brill's disease was a form of typhus.

During the period from 1917 to 1932 the work of several investigators established the existence of two distinct varieties of typhus fever: the first caused by *Rickettsia prowazeki,* classic epidemic typhus, spread from man to man by the human body louse; the second caused by *R. mooseri,* the murine variety, a disease in rats spread from rat to rat by the rat louse and the rat flea and occasionally transmitted from rat to man by the rat flea. Since "Brill's disease" could not be ascribed to human lice or to rat fleas, however, this differentiation of typhus fever into louse-borne epidemic and flea-borne murine did not establish the position of Brill's disease as either one or the other. It is unfortunate that many authors have erroneously used the term "Brill's disease" to describe sporadic cases of murine typhus.

Etiology and Transmission. In 1934, Zinsser and Ruïz Castaneda isolated typhus rickettsiae from three "Brill's disease" patients. Their strains were similar to classic epidemic strains, using the tests available for differentiation at that time. On the basis of this information and his analysis of 538 cases of "Brill's disease" in Boston and New York, Zinsser advanced his hypothesis that "Brill's disease" represents a recrudescence of an old typhus infection, implying that the epidemic typhus rickettsiae, once acquired,

Murray and co-workers (1951) showed that Brill-Zinsser disease occurred in Yugoslavia under conditions which precluded its explanation on the basis of transmission by body lice.

The main differences between primary epidemic typhus and Brill-Zinsser disease are listed below (from Murray and Snyder 1953).

	BRILL-ZINSSER DISEASE	EPIDEMIC LOUSE-BORNE TYPHUS
Past history of typhus	Yes	No
Occurrence of cases	Sporadic	Epidemic
Transmission	Cases can occur *without* lice	By infected lice
Usual duration of fever	7 to 11 days	12 to 18 days
Complement-fixing antibody with specific *epidemic* antigen:		
(a) On 8th day of illness:	More than 1000	Less than 100*
(b) Maximal titer occurs:	Between 8th and 10th day	Later than 12th day
Complement-fixing antibody with specific *murine* antigen	Titer moderately high (usually 2 to 8 fold less than titer with epidemic)	Absent or low titer (at least 32 to 64 fold less than titer with epidemic)
Proteus OX 19 titers†	Usually less than 160	Usually from 320 to 5000

* Titers refer to denominators of serum dilutions.

† By the concentrated antigen method (U. S. Army Medical Service Graduate School).

remained latent for many years somewhere in the tissues of infected human beings. According to Zinsser, "Brill's disease" cases, when occurring in louse-infested communities, might become foci of outbreaks of epidemic typhus; thus, over the centuries, man might be the reservoir, serving to maintain the disease between epidemics.

Zinsser's hypothesis has received support from recent studies. The serums of Brill's disease patients have higher titers to epidemic antigen than to murine antigen in complement fixation tests (Plotz; Mooser and Loeffler). Murray and Snyder have obtained seven new strains of typhus rickettsiae from cases of Brill's disease in New York, Boston and Philadelphia. By means of several laboratory procedures not available at the time of Zinsser's studies, it has been conclusively shown that all seven new strains of Brill's disease rickettsiae are indistinguishable from classic epidemic strains. Furthermore, it has been clearly shown that human body lice become typhus-infected by feeding on "Brill's disease" patients early in the disease.

Loeffler and Mooser (1952) suggested the name Brill-Zinsser disease in recognition of Zinsser's brilliant contribution to knowledge of this disease.

Morbid Anatomy, Pathologic Physiology and Chemistry, Symptoms and Clinical Course. The findings in Brill-Zinsser disease under these headings are the same as those described under Epidemic Typhus with the exception that the illness is somewhat milder and definitely shorter in duration.

Diagnosis. The clinical diagnosis of Brill-Zinsser disease should be made when a fever of unknown origin occurs in a foreign-born patient who has lived at some previous time in an area where typhus fever occurs in epidemic form, who complains of an intense persistent headache, and who has a macular or maculopapular rash on the fourth to the sixth day of the disease.

The laboratory diagnosis should be made by the complement fixation test (or the rickettsial agglutination test). Recent studies have shown that the Weil-Felix test should be ignored if negative.

Prognosis and Treatment. The statements in the paragraphs on Prognosis and Treatment of Epidemic Typhus apply to Brill-Zinsser disease as well.

Prevention and Control. Since the factor or factors which precipitate an attack of Brill-Zinsser disease are not known, nothing can be said in regard to prevention and control of this illness.

MURINE FLEA-BORNE TYPHUS FEVER

(*Endemic Typhus, Rat Typhus, Flea Typhus, Urban or Shop Typhus of Malaya, etc.*)

History. Murine typhus fever probably has occurred for centuries as a sporadic or endemic disease, but only since 1931 has it been clearly distinguished from classic epidemic louse-borne typhus. Sporadic cases of typhus were reported occasionally in Europe

rat fleas in Baltimore (1931), and Mooser, Zinsser and Ruïz Castaneda found the agent in rats in Mexico City. Mooser then named the disease "murine typhus" to indicate its presence as a natural infection of rats. Reports rapidly accumulated, showing the worldwide distribution of murine typhus. The distribution of the disease in the United States is shown in Figure 19, which indicates the rate per million population. It is evident that murine typhus has been

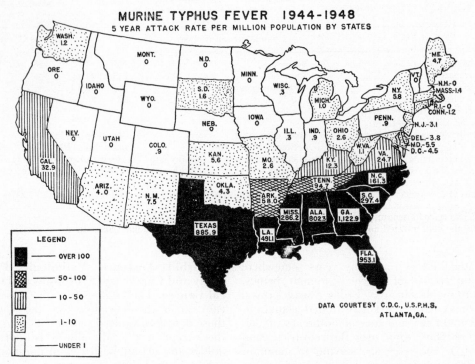

MURINE TYPHUS FEVER 1944-1948
5 YEAR ATTACK RATE PER MILLION POPULATION BY STATES

LEGEND

■ —— OVER 100

▩ —— 50 - 100

▥ —— 10 - 50

▦ —— 1 - 10

□ —— UNDER 1

DATA COURTESY C.D.C., U.S.P.H.S.,
ATLANTA, GA.

Fig. 19. This map was prepared for comparison with the map of Rocky Mountain spotted fever (p. 105). It shows the distribution and incidence of murine typhus in the United States during the five-year period, 1944–1948, inclusive, per million population (based on 1940 census). The data were furnished by Dr. A. Langmuir, Communicable Disease Center, U.S. Public Health Service, Atlanta, Georgia.

in the medical literature before Brill's disease was defined as an entity. Attention has already been called to the erroneous use of the term "Brill's disease" for cases of murine typhus, a point which is again emphasized in the interest of clarity. Indeed, several of the papers which prepared the way for the final differentiation of epidemic from murine typhus refer by title to "Brill's disease," although the cases under discussion were murine flea-borne typhus.

In 1922, Hone reported several isolated cases from Australia, and Wheatland described a noncontagious typhus-like fever in the farm population of Queensland at a time when a plague of mice afflicted that part of Australia. Maxcy concluded that typhus in the southeastern United States must have a reservoir other than man, and he mentioned mice and rats specifically. He further suggested that fleas, mites or ticks could be the vector. Mooser in 1928 observed a basic difference in behavior of certain strains of typhus rickettsiae in the tissues of guinea pigs. Dyer and his colleagues isolated typhus rickettsiae from

reported from most of the United States. The total number of cases between 1931 and 1949 exceeds 40,000. The reported incidence was increasing up to 1946; the decrease since 1946 has been attributed in part to the control measures which have been vigorously applied in certain states.

Etiology and Transmission. Murine typhus fever is caused by *Rickettsia mooseri*. This micro-organism is similar to *R. prowazeki* in size, shape and staining properties. The disease is maintained in nature as a mild infection of rats transmitted from rat to rat by the rat louse or the rat flea. Neither the health nor the life span of the rat flea, *Xenopsylla cheopis,* is impaired by *R. mooseri;* once infected, the rat flea probably continues to excrete *R. mooseri* in its feces for the rest of its life. The eggs laid by infected female fleas do not transmit *R. mooseri* to the next generation of fleas. Man usually acquires the disease when bitten by an infected flea. In certain circumstances it is also possible that the ingestion of food recently contaminated by infected rat urine or flea feces may result in murine typhus.

Unlike epidemic typhus, murine typhus is maintained in nature independently of man by the rat-flea-rat transmission cycle. The disease is not spread from one patient to another. It has been reported that human body lice have been responsible for small outbreaks of murine typhus in which *R. mooseri* has been transmitted from man to man in the same manner as described for *R. prowazeki*. This point cannot be settled until the more recently developed techniques for differentiation of epidemic from murine typhus rickettsiae are applied to the micro-organisms involved in such outbreaks of presumed louseborne murine typhus. The point is of great interest, however, since it has been postulated that murine typhus rickettsiae may change to the epidemic variety as a consequence of man-louse-man passage. This must likewise be studied further before conclusions are justified.

Morbid Anatomy. Information on the morbid anatomy of murine typhus is limited, but it is usually assumed that the lesions are essentially the same as those in epidemic typhus.

Pathologic Physiology and Chemistry. Murine typhus has been even less well studied than epidemic typhus as regards abnormalities in physiology and chemistry. No important qualitative differences between the two diseases are recognized, the deviations from normal in murine typhus being relatively infrequent and small in extent.

Symptoms and Clinical Course. The incubation period of murine typhus lasts from six to fourteen days, most often twelve days. The symptoms are similar to those of epidemic typhus. The principal differences between the clinical course of the two diseases are that murine typhus is milder and shorter; the rash is less extensive and persists for shorter periods; there are fewer complications; and the case fatality rate is lower (less than 5 per cent for all groups).

It is impossible to distinguish an ordinary case of murine from a mild case of epidemic typhus solely on clinical evidence. Although epidemiologic considerations are valuable, it should be emphasized that murine typhus is world-wide in distribution and may occur in the same localities as epidemic typhus.

Diagnosis. *Clinical Diagnosis.* The diagnosis of murine typhus is suspected when a patient has a sustained fever of several days' duration accompanied by headache, generalized aches and pains, and a macular rash appearing on the fifth or sixth day after onset of the fever. The rash is first noted on the trunk and later spreads to the extremities; the face, palms and soles are not involved. Since murine typhus is present in many of the places where Rocky Mountain spotted fever occurs, it is helpful to recall that the rash of the latter disease usually appears on the exposed extremities first, later involving the body, and that it often appears on the face, palms and soles. The patient with murine typhus usually gives a history of activities likely to bring him into contact with places where rats are numerous, a feature which is valuable in directing attention to the possibility of murine typhus. Nevertheless, a definite recollection of a flea bite is often absent.

Laboratory Diagnosis. The diagnosis of murine typhus is usually established by serologic tests, as indicated in the section on Epidemic Typhus. The use of washed specific rickettsial antigens, either in the complement fixation test or the rickettsial agglutination test, permits the differentiation of epidemic from murine typhus. Usually there is more than a twofold difference in the titer of the patient's serum against the two antigens, the higher value being found against the homologous antigen. Some difficulty may arise if the patient, previous to the attack of typhus, had received antityphus vaccine. In such cases the titers may be identical. Specific antibodies appear early in the second week of the disease, increase in amount during the first part of convalescence, and then subside slowly over a period of months. Some persons have demonstrable antibodies for years after an attack of typhus.

The Weil-Felix test, described earlier, does not distinguish between murine typhus and Rocky Mountain spotted fever. Consequently, the more specific rickettsial tests are preferred.

Rickettsia mooseri may be isolated from the blood of patients early in the disease by the inoculation of guinea pigs or rats. The scrotum of male guinea pigs often becomes enlarged a few days after inoculation with *R. mooseri,* and the testes cannot be pushed back into the abdomen because there are adhesions between the layers of the tunica vaginalis. This is called the Neill-Mooser or the tunica reaction. It is not specific for murine typhus, however, and is no longer regarded as the principal criterion for the differentiation of epidemic from murine typhus.

Prognosis. Murine typhus is usually mild, with fatalities only in the older age groups. The use of specific treatment is expected to reduce the severity of the illness.

Treatment. The comments on treatment as given in the section on Epidemic Typhus apply equally well to murine typhus.

Prevention and Control. The measures to prevent and control murine typhus are (1) use of DDT dust on rat runs to reduce the flea population of the rat colonies, followed by (2) reduction of the rat population by poisoning, trapping, rat-proofing buildings, eliminating rat harborages such as trash or rubbish piles and the like.

Vaccine suitable for human immunization is available and is recommended for persons who are likely to be exposed to murine typhus—for example, personnel engaged in rat control programs or laboratory workers. There is no justification for immunization of the general population, since the attack rate is low and the measures for specific treatment are effective. It should be noted that *murine* typhus vaccine is not effective against *epidemic* typhus, and vice versa. However, an attack of either disease protects man against an attack of the other in most instances.

JOHN C. SNYDER

References

American Association for the Advancement of Science: Rickettsial Diseases of Man. A.A.A.S., Washington, D.C., 1948.

Cox, H. R.: Cultivation of Rickettsiae of the Rocky Mountain Spotted Fever, Typhus, and Q Fever Groups in the Embryonic Tissues of Developing Chicks. Science, 94:399, 1941.

Loeffler, W., and Mooser, H.: Ein weiterer Fall von Brill-Zinsserscher Krankheit in Zurich. Schweiz. med. Wchnschr., 82:493, 1952.

McAllister, W. B.: The Pathology of Louse-Borne Typhus Fever from the Epidemic of 1943–1945 in Egypt. Nav. Med. Res. Inst., Proj. NM 007 017 (X-696), Rep. #1, 25 January 1949.

Mooser, H.: Experiments Relating to the Pathology and the Etiology of Mexican Typhus (Tabardillo). J. Infect. Dis., 43:241, 1928.

———: Die Beziehungen des murinen Fleckfiebers zum klassichen Fleckfieber. Acta Tropica, Supplementum 4. Basel, Switzerland, A. G. Reinhardt, 1945.

———: Twenty Years of Research in Typhus Fever. Schweiz. med. Wchnschr., 76:877, 1946.

Murchison, C.: A Treatise on the Continued Fevers of Great Britain. 3rd ed. London, Longmans, Green and Co., 1884.

Murray, E. S., and others: Brill's Disease. IV. Study of 26 Cases in Yugoslavia. Am. J. Pub. Health., 41:1359, 1951.

———, and Snyder, J. C.: Brill-Zinsser Disease: the Interepidemic Reservoir of Epidemic Louse-Borne Typhus Fever. Presented at the Sixth International Congress of Microbiology in Rome, September 1953.

da Rocha-Lima, H.: Zur Aetiologie des Fleckfiebers. Kriegspathol. Tagung, April 26, 1916; pp. 45–50, Beiheft zu Band 27, Zentralbl. f. allg. Path. u. path. Anat.

Smadel, J. E.: Evaluation of New Drugs in the Treatment of Rickettsial Diseases. Boletin de la Oficina Sanitaria Panamericana, 28:1, 1949.

Snyder, J. C., and others: Further Observations on the Treatment of Typhus Fever with Para-aminobenzoic Acid. Ann. Int. Med., 27:1, 1947.

Wolbach, S. B., Todd, J. L., and Palfrey, F. W.: The Etiology and Pathology of Typhus. Cambridge, Harvard University Press, 1922.

Yeomans, A.: Typhus Fever, in Christian: Oxford Medicine. New York, Oxford University Press, 1947, Vol. 5, p. 439.

Zinsser, H.: Rats, Lice, and History. Boston, Little, Brown and Co., 1935.

Q FEVER

Definition. Q fever is an acute, self-limited illness characterized by abrupt onset, high but somewhat irregular fever, headache and, in many instances, pneumonitis similar to that of primary atypical pneumonia. The first few cases of this disease were called "Query fever," and from this designation the final name "Q fever" evolved (Derrick).

Etiology. Q fever is caused by the microorganism *Coxiella burneti,* which is named for Burnet, who first recognized it in Australia, and for Cox, who described it in the United States. *Coxiella burneti* resembles the other rickettsiae in size, shape and staining properties, but it differs in certain respects; for example, it is more resistant to adverse physical and chemical factors than the other rickettsiae. An important feature is that *C. burneti* is the only rickettsial species which infects man without producing a macular or maculopapular rash. Furthermore, agglutinins for the Proteus group do not appear in human or animal serums as a consequence of infection with *C. burneti.* In the febrile stage of Q fever the micro-organisms have been recovered from the blood, urine and sputum of patients by appropriate laboratory procedures.

Distribution and Transmission. Q fever has been reported from Australia, the United States, Panama, Europe, the Middle East, North and Central Africa, possibly India and China. It is, therefore, potentially worldwide in distribution. The manner in which the disease is usually acquired by man is probably by inhalation of desiccated Q fever rickettsiae derived from various sources.

Q fever rickettsiae have been found in the milk of naturally infected cattle, sheep and goats, in the placentas of cattle and sheep and in the feces of sheep. The presence of huge numbers of Q fever rickettsiae in these locations usually is not associated with any evidence of illness of the animal. Pasteurization of milk is not completely effective in destroying the viability of Q fever rickettsiae in milk which has been heavily contaminated. Furthermore, Q fever rickettsiae have been demonstrated in dust-laden air at dairies in California. Butter made from contaminated milk may contain viable Q fever rickettsiae.

In the United States, human infections have been reported from many areas, particularly California, Montana, Texas and Illinois. Occupational exposure has been related to the occurrence of cases, for example in laboratories where the Q fever rickettsiae are cultivated, and in dusty environments where wool is processed. On the basis of serologic tests it is estimated that several thousand persons had Q fever in southern California in recent years. The disease is only rarely acquired by contact with patients suffering from Q fever; this fact is remarkable in view of the pneumonitis which is a feature of many of the cases. It should be noted that *C. burneti* has been found in certain ticks, but that only a few human cases of Q fever have been attributed to contact with infected ticks.

Morbid Anatomy. Few fatal cases of Q fever have been reported, and, in most of these, autopsies were not performed. Consequently, satisfactory data are not available for general remarks on the pathology of Q fever. The reader is referred to the articles by Lillie, Perrin and Armstrong, and Whittick.

Pathologic Physiology and Chemistry. The abnormalities in physiology and chemistry noted in Q fever are those which usually accompany mild fevers of diverse etiology.

Transient albuminuria and elevated sedimentation rates have been reported. The erythrocyte count and concentration of hemoglobin are usually normal, and the total leukocyte count is often within normal limits. Changes in the differential count have been noted, but are without diagnostic significance.

Symptoms and Clinical Course. The incubation period of Q fever is two to three weeks. In several outbreaks the onset occurred abruptly, but there are numerous cases in which the disease began insidiously. Malaise, chilly sensations, headache, anorexia and weakness are usually the first symptoms noted. The *temperature* rises more or less abruptly to 39° C. or higher. There are usually wide fluctuations in temperature, particularly if salicylates are administered. The fever persists for a few days in mild cases, or it may last for two weeks in severe cases. The *pulse rate* tends to be somewhat elevated, more or less in proportion to the fever. Generalized muscular aching is frequent. Retro-orbital pain is usually noted and is sometimes accompanied by photophobia. In some cases there may be severe and sharply localized pain which either shifts from one site to another, or persists for only a few hours.

Toward the end of the first week of illness a dry cough develops in more than half the patients. This may be accompanied by mild to moderate chest pain. In a few patients the cough may become productive of small amounts of sputum, occasionally blood-streaked. Despite the cough and chest pain, few patients have symptoms or signs of upper respiratory involvement as part of the Q fever syndrome. The rate of respiration ordinarily is not elevated. Furthermore, physical examination of the chest may reveal nothing to indicate the presence of pneumonitis, which is the characteristic feature of Q fever, although fine crepitant rales may reward a careful search. In nearly all cases roentgenographic examination, however, indicates the presence of patchy areas of consolidation involving only small portions of the lobe. A single lesion is the usual finding, but multiple involvement has been noted. Ordinarily, the lesions are in the lower lobes, but they may occur in any lobe. It is difficult or impossible to distinguish these findings from those which are present in atypical pneumonia or psittacosis (see p. 49). No correlation has been observed between the extent of pulmonary involvement as judged from the roentgenogram and the severity of the clinical course. The pulmonary lesions sometimes may be found by roentgenogram when the patient is convalescent.

The illness usually ends with complete recovery and the period of convalescence ordinarily is brief, but relapses have occurred in several instances; they are similar to the primary disease and may be mild or severe. The possibility of chronic infection with Q fever has been raised; this question needs careful study. It is probable that there have been many human cases of Q fever so mild as to escape medical attention.

Diagnosis. The clinical diagnosis of Q fever should be considered when a patient has a febrile illness with anorexia, weakness, severe headache and roentgenographic evidence of a patchy pneumonitis. The absence of symptoms or signs of upper respiratory tract involvement is helpful. The presence of pain in the eyes or of photophobia is a further aid. A prompt response to specific therapy with tetracycline or chloramphenicol may assist the clinical diagnosis. The final diagnosis is usually established by laboratory tests, however, particularly by a rise in titer of complement-fixing antibodies in the patient's serum early in convalescence. It is *not* advisable to attempt isolation of *Coxiella burneti* from a patient by inoculation of animals, since this procedure usually results in infection among the laboratory personnel. The Weil-Felix reaction and the cold agglutinin test are negative in Q fever.

Prognosis. The case fatality rate in Q fever is very low. The appropriate use of a tetracycline or chloramphenicol early in the illness should improve the prognosis.

Treatment. The tetracyclines (Aureomycin, Terramycin) or chloramphenicol may be used for Q fever. On the basis of present evidence, any of these drugs may be expected to arrest the illness promptly. Relapses may be anticipated if therapy is terminated too soon after the fall in temperature. These agents should be given in the same dosage for Q fever as for Rocky Mountain spotted fever or epidemic typhus (see p. 111).

Prevention. Preventive measures include the pasteurization or boiling of milk from cows, goats and sheep. Vaccine prepared from killed *Coxiella burneti* is in the trial stage, being used for laboratory workers at present. Its use is not recommended on a community-wide scale. For the infected patient, only one precaution is recommended, namely, the sterilization of sputum and excreta.

JOHN C. SNYDER

References

Berge, T. O., and Lennette, E. H.: World Distribution of Q Fever: Human, Animal and Arthropod Infection. Am. J. Hyg., 57:125, 1953.

Burnet, F. M., and Freeman, M.: Experimental Studies on the Virus of "Q" Fever. M. J. Australia, 2:299, 1937.

Cox, H. R.: *Rickettsia diaporica* and American Q Fever. Am. J. Trop. Med., 20:463, 1940.

————: Cultivation of Rickettsiae of the Rocky Mountain Spotted Fever, Typhus and Q Fever Groups in the Embryonic Tissues of Developing Chicks. Science, 94:399, 1941.

Derrick, E. H.: "Q" Fever, a New Fever Entity: Clinical Features, Diagnosis and Laboratory Investigations. M. J. Australia, 2:281, 1937.

————: The Epidemiology of "Q" Fever: A Review. M. J. Australia, 1953, page 245.

Lillie, R. D., Perrin, T. L., and Armstrong, C.: An Institutional Outbreak of Pneumonitis. III. Histopathology in Man and Rhesus Monkeys in the Pneumonitis Due to the Virus of "Q" Fever. Pub. Health Rep., 56:149, 1941.

Robbins, F. C.: Q Fever, Clinical Features, in Rickettsial Diseases of Man. American Association for the Advancement of Science, 1948, p. 160.

Whittick, J. W.: Necropsy Findings in a Case of Q Fever in Britain. Brit. M. J., 1:979, 1950.

ROCKY MOUNTAIN SPOTTED FEVER

(Spotted Fever, Tick Fever, Tick Typhus [England], Fiebre Manchada [Mexico], Fiebre Petequial [Colombia], Febre Maculosa [Brazil])

Definition. Rocky Mountain spotted fever is an acute, specific infectious endangiitis, chiefly of the peripheral blood vessels, caused by *Rickettsia rickettsii* and transmitted by ticks. It is characterized by an onset with chills; continued fever of almost two weeks' duration, terminating in lysis; severe pains in the bones and muscles; headache; and a macular eruption, becoming petechial, which appears after the middle of the first week on the wrists, ankles and back, and then spreads over the whole surface of the body.

History. The disease has probably existed in Idaho and Montana since the first settlement by white men, and seems to have been known to the Indians before that time. It was first described by Surgeon Major W. W. Wood, in 1896, in a report to the Surgeon-General. Maxcy of Idaho and McCullough of Montana gave the earliest clinical descriptions of the disease. Important laboratory and field investigations were made by Wilson and Chowning, and by Ricketts and his associates. Ricketts established the transmission of the disease by the tick, and defined most of the problems which have resulted in our present knowledge of the disease and its causation.

Distribution, Transmission and Incidence. Rocky Mountain spotted fever is limited to the western hemisphere. However,

Since the rickettsiae are transmitted transovarially by certain ticks, these vectors probably serve also as reservoirs.

Ten species of ixodid ticks have been found infected in nature in the western hemisphere; this by no means exhausts the list of potential vectors of the disease. The seasonal periodicity of spotted fever in man in a given area is related to the life cycle of the local

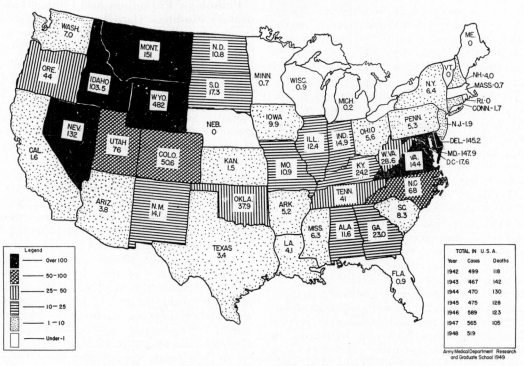

SPOTTED FEVER 1942-1946
5 YEAR ATTACK RATE PER MILLION POPULATION BY STATES

Legend

- Over 100
- 50—100
- 25— 50
- 10— 25
- 1 — 10
- Under—1

TOTAL IN U.S.A.		
Year	Cases	Deaths
1942	499	118
1943	467	142
1944	470	130
1945	475	128
1946	589	123
1947	565	105
1948	519	

Army Medical Department Research and Graduate School 1949

Fig. 20. Incidence of spotted fever in the United States in recent years.

closely related diseases occur throughout the world wherever *Ixodidae* have opportunity to feed on man; these include boutonneuse fever of the Mediterranean basin, South African tick-bite fever, North Queensland tick typhus, and perhaps the tick-borne rickettsioses of India and Russia. Although the term "Rocky Mountain" is firmly fixed as part of the name for American spotted fever, it now implies too restrictive a distribution of the disease. This malady has been recognized throughout the United States, except in Maine and Vermont, as well as in Canada, Mexico, Colombia and Brazil. No animal has been definitely incriminated as the reservoir for *Rickettsia rickettsii,* but all small mammal hosts are suspect, particularly rabbits.

vector tick; however, the majority of cases occur in late spring and early summer.

The annual incidence of cases of spotted fever in the United States from 1942 to 1948 is given in figure 20. About 500 cases occurred each year, and the case mortality was about 20 per cent. Figure 20 also presents graphically the attack rate per million population by states for the five year period 1942–1946. About two fifths of all the cases in the United States during this period occurred in the Middle Atlantic seaboard states of Delaware, Maryland, Virginia and North Carolina. The mountain states of Montana, Idaho, Wyoming, Colorado, Utah and Nevada contributed only two thirds as many cases as the eastern group, but Wyoming's rate was the highest in the country. In the West, where the wood tick (*Dermacentor andersoni*) is the vector, a relatively higher proportion of adult males contract the disease. On the other hand, in the East, where the dog tick (*Dermacentor variabilis*) is mainly responsible for transmission, children and women are mainly affected. Occupational propinquity to the vector is responsible for this distribution, not variations in susceptibility of different ages and sexes.

The mortality varies with age, being higher in adults than in children. Before the advent of specific chemotherapeutic measures, the mortality rate for nonvaccinated adults in the Bitter Root Valley of Montana was about 80 per cent, in contrast to 37.5 per cent for children. Topping pointed out that approximately half the patients in the western states were over 40 years of age, whereas in the East about this same proportion were under 15 years. Little difference was noted in the fatality rates when patients from the two regions were compared on the basis of age.

Etiology. *Rickettsia rickettsii* (Wolbach) Brumpt, the proved cause of Rocky Mountain spotted fever, has a number of characteristics which distinguish it from the rickettsiae of the typhus and tsutsugamushi groups, in addition to immunologic differences. Prominent among these are its cyclic morphology in ticks, its hereditary transmission in ticks and its intranuclear as well as intracytoplasmic growth in tick and mammalian tissues. It is distinguished from other rickettsiae of the spotted fever group by several types of immunologic procedures. Strains of *R. rickettsii* vary considerably in their virulence for man and animals. A toxin associated with the etiologic agent is capable of killing mice within a few hours; it is similar in many respects to the toxins of the typhus rickettsiae.

Morbid Anatomy. The distinctive pathologic changes of spotted fever are found in the small vessels and are observed microscopically. The gross changes often are unimpressive and usually add little to the clinical findings. The following description of the histopathology is taken from Wolbach's classical studies.

The blood vessel lesions consist at first of a proliferative reaction of the endothelium, followed by thrombosis, either mural or occluding. A considerable degree of perivascular infiltration occurs, but the perivascular nodules of typhus do not develop.

The causal agent of the disease is found in endothelial cells and also in smooth muscle cells of blood vessel walls. Arteries, veins and capillaries are affected. Minute focal lesions of the central nervous system, resembling those of typhus, but accompanied by more conspicuous infarction of arterioles, are common in patients who survive more than twelve days. In addition to lesions of small blood vessels, diffuse infiltrations by mononuclear cells, chiefly monocytes, are found in the heart, liver, spleen and in the alveolar walls of the lungs. Small areas of necrosis and considerable damage to the endothelium of the sinusoids are found in the liver.

Pathologic Physiology and Clinical Laboratory Findings. Harrell points out that in fulminating disease with death early in the first week, the picture is that of peripheral vascular collapse. There is marked dilatation of capillaries and pooling of blood without increased capillary permeability or loss of fluid into extravascular spaces. As the proliferative and thrombotic lesions develop in the small vessels, anoxia occurs in the areas supplied with the usual resultant effects, including necrosis. In severe infections there is increasing capillary permeability with loss of water, electrolytes, proteins and erythrocytes. This and other contributing factors result in a decrease in plasma volume and in serum proteins and chlorides along with an increase in thiocyanate space and even clinical edema. Electrocardiographic changes consistent with edema and anoxia of the myocardium are found. Liver function is diminished, as evidenced by slight elevation of serum bilirubin and marked reduction of hippuric acid excretion after benzoic acid administration. The elevated nonprotein nitrogen appears to be an extrarenal type of azotemia. These various abnormalities intensify one another and set the stage for the development of terminal peripheral vascular collapse. With recovery, whether natural or induced by specific antimicrobial therapy, most of the physiologic abnormalities are rapidly corrected; however, loss of edema fluid and restoration of serum proteins may take several weeks in the patient who suffered severe disease. In the milder cases or in those given specific treatment early, the physiologic observations are minimal.

The urine is that of any febrile disease. Moderate leukopenia with neutropenia is frequent during the first few days; eosinophils are decreased or absent. Subsequently, a mild leukocytosis appears with an increase in polymorphonuclear cells and a shift toward the left in the Schilling hemogram. During the second week a normochromic, normocytic anemia generally appears; hemoglobin values of 9 grams and erythrocyte counts of 3,000,000 per cubic milliliter are common. The blood platelets remain within normal limits but the prothrombin time may become somewhat elevated late in the disease. Increased capillary fragility is usually demon-

evident in cases which prove to be relatively mild. The onset is usually accompanied by a chill, and there are severe general pains referred to the bones, muscles, back and joints, particularly in the calf muscles, large joints and lumbar region of the back. Headache is common and severe. The face is flushed, the conjunctivas injected, and the tongue white-

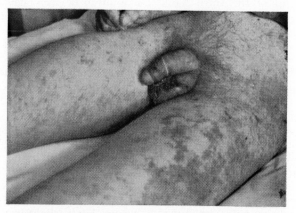

Fig. 21. Rocky Mountain spotted fever. Photograph of skin lesions taken two days before death. (Courtesy of Dr. George E. Baker, Casper, Wyoming.)

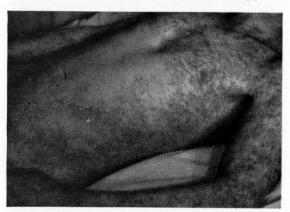

Fig. 22. Same patient as in Figure 21, illustrating coalescence of skin lesions, which have become purpuric. Localized areas of necrosis are evident. (Courtesy of Dr. George E. Baker, Casper, Wyoming.)

strable by the tourniquet test. The cerebrospinal fluid may be under slightly increased pressure and show a slight pleocytosis, especially in patients with severe cerebral involvement. Serologic findings are discussed in the section on Diagnosis.

Symptoms. *Incubation.* The incubation period of the more severe infections is two to five days, and of the milder ones from three to fourteen days.

Prodromal Stage. Before the definite onset of the disease there may be a few days of malaise, accompanied by chilly sensations and loss of appetite. A prodromal stage is more

coated with moist edges and tip. Constipation is usual. There is usually photophobia, and there may be epistaxis. A short dry cough is common. The patient is frequently ill enough to take to bed on the second day of symptoms.

Temperature. Before the initial chill there may be a slight evening elevation of temperature. After the chill the temperature rises fairly rapidly and reaches 102° to 104° F. (38.8° to 40° C.) by the second day. In nonvaccinated persons who contract the disease and do not receive specific therapy the fever continues to rise gradually to a maximum of 104° to 105° F. (40 to 40.5° C.) during the second week. In very severe cases in the Bitter Root Valley, temperatures from 106° to 107° F. have been recorded. The maximum temperature persists in untreated patients throughout the second week of the disease, with slight morning drops, then falls by lysis, so that normal temperature is reached before the end of the third week. After recovery the temperature may be slightly subnormal for a few days. In fatal cases the temperature may drop to normal or subnormal and then rise eighteen to twenty-four hours before death, which in severe cases usually takes place between the sixth and twelfth days of the disease.

The *pulse* is at first full and strong, but gradually loses volume and strength, and increases in rapidity out of proportion to the fever. During the height of the fever the blood pressure is markedly lowered as in typhus fever. The pulse rate ranges from 110 to 140, and may reach 150 a few days before death. A pulse rate of 120 with a temperature of 102° F. is not uncommon. Electrocardiographic changes occur (see section on Pathologic Physiology).

The *respirations* behave very much as does the pulse. They are rapid and out of proportion to the apparent severity of the illness, usually 30 to 40 a minute, but increasing occasionally to 60 before death.

Eruption. The rash appears most often on the third day of fever, but may occur later during the first week, or rarely on the second day. Occasionally it may be preceded by a mottled appearance of the skin of the face, neck and upper chest, inconstant in appearance, sometimes suggesting the onset of measles. It appears first on the flexor surfaces of the wrists and ankles and back, then on the forehead, arms, legs, chest and abdomen. The efflorescence requires twenty-four to thirty-six hours, although the eruption may appear still later than this on the palms of the hands, soles of the feet, and scalp. The mucosa of the cheeks, palate, fauces and pharynx may show the eruption. The temperature is not appreciably affected at the time of the eruption, but the subjective symptoms ameliorate. The rash at first is in the form of rose-colored macules 1 to 4 or 5 mm. in diameter, not elevated, not palpable, and disappearing upon pressure. The skin may be tender at the site of the spots. The macules soon become deep red or purplish and increase in size, often becoming confluent. After a few

days the rash begins to persist upon pressure, and then becomes generally petechial. Cutaneous and subcutaneous hemorrhages of considerable size occur frequently in severe cases, and the skin in the second week of the disease may assume a glazed appearance. Where the skin is thin, as over the thighs, a peculiar dusky reddish or bluish mottling may often be seen, which is due to stasis of blood in the subcutaneous vessels because of thrombosis. In mild cases the rash does not become confluent, and the petechiae, remaining small, give a peculiar mottling which several Idaho physicians have compared to the markings of turkeys' eggs. Slight icterus may appear in the second week of the disease.

The rash begins to disappear with the subsidence of fever, but may long be indicated by the persistence of pigmented spots. Necrosis of the skin of the scrotum, prepuce, fingers, toes, vulva, lobes of the ear and mucous membrane of the soft palate may occur in the third week. *Desquamation* follows recovery, but is slight except where the lesions have been most marked. Minute cicatrices in the skin may persist for a long time after recovery. In very mild cases the rash may be limited to one extremity. In persons previously vaccinated the rash may be entirely absent.

Neurologic Symptoms. Restlessness and insomnia are common throughout the disease, constituting its most distressing features. Hyperesthesia may be severe. Delirium is usual in severe cases during the height of the fever, and coma usually precedes death by a few hours or a day. Rarely, convulsions, muscular rigidity and opisthotonus occur. After recovery, deafness, visual disturbances, slurring speech and mental confusion have been noted for a few weeks.

Complications and Sequelae. Secondary pneumonia is the one important complication and it is infrequent. Circulatory failure and necrosis of tissue may be looked upon as resulting directly from severe pathologic changes characteristic of the infection rather than as complications. Harrell (1952) has drawn attention to evidence of residual damage in the heart and brain of certain recovered patients.

Immunity. Recovery from Rocky Mountain spotted fever is accompanied by complete immunity for a long period of years. According to Parker (1938), second infections have been reported eight or more years after the first, in some instances ending fatally.

Guinea pigs recovered from feebly virulent strains are not fully protected against highly virulent strains. Recovery from virulent strains does confer complete and lasting immunity in animals.

A brief period of passive immunity may be conferred by the injection of blood from an immune animal.

Active immunity can be produced by the injection of chemically killed rickettsiae; the use of vaccine is discussed under Prophylaxis.

Diagnosis. Theoretically, the same diseases must be considered in the differential diagnosis of Rocky Mountain spotted fever as in typhus, but practically, the seasonal incidence of the disease and its prevalence in certain geographic areas eliminate a number of possibilities. *Meningococcal infections* and *measles* are the two diseases most liable to be temporarily mistaken for Rocky Mountain spotted fever. Spinal puncture should be resorted to when there is a question of meningococcal infection, since the rash may simulate that of Rocky Mountain spotted fever. Usually the more severe nervous symptoms, with early rigidity of the neck, and the character of the onset of meningococcal infection with meningitis should serve to differentiate the two. Measles at its height in children presents difficulty, for the rash may closely resemble the early rash of spotted fever. The history of slower onset, with coryza and lacrimation, the presence of Koplik's spots, the absence of severe muscular pains, and the papular character and sequence of distribution of the rash are the most important differential data. Typhoid fever, with a pronounced rash, may also have to be excluded. The rash in typhoid fever, however, is more palpable and elevated than in Rocky Mountain spotted fever, and is generally more restricted to the trunk. A slower pulse rate, lower fever, diarrhea, and positive blood cultures, or a positive Widal reaction, make final exclusion simple.

Since Rocky Mountain spotted fever and endemic (murine) typhus coexist in at least twenty-three states, the problem of differential diagnosis often arises.

Spotted fever is essentially a rural disease, and exposure to ticks is important. Most cases occur in the spring and early summer. Endemic typhus, transmitted by the rat flea, is predominantly an urban disease in the United States, but has a rural distribution in certain areas of the South where peanuts are cultivated. It occurs most often in food handlers and peanut farmers whose premises are heavily infested with rats. In contrast with spotted fever, endemic typhus is more likely to occur in late summer and autumn.

The outstanding clinical difference is in the evolution and distribution of the rash. In endemic typhus it appears first on the chest and upper abdomen, usually spares the palms and soles and rarely involves the face and neck, wrists and ankles.

Final differentiation of spotted fever from endemic typhus, and also from epidemic typhus in some Latin American countries, often requires the use of specific complement fixation tests. This has become especially true since the introduction in 1948 of treatment with the antimicrobial drugs chloramphenicol and the tetracyclines; now these diseases may be cut short so early in their courses that the typical clinical picture never develops.

The Weil-Felix reaction is of some value in the diagnosis of spotted fever. All three types of *Proteus vulgaris* used (OX-19, OX-2 and OX-K stains) may be agglutinated by the patient's serum; most often the highest titer is obtained with the OX-19 strain, but occasionally with the OX-2 strain. A titer of 1:320 with a single convalescent serum is the lowest that can be considered of diagnostic importance, but, as in typhus, a rising titer during the course of the disease is of greatest significance. A test should be made as early as possible in the disease and repeated after the tenth day. A significant reaction may not be obtained until convalescence has begun.

A differential diagnosis between Rocky Mountain spotted fever and the other rickettsial diseases should not be attempted by means of the Weil-Felix reaction.*

The complement fixation technique using *Rickettsia rickettsii* as antigen provides a specific diagnostic test. Complement-fixing antibodies usually appear during the second or third week in patients who receive no specific therapy but may be delayed a week or so in those treated early in the disease. No cross-reactions are obtained with the typhus group, but an appreciable number of cross-reactions occurs with diseases of the spotted fever group, including mite-borne rickettsialpox. The more highly purified antigens give fewer cross-reactions.

Prognosis. The prognosis has changed radically since the introduction of treatment with chloramphenicol and the tetracyclines.

* See Typhus Fever for further consideration of the Weil-Felix reaction.

Previously the over-all mortality was about 20 per cent, now deaths are rare in treated patients and are limited essentially to those who first receive specific therapy late in the course of the disease. The prognosis in patients given only supportive treatment is best in vaccinated persons and in children and becomes progressively worse with advancing age or with secondary bacterial pneumonia.

Harrell (1949) indicates the difficulty of estimating the prognosis in an individual early case, but his classification of stages of severity of the disease is of interest. Mild cases are those with negative tourniquet tests throughout the illness, no edema, and stable pulse and blood pressure. Moderate cases show increased capillary fragility, slight clinical edema, tachycardia and toxic symptoms. Severely ill patients exhibit marked purpura, moderate edema, delirium, toxemia and vasomotor instability.

Prophylaxis. General measures for control of the disease are directed toward reducing the chance of contact with infected vector ticks and immunization against the rickettsial agent.

Recent advances have made personal prophylaxis, the avoidance of tick bites, more practicable than heretofore. Brennan has found that clothing treated with N-n-butyl-acetanilide gives excellent protection against nymphs and adults of *Amblyomma americanum*. Dimethyl-phthalate, one of the standard Army insect repellents, has only a slight effect against ticks.

Persons exposed in endemic tick-infested areas should preferably wear high boots and one-piece outer clothing. When camping, clothes and bedding should be carefully examined for ticks before use. Daily stripping and thoroughly inspecting the entire body for ticks, particularly about the hairline of the neck and the perineum, is strongly recommended; a shaving mirror will assist lone adults. Children should be inspected twice daily. The tick is slow to attach and ordinarily remains attached for a short time before beginning the act of feeding. Furthermore, at times the tick apparently cannot readily transmit the disease without having been attached for some hours.

Ticks which have attached should be removed with care. Applying ether, chloroform or kerosene to a tick or holding a lighted cigarette near it may cause the arthropod to detach. Otherwise forceps or tweezers should be used, grasping the tick as close as possible to the point of attachment and applying gentle traction lest the mouth parts remain embedded in the skin. Every effort should be made to avoid crushing the tick and contaminating the bite site with its contents. Disinfect the area of attachment with soap and water and the wound proper with a toothpick dipped in crude phenol. Silver nitrate and iodine are less effective.

Removal of engorged ticks with bare fingers from human beings or animals is dangerous, since infection through the unbroken skin is apparently possible.

Measures for reducing the tick population have definite prophylactic value, but, because of their cost, are rarely used primarily for the prevention of spotted fever in man. Clearing and cultivation of infested land renders such areas safe. Removal of ticks from live stock and dogs is an important control measure because these animals are regular hosts of adult *Dermacentor*. This should not be done by hand. A satisfactory dip for these animals is either 0.5 per cent chlordane or a combination of 0.025 per cent gamma isomer benzene hexachloride and 0.5 per cent DDT. Dust sprays containing these insecticides may also be used. None of these residual insecticides should be applied to cats, which lick their fur and hence may be poisoned. Campaigns for the destruction of small mammals which serve as hosts for the larval and nymphal ticks may be practicable in special circumstances, particularly when directed against cottontail rabbits. The rodenticide sodium monofluoracetate (Compound 1080) is most effective for this purpose, but its high toxicity for men restricts its use to specialized personnel.

Direct attack on the tick vectors by chemical means is feasible in selected instances. Both DDT and chlordane give excellent control of *Dermacentor* and *Amblyomma* ticks when applied directly to the ground and to low vegetation in the form of solutions, dusts or emulsions at the rate of about $2\frac{1}{2}$ pounds of either chemical to the acre. In certain areas, as in the northeastern United States, 90 per cent of the local *Dermacentor* population is frequently found within 4 feet of roads and trails. Most of this assemblage of ticks is often concentrated within a few inches of the trail margin.

Vaccines containing chemically killed *Rickettsia rickettsii* are of value. These were originally prepared from infected ticks (Spencer and Parker); more recently, from infected yolk sacs of embryonated eggs (Cox). The latter type is now produced commercially. Immunization comprises a course of three injections given in the spring before ticks become plentiful. The protective effect is sufficient to prevent or ameliorate the disease but is transient, and vaccination must be repeated annually. Vaccination has been one of the most important prophylactic measures for those habitually or occasionally exposed to spotted fever. It will no doubt continue to be useful for those at great risk, but the availability of highly satisfactory therapeutic agents may be expected to reduce its need in those subjected to only slight risk of infection.

Treatment. The introduction since 1947 of the antimicrobial drugs chloramphenicol and the tetracyclines, which are markedly effective in the treatment of rickettsial diseases, including spotted fever, has radically altered concepts of the therapy of this disease. Early diagnosis and the proper use of these new antimicrobials generally render the patient afebrile in a few days, and the severe disturbances of physiologic mechanisms associated with the classical disease are prevented or minimized. General supportive measures remain important, however, and their proper use in dangerously ill patients may tip the scale toward survival. Harrell has emphasized the similarity between the peripheral circulatory collapse of spotted fever and shock associated with burns and trauma. When such shock is present it should be treated vigorously in the usual manner; replacement of blood proteins by administration of plasma and by whole blood transfusions and restoration of blood volume with saline and glucose solutions are indicated. As in other forms of shock, these procedures should be carefully regulated on the basis of results of frequent chemical studies of the blood. Other general measures include those used for continuous fevers. The barbiturates are indicated if restlessness and insomnia contribute to exhaustion. Digitalis is rarely of value, since the major circulatory disturbances are of extracardiac origin. Penicillin is indicated in the presence of secondary bacterial pneumonia.

Pincoffs and his associates, who first demonstrated the specific therapeutic effect of chloramphenicol in spotted fever, observed that, irrespective of the height of the preceding fever, the age of the patient or the duration of the disease, all fifteen of their treated patients survived and their temperatures fell to normal within three days of initiating therapy (average 2.2 days). Although the eruption does not spread after treatment, clinical improvement is not striking until after the first day. Ross and his co-workers clearly demonstrated that oxytetracycline (Aureomycin) was also a highly satisfactory therapeutic agent in spotted fever and Bauer and his colleagues did the same for chlortetracycline (Terramycin). As for arresting the disease, there appears to be little choice between these three antimicrobial drugs. Each is vastly superior to para-aminobenzoic acid which was used before their introduction.

Chloramphenicol or a tetracycline is given orally in 2 to 4 gm. amounts as a "loading dose" over a few hours, followed by 2 to 4 gm. daily in divided doses at 6- to 8-hour intervals until the patient has been afebrile for a day or so. In patients too ill to take oral medication an intravenous preparation of one of the antimicrobials may be employed for the loading dose. Recent studies by Woodward's group at the University of Maryland and others (see Harrell, 1952) indicate that addition of cortisone to the usual chloramphenicol regimen produces a more rapid subsidence of fever and toxemia than antimicrobial therapy alone. Although still under investigation, this combined therapy should be considered for critically ill patients. A regimen of 200 mg. of cortisone, orally or intramuscularly, followed by 100 mg. doses at 6-hour intervals, has been used for this purpose but cortisone should not be continued after the patient becomes afebrile or for longer than 36 hours. The minor untoward manifestations of treatment with the tetracyclines and chloramphenicol are well known as are the rare but serious blood dyscrasias associated with use of chloramphenicol. Fear of neither type of toxic response should inhibit the physician from using these life-saving drugs in spotted fever which, if untreated, has a high mortality, a long convalescence and occasional sequelae.

JOSEPH E. SMADEL

References

Ash, J. E., and Spitz, S.: Pathology of Tropical Diseases; An Atlas. Philadelphia, W. B. Saunders Company, 1945, pp. 32–33, 47–49.

Bauer, R. E., and others: Clinical and Experimental Observations with Terramycin in Certain Rickettsial and Bacterial Infections. Ann. N. Y. Acad. Sci., 53:395, 1950.

Bell, E. J., and Pickens, E. G.: A Toxic Substance Associated with the Rickettsias of the Spotted Fever Group. J. Immunol., 70:461, 1953.

Bustamante, M. E., and Varela, G.: Caracteristicas de la Fiebre Manchada de las Montañas Rocosas en Sonora y Sinaloa, México. Rev. d. Inst. Salub. y Enferm. Trop., 5:129, 1944.

Cox, H. R.: The Spotted-Fever Group, in Rivers, T. M.: Viral and Rickettsial Infections of Man. 2nd ed. Philadelphia, J. B. Lippincott Company, 1952, pp. 611–637.

Harrell, G. T.: Rocky Mountain Spotted Fever. Medicine, 28:333, 1949.

————: Treatment of Rocky Mountain Spotted Fever with Antibiotics. Ann. N. Y. Acad. Sci., 55: 1027, 1952.

Pincoffs, M. C., and others: The Treatment of Rocky Mountain Spotted Fever with Chloromycetin. Ann. Int. Med., 29:656, 1948.

Ricketts, H. T.: Contributions to Medical Science by Howard Taylor Ricketts, 1870–1910. Chicago, University of Chicago Press, 1911.

Ross, S., and others: Aureomycin Therapy of Rocky Mountain Spotted Fever. J.A.M.A., 138:1213, 1948.

Wolbach, S. B.: Studies on Rocky Mountain Spotted Fever. J. Med. Res., 41:1, 1919.

SCRUB TYPHUS

(Tsutsugamushi Disease, Mite-Borne Typhus, Japanese River Fever, Tropical Typhus, Rural Typhus)

Definition. Scrub typhus is a self-limited febrile illness of two weeks' duration caused by *Rickettsia tsutsugamushi,* transmitted by chiggers and distributed widely in the Asiatic-Pacific area. It is characterized by sudden onset of fever accompanied by a primary skin lesion (eschar) and by the development of rash on about the fifth day.

History. Scrub typhus may have been known in South China during the sixteenth century, but the earliest recognizable description of the disease was by Hashimoto in 1810. He noted that the disease (tsutsuga) occurred along the banks of the Shinano River in Japan and that the natives of the area believed it to be caused by the bite of a minute insect or mite (mushi). Although it was extensively studied by Japanese investigators after its original description, the interest of Western physicians remained dormant until the disease was recognized in Sumatra and Malaya about twenty-five years ago.

During World War II, scrub typhus emerged from obscurity to occupy a position of great importance in military medicine. Philip tabulated the cases in the Allied Armies in the Pacific-Southeast Asia-India areas during 1942–1945 and found 18,450 incidents of scrub typhus; this tabulation is by no means complete. The United States Army had 243 deaths among its 6685 men who contracted the disease.

Distribution and Incidence. Scrub typhus continues to occur in a number of sharply defined areas in river valleys of northwest Honshu Island, Japan. It is present in Formosa, the Pescadores, the Philippines, and on south through the island chains to the northern shore of Australia. To the west it is found in Java, Sumatra, Malaya, Siam, Indo-China, Burma, India, Ceylon and a number of the island groups in the Indian Ocean.

There are no reliable statistics on incidence of the disease in civilian populations in the Asiatic-Pacific area; however, it is possible to arrive at certain estimates. In the Shinano River area of Japan a survey was made in 1947 of the history of previous attacks of scrub typhus among 2300 farmers whose occupation exposed them in infected fields during the mite season each year; the average period of exposure was nine years. There were 247 attacks among these farmers during a total of 20,692 person-years' exposure. This gives an attack rate, in which the patient recovered, of twelve cases per thousand farmers per year. Because of limited geographic distribution of the disease in Japan, the total number of cases is probably only a few hundred each year.

The disease is more common in parts of Southeast Asia than in Japan. Selangor, one of the states of the Federation of Malaya, with an area about two-thirds that of Connecticut and a population of about 400,000, reported 162 cases of typhus with 3 deaths in the first eight months of 1948. The U. S. Army Scrub Typhus Research Unit working there during three months of this period diagnosed and treated forty-three of the 162 cases. Forty of the group were proved to have scrub typhus, and one of these died; the remaining three had murine typhus. On the basis of these data there were 565 cases of scrub typhus per million population in Selangor during 1948. This is appreciably higher than for Malaya as a whole or for any known general civil population on which even an estimated rate can be made.

High attack rates were attained during brief periods in certain Allied military groups during World War II. Among Americans at the Sansapor beach head, in the Southwest Pacific, 403 men of one regiment suffered the disease between the sixth and twentieth days after landing; moreover, the attack rate during the second week at Sansapor reached 900 cases per thousand troops per year.

Similarly, 18 per cent of one British battalion contracted scrub typhus during two months in Burma in 1944, and 5 per cent of the total strength died of the disease.

The mortality in scrub typhus has varied widely in different geographic areas and in different populations. The highest rates have been in Japan, where 40 to 60 per cent of the diagnosed patients have succumbed. In Malaya, during the past twenty years, about 7 per cent of the cases terminated fatally. Even in the same general area and in a relatively homogeneous population, viz., United States Army personnel in the Southwest Pacific, the case fatality ranged between 0.6 and 35 per cent for the outbreaks at Owi-Biak and Finchaven, respectively. Many factors undoubtedly contribute to the variations in mortality of scrub typhus, but it is well established that certain strains of *Rickettsia tsutsugamushi* are more virulent than others for laboratory animals, and presumably this is also true for man.

Epidemiology. Scrub typhus is transmitted to man by at least two species of mites, *Trombicula akamushi* and *T. deliensis*. Only the six-legged larvae are parasitic on mammals and birds. The nymphs and adults, both of which have eight legs, also live in soil and vegetation, but presumably feed on eggs of mosquitoes and other insects. The tiny (0.15 to 0.4 mm.) red larvae attach themselves to the skin of the host and obtain a feeding of lymph or tissue juice. During the attachment infected larvae may transmit *Rickettsia tsutsugamushi* to the host, or uninfected larvae may acquire rickettsiae from a host with active disease. The rickettsiae apparently maintain a symbiotic existence in the mite, since their presence does not interfere with the development and propagation of the arthropod. In *T. deliensis* at least, the rickettsiae are transmitted transovarially from one generation to the next. Thus the mite serves both as the vector and as a reservoir of the causal agent. Various small rodents constitute the animal reservoir. In different regions these include rats, voles, shrews and field mice.

Endemic areas of scrub typhus occur in different types of terrain, but are found most often in fields which, through neglect, have been permitted to become overgrown with scrub vegetation. The essential features of an endemic focus are (1) adequate ground moisture and warmth for the propagation and emergence of vector mites, (2) suitable rodent population and (3) the presence of *R. tsutsugamushi* in rodent hosts and vectors of the area. Because of the exacting requirements for a focus, the endemic areas are often sharply delimited small islands of infection which present the same general appearance as surrounding uninfected terrain. Birds serve as hosts for vector mites and may help seed infection in nearby or distant areas.

Man is an incidental host for *Trombicula*. He contributes to the cycle of scrub typhus in nature by modifying the ecology of the region and thus influencing the rodent and mite populations. His occasional inadvertent infection with *R. tsutsugamushi* is unimportant in the maintenance of either the disease or endemic areas.

The seasonal incidence of human disease is dependent on the prevalence of mites. In Japan, cases occur during the summer months, when mites emerge and become numerous. In the subtropics and tropics, cases occur throughout the year whenever susceptibles are introduced into an endemic area. However, infections are more prevalent during the wet seasons, when vector mites are more abundant.

Etiology. *Rickettsia tsutsugamushi* (Hayashi) Ogata, the etiologic agent of scrub typhus, is an intracellular obligate parasitic micro-organism. It has the general properties of other rickettsiae pathogenic for man, but is distinguished from them by its host range and by its specific immunologic properties. Strains of *R. tsutsugamushi* vary in their virulence for animals, and at least one strain yields a toxic material which, in concentrated form, kills mice within a few hours. All strains have certain specific antigens in common, but the results obtained with a variety of immunologic techniques indicate that the species *R. tsutsugamushi* is not antigenically homogeneous. The growth of *R. tsutsugamushi* in experimental animals is inhibited by a number of chemical substances. The four which have proved of value in the treatment of patients with scrub typhus are para-aminobenzoic acid, chloramphenicol and the tetracyclines (Aureomycin and Terramycin).

Morbid Anatomy. Macroscopic changes found at autopsy are not striking. The primary eschar may be present, but no rash is seen. The body cavities contain moderate amount of serofibrinous fluid, and the parenchymatous organs show cloudy swelling. The spleen is enlarged, and there is generalized lymphadenopathy. Hemorrhagic pneumonia is usually present with superimposed secondary bronchopneumonia.

The basic histologic lesions in scrub typhus, as in other rickettsial diseases, are associated with the vascular tree. There is a disseminated focal vasculitis and a perivasculitis consisting of accumulations of monocytes, plasma cells and lymphocytes. The lesions are less severe than those of epidemic typhus, and involvement of the muscular coat of small arteries, such as occurs in spotted fever, is limited to the eschar. Vascular changes with resultant lesions in adjacent parenchymatous tissue are most prominent in the heart, lung, brain and kidney. Acute nonsuppurative myocarditis and encephalitis and an interstitial pneumonitis are found in almost all fatal cases.

Clinical Laboratory Findings. There are no specific cytologic or chemical changes in the blood in scrub typhus. During the first week of illness the total leukocyte count is normal, or moderate leukopenia occurs; leukocytosis generally indicates secondary bacterial infections. Anemia is rare, but the erythrocyte count often becomes reduced slightly during the disease. In severely ill patients the plasma proteins may be moderately reduced. Plasma fibrinogen may be decreased in cases with impairment of hepatic function, and the serum bilirubin may be slightly elevated. Profuse sweating and an inadequate intake of water and salts may produce disturbances of acid-base equilibrium.

Rickettsia tsutsugamushi can be recovered from the blood of patients throughout the first ten or twelve days of fever. The agent is demonstrated indirectly; white mice inoculated intraperitoneally with the blood sample acquire typical disease, and rickettsiae are found on microscopic examination of stained smears of their peritoneal scrapings. Late in the second week, agglutinins for the OX-K strain of *Bacillus proteus* appear in the patients' blood.

Symptoms. After an incubation period of six to eighteen days, generally ten to twelve, illness begins suddenly with headache, feverishness and intermittent chilliness. The conjunctivas are injected; there is generalized lymphadenopathy; and, in the majority of Caucasians, a primary lesion or eschar at the site of attachment of the infected mite may be found. The fever may increase stepwise during the first week to levels of 104° to 105° F., or it may rise abruptly to such levels on the first or second

day and remain elevated. About the fifth day a red macular rash appears on the trunk and may extend to the arms and legs. It usually persists for several days, but may disappear within a few hours. The rash, like the eschar, is more often absent than present in Asian patients with scrub typhus.

The pulse during the first week is relatively slow, usually 70 to 100 per minute. Nonproductive cough is commonly present, and rales and rhonchi are generally heard. Roentgenographic evidence of pneumonitis is found in about one fifth of the patients. Despite the sustained high fever, the severe discomfort from headache and the apathy, patients rarely appear dangerously ill during the first week.

The temperature remains elevated during the second week, and even the less severely affected persons begin to show the debilitating effects of sustained illness. The relative bradycardia is often replaced by a pulse rate in proportion to the fever, or even higher, and the systolic blood pressure drops below 100 mm. of mercury. These findings, together with evidence of peripheral circulatory failure, are bad prognostic signs. Other manifestations of severe disease are signs of involvement of the central nervous system, such as delirium, stupor and muscular twitchings. Frank signs of pneumonia may develop.

At the end of the second week the temperature falls by lysis and remains normal after the fourteenth or fifteenth day. With the reduction in fever, the pulse rate and blood pressure return to normal levels. The eschar is practically healed. Convalescence is protracted in patients who failed to receive specific antimicrobial therapy, and full return to mental and physical vigor is usually delayed for several months. Sequelae in the form of nervous or psychiatric disorders and permanent damage to the heart are rare.

Immunity. Patients who recover from scrub typhus are resistant to reinfection with the homologous strain of *R. tsutsugamushi* for some years. However, within two months after recovery reinfection with a heterologous strain causes mild disease and after one year typical scrub typhus. Among the 223 Japanese farmers who gave a history of scrub typhus in the survey mentioned previously, 19 suffered a second attack and five had a third attack. The interval between attacks varied from two to forty-four years, with an average of seven years. Convalescent patients exhibit specific neutralizing and complement-fixing antibodies. Despite their presence, however, *Rickettsiae tsutsugamushi* persist in the tissues of mice and men for months after clinical recovery.

Diagnosis. The geographic distribution of scrub typhus assists in differentiating this disease from other rickettsial infections. Epidemic typhus is absent from the warm regions where most scrub typhus is found. In Japan, where both diseases exist, the louse-borne variety occurs in winter and the mite-borne type in summer. Relatively little is known about the spotted fever group of diseases which may be found in the Asiatic-Pacific area. In Southeast Asia, murine typhus (flea-borne, urban typhus) is the rickettsial infection most apt to be confused with scrub (rural) typhus. The history of recent exposure in town or country, the finding of the scrub typhus eschar, and the results of serologic tests during the second and third week serve to differentiate these two diseases. Agglutinins against the OX-K strain of *Proteus vulgaris* appear in the serum of patients with scrub typhus and against the OX-19 strain in murine typhus. Finally, negative results with the specific complement fixation tests for epidemic and murine typhus and for spotted fever, and recovery of *Rickettsia tsutsugamushi* from the blood of the scrub typhus patient, confirm the diagnosis. The presence in convalescent serum of specific complement-fixing antibodies which react with antigens containing *R. tsutsugamushi* is of diagnostic importance. Negative results are of no significance, however, since the antigenic heterogenicity of strains of scrub typhus is such that only a proportion of patients exhibit antibodies which fix complement with the available antigens.

Differentiation of scrub typhus during the first week of illness from typhoid fever, malaria, dengue, infectious hepatitis, leptospirosis and fevers of unknown origin is difficult. Headache, conjunctival injection and lymphadenopathy are more conspicuous in scrub typhus. The eschar and rash, if present, are of some aid, but the early primary lesion may be confused with cutaneous infections which are common in the tropics. The sustained fever in the second week, the development of the black necrotic center in the eschar, and negative results in laboratory tests for typhoid fever and malaria point to scrub typhus. The dramatic improvement within a matter of hours after chloramphenicol or a tetracycline is given to scrub typhus patients is helpful in eliminating most of the nonrickettsial diseases under consideration.

Prognosis. Patients with evidence of circulatory failure, encephalitis or frank pneumonia should be considered gravely affected. Death, when it occurs, usually happens during the second week and is attributable in about equal numbers of cases to the three manifestations just mentioned. The disease is rarely lethal for children, but fatalities increase in proportion to age, and elderly persons usually die. The variations in mortality in different areas have already been discussed.

The prognosis has changed radically since the introduction of chloramphenicol and the tetracyclines (Aureomycin and Terramycin) in the therapy of this disease. Even the gravely ill and the aged patients now recover under treatment.

Prophylaxis. Vaccines containing killed *Rickettsia tsutsugamushi* have not been successful in preventing disease in persons exposed under field conditions. It is assumed that the antigenic variations in strains of scrub typhus organisms are mainly responsible for the failure to protect man during field exposure.

Personal prophylaxis by avoidance of mites depends primarily on the use of mite repellents and miticidal agents such as dimethyl or dibutyl phthalate or benzyl benzoate. The phthalates are smeared by hand on the clothes and exposed surfaces of the skin (avoiding the eyes and crotch because of the burning sensation produced by the chemical). Impregnation of clothes with benzyl benzoate is attained by dipping the garment in an aqueous emulsion of the substance. When properly used, the mite repellents are highly effective in preventing scrub typhus. They are relatively expensive and require constant intelligent use; short periods of carelessness during exposure in hyperendemic areas result in infection.

Clearing and cultivation of endemic areas of scrub typhus eventually free them of hazard by reducing or destroying the vector mites and rodent reservoirs.

Chemoprophylaxis with 3 gm. oral doses of chloramphenicol at four- to six-day intervals for twenty-eight days after exposure of volunteers suppressed infection below clinical levels. Active immunization of man resulted when a few infectious doses of *R. tsutsugamushi* were injected intradermally and followed by this chemoprophylactic regimen. Both procedures have limited applicability.

Treatment. Chloramphenicol and the tetracycline drugs (Aureomycin and Terramycin) are highly effective in scrub typhus. There is no choice between them and each is given orally as follows: a "loading dose" of 3 to 4 gm. is administered, either at one time or over a few hours, and followed by 1 gm. amounts at eight-hour intervals until the patient is afebrile. On this regimen general improvement is evident in twelve hours and the patients are afebrile in thirty hours, on the average. As the temperature becomes normal, headache disappears, appetite returns and the mental apathy is lost. Critically ill patients may not become permanently fever-free for forty-eight to ninety-six hours.

If treatment is begun within the first few days of disease, a 3 gm. supplementary dose of the drug used should be given about the eighth day after onset to prevent relapse which occurs in about three fourths of such patients. A supplementary dose is not required in patients who are first treated on the seventh day or later, since immunity in scrub typhus, which begins to develop late in the second week, is adequate in these patients by the time the drug effect is lost. While mild untoward manifestations not infrequently result from administration of the tetracyclines and chloramphenicol and severe blood dyscrasias may occur very rarely, the value of these drugs in scrub typhus is so great and the disease so severe that they should be employed without hesitation.

Since the introduction of specific therapy the severe manifestations of scrub typhus are generally brought under control so rapidly that little is needed in the way of supporting therapy. For those in extremis at the time of admission to the hospital, parenteral fluids, transfusions or oxygen therapy may be indicated. Treated patients are now given a full hospital diet within a few days after becoming afebrile, are allowed to sit up a few days later, and are usually discharged after a week of normal temperature. They are permitted to return to light work shortly thereafter. Before the introduction of specific treatment, military patients were allowed to convalesce from one to four months before being returned to duty.

JOSEPH E. SMADEL

References

Allen, A. C., and Spitz, S.: Comparative Study of Pathology of Scrub Typhus (Tsutsugamushi Disease) and Other Rickettsial Diseases. Am. J. Path., 21:603, 1945.

Bailey, C. A., and Ley, H. L., Jr.: The Treatment and Prophylaxis of Scrub Typhus with Antibiotics. Ann. N. Y. Acad. Sci., 55:983, 1952.

Blake, F. G., and others: Studies on Tsutsugamushi Disease (Scrub Typhus, Mite-Borne Typhus) in New Guinea and Adjacent Islands: Epidemiology, Clinical Observations, and Etiology in the Dobadura Area. Am. J. Hyg., 41:243, 1945.

Ley, H. L., Jr., and others: Immunization Against Scrub Typhus. IV. Living Karp Vaccine and Chemoprophylaxis in Volunteers. Am. J. Hyg., 56:303, 1952.

Smadel, J. E.: Scrub Typhus, in Rivers, T. M.; Viral and Rickettsial Infections of Man. Philadelphia, J. B. Lippincott Company, 1948, pp. 516–528.

———, Woodward, T. E., Ley, H. L., Jr., and Lewthwaite, R.: Chloramphenicol (Chloromycetin) in the Treatment of Tsutsugamushi Disease (Scrub Typhus). J. Clin. Investigation, 28:1196, 1949.

RICKETTSIALPOX

Definition. Rickettsialpox is a mild, self-limited, acute febrile illness caused by *Rickettsia akari* and characterized by an initial skin lesion developing at the site of infection, fever of about one week's duration and a papulovesicular rash.

History, Distribution and Epidemiology. Rickettsialpox was first recognized in New York City in 1946, although it undoubtedly existed there earlier. From 140 to 180 cases have been reported annually in New York City since that time. A few cases have been diagnosed recently in Boston and Hartford; it is unlikely that the disease is restricted to these few areas.

The brilliant work of members of the U. S. Public Health Service and the New York City Department of Health resulted in prompt isolation of the causal agent from the blood of patients and its identification as a distinct rickettsial species, and in the elucidation of the epidemiology of the disease. Rickettsialpox is transmitted by a small colorless mite, *Allodermanyssus sanguineus* (Hirst), which normally infests mice and small rodents. House mice serve as a reservoir of infection. The etiologic agent has been recovered from mice and mites collected from houses in which patients acquired the disease.

Etiology. *Rickettsia akari,* the etiologic agent of rickettsialpox, has the general morphologic and biologic characteristics of other rickettsiae. It is antigenically related to, but distinct from, *R. rickettsii,* which causes Rocky Mountain spotted fever. White mice, guinea pigs and embryonated eggs are susceptible to experimental infection. Diagnostic antigen for use in the complement fixation test with human serum is prepared from yolk sacs of infected chick embryo.

Morbid Anatomy. No deaths have been attributed to rickettsialpox; however, skin lesions have been removed surgically for histologic examination. The initial lesion of rickettsialpox, which resembles the primary lesion of scrub typhus, is characterized by a superficial pustule with polymorphonuclear infiltration in the adjacent epithelium and changes in the vascular endothelium, together with perivascular cellular infiltrations in the corium. The histopathology of the early maculopapular rash of rickettsialpox is similar to that of other rickettsial exanthems and consists in changes in the vessels of the corium and perivascular accumulations of mononuclear cells. The vesiculation, which develops in the maculopapular lesions of rickettsialpox, is unique among the rickettsial diseases. Necrosis of epithelial cells results in an intra-epidermal vesicle superimposed on the papule. Some polymorphonuclear cells wander into the corium beneath the vesicle, but healing occurs without scarring.

Symptoms. The period between the bite of the infected mite and the appearance of the initial lesion at this site is from one to two weeks. Three to seven days after the lesion develops, the febrile phase begins. The rash may accompany the fever, but more frequently appears several days later.

The initial lesion begins as a firm red papule which increases to a diameter of 1 to 1.5 cm. After a few days the center becomes vesiculated, the papule is surrounded by a zone of erythema, and the regional lymph nodes are moderately enlarged. The clear vesicular fluid becomes cloudy and dries, and a black eschar is formed. The lesion, which is not painful, heals slowly; the scab drops off about the third week, leaving a small scar.

The febrile phase begins with sudden onset of chills or chilly sensations, sweats, headache, muscle pains, anorexia and photophobia. The temperature frequently reaches 103° to 104° F. and remains elevated, with morning remissions, for approximately one week.

The maculopapular-vesicular rash is generalized in distribution and may be abundant or scanty. Lesions occasionally involve the oral mucosa, but rarely the palms and soles. The exanthem runs its course in about a week; the vesicles dry and the scabs fall off, leaving a transient discoloration, but no scar.

Other findings are essentially limited to those associated with a febrile disease, although the spleen is palpable in some cases. Complications are rare.

Laboratory Findings. The usual laboratory examinations reveal a moderate leukopenia and the findings which are associated with a febrile illness. The erythrocyte sedimentation rate may be slightly elevated.

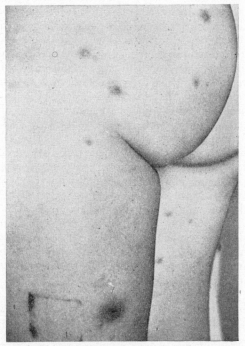

Fig. 23. Vesicular eruption of rickettsialpox, with initial lesion visible on posterior aspect of left thigh. (Courtesy of Dr. Harry M. Rose.)

During convalescence specific complement-fixing antibodies which react with antigens containing *Rickettsia akari* appear in the serum of patients. The Weil-Felix test, which becomes positive in patients with most rickettsial diseases, remains negative in rickettsialpox.

Diagnosis. Chickenpox has been most frequently confused with rickettsialpox. The following points help to differentiate the two diseases. Rickettsialpox occurs in persons of all ages and has an initial lesion, fever generally precedes the rash, the vesicle surmounts the papule which is discernible throughout the exanthem, and finally diagnosis can be established by a specific serologic test. In contrast, chickenpox is usually a childhood disease and has no initial lesion, the rash appears at the height of the fever, and the papular cutaneous lesion is entirely transformed into a vesicle.

The lesion of the papulovesicular stage of smallpox resembles that of rickettsialpox, but the exanthem is generally more abundant in variola. The constitutional reaction in smallpox is greater than in rickettsialpox, but it also precedes the rash. Finally, the variolar vesicles progress to pustules.

The rashes of the typhus fevers and of the other members of the spotted fever group of the rickettsial diseases are not vesicular, the febrile periods of these diseases are more prolonged than in rickettsialpox, and the illnesses are more severe, with appreciable mortality rates. The Weil-Felix reaction and specific complement fixation tests using rickettsial antigens are positive. Cross-reactions are obtained with serums from patients with Rocky Mountain spotted fever and rickettsialpox when complement fixation tests are used. However, if highly purified and washed rickettsial antigens prepared from the two causal rickettsiae are used in the test, a definite serologic diagnosis can be made.

Prophylaxis. Control measures consisting in elimination of house mice and vector mites have been attempted in certain of the housing projects in New York City where multiple cases occurred.

Treatment. Symptomatic treatment has been used in this mild, self-limiting disease. Dramatic improvement follows the use of chloramphenicol or the tetracyclines (Aureomycin or Terramycin); oral doses of 2 to 4 gm. daily render the patient afebrile and essentially free of complaints in 48 hours.

JOSEPH E. SMADEL

References

Dolgopol, V. B.: Histologic Changes in Rickettsialpox. Am. J. Path., 24:119, 1948.
Franklin, J., Wasserman, E., and Fuller, H. S.: Rickettsialpox in Boston. New England J. Med., 244:509, 1951.
Greenberg, M.: Rickettsialpox in New York City. Am. J. Med., 4:866, 1948.
Huebner, R. J., Jellison, W. L., and Armstrong, C.: Rickettsialpox, a Newly Recognized Rickettsial Disease. V. Recovery of *Rickettsia akari* from a House Mouse (*Mus musculus*). Pub. Health Rep., 62:777, 1947.
Huebner, R. J., Jellison, W. L., and Pomerantz, C.: Rickettsialpox, a Newly Recognized Rickettsial Disease. IV. Isolation of a Rickettsia, Apparently Identical with the Causative Agent of Rickettsialpox from *Allodermanyssus sanguineus,* a Rodent Mite. Pub. Health Rep., 61:1677, 1946.
Huebner, R. J., Stamps, P., and Armstrong, C.: Rickettsialpox, a Newly Recognized Rickettsial Disease. I. Isolation of the Etiological Agent. Pub. Health Rep., 61:1604, 1946.
Rose, H. M.: The Treatment of Rickettsialpox with Antibiotics. Ann. N. Y. Acad. Sci., 55:1019, 1952.

TRENCH FEVER

(Quintan Fever, Shin Bone Fever, Wolhynian Fever, His-Werner Disease, etc.)

Definition. Trench fever is a specific, exanthematic louse-borne infection, characterized usually by a sudden febrile onset with pain and soreness in muscles, bones and joints. The disease is never fatal.

History. The disease was first recognized in 1915, when it appeared on the Western and Eastern fronts during World War I. It constituted one of the major medical problems of World War I and was investigated intensively by a British and by an American commission. After demobilization the disease practically disappeared. It reappeared during World War II, but on a relatively small scale.

Epidemiology and Etiology. The responsibility of the body louse in transmitting the disease to man was established by both British and American commissions, as a result of well controlled louse-feeding experiments upon human volunteers. The infective agent is present in the excreta of lice, where it may remain infective for several months. The disease is transferable from man to man by intravenous inoculation of blood.

As for the etiologic agent, there is strong but perhaps not conclusive evidence incriminating an organism (*Rickettsia wolhynica, R. pediculi, R. quintana*) the presence of which in the intestines and feces of lice was definitely correlated with infectivity by Bacot, Arkwright and Duncan. The organism occurs extracellularly in the gut of the louse, thus differing from other pathogenic rickettsiae. Recently Mooser and Weyer have transmitted the infection to *Rhesus* monkeys, in which it is subclinical, and demonstrable only by the fact that lice fed on infected monkeys develop the etiologic organism in their intestinal tracts. No other experimental animal has been shown to be susceptible.

Morbid Anatomy. Postmortem studies have not been made, since the disease is never fatal. Examinations of excised macules from the skin have apparently shown no important specific changes. The spleen is usually enlarged and firm to palpation. Rickettsia have not been satisfactory demonstrated in human tissues.

Symptoms. *Incubation Period.* Experimental evidence indicates that the usual incubation period is from ten to twenty days, with extreme limits of five to thirty-eight days.

Onset. The onset is usually acute, with chills and a rise in temperature to 102° or 103° F. Severe headache, usually behind the eyeballs, and complete anorexia are almost constant at this stage. Nausea and vomiting sometimes occur. Laryngitis and bronchitis may be present, but are rarely severe. Perhaps the most characteristic symptom is severe "myalgic" pain in various parts of the body, but most prominent in the lumbar region, and legs. There is also muscular soreness, pain on rotating the eyeballs, conjunctivitis and photophobia. Occasionally the onset is insidious, with symptoms of neurasthenia and tachycardia.

Course of the Disease. The progress of the disease is remarkably variable. The fever and symptoms may last only two or three days or may be typhoidal in character, lasting two or three weeks. A common form is that in which there are two febrile periods, of three to five days each, with twelve to twenty-four hours of remission between them. Again, there may be short febrile periods of only twenty-four to thirty hours, recurring regularly every five days for a variable period of time. Relapses are prone to occur several weeks or months after apparent recovery.

The characteristic *rash* usually appears during the first twenty-four hours, and thereafter comes and goes with fever, even in the case of late relapse. It is composed of red macules, 2 to 10 mm. in diameter, appearing first on the chest and abdomen, and usually confined to those regions, although they may involve the entire trunk. The extremities are occasionally involved, but the face always escapes.

The pulse rate during the initial acute attack is increased in proportion to the fever, but may be relatively much higher in late relapses. A sharp increase in the pulse rate often precedes and may be the only objective evidence of a relapse.

Pain and soreness in the muscles usually recur with each febrile relapse. Lumbar pain is most apt to persist in the chronic stage of the disease. Abdominal pain and tenderness, probably of muscular origin, are usually bilateral and more pronounced on gentle than on firm pressure. This fact, together with the palpable spleen, rash, and generalized pain and tenderness, usually serves to differentiate the condition from appendicitis.

Prognosis. The disease has no mortality. Its duration is extraordinarily variable, but about 85 per cent of all patients are able to return to work within two months of the time of onset. It is believed that in about 5 per cent of all cases the disease becomes chronic, necessitating a much longer period of time for complete recovery. Recovery is apt to be delayed in the aged and in the debilitated.

Diagnosis. During epidemics typical cases are readily diagnosed on the basis of the symptomatology. The atypical abortive cases may be confused with influenza in the absence of the characteristic rash. The mild respiratory symptoms and the enlarged hard spleen of trench fever are valuable differential criteria in such cases. The typhoidal type is differentiated from true typhoid by the negative Widal reaction and by the almost constant presence of mild to moderate leukocytosis rather than leukopenia. In typhoid, typhus and dengue fever the onset is more gradual than in trench fever, and the rash usually appears several days later. Spirochetal relapsing fever and malaria may be excluded by examination of the blood for their specific etiologic agents. In cases of the chronic type, with tachycardia, fatigue, loss of weight and symptoms of neurasthenia, diagnosis may be most difficult. It is theoretically possible to establish strong presumptive evidence of trench fever by feeding carefully controlled lice on such patients and finding that they acquire *Rickettsia wolhynica.*

Treatment. No reliable information is available concerning the value of the new antirickettsial agents (chloramphenicol and the tetracyclines) in trench fever. Pain and discomfort should, whenever possible, be controlled by such drugs as acetylsalicyclic acid and phenacetin rather than by opiates. Codeine is useful in severe pain. Insomnia can usually be controlled by hypnotics. The patient should remain in bed under the best available hygienic and dietary conditions for a week or more after complete cessation of subjective and objective evidence of infection. He should be kept under observation for several months, and returned to bed at the first sign of relapse.

Prophylaxis. Prevention of the disease is largely a question of efficient delousing by the chemical techniques developed during World War II (see Typhus Fever, page 98). Destruction of the infective agent on clothing contaminated by louse excreta is also of primary importance. Autoclaving is probably the most satisfactory method. Disinfection of urine and sputum may be carried out by chemical methods or by heat. Louse-proof garments and rubber gloves should be worn by those attending patients or handling clothing. Trench fever patients are best treated in separate wards.

HENRY PINKERTON

References

Bacot, A.: On the Probable Identity of *Rickettsia Pediculi* with *Rickettsia Quintana*. Brit. M. J., *1*:156, 1921.

———, Arkwright, J. A., and Duncan, F. M.: Association of Rickettsia with Trench Fever. J. Hygiene, *18*:76, 1919.

British Investigation Committee. Brit. M. J., *1*:91, 296, 1918.

McNee, J. W., Brunt, A., and Renshaw, E. H.: Trench Fever. Brit. M. J., *1*:225, 1916.

Mooser, H., and Weyer, F.: Experimental Infection of Macacus Rhesus with *Rickettsia quintana* (Trench Fever). Proc. Soc. Exper. Biol. & Med. 83:699, 1953.

Strong, R. P.: Stitt's Diagnosis, Prevention and Treatment of Tropical Diseases. 7th ed. Philadelphia, Blakiston Co., 1944.

Swift, H. F.: Trench Fever. Harvey Society Lectures, *15*:58, 1919–1920.

Trench Fever: Report of Commission on Trench Fever. American Red Cross Med. Res. Committee. London, Oxford University Press, 1918.

BACTERIAL DISEASES

INTRODUCTION TO BACTERIAL DISEASES

An understanding of the general principles of bacteriology and immunity is of the highest importance in the interpretation of the symptoms and signs of infection. In this introduction, a few aspects of bacteriology, immunology and pathology will be presented.

Pathogenic and Virulent Bacteria. *Pathogenic* organisms are defined as those which are capable of invading and multiplying within the human body, where they produce harmful effects. By and large, microorganisms must penetrate some protective covering layer, such as the skin or mucous membranes, and multiply in the tissues before they become capable of producing damage. The ability to penetrate tissues, apart from mechanical injuries to the tissues, probably depends upon the capacity of the organisms to survive long enough in a given environment so that they gain contact with a surface from which they can penetrate the lymphatics or the subepithelial tissues.

Once pathogenic organisms have entered the tissues, they may remain localized to a relatively small area or they may multiply rapidly and invade the tissues widely. Some organisms which remain in a local area produce their harmful effects by the generation of toxic substances which are absorbed by and poison tissue cells remote from the local area of infection (diphtheria, tetanus); others are rapidly disseminated through the blood stream to various organs of the body; and a third type combines the properties of both a toxigenic and an invasive organism.

A *virulent* organism can be defined as one which produces harmful effects in the tissues whether it is capable of widespread invasion or not. An organism possessing the properties of invading the tissues widely is most certainly virulent, but it is well to separate and define invasive and virulent organisms.

Once virulent organisms break through the normal protective barriers, they may invade tissues rapidly and produce *bacteremia.* Whether this occurs depends upon the balance of a number of factors, including the site of the initial infection, the dose, the vegetative activity and species of bacteria, as well as the defense mechanism of the host. The factors determining the resistance of the host to widespread invasion depend upon the character and location of the local inflammatory reaction and the patient's immune mechanism. The immune mechanism, in turn, is conditioned by natural responses to injury and by the patient's previous reaction to the organisms in question. This reaction may have been acquired as a result of a previous natural infection, from artificial immunization, or from contact with the organism or its related antigenic components, so that antibodies have been produced.

Normal Bacterial Flora. The interpretation of bacteriologic findings necessitates familiarity with the normal bacterial flora of various parts of the body and ability to detect and interpret the so-called carrier state in its proper light.

It is widely recognized that the skin and mucous membrane surfaces have a "normal" bacteriologic flora where organisms thrive without doing any harm. Once they leave their normal habitat and multiply in other tissues, harmful effects are frequently produced. For example, *E. coli* grows freely on the surface of the mucous membrane of the large bowel and produces no harmful effects. If it leaves the intestine and focalizes in the kidney, pyelonephritis results. It is necessary, then, to be familiar with the normal flora of various areas in order to make the proper interpretation of bacteriologic findings. It is well worth remembering that the surface of the skin and mucous membranes has provided itself with defense mechanisms for making it difficult for some bacteria to gain a foothold. Many bacteria are eliminated, whereas others are capable of surviving. The result of these variations is that each region has developed a very distinctive flora. These flora may exhibit seasonal variations, or may depend upon contact with patients with disease, or the use of antimicrobial drugs. (See table.)

Normal Bacterial Flora

ORGANS	BACTERIA
Skin	Staphylococci
	Diphtheroids
Mouth and	Nonhemolytic streptococci
throat	Gram-negative cocci
	Influenza bacilli
Less often {	Diphtheroids
than {	Pneumococci
others {	Hemolytic streptococci
Stomach	None
Small intestine	Gram-positive cocci
	Colon bacilli
	Various aerobic and anaerobic bacteria
Nose	Diphtheroids
	Staphylococcus albus and *aureus*
	Streptococcus viridans
	Hemophilic bacilli
Vagina	Döderlein bacilli
Colon	Mixed flora
	E. coli
	Aero. aerogenes
	Friedländer bacillus
	Enterococci
	Staph. aureus
	Anaerobic organisms

The Carrier State. It is well known that some persons carry pathogenic organisms in the bacterial flora of the throat or intestinal tract, where the bacteria lead a parasitic existence, but when they are transferred to other human hosts, acute disease may follow. This carrier state may be temporary or permanent. It may follow an acute disease or it may come into being from contact with an acute disease without producing symptoms. Its recognition is of importance in tracing infection to its source and in the proper assessment of the bacteriologic findings.

The Factors Concerned in the Invasion of Bacteria. While it is not possible to state why some organisms invade the tissues freely and others remain localized, there is some information available that assists in understanding the determining factors in many cases. One of the problems is to determine the factors which influence the immobilization of bacteria, the suppression of their growth and their final destruction.

From the experimental work in animals, it is clearly evident that the prevention of the spread of organisms depends upon the summation and balance of a number of factors. Controversy exists when the relative importance of various reactions and responses

is assessed and interpreted. Such host factors as the portal of entry, the anatomy of the particular region, the influence of nonspecific inflammation, the thrombosis of lymphatics, cellular and humoral immunity, the activity of phagocytes, cellular aggregation, allergic inflammation and other changes in the environment have all been called into account to explain the various phenomena influencing the spread of bacteria. Parasite factors such as the peculiar characteristics of various species of bacteria, the infecting dose, vegetative activity and the virulence of the infecting organism must be taken into account.

With the widespread use of anti-infective agents the bacterial flora of various regions of the body may change, and this is true not only of persons who receive anti-infective agents but also of those who are in contact with them. The flora of the nose and throat in hospital personnel may be quite different from those in the general population.

Anatomy of the Region. The invasion of the body by bacteria depends to some extent upon the anatomy of the region where organisms first enter the body. When the skin is broken and actively growing, virulent organs gain an entrance, they are taken up by the lymphatics very freely and carried to the neighboring lymph nodes. They may be removed at this point or they may progress further and enter the general circulation for removal elsewhere. When there is an infection of the peritoneum, on the other hand, there is an exudation of plasma and leukocytes with an outpouring and precipitation of fibrin. Some of the organisms are aggregated on the surface of the omentum in preparation for lysis or phagocytosis; others enter the lymphatics and are rapidly carried to the mesenteric lymph nodes and general circulation, so that bacteremia results much more quickly following peritoneal infection than following infections of the skin. One could illustrate these differences in the clearing mechanism in various organs, but the two examples given serve to indicate that the anatomy of a region is a most important factor in studying the question of invasion.

Portal of Entry. Once virulent organisms penetrate the normal skin or mucous membranes, they may either spread directly through the tissues or be carried to distant points by way of the lymphatics or blood stream. Information regarding the portal of entry is frequently helpful in localizing infection that appears at some distance from the primary infection. It also suggests the type of infecting organism. Knowing the portal of entry is particularly helpful in the diagnosis of infection of various internal organs at a time when the primary focus has healed entirely. The history of an infection of the skin or mucous membranes occurring some days or weeks, or even several months, before the onset of the symptoms of infection may be exceedingly important in giving a lead as to the possible type of infection; it may also suggest the possible location of a lesion that is giving rise to symptoms and signs. The customary portal of entry for the various organisms is listed under "organs" in the table.

Skin. The types of infection that arise in the skin are commonly staphylococcal and streptococcal infections. These naturally give rise to localized abscesses or lymphangitis with regional lymphadenitis. Streptococcal infections invade the lymphatics rapidly and freely and are disseminated through the course of the lymphatics draining the particular area. Staphylococci are more likely than streptococci to produce localized abscesses with regional lymphadenitis. Both of these organisms may cause primary infections which heal only to have localized abscesses develop elsewhere in the body. For example, following an infection of the hand or forearm which heals, one may find a localized lymphadenitis in the axilla or in the subpectoral region. This may be the source for an obscure sepsis. In lesions of the left arm the infection may spread through the lymphatics to involve the thoracic duct and in this way cause retrograde peritonitis. This has been observed in a few instances of hemolytic streptococcal infection. Infections of the arms may likewise produce an abscess in the mediastinum due to spread of organisms to the lymph nodes in the anterior mediastinum. In these cases the organisms spread directly through the lymphatics to the lymph nodes, which suppurate and spread infection. Staphlococci may invade the blood stream from local infections of the skin and be disseminated throughout the body, focalizing in such areas as the kidney, muscles, bone and the organs in general. The symptoms of an infection may not appear for some weeks or months after the primary infection, so that it is highly important to obtain a good history regarding the presence of a previous infection, no matter how insignificant it may seem.

Nasopharynx and Throat. The common organisms causing infection in the nasopharynx or throat are hemolytic streptococci, the pneumococci and the hemolytic *Staphylococcus aureus.* The nose and throat may serve as portals of entry for generalized infection or localized areas of suppuration in the immediate neighborhood. Lymphadenitis of the cervical lymph nodes, otitis media and mastoiditis, lateral sinus thrombosis, brain abscess and meningitis may all have their origin in a nose or throat infection. Thrombophlebitis of the peritonsillar veins and mediastinal abscess may also follow these local infections. A history of tonsillitis or nasopharyngeal infection is of definite assistance in suggesting the possible localization of the above infections.

Lungs. From the lungs, hemolytic streptococci, pneumococci or other pyogenic organisms may be disseminated to other tissues. The brain, the endocardium, the spleen, and the muscles, bones and joints may be the site of abscess formation. These areas of suppuration or infection are observed following acute or chronic pulmonary infection.

Gastrointestinal Tract. The organisms disseminated from the gastrointestinal tract are usually the typhoid-paratyphoid group of organisms, *Brucella abortus,* the colon bacillus, enterococci, Friedländer's bacilli, and rarely pneumococci. In a number of these cases there has been no previous evidence of a disturbance of the gastrointestinal tract due to the presence of these organisms.

Genitourinary Tract. E. *coli,* staphylococci, Friedländer's bacilli, various strains of the typhoid-paratyphoid group of organisms, *B. proteus, Pseudomonas aeruginosa* and *H. influenzae* may invade tissues from the genitourinary tract. By and large, organisms invade the blood stream from the urinary tract following a rupture of the local defense mechanism by passing sounds, cystoscopes or catheters or following operations. Spontaneous invasion is much less common, and when it occurs should always lead one to suspect a thrombophlebitis of the renal veins.

Phlebitis of the veins of the bladder wall in elderly individuals with cystitis may serve as a focus for bacteremia and sepsis and, indeed, such infections may rarely cause peritonitis with or without perforation of the bladder.

From the genital tract, various organisms invade the blood stream such as hemolytic streptococci, gonococci and anaerobic organisms, mostly following puerperal infections or venereal disease.

Bacterial Spread; the Significance of Bacteremia. Once pathogenic organisms have broken through the normal barriers, they may invade the circulating blood. From the blood they are often rapidly removed by a very effective clearing mechanism. This mechanism has been studied most effectively in animals, but from studies in man there is every reason to believe that the same fundamental process goes on. An understanding of this process is helpful in assessing clinical findings. What, then, is the significance of bacteremia when it exists?

Speaking broadly, bacteremia is the result of a loss of equilibrium between the normal clearing mechanism and the rapid overflow of bacteria from one or more foci of infection. It follows, then, that the presence or absence of bacteria in the blood will depend upon a balance of these two factors. If organisms are growing rapidly and overflowing into the blood faster than the clearing mechanism can eliminate them, bacteremia will follow or, if there is an overflow of organisms when the clearing mechanism has ceased to operate, bacteremia will be present. Bacteremia may be temporary or it may be of long duration.

From numerous observations, it is known that bacteria are removed from the circulating blood in the same manner as any foreign substance, and that the circulating and fixed phagocytes of the reticuloendothelial system are in large measure responsible for the phagocytosis. Bacteria are agglutinated in cell masses and filtered off in the capillaries, where they become entangled with fibrin and platelets. They may be phagocytized or they may be carried off to other areas such as the liver, spleen and bone marrow, where they are disposed of by the action of powerful phagocytic cells. When bacteria lodge in areas where the defense mechanism operates at a low level of efficiency, or where the environment is favorable for their growth, foci of infection develop which may localize temporarily and then again overflow into the blood stream. The clearing mechanism operates at a much higher level of efficiency and prevents the growth and reinvasion of the blood by organisms if there are antibodies present in the tissues or circulating blood. These antibodies may have been produced as a result of previous experience with the organisms or they may be natural to the host. By and large, localized areas of suppuration without bacteremia usually mean that antibodies are present and the mechanism for the prevention of the spread of bacteria is operating effectively. The mechanism for their complete destruction may be ineffective unless the local infection is treated adequately.

Bacteria enter the circulating blood when the lymphatics are free or following an infective thrombophlebitis of the vessels. The frequency of this invasion depends in large measure on the type of infecting organism and the site of the infection. The commonest organisms to invade the blood are pneumococci, meningococci, streptococci and staphylococci; less frequently colon bacilli and occasionally, gonococci. The commonest sites for infection followed by bacteremia are the skin and subcutaneous tissues, the peritoneum, the nose and throat, and the intestinal tract. When organisms, such as typhoid bacilli, enter the gastrointestinal tract they are filtered out by the lymphoid tissue of the small intestine, especially in Peyer's patches, and are carried to the mesenteric lymph nodes, then to the thoracic duct, and enter the circulation. From the general circulation these organisms focalize in the various tissues which are abundant in reticuloendothelial cells, namely the liver, spleen, bone marrow and lungs.

In the secondary foci of infection the organisms continue to grow and overflow into the general circulation. Some of the organisms are excreted into the bile and, in this way, reenter the gastrointestinal tract.

As antibodies begin to appear in the blood, the organisms become fewer and fewer, and their growth seems to be suppressed in the localized foci of infection.

When micro-organisms infect the skin or subcutaneous tissues, they commonly invade the lymphatics and are carried to the regional lymph nodes. From here they enter the general circulation, usually by way of the lymphatics and the thoracic ducts. In many cases, however, the infection remains localized in the skin and the adjacent lymph nodes. This depends to some extent upon the type and virulence of the infecting organism, together with the response on the part of the tissues to the particular organism in question. Staphylococci localize more readily than hemolytic streptococci. This is due, in part, to the type of tissue reaction, which in the case of staphylococci seems to bring about a marked precipitation of fibrin with rapid thrombosis of the neighboring lymphatics. In this way the organisms are prevented from spreading from the local area. In the case of the hemolytic streptococcus, focalization takes place less readily. This seems to be due to the fact that the lymphatics are thrombosed less rapidly and the organisms are capable of producing fibrinolysin, which dissolves fibrin or prevents its formation. When bacteria invade the blood vessels and produce infective thrombi, they are able to survive because it is difficult for the normal clearing mechanism to become operative in such a location. The same is true when bacteria localize on the heart valves. It is well to recall, then, that the presence of bacteria in the circulating blood over a long period of time should lead one to suspect the growth and overflow of organisms from a focus of infection which has free access to the general circulation.

Once an infection becomes localized and organisms are not present in the circulating blood, any traumatic lesion to the infected focus may lead to bacteremia. In these cases the normal barriers are disturbed and organisms can enter the circulation freely once again. Bacteremia following cystoscopy or catheterization in an individual with a urinary tract infection is an example of this situation.

The presence of bacteria in the circulating blood indicates a focus of infection which is not localized or walled off so that organisms are prevented from entering the blood stream, or it may mean that the normal clearing mechanism is ineffective. If the blood culture has been positive and then becomes negative, it may be taken as an indication of localization of the infection or an increase in the efficiency of the normal clearing mechanism. The latter state of affairs usually develops as a result of passive immunization or from the active development of antibody. Summing up, then, bacteremia indicates a loss of equilibrium between the clearing mechanism and the overflow of organisms from one or more active foci of infection. It may also mean that the clearing mechanism itself has broken down.

Practically speaking, bacteremia is of value in the clinic both as a diagnostic and a prognostic test. When it is recalled that bacteria do not multiply in the circulating blood but are there as a result of an overflow from a focus of infection, the presence of bacteremia may supply the diagnosis when the signs of a localized infection are obscure or absent, or it may indicate a serious state of affairs when there exists a recognizable infection which is no longer localized.

The common conditions in which bacteremia may be present without localizing signs are:

(1) Typhoid-paratyphoid group.
(2) *Brucella* infections.
(3) Chronic meningococcal and gonococcal infections.
(4) Obscure staphylococcal and streptococcal infections.

It is in these diseases that bacteremia is of great diagnostic importance.

Conversely, the absence of bacteremia in fevers of infectious origin with or without localizing signs is helpful in excluding certain etiologic agents and suggesting others. It may be an indication of a well localized infection with an effective clearing mechanism, or it may suggest noninfectious conditions which are commonly accompanied by fever.

Selective Localization of Bacteria. It is generally recognized that many virulent bacteria tend to lodge and multiply in tissues remote from their portal of entry; and for some reasons, as yet not well understood, they differ in regard to the particular organ or tissue in which they localize. The site of the primary lesion and the direction of the initial spread are determined by the portal of entry, the local anatomy and the direction of the lymph flow. As mentioned previously, the portal of entry is determined by the natural habitat of the organism and this, in turn, is determined by its ability to survive in a particular environment. While very little is known regarding the factors that favor the localization of bacteria in various tissues, it would appear that the organism's ability to survive in a given environment, the type of tissue, the duration of illness and the presence of specific antibodies must be of significance. Clinical and bacteriologic experience teaches us that the predilection of some organisms to focalize in certain tissues is common. The more important ones are summarized in the table.

One of the factors concerned in the development of bacteremia is the species of the infecting organism. Some species of bacteria

secondary to injury of the respiratory mucosa by viral infections such as influenza and the common cold.

The types of pneumococci that most commonly cause pneumonia in adults are types I, III, VII, II, VIII, IV, XI, X, XIX and XIV, in the order listed. Together, these ten types account for three quarters of all cases. Type XIV is particularly common in childhood infections. Other types are occasionally isolated from pneumonic sputum, but their comparative rarity suggests that they are of less virulence for man than the more commonly encountered types.

Pneumococci, particularly of the higher types, are frequently present in the respiratory tracts of normal subjects. Ordinarily the incidence of carriers of highly pathogenic types, such as I and II, is relatively low, except for type III, which is a common inhabitant of the normal pharynx. Nevertheless, there is evidence that normal carriers play a more important role in the dissemination of infective types than do patients ill with pneumonia. Occasionally, in relatively closed communities, high carrier rates of pathogenic types are encountered. In such circumstances the occurrence of widespread viral disease of the respiratory tract may result in an epidemic of pneumococcal pneumonia. Except for these rare epidemics, most of which occur in hospitals or custodial institutions, the disease is sporadic.

Pneumococcal pneumonia is slightly more common in Negroes than in whites and is particularly frequent among workers in steel mills and coal mines. It may occur at any age, but is of highest incidence in the second, third and fourth decades. The ratio of male to female patients is approximately three to two, the difference probably being due to occupational factors involving frequency of exposure.

Pathogenesis and Morbid Anatomy. The lung is the only major viscus of the body exposed to the air. Since the atmosphere, particularly in congested places, contains many bacteria, it is remarkable that pneumonia is not an almost universal disease. The failure of normal subjects to acquire acute bacterial pneumonia as an air-borne infection is due to the extraordinarily efficient defense-barriers of the lower respiratory tract. These defenses include (1) the epiglottis reflex, which prevents gross aspiration of infected secretions from the pharynx; (2) the sticky mucus which lines the bronchial tree and to which air-borne organisms adhere; (3) the cilia of the respiratory epithelium which keep the infected mucus moving constantly upward toward the pharynx (at a rate of 1 to 3 cm. per hour); (4) the cough reflex, which serves to propel the mucus out of the lower tract; (5) the lymphatics which drain the terminal bronchi and bronchioles; and (6) the mononuclear phagocytes (dust cells) which are ever present in the normal alveoli. In addition, the alveoli themselves are relatively dry and thus offer a poor medium for growth to the few bacteria that succeed in reaching them. Only when the defense barriers of the normal respiratory tract are disturbed does acute bacterial pneumonia result.

The thesis that bacterial pneumonia frequently results from aspiration of infected secretions from the upper respiratory tract is strongly supported by both experimental and clinical observations. Rats infected with pneumococci in the nasopharynx regularly exhibit pulmonary lesions only when subjected to experimental procedures involving chilling of the body, anesthesia, administration of morphine and alcoholic intoxication, all of which are common predisposing factors in human pneumonia and have been shown in the experimental animal to slow the epiglottal reflex and thus to facilitate aspiration. Experimental pneumonia can best be produced by intrabronchial inoculation of organisms suspended in mixtures of gastric mucin or starch having viscosities similar to that of mucus. Viral infection of the upper respiratory tract in man usually precedes the onset of acute bacterial pneumonia by several days. Not only is the volume of secretion from the nasopharynx greater than normal during viral infections such as the common cold, but also the number of pathogenic micro-organisms in the secretions is significantly increased. Thus the stage is set for aspiration of infected mucus. That such aspiration often occurs at the onset of human pneumonia is suggested by the usual sites of initial involvement of the lung. As shown in Figure 24, the earliest lesions of bacterial pneumonia usually appear in those parts of the lungs into which aspirated fluid is most likely to drain. Whereas most air-borne bacteria are caught on the sticky surfaces of the bronchial tree and never reach the alveoli, organisms contained in thin nasopharyngeal secretions are readily carried into the alveoli by the liquid mucus. The latter, like Lipiodol, cannot all be ejected by ciliary action, and much of it penetrates to the farthest reaches of the bronchial tree, where it establishes the initial focus of infection.

Other factors known to predispose patients to acute bacterial pneumonia include exposure to noxious gases and anesthetics, cardiac failure, influenzal virus infection of lungs, trauma to the thorax and pulmonary stasis

(Fig. 25, *b*), but later in such quantities as to fill each alveolus and thus render the area completely consolidated (Fig. 25, *c*). Once the infected alveoli become crowded with leukocytes, phagocytosis of bacteria takes place, and the invading organisms are destroyed. Macrophages appear in the exudate, and resolution begins only after most of the organisms have been ingested. The macrophages which accomplish the final clearing of

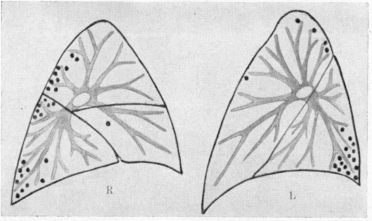

Fig. 24. Site of initial lesions in pneumococcal pneumonia. (From H. Loeschcke; Beitr. z. path. Anat., Vol. 86.)

resulting from prolonged bed rest. A feature common to all these conditions is the accumulation of fluid in the alveoli. Harford has shown that the dry lungs of normal mice are able to rid themselves of large numbers of inspired bacteria, whereas lungs containing fluid are readily infected. This observation suggests that pulmonary edema, by providing a suitable culture medium for the bacteria, may facilitate the establishment of active infection within the alveoli.

Early Lesion. Once the infection has gained a foothold within the alveoli, the lesion evolves in a characteristic manner. The first response of the lung to bacterial invasion is an outpouring of edema fluid into the alveoli. This serous fluid not only serves as a suitable culture medium for the organisms, but also "floats" them into new alveoli through the pores of Cohn and terminal bronchioles (Fig. 25, *a*). Centrifugal spread of the alveolar fluid is enhanced by motion of the pulmonary parenchyma caused by respiration and cough. After the outpouring of edema fluid, polymorphonuclear leukocytes and some erythrocytes accumulate in the infected alveoli, first in small numbers

cellular debris from the resolving lesion appear to be derived both from monocytes of the blood and from the septal cells of the alveolar walls, which become characteristically thickened during the process of resolution (Fig. 25, *d*).

Spreading Lesion. These stages in the inflammatory reaction account for the distinguishing histologic features of the spreading pneumonic lesion. In the outermost portion there appears an "edema zone" in which the alveoli are filled with acellular serous fluid containing many bacteria. Inside the edema zone a second zone may be identified in which there are signs of early consolidation with leukocytes in most of the alveoli. Here phagocytosis is often noted. Still more centrally a third transition to a "zone of advanced consolidation" is noted where the alveoli are packed with cells and where beginning resolution may be evident. In the central zone of advanced consolidation, fibrin is often noted in the alveolar exudate, the large fibrinogen molecules having passed through the injured walls of the alveolar capillaries along with erythrocytes.

From the foregoing description it is clear

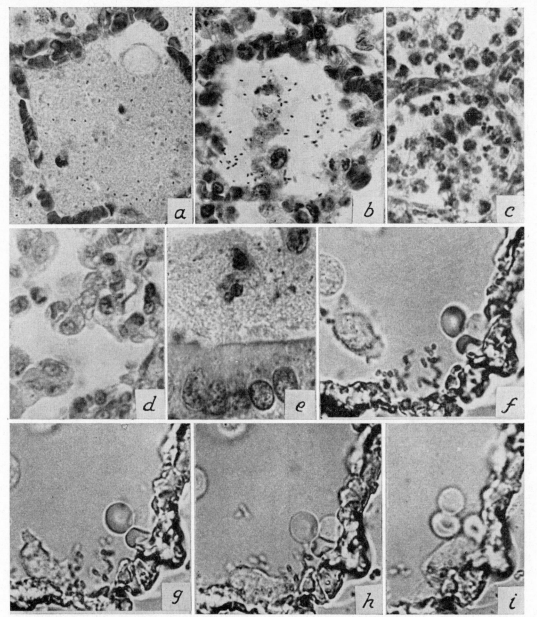

Fig. 25. *a,* Pneumococci in edema-filled alveoli at margin of spreading pneumonic lesion (× 800).

b, Beginning stage of polymorphonuclear exudation in zone of early consolidation. Note leukocytes in alveolar capillaries, some in process of diapedesis (× 800).

c, Leukocytic exudate (still predominantly polymorphonuclear) in inner zone of advanced consolidation. Pneumococci have been phagocyted and destroyed (× 800).

d, Alveolar macrophage reaction characteristic of late stage of resolution (× 800).

e, Pneumococci in edema fluid contained within lumen of a large bronchus. Such infected bronchial fluid causes spread of pneumonia to other lobes of the lungs (× 1250).

f–i, Surface phagocytosis of encapsulated microorganisms in formalin fixed rat lung (× 1250). Bacteria shown in these photomicrographs are Friedländer's bacilli, but same results have been obtained with pneumococci.

f, Polymorphonuclear leukocyte is seen approaching bacteria near alveolar wall. Time 12:30.

g, Leukocyte has reached alveolar wall and is about to trap organisms against the tissue surface. Time 12:31.

h, Cell has trapped some of the encapsulated bacteria against the wall and is in the process of phagocyting them. Time 12:32.

i, Having ingested several of the organisms, the leukocyte is moving up the alveolar wall. Time 12:35.

(Photomicrographs from studies on experimental pneumonia. W. B. Wood, et al.; J. Exper. Med., Vol. 73, and Smith and Wood; *ibid.,* Vol. 86.)

that all stages of inflammation can be found in a spreading lesion. In the most recently invaded areas at the periphery, edema and hemorrhage predominate, causing "red hepatization," whereas in the older, more central parts of the lesion, dense consolidation with leukocytes accounts for the characteristic color of "gray hepatization." Only if the infection has stopped spreading hours before necropsy will the entire lesion be in "the stage of gray hepatization." Thus the spread of pneumococcal pneumonia may be likened to that of grass fire where the flames, having spread centrifugally, are concentrated at the periphery, leaving behind a charred and burned-out center.

Not all pneumococcal pneumonia causes lobar consolidation. Less malignant lesions may be patchy in distribution and concentrated particularly about the bronchi. Since a clear-cut distinction between pneumococcal bronchopneumonia and lobar pneumonia cannot always be made even by the pathologist, and since management of the two conditions is essentially the same, it is rarely important for the clinician to differentiate them. The etiology rather than the anatomy of the lesion determines therapy.

Interlobar Spread. If the pneumonic process has involved all the parenchyma of a single lobe, its spread may be stopped by the pleural boundaries of the lobe and spontaneous recovery may then ensue. Often, however, the infection spreads to other lobes of the lungs. Interlobar spread has been shown in experimental pneumonia to result from the flow of infected edema fluid (Fig. 25, *e*) from bronchi of the involved lung into the bronchial tree of a new lobe. Spread to a given lobe may be brought about by suspending the infected animal in such a way that gravity will carry the bronchial fluid into the desired lobe. It may be assumed that a similar mechanism operates in human patients with multilobar lesions. The fact that the commonest spread in human pneumonia is from one lower lobe to another is in keeping with the assumption that organisms are carried to the new lobe by infected bronchial fluid, the flow of which is influenced by cough, respiration and the force of gravity.

Bacteremia. Bacteremia frequently occurs during the course of pneumococcal pneumonia, particularly when the infection is fulminating. The fact that organisms appear in the thoracic duct in experimental pneumonia before they appear in the systemic circulation suggests that many of the organisms reach the blood stream via the lymphatics. It is well known that particles introduced experimentally into the alveoli are cleared primarily by lymphatic drainage. At least some of the bacteria in the spreading lesion appear to be removed from the lung by a similar mechanism. Their presence in regional mediastinal lymph nodes during experimental pneumonia has been repeatedly demonstrated. Whether bacteria gain access to the blood stream by penetrating the alveolar capillaries directly is not known.

Invasion of Pleura and Pericardium. The exact mechanism whereby pneumococci invade the pleura or pericardium is also unknown. Since the lymphatics at the periphery of the lung drain outward toward the pleura, it is possible that pleural invasion results from lymphangitic spread. On the other hand, it is also possible that organisms are carried through the visceral pleura along with edema fluid which accumulates in infected subpleural alveoli. When infection of a pleural or pericardial cavity occurs, there results an outpouring of serous fluid followed by the deposit of fibrin. Later, leukocytes accumulate in the infected cavity, and, if infection persists, a purulent focus results. The pus in such cavities is at first thin, but later becomes thick and stringy as a result, not only of fibrin formation, but also of the precipitation of desoxyribonucleic acid derived from the nuclei of disintegrating leukocytes. Finally, the thick fibrinous pus becomes walled off, forming loculated foci of chronic suppuration.

Similar purulent foci may occur in the meninges or joints, probably as a result of hematogenous metastasis. Acute vegetations on the endocardium of the heart valves are sometimes encountered, and acute splenic tumor indicative of systemic infection is a common finding in fatal cases observed at necropsy. Degeneration of renal tubules is also occasionally noted, and, since identical changes can be produced in the kidneys of laboratory animals by repeated injections of killed pneumococci, the lesions are assumed to be of pneumococcal origin.

Mechanism of Recovery. *Surface Phagocytosis.* Because of the antiphagocytic properties of their capsules, virulent, fully encapsulated pneumococci are resistant to phagocytosis when suspended in a fluid medium, as in ordinary opsonocytophagic tests performed in the laboratory. Such is not the case, however, within consolidated lesions *in vivo,* where phagocytosis of fully encapsulated bacteria readily occurs. This important difference in phagocytic efficiency has been shown to be due to the presence in tissues of suitable surfaces against which the leukocytes are able to trap the encapsulated organisms and thus ingest them without the aid of opsonizing antibody (see Fig. 25, p. 130). The efficiency of this "surface phagocytosis," which operates also within the interstices of fibrin clots, depends in large measure upon the amount of fluid present in the lesion. In the outer edema zone, where fluid is abundant and leukocytes relatively scarce, little phagocytosis occurs. In areas of more advanced consolidation, however, where actively motile leukocytes are packed closely together, the bacteria are not only effectively trapped against tissue surfaces and fibrin strands within the exudate, but are also caught between the surfaces of the phagocytic cells themselves and are thus ingested. This efficient mechanism of natural defense, operating in the absence of immune bodies, explains the prompt destruction of bacteria which is characteristic of the central portions of even the spreading pneumonic lesion. Recent studies on experimental bacteremia have also shown that surface phagocytosis plays an important role in disposing of pneumococci which have invaded the blood stream.

Likewise, when spread of the lesion is controlled by antimicrobial drugs such as penicillin, surface phagocytosis promptly disposes of the bacteria that are not destroyed outright by the drug or by autolysis. Consequently, it is not surprising that, with adequate chemotherapy, experimental pneumococcal lesions may clear completely and patients with pneumococcal pneumonia may experience dramatic defervescence many hours before opsonizing immune bodies can be detected in either the serum or the lesion. When a patient is treated sufficiently late in the course of the disease, antibody may be present in the serum and may then contribute to recovery by accelerating phagocytosis.

Macrophage Reaction. The exact role of the "macrophage reaction" in the recovery process is not entirely clear. Because the appearance of macrophages in the alveolar exudate coincides in general with the disappearance of organisms from the lesion, it has long been assumed that these large mononuclear phagocytes take an active part in destroying the bacteria and in the final analysis tip the

scales in favor of the cellular defenses of the host. Recent studies relating to experimental lymphadenitis cast some doubt upon this assumption. The "macrophage reaction" in a regional lymph node draining an area of active infection can be artificially initiated at any stage of the nodal inflammation by merely cutting the afferent lymph vessels bringing bacteria to the node. Thus it appears that macrophages accumulate in the exudate only when the active stimulus of direct bacterial invasion has been eliminated. If this interpretation is correct, the polymorphonuclear leukocytes may be looked upon as the "shock troops" that play the major role in controlling the infection, whereas the macrophages serve primarily to remove the particulate debris from the resolving exudate and thus promote clearing of the lesion.

Resolution. One of the most remarkable features of pneumococcal pneumonia is the completeness with which it resolves. Even when several lobes are completely consolidated at the height of the illness, recovery usually results in restoration of the entire pulmonary parenchyma to its normal state within a few weeks. Not all the processes that take part in this dramatic resolution have been identified, but they appear to include (*a*) the action of cytolytic ferments upon disintegrating leukocytes; (*b*) increased acidity of the exudate; (*c*) transport of cells from the lesion via lymphatics; and (*d*) phagocytosis and digestion of cellular debris by macrophages. The rarity with which tissue necrosis occurs in pneumococcal pneumonia, despite the violence of the inflammatory response, appears to account for the completeness of the healing. Occasionally recovery proceeds more slowly than usual and leads to "delayed resolution." The factors responsible for delaying the removal of exudate from the lesion in such cases are not known. In rare instances, as the result of irreversible damage to the pulmonary parenchyma, resolution fails to take place altogether, and the lesion becomes the site of intense fibroblastic activity which leads to the permanent scarring of "organized pneumonia."

Although resolution is usually complete in pneumococcal pneumonia, infection with type III pneumococcus may occasionally lead to pulmonary suppuration. This particular type of pneumococcus, in its most virulent form, has a large capsular "slime layer" which interferes with surface phagocytosis and accounts, at least in part, for its extraordinary pathogenicity. Type III pneumococci may accumulate in huge numbers in infected alveoli and on occasion cause necrosis, not only of leukocytes, but also of the alveolar walls. If the necrosis is sufficiently widespread, chronic lung abscesses result.

Suppurative Extrapulmonary Foci. Suppurative pneumococcal lesions, which usually occur in such extrapulmonary sites as the pleura, pericardium, mastoids or accessory sinuses, resolve much less readily, even with intensive chemotherapy, than does uncomplicated pneumococcal pneumonia. In such areas of suppuration, phagocytosis is relatively inefficient, first, because of the fluid present in the lesion, secondly, because of the absence of such extensive tissue surfaces as are afforded by the alveoli of the lung, and, thirdly, because many, if not most, of the leukocytes in the exudate are nonviable. In addition, chemotherapeutic agents administered systemically probably do not penetrate subacute or chronic suppurating lesions as readily as they do areas of acute pneumonia. Even when a drug such as penicillin reaches the organisms in a purulent focus, it may not necessarily destroy them. Pneumococci do not multiply rapidly in pus of long standing, and it is well known that "resting" bacteria are not susceptible to the antibacterial action of penicillin. Thus it is not surprising that clinical experience has demonstrated that purulent pneumococcal infections, such as an empyema, respond satisfactorily only when chemotherapy is combined with some form of drainage which removes the bulk of the necrotic exudate.

Symptoms. Victims of pneumococcal pneumonia are often seriously ill when first seen. The degree of prostration may be such that an adequate history can be obtained only from the family or some other close associate of the patient. The story of a *mild nasopharyngitis* preceding by several days the onset of major symptoms is frequently elicited by careful questioning. The first distressing symptom is usually a *shaking chill* lasting for several minutes to a half hour. More than 80 per cent of patients with pneumococcal pneumonia experience one or more chills during the earliest stages of the disease. The initial rigor is often so violent as to cause the bed to shake and the patient's teeth to chatter. It is followed in about one case in three by vomiting. The exact cause of the initial chill is not known, but it usually coincides with bacterial invasion of the lung and marks the onset of fever. Several chills may occur at the start of pneumococcal pneumonia, but repeated attacks of rigor late in the disease suggest an extrapulmonary complication such as endocarditis or empyema.

Chest Pain. In approximately 70 per cent of cases severe chest pain occurs at the onset and may even precede the rigor. The pain, which is "stabbing" in character and is exaggerated by cough and respiration, is caused by inflammation of the pleura resulting from the characteristically peripheral location of the initial lesion (see Fig. 24). There may be local tenderness in the chest wall at the site of the pleurisy. When the diaphragmatic surfaces of the pleura are affected, the pain is referred either to the corresponding side of the abdomen or to the shoulder, depending upon whether the peripheral (intercostal innervation) or central (phrenic innervation) part of the diaphragm is involved. The patient may gain some relief from the knifelike pain by lying on the affected side, thereby partially splinting that half of the thorax.

Cough may be absent at the onset, but usually is a prominent symptom during the course of the disease. Stimulation of the cough reflex results from irritation of the lower respiratory tract and from accumulation of mucus and exudate within the bronchial tree. Approximately 75 per cent of patients raise diffusely bloody or "rusty" sputum in contrast to "blood-streaked" sputum. The thorough mixing of the blood and mucus appears to be due to the fact that bleeding occurs directly into the alveolar exudate and thus constitutes an integral part of the inflammatory response to the infection. When the sputum is particularly sticky or jelly-like, type III pneumococcus or Friedländer's bacillus should be suspected as the cause of the pneumonia, since both these organisms produce, during growth, an inordinate amount of capsular polysaccharide which causes the exudate to be highly viscous.

Fever and *toxemia* are constant features of the disease, the temperature usually ranging between 103° and 106° F. During the febrile period complaints of malaise, weakness, myalgia and general prostration are extremely common.

Physical Signs. Since pneumococcal pneumonia may occasionally progress with great rapidity and the general condition of the patient may deteriorate alarmingly within a few hours, it is essential that the initial physical examination be as thorough as possible.

The temperature, pulse rate and respiratory rate are usually elevated by the time the patient seeks the aid of a physician. The temperature should be taken by rectum, since oral measurement with the subject breathing rapidly through the mouth is likely to be inaccurate. The pulse pressure is characteristically widened, as in any high fever, and the pulse at the wrist may be collapsing in quality. Subnormal blood pressure indicates shock and a poor prognosis.

Patients with well established pneumococcal pneumonia appear acutely ill. There is moderate to severe respiratory distress. The nostrils dilate with each inspiration. Paroxysms of hacking cough, often productive of bloody or rusty sputum, occur during the examination. The chest pain, which is usually unilateral, may be so severe as to interfere with the patient's breathing and coughing; in these circumstances grunting expiration results. The location of the pain indicates immediately the approximate site of at least part of the lesion. The patient occasionally appears apprehensive and may even be delirious.

The skin is usually hot and moist with beads of perspiration visible on the face and forehead. Cold extremities may indicate impending shock. Herpetic blisters are frequently noted about the mouth. The lips, mucous membranes and nail beds are often cyanotic as a result of blood passing through involved lung. The cyanosis may be exaggerated by poor respiratory exchange caused by severe pleural pain. Icterus of the sclerae should be carefully looked for because of the prognostic significance of jaundice in pneumonia. Occasionally petechiae are found in the skin of patients suffering from complicating pneumococcal endocarditis.

The ears should always be examined with an otoscope to rule out the presence of active otitis. Tenderness over a mastoid process or over an accessory nasal sinus should also be noted. The presence of exudate in the pharynx or over the tonsils suggests the possibility of streptococcal pneumonia. Definite nuchal rigidity is usually indicative of pneumococcal meningitis, a serious and not too infrequent complication of pneumonia. The neck veins must be carefully examined to detect the presence of increased venous pressure caused by complicating congestive heart failure. Deviation of the trachea constitutes an important sign of either atelectasis (toward the involved side) or pleural effusion (away from the involved side).

Examination of the Chest. The thorax must be examined with the utmost care. Diminished respiratory excursion or a slight inspiratory lag of one side of the chest often reveals the site of the principal lesion. A localized area of tenderness in the chest wall, noted during percussion, may be one of the earliest signs of pleural invasion. The presence of a large pleural effusion sometimes causes a noticeable fullness of intercostal spaces. Careful percussion and auscultation do not invariably reveal signs of consolidation. In early cases, particularly, there may be no conclusive physical signs. Lesions at a distance from the chest wall are difficult to outline by percussion. Breath sounds may be only slightly depressed if normal lung tissue separates the lesion from the large bronchi. When consolidation is extensive, the typical findings of dullness to percussion, bronchial or tubular breath sounds and fine crackling rales are easily elicited, except in the presence of complicating bronchial obstruction or extensive pleural effusion. A coarse "leathery" friction rub is frequently audible in the region of consolidation.

Examination of the heart may be difficult because of loud respiratory sounds. Its position and size should be carefully determined by palpation and percussion. A later shift in the position of the left cardiac border may indicate any one of the following complications: cardiac enlargement from heart failure, invasion of the pericardial cavity, atelectasis or pleural effusion. An apical systolic murmur is frequently heard during high fever and is often of no significance, although it may be due to bacterial vegetation. Diastolic murmurs, on the other hand, arising from either the mitral or aortic valve are usually indicative of underlying organic heart disease or complicating pneumococcal endocarditis. A pericardial friction rub often constitutes the first sign of spread of the pneumococcal infection to the pericardial cavity. Ventricular premature contractions are not uncommon in the presence of any moderate or severe infection.

Abdominal Distention. Distention of the abdomen is frequently encountered in advanced bacterial pneumonia. Its presence is due to paralytic ileus. Occasionally the examiner will note rigidity and even tenderness in one or both upper quadrants of the

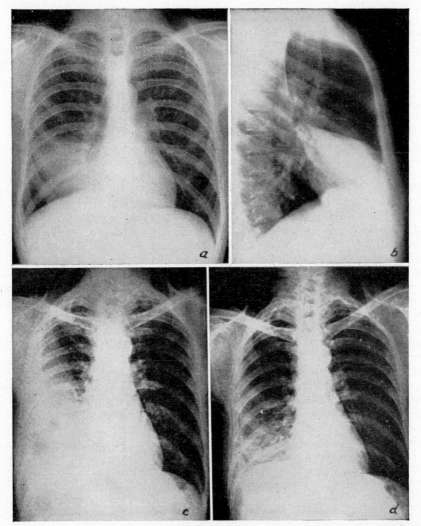

Fig. 26, *a*, Postero-anterior roentgenogram of chest of fifty-year-old man with pneumococcal type VI pneumonia of five days' duration. Note narrowed intercostal spaces on right and increased density in right lower lung field. Such a pulmonary shadow might be due to pneumonia in either the middle (anterior) or the lower (posterior) lobe, or in both.

b, Lateral view reveals that consolidation is confined to middle lobe, except for a few small patches in the lower. The sharpness and density of the upper border of the middle lobe shadow suggest the presence of a pleural effusion in the interlobar fissure between the upper and middle lobes. Sterile pleural fluid was obtained from the interlobar space by thoracentesis. The patient recovered promptly with penicillin therapy.

c, Loculated postpneumonic empyema in a forty-year-old white man admitted to the Bellevue Hospital, New York, on the nineteenth day of pneumococcal pneumonia. Only 50 ml. of thick greenish pus could be removed from the right chest by aspiration. Cultures were sterile. Pleural loculations are visible in the roentgenogram. Ten milliliters of a preparation containing 100,000 units of streptokinase and 25 units of streptodornase were introduced through the thoracentesis needle. Twenty-four hours later 465 ml. of cloudy, thin, blood-tinged fluid were removed.

d, Roentgenogram taken after the second thoracentesis, performed twenty-four hours after enzyme treatment. Temperature fell to normal, and patient made a rapid recovery. No further aspirations were necessary.

(*c* and *d* from W. S. Tillett et al.: Ann. Surg., Vol. 131.)

abdomen, suggesting a subdiaphragmatic lesion. This sign is usually due to referred pain resulting from involvement of the parietal pleura over the outer part of the diaphragm. The right upper quadrant should always be carefully examined for signs of enlargement or tenderness of the liver resulting from congestive heart failure.

In addition to edema from heart failure, the most important physical signs encountered in the extremities are those of phlebothrombosis. Since pulmonary infarction may closely resemble acute bacterial pneumonia, it is of the utmost importance to look for evidence of venous thrombosis in the legs.

The neurologic examination is rarely abnormal in pneumococcal pneumonia except in the presence of meningitis or brain abscess. Digital examination of the rectum may be postponed if the patient is acutely ill, but in women a sufficiently complete pelvic examination should be performed to rule out the possibility of an infected abortion, which often leads to metastatic bacterial pneumonia.

Laboratory Findings. The most important laboratory findings in pneumococcal pneumonia may be grouped under the following headings:

1. *Findings Indicating the Presence of an Acute Infection.* As in most acute infections of bacterial etiology, the total leukocyte count in pneumococcal pneumonia is elevated and there is a "shift to the left" in the differential count; the erythrocyte sedimentation rate is also increased. The number of leukocytes in the peripheral blood during the active infection usually ranges from 15,000 to 40,000 per cubic millimeter; counts above 40,000 are occasionally encountered. Leukopenia (with a "shift to the left") is observed in fulminating pneumococcal infections, particularly in the presence of bacteremia.

2. *Findings Indicating Pulmonary Consolidation.* Although the presence and location of the pulmonary lesion can usually be determined by physical examination, confirmatory roentgenographic evidence is often helpful. Patients seen in the hospital should either be fluoroscoped (on a stretcher, if necessary) or subjected to roentgenographic examination. Both postero-anterior and lateral views of the chest should be taken. The lateral film may be of great value in (a) detecting retrocardiac consolidation in the left lower lobe, (b) indicating whether a lesion visible in the postero-anterior view is located anteriorly or posteriorly and thus in what

lobe it is situated, and (c) identifying interlobar accumulations of fluid (Fig. 26, a, b). If the patient is too ill to be subjected to such a complete examination, a portable chest film should be taken at the bedside. Proper management of pneumococcal pneumonia in the home does not necessarily require roentgenographic examination.

3. *Findings Indicating Etiology.* Whenever the diagnosis of pneumococcal pneumonia is suspected, blood should be drawn for culture. Anaerobic (thioglycollate broth) as well as aerobic cultures are recommended, since many strains of pneumococci multiply most readily at a reduced oxygen tension. A positive blood culture not only affords clear-cut evidence regarding etiology, but also gives valuable information concerning prognosis. The physician should make a real effort to obtain a suitable specimen of sputum. Whenever possible, the patient should be made to expectorate mucus raised directly from the bronchial tree; secretions from the nasopharynx may be unsatisfactory. The specimen should be taken to the laboratory immediately to be cultured, inoculated intraperitoneally in a mouse, and smeared for Gram stain. When typing serums are available, direct typing of the sputum should be attempted, and, if unsuccessful, the pneumococci isolated by culture or mouse inoculation should be identified by the quellung technique. The practical importance of pneumococcal typing today is limited, but is of some value in differential diagnosis, as noted below. In the days of serum therapy, however, specific treatment could not be begun until the type of the infecting organism had been determined. When no sputum specimen can be obtained from the patient, a throat swab may be cultured. Although it is not a hazardous procedure, lung puncture is now rarely used to determine the etiology of acute bacterial pneumonia.

Other laboratory examinations which may be of value in the management of the patient include the measurement of serum sodium and chloride. During the acute phase of bacterial pneumonia there may be a profound disturbance in electrolyte metabolism characterized by (a) depressed urinary excretion of sodium chloride and (b) decrease in the concentration of sodium and chloride in the serum. Both these changes appear to be due to transfer of sodium chloride from plasma and extracellular fluid. In particularly severe infections hyponatremia and hypochloremia may be associated with "prerenal" azotemia and shock. The exact mechanism of the electrolyte disturbance is at present not known.

Clinical Course. During the course of the disease the patient should be examined carefully once a day. More frequent physical examinations may unduly exhaust an acutely ill subject. The common complications of pneumococcal pneumonia should be specific-

provement in general appearance. Physical signs in the chest also change within a few days, coarse sticky rales of resolution replacing the fine crepitant rales and tubular breath sounds of consolidation. Complete clearing of the pulmonary lesion may occur within a few days, but usually the auscultatory signs of resolution persist for a week or more after defervescence. If resolution is not complete

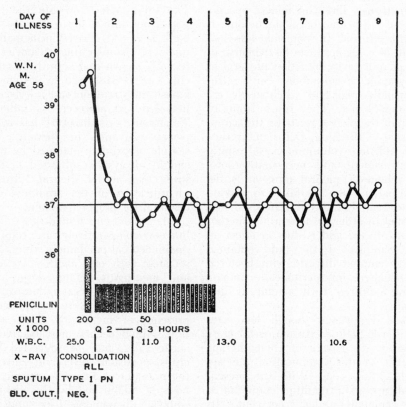

Fig. 27. Response of uncomplicated pneumococcal pneumonia to oral treatment with penicillin. (From W. McDermott; Nelson's Loose Leaf System of Medicine, Vol. I, Chap. 6.)

ally looked for during each examination, particularly when fever persists.

Defervescence. The fever of untreated pneumococcal pneumonia may either terminate abruptly by "crisis" five to ten days after the onset or may gradually subside by lysis. When effective antibacterial therapy is used, a dramatic crisis often ensues within twenty-four hours (Fig. 27). Sometimes a slight secondary rise in temperature occurs after the crisis, and low grade fever may persist during the first few days of recovery. Not only does defervescence occur promptly after effective therapy, but the patient experiences striking relief of symptoms and exhibits a marked im-

within twenty-one days, it is arbitrarily classified as delayed. The speed of resolution is in general inversely proportional to the age and extent of the lesion at the time treatment is begun.

Crisis marking the start of recovery must be differentiated from the "pseudocrisis" occasionally noted at the onset of peripheral vascular collapse or at the time of interlobar spread of the infection. Although the temperature may fall precipitously during a pseudo-crisis, the pulse rate remains elevated and the patient's general condition fails to improve.

Relapse may occur in pneumococcal pneumonia, particularly when chemotherapy is discontinued too soon. If fever, tachycardia and other signs of active infection recur while the patient is still receiving intensive penicillin therapy, it may usually be assumed either that a previously unrecognized purulent complication of the pneumococcal infection (such as empyema) exists or that a drug-resistant secondary invader has gained a foothold in the lung.

Complications. The commonest specific complication of pneumococcal pneumonia is pleurisy with effusion. In somewhat less than 10 per cent of cases fluid can be demonstrated in the pleural cavity by either physical or roentgenographic examination. Such effusions are usually small and, when sterile, are rarely of significance. They result from inflammation of the pleura overlying the parenchymal lesion of the lung. Occasionally they may be of sufficient volume to cause respiratory embarrassment and necessitate thoracentesis. Whenever pleural effusion is detected in a patient who has failed to respond promptly to treatment, a thoracentesis should be performed in order to determine whether the fluid is infected and is thus in effect an empyema. Samples of the fluid obtained should be examined directly with bacterial stains, inoculated intraperitoneally into a mouse, and cultured both aerobically and anaerobically.

Empyema. Empyema, though less common than sterile pleural effusion, is far more serious. Before the advent of chemotherapy the incidence of this complication was approximately 5 per cent. With the present widespread use of penicillin, empyema is much less common (under 2 per cent). Its presence is indicated by continued fever (often irregular), persistent leukocytosis, repeated sweats and signs of pleural effusion (Fig. 26, c). Localized tenderness is frequently noted in the chest wall overlying the site of the lesion. The exudate in the pleural cavity may become loculated by thick, fibrinous adhesions. If it is present in sufficient quantity, it may cause fullness of intercostal spaces and a shift of the trachea and mediastinum away from the side of the lesion. When the lesion is confined to an interlobar fissure or located in the thoracic "gutter" adjacent to the spine, it may be detectable only by roentgenographic methods. Repeated exploratory thoracenteses may be required to prove the presence of empyema. Its detection is of the greatest importance, since, once dis-

covered, it is amenable to proper therapy; whereas, if left untreated, it may eventually drain exteriorly through the chest wall (empyema necessitatis) or rupture into a bronchus and cause a bronchopleural fistula. Rarely, empyema heals spontaneously, causing calcification of the pleura. The fluid contained within an empyema cavity is at first thin, but soon becomes so thick and "stringy" that aspiration through a needle is difficult. The solid material within the pus is composed, not only of fibrin, but also of desoxyribonucleic acid derived principally from the nuclei of disintegrating leukocytes. Tillett has recently shown that both these solid components can be dissolved by enzymes (streptokinase and streptodornase) derived from beta-hemolytic streptococci. As indicated under Treatment, this discovery has led to an important advance in therapy. The initial sample of exudate obtained by thoracentesis should always be subjected to bacteriologic study (see under Pleural Effusion), since identification of the offending organism is essential for proper treatment.

Meningitis and Endocarditis. Two serious, but now comparatively rare, complications of pneumococcal pneumonia which are often associated with one another are endocarditis and meningitis. Eighteen out of nineteen cases of pneumococcal endocarditis described by Ruegesegger were complicated by the presence of meningitis. Endocardial infection, which occurs most commonly on the aortic valve, may be suggested by repeated chills, persistent fever and leukocytosis and the presence of a cardiac murmur. The diagnosis is established by the identification of embolic phenomena (see under Bacterial Endocarditis) and by the demonstration of persistent bacteremia. Only rarely does recovery occur without treatment. Equally serious is pneumococcal meningitis resulting from blood-borne metastasis to the meninges. Its presence is indicated by the usual manifestations of meningitis (headache, nausea and vomiting, stiff neck, positive Kernig's sign, stupor, and so forth), and the diagnosis is established by the demonstration of purulent cerebrospinal fluid containing pneumococci. The meningitis is characterized by the presence in the pia-arachnoid of a heavily infected exudate, which may cause subarachnoid block or lead to localized subarachnoid abscesses. Unless vigorous therapy is instituted promptly, the prognosis is hopeless.

Pericarditis. Like the other complications

of pneumococcal pneumonia, pericarditis has also become relatively rare since the introduction of potent antimicrobial drugs. When the pericardium is invaded, the patient usually experiences precordial pain, and a leathery friction rub may be heard over the heart. Pericardial effusion usually results, causing a "dampening" of the heart sounds. If the fluid is sterile, the condition is benign, unless so large a volume accumulates as to cause cardiac tamponade. Empyema of the pericardium, on the other hand, is a serious complication requiring prompt and vigorous treatment. If it is allowed to persist untreated, purulent pericarditis may gradually heal, but will often lead to pericardial calcification. Years later serious and even fatal constriction of the heart may result from contraction of the healed lesion.

Other Specific Complications. Still rarer specific complications include peritonitis, pyogenic arthritis, metastatic cutaneous abscesses and nephritis. The last of these usually occurs several weeks after the pneumonia, the latent period appearing to be similar to that in nephritis following group A streptococcal infection. Occasionally the pulmonary lesion of pneumococcal pneumonia fails to resolve even after many weeks and finally becomes replaced by fibrous tissue. This complication is termed organized pneumonia and rarely causes serious disability unless accompanied by suppuration.

Nonspecific Complications. Three nonspecific complications of importance occur not infrequently during the acute phase of pneumococcal pneumonia: paralytic ileus, peripheral vascular collapse (shock) and congestive heart failure. *Ileus* occurs particularly in patients suffering from anoxia and severe toxemia and gives rise to gaseous distention of the abdomen (tympanites) which causes discomfort and often increases respiratory embarrassment. *Shock,* likewise, is a complication of severe toxemia and indicates a serious prognosis. The circulatory disturbance is characterized by hemoconcentration, an increased rather than a depressed cardiac output, and peripheral vasodilatation. Whether "toxic myocarditis" also plays a role is uncertain. The skin, particularly of the extremities, is cold and moist and exhibits a characteristic gray cyanosis. Peripheral vascular failure, when present for a sufficient length of time, becomes irreversible, and the patient eventually dies in shock despite the fact that the infection in the meantime may have been adequately controlled by chemotherapy. *Congestive heart failure,* which also occurs not infrequently as a complication of severe pneumonia, particularly in patients with underlying heart disease, must be differentiated from peripheral vascular collapse, for the proper methods of treating the two conditions are different. Since congestive heart failure is an important predisposing factor in bacterial pneumonia, it is not surprising that they are often associated, and obviously both must be treated. The diagnosis of congestive heart failure in the presence of pneumonia may at times be difficult, but should be considered in any patient with abnormal distention of neck veins, peripheral edema, an enlarged tender liver, elevated venous pressure and a prolonged circulation time. Pulmonary signs of congestion may be unreliable, particularly if the pneumonia is bilateral.

Jaundice, the pathogenesis of which appears to be related to increased hemolysis of the erythrocytes in the pneumonic lesion and depressed liver function resulting from anoxia, occurs most often in patients who have severe pneumonia and have had a poor diet. The presence of icterus usually indicates a poor prognosis. As in any bedridden patient, phlebothrombosis may occur during pneumonia. Its presence should suggest the possibility that the pulmonary lesion is due to infarction of the lung rather than to primary pneumonia. *Herpes labialis* occurs in from 5 to 40 per cent of patients with pneumococcal pneumonia and constitutes an essentially benign complication. Occasionally the herpetic lesions become secondarily infected, causing mild pyoderma.

Differential Diagnosis. The symptoms and signs of pneumococcal pneumonia are usually so characteristic as to make the diagnosis relatively simple. Atypical cases occasionally occur in which a definitive diagnosis cannot be made and in which antimicrobial treatment on suspicion is justified. Sometimes the disease is mistaken for less serious forms of respiratory tract infection, such as acute tracheobronchitis or "grippe." This error can often be avoided if proper significance is attached to the history of chills, bloody sputum and chest pain, if the lungs are carefully examined at frequent intervals for signs of pulmonary consolidation, and if postero-anterior and lateral roentgenograms are made of the chest.

Pneumonia due to organisms other than pneumococcus may at times be difficult to differentiate from pneumococcal pneumonia. Only by bacteriologic study of the sputum can pneumonia due to Friedländer's bacillus, *Staphylococcus aureus* or group A beta-hemolytic streptococcus be identified. Tuberculous pneumonia rarely causes the acute prostration characteristic of coccal infection, and the leukocyte count is usually normal or only slightly elevated. *Primary atypical pneumonia* and other viral and rickettsial infections of the lungs, such as psittacosis and Q fever, do not often cause shaking chills, diffusely bloody sputum, severe pleural pain or a marked leukocytosis, although they may at times be confused with acute bacterial pneumonia (see p. 152). Tularemic pneumonia must also be considered. When the diagnosis is in doubt, repeated examinations of the sputum should be made, using both the Gram and Ziehl-Neelsen stains. Sputum specimens should not only be cultured, but should be injected into mice. The identification of one of the lower types of pneumococcus (excluding type III) constitutes strong circumstantial evidence in favor of the diagnosis of pneumococcal pneumonia. Specific diagnosis of pneumonia is of great practical importance, because of therapy. Whereas tuberculous, tularemic and Friedländer's bacillus pneumonia respond to streptomycin and individual instances of primary atypical pneumonia might be influenced by the tetracycline drugs, most other forms of acute pneumonia are best treated with penicillin.

Nonpulmonary Bacterial Infections. Bacterial infections other than pneumonia must be considered in the differential diagnosis. Pleurisy involving the outer part of the diaphragm and resulting from right lower lobe pneumonia often causes referred pain to the right side of the abdomen, thus simulating acute appendicitis. Subdiaphragmatic abscess arising from perforation of the appendix conversely may simulate pneumonia. Acute pyelonephritis with chills, fever, flank pain and leukocytosis must not be confused with pneumonia; the diagnosis is usually established by examination of the urine and by the absence of signs of frank consolidation in the lungs. Differentiation of acute pyelonephritis from pneumococcal pneumonia is of primary importance, since most urinary tract infections are caused by organisms that are not susceptible to penicillin.

Noninfectious Diseases. Among the essentially noninfectious processes which must be differentiated from pneumococcal pneumonia are congestive heart failure, pulmonary infarction, and atelectasis. That *congestive heart failure* predisposes to acute bacterial pneumonia has already been emphasized. The two conditions not infrequently coexist, but occasionally congestive heart failure is mistaken for pneumococcal pneumonia. This error is most frequently made in cases with dyspnea, cough, blood-streaked sputum, and signs in the chest which simulate those of consolidation, but in reality are due to pleural effusion. In such cases the absence of high fever and leukocytosis and the presence of distended neck veins and peripheral edema usually suggest the correct diagnosis.

Pulmonary infarction, on the other hand, is more difficult to differentiate from pneumonia. The dyspnea, pleural pain, hemoptysis, fever, physical signs of pulmonary consolidation, roentgenographic findings, and leukocytosis are all in keeping with an acute infection of the lungs. Not infrequently, however, the initial symptom is intense pleural pain of explosive onset; shaking chills rarely occur; there is no preceding history of respiratory infection; the fever usually is not high; frank hemoptysis is common; pulmonary signs, when present, appear early; and the total leukocyte count rarely reaches 20,000 per cubic millimeter. When a pulmonary infarct becomes infected, as not infrequently happens, differentiation from primary bacterial pneumonia may be extremely difficult. Although in such cases the patients should receive antimicrobial treatment as in pneumonia, recognition of the infarction is of importance because of the need for anti-coagulant therapy.

Pulmonary atelectasis, resulting from bronchial obstruction, not only may simulate pneumonia, but often leads to serious infection of the lung if the bronchial obstruction is not relieved. Aspiration of mucus during or after surgical anesthesia is a common cause of atelectasis. Dyspnea, cough, chest pain, splinting of one side of the thorax, dullness to percussion and suppressed breath sounds may all suggest primary pneumonia. Fever and leukocytosis also are noted when infection is present. Since pulmonary atelectasis may be relieved by forced coughing and postural drainage or, if necessary, by bronchoscopy, it is important to differentiate it from primary pneumonia. Occasionally, sufficient shift of the mediastinum occurs to make the diagnosis obvious. Collapse of a segment of the lung may also result from chronic bronchial obstruction due to bronchogenic carcinoma or aortic aneurysm.

Even when the diagnosis of pneumococcal pneumonia is established beyond doubt, the possibility of a second underlying lesion of the lung must be borne in mind. Bronchiectasis may lead to repeated attacks of bacterial pneumonia and often becomes evident only after the pneumonic consolidation has resolved. Bronchogenic carcinoma, as well as pulmonary tuberculosis, must likewise be looked for during the follow-up examination.

Treatment. The treatment of pneumococcal pneumonia may best be discussed under three headings: (a) antimicrobial therapy, (b) supportive measures and (c) the treatment of complications. Before the advent of effective antibacterial therapy, supportive treatment was of the greatest importance. The introduction, first of antipneumococcal serum and later of sulfonamides, penicillin and the other antimicrobial drugs, has so altered the management of pneumococcal pneumonia that today supportive treatment is rarely crucial, and serious complications are only occasionally encountered.

Antibacterial Therapy. PENICILLIN. Penicillin is at present the drug of choice in the treatment of pneumococcal pneumonia. Most strains of the organism are extremely sensitive to penicillin and are inhibited in broth culture by concentrations of less than 0.01 unit per milliliter. The effectiveness of antimicrobial treatment is due in part to the natural resistance of the host, which accounts for the destruction of a large proportion of the invading bacteria. Host resistance, which results primarily from the activity of phagocytic cells in the lung, when combined with the bacteriostatic and bactericidal effects of drug therapy, controls promptly all but the most malignant pneumonia. Even with no treatment at all, approximately seven of every ten patients with pneumococcal pneumonia eventually recover.

Conventional penicillin therapy involves the intramuscular administration of 10,000 to 100,000 units every three hours, depending upon the severity of the infection. A fairly large initial dose, 50,000 to 100,000 units, is often advisable. Treatment should be maintained until the temperature has been normal for seventy-two hours; if treatment is discontinued too soon, relapse of the infection occurs. Since penicillin continues to exert a bacteriostatic effect for several hours after the drug has been removed from the site of infection, it is possible to lengthen the interval between doses to eight or even twelve hours, provided large enough doses are given. In severe infections, however, it is safest to give the drug at least every six and preferably every four hours.

Penicillin may be given either intramuscularly or orally. When oral penicillin is used, it must be prescribed in doses five times as large as those used intramuscularly, since only 20 to 30 per cent is absorbed from the gastrointestinal tract. Slowly absorbed ("depot") penicillin, in the form of the procaine salt, may be injected intramuscularly in doses of 300,000 units once or twice a day. This form of treatment, though convenient to both patient and physician, should not be relied upon in severe infections, since the blood levels attained are considerably lower than those resulting from multiple injections of aqueous penicillin.

Response to penicillin therapy is usually dramatic (Fig. 27). Bacteremia, when present at the start of treatment, clears within a few hours. A crisis, characterized by rapid defervescence and a striking subsidence of symptoms, occurs in less than 48 hours in approximately 85 per cent of patients. The remaining 15 per cent experience a more gradual recovery, the temperature falling by lysis over a period of three to seven days. Not infrequently a secondary rise in temperature occurs after the crisis. This elevation is usually low grade and subsides spontaneously within a few hours, or at most a few days. Such secondary fever must be distinguished from that caused by complications or continued pulmonary infection, and can usually be recognized by the fact that it is accompanied neither by symptoms of continued toxicity nor by significant leukocytosis.

When a patient fails to respond within forty-eight hours to penicillin therapy, two possible explanations should be considered: (a) that the patient is suffering from a serious complication such as empyema, endocarditis or meningitis, or (b) that the primary infection is of nonpneumococcal etiology and is due to an agent that is resistant to the antimicrobial action of penicillin. Lack of response to penicillin cannot be explained on the basis of a penicillin-resistant strain of pneumococcus, since such strains are rarely, if ever, encountered in human pneumonia. Occasionally patients will respond initially to treatment only to have unmistakable signs of persistent pneumonia subsequently develop, in spite of continued therapy. This sequence of events is usually due to the presence of a mixed infection, the initial response to treatment resulting from control of penicillin-sensitive organisms, and the relapse occurring as a result of secondary invasion by penicillin-resistant species. Immediate institution of combined therapy, with streptomycin, erythromycin or a tetracycline drug (Aureomycin, Terramycin) is indicated in all such cases.

Toxic reactions to penicillin are rarely of sufficient severity to warrant discontinuation of treatment. Urticaria may be bothersome, and a combination of symptoms and signs suggesting "serum sickness" occasionally occurs. Patients with dermatophytosis may experience an exacerbation of the lesions during penicillin therapy.

SULFONAMIDES. Sulfonamides such as sulfathiazole, sulfadiazine and sulfamerazine are highly effective in the treatment of pneumococcal pneumonia, may be given by mouth, and are less expensive to the patient than penicillin. In addition, the drugs have a somewhat wider range of antibacterial activity than does penicillin. In general, however, sulfonamides should not be used in the treatment of pneumococcal pneumonia for the following reasons: (1) Penicillin is a more potent antibacterial agent than the sulfonamides, it causes more prompt destruction of the bacteria, and it is far more effective in controlling purulent complications; and (2) toxic reactions to sulfonamides (particularly to sulfathiazole) are significantly more common than to penicillin and include such conditions as toxic nephritis and periarteritis nodosa, which may terminate fatally. There is no conclusive evidence that combined penicillin-sulfonamide therapy is any more effective than treatment with penicillin alone, except possibly in the presence of meningitis or in the case of mixed infections involving penicillin-resistant organisms. In the latter situation other antimicrobial drugs (see above) rather than sulfonamides should be combined with penicillin.

When sulfonamides are used, they should be administered orally to adult patients as follows: An initial dose of 4 to 6 gm. should be followed by maintenance doses of 1 to 2 gm. every four hours, and continued until the temperature has been normal for three to five days. The concentration of sulfonamide in the blood should be measured at daily inter-vals, if possible, and dosage should be regulated to maintain the concentration at approximately 10 mg. per 100 cc. Fluid intake should be such as to maintain a daily urinary output of 800 to 1200 ml. In noncardiac patients sodium bicarbonate may be given (in a dosage 2.5 times that of sulfonamide) to maintain an alkaline urine and thus lessen the likelihood of precipitation of sulfonamide crystals in the urinary tract.

ANTISERUM. Type-specific antiserum is no longer used in the treatment of pneumococcal pneumonia.

The TETRACYCLINE DRUGS (e.g., Aureomycin, Terramycin) and CHLORAMPHENICOL may be used in the treatment of acute bacterial pneumonia. When the diagnosis of pneumococcal pneumonia is not clearly established, it may be advisable to use a tetracycline (0.5 to 1 gm. by mouth every six hours) because of their broader antibacterial action and their possibly beneficial effect in primary atypical pneumonia. Erythromycin is less effective than penicillin or the tetracyclines in pneumococcal pneumonia and should be used (0.3–0.5 gm. every 6 hours) only when the lesion is suspected of harboring penicillin-resistant staphylococci.

Supportive Treatment. Patients suffering from pneumococcal pneumonia should be kept at bed rest, and visitors to the sick room should be limited to the immediate family. Pleural pain, if mild, may be treated with codeine sulfate (30 to 60 mg.) orally, and, if severe, with subcutaneous morphine sulfate (10 to 15 mg.) or an equivalent analgesic such as methadone hydrochloride (5 to 10 mg., subcutaneously). A tight chest-binder is sometimes helpful in providing "something to cough against." Restlessness and insomnia, which are most commonly associated with delirium, are best controlled by paraldehyde (4 to 12 cc. by mouth or 10 to 20 cc. in 20 to 30 cc. of olive oil by rectum). Dyspnea and cyanosis should be treated with oxygen, administered by tent (40 to 60 per cent oxygen) or by nasal catheter (35 to 50 per cent oxygen, when gas is delivered at 4 to 7 liters per minute). Oxygen masks are usually unsuitable because of the patient's cough and expectoration.

FLUID AND ELECTROLYTES. During the acute stage of pneumococcal pneumonia considerable fluid is lost from the body, chiefly through the skin as the result of high fever. Dehydration may develop rapidly and, if severe, may become a contributing factor in the development of shock. Most patients require between 3 and 4 liters of fluid a day when the fever is high. Because of the loss of salt through the skin and the tendency for the serum sodium to be low during the acute phase of the infection, it is advisable to supplement the intake of sodium chloride with 1 per cent salty broth. A total daily intake of 6 to 10 gm. of salt is usually sufficient. Intravenous saline may be used if the patient is unable to take fluid by mouth. In the presence of congestive heart failure the use of supplementary sodium chloride is contraindicated. In the absence of renal disease, glycosuria or congestive heart failure, the patient's state of hydration may be estimated by the specific gravity of the urine. When hydration is adequate, the specific gravity should remain below 1.020.

DIET. Many patients with pneumococcal pneumonia are too ill to tolerate a full diet and should receive only liquids during the height of the fever. Fruit juices, ginger ale and soups are well tolerated. After the crisis a regular diet may be prescribed.

The patient should be kept in bed until the temperature has been normal for several days and should be observed closely until the pneumonic lesion has resolved. As already emphasized, all patients should be subjected to a follow-up roentgenographic examination three to four weeks after recovery.

Treatment of Complications. SHOCK. Patients with peripheral vascular collapse (shock) resulting from severe pneumococcal pneumonia usually respond poorly to the accepted forms of antishock therapy. The prognosis is almost invariably grave when this complication develops. Oxygen therapy should be begun immediately even if cyanosis is absent. Norepinephrine is at present the best drug available for combating peripheral vascular collapse. It should be given continuously by intravenous drip in sufficient amounts to maintain the systolic pressure at levels between 100 and 110. Enough norepinephrine (one vial contains 4 mg.) must be added to each liter of salt solution so that the hypotension can be controlled by the administration of not more than 2000 to 3000 ml. of fluid in 24 hours. Adrenocortical extract (30 to 50 cc. intravenously, followed by 10 cc. intramuscularly every four to eight hours) is occasionally used, although its effectiveness is not established. These measures should be used only with the greatest caution if signs of congestive heart failure are

also present. The treatment of congestive heart failure in patients with pneumococcal pneumonia is essentially the same as the treatment of heart failure under other conditions (see The Treatment of Congestive Heart Failure).

ABDOMINAL DISTENTION. Abdominal distention (paralytic ileus) is best managed by the use of daily enemas, the insertion of a rectal tube, the administration of oxygen, the application of heat to the abdomen (warm turpentine stupes) and repeated hypodermic injections of prostigmine methylsulfate (0.5 mg.). The prostigmine injections should be repeated every hour until a definite effect is obtained; subsequent doses should be spaced at intervals of two to four hours and maintained as long as is necessary.

Delirium may sometimes be difficult to control, particularly in patients with a history of chronic alcoholism. The use of 30 to 90 cc. of whisky per day may quiet alcoholic patients during the acute phase of the disease. The safest hypnotic to use is paraldehyde. A restraining net over the bed is often required to prevent the patient from climbing out of bed and injuring himself.

EMPYEMA AND PERICARDITIS. The treatment of empyema and of purulent pericarditis until recently has always been surgical. During World War I, Graham demonstrated that open thoracotomy must always be delayed until the pus aspirated from the chest is relatively thick and the area of infection is sufficiently well walled off to prevent marked shift of the mediastinum. Since the advent of penicillin, cases of both empyema and pericarditis have been successfully treated by repeated aspiration and injection of aqueous penicillin (50,000 to 200,000 units daily) through a thoracentesis needle. More recently, Tillett and his co-workers have demonstrated that the treatment of empyema without surgical drainage is greatly facilitated by the use of two enzyme preparations obtained from filtrates of beta-hemolytic streptococci. The first of these enzymes, *streptokinase,* activates the the fibrinolytic system in plasma and thereby causes lysis of the fibrin contained in purulent exudates. The second enzyme, known as *streptodornase* (abbreviation for streptococcal desoxyribonuclease), brings about depolymerization of the desoxyribonucleoprotein. By lysing both the fibrin and the nucleoprotein, the streptococcal enzymes cause a dramatic liquefaction of longstanding purulent exudates, which otherwise would be too thick to aspirate through even the largest thoracentesis needle. Loculation also is broken up by the "enzymatic débridement." Because of their large molecular dimensions, the streptococcal enzymes do not penetrate living cells and therefore are not injurious to tissue or to viable phagocytes. The streptokinase and streptodornase are injected directly into the pleural (or pericardial) space in doses of 200,000 to 400,000 units and 50,000 to 100,000 units, respectively. A mild and transient febrile reaction often occurs within a few hours. Several injections may be necessary, particularly when the empyema has become loculated. By the use of the streptococcal enzymes, combined with daily aspiration and the local injection of penicillin, prompt and permanent cures of both acute and relatively chronic empyemas have been effected (Fig. 26, c, d).

The treatment of the remaining two major complications of pneumococcal pneumonia, namely, meningitis and endocarditis, are discussed elsewhere (see Meningitis and Bacterial Endocarditis).

Prognosis. The case fatality rate in untreated pneumococcal pneumonia ranges from 20 to 40 per cent. The widespread use of sulfonamide drugs in the late 1930's resulted in a lowering of the fatality rate among treated patients to approximately 10 per cent. Penicillin therapy has lowered the rate still further. At present approximately 95 per cent of patients with pneumococcal pneumonia recover when properly treated with penicillin.

The prognosis in pneumococcal pneumonia is influenced adversely by each of the following: (1) old age (and also infancy), (2) late treatment, (3) infection with certain types of pneumococci (particularly types II and III), (4) involvement of more than one lobe of the lung, (5) leukopenia, (6) bacteremia, (7) jaundice, (8) the presence of complications (notably shock and meningitis), (9) pregnancy (particularly in the third trimester), (10) the presence of other disease (i.e., heart disease, cirrhosis of liver, and so forth), (11) alcoholism. Through a consideration of these factors a rough estimate may be made of the severity of the infection in each individual case, and therapy may be modified accordingly.

Prevention. Since pneumococcal pneumonia is not highly contagious and since it responds promptly to early therapy, prophylaxis constitutes less of a problem than it does in many other infectious diseases. It is estimated that only one in every 500 persons of all ages in the United States may be expected to contract the disease in any one year. In certain closed communities, however, and in areas where the pneumococcal carrier rate is particularly high, epidemics occasionally occur. Under such conditions, immunization with pneumococcal polysaccharide may be indicated. During World War II the effectiveness of polyvalent pneumococcal vaccine in preventing pneumonia and in lowering the pneumococcal carrier rate was clearly demonstrated in a controlled experiment on Army personnel. Although immunization may prove to be of value in military medicine, its application to the general population is not indicated because the incidence of the disease in ordinary circumstances is too low to justify vaccination. Likewise, the use of methods of "air sterilization" by ultraviolet radiation and by aerosols is of limited applicability.

Although pneumococcal pneumonia can undoubtedly be prevented (or at least aborted) in many patients by the intensive treatment of every upper respiratory tract infection with antimicrobial drugs, their indiscriminate use for this purpose should be avoided. The possible inconvenience to the patient of hypersensitivity reactions and the theoretic danger of producing drug-fast strains of bacteria outweigh the advantages to be gained in preventing such a relatively uncommon and readily treatable disease as pneumococcal pneumonia. Such chemoprophylaxis during outbreaks of epidemic influenza, on the other hand, may be indicated.

Isolation Procedures. Ideally, every patient with pneumococcal pneumonia should be placed in respiratory isolation, all attendants and visitors being required to wear masks when in the patient's room. The isolation precautions should be enforced until the patient has been afebrile for several days. The cross-infection rate in pneumococcal pneumonia is low and patients receiving chemotherapy are probably not highly infectious. Hence isolation rules are often disregarded without apparent ill effect. The danger of cross infection in a general hospital, particularly among patients with congestive heart failure, pulmonary edema or other severe debilitating diseases, may be greater than in the general population.

W. BARRY WOOD, JR.

References

Harford, C. G., and Hara, M.: Pulmonary Edema in Influenzal Pneumonia of the Mouse and the Relation of Fluid in the Lung to the Inception of Pneumococcal Pneumonia. J. Exper. Med., *91:* 245, 1950.

Heffron, R.: Pneumonia, with Special Reference to Pneumococcus Lobar Pneumonia. New York, Commonwealth Fund, 1939.

Loosli, C. G.: The Pathogenesis and Pathology of Experimental Type I Pneumococcic Pneumonia in the Monkey. J. Exper. Med., 76:79, 1942.

MacLeod, C. M.: The Pneumococci, in Dubos, R. J.: Bacterial and Mycotic Infections of Man. 2nd ed. Philadelphia, J. B. Lippincott Company, 1952, Chap. 10.

McDermott, W.: Pneumococcus Pneumonia. New York, Nelson's Loose Leaf System of Medicine, Vol. 1, Chap. 6.

Robertson, O. H.: Recent Studies on Experimental Lobar Pneumonia: Pathogenesis, Recovery, and Immunity. J.A.M.A., *111:*1432, 1938.

Tillett, W. S.: Studies on the Enzymatic Lysis of Fibrin and Inflammatory Exudates by Products of Hemolytic Streptococci. Harvey Lecture Series 1949–1950. Springfield, Illinois, Charles C Thomas, 1951.

Wood, W. B., and others: Studies on the Mechanism of Recovery in Pneumococcal Pneumonia. J. Exper. Med., 73:201, 1941; 84:365, 1946.

———: Studies on The Cellular Immunology of Acute Bacterial Infections. The Harvey Lectures, Series 47, 1951–52.

———, and Smith, M. R.: Host-Parasite Relationships in Experimental Pneumonia Due to Pneumococcus Type III. J. Exper. Med., 92:85, 1950.

OTHER FORMS OF ACUTE BACTERIAL PNEUMONIA

The bacteria, other than pneumococcus, that most commonly cause acute pneumonia are Friedländer's bacillus, beta-hemolytic streptococcus (group A) and *Staphylococcus aureus*. Each accounts for approximately 1 to 2 per cent of cases. Rarely the influenza bacillus may be involved, although usually, when present, it acts only as a secondary invader. Except as set forth below, the pneumonias due to these organisms are essentially the same as pneumococcal pneumonia.

FRIEDLÄNDER'S BACILLUS PNEUMONIA

Early recognition of acute Friedländer's pneumonia is of particular importance because (*a*) it is a highly malignant infection which is fatal in eight out of ten cases, if untreated; (*b*) it frequently causes irreversible suppuration of the lung; and (*c*) it does not respond to treatment with penicillin. The diagnosis is established by the demonstration of encapsulated gram-negative bacilli in the sputum, pleural fluid or blood. Because the Friedländer's bacillus is a short, stubby rod with a prominent capsule, it may be mistaken for a pneumococcus, unless the sputum is stained by the Gram technique. Accordingly, the Gram stain should be used routinely in the examination of sputums from all patients suspected of having acute bacterial pneumonia. For further discussion see Klebsiella Pneumonia (p. 236).

STREPTOCOCCAL PNEUMONIA

Streptococcal pneumonia usually occurs as a complication of viral infections involving the respiratory tract, particularly influenza and measles. It may occasionally occur also as a complication of severe streptococcal pharyngitis, erysipelas or scarlet fever. The pneumonic lesion produced may be predominantly interstitial or lobular and not infrequently leads to pulmonary suppuration and organization. Early invasion of the pleural space is characteristic of streptococcal pneumonia, and, since the pleural exudate is thin and pleural adhesions sparse during the first few days, early open drainage of the thorax should be avoided (see Pneumococcal Pneumonia, Treatment of Complications, p. 143).

Diagnosis. The diagnosis of streptococcal pneumonia is made difficult by the fact that beta-hemolytic streptococci are frequently present in the respiratory secretions of patients with nonstreptococcal respiratory infections. Only if mucoid or matt group A streptococci are found in large numbers in the sputum or are cultured directly from the lung (lung puncture), blood or pleural fluid, can the disease be identified with certainty. A rising antistreptolysin or antifibrinolysin titer during convalescence provides suggestive, though not always conclusive, evidence regarding etiology. The presence of exudative tonsillitis does not establish the diagnosis, since a large proportion of such infections are of nonstreptococcal etiology.

Treatment. Treatment is essentially the same as that for pneumococcal pneumonia, except that antimicrobial therapy should be continued for at least fourteen to twenty-one days because of the tendency of beta-hemolytic streptococci to cause irreversible damage to the lung. The incidence of the disease may be lowered by the use of prophylactic chemotherapy in patients with measles and influenza.

STAPHYLOCOCCAL PNEUMONIA

Staphylococcal pneumonia likewise occurs primarily as a complication of influenzal infection of the lungs, although occasionally it may result from staphylococcal septicemia of extrapulmonary origin (i.e., acute osteomyelitis or infected abortion). In infants, staphylococci may cause primary tracheobronchitis. The strains isolated from patients with staphylococcal pneumonia are usually of the aureus variety and coagulase-positive. Some are avirulent for mice, and many are "resistant" to one or more of the antimicrobials usually employed in the treatment of bacterial pneumonia. Since staphylococci are commonly present in the normal nasopharynx, the same difficulty obtains as in streptococcal pneumonia regarding diagnosis from sputum examinations. The acute pneumonic lesion involves principally the bronchi and interstitial tissues. Like the hemolytic streptococcus and the Friedländer's bacillus, *Staphylococcus aureus* frequently causes irreversible damage to the lung resulting in multiple abscesses, bronchiectasis and eventual organization and pulmonary fibrosis. Accordingly, recovery is less prompt than in pneumococcal pneumonia, and prolonged and intensive antimicrobial therapy is indicated. For further discussion of this subject, see Staphylococcal Infections (p. 181).

W. BARRY WOOD, JR.

References

Dowling, H. F., Lepper, M. H., and Jackson, G. S.: Observations on the Epidemiological Spread of Antibiotic-Resistant Staphylococci, with Measurements of the Changes in Sensitivity to Penicillin and Aureomycin. Am. J. Pub. Health, 43:860, 1953.

Finland, M., Peterson, O. L., and Strauss, E.: Staphylococcic Pneumonia Occurring during an Epidemic of Influenza. Arch. Int. Med., 70:183, 1942.

Keefer, C. S., Rantz, L. A., and Rammelkamp, C. H.: Hemolytic Streptococcal Pneumonia and Empyema: A Study of 55 Cases with Special Reference to Treatment. Ann. Int. Med., 14:1553, 1941.

McDermott, W.: Streptococcal Pneumonia, Staphylococcal Pneumonia, and Friedländer's Bacillus Pneumonia. New York, Nelson's Loose Leaf System of Medicine, Vol. 1, Chaps. 8, 11, 22.

Sale, L., Jr., Smith, M. R., and Wood, W. B., Jr.: Studies on the Mechanism of Recovery in Pneumonia Due to Friedländer's Bacillus. J. Exper. Med., 86:239, 249, 257, 1947.

PNEUMONIA DUE TO FILTERABLE AGENTS

A primary type of bronchopneumonia may be caused by a variety of filterable agents, including at least one species of Rickettsia, several of the known viruses and a number of as yet unidentified agents which are presumably viral. These diverse etiologic forms of nonbacterial pneumonia have become increasingly prominent and important during the past few years, especially since the introduction of the sulfonamide drugs and penicillin. The phenomenal success of these chemotherapeutic compounds in the control of pneumococcal and other types of bacterial pneumonia focused attention on pulmonary infections which did not respond to their use, and thereby aided the recent differentiation of several viral infections, particularly primary atypical pneumonia. Other contributing factors have been the greater frequency of roentgenographic examination in diseases of the respiratory tract and the increased perfection and wider use of laboratory methods for the diagnosis of viral and rickettsial infections.

For a general review of the literature the reader is referred to the article by Reimann.

PNEUMONIA CAUSED BY KNOWN VIRUSES AND RICKETTSIAE

PSITTACOSIS

(*Ornithosis*)

A pneumonia which is clinically and roentgenologically indistinguishable from primary atypical pneumonia may be caused by several closely related viruses of the psittacosis-lymphogranuloma group. This form of pneumonia is discussed under Psittacosis (p. 48).

VIRUS INFLUENZAL PNEUMONIA

Since the identification of the virus of influenza by Smith, Andrewes and Laidlaw in 1933, widespread epidemics, localized outbreaks and sporadic cases of this disease have been repeatedly recognized in nearly all parts of the world. Influenza is now known to be caused by a group of filterable agents most of which can be classified as either influenza A or influenza B virus, according to their antigenic characteristics. There is evidence of still other types of the virus. The infection typically causes a grippelike syndrome with sudden onset, symptoms of catarrhal inflammation of the upper respiratory tract and a more or less severe febrile reaction accompanied by malaise, headache and muscular aching.

Unlike pandemic influenza, as seen in 1918–1919, the case mortality rate of epidemic influenza is low and secondary bacterial pneumonia is uncommon. During recent years a small number of cases of associated staphylococcal pneumonia have occurred in some outbreaks. The incidence of pulmonary involvement attributable to the virus alone has varied considerably in different epidemics, but in the majority it has been small. The pulmonary lesions are usually lobular in distribution and, in contrast with primary atypical pneumonia, the roentgenographic findings are ordinarily less in extent than would be expected from the nature of the physical signs.

For further information on influenzal pneumonia, see the chapter on Influenza (p. 12).

Q FEVER PNEUMONIA

Q fever was first identified as a clinical entity in Australia in 1937, but during the past few years it has been found to have virtually a world-wide distribution. Since 1946 the disease has been found in Arizona, California, Illinois, Montana and Texas, while serologic surveys have revealed evidence of its presence in nearly all parts of the United States. The etiologic agent is a filter-passing species of rickettsia, *Coxiella burneti*. Although the infection is essentially systemic, it is usually but not always accompanied by a more or less extensive pneumonitis. Cases with pulmonary involvement present a clinical picture and roentgenographic findings indistinguishable from those of primary atypical pneumonia. The only means of diagnosis are by isolation of the causative agent or by serologic tests for specific antibodies which develop during convalescence. The disease responds readily to treatment with a tetracycline drug.

For further information on Q fever, see the section on Rickettsial Diseases (p. 102).

PNEUMONIA IN SMALLPOX

It is not generally appreciated that pulmonary lesions occur frequently in smallpox. Variola virus produces a specific bronchopneumonia with characteristic inclusion bodies in many of the affected cells. The pneumonia may be a serious complication,

since there is a pronounced predisposition to secondary invasion by pyogenic bacteria, particularly staphylococci.

PNEUMONIA IN CHICKENPOX

A diffuse and occasionally fatal bronchopneumonia occurs rarely in chickenpox, especially among adult patients. In several autopsied cases the absence of demonstrable bacteria and the character of the pathologic findings indicated that the pulmonary lesions may be caused entirely by the viral agent.

PNEUMONIA IN MEASLES

Bronchopneumonia occurs frequently in measles and has been demonstrated in 20 to 60 per cent of patients in several series studied roentgenographically. The pneumonitis resembles other forms of viral pneumonia and is often caused solely by a specific reaction to the measles virus. Superimposed bacterial infection is common, however, and accounts for the majority of the severe or fatal cases. *Streptococcus haemolyticus, Staphylococcus aureus* and *Hemophilus influenzae* are the usual secondary invaders. In recent years the mortality rate from measles pneumonia has been markedly reduced by treatment with antimicrobial drugs. Penicillin is the agent of choice in most instances.

PNEUMONIA IN LYMPHOCYTIC CHORIOMENINGITIS

Lymphocytic choriomeningitis is caused by a specific viral agent. The disease in man is usually characterized as an acute aseptic meningitis, but occasionally a grippelike syndrome is produced without clinical evidence of central nervous system involvement. Several cases with pulmonary involvement have also been described, and the virus has been isolated from the lung at necropsy. Pulmonary lesions occur frequently in experimentally infected animals and, if searched for, would probably be found more often in human cases.

PNEUMONIA CAUSED BY UNIDENTIFIED FILTERABLE AGENTS OR AGENTS PRESUMED TO BE VIRUSES

PRIMARY PNEUMONITIS OF INFANCY

Adams and his co-workers have described the epidemic occurrence of nonbacterial pneumonia in newborn and premature infants. Sporadic cases of the disease have also been recognized. The onset is usually abrupt, with sneezing, cough, abundant tenacious pharyngeal exudate and fever. Severe cases may show marked dyspnea and some cyanosis. Rales may be heard over the lungs, and the roentgenograms reveal diffuse or localized areas of pulmonary infiltration. Although no specific viral agent has been isolated, smears of the pharyngeal exudate usually show many epithelial cells containing eosinophilic intracytoplasmic inclusion bodies. Similar inclusion bodies have been regularly demonstrated in the epithelium of the nose, pharynx, trachea and bronchi at necropsy. In typical sporadic cases a history of antecedent upper respiratory tract infection in the parents is frequently elicited. The morbidity and mortality rates are higher in prematurely born babies than in normal full term infants. The over-all mortality rate was 28 per cent in one outbreak of the disease.

PNEUMONIA IN INFECTIOUS MONONUCLEOSIS

Infectious mononucleosis is generally considered to be a viral disease, although the etiologic agent has not been isolated and identified. A more or less extensive bronchopneumonia may sometimes accompany the infection, though it is rarely a dominant feature. Respiratory symptoms are usually mild or absent, and the pulmonary involvement may be discovered only incidentally on roentgenographic examination.

PNEUMONIA IN ERYTHEMA EXUDATIVUM MULTIFORME

A nonbacterial pneumonia occurs frequently in the more severe forms of erythema exudativum multiforme (Stevens-Johnson syndrome), although it rarely occurs in milder forms of the disease as originally described by Hebra. The pneumonia is considered to be an integral part of the disease and in its clinical features closely resembles primary atypical pneumonia. The etiology has not been determined but it is generally believed that the causative agent is a virus. In some cases there is evidence that infection with the virus of herpes simplex may have been responsible.

PRIMARY ATYPICAL PNEUMONIA

Definition. Primary atypical pneumonia is an acute infectious disease of the human respiratory tract in which pulmonary infiltration of varying degree is a prominent feature. The causative agent is in all probability a virus, although it has not been definitely isolated and identified. Certain other viral and rickettsial diseases of known etiology may clinically resemble primary atypical pneumonia, including psittacosis or ornithosis, influenza, lymphocytic choriomeningitis and Q fever.

History. There is some indication that primary atypical pneumonia is not a disease of recent origin, but possibly has existed for a century or more. However, in the older literature it is impossible to distinguish this form of pneumonia from influenza and many other infections of the respiratory tract. Contemporary knowledge began to accumulate between 1930 and 1940, when a series of reports were published which described localized outbreaks of the disease, emphasized its apparently rising incidence, defined its clinical characteristics and presented evidence that none of the usual bacteria were etiologic factors. The literature of this period has been well reviewed in articles by Dingle and Finland. An important factor in the recognition of primary atypical pneumonia was the introduction, between 1938 and 1940, of sulfonamide derivatives for the successful chemotherapy of pneumococcal and streptococcal pneumonia. The failure of primary atypical pneumonia to respond to treatment with these drugs, and later to the even more effective antibiotic penicillin, clearly established its distinction from the common bacterial pneumonias and contributed greatly to its present classification as a clinical and etiologic entity. Over the past decade the high incidence of the disease and the intriguing new problems of its natural history, diagnosis and control have attracted wide study by many groups of investigators.

Etiology. There seems little reason to doubt that primary atypical pneumonia is caused either by a single virus or by a group of closely related viruses. During World War II carefully controlled experiments by the Commission on Acute Respiratory Diseases showed that the disease could be transmitted from man to man by spraying the nose and throat of healthy human volunteers with pooled sputum and throat washings collected from active cases. Transmission was effected, not only with these untreated inocula, but also with the same materials freed of bacteria by passage through sintered-glass or Seitz filters. The characteristic illness which resulted in a considerable proportion of the subjects was again successfully passed from them to fresh volunteers by the same method. Of great interest was the fact that minor respiratory illnesses differing from primary atypical pneumonia also developed in other subjects of the same experimental group. This raised the question whether the same filterable agent could be responsible for several clinical varieties of infection, or whether the inocula actually contained more than one type of virus. The results of later studies by the Commission indicated that the latter possibility was probably correct, although it is still uncertain whether all cases of primary atypical pneumonia are caused by a single infectious agent.

In 1953, by direct inoculation of tissue cultures, a group of closely related viruses were isolated from patients with atypical pneumonia and minor respiratory illnesses (Hilleman and Werner) and from excised adenoidal tissue (Huebner et al.). The precise role of this virus group in atypical pneumonia has not yet been defined but they appear to bear some relationship to the disease.

Many attempts have been made in the laboratory to transfer the infection from man to a wide variety of mammalian and avian species. None have been unequivocally successful. Eaton and his associates claimed the isolation of a virus which produces pulmonary lesions in cotton rats and hamsters, can be propagated in the developing chick embryo, and is specifically neutralized by the convalescent serums of patients. Other observers have failed to confirm these findings, however, and Horsfall has shown that the neutralization of Eaton's virus by convalescent serums may well be due to nonspecific and unrelated antigen-antibody reactions.

No bacteria have been identified as etiologic factors, although pneumococci, hemolytic streptococci, staphylococci and more rarely other pathogens may be recovered in cultures of the throat or sputum early in the disease. Thomas and his co-workers isolated a serologically distinct, nonhemolytic streptococcus (streptococcus MG) from the lungs of fatal cases of primary atypical pneumonia and demonstrated specific antibodies to this micro-organism in the blood of about 50 per cent of patients during their convalescence. These observations led to the hypothesis that streptococcus MG might play an etiologic role by functioning as a symbiont, together with a virus, in a manner analogous to the role of *Hemophilus influenzae* in swine influenza. Later studies have shown, however, that streptococcus MG occurs not infrequently in the upper respiratory tract of normal persons and of those suffering from acute infections of the respiratory tract without pulmonary involvement. Moreover, in the transmission experiments previously mentioned, the micro-organism was isolated from human volunteers with equal frequency both before and after successful inoculation. It should also be noted that streptococcus MG is quite sensitive to penicillin, whereas penicillin has no effect on the course of primary atypical pneumonia.

Epidemiology. Primary atypical pneumonia is widely prevalent, but its incidence in the general population is unknown. The disease tends to occur in sporadic form, but numerous localized outbreaks have been reported, especially in semiclosed and crowded population groups, such as schools and military establishments. Among personnel of the armed forces it was more common than all other forms of pneumonia during World War II. Epidemiologic studies and transmission experiments indicate that the disease is spread directly from person to person via the respiratory route by infected discharges from the nose and mouth. There is no evidence that food, water or insects may be vectors. The communicability is often low, and there is usually no history of contact. In early epidemiologic surveys the frequent failure to establish a history of contact was puzzling until it became apparent that there are many mild or unrecognized cases of the disease. Patients hospitalized on open wards rarely transmit their infection to other patients, but the relatively high incidence among physicians, nurses and other hospital personnel serves to emphasize the importance of contact as well as the frequency of exposure in transmission. Occasionally the disease seems to have an enhanced communicability, in which case the history of antecedent contact may be readily obtained and the patients appear to transmit their disease more easily to other persons. The factors responsible for this phenomenon have not been determined.

All age groups are affected, but the disease is recognized most frequently among persons in early or middle adult life. There is no predilection for sex, race or color. The disease is widespread in the northern temperate zone and is relatively rare in the tropics. Cases occur throughout the year, although the greatest incidence is during the winter months. In some years the disease has been prevalent during middle and late summer, but in general it tends to parallel the combined incidence of upper respiratory tract infections. The factors which influence susceptibility and resistance have not been established.

The period of communicability is unknown. One attack appears to confer at least temporary resistance to reinfection, but the duration and quality of such immunity have not been determined. The occasional occurrence of second attacks after an interval of apparent health indicates that immunity does not persist indefinitely in all patients.

Morbid Anatomy. Since the mortality rate is low, there has been relatively little opportunity to study pathologic changes in the lungs or elsewhere in the body. The available postmortem studies indicate that the pulmonary lesions are not distinctive and probably cannot be differentiated from those of psittacosis, Q fever and other nonbacterial pneumonias. Characteristically, there is a more or less extensive patchy bronchopneumonia with areas of hemorrhagic consolidation in various stages of evolution. The bronchi appear inflamed and contain mucoid or mucopurulent exudate. Localized atelectasis or emphysema may be present as the result of bronchial obstruction. The pleura may show patches of fibrinous exudate, and occasionally the pleural cavity contains small amounts of fluid. Large pleural effusions are uncommon. Enlargement of the tracheobronchial lymph nodes has been observed in some cases.

Microscopic examination generally reveals an interstitial type of pneumonia most prominent in regions adjacent to bronchi and bronchioles. The alveolar septums appear thickened, with dilatation of the capillaries, infiltration by lymphocytes and monocytes, and varying degrees of edema. Polymorphonuclear leukocytes are relatively few. The alveolar spaces contain some edema fluid or a scanty exudate in which either mononuclear cells or erythrocytes may predominate. Bacteria appear to be absent or are few in number. Occasionally the alveoli and smaller bronchioles may be lined by hyaline membranes. Peribronchial and perivascular infiltration by mononuclear cells is sometimes marked in extent. The epithelium of the bronchi is usually intact, although areas of necrosis and sloughing may be seen, particularly in the smaller bronchi and bronchioles. In these areas of necrosis, polymorphonuclear cells are numerous. Large numbers of polymorphonuclear cells are also seen in the exudate within bronchial lumina. Intracellular inclusion bodies and elementary bodies have not been demonstrated.

In some cases clinical evidence of encephalitis has been accompanied by demonstrable lesions of the brain. Microscopic examination has shown focal hemorrhages, perivascular cuffing with mononuclear cells and proliferation of astrocytes and glial cells. There is some question whether these changes are directly caused by the viral agent, or whether they represent a nonspecific tissue reaction which has been seen occasionally in other infectious diseases.

No pathologic alterations of note have been described in other organs or tissues.

Symptoms. The incubation period usually varies from two to three weeks. In most cases the onset is gradual, although occasionally it may be abrupt. During early stages of the illness the symptoms are not distinctive and generally consist of fever, cough, headache, malaise and chilly sensations. Headache is often distressing or severe. Shaking chills and sweats sometimes occur. Sore throat is not uncommon. *Cough is an outstanding feature, and its absence makes the diagnosis questionable.* The cough at first is dry and paroxysmal, but later it usually becomes productive of mucoid or mucopurulent sputum. The sputum is not infrequently blood-streaked and in rare instances may be frankly bloody or rusty in appearance. Pain in the chest, usually substernal in location and aggravated by cough, occurs in many cases. However, typical pleuritic pain is relatively uncommon. Anorexia is often complained of, and some patients have nausea and vomiting.

Physical Findings. Most patients appear to be acutely but not seriously ill, although exceptions to this rule occur. The temperature may range from 99° F. to over 105° F., but is usually between 102° F. and 104° F., at the height of the disease. The fever curve may be either sustained or remittent in type.

A relative bradycardia is observed in more than 50 per cent of patients and is of some diagnostic value. The respirations are usually either normal or only moderately increased, but in severe cases there may be dyspnea and cyanosis. The nasal and pharyngeal mucous membranes often appear inflamed. Examination of the chest almost always reveals fewer abnormal signs than would be expected from the roentgenographic findings. Some dullness on percussion may be found over the affected pulmonary area. Harshness or diminution of the breath sounds may be detected. Fine or medium rales are usually present and may be the only abnormal signs; as the disease progresses they frequently become coarse and moist. Rhonchi are sometimes heard and occasionally may be sharply localized and intensified on forced expiration, indicating bronchial obstruction. Pleural rub and signs of pleural effusion are uncommon. The spleen becomes palpable in rare instances.

Roentgenographic Findings. The pulmonary lesions as seen on roentgenograms vary widely in character and distribution. The abnormal shadows may appear mottled, feathery or uniformly opaque with differing degrees of density. In the majority of cases the lesions are most dense in the hilar region and become less dense toward the periphery of the lung field. The margins of the pneumonic areas are usually poorly defined. The lower lobes are most frequently involved, although any part of the lungs may be affected. In about 50 per cent of patients the disease is confined to one lobe, but in the remainder more than one lobe is affected. Occasionally the pneumonia is migratory and spreads from lobe to lobe, with clearing in one area as extension occurs in another. There is nothing characteristic about the roentgenographic changes, and a similar picture may be produced by many other infections of the lung, including pulmonary tuberculosis.

Laboratory Findings. In the majority of cases the total leukocyte count is within normal limits, although a slight leukopenia or a moderate leukocytosis may be found. The differential count may show a moderate increase in polymorphonuclear leukocytes, but rarely to the degree seen in bacterial pneumonias. Occasionally a brisk leukocytosis is seen during convalescence in the absence of a detectable secondary bacterial infection. The erythrocyte count and hemoglobin values are seldom reduced except in severe, prolonged cases or in rare instances of acute hemolytic anemia. The urine may contain a little protein and a few cellular elements, as in other infectious diseases. The erythrocyte sedimentation rate usually is moderately elevated at the height of the disease, but falls slowly to normal during convalescence. Bacteriologic examination of the sputum ordinarily reveals only those micro-organisms found normally in the upper respiratory tract. Pneumococci of the higher types may be present. In many cases the bacterial content of the sputum is remarkably scanty. Unlike pneumococcal pneumonia, the serum chloride levels, as well as the chloride excretion, remain within the normal range. Transitory weakly positive Wassermann and other serologic tests for syphilis may be obtained with the acute or convalescent phase serums of some patients. During or after the illness the serums of the majority of patients contain increased titers of cold hemagglutinins or of agglutinins for streptococcus MG.

Clinical Course. The clinical course of primary atypical pneumonia is variable, ranging from a mild febrile illness of a few days' duration to a severe disease with high temperature which may continue for several weeks. In the average case of moderate severity the temperature is elevated for about ten days and falls to normal by lysis. Symptoms usually abate as the fever declines, although physical and roentgenographic signs of pulmonary involvement usually do not resolve completely until the temperature has been normal for several days. Cough sometimes persists until the pulmonary lesion has cleared entirely. The patient's convalescence may be prolonged by sensations of weariness and ease of fatigue.

Complications are relatively uncommon. Secondary bacterial infection occurs so infrequently that the disease seems almost to predispose against it. Large pleural effusions are rare. Otitis media, sinusitis, stomatitis, tonsillitis, bronchiectasis, empyema, pericarditis and myocarditis have been described. Peripheral circulatory collapse has been noted. Meningo-encephalitis has been observed clinically and at necropsy. In a few cases, especially those with high titers of cold agglutinins, an acute hemolytic anemia has developed. The anemia has appeared usually in patients treated with the sulfonamide drugs, but has also been seen in patients who received symptomatic therapy alone; its mechanism is not well understood.

Prognosis. The prognosis in primary atypical pneumonia is excellent. Although a few instances of death have been reported, the uncomplicated disease is self-limited in the vast majority of patients, including those who may appear severely or even critically ill.

Diagnosis. No specific diagnostic procedures are available, but in most cases the diagnosis can be established with reasonable certainty by adequate clinical, roentgenographic and laboratory studies. The disease may be strongly suspected from the following features: gradual onset, fever, relative bradycardia, normal respiratory rate, paroxysmal cough and roentgenographic evidence of pneumonia with absent or few physical signs. Failure to respond to treatment with penicillin or the sulfonamides adds support to the diagnosis, but is not a completely reliable criterion. Corroborative laboratory findings are a normal or only slightly elevated leukocyte count and normal bacterial flora on culture of the throat or sputum. Tests for cold hemagglutinins are helpful in making a definite diagnosis, since these peculiar antibodies appear exceptionally in diseases other than primary atypical pneumonia. Cold hemagglutination may be demonstrated in approximately 55 per cent of patients, although the incidence and magnitude of the titer varies according to the severity and duration of the illness. For example, the reaction becomes positive in over 90 per cent of patients in whom the disease is severe or prolonged, atypical pneumonia. Pneumococcal pneumonia and other acute bacterial infections of the lung not infrequently present similar clinical manifestations, especially during the onset and early stages of their development. In some cases pulmonary tuberculosis and mycotic infections of the lung must also be considered. These diseases can nearly always be identified, however, either by isolation of the responsible agent or by the eventual demonstration of specific antibodies in the pa-

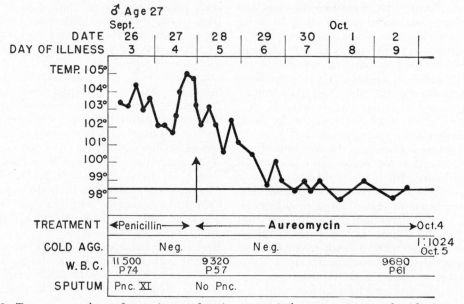

Fig. 28. Temperature chart of a patient with primary atypical pneumonia treated with Aureomycin. (Kneeland, Rose and Gibson: Am. J. Med., Vol. 6.)

but is positive in only about 20 per cent of mild cases. The hemagglutinins do not appear in the serum until the second or third week after onset and the test is therefore of value only in making a late or retrospective diagnosis. It is advisable to examine the patient's serum repeatedly for cold hemagglutinins at intervals of five to seven days, since a significant rise in titer is more important than a single positive test. Tests for agglutinins of streptococcus MG may also be made, although these antibodies develop somewhat less frequently than do cold hemagglutinins. If either or both of the tests become positive, the patient almost certainly has suffered from primary atypical pneumonia, but if both are negative it may be difficult or impossible to reach a definite diagnosis.

Psittacosis, Q fever, influenza and lymphocytic choriomeningitis with pulmonary involvement may closely resemble primary tient's blood. Bronchogenic carcinoma, pulmonary infarction and bronchiectasis occasionally must be included in the differential diagnosis.

Treatment. Studies by several groups of investigators have indicated that most patients recover rapidly after a tetracycline drug (Aureomycin or Terramycin) is administered, and that the average course of the disease is shorter than when either penicillin is given or the patient receives symptomatic therapy alone. While there is some controversy in the literature concerning the validity of these observations, it is the opinion of the writer that broad-spectrum drugs of the tetracycline series favorably affect the fundamental disease process. Usually within 24 to 48 hours after treatment is begun the temperature approaches normal, cough is considerably diminished or absent and the patient notes a striking increase in the sense of well-being. The characteristic fever chart of a treated case of primary atypical pneumonia is illustrated in Figure 28. The recommended dose of a tetracycline is 0.5 gm. by mouth every 6 hours and this should be continued for at least three days after the temperature reaches normal, since relapse may be expected when treatment is stopped too soon. If side reactions such as diarrhea, nausea and vomiting occur, it may be necessary to reduce dosage and in rare instances to discontinue therapy. There is some evidence that treatment with a tetracycline drug may suppress the development of cold agglutinins and thereby reduce the utility of this serologic phenomenon in the diagnosis of the disease. No information is available concerning the possible effect of chemotherapy on residual immunity to reinfection.

Symptomatic therapy may include codeine in doses of 0.03 to 0.06 gm. to control cough. Inhalations of steam are helpful in relieving soreness and dryness of the upper respiratory passages. Salicylate compounds should be used cautiously, since some patients respond badly to their use. When the disease is severe with respiratory embarrassment, oxygen therapy is usually indicated. During convalescence it is recommended that the patient be kept at bed rest for several days after the temperature is normal, since early ambulation may be followed by prolonged symptoms of weakness, lassitude and easily induced fatigue.

HARRY M. ROSE

References

Adams, J. M.: Primary Pneumonitis in Infancy. J.A.M.A., *138*:1142, 1948.
Berge, T. O., and Lennette, E. H.: World Distribution of Q Fever: Human, Animal and Arthropod Infection. Am. J. Hyg., 57:125, 1953.
Commission on Acute Respiratory Diseases: The Transmission of Primary Atypical Pneumonia to Human Volunteers. Bull. Johns Hopkins Hosp., 79:97, 1946.
Dingle, J. H., and Finland, M.: Virus Pneumonias. II. Primary Atypical Pneumonias of Unknown Etiology. New England J. Med., 227:378, 1942.
——, and others: Evidence for the Specific Etiology of "Acute Respiratory Disease (ARD)." Tr. A. Am. Physicians, 67, 1954 (May).
Finland, M., and Dingle, J. H.: Virus Pneumonias. I. Pneumonias Associated with Known Nonbacterial Agents: Influenza, Psittacosis and Q Fever. New England J. Med., 277:342, 1942.
Hilleman, M. R., and Werner, J. H.: Recovery of New Agent from Patients with Acute Respiratory Illness. Proc. Soc. Exper. Biol. & Med., 85:183, 1954.
Horsfall, F. L., Jr. ed.: The Diagnosis of Primary Atypical Pneumonia. Symposia of the Section on Microbiology. The New York Academy of Medicine, Number I: The Diagnosis of Viral and Rickettsial Infections. New York, Columbia University Press, 1949, pp. 42–56.
Jordan, W. S., Jr., Albright, R. W., McCain, F. H., and Dingle, J. H.: Clinical Variations in Primary Atypical Pneumonia. Am. J. Med., *10*:3, 1951.
Kneeland, Y., Jr., Rose, H. M., and Gibson, C. D.: Aureomycin in the Treatment of Primary Atypical Pneumonia. Am. J. Med., 6:41, 1949.
Reimann, H. A.: The Viral Pneumonias and Pneumonias of Probable Viral Origin. Medicine, *26*: 167, 1947.
Rowe, W. P., and others: Isolation of Cytopathogenic Agent from Human Adenoids Undergoing Spontaneous Degeneration in Tissue Culture. Proc. Soc. Exper. Biol. & Med., *84*:570, 1953.
Thomas, L., and others: Studies on Primary Atypical Pneumonia. II. Observations Concerning the Relationship of a Non-Hemolytic Streptococcus to the Disease. J. Clin. Investigation, *24*:227, 1945.
Womack, C. R., and Randall, C. C.: Erythema Exudativum Multiforme. Am. J. Med., *15*:633, 1953.

STREPTOCOCCAL INFECTIONS

INTRODUCTION

Acute infections due to streptococci constitute one of the most important groups of diseases in the temperate zones. It has been estimated that up to 20 per cent of all respiratory infections in a civilian population are caused by hemolytic streptococci. In time of war the incidence is often much higher among freshly mobilized military personnel. Streptococcal diseases are also of importance because of serious sequelae that follow the acute illness. During the past decade or two significant advancements have been made which have contributed to the control and management of streptococcal illness. Most outstanding are the precise serologic methods developed for the classification of streptococci, which have been successfully used in epidemiologic investigations; and the introduction of antimicrobial drugs for the prevention and treatment of streptococcal diseases.

Classification of the Streptococci. A widely accepted method for classifying streptococci, described in 1919 by Brown, is based upon the effect of the bacteria upon erythrocytes when grown in blood agar plates. Growth of the *alpha* group is associated with two types of reactions against the erythrocytes. One is a zone of green pigment formed around the colonies, and the second results in hemolysis of the erythrocytes, but close inspection reveals unhemolyzed cells adjacent to the colony. The *beta* group of streptococci have a clear-cut zone of hemolysis right up to the edge of the colony. The nonhemolytic streptococci cause no hemolysis and have been designated by Brown as the *gamma* group. Further advancement in the classification of streptococci was made by Lancefield, who has separated strains of streptococci into several groups by means of serologic methods. This differentiation depends upon a group-specific carbohydrate being present in the bacterial cells, against which specific antiserum may be prepared. Twelve main groups have been identified and designated by the letters A, B, C, D, E, F, G, H, K, L, M and N. As far as human infections are concerned, *group A streptococci* are the most significant and, with but rare exceptions, produce the *beta* type of hemolysis. Though the remaining groups may include *beta* hemolytic strains, they frequently produce no hemolysis and often cause greening of blood agar.

Group B hemolytic and nonhemolytic strains cause bovine mastitis and, occasionally, serious human infections. *Streptococci in group C* are mainly pathogenic for animals, and infrequently are associated with respiratory disease in human beings. *Group D streptococci include the enterococci* such as *Streptococcus faecalis* and are the frequent cause of human urinary tract infections and, less often, of subacute bacterial endocarditis (see chapter on Bacterial Endocarditis). The other groups are of less significance in human disease.

Another achievement in the classification of streptococci was the contribution of Griffiths and Lancefield whereby group A hemolytic streptococci may be divided into specific types by serologic means. The separation into types has been made possible because the bacterial cells have a type-specific agglutinogen and a type-specific protein against which specific antiserums can be prepared. Lancefield found that there are over forty types of group A hemolytic streptococci which are responsible for human disease. The grouping and typing of hemolytic streptococci have been used in the epidemiologic study of streptococcal diseases, and have afforded a means whereby the biologic characteristics of the organisms in relation to human illness may be more precisely investigated.

Epidemiology of Streptococcal Infection. In the following discussions particular emphasis is placed upon disease caused by group A hemolytic streptococci. The maintenance and spread of hemolytic streptococcal infections are due to persons who harbor the organisms in the pharynx or exudative lesions. The most important reservoir of pathogenic hemolytic streptococci is the pharynx of the asymptomatic carrier. The immediate environment of an actually ill patient with a hemolytic streptococcal infection is usually contaminated with microbes. This includes personal effects and bed clothing. Contamination of the hands of an attendant in an acute case may result in the subsequent infection of the burns and wounds of other patients, and the spread of streptococcal disease has been traced to the indiscriminate interchange among patients of urinals, bed pans, warming pads and hot water bottles. Hemolytic streptococcal infections of the upper respiratory tract are very likely air-borne, though the ingestion of contaminated food and milk has precipitated epidemics. Symptomless carriers of hemolytic streptococci, acutely ill patients and those convalescing from streptococcal disease expel minute droplets of secretions from the nose and throat containing hemolytic streptococci; and people coming in close contact with those disseminating the bacteria may inhale the streptococci. These people in turn may become acutely ill or become carriers. In summary, the basic principle involved in the transmission of streptococci from human to human is *intimate contact* of susceptible persons with either healthy carriers or acutely ill patients. Of less significance is an indirect transmission of organisms in which droplets containing streptococci adhere to dust particles and remain viable in bed clothing and on the floor. The subsequent disturbance of the bed clothing or the raising of dust may distribute the streptococci into the air. The inhalation of streptococci is then made possible.

Factors to be considered in the genesis of streptococcal respiratory infections include the association of susceptible persons under crowded conditions with carriers or those with acute illness; the presence of other types of respiratory disease, such as the common cold or influenza; the numbers of organisms invading the tissues; and the type of group A hemolytic streptococci being disseminated.

Pathogenesis of Streptococcal Diseases. Invasion of the tissues by hemolytic streptococci is followed by variable clinical manifestations, but in most instances a definite clinical pattern may be recognized. Powers and his associates have emphasized the influence of age upon the clinical course of streptococcal disease. They coined the term *streptococcosis* to include all human disease caused by group A beta-hemolytic streptococci and drew similarities between the clinical patterns of streptococcosis and tuberculosis: namely, childhood, intermediate, adult and latent types of response to the hemolytic streptococci. Suppuration is more commonly associated with streptococcal disease in childhood, while nonsuppurative sequelae occur more often in older children and adults.

Keefer called attention to four phases in the clinical course of hemolytic streptococcal infections. The first phase is one of toxemia and is associated with fever, constitutional symptoms and a rash in susceptible persons. The second phase, linked closely with the first, comprises septic manifestations with signs of *local suppuration* with and without bacteremia. The third phase involves a latent or a symptomatic period averaging two to three weeks, which may be followed by the fourth phase of *nonsuppurative lesions,* or *Nachkrankheiten,* and may include fever, lymphadenitis, nephritis, arthritis, edema, acute rheumatic fever and skin lesions such as erythema nodosum, erythema multiforme and scleredema adultorum. These latter disturbances may be only transitory, or may be the manifestations of a progressive systemic disease ending ultimately in death. The work of Rammelkamp and his associates has demonstrated that only a certain few of the serologic types of group A streptococci are associated with the nonsuppurative complication of acute glomerulonephritis, whereas any of the types are probably involved in the development of rheumatic fever.

Depending upon the severity of the infection, there is evidence that widespread tissue reactions appear early in the course of streptococcal disease. Mallory and Keefer observed anatomic changes in the heart, kidneys, liver, spleen and pancreas of patients dying during the early stages of such streptococcal diseases as scarlet fever, erysipelas, wound infections and puerperal sepsis. More severe lesions were noted in the organs of patients expiring in the later stages of the infections.

These tissue reactions are commonly reflected in abnormal laboratory findings, many of them being transitory, such as albuminuria and an increase in the formed elements in the urine, electrocardiographic changes, leukocytosis and an acceleration of the sedimentation rate of the erythrocytes. The interpretation of these changes becomes increasingly difficult when they persist and the patient fails to recover completely from his illness.

Prophylaxis and Treatment of Hemolytic Streptococcal Infections. Before the epoch-making announcement of Domagk in 1935 that prontosil was a specific antibacterial agent for hemolytic streptococci, no specific therapy was available for streptococcal diseases with the exception of antitoxin, used in the treatment of scarlet fever. Prontosil was soon succeeded by sulfanilamide and its various derivatives, notably, sulfadiazine and sulfamerazine. Moreover, it was subsequently demonstrated that penicillin, streptomycin, the tetracyclines, chloramphenicol and erythromycin are all active in the treatment of streptococcal infections.

In considering the use of these various drugs in the chemoprophylaxis and treatment of streptococcal infections, it is of the greatest importance to distinguish between (*a*) the prevention of *streptococcal infection* in a healthy person; (*b*) the prevention of *suppurative complications* in a person already infected with group A hemolytic streptococci; and (*c*) the prevention of *nonsuppurative complications,* e.g., rheumatic fever and glomerulonephritis, in a person already infected with group A hemolytic streptococci. The choice of drug and the intensity and duration of therapy are considerably different for the attainment of these three separate goals.

Prevention of Streptococcal Infection in a Healthy Person. Experience during World War II demonstrated that sulfadiazine administered to large numbers of military personnel was associated with a reduction of streptococcal respiratory disease; this practice also was accompanied by the appearance of sulfadiazine-resistant strains of streptococci. Sulfadiazine has also been used in considerable numbers of children as a prophylactic against recurrent attacks of rheumatic fever. Because streptococci do not appear to display resistance so readily to the action of penicillin, this drug is recommended instead of a sulfonamide in any prophylactic programs for streptococcal respiratory disease. The details of dosage and timing of administration are discussed in the chapter on Rheumatic Fever.

Prevention of Suppurative Complications in a Person Already Infected with Group A Hemolytic Streptococci. The administration of penicillin, the tetracyclines, chloramphenicol, erythromycin or the sulfonamides will interrupt the natural course of streptococcal diseases in favor of the patient. Moreover, unless abscess formation has already occurred (see Peritonsillar Abscess), the proper use of any of these drugs will virtually eliminate the development of the *suppurative* complications of group A hemolytic streptococcal infections.

The use of sulfonamide for this purpose has largely been abandoned because of the superiority of the other drugs. Penicillin may be administered intramuscularly in a single daily injection of 300,000 units of the procaine salt or in aqueous solution in 100,000 to 200,000 unit doses at eight to twelve hour intervals. After the first one or two days the latter regimen may be changed to the oral administration of 100,000 units of penicillin four times each day. Other repository types of penicillin preparations are available so that only one or two injections a week are necessary. Oxytetracycline, chlortetracycline or tetracycline may be administered orally in a total daily dose of 20 to 30 mg. per kilogram of body weight. This dose should be given in four equally divided doses, each administered every six hours. Except under rare conditions, it is not necessary to exceed a total daily dose of 2 gm. in adults. Oxytetracycline hydrochloride or chlortetracycline hydrochloride may be given intravenously in a dose of 5 to 10 mg. per kilogram of body weight, administered every eight to twelve hours. With any of these drugs it is essential to continue treatment after recovery has apparently taken place in order to prevent relapses. In general, the total duration of antimicrobial therapy should be seven to ten days. Moreover, it should be emphasized that some of the regimens outlined here, though entirely satisfactory for control of the suppurative aspects of the disease, might not afford maximal protection against the possibility of the development of rheumatic fever or other nonsuppurative complications.

Prevention of Nonsuppurative Complications in a Person Already Infected with Group A Hemolytic Streptococci. The investigations of Weinstein, Kilbourne and Loge, and of Rammelkamp and his associates, provide strong evidence that the likelihood of the development of poststreptococcal rheumatic fever can be drastically reduced if group A hemolytic streptococcal infections are treated promptly, for a sufficient period, with proper amounts of penicillin. Consequently, whenever it is desirable to attempt to afford maximal protection against the development of rheumatic fever, penicillin should be administered daily for a seven to ten day period. The drug may be given intramuscularly either in a single daily injection of 300,000 units of the procaine salt, or in individual divided doses of 20,000 to 50,000 units of the aqueous solution administered at no greater than three hour intervals throughout the entire twenty-four hour period. Slowly absorbed penicillin preparations may be used for this purpose so that only one or two injections a week are necessary. Presumably the earlier in the course of the streptococcal infection that penicillin is started, the better the chance that the therapy might protect against rheumatic fever.

It is possible that the tetracyclines or erythromycin might be as satisfactory as intensive penicillin therapy for the attainment of this purpose. It is known, however, that sulfonamide therapy and the intramuscular administration of penicillin in aqueous solution at eight to twelve hour intervals are *not* sufficiently powerful to protect against rheumatic fever.

WESLEY W. SPINK

References

Aerobiology. Publication of the American Association for the Advancement of Science. No. 17. Washington, D. C., 1942.

Brown, J. H.: The Use of Blood Agar for the Study of Streptococci. Monograph No. 9, 1919. Rockefeller Institute for Medical Research.

Coburn, A. F., and Young, D. C.: The Epidemiology of Hemolytic Streptococcus During World War II in the United States Navy. Baltimore, Williams and Wilkins Co., 1949.

Griffith, F.: The Serological Classification of *Streptococcus pyogenes*. J. Hyg., 34:542, 1934.

Keefer, C. S.: The Late Non-Suppurative Disorders of Hemolytic Streptococcal Diseases. Texas State J. Med., 35:457, 1939.

Lancefield, R. C.: A Serological Differentiation of Human and Other Groups of Hemolytic Streptococci. J. Exper. Med., 57:571, 1933.

Mallory, G. K., and Keefer, C. S.: Tissue Reactions

in Fatal Cases of Streptococcus Haemolyticus Infection. Arch. Path., 32:334, 1941.

Powers, G. F., and Biosvert, P. L.: Age as a Factor in Streptococcosis. J. Pediat., 25:504, 1944.

Rammelkamp, C. H., Jr., Wannamaker, L. W., and Denny, F. W.: Epidemiology and Prevention of Rheumatic Fever. Bull. New York Acad. Med., 28:321, 1952.

——, Weaver, R. S., and Dingle, J. H.: Significance of the Epidemiological Difference Between Acute Nephritis and Acute Rheumatic Fever. Tr. A. Am. Physicians, 65:168, 1952.

ACUTE TONSILLITIS

Definition. Acute tonsillitis is an infection of the lymphatic tissue of the pharynx, involving especially the palatine or faucial tonsils. The disease is contagious and is usually caused by group A hemolytic streptococci.

Etiology. Most cases of acute tonsillitis are caused by group A hemolytic streptococci. Groups B, E, F and G have occasionally been implicated in mild attacks. There is little to support the view that staphylococci or pneumococci give rise to tonsillitis.

Many strains of group A hemolytic streptococci produce potent erythrogenic toxins. Acute tonsillitis caused by one of these toxin-producing strains in a person without circulating antitoxin may be associated with a rash, and the disease is called scarlet fever. If a person has adequate antitoxin to neutralize the toxin produced by the same strain, the diagnosis of acute tonsillitis is made, or *scarlatina sine eruptione.*

Anatomy. The "ring of Waldeyer" consists of groups of tonsils joined together by lymphoid tissue. The palatine or faucial tonsils are situated between the pillars of the fauces. At the roof of the nasopharynx in the midline is the pharyngeal tonsil or adenoids. The lingual tonsils are at the base of the tongue, one on each side of the midline. On the posterior wall of the eustachian tube there is the tubal or eustachian tonsil. Extending down from the eustachian opening on the walls of the pharynx are strands of lymphatic tissue. It is apparent that an infection of the pharynx may involve more than one tonsil, as well as the wall of the pharynx.

Epidemiology. Sporadic and epidemic forms of the disease occur. Sporadic cases very likely arise as a result of close contact with an asymptomatic carrier of hemolytic streptococci or with one who has an acute illness. Epidemics of acute tonsillitis usually appear in groups of people living together where there is a high rate of healthy carriers coming in contact with susceptible persons. In addition, there are environmental factors such as overcrowded and dusty living quarters and poor ventilation.

Epidemics of acute tonsillitis have also been food-borne and milk-borne. The transmission of the disease by the latter route has given rise to the use of such terms as *epidemic sore throat* or *septic sore throat.* Though an epidemiologic differentiation is desirable, it is superfluous to distinguish these cases on clinical grounds, except that in these circumstances more severe cases of acute tonsillitis may be encountered.

During an epidemic of respiratory illness, hemolytic streptococci of the same type produce a variable clinical picture, as Glover and Griffith demonstrated. There is a group of persons whose pharynx is invaded without any signs of disease and who become healthy carriers. The second group suffer acute tonsillitis. A third group will have scarlet fever, and a fourth group will have a pharyngitis without a significant sore throat. All four groups are reservoirs for the further spread of disease.

Age Incidence. Acute tonsillitis has its highest incidence in childhood, especially between five and fifteen years of age. The disease is uncommon in infants and younger children, and there is a low incidence in elderly persons.

Seasonal Incidence. In the temperate zones the incidence of acute tonsillitis parallels the attack rate of all upper respiratory diseases. The incidence is highest during the winter and spring months.

Pathology. The crypts of the tonsils are filled with leukocytes, epithelial cells, fibrin and bacteria, all of which form amorphous masses seen at the orifices of the crypts as an exudate. The gland is congested; there is a leukocytic infiltration of the lymphatic nodules; and small suppurative foci may be noted in the follicles.

Symptoms. The onset is sudden, beginning frequently with chilly sensations or chills. Headache may be a prominent symptom, accompanied by pains and aches in the back and extremities. Occasionally, nausea, vomiting and diarrhea may occur. Shortly after the onset the temperature rises to 103° or 105° F., and the pulse is rapid with a rate of 100 to 120 per minute. The throat feels full, and on the affected side there is pain on deglutition, with the pain often radiating to the ear. With involvement of both palatine tonsils, the pain is bilateral. There is an attempt to swallow frequently which is associated with pain. In severe cases the patient looks and feels miserable during the first twenty-four to forty-eight hours. An invariable part of the clinical picture is a unilateral or bilateral tender swelling at the angle of the jaw, representing cervical adenitis. There may be a transitory albuminuria and an increase in the formed elements of the urine. Leukocytosis is usually found.

On examination, the inflamed tonsils appear red, projecting medially from the injected anterior and posterior pillars of the fauces. The openings of the crypts contain a yellowish exudate which may cover the surface of the tonsils like a membrane. This can be readily removed with an applicator. The uvula is commonly reddened, edematous and elongated. The posterior wall of the pharynx is red and edematous and covered with thick mucus.

At the end of the fourth or fifth day of the disease the temperature approaches normal and the patient is markedly improved. Coincident with subjective improvement there is a diminution in the inflammatory reaction of the tonsils.

Complications. Two general groups of complications may follow acute tonsillitis. The first group comprises suppurative lesions such as *sinusitis, otitis media, mastoiditis, cervical adenitis, peritonsillar abscess* and *bacteremia with metastatic lesions.* An uncommon but serious complication is *postanginal sepsis,* originating in the parapharyngeal space with a septic phlebitis of the tonsillar, facial or internal jugular veins. The *late nonsuppurative lesions* are described in the introductory section and also in the chapter on Scarlet Fever.

Diagnosis. The diagnosis of acute tonsillitis is not difficult on clinical grounds, but a differentiation must be made occasionally on an etiologic basis. *Diphtheria* may simulate acute tonsillitis of streptococcal origin. The onset of diphtheria is usually gradual; chills are rare; and the diphtheritic membrane on the tonsils or pharynx is very adherent, and, when it is removed, the denuded surface bleeds. Whenever there is doubt about the presence of diphtheria, the exudate should be cultured for the identification of *Corynebacterium diphtheriae.* Streptococcal tonsillitis or pharyngitis may co-exist with diphtheria.

Infectious mononucleosis may simulate the clinical features of streptococcal tonsillitis so closely that only the subsequent course of the disease along with hematologic and serologic information will establish the diagnosis. *Vincent's angina* usually causes a visible ulceration covered with an adherent membrane. In an uncomplicated case constitutional symptoms are minimal. Typical organisms may be demonstrated in appropriately stained smears of the exudate. A streptococcal infection may be superimposed upon a Vincent's infection.

The Commission on Acute Respiratory Diseases of the U. S. Army has described the clinical features and the bacteriologic and immunologic data of a group of cases under the heading of *endemic exudative pharyngitis and tonsillitis.* In most of the patients observed by this group the illness was not caused by streptococci, and the etiology remained unknown. In general, the disease of unknown etiology appeared to be less severe than that proved to be due to hemolytic streptococci. Another significant conclusion of the study was that, just as normal persons may be healthy carriers of group A hemolytic streptococci, so may patients with exudative disease of the pharynx of unknown etiology harbor pathogenic streptococci unrelated to their illness.

Treatment. The patients should be kept in bed; a liquid diet should be administered; and they should be encouraged to take fluid by mouth at frequent intervals. Antipyretics such as acetylsalicylic acid may be administered every three to four hours in doses of 0.3 to 0.6 gm. Dover's powders in doses of 0.6 gm. may allay the discomfort and restlessness. Cold applications to the neck in the form of an ice collar may afford some relief of the local pain. Throat gargles frequently induce more discomfort than relief. Irrigation of the throat with a hot solution of 2 per cent sodium bicarbonate is to be preferred. In the more severe cases, codeine sulfate should be administered for the general discomfort and local pain in doses of 0.03 to 0.065 gm. every six to eight hours if necessary.

The sulfonamides have been widely used in the treatment of acute tonsillitis, but without outstanding results. Such therapy may prevent suppurative complications, but it will not eradicate the streptococci from the throat or prevent the onset of the late nonsuppurative complications. Though the clinical course is generally not shortened with sulfonamide therapy, the more severe cases may reveal subjective improvement more promptly than untreated subjects. In older children and adults, sulfadiazine may be administered in an initial dose of 3 to 4 gm., and then 1 gm. every four to six hours night and day until the temperature subsides and the patient is improved. Then therapy may be discontinued or continued for a few days longer with the doses reduced by one half. An alkaline urine should be maintained. The drug of choice in the treatment of streptococcic tonsillitis is penicillin, unless there are contraindications, such as drug hypersensitivity. Other effective agents include the tetracyclines and erythromycin.

After patients have recovered from the acute phase of the illness they should be observed for possible subsequent development of late complications, especially nephritis and rheumatic fever.

WESLEY W. SPINK

References

Boharas, S.: Postanginal Sepsis. Arch. Int. Med., 71:844, 1943.
Commission on Acute Respiratory Diseases: Endemic Exudative Pharyngitis and Tonsillitis: Etiology and Clinical Characteristics. J.A.M.A., 125:1163, 1944.
Glover, J. A., and Griffith, F.: Acute Tonsillitis and Some of Its Sequels: Epidemiological and Bacteriological Observations. Brit. M. J., 2:521, 1931.

PERITONSILLAR ABSCESS

(Quinsy Sore Throat)

Peritonsillar abscess in practically all instances follows acute tonsillitis. This complication is not seen in infancy; it occurs occasionally in childhood, rarely in elderly people, the highest age incidence being between 15 and 35 years. The seasonal incidence is the same as that of tonsillitis.

Etiology. The usual cause of acute tonsillitis is group A hemolytic streptococci, and this may be considered to be the initiating factor for the development of peritonsillar abscess. However, even in these circumstances, streptococci may not be cultured from the exudate. The factors whereby a peritonsillar abscess develops as a complication of tonsillitis in some persons are not known.

Pathology. Suppuration extends through the capsule of the palatine tonsils into the loose connective tissue surrounding it. In most cases the process extends upward into the soft palate, being limited at the midline at the median raphe. This is associated with marked distention of the tissues by the exudate. Spontaneous rupture of the abscess takes place in the supratonsillar fossa. Occasionally the infection may extend down the posterior pillar of the fauces and along the wall of the pharynx, and rarely into the tonsillar tissue.

Symptoms. During the course of an attack of acute tonsillitis there may be an increase in the severity of pain radiating up to the ear; the appearance of chills and a rise in temperature; and considerable difficulty with deglutition, so that swallowing is impossible and saliva and mucus drool from the mouth of the patient. The neck is stiff, and the head is turned to the affected side. At the end of two or three days, opening the mouth even to the slightest degree is a painful task. There is marked enlargement and tenderness of the cervical lymph nodes on the affected side. The voice is guttural, a fact which may first call attention to the presence of peritonsillar abscess.

Examination reveals marked swelling of the soft palate just lateral to the uvula, with a purple-red discoloration of the mucosa. The inflamed anterior pillar and tonsil are projected to the midline, and they also extend forward in the mouth. The surface of the tonsil may be covered with exudate or a thick mucus. The uvula is edematous and elongated and clings to the enlarged tonsil. In a fully developed case, palpation of the supratonsillar fossa with the gloved finger discloses an area of fluctuation. The cervical lymph nodes are enlarged and tender.

Complications. If spontaneous rupture of the abscess should occur during sleep with aspiration of the purulent exudate, serious pulmonary complications may ensue. In the less usual type of lesion that extends down the lateral wall of the pharynx, edema of the larynx may occur. Thrombosis of the deep cervical vessels may result in a pyemia. Recurrent abscesses may follow subsequent attacks of tonsillitis.

Treatment. Acetylsalicylic acid and codeine or morphine sulfate may be necessary to allay the discomfort and pain. Sulfonamide therapy or, preferably, parenteral therapy with penicillin will at times prevent the progressive development of an abscess if treatment is started early in the course of the disease. However, with the establishment of purulent exudate in the peritonsillar tissues, treatment with sulfadiazine or penicillin is of limited value, although it should be continued (the reader is referred to the Introduction to Streptococcal Diseases, p. 155, for a detailed discussion of this subject). After a lapse of several days, suppuration will progress to a point where the spontaneous rupture of the abscess affords immediate and dramatic improvement in the patient's condition. If, by this time, spontaneous rupture of the abscess has not occurred, incision of the fluctuant area should be made. After the liberation of the pus, the fever abates, the pain subsides, and the patient is able to swallow with but little discomfort. After this procedure, irrigations with warm saline solution should be instituted at frequent intervals for a day or two. Mouth washes also aid in maintaining oral hygiene. Several months later, after all signs of inflammation have subsided, tonsillectomy should be seriously considered.

WESLEY W. SPINK

ERYSIPELAS

Definition. Erysipelas is an acute infection of the skin, caused by the hemolytic streptococcus. The face is involved in the majority of cases; less frequently, the body and extremities. The disease is characterized by localized redness and swelling, with fever and systemic manifestations.

History. The disease was probably described by Hippocrates. In the Middle Ages erysipelas was confused with acute ergot poisoning (St. Anthony's fire). The contagious nature of the illness was suspected long before the etiology was established by Fehleisen in 1882, when he isolated streptococci from the skin lesions and reproduced the disease in animals and in man.

Etiology. Erysipelas is not due to a specific strain of streptococcus such as *Streptococcus erysipelatis*. It is now well established that the disease may be caused by several different types of group A hemolytic streptococci, which are capable of producing other forms of streptococcal illness. There is no reason for believing that strains giving rise to erysipelas yield a specific toxin for this disease. Streptococci which cause erysipelas may produce potent erythrogenic toxins and thus initiate scarlet fever in other susceptible persons.

Epidemiology and Pathogenesis. Like other streptococcal infections, erysipelas is most prevalent in the temperate zones. The highest incidence occurs during the winter and early spring months. The disease is most prevalent after twenty years of age, though it appears among young infants as well as in the aged. Cases of erysipelas usually occur sporadically, even in the midst of epidemics of streptococcal disease. It is not uncommon for the same type of hemolytic streptococcus to cause various manifestations of streptococcal disease among persons in close contact with each other. Accordingly, some may have acute tonsillitis, others scarlet fever, another erysipelas, and still others may remain healthy pharyngeal carriers of streptococci. Factors responsible for the spread of streptococci, as already described, also apply to erysipelas.

It is not entirely clear why some persons express a susceptibility to hemolytic streptococci in the form of erysipelas. It is not unlikely that the bacteria gain entrance to the skin through small abrasions and, more obviously, through previously established wounds. In an analysis of 1400 cases of erysipelas at the Boston City Hospital, Keefer and Spink concluded that contributing factors in the genesis of erysipelas included debilitating diseases such as chronic alcoholism, cirrhosis of the liver, carcinoma and chronic cardiac and renal disease. Erysipelas was also found to be a complication of acute tonsillitis, acute sinusitis, acute otitis media or mastoiditis, puerperal sepsis, streptococcal empyema and streptococcal infections of the umbilicus. In the majority of cases of erysipelas, hemolytic streptococci can be readily obtained from the nasal orifices of patients, indicating that the organisms may enter the adjacent skin through small abrasions. The writer has frequently observed that erysipelas begins at the inner canthus of the eye. Hemolytic streptococci could be cultured with ease from the nasal and oral passages of these patients. This suggested that streptococci invaded the lacrimal duct from the cavity of the nose and that infection of the skin took place at the orifice of the lacrimal duct.

Morbid Anatomy. The disease causes an acute inflammatory reaction of the skin and subcutaneous tissue. The outstanding feature is edema with dilatation of the vessels and an infiltration of polymorphonuclear leukocytes. This gives the skin the characteristic red, shiny and swollen appearance.

The edema may result in bullae in the sub-epidermal spaces. Streptococci are present in the vessels and tissues, particularly in the central and marginal areas of the inflammation.

Symptoms. As with many other streptococcal illnesses, erysipelas may start with prodromata such as general malaise, chilly sensations or chills, fever, and nausea and vomiting twenty-four hours before any localizing signs appear. Not infrequently there may be a preceding upper respiratory infection. In the facial type the lesion appears as a well circumscribed, small, reddened, elevated area of skin with a shiny surface. The inflammation may be localized to one side of the face, but more often it progresses so that the skin of both cheeks, the eyelids, the nose and the ears may be involved. In more serious cases the scalp may be included. The swollen eyelids may approximate each other. Small blebs containing serous fluid may appear. From the beginning of the illness the patient is febrile; temperatures of 104° to 105° F. may persist for a week, and then approach normal. About the fourth or fifth day of the illness the tissues assume a purplish-red color, and in a week, desquamation of the skin appears. The bullae rupture or are absorbed, and the edema subsides. The mucous membrane of the nose may be encrusted and tender. The conjunctivas are injected. In a week to ten days the constitutional symptoms abate, leaving the patient in a weakened state. The skin usually heals with no residual scarring.

The manifestations of the illness and the severity of the disease are increased when larger areas of the body are involved, such as the trunk or extremities.

Complications. The most serious complication is a bacteremia due to hemolytic streptococcus. Unless this is prevented or treated with specific therapeutic agents, the mortality rate is high. Pneumonia is another serious complication. Suppuration and necrosis, especially of the tissues of the eyelids and scalp, occur. This complication is frequently due to secondary invasion of the tissues by *Staphylococcus aureus*. In summarizing the ocular complications of erysipelas, Bellows states that orbital cellulitis is not infrequent and may be the major manifestation. Loss of vision may follow orbital cellulitis or corneal involvement, and, more rarely, metastatic iridocyclitis or abscess of the vitreous.

The late nonsuppurative manifestations of streptococcal disease, such as glomerular nephritis, are infrequently encountered. During the acute illness there may be a transient albuminuria. Erysipelas in children is rarely followed by acute rheumatic fever.

Diagnosis. The facial type of erysipelas is readily recognized by the characteristic elevated, reddened glazed skin with its rapidly advancing border and accompanying acute febrile state with constitutional reactions. There is a leukocytosis and an increase in the polymorphonuclear leukocytes. Beta hemolytic streptococci are usually obtained from the nasal and oral pharynx and, in doubtful cases, from the margins of the advancing lesions by the aspiration of a small amount of serous fluid. Blood cultures are usually sterile, except in the progressive and fatal cases. Bacteremia is more likely to occur in small infants and in elderly patients.

Erysipelas must be distinguished from an *erythematous eczema,* which does not have the characteristic lesion of erysipelas and is not associated with an acute febrile state. *Erysipeloid* affects the skin of the fingers and hands, and the violaceous lesion spreads slowly.

Recurrent Erysipelas. In contrast to scarlet fever, one attack of erysipelas predisposes a patient to subsequent attacks. There are two types of recurrent erysipelas. Within a few weeks after recovery from an initial attack the patient may have a recurrence with involvement of the same area of skin. The clinical course is usually less severe, but hemolytic streptococci may be recovered from the local lesions. The second type of recurrence consists in repeated explosive onsets of a febrile illness with localized redness and swelling of a previously involved region of the face. The illness lasts only a few days, and streptococci cannot be recovered from the lesion. However, organisms may be obtained from the paranasal sinuses or other foci. Filtrates of a culture of the inciting strain may precipitate a recurrent attack of erysipelas when injected into a distant part of the body. There may be no reaction at the site of the injection. It would appear that the recurrences of this second type are an expression of local tissue hypersensitivity to the products of the hemolytic streptococci. Permanent local elephantiasis of the tissues, particularly the eyelids, may follow repeated attacks.

Prognosis. Before the introduction of ef-

The distinctive signs are limited to the pharynx, the cervical lymph nodes and the skin. In typical cases the mucous membrane of the throat is fiery red. The tonsils are swollen and covered with patchy exudate. Marked edema of the other tissues of the fauces is present, the uvula and soft palate and pillars often being several times normal size. The tongue may be bright and the papillae large, the *raspberry tongue;* or coated with the red papillae protruding, the *strawberry tongue.* These manifestations of the disease are rarely seen in adults. Tender anterior cervical adenitis is regularly present, even if the disease is mild. Atypical cases are common, particularly in persons in whom the tonsils have been removed. Tonsillar and pharyngeal exudate, edema and redness may be minimal or absent.

The *rash* usually appears on the second day. It consists of a diffuse, bright scarlet erythema with many points of deeper red. The distribution is variable, but the trunk and inner aspects of the arms and thighs are most often affected. In many cases the rash is well marked only in the axillae and groins. The face is flushed and red, but a pale area, the *circumoral pallor,* is often seen around the mouth. The palms and soles are not erythematous. Petechiae and occasionally ecchymoses are observed, especially in severely ill patients. The application of a tourniquet to the arm for five minutes will be associated with the appearance of large numbers of petechiae distal to the obstruction in nearly all cases. This is *Rumpel-Leede's sign;* it is not specific for scarlet fever.

Course. The rash reaches its height, as do the other manifestations of the disease, on the third or fourth day, after which there is a defervescence, the erythema disappearing by the sixth to ninth day in association with a return of the temperature and of the throat to normal.

Desquamation begins as a fine scaling of the face and body which is usually completed during the second week. About this time the extensive and characteristic desquamation of the palms and soles starts and continues for one or two weeks.

The course and clinical features of scarlet fever vary greatly with the severity of the disease. Many mild cases are observed in which constitutional symptoms and sore throat are minimal, fever is low grade and of short duration, and the rash is evanescent. A florid eruption is sometimes seen in persons in whom all other evidences of the disease are slight, indicating that the reaction to the erythrogenic toxin per se is not primarily responsible for the systemic manifestations of scarlet fever.

As the disease becomes more severe, there is a general increase in the intensity of all symptoms and signs. The maximum temperature in individual cases of the more severe forms will be from 101° to 106° F. The angina will be distressing and marked prostration evident. The rash will usually be prominent, but severe cases with little erythema are often seen.

Malignant Scarlet Fever. A toxic or malignant type of scarlet fever has been regularly described in earlier studies of this disease. A fulminating course was associated with delirium, collapse and death, often within forty-eight hours. The short duration of the disease did not permit the development of a typical erythema, but hemorrhages in the skin were observed. Such cases, in which death occurred quickly without dissemination of the streptococci from the local focus in the throat, are now rare. Occasional examples of the disease are observed in which high and prolonged fever, delirium or coma, and hemorrhagic rash are observed, but death has become an unusual event since the introduction of antimicrobial therapy. Similarly, septic scarlet fever with bacteremia, metastatic suppuration in the joints and elsewhere, and a prolonged and often fatal course has disappeared in properly treated cases.

Complications. The complications of scarlet fever are those common to all forms of hemolytic streptococcal upper respiratory infection with or without a skin rash, and are of two types.

Suppurative Complications. Suppurative complications are the result of the direct extension of the infectious process in the pharynx to the contiguous structures. Rhinitis and sinusitis and otitis media are the most common of these and occur frequently in children, but rarely in adults. Mastoiditis may follow extension of the infection to the middle ear. Peritonsillar abscess, or quinsy, and retropharyngeal abscess are less common. Streptococcal pneumonia is rare. These septic complications may be largely prevented or, should they appear, effectively treated by the administration of proper antimicrobial therapy. Cervical adenitis is regularly present and is not to be regarded as a complication unless the nodes become very large and liquefaction is imminent.

Types of Hemolytic Streptococci to Produc
let Fever. J.A.M.A., *124*:564, 1944.

Rantz, L. A., Boisvert, P. L., and Spink, W
Hemolytic Streptococcic and Nonstrepto
Diseases of the Respiratory Tract. Arch. Int.
78:369, 1946.

Schwenkter, F. F., Janney, J. H., and Gordon,
The Epidemiology of Scarlet Fever. Am. J.
38:27, 1943.

Trask, J. D., and Boisvert, P. L.: Scarlet Feve
ford Medicine. New York, Oxford Uni
Press, 1947.

Wesselhoeft, C., and Weinstein, L.: Scarlet
New England J. Med., 232:500, 531, 194!

RHEUMATIC FEVER

Definition. Rheumatic fever is a f
disease which occurs as a delayed sequ
infections with group A hemolytic str
cocci. It is characterized by the occurren
multiple focal inflammatory lesions in
parts of the body, notably in the heart,
vessels and joints. Among the diverse i
festations of the disease, those with the
serious clinical implications are conce
with involvement of the heart. Thus
name rheumatic fever, which emphasize
occurrence of inflammation of the joints,
to convey anything with regard to the r
festations of primary importance.

Etiology. In recent decades it has be
increasingly clear as the result of severa
dependent lines of evidence that grou
hemolytic streptococci are intimately
cerned in the pathogenesis of rheumatic f
Numerous clinical and epidemiological
ies pointed to a relationship between str
coccal sore throat and rheumatic fever. T
observations have been strongly supporte
an increasing body of immunologic
which demonstrate the occurrence of
bodies to streptococcal antigens in the co
of rheumatic fever. Indirect confirmatic
provided by the fact that the disease ca
prevented by the antimicrobial therap
prophylaxis of streptococcal infections.

While the importance of streptococca
fections in rheumatic fever appears to
established, the mechanism by which
hemolytic streptococcus initiates the dis
process remains obscure. The disease is
comparable to those bacterial infection
which the organism is readily demonstr
in the lesions. The symptoms of rheum
fever first become manifest after an inte
of several days to several weeks following

Nonsuppurative Complications. Nonsuppurative complications of scarlet fever and the other types of hemolytic streptococcal disease are of great interest. They may be precipitated by initial infections of all grades of severity. The acute respiratory illness subsides uneventfully and convalescence is well established when there may be the explosive appearance of a new disease of different pathology and not associated with the presence of the streptococcus in the involved tissue.

RHEUMATIC FEVER. The most common syndrome consists of fever, arthritis and carditis in varying severity and combinations, and is observed in 3 to 4 per cent of cases of scarlet fever. It is indistinguishable from and presumably identical with classic rheumatic fever. The disorder is readily recognized when the joints are involved, but it is important to bear in mind that nonarthritic poststreptococcal disorders of this type are common.

Occasionally erythema marginatum or nodosum will be observed.

LYMPHADENITIS. Reappearance of cervical lymphadenitis during convalescence is regarded as another type of nonsuppurative disorder. An episode of abdominal pain may indicate that the mesenteric lymph nodes have been involved. A condition requiring surgical intervention will often be suggested in such cases, and the differential diagnosis may be difficult. Needless laparotomies will be avoided if the possibility of mesenteric adenitis is borne in mind in persons recovering from streptococcal infection.

GLOMERULONEPHRITIS. Acute glomerulonephritis is a rare but dramatic nonsuppurative complication of streptococcal respiratory infection. It is most likely to be a sequel of cases in which septic complications have supervened. The abrupt appearance of hematuria, edema and hypertension during an uneventful convalescence from scarlet fever permits the ready recognition of the typical disorder. Mild and atypical forms of hemorrhagic Bright's disease will not be recognized unless urine examinations are performed frequently for two to three weeks after the termination of the initial respiratory disease.

RELAPSE. Relapse is unusual in untreated scarlet fever, but reinfection with a new serologic type of hemolytic streptococcus may occur at any time during convalescence and lead to an apparent exacerbation of tonsillitis and pharyngitis. Recovery from scarlet fever

is usually associated with a permanent immunity to the rash toxin, and second attacks are rare. It must be emphasized again that protection against subsequent infections by other types of hemolytic streptococci is not conferred, and episodes of tonsillitis and pharyngitis are very likely to occur in persons who have had scarlet fever.

Diagnosis. The recognition of scarlet fever in its characteristic form is not difficult. The presence of angina, tonsillitis, anterior cervical adenitis and erythema permits a clinical diagnosis in many instances. Cultural examination of material obtained from the nasopharynx is essential in atypical cases. Large numbers of hemolytic streptococci will be isolated if the illness is scarlet fever. The absence of these organisms excludes the disease. Their presence in small numbers does not present conclusive diagnostic evidence, since 5 to 10 per cent of the population are nasopharyngeal carriers of hemolytic streptococci.

The injection of 0.1 cc. of scarlet fever antitoxin, or of 0.2 to 0.3 cc. of convalescent human serum, into an area where the rash is florid will be followed by blanching of an area around the site of injection in eight to twelve hours. This is the *Schultz-Charlton reaction,* and is of diagnostic value if positive. Polymorphonuclear leukocytosis is the rule in moderately severe and severe scarlet fever, but is often absent in mild cases.

The local pharyngeal lesion in scarlet fever may resemble that of *diphtheria.* No rash is seen in the latter disease, but it must be remembered that the two may occur simultaneously. The erythema of *rubella* (German measles) and *rubeola* (measles) must be distinguished from that of scarlet fever. *Infectious mononucleosis* with angina and a rash may easily be mistaken for scarlet fever if appropriate cultural and hematologic studies are not carried out. The erythematous rashes of drug sensitivity are often similar to the dermal lesion of streptococcal disease. The absence of other characteristic symptoms and signs of scarlet fever should permit their recognition in other than the most unusual case.

Prognosis. Scarlet fever in the United States at the present time is a relatively mild disease, and the prognosis without antimicrobial therapy is uniformly good. Suppurative complications are common in younger children, but are well controlled by proper treat-

ment. Serious late, nonsuppurat
tions must be anticipated duri
ence regardless of the severity
illness. Rheumatic fever is m
supervene in patients with a p
the disease.

Prophylaxis. Satisfactory te
the prevention of scarlet fever
able. It has been customary to is
persons, but this procedure has r
the spread of hemolytic streptoc
tory infection in the population
numbers of carriers and cases
and pharyngitis without rash a
reservoirs for the disseminati
organisms. Many state and loc
partments have abandoned q
scarlet fever. It is important t
hemolytic streptococci rapidly di
the respiratory passages after tl
of penicillin therapy. This fa
simple means for the protectio
mediate potential contacts of
streptococcal disease, since thes
unable to transmit infection af
is begun.

Active immunity to the eryth
may be attained in Dick-positiv
repeated injections of increasin
the active material. This proc
recommended, since protection
only against the development o
not against infection by hemo
cocci. Furthermore, reactions
munization are common and oft

Prophylactic administration o
per day of sulfadiazine or of 2
of penicillin twice daily has
utilized. Such regimens will prev
by hemolytic streptococci unles
ant strains of these organisms ap
of value in special situations. Th
most often in institutions threa
demics of streptococcal infectic
management of the rheumatic s

Treatment. The manageme
fever should include those gene
that are applied in all the acu
Bed rest, light or liquid diet if
severe, and adequate but not e
intake are indicated. Gargles
value, but considerable relief o
may be obtained by the use o
throat irrigations. Acetylsalicylic
of 0.3 to 0.9 gm. every three to
often of great symptomatic bene

related to the high incidence of streptococcal infections during this period of life. When unusual conditions result in an increase in the attack rate of streptococcal disease in adult populations, as has occurred in the case of certain military establishments, the incidence of rheumatic fever appears to be comparable with that seen in childhood.

For many reasons there are no reliable figures which give an accurate picture of the general incidence of rheumatic fever. The disease is not reportable in most communities and even if it were, the difficulties of diagnosis would seriously affect the accuracy of the data. Special surveys in individual communities have yielded figures for the incidence which vary over a wide range from 0.1 per cent to more than 5 per cent. As a result of recent studies, somewhat more consistent figures are available for the frequency with which rheumatic fever occurs following streptococcal infections. In a number of epidemics of streptococcal disease in different localities of the United States, the incidence of rheumatic fever was approximately 3 per cent. While the attack rate may be appreciably greater or smaller in certain epidemics, this figure provides a reasonable index of the risk of rheumatic fever in untreated streptococcal infections. In contrast to these findings, the incidence of recurrences of the disease in known rheumatic subjects has been reported to be as high as 30 to 50 per cent following streptococcal infection.

Despite the inadequacy of statistical information, it is generally believed that the incidence of rheumatic fever, like that of streptococcal sore throat and scarlet fever, has been decreasing for several years. It is possible that the rate of decrease has recently been accelerated by the wide use of antimicrobial drugs. However, rheumatic fever remains one of the most important of the serious diseases of childhood.

It is evident from the close relationship between the two diseases that the epidemiology of rheumatic fever may be considered as a special branch of the epidemiology of streptococcal infections. The parallelism between the two diseases is illustrated by the geographical and seasonal variations in their occurrence. In the United States both have their peak incidence during the late winter and early spring, and they are encountered with considerably greater frequency in the northern than in the southern states. In

individual epidemics the peak incidence of streptococcal disease precedes that of rheumatic fever by one to three weeks, as would be expected on the basis of the time interval separating them in individual cases of rheumatic fever.

Rheumatic fever appears to be more common among families in the lower economic group. The effect of poverty is probably dependent upon such factors as malnutrition, overcrowding and substandard housing, which in turn lead to an increased incidence of streptococcal disease. There is, in addition, evidence for an hereditary predisposition to the disease, and it is common to obtain a family history of rheumatic fever as well as to encounter multiple cases among the siblings of a single family. No data are available to determine whether this hereditary predisposition is associated with an increased susceptibility to streptococcal infection.

Morbid Anatomy. Histologic examination of the tissues in rheumatic fever reveals multiple areas of focal inflammation which are disseminated widely throughout the body with special predilection for connective tissue. The basis for the focal nature of the lesions is not determined, although it is known that the small blood vessels are extensively involved. The detailed microscopic appearance of the inflammatory lesion varies with its location, and the most characteristic and specific pattern is found in the myocardial Aschoff body. This lesion, when present in its classic form, is generally considered to be pathognomonic of rheumatic fever. In many areas the inflammatory lesion is accompanied by an alteration in the staining properties of the ground substance of the connective tissue. This change is described as "fibrinoid degeneration of collagen," but its chemical basis has not been established. Valvulitis, which leads to the most serious permanent damage, is characterized during the acute stage by interstitial inflammation and the appearance of minute vegetations on the surface of the valve near its margin.

Pathologic Physiology and Chemistry. In many respects the alterations in chemical constitution of the body which occur in the course of rheumatic fever are similar to those encountered in other acute febrile diseases. This is particularly true of the numerous changes in the peripheral blood. It has been demonstrated by chemical and electrophoretic analysis that increases in concentration occur in several of the protein fractions of the blood, including fibrinogen and alpha and gamma globulins. These increases in protein concentration are accompanied by a variety of changes in the properties of the blood which are dependent upon an increased concentration of certain individual components. Thus, the erythrocyte sedimentation rate is markedly elevated, and abnormally high concentrations of such constituents as complement, mucoprotein and nonspecific hyaluronidase inhibitor are found. In addition, new substances appear which are not normally present in blood. These latter are exemplified by the so-called C-reactive protein and by substances which are bactericidal for a variety of microorganisms.

It should be emphasized that these changes in constituents of the blood are not limited to rheumatic fever but are found in numerous disease states. Somewhat more specific alterations occur as the result of the appearance of antibodies directed against various components of the hemolytic streptococcus. These antibodies are responsible for at least part of the observed increase in gamma globulin concentration. They have been demonstrated for several extracellular products of the streptococcal cell, such as streptolysin O, streptokinase, streptococcal hyaluronidase and desoxyribonuclease, as well as for cellular components such as the type-specific M-protein. The anti-streptococcal antibodies usually become detectable in the blood about one week after a streptococcal infection and increase in titer for three or four weeks. Because of the time relationships between precursory streptococcal infection and rheumatic fever, the antibody titers are generally still increasing at the time of appearance of rheumatic symptoms. The level of circulating body declines gradually after the peak has been reached.

Numerous comparisons have been made in recent years between the antibody response shown by patients with uncomplicated streptococcal infections and those who develop rheumatic fever as a late complication. It has been found that while there is no consistent qualitative difference between the two groups, the proportion of rheumatic patients who develop significant antibody responses to a given antigen is higher than that of patients with uncomplicated streptococcal disease. In individual epidemics of streptococcal infection, the mean antibody response of those who develop rheumatic fever is consistently greater than the mean response of the great majority who suffer no complications. The significance of this immunologic hyperreactivity of the rheumatic subject in relation to the pathogenesis of the disease has not been established.

Gross changes in the respiratory and cardiac physiology during acute rheumatic fever are dependent to a large extent on the degree of involvement of the heart. When myocarditis is extensive, cardiac failure may intervene early in the disease, and the alterations dependent on the acute febrile nature of rheumatic fever are complicated by those arising from cardiac decompensation. More subtle disturbances in cardiac physiology frequently result from interference with the conduction system, so that alterations in rhythm and various types of heart block are encountered.

Symptoms and Signs. The symptoms of rheumatic fever are diverse and cover an extremely wide range, both with respect to the variety of manifestations and the degree of intensity with which they occur. In part, this is a reflection of the fact that it is not a disease of a single circumscribed organ but appears to involve the mesenchymatous connective tissue, so that numerous areas of the body may be affected. The major symptoms include fever, pain arising from inflammation of the joints, various manifestations of involvement of the heart and pericardium, abdominal pain, skin changes and chorea. The general symptoms of anorexia, loss of weight, weakness and fatigability are almost invariably present.

The onset of the disease may be insidious and gradual or acute. The relationship to a preceding streptococcal infection is not always clear, since the infection can be so mild as to escape notice completely. During the interval between the streptococcal infection and the onset of rheumatic fever, usually a period of one to four weeks, the patient may appear to be entirely well and be able to engage in his normal activity. On some occasions, however, laboratory examinations will reveal evidence of disease activity during this so-called latent interval.

The most common type of onset of rheumatic fever is characterized by the sudden occurrence of fever and joint pain. While the fever may be high and sustained in severe cases, it is more frequently moderate and often low grade. The patient may complain of sore throat, even though examination reveals minimal evidence of acute inflammation and significant bacterial infection may not be demonstrable. Epistaxis occurs commonly both at the onset and throughout the acute stage of the disease, and in some cases results in serious loss of blood.

Joint Involvement. The manifestations of *polyarthritis* vary from vague discomfort in the extremities to the exquisite pain associated with acutely inflamed and swollen joints. In the former instance there is little or no objective evidence to confirm the presence of inflammation of the articular surfaces. On the other hand, in the case of the severely involved joint the skin shows local redness and heat, the joint is markedly swollen with obliteration of the normal configuration, and fluid is obviously present within the joint cavity. Passive or active movement of the joint is extremely painful. The fluid in joints of this type is turbid and contains inflammatory leukocytes but is sterile on bacteriologic culture. A single joint may be affected or most of the large joints in the body may be involved at one time. Characteristically, however, the arthritis is migratory in nature and as the pain and swelling subsides in one area, others become involved. The large joints of the extremities are most frequently affected, but no area appears to be immune and one may find arthritis of the hands, feet, spine or of such joints as the sternoclavicular and temporomandibular.

There appears to be some variation with age in the pattern of joint involvement most frequently encountered. In the youngest age group in which rheumatic fever is regularly recognized, from 4 to 6 years, frank arthritis is a less common feature of the disease. These small children may complain of mild joint pains or merely vaguely localized aching of the extremities. This type of complaint, at one time discounted as "growing pains," is usually associated with only low grade fever but, despite the benign character of the overt symptomatology, can be associated with serious involvement of the heart. Rheumatic fever in older children and young adults is more often associated with the classic migratory polyarthritis, although even in this group the manifestations are diverse. It should be emphasized that rheumatic fever can occur without any evidence of joint involvement whatever.

Cardiac Involvement. In the course of acute rheumatic fever the patient may have little in the way of symptoms referable to cardiac involvement, and it is usually necessary to depend on clinical, roentgenographic and electrocardiographic examinations to determine the extent and seriousness of this manifestation of the disease. Since all of the major anatomic divisions of the heart are subject to the disease, the manifestations vary depending on the relative concentration of lesions in the different areas of the heart. *Myocarditis* and *pericarditis* are responsible for most of the abnormal findings during the acute stage of the disease, and the presence of *endocarditis* is not readily demonstrated even in those cases in which the subsequent course of events makes it obvious that endocarditis was extensive. Endocarditis involving the leaflets of the valves is responsible for the scarring and distortion which lead to permanent valvular heart disease.

Precordial pain or discomfort is one symptom which is often encountered, and it is usually a reflection of myocardial disease rather than of pericarditis. The patient may also complain of palpitation or unpleasant consciousness of the rapid action of the heart. If the disease is sufficiently extensive to cause serious impairment of the function of the heart, the usual symptoms of cardiac failure will be superimposed on those of the acute rheumatic process.

The findings on physical examination reflect the same wide variation in severity of disease that the symptoms display. In the simple, relatively benign case there may be nothing more than a tachycardia which cannot be interpreted as unequivocal evidence of cardiac involvement. In the more severe cases, one may detect generalized cardiac enlargement, and, in addition to the rapid heart rate, the heart sounds in the apical area may be muffled, indistinct and of poor muscular quality. The latter findings are often associated with a diffuse precordial impulse. The second sound in the pulmonic area is commonly greatly accentuated in comparison with the second aortic sound. Gallop rhythm may occur and is usually an indication of serious myocardial disease.

The cardiac murmurs which appear during the acute phase of initial attacks of rheumatic fever are most frequently blowing systolic murmurs best heard in the apical area, and are considered to be caused by dilatation of the valve rings as a result of general dilatation of the heart. Less commonly, soft diastolic murmurs will be heard along the left sternal border in the third and fourth interspaces. It is difficult to determine whether inflammation of the valve leaflets contributes significantly to these murmurs. As the murmurs may disappear permanently on recovery, their final significance cannot be determined except by repeated examination during and after convalescence.

When the pericardial component of carditis becomes extensive, the classical to-and-fro friction rub will be heard over the precordium. This physical sign may be of brief duration or may persist for days, and it will sometimes disappear with the accumulation of fluid in the pericardial sac.

Disturbances in the conduction system of the heart are best detected by the use of electrocardiography. Occasionally, however, irregularities in the rhythm resulting from second degree heart block can be recognized clinically. The most common manifestation of interference with conduction in rheumatic fever is prolongation of the P-R interval in the electrocardiogram, reflecting a delay in transmission of the excitation wave from auricle to ventricle. The interference with conduction may be increased to the point where dropped beats result, and the rhythm may assume a regular pattern with the beats occurring in couplets or triplets. Complete auriculo-ventricular dissociation may also occur, with the ventricles assuming a rhythm independent of that of the auricles. More rarely, auricular fibrillation will make its first appearance during acute rheumatic fever. In addition to these conduction anomalies, the electrocardiogram may show T wave abnormalities, most commonly inversion of the wave in one or more leads. In the presence of pericarditis elevation of the S-T segment may occur in the acute phase with subsequent alterations in the configuration of the T wave which simulate those seen in coronary disease.

The roentgenographic findings may be unremarkable in acute rheumatic fever unless the myocarditis is sufficiently severe to give rise to dilatation of the chambers of the heart. When dilatation occurs, generalized enlargement of the heart is apparent on roentgenography, and changes in size may occur quite rapidly as a result of changes in the activity of the disease process.

The foregoing description of the findings referable to cardiac involvement is applicable to those cases of acute rheumatic fever in which previous damage to the heart has not occurred. However, since rheumatic fever is characteristically a recurrent disease, it is common to encounter the acute disease in patients with well-established rheumatic valvular disease. This may occur even in the absence of a history of previous attacks of rheumatic fever. In cases of this type, the manifestations of acute rheumatic carditis are superimposed on those of chronic valvular disease. The character of established murmurs may be modified by the acute myocardial disease, and the reserve of the heart is diminished so that cardiac failure is a greater threat. If the status of the patient prior to the onset of the acute attack is unknown, it is frequently difficult to distinguish between the effects of the acute process and those of chronic disease until convalescence is complete.

Miscellaneous Clinical Manifestations. Involvement of the lung in rheumatic fever leads to a type of pneumonitis which is very difficult to detect clinically. The existence of rheumatic pneumonia was first established by the pathologic examination of postmortem material. It is most common in the severe and fulminating cases in which any clinical or roentgenographic evidence of a pneumonic process may be obscured by acute congestion of the lungs resulting from cardiac failure. *Pleurisy,* which at one time occurred quite frequently in rheumatic fever, appears to be an unusual manifestation of the disease at the present time.

Abdominal pain, unassociated with arthralgia or arthritis, may be the presenting complaint at the time of onset of the disease. This symptom is most commonly encountered in children, and although the pain and associated tenderness are usually not well localized, their significance is frequently misinterpreted. In some instances, bouts of abdominal discomfort or pain persist throughout the period of activity of the disease. The precise origin of these abdominal symptoms has not been established.

The characteristic manifestation of *skin involvement* in acute rheumatic fever, occurring in about one fourth of childhood cases, is a multiform type of erythema commonly designated as *erythema marginatum* or *circinatum.* It consists of roughly circular lesions which may be distributed over the extremities, trunk and sometimes the face and which spread centrifugally leaving a clear center. The lesions tend to coalesce so that, although individual areas are iris-like, the larger areas are serpiginous in outline. The erythema blanches on pressure, and may be quite evanescent, disappearing and later reappearing at the same sites. The lesions are usually not elevated, although in some cases a slight papular quality may be detected. In the vast majority of instances the rash occasions no discomfort, but well authenticated cases have occurred in which itching has been a troublesome factor. Erythema marginatum is not pathognomonic of rheumatic fever and similar rashes may occur in association with other diseases. Rarely, purpura is seen in rheumatic fever.

Erythema nodosum is another skin disorder which appears to be a manifestation of the acute rheumatic process. However, it is not nearly so frequent in occurrence as erythema marginatum, and often occurs when other evidence of rheumatic disease is equivocal or lacking. It would appear that only a portion of the cases of erythema nodosum are referable to rheumatic fever. The dull red, nodular lesions occur most frequently on the extensor surfaces of the extremities and vary in size from less than one centimeter to many centimeters in diameter. They are extremely tender on pressure, and the pain is aggravated by movement of the extremities.

Subcutaneous rheumatic nodules represent a quite different type of lesion. These are firm, insensitive nodules which occur over the bony prominences of the various joints and tendons of the extremities, the spine and the back of the head. They appear to be loosely attached to the underlying tissue and the skin is freely movable over them. Increasing the tension of the skin by flexion of the joints makes the nodules more readily apparent, and it is often necessary to use this procedure in order to detect the presence of small nodules. When nodules are numerous, there is a tendency for them to be symmetrical in distribution. Subcutaneous nodules are most frequently encountered in the more severe cases of rheumatic fever with serious cardiac involvement. In part, this may be due to the fact that the presence of nodules is much more readily detectable when there is loss of subcutaneous tissue as the result of chronic rheumatic disease. Thus, patients with nodules usually also show marked evidence of wasting and loss of weight.

Chorea may occur as a manifestation of rheumatic fever either alone or in combination with other symptoms of the disease. While there is some question whether all cases of pure chorea, without other evidence of rheumatic disease, are related to rheumatic fever, there is no doubt that it occurs as the sole manifestation of the disease in some cases. When chorea is unassociated with other rheumatic symptoms, fever and other systemic changes, reflected by such tests as the erythrocyte sedimentation rate, are usually absent. It would appear that when rheumatic involvement is confined to the central nervous system, the characteristic general systemic response is reduced to a minimum.

The onset of chorea is usually insidious, and the parents of a child with chorea may first note only increased awkwardness and a tendency to spill food or drop objects which is attributed to carelessness. Even the appearance of involuntary purposeless movements of the extremities may be discounted as "nervousness." However, with further progression of the disease, the irregular and uncontrollable movements become obvious. These may be extensive and involve not only the hands, feet, arms and legs but the tongue and facial muscles. The severity may range from cases in which the movements are detectable only after close observation to those in which violent continual activity totally incapacitates the patient and necessitates protection from self-injury. In moderate cases, it is common for chorea to interfere with all coordinated operations, such as writing and eating. In some cases chorea may be limited to one side of the body. The disease appears to affect females somewhat more frequently than males, although this sex preponderance probably has been overstressed in the past.

Laboratory Findings. *Hematology.* Alterations in the leukocytes during acute rheumatic fever are similar to those encountered in an acute streptococcal infection. A definite leukocytosis is usually encountered with total leukocyte counts ranging from 12,000 to 24,000 per cubic millimeter. This is associated with an increase in the percentage of polymorphonuclear elements.

A moderate degree of anemia is found in the majority of cases. This anemia is usually normocytic in type with proportional decreases in the hemoglobin concentration and erythrocyte count. It is similar to the anemia encountered in infections and to some extent may have its origin in the precursory streptococcal infection. However, the anemia does not tend to improve while the rheumatic process remains active. In many cases, the anemia is superimposed on a pre-existing nutritional anemia and may be more severe in degree. The most severe anemias encountered in rheumatic fever are those associated with loss of blood resulting from epistaxis.

Urinary Findings. A high percentage of patients with rheumatic fever show the presence of some proteinuria and an increase in the numbers of formed elements in the urine during the acute phase of the disease. However, the changes are rarely as marked as those characteristically encountered in acute hemorrhagic nephritis, and it is uncommon to find the two diseases simultaneously in the same patient, despite the fact that both follow infection with hemolytic streptococci.

Diagnosis. In the classic case of rheumatic fever, diagnosis presents no problems. Thus, when one is confronted with a patient who develops fever, migratory polyarthritis, unequivocal evidence of carditis and erythema marginatum three weeks following a severe sore throat, there is little doubt concerning the correctness of the diagnosis. This type of case is relatively unusual, however, and it is more often necessary to rely on careful evaluation of all available lines of evidence, including history, symptoms, signs and laboratory data. Criteria for diagnosis of rheumatic fever have been suggested on the basis of the combination of major and minor manifestations of the disease which should be considered as the minimal requirement, but in practice it is not possible to adhere rigidly to any formula for diagnosis. Not only do the symptoms of certain other diseases simulate those of rheumatic fever, but the overt manifestations of rheumatic fever may be so atypical or minimal as to mislead the diagnostician. In this connection, it is pertinent to note that in routine examination of school populations, cases of unequivocal rheumatic heart disease with no history of an attack of acute rheumatic fever are frequently encountered, and it must be assumed that the acute disease occurred as an undiagnosed illness. When one considers the mildness or the bizarre character of certain cases of known rheumatic fever, it is not difficult to understand how the disease frequently escapes recognition.

It is important to inquire carefully for family history of rheumatic fever and for past illnesses that may have represented previous attacks of the disease. The history of sore throat in the weeks prior to the onset of the disease may be helpful as an indication of a precursory streptococcal infection. However, it should be noted that a negative history in this regard is inconclusive, since mild or relatively asymptomatic infections may be disregarded or forgotten by the patient. Evaluation of the various symptoms presented by the patient often requires close questioning concerning their exact nature and timing. Arthralgia and vague pain or discomfort in the extremities, especially in the young child, must be given serious consideration as possible manifestations of the disease. In the doubtful case, in which objective joint involvement is lacking, physical examination centers on the attempt to determine whether carditis is present. When recurrence of the disease is suspected in a known rheumatic patient, it is necessary to distinguish between the manifestations of acute carditis and those of established valvular disease.

The difficulties involved in recognition of the disease are increased by the fact that there is no specific diagnostic laboratory test. The laboratory procedures that provide the most assistance in diagnosis are those concerned with the measurement of antibodies to streptococcal antigens, but the most that can be expected of these tests is that they will supply evidence of a recent streptococcal infection. The limitations of this type of evidence are twofold. In the first place, all persons do not show significant antibody responses to a single streptococcal antigen, and consequently a negative result does not eliminate the possibility of a recent streptococcal infection. Secondly, patients with nonrheumatic disease may also show evidence of an antibody response to a streptococcal infection which is unrelated to their presenting illness, particularly during periods of high incidence of streptococcal disease. Despite these limitations, the antibody tests are valuable additions to the total collection of facts which must be evaluated in reaching a diagnosis.

Among these tests, the most widely employed and the most practical for general use is the measurement of antibody against streptolysin O. The *antistreptolysin O titer* is significantly elevated (above 150 units per cubic centimeter) in 85 per cent or more of rheumatic fever patients. The significance of the antibody information can be increased by carrying out determinations of more than one antibody, and in some cases it is helpful, if facilities are available, to measure antistreptokinase and antihyaluronidase in addition to antistreptolysin O. The absence of a significant elevation in titer of any of the three antibodies would render the diagnosis of rheumatic fever doubtful.

Other laboratory tests used in rheumatic fever, such as the erythrocyte sedimentation rate, offer relatively little assistance in diagnosis and are of value chiefly in following the activity of the disease process once the diagnosis has been established.

Differential Diagnosis. Because of the protean manifestations of rheumatic fever a wide variety of clinical conditions must be considered in differential diagnosis. Low grade febrile illnesses of undetermined origin frequently present the most difficult diagnostic problems. The possibility that illnesses of this type represent subclinical or smouldering rheumatic activity must be considered, and this is especially true when the common symptom of pain or discomfort in the extremities is present. The problem becomes even more pressing when low grade febrile disease occurs in a person known to have previously suffered one or more attacks of rheumatic fever. In this instance, the marked tendency of rheumatic fever to recur increases the likelihood that the obscure disorder represents rheumatic activity. The problem can be resolved only by close observation and careful study to uncover additional evidence for or against the diagnosis. *Chronic upper respiratory disease, chronic tonsillitis, brucellosis* and *infectious mononucleosis* are among the diseases which must be considered in this connection.

Intercurrent respiratory disease or other febrile illness in children with previously undiagnosed congenital heart disease may be confused with rheumatic fever, if cardiac murmurs arising from the congenital defect are misinterpreted as rheumatic in origin. Thorough study of the cardiac abnormality will usually reveal its nature.

Acute septic arthritis, for example streptococcal or gonococcal arthritis, will simulate rheumatic arthritis, especially in the early stages when the inflammation of the joint is indistinguishable from that seen in the severely involved joint in rheumatic fever. As the disease progresses, the manifestations of the septic joint are more severe than observed in rheumatic fever, and there is a marked tendency for inflammation and edema to extend into the soft tissues at some distance from the joint. The diagnosis can be readily established by removal of fluid from the involved joint for bacteriologic examination. Among other acute bacterial infections, *acute staphylococcal bacteremia* may also simulate rheumatic fever in its early stages, since wide dissemination of the organisms may lead to transient symptoms of multiple joint involvement as well as to pleurisy and pericarditis. In addition, before the pain of *staphylococcal osteomyelitis* becomes sharply localized this disease may be confused with rheumatic fever. When joint involvement occurs in *serum disease,* the clinical picture is similar to that of certain cases of rheumatic fever.

Chronic rheumatoid arthritis, especially in the early months of the disease before the chronicity of the process and the extensive nature of the articular damage become apparent, must be distinguished from rheumatic fever. Although cardiac signs and symptoms and other stigmata of rheumatic fever are usually absent, continued observation for many weeks is sometimes required before the diagnosis can be eliminated as a possibility. Similarly, the arthritis due to *gout* must be considered in the differential diagnosis in the adult. Among rarer disease states, certain cases of *periarteritis nodosa* and *disseminated lupus erythematosus* may be difficult to differentiate from rheumatic fever in early stages of the disease.

Subacute bacterial endocarditis occurs most commonly in persons with valves previously damaged by rheumatic fever, and it often presents a clinical picture which is not readily distinguishable from a rheumatic recurrence. Vague pains in the extremities are more common than overt arthritis, but these symptoms together with fever and debility in a known rheumatic individual are sufficient to suggest a rheumatic recurrence. The difficulties are increased by the fact that in some cases it is not possible to recover the offending organism in blood culture. The characteristic petechiae and painful septic emboli of endocarditis are helpful in differential diagnosis. (See section on Bacterial Endocarditis, in Diseases of the Cardiovascular System.)

When abdominal pain is the initial symptom in acute rheumatic fever, the illness is frequently mistaken for *appendicitis* and all too frequently an unnecessary appendectomy is performed. The highly localizing signs characteristic of classic appendicitis are not found, but because of the fact that appendicitis in children is often atypical, the lack of these findings is not conclusive. However, if a brief period for observation is allowed in doubtful cases other manifestations of rheumatic fever may become apparent.

The so-called *benign idiopathic pericarditis,* which is apparently not rheumatic in origin, is indistinguishable in the acute phase from those cases of rheumatic fever in which pericarditis is the major detectable manifestation. The diagnosis of idiopathic pericarditis is dependent primarily on elimination of other possibilities and on the subsequent course of the disease, which is characterized by complete recovery without residual damage. Thus, the final conclusion is often reached only in retrospect, and must remain somewhat uncertain since rheumatic pericarditis with minimal involvement of the myocardium and endocardium could conceivably behave in a similar fashion.

Acute aleukemic leukemia may occasionally mimic rheumatic fever closely with fever and extremity pain. The nature of the disease may not be suspected until the failure of therapeutic measures suggests the possibility. Examination of the peripheral blood and the bone marrow will serve to suggest the correct diagnosis. *Sickle cell anemia* represents a second disease of the blood which can simulate rheumatic fever. It is advisable to examine the blood for sickling in all cases of suspected rheumatic fever in members of the Negro race.

When uncertainty concerning the diagnosis exists, it is often useful to employ a therapeutic test with salicylates. The rapidity with which the symptoms of rheumatic fever are controlled by these drugs in many cases is in sharp contrast to its lack of effect in most of the diseases that cause confusion in the diagnosis.

Prognosis. The course of rheumatic fever does not follow any single well defined pattern. Some patients who appear quite ill at the onset of the disease become symptom-free in a few days and proceed to rapid and complete recovery, so that the total duration of the illness is not longer than three to four weeks. In contrast to this type of illness, fulminating attacks may be so overwhelming that death occurs early in the acute phase. At the other extreme there are patients who show persisting evidence of rheumatic activity for many months or perhaps years. Any of the various symptoms of the disease may occur during the course of this protracted form of the disease. In some instances, the subacute and chronic type of rheumatic fever is characterized by recurring cycles of activity with intervening periods of relative freedom from symptoms. The importance of these characteristics of the disease from the point of view of prognosis lies in the fact that the course which the disease will follow is totally unpredictable, and there is nothing in its pattern during the early stages which can be relied upon to indicate the probable duration of the illness or the likelihood of the appearance of permanent cardiac damage.

Death in the acute phase of the first attack is rare, but the incidence of fatality increases in recurrences of the disease in which the acute process is superimposed on permanent cardiac damage resulting from previous bouts of rheumatic fever. Cardiac failure appears to be the immediate cause of death in these patients. The clinical impression that the severity of rheumatic fever has tended to decline in recent decades is supported by figures indicating that the fatality rate has decreased.

The long-term prognosis is dependent primarily on the nature and degree of cardiac involvement. Extensive malformation of one or more of the valves, leading to serious interference with the efficient functioning of the heart, greatly decreases the life expectancy of the patient. Follow-up studies on large groups of rheumatic patients have shown that the majority of those with severe cardiac involvement, as indicated by marked enlargement of the heart or congestive failure, succumb within ten years. The prognosis is also affected by the fact that a new attack of rheumatic fever may contribute further damage. Recurrences of the disease are most frequent in the first five years following the initial attack of the disease, and the danger appears to diminish with advancing age. However, there is no age at which the rheumatic subject can be considered free from the threat of recurrence following an infection with hemolytic streptococci.

The predisposition to bacterial endocarditis is another factor which affects the long-term prognosis in rheumatic fever. Prior to the introduction of effective antimicrobial therapy, endocarditis was a uniformly fatal disease and second only to congestive heart failure as a cause of death among rheumatic subjects. The present success in curing a high percentage of cases of endocarditis does not completely remove the serious prognostic implications of the disease, however, since the bacterial infection frequently results in further damage to the affected valves before it is eliminated.

Recently, as a result of the widespread use of mitral commissurotomy for surgical correction of stenotic mitral valves, biopsy fragments of the auricular appendage have become available for pathologic examination. It has been found that Aschoff bodies are present in the auricular tissue of at least 40 per cent of patients coming to operation, even though care has been taken to eliminate all patients with clinical or laboratory evidence of rheumatic activity. This finding again raises the question of whether rheumatic activity continues at a subclinical level for many years in a high percentage of cases. However, at the present time the significance of the Aschoff body is not sufficiently well established to draw final conclusions concerning the persistence of rheumatic activity on the basis of this finding alone.

Treatment. During the acute febrile phase of rheumatic fever, general care is like that of other febrile diseases with emphasis on maintenance of an adequate fluid intake. Conservative management of the disease requires that bed rest be continued as long as evidence of the disease activity persists. Because of the prolonged nature of the disease in many cases, this requirement poses a special problem in the maintenance of the patients' morale. Therapeutic measures will usually eliminate all symptoms of the disease, and consequently it is difficult to reconcile the patient to the necessity of remaining in bed. Planned recreation and occupational therapy, adjusted to the interests and capabilities of the patient, are essential; at the same time it is advisable to attempt education concerning the nature of this disease. Education must be continued into the period of convalescence, since the concept of the variability of the outcome of rheumatic fever is often poorly grasped and one must guard against both unnecessary anxiety and unfounded complacency. It is possible for a patient without significant residual heart damage to become psychologically crippled by exaggerated fear of the disease, and on the other hand an individual with serious cardiac involvement may discount the dangers and attempt to carry on all the activities of a normal healthy person. In childhood rheumatic fever, education of the parents assumes first importance.

The necessity for prolonged bed rest has been challenged by some clinicians, and it must be admitted that proof of its value has not been established by controlled experiment. However, it has been repeatedly observed that the most unfavorable results in rheumatic fever occur when intermittent or semi-ambulatory care is practiced. It is permissible to modify the regimen by allowing bathroom privileges, and exceptions to the rule that bed rest must be continued until all evidence of disease activity is gone may occasionally be made when a minor manifestation of the disease persists in the absence of all other symptoms or signs. Thus, it is difficult to justify keeping a patient in bed solely because of the presence of erythema marginatum.

After rheumatic fever is first diagnosed, a course of penicillin should be given to eliminate hemolytic streptococci. This is advisable even if bacteriologic examination yields negative throat cultures for streptococci, since the organisms may remain in inaccessible areas. It is preferable to administer the penicillin parenterally, and 300,000 units of procaine penicillin once a day in children and twice a day in adults for seven to ten days represents an effective dose. Whether the patient is cared for in the home or in the hospital, it is important to provide continuous protection from reinfection with hemolytic streptococci. In addition to employing isolation techniques and general procedures to prevent exposure, one can institute a program of prophylactic drug treatment according to one of the regimens discussed below.

The *symptomatic treatment* of rheumatic fever at the present time is generally carried out with salicylates or with one of the hormone products: cortisone, hydrocortisone or corticotropin. The relative merits of these agents in controlling the various manifestations of the disease are still under investigation, and it is not yet possible to define an order of preference. The opinion is widely held that the hormones are able to bring about more rapid control of the symptoms, especially the manifestation of carditis, but it is clear that patients vary in their response to the several drugs so that even this generalization has its limitations. An important practical consideration in therapy is that both salicylates and the hormones suppress the overt manifestations of rheumatic fever without eliminating the underlying disease process. Thus, they cannot be considered as therapeutic agents in the same sense that an antimicrobial drug is a therapeutic agent in bacterial infections.

When the antirheumatic drugs are given in adequate dosage not only do the signs and symptoms of the disease tend to disappear, but the changes in the blood responsible for the various tests for rheumatic activity, such as the erythrocyte sedimentation rate, revert to normal. Under full treatment, therefore, the patient may appear to have recovered completely. However, upon withdrawal of therapy all the symptoms and abnormalities may rapidly reappear with an intensity as great as that which existed prior to the initiation of therapy.

The current concept of the action of these drugs is that they interfere with the tissue reaction to the abnormal process but do little to accelerate its elimination from the body. They serve the purpose, therefore, of reducing the inflammatory response and maintaining the patient in a state of relative well-being while the body gradually disposes of the substances responsible for the disease.

Salicylates may be given in the form of acetylsalicylic acid or sodium salicylate in a total daily dose of 0.064 gm. (1 grain) per pound of body weight (1.5 gram per kilogram), varying from 3 gm. in young children to 10 gm. or more in adults, given in equally divided doses at 4-hour intervals. Individual variation in the efficiency of absorption or excretion of the drug and in its therapeutic effectiveness requires readjustment of the dose in many cases. The aim is to give the minimum dose that results in full control of symptoms and to avoid serious toxic side reactions. Studies on the concentration of salicylates in the blood have shown that it is usually necessary to attain a level of at least 25 mg. per 100 ml. to obtain full effect, and that this concentration is sometimes reached with less than 0.064 gm. per pound while at other times more is required.

The most common toxic manifestations of salicylate therapy are nausea, vomiting and gastric distress. Tinnitus and some degree of temporary impairment of hearing usually occur at full therapeutic dosage. Hyperpnea is commonly seen, but the severe acidosis characteristic of intoxication with methyl salicylate rarely occurs in the course of treatment of rheumatic fever. Occasionally, mental disorientation and delirium may be seen as a manifestation of salicylate toxicity. In practice, nausea and vomiting are the most frequent causes of difficulty in maintaining an adequate dosage of the drug. Although this toxic effect is not due solely to local action on the gastric mucosa, it is sometimes beneficial to use enteric-coated drug. In addition, better tolerance of the drug is established if the initial dosage is somewhat below the optimum and gradually increased over a period of a few days. The use of sodium bicarbonate is contraindicated because it reduces the efficiency of absorption of salicylate.

Hormonal Therapy. Ideal dosage schedules for the use of the hormone products in rheumatic fever have not yet been determined. The most generally accepted procedure at the present time is to begin with relatively large doses until the activity of the disease appears to be under control and then to reduce the dosage to the minimum amount which will maintain full effect. In the case of *corticotropin* the initial dose is 1 to 2 mg. per pound per day given intramuscularly in four equal doses at 6-hour intervals. The use of *cortisone* offers the advantage of oral administration of the drug. The initial dose is 2 to 4 mg. per pound per day divided in equal doses given at 4- or 6-hour intervals. With any of these hormones the amount of drug which is required for continued treatment once the desired effect has been obtained varies from case to case, and can only be determined empirically. Because of the unpleasant side effects associated with hyperadrenalism, however, it is important to use no more than the amount required to control the manifestations of the disease.

In two separate areas auxiliary therapy is required to counteract certain effects of the adrenal hormones unrelated to control of the rheumatic process. Because of the effect of the hormones on the salt and water balance of the body, a *low sodium* diet should be provided. This is of particular importance in the presence of extensive carditis when accumulation of fluid may increase the risk of cardiac failure. Secondly, since the hormones may completely suppress the overt manifestations of bacterial infections, it is important to give suitable *antimicrobial therapy* during long-continued hormone administration. Penicillin can be used for this purpose at dosage levels recommended for prophylaxis of streptococcal infections. Theoretically, one of the broad spectrum drugs such as the tetracyclines would provide protection against a wider variety of infections, but their effectiveness in patients receiving hormone therapy is less well established.

Other drugs, such as aminopyrine, hydroxyphenylcinchoninic acid and gentisate, have been employed for symptomatic control of rheumatic fever, but at the present time salicylates and the hormones appear to be the drugs of choice.

When cardiac failure supervenes in the course of acute rheumatic fever, the general measures employed for the treatment of congestive failure must be added to those for management of the acute disease. Digitalis should be administered according to the dosage schedule outlined in the chapter on valvular heart disease.

Duration of Therapy. The difficult problem of determining how long therapy should be maintained is the same regardless of the agent employed. Since the various changes in the blood revert to normal under suppressive therapy, there is no laboratory test which serves as a reliable guide to the persistence of the active rheumatic process. The best that can be done, once the general improvement of the patient suggests that recovery may have occurred, is to withdraw the therapeutic agent gradually and to observe carefully for the return of symptoms or signs of rheumatic fever. If unmistakable signs of severe activity reappear, there is no alternative but to reinstitute therapy. In this connection, it is important to differentiate between a true recrudescence of rheumatic activity and the so-called *rebound phenomenon.* The latter phenomenon occurs to some degree in a high percentage of patients upon withdrawal of therapy and is a self-limited episode characterized by the return of certain manifestations of the disease. Thus, there may be a change in the laboratory tests, specifically some elevation in the sedimentation rate and reappearance of C-reactive protein in the blood, and on some occasions symptoms such as low grade fever or arthralgia may occur.

Since these mild manifestations disappear spontaneously in one to three weeks, it is unnecessary to resume therapy. However, when unmistakable evidence of carditis recurs, it is not advisable to withhold treatment regardless of the mildness of the symptoms.

Prophylaxis. *Prevention of Recurrence in a Rheumatic Subject.* The prevention of recurrences of rheumatic fever depends on the prevention of streptococcal infections, and every rheumatic patient should receive continuous prophylactic therapy through the school age and for at least five years following the last attack of the disease. The most practical regimens involve the use of sulfadiazine or oral penicillin. The dose of sulfadiazine is 0.5 gm. for children under 60 pounds and 1.0 gm. for older children and adults, given once daily. Because of the more rapid elimination of penicillin, it is advisable to give this drug twice daily in doses of 100,000 to 2000,000 units. Penicillin should be given on an empty stomach, preferably before breakfast and at bedtime. With either of these drugs the patient must be kept under periodic observation for the possible occurrence of toxic reactions. Although adequate experience with the tetracyclines for prophylaxis has not yet been obtained, it appears possible that any one of this group (e.g., Aureomycin or Terramycin) in a single daily dose of 0.5 to 1.0 gm. might be effective.

Prevention of Rheumatic Fever in a Nonrheumatic Subject. In addition to this prophylactic effect of antimicrobial drugs, it has been shown that prompt and intensive penicillin treatment of established streptococcal infections greatly reduces the risk of the subsequent development of rheumatic fever (see chapter on Streptococcal Infections). This fact stresses the importance of accurate and early diagnosis of streptococcal disease in all patients regardless of whether there is previous history of rheumatic fever.

MACLYN McCARTY

References

Coburn, A. F.: The Factor of Infection in the Rheumatic State. Baltimore, Williams and Wilkins Co., 1931.
Lancefield, R. C.:: Specific Relationship of Cell Composition to Biological Activity of Hemolytic Streptococci. The Harvey Lectures. Lancaster, The Science Press Printing Co., Series 36:251, 1940–41.
McCarty, M.: Present State of Knowledge Concern-

ing Pathogenesis and Treatment of Rheumatic Fever. Bull. N. Y. Acad. Med., 28:307, 1952.

Paul, J. R.: The Epidemiology of Rheumatic Fever. 2nd ed. Metropolitan Life Insurance Co., 1943.

Swift, H. F.: The Etiology of Rheumatic Fever. Ann. Int. Med., 31:715, 1949.

Swift, H. F.: The Streptococci, in Dubos, R.: Bacterial and Mycotic Infections in Man. 2nd ed. Philadelphia, J. B. Lippincott Co., 1952, Chap. 11.

Thomas, L.: Rheumatic Fever, A Symposium. Minneapolis, University of Minnesota Press, 1952.

Wannamaker, L. W., and others: Prophylaxis of Acute Rheumatic Fever by Treatment of the Preceding Streptococcal Infection with Various Amounts of Depot Penicillin. Am. J. Med., 10: 673, 1951.

Wilson, M. G.: Rheumatic Fever. New York, The Commonwealth Fund, 1940.

STAPHYLOCOCCAL INFECTIONS

INTRODUCTION

Staphylococci are responsible for most suppurative infections of the skin and not infrequently cause infection of the lungs, bones, kidneys and other organs. Typically, such infections are associated with abscess formation.

Staphylococci may be divided into three species according to the color of pigment produced. Pigment production is best demonstrated in freshly isolated strains grown on solid medium at 22° C. *Staphylococcus aureus* is golden yellow, *S. albus* is white and *S. citreus* forms a lemon-yellow pigment. Strains of *S. aureus* are responsible for the majority of infections in man; *S. albus* may occasionally cause mild infections; *S. citreus* rarely infects man.

Staphylococcus aureus produces toxic substances with hemolytic, necrotizing, leukocytolytic and lethal properties. A small number of staphylococci produce an enterotoxin which is responsible for most cases of food poisoning. In addition they produce an enzyme, hyaluronidase or "spreading factor," which hydrolyzes hyaluronic acid. Although antiserums to some of these toxic substances have been prepared, they have not proved especially useful in the treatment of infections in man.

Pathogenic strains of staphylococci may be recognized by several methods. Most strains isolated from infections ferment mannite. By means of acid extraction Julianelle has isolated two polysaccharides from staphylococci and has demonstrated that pathogenic strains contain type A polysaccharide and nonpathogens, type B. Antiserums to type A staphylococci have been prepared, but have failed to alter the natural course of infections in man appreciably. The pathogenic strain, type A, may be recognized by precipitation tests using the specific carbohydrate and antiserum. Another characteristic of pathogenic strains is their ability to grow in human whole blood, whereas nonpathogenic strains are easily killed in the bactericidal test.

The ability of certain staphylococci to coagulate plasma has long been recognized and used as a laboratory test for pathogenicity. Recently the mechanism of this reaction has been elucidated. Staphylococcal coagulase reacts in some way with a factor (reacting factor) present in blood to produce a clotting substance. Coagulase is antigenic, and after infection an antibody develops which inhibits the coagulase reaction. In order to demonstrate such antibodies, the specific coagulase produced by the infecting strain must be utilized.

Pathogenesis. Invasion of the tissues by pathogenic staphylococci follows a rather characteristic course. The organism multiplies locally and is probably facilitated in its spread by the production of hyaluronidase, which increases the permeability of the connective tissues. The organism may be protected from the phagocytic cells by the deposition of a thin barrier of fibrin at its periphery through the production of coagulase. The organisms multiply locally and produce toxins and more coagulase. Presumably coagulase diffuses into the surrounding tissues and accounts for local thrombosis in the blood vessels. The toxins meanwhile cause marked inflammatory changes in the tissues, and necrosis occurs centrally. Eventually the abscess ruptures and repair of the tissues begins. Occasionally, when the organism is especially virulent, the local barriers break down and bacteremia becomes evident. Certain animals, notably birds, do not develop abscesses when pathogenic strains of staphylococci are injected. This may be due to the fact that coagulase fails to act on plasma of birds because of an apparent deficiency in the amount of reacting factor in the blood.

Epidemiology. By means of bacteriophage

typing the epidemiology of staphylococcal infections has been clarified to some extent. It has long been recognized that staphylococci may be cultivated from various parts of the body. More than half of the population carry *Staphylococcus aureus* in the nasal secretions, and most persons harbor the same organism on the skin. Nasal carriers are especially likely to be skin carriers. The fact that the bacteriophage type of the organisms isolated from the nose and skin of one person is the same, suggests a common source. Apparently the skin is being continuously contaminated by the nasal secretions. Staphylococci are most frequently found on the back of the hands, over the forearm, and back of the neck, and somewhat less commonly along the midline of the body and in the inguinal folds.

Treatment. Certain general principles should be followed in the treatment of all staphylococcal infections. Of primary importance is the surgical drainage of abscesses, since the available antistaphylococcal drugs are markedly reduced in effectiveness in the presence of pus. Before the days of antimicrobial therapy patients with bacteremia were occasionally cured by the drainage of an abscess.

In general, the drugs useful in the treatment of staphylococcal infections include penicillin, erythromycin, bacitracin, the tetracyclines, chloramphenicol and streptomycin. Treatment must be prolonged since the organisms are killed slowly. This is in striking contrast to the rapid bactericidal action of certain of these drugs, notably penicillin, on pneumococci or group A streptococci. It is difficult, if not impossible, to recommend a single therapeutic regimen for all staphylococcal infections. This is due to the fact that the susceptibility of the various strains of staphylococci to each antimicrobial drug appears to be changing rapidly. Indeed, the drug of choice in certain geographic areas may be relatively ineffective in others. Furthermore, the nature and location of the infection also alters the method of treatment. Sufficient data are not available to allow critical evaluation of the use of combinations of antimicrobial drugs in the treatment of staphylococcal infections.

Drug-susceptibility tests of the infecting strain of staphylococcus are invaluable in guidance of therapy. In areas where such tests cannot be obtained, either penicillin, streptomycin with penicillin, or erythromycin should be administered in full dosage, and if a favorable response is not observed after a few days, therapy should be altered. In severe infections initial therapy should include penicillin or erythromycin in combination with either streptomycin or bacitracin. The latter drug should be given in doses of 15,000 to 20,000 units four times daily and should not be employed if there are signs of renal failure. The choice of drug or combination of drugs after the first few days of treatment should be governed by the results of the drug-susceptibility studies of the strain of staphylococcus involved.

CHARLES H. RAMMELKAMP, JR.

FURUNCLES AND CARBUNCLES

Definition. A *furuncle* or boil is a circumscribed, suppurative, inflammatory lesion of the skin and the immediate subcutaneous tissues. A *carbuncle,* which may be considered a furuncle with multiple foci, develops when a suppurative infection occurs in thick inelastic skin and extends into the deeper layers of fibrous tissue.

Etiology. Furuncles and carbuncles are most commonly caused by *Staphylococcus aureus.*

Symptoms. Although furuncles occur in any location, they are especially prone to occur on the face, neck, forearms, axillae, midline and upper part of the back, breasts, groins and legs. Carbuncles are essentially limited to the nape of the neck and back.

Careful observation will show that most of these infections begin with a small pustule at the base of a hair follicle. At this stage there is no pain, perhaps only an itching sensation. Within a few hours swelling and redness occur, and some pain is experienced. Gradually, over a period of three to five days, the boil becomes elevated, the involved area is exquisitely tender, and movement of the involved part causes pain. At the apex of the swelling the skin glistens and becomes thinned, and a yellow spot appears. The boil is now said to be "pointing" and shortly will drain spontaneously. The pus is creamy yellow in color, and at the center of the boil a hard core may be evident.

At the time of rupture of the abscess, pain is relieved almost immediately. The abscess continues to drain a serosanguineous fluid, swelling decreases, and within a few hours to days the discharge ceases. Redness may persist for several days or weeks, but eventually all signs of the abscess disappear.

Although this description applies to the majority of boils, certain features of these infections deserve emphasis. Infections of the hair follicles which never involve the surrounding tissues are known as simple *folliculitis*. They are apt to occur in persons who are in constant contact with oil, grease and other skin irritants. People with prominent sebaceous glands are prone to suffer staphylococcal infection which the dermatologists designate as *pustular acne vulgaris*. These infections are seen over the face and the upper part of the back.

Furuncles occasionally occur in the axilla, but most infections in this region arise in the sweat glands; hence the name *hidradenitis*. These infections start as small inflammatory nodules which cause considerable discomfort. When the abscess discharges, the organisms invade other sweat glands and hair follicles with subsequent scarring of the tissues.

A single boil may be followed by multiple infections of the surrounding skin, i.e., *furunculosis*. The secondary infections are due to the purulent discharge from the abscess invading other hair follicles in the adjacent skin. Boils around the nose and lips are especially dangerous, since local trauma may result in the invasion of the venous sinuses within the skull.

Characteristically, the *carbuncle* occurs at the nape of the neck and begins with infection of one or, usually, several hair follicles. As a result, the area of swelling and redness is wide and the surface is covered with multiple pustules. As the infection spreads, the center becomes a grayish-yellow crater with ragged edges. Most carbuncles are extremely painful, although occasionally they cause little discomfort. The patient's head is usually held rigidly. Older persons may be critically ill, and bacteremia is common.

Diagnosis. Simple *folliculitis* is frequently caused by *Staphylococcus albus* and is easily recognized because of the lack of redness and induration around the hair follicle. *Pustular acne vulgaris* is always associated with an oily skin. Most furuncles are not associated with a constitutional reaction, whereas a person with a carbuncle frequently has fever and leukocytosis. Cultures of the boil or carbuncle show coagulase-positive *S. aureus*. Since diabetics are subject to carbuncles and boils, the urine should be examined for sugar in all patients with these infections.

Treatment. When a furuncle or carbuncle is observed before there are signs of abscess formation, the daily intramuscular injection of 600,000 units of procaine penicillin and/or the administration of 0.5 gm. of erythromycin every six hours may abort the process. Usually treatment must be given for at least one week. In the presence of fever a blood culture should be obtained and the dose of penicillin increased. The application of hot packs to the infected area may relieve pain and aid in the localization of the infection. In all severe infections the involved part should be immobilized and the patient kept in bed.

In well localized abscesses the cavity should be drained and antimicrobial therapy continued until signs of inflammation have disappeared. Moist dressings should not be applied to the skin after the abscess drains, since moisture tends to macerate the skin and facilitates the implantation of organisms. The skin around draining sinuses should be protected by a thick layer of penicillin or tyrothricin cream.

The prevention of furuncles or carbuncles is difficult, probably because the skin is being continuously contaminated via the hands with virulent staphylococci from the nasal secretions. The patient should be cautioned not to traumatize the skin, and to avoid oils, dirt and other skin irritants, and to use mild soaps and cool water when washing. Such procedures decrease the opportunity for invasion of hair follicles and sebaceous or sweat glands. When infections recur frequently, the daily application of tyrothricin cream is recommended. Such advice is especially indicated in diabetic patients, since recurrent boils are common.

CHARLES H. RAMMELKAMP, JR.

STAPHYLOCOCCAL PNEUMONIA

Definition. Pneumonia caused by *Staphylococcus aureus* is characterized by abscess formation.

Etiology. Staphylococcal pneumonia is relatively rare except during periods when there are epidemics of influenza, measles or whooping cough. The exact cause for this relationship is unknown. Both in the primary form and in pneumonia secondary to other respiratory infections, staphylococci probably invade the parenchyma of the lung through the bronchial and bronchiolar walls. Isolated areas of pneumonia with abscess formation are a common complication of staphylococcal bacteremia. *Cystic disease of the pancreas* is often complicated by chronic staphylococcal infections of the lung.

Morbid Anatomy. The mucosa of the trachea and bronchi is ulcerated and intensely inflamed, and is covered with thick, purulent secretions. Around the bronchi the alveoli are filled with an inflammatory exudate containing blood and fibrin. Multiple small abscess pockets are observed, some communicating with bronchi. Necrosis of the lung parenchyma is prominent.

Symptoms. Staphylococcal pneumonia is usually preceded by a respiratory infection, the symptoms of which may include sore throat, cough or generalized malaise and fever. After a variable period of one to several days the patient suddenly becomes quite ill. The temperature increases; there may be a rigor; and the cough becomes aggravated and productive of purulent sputum. At times the sputum may be streaked with blood or is brownish or yellowish in color. Pleuritic pain is common.

In some patients the course of the disease may be rapidly fatal, with a sudden onset, prostration, a peculiar reddish-blue cyanosis, rapid respirations and high fever. In others the disease appears to be more chronic, with remittent fever but moderately rapid pulse.

The physical signs in patients with staphylococcal pneumonia are not characteristic, but are variable. Early, there may be no change in the percussion note; later, dullness to percussion is exhibited. Rales, both coarse and fine, may be elicited over the involved area of the lung. Since pleural effusion and empyema are common, dullness and other signs of fluid may be found.

The leukocyte count is elevated to between 15,000 and 25,000 per cubic millimeter; rarely is it low or normal. Roentgenograms of the chest show one or more areas of consolidation near the hilum of the lung. Later, cavities may develop, and their fluid levels can be easily demonstrated in the roentgenogram. Pleural fluid is common.

Diagnosis. Cyanosis, remittent fever and purulent sputum should lead one to suspect staphylococcal pneumonia. The diagnosis is dependent on the isolation of *S. aureus* in relatively pure culture from the sputum. The development of empyema, from the fluid of which staphylococci may be cultured, aids in the establishment of the diagnosis. Abscess formation, as shown by the roentgenogram, is characteristic. The blood culture, which should be made in each case, is usually sterile. When bacteremia is present, the pneumonia may be secondary to a focus elsewhere in the body.

Differential Diagnosis. One must consider all other forms of bacterial pneumonia and primary atypical pneumonia in the differential diagnosis. Abscess formation is most apt to occur in staphylococcal, streptococcal and Friedländer's bacillus pneumonia. Pneumonia caused by the Friedländer bacillus is confused with staphylococcal pneumonia because of the remittent character of the temperature. Careful culture of the sputum is the only method of establishing the diagnosis.

Prognosis. Most patients recover from staphylococcal pneumonia, but a few succumb. The illness in those who recover usually lasts three or four weeks, and recovery is gradual.

Treatment. As in all severe infections, the staphylococcus isolated from the patient should be tested for susceptibility to the various antimicrobial drugs. If the organism is susceptible to penicillin, 2 to 4 million units should be administered in divided doses every four hours. It is also advisable to administer streptomycin. Bacitracin or erythromycin may be substituted for streptomycin if the organism is susceptible to one or another of these drugs. Treatment should be maintained for at least one week after the temperature returns to normal. As in other staphylococcal infections, the temperature falls slowly after institution of specific therapy. Empyema should be treated early by the intrapleural injection of 50,000 to 100,000 units of penicillin every 24 to 48 hours. The intrapleural instillation of the enzymes streptokinase and streptodornase is advisable, as discussed in a later chapter on Empyema. If the intrapleural fluid is thick, surgical drainage may be required in addition to penicillin therapy.

The subject of staphylococcal pneumonia is also discussed in the section on Bacterial Pneumonia (p. 146).

CHARLES H. RAMMELKAMP, JR.

OSTEOMYELITIS

Definition. Osteomyelitis is an infection of the bone most frequently caused by *Staphylococcus aureus*.

Etiology. Staphylococci reach the bone after invasion of the blood stream. The usual focus is a wound, furuncle or other external infection. The initial, acute infection is practically confined to children and is more frequent in boys than in girls. The usual explanation for localization in the bone is the fact that the diaphysis of the child gets its blood supply through terminal capillary loops. The bacteria tend to settle out in this area. The fact that the blood of the young child contains little coagulase-reacting factor as compared to that of the adult may possibly account for the initial blood stream invasion in the younger age groups.

Pathogenesis and Morbid Anatomy. The staphylococci set up an acute inflammatory reaction with necrosis of the bone. The initial infection occurs at the diaphysis and seldom crosses the epiphysis; instead, as the infection progresses, the pus emerges to the surface of the bone, raising the periosteum. Although purulent material is present at an early stage, the bone is not destroyed immediately. As the bone dies, *sequestra* are formed. Repair begins after drainage of the abscess; small sequestra may be absorbed, and new bone is laid down by the osteoblasts forming the *involucrum*. Not infrequently a chronic infection of the bone is established which intermittently results in an acute inflammatory process.

Symptoms. Acute osteomyelitis is usually ushered in by fever, chills, pain and, in the very young patient, by nausea and vomiting. Careful examination may reveal a recently healed wound, pustule or furuncle. Pain over the bone may be the only early sign of localization of the infection. Tapping on the bone may cause pain referred to the involved area. Pain sometimes skips around to various bones before it finally localizes. Muscle spasm around the involved bone is a common and frequently early sign of osteomyelitis. At this stage of the disease, roentgenograms of the bone reveal no abnormality.

As the infection progresses, redness and swelling occur over the involved bone. The patient splints the limb or affected part, for movement causes pain. When the infection is near a joint, swelling of the periarticular tissues occurs and effusion into the joint is common. The temperature is likely to be high and the patient critically ill. By ten days to two weeks after the onset the roentgenogram may show some rarefaction of the bone. Subsequently, periosteal reaction is exhibited by new bone formation. As the bone dies, dead bone or sequestrum may be observed in the roentgenogram.

Chronic osteomyelitis is especially likely to occur if sequestra remain unabsorbed, or if adequate drainage is not established. Repeated attacks of acute osteomyelitis with the establishment of chronic draining sinuses characterize this phase of the disease. Amyloidosis is a complication of the prolonged suppurative process.

Diagnosis. During the first few days of the disease the history of fever, chills, and pain over long bones is enough to suggest the diagnosis of acute osteomyelitis. There is usually a leukocytosis of 20,000 or more cells per cubic millimeter, and the blood culture frequently shows *Staphylococcus aureus*. As the disease progresses, anemia develops. After ten days the roentgenogram exhibits diagnostic abnormalities, such as periosteal new bone formation and sequestra.

Acute osteomyelitis must be differentiated from other bacterial infections and erythema nodosum. Usually the diagnosis is not difficult. A serious error can be made, however, if a patient with acute osteomyelitis is mistakenly considered to be suffering from *acute rheumatic fever*. A history of recent furunculosis with or without trauma, the usual monoarticular involvement, the degree of leukocytosis (20,000 or more cells per cubic millimeter), the response to penicillin, and, in some cases, the demonstration of staphylococcemia, all serve to establish the presence of acute osteomyelitis. This question of the differences between rheumatic fever and osteomyelitis is also discussed in the chapter on Rheumatic Fever (p. 174).

Treatment and Prognosis. Before the introduction of penicillin the case fatality rate for patients with acute osteomyelitis was about 15 per cent in the absence of bacteremia, and 25 to 50 per cent in the presence of bacteremia. If the patients survived the initial infection, a chronic infection was usually established and metastatic foci in other bones were common. Today, death from acute osteomyelitis is rare and chronic osteomyelitis is uncommon.

Acute Osteomyelitis. In order to avoid surgical intervention, early treatment of acute osteomyelitis is required. For this reason it is advisable not to wait for bacteriologic or roentgenographic confirmation of the diagnosis before starting antimicrobial therapy. Penicillin is instituted in doses of at least 200,-000 units intramuscularly every three hours throughout the entire 24-hour period. It is also advisable to administer 2 or 3 gm. of erythromycin in divided doses each day. Bacitracin may likewise prove beneficial in those patients with normal kidney function. Doses of 15,000 units every four hours are well tolerated. Every effort should be made to isolate the infecting organism so that therapy may be altered according to the results of sensitivity tests. Treatment is continued for a minimum period of three weeks. During the later period of therapy, procaine penicillin may be substituted for the sodium salt in dosages of 600,000 units daily. Such therapy, instituted within four days of onset, usually results in the subsidence of signs of inflammation within two to four days, and minimal or no damage to the bone can be demonstrated in the roentgenogram. In those patients whose disease has been present for four days or longer, localized abscesses may form and damage to the bone is more extensive. Small sequestra usually absorb, but larger pieces of dead bone may require removal. In addition to these measures, the fluid balance is to be maintained, and anemia corrected by transfusion.

Chronic Osteomyelitis. The treatment of chronic osteomyelitis usually requires sequestrectomy, saucerization of the infected bone and removal of the sinus tract. The antimicrobial drugs, in the amounts already indicated, should be administered before and after operation. In a few patients intensive penicillin treatment alone results in eradication of the disease.

CHARLES H. RAMMELKAMP, JR.

STAPHYLOCOCCAL BACTEREMIA

Pathogenesis. Staphylococci may invade the blood stream from abscesses in any location. The studies of Skinner and Keefer have demonstrated that infections of the skin account for the primary focus in about 40 per cent of the cases. Infections of the bone and respiratory tract account for another 40 per cent, and in the remainder the bacteria are fed into the blood stream from the genitourinary tract or from an unknown focus.

Factors which contribute to the frequency of blood stream invasion are trauma and the presence of debilitating disease. Early incision of an abscess or attempts to evacuate the pus by squeezing may result in bacteremia. Such procedures are especially dangerous when the boil is located about the face. Bacteremia occurs frequently in patients with diabetes, arteriolosclerosis, cancer and other debilitating diseases. Virulent staphylococci are more likely to produce a fatal bacteremia than nonvirulent organisms belonging to the coagulase-negative group. Fortunately, bacteremia following infections of the skin is rare. In 11,568 patients seen with carbuncles and furuncles, Sutherland observed only 7 instances of bacteremia.

Symptoms. Typically, the patient has chills and fever after invasion of the blood from a boil or carbuncle. The fever may be high and remittent in type or, less frequently, intermittent. In a few cases the fever is low and continuous. Rigor is observed in about 25 per cent of patients. Marked perspiration is common. Complaints such as headache and malaise are frequent, but not characteristic of the disease.

One of the characteristic features of *Staphylococcus aureus* bacteremia is the production of metastatic abscesses, whereas *S. albus* does not produce such lesions. Patients who survive *S. aureus* bacteremia more than a few days get abscesses. The most frequent sites of these metastatic abscesses are the skin, subcutaneous tissues and the lungs.

Infection of the lung is a common complication of staphylococcal bacteremia. For this reason every effort should be made to locate the portal of entry of the staphylococcus in patients with pneumonia and a positive blood culture. It will be recalled that primary staphylococcal pneumonia is not commonly associated with bacteremia.

Superficial abscesses of the skin, joints and muscles account for 30 per cent of the metastatic complications. Petechiae and purpura are occasionally seen. Internal abscesses of the kidneys, brain and spinal cord are not uncommon.

Infection of the pleural, peritoneal and pericardial cavities occurs in less than 10 per cent of cases. Sinus thrombosis and meningitis are rare and usually occur as the result of direct extension of the infection. Endocarditis should be suspected when there are cardiac murmurs which change in character or whenever bacteremia persists in the absence of an obvious extracardiac focus.

Diagnosis and Prognosis. The history of a preceding staphylococcal infection in a patient with intermittent fever should suggest the diagnosis of staphylococcal bacteremia. The finding of multiple peripheral abscesses also suggests such a diagnosis. Most patients exhibit a high leukocyte count and anemia. The diagnosis is established by the isolation of the organism from the blood stream.

Before the introduction of modern chemotherapy the case fatality rate was 80 per cent.

Treatment. The therapy of staphylococcal bacteremia is still unsatisfactory. Every effort should be made to drain all abscesses promptly and treatment should be guided by drug-susceptibility tests. In general, combinations of drugs are usually employed. The compounds most frequently used are penicillin, erythromycin and bacitracin. The tetracycline drugs or chloramphenicol are given if the organism is susceptible to their action. Each drug should be given in the maximum dose that can be tolerated. In patients with anemia blood transfusions should be given.

CHARLES H. RAMMELKAMP, JR.

References

Finland, M., Peterson, O. L., and Strauss, E.: Staphylococcic Pneumonia Occurring During an Epidemic of Influenza. Arch. Int. Med., 70:183, 1942.
Herrell, W. E., Nichols, D. R., and Martin, W. J.: Erthromycin for Infections Due to Micrococcus Pyogenes. J.A.M.A., 152:1601, 1953.
Price, R. B.: Cause and Treatment of Furunculosis. J.A.M.A., 124:1189, 1944.
Rammelkamp, C. H., Jr., Hezebicks, M. M., and Dingle, J. H.: Specific Coagulases of Staphylococcus Aureus. J. Exper. Med., 91:295, 1950.
Skinner, D., and Keefer, C. S.: Significance of Bacteremia Caused by Staphylococcus Aureus. A Study of One Hundred and Twenty-two Cases and a Review of the Literature Concerned with Experimental Infection in Animals. Arch. Int. Med., 68:851, 1941.
Smith, W., and Hale, J. H.: The Influence of Coagulase on the Phagocytosis of Staphylococci. Brit. J. Exper. Path., 26:209, 1945.
Sutherland, R. T.: Staphylococcic Septicemia. Arch. Int. Med., 66:1, 1940.
Williams, R. E. O.: Skin and Nose Carriage of Bacteriophage Types of Staphylococcal Aureus. J. Path. and Bact., 58:259, 1946.

GONOCOCCAL INFECTIONS

Definition. Gonorrhea, commonest of the venereal diseases, is the principal infection caused by the gonococcus (*Neisseria gonorrhoeae*). From the primary focus in the genital tract, the organism may spread to involve other parts of the body, particularly synovial tissues and serosal surfaces, causing a variety of clinical entities such as arthritis, endocarditis and meningitis. Formerly common and important, extragenital infections with the gonococcus have become rare since the advent of penicillin.

Etiology and Bacteriology. As seen in smears of purulent exudates the gonococcus is a gram-negative, kidney-shaped diplococcus, often located within the cytoplasm of polymorphonuclear leukocytes. This characteristic appearance was first observed in urethral pus by Neisser in 1897. In cultures, single cells tend to predominate and the flattening of one surface of the oval coccus is often absent.

Primary cultivation of the gonococcus is difficult because of its fastidious growth requirements and its susceptibility to toxic substances often present in culture media. Blood is commonly used for enrichment, and the deleterious effects of certain amino acids are reduced by heating the medium after the blood is added (chocolate agar). Toxic materials present in agar can be neutralized by the addition of starch or charcoal. Dyes such as Nile blue inhibit the growth of contaminating bacteria but do not affect the growth of the gonococcus. Media are commercially available which take advantage of all the known facts concerning growth requirements, so that routine cultural techniques are now quite simple. The results still leave much to be desired, however, since the reproducibility in different laboratories using the same cultural techniques is not greater than 75 per cent. The growth of most strains is enhanced by incubating the cultures in an atmosphere containing 2 to 10 per cent carbon dioxide.

Colonies of N. gonorrhoeae are gray and translucent, and their recognition is aided by performing the oxidase test. A 1 per cent solution of p-aminodimethylaniline monohydrochloride is poured over the surface of the agar plate, and within a few minutes colonies of the gonococcus turn pink, then purple. A positive test occurs with all members of the genus *Neisseria,* and occasionally with certain other bacteria. With cultures from the genital tract a positive oxidase reaction, together with characteristic colonial morphology and the presence of gram-negative diplococci, constitutes presumptive evidence that the organism is a gonococcus. However, since saprophytic *Neisseria* and other bacteria are known to produce false-positive results, particularly in women, confirmatory fermentation reactions with glucose, maltose and sucrose should always be performed. Carbohydrate reactions are also used to differentiate gonococci from meningococci when positive cultures are obtained from blood, cerebrospinal or joint fluid. Meningococci ferment both dextrose and maltose, while the gonococcus gives a positive reaction only with dextrose. Differentiation can also be accomplished by agglutination tests.

Since the gonococcus is quickly killed by drying, exudates from the genital tract should be cultured directly on agar plates, or the swab should be placed in a small amount of broth while it is transported to the laboratory. Urine should be centrifuged and the sediment inoculated on the culture plate. With cerebrospinal fluid, blood and synovial fluid, in which the number of organisms may be small and contaminating bacteria are usually not present, the best results are often obtained by culturing the specimens in shallow layers of broth enriched with plasma or ascitic fluid, using an increased tension of carbon dioxide.

Epidemiology and Pathogenesis. Gonorrhea is world-wide in distribution, and all races appear to be equally susceptible. There is considerable individual variation in resistance to infection, however, the nature of which is not known. Even when massive numbers of gonococci are instilled directly into the urethral canal, less than half the males so inoculated contract the disease. Similarly, the relatively low incidence of infection among professional prostitutes is probably an expression of natural resistance.

Accurate information concerning the incidence of gonorrhea is difficult to obtain, since reporting is poor, and penicillin is so easily obtainable that many cases are treated by persons other than physicians. The evidence available indicates that there probably has been a marked decline in the total number of infections since 1945. The disease is still widespread, however, and is prevalent chiefly among lower income groups. The incidence of syphilis appears to have declined more rapidly, partly because gonorrhea seems to be more easily acquired as a result of a single exposure to both infections simultaneously. Moreover, the lack of immunity following a gonococcal infection makes it possible for an individual to have a number of attacks. Analysis of such "repeaters" indicates that in most instances they are either indifferent or are unable to comprehend the facts of prevention and treatment. Transmission of gonorrhea by asymptomatic carriers also tends to propagate the disease. This problem is aggravated by the difficulty of detecting the carrier state, especially in women.

The resistance of stratified squamous epithelium to infection by the gonococcus explains the lack of lesions on the external genitalia of both sexes, and in the vagina. The susceptibility of columnar epithelium permits infection of the urethra, prostate, seminal vesicles, epididymis and glands associated with these structures in the male. In women, infection occurs chiefly in the urethra, Skene's and Bartholin's glands, endocervix and Fallopian tubes. Once established, the infection tends to persist for weeks or months in the genital tract unless treatment is given. This tendency towards chronicity was one of the factors chiefly responsible for the spread of the disease before effective chemotherapy became available. Persistence of the infection is associated with tissue destruction and abscess formation, leading to urethral strictures in the male, and chronic inflammation and sterility in the female. In a small percentage of cases the organisms find their way into the blood stream and set up metastatic foci in distant organs such as the joints and endocardium.

Nonvenereal transmission of infection by the gonococcus occurs rarely if at all. Instillation of penicillin or silver compounds into the eyes of newborn babies has virtually eliminated ophthalmia neonatorum, formerly an important cause of blindness. Epidemics of vulvovaginitis in young girls were once thought to be neisserian in nature, and to be transmitted by bedclothes and towels. It is now realized, however, that in most instances the gonococcus is not the causative agent, and when it is, sexual contact has occurred.

Symptoms and Signs. From two days to two weeks following sexual exposure, burning on urination is the first symptom of gonorrhea usually noted in the *male,* and is followed by the appearance of a purulent urethral discharge. The infection tends to spread posteriorly and involvement of the posterior urethra is indicated by cloudiness in the second glass of voided urine. Urinary retention may occur if the prostate is involved, and infection of the seminal vesicles usually causes fever and pain which may radiate to various parts of the pelvis. Acute epididymitis is associated with severe pain and tenderness, and the testicle may become swollen. Involvement of the epididymis is a serious complication which often leads to sterility. Following treatment the signs and symptoms gradually subside, but a slight mucoid discharge may persist for several weeks.

In the *female* painful urination and vaginal discharge are the commonest early symptoms. Involvement of Skene's or Bartholin's glands is usually indicated by reddening at the orifices, but may lead to the formation of large, painful abscesses. The notion that most Bartholin gland abscesses are gonococcal in origin has been disproved; in most instances they are caused by other organisms such as streptococci. Lower abdominal pain characteristically appears when the infection spreads from the cervix into the Fallopian tubes. The symptoms of acute salpingitis often appear quite abruptly, and must be differentiated from those of appendicitis, pyelonephritis and ectopic pregnancy. Acute pelvic inflammatory disease is readily diagnosed when there is a history of recent sexual exposure, tender adnexal masses are present bilaterally, and gonococci can be demonstrated on cervical smears. These aids are often not present, however, and differentiation of this condition from other causes of lower abdominal pain may be very difficult. Surgical exploration is sometimes necessary to exclude conditions which require surgical management. Salpingitis tends to recur, causing fibrosis and destruction of the pelvic structures. Abscesses form, and pain and fever are present intermittently. The patient is usually sterile, and surgical removal of all the pelvic organs may eventually be necessary.

Complications. The establishment of metastatic foci secondary to invasion of the blood stream by gonococci is relatively uncommon at the present time. Awareness that it can occur is important, however, since prompt recognition and adequate therapy often lead to complete recovery. Transient bacteremia may occur without causing symptoms, or there may be a shaking chill followed by a silent period prior to the appearance of symptoms caused by metastatic lesions. Occasionally, gonococci may invade the blood stream repeatedly over a period of weeks or months causing fever, chills, arthralgia and a variable skin rash. This syndrome of *gonococcemia* is difficult to differentiate clinically from the commoner entity of *meningococcemia.* Rarely *endocarditis* occurs, and runs the malignant course characteristic of acute rather than subacute bacterial endocarditis. In most cases there is no pre-existing valvular damage. The aortic valves are the commonest site, but next in order of frequency are the valves of the right side of the heart. It is often difficult to obtain positive blood cultures, and too few proved cases have been reported in the past decade to assess accurately the results of penicillin therapy.

Arthritis is the commonest extragenital complication of gonorrhea. Formerly a common and crippling disease, this condition is now so rare that only a few cases are seen each year even in the larger city hospitals. Arthritis occurred in 3 to 5 per cent of patients with gonorrhea in the pre-penicillin days, but the incidence is now probably not greater than one-tenth of one per cent. The onset is usually sudden, consisting of an acute migratory polyarthritis, which occurs from one to four weeks following the initial infection. The knees, wrists and ankles are most commonly affected, but any of the joints in the arms and legs may be involved. Rarely, the infection may be limited to one of the less commonly involved joints such as the sternoclavicular or temporomandibular. Tenosynovitis occurs more frequently than in any other type of arthritis, and is present usually about the wrists, hands and feet.

The course of gonococcal arthritis is extremely variable. Thin serous fluid may accumulate in several joints, and in these cases it is often difficult to demonstrate bacteria in the joint fluid. There is usually a prompt response to penicillin therapy, however, and complete recovery occurs within a few weeks. In other instances the arthritis becomes monarticular after several days, and the joint fluid is then more likely to be purulent and to contain gonococci which are demonstrable sometimes on smear but more often by culture. Prognosis in this type of case is likely to be poor, particularly when treatment is delayed. Return of function to normal is unusual, and limitation of motion, which may progress to bony ankylosis, is common especially when the wrist and hand joints are involved. Finally, there is a group of patients in whom the onset and clinical course are indistinguishable from that of rheumatoid arthritis. The gonococcal infection may provide a "trigger mechanism" for the initiation of this disease. However, some authorities have elicited histories of previous attacks on careful questioning, and feel that the gonococcal infection is usually an incidental occurrence in rheumatoid subjects.

Differentiation of gonococcal arthritis from rheumatoid arthritis and acute rheumatic fever is in many instances very difficult. A clear-cut history of gonorrhea may be unobtainable, and it is often impossible to culture gonococci either from the genital tract or the joint fluid. The gonococcal *complement fixation test* is helpful in some cases, particularly when it is negative initially and there is a rising antibody titer after several weeks. This test, which requires carefully prepared and standardized reagents, is not performed in the ordinary laboratory but is available through most state laboratories. *Reiter's disease,* characterized by urethritis, arthritis and conjunctivitis, also offers serious diagnostic difficulties, especially since a catarrhal form of conjunctivitis occurs in 10 per cent of patients with gonococcal arthritis. Penicillin reactions and gout are other disorders which can cause confusion. Since a precise diagnosis is often impossible during the early stages, therapy must be started empirically, and the response to salicylates or to penicillin is often helpful in establishing the true cause.

Other complications, such as meningitis, myelitis, liver abscesses and keratodermia blennorrhagica, are now so rare that they have become medical curiosities.

Diagnosis. Gonococcal urethritis is readily diagnosed in both sexes when the typical clinical picture is present and gram-negative intracellular diplococci are seen on smears of the urethral discharge. Symptoms are sometimes mild and transient in the male, however, and endocervicitis may pass unnoticed in the female. Unfortunately, there is no reliable method available, especially in females, for detecting the carrier state. Negative cultures do not provide adequate evidence that an individual is unable to transmit the disease. Aside from genital infections, the main problems in diagnosis occur with

arthritis and salpingitis, and the salient differential features have been covered in the preceding section.

Treatment and Prognosis. Penicillin is the drug of choice for the treatment of gonococcal infections. In gonococcal *urethritis* a single intramuscular injection of 600,000 units of procaine penicillin will cure over 95 per cent of cases in both males and females. This dose is also adequate to abort syphilis. Longer acting forms of penicillin, either the aluminum monostearate form of procaine penicillin or the newer dibenzylethylenediamine dipenicillin G, may also be used in the same dosage. The more prolonged drug concentrations in the blood produced by these preparations are theoretically advantageous, although their superiority in the treatment of acute gonorrhea and in the prevention of syphilis has not been clearly demonstrated. Cultures should be performed at weekly intervals for three or four weeks, and if these are negative the patient can be considered cured. It is common, especially in males, to have a slight mucoid urethral discharge for weeks or months, even when the cultures are negative. This is regarded by some authorities as a nonspecific form of urethritis which is acquired at the same time as the gonococcal infection, and it is said to respond to therapy with oxytetracycline. Until this view is better substantiated it is probably best to regard the persistent discharge as a manifestation of subsiding inflammation which usually disappears spontaneously and requires no therapy. Retreatment is indicated in the small number of patients whose cultures remain positive. Treatment failures are not due to the development of penicillin-resistant gonococci, and few if any cases fail to respond to a second course of therapy consisting of two to four daily injections. To be certain that the therapy has been effective in preventing syphilis, serologic tests should be performed for four months.

If the prostate, seminal vesicles or epididymis is involved the patient should be put to bed, and should receive 600,000 units of procaine penicillin two or three times daily for one or two weeks. When abscesses form in the prostate or epididymis or there is a failure to respond to penicillin after two or three weeks, surgery may be indicated. The same general principles are applicable in the management of acute *salpingitis.* There is usually a prompt response to penicillin, with subsidence of pain and a return of the temperature to normal within 48 hours. Except for the drainage of abscesses, surgery is not indicated in the acute stage. Resection of infected tissues including all pelvic organs is performed in chronic cases only when there is failure to respond to conservative management over a period of eight to twelve months. Penicillin, either crystalline or procaine, is often administered in doses much larger than those specified. In the opinion of the writer, this is rarely necessary. For patients who cannot be treated with penicillin because of sensitivity reactions, tetracycline or one of its derivatives is effective. Two grams (0.5 gm. every 6 hours by mouth) is adequate for uncomplicated gonorrhea, and the same dosage may be continued for one or two weeks when complications are present.

Gonococcal *arthritis* usually responds well to rest and penicillin if treatment is started early, before the joint fluid becomes thick and purulent and tissue destruction has occurred. Because of the diffusibility of penicillin, it is not necessary to inject the drug into the joint cavity. The involved joints should be kept in good position but prolonged immobilization is rarely indicated. The temperature usually remains elevated for seven to ten days, but pain may persist for several weeks. Penicillin should be administered for about two weeks in most cases. Occasionally thick pus persists despite intensive therapy, and surgical drainage may be necessary. Physical therapy is a valuable adjunct in promoting return of function in the convalescent stage. Failure to respond to penicillin is often helpful from a diagnostic standpoint for, as has been pointed out, the differentiation of gonococcal arthritis from other forms of acute arthritis is often difficult. Large doses of crystalline penicillin G (5 to 10 million units daily) should be used in the treatment of gonococcal *endocarditis* and *meningitis*.

Prevention. Programs of case finding and education have not been very successful. Gonorrhea can be prevented by ingesting a single penicillin tablet (250,000 units) within 3 or 4 hours after exposure. Unfortunately, this simple remedy has not been widely used so far by those who need it most.

WILLIAM M. M. KIRBY

References

Babione, R. W., Hedgecock, L. E., and Ray, J. P.: Navy Experience with the Oral Use of Penicillin as a Prophylaxis. U. S. Armed Forces M. J., 3: 973, 1952.

Keefer, C. S., and Spink, W. W.: Gonococcic Arthritis; Pathogenesis, Mechanism of Recovery, and Treatment. J.A.M.A., 109:1448, 1937.

Mahoney, J. F., and Thayer, J. D.: The Gonococci, in Dubos, R.: Bacterial and Mycotic Infections of Man. 2nd ed. Philadelphia, J. B. Lippincott Co., 1952, Chap. 26.

Marcussen, Paul V.: Variations in the Stability of Sexual Relations as Explanation of Differences in the Spread of Syphilis and Gonorrhea. Am. J. Syph., Gonor. & Ven. Dis., 37:355, 1953.

Spitzer, N., and Steinbrocker, O.: The Treatment of Gonorrheal Arthritis with Penicillin. Am. J. M. Sc., 218:138, 1949.

Williams, R. H.: Gonococcic Endocarditis. Arch. Int. Med., 61:26, 1938.

MENINGOCOCCAL INFECTIONS

Definition. Meningococcal infections are manifestations of a specific infectious disease characterized by infection of the upper respiratory tract, invasion of the blood stream (meningococcemia), and focal involvement of various sites, notably the central nervous system (meningococcal meningitis, cerebrospinal fever, spotted fever or epidemic cerebrospinal meningitis). One or all of these features may be exhibited in a single patient. Meningitis has occurred sporadically and epidemically since its first recognition in Geneva in 1805 by Vieusseux and in the United States by Danielson and Mann in 1806.

Etiology. The meningococcus (*Neisseria intracellularis, Diplococcus intracellularis meningitidis*) was established as the causative agent by Weichselbaum in 1887. It is a gram-negative coccus, variable in size and occurring singly or as biscuit-shaped diplococci. Certain strains are encapsulated. The organism is fastidious in its metabolic requirements and will grow only on enriched laboratory media at body temperature. Meat infusion broth or agar containing 5 to 10 per cent of blood (rabbit, sheep or horse) or human ascitic fluid is an adequate medium. Chocolate agar, prepared by heating fresh blood agar, is especially suitable for initial isolation. Growth is augmented by incubating the cultures in an atmosphere containing 5 to 10 per cent of carbon dioxide.

Meningococci are easily killed by chilling or drying, so that prompt inoculation and incubation of all cultures is desirable. Because of the extreme susceptibility of meningococci to the sulfonamides, para-aminobenzoic acid in concentration of 5 mg. per 100 ml. should be added to media used for the culture of specimens from patients.

Identification of meningococci is based on morphology, fermentation of glucose and maltose, and immunologic reactions. Four immunologic types have been differentiated in the past by agglutination with specific antiserums, but cross-reactions are frequent, particularly between types I and III. For practical purposes, therefore, it seems advisable to consider only two immunologic groups of meningococci: *group I* to include the old types I and III, and *group II* to include the remaining types and atypical strains. Group I strains are encapsulated and may readily be identified immunologically by capsular swelling with homologous type-specific antiserum. One strain in group II, termed group IIα, is likewise encapsulated and thus may be similarly identified. Other serologic methods of identification, such as precipitation and complement fixation, may be used, but are generally less simple and satisfactory than agglutination and capsular swelling.

Substances termed "endotoxins" may be extracted from living or dead meningococci. Although the toxicity of such extracts for animals has been demonstrated, there is little evidence of type or group specificity. The production of a true, type-specific toxin, or "exotoxin," by the meningococcus has been reported, but most authorities question its existence.

Epidemiology. Sporadic meningococcal infections occur almost constantly throughout the world. Epidemics tend to recur irregularly in five- to ten-year cycles, superimposed on an annual seasonal increase, the peak month of which is usually March in temperate zones. In the United States and Canada, the reported incidence of meningitis has been slowly rising annually since 1948 (Hedrich). The susceptibility of the general population is low, and morbidity rates for clinically apparent disease are seldom higher than 10 to 1000 per 100,000 in the exposed population during epidemic periods. Infants and children are most frequently attacked; in one series of 3557 cases, 27 per cent of the patients were less than 5 years of age and 45 per cent were less than 15 (Beeson and

Westerman). The incidence is usually higher in males than in females. Race and color have no known influence on incidence or susceptibility. The higher rates reported among Negroes in certain urban areas have been attributed primarily to crowding. The exact incubation period is unknown, but probably is between one and ten days.

The portal of entry of the organisms is the upper respiratory passages, and transmission from person to person presumably may occur by direct or intimate contact, by airborne droplets, or by articles contaminated with secretions of the respiratory tract. Even during severe epidemics, however, the majority of clinical infections have no apparent connection with one another, and case-to-case spread is usually impossible to trace. Cultural surveys during periods of high incidence have shown that more than 90 per cent of the population harbor meningococci in the nasopharynx, either constantly or intermittently during an outbreak, without clinical evidence of infection (carriers). During interepidemic periods the organism may be recovered from less than 5 per cent of persons examined. Even under conditions of low carrier prevalence, however, a considerable proportion of the population will harbor meningococci at some time during a period of weeks or months, since the respiratory tract flora is not static, but changes constantly through acquisition of new bacteria and their subsequent loss.

Morbid Anatomy. In carriers, or *inapparent infections,* abnormal reactions are ordinarily not found. *Meningococcemia* is characterized by focal hemorrhages into the cutaneous, subcutaneous, submucosal and synovial tissues. The fundamental lesion is vascular in character, with endothelial damage, inflammation of the vessel wall, necrosis and thrombosis (Hill and Kinney). The classic finding in rapidly *fulminating meningococcemia,* the *Waterhouse-Friderichsen syndrome,* is bilateral adrenal hemorrhage. Damage to the adrenal cortex, however, may occur without hemorrhage (Banks; Rich).

Involvement of the central nervous system is characterized chiefly by *meningitis* which progresses from hyperemia and an increased amount of cerebrospinal fluid to a yellowish, purulent exudate, becoming organized if the disease persists into a chronic phase.

Pathologic Physiology and Chemistry. The present theory of the pathogenesis of meningococcal infections is that the bacteria enter the body through the upper respiratory passages and become implanted in the membranes of the nasopharynx and adjoining structures. Symptoms and signs of acute upper respiratory infection may then result. Direct invasion of the blood stream takes place from these sites and the evidences of bacteremia appear. Dissemination of the meningococci is followed by metastatic lesions in various sites, such as skin, meninges, joints, eyes, ears and lungs. The symptoms and signs are dependent on the site of localization. In meningitis, two factors—increased intracranial pressure and meningeal inflammation—are responsible for most of the characteristic clinical findings.

The reasons for limitation of meningococcal infection to the nasopharynx and the blood in some persons, or for its extension to other sites of the body, particularly the meninges, in other persons, are not clear.

Chemical alterations in meningococcal infections may be profound. Presumably they are initiated and maintained by metabolic and endotoxic substances from the bacterial cells, together with the chemical by-products of damaged tissue cells responsible for the phenomena of inflammation. The hemorrhagic manifestations are due to vascular damage. Other changes are similar to those in acute sepsis: namely, dehydration, reduction in blood volume, altered acid-base equilibrium from differential loss of acid or base, negative nitrogen balance, and fever. Meningismus may develop coincident with a relative increase in the ratio of the chlorides in the cerebrospinal fluid to the blood chlorides. In severe or overwhelming infections, cyanosis, circulatory collapse and other signs of shock may develop, probably because of the combined action of bacterial endotoxins and tissue anoxia. If fluid intake is adequate, there is no decrease in plasma volume, no fall in plasma protein concentration, and no abnormal increase in capillary permeability to protein (Ebert and Stead). Alterations in the blood similar to those of adrenal insufficiency, such as low sodium, elevated potassium, low chloride and hypoglycemia, may be found and are consistent with an inadequacy of cortical secretion resulting from damage to the adrenal cortex.

Symptoms. The clinical manifestations of meningococcal infections can most conveniently be described by considering successive stages in the pathogenetic sequence: namely,

infection of the upper respiratory tract, bacteremia, and meningitis or other metastatic localization. It should be emphasized, however, that this sequence of infection may not always be apparent clinically; the infection may extend so rapidly that the symptoms and signs of all the stages coexist in a given patient at the time he is first examined, or there may be such variations in the intensity of the symptoms referable to a single aspect of the disease that other aspects are overlooked.

Infection of the upper respiratory tract is numerically the most frequent type of meningococcal infection. In the majority of patients, however, symptoms are absent or inconsequential and infection can be detected only by culture of the nasopharynx. In the remainder, dryness or slight discharge from the nose, postnasal drip, soreness of the throat and suffusion of the conjunctivas may be present. Physical examination reveals congestion or injection of the mucous membranes of the nose and pharynx, discharge from the sinuses and rarely redness and edema of the tonsils. Exudate and regional adenopathy are ordinarily absent. Approximately 75 per cent of patients with generalized meningococcal infection give a history of preceding or coexisting nasopharyngitis. It has been postulated that in some of these patients the symptoms are due to infection with a virus, although the nature of such a virus has not been determined.

Meningococcemia. Bacteremic forms of meningococcal infections vary greatly from acute fulminating illnesses of a few hours' duration to indolent, chronic infections lasting weeks, months or even years. The progress of the infection may be steady and constant, or there may be relapses and recrudescences at varying intervals.

The commonest type of meningococcemia is a relatively mild, acute or subacute infection. Prodromal *symptoms* are ordinarily absent, with the possible exception of those of a mild upper respiratory infection. The onset is usually sudden with feverishness, chilliness, occasionally frank chills which may be recurrent, malaise, myalgia and apathy. The presenting symptoms may be any of the above, but not infrequently the initial complaint will be recurrent fever, rash, arthralgia, acute polyarthritis, gastrointestinal upsets characterized by nausea and vomiting, or occasionally monarthritis or conjunctivitis. The symptoms persist and often become exaggerated as the disease progresses. The fever may be remittent and irregular with "spikes" to 102° or 103° F., or it may be intermittent in quotidian, tertian or quartan fashion (Fig. 29). The pulse is full and strong with a rate proportionate to the fever. Respirations are usually normal or only slightly elevated.

The most striking feature *on physical examination* is the rash which is present in the

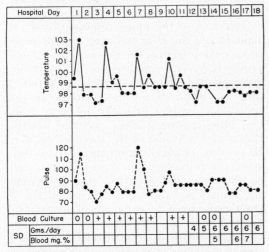

Fig. 29. Meningococcemia without meningitis in a 24 year old male due to *Neisseria intracellularis*, group II, treated with sulfadiazine.

majority of patients, particularly during epidemics. It appears soon after onset and may take a variety of forms, although the commonest lesions are petechial or purpuric, measuring in diameter from 1 or 2 mm. to a centimeter and are pink to reddish-blue in color (Fig. 30). Early in the disease there may be a generalized, mottled erythema which appears dusky if the patient is slightly cyanotic. Yellowish pink macules simulating the "rose spots" of typhoid, wheals, or nodules resembling erythema nodosum may appear before petechiae and ecchymoses. Careful search in strong daylight may be necessary to detect the early lesions. Occasionally, vesicular, pustular or bullous lesions are present; superficial or deep ulcerations may result. A common site for the lesions first to appear is about the wrists and ankles, but any area of the body may be involved, including the conjunctivas and the mucous membranes. The hemorrhagic lesions fade to a brown, rusty color three or four days after their appearance, and new crops may appear, often following chills, so that the rash may present a varied appearance.

Other physical findings, with the exception of splenomegaly, are inconstant. *Herpes labialis* is found in about 10 per cent of the cases. Unless meningismus develops, symptoms referable to involvement of the central nervous system are absent. The symptoms of metastatic localizations are usually self-evident, depending on the site involved.

Laboratory examinations serve to establish the final diagnosis. Leukocytosis, varying from 12,000 to 40,000 cells per cubic millimeter, is almost constantly present. From 80 to 90 per cent of the cells are neutrophils. Occasionally, intracellular diplococci may be seen within the cells on a stained smear of capillary blood or of blood obtained directly from a skin lesion. Cultivation of meningococci from the blood furnishes final etiologic proof. It should be emphasized that repeated cultures of the blood may be necessary to detect the meningococcus and that growth of the organism in liquid culture medium may be delayed. Other laboratory examinations give normal findings or results compatible with any febrile illness.

The subsequent course is dependent on therapy, although approximately 20 per cent of the patients recover spontaneously after several weeks or months. Any of the complications and sequelae of meningococcal infections may develop.

Acute fulminating meningococcemia differs from the milder form chiefly in the rapidity of its progress and its overwhelming character. The onset is often abrupt and represents a dramatic departure from normal health with a shaking chill, severe headache, dizziness or vertigo, collapse or unconsciousness. Three forms may be differentiated (Banks): (1) The *adrenal* form is characterized by massive purpura, low blood pressure, clear mental condition, rapid, quiet respiration and overwhelming bacteremia. The extensive rash (Fig. 31) involves skin and mucous membranes as well as internal organs, classically the adrenals. The temperature may be subnormal, normal or slightly elevated. Within a few hours circulatory collapse develops. Adrenal hormone replacement therapy may help to sustain these patients. (2) The *encephalitic* form is characterized by rapidly developing coma, rapid stertorous breathing, a petechial but not massive purpuric rash and normal blood pressure. (3) The *mixed encephalitic-adrenal* form is a combination of the two forms, characterized by early deep coma, purpura and

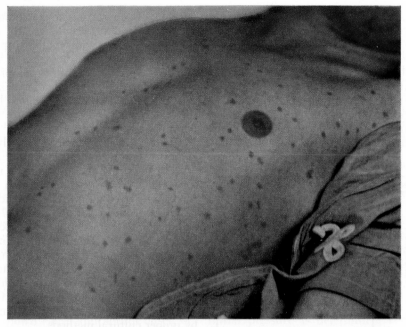

Fig. 30. Common skin lesions in meningococcal infection. (Courtesy of Dr. Worth B. Daniels.)

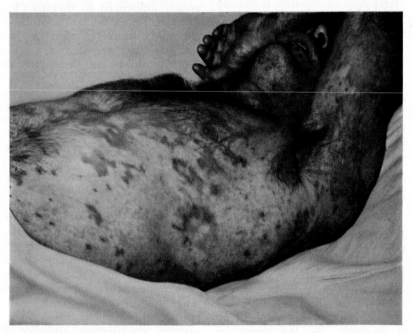

Fig. 31. Skin lesions in fulminating meningococcemia. (Courtesy of Dr. Worth B. Daniels.)

low blood pressure. Occasionally the pituitary gland may be damaged. Despite all efforts, these illnesses usually are rapidly fatal.

Chronic meningococcemia is an infrequent form of meningococcal infection in which episodes of fever of a few days' duration recur at intervals of days, weeks or months. Chills and arthralgic symptoms may accompany the bouts. Lesions of the skin or other characteristic signs may be absent or evanescent, making diagnosis difficult. Repeated cultures of the blood may be necessary before the meningococcus is recovered. Unless recognized and treated, meningitis or endocarditis may develop.

Meningitis. This is the most characteristic

cate meningococci from the nasopharynx. Mass administration of the drug to small closed populations has accordingly been advocated as a control measure during epidemic periods and has apparently been successful. Isolation of patients with meningococcal infections is not necessary after 24 hours of adequate therapy with sulfonamide drugs, since the organisms are eradicated from the respiratory tract within this period. Such is not the case, however, when the other antimicrobial drugs are used.

JOHN H. DINGLE

References

Ballard, S. I., and Miller, H. G.: Sequelae of Cerebrospinal Meningitis: Analysis of 60 Cases. Lancet, 2:273, 1945.

Banks, H. S.: Meningococcosis: a Protean Disease. Lancet, 2:635, 677, 1948.

Beeson, P. B., and Westerman, E.: Cerebrospinal Fever; Analysis of 3,575 Case Reports, with Special Reference to Sulfonamide Therapy. Brit. M. J., 1:497, 1943.

Browne, M. P., Waddy, B. B., and Tudor, R. W.: Cerebrospinal Meningitis in the Gold Coast: a Review of 9864 Cases. Lancet, 1:741, 1947.

Daniels, W. B.: Meningococcic Bacteremia. Arch. Int. Med., 81:145, 1948.

Dingle, J. H., and Finland, M.: Diagnosis, Treatment and Prevention of Meningococcic Meningitis. War Med., 2:1, 1942.

Ebert, R. V., and Stead, E. A., Jr.: Circulatory Failure in Acute Infections. J. Clin. Investigation, 20: 671, 1941.

Hedrich, A. W.: Recent Trends in Meningococcal Disease. Pub. Health Rep., 67:411, 1952.

Hill, W. R., and Kinney, T. D.: The Cutaneous Lesions in Acute Meningococcemia. J.A.M.A., 134:513, 1947.

Kinsman, J. M., and D'Alanzo, C. A.: Meningococcemia: a Description of the Clinical Picture and a Comparison of the Efficacy of Sulfadiazine and Penicillin in the Treatment of Thirty Cases. Ann. Int. Med., 24:607, 1946.

Lepper, M. H., and others: Meningococcic Meningitis: Treatment with Large Doses of Penicillin Compared to Treatment with Gantrisin. J. Lab. Clin. Med., 40:891, 1952.

McKay, R. J., Jr., Ingraham, F. D., and Matson, D. D.: Subdural Fluid Complicating Bacterial Meningitis. J.A.M.A., 152:387, 1953.

Meads, M., Harris, H. W., Samper, B. A., and Finland, M.: Treatment of Meningococcal Meningitis with Penicillin. New England J. Med., 231: 509, 1944.

Rich, A. R.: A Peculiar Type of Adrenal Cortical Damage Associated with Acute Infection, and Its Possible Relation to Circulatory Collapse. Bull. Johns Hopkins Hosp., 74:1, 1944.

BACILLARY DISEASES

HEMOPHILUS INFECTIONS

PERTUSSIS

(Whooping Cough)

Definition. Pertussis is an acute infectious disease of the respiratory tract characterized, in its typical form, by a series of repeated spasmodic coughs followed by a sudden forceful inspiration (the whoop) and sometimes by vomiting. Since the disease may exist without the whoop, and since other infections of the respiratory tract may exhibit this symptom, the name "pertussis" is preferred to that of "whooping cough."

History. Although the earliest reference to the disease was probably made by Moulton in 1540, De-Baillou in 1578 is credited with the first classical description of pertussis.

Incidence. Pertussis is sporadic and endemic to the more thickly populated communities throughout the world. Epidemics prevail at intervals of two to four years. Though cases occur regularly during the summer months, they are more numerous in winter and spring, when complications are likewise more frequent. The peak of the incidence in the southern states occurs in May; in the North, in January or February. It appears to be more frequent among females. The communicability rate is high, resembling that of measles and varicella. In family exposures it approximates 85 per cent.

Although pertussis occurs at all ages, it is decidedly a disease of early life. About 85 per cent of all cases occur in children less than 7 years of age, and about one half of these is found in infants less than 2 years of age. Though maternal immunity may be passively conferred upon the newborn in certain instances, infants younger than 6 months of age are very susceptible and are subject to a high mortality.

Etiology. *Hemophilus pertussis,* discovered by Bordet in 1906, is the causative agent. It is a small, gram-negative, ovoid bacillus about 0.5 micron in length. It occurs in the respiratory tract in great numbers during the catarrhal stage of the disease, but rapidly disappears during convalescence. Carriers are rare.

The disease has been produced experimentally by inoculation of suitable animals and man with pure cultures of the organism. Specific humoral antibodies result from the natural infection and from injection of specific vaccine. Immunity usually follows an attack of pertussis, but a few bacteriologically proved instances of second attacks have been observed.

Other organisms such as *Hemophilus influenzae, Brucella bronchiseptica* and *H. parapertussis* may cause infections resembling whooping cough. The last two of these are related to *H. pertussis* on the basis of a common minor antigen.

Morbid Anatomy. Catarrhal infection of the epithelium of the larynx, trachea and bronchi is always present. Numerous clumps of *H. pertussis* may be demonstrated here. The essential lesion probably consists of necrosis of the midzonal and basal portions of the bronchial epithelium, with infiltration of this area by polymorphonuclear leukocytes. Peribronchiolitis, extending from the hilum along the bronchial-vascular rays to the middle or even the outer zones of the lung, occurs. As the lesion progresses, typical interstitial pneumonia develops. Edema and hemorrhage mark the early stage of parenchymal involvement. Accumulation of mucus, pus and cellular debris within the alveolar spaces results chiefly from infection by secondary invading organisms. It is probable that *H. pertussis* is responsible for the lung lesion to a considerable degree.

In cases characterized by severe paroxysms or convulsions the brain is intensely congested and may reveal punctate or even large hemorrhages. In rare instances encephalitis with degeneration and atrophy of the cortex has been described.

Pathologic Physiology. The essential departures from the normal physiologic state observed in pertussis are (1) those related to disturbances in nutrition; (2) those resulting from changes in the pulmonic circulatory system; and (3) those referable to the central nervous system.

Loss of appetite and vomiting cause weight loss. Excessive vomiting may produce gastric tetany. In infants, diarrhea frequently occurs. Dehydration, starvation and emaciation impair nutrition to the extent that fatal secondary infections develop.

Irritation of the mucous membranes of the trachea and bronchi provokes the paroxysm. Obstruction of the lower air passages by mucous plugs induces atelectasis, which, along with interstitial pneumonia, prevents proper oxygenation of the blood. According to Regan and Tolstoouhov a state of uncompensated acidosis results. Enlargement of the right side of the heart may result from increased impediment of the pulmonary circulation.

Anoxemia probably causes convulsions in many instances. Infancy, pneumonia, and severity of the paroxysms are important factors. Cerebral congestion, edema, hemorrhage and encephalitis are responsible for convulsive and other types of disturbances in the central nervous system. In rachitic infants, convulsions may be due to tetany.

Symptoms. The incubation period, though variable, is usually from seven to fourteen days. In a series of 1123 cases, Lawson found the mean duration of the period to be thirteen days. The course of the typical disease is six weeks in length, representing three stages: the catarrhal, spasmodic and convalescent, each lasting approximately two weeks.

Catarrhal Stage. This period begins with a mild cough, usually nocturnal, which progresses in intensity and soon becomes diurnal. The mean duration of this period, according to Lawson, is eleven days. Coryza and sneezing are usually present, and the appetite fails. The cough later resembles that of bronchitis. At this stage the physician is frequently consulted. In rare instances hoarseness is present, and occasionally the disease begins with the features of acute obstructive laryngitis. There is often suffusion of the conjunctiva.

Spasmodic Stage. After about ten to fourteen days the cough becomes so aggravated that it occurs in series of explosive efforts in which the face becomes congested, often cyanotic, the tongue protrudes with each cough, and the patient appears to strangle. Finally the attack ends with a sudden forceful inspiratory crow or whoop. Large amounts of thick, ropy, mucoid material are coughed up, swallowed or vomited. Perspiration, congestion of the neck and scalp veins, mental confusion and exhaustion may follow the more severe paroxysms. Infants particularly may become so cyanotic and exhausted that they may require artificial respiration.

Excitement, sudden thermal changes, swallowing, inhalation of irritating fumes, tobacco smoke or even the occurrence of a paroxysm in a nearby patient may excite a spell of coughing. If a plug of mucus remains in contact with the hyperesthetic mucous membrane of the respiratory tract, recurrent paroxysms very likely follow until it is dislodged. Epistaxis often occurs when the spasms are severe. Subconjunctival hemorrhages and edema of the lower eyelids occur frequently in cases with severe coughing.

Convalescent Stage. The number and severity of the paroxysms gradually decrease, vomiting becomes less frequent, and the disease thus progresses into the stage of decline or convalescence. During this period the hilar and basilar rhonchi gradually disappear. For a period of weeks or months an intercurrent infection may cause the major symptoms to reappear even to the point of resembling a new attack.

It must be remembered that pertussis is a variable disease and may exist in a mild, atypical form. The entire course may last only a few days. Proved cases have been known to last but from seven to fourteen days. Vomiting and the classic whoop may never occur. Very young infants, particularly, may have choking and cyanotic spells without the whoop.

Complications and Sequelae. Bronchopneumonia is by far the most important complication. This is usually interstitial in type. Lobar pneumonia is rarely seen, but occasionally confluent bronchopneumonia produces a lesion which clinically resembles that seen in the lobar type. Atelectasis is common because the blocking of a bronchus with mucus, resulting in collapse of a portion of the lung and frequently leading to the erroneous diagnosis of pneumonia. Vesicular and interstitial emphysema occurs in practically all severe cases. Emphysema of the cellular tissue of the mediastinum may result from rupture of air blebs on the surface of the lung. From the mediastinum the air may find its way into the subcutaneous tissues of the neck and even spread to other parts of the body. Cases with widespread subcutaneous emphysema are usually fatal. In one case of this type which later came to anatomic examination there was hyperleukocytosis of 257,000 cells per cubic millimeter. Pneumothorax may occur. Bronchial asthma and bronchiectasis may result from an attack of pertussis. An existing tuberculous lesion may spread during the disease, although the effect of pertussis on tuberculosis is probably not as disastrous as was formerly believed. Unresolved pneumonia and pulmonary fibrosis are of common occurrence.

Cardiac dilatation, particularly of the right side, is observed. It is most commonly associated with diffuse pneumonic involvement.

Otitis media is frequently encountered and is due to secondary invading organisms. Because of the tendency to suppurate, the ears require the careful attention of the attending physician.

The hemorrhages of pertussis are mechanical in origin, resulting from the venous congestion associated with severe coughing. Epistaxis and hemorrhage of the bulbar conjunctivas are common. Blood-tinged sputum is a result of small erosive lesions in the trachea which occur during a paroxysm. Hemorrhage of the brain has been reported.

The most common neurologic complication of pertussis is convulsions. They occur in about 8 per cent of hospitalized cases and are especially common in infants. The cerebrospinal fluid of those suffering from convulsions is usually normal.

Other neurologic complications of pertussis are epilepsy, mental retardation, spastic paralysis, myelitis and temporary or permanent visual disturbances.

Hernia, usually umbilical, and prolapse of the rectum are results of severe straining associated with the cough. Ulcer of the frenum occasionally results when the tongue is repeatedly thrust over the edge of the lower incisor teeth during the paroxysms.

Diagnosis. Typical pertussis in the paroxysmal stage can be readily recognized. In the catarrhal period and in the atypical abortive form it is difficult to diagnose. Pertussis should be suspected in a person suffering from a cough of a week's duration if examination of the nose, throat and chest reveals no apparent cause for it. History of exposure may not be elicited. The physician may be obliged to defer diagnosis until the cough becomes more definite. In such instances the patient should be isolated and a culture taken if the facilities are available. In doubtful cases inquiry should be made concerning previous injections of vaccine, since mild, atypical cases may occur as a result of the partial immunity thus conferred.

The most valuable of the laboratory diagnostic tests consists in the isolation of the organism from the upper respiratory tract. This may be accomplished by the cough-plate technique or by the nasal swab method. Bacteriologic diagnosis is particularly applicable during the catarrhal period, when positive cultures may be expected in from 70 to 90 per cent of the cases. Only positive cultures are significant. A single negative culture does not exclude the disease.

A characteristic change in the leukocytes occurs during the late catarrhal or early spasmodic stage. This consists in a definite leukocytosis of from 15,000 to 40,000 white blood cells per cubic millimeter, reflecting progressive increase in the absolute number of lymphocytes. Occasionally, extreme degrees of hyperleukocytosis occur, usually in cases complicated by pneumonia. This change in the leukocytes is probably due to direct stimulation of the hematopoietic tissues by *H. pertussis*. Failure to find this blood change does not constitute conclusive evidence against the existence of the disease.

In certain instances the finding of a significant titer of humoral antibodies in an unvaccinated patient may suggest recent infection with *H. pertussis*. Tests for agglutinins, and complement-fixing and mouse-protective antibodies, may be made with the patient's serum. Unfortunately, humoral antibodies do not appear until the paroxysmal stage; hence they are of little diagnostic value early in the disease. Attempts to develop a diagnostic skin reaction with various toxins and fractions of the organism have not been entirely successful.

Prognosis. During the period from 1909 to 1949 the mortality from pertussis in the United States decreased from 11.3 to 1.6 per 100,000 population. In 1950 there were 120,718 cases reported from the United States Registration Area with 1118 deaths— a fatality rate of 0.93 per cent or 0.7 deaths per 100,000 population.

The younger the patient the more grave is the prognosis. About 5 per cent of the hospitalized patients under one year of age die. The highest death rate now occurs in rural, rather than urban, areas.

Consideration of the prognosis in pertussis should include recognition of the more serious sequelae, especially the pulmonary and cerebral complications, as well as the immediate fatality rate.

Treatment. *General Measures.* Normal room temperature and bed rest are desirable. Good nursing and hospital care are important in the care of seriously ill infants. Excitement and extreme changes in temperature provoke coughing. When vomiting is excessive, small frequent feedings are advisable. Obstruction of the respiratory tract by excessive mucus may be relieved by careful suction.

Oxygen should be given to all patients with increased respiratory rates with or without cyanosis, for it is one of the most important therapeutic agents for this disease. Small blood tranfusions are indicated in cases complicated by anemia, convulsions or pneumonia. A roentgenogram of the lungs and a tuberculin test should be obtained during convalescence.

Medication. Codeine, paregoric and phenobarbital are useful sedatives. Rectal instillations of a mixture of 2 to 8 cc. of ether in 15 cc. of olive oil, every 6 to 8 hours as necessary, are effective for the control of severe paroxysms. The subcutaneous injection of 0.008 to 0.016 gm. of sodium phenobarbital may prove helpful for the control of convulsions. Magnesium sulfate (0.06 gm. per kilogram of body weight) may be injected intramuscularly for the same purpose.

Specific Therapy. Hyperimmune serum is indicated in severe cases. Immune rabbit serum (5 to 10 cc.) may be injected intramuscularly after preliminary testing for serum sensitivity. Hyperimmune human serum (20 to 40 cc.) or the gamma globulin (5 to 10 cc.) prepared from it serves similar purposes.

Chloramphenicol and the tetracyclines (Aureomycin, Terramycin) are about equally effective in dosages of 50 mg. per kilogram of body weight per day divided into four doses. Because of its potential toxic effect on the bone marrow, chloramphenicol should be used only in severe cases with careful observations of the blood count.

Penicillin is obviously indicated for the treatment of pyogenic complications.

In a previously vaccinated person, additional injection of vaccine early in the disease is immunologically sound treatment.

Prevention. Young infants should be carefully protected from exposure to pertussis. The period of infectivity is about six weeks, but the catarrhal stage is most dangerous.

Active immunization should start at or before the third month of age. The initial course of vaccine should be given in three monthly injections. The total dose should be 12 units contained in not more than 96 billion organisms in saline or 48 billion organisms in alum-precipitated preparations. Stimulating injections (2 units each) should be given every two years until school age.

To the exposed, nonimmunized infant, passive protection may be given by the intramuscular injection of immune rabbit serum

(2.5 to 5 cc.), hyperimmune human serum (10 to 20 cc.) or gamma globulin, prepared from hyperimmune human serum (2.5 to 5 cc.).

WILLIAM L. BRADFORD

References

Ames, R. G., and others: Comparison of the Therapeutic Efficiency of Four Agents in Pertussis. Pediatrics, *11:*323, 1953.

Booher, C. E., Farrell, J. B., and West, E. J.: Pertussis: Clinical Comparison of the Newer Antibiotics. J. Pediat., 38:411, 1951.

Bradford, W. L.: Recent Contributions to the Diagnosis and Treatment of Pertussis. New York State J. Med., *49:*397, 1949.

————, Brooks, Anne M., and Katsampes, C. P.: The Therapeutic Effect of Sulfadiazine and Immune Rabbit Serum in Experimental Murine Pertussis. Yale J. Biol. & Med., *16:*435, 1944.

Brooks, A. M., Bradford, W. L., and Berry, G. P.: The Method of Nasopharyngeal Culture in the Diagnosis of Whooping Cough. J.A.M.A., *120:*883, 1942.

Felton, H. M., and Willard, C. Y.: Current Status of Prophylaxis by Hemophilus Pertussis Vaccine. J.A.M.A., *126:*294, 1944.

Gallavan, M., and Goodpasture, E. W.: Infection of Chick Embryos with H. Pertussis Reproducing Pulmonary Lesions of Whooping Cough. Am. J. Path., *13:*927, 1937.

Katsampes, C. P., McGuinness, A. C., and Bradford, W. L.: Effect of Hyperimmune Human Serum (Lyophile) on the Humoral Antibody Titer in Pertussis. Am. J. Dis. Child., *58:*1234, 1939.

Nelson, R. L.: Neurological Complications of Whooping Cough. Review of Literature with Respect to 2 Cases of Pertussis Encephalitis. J. Pediat., *14:*39, 1939.

Sako, W., Trenting, W. L., Witt, D. B., and Nichamin, S. J.: Early Immunization against Pertussis with Alum Precipitated Vaccine. J.A.M.A., *127:*379, 1945.

HEMOPHILUS INFLUENZAE INFECTIONS

The influenza bacillus has played two major roles in human infections: (1) as a secondary invader in the influenza virus pandemic of 1918—Jordan has summarized the evidence for this influence; and (2) as a primary agent in pyogenic infections.

PRIMARY H. INFLUENZAE INFECTIONS

Encepsulated H. influenzae. Although six specific types of *H. influenzae,* a, b, c, d, e and f, were differentiated by Pittman, type b is responsible for almost all primary severe infections caused by influenza bacilli. The pathogenic potentialities of encapsulated *H. influenzae* as a primary agent are greatly modified by the age of the host. The severe pyogenic infections occur almost exclusively in infants and children. The decline in incidence with increasing age has been shown by Fothergill and Wright to be closely related to a greater bactericidal power of the blood of older subjects. This immunity is apparently the result of past contact with the organism.

In Childhood. Type b *H. influenzae* is one of the commonest causes of severe infections in infants and children (Alexander et al., 1942). Pediatricians are now familiar with several patterns of illness, all of which are preceded by a nasopharyngitis. The complications result from remote seeding, consequent to a bacteremia, as well as from spread to the ears, paranasal sinuses, larynx and lungs. Of the severe infections, meningitis, obstructive laryngitis, pyarthrosis and pneumonia occur most frequently.

In Adults. Immunity to these severe *H. influenzae* infections, while exhibited by most adults, is not uniformly present. Type b *H. influenzae* pneumonia, meningitis, obstructive laryngitis and pyarthrosis are seen in adults but they occur very rarely.

PNEUMONIA. *H. influenzae* type b pneumonia cannot be differentiated from pneumococcal pneumonia by clinical signs or the ordinary laboratory examinations. The lesion may be lobar in distribution, the blood shows a moderate leukocytosis and the erythrocyte sedimentation rate is significantly elevated. Following adequate sulfonamide therapy the subsidence of infection is as prompt as in the average patient with pneumococcal pneumonia. Penicillin in the usual dosage is not effective, and on this basis *H. influenzae* pneumonia may at times be erroneously classified as "virus pneumonia."

MENINGITIS. *H. influenzae* is the most frequent cause of meningitis in infants and children. Prior to 1938 the mortality rate was virtually 100 per cent. Patients with *H. influenzae* meningitis do not exhibit clinical signs which can be distinguished from those of other varieties of pyogenic meningitis. The clinical signs and changes in the cerebrospinal fluid vary with the stage of the disease and the severity of infection. However, prompt identification of the etiologic agent can be made by bacteriologic and serologic procedures.

OBSTRUCTIVE LARYNGITIS WITH EPIGLOTTITIS. One form of severe, rapidly progressing laryngeal obstruction is caused by *H. influenzae.* Lemierre was the first to separate influenzal laryngitis from other forms of croup; he reported its occurrence in both children and adults. In children, *H. influenzae* laryngitis presents a characteristic history and the patient a characteristic appearance. The onset is sudden and the course fulminating. Mild fever and dysphagia develop during an apparently innocuous respiratory infection. Dyspnea starts abruptly and increases within a few hours to such a degree as to make hospitalization imperative. The picture is that of a prostrated child with severe laryngeal obstruction, usually demanding tracheotomy. The temperature is high. On examination of the pharynx there is diffuse erythema, often with evident edema, and when the tongue is pressed downward, the enlarged, red and edematous epiglottis is easily seen.

Bacteriologic Diagnosis. H. influenzae may usually be identified within thirty minutes when the infection is severe, by the demonstration of capsular swelling of bacterial cells found in the appropriate biologic fluid. In patients with pneumonia or obstructive laryngitis the organisms should be sought for in a concentrated suspension of nasopharyngeal mucus; they are found in cerebrospinal fluid in patients with meningitis, in joint exudate in those with pyarthrosis and in the pleural exudate in empyema. When such direct identification is impossible, growth in special media can usually be obtained in 12 hours (Dubos). In children bacteremia is a constant feature in all varieties of severe *H. influenzae* infections.

Nonencapsulated H. influenzae. A primary pathogenic role of nonencapsulated *H. influenzae* can seldom be established; this organism in fact is found frequently (30 to 50 per cent) in the nasopharynx of normal persons of all age groups. In infants it may occasionally cause meningitis or pneumonia. In adults it is a rare cause of subacute bacterial endocarditis and brain abscess. The Koch-Weeks bacillus (which cannot be differentiated from *H. influenzae*) has been reported as the primary agent in epidemics of conjunctivitis.

Treatment of H. influenzae infections. The therapeutic efficacy of sulfonamides, specific rabbit antiserum streptomycin and chloramphenicol against *H. influenzae* is now well established. When the infection is sufficiently mild, each of these agents can bring about recovery. On the other hand if the infection is severe, each is limited in its therapeutic capacity; the combined action of two or three is required for successful treatment.

The location, duration and severity of infection govern the number of agents which should be used simultaneously in a given patient. Experience with these agents in the various *H. influenzae* clinical patterns is well documented in childhood infections only, but there is every reason to believe that the methods of treatment in this age group are applicable to adults (Alexander and Leidy).

In obstructive laryngitis sulfadiazine alone can cure most patients after an adequate airway is established by tracheotomy. Pneumonia can also be successfully treated with sulfadiazine alone. However, the risk of therapeutic failure is virtually eliminated by the initial use of a second effective agent; chloramphenicol is the drug of choice. In meningitis, pyarthrosis and empyema the combined action of two drugs is indicated. There are now sufficient data for comparison of three different therapeutic programs in meningitis: (1) type-specific rabbit antiserum and sulfonamides; (2) streptomycin and sulfadiazine; and (3) chloramphenicol and sulfadiazine. Any of the three can be expected to cure virtually 100 per cent of the patients who are treated early in the course of the disease. It has not been possible to show a significant difference between the efficacy of these three pairs of agents. The ease with which optimal concentrations can be maintained in the cerebrospinal fluid by either the oral or parenteral routes, and the rarity of injurious effects, make the combined action of chloramphenicol and sulfadiazine the treatment of choice for meningitis and all other severe varieties of *H. influenzae* infections. When the oral route is used for chloramphenicol, 200 mg. per kilogram is given daily in four doses (not to exceed 3 gm.); when parenteral administration is necessary, 100 mg. per kilogram (not to exceed 2 gm.) is given each 24 hours, in three doses. The dose in adults should not exceed 5 gm. orally or 3 gm. parenterally.

H. E. ALEXANDER

References

Alexander, H. E., in Dubos, R.: Bacterial and Mycotic Infections of Man. 2nd ed. Philadelphia, J. B. Lippincott Co., 1952, Chap. 23, pp. 472–492.
——, Ellis, C., and Leidy, G.: Treatment of Type-Specific Hemophilus Influenzae Infections in Infancy and Childhood. J. Pediat., 20:673, 1942.
——, and Leidy, G.: The Present Status of Treatment for Influenzal Meningitis. Am. J. Med., 2:

457, 1947. Hemophilus influenzae infections in children. Conn. State Med. J., 13:713, 1949.

————, Leidy, G., and Redman, W.: Comparison of the Action of Streptomycin, Polymyxin B, Aureomycin and Chloromycetin on H. pertussis, H. parapertussis, H. influenzae and Five Enteric Strains of Gram Negative Bacilli. J. Clin. Investigation, 28:867, 1949.

Fothergill, L. D., and Wright, J.: Influenzal Meningitis; Relation of Age Incidence to Bactericidal Power of Blood against Causal Organisms. J. Immunol., 24:273, 1933.

Jordan, E. O., Epidemic Influenza. Chicago, American Medical Association, 1927.

Lemierre, A., Meyer, A., and Laplane, R.: Les septicémies à bacille de Pfeiffer. Ann. de méd., 39: 97, 1936.

Pittman, M.: Variation and Type Specificity in Bacterial Species Hemophilus influenzae. J. Exper. Med., 53:471, 1931.

HEMOPHILUS DUCREYI INFECTIONS

(Chancroid)

Hemophilus ducreyi was first described by Ducrey in 1889 in stained purulent material from soft chancres as minute gram-negative bacilli, 1 to 2 microns in length, arranged in pairs, chains or "fish school" formations. The microorganism cannot be cultivated on ordinary media. By special methods, however, growth of *H. ducreyi* is usually obtained from pus derived from infected patients, provided that the lesion is not grossly contaminated by secondary invaders. Typical morphology on stained smear and characteristic growth are accepted by some as adequate evidence for diagnosis of *H. ducreyi* as the etiologic agent. Others require in addition a positive skin test, autoinoculations by rubbing the lesion fluid into the scarified skin of the forearm, and typical histologic changes on biopsy. The reliability of any one of these tests for diagnosis in a particular patient is open to question. The presence of characteristic clinical features, and exclusion of syphilis, lymphogranuloma venereum, granuloma inguinale and herpetic infections, by specific laboratory tests, are necessary prerequisites for diagnosis of *H. ducreyi* as the causative agent.

H. ducreyi infection has assumed an important role as a venereal disease in the southern part of this country and in tropical regions of the world. During World War I about 10 per cent of all chancres were caused by *H. ducreyi*. Soft chancre, or chancroid, produced by *H. ducreyi* has a characteristic clinical appearance and history. After an incubation period of two to fourteen days following sexual intercourse, there appears a small red papule, on the genitals or surrounding skin, which in a period of a few days goes through a purulent and then necrotic stage followed by ulceration. The ulcer is characterized by surrounding erythema and edema and by edges which become irregularly undermined. The induration which is typical of the syphilitic chancre is absent in chancroid. The lesions produced by *H. ducreyi* are frequently multiple as the result of autoinoculation. When untreated, abscesses of the inguinal lymph nodes follow and are associated with constitutional signs.

Sulfonamides are effective treatment for *H. ducreyi* lesions; the tetracyclines, streptomycin and chloramphenicol have also been used with success. However, as each of the latter agents shows some action against *Treponema pallidum,* their use is contraindicated unless the lesion proves resistant to sulfonamides and daily darkfield examinations on four successive days fail to demonstrate *Treponema pallidum*.

H. E. ALEXANDER

References

Dienst, R. B.: New Preparation of Antigen for Intracutaneous Diagnosis of Chancroidal Infection. Am. J. Syph., Gonor. & Ven. Dis., 26:201, 1942.

Ducrey, A.: Recherches expérimentales sur la nature intime du principe contagieux du chancre mou. Ann. de dermat. et syph. 3e Sér., 1:56, 1890.

Greenwald, E.: Chancroidal Infection: Treatment and Diagnosis. J.A.M.A., 121:9, 1943.

Heyman, A., Beeson, P. B., and Sheldon, W. H.: Diagnosis of Chancroid; Relative Efficiency of Biopsies, Cultures, Smears, Autoinoculations and Skin Tests. J.A.M.A., 129:935, 1945.

Satulsky, E. M.: Management of Chancroid in a Tropical Theater; Report of 1,555 Cases. J.A.M.A., 127:259, 1945.

Taggart, S. R., and others: The Treatment of Chancroid with Streptomycin. Am. J. Syph., Gonor. & Ven. Dis. 33:180, 1949.

Willcox, R. R.: Aureomycin and Chloramphenicol in Chancroid. Brit. M. J., 1:509, 1951.

Zheutlin, H. E. C., and Robinson, R. C. V.: Aureomycin in Treatment of Chancroid; Report of 3 Cases. Am. J. Syph., Gonor. & Ven. Dis., 34:71, 1950.

DIPHTHERIA

Definition. Diphtheria is an acute infectious disease caused by a bacillus, *Corynebacterium diphtheriae*. The primary lesion is usually located in the pharyngeal area (fauces, nasopharynx or larynx) and is characterized by the formation of a grayish pseudomembrane. The organism elaborates a specific soluble exotoxin which is responsible for the local cellular injury and the systemic manifestations of the disease.

History. Although a diphtheria-like disease was described by medical writers as early as the second century A.D., diphtheria was first established as a clinical entity by the publication of Pierre Bretonneau's classical monograph in 1826. In 1883 Klebs described the diphtheria bacillus; a year later Loeffler demonstrated its etiologic relationship to the disease, and in 1888 Roux and Yersin clarified the pathogenesis of the disease by their discovery of the specific exotoxin. The first effective antitoxin was produced by von Behring in 1890. Schick introduced his skin test for determining susceptibility in 1913. Active immunization, first introduced by Theobald Smith and by von Behring, received its greatest impetus from Ramon's demonstration in 1923 that formalin-treated toxin (i.e., toxoid) represented a nontoxic, antigenically effective immunizing agent.

Etiology. The causative agent of diphtheria, *Corynebacterium diphtheriae,* is a gram-positive, nonmotile, nonsporulating bacillus which is characteristically club-shaped and frequently beaded in appearance. In stained smears the organisms are usually found arranged so as to form sharp angles with each other, giving the characteristic Chinese letter appearance. Diphtheria bacilli grow well on ordinary laboratory media containing "peptones" or tissue extracts. The commonest media used are Loeffler's coagulated blood serum and potassium tellurite agar. Virulent diphtheria bacilli are distinguished by the ability to elaborate and secrete a specific poisonous substance, diphtheria toxin, which is a true exotoxin. It is the cause of the tissue necrosis occurring in the course of the clinical disease. Chemically it is a complex protein but the mechanism of its action is obscure. So-called nonvirulent strains of C. *diphtheriae* fail to produce this toxin. Three types of C. *diphtheriae* are recognized, largely on the basis of their characteristic colonial formation on potassium tellurite medium and their distinctive fermentation reactions. All three types, *gravis, mitis* and *intermedius,* produce the same toxin and the same clinical picture. The weight of evidence at the moment suggests that *gravis* strains are found associated most frequently with epidemic diphtheria, and *mitis* and *intermedius* strains with the endemic disease.

Geographic Distribution and Incidence. Although diphtheritic infections occur throughout the world, the clinical disease is recognized more frequently in the temperate zones as compared to the tropics. During the last half of the nineteenth century diphtheria occurred in epidemic form in both Western Europe and the United States. Since approximately 1890 there has been a marked downward trend in the incidence of the disease in these areas. Although the introduction of active immunization on a broad scale in recent years has increased this trend, it seems obvious that other factors as well are playing a significant role in this steady decline. During World War II there was a sharp increase in the amount of diphtheria experienced by the occupied countries of Northwestern Europe, and smaller increases were noted in certain neutral countries and in the United States. Following the cessation of hostilities the incidence rates fell to their prewar levels. In the United States, 2960 cases with 217 deaths were reported in 1952, giving an incidence rate of 1.9 per 100,000 and a case fatality rate of 7.3 per cent. The disease occurs most commonly during the fall and winter months; unimmunized children under 5 years of age are particularly at risk.

Epidemiology and Immunity. *Corynebacterium diphtheria* is essentially an obligate parasite of man; hence the human host represents the only significant reservoir of diphtheritic infections. The organism may be transmitted directly or indirectly from one person to another. As the usual habitat of the organism is the upper respiratory tract, droplet infection is probably the commonest method of spread although contamination of the hands, handkerchiefs and similar objects may play an important role. Discharges from extrarespiratory sites of infection (such as superficial ulcers of the skin) are infectious. Although the organism may survive for a brief period outside the human body, spread of infection by contaminated dust appears to be a rare occurrence. A few milk-borne outbreaks have been reported.

Invasion and infection of the human body by the diphtheria bacillus is not always followed by the development of clinical disease. More frequently the organism multiplies in the mucous membrane linings of the air passages for a shorter or longer period without causing signs of illness. Presumably in such a case the "carrier" possesses a pre-existing immunity of greater or lesser degree, which, although it does not prevent the actual implantation of the organism, does limit the amount of damage to the host's cells so markedly that no clinical manifestations develop.

Immunity against the clinical disease depends primarily upon the presence of antitoxin in the blood of the infected person. Although it is probable that upon occasion antibacterial mechanisms play a role in preventing the diphtheria bacillus from actually establishing itself in the throat of the human subject, nothing is known concerning the nature or specificity of the reaction. On the other hand, recovery from an attack of clinical diphtheria is associated with the appearance of appreciable amounts of antitoxin in the blood.

This antitoxin is formed in response to the direct stimulation of diphtheria toxin. It has the characteristics of a true antibody: it may be formed in response to either clinical or subclinical infection or as a result of artificial active immunization; although it is produced relatively slowly in response to the primary stimulation, it appears rapidly and in large amounts following secondary stimuli, even though little or no antitoxin can be demonstrated at the time of the secondary stimulation; it may be transferred to other persons (naturally by transplacental passage *in utero,* artificially by transfusion) thereby conferring temporary passive immunity upon the recipient.

Schick Test. Although the accurate determination of antitoxin levels is a laboratory procedure, the Schick test will usually yield valuable information concerning the immune status of an individual. This test is performed by injecting into the skin of the forearm 0.1 ml. of diluted diphtheria toxin. A positive reaction is characterized by the development of a variable area of redness at the site of inoculation over a period of 72 to 120 hours. The reaction reaches its height on about the fifth day; after this it gradually fades, leaving an area of brownish pigmentation which may persist for some weeks. Such a positive reaction is associated with an antitoxin level in the circulating blood of less than 0.03 units of antitoxin per milliliter, and is interpreted to mean that the patient is susceptible to the clinical disease. A negative Schick reaction signifies that the blood antitoxin level exceeds 0.03 units per milliliter, and that the subject's chances of contracting clinical diphtheria are comparatively slight. The occasional negative reactor who does develop clinical illness usually has a mild attack.

In actual practice the diluted toxin is injected in one forearm while the other forearm is injected with a similar amount of the same material which, however, has been heated to 60° C. for 30 minutes in order to destroy the toxin. This control is necessary in order to detect *pseudo-Schick reactions,* reactions due to products of growth of the diphtheria bacillus other than the toxin itself. The pseudo-Schick reaction is characterized by the development of erythema at the site of inoculation about 18 hours after injection. This increases to reach its maximum intensity at 24 to 36 hours, and then fades gradually to disappear completely within the next 72 hours. Such a reaction connotes allergy to some component of the injected material rather than absence of circulating antitoxin in quantities adequate to confer immunity. Thus, four types of reaction are possible as is indicated in the accompanying table.

Babies born to immune mothers will give negative Schick reactions at birth, owing to the transplacental transfer of antitoxin. This passive immunity wears off rapidly, and by the sixth month in the absence of artificial immunization nearly all infants are susceptible to the disease as evidenced by the demonstration of a positive Schick reaction. From this point on there is a gradual rise in the proportion of persons giving Schick-negative reactions as a result of natural im-

Reactions to Schick Test

TYPE OF REACTION	OBSERVATION				INTERPRETATION	
	Test 36 hr.	Test 120 hr.	Arm Control Arm 36 hr.	Arm Control Arm 120 hr.	Immunity	Sensitivity
Positive	−	+	−	−	Absent	Absent
Negative	−	−	−	−	Present	Absent
Pseudo	+	−	+	−	Present	Present
Combined	+	+	+	−	Absent	Present

munization usually following subclinical infection. In the absence of continued contacts with the diphtheria bacillus, the antitoxin level falls to a point where the individual is again susceptible to the disease.

Pathogenesis and Pathologic Physiology. The usual habitat of the diphtheria bacillus is the upper respiratory tract of man. In a susceptible individual the organism multiplies in the superficial epithelial cells of the pharynx, elaborating and secreting the specific toxin in the process. The absorption of this toxin by neighboring cells initiates a process of tissue necrosis, which furnishes conditions favorable to the growth of the organism which in turn produces more of the toxin. As the process continues it stimulates an inflammatory reaction on the part of the body, leading to the formation of the typical diphtheritic membrane. The absorption of toxin into the general circulation results in a degree of prostration usually out of proportion to the relatively mild appearance of the local lesion at this stage. If the membrane involves the larynx and trachea, either primarily or secondarily, mechanical obstruction to the airway may develop, and death due to suffocation may occur unless the oxygen lack is corrected by intubation or tracheotomy. The soluble toxin is carried in the general circulation to susceptible organs such as the heart and cranial or peripheral nerves. Cardiac failure may be the result of specific necrotic injury to the myocardium or it may be secondary to peripheral circulatory disturbances. The cranial or peripheral nerve involvement is presumably due to the direct action of the toxin on the nerve cells. The explanation of the relatively selective action of the toxin remains obscure.

Aside from the striking picture of the local lesion, the pathologic changes noted in fatal cases of diphtheria are relatively nonspecific. Grossly the heart, liver, kidneys and adrenal glands may show degenerative changes characterized microscopically by necrosis, fatty infiltration and parenchymatous degeneration.

Clinical Manifestations. Diphtheria is characterized by a relatively short incubation period—one to four days on the average with an outside limit of one week. The clinical manifestations depend *first* upon the severity of the process (which may show every gradation between a mild, nearly inapparent infection and a highly malignant progressive one), and *second* upon the anatomic location of the primary lesion. The more important clinical types are faucial (or tonsillar), nasopharyngeal and laryngeal. Extrarespiratory forms of the disease such as ocular, aural and cutaneous diphtheria do occur but in general are of less importance.

In *faucial diphtheria* the process is limited essentially to the tonsillar area. The onset is abrupt and is characterized by moderate fever, chilliness, general malaise and mild sore throat. Swallowing is relatively painless. The pharynx is moderately injected and dull red in appearance. The pseudo-membrane first appears as a thick gelatinous exudate confined to one tonsil. This spreads to the other tonsil and thickens up so as to give the typical dirty white or grayish yellow diphtheritic membrane. If the pseudo-membrane is forcibly removed a raw, bleeding surface is exposed beneath, over which the membrane rapidly forms anew. Tonsillar swelling is usually present and frequently there is some enlargement of the cervical lymph nodes. If the tonsils are absent the membrane may be less characteristic. Often the process spreads to involve the uvula and soft palate which become edematous. If the process remains limited to the tonsillar area, the clinical manifestations may be so mild that a definite diagnosis can be made only by isolation of the organism.

Nasopharyngeal diphtheria represents a spread of the original process from the faucial area to the uvula, soft palate, posterior pharyngeal wall and nasal mucosa. The membrane covering these areas presents a dirty yellow appearance; in some instances it invades the anterior nares and actually protrudes through the external opening. Occasionally the middle ear may be invaded as well. Faucial edema is marked and there is usually a sero-sanguineous nasal discharge. Enlargement of the cervical lymph nodes is almost invariably present; the swelling may be so marked as to deserve the name "bullneck." A characteristic diphtheritic odor is usually present as well as pallor and cyanosis. Marked toxemia is the rule, and the patient is almost always prostrated. Oliguria, albuminuria, weak, rapid pulse and high fever are prominent features. If recovery ensues, sequelae are common. This form of the disease should not be confused with anterior nasal diphtheria, in which the disease process is limited to the anterior nares. This latter is a relatively benign process with minimal toxemia, and its importance is chiefly epidemiologic rather than clinical.

Laryngeal diphtheria usually results from the spread of infection downward from the nasopharynx, although the primary lesion may be in the larynx itself. It is a particularly dangerous form of the disease, since the membrane and accompanying edema produce mechanical obstruction of the airway, giving rise to the classic diphtheritic croup. The first symptoms are hoarseness, dyspnea and a characteristic brassy cough. As the obstruction increases, dyspnea becomes more marked and ultimately cyanosis appears together with aphonia and expiratory and inspiratory stridor. As bronchial secretions accumulate behind the obstruction the accessory muscles of respiration are brought into play, and the spasmodic attacks of severe dyspnea gradually become frequent and persistent. Unless the airway is restored by intubation or tracheotomy, death by suffocation ensues. Rarely the process involves the bronchial tree as well.

Extrarespiratory Diphtheria. Although diphtheria is usually a disease of the upper respiratory tract, other parts of the body may be the site of primary or secondary diphtheritic lesions. Thus, wounds, sores and abrasions of the skin may become secondarily infected. During World War II a number of skin infections occurred among men serving in the tropics. These took the form of chronic, nonhealing ulcers which developed at the site of minor abrasions. In the course of time a dirty grayish membrane appeared. The majority of these infections yielded *mitis* strains on culture. The relatively low percentage of sequelae suggests that the absorption of toxin from such wounds was not marked, while the fact that antitoxin usually gave disappointing results raises the possibility that these so-called "tropical sores" had a complex etiology.

Ocular diphtheria is a rare form of the disease; the conjunctivae are chiefly involved.

Diagnosis. The *presumptive diagnosis* of

diphtheria must be made on clinical grounds without waiting for laboratory confirmation, since the importance of early specific therapy of the disease is so paramount. The cardinal features pointing to the diagnosis are: (1) a comparatively painless pharyngitis involving the tonsils (or tonsillar beds) and frequently the uvula and soft palate as well; (2) a relative lack of redness in spite of the presence of a significant degree of edema; (3) the appearance of the characteristic membrane in the tonsillar area; and (4) moderate pyrexia. In severe cases, significant systemic manifestations occur; in mild cases, however, the patient may feel well throughout while the throat may appear comparatively innocuous.

The *laboratory diagnosis* depends upon the isolation and identification of the causative organism from the lesion. The throat or wound swab should be taken by an experienced person and sent to the laboratory without delay. Here a Loeffler's slant, a tellurite plate and a blood agar plate should be inoculated promptly. Although experienced workers can recognize the organism in a fair percentage of cases by smears made directly from the wound or throat swab, this procedure is not recommended for the average laboratory. The inoculated cultures may be inspected at the end of 16 to 24 hours and a presumptive diagnosis made on the basis of characteristic colony formation and cellular morphology. Confirmatory evidence may be obtained by a study of fermentation reactions, and whenever indicated, virulence tests should be carried out. Other laboratory findings include a moderate leukocytosis and a transient albuminuria in all but the mildest cases.

Streptococcal tonsillitis and pharyngitis are most often confused with diphtheria. In the former conditions the throat is usually a fiery red, the tonsillar exudate thinner and lighter colored, the fever higher and swallowing is markedly painful. Frequently the follicles in the faucial area are quite prominent. Upon occasion it may be impossible to differentiate the two infections without resort to laboratory means. Rarely a concomitant streptococcal infection may mask the underlying diphtheritic process. Other conditions which must be considered in the differential diagnosis are *Vincent's angina, agranulocytic angina, infectious mononucleosis* and *posttonsillectomy throat.*

Complications. The most important complications are related to the *myocardium* and the *nervous system.* Signs of myocarditis may appear as early as the second week of the disease, although the usual time of onset is somewhat later. They are characteristically associated with the severer forms of respiratory diphtheria. In general, those cases showing early myocardial involvement tend to run a graver course. The onset may be insidious, with rising pulse of poor quality, distant heart sounds, premature contractions and gradual cardiac enlargement. Less often cardiac failure may appear with little warning. Pallor, epigastric pain, vomiting and circulatory collapse are the usual signs and symptoms. Inversion of the T waves, delayed conduction time, bundle branch block and terminally ventricular flutter or fibrillation are the commonest electrocardiographic changes noted. Occasionally peripheral circulatory collapse occurs in the absence of demonstrable cardiac damage. Recovery, when it takes place, is usually complete.

Postdiphtheritic paralysis affecting the cranial or peripheral nerves is a relatively frequent complication. The commonest form of cranial nerve palsy is *paralysis of the soft palate.* This makes its appearance in the third to fifth week of the disease, and is ushered in by the development of a nasal twang to the voice and regurgitation of fluid through the nose upon attempted swallowing. Although the course is usually mild, occasionally tube feeding may be required. The condition tends to clear up completely in the course of a week or ten days. *Ocular paralysis* may occur in the fourth to sixth week of the disease. The two commonest types are *oculomotor,* affecting the external rectus of one or both sides, thus resulting in a convergent squint, and *ciliary,* in which the power of accommodation is weakened or lost. Spontaneous recovery in the course of a week is the general rule. Rarer forms of cranial nerve palsies are *facial, pharyngeal* and *laryngeal* paralysis. The prognosis in these forms is good unless there is concomitant involvement of the respiratory muscles.

Paralysis of the peripheral nerves appears somewhat later than do the cranial nerve palsies; the usual time of occurrence for the former is between the fifth and eighth week of the disease. The commonest form is a polyneuritis of the lower extremities, as evidenced by weakness or paralysis of certain muscle groups. Total loss of function is rare and sensation is unimpaired. Complete recovery over a period of a few weeks is the general rule. Less commonly the upper extremities, the neck and the trunk may be involved. Again, in general the prognosis is good; if, however, the intercostal muscles are involved there is danger of serious respiratory embarrassment, particularly in the presence of diaphragmatic weakness or paralysis.

Treatment. The prompt administration of diphtheria antitoxin in adequate amounts is the first and most important step. Laboratory studies and clinical experience have demonstrated the importance of administering antitoxin as early as possible in the course of the disease. Presumably, the union between toxin and cell is a stable one which cannot be broken down by any practicable amount of antitoxin; the role of the latter is confined therefore to neutralizing unbound toxin circulating in the blood stream and other body fluids, thereby protecting the undamaged cells which have not come into intimate contact with the toxin as yet. Antitoxin should be administered as soon as diphtheria is suspected on clinical grounds without waiting for confirmation from the laboratory. Attainment of the early treatment of the actual case of diphtheria is well worth the price of administering antitoxin unnecessarily to an occasional individual. In a severe case of diphtheria the prognosis depends largely upon how early an adequate amount of antitoxin can be administered.

There is no agreement among clinicians as to the amount of antitoxin that should be administered. A conservative scheme calls for 10,000 to 20,000 units for mild cases, 25,000 to 50,000 units for moderate cases and 50,000 to 100,000 units for severe cases. These figures are for the average adult, but in actual practice age and weight are not often taken into account except among the very young. The total dose required should be administered at one occasion if possible. The route of administration may be intramuscular or intravenous. The latter route has the advantage of speedier absorption but in theory gives a greater risk of an overwhelming anaphylactic reaction. In general, the intramuscular route is preferred for doses up to 20,000 units and the intravenous route for amounts above this. The subcutaneous route should not be used, since absorption is relatively slow.

As diphtheria antitoxin is a foreign protein (horse serum), precautions should be observed against the occurrence of hypersensitivity reactions (i.e., anaphylaxis). These are (1)

inquiry of the patient or of his family as regards a history of sensitivity to horses (or horse products such as dander, etc.) or of previous exposure to horse serum, and (2) performance of ophthalmic and intradermal sensitivity tests. In both tests a 1:10 dilution of antitoxin in saline is used. In the first method one drop of this dilution is dropped into the conjunctival sac, and the eye is observed for the development of redness during the next 30 minutes. In the second method, 0.1 ml. of the 1:10 dilution is injected intracutaneously in the forearm, and the area is observed for the development of erythema, wheals, and similar reactions for the next half hour. If a positive reaction is obtained by either method it is prima facie evidence of sensitivity to the horse serum, and hence antitoxin should be administered with caution. Desensitization is carried out by giving small doses of highly diluted antitoxin by the subcutaneous route at first and then gradually working up to the intramuscular and intravenous routes until the full dose has been given. Desensitization may be a tedious and nerve-racking task, but as antitoxin is the only specific therapeutic weapon available it is a process which must be carried out in cases in which sensitivity exists. Epinephrine must be at hand before antitoxin is administered by any route.

Since diphtheria bacilli are susceptible to the action of penicillin *in vitro,* there has been an understandable tendency toward the routine administration of penicillin to all cases of diphtheria. Although it has been shown that penicillin in daily doses of 240,000 units helps to eliminate the causative organisms from the nasopharynx, the drug has no neutralizing effect upon the toxin. Penicillin finds its chief value in the prevention of secondary infections and in the treatment of the chronic carrier.

General Management. Complete bed rest is the first requirement. The period over which this should be maintained depends upon the degree of toxemia and the presence or absence of cardiac complications. In any event the return to activity should be gradual and guided by the careful observations of the physician. Local therapy of the throat is rarely needed in the absence of secondary infection, although hot saline irrigations may be comforting. Dehydration should be treated with parenteral fluids containing dextrose. Careful watch must be kept for signs of developing cardiac or neurologic complications.

In these, adequate rest is also the keynote of expectant therapy. Digitalis appears to be without benefit in the treatment of cardiac complications. The patient should be kept isolated until two successive daily cultures are negative for the presence of virulent diphtheria bacilli.

Prevention. *Active immunization* represents the basic means at hand with which to control the occurrence of clinical diphtheria. Of the various preparations available, two, fluid toxoid and alum-precipitated toxoid, are the most widely used in the United States. Both preparations consist of a filtrate of a broth culture of diphtheria bacilli (i.e., diphtheria toxin) which has been treated with 0.3 to 0.5 per cent formalin at a temperature of 37° C. until toxicity has disappeared. The resulting fluid toxoid is given in a primary course consisting of three injections (0.5 ml., 1.0 ml., 1.0 ml.) at weekly intervals. If suitable amounts of alum are added to the fluid toxoid, a precipitate forms. This alum-precipitated toxoid may be resuspended giving a relatively purified immunizing preparation with a slightly superior antigenic potency because of a local stimulating effect of the alum on the tissues. A primary course consists of two 1 ml. injections spaced a month apart. Against this obvious advantage must be weighed the fact that the greater sensitizing ability of the alum-precipitated toxoid may lead to unpleasant reactions upon subsequent reinjection. In addition, a sterile abscess occasionally develops at the inoculation site as a result of the irritating action of the alum. Both fluid and alum-precipitated toxoid are excellent immunizing agents; at least 85 per cent of individuals receiving a primary course may be expected to become Schick-negative.

The primary course of active immunization should be administered within the first year of life, preferably at about the third month. It may be combined with immunizations against tetanus and pertussis. One stimulating dose should be administered two years later and another at the time the child enters school. In the case of susceptible older children or adults, the possibility of a sensitivity reaction to the toxoid should be guarded against by the prior administration of 0.1 ml. of a 1:10 dilution of fluid toxoid intradermally (the *Moloney test*). The development of a local reaction (best described as a severe pseudo-Schick reaction) is warning that toxoid must be administered cautiously in multiple, small, suitably diluted doses. These reactions, fortunately almost unknown before adolescence, represent the great problem in immunizing adult population groups. Presumably they represent some degree of immunity, and the mere carrying out of a Moloney test in a person giving a positive reaction may serve as an adequate antigenic booster.

Passive immunization is possible since the administration of relatively small amounts of antitoxin (1000 units) will confer protection for a period of two to three weeks. Because of the danger of inducing sensitization or of eliciting anaphylactic shock in a person already sensitized to the foreign protein, its use should be limited to immunization of persons peculiarly at risk of infection, as for example in the case of nonimmunized children heavily exposed to virulent diphtheria bacilli. Inasmuch as the protection conferred by antitoxin is of such short duration, active immunization with one of the toxoid preparations should be carried out at the same time.

In the event of an outbreak of diphtheria in a closed community (such as a school), the exposed persons should be observed closely in order that antitoxin may be administered at the first sign of suspicious illness. Routine throat cultures usually yield little information of practical value. The exposed persons should be given Schick and Moloney tests and those found susceptible and not sensitive should be immunized promptly with one of the toxoid preparations. Under special circumstances the administration of prophylactic antitoxin may be indicated.

F. S. CHEEVER

References

von Behring, E.: Zur Behandlung der Diphtherie mit Diphtherieheilserum. Deutsche med. Wchnschr., 19:543, 1893.

Dudley, S. F.: Schick's Test and Its Application. A Critical Review. Quart. J. Med., 22:321, 1929.

Frost, W. H.: Infection, Immunity and Disease in the Epidemiology of Diphtheria, with Special Reference to Some Studies in Baltimore. J. Prev. Med., 2:325, 1928. (Reprinted in Maxcy, K. F., ed.: Papers of Wade Hampton Frost. New York, The Commonwealth Fund, 1941, pp. 447–466.)

Holmes, W. H.: Bacillary and Rickettsial Infections. New York, The Macmillan Company, 1944, Chapters 18–20 inclusive.

McLeod, J. W.: The Types Mitis, Intermedius and Gravis of Corynebacterium diphtheriae. Bact. Rev., 7:1, 1943.

Mueller, J. H.: The Diphtheria Bacilli and Diph-

theroids, in Dubos, R. J. ed.: Bacterial and Mycotic Infections of Man. 2nd ed. Philadelphia, J.
B. Lippincott Company, 1952, Chap. 9.

Schick, B.: Die Diphtherietoxin-Hautreaktion des
Menschen als Vorprobe der prophylaktischen
Diphtherieheilseruminjektion. München. med.
Wchnschr., 60:2608, 1913.

Semple, R. H. (Translator): Memoirs on Diphtheria
from the writings of Bretonneau, Guersant, Trousseau, Bouchat, Empis and Davoit. London, The
New Sydenham Society, 1859.

Weinstein, L.: The Treatment of Acute Diphtheria
and the Chronic Carrier State with Penicillin.
Am. J. Sc., 213:508, 1947.

Worcester, Jane, and Cheever, F. S.: The Schick
Status of 18,000 Young Adult Males. New England J. Med., 240:954, 1949.

CLOSTRIDIUM INFECTIONS

General Considerations. The clostridia, that is the anaerobic gram-positive spore-bearing bacilli, are so widely distributed in nature—in soil and garbage, in dust of all kinds and in the intestinal tracts of most animals—that they are frequently found in pathologic lesions. Although, as might be expected, they are particularly common in open wounds, where they may produce various severe infections, these organisms can, under suitable circumstances, attack almost any tissue of the body. Nevertheless, their mere presence in a lesion is of little significance, for the clostridia require special and delicately adjusted environmental conditions before they can produce manifestations of disease. In other words, and this cannot be too strongly emphasized, the clostridial infections of man are *clinical* and not *bacteriologic* entities.

This fact has given rise to some difficulty in assessing the relationship of these organisms to disease, but, in a broad way, the many and varied pathologic conditions due to the clostridia may be divided into two main groups: *neurotoxic,* which includes botulism and tetanus, and *histotoxic,* in which various tissues of the body, particularly the muscles, are invaded and destroyed. Although it is primarily the histotoxic infections of man with which this section is concerned, it should be pointed out that simultaneous infections with both histotoxic and neurotoxic clostridia can occur. Thus, particularly in war time, the association of gas gangrene and tetanus is not uncommon. *Cl. botulinum* has also been recovered from infected wounds and on at least three occasions has produced a fatal and clinically typical infection in this way. Finally, it should be mentioned that in addition to infection of traumatized tissues, one species, *Cl. perfringens,* has been implicated in the syndrome of acute gastrointestinal disease.

HISTOTOXIC INFECTIONS

GAS GANGRENE

Of the many different species of clostridia, only a small number are truly histotoxic and capable, on their own, of initiating severe and frequently fatal infections. Of this limited group of organisms the most important are *Clostridium perfringens, Cl. novyi, Cl. septicum, Cl. histolyticum* and *Cl. bifermentans* (*sordellii*).

Toxin Production. All of these species of Clostridia owe their pathogenic powers to the production of one or more potent exotoxins. These exotoxins are among the most powerful poisons known and are (with one minor and unimportant exception) entirely species-specific. This point is of considerable practical importance in that the antitoxin prepared against *Cl. perfringens* is quite useless in combating an infection with *Cl. novyi.* Moreover, all the clostridia mentioned probably produce several different toxins; *Cl. perfringens* elaborates no less than twelve, *Cl. novyi* at least six and *Cl. histolyticum* three, and there can be little doubt that more toxins remain to be discovered. However, it is fortunate from a practical point of view that in any one species there appears to be but one single toxin of overriding importance in the genesis and progression of the disease, and it is against this toxin that the appropriate antiserum is prepared. It should be mentioned here that a classification of *Cl. perfringens* and *Cl. novyi* into subspecies has been made in recent years on the basis of the various toxins produced or the different combinations of the same toxins: thus six types of *Cl. perfringens,* A, B, C, D, E and F, and three types of *Cl. novyi,* A, B and C, are now recognized. So far as human infections are concerned, only *Cl. perfringens,* types A and F, and *Cl. novyi,* types A and B, are of interest to us. Finally, it must be pointed out that certain of these toxins, including some of great importance, have been shown to be enzymes and that their specific substrates have been identified. This, of course, is a discovery of the greatest importance, not only for our understanding of clostridial infections, but for our investigation of disease processes in general.

Mechanism of Production of Gas Gangrene. It has already been stated that clostridia require special environmental conditions within the host before they can produce their pathologic effects—indeed, before they can even grow. Although it is known in a broad way what these essential factors are, detailed knowledge of this complex problem is still meager. The fundamental point to be borne in mind is that all these organisms are strictly anaerobic and will grow and produce their toxins only under conditions of markedly reduced oxygen tension. In the animal body such conditions may be achieved by various means: the prolonged application of a tourniquet, the pressure of a tight plaster, slight trauma, the presence of necrotic tissue in a wound, the occurrence of foreign bodies, such as earth, shell fragments or clothing, and even necrotizing lesions due to aerobic organisms. Any of these situations is sufficient to permit germination of clostridial spores, the multiplication of the clostridia and the elaboration of toxins. Once the toxins have been produced, the process is relatively simple. The toxin diffuses out into the surrounding tissues, kills them, and so permits the organisms themselves to spread into new areas of reduced oxidation-reduction potential. There the process is repeated, and so the disease continues to spread, gaining momentum and severity as it progresses.

That is the process in broad outline; of the details we are far less certain. In the case of *Cl. perfringens*, the organism most studied, it seems clear that the alpha toxin is the element of prime importance. This has been shown to be a *lecithinase*, which can readily kill tissue cells by attacking the lecithin present in the cell wall. Diffusion through the entire infected area is aided by the production of a *collagenase*, a *hyaluronidase* and a *fibrinolysin,* each of which can break down certain of the binding elements in the tissues. Although fully toxigenic strains of clostridia may be found multiplying in the depths of many wounds, only when these organisms invade muscle tissue do they become really dangerous. The reason for this anomaly is far from being understood, though various hypotheses have been advanced in recent years. Indeed, we are as yet uncertain of the ultimate cause of death in gas gangrene.

Destruction of muscle tissue should not in itself be fatal, yet it may be safely said that every untreated patient with gas gangrene will surely die. For this reason it has generally been assumed that death has been due to the toxins gaining access to the blood stream and then lodging in various ill defined "vital centers." There is little evidence of such a process, and it has been suggested that the lesion is essentially a local one, analogous to the "crush syndrome" and similar sterile destructive lesions of muscle. Final proof of this thesis is lacking.

Pathologic and Clinical Features. Pathogenic clostridia may be found in any traumatic lesion, but so far as man is concerned, three main types of infections may be discerned: *simple contamination, anaerobic cellulitis* and *anaerobic myositis.* However, these are not strictly circumscribed clinical entities; they are rather the most obvious stages in a continuous infectious process.

Little need be said of *simple contamination,* for in the majority of wounds the presence of clostridia is quite unsuspected on clinical grounds. In *anaerobic cellulitis,* on the other hand, the anaerobic bacteria find conditions more suited to their needs and proliferate more widely, producing gas in the tissues both by a proteolytic and a saccharolytic process. The muscles, as the name indicates, are not invaded. The condition usually develops three to six days after injury, is of gradual onset and is unaccompanied by any severe signs of systemic upset. Pain is usually absent. Indeed, by far the most obvious clinical signs are the presence of gas, foul odor and a thin, brownish seropurulent discharge.

In *anaerobic myositis,* or true gas gangrene, the process is far more acute, the reaction far more severe. The onset is sudden and usually occurs within 12 to 36 hours of wounding. The first symptom is almost invariably severe pain in the infected area; this pain progresses with the disease, disappearing only shortly before death in untreated cases. There is also a rise in the pulse and respiratory rate and a fall in the blood pressure. The temperature, apart from septicemic cases, is not as a rule much raised. Locally, one finds gross edema of the infected area and a profuse yellow or blood-stained serous discharge from the wound. This edema is frequently massive enough to mask any gas production in the tissues; indeed, gas is rarely as pronounced a feature of the disease as the name would indicate. The odor of the infection is sometimes stated to be entirely typical, but this has not been the writer's experience—both in quality and degree the smell may be variable. As the disease progresses, the skin over the infected muscles, at first pale from the edema, assumes a bronze color, which, if the patient lives long enough, may become dark purple or black and covered with dark red bullae. In the rare septicemic cases, jaundice, hemoglobinemia and hemoglobinuria develop.

In the later stage of the disease there is a condition of profound shock, frequently associated with a peculiar and distressing mental reaction. The patient is unnaturally alert, fully aware of the seriousness of his condition, and filled with terror of impending death.

It is only at operation that the changes in the infected muscles may be seen; essentially these consist of edema, loss of contractility, and discoloration, varying from increased pallor to reddening and finally to dark purple mottling. On squeezing, bubbles of gas can frequently be expressed.

Uterine infections, particularly with *Cl. perfringens,* are today probably the commonest form of gas gangrene seen in civilian practice. Usually they result from attempts at criminal abortion, but they may also occur following prolonged labor or instrumental delivery. Neither pathologically nor clinically do they differ from the classic form of the disease, with the important exception that septicemia is a far commoner complication. This is still a highly fatal type of infection, for cases which survive the acute stage frequently succumb to anuria. This anuria is due to a lower nephron nephrosis which is, presumably, of similar origin to that seen in the *"crush syndrome."* The suggestion has recently been made that all postabortal nephroses are due to *Cl. perfringens* infection, but adequate proof is lacking.

Diagnosis. The diagnosis of gas gangrene is essentially a clinical problem and rarely presents much difficulty. Indeed, it is possible that more harm has been done in the past by the too ready diagnosis of gas gangrene than by any failure to recognize it. The mere presence of clostridia in a wound is of no significance, and, in the absence of other good evidence, the presence of gas is of relatively small importance. Within limits, the more obvious and extensive the gas, the less likely is the condition to be gas gangrene. For the diagnosis of gas gangrene, much more importance should be attached to the occurrence of local pain and edema and to the general condition of the patient. As the appearance and reaction of the muscles and, indeed, of all the infected tissues varies somewhat according to the species of clostridium involved, it is, with experience, often possible to arrive at a presumptive bacteriologic diagnosis on clinical grounds alone. Various serologic tests have also been devised to this end but have not proved satisfactory. However, it is doubtful whether such refinements have much practical value.

Prevention. Prophylaxis is primarily a surgical problem. It is doubtful whether, without effective surgical cleaning of a wound, any of the newer antimicrobial agents will by themselves prevent the onset of gas gangrene, nor will the administration of gas gangrene antiserum. There is some evidence, however, that the antiserum will prolong the incubation period—a point of some importance in wartime. Much progress has been made in developing specific toxoids against some of the clostridial toxins, but their evaluation has not progressed beyond the experimental laboratory. In handling casualties, care must also be taken to avoid poor circulation, whether by the prolonged application of a tourniquet or by the use of tight plaster or bandages.

Treatment. Treatment is even more a matter for the surgeon. It can safely be said that unless all the infected tissues have been excised, there is little chance of recovery from gas gangrene, no matter what the ancillary treatment has been.

Of these secondary therapeutic measures, probably the most important is the transfusion of plasma or whole blood. Polyvalent antitoxin—active against all the organisms mentioned—should be administered intravenously with the transfused blood in doses of 100,000 International Units or more, and repeated in 8 to 12 hours if the patient's condition warrants it. Finally, some antimicrobial drug should be administered, both locally into the wound and systematically. Although many of the newer antimicrobial drugs have been used with apparent success in the treatment of individual cases of gas gangrene, none appears to be in any way superior to penicillin and this must still be regarded as the agent of choice. However, all these techniques are secondary to radical surgery.

NONTRAUMATIC CLOSTRIDIAL GASTROENTERITIS

Quite apart from these traumatic infections, it has recently been established that *Cl. perfringens* may also be involved in various gastrointestinal diseases.

The simplest of these is a mild gastroenteritis, differing in no way from food poisoning due to other bacterial species. An aberrant form of *Cl. perfringens* type A has been implicated in this condition: it has been isolated from the suspected foods, from the stools of patients and, in volunteers, has produced a similar clinical picture.

A much more severe infection is *enteritis necroticans*—the "Darmbrand" of the German writers—in which, as the name indicates, there is an acute regional gangrene of the small intestine, particularly of the jejunum. This disease first appeared in Northwest Germany towards the end of World War II and by 1946 several hundred cases were known to have occurred in this area. Today the infection has almost disappeared; however, essentially similar cases have since been reported both in England and the Americas. The exact pathology of *enteritis necroticans* is obscure, but it has been suggested, with some reason, that malnutrition may be an important predisposing cause. There can be little doubt that the exciting agent is *Cl. perfringens* type F. This organism differs from the classical type A in producing relatively little of the alpha toxin (the lecithinase), but large amounts of the beta toxin. The beta toxin, it may be added, is a hemolytic, necrotizing and lethal factor known to be of importance in various enterotoxemic diseases of domestic animals. Infection apparently occurs by the ingestion of contaminated food stuffs, of which by far the commonest have been canned or preserved fish and meat. The signs and symptoms of the disease are those of any similar acute lesion of the small intestine, so that the specific diagnosis has as a rule been made only at operation or, more commonly, at autopsy. The fatality rate is high and treatment has usually consisted of supportive measures together with the oral administration of various sulfonamide preparations. Serum therapy appears to have been of little value, but the data are insufficient for a final evaluation. Much the best results have been obtained by surgical resection of the affected areas of the gut, but for technical reasons this is not always possible.

Several reports have also been published of acute necrotizing gastritis and enteritis following total or partial gastrectomy. In many of these cases *Cl. perfringens* has been recovered in large numbers from the affected areas, but the exact relationship of the organism to the infectious process has not been fully established. The strains of *Cl. perfringens* have not been typed and the relationship (if any) of this condition to *enteritis necroticans* remains to be determined.

JOHN D. MACLENNAN

References

Clinical

Douglas, G. W., Carney, B. H., and Pellillo, D.: Postabortal Sepsis Due to *Cl. welchii.* Surg., Gynec. & Obst., 97:490, 1953.

Hobbs, Betty C., Smith, Muriel E., Oakley, C. L., Warrack, G. Harriet, and Cruickshank, J. C.: *Cl. welchii* Food Poisoning. J. Hyg., 51:75, 1953.

MacLennan, J. D.: Anaerobic Infections of War Wounds in the Middle East. Lancet, 2:63, 94, 123, 1943.

Thomas, C. G., Keleher, M. F., and McKee, A. P.: Botulism, a Complication of *Cl. botulinum* Wound Infection. A.M.A. Arch. Path., 51:623, 1951.

Zeissler, J., and Rassfeld-Sternberg, L.: Enteritis Necroticans Due to *Cl. welchii* Type F. Brit. M. J., 1:267, 1949.

Bacteriological

Smith, L. DeS.: Clostridia in Gas Gangrene. Bact. Rev., 13:233, 1949.

Toxicological

MacLennan, J. D.: Recent Advances in Bacteriology. 3rd ed. Philadelphia, The Blakiston Co., 1951.

Oakley, C. L.: The Toxins of *Cl. welchii* Type F. Brit. M. J., 1:269, 1949.

NEUROTOXIC INFECTIONS

TETANUS

Definition. Tetanus is a neuromuscular disorder, often referred to colloquially as lockjaw, which is caused by a specific exotoxin of the infectious agent, *Clostridium tetani.*

History. The disease has been recognized as a clinical entity since antiquity, especially as a sequel to wounds sustained in combat, but definitive knowledge of its nature and of means for its prevention and treatment was not acquired until the close of the nineteenth century. Nicolaier in 1884 produced tetanus by injecting animals with samples of garden soil and described a bacillus resembling *Cl. tetani* at the loci of inoculation. However, the micro-organism was not isolated in pure culture until 1889 by

Kitasato. In 1890 von Behring and Kitasato published their classic report of successful immunization by repeated small doses of toxin and the neutralization of toxin by specific antiserum; this great discovery laid the foundation for all subsequent work on immunologic methods of prophylaxis and treatment. Evidence for the central action of tetanus toxin advanced by Marie and Morax in 1902 and by Meyer and Ransom in 1903 was subsequently challenged by Abel and his associates, but recent studies by Wright and his colleagues have fortified the earlier views. Ramon was responsible for the introduction, in 1925, of tetanus toxoid for active immunization and for procedures whereby toxoid and antitoxin may be standardized.

Etiologic Agent. *Clostridium tetani* is a strict anaerobe and one of the few pathogenic microorganisms which may be identified with reasonable certainty on morphologic grounds alone. This is owing to the fact that in sporulating forms the spore is located terminally, thus giving a characteristic "drumstick" or "squash racket" appearance to the cell.

The many studies on resistance of tetanus spores to heat and chemical agents have given varying results. It may be concluded, however, that none of the antiseptic agents employed clinically can be relied on to devitalize spores, nor is simple boiling an entirely safe procedure. Autoclaving at 120° C. for 15 minutes is the best method for sterilizing potentially contaminated instruments and equipment.

Although ten distinct antigenic types of *Cl. tetani* have been recognized by differences in their flagellar antigens, all of them fortunately elaborate the same antigenic type of exotoxin which may be neutralized by a single antitoxin. The toxin has been isolated in crystalline form and is a protein with a molecular weight of approximately 67,000. Next to botulinum toxin it is the most powerful poison known, each milligram of nitrogen corresponding to about 75,000,000 guinea pig M.L.D. units. In solution the toxin is unstable and converts spontaneously to toxoid, apparently by molecular dimerization; this conversion is accelerated and driven to completion by 0.4 per cent formalin.

Epidemiology. Although tetanus is relatively uncommon the responsible agent is widely found in nature, its chief distribution being in the soil and in the gastrointestinal tract of man and a wide variety of animals. In fact, its occurrence elsewhere may be said generally to depend on contamination from either of these two sources. There seems to be little doubt that a direct relationship exists between the extent to which soil is cultivated and its degree of contamination by tetanus spores. The population density of man and animals, as well as climatic conditions, terrain and types of soil, is also an important factor. These points are exemplified by the fact that *Cl. tetani* has rarely been recovered from virgin soil or from areas of wasteland, while a high percentage of positive results has usually attended the investigation of samples from urban and agricultural communities.

Studies of the carrier rate of *Cl. tetani* in the intestinal tract of man have yielded widely divergent results but have served to show that rural inhabitants, especially farm workers, harbor the micro-organism much more frequently than do city dwellers or persons of sedentary occupation. These findings illustrate the epidemiologic significance of sanitary conditions and of contact with horses and cattle. It is of interest in this latter connection that some of the highest carrier rates have been discovered in hostlers and cavalrymen.

As might be expected from its natural habitat and general distribution, *Cl. tetani* has been frequently isolated from the surface of the human body and occasionally from the oral cavity. It exists not uncommonly in house dust and has been recovered with disturbing ease from the floors of operating rooms, where it probably was introduced by footwear. Plaster of paris and surgical dusting powders have also been found to be contaminated.

In spite of the ubiquity of the etiologic agent the incidence of tetanus is, for the most part, remarkably low. For example, during the five-year period ending in 1952 an average of approximately 500 cases were recorded annually in the United States, although doubtless many others were not reported. This represents a considerable decline in incidence over the last two decades which probably reflects the shift of population toward cities, the general improvement in medical and surgical care of injuries, and the greater use of tetanus toxoid as part of the immunization program in childhood.

Tetanus continues to be a problem of considerable magnitude in world areas where sanitation is poor, population density is high and medical services are inadequate.

Pathogenesis. It is well known that tetanus almost always results from some sort of injury, occasionally of the most trivial nature. For instance, in addition to tetanus following war wounds, highway accidents, burns and other major types of trauma, the disease has supervened after hypodermic injections, smallpox vaccination, the peck of a hen, an insect bite, and so on. In occasional cases, particularly among children, it may be impossible to determine which of several minor injuries may have been responsible, while in some patients no wound at all may be discovered.

The all-important feature of the initial event is that spores of *Cl. tetani* must be deposited, or exist already, in tissues where the conditions are properly altered to suit its exacting metabolic requirements. In general this means an area where the tissue has been devitalized and the oxidation-reduction potential is properly poised to permit multiplication and toxigenesis. The infection itself, once started, remains remarkably well localized at the original site, since the invasive powers of the micro-organism appear to be even feebler than those of *Corynebacterium diphtheriae*. This fact, incidentally, is responsible for the former advocacy, now outmoded, of local excision or even amputation as a part of treatment.

The disease proper is unquestionably caused by tetanus toxin but the mechanisms whereby it is absorbed and produces its effects are still largely unknown. The early work of Marie and Morax and of Meyer and Ransom led to the theory that the toxin acted centrally in the nervous system rather than peripherally in the affected muscles, and that it gained access to motor cells of the spinal cord by a centripetal spread via regional nerve trunks. In cases of local tetanus it was assumed that the amount of toxin released was relatively small and that involvement of the cord was confined to the anterior horn cells mediating the regional reflex arcs. It was also assumed that generalized tetanus represented a further spread of toxin by neural pathways in the cord itself to involve the motor areas more widely. These concepts were challenged by Abel and his associates in a series of papers, about 1935, in which experimental evidence was adduced that the toxin had a peripheral rather than a central action and was distributed by the blood stream rather than by nervous channels. Since then additional support for both points of view has been brought forward from various sources, but during the past few years the work of Wright and his colleagues has more and more convincingly shown the probable correctness of the first theory. This work is too extensive to be described here and the reader is therefore referred to the original references.

The mode of action of tetanus toxin is entirely unknown. No substrate for the toxin has been found, attempts to demonstrate anticholinesterase activity have given negative results, and no effect on production of acetylcholine has been clearly shown. Certain investigators have claimed that the toxin acts as an enzyme to release a hypothetical substance with strychnine-like activity, but this suggestion does not seem to deserve serious consideration.

Morbid Anatomy. Tetanus toxin fails to produce any recognizable pathologic lesions in the tissues it affects, nor do any specific changes occur at the site of infection by *Cl. tetani*. In certain cases fractures or muscle disruptions may occur as the result of tetanic spasms.

Incubation Period. The incubation period in tetanus ranges from about three days up to four weeks and, in exceptional cases, even longer. It should be stressed that the severity of tetanus and, hence, its outcome, are related to the period of incubation, cases with onset less than one week after injury having, in general, a more fulminating course. This fact should be borne in mind in anticipating the therapeutic management of patients.

It should also be noted that the incubation period may sometimes be extremely protracted, in the sense that infection may be regenerated from spores which have resided in tissues for months, or even years. A case is on record in which tetanus developed fourteen years after an original war injury, and in another *Cl. tetani* was recovered from a hysterectomy scar ten years following postoperative tetanus. Numerous accounts of shorter periods of latent infection have appeared. In traumatic surgery, especially of war wounds, reoperation at the site of earlier injury may reactivate dormant spores, and care should be taken in all such cases to ensure adequate immunologic prophylaxis beforehand.

Clinical Manifestations. Tetanus may occur in a localized form but more frequently the neuromuscular disturbance is generalized. Local tetanus is seen chiefly in persons who develop symptoms despite the prophylactic administration of antitoxin, and consists usually of persistent spasm in muscle groups near the site where the injury or wound was incurred. The spasm may last, in diminishing intensity, for several weeks. In rare cases of head injury a cephalic type of local tetanus has been described with bizarre combinations of motor phenomena, depending on the involvement of one or more cranial nerves.

More typically the onset of tetanus begins with an increase in tone of various muscle groups, often accompanied by restlessness, irritability and difficulty in swallowing. Spasm of the masseter muscles which interferes with opening the jaws (trismus) is the most common initial symptom, and its recognition should always suggest the possibility of tetanus to the physician. As the disease progresses, stiffness and rigidity of the neck, back, abdomen and extremities become more pronounced and involvement of the facial muscles may cause a grotesque grinning expression, classically referred to as *risus sardonicus*. Tonic spasms usually ensue in which the teeth are tightly clenched, the neck and back are arched (*opisthotonos*), the abdomen is taut and the extremities are rigidly extended. These spasms can be precipitated by the very slightest stimuli, such as noise, a draft of cold air, jarring of the patient's bed, sudden illumination of the room, and so on; in severe cases they recur frequently and apparently develop spontaneously. Although duration of the individual tetanic episodes is ordinarily quite short, their persistence is sometimes long enough to interfere seriously with the mechanics of respiration, thus leading to anoxia and cyanosis, and even to sudden death. However, the cause of death is usually less readily apparent and is generally attributed to exhaustion. Throughout the disease the sensorium remains clear and therefore, unfortunately, the patient may be altogether conscious of the severe pain which invariably accompanies each tetanic spasm. As a rule there is some degree of fever, with temperatures exceeding 103° F. in occasional cases, as well as elevation of the pulse and respiratory rates. In patients who recover, the signs and symptoms abate gradually after reaching their maximal intensity.

It should be noted that many variations in symptomatology may be observed, especially during onset of the disease. By way of example, the following initial manifestations have been described: fever and chilliness, headache, stiffness of gait, abdominal pain caused by muscular spasm, difficulty in swallowing, pain in the neck and back, and biting of the tongue.

Laboratory Findings. There are no laboratory procedures which are helpful in the specific diagnosis or management of tetanus. It has been suggested that electromyograms may aid in distinguishing the incipient disease from other disorders of neuromuscular function, but from the practical standpoint they are of little value. The electroencephalogram shows no abnormal changes even in fully developed cases, thus indicating that the tetanic spasms are probably not cortical in origin.

Bacteriologic examination as a means of diagnosis not only is almost worthless but also may be dangerously misleading. To isolate and accurately identify *Cl. tetani* from a wound requires a minimum of two or three days, and the microorganism cannot be recovered in a considerable proportion of cases. Moreover, although *Cl. tetani* characteristically shows a terminal spore, other terminally-spored nonpathogenic anaerobes exist and may be present as incidental contaminants. The direct microscopic examination of wound material from a suspected case of tetanus should therefore be undertaken only by an expert. It is also important to point out that *Cl. tetani* may be found among the bacterial flora of many surface infections without evidence of harm to the patient. Consequently, the chance discovery of *Cl. tetani* on routine bacteriologic study does not imply that the disease will necessarily follow.

Differential Diagnosis. Once tetanus has developed the diagnosis is usually regrettably simple, but in the early stages it may be confused with several other disorders. Local infections in the mouth may cause trismus, especially when molar teeth are involved. The diagnosis in such cases ordinarily is obvious, but the possibility of tetanus originating from such foci should always be borne in mind. Meningitis and encephalitis must also be differentiated at times, although it is rarely possible for the alert physician to be seriously misled. Trismus and muscular spasms occur in certain cases of encephalitis but characteristically the sensorium is clouded and other neurologic signs exist. In tetany the typical carpopedal spasm and absence of trismus should suffice to indicate the correct diagnosis. The writer has observed a case of hysterical trismus following a lacerated wound in a person familiar with the natural history of tetanus.

Prognosis. In severe cases of generalized tetanus the outlook is grave and the mortality rate still approximates 50 per cent despite recent advances in therapy. The unfavorable features to be stressed are a short incubation period and the rapid progression of symptoms after onset. Patients with an incubation period exceeding ten days generally have a more benign course and recover more frequently. The disease also is apt to be less dangerous and severe in cases with no evident focus of infection, and in persons who develop tetanus even though antitoxin has been given prophylactically.

Treatment. The treatment of tetanus varies widely according to the severity of the disease and the needs of the individual patient. In general, however, therapy is designed to prevent further elaboration and absorption of toxin, to control tetanic spasms and to provide supportive measures which will maintain respiration, nutrition and fluid balance.

The usual dose of antitoxin in adults is 200,000 units intravenously, to be given only after a preliminary test to determine whether the patient is hypersensitive to horse serum. If sensitivity is found to exist, desensitization by the standard method will have to be carried out before the total dose of antitoxin is administered. This amount of antitoxin should suffice to neutralize any preformed toxin which has not been absorbed as well as toxin liberated subsequently at the focus of infection; it will not affect toxin which already has been bound by nervous tissue. Local injections of antitoxin around the site of the wound or injury, totaling 10,000 to 20,000 units, may also be made although their efficacy is doubtful. The intrathecal use of antitoxin is not recommended.

Prompt surgical attention to the wounded or injured tissues is essential, with special reference to careful débridement and the removal of foreign bodies. However, it is important not to undertake these procedures until antitoxin has been given, in order that any toxin which is released by manipulation may be neutralized before it reaches the central nervous system. Penicillin should also be given, since it has been shown to eliminate *Cl. tetani* rapidly in most, but not all, cases; it also aids in controlling secondary wound infections and serves as a prophylactic agent against the otherwise common complication of pneumonia. In most instances 400,000 units of fortified procaine penicillin (sodium penicillin 100,000 units plus procaine penicillin 300,000 units) given every 12 hours will be adequate, but in some cases larger amounts of penicillin and the additional use of other antimicrobial drugs with broader antibacterial spectrums may be required.

Management of Muscular Spasm. The management of muscular spasms is of vital importance and may be extremely difficult, especially if the patient is suffering from severe, generalized tetanus. Treatment must be suited to the individual case but it is essential that continuous nursing care be provided and that a physician always be in immediate attendance. Since therapy will not actually shorten the illness, even though the course is greatly modified, it must be continued until muscular spasms and rigidity have largely disappeared. The common procedure is to combine the use of sedatives, in heavy dosage, with a muscle relaxant drug. In order to administer these agents, as well as to provide means for the intravenous administration of fluids, electrolytes and nutrients, it is advisable to place at least one indwelling needle near the wrist or ankle. Two such needles are better for plugging may occur or it may be necessary to infuse immiscible drugs simultaneously, e.g., *d*-tubocurarine and thiopental sodium (Pentothal); furthermore, the dosage of two drugs used concurrently by this route can be more accurately controlled if they are given separately. Sedation sufficient to cause loss of consciousness is usually required and thiopental sodium has generally been recommended as the drug of choice. A 2.5 per cent solution is given by vein in doses which can only be determined by the response of the patient. The objective is to cause relief of pain and spasm without dangerous depression of respiration. Since treatment must often be continued for a number of days, it is important to bear in mind that thiopental sodium has a cumulative action when administered repeatedly. In many cases phenobarbital sodium and paraldehyde, intramuscularly, will be helpful adjuncts. Tribromoethanol (Avertin) given rectally has been used but is not recommended. Chloral hydrate, also per rectum, has been employed with satisfactory results in some patients, but its irritative properties sharply limit the length of time it can be used by this route.

For muscle relaxation a number of drugs are available, and the literature is conflicting as regards their relative efficacy and the extent to which they should be employed. *Curare* and curare-like compounds have been most frequently used and probably represent the agents of choice if they are intelligently and carefully administered. Their pharmacologic effects are considered to result from a direct competition with acetylcholine which leads to a depression of excitatory action at the motor end-plate. Thus they differ markedly from drugs like mephenesin (Myanesin, Tolserol), which causes central depression of reflex activity, and from compounds producing persistent end-plate depolarization by an acetylcholine-like effect, e.g., succinylcholine. D-tubocurarine chloride may be used as a repository preparation in oil and wax containing 30 mg. per cubic centimeter. The usual initial dose is 0.5 cc. and later doses may be increased to 1.0 cc. or more depending on the response of the patient. Since the rapidity of absorption from this depot form of curare is usually slow but may vary considerably, it may be found advisable to employ *d*-tubocurarine chloride intravenously in an isotonic aqueous solution containing 3 mg. per cubic centimeter, the initial dose generally being 3 mg. for each 40 pounds of body weight. Larger amounts may be required according to the needs of the patient, but the drug must always be given under constant supervision with the knowledge that successive doses tend to show a cumulative type of effect. The respiratory difficulty sometimes observed in patients receiving curare, which results not from muscular paralysis but from bronchiolar spasm, may be controlled by antihistaminic therapy. Another compound similar to curare in its action is tri-(diethylaminoethoxy) benzene triethyliodide (*Flaxedil*), which is claimed not to cause histamine-like side reactions. The initial intravenous dose of Flaxedil is approximately 1 mg. per kilogram of body weight. If the use of a curariform compound is not desired, *mephenesin* may be given by vein in a 2 per cent solution. This drug must be diluted in isotonic glucose or saline since it readily provokes phlebitis; it is also a hemolytic agent and hemoglobinuria has been seen following its use. Mephenesin is short-acting and its dosage varies considerably, from 1 to 6 gm. being given over a one hour period. Succinylcholine, decamethonium and other muscle relaxants of a similar type are contraindicated in the treatment of tetanus because of the possible dangers that attend prolonged depolarization of the motor end-plate and adjacent areas of muscle fiber.

Tracheotomy. In all cases it is essential that provision be made for the immediate treatment of respiratory arrest and for the maintenance of the patient's airway. Cumulative experience has indicated more and more that early tracheotomy should be performed in severe cases in order to circumvent the problem created by laryngeal spasm and to permit the easy use of tracheal suction for removing secretions. In addition, tracheotomy will permit emergency oxygen therapy under intermittent positive pressure, using the apparatus described by Harris and her associates. In some cases a mechanical respirator will be necessary.

Tetanic spasms are usually accompanied by profuse sweating, and throughout the illness proper attention must be devoted to maintenance of the fluid and electrolyte balance and the nutrition of the patient. In severe cases under heavy sedation a nasogastric tube may be inserted for feeding by this route, but it should be borne in mind that the use of muscle relaxant drugs also may cause relaxation of the cardiac sphincter with a tendency to regurgitation. Intravenous fluids containing glucose, balanced electrolytes and amino acids should be used as in any situation in which prolonged parenteral alimentation is required, and periodic chemical examinations of the blood should be carried out to aid in guiding this phase of therapy.

Following recovery from tetanus the patient should always be actively immunized in order to prevent possible recurrence of infection from retained spores of *Cl. tetani*. There is no evidence that the disease itself confers subsequently immunity and second attacks have been described.

Prevention. The greatest single advance in the management of tetanus has been the development of methods for specific immunization against the toxin. When such methods are properly employed the disease is almost entirely preventable. It should be emphasized that *antimicrobial drugs are not effective preventive agents and must never be used alone in tetanus prophylaxis.*

Temporary immunity may be passively transferred by the subcutaneous injection of tetanus antitoxin, the usual dose being 1500 units regardless of the age or weight of the patient. The antitoxin is actually standardized immune horse serum and can cause severe or even fatal anaphylactic reactions in persons previously sensitized or allergic to horse protein. Whenever possible, therefore, a history of earlier immunizing procedures and allergic symptoms should be carefully sought and, even when this is negative, injection must be preceded by an intradermal test with 0.01 ml. of the antiserum. Positive reactions to the test, indicating hypersensitivity, are of the immediate wheal-and-flare type, occurring within less than 15 minutes.

The great value of antitoxin was first conclusively demonstrated during World War I and today it is still the only reliable means of preventing tetanus in persons who have not been actively immunized. However, it has many shortcomings, most but not all of which result from the fact that it is a foreign protein. In addition to the hazards of its use in patients who are already allergic, a prophylactic dose of antitoxin may itself engender sensitivity to horse serum, thus creating a difficult problem if readministration becomes necessary, as well as a dangerous situation if other types of therapeutic horse antiserums should be given subsequently. The writer has seen sudden anaphylactic death in a patient who incautiously was given gas gangrene antitoxin ten days following the prophylactic use of tetanus antitoxin. Besides reactions of this sort, antitoxin may cause either general or local serum disease of varying severity; it is also responsible in rare instances for a peculiar form of peripheral neuritis, predominantly involving the brachial plexus, the mechanism of which, although not well understood, presumably has an immunologic basis. Passive immunization against tetanus also has other drawbacks, the most notable being that antitoxin obviously cannot be given after every traumatic event, while the physician has no way of predetermining when its use will be essential.

Tetanus prophylaxis is more readily and more safely achieved by active immunization with *toxoid,* which fortunately is being practiced on an ever-widening scale. Toxoid is available in two forms, fluid and alum-precipitated, the latter type being more slowly absorbed and providing a longer antigenic stimulus. Experiment has revealed in man that one injection of either toxoid causes little or no antitoxin to appear in the blood. A second injection three to four weeks later usually results in the development of measurable antitoxin equal to or exceeding 0.1 standard unit per milliliter of serum, which is generally accepted as the protective level.

A third injection after another three to six months stimulates an even more marked antibody response, and thereafter adequate amounts of circulating antitoxin can be readily maintained by booster doses at intervals of one to three years. At the time any injury is sustained that warrants tetanus prophylaxis, the individual who has completed the basic course of immunization and has continued to receive stimulating injections is merely given another dose of toxoid; antitoxin is not administered. Immunization in this manner was extraordinarily successful in preventing tetanus among the armed forces of the United States during World War II, only 6 cases occurring in the Army and 2 in the Navy among personnel who had received the basic course of injections. All these cases had short incubation periods and hence probably represented massive infections; in addition, it is possible that some of them had low serum titers of antitoxin since not all persons are good antibody formers.

It is generally recommended that children or adults be immunized by giving three subcutaneous injections of 0.5 ml. fluid toxoid at intervals of three to four weeks, or two injections of 0.5 ml. alum-precipitated toxoid four to six weeks apart. Another injection of 0.5 ml. of either toxoid should be given six months to one year later. Thereafter stimulating doses of 0.5 ml. should be administered every three years. In the event that prophylaxis becomes desirable, a stimulating injection of 0.5 ml. of *fluid* toxoid is given, since this induces a more rapid rise in antitoxin than does alum-precipitated toxoid. If a previously immunized patient has not received toxoid for more than three years, it is advisable to give both antitoxin, 1500 units, and fluid toxoid, 0.5 ml. Separate syringes must be used since mixture in the same syringe will result in partial or complete neutralization. There is experimental evidence that the combined use of antitoxin and toxoid causes an initial sharp rise in the blood level of antitoxin, provided by the passively transferred antibody, which is overlapped by a secondary sustained elevation resulting from the antigenic stimulus of the toxoid. In patients who are seriously injured, with shock, compound fractures or large, massively contaminated wounds, some authorities advocate that both antitoxin and toxoid be used regardless of the status of antecedent immunization.

Proper surgical care is also essential in

the prevention of tetanus. In all types of trauma, whether suffered in military or civilian life, the well known principles of prompt treatment, adequate débridement of wounds and the control of shock and secondary infection, are of paramount importance.

HARRY M. ROSE

References

Abel, J. J., Firor, W. M., and Chalian, W.: Researches on Tetanus, IX. Further Evidence to Show That Tetanus Toxin Is Not Carried to Central Neurons by Way of the Axis Cylinders of Motor Nerves. Bull. Johns Hopkins Hosp., 63: 373, 1938.

von Behring, E., and Kitasato, S.: Ueber das Zustandekommen der Diphtherie-Immunität und der Tetanus-Immunität bei Thieren. Deutsche med. Wchnschr., 16:1113, 1890.

Diaz-Rivera, R. S., Ramirez, E., Pons, E. R., Jr., and Torregrosa, M. V.: Management of Tetanus. J.A. M.A., 147:1635, 1951.

Edsall, G.: Immunization of Adults against Diphtheria and Tetanus. Am. J. Pub. Health, 42:393, 1952.

Harris, R. C., McDermott, T. F., and Montreuil, F. L.: The Treatment of Tetanus. Pediatrics, 2:175, 1948.

Kitasato, S.: Ueber den Tetanusbacillus. Ztschr. f. Hyg., 7:225, 1889.

Marie, A., and Morax, V.: Recherches sur l'absorption de la toxine tétanique. Ann. Inst. Past., 16: 818, 1902.

Meyer, H., and Ransom, F.: Untersuchungen über den Tetanus. Arch. f. exp. Path. u. Pharmakol., 49:369, 1903.

Miller, J. J., and Ryan, M. L.: Combined Active-Passive Re-immunization against Tetanus in Previously Immunized Individuals. J. Immunol., 65: 143, 1950.

Nicolaier, A.: Ueber infectiösen Tetanus. Deutsche med. Wchnschr., 10:842, 1884.

Ramon, G.: Sur l'anatoxine diphthérique et sur les anatoxines en général. Ann. Inst. Past., 39:1 1925.

Wright, E. A., Morgan, R. S., and Wright, G. P.: Tetanus Intoxication of the Brain Stem in Rabbits. J. Path. & Bact., 62:569, 1950.

Wright, E. A., Morgan, R. S., and Wright, G. P.: The Site of Action of the Toxin in Local Tetanus. Lancet, 2:316, 1952.

Wright, E. A.: The Effect of the Injection of Tetanus Toxin into the Central Nervous System of Rabbits. J. Immunol., 71:41, 1953.

BOTULISM

Botulism is a form of food poisoning produced by the toxins of *Clostridium botulinum*. For a description of this disease, the reader is referred to the chapter on Food Poisoning (p. 584).

SALMONELLA INFECTIONS

TYPHOID FEVER

Definition. Typhoid fever is an acute illness lasting several weeks, caused by *Salmonella typhosa* and characterized by sustained fever with headache and apathy, cough, splenomegaly, a sparse maculopapular eruption and leukopenia.

Etiology. *Salmonella typhosa* is a motile gram-negative bacillus which grows readily on simple infusion media. Formerly called *Eberthella typhosa,* it is now classified in the Salmonella group by most authorities, because of similarities in biochemical properties, antigenicity and pathogenicity. Unlike most salmonellas, it fails to produce gas during fermentation of sugars. Final identification is made by agglutination with specific serum.

The principal antigenic components of the typhoid bacillus are the flagellar, or H, antigen, which is heat-labile, and the O, or somatic, antigen, which is heat-stable. Virulent forms have another antigen, located on the surface of the cell, called the Vi antigen.

At least twenty strains of S. *typhosa* have been differentiated on the basis of susceptibility to lysis by bacteriophages. This procedure has been helpful in studies of the epidemiology of typhoid but is not useful in clinical practice, since there is no significant variation in the disease produced by different strains.

Epidemiology. *Salmonella typhosa* is a parasite of man and does not cause disease of other animals in nature. The organisms are excreted in the urine and feces by patients with typhoid fever, usually disappearing from the urine during the acute illness, but sometimes persisting in the stools during convalescence. Occasional patients become permanent *carriers,* continuing to excrete bacilli in the stools for years after recovery from the disease. Urinary carriers are rare, except when there is coexistent disease of the urinary tract; for example patients with schistosomiasis become urinary typhoid carriers rather commonly. The bacilli do not multiply significantly outside the human body, but may survive for weeks or months under natural conditions. The danger from excreta of typhoid patients is well recognized, and simple precautions are effective in preventing infection of other persons. Much more difficult to control is spread of the disease by apparently healthy carriers, who are responsible for its perpetuation.

Infection of man invariably occurs by ingestion or fecally contaminated material. Direct contamination of uncooked foods such as salads and raw milk by the soiled hands of a carrier has been the cause of many outbreaks, while epidemics have occurred from sewage contamination of water or shellfish. Flies may transmit the bacilli from feces to food. Modern municipal methods of water supply and sewage disposal, together with pasteurization of milk, have almost eliminated large epidemics of typhoid fever. As a result of these measures supplemented by improved sanitation in rural areas and active immunization, the prevalence of typhoid fever has declined greatly in the United States since 1900. Although formerly occurring in huge summer epidemics, the disease is now seen sporadically throughout the year. Cases appear singly or in small groups, and most of them are traceable to contamination of food by typhoid carriers.

Pathogenesis. Typhoid bacilli enter the body through the mouth. It has been suggested that the organisms may lodge in the tonsils or pharynx, and invade the interior of the body from there. It seems more probable, however, that they pass through the stomach into the small intestine, penetrate the lymphoid tissue in its wall, and are transported to the mesenteric lymph nodes. Multiplying in these locations, the organisms then pass, probably via the thoracic duct, into the blood stream, where they can regularly be demonstrated in cultures taken during the first week or ten days of illness. The bacilli localize in lymph nodes, spleen, lungs, bone marrow and liver. Since bile is a good culture medium for *S. typhosa,* luxuriant growth takes place in the biliary tract; this provides a continuous discharge of organisms into the small intestine and contributes to the heavy involvement of the Peyer's patches which occurs during the second and third weeks of the disease. The infection of the biliary tract also accounts for the positive stool cultures usually found at this stage. Cultural studies on persons who die during the second or third week of typhoid fever have shown that the greatest concentration of the bacilli is in the biliary tract and duodenum, with progressive diminution in the number of organisms in the remainder of the small bowel and the colon.

Antibodies for the typhoid bacillus generally appear in the blood during the second week of the disease, and at about the same time bacteremia usually ceases. There is no slackening, however, in the clinical manifestations. The role played by antibodies in recovery is uncertain, as is the reason for gradual regression of the infection. There is some evidence, however, that typhoid bacilli can grow within cells, particularly in plasma cells, where they may be protected until the death of the sheltering host cells exposes them to the combined assault of antibodies and phagocytes. Such a process might explain the slow defervescence of the disease.

Second attacks of typhoid fever have been observed, but as a general rule one attack confers lifelong immunity.

Morbid Anatomy. In nearly all tissues of the body there is proliferation of large mononuclear cells, derived from reticuloendothelial tissue. Lymphoid hyperplasia is notable everywhere, but especially in the Peyer's patches of the ileum, the mesenteric lymph nodes, and the spleen. The Peyer's patches may undergo necrosis, leading to intestinal perforation or to hemorrhage. The liver is usually enlarged, and local areas of necrosis can be seen microscopically. There may be a diffuse patchy pneumonitis.

Symptoms. The clinical manifestations of typhoid fever are subject to great variation in character and intensity. The disease may take the form of a mild illness lasting only a week or two, or it may last six to eight weeks. Occasionally it is a fulminating process which overwhelms the patient within a period of ten days. The description to follow will pertain to cases of average severity, lasting four to five weeks.

The incubation period is ten to twelve days. Abrupt onset is unusual; more often there is gradual development of malaise, headache and feverishness, causing the patient to take to his bed about the third or fourth day. The *fever* is remittent in type, tending to be higher each day. During the first ten days *headache* is likely to be the most prominent symptom, accompanied by *general malaise* and a nonproductive *cough*. *Anorexia* is the rule, occasionally with *nausea* and *vomiting*. *Constipation* is common during the first two weeks of illness, and there is often generalized abdominal discomfort and distention. *Epistaxis* is an early symptom in about one fifth of all cases. By the third week the fever is generally high, varying from 102° to 104° or 105° F. each day. There are periods of profuse sweats and occasional chills associated with the temperature variations. Administration of an anti-pyretic drug is likely to result in a precipitous fall in temperature, followed in a few hours by a chill and rapid return to the previous level. There may be *delirium* at the peaks of fever. The sensorium is dulled; the patient often has a blank, staring expression and may pick aimlessly at the bedclothes. At this stage, *diarrhea* may supervene, and several watery grayish or greenish stools may be passed each day.

Once the fever reaches a plateau, it is sustained for a week or two, then gradually begins to lessen. Each day the remission is greater, and the elevation a little less, normal temperature being attained after about thirty days of illness.

Physical Signs. Physical findings vary according to the stage of the disease. In the first week, aside from feverishness and perhaps slight abdominal distention, there are no helpful physical signs. During the second week the *spleen* becomes palpable in about three fourths of all cases. It is soft, not greatly enlarged, and may not be felt if palpation is carried out too firmly. The *rash* appears during the second and third week. It can be seen in about 90 per cent of white patients, but is difficult to detect in the Negro. It consists of crops of round, slightly elevated *"rose spots,"* 2 to 3 mm. in diameter, which blanch under tension, and persist two to five days. The lesions are seldom numerous; often less than a dozen can be seen at a time. They are found principally on the trunk, especially on the upper abdomen and lower chest; rarely they are found on the face and extremities. Examination of the lungs may reveal scattered *moist rales,* evidence of the bronchitis which is commonly present in typhoid fever. During the first two weeks of illness the *pulse rate* may be comparatively slow in relation to the fever, e.g., 85 per minute at a temperature of 104° F.; but subsequently the pulse rate is usually proportional to the fever. At the height of the illness *abdominal distention* may be severe and there may be moderate *generalized abdominal tenderness,* most pronounced on the right side. All these signs subside as the fever diminishes, and by the time the temperature has returned to normal the rash, splenomegaly, abdominal distention and bronchitis have usually also disappeared. Convalescence is slow; the patient is seldom able to resume former activity within a month after the fever subsides.

Older descriptions of typhoid fever based upon the clinical picture seen around 1900 stressed the remarkable wasting which occurred, as well as changes in the mouth and tongue, sordes on the lips and teeth, and parotitis. With good nursing care, administration of adequate fluids and nutriment, these developments are now rarely encountered, and will not be described in detail.

Laboratory Findings. During the course of the illness a normochromic *anemia* develops. This may be aggravated by extensive bleeding into the bowel. As a rule the *leukocyte count* is normal during the first two weeks of illness; in the third and fourth weeks there is usually a neutrophilic *leukopenia,* the total count ranging from 3000 to 6000 cells per cubic millimeter. *Albuminuria* of moderate degree is common when the fever is high. The *feces* usually give a positive reaction for *occult blood* during the third and fourth weeks of the illness, and sometimes they contain gross blood.

Isolation of S. typhosa *from the Blood.* It is possible to isolate S. *typhosa* from the blood in nearly all cases during the first week of illness, but with diminishing frequency thereafter. Blood culture is rarely positive after the third or fourth week unless the patient remains acutely febrile. The organisms can often be cultivated from sternal *marrow,* however, until the fourth or fifth week of illness. Typhoid bacilli do not appear in the feces until the second or third week, but by the fourth week *stool culture* is positive in approximately 85 per cent of cases. The frequency of positive cultures declines rapidly thereafter and by the sixth or seventh week is less than 5 per cent. In approximately 2 to 3 per cent of cases the organisms continue to be excreted in the feces long after clinical recovery; i.e., the patient becomes a typhoid carrier. This state may continue for as long as twenty or thirty years, or may cease spontaneously at any time. The *urine culture* reveals S. *typhosa* during the third or fourth week in about 25 per cent of cases, but persistent excretion of the bacilli is rare.

Serologic Tests. Demonstration of development of H and O agglutinins (Widal reaction) during the course of an illness is strong evidence in support of the diagnosis of typhoid. However, two sources of misinterpretation should be recognized. Persons inoculated with *typhoid vaccine* within the previous six to twelve months may have agglutinins. Moreover, persons who have previously had the disease or been vaccinated may exhibit an *anamnestic reaction* with reappearance of typhoid antibodies during some other febrile illness, especially typhus fever or brucellosis. Recent vaccination can usually be ascertained from the history. The anamnestic response is characterized by early rise and fall in titer and by the fact that serologic reactions for the responsible disease rise to even higher titers and persist longer than the typhoid antibodies. It is useful to test for both O and H antibodies in the Widal reaction, since infections with serologically related salmonella organisms may serve as antigenic stimulus for one or the other of these. The H titer usually is higher than the O. No arbitrary level can be given as diagnostic; occasional patients never have antibody titers higher than 1:40 or 1:80. Demonstration of a rising titer is more significant than any single level, although titers of 1:160 or greater, especially for antibodies to the O antigen, are strongly suggestive of active infection. Tests for Vi antibodies are technically more difficult, but a positive result is especially significant because typhoid vaccine does not usually cause development of Vi antibodies.

Complications. The most frequent serious complication is *hemorrhage* from the small bowel, which results from erosion of blood vessels in the ulcerated Peyer's patches. As already noted, bleeding sufficient to give a positive test for occult blood in the feces occurs in nearly every case of typhoid fever during the third and fourth week. Gross blood is present in 10 to 20 per cent of all cases. Profuse bleeding is sometimes fatal. Serious blood loss is evidenced by pallor, shortness of breath, tachycardia and fall in blood pressure. In some instances there is also an abrupt fall in body temperature. *Perforation* of the intestine is less frequent (about 2 per cent of cases), but is an even more serious complication, often resulting in death. Gross intestinal hemorrhage sometimes precedes perforation. The clinical signs of perforation are often obscured by preexisting abdominal distention, pain and tenderness. Usually, however, sudden intensification of pain occurs in the right lower abdomen, with localized tenderness, and diminished or absent peristalsis. Free air within the peritoneal cavity may be demonstrable on a roentgenogram. The pulse rate often increases, and a rise in leukocyte count

is a helpful diagnostic sign. *Pneumonia* may occur as an extension of the bronchitis which usually accompanies typhoid fever, but occasionally it is caused by pneumococcus or some other micro-organism. *Cholecystitis* occurs in 2 to 3 per cent of patients, and is characterized by pain and tenderness in the right upper quadrant. Cholelithiasis may develop as a late sequel. *Periostitis* occasionally occurs during or after the febrile period. It is usually situated near the end of a long bone, or in one of the vertebrae. The lesion tends to flare up and subside at irregular intervals over long periods of time. Typhoid *pyonephrosis* has been described. *Thrombophlebitis* is uncommon. *Meningitis* is rare. *Arthritis* is also a rare complication, the large joints being the ones affected. *Abortion* or *premature delivery* almost always occurs in pregnant women.

Relapse. Relapse occurs during convalescence in about 10 per cent of cases. This may amount to only a few days of fever, or there may be a reappearance of all manifestations, including bacteremia and "rose spots." The course is usually short, however, and the clinical illness milder than the initial attack.

Diagnosis. During the first week of illness the diagnosis can be established by blood culture. The appearance of "rose spots" and enlarged spleen during the second week is suggestive, and at this time a rising titer of antibodies is usually demonstrable. During the third and fourth weeks the causative organisms can nearly always be isolated from the feces. Culture of sternal bone marrow may be resorted to at any time during the first four or five weeks.

Differential Diagnosis. Because of the insidious onset with cough, typhoid fever can be confused with *primary atypical pneumonia*. Demonstration of pulmonary consolidation within the first week and development of cold agglutinins point to the correct diagnosis. *Murine typhus fever* may be difficult to distinguish from typhoid. Typhus fever is more likely to have a sudden onset with chills and a more profuse skin eruption. Laboratory tests include a positive Weil-Felix reaction and positive complement fixation reaction with typhus rickettsiae. Clinical improvement with a tetracycline drug such as Aureomycin would favor typhus fever. In *tularemia* there may be a history of handling wild rodents or of tick bite, and an ulcer with regional lymphadenopathy may be found. Clinical improvement with streptomycin or a tetracycline drug would suggest this diagnosis, and development of agglutinins for *Pasteurella tularensis* would confirm it. In *Rocky Mountain spotted fever* the onset is abrupt, there may be a leukocytosis, and the hemorrhagic eruption is usually heaviest on the wrists and ankles. The Weil-Felix reaction and complement fixation test are positive after ten days. This illness also responds dramatically to therapy with one of the tetracyclines (e.g., Aureomycin, Terramycin). *Pulmonary tuberculosis* can usually be differentiated by roentgenographic studies, but the presence of *miliary tuberculosis* is more difficult to exclude, since lesions are demonstrable on the roentgenograms in only half the cases. In such instances the diagnosis may be established by the appearance of choroidal tubercles, the finding of tubercles in sternal marrow, or the development of meningitis. *Hodgkin's disease,* localized chiefly in the abdomen, may resemble typhoid fever, but can be differentiated by negative bacteriologic and serologic tests for typhoid and eventual development of characteristic lesions in the mediastinal or superficial lymph nodes. *Brucellosis* may be clinically similar, but in those cases which resemble typhoid, antibodies against brucella or the micro-organisms themselves should be demonstrable in the blood. *Malaria* may have an onset similar to that of typhoid, but the typical relapsing course usually becomes established after a few days, and the plasmodia can be demonstrated in the blood smear. The *paratyphoid fevers* simulate typhoid fever in all respects, but are usually milder. They can be differentiated only by serologic and bacteriologic methods.

Prognosis. Before the introduction of chloramphenicol the over-all case fatality rate of typhoid fever was 8 to 10 per cent. The prognosis is especially grave in cases with profuse hemorrhage or perforation. It appears probable that with chloramphenicol therapy the fatality rate in typhoid fever can be reduced to less than 1 or 2 per cent.

Treatment. Attendants should be immunized against the disease. They should wear gowns and should wash their hands with soap and water after contact with the patient or anything he may have touched. Eating utensils should be boiled. Bedding, towels and so forth should be boiled. The stools and urine can safely be disposed of in municipal sewage systems.

Until 1948 there was no specific treatment for typhoid fever, and patients with the disease had to go through a prolonged, severe febrile illness. Careful nursing, various supportive measures, and maintenance of fluid balance and nutrition were of utmost importance. With the introduction of chloramphenicol (Chloromycetin) the situation has been altered. This drug terminates the febrile period so quickly that the relative importance of nursing and general supportive measures has lessened.

The optimal dosage schedule for *chloramphenicol* remains to be determined. It is advisable to administer 2 or 3 gm. daily during the first few days until the temperature is normal. Thereafter, a total daily dose of 1 to 1.5 gm. is apparently adequate. The daily dose can be divided into two or four parts and given at twelve- or six-hour intervals. The pattern of response is remarkably uniform. During the first two days there is little or no apparent change in the clinical condition; fever continues and the symptoms are not modified. Blood cultures reveal, however, that the bacteremia terminates within the first few hours after starting treatment. During the third day dramatic improvement usually takes place. The temperature subsides, the symptoms abate, the appetite improves, and the patient enters the convalescent stage.

It has been shown that an even more dramatic clinical improvement can be obtained by giving cortisone as an adjunct to chloramphenicol therapy. Cortisone, in a dose of 200 mg. daily for four or five days, causes a rapid defervescence and lessening of the symptoms. It can be discontinued at the time chloramphenicol would be expected to have the infection controlled. So far as has been determined, this use of cortisone has not been harmful to the patient.

Relapses have been encountered in patients treated with chloramphenicol for only seven to ten days, but resumption of the chemotherapy brings about rapid improvement. Relapses can probably be prevented by continuing drug administration (in a dose of 1 gm. daily) for three to four weeks. Complications such as hemorrhage or perforation of the bowel may also occur even though the patient is afebrile and otherwise asymptomatic after chloramphenicol treatment, and indicate the need for prolonged rest and careful observation. Probably these complications can be reduced to a minimum by continuing chloramphenicol therapy for three to four weeks in all cases.

Should a large hemorrhage occur, blood transfusions are indicated. The treatment recommended for perforation of the bowel formerly was surgical drainage, but conservative treatment with penicillin and chloramphenicol is now probably preferable.

Treatment of Carriers. Persons known to be carriers should not be permitted to work as food handlers. The members of their households should be immunized against the disease. Chloramphenicol is not effective in eliminating the carrier state. Cholecystectomy will eradicate the carrier state in about 90 per cent of cases. Before resorting to surgery, however, a trial of penicillin therapy in large doses should be given, i.e., 10,000,000 units daily for 10 days. This occasionally succeeds in terminating the carrier state.

Prophylaxis. Immunization against typhoid fever is practicable and effective. The vaccine usually used contains 1 billion heat-killed organisms per milliliter. In some parts of the world paratyphoid A or B bacilli are also included. A course of immunization usually consists of three subcutaneous injections, given at weekly intervals, the individual doses being 0.5, 1.0 and 1.0 ml. The injection often causes some local soreness, and there may be fever during the succeeding six to twelve hours. The vaccine can be inoculated intracutaneously, in doses of 0.1 ml. This method reduces the likelihood of systemic reaction, but the local pain and tenderness are as uncomfortable as with subcutaneous injection of the larger quantities. Except with massive exposure, the immunity conferred is reasonably sure for twelve months, and in many persons for considerably longer periods of time.

PAUL B. BEESON

References

Knight, V., and others: Antimicrobial Therapy in Typhoid. Arch. Int. Med., 85:44, 1950.
Morgan, H. R.: The Salmonella, in Dubos, R. J., ed.: Bacterial and Mycotic Infections of Man. 2nd ed. Philadelphia, J. B. Lippincott Co., 1948.
Stuart, B. M., and Pullen, R. L.: Typhoid. Clinical Analysis of Three Hundred and Sixty Cases. Arch. Int. Med., 78:629, 1946.
Woodward, T. E., and others: Treatment of Typhoid

Fever: Combined Therapy with Cortisone and Chloramphenicol. Ann. Int. Med., 34:1, 1951.

SALMONELLOSIS OTHER THAN TYPHOID FEVER

Definition. Salmonella infections are a group of acute illnesses caused by the numerous members of the genus *Salmonella*. The clinical picture may cover a spectrum ranging from severe enteric fever, closely resembling typhoid, to mild gastroenteritis.

History. The typhoid bacillus, observed in tissue sections by Eberth in 1880 and isolated by Gaffky in 1884, was the first of a series of related organisms found to produce enteric infection in man. *Salmonella entertidis* was isolated by Gaertner in 1888 and *S. typhimurium* shortly thereafter, both from cases resulting from the ingestion of infected meat. *S. schottmuelleri* was obtained by Gwyn from the blood of a patient with paratyphoid fever in 1898, *S. paratyphi* from contaminated water by Paladino-Blandino in 1903, and *S. hirschfeldii* by Hirschfeld from cases of paratyphoid in Mesopotamia during the First World War among troops who had been immunized with TAB vaccine. *Salmonella choleraesuis,* isolated in 1885 by Salmon and Smith from swine and from cases of enteric fever in man by Longcope in 1902, was originally thought to be the cause of hog cholera, but subsequent work has shown that it is only a frequent secondary invader in a disease caused by a virus. The work of a large number of medical and veterinary bacteriologists has led to our present knowledge of this ubiquitous and important group of enteric organisms, which now comprises over 150 species.

Etiology. The salmonellas are gram-negative motile bacilli which may be distinguished from the bacilli of the coli-aerogenes group by their inability to ferment lactose and by their capacity for growth in the presence of certain compounds which inhibit the latter organisms, such as sodium citrate, sodium tetrathionate, selenium salts, sodium desoxycholate and brilliant green. These two characteristics form the basis for the methods, using enrichment and differential media, which have been devised for their isolation from feces. As a group the salmonellas do not produce indol or liquefy gelatin, do not ferment sucrose, lactose or salicin, but produce acid and gas when grown in the presence of glucose, mannitol and maltose, with two exceptions—*S. typhosa* (typhoid bacillus, which is now usually grouped with the salmonellas) and *S. pullorum,* which produce acid but no gas. Identification of individual strains is usually made on the basis of biochemical reactions, particularly sugar fermentations, and serologic reactions in properly prepared antiserums.

The modern serologic classification of the salmonellas is based on studies of their antigenic structure by Kauffmann and White. They may be divided into seven groups on the basis of their O (somatic, or heat-stable)

the strains which they isolate to one of the Salmonella Centers for final identification.*

Epidemiology. The salmonellas are natural pathogens for a wide variety of animals and birds. The number of species capable of causing disease in man is constantly increasing. In general, the group may be di-

Important Members of the Salmonella Group

GROUP	TYPE	CHIEF O ANTIGENS	H ANTIGENS		NATURAL SOURCES
			Phase I	Phase II	
A	S. paratyphosa (paratyphoid A bacillus)	II, XII	a	....	Man
B	S. schottmuelleri (paratyphoid B bacillus)	IV, XII	b	1, 2	Man
	S. typhimurium (Bact. aertrycke)	IV, XII	i	1, 2, 3	Rodents
C$_1$	S. hirschfeldii (paratyphoid C bacillus)	VI$_1$, VI$_2$, VII	c	1, 5	Man
	S. choleraesuis (S. suipestifer American type)	VI$_1$, VII	c	1, 5	Swine, cattle, sheep
	S. oranienburg	VI$_1$, VI$_2$, VII	m, t	....	Quail, chickens
	S. montevideo	VI$_1$, VII	g, m, s	....	Monkeys, swine, turkeys, chickens
C$_2$	S. newport	VI, VIII	e, h	1, 2, 3	Rodents, swine, chickens, turkeys
D	S. typhosa (typhoid bacillus)	IX, XII	d	....	Man
	S. enteritidis (Gaertner's bacillus)	IX, XII	g, m	....	Horses, swine, rodents, ducks
	S. pullorum	IX, XII	nonmotile		Chickens
E	S. anatum	III, X, XXVI	e, h	1, 6	Swine, ducks, chickens, turkeys

Adapted from Bacterial and Mycotic Infections of Man, edited by R. J. Dubos, published by J. B. Lippincott Company and printed with permission of the publisher.

antigens, while within these groups the individual types or species may be identified by their H (flagellar, or heat-labile) antigens. The situation is confused by the sharing of certain O antigens among different groups and by phase variation of the H antigens. In phase 1 the H antigens are relatively specific—that is, they are found in one or only a few species—but in phase 2 or the group phase, which certain species may exhibit at times, the flagellar antigens may be common to other species in the group phase. These complexities are illustrated in the accompanying table. Few laboratories are equipped for more than isolation of salmonellas and tentative identification of one of the common types. Correct identification is important in tracing the epidemiology of these infections; consequently, most public health laboratories and many hospital laboratories now forward

vided into (1) those species found only in man, (2) those usually found in animals or birds, but capable of causing disease in man, and (3) those found only in animals or birds. The first group is small, including S. typhosa, S. paratyphosa, S. schottmuelleri and S. hirschfeldii—in other words, the typhoid and paratyphoid A, B and C bacilli. All these organisms may cause enteric fever, in general with somewhat diminishing frequency and severity as one moves down the list, while the frequency with which sepsis with focal complications or severe gastroenteritis characterizes the infection becomes more common. The second group is the largest and is constantly growing, while the third

* Salmonella Typing Center, Agricultural Experiment Station, University of Kentucky, Lexington, Kentucky, or Salmonella Center, Beth Israel Hospital, New York City.

is shrinking, with more thorough bacteriologic studies of sporadic cases and outbreaks of food poisoning. Organisms of the second group rarely cause enteric fever, but most often gastroenteritis or septicemia.

Human infections with salmonellas are occasionally acquired as a result of direct contact with infected animals, but usually by ingestion of contaminated water or food. The latter may be contaminated from infection in the animal from which the food was obtained, or as a result of contamination by the excreta of other animals, such as rodents, by flies, or by human beings who are sick or are carriers. Meat, milk and eggs are the foods most frequently involved in transmission, since the organisms may multiply in them before ingestion. This rapid growth results in a large dose of bacteria and thus increases the likelihood of infection with those *Salmonella* types which are of low pathogenicity for man.

Important factors in the spread of these infections are the relative resistance of the organisms to physical and chemical agents, their ability to multiply outside the bodies of their hosts, their widespread distribution in rodents, domestic animals and fowls, and the frequency of human carriers, who probably play an important role in human infections. Approximately 3 per cent of typhoid patients become permanent carriers after the illness. Although the percentage of permanent carriers is lower after paratyphoid infection, a considerable number may carry the organisms for weeks or months, and, with the less pathogenic types, inapparent infections occur frequently.

Pathogenesis. Much of our knowledge of the pathogenesis of enteric fever is derived from studies on typhoid fever by Goodpasture and Adams, based on correlation of postmortem findings with experimental work in the chick embryo.

The pathogenesis of infection with *Salmonella typhosa* is described in the immediately preceding section on Typhoid Fever. Presumably the general features of infection with other salmonellas are similar, but permanent localization within the biliary system is much less common, as is deep ulceration of the lymphoid tissue of the bowel. Relapses and recrudescences appear to be due to reinvasion of the blood from secondary foci of infection.

Immunity. The degree to which an attack of infection with one *Salmonella* species confers protection against subsequent attacks with the homologous species or others of the same group is largely unknown. Presumably the degree of immunity conferred by the disease will depend upon the intensity of the antigenic response evoked by the attack, the interval before reexposure, and the dose of infecting organisms. This is borne out by experimental feeding of volunteers and by studies on actively immunized persons which indicate that the protection conferred by prophylactic vaccination is relative, not absolute, immunity being definitely inferior in those receiving less than the full course of injections and infection occurring in a small but definite percentage of immunized persons after exposure.

Morbid Anatomy. The pathologic lesions found in these infections are not particularly specific. Death seldom occurs except in severe enteric fever or in the septic cases. The findings in the former are those of typhoid fever, although the involvement of Peyer's patches is less prominent and ulceration much less frequent. In the septicemic forms of infection, intestinal lesions are usually absent and the findings are those of any acute generalized infection—acute splenic tumor, focal necrosis of the liver, cloudy swelling of the kidneys, widespread petechial hemorrhages, and occasional purulent foci in which the exudate consists of mixed polymorphonuclears, lymphocytes, plasma cells and macrophages.

Pathologic Physiology and Chemistry. Like other gram-negative organisms of the enteric groups, the O or somatic antigens of the *Salmonella* are polysaccharide-lipid-protein complexes. The protein portion appears to be identical in the various salmonellas and shigellas while the polysaccharide, which is a haptene, confers specificity. These antigens presumably are the heat-stable endotoxins, released as the result of autolysis and destruction of organisms in the body, which give rise to most of the manifestations of the infection. This statement is based on the result of clinical and experimental studies with purified endotoxins. Their intravenous injection into human beings in minute amounts is followed, after a latent period of thirty minutes to an hour, by chill, fever, headache, nausea, malaise and leukopenia. Antibodies against the O antigen develop after a week or two for the organisms from which the endotoxin was derived, and the patient shows a steady increase in tolerance, requiring constantly increasing doses to elicit the effect on each succeeding injection. This phenomenon, which is characteristic of the response to intravenous typhoid vaccine, is not specific; that is, the tolerance is increased for endotoxins derived from any of the organisms of the enteric group, and appears to be related to hyperplasia of the reticuloendothelial system.

Incidence. The incidence of salmonella infections bears a general relation to the degree of sanitation. However, in the United States, despite the low incidence of typhoid fever in all but certain rural areas, other salmonella infections occur with greater frequency. The New York Salmonella Center collected 2916 cultures of *Salmonella,* excluding *S. typhosa,* in the period from 1939 to 1945. These had the following distribution:

closely resembles typhoid fever, but tends to be shorter in duration and milder, and to have fewer complications, although it can be a severe and serious disease. The incubation period is shorter (one to ten days), rose spots are less frequently seen than in typhoid, diarrhea is more common, and there is considerably less ulceration of the small bowel, so that hemorrhage and perforation, although they may occur, are less often observed. Relapses and recrudescences are common, and, although the permanent carrier state occurs rarely, as many as 20 per cent of patients may have positive stool cultures for several months after *S. schottmuelleri* infection. The differences between paratyphoid fever and typhoid fever are quantitative rather than qualitative, and these two infections can be distinguished only by bacteriologic methods.

Frequency of Salmonella Organisms

GROUP	NO. OF TYPES ISOLATED	FREQUENCY	COMMONEST TYPES
A	1	21	*S. paratyphi*, 21
B	11	950	*S. schottmuelleri*, 148 *S. typhimurium*, 795 *S. derby*, 71
C_1	11	1157	*S. choleraesuis*, 144 *S. oranienburg*, 709 *S. montevideo*, 134
C_2	7	321	*S. newport*, 270
D	5	155	*S. enteritidis*, 44 *S. panama*, 95
E	8	263	*S. anatum*, 181
F	10	49	
7 groups	53 types	2916 cultures	

Compiled from figures in Seligmann, E., Saphra, I., and Wassermann, M.: J. Immunology, Vol. 54.

Symptoms. These organisms cause three major syndromes in man: *enteric fever, septicemia,* and *acute gastroenteritis.* Although any of the pathogenic salmonellas may produce any of these three types of disease, each syndrome tends to be associated with certain species. The clinical pictures of these three syndromes are not completely distinct, and many cases are seen in which the picture of one syndrome shades into the other.

Enteric fever, caused by *S. paratyphosa, S. schottmuelleri* or *S. hirchfeldii,* and occasionally by other members of the group,

The *septicemic type of infection* is seen most often when *S. choleraesuis* (*B. suipestifer*) is the infecting organism. This type of infection occurs sporadically and is usually seen in children or in adults debilitated by other diseases, surgical operations or malnutrition. The illness begins with an acute onset of high fever, occasionally preceded by a chill. In a few cases the onset is more gradual. The bacteremia is uncomplicated by the development of focal lesions in about two thirds of these cases, and the course is that of a typhoid-like febrile disease, with leukopenia and fever lasting one to three weeks. Tachycardia is much more common than bradycardia, and although cough, coryza, headache, delirium, stupor, vomiting, constipation and diarrhea all may occur as in typhoid fever, they are much less frequent symptoms. Intestinal hemorrhages and perforation have not been described.

Focal complications are more frequently observed than in typhoid and paratyphoid fever. Pulmonary lesions, particularly bron-

The characteristic laboratory findings are a mild anemia, which progresses during the disease, and leukopenia, which may be followed by the development of a leukocytosis when focal complications appear. Bacteremia occurs in a high percentage of cases and persists throughout most of the febrile course. The agglutination reaction becomes positive to a high titer in most cases. Positive urine cultures are frequently obtained, but positive stool cultures are rare.

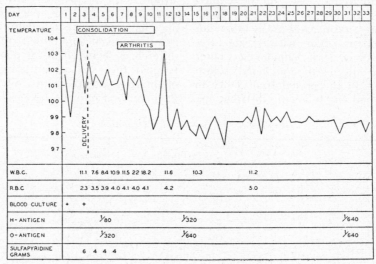

Fig. 33. Clinical course of septic type of infection due to *S. choleraesuis* in a 21 year old primiparous woman who had had a spontaneous delivery during the disease and who acquired pneumonia and arthritis of the sacroiliac joint as focal complications. The baby appeared ill for the first week, but recovered. *S. choleraesuis* was isolated from its stools on the twentieth day of life. (Goulder, Kingsland and Janeway: New England J. Med., Vol. 226.)

chopneumonia, have been noted in about one third of the cases. Lobar pneumonia, pleural effusion, empyema and pericardial effusion have been observed. In some cases the organisms have been isolated from the sputum or from the lung at autopsy.

Bone and particularly joint lesions occur in about 20 per cent of cases, according to Harvey. The lesion is usually a pyarthrosis, with organisms present in the greenish fluid which accumulates in the joint space, and with involvement of the adjacent bone. Any joint may be involved, and the lesions frequently occur after the acute systemic infection has subsided.

Purulent meningitis, particularly in infants and children, bacterial endocarditis superimposed on damaged valves, pyelonephritis, and abscesses in various parts of the body have all been described as complications of *S. choleraesuis* infection.

Acute gastroenteritis usually occurs in epidemics and may be caused by any of the salmonellas, but *S. typhimurium, S. oranienburg* and *S. newport* are probably most often implicated in this country. It results from the ingestion of heavily contaminated food and begins abruptly with fever, headache, abdominal pains, nausea, vomiting and diarrhea after an incubation period of 6 to 48 hours. In a few cases in any outbreak, bacteremia may occur with high fever and chills, or, in children, convulsions and drowsiness at onset, cough, pneumonitis, splenomegaly, muscle pains and weakness. The course is brief, usually lasting two to five days, and the mortality low. Generally there is leukopenia, although leukocytosis often occurs, particularly at the onset. The clinical picture in such outbreaks depends to a considerable extent on the dose and pathogenicity of the infecting species. In many instances, when the dose is small or the infection due to organisms of low virulence for man such as *S. pullorum* or *S. anatum,* gastroenteritis may be mild, so that diarrhea, cramps and slight fever are the only manifestations of infection. In any outbreak a number of persons are found in whom positive stool cultures are obtained although they have no symptoms.

Complications. The complications of paratyphoid fever are those of typhoid fever, but they occur somewhat less frequently— hemorrhage, perforation, urinary tract infections and, in older patients, circulatory collapse, bronchopneumonia, or thrombophlebitis with pulmonary embolism. The septicemic forms of infection, often due to organisms of the suipestifer (C_1) group, may result in the development of purulent foci of infection, particularly in the bones and joints, but also in the kidneys, meninges or the soft tissues. Gastroenteritis may result in dehydration and acidosis, with serious results in the infant or debilitated elderly patients. It may be followed, in occasional cases, by urinary tract infection or infection of bones or joints which may be the first signs of disease to attract attention.

Diagnosis. The diagnosis of salmonella infection is a bacteriologic one which can only be made by isolation of the organisms from blood, feces, urine or some local focus of infection. It may be suspected from a rise in the titer of O agglutinins for any organism of the homologous group, or of H agglutinins for the infecting or a serologically related strain. Caution must be used in interpreting the results of agglutination tests, since rises may occur during infections with antigenically related organisms, in such diseases as typhus fever, or as an anamnestic reaction in previously immunized persons. The agglutination reaction is of more value in those cases with blood stream invasion than in gastroenteritis. Invasion of the blood occurs in the early stages of paratyphoid fever, with the later appearance of organisms in the stools, while in most septicemic cases the organism may be isolated from the blood, urine or from local foci of infection, but rarely from the stool. In gastroenteritis due to salmonella in contrast to bacillary dysentery, organisms are more readily isolated later in the disease than at onset and frequently persist into convalescence.

Although a definite diagnosis can only be made bacteriologically, salmonella infection should be suspected in any case of unexplained fever, particularly one in which leukopenia or gastrointestinal or joint symptoms occur. In such cases, differentiation from brucellosis may be difficult, or, if rose spots are seen, from one of the rickettsial diseases. Meningitis and pneumonia may be confused with salmonella infections, since leukocytosis, meningismus and cough frequently occur in cases with a rapid onset. Salmonella gastroenteritis must be distinguished from epidemic nausea, vomiting and diarrhea ("intestinal flu"), which is probably a virus disease, from poisoning from toxins elaborated by staphylococci, streptococci or other organisms in the food before ingestion. The first can only be distinguished on epidemiologic grounds as a cold weather disease with a short incubation period, apparently spread by droplet infection. Food poisoning develops in a few hours after ingestion of the food. Bacillary dysentery may be indistinguishable except bacteriologically, and in all instances of gastroenteritis in which abdominal pain is severe, differentiation of salmonella infections from acute appendicitis may be difficult, particularly when diarrhea occurs, as it may when the appendix is retrocecal. Elevation of the leukocyte count and localized pain and tenderness are the most helpful leads and suggest the need for a surgical approach. Instances of appendicitis with rupture due to salmonella infection have been described.

Prognosis. The prognosis of salmonella infections depends on the virulence of the infecting organism and the condition of the patient. Septic infections due to *S. cholerae-suis* have a high case fatality rate (26 per cent in Seligmann's last series). This is nearly five times as high as the case fatality rate of 5.1 per cent for all salmonella infections in his 1107 civilian cases, which should be contrasted with a rate of 0.12 per cent in 809 Army cases. Age has an important bearing on mortality as in many other infections. Most of the deaths occur in older people. In children, the infection, though frequent, is apt to be relatively benign, except in very young infants.

Treatment. Acute gastroenteritis seldom requires more than symptomatic treatment— restriction of food intake to liquids and bland soft solids, and, if necessary, repair of dehydration and provision of fluid by the parenteral route. In a few instances the use of antispasmodics, such as tincture of belladonna or atropine, or such time-honored remedies as bismuth subcarbonate and paregoric, may be necessary to control severe cramps.

Enteric fever, septicemia and severe gastroenteritis should be treated with chloramphenicol or one of the tetracyclines which, at the present time, appears to be the most effective of the newer drugs in salmonella infections. The drugs should be given in full doses (50 to 60 mg. per kilogram in adults per 24 hours in four to six divided doses) and continued for at least seven to ten days after the patient has become afebrile.

Prevention. Sanitation is the key to control of these infections. However, the fact that many persons may be temporary carriers without symptoms of infection or even contact with other known cases makes the problem of control of gastroenteritis difficult. If meat and eggs are properly cooked, water and milk supplies controlled and fresh food is properly handled, those infections which depend on a heavy dose of organisms should seldom occur. Paratyphoid fever may occur as a result of a small infecting dose. In view of the frequency of infections due to group C in this country, its is rather surprising that the latter have not been included in the standard typhoid, paratyphoid A and B vaccine. However, protection by vaccination is only relative, and under conditions of heavy exposure infections may occur despite immunization.

CHARLES A. JANEWAY

References

Adams, J. W., Jr.: Intracellular Bacilli in Intestinal and Mesenteric Lesions of Typhoid Fever. Am. J. Path., 15:561, 1939.

Beeson, P. B.: Development of Tolerance to Typhoid Bacterial Pyrogen and its Abolition by Reticulo-Endothelial Blockade. Proc. Soc. Exp. Biol. & Med., 61:248, 1946.

Goulder, N. E., Kingsland, M. F., and Janeway, C. A.: Salmonella Suipestifer Infection in Boston. New England J. Med., 226:127, 1942.

Harvey, A. M.: Salmonella Suipestifer Infection in Human Beings. Arch. Int. Med., 59:118, 1937.

Kunstadter, R. H., Milzer, A., and Kagan, B. M.: Chloramphenicol and Terramycin in the Treatment of Salmonella and Shigella Infections. J. Pediat., 39:687, 1951.

McCullough, N. B., and Eisele, C. W.: Experimental Human Salmonellosis. II. Immunity Studies following Experimental Illness with *Salmonella mekagridis* and *Salmonella anatum*. J. Immunol., 66:595, 1951.

Morgan, H. R.: Resistance to the Action of the Endotoxins of Enteric Bacilli in Man. J. Clin. Investigation, 27:706, 1948.

————: The Salmonella, in Dubos, R. J.: Bacterial and Mycotic Infections of Man. 2nd ed. Philadelphia, J. B. Lippincott Company, 1952, Chap. 17.

Rubenstein, A. D., Feemster, R. F., and Smith, H. N.: Salmonellosis as a Public Health Problem in War Time. Am. J. Pub. Health, 34:841, 1944.

Seligmann, E., Saphra, I., and Wassermann, M.: Salmonella Infections in the U. S. A. J. Immunol., 54:69, 1946.

Syverton, J. T., Ching, R. E., Cheever, F. S., and Smith, A. B.: Typhoid and Paratyphoid A in Immunized Military Personnel. J.A.M.A., 131:507, 1946.

INFECTIONS WITH THE COLIFORM, PROTEUS AND PSEUDOMONAS GROUPS OF BACILLI

Definition. The various forms of infection caused by the gram-negative aerobic bacilli normally present in the intestinal tract may be considered together under this heading.

Bacteriology. The coliform bacilli, most of which are motile, are differentiated from the salmonellas by their ability to ferment lactose with the production of acid and gas. There are two main types: *Escherichia coli* (*B. coli*), the predominant organism in the gastrointestinal tract of man and animals, and *Aerobacter aerogenes* (*B. lactis aerogenes*), usually capsulated, which is also found in the bowel, but derived primarily from vegetable sources. Strains intermediate between the two classic representatives of the colon-aerogenes group have been described, while the *paracolon bacilli,* which ferment lactose slowly, occupy a position between them and the salmonellas. The concept of a whole spectrum of organisms in the enteric group is further strengthened by the finding of some of the somatic antigens of the salmonellas in certain strains of coliform bacteria.

Klebsiella pneumoniae (*Friedländer's bacillus*), a variable lactose fermenter, is morphologically similar to *Aerobacter aerogenes,* but is more virulent and may be isolated from the respiratory tract or from the bowel in a small percentage of normal people. It occasionally produces gastroenteritis, but is known chiefly as the cause of severe pulmonary infections. *Alcaligenes faecalis,* a motile organism found in normal stools, may be confused with the enteric pathogens by its failure to ferment lactose in differential media, but is identified by the lack of fermentation when grown in media containing the standard sugars. This organism has occasionally been isolated in urinary tract infections and in cases of gastroenteritis, bacteremia or meningitis in infancy.

The *Proteus bacilli* are pleomorphic, non-lactose-fermenting organisms, characterized by active motility, which gives rise to spreading growth on solid media. These organisms, although widely disseminated in decaying organic matter and feces, are only present in large numbers in stools in abnormal circumstances. *Proteus vulgaris* and *P. morgani,* the two species usually isolated from human infections, are active urea splitters, with the liberation of ammonia.

Pseudomonas aeruginosa (*B. pyocyaneus*) is a motile, aerobic bacillus capable of producing two water-soluble pigments which diffuse into the medium used for cultivation —pyocyanin, a bluish color, and fluorescein, which is yellowish-green and fluorescent. Strains vary in their production of these pigments, and some variants do not produce color. This organism is occasionally recovered in small numbers from normal stools, but more often is found on the skin. It has been isolated from water, sewage and air, and from improperly sterilized instruments, solutions and surgical dressings.

Etiology. Recent work has implicated two specific types of *E. coli* (111, B4 and 55, B5) as the cause of epidemic diarrhea in hospitalized infants and has suggested that ingestion of these same types may occasionally produce gastrointestinal upsets in adults. However, since normally the coliform organisms are saprophytic inhabitants of the intestinal tract, it is only under special conditions that they gain access to the body cavities or tissue spaces where they may initiate infection.

In infancy resistance may be inadequate, and these organisms may invade widely from foci in the respiratory or gastrointestinal tracts, or in the newborn as a result of infection of the umbilical stump. Elderly patients likewise may suffer from bacteremia due to these organisms, usually as a result of some complicating factor, such as carcinoma, gallstones or renal calculi.

In the abdominal cavity surgical infections arise as a result of obstruction to or perforation of a hollow viscus or from interference with its blood supply. Puerperal infections due to colon bacilli may occur as a consequence of poor obstetrical technique or difficult labor.

Open wounds, chronic infections of the middle ear, and ulcerations, such as bed sores, in areas of poor circulation, may become secondarily infected with gram-negative bacilli, particularly *Proteus* or *Ps. aeruginosa.* The latter organism may be introduced accidentally into the thecal space or the urinary passages as a result of lumbar puncture or instrumentation. Indeed the development of meningitis following intraspinal anesthesia is almost invariably caused by *Ps. aeruginosa.*

Recently the prolonged or intensive use of antimicrobial drugs has created a biologic imbalance, leading to the elimination of susceptible strains of bacteria and their replacement by more resistant ones. This phenomenon may not only occur in the individual patient during therapy, but also in the hospital environment, where the presence of a large number of patients under treatment with antimicrobials may lead to a marked increase in the population of drug-resistant micro-organisms in human carriers and in the dust. Coliform organisms and *Staphylococcus aureus* seem particularly prone to develop resistance during the course of treatment, while *Pseudomonas aeruginosa,* which is unusually resistant to the ordinary antimicrobial drugs, has become an important cause of superinfection in treated patients.

The most common disease produced by colon bacilli is urinary tract infection. It often arises as a complication of diarrheal disease, when the enteric organisms seem to gain more ready access to the lymphatics and blood stream, and is frequently seen in elderly patients with constipation. Trauma to the urinary passages, as from an inlying catheter, stasis in the bladder or obstruction to the ureters, predisposes to infection. Urinary tract infections may be caused by any of the coliform bacilli in pure or mixed culture, but the majority are due to *E. coli,* often in combination with the *Enterococcus* (*Streptococcus faecalis*). *Proteus* and *Pseudomonas aeruginosa* are usually encountered as secondary invaders in chronic urinary tract infections, particularly after instrumentation, and in chronic pulmonary infections.

The incidence of urinary tract infection is considerably higher in women than men, and diabetics are particularly subject to the disease. In men some obvious mechanical difficulty such as neurologic bladder, prostatic hypetrophy, urethral stricture or calculus can usually be found to account for the infection.

Morbid Anatomy. Acute infection with these organisms produces purulent inflammation. In cases of bacteremia in infants there is a tendency to localization in the kidneys, meninges, lungs and serous cavities. Contrary to earlier opinion, the lesion in "pyelitis" has been found to involve the renal parenchyma as well as the pelvis and ureters; so the term "pyelonephritis" has come into common use for this condition.

The characteristic local lesions of the skin and gastrointestinal tract which occur in infections due to *Ps. aeruginosa* are ulcerative or gangrenous. On microscopic examination there is necrosis around a thrombosed small blood vessel with large numbers of bacilli in the surrounding tissue and relatively little reaction. Leukopenia and hypoplasia of the bone marrow have been observed in some cases of severe infections.

Pathologic Physiology and Chemistry. All the gram-negative enteric bacilli have potent endotoxins, associated with their somatic antigens. Consequently, invasion of the blood stream by these organisms or absorption of their breakdown products gives rise to the same symptoms as those which follow the intravenous injection of typhoid vaccine: chills, fever, headache, nausea and malaise.

Certain of these organisms, particularly *Proteus,* produce large amounts of ammonia from urea, which results in an alkaline urine and a tendency to the formation of calculi containing calcium, magnesium, carbonate and phosphate.

Symptoms. The symptoms of colon bacillus infection are of two types, local and constitutional. The *local symptoms* are determined by the particular organ infected—gallbladder, bile ducts, appendix, urinary bladder, kidney—more than by the organism concerned, and detailed descriptions of these conditions will be found in appropriate sections of this book. The *constitutional* symptoms are most marked in cases of peritonitis, suppurative pylephlebitis, cholangitis, acute pyelonephritis, or whenever there is bacteremia. In children and adults severe shaking chills followed by episodes of high fever, malaise, headache, nausea and sometimes vomiting are the rule. Relative bradycardia may be seen. Where there are purulent foci, leukocytosis with a predominance of polymorphonuclear cells is marked, and anemia develops rapidly. In newborn infants the picture of sepsis with these organisms, which may involve middle ears, lungs, kidneys and meninges, may be one of prostration, with subnormal temperature, vomiting, diarrhea and

convulsions, although fever, leukocytosis, jaundice and hepatosplenomegaly are usually seen in instances of ascending infection from the umbilical stump. Although acute pyelonephritis is generally associated with prominent constitutional symptoms, many urinary tract infections remain chronic throughout and may manifest themselves only by fatigue, backache and slight malaise.

Superficial infections with *Ps. aeruginosa* are relatively asymptomatic, but when invasion occurs, this organism produces serious toxic manifestations, even more marked than those observed in infections with the colonaerogenes group. In infants, in whom infection of the gastrointestinal tract may cause ulceration at any point along its course from mouth to anus, prostration, vomiting, diarrhea, abdominal distention with paralytic ileus, and a tendency to pancytopenia may be observed. In bacteremic cases, skin lesions may occur as primary or metastatic foci. Most characteristically these consist of a bright pinkish areola surrounding a gangrenous center (ecthyma gangrenosum). Other types of rashes, including rose spots, have been observed, particularly in certain cases where the clinical picture has resembled that of typhoid fever. In adults, bed sores or chronic foci of infection in the genitourinary tract may serve as the sources of bacteremia, which is apt to give severe chills, high fever and prostration. Meningitis is the commonest metastatic complication of bacteremia, but may also develop as a result of the accidental introduction of organisms at lumbar puncture or spinal anesthesia. Pneumonia and arthritis are also seen as local manifestations of *Pseudomonas* infection. Infection of the cornea with ulceration due to *Ps. aeruginosa* usually leads to a destructive panophthalmitis unless vigorously treated. Although leukopenia, anemia and thrombocytopenia have been observed in severe cases of *Pseudomonas* infection, moderate leukocytosis occurs more frequently.

Diagnosis. In local infections, colon bacillus infection may be suspected from the fecal odor and greenish color of the pus, whereas *Pseudomonas* infection should be considered whenever pus or discharges have a bluish or greenish-yellow color. Diagnosis can be made only by bacteriologic methods, the findings of gram-negative bacilli on smear and their isolation on culture of the local lesion. Blood culture should be performed in cases with high fever, and a fresh specimen of urine examined and cultured in all cases of suspected urinary tract infection. In women the urine must be obtained by catheter in order to be certain that extraneous organisms are excluded.

Prognosis. In severe infections due to the colon group, prognosis depends on several factors. First, pure colon bacillus infections have a better prognosis than mixed infections, particularly in the abdomen, where the presence of pyogenic cocci and anaerobic bacilli adds greatly to the severity of the disease. Second, the age and condition of the patient make a tremendous difference; infants and elderly patients do badly. Third, the type of anatomic difficulty which gives rise to the infection has a marked bearing on prognosis.

In the urinary tract the degree of destruction of the renal parenchyma and the possibility of remedying the obstruction to urinary flow will influence the outcome of the acute attack and the ultimate course of the disease. Urinary infections in diabetic patients and infections due to *Proteus* or *Pyocyaneus* are apt to be resistant to therapy.

Treatment. The treatment of these infections should be of three types: first, general supportive measures; second, antimicrobial therapy; and third, therapy of the local infection. The last frequently calls for surgical intervention in the case of intra-abdominal infection. In such cases, as in other types of generalized or severe infections with the gram-negative bacilli, intensive chemotherapy is essential.

The intelligent use of antimicrobial therapy in gram-negative bacillary infections demands close collaboration between the physician and the laboratory because of the varied drug susceptibilities of members of this group of organisms, their tendency to develop resistance during treatment, and their capacity for producing superinfection. For these reasons, cultures should be obtained, and the effect of the available drugs upon the strain in question determined *in vitro* whenever possible. In severe infections of the abdominal or pelvic viscera, which are apt to be mixed infections, the combination of penicillin and one of the drugs effective against bacteria of the coliform group (streptomycin, chloramphenicol, or one of the tetracyclines in doses of approximately 30 to 50 mg. per kilogram) should be used until an accurate bacteriologic diagnosis can be made. A tetracycline drug or streptomycin and a sulfonamide represent

probably the best drug regimens for the early treatment of known infections due to *E. coli* or *Aerobacter,* in the absence of laboratory data on drug susceptibility. With *Proteus* infections the situation is more difficult and streptomycin with chloramphenicol (or a sulfonamide) probably represents the most reasonable initial therapy. In any of these situations, however, if a therapeutic response is not obtained after 48 hours of adequate dosage, another drug of the group listed above should be tried. Polymyxin B (Aerosporin) is at present the most effective antimicrobial drug for the treatment of systemic infections due to *Pseudomonas aeruginosa,* but because of its potential toxicity, it should not be used unless a specific bacteriologic diagnosis has been made. Average dosage is 2.5 mg. per kilogram.

Management of urinary tract infections should include the following:

1. Evaluation of the anatomic situation;
2. Relief of obstruction, if possible, and care of disease of the large bowel;
3. Forcing of fluids to maintain a free flow of urine, thus washing out pus and cellular debris, whenever this is compatible with chemotherapy;
4. Adequate chemotherapy to relieve acute symptoms and cure the infection, if possible;
5. Careful follow-up study in order to recognize and treat recurrences promptly.

The treatment of chronic urinary tract infections should be carried out in cooperation with a skilled urologist and planned after careful bacteriologic studies of the organisms involved, because of the tendency to recurrence or the development of resistant organisms, unless the mechanical factors responsible for the infection can be controlled. In general, continued prophylactic administration of broad spectrum antimicrobials in chronic pulmonary or urinary tract infections, in which the anatomic changes preclude permanent cure, would seem more likely to lead to the development of a resistant flora than their intermittent administration for the treatment of exacerbations of infection.

The local treatment of chronic infections involving the skin, wounds, ears and bronchial tree in which gram-negative bacilli may be involved cannot be considered in detail here, but methods are constantly improving. The development of enzymatic therapy with streptodornase and streptokinase has represented an important advance in this field, particularly in the treatment of *Pseudomonas* infections. Application of sulfonamides or penicillin to the skin should be avoided, because of the danger of sensitization of the patient to their subsequent systemic administration.

Prevention. The prevention of serious infections of this type consists mainly in the prompt recognition and treatment of abdominal disease such as appendicitis and cholecystitis, the proper handling of labor, scrupulous cleanliness in the handling of open wounds, and prompt institution of tidal drainage in neurologic conditions in which control of the sphincters is lost for more than a few days. Above all, it is important to consider infections of the urinary tract as potentially serious, since they are prone to recur, to induce the formation of calculi, and to produce renal damage and even severe hypertension in some cases.

CHARLES A. JANEWAY

References

Bowers, W. F.: Appendicitis, with Especial Reference to Pathogenesis, Bacteriology, and Healing. Arch. Surg., 39:362, 1939.

Ferguson, W. W., and June, R. C.: Experiments in Feeding Adult Volunteers with *Escherichia coli* 111 B₄, a Coliform Organism Associated with Infant Diarrhoea. Am. J. Hyg., 55:155, 1952.

Morgan, H. R., and Cheever, F. S.: The Enteric Bacteria, in Dubos, R. J.: Bacterial and Mycotic Infections of Man. 2nd ed. Philadelphia, J. B. Lippincott Company, 1952, Chapter 16.

Stanley, M. M.: Bacillus Pyocyaneus Infections. Am. J. Med., 2:253, 347, 1947.

Taylor, J.: Discussion of Infantile Gastroenteritis. Proc. Roy. Soc. Med., 44:516, 1951.

Yow, E. M.: Development of Proteus and Pseudomonas Infections during Antibiotic Therapy. J.A.M.A., 149:1184, 1952.

KLEBSIELLA INFECTIONS (FRIEDLÄNDER'S BACILLUS)

History. The organism was discovered by Friedländer in 1882. It was first described as a coccus and as the cause of pneumonia. This gave rise to considerable confusion and to a bitter controversy, especially with Fraenkel. The controversy was essentially resolved in 1886 by Weichselbaum, who came around to the view now generally held, namely, that pneumococcus is the chief etiologic agent of pneumonia and that Friedländer's bacillus may be the cause in a small percentage of cases.

Bacteriology. Friedländer's bacillus, *Klebsiella pneumoniae* (synonyms: *Bacillus mucosus capsulatus, B. friedländeri, B. pneumoniae, Pneumobacillus, Encapsulatus mucosus*), is an encapsulated, short, plump, nonmotile, gram-negative rod which grows to form mucoid gelatinous colonies on agar and a slimy surface pellicle in broth. Organisms of the genus *Klebsiella* are often difficult to differentiate from other encapsulated species of the tribe Escherichia, particularly those of the genus *Aerobacter*. There is considerable overlapping not only in the biochemical reactions, which are still the most useful for clinical purposes, but also in the "groups," which are based on the O or somatic antigens and in the "types," based on capsular antigens. More than 41 capsular types have already been identified.

Occurrence and Pathogenicity. *Klebsiella* occurs in the respiratory passages of from 2 to 25 per cent of normal persons, in the normal intestinal tract even in infants, and in the respiratory tract of mice, guinea pigs and rabbits. They have been found in soil, dust, air and water. They are pathogenic for man, producing characteristic acute and chronic pulmonary infections and also suppurative infections in the upper respiratory passages; in the intestinal, biliary, genital and urinary tracts; and in serous cavities and meninges. They give rise to septicemia and pyemia. They produce septicemia and widespread lesions when injected into mice, guinea pigs and rabbits.

KLEBSIELLA PNEUMONIA

Definition. Klebsiella pneumonia is a specific acute infectious disease caused by *Klebsiella pneumoniae* and characterized by massive mucoid inflammatory exudate of lobar or confluent lobular distribution in one or more lobes of the lung, with a tendency to necrosis and abscess formation.

Incidence and Distribution. Klebsiella pneumonia constitutes from 0.6 to 13 per cent of all cases of pneumonia in different series, averaging 1.1 per cent in over 17,000 cases (Julianelle). It has been encountered in most parts of the world and in all seasons. The disease is usually sporadic, but contact cases and epidemics have occurred.

Bacteriology. *Klebsiella* has been found in pure culture during the first days of the disease in sputum, lung and pleural fluids and in blood cultures, and in direct smears and cultures from the blood and lungs at autopsy in rapidly fatal cases. The pneumonias are caused predominantly by type A strains, which are found in about two thirds of the cases. Type B is next in frequency.

Predisposing Factors. Pneumonia due to *Klebsiella* has its greatest incidence between the ages of 40 and 60 years. Chronic alcoholism, malnutrition and general debility are encountered frequently in these cases. Antecedent simple upper respiratory infections are relatively infrequent. The disease may occur as a secondary infection following pneumonia due to other organisms, particularly pneumococci, or, contrariwise, it may be followed by infections with other organisms.

Morbid Anatomy. The involved lung is heavy, voluminous and noncrepitant with massive consolidation (lobar or confluent lobular) of one or more entire lobes. Plaques of fibrin are found on the pleural surfaces. The cut section usually has a smooth but mottled gray-red or red-brown surface from which thick, stringy mucinous exudate often oozes as if under pressure. The underlying lung often reveals soft areas in which alveoli appear liquefied and replaced by the mucinous exudate. In older lesions there may be gray-green purulent exudate with large areas of abscess formation. Histologically, the outstanding features are the necrosis of alveolar tissue, the enormous numbers of encapsulated bacilli, and the exudate, consisting of polymorphonuclear, large mononuclear (alveolar epithelial cells or monocytes) and erythrocytes in varying proportions with only a small amount of fibrin. The phagocytosis of *Klebsiella* in an experimental pneumonic lesion may be seen in Figure 25 in the section on Pneumococcal Pneumonia.

Symptoms and Course. The onset is usually with chill, pleuritic pain, cough and bloody sputum. Profound prostration sets in early, and delirium and distention are common. Dyspnea and cyanosis also occur early and may be intense. Sputum is usually copious, but is often raised with difficulty because of its mucoid and sticky character; it may appear rusty, but is more often brick-red or bloody and gelatinous, resembling currant jelly. Organisms are abundant in smears of such sputum. Hemoptysis, vomiting and diarrhea are frequent, and jaundice is present in many of the severe cases. Erythemas, sometimes scarlatiniform, occur, and patients with bacteremia may have petechiae. Herpes rarely occurs.

Signs of consolidation may be made out early, but more often the classic signs are absent and there may be only dullness and muffled breath sounds even when massive density is visible in the roentgenogram. This is presumably due to plugging of bronchi with viscid exudate. Moist rales may be heard over some areas of the lung. Involvement of the upper lobes or of multiple lobes is more frequent than in pneumococcal pneumonia. The fever may be sustained or irregular, but usually ranges lower than in cases due to pneumococci.

The disease may run a fulminating course, ending fatally in 24 to 36 hours. The average duration in Bullowa's cases was about five and a half days. Death is usually associated with peripheral vascular collapse, pulmonary edema, or extreme respiratory distress without pulmonary edema. Recovery is sometimes by crisis, but more often it is by lysis, and then may frequently be followed by the chronic type of pulmonary infections to be described later.

Laboratory Findings. The chief distinctive finding is the large number of characteristic bacilli in smears of the sputum. Agar cultures made of the sputum directly yield the characteristic mucoid colonies, usually in pure culture. Blood cultures yield the same organisms in more than half of the cases, and the organisms may be obtained almost regularly in pure culture by lung puncture or from pleural exudates, even when the blood culture is sterile. Total leukocyte counts below 6000 per cubic millimeter occur in more than one third of the cases. In other cases there is a moderate leukocytosis, with total counts reaching 25,000 or 30,000 per cubic millimeter in the presence of purulent complications.

Roentgenograms usually show marked density developing early. Areas of rarefaction may appear later, indicating abscess and cavity formation, which, in patients who survive long enough, then shows evidence of healing and fibrosis.

Complications. The commonest complication is delayed resolution with abscess formation and fibrosis of the lung (see below). Pleurisy is frequent. Empyema, pericarditis, meningitis, nonsuppurative arthritis and superinfections with other organisms, notably pneumococci and hemolytic streptococci, have been noted. Empyema and lung abscess which does not drain properly may require surgical intervention, but this should be avoided in the latter instance if possible because a chronic sinus may result.

Diagnosis. Klebsiella pneumonia is suspected in any case of acute pneumonia with severe prostration occurring early, especially if there is bloody gelatinous sputum. The diagnosis is based on demonstrating the characteristic encapsulated bacilli in smears and cultures of sputum as the only or predominant organism. They may be typed directly by the Neufeld method. The disease in some of its stages may simulate acute pneumonias due to other organisms, particularly pneumococcus, pulmonary tuberculosis, "influenza" pneumonia, acute pulmonary infarction and bronchiectasis.

Prognosis. The mortality in primary acute cases when untreated averages about 80 per cent, regardless of whether or not bacteremia is demonstrated; this has been reduced to about 40 per cent in patients treated adequately with antimicrobial drugs. The mortality in chronic or recurrent cases is appreciably lower.

Treatment. The general and symptomatic treatment is the same as for severe cases of lobar pneumonia due to pneumococcus. Specific antiserums have been disappointing. Sulfadiazine has proved effective in many cases; it should be used in full doses for ten days or longer. Penicillin is not effective, although some cures have been ascribed to it. Streptomycin is the agent of choice for starting treatment but resistant organisms may develop rapidly. One of the tetracyclines (Aureomycin, Terramycin or Achromycin) or chloramphenicol may be substituted for streptomycin, or given along with it, particularly after the first three or four days of treatment.

CHRONIC KLEBSIELLA INFECTIONS OF THE LUNGS

Definition. These are subacute or chronic infections of the lung caused by *Klebsiella pneumonia,* with a protracted and relatively benign course and expectoration of purulent, nonputrid and sometimes bloody sputum. Characteristically, they are accompanied by abscess formation, bronchiectasis and pulmonary fibrosis, and exhibit a tendency to exacerbations of acute pneumonia.

Occurrence, Etiology and Pathogenesis. The exact incidence of these chronic forms is difficult to establish, but they are much less frequent than the acute Klebsiella pneumonias. Probably many cases go unrecognized and are included as tuberculosis or as other chronic pulmonary infections. The relation of the *Klebsiella* to the disease is based upon finding the organism in large numbers and often in pure culture in sputum, in abscess or pleural fluid or in blood cultures during acute phases. Other organisms are also found in varying numbers in the later stages.

Morbid Anatomy. Grossly, the lungs present a picture of confluent bronchopneumonia with fibrosis, bronchiectasis and abscess formation. The walls of the cavities consist of bundles of collagen fibers bearing connective tissue cells without the remains of alveolar walls. Bronchi showing bronchiectatic changes often blend with foci of acute inflammation and with abscesses.

Symptoms and Course. The disease usually begins as an acute Klebsiella pneumonia with slow lysis over a period of weeks, during which abscess formation and fibrosis of the lung occur. In some cases there is a milder course from the start, with low grade persistent fever, cough with copious purulent sputum, loss of weight, and recurrent pleurisy. The sputum is not foul, unless there is a mixed infection, and intermittently becomes blood-streaked, brick-red or grossly bloody. The disease may go on for several weeks and end in complete symptomatic recovery with apparent clearing of the lesions on the roentgenogram, or it may persist for many months or years. Chronic abscess formation and bronchiectasis with fibrosis tend to reproduce the disease and give rise to relapses and frequent hemoptysis, particularly after acute respiratory infections. In more than three fourths of the cases one or both upper lobes are involved.

Laboratory Findings. The typical encapsulated bacilli are always present in large numbers. Secondary organisms, including pneumococci, staphylococci, influenza bacilli and other common mouth inhabitants, may also be abundant. Bacteremia is less common in these cases, but positive blood cultures have been obtained during the original acute pneumonia and during exacerbations. Specific antibodies may be demonstrated early and persist for a few weeks. Low grade leukocytosis is the rule except during acute phases, when there may be a leukopenia. Roentgenograms of the chest show thin-walled cavities with or without fluid, and later there is fibrosis and retraction of the upper lobes, simulating tuberculosis.

Complications. Recurrent pleurisy is frequent. Empyema, usually encapsulated, with thick mucoid pus, may occur with or without relation to abscess formation in the lung. Serous effusions are encountered, which may be sterile or infected, and may occur in patients who have purulent empyema elsewhere. Recurrences of acute pneumonia and hemoptyses are the rule. Axillary thrombophlebitis with acute arthritis has been encountered. Pericarditis and meningitis may occur as terminal events.

Diagnosis. In cases seen during the acute phase the diagnosis is made when there is slow lysis and evidence of abscess formation with copious sputum. The disease may be simulated by *pulmonary tuberculosis with cavitation.* Many patients with the latter diagnosis, in whom tubercle bacilli are not found, are shown to have chronic *Klebsiella* infections. The diagnosis depends on repeatedly demonstrating the characteristic encapsulated bacilli as the only or predominant organism in smears and cultures. Staphylococcal pneumonias, bronchomycoses, lung abscess, bronchiectasis and tumors of the lung must be considered in the differential diagnosis.

Prognosis. The mortality is said to be about 25 per cent. Death may occur in the original attack after a slowly progressive illness of several weeks or months, or it may occur during an acute exacerbation of pneumonia with the same or other organisms, or as a result of complications such as pericarditis, meningitis, or after operation for empyema or lung abscesses. Some patients apparently recover completely, while most of the others continue to have signs and symptoms for many years.

Treatment. Cases are recorded in which the use of sulfonamide drugs during a relapse resulted in apparent clearing up of the infected focus, but the results on the whole are unsatisfactory. Empyema usually necessitates rib resection, which may also be necessary for large pulmonary abscesses which fail to drain. Conservative treatment is recommended for abscesses in general, in the hope that they will eventually drain into a bronchus. Streptomycin parenterally, along with a sulfonamide is the treatment of choice. If the bacilli are streptomycin-resistant, one of the tetracyclines or chloramphenicol should be administered in large doses. In cases in which the chronic *Klebsiella* infection is localized to a lobe or pulmonary segment, some form of excisional surgery should be considered.

KLEBSIELLA SEPSIS

Definition. This is a local or generalized infection caused by the *Klebsiella pneumoniae,* frequently accompanied by bacteremia and associated with localized purulent infections in one or more organs.

Septicemia with this organism is relatively uncommon and is less frequent than with the streptococci, staphylococci, colon bacilli, meningococci or pneumococci. Several types are described: (1) a pure septicemic type which has an acute and rapidly fatal course; (2) a pyemic type with multiple abscesses in many organs; (3) a septicemia with symptoms referable predominantly to one organ; and (4) one which is secondary to infection with other organisms.

Portal of Entry. The organisms may gain access to the blood stream from any of the following foci: the middle ear; the lungs, particularly when there is thrombophlebitis of the pulmonary vein; the intestinal tract, commonly in infants; the liver, especially when there is thrombophlebitis of the hepatic or portal vein; the urinary tract; the genital tract, notably the prostate in males; the adnexa or the puerperal uterus in females. A large proportion of the cases are so-called cryptogenic, and the original focus cannot be determined even at autopsy. Little is known concerning the type distribution of *Klebsiella* in these cases. The organism is recovered in pure culture from the blood and from foci of suppuration, and frequently from the urine.

Occurrence and Predisposing Factors. Many of the cases occur in infants, children and young adults of both sexes, differing in these respects from the pneumonias. Alcoholism, cirrhosis of the liver and diabetes are particularly frequent in the adult cases.

Morbid Anatomy. The dominant feature is the finding of metastatic abscesses in the liver, lungs and kidneys. Only those in the lungs are characteristic. The pus in the abscesses is usually mucoid and tenacious, and the characteristic organisms are readily found in large numbers in smears and are usually in pure culture. Ulcerative endocarditis, meningitis and involvement of serous cavities are sometimes encountered.

Symptoms and Course. The onset may be abrupt with severe chills or may be insidious with high continuous or intermittent fever and general malaise, with or without chills. Vomiting and diarrhea are common. Rashes occur and may be scarlatiniform, maculopapular or petechial in character. There is an acute fulminating type described (Blumer and Laird) with a hemorrhagic septicemia, in which intestinal symptoms predominate and in which changes in the intestine similar to those of typhoid fever are found at autopsy. In some cases, particularly in adolescents, the course may simulate that of typhoid fever in every respect, including the leukopenia. In others the picture is dominated by some local lesion, such as abscesses of the kidney, lungs, prostate or liver, or by a cholecystitis with ascending infection, or there may be perforation of the intestine with peritonitis. In the cases with liver abscesses, jaundice may be prominent. The disease may be of short duration or last for several weeks. Meningitis or endocarditis may occur terminally.

Diagnosis. This depends on finding the *Klebsiella* in blood cultures or on demonstrating the organisms in characteristic pus from metastatic lesions.

Prognosis. The mortality is high, but, except in cases with pyemia, recoveries are recorded in all types of cases, including some which have shown a persistent bacteremia for some time. The prognosis is particularly favorable in cases in which there is a predominant focus, such as the prostate, which is accessible to surgical drainage.

Treatment. Streptomycin, along with sulfonamide, one of the tetracyclines or chloramphenicol, should be given in full doses as in the cases of pneumonia. Accessible foci should be drained surgically.

FOCAL INFECTIONS DUE TO KLEBSIELLA

Occurrence. According to some writers, notably Baehr and his colleagues, these represent the bulk of infections with *Klebsiella*, and they assign only a secondary role to the pulmonary infections. They consider the most common infections caused by the Friedländer's bacillus to be in the abdomen and to originate in the intestinal tract. These include appendiceal and subphrenic abscesses and peritonitis. In most of the cases the organisms are obtained in pure culture, but in a large proportion they are found together with colon bacilli. An epidemic form of diarrhea in children has been ascribed to *Klebsiella*. The urinary tract is the next most frequent site of infection. Here and in infections of the gallbladder and bile ducts, associated defects, particularly those causing obstruction, are present in almost all cases

in which suppuration occurs. Positive cultures may be obtained from the duodenal bile in some of the cases of biliary tract infections. Occasional cases have a course simulating that of catarrhal jaundice. Prostatitis, salpingitis, infections of the skin and of the uterus and vagina have been encountered. Suppurative arthritis is usually a metastatic lesion, and ulcerative endocarditis occurs in cases with associated bacteremia. Meningitis may occur after sinusitis, otitis media or trauma.

Course and Treatment. The course depends on the site of the lesion. Transient bacteremia may occur in any of these cases. In acute severe cases, especially those with bacteremia, intensive chemotherapy should be used. Surgical drainage is indicated whenever collections of pus become accessible. Urinary tract infections are amenable to treatment with the tetracyclines, streptomycin, chloramphenicol or a sulfonamide. When obstructive lesions of the intestinal, biliary or urinary tract are present, the obstruction must be relieved, if possible, in order to bring about a cure of the infection.

MAXWELL FINLAND

References

Baehr, G., Schwartzman, G., and Greenspon, E. B.: *Bacillus Friedländer* Infections. Ann. Int. Med., 10:1788, 1937.

Felsen, B., Rosenberg, L. S., and Hamburger, M.: Roentgen Findings in Acute Friedländer's Pneumonia. Radiology, 53:559, 1949.

Friedländer, C.: Ueber die Schizomyceten bei der acuten fibrinösen Pneumonie. Virchows Arch. f. path. Anat., 87:319, 1882.

Henriksen, S. D.: Classification of the Klebsiella Group. Acta Path., 30:230, 1953.

Jaffe, S. A.: Extrapulmonary *Klebsiella pneumoniae* Infections. J.A.M.A., 122:292, 1943.

Julianelle, L. A.: A Biological Classification of *Encapsulatus pneumoniae* (Friedländer's Bacillus). J. Exper. Med., 44:113, 1926.

Kinney, T. D., and Ginsberg, H. S.: Pyogenic Liver Abscesses Due to *Klebsiella pneumoniae* (Friedländer's Bacillus). New England J. Med., 228:145, 1943.

Kornblum, K.: The Roentgen-Ray Diagnosis of Pulmonary Infections with the Friedländer Bacillus. Am. J. Roentgenol., 9:513, 1928.

Obrinsky, W., and others: Friedländer-Aerogenes Infections in Infancy. Am. J. Dis. Child., 80:621, 1950.

Olcott, C. T.: Pneumonia Due to Friedländer's Bacillus. Arch. Path., 16:471, 1933.

Perlman, E., and Bullowa, J. G. M.: Primary Bacillus Friedländer (*Klebsiella pneumoniae*) Pneumonia. Arch. Int. Med., 67:907, 1941.

Rolly, F.: Beitrag zur Klinik der durch den Bacillus Friedländer erzeugten Sepsis. Muench. med. Wchnschr., 58:17, 1911.

Solomon, S.: Chronic Friedländer Infections of the Lung. J.A.M.A., 115:1527, 1940.

Thompson, A. J., and others: Klebsiella pneumoniae Meningitis. Review of the Literature and Report of a Case with Bacteremia and Pneumonia, with Recovery, A.M.A. Arch. Int. Med., 89:405, 1953.

Weichselbaum, A.: Ueber die Aetiologie der acuten Lungen- und Rippenfellentzündungen. Med. Jahrb., 1:483, 1886.

Wylie, R. H., and Kirschner, P. A.: Friedländer's Pneumonia. Am. Rev. Tuberc., 61:465, 1950.

BACILLARY DYSENTERY

Definition. Bacillary dysentery is an infectious disease characterized by pyogenic inflammatory lesions of the large bowel. The cardinal clinical symptoms are diarrhea, tenesmus and abdominal cramps. In severe cases mucus and pus are characteristically found in the stools. Blood may or may not be present. The causative organisms belong to the genus *Shigella,* hence the use of the term "Shigellosis" to include all types of infection caused by them. The disease is widespread throughout the world, but is particularly prone to appear in epidemic form in the tropics.

History. Bloody diarrhea accompanied by tenesmus and abdominal pain was recognized as a clinical entity by Hippocrates in the fourth century B.C. Herodotus attributed the defeat of the Persian Army in 380 B.C. in part to dysentery, and since that time it has been an important scourge of military campaigns. Only in World War II was field sanitation sufficiently developed to prevent epidemic outbreaks of the disease. The separation of amebic and bacillary dysentery on clinical, epidemiologic and pathologic grounds took place in the latter part of the nineteenth century. In 1898 Shiga identified *Shigella dysenteriae* as the causative agent in an outbreak of the disease occurring in Japan, and in the course of the next twenty years Flexner, Sonne and Schmitz isolated related organisms from patients suffering from dysentery in other parts of the world.

Etiology. The causative agents of bacillary dysentery are bacteria belonging to the genus *Shigella.* These organisms are slender, nonsporulating, gram-negative rods which are neither motile nor encapsulated. They are facultative anaerobes which show optimum growth at 37° C. and are not fastidious in their growth requirements. On the basis of biochemical and antigenic studies several distinct species have been recognized within the genus.

The four main groups are: A, nonmannitol and nonlactose fermenting organisms, B and C, mannitol fermenting and nonlactose fermenting organisms, and D, mannitol and late lactose fermenting organisms. The more important pathogens are:

Group A
   1. *Shigella dysenteriae,* Type 1 (Shiga bacillus)
   2. *Shigella dysenteriae,* Type 2 (Schmitz bacillus)
Group B
   1. *Shigella flexneri* (Flexner subgroup of paradysentery bacilli, multiple antigenic types)
Group C
   1. *Shigella boydii* (Boyd subgroup of paradysentery bacilli, multiple antigenic types)
Group D
   1. *Shigella sonnei* (Sonne bacillus, two antigenic types)

Of these species only *Shigella dysenteriae* produces a soluble heat-labile exotoxin. This is neurotoxic in nature, and its relation to the pathogenesis of the disease remains uncertain. The cell substance of dysentery bacilli (in common with other gram-negative organisms) contains a relatively heat-stable endotoxin which, when injected parenterally into small mammals, causes diarrhea, weight loss and inflammation of the gastrointestinal wall which may progress to actual ulceration. While it is plausible to assume that the release of this endotoxin in the gut wall as a result of autolysis of the bacterial cells is related to the production of the specific lesions, direct proof of this is lacking. The pathogenesis of the disease process is not clear.

Epidemiology. The portal of entry for the dysentery bacillus is the gastrointestinal tract; the usual vehicle is contaminated food or water. During the acute stage of the disease the organisms are excreted in large numbers in the liquid stools. This process may continue during convalescence or even into the period when the patient has become asymptomatic. Dysentery in epidemic form is likely to occur at times when large groups of people are massed together under conditions of defective sanitation: e.g., armies in the field, refugee camps, overcrowded asylums for the mentally deficient. Tropical conditions, by favoring the mechanical spread of the disease by flies and other arthropods, are propitious for the development of epidemic disease. Although in temperate climates the disease tends to appear in endemic rather than epidemic form, it is nonetheless widespread. In these conditions the symptomless carrier is presumed to represent the usual source of infection. The incidence of the disease in these areas is usually greater in the warmer months of the year. For the year 1952, 23,197 cases of bacillary dysentery with 334 deaths were reported in the United States, giving a morbidity rate of 14.9 per 100,000 and a case fatality rate of 1.4 per cent.

Morbid Anatomy. Bacillary dysentery is a pyogenic inflammation of the mucous membrane of the large bowel which may extend to involve the lower ileum as well. The earliest changes are generalized hyperemia and edema of the mucosa. Focal ulceration occurs as the surface tissue becomes necrotic and sloughs off. These ulcers show sharp, well defined margins in contrast to the undermining lesions of amebic dysentery. In bacillary dysentery, the ulcers do not extend as a rule beyond the muscularis mucosae and only rarely go on to perforation. The infectious process is essentially *local,* being limited to the gut wall, and invasion of the blood stream is an uncommon finding. Healing takes place by the formation of granulation tissue which is often pigmented. Scar tissue formation is common only if the ulcers are unusually deep and extensive.

Pathologic Physiology and Biochemistry. The frequent passage of copious liquid stools as a result of the inflammatory process involving the large bowel causes a significant loss of both water and electrolytes. As a result of the relatively greater loss of base (sodium and potassium) in the form of intestinal secretions, acidosis develops which is accentuated if the patient is unable to take food by mouth. If fever is present, the insensible loss of water increases, and dehydration is correspondingly more marked. In severe cases appreciable amounts of blood may be lost with the stools, but in the uncomplicated infection it is rare for this to progress to the point where significant anemia develops. In interfering with the proper absorption of foodstuffs, long-continued diarrhea results in significant malnutrition.

Clinical Manifestations. The incubation period probably varies from one to six days, with a median of approximately 48 hours. Incubation periods of less than 24 hours have been reported, but are rare. The magnitude of the infecting dose and the general physical condition of the patient are factors which probably affect it.

The clinical severity of bacillary dysentery varies greatly from the very acute case in which the severity of the diarrhea and the prostration of the patient simulate cholera to the mild one in which there may be no more than slight diarrhea for a few hours, with the passage of no blood and but little mucus. The average case falls between these extremes and is the one most commonly seen.

The *onset* is usually abrupt. Fever and abdominal cramps are the initial complaints. Chilly sensations and even frank chills are occasional symptoms at this stage. Diarrhea follows within a few hours. The stools, semisolid at first, rapidly become watery and in all but mild cases are accompanied by the passage of mucus and pus and, less frequently, blood. The patient may have watery bowel movements as often as four to five times an hour. After a few hours the frequency of movement becomes less, generalized abdominal cramps are succeeded by tenesmus, and the relatively scanty movements may begin to show gross blood. Headache, lassitude and general prostration are prominent features of the severer cases. Nausea is a common complaint. Vomiting may occur, but is rarely protracted.

Physical examination at this time shows an anxious patient complaining of generalized abdominal discomfort and scalding bowel movements. Evidence of dehydration, dry tongue and skin and drawn facies, may be apparent in the more severe cases. Abdominal tenderness, most marked in the lower quadrants, is usually found and at times is accompanied by generalized muscle spasm. Occasionally this is sufficiently localized in the right lower quadrant to suggest acute appendicitis. Sigmoidoscopic examination reveals hyperemia and edema of the bowel wall accompanied by spasm and rigidity. Injection of the lymph follicles and areas of purulent exudate may often be seen as well. A normal or moderately elevated leukocyte count (10,000 to 15,000 cells per cubic millimeter) is the usual finding. Leukopenia is occasionally encountered; if this is marked and primarily granulocytic, the prognosis must be guarded.

In the case of average severity to which supportive therapy is given the disease runs its course over a period of a week or ten days. Concomitant with a diminution in the daily number of stools is a decrease of tenesmus, and a return of appetite and a sense of well-being. Mild diarrhea may continue for some days after the tenesmus and anorexia have disappeared. In light cases, strength and weight are regained in a matter of days; if the attack has been severe, the return to the normal state of well-being may take several weeks. If the infection is complicated by preexisting malnutrition or debility, or if opportunity for supportive therapy is not available at the onset, convalescence is correspondingly prolonged.

Conjunctivitis, upper respiratory symptoms and signs of meningeal irritation are occasionally met with during the acute stage of the disease. In the last instance lumbar puncture reveals a normal cerebrospinal fluid. Toxic encephalitis and peripheral neuritis have been reported as rare complications of *Shigella dysenteriae* infections.

Arthritis has been reported as a late complication in a small (1 per cent) proportion of cases. It usually occurs during the second or third week after onset of the acute disease, at a time when complete recovery is about to be attained. The process involves the larger joints in single or multiple fashion. Migratory polyarthritis is less common. Usually the inflammatory condition subsides completely and spontaneously within the course of a fortnight.

In a minority of instances the disease may progress from the acute to the chronic state. Low grade irregular fever may persist for some weeks, accompanied by intermittent bouts of mild diarrhea during which the stools show mucus in varying quantities, but rarely significant amounts of blood. Felsen feels that these cases are particularly prone to develop chronic ulcerative colitis and ileitis. The etiologic relationship between acute bacillary dysentery and these conditions remains unclear.

Diagnosis. The abrupt onset of fever, abdominal pain and diarrhea, accompanied by the passage of mucus and blood, strongly suggests the diagnosis of bacillary dysentery, particularly if similar cases are encountered simultaneously in the same household or community. Atypical cases present more difficulty. Microscopic examination of the stool should always be done if possible. The gross findings of mucus and blood may be confirmed by examination of coverslip preparations of mucus previously emulsified in saline. The exudate of bacillary dysentery is highly cellular with a great predominance of polymorphonuclear cells, as opposed to the mononuclear exudate characteristic of protozoal infections. The failure to find motile trophozoites of *Endamoeba histolytica* after prolonged and repeated search tends to exclude the presence of amebic dysentery.

The specific diagnosis is made by the isolation and identification of the etiologic agent. Cultures are best taken either by sigmoidoscopy or by means of the rectal swab technique as outlined by Hardy, Mason, Hamerick and Mitchell. If stool culture must be resorted to, the specimen should be brought promptly to the laboratory and cultured as soon as possible. Since the organisms are found in greatest numbers in the mucous exudate, flecks of this material should be selected for culture. Of the various differential media used for the isolation of dysentery bacilli, S.S. agar (Difco) and desoxycholate citrate agar are the most useful. Once suspected colonies have been isolated, they may be identified by the proper biochemical and serologic techniques, notably fermentation of carbohydrates, and agglutination by specific antiserums. Since even in the best of circumstances it is not always possible to isolate dysentery bacilli from clinical cases that are otherwise typical, a negative culture does not exclude the diagnosis.

During the second week of the disease, agglutinins appear in the patient's blood. The serologic diagnosis by the demonstration of these antibodies is unsatisfactory, however, since they develop irregularly and relatively late in the course of the disease. In addition, many healthy persons have significant agglutinin titers as a result of previous contact with the organisms. This is particularly true in areas in which the dysentery is widespread, as in the tropics.

Differential Diagnosis. The differential diagnosis must include other infections characterized by diarrhea. In contrast to bacillary dysentery, amebic dysentery usually occurs sporadically, the onset is insidious, and the patient is not incapacitated in the early stages of the disease, which, however, usually progresses to chronicity. Sigmoidoscopic examination reveals the typical lesions, while the finding of the specific amebas in the stools confirms the diagnosis. Cholera may usually be excluded on epidemiologic grounds, as well as by the absence of excessive vomiting and of typical "ricewater" stools containing cholera vibrios. Occasionally typhoid and paratyphoid fevers may be accompanied in their early stages by diarrhea, but the onset is usually much less abrupt. The diarrhea caused by *Salmonella* food infections comes on suddenly and is often severe; in addition, the cellular exudate may resemble that of bacillary dysentery. In such cases the differential diagnosis depends upon the isolation and identification of the etiologic agent. Food infection due to streptococci or staphylococci may usually be differentiated on the basis of the shorter incubation period, more vomiting, and the absence of mucus and cellular exudate in the stools.

Prognosis. In ordinary circumstances bacillary dysentery tends to be an acute self-limited disease which usually runs its course over a period of ten days without an appreciable case fatality rate. Outbreaks of bacillary dysentery have been reported, however, in which the case fatality rate has been as high as 30 per cent. In general, prognosis in any individual case depends upon three factors: (1) the species of infecting organism, (2) the age and general physical condition of the patient at the time of infection, and (3) the opportunities for supportive treatment and chemotherapy.

Shigella dysenteriae has long been credited with causing a particularly virulent type of the disease, which in Japan and India has been attended by a high mortality rate. Infections with this organism are fortunately rare in the United States and Canada. In these countries the predominating bacteria, various types of *Shigella flexneri* and *Shigella sonnei*, generally give rise to a milder form of the disease.

Persons in the extremes of life, infants and the aged, are less resistant to the disease, and in them the case fatality rate is appreciably higher. Further, persons debilitated by acute or chronic malnutrition, hardship, privations or other unfavorable conditions of living are particularly susceptible to its ravages. These environmental factors are undoubtedly responsible in part at least for the high case fatality rate accompanying epidemics of bacillary dysentery in the Far East.

If adequate supportive therapy is made available for the patient early in the course of his disease, the prognosis is greatly improved. Under favorable conditions chemotherapy may play an important role in controlling the infection.

The importance of all these factors is borne out by the remarkably low case fatality rates observed in the British and American Armed Forces during the latter part of World War II.

Treatment. The rational aims of the treatment of bacillary dysentery are (1) suppor-

tive and symptomatic, to maintain the patient's strength and to relieve his symptoms; (2) correction of the pathologic disturbances of salt, water and protein metabolism; (3) eradication of the infectious agent by means of antimicrobial agents.

General Management. During the acute phase of the disease, complete bed rest is indicated. The use of a diaper of absorbent cotton or cellulose instead of a bedpan saves the patient from unnecessary exertion. Purging should be avoided, since it merely increases the patient's discomfort. In severe cases expert nursing care is of vital importance. The patient should be isolated, kept warm and screened from flies. Sanitary precautions as for any enteric infection must be maintained, and particular attention should be paid to the sterilization of excreta and of soiled bed linen.

The abdominal pain and discomfort may usually be relieved by the application of heat (hot water bottles, stupes, and so forth) to the abdomen plus the judicious use of sedatives and antispasmodic drugs. According to Thompson, White and Schafer, the following prescription is particularly useful:

	Gm. or cc.
Tincture of belladonna	8
Sodium bromide	10
Elixir phenobarbital, to make	60
Directions: 1 teaspoonful every four hours.	

In some instances these measures will not control the discomfort. Though the routine use of paregoric and other opiates is contraindicated because of the artificial intestinal stasis that they cause, a gravely ill patient can occasionally be tided over the acute episode by the parenteral administration of codeine (45 mg.) or morphine sulfate (10 mg.), which will usually give him a few hours' comfort.

Dehydration, and acidosis resulting from loss of base in the intestinal secretions must be combated vigorously by use of supplemental parenteral fluids if an oral intake adequate to produce a daily urinary output of 1500 to 2000 ml. cannot be maintained. In the average case the daily intravenous administration of 1500 ml. of physiologic saline (9 gm. of sodium chloride per liter), to which 75 gm. of dextrose has been added, suffices to correct the electrolyte balance and adds much to the patient's comfort. Severe cases require more parenteral fluid, which should be given in the form of 5 per cent dextrose in distilled water. Rarely is the acidosis so severe as to require the use of supplementary sodium lactate.

If the patient shows evidence of incipient vasomotor collapse or shock coupled with hemoconcentration, plasma should be given in amounts adequate to restore the hematocrit reading to normal. It is rarely necessary to give more than 500 ml. for this purpose. It is important that dehydration be relieved *before* or at least *simultaneously* with the administration of plasma. In the occasional patient who develops a significant anemia secondary to blood loss in the stools, whole blood transfusions are indicated.

The diet during the acute stage of the disease is best limited to clear fluids, given warmed and in small quantities. With the return of appetite and feeling of well-being a bland low residue diet containing adequate protein and vitamins is given. The return to a full diet should be made gradually and cautiously. In severe, protracted cases the oral or parenteral administration of supplementary vitamins may be advantageous.

Antimicrobial Therapy. The broad spectrum drugs oxytetracycline (Terramycin), chlortetracycline (Aureomycin) and chloramphenicol (Chloromycetin) are markedly effective in the treatment of bacillary dysentery. In the extensive field trials reported by Hardy and his associates, the administration of any of these drugs in 4 gm. amounts over a period of 24 hours resulted in the prompt disappearance of clinical manifestations and a rapid conversion from positive to negative cultures in nearly all cases. The recommended dosage schedule is 2 gm. initially, followed by 1 gm. at 12 and 24 hours. In severe cases it is probably wise to continue specific therapy for another 24 hours. The occurrence of relapses and of drug-resistant organisms has not constituted a significant problem as yet. Of the three agents oxytetracycline appears to be the drug of choice since it gives rise to practically no troublesome side reactions. This drug has the added advantage of being effective in the therapy of amebic dysentery, a point worth considering in cases in which the etiologic agent has not been identified.

The effectiveness of the sulfonamides in the treatment of bacillary dysentery has been considerably reduced in recent years by the frequent occurrence of drug-resistant strains. In the past, sulfadiazine has proven to be the most effective of these compounds; an initial dose of 2 gm. should be followed by 1 gm. every 6 hours until the patient is symptom-free and, ideally, until three successive daily cultures are negative. During the period of sulfonamide therapy, an adequate urinary output (2000 ml. daily) must be maintained in order to avoid the possibility of renal complications. Streptomycin and polymyxin appear to be less effective while penicillin has no demonstrable therapeutic value.

Bacteriophage therapy has been ineffective in actual practice. With the possible exception of specific antitoxin in infection with *Shigella dysenteriae,* there is no evidence that antiserums are of practical use.

Prevention. The prevention of bacillary dysentery depends upon the detection, isolation and treatment of all cases of the disease, and, in addition, upon the detection and treatment of asymptomatic carriers of dysentery bacilli. This is particularly important in food handlers. Since healthy carriers of dysentery bacilli may excrete the organisms intermittently, repeated cultures may be necessary in order to detect them. Strict attention to personal hygiene is most important. Adequate sanitation with the proper safeguarding of food and water supplies and effective disposal of sewage coupled with fly control are the most valuable public health measures. Bacterial vaccines have not been effective. As yet no adequate trials of the broad spectrum drugs, the tetracyclines or chloramphenicol, as chemoprophylactic agents have been reported; in theory they should be effective. Prophylactic sulfadiazine, 1 or 2 gm. daily, has been tried with indifferent success, largely because of the rapid development of drug-resistant strains.

F. S. CHEEVER

References

Cheever, F. S.: Bacillary Dysentery and the Shigella, in Dubos, R. J.: Bacterial and Mycotic Infections of Man. Philadelphia, J. B. Lippincott Company, 1952, Chapter 18.
———: The Treatment of Shigellosis with Antibiotics. Ann. N. Y. Acad. Sci., 55:1063, 1952.
Felsen, J., and Wolarsky, W.: Acute and Chronic Bacillary Dysentery and Ulcerative Colitis. J.A.M.A., 153:1069, 1953.
Garfinkel, B. T., and others: Antibiotics in Acute Bacillary Dysentery: Observations in 1,408 Cases with Positive Cultures. J.A.M.A., 51:1157, 1953.
Hardy, A. V., Mason, R. P., and Martin, G. A.: The Antibiotics in Acute Bacillary Dysentery. Ann. N. Y. Acad. Sci., 55:1070, 1952
———, Mason, R. P., Hamerick, D., and Mitchell,

R. B.: The Bacteriologic Diagnosis of Enteric Infections. U. S. Armed Forces M. J., 4:541, 1953.

———, and Watt, J.: Studies of the Acute Diarrheal Diseases. XIV. Clinical Observations. Pub. Health Rep., 60:521, 1945.

———, and Watt, J.: Studies of the Acute Diarrheal Diseases. XVIII. Epidemiology. Pub. Health Rep., 63:363, 1948.

Holmes, W. H.: Bacillary and Rickettsial Infections, Acute and Chronic. New York, The Macmillan Co., 1944, Chapter 17.

Rogers, Sir Leonard: Dysenteries: Their Differentiation and Treatment. London, Oxford Medical Publications. 1913.

Shiga, Keyoshi: The Trend of Prevention, Therapy and Epidemiology of Dysentery Since the Discovery of the Causative Organism. New England J. Med., 215:1205, 1936.

Thompson, C. M., White, B. V., and Schafer, W. L.: Shigellosis Studies: I. Etiology and Clinical Features. U. S. Nav. Med. Bull., 46:528, 1946.

CHOLERA

Definition. Cholera is an acute infectious disease caused by *Vibrio comma,* in which the primary seat of the infection is in the gastrointestinal tract. It is characterized by diarrhea, vomiting and dehydration, which are extremely severe in typical cases.

History and Geographic Distribution. Cholera has been known for centuries in India, whence it spread to China in the seventeenth century. A number of pandemics occurred during the nineteenth and early twentieth centuries. The United States was invaded repeatedly, but after 1873 practically all cases were stopped at seaports. In recent years few cases have been brought to this country. During and after World War I, epidemics occurred in Europe. Although World War II was associated with extensive epidemics in the Far East and with smaller outbreaks in the Near East, the disease did not reach Europe or the Americas.

Cholera is always present in the region of the lower Ganges River in India and frequently spreads from that area both to the east and to the west. It often appears in Thailand, Indo-China, the Chinese ports and the Yang-tse River Valley. Cholera should be regarded as potentially having a world-wide distribution, against which constant sanitary vigilance is needed.

Etiology. The specific cause of cholera is the *Vibrio comma (V. cholerae)* of Koch (1883). The organism is a short, curved bacillus, with a terminal flagellum. It is aerobic, grows on ordinary media, is motile, easily stained by the usual methods, and is gram-negative. It is readily dissociated into R and S forms. Both H and O antigens are present. The cholera bacillus is one of a large group of vibrios, and its identification necessitates the use of a specific agglutinating serum or of special cultural procedures when agglutination fails, as occasionally happens.

Epidemiology. The etiologic agent may persist in nature in favorable circumstances for a few days, but it dies out in stools in one or two days. For this reason, infection generally can be traced to patients in the immediate neighborhood. The existence of subclinical infections in the community probably explains the often apparently haphazard distribution of clinical cases. It is doubtful that true carriers exist, although convalescent patients may pass virulent organisms for a short time. The most important sources of infection are patients in the incubation stage and those with mild symptoms. Cholera is acquired by the ingestion of food or drink contaminated by feces which contain the vibrio. Contaminated water is one of the most important means of spreading the disease. Flies may play an important role. The development of epidemics is seasonal, being favored as a rule by high temperature, high relative humidity and intermittent rains. Unless effective control is exercised, an epidemic rapidly spreads through an unprotected population, moving along lines of communication, such as railway, steamship and air routes. Cholera is not, however, as readily communicable as was formerly thought, for many exposed persons escape infection.

Morbid Anatomy. The striking changes are the result of extreme dehydration. Rigor mortis is unusually marked. Dryness and shrinkage are everywhere apparent, but in general inflammatory changes are conspicuous by their absence. The blood is thick and scanty. The serous membranes have the look of ground glass and are somewhat sticky. The intestinal wall is cyanotic and congested. The lumen contains much grayish opalescent liquid, often with no trace of fecal matter. Large areas of mucosa may be lost, but localized ulceration is not present. The lymphoid tissue of the ileum is somewhat prominent. The kidneys may show marked congestion.

Pathologic Physiology and Chemistry. The cholera vibrio has its principal localization in the ileum. Organisms may be found in small numbers in the lungs and other organs, but they are seldom if ever demonstrated in the blood. Cholera vibrios produce no exotoxin so far as is known. Hence their effects must be attributed to the liberation of a powerful endotoxin when they die. The principal immediate effect of the infection is precipitate loss by the body of large amounts of fluid and salts, as the result of profuse diarrhea and vomiting. The extraction of fluid from blood, tissue spaces and tissues in turn is rarely equalled in any other condition, except some cases of infantile diarrhea and extreme hemorrhage. The tissues become desiccated and the blood is concentrated to a high degree. Such extreme values may be encountered as 1.070 for specific gravity, 20 gm. per 100 ml. for hemoglobin concentration, 7.0 million per cubic millimeter for erythrocyte count, and 75 for erythrocyte volume percentage. The concentration of plasma proteins is also increased. These alterations in the blood have a profound effect on the circulation. The blood pressure is greatly reduced and the cardiac output is much decreased. In part, at least, because of these circulatory changes, renal function is gravely impaired.

Chlorides are lost with the fluid of vomitus, but this loss is overbalanced by that of bases, principally sodium, from the bowel. The resulting shift in the acid-base balance is accentuated by the retention of acid which results from renal insufficiency. Values as low as 7.1 have been recorded for pH, and 138 milliequivalents per liter for total base in the blood. Urea and other nitrogenous substances are also retained as a result of renal insufficiency. After the liberal intravenous administration of fluids, even though no alkaline solution is given, alkalosis tends to be present for a time during recovery. In most cases death in the early stage is chiefly the result of dehydration, while in the later stages it is due to renal insufficiency. An attack of cholera confers only limited immunity to subsequent infection.

Symptoms. The incubation period is usually only one to three days, sometimes as many as five. In occasional instances premonitory symptoms of depression, lack of energy and simple diarrhea occur. The onset is usually sudden. It is characterized by voluminous watery stools, copious vomiting and great prostration. In many cases the speed with which the symptoms attain overwhelming proportions is striking. Stools are passed with great frequency and soon lose all fecal character. They are grayish and contain clumps of degenerating epithelial cells and mucus, but little if any blood and no pus. The absence of tenesmus is often noted. Vomiting may occur suddenly, without nausea or retching. After a time the vomitus resembles the stools. As dehydration becomes marked, there is great thirst, but almost nothing taken by mouth can be retained. The features become gaunt and pinched and the eyes sunken. The skin is cyanotic and shriveled. Muscular cramps may be widespread and exceedingly painful. The voice becomes thick and feeble. A marked tachycardia develops and the pulse may be hardly perceptible. The blood pressure falls, the systolic level often reaching values below 60 mm. of mercury. Venesection may result in only slight bleeding. The excretion of urine is diminished and may cease. In severe cases uremia often develops. The skin temperature usually falls below normal, although the rectal temperature may be normal or even elevated unless the patient is in a state of complete collapse. Unless uremia develops, the mind remains clear, although patients are usually extremely apathetic. Complications other than those directly related to the disease are not common or characteristic. They are usually related to the previous poor health of the patient, as in the instances in which clinical signs of avitaminoses appear, or to poor treatment. Occasionally secondary infections may occur, such as those causing parotitis.

Of great practical importance is the fact that, in epidemics, cases occur in which only malaise and simple diarrhea are present throughout the course.

Diagnosis. Information that there is cholera in the area in which a patient lives or from which he has recently come should suggest the possibility of cholera. The clinical picture is highly characteristic in ordinary cases, and typical stools are highly suggestive. In differential diagnosis confusion may arise over acute bacillary dysentery, food poisoning, heat exhaustion, some forms of malaria (especially *falciparum* malaria), and other conditions associated with diarrhea and shock. Mild cases of cholera masquerading as dysentery or food poisoning may be overlooked. They are extremely dangerous for the public health. The ordinary clinical laboratory examinations of blood, urine and stool are not very helpful.

The specific diagnosis of cholera is made by identification by agglutination of *V. comma* derived from passed stools or, better, from samples obtained from the rectum. Characteristic forms seen in smears stained with dilute carbolfuchsin are suggestive, but the finding requires confirmation. The organism may grow poorly or not at all on media usually used for other intestinal pathogens. Cultures should be made from fresh specimens, using peptone water at pH 8.0 to 8.4. After incubation at 37° C. for six to eight hours, the surface growth, in which vibrios are concentrated if present, should be examined microscopically. If suggestive forms are found, subcultures are made by streaking on nutrient or infusion agar. After 24 hours, suggestive colonies should be tested by the slide method with agglutinating serum specific for *V. comma.* When positive tests are obtained, the colonies should be isolated and further confirmation should be sought in the biochemical reactions of the organisms and by macroscopic tube agglutination tests.

Prognosis. The outcome depends greatly on the patient's previous state of health and on the promptitude and quality of medical care. The course is usually short, averaging three to five days. Death may take place, however, in a few hours or only after many days. The case fatality rate in epidemics among poorly treated patients is often 60 per cent. On the other hand, when adequate treatment is promptly given, it may be as low as 5 per cent.

Treatment. Strict isolation is indicated for both patients and proved carriers. Clothing, bedding and eating utensils should be boiled. Stools, vomitus and (because of the danger of their being contaminated) urines should be thoroughly disinfected as for typhoid fever. While stools are frequent, patients may be kept on cots with holes cut in the center, so that they defecate directly into pans containing a suitable disinfectant, such as 1 per cent cresol. Because of the brevity of the acute stage, the diet during that period is relatively unimportant. At best, patients can retain only small quantities of fluid at this time. A soft diet may be given as soon as the patient desires it. When the temperature is below normal, the patient should be kept warm. Such drugs as sedatives, hypnotics, laxatives, epinephrine and digitalis have no place in the treatment of the usual patient. The value of cholera bacteriophage is controversial. No therapeutic serum which is known to be effective is available. The use of antimicrobial agents is discussed later.

Replacement Therapy. The prompt parenteral administration of adequate amounts of solutions suitable to replace the lost water and electrolytes is crucial. Failure to recognize this need or delay in action may result in loss of the patient. The intravenous route is best. Whole blood is not indicated in cholera. The value of plasma is uncertain, and the rationale of its use is obscure. The main reliance should be placed on physiologic saline solution, but it is customary in early cases to give limited amounts (500 to 1000 ml.) of a hypertonic saline solution (sodium chloride, 14 gm. per liter). Only sterile distilled water which is free of pyrogens should be used to make solutions for intravenous injection. It is desirable to add to any solution given sufficient dextrose to make a 5 per cent solution, and 1 mg. of thiamine chloride for each 25 gm. of dextrose, but this should be done so that not more than 50 gm. of dextrose are given in one hour or 400 gm. in 24 hours. Solutions should be given at body temperature.

No rule can be given for the amount of saline solution which may be required or the period over which its administration may be necessary. Patients with cholera generally need amounts of fluid rarely given for other diseases. On the other hand, too much fluid of any type may precipitate a fatal issue. The patient must be closely and continuously observed. The blood pressure is the most important single guide to clinical judgment. Other helpful guides are the pulse rate, the color and consistency of the blood, and the volume of urine. Signs that too much fluid has already been given are restlessness, palpitation, pain in the chest, coughing and edema. The best objective guide to treatment is the specific gravity of the blood. The most convenient suitable method is the copper sulfate procedure of Phillips and his co-workers. The higher this value is at the start of treatment, the greater is the total volume of fluid required. As the specific gravity approaches its normal value (1.056 to 1.058), the rate of administration of fluid should be retarded. As a rule, 2 liters of fluid are needed in the first 2 hours and more fluid every 3 or 4 hours for sometime thereafter. In the first 24 hours, 4 to 8 liters are often required, and injections may have to be continued through the second 24 hours or longer.

In many cases the loss of alkali is so great that replacement is indicated. The acidosis of cholera differs from that of diabetes or nephritis. In the acute stage the respiration is not a good guide to the condition. Ketone bodies are not to be expected in the urine because of cholera itself. The volume and reaction of the urine are important indications. If practicable, determinations of the blood pH, carbon dioxide-combining power and nonprotein nitrogen are helpful. Alkali replacement may be made by the intravenous injection of a solution of sodium bicarbonate, 18 gm., and sodium chloride, 6 gm. per liter, which should be prepared with the usual precautions. Certain advantages, including greater ease of preparation, are offered by one-sixth molar solution of racemic sodium lactate. A good many patients need 500 ml. of alkaline solution, but this amount often suffices. Care should be taken not to overdo the alkaline treatment. In addition to sodium, other electrolytes are undoubtedly lost, especially phosphate and potassium. The ideal replacement solution should contain such additional electrolytes as may be depleted. A detailed statement, however, can be made only when more information about electrolyte balances in cholera and experience with the use of complex solutions become available.

Chemotherapy. No drug treatment should be used in cholera to the neglect of replacement therapy. The good results obtainable without using antimicrobial agents render difficult the evaluation of such agents. So far, none of these agents has been proved to produce significantly lower fatality rates than those seen following good replacement therapy. A few observers have felt that the use of sulfonamides shortened the course (it is usually very short with replacement therapy alone). When chloramphenicol or oxytetracycline is given, organisms disappear early from the stools but without clinical benefit. The general conclusion is that antimicrobial agents add nothing significant to what is accomplished by replacement therapy.

Prevention. Since the spread of cholera is always closely associated with patients suffering from the disease, the isolation of such patients and the proper disposal of their excreta and vomitus are essential. Cholera is one of the few diseases subject to foreign quarantine. Strict control of the water supply, of food and food handlers, and of flies is necessary for cholera control. If the water supply is not subject to general control, it should be boiled and then chlorinated. In areas where cholera is present, raw food should not be eaten and all handlers of food should be frequently examined and closely supervised. All food should be thoroughly protected from flies and other insects. Insects should be controlled by proper use of appropriate preparations of DDT.

Immunization. Control measures should not be neglected because of immunization. Vaccination against cholera affords partial immunity which lasts only three to six months. It is recommended only for persons through an area where cholera is known to be present. Two doses (0.5 cc. and then 1 cc.) of a reliable vaccine should be given at an interval of seven to ten days. If exposure continues, a stimulating dose of 1 cc. is given every four to six months.

FRANCIS R. DIEUAIDE

References

Chaudhuri, R. N., and others: Treatment of Cholera with Oral and Intravenous Chloromycetin. Indian Med. Gaz., 87:455, 1952.
Das, A., and others: Terramycin in Cholera. J. Indian M. A., 22:268, 272, 1953.
Ghanem, M. H., and Mikhail, M. N.: Clinical and Biochemical Studies in Cholera and the Rationale of Treatment. Tr. Roy. Soc. Trop. Med. & Hyg., 43:81, 1949.
Lahiri, S. C.: Chemotherapy in Cholera. Brit. M. J., 1:500, 1951.
Mackie, T. T., Hunter, G. W., and Worth, C. B.: Manual of Tropical Medicine. 2nd ed. Philadelphia, W. B. Saunders Company, 1954.
Phillips, R. A., and others: Copper Sulfate Method for Measuring Specific Gravities of Whole Blood and Plasma. Bull. U. S. Army Med. Dept., 71:66, 1943.
Reimann, H. A., and others: Asiatic Cholera. Clinical Study and Experimental Therapy with Streptomycin. Am. J. Trop. Med., 26:631, 1946.
Rogers, L.: Cholera Incidence in India . . . Inoculation of Pilgrims as a Preventive Measure. Tr. Roy. Soc Trop. Med. & Hyg., 38:73, 1944.
Saha, H., and Das, A.: Observations on Biochemical Findings of the Blood in Cholera. J. Indian M. A., 20:427, 1951.

BRUCELLOSIS
(Undulant Fever, Malta Fever)

Definition. Brucellosis is an infectious disease due to organisms belonging to the genus *Brucella,* the disease being transmitted to man from lower animals. The acute stage is characterized by fever, sweats, weakness, pains and aches, and few or no localizing physical abnormalities. Occasionally the same manifestations predominate in a chronic illness enduring for months or years.

History. Brucellosis constituted a febrile illness which puzzled the medical personnel of the British Army and Navy stationed in the Mediterranean area during the latter part of the nineteenth century. It appeared to differ from paludism (malaria) and enteric fever (typhoid). Marston, a Royal Army

Surgeon, presented a report of his own illness in 1863, which was an accurate clinical description of brucellosis. The etiologic agent was described by David Bruce in 1887. Bang in Denmark reported in 1897 the recovery of another species, *Brucella abortus,* from aborting cattle, while Traum isolated a third species, *Br. suis,* from aborting sows in 1914. Alice Evans differentiated strains of *Br. melitensis* from *Br. abortus* by serologic methods and predicted correctly that human disease would result from drinking raw cow's milk. The classic monograph, "Mediterranean, Malta or Undulant Fever," by Hughes, appeared in 1897. Wright and Semple described the agglutination test for brucellosis in 1897. The epidemiology of brucellosis on the Island of Malta was clearly defined by the brilliant reports of the Mediterranean Fever Commission issued between 1905 and 1907.

Etiology. At least three species of *Brucella* are known, each of which is commonly identified with one of three animal species. They are *Br. melitensis* (goat), *Br. suis* (hog) and *Br. abortus* (cattle). *Brucella* are small, gram-negative rods which are nonmotile and do not form spores. Growth is supported in liver infusion broth, tryptose phosphate broth or trypticase soy broth. The combined liquid-solid medium of Castaneda with tryptose phosphate broth contained in a rectangular flask and tryptose phosphate agar distributed along one of the sides of the bottle affords a simple and safe method of handling *Brucella* cultures. Primary isolation of *Br. abortus* requires about a 10 per cent displacement of air by carbon dioxide. Differentiation of the three species is based upon biochemical reactions, serologic tests and the resistance of the organisms to the bacteriostatic action of various dyes.

Morbid Anatomy. *Brucella* localizes intracellularly in the tissues of the reticuloendothelial system, particularly the lymph nodes, bone marrow, liver and spleen. The initial cellular response to the organisms is the appearance of mononuclear and epithelioid cells, and then the formation of tubercles or granulomas having foreign body and Langhans' types of giant cells. This pattern of tissue reaction is characteristic of brucellosis, but is not specific. A similar type of cellular response may be encountered in some instances of sarcoidosis, tuberculosis and syphilis. Sometimes *Brucella* induces necrosis of the tissues and small abscesses may be seen in the parenchyma of the liver, spleen and, occasionally, in the osseous tissue of the vertebrae and long bones. Caseation is not a feature of brucellosis. *Brucella* may localize in other organs or tissues such as the testicles, ovaries, meninges and endocardium.

Epidemiology and Pathogenesis. The natural reservoir of brucellosis is in domestic animals, especially cattle, hogs and goats. In animals, *Brucella* tends to localize more abundantly in the mammary gland and in the pregnant uterus. Healthy-appearing animals may shed large numbers of organisms in the milk for months or years, and the disease may provoke abortions in pregnant animals. Man contracts the disease by direct contact with infected animals or contaminated secretions and excretions. The organisms gain entrance through small abrasions of the skin. Human disease is also acquired through the ingestion of raw milk and fresh cheese prepared from unpasteurized milk. The disease is rarely transmitted from human to human. Brucellosis is primarily an occupational disease and involves rural populations much more frequently than city dwellers. The disease occurs most often in farmers, livestock producers, meat packing plant employees and veterinarians. Children are more resistant to brucellosis than are adults.

In general, *Br. abortus* produces a milder disease than that caused by *Br. suis* or *Br. melitensis.* Not infrequently, however, *Br. abortus* may produce a severe, even a fatal, illness. While the principal habitat of *Br. abortus* is cattle, it has been recently established that this species occurs in hogs under natural conditions. The more invasive *Br. melitensis* is traditionally associated with goats, but in recent years naturally infected hogs have been found infected with this species in the midwestern area of the United States, and an increasing number of human cases have occurred as a result of contact with infected porcine tissues. Much less frequently, *Br. melitensis* resides in cattle. *Brucella suis* is most often found in hogs, but invasion of cattle has occurred. Epidemics of human brucellosis have been traced to raw cow's milk containing *Br. suis.* Except for unusual circumstances, human brucellosis is a sporadic disease. Because different degrees of illness are caused by the three species of *Brucella,* it is well for physicians in any given geographic area to know what species of domestic animal is harboring the organisms and what species of *Brucella* is causing human disease. In Minnesota and in Wisconsin most human cases are due to *Br. abortus,* but in Iowa, *Br. suis* is more commonly the cause of human disease. In Mexico, human brucellosis exists almost as an epidemic disease, being due entirely to *Br. melitensis*. However, in Puerto Rico, *Br. abortus* is the cause of human disease.

Little is known about the invasive properties of *Brucella*. The bacterial cells produce no exotoxin, and scant information is available about the so-called endotoxins. After invasion of the tissues, the organisms reside, and very likely proliferate, within the host's cells. This intracytoplasmic parasitization may account for the chronicity of the disease, both in animals and in man. Hypersensitivity to *Brucella* antigens is an outstanding feature of brucellosis, which probably contributes to the symptomatology of the disease.

Symptoms and Signs. The incubation period is usually between five and twenty-one days, but in an occasional patient the latent period between the entrance of *Brucella* into the body and the appearance of symptoms may be as long as six to nine months. Brucellosis may have an abrupt onset with chills, fever and sweats indistinguishable from many other febrile conditions. In many instances the disease begins insidiously, and it is only after days or weeks that an apprehensive patient seeks medical advice because of an ill defined incapacitating illness. An almost constant symptom of brucellosis is weakness. Patients may feel reasonably comfortable while in a resting state, but even the slightest physical exertion may induce extreme fatigue and exhaustion. A feeling of chilliness and, less often, frank chills may precede a rise in temperature. Profuse nocturnal sweats are a common manifestation. Generalized aches and pains occur frequently, and often there are headaches, and pain over the thoracolumbar spine. Abdominal pain may be generalized or localized to any one of the quadrants. Arthralgia may occur with periarticular swelling, but rarely is the tissue over the joints reddened and hot. Anorexia and constipation are predominant gastrointestinal complaints, though the illness may be ushered in with diarrhea. A nonproductive cough may be present, but symptoms referable to the upper respiratory tract are not prominent. Table 1 summarizes the symptomatology in brucellosis due to *Br. abortus*. Examination of the patient may reveal few or no physical abnormalities. Table 2 reveals the physical findings in cases of brucellosis due to *Br. abortus*. Almost one half of the patients have enlarged

peripheral lymph nodes or splenomegaly. Hepatomegaly is often present, though jaundice is rare.

As the illness extends beyond the first few days, the manifestations of the disease become

Table 1. Symptomatology in 94 cases of bacteriologically proved disease due to Br. abortus (University of Minnesota series).

	NO. OF CASES	PER CENT OF CASES
Weakness	86	91.5
Sweats	72	76.5
Chills	71	75.5
Anorexia	66	70.0
Generalized aches	65	69.0
Headache	60	63.8
Rigors	52	56.3
Nervousness	49	52.0
Backache	48	51.0
Joint pain	41	43.6
Depression	38	40.0
Insomnia	36	38.3
Pain back of neck	34	36.1
Cough	28	30.0
Abdominal pain	20	21.0
Constipation	11	11.6
Visual disturbances	11	11.6
Nausea and vomiting	9	9.6
Diarrhea	9	9.6
Genitourinary disturbances	7	7.4
Neuralgia	5	5.3

Table 2. Physical findings in 94 cases of bacteriologically proved disease due to Br. abortus (University of Minnesota series).

	NO. OF CASES	PER CENT OF CASES
Fever	92	97.9
Lymphadenopathy	43	45.7
Palpable spleen	42	44.7
Palpable liver	24	25.5
Abdominal tenderness	8	8.5
Skin lesions	8	8.5
Neurologic changes	7	7.5
Cardiac abnormalities	7	7.5
Tenderness over spine	6	6.4
Funduscopic changes	3	3.2
Orchitis	2	2.1
Pain over hip joint	2	2.1
Jaundice	1	1.0
Pain over sacroiliac joint	1	1.0

established in a fairly characteristic pattern. Contrary to classic descriptions of the disease, the temperature curve does not usually exhibit a remittent or undulating type of fever. This may occur in the more chronic case or in infections due to *Br. melitensis*. The usual course is that of an intermittent fever with diurnal variations from 98° up to 100° to 104° F. Occasionally a sustained fever may take place, as observed in typhoid fever. The patients may feel better in the early morning hours, but, as evening draws on, the face may feel flushed, and a rise in temperature is associated with the onset of a headache. Nights are marked by discomforting sweats and insomnia. Pain involving the muscles of the back of the neck is a common complaint. Persistent anorexia results in weight loss. Vasomotor disturbances are reflected by the presence of an intermittent tachycardia, labile blood pressure, and cold and moist palms of the hands and soles of the feet. Amenorrhea may appear in young women, and the sexual drive in both sexes is greatly diminished. Nervousness is a constant feature with the display of gross tremors of the extended fingers and tongue. The patients become irritable and mentally depressed. Visual disturbances are not uncommon. Brucellosis does not cause a greater number of abortions or miscarriages in pregnancy than many other bacteremic and febrile diseases.

Complications. Serious complications occasionally occur and depend in part upon the species of *Brucella* causing the disease. Organic disturbance of the *central nervous system* may be manifested by encephalitis and meningitis, which are usually chronic and are frequently associated with ocular complaints and diminution in hearing. *Peripheral neuritis* is not an uncommon complication, especially in disease due to *Br. melitensis*. An excruciating type of pain over the course of the sciatic nerve, either unilateral or bilateral, is encountered. *Radiculoneuritis* is often associated with spondylitis. Destructive *bone* lesions are occasionally seen with involvement of the spine. The *spondylitis* of brucellosis most often involves the thoracolumbar area and is characterized by a destruction of the intervertebral disks and the adjoining vertebral bodies. Brucellosis causes a destructive suppurative *arthritis,* usually attacking but a single joint. A deforming and chronic polyarthritis is extremely rare, if it ever does occur as a complication of brucellosis. Single *osteolytic lesions of the long bones* occasionally appear, similar to the Brodie's abscess caused by typhoid bacilli. A more serious complication is *vegetative bacterial endocarditis.* *Pulmonary infiltration* and

pleural effusions have been described. Though *Brucellae* uniformly localize in the liver in bacteremic cases with the formation of granulomas, serious *hepatitis* is a rare complication. However, there is evidence that brucellosis may at least be a participating factor in the genesis of some cases of *cirrhosis of the liver.* An occasional complication of brucellosis due to *Br. melitensis* is orchitis. *Cystitis* and *nephritis* have been reported as rare complications.

Duration of Acute Illness. In a few instances brucellosis may remain active for many years with either an intermittent or continuous state of debility. In discussing the duration of infections due to *Br. melitensis* and summing up the experience of the Mediterranean Fever Commission, Eyre stated that 85 per cent of the patients had recovered within three months. Observations at the University of Minnesota Hospitals between 1937 and 1953 on cases infected with *Br. abortus* revealed that the majority of patients had recovered within three to six months and that less than 20 per cent had residuals of their disease after one year. Now that highly effective therapy has become available, the duration of the disease has been shortened considerably.

Chronic Brucellosis. Patients with chronic brucellosis must be carefully differentiated from patients with personality aberrations or neurologic disorders, especially if immunologic evidence points to past contact with *Brucella.* Acute brucellosis in most patients has a marked impact upon the central nervous system and disturbs the equilibrium of the autonomic nervous system. The main symptomatology of weakness, headaches, sweats, anorexia, constipation, insomnia, irritability, nervousness and depression emphasizes the neurogenic features of the disease. If active disease persists for weeks, these manifestations become deeply entrenched as an emotional pattern of the patient. It is readily seen why, in unstable persons or in those with an underlying psychoneurosis, brucellosis may have serious repercussions in the ensuing years. Long after the infection has subsided, a few patients flounder in a state of ill health, they and their physicians explaining this lack of well being on the misconstrued basis of chronic brucellosis. In endemic areas, especially, many persons have been exposed to brucellosis without serious consequences. A considerable number have had their tissues invaded by *Brucella* without having had any demonstrable clinical evidence of active disease. Included in this group have been those with psychoneurosis, asthenia and anxiety states. On the basis of inconclusive laboratory and immunologic data, an erroneous diagnosis of chronic brucellosis may be pinned on these emotionally disturbed people.

Diagnosis. The diagnosis of brucellosis can be made with certainty only on the basis of laboratory procedures. Epidemiologic information of a possible exposure to the disease, coupled with a symptomatology consistent with brucellosis, should lead the physician to make a presumptive diagnosis, which then should be followed up with appropriate diagnostic procedures. In a febrile patient the *leukocyte* count of the peripheral blood may be helpful in the rapid detection or elimination of brucellosis. The total number of leukocytes is usually normal or reduced. It is most unusual to have a count exceeding 10,000 cells per cubic millimeter in an uncomplicated acute case. The differential count usually shows a relative lymphocytosis. The *erythrocyte sedimentation* rate may be normal or accelerated and is of no diagnostic value. It may be of some prognostic aid when the rate is rapid, in the sense that a persistently abnormal value may indicate the presence of active disease. Aspirated sternal *bone marrow* may reveal the presence of granulomas, which are characteristic but not specific for brucellosis.

Agglutination Reaction. The agglutination test provides a dependable laboratory method for making a diagnosis of brucellosis. Consistent success with the agglutination reaction is dependent upon a reliable antigen and upon the techniques which are used. Rapid slide agglutination tests are valuable for bedside or office use. For this purpose Castaneda's antigen and techniques have been utilized at the University of Minnesota Hospitals. The antigen is a formalized aqueous suspension of *Brucella* cells stained with methylene blue and titrated so that positive reactions are obtained only when the peripheral blood has agglutinins in a titer of 1:100 or higher, as determined by the multiple dilution tube method. In Castaneda's test, when a drop of blood from the finger is mixed with a drop of the antigen on the slide, the blue peripheral ring of agglutinated antigen may be demonstrated within 30 seconds. The multiple dilution tube method should also be used. In the laboratories of the University Hospitals

and of the Minnesota State Department of Health a satisfactory antigen has been that supplied by the United States Bureau of Animal Industry. When the agglutination test is properly performed with a sensitive antigen, agglutinins are uniformly demonstrated in acute or chronic cases of brucellosis, with but rare exceptions. Agglutinins were observed in 267 of 268 consecutive bacteriologically proved cases of brucellosis in Minnesota. Over 90 per cent of the patients exhibited titers of 1:320 or above. The higher the titer of agglutinins, the more likely that cultures of blood will be positive. At the University Hospitals, not one bacteriologically proved case of brucellosis has failed to show agglutinins in the blood in a period of twelve years. If the titer is 1:100 or above, serious consideration must be given to the diagnosis of brucellosis. As in typhoid fever, a rising titer of agglutinins during an acute febrile illness is of considerable diagnostic importance. It is the exceptional case in which a dilution under 1:100 is a reliable index of active disease. Agglutinins may be demonstrated in the blood months and years after patients have recovered from their illness. Agglutinins for *Brucella* may be stimulated by *P. tularensis* and after vaccination for cholera with *Vibrio cholerae*. A technical point to be recalled is that in the macroscopic tube method a prozone phenomenon may be present in which the lower dilutions of serum show no agglutination of the antigen. Rarely, a blocking of the antigen-antibody reaction may occur.

As a practical procedure there is no advantage in using the more technical *complement fixation* test. The *opsonocytophagic* test is a measurement of the phagocytosis of *Brucella* by polymorphonuclear neutrophile leukocytes. The test yields such meager and indecisive information in the sporadic cases of suspected brucellosis that it is not advocated as a diagnostic procedure. A *culture* of venous blood, preferably several, should be undertaken in every patient suspected of having brucellosis. This applies particularly to persons having a positive agglutination reaction. Bacteremia is more likely to be demonstrated in febrile patients with a high titer of *Brucella* agglutinins and an enlarged and tender spleen. In a period of twelve years at the University Hospitals, positive blood cultures have been obtained in about 50 per cent of all the cases of brucellosis. Most of these patients had infections due to *Br. abortus*. In an occasional case, *Brucella* may be cultured from aspirated sternal bone marrow when simultaneous cultures of venous blood remain sterile. The organisms have been isolated from the bile, urine and cerebrospinal fluid.

Cutaneous Tests. Intradermal reactions following the injection of *Brucella* antigens indicate a specific state of hypersensitivity to *Brucella*. Like the tuberculin reaction in tuberculosis, a positive *Brucella* skin test indicates past invasion of the body by organisms, but it does not mean that active disease is present. Intradermal tests may be performed with heat-killed *Brucella* cells, a nucleoprotein fraction (brucellergin), and purified protein fraction, all of which yield a delayed type of reaction reaching their maximum in 24 to 48 hours. The carbohydrate fraction of *Brucella* results in an immediate cutaneous reaction. The great majority of acute and chronic cases of brucellosis demonstrate positive skin tests. Exceptions include the acute cases of only a few days' duration, and the seriously ill patients. Patients with *Brucella* subacute bacterial endocarditis have a high titer of agglutinins and negative skin tests, and recovery is associated with the appearance of positive skin tests. Dermal hypersensitivity may persist for years after the patient has recovered from the disease. It should be emphasized that all the antigens may provoke the appearance of *Brucella* agglutinins in normal persons a week or two after an injection. In these circumstances, titers well over 1:100 may be achieved.

The skin test is an unreliable method for detecting active cases of brucellosis, and its routine use is not recommended. If agglutinins are absent from the blood and blood cultures remain sterile, a diagnosis of active brucellosis is not justified. If in a particular case there is a history of possible exposure to the disease, and the illness is consistent with the characteristic pattern of brucellosis, and agglutinins are present in a titer of 1:100 or above, no further information is to be gained by performing a skin test. If, in such a case, agglutinins are consistently absent and blood cultures remain sterile, a positive or negative skin test cannot decide the issue.

Differential Diagnosis. In the differential diagnosis of acute brucellosis other febrile diseases must be considered. Brucellosis is commonly mistaken for *influenza,* but the latter disease is a self-limited illness of short duration and may be associated with upper respiratory symptoms. *Infectious mononucleosis* is differentiated from brucellosis on the basis of hematologic and serologic evidence. Where *malaria* and brucellosis occur together, the diagnosis of the former is resolved by finding plasmodia in blood films. Serologic and cultural studies should differentiate brucellosis from *Hodgkin's disease, lymphoblastoma* and *tuberculosis. Typhoid fever* is differentiated by isolating *S. typhosa* from the blood, and by the agglutination test. The more chronic cases of brucellosis may be differentiated only with considerable difficulty from *psychoneurosis* or an *anxiety state.* Not infrequently, an attack of brucellosis may be the "trigger" mechanism for displaying an underlying neurosis, and neurotic symptoms may persist long after the infection has subsided.

Prognosis. The natural course of brucellosis will depend upon the geographic area where the disease is being observed, and the species of *Brucella* causing illness. In a locality where a population is malnourished and parasitized by other diseases, *Br. melitensis* will cause more chronic disabling illness than in a community where good health and nutrition abound and where brucellosis is caused by *Br. abortus.* In general, the case mortality rate of the disease is not greater than 2 to 3 per cent, and up to 75 per cent of the patients recover within three to six months. Now that highly effective treatment is available, the incidence of chronic illness should be considerably reduced. In a small number of cases a relapsing type of febrile illness is observed. Reinfections may also occur. Where there is repeated exposure to the disease it is not always possible to distinguish between a relapse and a reinfection.

Treatment. *General Management.* It is of primary importance that the physician reassure any patient having either acute or chronic brucellosis that the disease is self-limited and that he will completely recover from his illness. Too often patients are informed that brucellosis is a chronic debilitating disease for which there is no satisfactory treatment. The patient then corroborates this dismal outlook by reading about the disease and consulting with his friends and other physicians. Finally, he is psychologically prepared to endure an illness of several years' duration. It is easy to see why a mistaken diagnosis of chronic brucellosis in the place of a correct diagnosis of psychoneurosis provides an escape mechanism for many persons and a needless infliction for others. It cannot be emphasized too strongly that vigorous reassurance by the physician that the patient will recover from this illness is essential, whether or not specific therapy is used. Another therapeutic recommendation of major value to the patient is rest, physical and mental. Since the outstanding symptoms of brucellosis are weakness and easy fatigability, the victims are unable to pursue their daily routines. Not infrequently, adequate rest is associated with a decline in temperature and permanent recovery. One need only consult the reports of the Mediterranean Fever Commission to appreciate the value of rest. Any specific therapy in brucellosis should be augmented by intelligent psychotherapy. There are few other diseases in which indecision or discouragement on the part of the physician is so detrimental to the welfare of the patient.

Antimicrobial Therapy. Treatment with antibrucella agents is recommended for either acute or chronic cases. Though an occasional patient has recovered coincidentally with the administration of a sulfonamide, such as sulfadiazine or sulfathiazole, sulfonamide therpay alone is not recommended. Streptomycin will alter the clinical course of brucellosis favorably in only a small number of patients, but when either streptomycin or dihydrostreptomycin is injected simultaneously with the oral administration of a sulfonamide such as sulfadiazine, an effective therapeutic response is observed more consistently. Streptomycin or dihydrostreptomycin is administered intramuscularly in a dose of 0.5 gm. every 8 hours for seven to ten days. At the same time, 1 gm. of sulfadiazine is given orally every 4 to 6 hours for two weeks. Though this combined therapy has proved satisfactory in a large number of patients, there are certain disadvantages in the method. Because of the need for parenteral injections and the dangers of toxic reactions from either the streptomycin or the sulfonamide, it is necessary for the patients to be treated and observed in a hospital. Furthermore, a number of patients have had a relapse of their illness after therapy has been completed. Combined streptomycin-sulfonamide therapy is not the treatment of choice for brucellosis.

Chlortetracycline or oxytetracycline has been used effectively in the treatment of acute and chronic brucellosis. Tetracycline appears to be equally as effective. The recommended dose for each of these drugs is 0.5 gm. every 6 hours for two to three weeks. In infections due to *Br. abortus* approximately 80 to 90 per cent have recovered after an initial course of treatment. Relapses can be treated favorably with a second or even a third course of chemotherapy. The foregoing treatment is recommended for the mildly ill patient, and especially for those having disease due to *Br. abortus.* For the more seriously ill patient, with or without complications, and particularly for those having infections caused by *Br. melitensis* or *Br. suis,* it is recommended that chlortetracycline, oxytetracycline or tetracycline should be administered in the doses already suggested along with dihydrostreptomycin, which is given intramuscularly in a dose of 2 gm. daily. The administration of the two drugs together should be prescribed for a minimum of fourteen to twenty-one days. Chloramphenicol is no longer employed in the University of Minnesota clinics for brucellosis.

Attempts at "Desensitization." It is common practice to treat the more chronic cases of brucellosis with *Brucella* antigens, such as heat-killed cells and filtrates (brucellin). Unless the injection of antigens is carefully controlled, disturbing local and systemic reactions may occur. Because of the dubious clinical results obtained with such a procedure, and because some patients are extremely sensitive to the antigen, this type of treatment has not been advocated at the University of Minnesota Hospitals. It is more logical and practicable to use an antibrucella drug or drugs as an aid to the tissues in eradicating the organisms, rather than subject patients to a prolonged period of "desensitization" or "immunization" with *Brucella* antigens.

Prevention. Brucellosis as a human disease will be eliminated only when the reservoir in domestic animals is eradicated. There is no established method for immunizing human beings against brucellosis. A significant segment of the population may be protected against the disease by legislation requiring that all milk destined for human consumption be pasteurized.

WESLEY W. SPINK

References

Brucellosis: A Symposium. Washington, D. C., American Association for the Advancement of Science, 1950.

Evans, A. C.: Further Studies on Bacterium Abortus and Related Bacteria. II. A Comparison of Bacterium Abortus with Bacterium Bronchisepticus and with the Organisms Which Cause Malta Fever. J. Infect. Dis., 22:576, 1918.

Hardy, A. V., Jordan, C. J., Borts, I. H., and Hardy, G. C.: Undulant Fever, with Special Reference to a Study of Brucella Infection in Iowa. Bull. No. 158, National Institute of Health, 1931.

Huddelson, I. F.: Brucellosis in Man and Animals. New York, The Commonwealth Fund, 1943.

Hughes, M. L.: Mediterranean, Malta or Undulant Fever. London, Macmillan and Co., Ltd., 1897.

Meyer, K. F.: Observations on the Pathogenesis of Undulant Fever. Essays in Biology. University of California Press, Berkeley and Los Angeles, 1943.

Reports of the Commission for the Investigation of Mediterranean Fever. London, Harrison and Sons, Parts 1 to 7, 1905–1907.

Spink, W. W.: The Laboratory in the Diagnosis of Brucellosis. Am. J. Clin. Path., 22:201, 1952.

———: Epidemiologic and Clinical Studies on Brucellosis, 1937–1952. Tr. & Stud., Coll. Physicians, Philadelphia, 21:51, 1953.

Third Inter-American Congress on Brucellosis. Washington, D. C., Pan American Sanitary Bureau, 1950.

PASTEURELLA INFECTIONS
PLAGUE

Definition. Plague is an acute infection caused by *Pasteurella pestis* and transmitted chiefly by certain fleas. It is enzoötic or epizoötic in many wild rodents and in "domestic" rats, from which it spreads to man. Plague is characterized by inflammation of the lymphatic and blood vascular system and by hemorrhages in the tissues. It is customary to divide the disease into three types, bubonic, septicemic and pneumonic. The disease, however, may be considered fundamentally a single entity. The septicemic type is characterized by wide extension and great severity. The bubonic and pneumonic types have important epidemiologic and clinical significance which is discussed later.

History. Plague constitutes the "black death" of history and literature (Boccaccio, Pepys). Epidemics swept in waves through Europe during the Middle Ages and up to the first part of the nineteenth century, often killing one in ten or more of the population. In 1894 plague began to spread from western China and in fifteen years had reached most parts of the world. It arrived in the United States in 1900. Although the total number of human cases in the

United States since then is only 500-odd, small outbreaks of pneumonic plague occurred in California in 1919 and 1924.

Geographic Distribution. The principal centers of human plague are China, Burma and India. The disease often appears in Ceylon, Indo-China, Thailand, Indonesia, the eastern and southern shores of the Mediterranean, the Azores, and parts of Africa and South America. A small number of cases occur nearly every year in the United States.

Many species of wild rodent are infected with plague in various parts of the world, including central and eastern Asia, Russia, South Africa, South America, Hawaii and the United States (sylvatic plague). Ground squirrels and prairie dogs have been found infected throughout the western part of the United States.

Etiology. *Pasteurella pestis* (Yersin and Kitasato, 1894) is a short thick bacillus with rounded ends. Its form varies greatly according to the conditions in which it is obtained or grown. A capsule is demonstrable. This organism is aerobic, grows well on usual media, is nonmotile, easily stained and gram-negative. Characteristic stained preparations show a marked bipolar configuration. Under favorable conditions in darkness and moisture it may live outside the body for months or even years. The bacillus is killed by thorough drying in air for two or three days. It may remain viable in dead bodies for weeks, in flea feces for a month, and in pus or sputum for one or two weeks. *Pasteurella pestis* may survive for some time in grain, cotton and gunny sacks. It is quickly killed by a temperature of 80° C., but is very resistant to cold, surviving almost indefinitely in frozen material.

Epidemiology. Plague may be transmitted from wild rodent to "domestic" rat, or vice versa, from either of these to man, and from man to man. Most human infections are acquired from rats. The disease is usually transmitted by rodent fleas. In man, transmission is ordinarily through rubbing into the skin the infected vomitus or feces of a rodent flea, many species of which are capable of carrying plague. In addition, the human flea, *Pulex irritans,* is considered a potential vector, and other insects have been incriminated. Man sometimes acquires plague by contact with the bodies of rodents or human beings sick or dead of the disease, or by handling tissues, blood or discharges derived from them. Apparently the disease can be acquired by ingestion. Inhalation is an uncommon but extremely dangerous method of spread, since it gives rise to fulminant primary plague pneumonia. Usually the inhaled infective material consists of droplets from the sputum of patients with plague pneumonia.

Plague is spread from place to place chiefly by migration or transportation (especially in ships) of infected rats or other rodents. It is occasionally transported by patients with mild disease and by infected fleas through their survival in grain sacks.

There is no evidence of any racial, age or sex variation in susceptibility. The development of human epidemics is determined largely by the following conditions: presence of the infection in rats or other rodents; size of the rodent population; infestation of rodents with fleas; and association of man with rodents. Bad housing and bad sanitation are favorable to rats. Moisture and temperatures between 50° and 80° F. are generally favorable to fleas. Human crowding and poor hygiene are important factors, especially in droplet transmission, which is also favored by cold temperatures.

The method of transmission has great epidemiologic and clinical significance. Inhalation is associated with severe pulmonary disease which is rapidly fatal. This form of the infection is called pneumonic plague. Other forms may be grouped as bubonic plague.

Morbid Anatomy. Rarely, a pustule is found at the site of entry of the infection. The most marked changes are in and about the lymphatics and lymph nodes, which are swollen, edematous and hemorrhagic. Buboes, or swollen nodes, may not be visible on the exterior. Although the changes are most marked in the drainage area of the portal of entry, they are usually found elsewhere as well. The characteristic processes are edema formation, hemorrhage and necrosis. The spleen is much swollen, grayish and soft. Acute hemorrhagic nephritis and meningitis are occasionally present. Inflammation of the endothelium of lymphatics and blood vessels, with small embolic lesions, is characteristic. Large numbers of bacilli are often found in plague lesions and even in the blood. Plague pneumonia, though it may occur in other cases, is the predominant finding in the pneumonic form of the disease in which there are usually no extensive changes in other parts of the body. In this condition the lungs generally show confluent lobular consolidation, but the distribution may be lobar. The appearance is one of engorgement, with little accumulation of fibrin or leukocytes.

Pathogenesis. In mild cases the bacilli remain for the most part localized in the lymphatic system, with only occasional organisms entering the blood. In severe cases they invade and multiply in the blood stream and may reach all parts of the body (septicemic plague). The formation of an exotoxin has not been demonstrated, nor have the physiologic and chemical changes produced by the infection been analyzed in detail. Except in very mild or extremely severe instances, a leukocytosis (usually 20,000 to 25,000 per cubic millimeter) develops, the increase being mainly in neutrophilic granulocytes. There is no anemia. The urine is scanty and usually contains albumin, casts and erythrocytes. Hematuria may occur. An attack of plague usually confers immunity against subsequent infection.

Symptoms. The incubation period varies from two to ten days. Apart from infections acquired by inhalation, the severity also varies. In mild cases with little extension of the disease there may be no constitutional symptoms and the patient may remain ambulant. In severe infections which spread rapidly and in pneumonic plague, prostration quickly occurs. Headache, dizziness and thirst are common complaints. Many patients are confused. As a rule, there is high, remittent fever and marked restlessness. The respirations are fast and shallow and the pulse is rapid and feeble. In a few cases a pustule may be found at the site of inoculation. Signs of lymphangitis may be visible. Enlarged lymph nodes, or buboes, begin to appear on the second day. Pain in them varies from slight to severe. They are usually red and tender. At first they are hard, but they generally suppurate and become soft and matted together. Buboes may rupture and discharge their contents, but sometimes they resolve without so doing. The surrounding tissue is inflamed and edematous. In septicemic cases, blebs, petechiae or purpuric spots may be seen in the skin. Rarely, areas of skin may become necrotic. Hemorrhages may take place from the nose, the stomach and the bowel, and in pneumonic cases from the lungs. In most so-called bubonic cases the lungs show little or nothing, though patches of pneumonia may be present; in such cases there is usually no sputum. In pneumonic plague the physical signs are usually minimal and consist mainly of scattered fine rales, but breathing is rapid and shallow and cyanosis is marked (the picture resembles that of certain cases of diffuse streptococcal pneumonia). In these cases the sputum is thin, at first watery and later bloody. It is loaded with bacilli. Although the spleen is usually enlarged in all types of plague, it is often not felt. At first apathetic, patients tend to become delirious. Convulsions and coma may develop. A few instances of subacute meningitis have been described. The principal complications are secondary infections which often arise in buboes and in the lungs, where they must be distinguished from plague pneumonia.

Diagnosis. The possibility of plague should be suggested by epidemiologic considerations and by the clinical picture. The difficulties in differential diagnosis vary with the stage and anatomic developments. Plague buboes must be separated from adenitis due to streptococcal infections, lymphogranuloma venereum, syphilis and filariasis. Septicemic plague might be confused with many forms of septicemia, tularemia, several forms of typhus, typhoid fever and malaria. Pneumonic plague should be distinguished from streptococcal pneumonia of the type sometimes associated with influenza.

The specific diagnosis of plague is made by demonstrating the presence of *P. pestis* in the contents of buboes (obtained by aspiration), in blood or in sputum. All material which is considered as possibly infected with plague must be handled with the greatest care. All animals inoculated for diagnosis must be free of fleas and other ectoparasites and must be kept in insect-proof cages in a room containing no other animals. Everyone who handles smears, cultures, cages or inoculated animals must wear gowns, masks and rubber gloves. Throughout all diagnostic procedures the strictest aseptic technique must be observed.

Smears should be stained with methylene blue and by Gram's method. Characteristic bacilli are usually seen in good preparations of bubo contents and, in pneumonic cases, in the sputum. Occasionally they are even found in blood smears. Cultures and animal inoculations are often necessary, however, and should always be made for confirmation of smear findings. The plague bacillus grows well on nutrient agar and in broth. The reaction should be approximately neutral, and the incubating temperature should be below 30° C. Mice, rats and guinea pigs are used for inoculation, which is done by intraperitoneal injection or by rubbing material into the scarified skin. If plague is inoculated, these animals die in twenty-four to seventy-two hours. Characteristic lesions should be found and *P. pestis* should be recovered by culture. Agglutination reactions cannot be used.

Prognosis. The course is usually run in five or six days at most. In very severe cases it is over within three days. The over-all fatality rate is not accurately known, because numerous mild cases are not counted. Before the use of chemotherapy, fatality rates in bubonic cases without wide extension of the disease ran from 25 to 75 per cent. Recovery was rare in severe septicemic cases, and pneumonic plague was regarded as uniformly fatal. Chemotherapy greatly improves the outlook.

Treatment. Patients should be confined to bed, and strict isolation should be maintained. Good general medical and nursing care is essential. The type of diet has little importance. The fluid intake should be such as to ensure a daily volume of urine of at least 1500 ml. Fluid, including glucose solution, should be given slowly by the intravenous route, if necessary. Restlessness and delirium are best treated with morphine (10 mg. for adults). With the exception of antimicrobial agents, other drugs have little if any place in the treatment of plague. Antiplague serum and serum globulin have been recommended, but their value remains uncertain and reliable preparations are not generally available.

Chemotherapy. Sulfadiazine, streptomycin, chloramphenicol and oxytetracycline have all been shown to be efficacious. In one series of 118 streptomycin-treated cases only 4 patients died. A number of recoveries from pneumonic plague are on record. Nevertheless, a wholly satisfactory treatment has not yet been achieved. Therapy must be adjusted to the severity of the disease and to its duration. The earlier chemotherapy is begun, the better will be the results. In severe and late cases, especially in pneumonic plague, full dosage of the best available drug is needed. The relative value of the antimicrobial agents mentioned is not yet clear. For most cases streptomycin is recommended as the first choice. It may be given intramuscularly in 0.5 gm. doses at intervals of 3 to 6 hours for 24 to 48 hours, followed by a total daily dosage of 1.5 to 3 gm. in divided doses for about six days in the usual case.

Experience with chloramphenicol and oxytetracycline in the treatment of plague is limited, but it is helpful to know that either of these drugs may be used as an alternative to streptomycin. The suggested schedule for each of these alternatives is three treatments at 3-hour intervals of 0.5 gm. orally and 0.5 gm. intravenously, followed by oral doses amounting to 4 gm. a day for two days and 2 to 3 gm. a day for four or five days. Unfortunately, the possibilities of toxic reactions to all three drugs must be borne in mind, as well as the possible development of drug-resistant organisms.

Sulfadiazine has proved so valuable in less severe cases that its availability should not be overlooked. In mild or very early cases it may be given by mouth in the initial dose of 4 gm., followed by 1.5 to 2 gm. every 4 hours until the temperature is normal. After the temperature is normal, the drug should be continued in doses of 0.5 gm. every 4 hours for about ten days. The usual precautions in the administration of sulfadiazine should be observed, particularly the maintenance of an alkaline urine which generally requires the oral administration of 2.4 gm. of sodium bicarbonate with each dose of sulfadiazine.

Complicating infections which may develop especially in buboes or in the respiratory tract should be treated with an antimicrobial drug to which the infecting organisms are susceptible.

Local Treatment. Hot, wet applications may decrease the discomfort of buboes. Incision should not be performed unless and until suppuration is clearly present.

Prevention. Patients with plague should be isolated in separate screened rooms. When a patient with pneumonic plague is found, known and suspected contacts should be isolated and their temperatures taken twice a day for one week. Attendants on patients with plague pneumonia suspected or established should wear coveralls, with hoods, goggles and rubber gloves. All articles contaminated by the patient or his discharges should be sterilized by boiling or autoclaving or burned. A room vacated by a plague patient and its contents should be thoroughly cleaned and dusted with DDT powder. The bodies of those who have died of the disease must be handled with strict aseptic technique.

Immunization. Vaccination is considered to afford partial protection for six months, but not longer. It is recommended only for those who must necessarily undergo serious exposure or the possibility of serious exposure. It is also used in the control of localized outbreaks of plague. For individual prophylaxis two injections (0.5 and 1 cc., respectively) of a reliable vaccine should be given with an interval of seven days. If necessary, stimulating doses of 1 cc. may be given at intervals of four to six months.

Rodent and Flea Control. Effective prevention of plague is achieved by adequate control of rodents, especially rats. The rat population should be watched for undue increases and for the presence of infected animals. Rodents that may have plague should be handled and disposed of with great care and with particular attention to the possibility that they may harbor fleas. In endemic areas trapping surveys are regularly made. To keep down the rat population, all buildings and ships should be rat-proofed. Adequate protection of food suplies and garbage collections against rats is essential. Rat extermination campaigns should be conducted by trained personnel. The rat poisons now recommended are sodium fluoroacetate and Warfarin. The older poisons such as red squill and thallium sulfate may also be used. All these chemicals are dangerous to man and must be used with great care. Cyanide or carbon disulfide is used in fumigation, but this process can be safely applied only by specially trained workers. Local antirat campaigns have only brief value, unless extensive rat-proofing is undertaken and rat harborages are destroyed. The destruction of fleas is important, especially in rat harborages. DDT is a very effective agent for this purpose. It is applied as a powder or in solution in kerosene.

FRANCIS R. DIEUAIDE

References

Ash, J. E., and Spitz, Sophie: Pathology of Tropical Diseases; An Atlas. Philadelphia, W. B. Saunders Company, 1945.

Hirst, L. F.: The Conquest of Plague: A Study of the Evolution of Epidemiology. New York, Oxford University Press, 1953.

Hoekenga, M. T.: Plague in the Americas. J. Trop. Med. & Hyg., 50:190, 1947.

McCrumb, F. R., Jr., and others: Chloramphenicol and Terramycin in the Treatment of Pneumonic Plague. Am. J. Med., *14:284,* 1953.

————: Chemotherapy of Experimental Plague in the Primate Host. J. Infect. Dis., 92:273, 1953

Meyer, K. F.: Modern Therapy of Plague. J.A.M.A., 144:982, 1950.

————: Ecology of Plague. Medicine, 21:143, 1942.

Pollitzer, R.: Plague. World Health Organization Monograph Ser., No. 22. New York, Columbia University Press, 1954.

Strong, R. P.: Stitt's Diagnosis, Prevention and Treatment of Tropical Diseases. 7th ed. Philadelphia, Blakiston Co., 1944.

Wagle, P. M.: Recent Advances in Treatment of Bubonic Plague. Ind. J. M. Sc., 2:489, 1948.

TULAREMIA

(Plaguelike Disease of Rodents, Deer Fly Fever, Tick Fever, Rabbit Fever)

Definition. Tularemia is a specific infectious disease caused by *Pasteurella tularensis.* It is a potent factor in the destruction of wild animal populations, acting as a heterogeneous infection-chain involving a great variety of rodents and insects. Man may enter the chain accidentally or occupationally by contaminating his hands, conjunctival sac or buccal cavity with the infected internal organs and body fluids of mammals, birds and insects; by the bite of an infected blood-sucking fly or tick; or by drinking contaminated domestic rural water (Parker et al., 1951). Wild rabbits and hares have been the principal sources for the disease in man.

Bacteriology. *Pasteurella tularensis* is an extremely polymorphous micro-organism. It has neither capsules nor flagella. It is nonmotile and gram-negative, but stains well with fuchsin or crystal violet. For routine cultures, cystine-beef heart agar is excellent. The guinea pig is used for laboratory tests and the mouse for testing specimens of sputum (Foshay, 1950).

Epidemiology. Tularemia occurs in nearly all of the United States, in Canada, Alaska, Mexico and Japan. With the endemic areas in central and south Russia are apparently associated the recent geographic extensions into Norway, Sweden, Czechoslovakia, Austria, Poland and, since 1946, France, Belgium and Germany. An increase in typical cases in Turkey and France is reflected in the number of publications that have emanated from these countries in recent years. The time of year when plague occurs depends on the habits of infected ticks, density of infected rabbit population and on the hunting season. More than 10,000 human

infections have been observed; the highest annual incidence was 261 cases in 1939. Sex, race and age are not factors in the incidence. The history and epidemiology of tularemia have been reviewed recently by Ayres and Feemster and Foshay.

Pasteurella tularensis requires no particular portal of entry for its penetration. The most important sources of human infections are (1) contact with infected rabbits (principally cotton-tail rabbits, *Sylvilagus floridans*); (2) bites of arthropods such as the deer fly (*Chrysops discalis*), the wood tick (*Dermacentor andersoni*) and dog tick (*D. variabilis*); (3) bites of such animals as cats, coyotes, dogs and skunks; (4) contact with sheep (fecal droplets of ticks in the wool of sheep); (5) skinning and dressing of mammals, such as muskrats and beavers, and handling pheasants; (6) laboratory infections, presumably by the aerogenic route; (7) ingestion of partially cooked rabbit meat (Amoss and Sprunt) or of water contaminated by water rats due to multiplication of the bacteria in the water-mud medium (Parker et al., 1951).

No proved human-to-human transmission of tularemia has been reported. Although *P. tularensis* is easily recoverable by nasal and pharyngeal swabs or from sputum in cases of tularemic pneumonia and in many without pneumonia, no secondary case has ever been recorded in bedside attendants exposed to droplet infection.

Morbid Anatomy. The autopsy reports (56) by Foshay, Lillie and Francis stress the presence of focal areas of necrosis in various phases of evolution throughout the body. Macroscopically, whitish yellow foci ranging in size from those hardly visible to the eye to those measuring 8 cm. in diameter are found in the lymph nodes, spleen, liver, kidneys and lungs.

Symptoms. The period of incubation in tularemia is from one to ten days. Only the typhoid type proceeds as a general disease without local processes. Since the *onset* is sudden, the patient usually remembers the hour at which he fell ill. Severe headache, vomiting, chills and fever with an initial rise in temperature above 104° F., accompanied by general aching and weakness, are followed by prostration, sweats and loss of weight. Delirium and stupor may be present in the more severe cases. The constancy of the sequence of initial rise in temperature, remission and secondary rise, is striking in the cryptogenic type of the disease. Continuous high temperature is noted in extreme toxemia. Ordinarily, the febrile period may last ten to fifteen days; in the more severe forms the disease usually runs a course of three to four weeks. Febrile periods or elevation of temperature of 1 degree may persist for three weeks. Papular exanthema on the palmar surfaces or roseola, pustules and petechiae on any part of the body may appear at any stage in all forms of tularemia. They heal by absorption or exfoliation.

Enlargement of the spleen is evident in about one quarter of the cases and is not great; on rare occasions it extends from three to four fingerbreadths below the costal margin. Tenderness and pain indicate the existence of a perisplenitis. A slight to moderate polymorphonuclear leukocytosis (12,000 to 15,000 cells per cubic millimeter) may be noted during the course of the disease. Anemia is common. The amount of urine is diminished and results of urinalysis suggest the presence of fever. Myalgia, arthralgia and neuralgia occur frequently.

Cutaneous Tularemia. Thirty-six to forty-eight hours after the onset of the disease with slight, painful enlargement of a lymph node, the patient usually notices that a previous cut or sore is inflamed and tender. This primary lesion evolves from a papular to a pustular stage with a necrotic plug. The pustule is supplanted by a punched-out ulcer with scanty serous discharge which ultimately is replaced by a scar. Not infrequently, painful lymphatics, with or without subcutaneous nodules (nodular lymphangitis) resembling mycotic lesions, extend from the ulcer to the regional epitrocheal or axillary lymph nodes. The nodes vary in size from that of an almond to that of a small orange. Sometimes several groups of nodes show reactions to a single primary lesion; for example, the axillary and supraclavicular nodes may react to a single ulcer on the shoulder. Some lymph nodes suppurate in one to twenty-four months; others remain hard, tender and palpable for periods up to twelve months and ultimately may require incision.

Ophthalmic Tularemia. The primary localization is in the conjunctival sac; it occurs unilaterally or, rarely, bilaterally. Itching, lacrimation, photophobia and pain are early subjective symptoms which are accompanied by swelling of the pre-auricular, parotid, submaxillary and cervical lymph nodes. The eyelids are swollen, and the chemotic, deep red conjunctivitis is studded with small, discrete yellow nodules. Occasionally both the palpebral and bulbar conjunctivas may be covered by a gray, translucent, organized exudate. Punched-out ulcers follow the breakdown of the necrotic nodules. A thin mucoid or purulent discharge accompanies the conjunctivitis for three to five weeks, after which the swelling recedes and complete recovery is the rule. Suppuration of the regional lymph nodes is fairly common in ophthalmic tularemia. Dacryocystitis, corneal ulcers, permanent impairment of vision, optic atrophy and blindness have been observed following perforation of the cornea.

Cryptogenic Tularemia. The symptoms of a general systemic infection are fever, profound toxemia with drowsiness or a typhoidal state, abdominal distress and prostration. Severe pulmonary symptoms in at least 50 per cent of the cases, or intestinal symptoms, may follow.

Pleuropulmonary Tularemia. The symptoms of pulmonary tularemia are variable, and the diagnosis without laboratory aids is difficult. The disease may begin as an inhalation infection with pulmonary symptoms or may develop on a hematogenous basis secondary to some primary focus on the skin or elsewhere. In the first group, pulmonary symptoms, less abrupt than in the pneumococcal types, initiate the disease; hacking, nonproductive cough, dyspnea, fever, malaise and occasional chills are present. Pleuritic pains may be a dominating symptom. Milder infections simulate atypical pneumonias in which the pulmonary lesions last for a month (see Primary Atypical Pneumonia, p. 148).

Primary tularemic pneumonia has been reported, but conclusive proof that it occurs is lacking. Pulmonary tularemia does develop in patients with other well recognized symptoms of tularemia such as ulcers or infections of the eye. Cases of this type offer no problem in diagnosis; as a rule, the sickest patients are most likely to have involvement of the lungs. Pleuritis usually is present, and the development of a pale yellow, slightly cloudy pleural effusion of high specific gravity but low cell count (2000 to 5000 per cubic millimeter) is of great diagnostic value. The pneumonic consolidation as parenchymal confluent or lobular bronchopneumonic infiltration consists of small patchy, later large, coalescing areas. The physical signs may vary from day to day, indicative of a migratory type of pneumonia, usually more extensive in one lung than in the other. When the process is predominantly necrotizing, gangrene, cavitation and pulmonic abscesses develop in the most severe cases. Despite large cavities or abscesses, the sputum is moderate in amount, mucopurulent and rarely blood-tinged or rusty. Roentgenograms taken a few days to two weeks after onset may reveal a slowly advancing, lobular type of consolidation. The mediastinal and peribronchial lymph nodes almost always are enlarged.

Oral and Abdominal Tularemia. Ingestion of insufficiently cooked wild rabbit meat or water contaminated with *P. tularensis* may cause a violent local process in the form of a necrotizing pharyngitis or angina, abscesses on the roof of the mouth, ulcers in the pharynx and nasopharynx, fever, enlargement of the submaxillary and anterior cervical lymph nodes and, in some cases, conjunctivitis. Vomiting, excruciating pains in the abdominal regions and diarrhea begin either during the febrile period or after the temperature has fallen. The course may be fulminant; children have had convulsions, become stuporous and died in the first week of illness.

Complications. Symptoms of general peritonitis with the findings of plastic exudate at autopsy (Francis, Fulmer), and persistent ascites requiring tapping three and five months after onset, have been reported. Appendicitis, diarrhea and intestinal hemorrhages may be present during the last days of illness. Occasionally pericarditis, pneumothorax, thrombosis of the veins or osteomyelitis complicates the convalescence. Meningeal or leptomeningeal localization and meningoencephalitis (Glass), demonstrated by the isolation of *P. tularensis* from the cerebrospinal fluid, usually are fatal.

Course and Prognosis. Many of the patients are ambulatory. In about one third of the cases recovery, even without complications, is slow; it confers a relative immunity. Reinfection has been reported (Green and Eigelsbach, 1950). According to Foshay, the mean duration of fever in untreated cases is twenty-six days, the duration of the adenopathy three to four months, and the duration of the disease five and one-half months. Even though clinical recovery is evident, *P. tularensis,* because of its facultative intracellular parasitism, may remain alive in the tissue for months and perhaps years (Blackford, Foshay and Mayer). Pulmonary tularemia

has had a high rate of fatality (62.5 per cent), while the average mortality for tularemia in the United States has been reported by the United States Public Health Service as 5.6 per cent (Foshay, 6.0; Simpson, 11.0 per cent). Death may occur within four days to nine months after onset.

Diagnosis. Tularemia should be considered in every doubtful case of fever or atypical pneumonia in which the patient may have been exposed by contact with some animal. The following immunologic and bacteriologic tests, in the order mentioned, are valuable diagnostic aids:

1. *Intracutaneous or percutaneous allergic skin tests* with detoxified formalin-killed *P. tularensis* as antigen (Foshay) may yield positive reactions on the third day of illness. Since hypersensitiveness of the skin is a notable feature of tularemia throughout the disease, this method deserves more frequent use than has been customary in the past. The inflammatory response is similar to the reaction to tuberculin, and the wheal attains maximal size 48 hours after injection or application on the scarified skin.

2. *Agglutination and Complement Fixation Tests.* Specific antibodies in the blood never appear before the tenth or twelfth day of the disease, and thus the agglutination test is of little help during the first period of the disease when it is most difficult to diagnose clinically. The serums of patients with brucellosis, furthermore, may give positive reactions with tularemic antigens. When repeatedly applied in order to determine a rise in the titer of the agglutinins, the test is valuable and irreplaceable for retrospective diagnosis.

3. *Cultures* on dextrose-cystine or thioglycolate blood agar, inoculation of guinea pigs or chick embryos with blood, pleural effusions and infected material, or of mice with sputum during life and with blood from the heart at autopsy should be made when agglutinins are absent and the course of the disease suggests tularemia. *Pasteurella tularensis* may be isolated from the sputum of persons suffering from tularemia who manifest no frank clinical signs of pulmonary involvement. The danger to the laboratory worker who makes use of direct cultivation or animal tests should be recognized.

Differential Diagnosis. Tularemia may masquerade in a variety of forms; the signs and symptoms are so similar to many other acute infectious diseases, notably influenza, psittacosis, atypical pneumonia, undulant fever, typhoid and septicemia, that differential diagnosis is difficult. The subcutaneous nodules and the enlarged lymph nodes have been erroneously attributed to sporotrichosis, and at autopsy tularemia has been mistaken for tuberculosis. In any locality where the infection is prevalent among rodents, the clinician must have tularemia in mind.

Treatment. Until Heilman proved streptomycin a specific chemotherapeutic agent in experimental infections with *P. tularensis,* the treatment of tularemia had been largely symptomatic. Chlortetracycline (Aureomycin) and chloramphenicol gave good experimental indications that they might be valuable, but patients treated with chlortetracycline had prompt remissions followed by recrudescence. All recent reports emphasize that streptomycin and dihydrostreptomycin are the drugs of choice and approximate the ideal therapeutic agent. The histories of 71 patients fully document this conclusion (Corwin and Stubbs, 1952). If the illness is acute and pursuing a stormy course, administration of 0.5 to 1.0 gm. of streptomycin or its dehydro derivative per day produces dramatic effects. Higher doses (2 to 4 gm.) are necessary in the highly fatal pneumonic or pleuropulmonary form than are required in the milder ulceroglandular and ophthalmic forms. As a rule, no benefit is derived from treatment with the drug for longer than ten to twelve days. The local cutaneous lesions should not be incised; they are best treated by hot, moist applications containing some germicide which makes the handling of the dressings less dangerous. Suppurating lymph nodes should be incised only after they show definite fluctuation. Since febrile reactions and even chills may follow such a procedure, surgical treatment of tularemia should be judicious.

Prevention. Tularemia, as an everlasting endemic and frequently epidemic disease of rodents and with a latent parasitism in insects, cannot be eradicated. There is a likelihood that an effective immunizing antigen may be prepared. Until the prophylactic value of vaccine has been established it is imperative that sportsmen, butchers and those who live in regions where the infection prevails should be educated to the dangers of this disease. Rubber gloves should be worn while dressing wild rabbits. Laboratory workers should use face masks. To render the meat of rabbits harmless, thorough cooking

is imperative. Some reduction in the incidence of tularemia would be accomplished by supervision of interstate shipments of wild hares and of their sale for food in markets and restaurants.

KARL F. MEYER

References

Ayres, J. C., and Feemster, R. F.: Epidemiology of Tularemia in Massachusetts with a Review of the Literature. New England J. Med., 238:187, 1948.

Corwin, W. C., and Stubbs, S. P.: Further Studies on Tularemia in the Ozarks. J.A.M.A., 149:343, 1952.

Foshay, L.: Tularemia: Summary of Certain Aspects of Disease, Including Methods for Early Diagnosis and Results of Serum Treatment in 600 Patients. Medicine, 19:11, 1940.

————: Tularemia. Ann. Rev. Microbiol., 4:313, 1950.

Glass, G. B. J.: An Epidemic of Tularemia Transmitted by Insects in Settlements of Deportation, Asino and Jaja, Siberia, Soviet Russia. A Report of 121 Cases. Am. J. M. Sc., 216:411, 1948.

McCoy, G. W.: A Plague-like Disease of Rodents. Pub. Health Bull., 43:53, 1911.

Meyer, K. F.: Tularemia. Bacterium tularense, in Dubos, R. J.: Bacterial and Mycotic Infections of Man. 2nd ed. Philadelphia, J. B. Lippincott Company, 1952, pp. 476–487.

Parker, R. R., Steinhaus, E. A., Kohls, G., and Jellison, W. L.: Contamination of Natural Waters and Mud with Pasteurella tularensis and Tularemia in Beavers and Muskrats in the Northwestern United States. National Institutes of Health Bull. No. 193, 1951, 61 pp.

GLANDERS
(Farcy, Morve, Rotz, Malleus, Hautwurm)

Definition. Glanders, an infectious disease of equines (horses, mules and donkeys) occasionally transmitted to man, is caused by a specific micro-organism, *Malleomyces mallei.* Under natural conditions wild catlike carnivores and dogs may contract the infection. The disease is characterized by nodular lesions in the internal organs and by ulcerative papules or nodes of the skin and subcutaneous tissues, and of the respiratory mucous membrane.

History. In ancient times certain diseases of the equine species were known as μηλις (malleus). Its transmissibility was proved in the eighteenth century; its microbic nature was recognized by Chauveau in 1868, and the organism was fully identified by Löffler and Schütz in 1882 and 1886. They isolated *Bacillus mallei* in pure culture and with these cultures produced typical glanders in horses. As a diagnostic agent, "mallein" was produced by Helman in 1891; serologic methods were developed by Schnürer (1905), and the complement fixation test by Schütz and Schubert (1909).

Etiology. In smears prepared from the viscid pus of the abscesses, M. *mallei* is seen in extracellular or intracellular location, usually in small numbers, as straight or slightly curved rods with rounded ends, 1.5 to 3.0 microns long and 0.5 micron broad, singly, sometimes in pairs or parallel bundles. It is nonmotile, noncapsulated and gram-negative, and stains distinctly with alkaline methylene blue or carbolthionin, exhibiting a characteristic beaded, granular or bipolar appearance. The organism produces a brownish coloration on potato media.

Since some other micro-organisms are similar to the glanders bacillus, it is advisable to test the pathogenicity of the isolated bacteria on male guinea pigs or male hamsters. After intraperitoneal or even subcutaneous injection the organism localizes in the serosa covering the tunica vaginalis and incites a thick purulent exudate. The testes are swollen (second to twelfth day), and the scrotal skin may become adherent and ulcerated; the animal usually dies between the tenth and the fourteenth days. This testicular reaction, first described by I. Straus (1889), is diagnostically significant, provided the exudate is controlled both microscopically and culturally. Several different species of bacteria (*Ps. aeruginosa, B. preisznocard, Brucella,* and others) and fungi (*Sporotrichum, Coccidiomyces* and others) produce a Straus reaction similar to that induced by M. *mallei.*

Melioidosis. Of particular importance is the fact that the organism of *melioidosis,* a disease of man which closely resembles glanders and is caused by M. *whitmori* (*M. pseudomallei*), produces a Straus reaction. *Malleomyces whitmori* differs from M. *mallei* in the following particulars: it is motile, forms a corrugated growth, attacks a larger range of carbohydrates, and decomposes sodium fumarate.

Spontaneous infections have been discovered in rodents, primarily in rats, in Burma. In recent studies in Indo-China not a single infection was found in 20,000 rats. Nor have any been found any place in the course of the many mass examinations of rats for *P. pestis.* Single, usually fatal infections in horses, cattle, hogs (Madagascar), dogs, cats and sheep (Queensland) are on record. The first 83 human cases were seen in Burma, the Malay States, India, Ceylon, Indo-China and Thailand. According to a report from Indo-China 19 of 38 infections ended fatally. The mode of transmission in these 38 is unknown; the increased disposition to infection and poor health of the Europeans in that area were emphasized. A report from England (Grant and Barwell) and one from the United States (Garry and Koch) indicate that the disease is not confined to Asia. In 1942 two fatalities were encountered in military personnel on Guam.

Epidemiology. *Equine Glanders.* In the United States and Canada, glanders was prevalent until 1905; suppressive measures have since almost freed these countries from the disease. Experience has taught that it spreads among equines by water supplies, e.g., drinking troughs soiled with the nasal discharge containing M. *mallei* in great numbers. Since the bacilli are also excreted from the skin and mouth, feed bags, harness, brushing and grooming utensils, and even bedding and fodder contaminated with such excretions are especially dangerous.

Glanders in Man. Today glanders in man is rare. Since 1936, 12 cases have been reported (Mendelson). As an occupational infection, it is seen in grooms, coachmen, veterinary surgeons, soldiers, farmers, and the like. Several cases have been reported in laboratory workers. Infection results most frequently from contamination of an abrasion or wound with a glanderous discharge, but primary invasion of the conjunctiva and possibly the respiratory and alimentary tract may occur.

Clinical Manifestations. Just as in the horse, glanders manifests itself in man in an acute and chronic form. It should be emphasized that chronic glanders frequently may terminate with acute symptoms, and in rare instances a case with typical acute onset may run a chronic course.

Acute Glanders. After an incubation time of a few hours to three weeks, on the average four days, general malaise, anorexia, chills, fever up to 104° F., vomiting, diarrhea and rheumatic pains accompany the local swelling and infiltration at the site of the cutaneous infection. Ulcers with irregular edges and sloughing, yellow-grayish bases appear, and multiple intramuscular and subcutaneous nodules along the lymphatics, the so-called "farcy buds," are gradually transformed into abscesses. They show little tendency to heal. When the primary lesions are in the nose, the sticky blood-tinged secretion gradually becomes converted into ropy, viscid, mucopurulent material which excoriates the skin over which it runs, forming crusts on the lips and mouth. Sometimes the onset suggests influenza, pneumonia or typhoid fever; one is then struck by the degree of prostration, which is entirely out of proportion to the clinical signs. With the development of localized purulent foci, bacteriologic examination may serve to identify the infection. An *exanthematous eruption*, brawny, purplish lentil-shaped spots, and pustules containing clear yellow-white matter, on the face, neck, trunk and limbs, indicates sepsis and is the precursor of death. Invariably, the glanders bacillus may be isolated in blood cultures. Delirium and coma precede the fatal termination, which may occur within one to seven weeks, owing to circulatory collapse.

Chronic Glanders. Negligible constitutional symptoms may appear at first. Fever may be absent, although general malaise, inertia and pains in the extremities are comparatively common. Within one to four weeks, however, irregular fever develops which tends to assume a septic character with deep remissions. The most constant lesions appear in the form of subcutaneous or intramuscular abscesses or tumors on the upper and lower extremities, on the head and neck, rarely on the trunk. As a rule the regional lymph nodes are enlarged. Earlier lesions are usually painful and tender; they may rapidly ulcerate, or on incision suppurate profusely, discharging a few specific organisms. Stubborn resistance to treatment, and partial healing with discharging sinuses and a tendency to spread are striking features of the disease. Involvement of the joints and periosteum is not rare. Pulmonary and pleural disturbances, bronchitis, consolidation and exudates are reported in about one quarter of the cases. Some patients present only symptoms of a minor ailment, but rapidly lose weight and strength. Emaciation usually accompanies the development of foci. Periods of irregular fever and profuse sweating may be followed by quiescent intervals during which the patient may regain his strength. This peculiar remittent disease may drag on for years; the duration, from six weeks to fifteen years, averages about one and one half years. Remissions at intervals of two to five years have been observed. The lesions may heal slowly, or a remission with rapid generalization resembling acute glanders may be fatal.

Many patients succumb to cachexia and amyloid disease. Chronic glanders may be latent at the beginning and during the entire course. A personal account of chronic relapsing glanders in a veterinarian vividly describes this distressing malady (Gaiger).

Diagnosis. The varied clinical picture renders diagnosis difficult. Any wound infection in a person with a history of contact with glandered horses, or with laboratory handling of *M. mallei,* should be regarded as gravely suspicious, however, and proper bacteriologic tests by culture and inoculation of hamsters should be instituted. Aside from bacteriologic tests, the newer *serologic procedures* are indispensable. The most specific reactions have been obtained with the complement fixation test; the technique is the same as that used in the recognition of latent equine glanders. Agglutination reactions in dilutions of 1:800 or a significant and sustained rise in the serum titer is diagnostic. In chronic glanders the antibodies persist for a long time, but the titer may fluctuate. It is advisable, therefore, to use and repeat several methods of examination (complement fixation and agglutination). The diagnostic *intradermal test* with commercial mallein (0.1 cc. of a 1:100,000 dilution) gives an acute positive reaction in human beings with glanders.

Melioidosis. The "glanders-like" disease melioidosis, described by Stanton and Fletscher, is not readily diagnosed or differentiated from glanders during life. At autopsy the causative organism can be readily isolated from the visceral lesions. Several cases of melioidosis without constitutional symptoms have been recorded.

Prognosis. Few patients recover from acute glanders; 30 to 50 per cent survive chronic glanders without treatment.

Treatment. The patient must be isolated and the discharges carefully disinfected. Iodine, hypochlorite and benzalkonium chloride (Roccal) are highly effective, but the phenol compounds are not. Aside from symptomatic treatment and complete rest, chemotherapy has yielded promising results. Sulfadiazine, sulfathiazole and streptomycin are effective for both glanders and melioidosis in experimentally infected hamsters. There are indications that human infections with *M. mallei* are amenable to treatment with sulfonamides, particularly sulfamethazine (Howe and Miller; A. M. A. Foreign Letters, 1952). Treatment with both sulfathiazole and penicillin has been claimed successful in

Yugoslavia. Streptomycin, not yet adequately evaluated, has been efficacious in one case (Womack and Wells). Chloramphenicol (Chloromycetin) inhibits the growth of *M. whitmori,* and its clinical use, either alone or with sulfonamides, has been suggested (Green and Mankikar). Chlortetracycline (Aureomycin) has shown experimental promise (Cruickshank).

Prevention. The prevention of glanders in man depends on the vigorous suppression and ultimate eradication of the disease in horses. Without accurate diagnostic methods, control of glanders was difficult, since mild, abortive and latent glanders are important factors in the spread of the infection in the crowded parts of cities. With the mallein test—intradermal, palpebral and ophthalmic —and the agglutination, complement fixation and conglutination tests, horses in infected or suspected stables can now be examined effectively. All animals proved to be infected with the disease, clinical or latent, must be destroyed and properly disposed of, and the stable and objects exposed to contamination thoroughly cleansed and disinfected with bleaching powder preparations. Horses in contact with infected animals, although considered healthy by allergic and serologic tests, must be reexamined every three weeks. Should there be no indication of the disease in these tests, the stable may be considered free from glanders. The education of persons who handle horses should call attention to the importance of rubber gloves, thorough disinfections and other methods of protection. Special care should be taken to prevent the spread of the disease through the discharges and contaminated fomites from human cases. Cultures of *M. mallei* and laboratory tests with the organism are dangerous and should not be entrusted to beginners.

KARL F. MEYER

References

American Medical Association (Foreign Letters): Effect of Streptomycin and Sulfonamides on Glanders. J.A.M.A., *149:*1051, 1952.
Gaiger, S. H.: Glanders in Man. J. Comp. Path. & Therap., *26:*223, 1913; *29:*26, 1916.
Garry, M. W., and Koch, M. L.: Chronic Melioidosis: Bacteriologic and Clinical Correlation in Diagnosis. J. Lab. & Clin. Med., 38:374, 1951.
Grant, A., and Barwell, C.: Chronic Melioidosis: Case Diagnosed in England. Lancet, *1:*199, 1943.
Howe, C., and Miller, W. R.: Human Glanders: Report of Six Cases. Ann. Int. Med., 26:93, 1947.
Mendelson, R. W.: Glanders. U. S. Armed Forces M. J., *1:*781, 1950.
Miller, W. R., Pannell, L., and Ingalls, M. S.: Experimental Chemotherapy in Glanders and Melioidosis. Am. J. Hyg., 47:205, 1948.
Mirick, G. S., Zimmerman, H. M., Maner, G. D., and Humphrey, A. A.: Melioidosis on Guam. J.A.M.A., *130:*1063, 1946.
Stanton, H. T., and Fletscher, W.: Melioidosis. Studies Inst. M. Research, Federated Malay States, Bull. No. 21, p. 59, 1932.

ANTHRAX

(Charbon, Maladie Charbonneuse, Milzbrand, Malignant Pustule or Cutaneous Anthrax, Woolsorters' Disease, Rag-Pickers' Disease or Pulmonary Anthrax)

Definition. Anthrax is an acute infectious disease, caused by the *Bacillus anthracis,* which attacks many species of animals, in particular herbivora, and is transmissible from them to man. Clinically, it takes the form of an external (malignant pustule and malignant edema) or internal (pulmonary and rarely intestinal) disease.

History. Anthrax has been known from antiquity; the name is derived from the Latin *anthrax,* a carbuncle. Maret (1752) and Fournier (1768) defined the clinical malignant pustule in man, while Chabert (1780) described anthrax in animals and Barthelémy (1823) proved its transmissibility by inoculation. Subsequently, Davaine (1863–1864) showed that anthrax was caused by a living organism that multiplied in the body, invaded the blood stream and produced death by septicemia. He found the same organism in the malignant pustule and thus demonstrated the etiologic identity of the disease in man and animals. The final proof of the causative role of *Bacillus anthracis* was furnished by R. Koch (1877) when he described the formation of spores, cultivation of the organism *in vitro,* reproduction of the disease by injection of pure cultures, and recovery of the bacillus at autopsy. Thus the study of anthrax established for the first time the specific relationship of a microbe to an infectious disease.

Etiology. *Bacillus anthracis,* so designated by Ferdinand Cohn (1875) and by many claimed as the "cornerstone" in modern bacteriology, is a nonmotile gram-positive rod which forms capsules in the tissues of man and animals. Under conditions of unfavorable growth outside the body it forms ellipsoid or oval spores quite resistant to heat (ten minutes' boiling) and to chemical disinfectants. The capsule formation, the inverted fir-tree growth in gelatin stab, and the pathogenicity for guinea pigs distinguish the microbe from those of anthrax-like or pseudoanthrax bacilli (*B. subtilis* and *B. megatherium*). The capsular polypeptide composed of glutamic acid, the virulence factor, neutralizes the normal defense mechanism of the host and thus incites infection. Apparently no conventional antigen-antibody type of protective mechanism is involved in acquired resistance to the anthrax bacillus (Raffel).

Epidemiology. Man contracts anthrax through direct or indirect exposure to animals or animal products; rarely is it spread from animal to animal. Infection occurs primarily or secondarily from feeding on contaminated pasture in low-lying marshy areas or on artificial foodstuffs such as bone, blood, fish and maize meal. In 1951, raw bone meal imported through Belgium from Asia and southern Europe was responsible for numerous outbreaks of anthrax in swine. Dried bones caused 13 cases of anthrax in England (Davies and Harvey). A mechanical transmission by biting flies occurs infrequently.

Anthrax infection exists in a few fairly well defined districts in the United States: (1) southeastern South Dakota, northeastern Nebraska, southern California and New York; (2) the delta regions of the lower Mississippi Valley; and (3) a belt along the Texas gulf coast. In these districts occasional serious outbreaks occur, but the incidence is kept down by appropriate preventive measures. The disease causes major epizoötics throughout the world, particularly in Asia, Africa and southern Europe.

Anthrax in man may be conveniently divided into two epidemiologic groups: agricultural and industrial. *Agricultural anthrax* is usually acquired by contact with infected livestock while handling, skinning or autopsying infected animals. Farmers, butchers, sheep herders, and veterinarians are the usual victims. The death rate, unfortunately, continues high because diagnosis and treatment are delayed. The lesion takes the form of a malignant pustule. *Industrial anthrax* arises from handling wool or animal hair, hides or skins and may take the form of cutaneous anthrax or pulmonary disease. It has recently increased in New England and the Middle Atlantic states owing to the handling of imported infected hair, wool, carpet wool and goat hair and skins from Asia and North Africa where the level of organization of the livestock industry is primitive (Wolff and Heimann, 1951; Steele).

Over 98 per cent of the cases of human anthrax in the United States are of the cutaneous type. Cutaneous anthrax has been caused by contact with horsehair shaving brushes, with anthrax meningitis as a frequent complication. Pulmonary infection was commoner than the malignant pustule fifty years ago, but, thanks to improvements in industrial hygiene, legislation and the introduction of exhaust ventilation, dust masks and proper clothing, this type is now infrequent.

From 1945 to 1951 inclusive, 372 cases of human anthrax occurred in the United States, most of them in seven northeastern states, where industrial exposure is usually stated to be the source of infection. In the remaining forty-one states, 63 cases were reported, of which 29 were due to agricultural exposure (21 farmers and 8 veterinarians). There are no records of human anthrax caused by ingestion of contaminated milk or meat in recent years. During 1952, according to provisional reports, there were 73 human cases of anthrax in the United States; there were 60 in 1951. The loss due to animal anthrax during 1945 to 1950 is estimated at 8504 head of livestock (Steele and Helvig).

The infection chain, animal-man, is, as a rule, broken. In 1948, however, a man-to-man transmission was proved (Reilly and Beeson). Moreover, healthy persons may carry spores in their clothing.

Symptomatology. *External Anthrax.* "MALIGNANT PUSTULE." The most common form (95 per cent) of cutaneous anthrax is seen by the physician when the carbuncle has already developed. From one to three days after infection, a reddened area of the skin on the arm, neck or face shows a fleabite-like patch transformed into a painless and insensible papule. Intense itching accompanies this primary lesion in its progress to a vesicle with a hard, dark purplish black center. Interestingly, the site of the lesions varies with the nature of the industry. Hide porters are frequently infected on the back of the neck, which is more open than other parts to excoriation. In butchers and veterinarians who handle carcasses the arms or hands are affected. As a rule, only one focus is present, although scratching may lead to autoinfection and the formation of several papules and multiple vesiculation with yellowish or hemorrhagic or even purulent content. Within a few hours after the papules appear, the soft tissues in the immediate vicinity become infiltrated and swollen. Coagulation necrosis, desiccation or scratching produces a dark bluish red, tough leathery eschar, which extends both in depth and width, and forms, with the densely edematous ring studded with small vesicles, the characteristic carbuncle. The term "pustule" is unfortunate, for pus formation is absent. The massive infiltration joins an extensive hemorrhagic edema which may extend along the neck to the face or chest or even to the abdomen and lead to extraordinary distortion of the involved parts. Reddened lymphatics spread from the carbuncle to the regional lymph nodes, which are painful, swollen and sometimes covered by an area of reddened and inflamed skin. In the mildest form, with but little swelling, the primary papule vesiculates rapidly and the resulting scab separates in a few days. Recovery in more severe cases is indicated by the gradually sloughing suppuration of the eschar at the end of the first week, recession of the edema and slow healing of the extensive defect by granulation, leaving a disfiguring scar.

Quite early, the general symptoms of headache, joint pains, nausea, malaise and fever may accompany the development of the carbuncle. The temperature varies, in the majority of cases it is elevated; on occasions it may be normal or even subnormal. The leukocyte count may show a slight increase (10,-000 to 13,000 cells per cubic millimeter) or leukopenia with 60 to 85 per cent polymorphonuclear leukocytes. Despite the alarming aspect of the carbuncle, the general manifestations of illness may be exceedingly slight. On the other hand, even the early stages of the local process may be accompanied by profound malaise, vomiting, circulatory collapse, cyanosis, profuse perspiration, diarrhea and subnormal temperatures. Death may take place in three to five days. Blood cultures usually reveal anthrax bacilli.

The presence of bacilli in the blood stream does not always constitute an unfavorable prognosis. In fact, the mode of action of the anthrax bacilli is by no means clearly understood. The invasion in the blood stream occurs late, remains confined to the blood vessels of the liver, lung, spleen and kidney, and is accompanied by severe toxic manifestations. Embolic bacillary occlusions of the capillaries and the formation of poisons in the extravasations of blood into the organs may be principally responsible for the severe symptoms and deaths. According to Szendey, cerebral hemorrhage is present in at least 40 per cent of the fatal cases. Cyanosis and respiratory distress are always grave symptoms.

MALIGNANT ANTHRAX EDÉMA. This is observed in the loose connective tissue of the eyelid, hand, neck, thigh and mucous membranes. It is characterized by a doughy, soft, transparent, faintly reddish or anemic infiltration and swelling without papules and vesicles, following rather than preceding constitutional symptoms. Rarely circumscribed, it spreads rapidly and is apt to terminate in extensive sloughing and gangrene. In general, the outcome of the edematous form is less favorable than that of the carbuncle.

Internal Anthrax. PULMONARY ANTHRAX. This presents no characteristic clinical symptoms. The onset is sudden with rigor and fever, slight or excessive. Aside from general malaise, headache and circulatory disturbance, the patients may complain of a feeling of tightness in the chest and difficulty in breathing, which in some may be accelerated to 40 to 50 respirations a minute. The sensorium is usually clear. The auscultating signs are usually those of bronchitis. The mucosa of the nose, larynx and pharynx becomes reddened and swollen. With increasing dyspnea, cough and pain in the chest, pneumonic infiltrations or even pleuritic exudates become discernible. Anthrax bacilli may be demonstrated in the frothy, occasionally blood-tinged sputum. Death may occur within 18 to 48 hours; when the disease lasts longer (up to ten days), delirium and unconsciousness govern the clinical picture. On the other hand, absence of the severe symptoms usually accompanying acute infections and the rapidity with which collapse sets in are characteristic features of this form of anthrax. Not infrequently the disease is suspected because the patient's occupation subjects him to inhalation of dust from hairs soiled with spores.

GASTROINTESTINAL ANTHRAX. This form, rare in the United States but frequent in Indonesia and southeast Asia, may result from ingestion of infected food or may follow the external type when the organisms are carried to the mouth from external lesions; it may occur as a secondary manifestation of anthrax in some other part of the body. The infection may be symptomless, as in Sinai's 38 patients who had eaten inadequately cooked meat from a calf that had succumbed to anthrax. The serums of 15 gave positive precipitin reactions with specific anthrax serum. Or, as in Soloweiff's 30 cases traced to infected sausage, the symptoms may include persistent vomiting, constipation and, rarely, diarrhea; an almost empty gastrointestinal tract with the occasional discharge of blood-tinged fecal material or pure blood; abdominal distention and tenderness; peritonitis and accumulation of exudates; and relatively little fever (maximal elevation: 102.2° F.). His patients were restless, anxiety-ridden and much concerned about their illness. Collapse, cyanosis and apoplectic death terminated the majority of infections within one to three days, and one patient died in eleven days. At autopsy, localized phlegmonous hemorrhagic infiltrations and carbuncles were noted in the ileum and cecum, and hemorrhages in the myocardium and brain.

Diagnosis. The diagnosis of anthrax is greatly facilitated when the cutaneous lesions are characteristic, and when the anamnesis and occupation of the patient suggest the nature of the infection. If no information is available, the differential diagnosis between an anthrax carbuncle and a simple coccal infection requires laboratory assistance. Any physician possessing a microscope

scopically in the sputum and in the pleural exudate. The vomitus should be inspected when gastrointestinal anthrax is suspected.

During the terminal stages of the disease and sometimes when severe general symptoms are present, the bacillus may be cultivated from blood if not less than 20 cc. is taken. Even in nonfatal cases and in the absence of symptoms indicative of generalization, the anthrax bacillus may be isolated from the blood. Blood or cerebrospinal fluid, after it

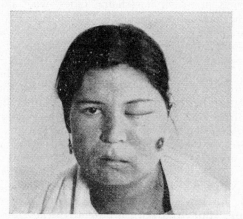

Fig. 34. Cutaneous anthrax with facial and orbital edema immediately preceding oxytetracycline therapy. Innumerable *B. anthracis* visible on stained smear of material from lesion. (Courtesy of Drs. Vernon Knight and A. Ruiz-Sanchez.)

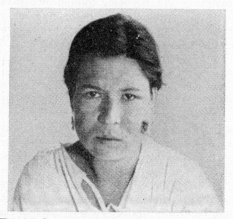

Fig. 35. Same patient as in Figure 34 seventy-two hours after start of oxytetracycline therapy. Note virtually complete disappearance of edema. *B. anthracis* no longer demonstrable in stained smears of exudate. (Courtesy of Drs. Vernon Knight and A. Ruiz-Sanchez.)

of medium power and some staining reagents can make an early diagnosis and thus reduce the risks attending the disease. If a vesicle has formed, films are made from the serum and stained. If it is already broken, gentle scraping of the pimple or puncture of the eschar will produce serum rich in typical encapsulated bacilli when stained with a polychrome eosin-methylene blue stain (Wright or Giemsa). Their direct cultivation on peptone agar should always be attempted. If the specimen has to be shipped, the tissue serum should be dried on silk threads or a sterile glass slide. On occasion, both the smear and the culture may show anthrax bacilli in small numbers or even none at all, while several varieties of cocci may grow in the culture. Repeated examinations and cultures are therefore indicated. In view of the occurrence of anthrax-like bacilli on the skin, it is imperative that all anthrax diagnoses should be confirmed by animal inoculations, preferably in guinea pigs or mice. In pulmonary anthrax the bacillus has been found micro-

has been treated with 3 per cent acetic acid solution, may be centrifuged and the sediment stained with Wright's stain and examined for bacilli. Estimation of the phagocytic power of the leukocytes by an expert may be of diagnostic and prognostic importance.

Prognosis. It is generally recognized that the prognosis in external cutaneous anthrax is favorable, provided the pustule is not on the neck or face and has not been irritated by physical and chemical procedures. Moreover, if the nature of the pustule is correctly and promptly diagnosed, the patient placed in bed and specific treatment instituted not later than the third day, the chances for recovery in most infections are favorable. To be sure, the statistics amply attest to the uneventful recovery without complications or sequelae without specific treatment. Individual susceptibility to anthrax varies considerably; cutaneous, even visceral, infections are not as deadly as popular belief would indicate. Thompson reports that only one of 20 veterinarians (18 with malignant pustule, one throat infection and one generalized infection) died. It is well to remember that the general fatality rate is around 20 per cent (Holland and the United States), but may be as high as 40 per cent. There is generally a low fatality rate for tannery anthrax, but a high rate for that resulting from animal contact. Septicemia with and without involvement of the viscera, and sometimes meningitis, are serious complications. In fact, double and multiple infections occur at times, and recurrences are possible, though not usual. When the eruption assumes the form of anthrax edema, indications of diminished resistance are obvious and the outcome may be in doubt. In respiratory and alimentary anthrax the prognosis is grave, largely because of the extensive visceral destruction and the presence of bacteremia (up to 300 to 400 bacilli per cubic centimeter). The presence of bacilli in the blood culture justifies an unfavorable prognosis, although dramatic cures may be achieved by modern therapeutic procedures. The true nature of mild cases may occasionally be suspected, but is rarely proved. An attack of the disease, if it produces immunity, induces a resistance of only short duration. Second attacks of cutaneous anthrax have occurred within a year.

The average hospital stay is about two weeks, and, provided the ulcer heals in two weeks, the patient returns to work within five to six weeks.

Treatment. Many forms of therapy have been used. The introduction of anti-anthrax serum made available a theoretically efficient approach. In combination with arsenical drugs and, in particular, with the "hands off" policy toward the local lesion, the therapeutic results reported by Lucchesi and Gildersleeve (1941) were excellent. During the past decade first sulfonamides and then penicillin have been successfully used. More recent experiences indicate that chloramphenicol and the tetracycline drugs (Aureomycin, Terramycin) are effective in cutaneous anthrax. All three agents in doses of about 750 mg. every 4 hours appear to be equally effective, but the exact dose schedules have not yet been investigated. Local edema and erythema disappear within 24 to 48 hours; pain and tenderness at the site of the lymph node involvement and all signs of systemic reaction subside rather promptly. Anthrax bacilli may be isolated from the lesions for two to three days; this rate of disappearance is not as rapid as that reported

after the administration of larger doses of penicillin. The advantage of oral administration, the nontoxicity, the complete freedom from side effects and the ambulatory method of treatment now make the tetracyclines the preferred drugs for the treatment of anthrax (Gold and Boger).

Prevention. The prevention of the disease in man must first be directed to a suppression of the infection in animals by veterinary control measures, disinfection of all raw materials in which horsehairs, hides, wool and other substances are liable to harbor the anthrax spore. Sick animals must be isolated or killed, and carcasses must be promptly disposed of by burial with lime (at least 3 feet deep) or by burning without skinning. The anthrax control measures proposed by the United States Public Health Service include annual vaccination of animals with a standardized potent spore vaccine in enzoötic areas (Steele); this prevents the disease from being a major economic problem.

The hair and wool from anthrax-infected or suspected areas may be disinfected by boiling for three hours or by steam under pressure. Hides and skins are treated in a hydrochloric acid and salt mixture at 40° C. for six hours. Workers in tanneries and wool factories may be protected by rubber gloves and aprons and by proper ventilation to carry off the dust. Active immunization of workers exposed to goat hair imported from China with a heat-killed anthrax vaccine was tried by Gold, but two persons who were so vaccinated were not protected.

KARL F. MEYER

References

Gold, H., and Boger, W. P.: Newer Antibiotics in the Treatment of Anthrax. New England J. Med., *244*:391, 1951.

Raffel, S.: Types of Acquired Immunity against Infectious Disease, in Clifton, C. E., Raffel, S., and Barker, H. A.: Annual Review of Microbiology. Stanford, Calif., Annual Reviews, Inc., 1949, pp. 222–229.

Sinai, G. J.: Symptomlose Milzbrandinfektion beim Menschen. Ztschr. f. Immunitätsforsch. u. exper. Therap., *79*:199, 1933.

Steele, J. H.: Veterinary Public Health. Advances in Veterinary Science, *1*:329, 1953.

———, and Helvig, R. J.: Anthrax in the United States. Pub. Health Rep. 68:616, 1953.

Symmers, D., and Cady, D. W.: Occurrence of Virulent Anthrax Bacilli in Cheap Shaving Brushes. J.A.M.A., 77:2120, 1921.

TUBERCULOSIS

Definition. Tuberculosis is an infectious disease caused by the tubercle bacillus. The disease is widespread among men and animals, uniformly fatal in some species, seldom if ever in others; acute and generalized in some persons, chronic and localized in others. Pathologically, the disease is characterized by inflammatory infiltrations, tubercles, caseous necrosis, abscesses, fibrosis and calcification.

History. Archeologic discovery of skeletons bearing the marks of tuberculous lesions indicate that the disease was present in remote antiquity. In the earliest medical records it was called consumption or phthisis because of its most conspicuous external feature, wasting. Long considered to be of many varieties and origins, the unity of the disease was first recognized by Laënnec. The correctness of his conceptions was not universally acknowledged until Koch in 1882 isolated the specific organism and reproduced the disease experimentally. The avian type of bacillus was isolated in 1890 by Maffucci, and the bovine type in 1898 by Theobald Smith.

Distribution. Under certain conditions, fish, amphibians, fowls and mammals may acquire tuberculosis, although in their wild state these classes are not very susceptible. Animals in captivity sometimes fall easy prey to the disease. Among domesticated animals it occurs in cattle, swine and gallinaceous birds and is seldom observed in dogs, horses and goats. In the United States, Norway, Sweden, Finland and Denmark, an active plan of eradication of tuberculosis from cattle has been highly successful. In some other countries the prevalence of infection among bovine herds is estimated to be as high as 40 per cent.

Incidence in Man. No branch of the human race has escaped the touch of tuberculosis. The severity of its effects, however, varies greatly in different communities. Although the infection is common, most people survive. The occurrence of infection, mortality and morbidity, therefore, must be analyzed separately. Formerly, in most communities, almost all adults reacted to the tuberculin test, and this is still true in some sections. In Guayaquil, Ecuador, for instance, a tuberculin testing survey in 1948 showed that about 50 per cent of the tested children under one year of age were reactors, while 90 per cent or more of those above 15 years revealed similar evidence of having been infected (Higgins). In the United States probably less than 50 per cent of the population is infected. Records of the American Student Health Association give figures for 105,633 students tested in ninety-one colleges during the year ending June, 1947. Nineteen per cent reacted to tuberculin; the male rate was 22.6 per cent, and the female, 9.4 per cent. In England and Wales the National Tuberculin Survey of 1949–50 included the testing of 94,221 persons. On the basis of the results, Simmonds estimates that there are about two and three-quarter million persons under 20 years of age who are tuberculin-positive, and probably about another 27 millions over that age.

Sensitivity to tuberculin may diminish as lesions become arrested, depending somewhat on the dose and the method of testing. As might be expected, therefore, more people bear lesions than the test would indicate.

Medlar, in 1947, after an extensive study of necropsy material in New York City, reported that evidence of tuberculous infection was present in approximately 35 per cent of persons 10 to 19 years old at the time of death. The incidence of infection rose to about 65 per cent in the 30 to 39 years age group, and to 85 per cent or more in the group above the age of 60 years. His comparative study of 17,196 necropsy protocols led him to conclude that the incidence of tuberculous lesions was approximately the same in 1940 to 1945 as it was in 1916 to 1920, in striking contrast to the steady diminution of deaths due directly to the disease. It may be inferred, therefore, that infection is still widely prevalent, but that the infected persons better resist the invasive effects of the resulting lesions. The increase of relatively resistant persons is presumably a result of the improvement in living conditions, nutrition and other hygienic standards. The potential threat of the disease is demonstrated by a rise in mortality whenever these standards are compromised.

Mortality from tuberculosis also varies greatly in different localities. It is estimated that it causes from 3 to 5 million deaths in the world each year. Areas with high rates include eastern Europe, Asia, Latin America, Alaska, Greenland, Newfoundland and Labrador. In the Philippine Islands tuberculosis is responsible for almost one of every 4 deaths, compared with one in 43 deaths in 1950 in the United States. England and Wales, the Netherlands, Sweden, Switzerland and Italy have death rates between 19 and 40 per 100,000 annually, while that of Denmark approaches 10. For many decades the rates in many nations have declined steadily, exceptions being noted in temporary upward trends during great wars.

In the United States the rate per 100,000 per year declined from 202 in 1900 to 153.8 in 1910, 113.1 in 1920, 45.8 in 1940, and to 13 or lower (estimated) in 1953. The most striking reductions have occurred in the early decades of life (Fig. 38). In this country tuberculosis now stands seventh among the leading causes of death, but is still the leading cause, except for accidents, between the ages of 15 and 34 years. Death is due to the pulmonary form of the disease in about 92 per cent of all cases and to nonpulmonary or generalized forms in 8 per cent. Morbidity can never be more than approximate, since there is no sharp division between active and inactive cases. In 1952 there were 24,195 (estimated) deaths from tuberculosis in the United States. Ten to 20 active cases are estimated for each annual death. Four to 6 new active cases are reported *each year for every death*. During World War II, among 18 million men examined in the United States for military service 20.1 out of every 1000 were found to have some form of tuberculosis; about one third of those rejected had the disease in an active phase (Smith, Reynolds and Hand).

Epidemiology. As man may be infected by the human or bovine type of the bacillus, the source is usually traced to another person with tuberculosis or to a tuberculous cow. Contaminated milk is seldom implicated in this country, but elsewhere it is considered responsible for much human disease, especially abdominal tuberculosis. In Scotland it has been estimated that as much as 8 per cent of the cases of pulmonary tuberculosis are due to the bovine type of bacillus, and the incidence is higher in lesions of the lymph nodes, bones and meninges. Much more often, however, human infection is the result of inhaling air contaminated by the person with "open" (i.e., cavitary) pulmonary tuberculosis as he coughs, sneezes and expectorates, heedless of hygienic care. Other lesions such as superficial tuberculous sinuses may constitute sources, and the possibility of transmission through contaminated urine or feces occasionally has to be considered. Direct mouth-to-mouth transmission may occur, particularly in nurslings. As would be expected, therefore, many new cases of tuberculosis are discovered near the abodes of people previously afflicted. In this sense the disease is frequently familial or household, and it is also somewhat more prevalent among the personnel of hospitals or other institutions caring for tuberculous patients. Infection has been shown to be almost inevitable among young children who in the home have close contact with the "open case," usually in an adult. Infrequently, infection occurs through the broken skin, e.g., among laboratory workers handling fresh tuberculous specimens. Rarely, a fetus is infected by way of the blood stream from a tuberculous placenta, or, less often, by aspiration of bacilliferous amniotic fluid into the lungs.

Bacteriology. *Mycobacterium tuberculosis* (the tubercle bacillus) exists in three types, *hominis, bovis* and *avium*. Man may be infected by the human or bovine types, seldom by the avian. Lower animals are infected most often by the bovine type. This varying pathogenicity may be used to help identify the type. Thus guinea pigs are susceptible to infection by the bovine and human types, but not the avian; rabbits are susceptible to the bovine and avian, much less to human; fowls usually are susceptible only to the avian. The bacillus is a rod-shaped organism distinguished particularly by its acid-fastness to stains. Granular forms have been described, but these may be artefacts (Yegian and Porter). The existence of a viral or zoogleal stage has been claimed, but is generally doubted. The bacillus grows slowly and aerobically on various culture media. R. J. Anderson particularly has studied the chemistry of the bacillus, which is made up mainly of lipids, waxes, polysaccharides and proteins. There is no capsule. Though the organism is tenacious of life and may survive many months in the dark or when refrigerated, it does not live long when exposed in rooms well supplied with unfiltered daylight (C. R. Smith), and it is killed by boiling in water for two minutes or pasteurization at 60° C.

Organisms isolated from human cases are with rare exceptions virulent in guinea pigs. The pathogenicity for these animals has been found to be reduced in strains recovered from patients treated with isoniazid; other drugs have not been reported to have this effect.

Resistance. Man is relatively resistant to tuberculosis. Infection is common, but less than 10 per cent of all those infected die of the disease. This bespeaks a native resistance which as a rule is highly effective. Its precise nature is not understood, and it cannot be clearly distinguished from the numerous other factors which influence the course of the infection. Natural resistance varies with age. Young infants may go on to acquire generalized tuberculosis soon after the first infection, and the case fatality rate at this time of life is relatively high. The mortality rate is generally low between the ages of 5 and adolescence, when there is an abrupt rise, reaching its peak in females in the early twenties, and somewhat later in males. This suggests strongly that biologic influences associated with puberty alter natural resistance. The relatively high death rate in old men as compared with old women may involve similar forces.

Allergy and Immunity. These factors, which begin to assert themselves shortly after the development of the first lesion, modify subsequent reactions. Koch demonstrated that a guinea pig infected with tubercle bacilli slowly suffers an indolent and sometimes ulcerating lesion at the site of inoculation and dies with progressive and generalized tuberculosis after a lapse of several months. Within a few weeks after the inoculation the tissues for the first time become sensitive to tuberculin. This altered reaction is known as tissue hypersensitivity, a form of allergy. Similarly, Koch found that a second inoculation of bacilli into the skin of a previously infected animal produces a lesion which behaves differently from the primary. The local reaction is rapid and intense with a tendency to abscess formation, ulceration, extrusion of the necrotic matter and subsequent healing. Dissemination of bacilli from this focus through the lymph and blood streams is much slower and less severe. This, the *Koch phenomenon,* is a manifestation of allergy and of acquired relative immunity, the nature of which has been identified only partly. Weakly concentrated humoral antibodies may be demonstrated. More important, however, as shown by Lurie, is the accelerated mobilization of phagocytic cells at the site of infection; these may form an effective barrier against further invasion. If the primary infection was not overwhelming or was accomplished with an attenuated strain of bacilli, the animal now may survive the effects of reinfection for many months. In the human being, tissue hypersensitivity, which usually develops within five or six weeks after the first infection, helps to explain certain intense inflammatory reactions such as serous pleurisy. Acquired immunity, which is never absolute,

seems to develop much more slowly, and in man may not reach its height for a year or more. Allergy, as indicated by the intensity of the reaction to tuberculin, is not a measure of immunity, but most workers believe that the two are closely associated.

Heredity. The superior resistance of certain groups such as Jewish people from certain geographic areas suggests that hundreds of years of experience with tuberculosis results in the elimination of the susceptible and the survival of relatively resistant members. It has been intimated that specific immunity may be inherited to a degree, but this has never been proved. The evidence is more suggestive that some racial stocks have a stronger or weaker natural resistance—a genetic character.

Constitution and Race. Clinicians have often described types of people thought to be susceptible to tuberculosis, e.g., the asthenic, thin-skinned, silken-haired, titian blond. However, adequate scientific estimates of the influences of constitutional factors remain for the future; recent work, such as that of Wolf and Ciocco, suggests their importance. Kallmann and Reisner, studying monozygotic and dizygotic pairs of twins, found that the chance of developing tuberculosis increases in direct proportion to the degree of genetic relationship to a tuberculous person. Lurie has been able to breed families of rabbits in which the greatly varying resistance is a function of their genetic constitution. The higher mortality among Negroes in many parts of the world is ascribed by some entirely to poor living conditions. However, the striking tendency of the lesions to undergo caseation rapidly and the greater liability to lymphohematogenous dissemination of the infection indicate that there is a real constitutional peculiarity in this race. In the United States the tuberculosis death rate for nonwhites is about three times that among whites; in 1910, 11 per cent of all deaths from tuberculosis occurred in nonwhite people, while in 1950 the proportion was 28.9 per cent. American Indians and Chinese in the United States have a death rate from the disease twice that of Negroes.

Age and *sex* influence the behavior of the disease, whether this originates in a recent primary infection or in a recent extension from remotely established lesions. Generalized tuberculosis is much more common in early childhood. Chronic pulmonary tuberculosis characteristically begins to appear in the second and third decades. When it first becomes manifest after the fourth decade it often tends to run a slow and indolent course. Figure 36 portrays the mortality experience with relation to sex and age. It will be noted that, in the United States, the prevalence of fatal tuberculosis is greatest among elderly men, a phenomenon which is duplicated in many other countries.

Physiologic and Psychologic Influences. Pregnancy aggravates tuberculosis in some women. Impaired nutrition, particularly when there has been a deprivation of essential vitamin and mineral elements, may lower resistance. The increase in fatal tuberculosis in Europe during both World Wars seems to have been related largely to the drastic reduction of food which permitted a reactivation of previously latent pulmonary lesions. In World War II the disease was rife in German concentration camps, such as Dachau and Buchenwald, as well as certain prisoner-of-war camps where the nutritional deficiencies of some inmates reached the edema level. Anxiety and tension created by psychologic maladjustments seem to lower resistance. There is some evidence that tuberculosis is more likely to develop in schizophrenics. The death rate is usually high in institutions for the mentally ill, but this seems now to be ascribable chiefly to intimate exposure and inadequate care and to be largely correctible by isolating the infectious cases.

Environment. Geographic location alone does not seem to be a major influence. Tuberculosis is a serious problem both in the Alaskan Indians and in Puerto Ricans. Social, economic and occupational factors are much more important. Ignorance, poor housing and overcrowding all are recognized as powerful evils. *Occupation,* which is a good index of social economic status, illustrates this strikingly. The death rate is highest among unskilled laborers and lowest among those in professions, including physicians. A specifically dangerous occupation with relation to tuberculosis is that which involves exposure to silicious dust: e.g., metal moulding, sandblasting, mining, stone cutting and polishing, and manufacturing of abrasive soaps. Meteorologic conditions have an influence, especially upon labile tuberculous lesions, and help to explain the trend to activation in the late winter and spring.

Trauma. Previously healthy traumatized tissue is not liable to be invaded by tuberculosis except by direct extension from an immediately adjacent lesion. Direct traumatization of tuberculous tissue, however, may be aggravating. Occasionally in pulmonary tuberculosis, a severe trauma of the chest may result in such manifestations as hemoptysis, bronchial dissemination of the infection or pleural rupture with secondary empyema.

Intercurrent Disease. Diabetes, if uncontrolled, especially in young people, predisposes to serious tuberculosis. The phenomenon was conspicuous before the discovery of insulin. Pulmonary tuberculosis is a frequent complication of congenital pulmonic stenosis, but, when present, usually runs a relatively mild course in association with mitral stenosis. Tuberculous patients frequently withstand pneumococcal pneumonia well unless the functional reserve has been almost depleted previously. Necrosing pneumonia or abscess, however, may lead to the breaking down of an arrested tuberculous focus and subsequent extension of the infection from it.

Morbid Anatomy. The earliest reaction of the body to infection with the tubercle bacillus is an accumulation of cells at the site. There is also some vascular congestion and exudation of fluid, but, as seen by Medlar, this is not usually intense. While some pathologists believe that this early accumulation consists almost or entirely of a proliferation of local tissue cells which may go on directly to form the classic histologic tubercle, Medlar submits experimental evidence that this is not the case, but rather that the neutrophilic leukocyte predominates. According to him, later developments depend on the rapidity of growth of tubercle bacilli. Leukocytes may continue to accumulate, forming an abscess which may heal or, if not, may proceed slowly to liquefaction—much more slowly, as a rule, than the abscess produced by most other bacteria. When the reaction is not so intense, the leukocytes may gradually be replaced by epithelioid cells (monocytes) and lymphocytes; these may be precursors or accompaniments of healing.

A frequent change in the early inflammatory lesion is *caseation,* a form of coagulative necrosis which, as the name implies, has the appearance and consistency of cheese. This rather dry necrotic matter may remain as such for many months, after which it may liquefy, or liquefaction may follow soon after caseation. The liquid collection is prone to break its bounds. In the lungs it frequently sloughs and empties its contents into the bronchi; a renal focus empties into the ureter. A necrotic superficial lymph node commonly sloughs through the skin or, if the node is deeply situated, may discharge into the trachea or some other passage; a vertebral abscess may dissect its way within the psoas sheath and rupture the skin of the groin. Whatever the outlet, sloughing and evacuation are accomplished,

may occur at various points. If the infection subsides in the early inflammatory phase, the exudation of cells and fluids ceases and resolution of the accumulated products follows, usually at a much slower rate than with other bacterial infections. If caseation has already set in, as it does in most lesions of material size and duration, resolution of the surround-

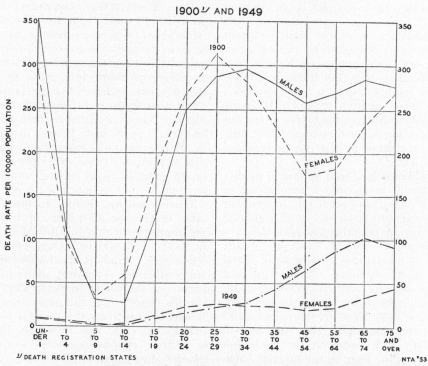

Fig. 36. (Courtesy of the National Tuberculosis Association.)

not primarily by the mechanical disruption of healthy tissue, but rather by necrosis and ulceration due to extension of the infection. It is the caseous necrosis of the wall of a pulmonary vein, for example, which often establishes a channel by which bacilli gain access to the blood stream.

After sloughing and excavation have occurred the damaged tissue is left with a defect which varies according to the structure of the particular part involved. In the larynx the defect is apt to be a superficial ulcer; in the middle ear, a perforated drum, and in the lung, a parenchymal cavity. Some of the defects, especially if the discharge from them does not drain freely, may be the seat of secondary infection with other bacteria.

Healing and *repair* of tuberculous lesions

ing non-necrotic exudate may occur, but the necrotic centers, still harboring bacilli, remain to be dealt with unless they have sloughed. Such caseous residues, if propitious conditions last, undergo slow fibrous organization with some drying and shrinkage. Eventually, the lesion may be converted into an irregular fibrocaseous mass or into a rounded structure enclosed wholly or in part by a fibrous envelope. This fibrosis may extend well beyond the center of the lesion. In time the caseous part of the fibrocaseous lesion may become infiltrated with mineral salts, chiefly calcium phosphate, from the body fluids. The process may proceed through a "chalky" phase to complete calcification or ossification. By this time the contained bacilli frequently die. At any time, if the bacilli survive, incompletely encapsulated caseous pulmonary lesions which maintain a communication with the bronchioles may slough and the disease may resume its progressive course. It is not uncommon to observe healing in one lesion while others progress. Ulcers and cavities can be repaired only by fibrous organization and contraction. The mucous membrane may grow back over a healed ulcer of the larynx, for instance, but destroyed alveoli of the lung are not restored. Large cavities, as of the lungs, seldom heal completely by natural processes.

An understanding of the time factor in healing is most important in clinical practice. Marked resolution may be observed within several months, but fibrous organization of the residual lesions is inevitably slow, requiring many months or years. In many cases, largely because of the extent of caseous necrosis, healing is incomplete and impermanent, and the status at best can be regarded only as "arrested."

Chemotherapy has been shown to modify tubercle bacilli in lesions; it may retard or halt active disease and accelerate healing but the essential processes of resolution and fibrous repair are not otherwise altered.

Pathogenesis. Present concepts of the evolution of tuberculosis from a small initial lesion to severe, disabling, chronic and fatal disease are derived from studies in epidemiology, clinical medicine and pathology. For many of the basic ideas we must look principally to the pathologist, since he observes most directly and completely the tracks followed through the body by the tubercle bacillus and the kind of damage it does. Interpretation of the findings is often difficult, and the terminology used has sometimes been confusing. In recent years there has been a tendency to discard such designations as *childhood type* and *adult type* of tuberculosis because they have no clear connotation. Likewise, *reactivation* or *exacerbation of disease* is suggested, instead of *endogenous reinfection,* to describe the renewed progression of lesions which previously had been inactive and perhaps partly healed.

The inflammation which appears at the site of the primary infection is known as the *primary lesion* (in the lung, sometimes called the Ghon focus in recognition of Ghon's important pathologic studies on tuberculosis in the early part of this century). The combination of the primary lesion and that which usually appears simultaneously or soon thereafter

in the tributary lymph nodes is the *primary complex* (Ranke). The complex may be incomplete in that the parenchymal or, less often, the lymph node focus may not be found, but this is unusual. A *reinfection lesion* is one caused by a new (exogenous) infection. Pathologic evidence of this is the finding, for example, of a recent lesion in the lung apparently unrelated to, but existing with, an old, well healed and calcified primary complex. The importance and frequency of reinfection (superinfection) in the presence of existing unhealed disease are not established. So long as there is an unhealed focus in the body, progressive disease is much more likely to originate from this than from an exogenous reinfection. After the primary complex has healed fully, the possibility of reinfection seems to be vastly greater. Thus, Medlar found at autopsy that progressive "minimal" pulmonary lesions in the bodies of 23 persons under 40 years of age were a part of primary disease in 91 per cent, while in 73 over 40 years of age similar lesions were due to reinfection in 72.6 per cent.

Dissemination. Before further consideration of the various phases of tuberculosis, the routes by which the infection is spread in the body should be recognized. Any such lesion may extend locally, i.e., by continuity and contiguity, depending somewhat on the nature of the tissue barriers. Thus it often spreads broadly over the pleural surface, but it seldom penetrates the parietal pleura and invades the chest wall unless the membrane is broken (e.g., by needle puncture). *Lymphatic** dissemination of the infection is observed most strikingly at the time of the primary infection, as indicated by the tributary lymphadenitis; it becomes lymphohemic if the bacilli are not retained in the nodes, but are carried with the lymph—through the thoracic duct, for instance—into the venous blood stream. Uncommonly, tuberculous lymphangitis may be set up along the route of spread. Retrograde lymphatic extension, i.e., against the lymph stream, seldom if ever occurs, according to the available evidence.

Two other common modes of dissemina-

---

* Certain terms, dignified by usage, are in their literal meaning quite incorrect as applied in pathogenesis. For clearness in these paragraphs, therefore, the terms *lymphatic, lymphohemic, hemic* and *bronchial* are used instead of *lymphogenous, lymphohematogenous, hematogenous* and *bronchogenic,* respectively.

tion depend on the tendency of lesions to slough and discharge after caseation. One is *hemic,* which is explained almost always by a caseous lesion invading and destroying the wall of a vein, thus allowing bacilli to enter the blood stream. The usual site is a pulmonary vein, but others are also recognized, such as a vein in a caseous prostate. The results of hemic dissemination vary according to a number of factors, the most important apparently being the mass and rate of discharge of bacilli from the caseous focus. Acute generalized miliary tuberculosis is usually interpreted as the result of an abrupt infection of the blood with an overwhelming mass of bacilli. Subacute and protracted generalized forms seem to be related to less severe infections of the blood which, however, may be continued over a period of time, perhaps with free intermissions. In this type of dissemination the natural clinical course, instead of being rapidly fatal, as in generalized miliary disease, may be protracted, while the lesions in their various sites, such as the lungs, lymph nodes, serous membranes, spleen, kidneys, and so on, may enlarge, caseate and show other local changes. Small and single or infrequent infections of the blood may set up one or a few isolated lesions which may heal or progress to local disease: e.g., in bone, eye, kidney, skin, and so forth. Frequently there is a long period of latency before some of these local lesions exacerbate and become manifest clinically. Ustvedt and his co-workers found that this period ranged from five to more than fifteen years in the case of renal tuberculosis, and was still longer with disease of the adrenal glands. Hemic dissemination due to the invasion of an artery occurs but rarely. The time of hemic dissemination bears some relationship to the phase of the disease and the age of the patient. In minor degree it is common as one of the terminal events in cases of fatal chronic tuberculosis. There are periods of relative frequency in infancy as an early result of primary infection and to a lesser degree in late life, especially among elderly men. The "time-table of tuberculosis," as Wallgren calls it, will be considered further in the clinical manifestations.

Another common route of dissemination is *intracanalicular,* a term suggested by the Germans to indicate channels such as the respiratory, alimentary and urinary canals (exclusive of lymph and blood vessels). The most familiar example is related to the presence of a tuberculous cavity in the lung. The bacilliferous discharge from this source passes through the bronchi and is for the most part expectorated, but sometimes is inhaled during breathing into healthy alveoli of one or both lungs, setting up new secondary lesions; this is known as *bronchial* dissemination. The severity of the secondary lesions varies greatly, depending somewhat on the rate of sloughing of the cavity, the amount, fluidity and bacillary content of the discharge, and the general resistance of the patient. Large and abrupt disseminations, such as may occur during a hemorrhage from the cavity, may lead to acute confluent tuberculous lobular or lobar pneumonia, but the more common pattern is a succession of smaller secondary lesions at intervals varying from days or weeks to many months. During periods of clinical arrest, when there are no freely discharging cavities, new secondary lesions seldom appear, but the exacerbation and sloughing of old arrested lesions often marks a reactivation of these mechanisms and is the usual explanation of relapse. In this way, sooner or later, chronic pulmonary tuberculosis often becomes established, the lungs and pleura showing old fibrous scars along with new inflammatory and caseous lesions.

Contact infection of the mucous membrane by the discharge from a pulmonary cavity may cause lesions in the bronchi, trachea or larynx, the last being a fairly common site. Other loci include the middle ear, infection here being carried more often via the eustachian tube than the blood stream, the tongue and the lip (usually through abrasions). Infection seems to favor places where bacilli have fairly long contact. Thus, when pus from the lungs is swallowed, as often in chronic cases, the alimentary organs usually escape until the lower ileum, cecum, and ascending colon are reached, and the passage of contents slows. Tuberculous ulcers are found there in many advanced pulmonary cases. By similar mechanisms the rectal crypts may be infected and an ischiorectal abscess may form.

Other manifestations of *intracanalicular* dissemination are from the kidney to the ureter and bladder and from prostate to epididymis. As implied, this mechanism is a common one after the disease has become confirmed and chronic in a visceral organ, usually the lungs.

From the foregoing it is easily seen that the lungs are peculiarly open to attack by the tubercle bacillus, which may find access through inhalational, hemic and bronchial routes.

Evolution of Primary Lesion. Ghon demonstrated that the primary lesion is to be found in the lungs of more than 90 per cent of infected persons, the bacillus having entered with inhaled air; many other pathologists have confirmed his findings. His pupil, Terplan, has amplified the studies in recent years. Other sites of primary lesions include the intestine (usually ascribed to the ingestion of contaminated raw milk), skin, tonsil and conjunctiva. In the lung the primary lesion is situated most often in a lower lobe or lower part of an upper lobe within 1 cm. of the pleura; almost always it is single, but occasionally two or three are found, rarely more. Medlar, from experimental and necropsy studies, believes that the primary lesion at its inception is a tiny focus of tuberculous pneumonia which undergoes some caseation by the time it reaches a size to be demonstrable macroscopically. The tracheobronchial lymph nodes in the line of drainage may also become enlarged and caseous. The disease may be arrested at this point and go on to healing, leaving a completely calcified primary complex. The time required for this healing must vary greatly according to the size of the lesions, the resistance of the host and other factors; it should be conceived in terms of many years, sometimes decades. There are numerous instances of only partly healed primary complexes remaining as such throughout the greater part of a lifetime.

Progressive disease from the primary lesions may occur at any age, immediately after the infection or after a long or short period of latency. Lesions acquired in childhood show a tendency to flare up during adolescence. In infants and young children there is a relatively strong tendency to severe involvement of the mediastinal lymph nodes and also to hemic dissemination with meningitis and generalized miliary tuberculosis. When primary infection is acquired in adolescence or adult life, there is a similar frequency of involvement of the nodes, but, as a rule, they do not become greatly enlarged. Hemic dissemination into abdominal organs is also common (26.8 to 76.4 per cent in Medlar's series), but the lesions usually are small and remain latent. In infants the tendency is much greater for the caseous nodes to perforate the bronchus. The primary parenchymal lesion may break down and ex-

cavate early, much more frequently in adults than in infants. Thus it is apparent that the pulmonary disease of adults, which accounts for more than 90 per cent of all disabling and fatal tuberculosis, may have originated from (a) the exacerbation of an old primary lesion; (b) from a recently acquired primary; or (c) from an exogenous reinfection. Whatever the origin, the implications are approximately the same except that reinfection lesions tend to run a mild course and do not often give rise to hemic disseminations.

In adolescents and adults the lesion which is observed later to go on to progressive pulmonary tuberculosis is usually a single focus of tuberculous pneumonia which roentgenographically appears to be 1 or 2 cm. in diameter. Actually, it is somewhat larger, and includes a necrotic part which has sloughed into a connecting bronchus sufficiently to give rise to adjacent small secondary lesions.

GENERAL CONSIDERATIONS IN CLINICAL DIAGNOSIS AND TREATMENT OF TUBERCULOSIS

Tuberculin Tests. A typical reaction to a standard tuberculin test is a specific indication of the presence of a tuberculous lesion somewhere in the body; beyond this fact there is always the implication that the lesion probably contains living tubercle bacilli.

Indications for Testing. The tuberculin test is a valuable means of determining the prevalence of infection in a community. It often is a tracer of sources of infection; e.g., a young child who reacts to tuberculin probably has been in contact at home or elsewhere with some person with tuberculosis in the infectious state. In such ways tuberculin testing is useful in communities where the disease is of low prevalence and is likely to exist in "nests." In clinical practice it is often distinctly helpful in diagnosis.

Materials and Techniques. Koch's Old Tuberculin (OT) and Seibert's Purified Protein Derivative (PPD and PPD–S, the latter being the more highly purified) are widely used, and there are other suitable tuberculins. The potency of OT has been found to vary considerably in different products, while PPD conforms to a standard. The test is performed usually on the volar surface of the forearm. The *cutaneous test* (von Pirquet) is made by lightly scarifying the skin for a few millimeters with a needle or special scarifier, and on this area a drop of undiluted OT is applied and allowed to dry in the open air. The *intracutaneous test* (Mantoux) is generally preferred over others and is made with a calibrated syringe by injecting 0.1 cc. of a measured dilution of tuberculin into the superficial layers of the skin, creating a wheal. If OT is used, the initial dose for apparently healthy persons is 0.1 mg. (10 "Tuberculin Units") (0.1 cc. of a 1:1000 dilution of OT in physiologic saline solution), while for patients with questionably active tuberculosis it is 0.01 mg. (one "Tuberculin Unit" or TU). If no reaction is elicited after 48 to 72 hours, repeated tests may be made with ten times the strength of the next preceding dose; as a rule the strongest dose used is 1.0 mg. of OT. For routine testing of apparently healthy persons a single dose of 0.001 mg. PPD in 0.1 cc. of diluent is generally used; if active disease is suspected one should start with a weaker dose, i.e., 0.00002 mg. A significant reaction to the cutaneous or intracutaneous test is indicated at the site of application by the appearance, usually within 48 to 72 hours, of an area of induration, 0.5 cm. or more in diameter, which may be appreciated by palpation, surrounded by a zone of redness. Severe reactions may result in the formation of a vesicle with slight necrosis of the tissues, and there may be pink streaks of lymphangitis extending up the forearm and palpable slightly tender nodes in the axilla. Atypical or false reactions, usually of short duration, are thought possibly to be due to nonpathogenic mycobacteria which may live in the body; these reactions are elicited only by relatively large doses of tuberculin, according to C. E. Palmer. A *percutaneous* or *patch test* is performed by applying to the skin a strip of adhesive tape on which a piece of gauze, saturated with dried tuberculin, is attached. The local reaction is represented, after 24 to 48 hours, by a red papular and occasionally slightly vesicular eruption. The patch test is said to approximate in accuracy the Mantoux test using 0.1 mg. of OT; dryness of the skin may interfere with a reaction to the patch. Its chief virtue is the simplicity of its application; it may be placed on the back, which is desirable for children. If no reaction occurs, the more dependable Mantoux test may be used.

In addition to the local reaction to any tuberculin test, there may be a constitutional reaction with fever and malaise and, less often, a focal reaction of inflammation about tuberculous lesions. These should be guarded against by carefully selecting the dose of tuberculin.

Interpretation of Cutaneous Hypersensitivity to Tuberculin. An infant who reacts to tuberculin is assumed to have an active tuberculous lesion due to a recent primary infection. In older persons the lesion may be old and fibrotic and, therefore, inactive. In the presence of manifest disease of uncertain causation a reaction is of little or no practical diagnostic value, but no reaction to the higher doses is significant, since the disease, in these circumstances, is unlikely to be tuberculous. The test is not a measure of immunity or of the degree of activity of the disease in the individual case. The reaction may be depressed or absent (1) if the disease is still in its incubation period (five or six weeks after the primary infection, sometimes longer); (2) if existing tuberculous lesions are thoroughly healed and calcified; (3) in some terminal cases of tuberculosis; (4) in the presence of severe acute attacks of measles or influenza; (5) during the latter months of pregnancy; and (6) if the dose of tuberculin is too small. Following the administration of cortisone or corticotropin the tuberculin sensitivity of the skin may be temporarily diminished.

Demonstrating the Tubercle Bacillus.*
When possible, the demonstration of the presence of tubercle bacilli is the final proof of the tuberculous nature of a lesion. Furthermore, in clinical practice the recovery of the bacillus may be taken in most instances as evidence that the lesion in question is active or only partly healed. The reason for this is the fact that the organism does not escape readily from the lesion until caseation, liquefaction and ulceration have occurred. Unlike most other bacterial pneumonias, for instance, the early tuberculous pneumonia is composed of an exudate which is relatively dry and possibly coagulated and on this account does not "leak" into the bronchus; moreover, at this time there is little or no tuberculous bronchitis. Bronchial discharges do not start until the parenchymal lesion sloughs; not until then are tubercle bacilli

* Various bacteriologic techniques, adapted especially for the problems of tuberculosis, are described in a booklet "Diagnostic Standards," which may be obtained from the National Tuberculosis Association, 1790 Broadway, New York City. A more comprehensive treatise is the book of Willis and Cummings, Diagnostic and Experimental Methods in Tuberculosis. Springfield, Charles C Thomas, 1952.

likely to be demonstrated in the sputum. According to the same principle the resulting defect or cavity cannot be said to have healed as long as bacilli are demonstrable. The same concept applies in other situations such as the finding of bacilli in the urine with respect to early tuberculosis of the kidney. Even after a lesion starts discharging its purulent contents it may do so slowly and in small quantities; bacilli may be recovered, therefore, only from isolated purulent particles or in a collection of the discharge, such as sputum, taken during several days. A few organisms from an early sloughing renal lesion may be greatly diluted in the urine and, therefore, hard to recover; consequently they must be concentrated again by centrifugation or some other method. Similarly, in serous effusions and in the pus of abscesses, there may also be great dilution, requiring artificial concentration before the bacilli can be demonstrated. In view of such circumstances, therefore, failure to detect the bacillus is not accepted as proof of its absence. However, there are particular relationships in which this failure is highly significant, such as a "negative" purulent sputum which is being expectorated in considerable quantities from a pulmonary cavity. In such circumstances the lesion is unlikely to be tuberculous.

Cultural methods and *animal inoculation* are of great assistance if the specimens are carefully prepared. The former are more convenient and, if skillful and meticulous techniques are used, they are as efficient as animal inoculation. In either case the results may not be known for six or eight weeks. Consequently, special methods have been developed to speed up bacterial growth. They include several media developed by Dubos and Middlebrook and a slide culture method proposed by Pryce. The characteristics of *virulence* of tubercle bacilli have been studied by Middlebrook, Dubos and Pierce, who observed the virulent forms growing on culture media in long serpentine cords. Dubos and Middlebrook have also described a cytochemical reaction with neutral red which appears characteristic of these forms. H. Bloch has identified a material of lipid character ("cord factor") which appears to coat the surface of the bacillus and to be closely related to its virulence. Such tests have not yet found any application in clinical practice. Presumably the tubercle bacilli growing in a lesion exist as a mixed population with varying individual potentialities.

One of the identifying marks of the tubercle bacillus, is its *acid-fast staining* by certain dyes. This characteristic is brought out by fixing the prepared specimen on a microscopic slide and applying the stain according to one of a number of techniques, usually the Ziehl-Neelsen. With this, a carbol fuchsin stain is applied, followed by acid alcohol to bleach all organisms except the mycobacteria, which retain the red color. With rare exceptions such acid-fast organisms in expectorated sputum are tubercle bacilli. However, gastric specimens, taken when the sputum is "negative," should be cultured, since these often contain nonpathogenic saprophytic mycobacteria ingested with food such as raw vegetables and fruits. Culturally these saprophytes grow more rapidly than the tubercle bacillus, and often at room temperature. Their colonies may be distinguished by their rich yellow or orange color, and when they are inoculated into animals, they do not cause disease. Similarly, acid-fast saprophytes, indigenous to the cerumen of the external auditory canal and the external genitalia (smegma bacillus), must be differentiated when specimens of pus or urine are taken for diagnosis. Rarely, acid-fast saprophytes may exist in the pus from a pulmonary abscess or bronchiectasis.

Secondary infection of tuberculous lesions, including effusions and abscesses, rarely occurs by way of the blood or lymph streams. Its presence usually is explained by communication with the respiratory or alimentary canals or with the external surface of the body after a sinus, fistula or cavity has formed; then the common pyogenic bacteria may gain access. Occasionally they are introduced by faulty technique, as in thoracentesis. The effect may be serious if drainage is poor or if there is a dead space causing a mechanical hindrance to healing (e.g., pleural empyema); or it may be inconsequential. Thus, a tuberculous pulmonary cavity is not usually aggravated by secondary infection unless a blockage of the bronchi interferes with free drainage of the discharges.

Surgical Biopsy and Diagnostic Aspiration. Biopsy or aspiration of an area may be indicated, especially to identify the nature of a lesion beneath the surface, such as an enlarged lymph node. The important principle here is to avoid breaking into the lesion, which may lead to infection of healthy local tissues and, rather rarely, to infection of the blood stream. It is undesirable to remove sections for diagnosis directly from lesions such as those located in the larynx or bronchus if these are suspected to be tuberculous, since this may be aggravating locally; as a rule the diagnosis can be made in other ways. The aspiration, with syringe and needle, of serous tuberculous effusions is usually harmless if good judgment and technique are used. If the effusion is purulent and teeming with tubercle bacilli, special precautions should be used to avoid infection of the needle track which sometimes leads to necrosis and the formation of sinuses and fistulas. The danger of reactivating or aggravating a local lesion by any of these procedures or of spreading the infection may be minimized by chemotherapy for a short time afterwards.

Changes in the Blood of Tuberculous Patients. In the early phases of tuberculosis significant changes in the cells of the blood are seldom detected. During insidious progression of the disease there may be no rise in the total number of *leukocytes,* though there may be some increase of the young forms and of monocytes, while lymphocytes may be relatively decreased. During acute exacerbations these tendencies may be greatly accentuated, the polymorphonuclear leukocytes may rise to 12,000 to 18,000 per cubic millimeter (seldom above 20,000), while the percentage of neutrophils also increases, but not often above 80 per cent. Higher ranges always raise the question of some other bacterial infection and, in this way, are often helpful in differential diagnosis. If and when the disease settles back to a quiescent, chronic or healed state, the numbers and proportions of leukocytes usually return almost or entirely to normal. The *erythrocytes* and their *hemoglobin* content usually remain normal until there has been considerable progression of the disease, when slight anemia may appear. Severe grades are observed in the late stages of the disease especially if it is complicated with intestinal involvement or amyloidosis. Electrophoretic studies of the *serum proteins* and *polysaccharides* have been reported by Seibert, Seibert, Atno and Campbell. They found in cases of minimal active pulmonary tuberculosis a significant rise in the gamma globulin with a corresponding decrease in the albumin fraction. As the disease advances, the alpha$_2$ globulin and polysaccharide content also increase; still later all the globulins. The mean total protein is normal. As the disease subsides and

improves, the albumin fraction is the last to return to normal.

The *sedimentation rate* of the erythrocytes is accelerated in almost all the febrile phases of tuberculosis. Also it may be accelerated in many of the afebrile phases and thus may be a more sensitive index of activity than the temperature curve. Its value is limited by the fact that it is not specific for tuberculosis and may be normal in the early active phases and also later when the lesions have become chronic, although not healed. The same limitation applies to other "activity" tests, of which there have been many. The *tuberculosis complement fixation test* is positive in varying titer in most cases, but has not been found helpful in clinical practice. A *hemagglutinin test* proposed by Middlebrook and Dubos has been observed to show some parallelism with phases of clinical activity and arrest of the disease. However it has not proved to be sufficiently sensitive and reliable to be of distinct clinical value. In the late stages of tuberculosis there may be other changes, including a lowering of the blood volume and of the content of mineral salts, enzymes and vitamins. *Bacteremia* must occur obviously during hemic disseminations and occasionally may be demonstrated culturally. Most efforts, however, are unsuccessful, probably because of the degree of dilution of the bacilli and their rapid disappearance into phagocytes which become immobilized.

There is no reliable specific test of resistance or immunity against tuberculosis, nor is there a good prognostic test. These factors are best judged by a summation and evaluation of accurate clinical, roentgenographic and laboratory data.

Toxemia of Tuberculosis. No true toxin has been identified as a product of the tubercle bacillus. Various chemical components of it and by-products of its growth in artificial culture media can be introduced into the tissues of a healthy animal without appreciable harm. If the tissues are allergic, because of previous infection, however, there may be definite and severe reactions, as with the tuberculin test. The mechanisms of this phenomenon are complex and unclear; one suggestion is that in the allergic patient toxic by-products of necrosis may be liberated during caseation. Whatever the explanation, the toxemia is characterized by its relative mildness. In the early phases of tuberculosis often enough there are no subjective general symptoms. Usually it is only after the disease has advanced and caused considerable involvement of tissues that loss of weight, malaise and fever occur. This disproportion between volume of disease and mildness of symptoms is almost unique and often gives a clue to the diagnosis. Even in acute phases, like tuberculous pneumonia and acute generalized miliary forms with high fever, the other toxemic symptoms often are only moderate. There may be no headache, no pains in the back or joints, some chilliness, but no shaking chills, and lassitude without great prostration. Herpetic eruptions rarely occur on the lips or elsewhere. These peculiarities explain in large part the ability of patients to keep working in spite of advanced active disease and their tardiness in seeking medical attention. Apparently it is also one reason why some patients are able to live on for years with more or less continuous toxemia from chronic disease.

In some cases chronic toxemia predisposes to the development of amyloidosis. However, the majority of fatal pulmonary cases are not associated with this complication. It is observed most often in secondarily infected lesions of the bones and joints, in mixed infection tuberculous empyema, and apparently also in cases of severe intestinal tuberculosis complicating pulmonary disease.

The symptomatology, local as well as general, is considered in more detail in the sections dealing with various forms of the disease. Emphasis is placed on the pulmonary form because this is the most frequent in clinical practice.

Likewise, the principles of treatment will be described with special reference to tuberculosis of the lungs and to problems related to other specific sites of the disease. Since the antituberculosis drugs have certain similar effects on all forms of tuberculosis, a general description of their actions will be given at this point. Particular applications will be mentioned in the separate discussions of each form.

SPECIFIC CHEMOTHERAPY FOR TUBERCULOSIS

"The *in vitro* growth of the tubercle bacillus is inhibited by an enormous range of organic compounds, few of which exhibit *in vivo* activity. To merit classification as a tuberculostat of interest, therefore, a compound should possess marked activity *in vivo*" (H. H. Fox). To be of practical value, it may be said in addition, the compound should not have serious toxic effects when administered in effective therapeutic doses.

The searches of investigators during the centuries have culminated in recent years in the discovery of several effective compounds, as well as recognition of the therapeutic properties in others which were known but not previously tested. In 1944 *streptomycin,* derived from *Streptomyces griseus,* was announced as a discovery by Schatz, Bugie and Waksman. Feldman and Hinshaw soon observed its tuberculostatic influence in experimental animals and treated patients. In 1946, Lehmann reported the favorable effects of para-aminosalicylic acid (PAS). The announcements of other discoveries followed; these included amithiozone (4-acetylaminobenzaldehyde thiosemicarbazone) and a number of other related compounds, and viomycin (derived from *Streptomyces puniceus* and *Streptomyces floridae*). Meanwhile, drugs which are distinguished for their action against other bacteria were also found to have some tuberculostatic effect; these include especially diaminodiphenylsulfone and its derivatives (Promin, Diasone, Sulphetrone and Promizole), and oxytetracycline (Terramycin). In 1952 Robitzek and Selikoff reported strikingly favorable effects of isoniazid (isonicotinic acid hydrazide) and iproniazid (1-isonicotinyl-2-isopropyl-hydrazine) in tuberculous humans. Their work was preceded by the experimental investigations of Grunberg and Schnitzer, Zieper and Lewis, Bernstein, Steenken and Wolinsky, Benson, Rubin and the associates of all these. Also in early 1952, the antituberculous activity of pyrazinamide, a derivative of nicotinic acid, was demonstrated in humans by Yeager and his associates after laboratory studies by Kushner and Malone and their respective associates.

As each of these agents became available they received extensive clinical testing in various parts of the world. The reports clearly indicated some merit in each compound. It was soon appreciated, however, because of the known wide variations in the natural course of tuberculosis and the complexity of the problems implicit in the new treatments, that organized studies of many hundreds of patients would have to be undertaken. Such organization in many cooperating hospitals was arranged by the United States Public Health Service, the United States Veterans Administration, Army and Navy Hospitals, and the British Medical Research Council, and this together with thousands of individual efforts has accomplished great progress.

The relatively high potencies of streptomycin and isoniazid have been satisfactorily demonstrated. PAS, while less effective, has retained an important place for reasons to be mentioned. The other drugs enumerated above have relatively limited effects, and several have all but fallen into disuse, especially since the advent of isoniazid. At the start each drug in its turn was tried singly; this had the virtue of demonstrating any toxic properties and the degree and range of therapeutic effects. It soon became evident that almost all the compounds and certainly the more potent of them, when given to patients, suppress the growth of offending tubercle bacilli except those which are drug-resistant; these resistant strains then may take over the field and escape the effects of any further therapy with the given drug. Such drug resistance becomes manifest at varying rates, but commonly within two to four months after the start of treatment. As a consequence the early favorable response frequently is followed by a relapse. Then it was found that the growth of resistant strains may be suppressed to a greater or lesser extent by exposing them to drugs of another class, and this was the genesis of combined therapy, i.e., administering two or more drugs simultaneously. Regimens employing two drugs are effective in preventing the proliferation of resistant strains for long periods of time, at least four months, and in most cases apparently for a year or more. It is questionable whether combinations of three drugs are superior in this respect to two, and there are reasons for holding one very potent drug in reserve in case of need during a late relapse of the disease. The approved practice now is not to give any specific drug alone under any circumstances except perhaps for the purpose of investigating unexplored fields, but rather to use one of a number of multiple regimens which are available and have been tested. This may be done with confidence that, in the majority of cases, therapeutic effects will be sustained for many months during which the administration is continued.

Common Effects of Chemotherapy. The mechanisms of antimycobacterial action of the drugs appear to be complex according to various studies. Whatever these may be, the outward manifestation is the failure of susceptible organisms to reproduce, at least at the usual rate, so long as they are exposed to effective quantities of the given drug. This interference with the reproductive cycle may continue in the tissues for many months; then, after discontinuance of treatment, bacterial activity may sooner or later resume its familiar course. Lesions removed surgically may yield organisms which grow in animals or in artificial media. In such instances, the effect is obviously more or less prolonged bacteriostasis. There is other evidence from the laboratory that in certain circumstances some of the bacteria actually may be killed by specific drugs, and this is thought by Middlebrook and others to apply especially to young forms. It has been found by many that more or less encapsulated lesions of solid caseous composition, removed surgically from the lungs of patients who have been treated with drugs for four months or longer, may contain numerous tubercle bacilli which take the acid-fast stain but fail to grow in artificial media or to produce disease in the usually susceptible animals. Whether some or all the bacilli are dead or whether the phenomenon indicates only a profound modification of their habits of growth and reproduction is not finally determined; there is much disagreement. The same phenomena have been identified in lesions from patients who have never had specific chemotherapy, but the time required for such modifications under natural conditions appears to be much longer. In contrast to this phenomenon, tubercle bacilli obtained from "open" cavities of the lung (i.e., with free bronchial communications) are found more often to be demonstrably viable and virulent; an exception with respect to isoniazid will be mentioned. From the clinical viewpoint, it is assumed that diseased tissues are never completely sterilized and, therefore, that treatment with drugs, rest and other measures should be applied for long periods of time so as to lessen and avoid the hazard of renewed bacterial activity and extension of the disease.

As mentioned before, the effects of specific chemotherapy on tuberculous lesions and clinical symptoms do not differ essentially from the effects of natural regression of the disease without such aid. However, with the relatively rapid bacteriostasis induced by chemotherapy, the favorable response is usually more surely predictable, more prompt and more consistently sustained. So far as known, chemotherapy does not directly stimulate the healing process, such as the production of fibrosis; it merely holds the infection effectively in abeyance and thus allows nature to take its course, unhindered by the continuing attack of actively growing tubercle bacilli. When the natural defenses are poor or entirely lacking, even the most potent drugs are unavailing. The well known but immeasurable variability of these defenses helps to account for differences in the behavior of individual cases and to support the concept that each patient is a law unto himself.

In most cases the early response to treatment (i.e., rest, supported by chemotherapy) is a cessation of exudation in and about lesions and a diminution of constitutional symptoms. As fever subsides, for instance, edematous swellings recede and the pain from this tissue tension eases and vanishes. Accumulated exudate then is removed by resolution, absorption and drainage; here again the rate is variable. Fibrous repair ensues and proceeds, its adequacy in the long run depending on the damage done beforehand by the necrosing effects of the infection. Eventually, as with any antituberculosis treatment, the outcome is determined not only by this healing but also by the persistence of partly repaired necrotic, ulcerous, excavated tissue which harbors tubercle bacilli, ready to renew the attack.

Action of Individual Drugs. *Streptomycin,* in a dilution of 1.56 micrograms per milliliter of artificial culture medium, completely inhibits the growth of almost all human and bovine strains of the tubercle bacillus; the avian strain is said to be more resistant. Resistant strains, assumed to exist in rare numbers in any bacterial colony, proliferate *in vitro* and *in vivo,* so that after about four weeks of exposure to the drug they begin to predominate. At the end of 120 days, 80 to 90 per cent of the cultures are found to be resistant to more than 10 micrograms of streptomycin per milliliter; many will resist the effects of 1000 micrograms or more. However, the virulence of resistant organisms is not appreciably altered. In clinical practice the emergence of resistance is found to depend more on the duration of treatment than on daily dosage; however, the rate of assuming predominance is slower if the drug is given only twice a week in 1 gm. doses.

Toxic effects, principally on the vestibular apparatus, are frequent when streptomycin is administered intramuscularly in doses amounting to 2 gm. daily for two to four months or longer; their incidence is much less when the dose is reduced to 1 gm. daily, and still less on a regimen of 1 gm. twice weekly. Vestibular dysfunction appears as vertigo, nausea, vomiting, ataxia and partial or complete loss of response to caloric stimulation; if severe, this loss may be permanent, but there may be partial recovery from mild damage. Less frequently, impairment of the auditory function may occur, usually preceded by tinnitus. Deafness is of the perceptive type, according to Winston. Other disturbances include dermatitis, which occasionally may be severe and exfoliative, eosinophilia and renal damage. Neurotoxic effects on the fetus have not been reported, and it is considered safe to give the drug during pregnancy. Streptomycin is now employed only in combination with some other active drug.

Dihydrostreptomycin has bacteriostatic effects similar to those of streptomycin and has been used in the same dosage. While dihydrostreptomycin causes less frequent disturbance of vestibular function, deafness is a more common result of its use; the onset of deafness may be rather abrupt and it may not appear until a few weeks after the treatment has been discontinued. Other toxic effects are much like those of streptomycin, though dihydrostreptomycin may be well tolerated by patients who are hypersensitive to streptomycin.

A combination of the two drugs in half the usual dose of each (0.5 gm. streptomycin plus 0.5 gm. dihydrostreptomycin) has been suggested to reduce neurotoxic effects. It must be remembered that this combination does not delay the proliferation of strains of tubercle bacilli which are resistant to either drug, so that this particular multiple drug preparation is not useful for prolonged treatment unless it is combined with a drug of another class, such as PAS.

Isoniazid and *iproniazid* compare very favorably with streptomycin against tuberculosis. As iproniazid produced troublesome toxic effects when given in therapeutic doses, it is not in general use at present. Other derivatives of this series are also receiving study. Isoniazid inhibits the growth of virulent tubercle bacilli in culture media in concentrations of 0.05 to 0.25 microgram per milliliter. Elmendorf and his associates found plasma concentrations of the drug five to ten times these concentrations at the end of three hours in patients given doses totalling 3 mg. per kilogram per day. The drug may be given parenterally. Isoniazid passes through tissue barriers readily and, when taken by mouth, it is found in considerable concentration in the cerebrospinal fluid. The drug penetrates caseous tuberculous lesions (R. W. Mathei, et al.) apparently more readily than streptomycin. It also inhibits the growth of tubercle bacilli within isolated rabbit macrophages in a concentration of 0.05 microgram per milliliter, compared with 25 micrograms of streptomycin required for a similar effect (Mackaness and Smith).

When isoniazid is administered alone for periods of six to seven months and tubercle bacilli are still present in the sputum, these are found to be resistant to 5 micrograms of the drug per milliliter of medium in 50 per cent or more of the cases (U. S. Public Health Service Study). A unique feature of some of these resistant strains is the loss of pathogenicity for guinea pigs; when inoculated they may cause only a small local lesion or none at all. In contrast many of these altered strains are fully pathogenic for mice. The significance of these phenomena is not clear, for the tuberculosis in patients yielding these strains sometimes continues to run a progressive course.

In clinical use the toxic effects of isoniazid are usually few and mild after the customary dosage of 2 to 5 mg. per kilogram of body weight daily (150 to 300 mg. daily for adults). These include muscular twitching, hyperreflexia (rarely clonic convulsions or temporary psychoses), difficulty in micturition and constipation. There have been a few isolated reports of agranulocytosis, eosinophilia, hemolytic anemia, and purpura. Doses up to 7 to 10 mg. of isoniazid per kilo per day have been given in cases of meningitis and generalized tuberculosis without significant evidence of toxicity, although large doses (25 mg. per kilo) may cause hepatic damage in animals. The principal toxic manifestation of isoniazid is *peripheral neuritis*. The occurrence of this reaction bears a rough relationship to dosage; it is rarely seen on a daily dosage of 5 mg. per kilogram; it has occurred in as many as 40 per cent of a group of patients receiving 20 mg. per kilogram each day. There is impressive evidence that *pyridoxine* in large doses (e.g., 300 mg. total daily dose) can prevent the appearance of isoniazid neuritis even when large doses of isoniazid are used. There is no evidence that the treatment of established isoniazid neuritis with pyridoxine is particularly useful. In general, however, the prognosis of isoniazid peripheral neuritis is excellent, although many weeks or even months may be required before recovery is absolutely complete. On withdrawing isoniazid there may be temporary disturbances such as bad dreams, nervousness, depression and digestive upsets.

Para-aminosalicylic acid is reported to inhibit the growth of tubercle bacilli in concentrations of 0.06 to 0.25 micrograms per milliliter of Dubos liquid culture medium. Resistant strains become predominant in many cultures after about four months. It is necessary for the therapeutic effects to administer the acid in doses of 12 to 15 mg. daily, divided and given orally after meals. These effects may be significant in some cases but are not generally equal to those of streptomycin or isoniazid. PAS in the usual dosage is ineffective in acute meningitis or generalized miliary tuberculosis, although some of the European clinicians are encouraged by the results of the intravenous use of the drug as a part of the chemotherapy of meningitis. Paraf advocates infusing 500 ml. of a 3 per cent solution slowly during two hours, once daily for about thirty days. The sodium salt can be given subcutaneously in 1 or 2 per cent solution. Because of its lesser potency PAS is not generally relied upon except as one of a combination with streptomycin or isoniazid in an effort to delay bacterial drug resistance.

The disadvantages of PAS are due largely to gastrointestinal irritation manifested by nausea, vomiting and diarrhea. Febrile and other reactions due to hypersensitivity occur, some of these possibly being related to impurities in the drug. Various devices are used to avoid these troubles, and some patients may tolerate the sodium salt more readily (15 to 20 gm. daily). PAS administration may lead to the development of goiter and has been reported to interfere with thyroxine production; it also causes some hypoprothrombinemia but this has not proved to be serious.

Viomycin is reported by Steenken and Wolinsky to have about 25 per cent of the potency of streptomycin in tuberculous animals. This drug is active against strains of tubercle bacilli which are resistant to other drugs, and may be used in situations where the effects of other chemotherapy have been exhausted. In daily doses of 50 mg. per kilogram it may have toxic effects including renal damage, hypokalemia and deafness. It is thought that a regimen providing for 2 gm. of viomycin twice or thrice weekly with 12 gm. of PAS daily may create a very useful place for this drug.

Oxytetracycline (Terramycin) has been used in combination with streptomycin and in this way has been reported to be effective in delaying the growth of streptomycin-resistant strains of tubercle bacilli. Doses of 2 to 3 gm. and more of oxytetracycline have been used, and it seems now that 1 or 2 gm. daily may suffice.

Amithiozone and the *sulfones* have relatively weak bacteriostatic effects in doses which can be tolerated by most patients. Amithiozone may cause disturbances of hepatic function and blood formation, although these usually correct themselves when the use of the drug is discontinued. Some have found this agent and also one of the sulfones to be of value in combination with one of the more potent drugs but they are not widely used.

Pyrazinamide when used alone exerts a substantial degree of antituberculous activity but the effects are usually of only short duration. Moreover, the use of this drug alone has been associated with the appearance of hepatitis (see below).

Neomycin is tuberculostatic but has highly toxic effects on the kidney and auditory function. Its clinical use, therefore, is precluded from antituberculosis regimens.

Combined regimens of proved value are several. In mild or moderately severe cases of pulmonary disease 1 gm. of streptomycin may be given every second or third day and 12 to 15 gm. of PAS daily. As prolonged administration is usually desirable, this may be continued six to twelve months or even longer. In more severe cases it may be indicated to administer 1 gm. of streptomycin daily for a few weeks, then reducing the schedule to twice or thrice weekly. If the situation warrants using the two most potent drugs at once, isoniazid in doses of 3 to 5 mg. per kilo daily may be substituted for PAS. Some prefer to avoid the possibility of exhausting the effects of these two simultaneously. Another alternative is a combination of isoniazid and PAS in the doses mentioned. Dosage may be varied within the chosen regimen, but the range is limited on one hand by bacteriostatic effectiveness and on the other by the possibility of toxicity. It will be seen, in reading the above account of the properties of the drugs, that other regimens are possible and may be selected especially when the problem of drug resistance is encountered.

Pyrazinamide-isoniazid has been subjected to extensive laboratory and clinical studies. McCune and Tompsett have found that the spleen and lungs of tuberculous mice may be sterilized by treatment with these two compounds simultaneously. McDermott and his associates have found the regimen studied to be likewise highly effective in humans but impractical as yet because of the high incidence of hepatitis (approximately 3 per cent). Nevertheless, the highly significant finding of apparent sterilization of the tissues in mice points to the possibility of a chemo-

therapy which may be superior to those in current use.

TUBERCULOSIS OF THE LUNGS

Viewed in broad perspective, pulmonary tuberculosis is the form dominating all others. To epitomize, the lung is the usual seat of the primary lesion and, later, if the primary heals, of the reinfection lesion. The pulmonary lesion is the common source of bronchial and other "intracanalicular" dissemination of the infection, and also of hemic dissemination leading to generalized disease. Pulmonary tuberculosis is numerically far in the lead of all other forms as a cause of death; epidemically, the pulmonary lesion is paramount because it is usually the source from which the tubercle bacillus is passed through the community.

Development and Clinical Course. The rather abrupt rise in the occurrence of pulmonary tuberculosis in adolescence and early adulthood and its subsequent prevalence seem to be related largely to constitutional or endocrine influences causing in some people a lowering of resistance, to the stress and strain of environment, and to the more frequent acquisition of infection as people circulate more freely and widely in the community. The onset of the disease at this time of life may be due to the exacerbation of old latent primary lesions or to the progression of those recently acquired. In the latter event, progressive disease is most likely to become manifest within approximately two years, after which a rising, specific immunity may help cope with the invader.

The Early Lesion. Characteristically, the first recognizable lesion of tuberculosis of the lungs is parenchymal, usually a bronchopneumonic focus which can be noticed in the roentgenogram because it casts a shadow approximately 1 cm., more or less, in diameter. Before this size is attained, as Medlar has shown, the lesion probably has undergone some caseation, sloughing and local bronchial extension which may have occurred within a few weeks or months, or perhaps at a much slower rate interrupted by periods of latency or retrogression. This inapparent evolution is not apt to produce symptoms, although, if it is a result of recently acquired primary infection, the rather rare occurrence of *erythema nodosum* is sometimes reported. Extension to the pleura may occur early, even before the lesion is detectable on the roentgenogram, followed by fibrinous or serofibrinous pleurisy. Likewise, while the lesion is still small and occult and especially when it is the result of a recent primary infection, it may be the source of hemic dissemination, the most serious manifestations of which are *meningitis* and *generalized miliary* disease.

Progression of the Lesion. The early lesion, having already progressed unseen, is likely to progress further, especially in young patients. If it does so, it is usually by further caseation, sloughing, ulceration and bronchial dissemination. The variety of progressions is infinite, and only a few will be mentioned. Most often the process is rather slow, and there will be a series of small extensions of the disease in one or both lungs. The clinical course is *insidious*. As sloughing occurs into the bronchial tubes, the purulent discharge mixes with bronchial mucus and the patient may have a slight cough, usually in the mornings, with scanty mucopurulent expectoration. Examination of the sputum will often reveal the presence of tubercle bacilli. After such ulceration, bleeding may occur, but, in the early phases, this seldom causes more than "streaking" of the sputum. The extensions in the lungs cause some toxemia, but this, too, is not usually severe. During a subsequent latency or even partial healing of the lesions these vague symptoms may all subside, to add to the deception of the victim. In such ways the disease may exacerbate and subside from time to time until both lungs are widely involved.

Acute Exacerbations. Acute exacerbations of pulmonary tuberculosis are explained by similar mechanisms and are symptomatically acute because of the suddenness and severity of bronchial dissemination. The parenchymal focus after caseation and liquefaction may empty rather abruptly into the bronchial tree a quantity of pus, highly charged with tubercle bacilli. This is readily inhaled into healthy alveoli. The irritating effects of the pus together with the massive infection give rise to an intense inflammatory reaction manifested as subacute or *acute tuberculous pneumonia,* usually of a confluent lobular distribution. In some cases, particularly in patients of low resistance, this goes on to *acute caseous pneumonia.* These acute forms are almost always related to a preexisting pulmonary lesion, as stated, but occasionally are caused by analogous mechanisms following the rupture of a caseous tracheobronchial lymph node

into a bronchus. The acute inflammation often produces profound toxemia. Such exacerbations may follow within 24 hours after a hemoptysis, obviously explained by the inhalation of blood issuing from a cavity and washing tubercle bacilli with it. This *acute posthemorrhagic tuberculous pneumonia* is usually in one or both lower lobes and may mark the transition from a limited disease with a single cavity into rapidly progressive and fatal bilateral disease.

Chronic Fibroid Lesions. Chronic fibroid pulmonary tuberculosis is seen most often in elderly people whose lungs bear the scars of repeated battles with the bacillus. The disease may have spread steadily but very slowly, or in a series of exacerbations with long intervals of quiescence. Areas of fibrosis may reflect good healing tendencies, but, as a rule, there are other areas in which cavities and necrotic foci persist in spite of this. With fibrosis goes emphysema, pleural adhesions, flattenings and immobilizations of the chest wall, and retractions of the mediastinum. Thus the elderly consumptive may far outlive his contemporaries; his range is limited by his shortness of breath, his chronic "bronchitis" and his feeling "poorly," but he is plenteously potent as a disseminator of infection in the community.

Onset of Pulmonary Tuberculosis. As indicated in the preceding paragraphs, the mode of onset varies greatly according to the susceptibility of the patient and the behavior of the pulmonary lesions. Commonly, the first manifestations lag behind the actual appearance of the lesions, and this *subclinical interval* may be short or long.

Acute tuberculous pneumonia may produce the first clinical symptoms. This form is uncommon although not rare, being observed most often in young people, in Negroes and in debilitated old people. A preexisting excavating lesion is almost always present, but the patient may not have been impressed with the mild symptoms caused by it. The acute attack may appear to be precipitated by exposure to inclement weather, by a common cold, by severe sunburn, by a hemoptysis or by some trivial influence. The patient may experience chilliness, prostration, pain in the chest and fever; this fever may rise quickly to 104° or 105° F. and the pulse rate to 100 or more per minute. The breathing is quickened at first (twenty to thirty respirations per minute), later becoming labored and more rapid as the lungs become further engorged. It is seldom noisy or grunting. A feeling of congestion in the chest increases and the lips and extremities become slightly or moderately cyanotic. The cough may not be severe at first and may be productive of only a few cubic centimeters of mucopurulent sputum daily; later, larger quantities of a greenish yellow purulent character appear. Unless hemoptysis occurred just before the onset, the sputum usually is not bloody. Because of the type of onset and the signs of lobar or lobular consolidation, the picture may resemble closely that of a pneumococcal infection (see Differential Diagnosis). Without proper treatment the course may be rapid, ending fatally in two or three months; in other cases it settles down to a subacute or chronic pace.

More often the onset is attended by *grippelike symptoms,* such as fever, weakness, fatigue and mild aching in the muscles which subside after a week or several weeks, perhaps to recur at intervals when the patient again undertakes exertion. In other cases, and this is common, there is an insidious, unexplained slow loss of weight, increasing fatigue and impairment of staying powers. These symptoms continue for weeks or months before the patient is aware of serious difficulty; then he may find an afternoon fever of a fraction of a degree to several degrees. The usual rest does not restore his energies, he finds his efficiency impaired, and he is puzzled by his inability to concentrate on his work. Other patients are disturbed by some particular constitutional symptoms such as *sweating* at night, *amenorrhea,* or *anorexia* and *indigestion.* Under any of these conditions it is learned usually that the patient previously has had some *cough* and *expectoration* or at least a clearing of the throat in the morning. Sometimes he will report that there has been a little blood in the sputum at irregular intervals. In other instances, *hemoptysis* may be the initial symptom so far as the patient is subjectively aware, and this may consist only of a few spots or streaks of blood in the sputum or free and profuse bleeding. He may find a small amount of blood accumulated in his throat upon awaking in the morning. *Pleurisy* may be the outstanding initial symptom (see Tuberculosis of the Pleura).

Hoarseness, dryness and tickling in the throat or other symptoms of acute or chronic *laryngitis* may be the first to arrest attention. Likewise, the pain or discharge of a perianal abscess may be the chief complaint, the mild pulmonary symptoms previously having been ignored.

Symptoms of Pulmonary Tuberculosis. *Fever.* Usually the temperature is normal or subnormal in the morning, the rectal reading sometimes being as low as 96.5° or 97° F., and there may be considerable prostration and weakness. Between 4 and 8 p.m. the fever reaches its height, which, in acute cases, may be 105° or 106° F. More commonly in subacute or mild cases it ranges up to two or three degrees above normal. Usually a low or moderate fever recurs each afternoon or evening for some days or weeks, and in the advanced case this may continue for many months. During grippelike episodes the temperature may rise to 103° or 104° F. daily for a week or so, then gradually subside by lysis until it is normal after several weeks.

Chilliness is sometimes a complaint associated with fever of 103° to 105° F., especially if this appears suddenly.

Sweating is not a feature of early tuberculosis and is not often a symptom except in the febrile and exhausted states. Then it occurs usually at the time of the temperature rise and immediately afterward. In some cases in which there is extensive excavation of the lungs and secondary suppurative infection the sweats are drenching and prostrating.

Malaise, lassitude and *fatigue* are the most common symptoms of tuberculous toxemia. At first they are noticed toward the end of the day's activity, when the patient may eschew his usual diversions or interests in order to get additional rest. If he is the type to disregard such mild symptoms, he may become irritable, grouchy and impatient. However, the symptoms are not always unpleasant and may be evidenced only as an urge to rest and sleep. If the toxemia increases, its effects become manifest earlier in the day, and the patient may even notice that, on awaking, his vigor and energy are not restored. In progressive disease the languor grows finally into a profound weakness and exhaustion.

Loss of weight and impairment of tissue tone are also common. At the true onset there may be no loss, and a few patients even report gaining when their disease is first discovered. The loss is usually gradual at first and may amount to only 4 or 5 pounds during several months. Young people may fail merely to gain at the expected rate. During acute and febrile phases the nutrition suffers much more rapidly and prominently.

Cardiocirculatory instability is also a usual symptom and may persist long after the temperature becomes normal. The usual manifestation is tachycardia; the rate is regular and accelerated to 80 or 90 per minute during the early phases and subsequently may be higher. After exertion or excitement the quickened rate does not subside as soon as might be expected. The pulse is soft and the systolic blood pressure may be low, frequently 90 to 100 mm. of mercury. The circulatory tone may be poor, and the patient may complain of clamminess and coldness of the hands or feet; the nails may be bluish. Clubbing of the digits may never develop, and only in advanced complicated cases is it occasionally extreme. Malar flushing and other local thermic disturbances are related to fever and vagosympathetic reflexes.

Digestive symptoms of a vague character are frequent and due particularly to the toxemia. Severe distress, such as dysphagia, is not observed unless there is extensive tuberculous involvement of the larynx or pharynx. Anorexia, manifested as an indifference to food or a capriciousness of the appetite, is frequent, but usually corrects itself as the toxemia abates, after which the patient, even though confined to bed, may eat heartily. Vomiting is unusual unless the patient has advanced disease of the lungs and a harassing cough. Intestinal symptoms, such as seizures of colicky pain and diarrhea, alternating with constipation, strongly suggest an ulcerative lesion in the bowel as a secondary complication.

The menarche may be delayed and menstruation may be irregular and scanty, but, as a rule, this is observed only after disease is well established. Amenorrhea is unusual except during the febrile stages. The *fertility* of tuberculous women is somewhat impaired, and, in the advanced stages of the disease, spontaneous *abortion* is not uncommon. A striking observation, however, is that chronically tuberculous women may bear a number of children. There is little or no impairment of the sexual functions otherwise. During the early and middle stages of the disease neither the *libido* nor *potentia coeundi* is appreciably reduced.

Nervous and *psychic disturbances* are mild or entirely lacking. In most of the early and moderately advanced and many of the far advanced cases there is no appreciable change, and the patient's reactions are normal in the circumstances. Later he may become rather neurotic, dependent, introverted and depressed (Schultz). This mood, however, is usually surprisingly mild, considering the discouragement which such a chronic illness often entails. Suicidal tendencies or attempts are most uncommon. Euphoria, which once was considered to characterize tuberculosis, is not often noticeable except during the late or terminal stages. *Toxic psychoses are rare.*

Dyspnea is not usually an early symptom. Slightly or moderately accelerated respiration may be noticeable during the febrile periods or in more advanced fibroid cases in which there is a good deal of secondary emphysema.

Cough is the most common local symptom and, like others of this class, seldom develops until the pulmonary lesion has broken down and ulcerated into the bronchi. In the earlier stages cough is most pronounced when the patient awakes in the morning and is due to irritation of the bronchial mucosa from the accumulated discharges. Occasionally cough is attributed to a reflex from irritation of the pleura, and later it may be traced partly to tuberculous involvement of the larynx. At first the symptom is usually slight and is quickly relieved after the small accumulation is cleared from the trachea and larynx. Later, especially if pulmonary excavation extends and the discharges increase, the symptom may become troublesome, interfering with eating and sleeping.

Expectoration. During the initial phases of the pulmonary infiltration there is seldom any expectoration, except perhaps a little clear glary mucus. Later, however, expectoration is a most common symptom. Its quantity and frequency are variable. Only a few particles of mucopurulent material may be brought up in the morning by clearing the throat or a few coughs; gradually this may increase. In other cases expectoration starts more abruptly and may soon amount to 1 ounce or so in a day. In any case, with progressive pulmonary excavation, the quantity usually increases until 30 or 60 cc. is produced each day, mainly in the morning. In advanced cases 300 to 350 cc. may be brought up daily, particularly after secondary infection of cavities has occurred. The sputum is not foul, except in the unusual case in which secondary anaerobic infection develops in the bronchi or pulmonary cavities. When expectoration is slight, the flecks of pus are seen in the clear mucus. In caseous pneumonic cases, particularly at the start of excavation, the sputum is purulent and of a greenish yellow color, but later this usually becomes yellow and the admixture of mucus is noted. In more chronic cases the mucopurulent material is of a coherent, sometimes tenacious, character. The sputum, on standing, retains its homogeneous mucopurulent character and does not separate into layers. The quantity and the character of the expectoration reflect to some extent the changes occurring in the pulmonary lesions. A daily production of 30 to 60 cc. of purulent green matter speaks for a caseous pneumonic liquefying lesion. A change to yellowish, more mucoid sputum suggests a subsidence of the ulcerative process, indicated further by a diminution of the amount and a continuing decrease of the purulent element. Sudden and marked variations in the quantity of the sputum may be due to bronchial occlusion or to the rupture into the lung of a localized fluid collection in the pleura.

Hemoptysis. Blood spitting occurs in more than one half of all cases of pulmonary tuberculosis. As a rule, the quantity is small, consisting of streaking, spotting or pinkishness of the sputum in the mornings, but copious bleeding is not rare. Hemoptysis usually is due to the ulceration or weakening and rupture of the walls of the vessels in tuberculosis cavities. Infrequently, in chronic healed cases, it may be traced to the mechanical rupture of superficial vessels in the walls of distorted bronchi. An ulcerative lesion in the trachea or bronchus also is an infrequent cause. As a rule, the symptom is obviously not an indication of early disease. Bleeding may start at any time during the day or night, but has been observed more frequently in the early hours of the morning. Exceptionally it is induced by a violent straining effort or by trauma. Staining or "streaking" of the sputum may occur without other sequels, but in other cases is a precursor of more copious hemoptyses. Frank hemoptyses, however, appear most often without forewarning. In women there may be a definite relationship with menstruation, and a few have recurrent hemoptyses monthly. During the bleeding the patient may notice boiling or bubbling sounds in his chest localized to one side or to the center. The blood may be raised easily or may flow so freely as to cause severe choking, coughing and gagging.

Immediately fatal hemoptyses occur only in a small minority of the cases, usually of longstanding fibroid cavernous tuberculosis in which vascular granulation and connective tissue have proliferated in the cavity walls; a vessel may undergo gradual aneurysmal dilatation (Rasmussen) until it finally gives way. As a rule, however, a single hemoptysis amounts to 30 or 60 cc.; occasionally, to as much as 300 cc. The bleeding is then usually arrested by the deposition of a clot at the site of the vascular rupture. Dark clots may be expectorated for several days, sometimes in the form of bronchial casts. This may be the end of it, but there may be a few or many recurrences at intervals of hours, days or longer periods. Then the loss of blood may cause anemia. The patient may become nervous and frightened, or may go into mild shock with fearfulness, pallor, coldness of the extremities, tachycardia and weakness, and sometimes sweating. Vomiting may occur soon after, especially if the patient has swallowed much blood. Within a day or two there may be a rise in temperature of several degrees, usually traceable to the aspiration of blood into the lower lobes of the lungs. The resulting tuberculous pneumonia has been described in previous paragraphs.

Pain in the chest is usually a symptom of inflamed pleura. It may be an early complaint, therefore, if the initial pulmonary infiltration is situated close beneath the pleura, facilitating such secondary extension. In cases associated with chronic adhesive pleurisy, a dullness, heaviness, soreness and aching of the side is a common complaint, and is particularly noticeable during fatigue and during cold damp weather. Such sensations may be noticeable for many years after all activity of the lesions has subsided. A sudden stabbing pain in one side or behind the sternum, followed immediately by shortness of breath and other manifestations, is usually indicative of collapse of the lung and acute pneumothorax. Persistent or recurrent localized pain may be referable to tuberculous lesions of the spine, costal cartilage or sternum, less often of the ribs or sternoclavicular joints; these may be associated with superficial swelling and redness.

Wheezing and stridulous breathing are occasionally complaints in cases of cavernous tuberculosis, less often in others. The wheezing may be noticeable behind the sternum, but more often is localized to one side of the chest, and is due usually to distortions or stenosis of the bronchus or trachea caused by tuberculous ulceration, granulomas or cicatrices. Rarely the trachea becomes so filled with granulations that suffocative attacks may occur. In old standing fibroid cases, wheezing may be referable to catarrhal accumulations in distorted bronchial tubes.

Hoarseness may be the result of temporary congestion of the larynx from incessant coughing. Persistent hoarseness, dryness and tickling of the throat are caused often by laryngeal tuberculosis.

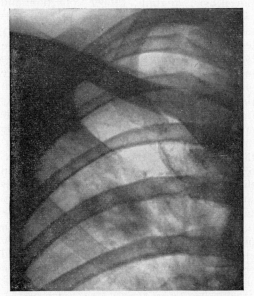

Fig. 37. Recently developed tuberculous lesion in right lung; moth-eaten appearance suggests softening and excavation.

Physical and Roentgenographic Examination in Pulmonary Tuberculosis. The physical examination of a patient for pulmonary tuberculosis should be thorough and complete. Fluoroscopy is useful and sufficient to visualize changes in respiratory mechanics and gross densities in the lungs which may be due to tuberculous lesions. However, the greater accuracy of the roentgenogram must be appreciated, particularly in detecting early lesions.

Physical Examination of the Patient with Limited or Early Pulmonary Tuberculosis. In the case of a relatively early lesion physical examination reveals no superficial abnormalities or perhaps only slight evidence of anemia and loss of weight. The temperature may be found normal or elevated a fraction of a degree to several degrees, and the pulse may be moderately accelerated. Careful examination of the chest may not reveal abnormal signs; or one may detect definite changes such as slight dullness, bronchovesicular breathing

and a few persistent crepitant or moderately coarse rales. Rales alone may be found in an area scarcely more than 1 or 2 cm. in diameter. The roentgenogram as a rule reveals evidence of the lesion more precisely as a soft cloudy mottling often associated with small honeycombed areas of rarefaction or larger round zones of similar translucency which represent cavities. (See Fig. 37.) It must be repeated that the early recognizable lesion frequently does not produce abnormal physical signs, but the roentgenogram almost always shows the characteristic shadows. Infrequently, in the case of a small tuberculous lesion, the roentgenographic findings are negative or indeterminate, while definite rales may be heard in a given spot. Oblique roentgenographic views or other special views then may reveal the mottling or rarefaction which, in the customary postero-anterior view, was concealed by the interposed density of the heart or some other structure. These evidences of the lesions are usually disclosed in the upper third of one lung, not infrequently beneath the level of the clavicle, but sometimes exclusively above it. Signs of similar or different intensity and variety may be detected sometimes in both lungs. These may be located on one side in the upper third, and at the apex of the opposite lung; or there may be other variations such as apical signs on one side, and basal signs in either one of the lower lobes. In a few cases the signs are limited to the middle or lower part of the interscapular region on one side; occasionally, even below this level. In some the original apical lesion is so slight as to give no definite signs either by physical or roentgenographic examination, while the obviously secondary lesions are easily detected.

Longstanding and fibroid lesions may betray their presence through the changes due to retraction and shrinkage of the fibrous tissue. Thus, a rather limited depression of the clavicular fossae on one side, slight or moderate atrophy of the muscles in this region, limitation of motion of the ribs, and deflection of the trachea give the main clue to the long duration of the lesion. Isolated nodular, fibrotic or calcified lesions, such as those of the primary complex, usually are not detected by physical examination, but cast characteristic dense, sharply circumscribed shadows in the roentgenogram.

Physical and Roentgenographic Signs of Advanced Lesions in Pulmonary Tuberculosis. There is no limit to the variety of signs which may be produced by extensive tuberculosis. If the disease remains confined chiefly to one lung, this may be converted into a fibrous shrunken mass with a variety of secondary effects such as flattening and immobilization of the hemithorax, atrophy of the muscles and skin on this side, inequality of the pupils from involvement of the sympathetic ganglia, flushing of one cheek from a similar cause, dilated superficial venules of the skin of the chest, marked deflection of the trachea and retraction of the heart. The roentgenogram may show a shrunken and opaque lung and the retractions associated with it, while physical examination may reveal dullness to flatness, bronchial and amphoric breathing, post-tussic suction, widely distributed rales and many other classical signs. In the case of advanced bilateral fibroid nodular tuberculosis, secondary emphysema may be conspicuous, and the physical signs of this, together with few rales, may leave one in doubt until the roentgenogram shows the typical distribution of nodular and streaky shadows throughout both lung fields.

Extensive bronchopneumonic or pneumonic lesions which have not existed long enough to produce such secondary changes give rise most constantly to widely distributed rales which vary from the crepitant quality in the early stages of infiltration to moderately coarse bubbling and consonanting rales after the lesions have caseated and undergone liquefaction and ulceration. With these are discovered varying signs of solidification and excavation, depending on the concentration of the lesions in a given lobe, and their state of degeneration. Physical signs then may be more informative than the roentgenogram, since, in the latter, the opacity may be so complete that detailed structure can no longer be made out. Smaller bronchopneumonic lesions, however, are usually depicted more faithfully by roentgenographic than by physical signs. In all these situations the findings may be associated with or modified by changes in the pleura or other adjacent structures. A large pleural effusion may obscure pulmonary lesions, while more chronic pleural changes may be well revealed by peripheral densities and retractions which stand out in contrast with the air-bearing lung.

Tomograms (planigrams, laminograms, selectoplanes) are helpful to supplement conventional roentgenograms, especially in defining more precisely the composition and location of individual lesions.

Complete examination of the body may also bring to light changes outside the thorax. Thus the discovery of an inflammatory thickening of one vocal cord, of a phlyctenule in the conjunctiva, of a nodule in the epididymis, or of a fistula-in-ano may be most important factors in constructing the complete picture of the disease.

Laboratory Findings in Pulmonary Tuberculosis. *Sputum.* Proper collection and examination of the sputum are most important. There may be none if the pulmonary lesion has not ulcerated. Even after ulceration has occurred the quantity of discharge may be so small that the patient is not aware of it and unconsciously may swallow it. In this case he is carefully instructed to collect in a suitable container any slight discharge appearing in the throat, particularly in the mornings. If he is unable to produce a satisfactory specimen, the *fasting stomach contents* are aspirated with a stomach tube when the patient first awakes in the morning. This specimen is treated by centrifugation, neutralization and inoculation on suitable cultural medium. *Laryngeal smears* have been used to recover small mucopurulent discharges for examination; this is quick and convenient, but not to be relied upon if no acid-fast organisms are demonstrated. *Bronchial lavage* (introducing 20 cc. of warm saline solution into the trachea and then collecting the expectorated material for examination) has been advocated, but is not to be recommended because of the hazard of bronchial dissemination of the infection. Occasionally bronchoscopic specimens contain demonstrable bacilli when expectorated material does not. Organisms may also be found in the feces.

Ordinarily the patient with a pulmonary cavity will be able to collect mucopurulent material upon awaking in the morning, and this is the specimen needed. Occasionally, bloody specimens or the blood from a hemoptysis will be suitable for examination. A great many elements may be searched for, such as elastic fibers, various types of cells, secondary organisms and albumin, but these have only subsidiary value unless some special point is to be determined. The most important items are an estimate of the character and daily volume of the sputum and an effort to detect tubercle bacilli in it. (See Demonstrating the Tubercle Bacillus, p. 279.) Appearance, consistency, possible layering and odor are noted.

Blood. Cell counts, estimation of the hemoglobin and the erythrocyte sedimentation rate are used routinely in clinical practice. Interpreted in combination with other data, they are valuable in diagnosis and in following the course of the disease. (See Changes in the Blood of Tuberculous Patients, p. 281).

Urine. In febrile tuberculosis the urine commonly shows slight traces of albumin. Protein loss through the kidney may become marked after amyloid changes have occurred. From the results of animal experimentation it has been suggested that tubercle bacilli, free in the blood stream, may be excreted through the intact and normal kidney and then may be discovered in the urine (excretory bacilluria). In human beings, however, experience indicates that this must be a rare happening, and the discovery of bacilluria is taken as presumptive evidence of a tuberculous lesion in the urinary tract or the genital organs. The discovery of pus cells and an abnormal number of erythrocytes or persistent albuminuria in a patient with pulmonary tuberculosis should always lead to a further investigation for the presence of a renal lesion.

Pleural Fluid. In some cases of pulmonary tuberculosis complicated by a pleural effusion the discovery of tubercle bacilli in the aspirated fluid may verify the diagnosis when this evidence is lacking on account of negative tests of the sputum.

Basal Metabolic Rate. In afebrile cases of pulmonary tuberculosis this is normal unless there is some independent cause for variation. In febrile cases the rate is elevated according to the degree of fever.

Respiratory Function. In the presence of limited lesions the respiratory function is not materially disturbed. In later stages functional impairment may become severe because of the invasion and destruction of pulmonary parenchyma, the shrinkage of fibrous tissue in the lung and the pleura, and the associated retraction of the heart and distortion of bronchi and blood vessels. Secondary emphysema may also be a serious functional handicap. The degree and significance of the impairment may be determined with considerable accuracy by the separate measurement of ventilation, the mixing of gases in the lungs, the adequacy of exchange of gases between the alveoli and the pulmonary capillaries and the efficiency of the pulmonary circulation. By using the bronchospirometer some of these measurements can be made separately for each lung. The tests are needed in certain cases to help determine the patient's probable tolerance of surgical procedures such as pulmonary resection.

Diagnosis of Pulmonary Tuberculosis. Tuberculosis should be considered as a possible cause (*a*) in any patient who presents vague symptoms of loss of weight, malaise and easy fatigue, particularly when this is associated with persistent cough; (*b*) in any patient, particularly a young person, who has recurrent or prolonged attacks simulating grippe or influenza; (*c*) in any patient who has atypical or unresolved pneumonia; (*d*) in any patient who has cough and expectoration persisting for more than several weeks, even though there may be little or no impairment of the general condition; (*e*) in any patient who spits blood; (*f*) in any patient who has pleurisy, especially with effusion; (*g*) in any patient with a persistent unexplained fever; (*h*) in any patient with other mild or obscure lesions such as persistent lymphadenopathy, fistula-in-ano and chronic laryngitis giving rise to chronic hoarseness. The diagnosis then depends particularly upon physical, roentgenographic and laboratory examinations. In such circumstances the finding of a lesion, usually in the upper half of the lung, which gives the characteristic roentgenographic appearance of an infiltration or fibrosis with or without cavity, and with or without demonstrable physical signs such as rales, warrants the presumptive diagnosis of tuberculosis. If there is no demonstrable cavity and no sputum, the diagnosis is confirmed by a period of observation during which the lesion persists or gradually changes; cultures of gastric fluid may grow tubercle bacilli. If excavation is demonstrated or suggested by the other examinations, the diagnosis should be verified by the finding of tubercle bacilli in the sputum. The failure to find bacilli in a case in which there is moderate or fairly copious mucopurulent sputum weighs heavily against the diagnosis of tuberculosis. The finding of tubercle bacilli in the discharges or material obtained from other lesions, such as pleural effusion or pus from a tuberculous fistula, strongly suggest that the pulmonary lesions are also tuberculous. The finding of rales in the upper third of the chest in a case in which the roentgenogram shows no parenchymal change and in which the sputum test is negative for tubercle bacilli leaves the diagnosis in doubt and raises the question whether the lesion is nontuberculous. The finding of physical and roentgenographic signs exclusively in the lower half of the chest does not exclude tuberculosis as a cause, but if, in addition, there is mucopurulent sputum devoid of tubercle bacilli, tuberculosis, as a rule, can be excluded. In doubtful or difficult cases the tuberculin test may be valuable, especially if negative.

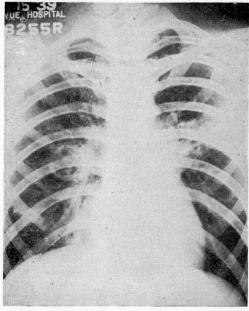

Fig. 38. Tuberculous cavity in the right lower lobe at the level of the eighth rib posteriorly. Exudative infiltrate in the middle of the left lung represents a bronchogenic extension from the cavity.

Modern methods of *tuberculosis case finding* among apparently healthy people afford another approach. These surveys are usually conducted by routine roentgenographic examination of the chest, with or without a preliminary tuberculin test. In about 2 per cent of apparently healthy people densities are discovered in the roentgenograms which may represent tuberculous disease. The lesions are usually in the upper half of the chest, often confined to one lung, and may be of a caseous or fibrous character. Discovery of such a shadow in the roentgenogram necessitates a complete history of the case, complete physical examination and study of the sputum. These tests, together with the necessary period of observation, usually confirm the tuberculous nature of the lesions.

Differential Diagnosis of Pulmonary Tuberculosis. The approach to differential diagnosis varies according to the presenting findings. Thorough and careful study of the

case usually enables one to arrive at a definite conclusion.

In a patient in whom unexplained fever develops and who is discovered to have a pneumonic lesion without demonstrable excavation, distinction often has to be made between early tuberculosis and *simple bronchopneumonia,* especially if the lesion is confined to an upper lobe. Demonstrably rapid changes in the lesions within a few days or a week and failure to find tubercle bacilli usually identify bronchopneumonia as such, while the failure of the lesion to clear in the expected time favors tuberculosis. Similar distinctions are of value in the differentiation of *eosinophilic infiltrates* of the lung, sometimes representing bronchopneumonia in a patient who gives a history of asthma or other allergy; the eosinophils of the blood may rise to 25 per cent or more of the leukocytes.

In *primary atypical (presumably viral) pneumonia* the pulmonary lesions sometimes may fail to resolve completely before several months have elapsed, as indicated by persistent shadows on the roentgenogram and rales. The acute onset and course, the absence of pulmonary cavity, the failure to demonstrate tubercle bacilli and the gradual and complete resolution of the lesions, even if delayed, exclude tuberculosis. Occasionally, acute caseous pneumonia occupying a large part of the lobe or lung may be confused with *pneumococcal lobar pneumonia,* and the confusion may be increased by the finding of pneumococci of a higher type in the sputum. While in a rare case of tuberculous pneumonia the leukocytes of the blood may rise to 20,000 per cubic millimeter, the count seldom attains the height commonly seen in lobar pneumonia, nor is there often such a pronounced relative increase of the polymorphonuclear neutrophils. Since caseous pneumonia usually represents an acute confluent bronchopneumonic extension from a tuberculous cavity, tubercle bacilli will be found on careful search of the sputum, which, as a rule, is not rusty, although it may be bloody. In caseous pneumonia the signs of cavity may be detected on physical and roentgenographic examinations. If not immediately, the diagnosis usually can be made in the space of a relatively few days. Acute bronchopneumonia due to organisms such as *streptococci* or *anaerobic bacteria,* which commonly goes on to abscess formation, may be confusing because of the pattern of the pulmonary lesions simulating tuberculosis. The acute onset, often with chills, the leukocytosis, the finding of an abscess or cavity, and the failure to demonstrate tubercle bacilli in the sputum are presumptive evidence against the tuberculous nature of the disease, while a great predominance of other specific organisms may give the real clue. One must be certain, however, that common pyogenic organisms are not merely contaminants from the mouth.

Foulness of the sputum shortly after the acute onset of the disease always speaks for *putrid lung abscess.* In longstanding cases of chronic lung abscess a cavity or fibrotic lesion may be discovered in the upper part of one lung, and this may give rise to suggestive symptoms such as hemoptysis. The history of onset, particularly the history of fetid expectoration, and the failure to demonstrate tubercle bacilli usually indicate the diagnosis.

When tuberculosis is suspected as the cause of a *protracted and obscure fever,* the failure to find a pulmonary lesion is presumptive evidence against this diagnosis, but it may be necessary still to exclude the presence of tuberculosis of other organs. The same is true in any chronic debilitated state in which tuberculosis may be suspected.

Bronchiectasis not infrequently must be differentiated in patients who give a history of chronic cough, possibly with foul and bloody sputum. The lesion is usually in the lower lobes, but occasionally is apical. Rales may be heard, but the roentgenogram fails to show the typical tuberculous infiltration and excavation, and, instead, there may only be strandlike densities suggesting interstitial or peribronchial fibrosis. This and the absence of tubercle bacilli from the sputum suggest bronchiectasis, which may be verified by the use of bronchography with iodized oil.

Cancer of the lung simulates tuberculosis because of the chronic cough, expectoration of pus and blood, febrile episodes, and gradual wasting. Physical and roentgenographic findings are more likely to be those of a bronchial lesion causing localized wheezing rhonchi or of suppurative pneumonia secondary to the bronchial occlusion. The failure to find tubercle bacilli in the purulent sputum is most important. Bronchoscopy, the biopsy of a superficial metastatic lesion in a lymph node, or the finding of other internal metastases may be diagnostic.

Special cytologic studies may reveal cancer cells in the sputum, and this may be a crucial finding in the case of peripheral, roentgenographically spherical lesions too distant to be reached by the bronchoscope. Such a density on the roentgenogram is also consistent with some benign tumors and with certain caseous or fibrocaseous lesions ("tuberculoma"). In doubtful cases of potentially serious import surgical exploration by thoracotomy may be indicated.

Pulmonary fibrosis and *emphysema* may have to be differentiated because of symptoms and because tuberculosis, particularly the chronic disseminated form, sometimes is a cause. Chronic cough, occasional blood spitting and increasing weakness may be particularly suggestive. In tuberculosis the fibrous changes are usually associated with calcifications identified by roentgenography. Extrapulmonary lesions may also be found, especially in the lymphatic system or in the abdomen. The history of some other possible cause such as chronic paranasal sinusitis or exposure to injurious dust may give the proper clue. In *silicosis* the nodular noncalcareous roentgenographic appearance of the lesions evenly distributed in both lungs, particularly in the central portions, is characteristic. Association of tuberculosis with silicosis, a not infrequent finding, may be suspected when there are confluent roentgenographic shadows in addition to nodular ones.

There is a sizable category of nodular and stringy lesions, revealed best in the roentgenogram, which may simulate tuberculosis of a disseminated distribution, particularly that due to hemic dissemination. In addition to silicosis this group includes sarcoidosis, metastatic carcinosis, and unusual or rare lesions such as the pulmonary granulomatosis of beryllium workers, and those associated with scleroderma, tuberous sclerosis and primary amyloidosis. Chronic pneumonia due to the inhalation of mineral or other oils may give a confusing picture, but is more likely to be unilateral, confluent and limited than widespread.

Mycoses may produce changes simulating tuberculosis, but these are unusual. The lesions may be of a subacute bronchopneumonic or chronic granulomatous and fibrous nature, and the pattern in the roentgenogram may simulate tuberculosis closely, even to cavity formation. In a patient suffering with a chronic cough, expectoration and general ill health, failure to demonstrate tubercle bacilli and the finding of specific fungi in the sputum by microscopic or cultural examinations may settle the diagnosis; other tests used include the serum antibody titer, skin sensitivity tests and virulence of the organisms for animals. It is important to know whether there has been an opportunity for infection with fungi and whether there have been systemic lesions.

In the desert section of southwestern United States infection with *Coccidioides immitis* is fairly common, and in a few of those infected acute pneumonic lesions develop, some with excavation. In less than 1 per cent of those infected the disease becomes generalized and fatal. The coccidioidin skin test, serologic and bacteriologic findings and the usually short clinical course are diagnostic features. *Histoplasmosis* also has been identified as a cause of chronic pulmonary lesions which may be followed by calcification, particularly in the eastern central part of the United States. Other mycoses, found more often in rural than in urban populations, which may involve the lungs and simulate tuberculosis include actinomycosis, blastomycosis and moniliasis. It is always important, when fungi are found in the sputum, to determine whether these are implicated in the pulmonary disease or are merely nonpathogenic inhabitants of the mouth. In the great majority of cases the diagnosis, uncertain at first, resolves itself into that of tuberculosis.

Pulmonary lesions secondary to cardiac disease sometimes create a confusing picture. The hemoptysis of mitral stenosis may be misleading at first because of the finding of rales and roentgenographic changes suggesting fibrosis and infiltration of the parenchyma. Demonstration of the cardiac lesion, the failure to demonstrate a cavity, the lack of sputum containing tubercle bacilli, and the distribution, character and behavior of the lesions lead correctly to the conclusion that the lesions are due to secondary fibrosis from congestion and stasis, to infarction or to edema. A pleural effusion clouding the picture may be found related to the same cause. Rarely a pulmonary *infarct* may become secondarily infected and break down to form an abscess, simulating a tuberculous cavity.

Suppurative lesions in other structures which may become connected with the lungs must be distinguished. Thus chronic pleural empyema which has ruptured into the lung may cause many symptoms common to pulmonary tuberculosis, and the same may be said of chronic hepatic or subphrenic abscess

which has perforated through the diaphragm into the lung. A searching history of previous illnesses and operations and failure to demonstrate tubercle bacilli in the sputum usually eliminate tuberculosis.

Unusual conditions such as Hodgkin's lymphoblastoma invading the lung from the mediastinum, esophagotracheal fistula, dermoid or parasitic cysts which have ruptured into the lung, and aortic aneurysm producing bronchial stenosis by pressure may necessitate ruling out tuberculosis because of the symptoms of chronic pulmonary disease. The clinical history, the failure to find tubercle bacilli and the demonstration of other lesions, especially in the mediastinum, exclude tuberculosis, as a rule, and suggest the proper diagnosis.

Prognosis of Pulmonary Tuberculosis. A favorable outcome is best assured by the detection of the disease in its early phases, the administration of proper treatment and the continuation of this procedure until healing processes are well established and a solid balance of vital resistance can be assumed to exist. There is a definite correlation between the *extent of the lesions* and the ultimate prognosis. Early "minimal" lesions without cavity formation almost always do well under suitable treatment. In such cases the life expectancy, as indicated by studies such as those conducted by Trudeau Sanatorium, is equal almost to that of groups of similar age in the general population. The more extensive the pulmonary lesions, the greater is the future hazard. Before the advent of chemotherapy patients with far advanced cavitary disease had an average life expectancy of two to five years and about a third of those in the moderately advanced stage were dead within five years. Chemotherapy has vastly improved the lot of such patients in prolonging life and raising the chances of satisfactory arrest of the disease. However, such benefits are far outweighed by the advantages of an early diagnosis.

The *character of the lesion* is of great and sometimes paramount importance. Lesions of a fibroid nodular character tend to run an indolent course and are more readily controlled by treatment; the tendency to excavation is less, while further healing by fibrosis is the rule. Exudative bronchopneumonic lesions may be resolved rather rapidly, but there is almost always an unresolved caseous center which sooner or later may liquefy and slough into the bronchial tree with secondary extensions into the healthy parenchyma. The instability of these lesions is striking, particularly during the first year or two after their discovery.

The *size and character of cavities* also have a prognostic bearing, particularly since these are sources of infectious discharge which frequently are responsible for secondary lesions in the lungs, larynx and intestine; there is also a liability to hemorrhage. Small cavities (up to about 2 cm. in diameter) often shrink, especially under the influence of chemotherapy. Larger cavities often become dried out under chemotherapy and tubercle bacilli may no longer be demonstrable in the sputum, but the lesions are likely, nevertheless, to be the seat of later exacerbations, leading to chronic disability, unless they can be dealt with surgically. The greater the amount of surrounding caseous pneumonic disease, the more precarious is the prognosis.

Clinical symptoms measure in an approximate degree the patient's reaction to the infection. Thus a young girl who reacts with prolonged fever usually does badly, while an older person with more tuberculosis but no fever may have a better prognosis. Another guide is the amount and character of the *sputum;* a patient who has only a small quantity, mucopurulent and coherent, may live for years without extension of the disease. On the other hand, a large amount of more liquid sputum favors early extension. In either case the number of tubercle bacilli in a given quantity of sputum may be approximately the same. Generally, however, the prognosis is better if tubercle bacilli are scarce, since this may be interpreted as evidence that the cavity walls are relatively clean and not undergoing active necrosis. *Complications* may alter or actually determine the prognosis.

The *age* of the patient is of great prognostic significance. Tuberculosis acquired during infancy or early childhood is of serious portent, as indicated by the careful studies of Wallgren, Miriam Brailey and Edith M. Lincoln. Adolescence is a serious time with relation to pulmonary disease. Young tuberculous girls have notoriously unstable lesions, and the mortality is relatively high; there is a similar trend, somewhat less striking, among young boys. Women past thirty have a relatively good prognosis, while men in the older age groups have a higher mortality. Most familiar prognostic criteria relate to the early behavior of the disease. The ultimate outcome is measured not only in terms of survival but

also in the frequency of chronic relapsing disease or freedom from it. This is determined, not only by the time and quality of treatment, but also by the later cooperation of the patient, the conditions under which he must live and constitutional factors over which he may have no control.

Treatment of Pulmonary Tuberculosis. The need of treatment is usually self-evident when the patient has overt symptoms of active disease. But, in addition, there is a large category of patients in whom the indications are not so clear-cut. Most of these are brought to notice by routine roentgenographic examination of the chest. Since the patient with a small active lesion often presents the vaguest of symptoms or none at all, the importance of determining the significance of the lesion cannot be overemphasized. The prompt and proper treatment of these cases yields results far superior to those achieved after more extensive invasion and destruction of tissue have occurred. The problem, therefore, is to distinguish these cases from those in which apparently healed and inactive lesions are found. It is simplified if certain data from previous examinations are available. An authentic negative tuberculin test within the previous several years is reliable evidence that the newly developed pulmonary lesion is of recent origin, presumably the result of a primary infection and, therefore, in need of treatment. Likewise, a roentgenogram taken several years previously and interpreted as normal has the same significance, except that no inference can be drawn as to the time of infection. Lacking such help, the physician must rely on his current findings. An adolescent or young adult patient, presenting a lesion without definite evidence of fibrosis and calcification, usually should have the benefit of treatment for, at this age, such lesions are almost always of recent origin and active; furthermore, this age carries with it a predisposition to rapidly progressive disease. For the same reason, young people with apparently fibrotic and calcified pulmonary lesions should be studied closely since these older foci usually harbor infection which sometimes becomes active at this time of life or later and may requires treatment for its control.

Older patients who appear healthy and whose lesions are judged to be densely fibrotic and calcified do not require treatment, but only a roentgenographic examination once every six to twelve months to detect possible instability. Others of less certain status, especially if the lesions are suspected to be poorly fibrosed, partly necrotic and possibly honey-combed with minute cavities, should be studied more thoroughly with all available diagnostic procedures, including cultures of the sputum and gastric fluid, to determine whether active treatment is needed. Some of these patients benefit by a period of hospitalization for this intensive study. This may clarify the situation and justify allowing some to continue an active life under the watchful eye of a physician. Others who have vague symptoms of undue fatigue and loss of weight may be assumed sometimes to suffer mild toxemia from partly healed but unstable pulmonary disease, and they may benefit from a period of simple rest treatment; such a precaution may prevent more serious exacerbations. Some, too, may have such symptoms from disease in other organs while the pulmonary lesions remain inactive; treatment may be indicated on this account.

There is also a group of patients who seem to have developed fairly good resistance and who have unawaredly coped with the disease with some success before a diagnosis is made. Many of these will be found to have partially fibroid lesions, containing small cavities, and mild symptoms, including scanty expectoration containing tubercle bacilli. Trouble is brewing for these patients and their management demands careful judgment. An elderly person may maintain the balance in his favor by limiting his activities under medical treatment, but a younger one should have the benefit of more active and radical treatment in view of the prospect of permanent recovery.

Patients with advanced bilateral cavitary disease can be helped at least temporarily with prolonged chemotherapy. Although they have chronic permanently disabling disease to which most of them eventually succumb, their lives often may be prolonged and made more comfortable.

Principles and Objectives of Treatment. Recognizing that tuberculosis of sufficient extent and activity to require treatment has already caused some necrosis and possible excavation of tissue, it is appreciated from the start that treatment is a long-term proposition. Fairly rapid resolution of exudative lesions may be promoted but the fibrous repair of necrotic residuals requires many months. Since there is no proof that infection can be completely eliminated by the use of drugs or other measures, the possibility of later re-crudescence of the disease must always be considered and treatment should be planned with the aim of averting this. Much time is required not only for fibrous healing of lesions but also to raise the patient's resistance to the infection to the highest possible level. When the diagnosis is made it may be possible to judge approximately the kinds of treatment which are likely to be most effective and to anticipate the probable outcome. However, the response varies from one patient to another, and valuable information is gained by observing the effects of a chosen regimen during the early weeks and months. In time it is learned, for instance, whether acute tuberculous pneumonia is to undergo extensive resolution or whether widespread necrosis prevents this and points to the eventual need of surgical resection. Similarly, during the early course small exudative lesions in one lung may resolve almost completely, leaving a major problem of advanced fibrocavitary disease in the opposite lung which may have to be treated by surgical collapse or resection. At the start the probable duration of treatment, though very important to the patient, is secondary to a consideration of the result which eventually it is hoped to achieve.

The first objective is to suppress bacterial activity and halt the progress of active and advancing disease. Bed rest alone accomplishes this in many cases. Improvement of symptoms may start immediately and there may be, for instance, a decided diminution of the amount of expectoration and, consequently, a decreasing risk of further spread of the disease through the lungs and elsewhere. While the mechanisms of the good effects of rest treatment are still somewhat obscure, many patients, even with advanced disease, recover with this alone. The diminution of the motion of the diseased lung, the alteration of circulatory mechanics by the recumbent posture and the general improvement of physiologic tone all may play a part.

The response to chemotherapy depends on its relatively prompt bacteriostatic action, the manifestations of which are essentially the same as those brought about by natural defenses of the body under rest treatment, though the rate is decidedly more rapid and predictable. The combination of rest and chemotherapy for active progressive disease usually exerts earlier and better control than either measure alone.

In the lungs, the first favorable local response to treatment is a diminution of exudation into and discharge from cavities, and a resolution of inflammatory products which have not undergone necrosis. Temporarily, sloughing may continue and cavities may enlarge, but at a slackening pace. Then slow fibrous repair is initiated and continues during many months and perhaps years, provided the infection remains controlled. When the lesion is small and the early response is good, well regulated living and discrete limitation of the patient's activities usually are sufficient to maintain the balance in his favor.

The ultimate objective after an initial good response to treatment is to ensure permanent recovery by establishing a heavy balance of resistance against the infection, and, if irreparable damage has been done, to recognize the inherent danger of such remaining foci and to deal with these in some suitable, if radical, manner. Under treatment virtually all symptoms may disappear and the patient may become outwardly healthy, but residual cavities and large solid necrotic pulmonary lesions are recognized as situations in which future exacerbations of the infection are almost inevitable. The timeliness of some measure to collapse the diseased lung or to remove these threatening foci must therefore be considered.

Very advanced disease may be brought to a halt by treatment but the result often is a quiescent or chronic state, a drawn battle between the host and the bacillus. Then the reasonable objective of treatment is to maintain the defenses of the patient as long as possible, realizing that the invader, perhaps after many years, will probably gain the upper hand.

Guides and Checks in Treatment. In order to apply the principles of treatment most effectively, the observation of the patient should be systematic. As a rule, relatively simple clinical data, supplemented by periodic examination of the sputum, roentgenography of the chest and study of the blood suffice. The temperature, preferably rectal, is recorded during the day at least every four hours. The pulse rate is recorded each time the temperature is taken; it is well to remember that the pulse may continue unstable after the temperature remains normal and therefore may be considered a more sensitive indicator of toxemia or other disturbances. The body weight is recorded every two weeks unless the patient is too sick. Note is made of the patient's appearance, his general feeling

and of his vegetative functions. Minor symptoms should not be ignored.

The sputum is collected during each 24 hours in a disposable container so that the amount and character may be estimated. If tubercle bacilli are found at the outset, later examinations at intervals of a month may show some change such as a diminution in the bacillary output, which, with a diminution in the quantity of expectoration, may be significant. If bacilli are not found at the start, frequently repeated examinations are indicated to verify the diagnosis and to detect early the evidence of an ulcerative process in the lung. When chemotherapy is employed it is desirable, in cultures, to test the susceptibility of the bacilli to each specific drug at intervals after the start of treatment. At the start, the erythrocyte sedimentation rate and a complete total and differential leukocyte count should be recorded. The milder the symptoms and the closer the approach to quiescence and arrest of the disease, the more likely are these estimations to be valuable. Then a series of observations at intervals of several weeks or months may help to determine the trend of the disease and, particularly, the degree of stability attained under treatment.

Though repeated physical examination is indispensable, its value is variable and it is not to be relied upon to detect early and slight changes in pulmonary lesions. For this purpose the roentgenogram is much more dependable. How often this examination should be made depends on the behavior of the case and one's judgment of the potentialities. In patients with exudative and unstable lesions, roentgenograms at intervals of a week may show definite extensions or regressions which are most important to recognize; in old fibroid cases, few or no changes may be shown during long periods.

Application and Duration of Treatment. Since any one of several regimens may promise satisfactory results, good judgment is important in adjusting the treatment of the individual patient. This is based on a preliminary study of the case and should take into consideration not only the overt manifestations of the disease but also its future potentialities. Since the level of vital resistance of the patient and the extent, distribution and composition of the lesions vary so widely from case to case, time must be allowed to observe the response to any chosen regimen. In some instances there will be a striking and

300   THE INFECTIOUS DISEASES

immediate change for the better, while in others the improvement may be slow and gradual, though still satisfactory.

Bed rest is one of the most successful means of improving the general condition of the patient and his resistance to the infection. It is indicated, at least at the start, for virtually all patients who require treatment of any kind, its strictness and duration being decided according to the urgency and individ-

complete healing which may indicate radical surgery. To illustrate current practices, several typical situations may be used as examples.

In acute and subacute tuberculous pneumonia, bacterial activity usually may be assumed to be rampant and the resistance of the patient often is low. There is urgent need, therefore, for vigorous chemotherapy. Following the principle that no drug should be

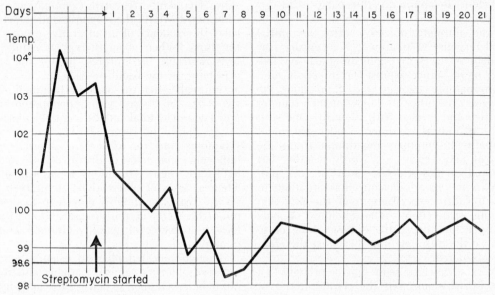

Fig. 39. Prompt defervescence in a case of tuberculous pneumonia treated with streptomycin.

ual needs. Twenty-four-hour bed rest is desirable for the active febrile case, continuing for at least several months, and frequently, in the more severe cases, for six months or longer. Some patients may be permitted to sit up in bed for meals and other periods and to have a bathroom privilege, while others require more rest even than this, including close nursing care. The behavior of symptoms is a guide but these usually subside before the lesions are safely controlled; consequently, the prolongation of rest of varying degrees is indicated until the pulmonary lesions are considered to be well arrested and started toward healing.

Specific *chemotherapy* is indicated in all symptomatically active cases, and in many without symptoms in which the disease is considered to be very unstable. The regimen is selected according to the severity of the disease, the anticipated time required for its control, and the possible need during future contingencies, such as in-

given alone, one of several combinations may be used with the expectation of good effects. Streptomycin, 1 gm. daily, and PAS, 12 to 15 gm. daily, is one of the standard regimens and is backed by the longest experience. Some prefer streptomycin, 1 gm. daily, and isoniazid, 200 to 500 mg. daily; another usually effective regimen is isoniazid, 200 to 500 mg. daily, and PAS, 12 to 15 gm. daily. The drugs chosen are continued in this way for a few weeks to several months, remembering that streptomycin may eventually cause neurotoxicity; consequently, when this drug is used along with another, its administration is usually reduced to 1 gm. three times weekly as soon as the acute symptoms have subsided and resolution of the inflammation has started. The combination is then continued for a period of many months, during which continued resolution may be anticipated, cavities may be reduced in size and fibrosis may be initiated. If the clinical course continues to be satisfactory and fibrosis promises to be sufficient to encapsulate caseous foci and to effect the closure of all cavities, the regimen frequently is continued for six months to a year and, in some cases, even longer. During the later months the dosage of streptomycin may be reduced to 1 gm. every third day, but smaller amounts of this drug are considered to be of little or no value. The duration and optimum time of termination of chemotherapy in these cases is difficult to determine and therefore is usually rather arbitrary. Some cases of symptomatically mild tuberculous pneumonia do very well with only three to six months of chemotherapy; others of more severe grade with extensive caseation require courses of a year or more and, even then, relapse may occur soon after terminating the use of the drugs. In either event symptoms may be well controlled. The prognosis therefore depends mainly on the number and extent of the cavities and necrotic residues which persist after the initial improvement. The more prominent these are, the greater is the length of disability and the likelihood that surgical resection may be indicated to minimize the prospect of later relapse.

Small pulmonary lesions which have originated within six months to a year are usually of a pneumonic character and have potentialities of great harm. Depending on the promptness of diagnosis and treatment, a great majority of these patients are known to do well under rest treatment alone, starting with a period of several months in bed. In most instances, twelve to eighteen months of rest with gradually increasing activity are required to ensure dependable and permanent recovery. However, since a variety of drugs is available, it seems best, especially for young patients, to employ chemotherapy from the start for the purpose of controlling the infection more promptly, avoiding extensive tissue destruction and possibly shortening the period of treatment. The chief reservation is to avoid the unnecessary treatment of lesions which are already in a good state of healing; a preliminary period of observation may be necessary for this determination. Employing one of the regimens described in the previous paragraph, the dose of streptomycin, if this is chosen, can usually be kept to 1 gm. two or three times a week. The course may be terminated in most cases after a period of three to six months. It is still a question whether a longer course might enable patients to return to work earlier with safety,

while still continuing chemotherapy. As most of these patients are free of symptoms from start to finish, the chief criterion is the judgment of the lesion and its potential threat. It seems wise, therefore, especially when dealing with adolescent and young adult patients, to continue a routine of extra rest and limited activity for at least a year after the inception of the disease. When light work is resumed it should usually be on a part-time basis at the start.

Chronic tuberculosis, consisting of more or less destructive (caseous and cavernous) lesions of mild or moderate activity, varies greatly in its prognosis and response to treatment. The same is true of chronic fibro-cavernous disease with recent subacute or acute pneumonic extensions. Each case is carefully analyzed and, as a rule, one of the regimens described in the first paragraph is started without delay. It must be anticipated that the old chronic changes may not be influenced greatly except perhaps for the drying out and possible reduction in the size of cavities, but there may be some resolution of exudative lesions, particularly those of recent origin. Depending on such considerations, continuous chemotherapy (maintaining the dose of streptomycin at 1 gm. two or three times weekly) is given for six to eighteen months or longer until the maximum response has been achieved. Then, if residual solid necrotic or cavitary lesions persist in a more or less stationary condition, some form of surgical treatment or collapse therapy is considered. In some of these cases artificial pneumoperitoneum, artificial pneumothorax or thoracoplasty may have distinct value relatively early in the course of treatment in addition to the other measures.

Chronic extensive bilateral cavitary tuberculosis does not have a good prognosis under any circumstances, although a trial of chemotherapy is justified. In most instances there is a temporary improvement, but drug-resistant tubercle bacilli may soon become predominant in the pulmonary cavities and explain the uncertainty and frequently short duration of the therapeutic effect. Some patients whose general condition is extremely poor do not show any perceptible response to any of the drugs and the disease continues to a fatal ending. In contrast, however, some respond surprisingly well and may become virtually free of symptoms in spite of the persistence of the pulmonary cavities. Combined therapy has been continued in a few of these patients with good effect for periods of two to five years. The patients may be greatly limited because of the extent of tissue destruction and the resulting functional impairment.

Associated lesions and complications outside the lungs may be a major consideration and may largely govern the course of treatment. The control of the pulmonary disease with chemotherapy often simplifies the treatment of other tuberculous foci which may respond simultaneously or may become so favorably altered as to permit radical surgical treatment. Control of pulmonary disease, for instance, may permit early operation for tuberculosis of the spine.

In patients who have latent or fibroid disease and who require treatment with cortisone or corticotropin for rheumatoid arthritis or some other condition, chemotherapy may add some protection against adverse effects upon the tuberculosis; nevertheless, such effects must be watched for, particularly if the tuberculous lesions are not old and fibrocalcific.

The better hospitals and sanatoriums offer special advantages to patients requiring treatment unless unusually suitable conditions permit their care at home. Institutional treatment is especially helpful during the early phases of the disease when close observation is important and the patient needs instruction and often a reorientation of his habits of living. The personality, intelligence, social, occupational and economic conditions should be taken into consideration. During a long rest cure a patient needs understanding attention, congenial and sympathetic companions and a pleasant environment in which to spend the time. Many sanatoriums provide suitable diversions and facilities for rehabilitation. An increasing number of patients are able with reasonable safety to leave institutions sooner than was formerly the rule, to return home for a continuation of their treatment.

Collapse Therapy. Mechanical therapy to bring about immobilization and collapse of the lung has proved beneficial in many cases. The procedures are used principally to collapse pulmonary cavities and promote their healing and obliteration by fibrosis. As a rule, these are the cavities which persist after preliminary treatment with chemotherapy has brought the infection under some control and improved the patient's condition.

Artifical Pneumothorax. Artificial pneumothorax is induced by injecting clean air in measured amounts from a special apparatus through a hollow needle into the pleural cavity. Provided the lung is not adherent, the introduction of air permits the lung to retract and collapse through its own elasticity. In the average case, however, the stiffness of the fibrotic cavity walls, the density of surrounding lesions or the presence of pleural adhesions interfere, so that, in ultimately successful cases, six months or more are usually required before the cavity is completely closed and tubercle bacilli disappear from the sputum. Barring complications, the treatment is then continued for two to four or five years, depending on the extent of the lesion, in order to ensure good healing. After this the lung is permitted to reexpand. In predominantly unilateral disease artificial pneumothorax is sufficiently effective in about one third of the cases attempted; in the remainder, adhesions are so extensive as to defeat the purpose. Sometimes these may be severed by Jacobaeus's *intrapleural pneumonolysis,* using a cautery guided under direct vision through the thoracoscope introduced between the ribs. Complications are encountered frequently in artificial pneumothorax. Air embolism may be avoided by careful technique. Serofibrinous pleurisy, usually tuberculous, occurs in 80 to 90 per cent of the cases. As a rule this is mild and the fluid may be absorbed spontaneously. If chronic, adhesions develop at the base of the lung, and the pneumothorax may be lost. Otherwise the visceral pleura becomes organized and fibrotic, and the lung may fail to reexpand. In a minority of cases the fluid becomes empyematous and the pleural disease chronic; amyloidosis then may be a result. Pleural perforation and secondary mixed infection empyema occur occasionally, more often in the active caseous forms of pulmonary tuberculosis. Because of these hazards and the wider use of other treatment, pneumothorax is not used as often as was formerly the case. It is contraindicated during acute phases of pulmonary tuberculosis except to control severe and repeated hemoptyses.

Paralysis of the hemidiaphragm may be accomplished by crushing the phrenic nerve in the neck; usually the nerve regenerates within six or eight months, and the diaphragm resumes its function. Diaphragmatic paralysis once was widely employed to give partial rest to the diseased lung but now is seldom used, except in conjunction with artificial pneumoperitoneum.

Pneumoperitoneum, induced by insufflating air into the peritoneal cavity, may be used with or without crushing and paralyzing the phrenic nerve on the more diseased side. Complications are few and only occasionally dangerous, and this measure may be helpful in advanced active bilateral cases in which pneumothorax offers little or no help. Pneumoperitoneum with phrenic paralysis may help control pulmonary lesions and pave the way for more effective surgical operations. This seems to be the chief value of the procedure.

When less drastic measures fail or offer little promise, *thoracoplasty* may be indicated. Sections of ribs are removed, usually from above downward, the number depending on the extent of the cavernous lesion. Two or more operations may be required. The ribs are removed subperiosteally, and eventually they regenerate partially in the collapsed position. This often results in approximation of the walls of the cavity and the release of tension, so that enveloping fibrosis may be effective for healing. The operation is indicated in well stabilized fibroid disease of one lung containing a cavity which has not healed or does not promise to heal under other treatment. If lesions are present in the opposite lung, they should be well arrested. As a preliminary to thoracoplasty a space may be created beneath the stripped ribs, and into this a plastic material may be inserted and left in order to obtain maximum collapse of the underlying diseased lung. There are several other operations designed for similar purposes; these procedures are generally designated as *plombage*.

Surgical resection of diseased lungs, lobes or segments of lobes is sometimes the treatment of choice if certain rigid conditions of selection can be satisfied. Inflammatory infiltrates which may resolve under chemotherapy and rest treatment are not resected. However, if these have gone on to produce extensive destruction of the parenchyma, with caseation and cavity formation, which is unlikely to be repaired adequately by fibrosis and portends chronic relapsing disease, excision is considered. Preferably, the resistance of the patient should be good, and the lesions should be somewhat stabilized, quiescent or chronic and anatomically well delimited. Perhaps this can be approximated by preliminary and preparatory treatment with rest and chemotherapy during many months. The presence of irreversible stenotic lesions of the draining bronchi may add to the indications

for surgery. If lobes or an entire lung are removed, thoracoplasty is usually performed to obliterate the dead space and prevent overdistention of the remaining lobes. It is not assumed that all the disease can be removed in this way. The patient is given the advantage of prolonged rest treatment so that he may obtain the maximum benefit from the drastic procedure.

Occasionally a tuberculous cavity is drained externally by thoracotomy and rib resection, but such a procedure is to be avoided if possible.

Treatment of Special Symptoms. *Cough and expectoration,* traceable usually to excavating lesions of the lungs and sometimes also to tuberculous laryngitis and bronchitis, are best controlled by rest treatment and chemotherapy. The patient is instructed to suppress coughing, if possible, and to expectorate by gentle clearing of the throat. However, it may be necessary to give sedatives such as codeine sulfate, 0.030 gm., at intervals of 3 or 4 hours or longer so that the patient may get sufficient rest; sometimes this may be supplemented with a hypnotic at night. For the distressing cough of patients who have considerable bronchitis, steam inhalations, perhaps with the addition of some medication like creosote or tincture of benzoin, may be alleviative.

Hemoptysis consisting only of slight streaks or spots of blood in the sputum requires no special treatment save rest in bed. Treatment of significant hemoptyses is designed to arrest the bleeding and to prevent a dissemination of the infection in the lungs by aspiration of contaminated blood. The patient should be in bed, and, in order to restore calm and quiet, may be reassured justifiably that the bleeding will subside. Violent coughing favors aspiration of the blood into healthy alveoli. If the patient is unable sufficiently to restrain the impulse, codeine sulfate, 0.030 to 0.060 gm., may be given hypodermically. Morphine is seldom indicated, and then only in small doses, 0.008 to 0.010 gm. Too much sedation depresses the reflexes unduly and may permit the retention of clots in the bronchi, which is undesirable. For a day or two after the initial hemoptysis, dark clots may be expelled, or fresh bleeding may recur, usually in diminishing amount. If the hemorrhages are large or frequently repeated, especially in cases in which the disease is predominantly unilateral, artificial pneumothorax is often indicated to relax the lung and, with it, the bleeding vessel; this, as a rule, is effective. Usually, however, pneumothorax is postponed for a few days or longer until accumulated blood has been cleared from the air passages, since this lessens the possibility of acute pneumonic reactions and serofibrinous pleurisy after the pneumothorax. If pneumothorax fails, other forms of collapse therapy may be considered in emergencies; occasionally thoracoplasty or resection of a cavity-bearing lobe is indicated without delay. Diaphragmatic paralysis is less effective. However, most hemoptyses subside after the loss of a small or moderate amount of blood, and treatment may then be continued according to the usual indications. During and for a few days after the hemoptysis the patient is given a soft or light diet, according to his desires, and it is not necessary usually to restrict this to fluids. The patient is encouraged to lie on the affected side, but during the waking hours he should change his position from time to time, since this aids in expelling clots of blood. Sometimes the patient goes into mild shock during the hemoptysis. This is treated by keeping him warm and giving him warm drinks and, if necessary, infusions of glucose in solution. Transfusion of 200 to 300 cc. of fresh blood may be helpful, but this measure should not be employed for slight indications because of the danger of serum hepatitis. Hemoptysis is relatively very infrequent while a patient is receiving chemotherapy; if bleeding does occur, new areas of pneumonic infiltration may follow, but the continued therapy usually prevents much caseation, and rapid resolution is often observed.

Dyspnea of sudden onset usually is due to acute pneumothorax or pleurisy and is treated accordingly. In advanced fibroid cases the symptom may become aggravated during attacks of acute bronchitis or bronchopneumonia when oxygen therapy is indicated for relief.

Pain in the chest is traceable most often to pleuritic involvement; strapping with adhesive plaster may give relief.

Night sweats are relieved usually by rest in bed and proper nursing. Drugs such as atropine or agaricin have little effect. The patient should not be covered too heavily with bed clothes, and the room should be airy and cool. Alcohol rubs or baths before retiring are helpful. After the sweat, the clothing should be changed and the patient should be given an alcohol rub.

Anemia is treated by a good general diet and, if necessary, the addition of ferrous sulfate. Often the most effective measure is the proper treatment of the complicating intestinal tuberculosis.

Rehabilitation, which consists in developing plans for good living, and suitable work after recovery, may be instituted as soon as conditions warrant. In many instances good morale and cooperation in treatment are promoted by encouraging the patient to see the goal of recovery ahead and by educating him to plan according to probable future opportunities and limitations. Early in his treatment his aptitudes may be estimated by approved testing; he may receive expert advice on vocations for which he is suited and, when able, begin study and training as he chooses. In many hospitals and sanatoriums, facilities and trained personnel are now available to render such services to patients.

Maintaining Arrest and Avoiding Relapse. In many advanced cases of tuberculosis the physician must recognize the impossibility of complete arrest of the disease and strive only to alleviate symptoms. But when there is a prospect of returning the patient to useful life, it is important to estimate when treatment has been sufficient to assure stability of the disease in the situations he is obliged to face later.

According to the standards of the National Tuberculosis Association, the disease is considered arrested when the lesions have remained apparently healed, tubercle bacilli have not been demonstrable, and the patient has been symptom-free under conditions of moderate physical activity for at least six months. As the lesions still harbor viable tubercle bacilli and relapse is possible, the gains are to be maintained and consolidated during the next several years. Experience shows that, if the patient goes through two years with continuing "arrest," the chance of relapse later is greatly minimized. During this time close and systematic medical observation and advice are important, as is the cooperation of the patient in following faithfully a prescribed daily routine. In most successfully treated cases, six months to a year of "arrest" should elapse before the patient returns to work. During the interval, as far as practicable, his daily schedule of activity should be increased gradually until it approximates that which he expects to continue at work. Patients who have followed light or sedentary occupations usually do best in returning to the same, particularly if the employer is willing to make some concessions pending complete rehabilitation. One-half day's work may be safe at first, to be gradually increased during the following months or years. Other patients often have to be educated for a new occupation, since laborious work under unfavorable conditions is always to be interdicted.

Periodic medical supervision is indicated indefinitely after recovery. At first the patient should be seen once a month; during this time he should be questioned about symptoms, the sputum should be searched for tubercle bacilli, and a roentgenogram should be made for comparison with those previously accumulated. Continued good general health, absence of tubercle bacilli and unchanging roentgenographic shadows (except perhaps for slight further contraction of the fibrotic lesions) permit, as a rule, continuation or expansion of the daily routine. After three or four months the interval between examinations may be gradually lengthened, but for the first two or three years the patient should be observed in this way every three to six months, and afterward at least once a year. The appearance of symptoms should always be the occasion for medical examination to determine the cause.

TUBERCULOSIS IN CHILDREN

In children the lesions of primary pulmonary infection have features which differ somewhat from the manifestations in adults. The primary parenchymal lesion is less likely in children to go on immediately to progressive caseation and excavation, while there is a pronounced tendency to gross involvement of the bronchopulmonary, tracheobronchial and other mediastinal lymph nodes, consequently, physical examination, though it should not be omitted, does not reveal the true nature of the lesion as well as it usually does in adults. Roentgenographic examination is a necessity. In children, more than in adults, enlarged lymph nodes may compress the bronchi in the root of the lung which in turn may lead to nonspecific changes distally in the parenchyma. Extension of the infection from the nodes may involve adjacent structures, eventually resulting in damage such as ulceration and stenosis of the bronchus and traction diverticula of the esophagus. On the other hand, inflammation of the nodes often subsides and their size diminishes strikingly, leaving relatively small calcific residues (Fig. 40). In infants there is a great frequency of hemic dissemination with generalized disease and meningitis. Wallgren has emphasized the occurrence of this within the first three months after the primary infection. After infancy and before adolescence there is a relative freedom from active tuberculosis, although it is by no

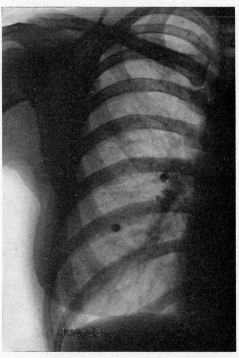

Fig. 40. Apparently calcified tuberculous lesions in the right lung and bronchopulmonary lymph nodes (primary complex).

means rare (see Fig. 38). During adolescence latent lesions have a tendency to flare up in the lungs, the frequency bearing some relationship to the extent of the primary disease after its onset perhaps many years before. The more caseous the primary lesions become, the greater is the likelihood of relapse later, especially in adolescence.

Treatment. The need of treatment in infants and children who have acquired primary infection is a matter of considerable confusion and uncertainty. The majority recover without disabling effects, although the exact number varies under different conditions of individual resistance and environmental conditions. A few have progressive disease of the lungs and serious complications, especially generalized miliary tuberculosis and meningitis. Whether or not these untoward consequences can be prevented by the routine chemotherapy of early symptomless primary disease remains to be proved. However, Edith M. Lincoln and her associates at Bellevue Hospital have demonstrated a great improvement of the prognosis of progressive disease with modern chemotherapeutic treatment.

TUBERCULOSIS OF THE LARYNX, TRACHEA AND BRONCHI

Tuberculous laryngitis is one of the common complications of chronic pulmonary tuberculosis. The lesions may be chronic and localized, or acute, exudative and diffuse. The lesion usually appears first at the level of the vocal cords or the arytenoids in the posterior part of the larynx. There may be a diffuse swelling or tubercle formation of the mucosa in the interarytenoid space, at the posterior end of one or both vocal cords, or in the region of one or both arytenoid cartilages. The inflammation may become almost completely resolved, or it may progress with caseation and ulceration. The irregular, ragged, shallow ulcers are found usually in the locations mentioned. Later, granulations may develop which have a serrated, granular or tubercular form. If extensive, fibrosis may cause slight stenosis of the larynx. The early symptoms are huskiness and hoarseness of the voice, dryness and slight soreness of the larynx. This may be noticed only on awaking or after talking, but usually continues beyond the time expected for simple catarrhal laryngitis. Laryngoscopic examination then may show the typical changes. Later, if the lesions progress, hoarseness becomes chronic and continuous, and the dryness and irritation may cause moderate or severe coughing. Pain is not usually a pronounced symptom unless deep invasion of the laryngeal cartilages occurs. One of these, the epiglottis, may become greatly enlarged, swollen, red and, finally, deeply ulcerated. Such extensive disease results in dysphonia, severe dysphagia and salivation, and the patient's nutrition may be seriously impaired. In treatment the most important principle is vocal rest, the patient being instructed to abstain from using the vocal cords. In most of these cases, specific chemotherapy is indicated not only for the laryngeal disease but also for the pulmonary tuberculosis, the regimens being

the same. The response of the laryngitis is usually very satisfactory, sometimes dramatically so. Painful symptoms often disappear rapidly.

The *bronchi* leading from a tuberculous pulmonary cavity usually are invaded, and, in some cases, lesions in the *larger bronchi* or *trachea* assume important clinical significance. Shallow lenticular ulcers of the mucosa are not uncommon, and more pronounced lesions develop occasionally in patients, especially women, with longstanding pulmonary disease. The bronchial wall may be attacked also by lesions in contiguous lymph nodes. The bronchial lesions consist of ulcers which are superficial or penetrate to or through the cartilage, or of granulomatous and fibrous formations which may partially occlude the lumen. Healing in the early stages leaves little or no scar, but more advanced lesions may be followed by extensive organization of the bronchial and peribronchial tissues, with contraction and cicatricial stenosis. Occasionally a bronchus is completely occluded. The affected bronchus may fail in its function as a drainage tube, and in this event the related segment of the lung becomes involved with secondary pyogenic infection, resulting in bronchopneumonia which may be necrotizing and associated with bronchiectasis. The diagnosis depends on eliciting the history of symptoms such as persistent severe coughing and wheezing, and the auscultation of rhonchi confined mostly to one side of the chest or to one lobe. Foulness of the sputum is suggestive of complicating anaerobic infection which often involves the parenchyma distal to the bronchial obstruction. Roentgenographic evidence of obstructive emphysema or cavities which appear distended and partly filled with fluid, or of diffuse pneumonia, is suggestive. Bronchoscopy may disclose the lesions. Chemotherapy for the pulmonary tuberculosis is often quite effective, in part because of the reduction of purulent discharge passing over the bronchial surfaces. At the same time the subsidence of bronchial edema allows better drainage of pulmonary cavities, thus favoring their healing. However, if the bronchus becomes narrowly constricted during its fibrous repair, lobectomy or even pneumonectomy may be necessary to prevent or remove the chronic destructive secondarily infected parenchymal disease which ensues almost inevitably.

TUBERCULOSIS OF THE ALIMENTARY TRACT

Tuberculosis of the mouth appears most often as ulceration of the tongue which becomes infected, as a rule, by extension from a laryngeal lesion or through an abrasion caused by biting or other trauma from the teeth. The lesion is situated most often on the margin, but may involve the dorsum, especially at the base. The ulcer at first is superficial, but progressive infiltration and caseation often follow with extensive destruction of the muscle. The chronic ulcers are often fissured, and yellow caseous or red granulating tubercles may be found in their depths. The indurated base is usually palpable. The ulcer is usually single, but others may appear. The diagnosis depends on the finding of such a lesion in a tuberculous patient and may be confirmed by demonstrating the organisms in curettings from the ulcer. Biopsy is to be avoided unless necessary. Specific chemotherapy may bring about partial or complete healing. Local heliotherapy may be helpful.

Tuberculosis of the lip is found usually under similar circumstances, the lesion appearing much the same as that of the tongue. An ulcer at the corner of the mouth may be fissure-like and penetrate deeply.

Tuberculosis of the salivary glands is rare, possibly because of the alkaline reaction of the tissue (Vivoli et al.).

Tuberculosis of the pharynx is found most often in association with lesions of the *tonsil*. Infection of the latter may be due to surface contamination or to hemic dissemination from a distant focus. Upon examining 2000 pairs of tonsils removed surgically, Long, Seibert and Gonzales found that the incidence of tuberculous lesions depends roughly on the prevalence of tuberculosis in the community; it was 6.5 per cent in specimens from American Indians; 2.5 and 0.25 per cent in those from Puerto Ricans and Philadelphians, respectively. The lesions are usually deep and focal. In cases recognized clinically the tonsil is slightly or moderately enlarged and may show yellow or whitish caseous areas beneath the shiny mucosa; later these break down, leaving ulcers of a grayish yellow ragged character. One or both tonsils may participate. When the pharynx becomes infected secondarily, the fauces, soft palate and uvula become thickly seeded with granular miliary tubercles, some of which have a minute yellowish center. These coalesce, break down, and form fissured ulcers, and the tissues may be slowly destroyed. The pain is severe, salivation profuse, and dysphagia marked. Such extensive disease is usually fatal unless it can be controlled early by specific treatment.

Tuberculosis of the esophagus is relatively rare. The upper end may be involved by direct extension from severe tuberculosis of the larynx. Tuberculous lymph nodes of the mediastinum, after caseation, may perforate the esophagus, discharging their contents, or the perinodal inflammation may involve the esophagus without perforation. In either event the cicatricial contraction may produce diverticula of the esophagus.

Tuberculosis of the stomach is reported in a few cases of pulmonary disease at autopsy (up to 2 per cent). The lesions usually extend to the stomach from a contiguous adherent lymph node, but they may result from surface contamination of the mucosa by swallowed discharges from the lungs. The gastric wall may be infiltrated, or there may be an ulcer, usually near the pylorus, which grossly resembles carcinoma.

The *intestine* is most frequently involved, the commonest site being the lower ileum and cecum. The mechanism of infection is principally from surface contamination with swallowed tubercle bacilli in patients with pulmonary tuberculosis (up to 70 per cent at autopsy). Much less often infection may be caused by primary invasion (e.g., contaminated milk), hemic dissemination or by extension from tuberculous peritonitis. Infiltration of the intestinal mucosa and lymphoid tissue usually is followed soon by superficial ulceration; the ulcers may extend rapidly or become localized and chronic with an organizing granulating base and overlying fibrinous or fibrous peritonitis. Sometimes, as in the cecum, the proliferative granulomatous changes become protracted, leading to great thickening of the wall, fibrous peritonitis and narrowing of the intestinal lumen, the whole forming a tumorous mass. Acutely progressive ulceration may involve several feet of the intestinal mucosa, enclosing small islands of intact tissue. Perforation of the wall by the ulcer is infrequent. Small ulcers may heal and the mucosa apparently regenerate.

The initial symptoms are indefinite, and considerable ulceration may be found in patients who have never had abdominal complaints. At first there is slight to moderate loss of weight, vague indigestion, loss of appetite, irritability and secondary anemia.

Local symptoms may appear early or late as a change in the usual rhythm of the stools. A short attack of mild diarrhea may be followed by constipation, and, after an apparently normal interval, this may recur. After many weeks or months diarrhea may become frequent, and, finally, the patient will have ten to twelve evacuations during the day and night, the diarrhea being watery and foul, seldom bloody. The diarrheal attacks are associated often with colicky pains in the lower half of the abdomen, aggravated perhaps by taking certain foods such as raw fruit. The patient may become anemic and emaciated. Physical examination usually reveals no palpable masses and frequently no tenderness, although the patient may complain of a little soreness on deep palpation, especially in the right lower quadrant. In certain mild chronic cases the recurrent pain simulates simple chronic appendicitis; in fact, the appendix may be involved in the tuberculous process. Sometimes this is not suspected until the lesions are discovered on routine histologic examination of the resected appendix. In cases of tuberculous enterocolitis roentgenographic examination after a barium meal or enema may reveal spasticity, filling defects and hypermotility of the lower ileum, cecum and ascending colon. Treatment consists first in proper general management and prescribed rest, since these patients almost always have chronic pulmonary tuberculosis. The diet should be bland; raw fruits, fruit juices and fat may have to be reduced or eliminated temporarily, and vitamins given parenterally. Medication to relieve pain and lessen the intestinal spasm may be indicated in the form of powdered opium or paregoric, bismuth subnitrate or bismuth subgallate by mouth, or calcium gluconate intravenously. Specific chemotherapy is highly effective.

Tuberculous ischiorectal abscess or *perianal abscess* and fistula are due usually to infection in a similar way and start with a localized painful perianal swelling which becomes acutely tender within a few days or several weeks. If not incised, this may perforate the skin to the exterior, less often the wall of the rectum, with the discharge of nonodorous pus in which tubercle bacilli may be demonstrated. The resulting fistula is apt to be chronic and later to require surgical treatment. However, if the original abscess was rather superficial and drains freely, it may heal satisfactorily with chemotherapy, administered in the usual way. Local applications of one or more of the drugs have been tried but this seldom seems to be necessary except following surgical resection of the fistula.

GENERALIZED FORMS OF TUBERCULOSIS

ACUTE GENERALIZED MILIARY TUBERCULOSIS

The disease occurs most frequently in young children or infants, and occasionally in adult life, especially in men over 60 years of age. The patient may have been in perfectly good health previously or may have had some clinical or other demonstrable evidence of tuberculosis, such as roentgenographic signs of mediastinal lymph node involvement (Fig. 40). The onset may be abrupt with chilliness, prostration, aching in the muscles, headache and drowsiness; or gradual with malaise, weakness and fatigue for a period of a few days or a week before the patient becomes prostrated. The temperature may rise at once to 103° or 104° F. in the afternoons, or attain this level gradually during a week or so. Night sweats may be profuse, the soft tissues waste rapidly, and the patient is overcome by weakness. Localizing symptoms depend on the predominant distribution of miliary tubercles. Dyspnea and cyanosis may become pronounced because of the extensive and rapid invasion of the lungs, but there is usually no cough or only a slight hacking. In other cases peritoneal symptoms such as pain, distention and constipation may predominate. Effusions may accumulate in the serous cavities with the well known clinical manifestations of their presence if they are profuse.

Physical examination initially shows only the general effects of the toxemia. After a week or more, fleeting rales may be heard in the lungs, later numerous and persisting; fluid may be demonstrated occasionally in the pleura or peritoneum, less often in the pericardium. The spleen becomes palpable in only a minority of the cases. Tubercles are seen somewhat less frequently in the choroid of adults than of children. The roentgenogram of the chest is indeterminate at first, but usually shows characteristic stippling of the pulmonary fields within several weeks. The leukocyte count usually remains within normal limits, but occasionally becomes moderately elevated, seldom above 20,000 per cubic millimeter. Leukemoid reactions and aplastic anemia, due presumably to invasion of the bone marrow, are rare complications. A biopsy of the bone marrow may show tuberculous changes, and sometimes tubercle bacilli may be grown in cultures seeded with the aspirated marrow. Occasionally the organisms are also grown from the blood, but they seem to disappear soon after dissemination from the focus of origin ceases. The situation may be aggravated by supervening meningitis, which may develop early or late in the course. In Debre's 170 cases of miliary disease in children, meningitis occurred in 88 per cent of the acute forms and in about 50 per cent of the subacute.

Treatment with combinations of specific drugs should be started as soon as the diagnosis is made. Initially streptomycin (2 gm. daily) and isoniazid (400 to 600 mg. daily) are administered to adult patients. Some prefer to add para-aminosalicylic acid (10 to 15 gm. daily) but it is doubtful whether this contributes any advantage. In early cases a symptomatic response with gradual lowering of the temperature to normal levels within two to eight weeks is the rule; at the same time a gradual fading of the miliary shadows from the roentgenogram of the lungs is observed. As the temperature becomes normal the dose of streptomycin is reduced to 1 gm. daily and that of isoniazid to 200 to 300 mg. daily, chiefly to avoid the toxic effects of the drugs; this regimen is continued for two or three months longer, after which streptomycin is further reduced to 1 gm. three times a week (every other day). This regimen then is maintained for a year or more, depending on the original severity of the case.

Under regimens of combined streptomycin and para-aminosalicylic acid, 106 cases of uncomplicated miliary tuberculosis were treated in the U.S. Veterans Administration and Military Hospitals and reported in 1952 by K. M. Smith; the survival rate at the end of three years was approximately 70 per cent; the rate was reduced to half this figure or less when meningitis supervened. Now, with the addition of isoniazid or its substitution for PAS, the prognosis for recovery is estimated to be about 90 per cent, assuming that treatment is started early.

SUBACUTE FORMS

The subacute forms are likewise observed most often in the early ages, but occasionally also in adults, particularly Negroes. Tubercle bacilli enter the lymph or blood stream, perhaps at recurring intervals, from a caseous focus. The number of lesions established in various organs is only moderate, and, since the patient does not die soon, time is sufficient to permit further local development with necrosis or partial healing. Many bacilli are picked up by the lymphatics and come to rest in various regional lymph nodes. The lungs are frequently involved, the lesions being particularly prominent in the upper parts. The spleen, kidneys, liver and serous membranes often participate.

The variety of clinical manifestations is great, but some are fairly constant. The patient may have obscure fever which has persisted for days or weeks without other obvious symptoms except loss of weight, malaise and fatigue. In time, peripheral lymphadenopathies may become apparent, as in the auricular, cervical, axillary, epitrochlear and inguinal regions. A roentgenogram of the chest may show only widening of the upper mediastinum from the lymphatic lesions. The spleen may become palpable within a few weeks or months. Other patients, with similar fever, reveal evidence only of an effusion in the pleura, peritoneum, or perhaps in several or all of the serous cavities. Still others may be found to have genitourinary tuberculosis, and occasionally papulonecrotic lesions of the skin give the first clue to the identity of the fever. Multiple lesions in the bones and joints and in the eye may be associated; some may become ulcerous or fistulous.

The natural course, unless interrupted by chemotherapy, is almost always progressively unfavorable; most patients die in three to six months, some with an acute miliary dissemination at the end. A few survive longer, when the disease may evolve in one or more local sites, usually the lungs; progressive cavitary lesions then may appear.

Treatment is the same as that for the acute form. Since the early course of the subacute forms is relatively mild and the diagnosis often uncertain, necrosis in many of the disseminated lesions may have occurred before treatment is started. Consequently the possibility of a late relapse may be greater than it is in the promptly treated acute case.

LATENT AND CHRONIC FORMS

It is not uncommon at autopsy to find tubercles, originating obviously in hemic dissemination of the infection perhaps many years before, distributed in such structures as the spleen, liver, kidneys, lungs and lymph nodes. These may be small, even microscopic, gray tubercles isolated in fibrous capsules. Others are represented by encapsulated round calcified nodules; sometimes they are so discrete and nonspecific in appearance that they are mistaken for simple phleboliths. Reichle and Work found such lesions in 20.1 per cent of 452 routine autopsies at the Cleveland City Hospital and, upon further investigation, demonstrated that most of them were tubercles. While these foci may never assume clinical significance, they are latent depots from which local active disease may develop after weeks, months or even many years.

Chronic generalized tuberculosis may be visualized as a stage between the subacute and the latent forms. Probably the most common clinical picture is mild chronic tuberculosis involving various lymph nodes, possibly one or more of the serous surfaces, and the lungs. Mild exudative or plastic inflammations may appear and recur in the serous membranes, and there may be slight or moderate recurrent swelling of lymph nodes which on roentgenographic examination appear partially calcified.

Among patients who recover from acute or subacute generalized tuberculosis it is to be expected that some may have local recurrences at sites where the lesions may not have healed sufficiently. The lungs then may be the site of numerous scattered fibroid lesions which cause some functional difficulty, and among them may be some small caseous lesions which progress, break down, and become the sources of bronchial dissemination. It has become apparent, however, that scattered pulmonary lesions of a chronic nature are almost always the result, not of blood-borne infection, but of bronchial dissemination from a sloughing local focus. Spain has produced pathologic evidence that tubercle bacilli in the blood stream are not completely filtered out in the lungs; when pulmonary lesions of this origin were identified, he always found lesions elsewhere, chiefly in the abdominal organs (see Pathogenesis, p. 276).

TUBERCULOSIS OF THE SEROUS MEMBRANES

Any of the serous membranes may become infected, usually singly, but sometimes in combination. The pleura is most commonly involved; secondly, the peritoneum; less often, the pericardium. The way of infection is by direct extension from some contiguous tuberculous lesion, less often by the blood or lymph streams. The lesions appear as isolated tubercles or as fibrinous or serofibrinous inflammations. Fibrinous changes usually are rather limited, while serofibrinous inflammations involve the whole membrane, which is edematous and red. The serous exudate may be absorbed, and fibrinous deposits may become partially or completely resolved. As a rule, however, some of the endothelial lining is destroyed, granulations develop and, eventually, are transformed into fibrous tissue; adjacent surfaces may be bound together by firm adhesions in which lymph and blood vessels may develop. In relatively few cases the effusion becomes purulent, deep inflammation and granulomatous thickening of the serosa occur, and this may undergo caseous degeneration. Subsequent organization and fibrosis leave behind permanent thickening and adhesions of the membranes with distortions and retractions of adjacent structures. The serous or purulent exudate may become loculated. After some years, if this is absorbed incompletely or slowly, free cholesterol accumulates in the fluid and the organizing walls of the pockets become infiltrated with calcium salts. Calcification of the pleura is seen occasionally, calcification of the pericardium less often; calcification of the peritoneum rarely.

Treatment of tuberculosis of the serous membranes should take into consideration that the infection is not primary here but originates most often in a local underlying focus. Infrequently, as a manifestation of hemic dissemination from a distant lesion, it is treated as a part of the generalized disease. Usually, however, attention is given to searching for the contiguous focus if this is not already manifest; common sites are mentioned below. The serositis may soon subside spontaneously or under treatment, but this should be given until the underlying infection, which obviously was active, is assumed to be controlled. Even though streptomycin, isoniazid or PAS, administered in the usual way, diffuses into serous and purulent effusions, the local therapeutic effects, if any, are usually slight. Given within a few days of the onset of the effusion, the acute general symptoms may be ameliorated and the accumulation of fluid may be limited.

TUBERCULOSIS OF THE PLEURA

The commonest form is fibrinous pleurisy, and this usually overlies a pulmonary lesion. Serofibrinous pleurisy develops in approximately 5 per cent of all cases of pulmonary tuberculosis; it may also be a manifestation of generalized tuberculosis. This is probably the case if both pleurae or other serous membranes are involved simultaneously or in close succession. Tuberculous empyema is uncommon except as a complication of pneumothorax, natural or induced, in which effusions are frequent; the most serious forms are caused by perforation of the pleura secondary to ulceration of an underlying pulmonary lesion. Isolated fibrous adhesions may be left behind; but after serofibrinous pleurisy heals, the pleura becomes widely or totally adherent, and the resulting organization and thickening may cause retraction of the mediastinum, diaphragm and chest wall. The same is true, to a more pronounced degree, of healing tuberculous empyema.

Fibrinous pleurisy may occur without localizing symptoms, but in a few cases is accompanied by the development of a severe, sharp pain in the side, immediately over the area of involvement or referred along the segmental distribution of the sensory nerves; thus diaphragmatic pleurisy may cause pain in the trapezius ridge and in the upper hypochondrium. The pain is usually aggravated by breathing and may last for a few hours to several days, occasionally longer. General symptoms of lassitude, possibly with low afternoon fever, may last for a few days to several weeks.

Serofibrinous pleurisy may develop as a complication of previously recognized pulmonary tuberculosis, in which case the clinical onset may not be distinguishable from the exacerbation of a pulmonary lesion. The preexisting pulmonary lesion may have been symptomless; it is often so small as to be indistinguishable, even by roentgenographic examination. Frequently the effusion is a sequel of the primary infection in which case it usually appears within six months after that event. In other cases the underlying source may be a focus in the spine, a rib or a mediastinal lymph node. Small effusions may collect and disappear, unknown to the patient. The onset may be insidious with malaise and fever, rising gradually to 101° or 102° F., or it may be acute with a sudden sharp pain in the side, chilliness, malaise and fever rising quickly to 104° or 105° F. The subsequent course may continue mildly or acutely. In its natural course a small effusion may be absorbed within a couple of weeks with complete subsidence of symptoms. In the acute cases, however, high fever frequently continues daily for four to six weeks, after which defervescence by lysis follows. During this time the patient may lose 10, 20 or more pounds in weight, become weak, and have severe sweats. Small effusions cause no local symptoms, but large collections may produce dyspnea and cyanosis on account of the displacement of the heart, blood vessels and lung. Convalescence usually starts after four to six weeks, but occasionally is delayed for three to six months; the fluid then becomes slowly absorbed, leaving behind varying degrees of thickening and retraction.

Diagnosis. The diagnosis of dry or fibrinous pleurisy is made by detecting a friction rub or pleural crepitus, but this may disappear soon or be entirely lacking. The diagnosis of serofibrinous pleurisy is indicated by the physical and roentgenographic signs of a basal effusion, possibly with associated signs of parenchymal tuberculosis and of displacement of the heart. In the early stages thoracentesis yields clear straw-colored fluid which has the characteristics of an exudate and contains cells of a mononuclear, occasionally polymorphonuclear type; infrequently it is sanguinolent. Tubercle bacilli usually are not discovered by microscopic examination because they are rather scarce. If possible, 500 cc. or more of fluid should be treated by centrifugation and the sediment inoculated on culture media and into a guinea pig; the organisms are usually demonstrated in this way. However, the failure to find tubercle bacilli, even on inoculation, does not necessarily exclude tuberculosis.

Treatment. The treatment of fibrinous or serofibrinous pleurisy is determined by the severity of the process and of any associated lesions. As a rule, fibrinous lesions remain localized and go on to resolution or fibrous organization. Occasionally after several weeks or months they are followed by a serous effusion. The treatment of serofibrinous pleurisy is more important. If the patient has pulmonary disease as well, the pleurisy is regarded as a problem in the general treatment already described. If no pulmonary lesions are demonstrated, it must be remembered, nevertheless, that many of these patients fall ill with pulmonary tuberculosis or some other form of the disease within five years. Among 141 young male adults, studied by Roper and Waring, after the occurrence of pleurisy with effusion, 92, or 65 per cent, subsequently developed tuberculosis in some form. Therefore the case should be treated as one of active tuberculosis, with rest in bed up to six months after the acute symptoms have subsided, to be followed by another three to six months' convalescence, preferably in a sanatorium. Chemotherapy is indicated; the regimen is based on the principles applying to pulmonary tuberculosis. The indications for withdrawing the fluid from the pleural cavity are (1) at the start, for diagnosis; (2) to relieve respiratory embarrassment from mechanical displacements; (3) to dispose of any residual collection after the febrile symptoms have subsided and absorption seems to be too slow; (4) to visualize the underlying lung if parenchymal lesions are suspected. For the last-mentioned purpose, 100 to 200 cc. of air is introduced with a pneumothorax apparatus during the evacuation of the fluid. The pulmonary parenchyma may then show much more clearly in the roentgenogram. Otherwise, pneumothorax should be avoided, since this interferes with healing and many prolong the exudation of fluid. The prognosis of uncomplicated tuberculous pleurisy with effusion is excellent if sufficient rest treatment is given. Among the patients of Roper's and Waring's study, the relapse rate was reduced to 31 per cent when six months or more of bed rest was taken. Mitchell followed 194 patients with pleurisy with effusion for five to twenty-five years after treatment in Trudeau Sanatorium; 85 per cent were well and working. Reactivation of tuberculosis had occurred in 24 per cent, usually within the first five years, and the mortality was 5 per cent. Because of the hazard of pulmonary tuberculosis developing later, roentgenographic examination of the chest every six to twelve months is advisable for any patient who has had tuberculous pleurisy.

Tuberculous empyema is related usually to some peculiar situation such as pleural ulceration and rupture or artificial pneumothorax, and is considered in this connection. The effusions complicating pneumothorax treatment are usually serous or serofibrinous, but in some cases there is a large output of polymorphonuclear leukocytes which rapidly undergo degeneration, giving the fluid at first a cloudy appearance and later a thick, light yellow or greenish, creamy consistency. Tubercle bacilli may be demonstrable easily microscopically and may appear in large clumps. A thick coating of fibrin and coagulated nucleoprotein is deposited on all the pleural surfaces. Unless the exudate is absorbed early, organizing pleurisy enveloping the collapsed lung may bind this down and prevent its reexpansion. Thoracotomy for drainage is contraindicated because of the danger of introducing secondary infection and creating a permanent sinus of the thoracic wall. Irrigations

of the pleura with solutions of streptomycin, dihydrostreptomycin (Ståhle) or isoniazid have been employed but these are difficult for the patient and are of doubtful value. Unless the lung reexpands readily while the fluid is removed by thoracentesis or by absorption, it may be necessary to open the chest surgically and strip off the "peel" (decortication).

Pneumothorax in tuberculous cases is related either to the ulceration of a subpleural caseous focus or to the rupture of a subpleural bulla which has developed secondary to the fibrosis. In the latter event the lung collapses, but, as a rule, the pleura does not become infected, nor is there any effusion. The tear heals readily and the lung expands within several months. In the former event, however, tubercle bacilli are invariably discharged into the pleura through the fistula, and acute serofibrinous pleurisy develops and often goes on rapidly to tuberculous empyema. Secondary infection with streptococci, staphylococci or pneumococci is common, creating a mixed infection empyema. After the lung collapses the fistula may operate as a valve mechanism, permitting the accumulation of air under great tension in the pleural space. The fistula is usually chronic and seldom heals except after operative intervention. Consequently the pleura is continually reinfected. Sometimes, too, the pleural effusion or empyema escapes through the fistula into the lung on the same or opposite side, causing acute tuberculous bronchopneumonia.

The symptoms of pneumothorax may develop in a known tuberculous patient or in one who previously appeared healthy. As a rule, a sudden sharp tearing pain in the chest is experienced, followed quickly by increasing shortness of breath and cyanosis. The patient seldom loses consciousness, but occasionally this accident may be the cause of sudden death. In other cases the event is symptomatically silent, particularly if the pleural perforation is tiny and the lung is partially anchored by adhesions which prevent its complete collapse; in the latter case the pneumothorax is detected as a localized pocket. If there is no infection, the symptoms may soon subside, with or without thoracentesis for the withdrawal of air, and the patient experiences no difficulty while the lung reexpands. With infection the symptoms of serofibrinous pleurisy develop acutely, and examination reveals hydropneumothorax with varying degrees of displacement of the yielding mediastinum, diaphragm and chest wall. Thoracentesis at the start reveals a clear or cloudy effusion in which tubercle bacilli may be found alone or in combination with pyogenic organisms.

Treatment is designed at first to relieve the acute mechanical displacement, by aspirating gas from the pleura at required intervals; or it may be withdrawn continuously through an indwelling tube connected with an aspirating apparatus. Fluid is aspirated to avoid drainage through the bronchopleural fistula into the lungs. As pyogenic infection usually continues and healing of the bronchopleural fistula seldom occurs spontaneously, thoracotomy for drainage is usually necessary. Eventually in some cases major surgery may be needed to remove the perforated lobe and to close the pleural space (thoracoplasty). The fatality rate is high because of the seriousness of the complication and frequently because of the extent of the underlying pulmonary tuberculosis.

Tuberculosis of the peritoneum may be the result of hemic infection or of extension from local lesions such as retroperitoneal lymph node involvement or salpingitis. Fibrinous inflammation in the visceral peritoneum at the site of intestinal ulcers is a common finding. General involvement may be miliary, serofibrinous or plastic and adhesive. Serofibrinous peritonitis may have an acute or insidious onset with constitutional symptoms like those described for serofibrinous pleurisy. Abdominal pain and tenderness are usually slight or moderate; occasionally, very intense. Initially there may be some vomiting and diarrhea, but, later, constipation is the rule. Abdominal distention may be great due to ascites and tympanites, but in other cases the wall is spastic and scaphoid. As adhesions develop, the exudate may become loculated in pockets and the omentum and intestine, matted.

Exudative peritonitis is most common in children and young adults, but may occur even in old people; it is observed more often in Negroes than in whites and in females than in males. Occasionally it is a complication of cirrhosis of the liver. Except when a part of generalized tuberculosis, the prognosis for healing is good, provided general rest treatment is instituted early and carried out long enough. Mechanical symptoms may require evacuation of the fluid; to avoid perforating the gut this is done best by a small surgical incision. Laparotomy is unnecessary in most cases. In female patients tuberculosis of the fallopian tube may prolong the peritonitis and favor chronicity; in such cases salpingectomy may later be indicated.

Plastic adhesive peritonitis usually is a later development of fibrinous or serofibrinous inflammation. Fibrous contraction may produce narrowing of the lumen of the bowel, the coils of which may be bound together in large inseparable tangles. Between the hyperplastic and caseous lesions tuberculous exudate, sometimes purulent, may be pocketed. Abdominal examination may reveal irregular masses of involved omentum, matted intestine, caseous deposits or enlarged lymph nodes. These may be numerous or confined to a single section such as the right lower quadrant surrounding the cecum. Aside from the manifestations of chronic toxemia, local symptoms may become distressing on account of the fixation and stenosis of the bowel. There may be constipation, obstipation or, occasionally, obstruction. Rarely the intestine is perforated and tuberculous pus may drain from the peritoneum into it.

Treatment is general and symptomatic unless the disease is localized and accessible, such as a hyperplastic process in and surrounding the cecum; this may be resected surgically. Postoperative abdominal fistulas which may be fecal are not uncommon. In most cases, especially those treated early, the course of the disease is arrested or favorably influenced by chemotherapy. Kahrs reports the outcome of 169 cases treated in Norway between 1930 and 1948 (mostly without chemotherapy). He found the serous type to have the most favorable outlook (20 deaths in 73 cases after 2.5 to 20.5 years), while the fibropurulent and purulent types (9 cases) all ended fatally.

Tuberculosis of the pericardium may represent an extension from the pleura, in which case the lesions are usually of a localized fibrinous, hyperplastic or adhesive character, giving rise to few or no symptoms. Serofibrinous pericarditis is caused by direct extension of the infection from adjacent caseous lymph nodes or, less often, by hemic infection. Among all cases of pericarditis, tuberculosis is identified as the cause in approximately 7 to 11 per cent (Reeves; Griffith and Wallace). Aside from the manifestations of toxemia, symptoms and signs referable to tamponade of the heart may be found; the embarrassment may be relieved by paracentesis. Because the infection often is systemic, the prognosis for recovery usually is poor. The effusion may continue reaccumulating, and after three to six weeks loculation may occur because of the formation of fibrinous adhesions. Caseation is observed occasionally, especially in Negroes, and may extend into the myocardium. In the few cases of recovery the layers of the pericardium may adhere completely, and in time the shrinkage may lead to chronic constrictive pericarditis with functional impairment. In this disabling situation the operation of pericardiectomy, or cardiolysis may effect partial or complete relief in 60 per cent of the cases (Heuer and Stewart).

Treatment is basically the same as that for tuberculous pleurisy and should take into consideration associated disease in the lungs and elsewhere. Chemotherapy is indicated and usually should be continued for a year or more.

TUBERCULOSIS OF THE LYMPH NODES

Lymph nodes may be infected by tubercle bacilli entering the lymphatic stream from a lesion in the tributary region or arriving by way of the blood stream. Most often the lesions are limited to a single chain, frequently the mediastinal system. However, in generalized forms of tuberculosis, multiple scattered lymphadenopathies are demonstrated commonly in the superficial and deep chains. The lesions may appear as acute, subacute or insidious inflammatory swelling of the nodes with gradual caseation and necrosis. Perinodal inflammation and agglutination with adjacent nodes may follow; later, liquefaction, rupture and sloughing of the contents through the overlying tissues, particularly in superficial involvement. As the inflammation subsides, calcification of the caseous residues may develop slowly during a period of years, and the lesions may remain as permanently enlarged, firm, usually discrete nodes. Sometimes chronic fistulas, usually superficial, persist and may burrow widely, causing extensive degeneration of the skin and subcutaneous tissues (scrofuloderma). Most often lymphadenitis is of a mild hyperplastic type with only a minimum of caseation. The lesions may be chronic, or may subside and become reactivated repeatedly after long or short intervals of time without any evidence of liquefaction or sloughing. Chronic caseous lymph node involvement, particularly in the mediastinum, is a potential source of danger even after long periods of latency. Despite partial calcification these lesions may be the source of disseminations in childhood, in adolescence and sometimes even in late adult life. In the chronic

systemic forms of tuberculosis the lymphatic system may harbor most of the lesions and account for the protracted ill health, including exacerbations of low fever from time to time.

Specific chemotherapy for tuberculosis of lymph nodes is subject to the same general principles previously discussed and to an estimation of the prognosis. Often the disease is a mild, self-limited process, and the important thing is to build up general resistance to avoid a recurrence. In acute cases specific therapy may help materially to halt the inflammation and promote resolution, but a lasting effect on the caseous components is not to be expected. These require a long time for natural healing, may liquefy in spite of specific therapy, and when accessible may eventually require surgical treatment.

Mediastinal and bronchopulmonary lymph node tuberculosis is observed most often in young children following the primary infection. Constitutional symptoms may be mild or entirely lacking. Massive lesions may produce pressure, giving a variety of symptoms such as stridulous cough simulating whooping cough, constant or intermittent wheezing respiration sometimes simulating asthma, less commonly stridor, dyspnea and cyanosis. Localized pressures on the bronchi may irritate and compress the tube, resulting in collapse of the lobe or the lung, or the development of nonspecific necrotizing bronchopneumonia and possibly bronchiectasis. Perforation of the nodes through the trachea, more often the bronchi, occurs most often during infancy and early childhood and very seldom during adult life; the tubercle bacilli thus discharged may then be aspirated into the lung, causing tuberculous bronchopneumonia. Calcified nodes similarly may ulcerate through the bronchi (broncholithiasis). Physical examination usually is not helpful unless the mass is very large; then it may be suspected by dullness and altered breath and voice sounds extending beyond the spine or sternum on one or both sides. The roentgenogram reveals the lesions unless they are small and concealed by other structures; the shadows include bulbous enlargements of the hilum, widening of the mediastinal density, and the round and oblong, homogenous or granular opacities of calcification. With few exceptions, the tuberculin test is positive, and often there are typical lesions also in the lungs or elsewhere. Occasionally, physical signs and symptoms of bronchial stenosis or tracheal and venous obturation may be elicited. The treatment is the general hygienic rest regimen together with pediatric supervision in children. Roentgen ray therapy has been tried, but usually is ill advised because of the possibility of aggravating necrosis. The same may be said of tuberculin therapy. Under rest treatment massive enlargements may gradually subside, eventually leaving little trace or possibly only calcified residues. The extent of these is in proportion to the amount of caseous degeneration which occurred previously. When the lymph node disease is a part of progressive primary tuberculosis, especially in children, chemotherapy is indicated. Combinations of isoniazid and streptomycin seem to be most efficacious. Surgical removal of massive diseased nodes has been accomplished but is seldom undertaken.

Cervical lymphadenitis is a common form, but in the United States has become much less prevalent since the early nineteen hundreds. The disease, which was known in earlier times as scrofula or king's evil, has been reduced through the elimination of tubercle bacilli from milk and the prevention of infection in childhood. The lesions may be confined to one or several nodes or may encircle the neck anteriorly from ear to ear. The upper deep cervical nodes are most frequently affected; as a rule, the lesions are more pronounced on one side. Infrequently the acute swelling is so marked as to impede the motion of the neck and to displace the trachea. If the onset is insidious, the lumps may be discovered purely accidentally. Tenderness is slight or moderate unless the overlying tissues become involved. The skin usually appears healthy, but may become red, tender and gradually thinned out until perforation occurs. A thick or nummular purulent discharge follows, and drainage may continue for a long time. Neglect of the condition may result in fistulas in various parts of the neck and in the upper thorax. Treatment during the acute stages includes bed rest and, often, the use of chemotherapy. This usually controls the active inflammation and dries discharging sinuses. Chronic lesions, usually composed of caseous matter, should be excised if the patient's general condition permits. Chemotherapy then is continued until healing is well established. Sloughing lesions sometimes are treated with lytic enzymes and allowed to granulate.

Abdominal lymphadenitis may be part of a generalized infection or result from lesions in the intestine, peritoneum or other adjacent organs. Usually there are no specifically localizing symptoms, but, when the involvement is moderate or extensive, vague abdominal pain, constipation and indigestion may be complaints. Sometimes the condition simulates chronic appendicitis. Advanced wasting disease in infants and young children is known as *tabes mesenterica*. Unless the lesions originally were extensive or part of generalized tuberculosis, the tendency to heal is striking. In chronic cases the infection may spread through adherent lymph nodes into the stomach, duodenum, pancreas, or liver. Adjacent iliac veins may become thrombosed; rarely a node perforates and discharges into the aorta.

TUBERCULOSIS OF THE URINARY TRACT

The kidney is the most frequent site of tuberculosis of the urinary tract, the infection usually being blood-borne. In males the infection sometimes extends to the urinary tract from the genitals. The disease is much more prevalent in adults than in children and is observed two to four times as frequently in males as in females. The finding of microscopic tubercles in the kidneys is common at autopsy, but gross lesions are detected in 10 per cent or less of all cases of chronic pulmonary tuberculosis. The disease often occurs in patients who have never suffered from pulmonary lesions, the presumption being that the infection was carried from a primary focus which subsequently healed. Renal lesions may be latent for a long time before causing clinical symptoms. The early lesion is usually in or near the glomerulus, and bacilli may pass from this through the tubules to the papilla. Caseation and ulceration may be limited or extensive, resulting in the formation of small fistulas and the discharge of bacilli into the renal pelvis and ureter. These more resistant structures also may be invaded. Often the kidney becomes more or less excavated. Occasionally the caseous lesions may be encapsulated or the ureters become sealed off; then calcareous changes may develop. The bladder may be infected with bacilli carried in the urine; tubercles and ulcers about the ureteral orifice appear, and, if the invasion is wide, later fibrous shrinkage may reduce the capacity greatly. It is to be assumed, on pathologic evidence, that the renal lesions are bilateral, but progressive destructive disease may be confined to one kidney.

The symptoms include polyuria, hematuria, pyuria, dysuria and strangury, but, at the inception, renal tuberculosis usually is symptomless. Similarly, physical examination at the start may be entirely negative. Later, slight tenderness may be elicited on palpation of the kidney or in the upper lumbar region posteriorly. Constitutional symptoms, if any, usually are slight. The condition is to be suspected, particularly in a patient with pulmonary tuberculosis, in the presence of unexplained albuminuria, hematuria or pyuria, especially the last two, even if the quantity of blood or pus is small. Dysuria or cystitis, not explained otherwise, should always be investigated. Examination of the urine may show small or moderate amounts of albumin, an abnormal number of erythrocytes and pus cells. Intensive search usually reveals the presence of tubercle bacilli (see Demonstrating the Tubercle Bacillus, p. 279). Pyelography, cystoscopy and ureteral catheterization are used to demonstrate the extent and location of the lesions.

Specific chemotherapy, using a combination such as streptomycin and PAS or streptomycin and isoniazid, administered for a year or more, usually abolishes symptoms and eliminates manifestations of pyuria, hematuria and bacilluria. Healing with fibrosis may be striking, and in the cases of limited destructive lesions this may result in a lasting arrest of the disease. If destruction is extensive, the experience thus far seems to indicate that the disease will usually be held in abeyance only temporarily. Therefore nephrectomy is usually considered to be indicated unless there is too much active disease in the other kidney. Before specific drugs became available, this operation in well selected cases led to lasting recovery in about 50 per cent. In recent years the Semb operation of partial nephrectomy has been performed successfully in a number of selected cases; in a few of these the opposite kidney had been removed previously.

TUBERCULOSIS OF THE GENITAL TRACT

Genital tuberculosis was found in 12.7 per cent of 1143 autopsies on tuberculous subjects by Auerbach at the Seaview Hospital; of these, 14.4 per cent were in males and 10.4 per cent in females. It is almost always caused by blood-borne infection from lesions elsewhere in the body. In 41 cases in females Auerbach found the fallopian tubes involved in 97.5 per cent, the uterus in 58.5 per cent and the ovaries in 31.7 per cent. The cervix

is seldom affected, the vagina and labia rarely. The most common sequel of salpingitis is localized or diffuse peritonitis. Both tubes may be involved, but the lesions are usually unilateral. There may be few or no localizing symptoms; if any, they appear as dull, vague pains in the lower abdomen, accentuated perhaps during menstruation. The menses may be scanty, irregular or absent. There may be slight or moderate leukorrhea; tubercle bacilli may be found in the discharge or in the menstrual blood. Curettage may bring away endometrial tissue, revealing tuberculous changes on microscopic examination. Pelvic and sometimes abdominal examination may reveal an elongated round mass a few centimeters in diameter in the pelvis. The lesions may heal spontaneously if they are not extensive, but, if they are chronic, surgical resection, after a prolonged course of chemotherapy, is favored sometimes to eliminate the focus and prevent extension to the peritoneum. Exacerbations of the disease, especially if the uterus is involved, may be caused by pregnancy; prolonged postpartum bleeding, not otherwise explained, should arouse the suspicion of tuberculosis. Chronic or healed tuberculous salpingitis may cause sterility.

Male genital tuberculosis usually is manifested first in the epididymis, but pathologic examinations suggest that the initial focus usually is in the prostate, the epididymal lesion being a secondary extension. In 105 cases examined at autopsy, Auerbach found the prostate involved in 95.2 per cent, the seminal vesicles in 61.9 per cent, the epididymis in 48.5 per cent, and the testes in 29.5 per cent. Ljunggren found associated involvement of the kidneys in 50 per cent of 60 cases of tuberculous epididymitis. As the lesions progress, extension to the opposite epididymis is common. The bladder also may be affected secondarily. Progressive disease may be followed by the establishment of sinus tracts perforating the scrotum and allowing the discharge of tuberculous pus to the outside.

The onset of *tuberculous epididymitis* may be insidious, with the development of a nodular or diffuse infiltration, and this may subside and remain latent for a time; or it may be acute with rapid swelling of the epididymis, possibly with a serous effusion in the scrotum. Later the testis may become swollen, painful, and even undergo softening. Usually the acute inflammation subsides after several weeks, leaving behind chronic lesions which may slowly progress. Examination then may reveal a thickened, more or less nodular epididymis; if the testicle participates, it may be enlarged to twice or more its natural size. The vas may be thickened and nodular, and rectal examination may reveal diffuse or nodular enlargement of the seminal vesicles and prostate. If any of the lesions have liquefied, limited fluctuant areas may be palpable. If fistulas develop, tubercle bacilli may be demonstrated in the discharging pus; they also may appear in the urine and the seminal fluid. While rest treatment is indicated in these cases, the lesions usually run a chronic course and the prognosis for ultimate healing is not good. Prolonged chemotherapy, i.e., for a year or more, using two specific drugs such as streptomycin and PAS in combination, may bring about great improvement and arrest the infection. Usually, the epididymis is excised if very necrotic; sometimes the testicle with it.

TUBERCULOSIS OF THE MENINGES AND CENTRAL NERVOUS SYSTEM

Tuberculosis of the meninges and central nervous system figures conspicuously among infected infants and children and is frequently the terminal event of fatal disease at this time of life. In adults, meningitis is a relatively infrequent cause of death even among those who have suffered from chronic pulmonary disease. Occasionally, however, it is a terminal event due to hemic dissemination as resistance breaks down. While leptomeningitis is the commonest manifestation, the dura may contain a few scattered tubercles or may become involved by extension from an adjacent bony focus, such as vertebral caries. Limited lesions, usually cortical, may appear also in the cerebrum, less often in the cerebellum or spinal cord. In rare cases these may heal eventually with calcification. Such tubercles may be of a chronic granulomatous character, gradually increasing in size and producing the clinical manifestations of tumor; the symptoms then depend on the location of the lesion.

Thus tuberculous meningitis may originate from a lesion previously established in the cortex, choroid plexus, pia or dura, or may develop as part of an acutely disseminated infection from some more remote source. The distribution of the tubercles, the perifocal congestion and the fibrinous exudate are characteristically basilar. The regions favored are those about the circle of Willis, the interpeduncular space, the fissures of Sylvius and the optic chiasm. Tubercles may be located in and close to the walls of arteries. The contiguous brain tissue is edematous or infiltrated for a short distance.

The patient may present the clinical picture of generalized miliary tuberculosis for several weeks before meningeal symptoms develop. In other cases obvious chronic tuberculous disease may have been present, usually in the chest. Not infrequently, however, the patient, especially if he is a child, previously may have appeared perfectly well. For no apparent reason the child becomes listless and irritable. The appetite fails and he loses weight. If he is too young to describe the headache, it may be eloquently indicated as he feels or fumbles his head with his hands and by the sharp so-called "hydrocephalic cry" or the unmistakable and sustained scream of pain. Vomiting is common, usually sudden, and often projectile; sometimes it is precipitated by a change of position in bed. The fever may rise to 103° F. or more in the afternoon. At first the pulse may be quick, but later it becomes slow in proportion to the fever. The pupils initially are contracted, later dilated. As the terminal or paralytic phase follows that of irritation, the restlessness, night terrors and outcries may give way to stupor, whimpering and muttering. The patient may be disoriented and wander from his bed. There may be clonic contractions of single groups of muscles, and, not infrequently, general convulsions. Photophobia is common, and there may be strabismus and blepharoptosis. Monoplegia or hemiplegia may be observed. The initial constipation and urinary retention usually are followed by incontinence.

Early in the disease the neck and the muscles of the back and extremities may be sore and stiff. Kernig's sign is usually positive, and there may be general hyperreflexia, ankle and patellar clonus and a positive Babinski sign. Later the muscles may become flaccid and reflexes diminished. As the coma deepens, the patient may execute athetoid movements. Finally he becomes completely motionless, the temperature varies widely and irregularly, and sweating may be profuse. In this unconscious state, his eyes half closed and jaw agape, he wearily breathes away his final hours.

The natural duration of the disease varies from three to six or eight weeks; occasionally deaths in children have been reported to occur in less than a week after the clinical onset. Actually the disease may exist some time before symptoms become manifest; occasionally during the course of generalized miliary tuberculosis a routine spinal puncture may yield fluid containing tubercle bacilli. Spontaneous recovery is rare.

Lumbar puncture yields fluid which is usually clear and under increased pressure; occasionally it is slightly turbid or xanthochromic. As the fluid stands in the tube, a thin coagulum develops, and tubercle bacilli may be found in this or in the sediment collected after centrifugation. Otherwise, culture or guinea pig inoculation usually proves positive. The number of cells in the fluid usually is 25 or more per cubic millimeter, lymphocytes predominating. The content of protein is found moderately or markedly increased; glucose is decreased.

Treatment. Specific chemotherapy has greatly improved the outlook of patients afflicted with tuberculous meningitis so that today, when the disease is diagnosed and treated in its early stages, the prospect of recovery is approximately 90 per cent. When experiences of statistical value started accumulating in 1948, it became apparent that about 20 to 25 per cent of the patients treated with streptomycin or dihydrostreptomycin alone (intramuscularly and intrathecally) for periods of a few months could be expected to survive two years or longer. Later the addition of PAS (orally and, in some clinics, intravenously) and the prolongation of such combined regimens for many months were found to improve the results substantially. Then the oral administration of isoniazid, which easily diffuses through normal tissue barriers into the cerebrospinal fluid, in combination with streptomycin, intramuscularly, proved that almost all patients will survive, at least for two years. Most experienced clinicians now consider it unnecessary to inject streptomycin intrathecally since, during the acute inflammatory phase of the disease, the drug enters the cerebrospinal fluid from the blood in quantities sufficient to be of therapeutic effectiveness; this also obviates the disadvantage of the local irritation caused by the drug when given intrathecally. Some add PAS, orally, to the other two drugs but it is not clear that this contributes any additional advantage.

In practice, when treating adult patients, isoniazid, 8 to 10 mg. per kilogram of body weight per day, is given in two or three divided doses orally, while streptomycin, 2 gm. daily, is injected intramuscularly, usually divided into two doses given 8 or 10 hours apart. The usual dose of PAS may also be given if desired. This regimen is continued up to six months, the results being judged by the subsidence of symptoms and the changes in the cerebrospinal fluid which, in the early weeks, should be estimated at least once a week. The glucose concentration is a good indicator of improvement as it rises to the normal; the protein and the cells usually diminish more slowly. Isoniazid is continued at the same dosage until the patient is obviously recovering, at which time it may be lowered to 5 mg. per kilo. Chemotherapy should be continued for at least a year, but the dose of streptomycin may have to be reduced because of neurotoxicity. If vertigo or impairment of hearing is manifested, the dose may be reduced after two to six months to 1 gm. daily; in some cases 1 gm. three times weekly or 2 gm. every third day has been considered sufficient. Des Autels and Pfuetze advocate continuing treatment for six months after the glucose and cells of the cerebrospinal fluid return to normal, and prefer continuing until the protein is normal or at least falling consistently toward the end of a total of eighteen or more months of treatment. The purpose of prolonged treatment is to guard against a recurrence, for this has been known to take place as long as five years after the early recovery under short-term therapy.*

When the disease is not treated until it has reached a late phase, the recovery rate is reduced to approximately 25 to 30 per cent. Before the advent of isoniazid, when meningitis was a complication of generalized miliary tuberculosis, recovery was less frequent by about 8 per cent (Lorber). Cortisone or hydrocortisone has been suggested as

* For tuberculous meningitis in children, the following regimen is carried out in the Children's Medical Service of Bellevue Hospital: Streptomycin, 1 gm. intramuscularly, for a minimum period of one month or until the cerebrospinal fluid glucose has been normal for one week, thereafter, 1 gm. twice weekly; isoniazid, orally, 10 mg./kg. daily, divided into two doses for four to six weeks, then 7 mg./kg.; sulfone (Promizole), orally, 0.25 to 8 gm. daily for two years.

a possible adjuvant to specific chemotherapy but clinical trials have not shown any significant advantages.

Sometimes, especially in cases diagnosed and treated in late phases of the disease, inflammatory exudate may accumulate to such an extent as to block the free circulation of fluid; this may be at the spinal, subtentorial or basal cisternal level. Lytic enzymes such as streptokinase, streptodornase and pancreatic dornase have been injected intrathecally and intraventricularly in an attempt to digest the coagulated exudate and break up the block. Occasional successes have been reported but some experienced clinicians do not consider the advantages to be significant. Tuberculin has been used for a similar effect, but has not been widely adopted. When there is evidence of abnormally increased intraventricular pressure, threatening hydrocephalus, especially in children, this sometimes is relieved through burr holes drilled through the frontal bone.

Following recovery there may occasionally be some residual damage including motor palsies, deafness (due mostly to streptomycin or dihydrostreptomycin given intrathecally), mental impairment and abnormal behavior. These are very infrequent with present chemotherapy.

TUBERCULOSIS OF THE SPECIAL STRUCTURES

The *breast* may be infected by way of the blood stream, but more often by extension from an adjacent lesion such as caries of a rib or tuberculous costal chondritis. The breast may be diffusely swollen and tender, but more commonly localized irregular nodular swellings, increasing in size, appear in one or more of the segments. The conglomerate tubercles usually become caseous, leading to the formation of abscesses from which cutaneous fistulas may originate. The infection may burrow widely under the pectoral tissues. If not too extensive, incision of the abscess followed by a course of combined chemotherapy may lead to healing. If the glandular tissue is extensively involved, mastectomy may be indicated.

Tuberculosis of the myocardium, while rare, may occur through infection extending into it from the epicardium; less often from the mediastinal lymph nodes or from the blood stream. The lesions may be numerous and isolated or diffuse and caseous. Alphonse described tuberculous phlebitis of the myocardial veins. An extremely rare lesion is tuberculous endocarditis with valvular vegetations.

Tuberculous arteritis of peripheral artries is also rare, sometimes due to the lodgment of infected emboli.

Tuberculosis of the hypophysis is rare; Kirschbaum and Levy studied the chronic granulomatous type, which may produce the symptoms of diabetes insipidus or of pituitary cachexia (Simmonds' disease).

Tuberculosis of the thyroid and the pancreas is rare and is observed only in generalized infection or as an extension from an adjacent lesion. Chronic thyroiditis and, less often, chronic pancreatitis on a tuberculous basis are occasionally reported.

Tuberculosis of the adrenals, if extensive, produces the Addisonian syndrome, which may be rapidly progressive and fatal. In these cases the adrenals are usually caseous. A few tubercles may be discovered in the adrenals in generalized miliary tuberculosis and, rarely, old calcifications may be found.

Tuberculosis of the Liver. Isolated gray tubercles in the capsule or substance of the liver are not uncommon findings at the autopsy of patients who have died of pulmonary tuberculosis, and they may be demonstrated in those who have never suffered from this disease. In subacute and chronic forms of generalized tuberculosis, particularly in young children and in Negroes, numerous caseous tubercles of various sizes may be found in the liver, but extensive abscess formation is uncommon. Infection of the gallbladder or duct is also infrequent; it is usually due to extension from an adjacent focus which may be in the lymph nodes.

At Seaview Hospital, Stemmerman found **tuberculosis of the bile ducts** in 3 per cent of 1500 autopsies on tuberculous subjects; usually the lesions were miliary or consisted of abscesses 1 to 20 mm. in diameter.

Tuberculosis of the spleen is a frequent sequel of hemic infection. A few or many miliary tubercles may be found in the capsule or in the parenchyma, or the organ may be enlarged and infiltrated with large caseous conglomerates; the latter, however, is uncommon. Nodular calcifications sometimes may be demonstrated roentgenographically.

Tuberculosis of the ear usually is a complication of cavitary pulmonary disease. The middle ear may be infected through the eustachian tube. The process is subacute or chronic, leading to abscess formation and slow perforation of the drum, after which a chronic fistula often persists. Secondary infection then may occur. The mastoid may become involved, but this is uncommon, at least in serious degrees. The diagnosis is suggested by gradually increasing painless deafness, tinnitus and a feeling of fullness in the ear of a patient with cavitary pulmonary tuberculosis. Perforation of the drum is usually painless also. Tubercle bacilli may be demonstrated in the discharging pus. The inflammation occasionally heals without perforation of the drum, leaving permanent partial deafness.

The *nose* may become involved in lupus vulgaris, the lesions of which may extend to the mucosa. Picking of the nose by a tuberculous patient is supposed sometimes to cause infection of the mucosa and development of a chronic perforating septal ulcer. **Tuberculosis of the paranasal sinuses** is observed rarely.

PREVENTION OF TUBERCULOSIS

The observations that some increase in resistance to tubercle bacilli may be conferred upon animals and that naturally acquired and limited tuberculous lesions have a similar effect in man have stimulated many attempts to develop means of prophylactic vaccination and passive transference of immune bodies. Killed, devitalized and attenuated bacilli have been tried as vaccines administered by various routes, as have fractions and products of the bacilli and of the lesions caused by them. It has been shown that relative immunity may develop, usually in slight degree, after the administration of living or dead, virulent or attenuated organisms. The duration of this may be a relatively few months or some years. Absolute protection against subsequent virulent infection has never been proved, and no plan has justified itself thus far for universal application. One of the better known vaccines, BCG, an attenuated living strain of the bovine type of bacillus prepared by Calmette and Guérin, is proved to have an immunizing capacity, and the degree of this is still under study. The reports of J. D. Aronson, who conducted a test of BCG among large groups of American Indians, and of R. G. Ferguson, who vaccinated the personnel of hospitals and sanatoria in Saskatchewan, Canada, are impressive because of the objective comparative methods

used. The tuberculosis attack and fatality rates were lower by at least 75 per cent in the groups vaccinated than in the unvaccinated. For the better protection of groups, especially the young, who do not react to tuberculin and therefore have presumably not been infected, and who are destined to have close and frequent contact with tuberculosis, as in poor economic areas and in hospitals, BCG is gaining some favor.

Measures which are assuredly effective for prevention include the following:

Elimination of tuberculous animals and pasteurization of milk

Improvement of living conditions and education in personal hygiene

Adequate medical examinations to detect lesions in their incipiency, usually in the preclinical phase

Sufficient and proper treatment of the early case to prevent excavation of the lesion and infection of "contacts"

Isolation of the infectious case

Rehabilitation of patients with arrested disease to prevent relapse.

J. BURNS AMBERSON

References

des Autels, E. J., and Pfuetze, K. H.: Chemotherapy of Miliary and Meningeal Tuberculosis in the Adult. Am. Rev. Tuberc., 68:912, 1953.

Debré, R.: Miliary Tuberculosis in Children. Lancet, 263:545, 1952.

Dubos, René J.: Unsolved Problems in the Control of Tuberculosis. Am. Rev. Tuberc., 70:391, 1954.

Editorial: Treatment of Renal Tuberculosis. Lancet, 1:1293, 1953.

Elmendorf, Dumont F., Jr., Cawthon, W. U., Muschenheim, Carl, and McDermott, Walsh: The Absorption, Distribution, Excretion and Shortterm Toxicity of Isonicotinic Acid Hydrazide (Nydrazid) in Man. Am. Rev. Tuberc., 65:429, 1952.

Fifth Report to the Medical Research Council by their Tuberculosis Chemotherapy Trials Committee: Isoniazid in Combination with Streptomycin or with P.A.S. in the Treatment of Pulmonary Tuberculosis. Brit. M. J., 2:1005, 1953.

Fox, H. H.: Newer Synthetic Structures of Interest in Tuberculostatic Drugs. Science, 118:497, 1953.

Francis, J.: Control of Infection with the Bovine Tubercle Bacillus. Lancet, 2:34, 1950.

Goyette, E. M., Overholt, E. L., and Rapaport, E.: The Treatment of Tuberculous Pericarditis. Circulation, 9:17, 1954.

Hobby, Gladys L., Auerbach, Oscar, Lenert, Tulita F., Small, Maurice J., and Comer, John V.: The Late Emergence of M. *Tuberculosis* in Liquid

Cultures of Pulmonary Lesions Resected from Humans. Am. Rev. Tuberc., 70:191, 1954.

Hughes, Hattie B., Biehl, J. Park, Jones, Audrey P., and Schmidt, L. H.: Metabolism of Isoniazid in Man as Related to the Occurrence of Peripheral Neuritis. Am. Rev. Tuberc., 70:266, 1954.

Kahrs, T.: Tuberculous Peritonitis: A Follow-up Study of 169 Cases. Tubercle, 33:132, 1952.

Koch, R.: Die Aetiologie der Tuberkulose. Berl. klin. Wchnschr., 19:221, 1882 (translation published by the National Tuberculosis Association, New York, 1932).

Laennec, R. T. H.: Traité de l'auscultation médiate et des maladies des poumons et du coeur. Paris. J. S. Chaudé, 1826.

Lincoln, Edith M.: The Effect of Antimicrobial Therapy on the Prognosis of Primary Tuberculosis in Children. Am. Rev. Tuberc., 69:682, 1954.

Lorber, J.: The Results of Treatment of 549 Cases of Tuberculous Meningitis. Am. Rev. Tuberc., 69: 13, 1954.

Lurie, M. B.: Native and Acquired Resistance to Tuberculosis. Am. J. Med., 9:591, 1950.

McDermott, Walsh, and others: Pyrazinamide-Isoniazid in Tuberculosis. Am. Rev. Tuberc., 69: 319, 1954.

Medical Research Council National Tuberculin Survey 1949–50, Lancet, 242:775, 1952.

Medlar, E. M.: Primary and Reinfection Tuberculosis as the Cause of Death in Adults. Am. Rev. Tuberc., 55:517, 1947; The Pathogenesis of Minimal Pulmonary Tuberculosis, ibid., 58:583, 1948.

———, Bernstein, S., and Stewart, Dorothy M.: A Bacteriologic Study of Resected Tuberculous Lesions. Am. Rev. Tuberc., 66:36, 1952.

Middlebrook, G., Dubos, R. J., and Pierce, Cynthia: Virulence and Morphologic Characteristics of Mammalian Tubercle Bacilli. J. Exper. Med., 86: 175, 1947.

Mitchell, R. S.: Late Results of the Treatment of Primary Tuberculous Pleurisy with Effusion with Modified Bed Rest. Am. Rev. Tuberc., 67:421, 1953.

Mount, Frank W., Jenkins, Barbara E., and Ferebee, Shirley H.: Control Study of Comparative Efficacy of Isoniazid, Streptomycin-Isoniazid, and Streptomycin-Para-Aminosalicylic Acid in Pulmonary Tuberculosis Therapy. IV. Report on Forty Week Observations on 583 Patients with Streptomycin-Susceptible Infections.. Am. Rev. Tuberc., 68: 264, 1953.

Progress Report on Therapeutic and Toxic Effects of Combinations of Isoniazid, Streptomycin, and Para-Aminosalicylic Acid. United States Public Health Service Cooperative Investigation of Antimicrobial Therapy of Tuberculosis, Am. Rev. Tuberc., 69:1, January, 1954.

Rich, A. R.: The Pathogenesis of Tuberculosis. Springfield, Illinois, Charles C Thomas, 1952.

Roper, W. H., and Waring, J. J.: Primary Serofibrinous Pleural Effusion. Tr. Nat. Tuberc. Assoc., 1952, p. 150.

Schatz, A., Bugie, E., and Waksman, S. A.: Streptomycin, a Substance Exhibiting Activity against Gram-Positive and Gram-Negative Bacteria. Proc. Soc. Exper. Biol. & Med., 55:66, 1944.

Seibert, Florence B., Seibert, Mabel V., Atno, A. Jane, and Campbell, H. W.: Variation in Protein and Polysaccharide Content of Serums in Chronic Diseases, Tuberculosis, Sarcoidosis and Carcinoma. J. Clin. Investigation, 26:90, 1947.

Smith, K. M.: Analysis of Tabulated Data Concerning Miliary and Meningeal Tuberculosis. Tr. Twelfth Conference on the Chemotherapy of Tuberculosis, U. S. Veterans Administration, Army, Navy, 1953, p. 146. (See also Tr. Thirteenth Conference, 1954.)

Smith, Michael, Reynolds, L. T., and Hand, M. E., Tuberculosis Among Selective Service Registrants. Am. Rev. Tuberc., 60:773, 1949.

Stein, S. C., and Aronson, J. D.: The Occurrence of Pulmonary Lesions in BCG-Vaccinated and Unvaccinated Persons. Am. Rev. Tuberc., 68:695, 1953.

Wilson, N. J., Armada, O., and Vindzberg, W. V.: Total Surgical Statistics in the Treatment of Pulmonary Tuberculosis. Am. Rev. Tuberc., 68:874, 1953.

LEPROSY

Definition. Leprosy is a chronic communicable disease with predilection for the skin and peripheral nerves. The tissue changes produced by the disease are those of an infectious granulomatous process.

History. Leprosy is undoubtedly of ancient origin, but all old records are invalidated by the collective sense in which the word "leprosy" was used. Conditions which probably included leprosy are described in the Egyptian Ebers Papyrus (c. 1350 B.C.), Vedas and Upanishads of India, Chinese writings of the time of Confucius, and in almost equally old Japanese chronicles. The account of Leviticus may have included leprosy. The disease was not known to physicians practicing in ancient Greece and was not described in the Roman Empire until the last century B.C. Spain is said to have been infected by Roman troops in the fifth and sixth centuries. Its further progress in Europe constitutes the most remarkable phase in the history of leprosy. It became widespread in northern and western Europe, reaching its height about the end of the thirteenth century.

In the nineteenth century Norway was the only northern European country in which the disease was a serious problem, and there it declined rapidly from about 1850. The Western Hemisphere probably owes its leprosy to early European colonizers and African slavers. Rapid spread occurred in the Pacific areas in the nineteenth century. About 1848 leprosy was introduced into Hawaii by the Chinese. In 1863 it reached New Caledonia and thence spread to the Loyalty Islands. Introduction into Nauru (Pleasant Island) from the Gilberts in 1912 resulted in no less than 30 per cent of the inhabitants being attacked within fifteen years.

Etiology. The leprosy bacillus (*Mycobacterium leprae*) was discovered by Hansen in 1874. It cannot be cultivated *in vitro* and does not produce disease in animals. Thus, Koch's postulates have not been fulfilled, but the constant presence of the mycobacterium in leprosy has led to the acceptance of *M. leprae* as the direct cause of the disease. It resembles *M. tuberculosis* in size, shape and staining properties.

Epidemiology. Leprosy is world-wide in prevalence, but occurs chiefly in the tropics and subtropics. The estimated world total is between three and five million cases. Areas of higher prevalence include tropical Africa, India and China; many of the Pacific islands, including Indonesia, Japan and the Philippines, but not Australia and New Zealand; the West Indies, and certain Central and South American countries. In Europe active foci remain along the Mediterranean. In the United States leprosy is indigenous only in Louisiana, Texas, Florida and Southern California, and the total number of cases is estimated at not more than 1500. The average patient population at the National Leprosarium is just under 400.

Leprosy is considered to be neither hereditary nor congenital, because removal of infants of leprous mothers immediately after birth apparently prevents infection. The disease is usually contracted in childhood, but adults may be infected. Approximately 32 United States soldiers, mostly from nonendemic states, acquired the disease during the Spanish-American War. Males are much more frequently attacked than females, especially by the lepromatous type of the disease. There is no racial immunity.

Studies in the Philippines have demonstrated that as a result of exposure to "open" cases in the household, 29 per cent of males and 14 per cent of females acquire the disease before reaching 25 years of age. Nevertheless, leprosy is much less infectious than tuberculosis. Apparently, intimate exposure is necessary. The bacilli escape from the body through abrasion or ulceration of affected cutaneous or mucous surfaces. They are commonly present in sputum and nasal discharges in patients with oral, nasal and laryngeal lesions. Though the portal of entry is unknown, it is generally considered to be either the injured skin or the mucous membranes of the nose and throat, or both. Several attempts to inoculate human volunteers through the skin have failed or had questionable results. Two cases have been reported in United States soldiers in which the first lesions were at the site of tattooing performed while on service in the Pacific during World War II. It seems unlikely that infection takes place by the gastrointestinal route or through the agency of insects. Similar diseases in animals such as so-called "rat leprosy" have no relationship to leprosy in man.

Classification. The older classification designated two clinical types: (1) *lepromatous,* nodular or cutaneous; and (2) *neural* or maculoanesthetic. A patient with lesions of both types was said to have "mixed leprosy." At Havana in 1948 the Fifth International Congress adopted a new classification based primarily on histopathology. Two polar types were recognized, *lepromatous* and *tuberculoid.* A group of cases of uncertain position and prognosis was called "indeterminate."

Pathogenesis and Morbid Anatomy. The pathogenesis of leprosy is not well understood. From some primary focus the bacilli lodge in the skin. Subsequent developments depend upon local and general resistance, which presumably vary in different persons.

Tuberculoid Type. If there is active tissue defense, but insufficient for complete healing, the *tuberculoid* type of disease follows. On the surface of the skin, major and minor tuberculoid macules are found, often with papular borders. Acid-fast bacilli are few. Round cells and macrophages are abundant. Foci of epithelioid cells are seen which frequently coalesce, forming giant cells of the Langhans type. Nerve endings in the corium show evidence of invasion, explaining the primary sensory changes in the macules. In certain cases the bacilli apparently pass up the sensory branches of the larger peripheral nerves, causing an intense cellular reaction followed by interstitial fibrosis and destruction of the fibers. Thickened nerve trunks may be surrounded by a dense fibrous sheath. Secondary polyneuritic lesions occur in the distal parts of the limbs with sensory changes, glossy skin, atrophies, contractures and trophic ulcers. The epithelioid cells is the characteristic cell of the tuberculoid type.

Lepromatous Type. When the tissue defense is less effective, the *lepromatous* type develops. The cutis and, to a lesser extent, the subcutis are filled with granulomatous masses which compress the epidermis and obliterate its papillae. These granulomas are composed of actively phagocytic macrophages, some of which become vacuolated and are known as lepra cells (foam cells, Virchow's cells). These lepra cells are frequently filled with acid-fast bacilli. Some epithelioid cells are seen, with lymphocytes and fibroblasts. In early lesions there is a characteristic clear zone between the epidermis and the granulomatous infiltration. Sometimes *M. leprae* are seen lying in cigar-shaped bundles. In advanced cases clumps of bacilli are surrounded by what appears to be capsular material (globi of Neisser). The bacilli spread to the lymphatics and blood stream, and lepromatous changes have been described in the spleen, liver and bone marrow. The larger peripheral nerves, especially the ulnar and peroneal, are invaded in nearly all advanced lepromatous cases, producing what was formerly called "mixed leprosy." Lepra cell infiltration is followed by formation of fibrous tissue, chiefly in the endoneurium, with subsequent destruction of nerve fibers. The lungs are not involved. The testicles are affected in a majority of advanced lepromatous cases, the ovaries much less frequently. The lepra cell is the characteristic cell of the lepromatous type.

Clinical Manifestations. The onset of leprosy is usually insidious and the early signs extremely variable. Consequently the duration of the incubation period is not known with preciseness. Muir considers that it averages about three and a half years and varies from a few months to five years. *In recent years much doubt has arisen regarding the extremely long incubation periods sometimes reported.* A definite nodule has been observed in a child of 19 months, and papular and flattened lesions, with epithelioid and tuberculoid structure and occasional acid-fast bacilli, have been described in children from 1 to 3 years of age exposed to their leprous parents at Culion, Philippine Islands.

Lepromatous Type. An evanescent eruption may be the first sign of lepromatous leprosy. This is followed by papules or macules which coalesce to cause a diffuse infiltration. Larger nodules appear on the thickened surfaces. The natural folds of the skin are accentuated by the infiltration. The forehead, cheeks, nose and chin change into masses of thickened folds and nodules, giving the face a "leonine" aspect (Fig. 41). The ear lobes become pendulous and nodular. The hair on the face, eyelashes and eyebrows is lost. In advanced stages practically all the surface of the body is involved except certain "protected areas," including the scalp, palms and soles, axillae and groins, antecubital, popliteal, orbital, retroauricular and interdigital spaces, and the hollow over the lumbar spine.

Mucosal leprosy involves principally the nasal, oral, pharyngeal and laryngeal surfaces. Infiltration of the nasal mucosa causes obstruction and hemorrhage and, in advanced cases, perforation and crumbling of the septum, with resulting saddle-back deformity. Laryngeal involvement may result in stenosis, requiring tracheotomy. A dry, hacking cough and huskiness of the voice point to invasion of the larynx.

The conjunctiva, cornea and uvea are often invaded. Leprous keratitis and repeated attacks of conjunctivitis and iridocyclitis lead to corneal opacities and ultimate blindness.

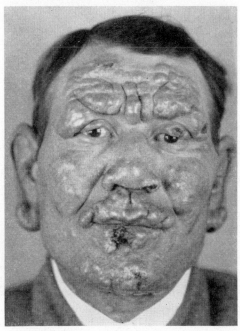

Fig. 41. Advanced lepromatous leprosy.

Tuberculoid Type. The characteristic early lesion is a macule which is slightly elevated above the level of the surrounding skin. The surface may be pebbled in appearance. As the patch enlarges, it flattens at the center, spreading with an irregular raised margin. Small "colonial" papules may appear beyond the margins. Lesions may coalesce and cover a large part of the body. The so-called "major leprides" are more sudden in their appearance, feel thicker to the fingers, and have a more erythematous appearance than the "minor leprides." Leprosy bacilli may be found in both varieties, but often are few in number. Preliminary hyperesthesia occurs followed by loss of sensation to light touch and to the pin point. Thermal sensation is also affected, the patient being unable to distinguish between test tubes filled with hot water and ice water. Anhidrosis is also an early sign. A rare type of major tuberculoid leprosy, first described in Mexico, is called "lazarine leprosy." The onset is frequently acute with fever which may last some weeks.

The lesions are widely scattered and ulcerate. Healing takes place with extensive scarring.

Neural Involvement. Secondary polyneuritic lesions are most severe in the tuberculoid type, but also occur almost always in ad-

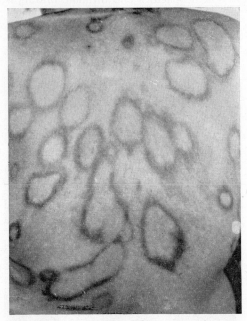

Fig. 42. Active macules of lepromatous leprosy.

vanced lepromatous leprosy (mixed leprosy). The inflammatory process in the affected nerve trunks causes marked sensory changes, anhidrosis, glossy skin, brittle nails, paralyses and wasting of muscles, perforating ulcers, and necrosis and absorption of bone with subsequent mutilations of the extremities. In the upper extremity wasting appears first in the thenar, hyperthenar and interosseous muscles, extending later to those of the forearm. The muscles of the feet and legs are similarly affected. Foot-drop is common. The classic *main en griffe,* or claw hand, results from contracture of the fingers (Fig. 43). Facial paralysis may occur, usually bilateral and limited to the upper half of the face and especially to the orbicular oculi. With complete facial paralysis, a masklike expression results. Bone absorption is confined chiefly to the small bones of the hands and feet.

Leprous Fever (Lepra Reaction). Systemic reactions with chills and intermittent or remittent fever, malaise, and protean skin eruptions occur in both lepromatous and tuberculoid types. The cause is unknown. Reactions may be severe, may last from a few days to four weeks, and tend to recur. Nodules

break down, discharging pus rich in bacilli, and new lesions appear with marked edematous swelling in surrounding areas. In reacting tuberculoid leprosy there may be ulceration of macules followed by healing with scar formation.

Lepromin Reaction. In 1916 Mitsuda injected patients and healthy persons intradermally with boiled, lepromatous tissue. A papule which sometimes ulcerated and which reached its maximum in three or four weeks constituted a positive result. In the lepromatous type the test was nearly always negative; in the tuberculoid type it was usually positive; and in normal persons it was either positive or negative. The reaction is considered to be allergic in nature, and a positive result may indicate resistance. The injection of lepromin may cause distant focal reactions.

Diagnosis. In most cases the diagnosis of leprosy is relatively simple, provided the disease is kept in mind. The whole body should be inspected in a good light. In the lepromatous type, acid-fast bacilli can always be demonstrated from skin lesions and often in scrapings from the nasal mucous membranes. In making skin smears a shallow incision is made and tissue juice free from blood is scraped from its edges for examination after staining by the Ziehl-Neelsen technique. Macules of tuberculoid leprosy show sensory disturbances, detected by use of a camel's hair brush, hot and ice water, and pin point. Biopsy sections may show acid-fast bacilli.

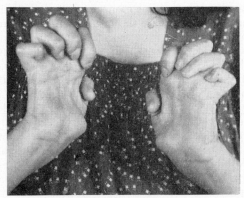

Fig. 43. Ulnar and median nerve involvement: "main en griffe," or claw hand.

Secondary polyneuritic lesions are usually accompanied by palpably enlarged and often tender peripheral nerves. In advanced cases the deformities and multilations are characteristic. Leprosy is frequently mistaken for syphilis. More than one third of the patients admitted to the National Leprosarium at Carville, Louisiana, have been treated for syphilis, in most instances erroneously. Not only may the skin lesions of the two diseases be similar, but serologic tests for syphilis are often positive in leprosy. Other diseases occasionally confused with leprosy are various forms of neuritis, ringworm, tuberculosis of the skin, yaws, Boeck's sarcoid, lupus erythematosus, von Recklinghausen's disease and syringomyelia.

The histamine test is useful in the diagnosis of leprides. The skin is punctured through a drop of 1:000 histamine phosphate. If leprous, a wheal appear without the normal hyperemia.

Prognosis. Because leprosy is a stubbornly chronic disease, the prognosis must always be guarded. The benign form of the disease does not necessarily shorten the normal span of life. Active advanced lepromatous leprosy generally reduces the life span, and death occurs from intercurrent diseases such as tuberculosis, pneumonia or nephritis. In this type of the disease, blindness occurs frequently, and where neural involvement is extensive, mutilations of the hands and feet are observed in a large number of cases.

Treatment. *Chemotherapy.* A number of chemical derivatives of diaminodiphenylsulfone, usually referred to as the sulfone drugs, have been developed in recent years as the treatment of choice in leprosy. Of these, Promin, Diasone and Sulphetrone are the ones most widely used. Leprologists who have had experience with these drugs universally uphold their therapeutic value.

Promin (sodium p,p-diaminodiphenylsulfone-N,N-didextrose sulfonate) is given intravenously in daily doses of 2 to 5 gm. Each course of two weeks' treatment (Sundays excepted) is separated by a week of rest. Rest periods seem to permit the hematopoietic system to keep pace with the hemolytic action of the drug, thus preventing or minimizing the anemia which sometimes accompanies administration of the drug. Iron salts and yeast must sometimes be given to counteract the development of anemia. In a situation where routine blood counts are not obtainable these antianemic substances should be administered routinely in the usual dosages. The intravenous administration of Promin together with the employment of rest periods seems to obviate any severe toxic reactions.

Diaminodiphenylsulfone, the "parent" sulfone, originally considered from animal experiments to be too toxic for human use, has been found to be quite safe for oral and parenteral use. Up to 200 mg. daily may be given by mouth. Subcutaneous injection of 300 mg. in pure neutral coconut oil once weekly has been found to give a satisfactory blood level. This drug has the great advantage of cheapness.

Diasone and Sulphetrone have the advantage over Promin of low toxicity by oral administration. Diasone is given in 0.3 gm. tablets from one to three times daily with meals. Sulphetrone is similarly administered, but in larger doses varying from 1 to 3 gm. To obviate possible intolerance to these drugs it is wise to begin treatment with small doses and increase to maximum doses slowly over a period of weeks. Rest periods of two weeks' duration should be instituted after each ten weeks' course of treatment. As with Promin, antianemic substances such as iron and yeast should be used routinely when routine blood counts are not done, for anemia will develop in a significant proportion of patients treated.

The results from the separate use of Promin, Diasone and Sulphetrone as far as therapeutic effects and toxicity are concerned are comparable. Combined or alternate use of the drugs remains to be evaluated by further clinical trial. There is evidence that streptomycin is of value although not superior to the sulfones.

Physical Therapy. The neural and muscular disabilities of leprosy may be limited by judicious usage of contrast baths, hot whirlpool baths, infra-red radiation, and diathermy followed by massage and passive and active motion. Painful neuritis sometimes responds to infra-red rays, diathermy or inductothermy. Ultraviolet light is helpful in the healing of resistant leprous ulcerations.

Treatment of Complications. All intercurrent diseases and complications of leprosy must be vigorously dealt with for the benefit of the patient.

The anemia of leprosy usually responds to large doses of iron and liver. Leprous ulcerations are indolent and require rest, control of secondary pyogenic infection, and stimulating applications to promote healing. Infections can be controlled by topical applications of an aqueous solution containing 200 to 1000 units of penicillin per cubic centimeter or a 5 per cent sulfathiazole ointment. At times the local therapy must be supplemented by 20,000 units of penicillin intramuscularly or

0.5 gm. of sulfadiazine orally three times a day. Balsam of Peru, cod liver oil, zinc oxide and byodine ointments are useful stimulating applications after pyogenic cutaneous infection has been eliminated.

In addition to the control of infection, trophic, plantar, foot or leg ulcers require for healing bed rest on the part of the patient, and some utilization of physical agents for stimulation of the peripheral blood circulation. The latter can be provided by the use of heat obtained from an ordinary electric light bulb installed in a wire cradle placed over the affected part.

When all else fails, the injection of 1 to 5 cc. of 6 per cent procaine around the affected nerve by means of the hypospray or with an ordinary needle and syringe generally succeeds in controlling the pain. Relief lasts from several hours to several days, after which the procedure must be repeated.

In leprous erythema nodosum, favorable results are generally obtained by the use of 0.45 gm. of antimony and potassium tartrate (tartar emetic, 1 per cent) intravenously every other day for three or four injections. Fuadin, intramuscularly, 3.5 to 5 cc. (0.22 to 0.315 gm.) daily or every other day for three or four injections, is equally effective and produces fewer undesirable toxic effects.

FREDERICK A. JOHANSEN

References

Cochrane, R. G.: Practical Textbook of Leprosy. New York, Oxford University Press, 1947.

Doull, J. A., Guinto, R. S., Rodriguez, J. N., and Bancroft, H.: The Incidence of Leprosy in Cordova and Talisay, P. I. Internat. J. Leprosy, 10: 107, 1942.

Faget, G. H., and Erickson, P. T.: Chemotherapy of Leprosy. J.A.M.A., 136:451, 1948.

Goodhue, W. J.: Leprosy in a Nineteen Months Old Child. Pub. Health Bull., 75:1916.

Hasseltine, H. E.: Leprosy in Men Who Served in United States Military Service. Internat. J. Leprosy, 8:501, 1940.

Johansen, F. A.: Benzocaine-Chaulmoogra Oil in the Treatment of Leprosy. Pub. Health Rep., 42 3005, 1927.

———: Leprosy as a Public Health Problem. Texas State J. Med., 35:629, 1940.

———: Endemic Foci of Leprosy in the State of Texas. Internat. J. Leprosy, 15:417, 1947.

———, and Erickson, P. T.: Antibiotics in the Treatment of Leprosy. Ann. New York Acad. Sci., 55:1154, 1952.

BARTONELLOSIS

(Carrión's Disease, Oroya Fever, Verruga)

Definition. Carrión's disease is a specific arthropod-borne infection caused by a minute rickettsia-like micro-organism and characterized clinically by an acute, febrile, anemic stage (Oroya fever) followed, several weeks later, by a nodular cutaneous eruption (verruga peruviana). Either of these stages may be inconspicuous or apparently absent, and for this reason the two clinical pictures were originally regarded as separate diseases.

Distribution and Epidemiology. The disease has been found chiefly in narrow valleys in the Andes Mountains at altitudes between 2000 and 9000 feet. It has been largely confined to Peru, with a few cases in Ecuador and Bolivia, but in 1939 a serious outbreak was reported in Columbia, suggesting that the distribution may be more widespread than has been supposed. The distribution of the disease corresponds in general to the habitat of its probable sandfly vectors, *Phlebotomus noguchii* and *P. verrucorum*, but in Colombia lice and ticks have been suggested as vectors. Many natives of the infected areas have asymptomatic infections, revealed only by blood culture. Severe epidemics in Peru have often been associated with the importation of railroad workers from noninfected regions. A reservoir for the infection in lower animals has been suspected but not found.

Etiology. The etiologic agent was first seen in the erythrocytes in the anemic form of the disease by Barton in 1909, and was named *Bartonella bacilliformis* by Strong and his co-workers in 1915. It was cultivated in Noguchi's leptospira medium by Noguchi and Battistini in 1926. Noguchi's original evidence of the etiologic identity of Oroya fever and verruga peruviana was further confirmed by new methods of approach by the Harvard 1937 Expedition to Peru, and the unity of the two conditions must be considered as established.

Rats, dogs and a number of other mammals suffer from latent bartonella infections, which, after splenectomy, evolve into a severe anemia comparable to Oroya fever. Cutaneous lesions apparently do not occur in lower animals. Except for the transmission of human bartonella infection to monkeys, each species of bartonella appears to be completely specific for the species of animals from which it is recovered.

Morbid Anatomy. Postmortem studies of fatal cases of the anemic form of the disease show pallor, enlargement of the spleen and lymph nodes, and a megaloblastic hyperplasia of the bone marrow. The endothelial cells lining small vessels in the lymph nodes, spleen, liver, bone marrow, adrenals, kidneys and many other organs are packed with small bacillary and coccoid organisms (bartonellae), often occurring in clusters. Organisms are also present in the erythrocytes. Cutaneous nodules are rarely seen at autopsy, since they commonly do not appear until convalescence from the anemic phase is well established. Microscopically, the cutaneous nodules have the appearance of rapidly growing capillary hemangiomas. Bartonellae may be demonstrated within the endothelial cells with suitable technique.

Symptoms and Course of the Disease. *Anemic Form (Oroya Fever).* The incubation period is believed to be fourteen to twenty-one days. In severe cases the onset is sudden, with intermittent fever ranging to 104° F., progressive pallor, emaciation, prostration, rapid pulse and dyspnea. Muscle and joint pains, headache and insomnia are also common symptoms, and delirium and coma are apt to be terminal manifestations. A petechial cutaneous eruption occasionally appears during the febrile period. The erythrocyte count may fall from normal to less than 1,000,000 per cubic millimeter in four or five days, more rapidly than in any other condition exclusive of actual hemorrhage. Examination of alcohol-fixed Giemsa-stained blood films shows bartonellae in the erythrocytes in large numbers, 90 per cent of the cells frequently containing from one to fifty or more organisms. Many reticulocytes and nucleated erythrocytes are present in the blood. In the severe form of the disease the mortality is 90 to 95 per cent. Secondary infection, particularly with organisms of the salmonella group, has been emphasized as an important factor in fatal cases. The average duration of this anemic stage of the disease is from one to three weeks; occasionally the condition of the patient remains critical for a period of eight to ten weeks. Convalescence is accompanied by a disappearance of the organisms from the erythrocytes and rapid blood regeneration, but blood cultures may be positive

for many months after apparent recovery. Reliable evidence indicates that most, if not all, of the patients who recover from this febrile anemic stage have cutaneous nodules (verrugas) during or even after apparently complete convalescence.

Cutaneous Form (Verruga Peruviana). This form of the disease, characterized by cherry-red hemangioma-like cutaneous nodules, may follow the severe anemic form, or may occur in patients who have had no

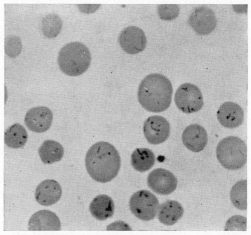

Fig. 44. Carrión's disease. Giemsa-stained blood films showing *Bartonella bacilliformis* in erythrocytes. Both bacillary and coccoid forms are seen.

previous symptoms. Intermediate cases are also frequently seen, in which there is moderate anemia, with rare bartonellae in the erythrocytes, slight or no fever, and only a few days of malaise, followed, weeks or months later, by the typical cutaneous eruption. The appearance of the cutaneous nodules may be immediately preceded by a few days of moderate fever with joint pains.

The cutaneous nodules (verrugas) are commonly 2 to 10 mm. in greatest diameter, but range up to 3 or 4 cm. They may be single or extremely numerous. These are most numerous on the head, hands, feet and lower arms and legs, and are rare on the thighs, abdomen or lower chest. Occasionally they are seen in large numbers on the mucous membrane of the mouth and pharynx. They are ovoid or spherical and usually half buried in the subcutaneous tissue and covered with thin bluish epidermis, which often breaks down, leading to ulceration and secondary infection. Healing occurs with little or no cicatrization, after a period of several weeks.

The cutaneous stage has no mortality *per se*. The possible complications are hemorrhage and local secondary infection, neither of which is apt to be serious.

Diagnosis. The diagnosis is made from a history of residence in an infected area and on the clinical pictures. Finding bartonellae in the erythrocytes in blood films establishes the diagnosis in the anemic stage. In the cutaneous stage a nodule may be excised, and bartonellae may be demonstrated in the endothelial cells. Blood cultures in Leptospira medium are positive in both stage. Rarely, the cutaneous nodules may appear a year or more after an uneventful visit to an infected area. Yaws, which may simulate verruga peruviana, can be differentiated by the demonstration of the specific organism.

The hematologic features of the disease, which are of particular interest, may be summarized briefly as follows. The anemia is of the macrocytic type, and the color index may be greater than one. The erythrocytes increase in both volume and hemoglobin content, but, since the increase in volume is proportionally greater, the anemia is classified as hypochromic. Anisocytosis, poikilocytosis and polychromatophilia are constantly present. Normoblasts are numerous, and megaloblasts are usually present. Reticulocytes may constitute more than 50 per cent of the erythrocytes. The leukocyte count is variable, but often high, and many immature forms are usually seen. The plasma volume is increased.

The blood bilirubin is usually moderately increased, but neither hemoglobinemia nor hemoglobinuria is present, even in the severely anemic cases.

Treatment. Recent evidence indicates that penicillin, streptomycin and chloramphenicol are all effective, causing disappearance of fever within 48 hours in most cases of the anemic form of the disease. The bartonellae disappear from the blood in a few days, but the cutaneous manifestations may not be prevented. The choice of an antimicrobial drug should depend on the presence of secondary bacterial infection, the reaction of the patient to the drug first chosen, and the effectiveness of the agent first used in causing bartonellae to disappear from the erythrocytes, as determined by Giemsa-stained blood films. Previous to disappearance, the organisms react by becoming coccoid rather than bacillary. Chloramphenicol may be given orally: 4 gm. the first day and 3 or 4 gm. daily thereafter, until a total of at least 20 gm. has been given. The recommended dose of penicillin is 200,000 units daily for ten days. The tetracycline drugs (Aureomycin and Terramycin) are effective in the related murine bartonellosis, but data concerning their use in man are not available. Transfusions may be given when indicated, and control of the electrolyte balance may be desirable in severely ill patients. Iron should be given during convalescence.

The cutaneous stage rarely requires treatment except for general cleanliness. Excision of large, necrotic, secondarily infected nodules occasionally may be indicated, but probably does not improve the final cosmetic result.

Prevention. Fine mesh screening (25 to 30 squares per inch) and DDT are most effective against the sandfly. These measures are most important during the night, when sandflies are active. The possibility of other insect vectors in Colombia has been mentioned.

HENRY PINKERTON

References

Barton, A. L.: Cron. Med. Lima, 26:7, 1909.
Hurtado, A., Pons, J., and Merino, C.: La Anemia de la Enfermedad de Carrion. Publication of the Faculty of Medical Sciences. Lima, Peru, 1938.
Noguchi, H., and Battistini, T. S.: Etiology of Oroya Fever. J. Exper. Med., 43:851, 1926.
Patino Camargo, L.: Estado Actual de la Bartonellosis (Fiebre Verrucosa, Verruga) en el Continente Americano. Rev. Fac. de Med. Bogota, 9:160, 1940.
Pinkerton, H., Weinman, D., and Hertig, H.: Carrión's Disease. Proc. Soc. Exper. Biol. & Med., 37:587, 1937.
Stanton, M. F., Laskowski, L., and Pinkerton, H.: Chemoprophylactic Effectiveness of Aureomycin and Terramycin in Murine Bartonellosis. Proc. Soc. Exper. Biol. & Med., 74:705, 1950.
Weiman, D.: Infectious Anemias Due to Bartonella and Related Parasites. Trans. Am. Philosoph. Soc., 33:243, 1944.
———: Bartonella Disease, in Kyser, F. A.: Therapeutics in Internal Medicine. New York, Paul B. Hoeber, 1953, p. 152.

THE MYCOSES

ACTINOMYCOSIS

Definition. Actinomycosis is a chronic granulomatous infection caused by several species of the genus *Actinomyces*. The disease is characterized by the development of numerous abscesses which break down and develop multiple sinuses. In the walls of the sinuses and in the discharge are found either the characteristic "sulfur granule" with its clubbed ends or small tangled masses of gram-positive branching filaments which may or may not be partially acid-fast.

History. In 1877 Bollinger found the ray fungus in a disease of cattle known as "lumpy jaw"; it was named *Actinomyces bovis* by Harz. J. Israel, in 1878, discovered the disease in man and pointed out the identity of the two infections. Lord, 1910, demonstrated that *Actinomyces* pathogenic for guinea pigs could be found in the gums and tonsils of apparently normal persons.

Etiology. Actinomycosis is widely disseminated and is the most common of the highly fatal mycoses. The disease occurs most frequently in males.

Mycology. The organism occurs in pus or tissues as lobulated or spherical granules, which vary in size from minute particles to forms about 1 mm. in diameter. Pure cultures are readily obtained from material aspirated from unopened abscesses, but isolation is difficult from draining sinuses because of the overgrowth from contaminating bacteria. *Actinomyces bovis* is anaerobic and grows best at 37° C. in glucose agar in a zone 5 to 10 mm. below the surface.

Nocardia asteroides (*Streptothrix asteroides,* atypical *Actinomyces,* or *Cladothrix*) is aerobic and grows on ordinary laboratory media at room and incubator temperatures. The colonies are chromogenic and have the consistency of tubercle bacilli. The granules are less compact than those of the true sulfur granule of *Actinomyces bovis*. The filaments are gram-positive, frequently show branching, and are more or less acid-fast. True club formation is absent, but club-shaped swelling of the terminal portion of the filaments may be observed. Pure cultures of some strains produce a rapidly fatal disease in guinea pigs in ten to twenty days.

Immunology. Not much is known about the serologic reactions of patients with actinomycosis.

Pathology. Actinomycosis may develop in any part of the body. A granulomatous lesion is produced which is surrounded and intersected by new connective tissue. The local lesions spread by direct extension through the connective tissue rather than by way of the lymphatics, although metastatic lesions appear in various parts of the body as a result of showers of infected emboli.

Clinical Manifestations. The clinical symptoms vary somewhat, depending upon the part of the body involved.

Cervicofacial actinomycosis accounts for more than 50 per cent of all instances of the disease. Infection takes place through the mucous membranes of the gums, mouth, pharynx or larynx. The whole infected area becomes indurated or "wooden" in consistency, and extends beyond the apparent area of inflammation. The overlying skin has a dark red or purplish color and a lumpy, uneven surface. As the infection spreads to the surface, multiple sinus tracts appear. With internal extension, the bones of the skull and even the meninges and brain may be involved. Trismus develops when the muscles of mastication are involved and dyspnea when there is pressure on the larynx. The lymph nodes of the neck usually are not involved. Pain is not a prominent feature, and the patient's general health is not much affected so long as the disease remains localized in the area of the face and neck.

Thoracic actinomycosis occurs in about 15 per cent of the cases and produces cough, sputum, increasing dyspnea, slight fever, loss of weight and strength, night sweats, pallor and emaciation. The sputum contains blood in about half the cases, and sometimes a fatal hemoptysis occurs. Pleural pain is common, and effusions not infrequent. After the disease has reached the pleura it usually involves the thoracic wall, extends through the subcutaneous tissues and produces localized areas of induration with suppurating foci and multiple sinus formation. There may be extension to the mediastinum, esophagus and pericardium.

Abdominal actinomycosis is found in 20 to 30 per cent of the cases and represents a highly fatal form of the disease. The earliest signs are usually in the ileocecal region and are associated with the development of an indistinct, irregular mass which is not painful as a rule and shows no characteristic features. This may be the first manifestation of the disease, or it may be preceded or accompanied by fever, chills, night sweats, intestinal colic and vomiting. As the disease progresses there is usually involvement of the liver and spleen, and symptoms of cystitis and pyelonephritis may appear. Jaundice may be present. Involvement of the central nervous system may occur in the terminal stages.

Actinomycotic mycetoma is occasionally encountered and usually is caused by *Nocardia asteroides*. (See Maduromycosis.)

Diagnosis. The diagnosis is based on the clinical syndrome, the finding of the sulfur granule in the exudate or lesion, or the cultivation of the organism. Biopsies of the sinus tract should be made when direct examination of the exudate fails to show granules. Frequent and repeated study of the exudate, both in fresh preparations and with the Gram stain, is imperative. Cultures are reliable in the yeastlike mycoses but not in actinomycosis. The cervicofacial forms must be differentiated from glanders, tularemia, tuberculosis and osteomyelitis. The pulmonary form simulates tuberculosis, pulmonary abscess, tularemia and other mycoses. The abdominal form may be mistaken for chronic appendicitis, amebiasis, typhoid fever, carcinoma of the intestines, tuberculosis, liver abscess, psoas abscess and sarcoma of the retroperitoneal tissue or of the iliac bones.

Prognosis. The prognosis is best in the localized skin and cervicofacial types, and becomes progressively worse with the thoracic, abdominal, generalized and neurologic types.

Treatment. The general resistance of the patient should be supported, as in tuberculosis, by rest in bed and good food, supplemented by vitamins and fruit juices. The cervicofacial form should be treated by surgical drainage, potassium iodide by mouth, and by sulfonamides. Potassium iodide should be administered by the method prescribed for blastomycosis.

Sulfonamides and penicillin have been used with some success in actinomycosis. The best therapy is the combination of sulfonamides or penicillin with iodides and radical surgery. This treatment offers the only hope for abdominal and generalized infections and should be continued for three to five months. Repeated surgical intervention may be required.

DAVID T. SMITH

References

Benbow, E. P., Jr., Smith, D. T., and Grimson, K. S.: Sulfonamide Therapy in Actinomycosis. Am. Rev. Tuberc., 49:395, 1944.

Brett, M. S.: Advanced Actinomycosis of the Spine Treated with Penicillin and Streptomycin. J. Bone & Joint Surg., 33B:215, 1951.

Conant, N. F., and others: Manual of Clinical Mycology. 2nd ed. Philadelphia, W. B. Saunders Company, 1954.

Cope, V. Z.: Actinomycosis of Bone with Special Reference to Infection of the Vertebral Column. J. Bone & Joint Surg., 33C:205, 1951.

Cruz, P. T., and Clancy, C. F.:: Nocardosis. Nocardial Osteomyelitis and Septicemia. Am. J. Path., 28:607, 1952.

Emmons, C. W.: Strains of Actinomyces Bovis Isolated from Tonsils. Puerto Rico J. Pub. Health & Trop. Med., 11:720, 1936.

Holm, P.: Studies on the Aetiology of Human Actinomycosis. I. The "Other Microbes" of Actinomycosis and Their Importance. Acta. Path. et Microbiol. Scandinav., 27:736, 1950.

Jacobson, J. R., and Cloward, R. B.: Actinomycosis of the Central Nervous System. J.A.M.A., 137: 769, 1948.

Lane, S. L., Kutscher, A. H., and Chavee, R.: Oxytetracycline (Terramycin) in the Treatment of Orocervical Facial Actinomycosis. Report of Seven Cases. J.A.M.A., 151:986, 1953.

Lord, F. T., and Trevett, L. D.: The Pathogenesis of Actinomycosis. Recovery of Actinomyces-like Organisms from the Normal Mouth. J. Infect. Dis., 58:115, 1936.

McVay, L. V., Jr., and Sprunt, D. H.: A Long Term Evaluation of Aureomycin in the Treatment of Actinomycosis. Ann. Int. Med., 38:955, 1953.

Strauss, R. E., Kligman, A. M., and Pillsbury, D. M.: The Chemotherapy of Actinomycosis and Nocardosis. Am. Rev. Tuberc., 63:441, 1951.

Weed, L. A., and Baggenstoss, A. H.: Actinomycosis. Am. J. Clin. Path., 19:201, 1949.

Wolff, F. M., and Israel, J.: Ueber Reincultur des Actinomyces und seine Uebertragbarkeit auf Thiere. Arch. f. path. Anat. u. Physiol., 126:11, 1891.

BLASTOMYCOSIS

Definition. Blastomycosis is a chronic granulomatous disease which may be confined either to the skin or lungs or disseminated throughout the body.

History. The disease was first described by Gilchrist in 1894 and by Gilchrist and Stokes in 1896. It is found frequently throughout the western hemisphere, but only sporadically in Europe, and is usually called American blastomycosis or Gilchrist's disease and should not be confused with European "blastomycosis," which is caused by *Cryptococcus neoformans* (*Torula histolytica*).

Etiology. Blastomycosis is prevalent in the Chicago area, Louisiana, Tennessee, North Carolina and other parts of the country. The disease is nine times as frequent in males as in females.

Mycology. The morphologic studies of Conant and the serologic investigations of Martin show that all strains of *Blastomyces dermatitidis* are morphologically and antigenically identical. Sputum, pus or biopsy material should be streaked heavily on Sabouraud's slants and on blood agar plates. The slants are kept at room temperature, but the blood agar plates should be incubated at 37° C. The primary growth may be slow, and cultures should be watched for two or three weeks. On blood agar the colonies are small, waxy and wrinkled and, when emulsified in water and examined fresh under the microscope, show typical budding, double-contoured yeastlike forms (7 to 10 microns) identical in appearance with those found in the lesions.

Immunology. Many patients acquire a sensitivity to the products of *B. dermatitidis* and give a skin test analogous to the tuberculin reaction. Martin found that patients with extensive involvement usually show a positive complement fixation when the whole yeast organism or certain of its extracts are used as the antigen. The test is negative when the lesions are small or well localized and becomes negative in the systemic cases after recovery.

Pathology. The primary skin lesions may be of a superficial verrucous type with little ulceration, or gummatous with open craters. The multiple subcutaneous abscesses found in the systemic type of blastomycosis are analogous to cold abscesses in tuberculosis. When the disease spreads from the skin, bones or other organs to the lungs, it produces the appearance in the roentgenogram, and at necropsy, of a miliary hematogenous tuberculosis.

The characteristic budding organisms are found in the giant cells, in the granulation tissue between the cells and about the edges of the necrotic areas.

Clinical Manifestations. *Cutaneous blastomycosis* occurs most frequently on the face, neck or extremities. The primary lesion usually begins as a small reddish papule or papular pustule which slowly increases in size and is soon capped with a crust. There is epithelial hyperplasia, giving the lesion a verrucous appearance. Minute epidermal abscesses appear about the edges of the lesions, and some lesions break down to form deep, crater-like ulcers with hard, raised edges. The subjective symptoms are mild, pain is minimal, and the patches are not sensitive to pressure. The regional lymph nodes usually are not enlarged, and the general health of the patient is not impaired so long as the disease is confined to the skin.

Systemic Blastomycosis. Patients with primary pulmonary blastomycosis have fever, night sweats, loss of weight, cough, sputum which is frequently bloody, leukocytosis, increased erythrocyte sedimentation rate and physical and roentgenographic evidence of extensive pulmonary disease. The lesion usually is incorrectly diagnosed as pulmonary tuberculosis, but it may be mistaken for primary bronchogenic carcinoma. Sinus formation is rare as long as the disease is confined to the lungs, but in the systemic cases, in which there are multiple lesions of the bones and involvement of the internal organs, it is frequent and characteristic.

Diagnosis. Cutaneous blastomycosis is readily diagnosed by its characteristic lesions, but the diagnosis should be confirmed by finding the organisms in the pus expressed from the small abscesses in the edge of the lesion, by culture or by biopsy. In the systemic form the organisms can usually be grown from the sputum or from pus aspirated from a subcutaneous lesion. A positive complement fixation reaction is diagnostic, but a negative result does not eliminate the possibility of the disease.

Prognosis. The prognosis is good in cutaneous blastomycosis, but poor for the pulmonary and systemic forms of the disease. Martin and Smith found that 92 per cent of the patients with the generalized form of the disease had died within two years. The prognosis in the pulmonary form can be improved by early diagnosis and prompt and adequate treatment.

Treatment. The introduction of stilbamidine and 2-hydroxystilbamidine has revolutionized the therapy of blastomycosis. Most of the previously incurable systemic infections can be cured and the response of the other types is more rapid than with the older vaccine-iodide regimen. Stilbamidine is the more potent but also the more toxic of the two drugs. Most systemic cases can be cured with maximum daily doses of 150 mg. a day for thirty days or with alternate periods of ten days of treatment and ten days of rest until the total dose of 4.5 to 6 gm. has been administered. The dose of 150 mg. should be diluted in 300 ml. of physiologic saline or in 5 per cent glucose in distilled water and administered intravenously over a 3-hour period. The drug should be protected from daylight both during preparation and during administration to prevent the development of toxic degeneration products. Most patients develop mild to severe symptoms of numbness and paresthesia of the face in three to six months after treatment has been discontinued. These symptoms usually disappear after a few months or a few years.

The hydroxystilbamidine is somewhat more stable and rarely produces facial neuropathy; the standard daily dose is 225 mg., the total dose 8 to 12 gm. and the period of treatment two to four months. Perhaps patients with cutaneous and other forms of localized infections should be treated with hydroxystilbamidine and the more severe generalized infections with stilbamidine.

Cutaneous blastomycosis usually responds satisfactorily to local x-ray therapy when given simultaneously with potassium iodide, and subsequently to desensitization of the sensitive patient. Many patients with pulmonary blastomycosis and a few with systemic infections have been cured with this therapy. If the patient is sensitive to a stock or autogenous vaccine, he should be desensitized by the injection of gradually increasing amounts of the vaccine at 48- to 72-hour intervals for ten to fifteen doses before potassium iodide is given. Both the nonsensitive patient and the desensitized patient should receive an initial dose of 3 drops three times a day of a saturated solution of potassium iodide after meals. The dose should be increased by 3 drops each day up to 30 to 40 drops three times a day. As much as 300 to 400 drops have been given in a single day. Sensitivity to iodides may develop and necessitate the discontinuance of the drug. After a rest period of seven to ten days it should be tried again.

DAVID T. SMITH

References

Baker, R. D.: Tissue Changes in Fungous Disease. Arch. Path., 44:459, 1947.

Baylin, G. J., and Wear, J. M.: Blastomycosis and Actinomycosis of the Spine. Am. J. Roentgenol., 69:395, 1953.

Conant, N. F., and others: Manual of Clinical Mycology. 2nd ed. Philadelphia, W. B. Saunders Company, 1954.

Gilchrist, T. C.: A Case of Blastomycetic Dermatitis in Man. Rep. Johns Hopkins Hosp., 1:269, 1896.

Martin, D. S.: Serologic Studies on North American Blastomycosis. J. Immunol., 71:192, 1953.

———, and Smith, D. T.: Blastomycosis (American Blastomycosis, Gilchrist's Disease). I. A Review of the Literature. II. A Report of Thirteen New Cases. Am. Rev. Tuberc., 39:275, 488, 1939.

Schoenbach, E. B., Miller, J. M., and Long, P. H.: The Treatment of Systemic Blastomycosis with Stilbamidine. Ann. Int. Med., 37:31, 1952.

Smith, D. T.: Immunologic Types of Blastomycosis: A Report on 40 Cases. Ann. Int. Med., 31:463, 1949.

———: Stilbamidine Therapy for Blastomycosis. General Practice, 8:69, 1953.

Snapper, I., and McVay, L. V., Jr.: The Treatment of North American Blastomycosis with 2-hydroxystilbamidine. Am. J. Med., 15:603, 1953.

GEOTRICHOSIS

The bronchi and lungs and occasionally the mouth and intestinal tract may be attacked by one or more species of the genus *Geotrichum*. The oral lesions resemble those of thrush, and the pulmonary infection simulates blastomycosis. Usually the patient has symptoms of bronchitis or of a rather mild but chronic type of bronchopneumonia. In the more severe forms of the disease, blood may be present in the sputum and cavities develop in the lungs. The *Geotrichum* is frequently a secondary invader in chronic Friedländer's bacillus infection of the lungs and occasionally in tuberculosis.

Mycology. The organism grows readily on Sabouraud's medium at room temperature and at 37° C. There is a budding form of *Geotrichum* which is readily confused with the budding form of *Blastomyces,* but this budding form is always accompanied by the rectangular conidia which are characteristic of the genus.

Treatment. The oral lesions respond to the gentian violet treatment described for *Candida albicans.* The intestinal form should receive oral doses of gentian violet in salol-coated capsules in doses of 32 mg. three times a day. The bronchial and pulmonary forms have a good prognosis when given the treatment described for blastomycosis.

DAVID T. SMITH

References

Bendove, R. A., and Ashe, B. I.: Geotrichum Septicemia. Arch. Int. Med., 89:107, 1952.

Conant, N. F., and others: Manual of Clinical Mycology. 2nd ed. Philadelphia, W. B. Saunders Company, 1954.

Kunstadler, R. H., Milzer, A., and Whitcomb, F.: Bronchopulmonary Geotrichosis in Children. Am. J. Dis. Child., 79:82, 1950.

Smith, D. T.: Oidiomycosis of the Lungs. J. Thoracic Surg., 3:241, 1934.

COCCIDIOIDOMYCOSIS

Definition. Primary coccidioidomycosis is an acute infection with a good prognosis, but may develop into progressive coccidioidomycosis, which is a generalized, granulomatous disease with a high mortality.

History. Posadas and Wernicke recognized the disease in Buenos Aires in 1892. Rixford reported a case from California in 1894, and Rixford and Gilchrist studied a series of cases in 1896. In 1900 Ophüls and Moffitt cultivated the organism and demonstrated that it was a fungus and not a protozoan.

Incidence. The disease is encountered most frequently in southern California, but may be found anywhere in the Southwest and appears to be spreading eastward. Thousands of soldiers in Army camps in the Southwest contracted the benign primary infection, and a few of them are now developing severe granulomatous disease five to eight years after the initial infection. The disease occurs at all ages from 3 months to 70 years, but is most prevalent between the ages of 25 and 55. In one series of 211 cases 83 per cent were in males.

Etiology. The causative agent is *Coccidioides immitis*. Emmons has shown that the organism is present in rodents in the endemic area, and Davis, Smith and Smith isolated the fungus from the soil. The organism may be introduced into man through a scratch or abrasion of the skin, although the more usual method is inhalation, which produces an atypical type of bronchopneumonia. The disease is not transmitted directly from man to man, but laboratory infections occur frequently from the accidental inhalation of arthrospores from cultures.

Mycology. *Coccidioides immitis* multiplies in the tissues by endosporulation. The organism is a spherule with a thick hyaline capsule, varies from 11 to 70 microns in diameter, and contains from 10 to 200 endospores. When infected tissues, sputum or other discharges are planted on Sabouraud's medium, the endospores germinate and grow out as mycelia.

Immunology. All strains of *C. immitis* apparently contain identical antigens. During the course of the primary infection the patient exhibits precipitins and complement-fixing antibodies and the skin becomes sensitive to coccidioidin. The precipitins and complement-fixing antibodies slowly disappear after recovery, but the skin sensitivity, like that to tuberculin, is relatively permanent.

Pathology. In chronic coccidioidomycosis the organisms are surrounded by epithelial cells, giant cells, lymphocytes and plasma cells. Abscess formation is more frequent than in tuberculosis, especially in the bones and subcutaneous tissues. Abbott and Cutler decribed three types of meningeal lesions: one is practically identical with tuberculous meningitis, a second has larger, more granulomatous lesions, and the third shows a thick accumulation of plastic exudate.

Clinical Manifestations. In some areas in the Southwest, positive skin tests with coccidioidin have been found in 50 to 84 per cent of the population, indicating that primary infection with *C. immitis* is common but usually asymptomatic. When the reaction to infection is severe enough to be recognized as a disease, the symptoms, signs, roentgenographic changes and course of the disease parallel that of primary tuberculous infection. The patients have malaise, anorexia, chills, fever, headache, backache, night sweats and pleurisy. The cough produces a scant amount of mucoid or mucopurulent sputum which contains the characteristic spherules of *C. immitis*. The organisms have been found in pleural fluid. Roentgenograms of the lungs may show thickening of the hilar region, peribronchial thickening or patches of nodular or bronchial pneumonitis. The larger, more solid lesions may break down and leave thin walled cavities which usually heal in a few weeks or months, but may persist for years. Sensitivity to coccidioidin appears after seven to fourteen days, and skin lesions resembling those of erythema nodosum or erythema multiforme develop in 20 per cent between the fifth and fourteenth days of the disease and persist for one to four weeks. This form of the disease has been known for years as "Valley fever," "Desert fever," "San Joaquin fever" or "the bumps."

Although recovery is usually rapid and complete, an occasional case passes into the progressive virulent type of the disease with involvement of bones, subcutaneous tissues and internal organs, including the brain.

Sometimes the organism gains entrance through the skin or possibly through the tonsils. Lesions of the cervical lymph nodes have been described which simulate those of tuberculous adenitis.

Diagnosis. One should suspect coccidioidomycosis in any obscure disease originating in a native of the endemic area and in persons who have visited such areas. *Coccidioides immitis* can be found in the sputum in the primary infection. In the progressive type the organisms are present in the sputum, in the subcutaneous abscesses and in the lesions of the internal organs. In progressive coccidioidomycosis there is a steady increase in the complement-fixing antibodies, while the skin sensitivity decreases or disappears.

Coccidioidomycosis must be differentiated from tuberculosis, syphilis, glanders, bacterial osteomyelitis, epithelioma and other mycoses.

Prognosis. The prognosis is excellent in primary pulmonary involvement, good in the dermal and lymph node types of the disease when they are a part of the primary infection, but most grave in the generalized and meningitic types.

Treatment. Most primary pulmonary infections heal rapidly in a few weeks without specific treatment. The primary cases which have persistent, thin-walled cavities present a difficult problem. If symptoms persist for more than six months, the infected area should be removed by segmental lobectomy.

The chronic generalized type of disease is difficult to treat. All the old drugs and many new ones have been tried without success. Some recoveries have been reported following the administration of actidione, ethyl vanillate, prodigiosin and 2-hydroxystilbamidine. Potassium iodide and vaccine therapy have been disappointing. Coccidioidin injections may serve to reduce the patient's sensitivity.

DAVID T. SMITH

References

Bass, H. E., Schomer, A., and Berke, R.: Question of Contagion in Coccidioidomycosis. Study of Contacts. Am. Rev. Tuberc., 59:632, 1949.

Buss, W. C., Gibson, T. E., and Gifford, M. A.: Coccidioidomycosis of the Meninges. Calif. Med., 72: 167, 1950.

Butt, E. M., and Hoffman, A. M.: Healed or Arrested Pulmonary Coccidioidomycosis. Am. J. Path., 21:485, 1945.

Clark, D., and Gilmore, J. H.: Study of 100 Cases with Positive Coccidioidin Skin Test. Ann. Int. Med., 24:40, 1946.

Conant, N. F., and others: Manual of Clinical Mycology. 2nd ed. Philadelphia, W. B. Saunders Company, 1954.

Cotton, B. H., and Birsner, J. W.: Surgical Treatment in Pulmonary Coccidioidomycosis. Preliminary Report of 30 Cases. J. Thoracic Surg., 20: 429, 1950.

Davis, B. L., Jr., Smith, R. T., and Smith, C. E.: Epidemic of Coccidioidal Infection (Coccidioidomycosis). J.A.M.A., 118:1182, 1942.

Emmons, C. W., and Ashburn, L. L.: The Isolation of *Haplosporangium parvum* N. Sp. and Coccidioides Immitis from Wild Rodents. Their Relationship to Coccidioidomycosis. Pub. Health Rep., 57:1715, 1942.

Forbus, W. D.: Coccidioidomycosis; A Study of 95 Cases of the Disseminated Type with Special Reference to the Pathogenesis of the Disease. Mil. Surgeon, 99:654, 1946.

Goldstein, D. M., and McDonald, J. B.: Primary Pulmonary Coccidioidomycosis. J.A.M.A., 124:557, 1944.

Kessel, J. F.: The Coccidioidin Skin Test. Am. J. Trop. Med., 19:199, 1939.

Rixford, E., and Gilchrist, T. C.: Two Cases of Protozoan (Coccidioidal) Infection of the Skin. Rep. Johns Hopkins Hosp., 1:209, 1896.

Smith, C. E., Beard, R. R., and Saito, M. T.: Pathogenesis of Coccidioidomycosis with Special Reference to Pulmonary Cavitation. Ann. Int. Med., 29:623, 1948.

Smith, C. E., and others: Histoplasmin Sensitivity and Coccidioidal Infection. 1. Occurrence of Cross-Reactions. Am. J. Pub. Health, 39:1949.

Smith, C. E., and associates: Serological Tests in the Diagnosis and Prognosis of Coccidioidomycosis. Am. J. Hyg., 52:1, 1950.

Smith, D. T., and Harrell, E. R., Jr.: Fatal Coccidioidomycosis; A Case of Laboratory Infection. Am. Rev. Tuberc., 57:368, 1948.

Taylor, A. B., and Briney, A. K.: Observations on Primary Coccidioidomycosis. Ann. Int. Med., 30: 1224, 1949.

Winn, W. A.: Pulmonary Mycoses, Coccidioidomycosis and Pulmonary Cavitation. Study of 92 Cases. Arch. Int. Med., 87:541, 1951.

SOUTH AMERICAN BLASTOMYCOSIS

South American blastomycosis is a chronic granulomatous disease quite similar in its clinical course to coccidioidomycosis.

At present the disease is confined to South America, where De Almeida has collected the reports of 255 cases. The portal of entry is frequently in the area about the mouth, and there is ulceration of the intestinal tract, and adenopathy severe enough to suggest Hodgkin's disease.

The organism is found in the tissues as a large (10 to 30 microns), round, doubly contoured form with multiple small buds about the periphery which were originally mistaken for endospores. It grows readily on Sabouraud's medium and on blood agar. Conant found that the method of growth and budding on blood agar was more like that of *Blastomyces dermatitidis* than of *Coccidioides immitis*.

The disease is usually fatal.

Sulfadiazine in daily doses of 2 to 4 gm. results in dramatic temporary improvement. Stilbamidine and 2-hydroxystilbamidine may prove to be useful in the treatment of this disease.

DAVID T. SMITH

References

Almeida, F. de: *Blastomyces* e Paracoccidioides. An. Fac. de ed. da Univ. de São Paulo, 22:61, 1946.

Conant, N. F., and others: Manual of Clinical Mycology. 2nd ed. Philadelphia, W. B. Saunders Company, 1954.

Conant, N. F., and Howell, A.: The Similarity of the Fungi Causing South American Blastomycosis (Paracoccidioidal Granuloma) and North American Blastomycosis (Gilchrist's Disease). I. Invest. Dermat., 5:353, 1942.

Jordon, J. W., and Weidman, F. D.: Coccidioidal Granuloma: Comparison of the North and South American Diseases with Special Reference to Paracoccidioides Brasiliensis. Arch. Dermat. & Syph., 33:31, 1936.

Versiani, O., and Bogliolo, L.: Lutz's Disease (South American Blastomycosis). Proceedings of the Fourth International Congress on Tropical Medicine and Malaria, Washington, D. C., May 10–18, 1948.

CRYPTOCOCCOSIS
(*Torulosis*)

Definition. Cryptococcosis is a subacute or chronic, highly fatal infection which may involve any part of the body, but has a marked predilection for the brain and meninges.

History. In 1894 Busse and Buschke isolated from a fatal case, with multiple lesions of skin and viscera, a yeastlike organism which they called *Saccharomyces*, but which has now been definitely identified as *Cryptococcus neoformans* (*Torula histolytica*). This disease is called "blastomycosis" in the European literature and "European blastomycosis" in America, to distinguish it from American blastomycosis, or Gilchrist's disease, which is caused by *Blastomyces dermatitidis*.

Etiology. Cryptococcosis occurs in all parts of this country and in scattered areas throughout the world. Benham found nonpathogenic strains and strains of low pathogenicity on human skin.

Mycology. *Cryptococcus neoformans* grows readily on Sabouraud's medium, the initial colonies appearing after four to twelve days' incubation at 37° C. The colonies are medium in size, soft, mucoid, with a creamy color. On examination the oval or slightly elongated cells, 5 to 6 microns in diameter, are surrounded by large capsules which are outlined clearly in india ink preparations. This fungus multiplies by budding; it does not form ascospores or mycelium. There are several immunologic types as determined by capsular swelling with specific serums.

Immunology. Patients usually exhibit no precipitins, agglutinins or complement-fixing antibodies, but filtrates from cultures have given positive skin tests of the delayed type.

Pathology. Mook and Moore described acneiform pustules, granuloma-like ulcers, deep-seated abscesses and nodules, which may increase in size and simulate "myxomatous tumors." Giant cells and "foam" cells are numerous, fibroblasts, lymphocytes and plasma cells are present; but there is a remarkable paucity of polymorphonuclear leukocytes. In several instances the tissue reaction was similar to that seen in Hodgkin's disease. The encapsulated organisms are present both in and outside of giant cells, but there is an almost complete absence of leukocytes.

Clinical Manifestations. The patient may present single isolated abscesses, subcutaneous tumor-like masses, or multiple subcutaneous abscesses, as in the original case of Busse and Buschke. The primary pulmonary lesions resemble those of primary carcinoma or reinfection tuberculosis.

In the more common cerebral type of infection the onset is insidious, with headache, dizziness, vertigo and stiffness of the neck. Occasionally the onset is sudden with violent and excruciating headache and vomiting. The patient has little or no fever, and the pulse and blood pressure remain normal. The disease often is mistaken for a rather chronic type of tuberculous meningitis. After several weeks or months, more severe symptoms and signs appear, such as neuroretinitis, papilledema, strabismus, nystagmus, ptosis, diplopia, ataxia or hemiplegia. The patient ultimately becomes comatose and dies of respiratory failure.

Diagnosis. The dermal, subcutaneous and lymph node lesions may be diagnosed by routine biopsies and cultures on Sabouraud's medium. The diagnosis of the pulmonary forms is made by growing the organism from the sputum. In the meningeal form of the disease the cerebrospinal fluid pressure is increased and the fluid usually contains 200 to 800 cells per cubic millimeter, which are chiefly mononuclear. The cerebrospinal fluid sugar is decreased. The cryptococci are present in small numbers and are readily mistaken for erythrocytes or lymphocytes. After centrifugalization, the sediment from the fluid should be planted on Sabouraud's medium and watched for three or four weeks. Not infrequently the organism can be found by direct examination if a drop of the sedimented material is mixed with india ink.

Prognosis. The prognosis is grave in all forms of the disease, especially the cerebral form, which until recently has been considered inevitably fatal.

Treatment. The local lesions are treated by surgical excision or drainage, supplemented by local x-ray therapy and potassium iodide by mouth (see Blastomycosis). Patients with hypersensitivity should be desensitized and treated with sulfadiazine and iodides. An occasional patient with cryptococcus meningitis has recovered following sulfadiazine or actidione therapy.

DAVID T. SMITH

References

Baker, R. D.: Resectable Mycotic Lesions and Acutely Fatal Mycoses. J.A.M.A., *150*:1579, 1952.

Benham, R. W.: Cryptococci—Their Identification by Morphology and by Serology. J. Infect. Dis., *57*:255, 1935.

Busse, O.: Ueber Saccharomycosis hominis. Virchows Arch. f. path. Anat., *140*:23, 1895.

Carton, C. A.: Treatment of Central Nervous System Cryptococcosis. A Review and Report of Four Cases Treated with Actidione. Ann. Int. Med., *37*:123, 1952.

Cawley, E. P., Grekin, R. H., and Curtis, A. C.: Torulosis. A Review of Cutaneous and Adjoining Mucous Membrane Manifestations. J. Invest. Dermat., *14*:327, 1950.

Conant, N. F., and others: Manual of Clinical Mycology. 2nd ed. Philadelphia, W. B. Saunders Company, 1954.

Cox, L. B., and Tolhurst, J. C.: Human Torulosis. Victoria, Melbourne University Press, 1946.

Emmons, C. W.: *Cryptococcus neoformans* Strains from a Severe Outbreak of Bovine Mastitis. Mycopath. et mycol. appl., 6:231, 1953.

Evans, E. E., and Thiriault, R. J.: The Antigenic Composition of *Cryptococcus neoformans* IV. J. Bact., *65*:571, 1953.

Mosberg, W. H., Jr., and Arnold, J. G., Jr.: Torulosis of the Central Nervous System. Review of 172 Cases. Ann. Int. Med., 32:1153, 1950.

Neill, J. M., Sugg, J. Y., and McCauley, D. W.: Serologically Reactive Material in Spinal Fluid, Blood and Urine from a Human Case of Cryptococcosis (Torulosis). Proc. Soc. Exper. Biol. & Med., 77:775, 1951.

HISTOPLASMOSIS

Definition. Histoplasmosis resembles coccidioidomycosis in having a benign primary pulmonary phase and a less common severe generalized form which involves the reticuloendothelial system.

History. In 1906 Darling, in Panama, found round or oval parasites, which he thought were protozoa, in the endothelial cells and monocytes of certain cases of splenomegaly. Dodd, Tompkins and De Monbreun, in 1934, isolated *Histoplasma capsulatum* from a typical clinical case in a child and discovered that the parasite was a fungus.

Etiology. Histoplasmosis occurs throughout the world and in all parts of the United States, but appears in greatest concentration in the Central Mississippi and the Ohio River valleys. All races are susceptible, and both sexes are attacked at all ages, but adult males seven times as frequently as females. Children seem to be relatively more susceptible than to other mycotic infections, and male and female children are infected in equal numbers. Spontaneous histoplasmosis has been found in dogs, rats, mice and skunks. The organisms grow in profusion in pigeon, bat and chicken dung and the inhalation of these dried materials has given rise to epidemics of histoplasmosis.

Mycology. The organism can be isolated directly from the blood, sputum, sternal bone marrow or from tissues at necropsy by planting the material in dextrose agar or dextrose broth at 37° C. Two types of colonies appear, one of them a mycelial type and the other a yeastlike type.

Pathology. Primary pulmonary histoplasmosis appears as multiple, small discrete spots in the lungs with associated infection and enlargement of the tracheobronchial lymph nodes. As healing occurs, the organism disappears, and the central portions of the lesions become caseous and later calcify. In rare instances, as shown by Dublin, the primary infection behaves like a primary progressive tuberculosis and kills the patient. Johnson has found several cases which showed the multiple calcification that is characteristic of healed primary infections in which reinfections have occurred with the development of cavities and of pulmonary fibrosis.

Histoplasma capsulatum is an intracellular parasite which, in progressive cases, invades the entire reticuloendothelial system.

Clinical Manifestations. The benign primary pulmonary infections are usually asymptomatic. Infections beginning in the mouth, larynx, pharynx and ears show local necrotic ulcerations and definite enlargement of the regional lymph nodes. The progressive form of the disease is characterized by splenomegaly, hepatomegaly, emaciation, irregular pyrexia, leukopenia and anemia. Not all patients present this complete syndrome; the liver and spleen may not be enlarged; the disease may be confined chiefly to the lungs or even to the skin, as in the case studied by Hansmann and Schenken.

Diagnosis. The disease should be suspected in every obscure infection in which there is enlargement of the lymph nodes, with or without accompanying enlargement of the liver and spleen. In most instances, within a few weeks after the initial infection, the patient has a tuberculin-like allergy which can be demonstrated by the intracutaneous injection of 0.1 cc. of a 1:1000 dilution of a standardized histoplasmin. The reaction is read like a tuberculin test after 48 to 72 hours, and has the same significance as the tuberculin. Most rapidly progressive cases never develop a histoplasmin reaction, and terminal cases, which formerly reacted, may become anergic.

Complement-fixing antibodies appear in the serum of patients with progressive infections and increase in titer as the disease progresses.

Histoplasma capsulatum shares a small amount of common antigen with *Blastomyces dermatitidis,* resulting in cross-reactions both to the skin tests and to the complement fixation. However, no confusion will arise if both tests are performed simultaneously. C. E.

Smith has found cross-reactions to histoplasmin in patients with *Coccidioides immitis* infections, although the reactions were always less in extent than to coccidioidin.

Prognosis. The prognosis is excellent with the primary pulmonary forms, dubious in the localized infections, and almost hopeless when the infection is generalized.

Treatment. The common antimicrobial agents including stilbamidine and 2-hydroxy-stilbamidine have been ineffective in the treatment of histoplasmosis. The compound β-diethylaminoethyl fencholate, called MRD-112, is fungicidal in the presence of serum, is nontoxic for dogs, monkeys and man and may prove to be useful in therapy.

DAVID T. SMITH

References

Bunnell, I. L., and Furculow, M. L.: Report on Ten Proven Cases of Histoplasmosis. Pub. Health Rep., 63:299, 1948.

Christie, A., and Peterson, J. C.: Benign Histoplasmosis and Pulmonary Calcification. Am. J. Dis. Child., 72:460, 1946.

Christie, A., and others: Treatment of Disseminated Histoplasmosis with Ethyl Vanillate. Pediatrics, 7:7, 1951.

Conant, N. F., and others: Manual of Clinical Mycology. 2nd ed. Philadelphia, W. B. Saunders Company, 1954.

Darling, S. T.: An Infection Resembling Kala Azar Found among Natives of Tropical America. Arch. Int. Med., 2:107, 1908.

De Monbreun, W. A.: The Cultivation and Cultural Characteristics of Darling's Histoplasma Capsulatum. Am. J. Trop. Med., 14:93, 1934.

Emmons, C. W.: Histoplasmosis. Animal Reservoirs and Other Sources in Nature of the Pathogenic Fungus Histoplasma. Am. J. Pub. Health., 40:436, 1950.

Furcolow, M. L., and Grayson, J. T.: Occurrence of Histoplasmosis in Epidemics. Etiologic Study. Am. Rev. Tuberc., 68:307, 1953.

———, Guntheroth, W. G., and Willis, M. J.: The Frequency of Laboratory Infections with Histoplasma capsulatum. J. Lab. & Clin. Med., 40:182, 1952.

Howell, A.: Studies on Histoplasma Capsulatum and Similar Form Species. I. Morphology and Development. Mycologia, 31:191, 1939.

Johnson, H. E., and Batson, R.: Benign Pulmonary Histoplasmosis. Dis. Chest., 14:517, 1948.

Moore, M., and Jorstad, L. H.: Histoplasmosis and Its Importance to Otorhinolaryngologists. Ann. Otol., Rhin. & Laryng., 52:779, 1943.

Palmer, C. E., and Peterson, O. S.: Studies of Pulmonary Findings and Antigenic Sensitivity Among Student Nurses. Pub. Health Rep., 65:1, 1950.

Parsons, R. J., and Zarafonetis, C. J. D.: Histoplasmosis in Man. A Review of Seventy-one Cases. Arch. Int. Med., 75:1, 1945.

Puckett, T. F.: Pulmonary Histoplasmosis. A Study of Twenty-two Cases with Identification of *H. capsulatum* in Resected Lesions. Am. Rev. Tuberc., 67:453, 1953.

Schulz, D. M.: Histoplasmosis of the Central Nervous System. J.A.M.A., *151*:549, 1953.

Schwartz, S. O., and Barsky, S.: Report of 193 Marrow Biopsy Specimens Cultured for *Histoplasma capsulatum*. Blood, 7:545, 1952.

MONILIASIS

Definition. Monilia may produce acute or subacute infections of the mouth, vagina, skin, nails, bronchi and lungs, and occasionally a septicemia, endocarditis or meningitis.

History. The organism now known as *Candida albicans* was discovered in oral thrush by Langenbeck in 1839.

Etiology. The disease is found in all parts of the world, at all ages, in all races and in both sexes. Oral thrush is most common in infants and in patients with wasting diseases. Pregnancy and diabetes predispose to vaginal moniliasis. Dermal lesions occur in bakers, waiters, fruit packers, bartenders, and housewives whose hands are macerated from frequent soaking in water. Poorly fitting artificial teeth predispose to infections of the tongue and mouth.

Benham isolated both pathogenic and nonpathogenic strains of Monilia from normal skin and showed by animal experiments that *C. albicans* is the only pathogenic species.

Mycology. Monilia grow readily on Sabouraud's medium after two to four days' incubation at room or incubator temperatures. The colonies are soft, moist, oval, white structures which have a distinct yeast-like odor. *Candida albicans* is lethal for rabbits, ferments certain sugars, agglutinates in specific serums, and forms typical chlamydospores on corn meal agar.

Immunology. Many normal persons have agglutinins in their blood and a positive skin reaction, while some patients with active infection have neither.

Pathology. Both budding cells and mycelial threads may be found in sputum and in scrapings from the dermal and mucosal lesions.

Clinical Manifestations. Monilia may produce *thrush, vaginal moniliasis, paronychia, onychia, intertriginous moniliasis, dyshydrosiform eruptions, generalized eruptions* and *chronic glossitis*. Certain of these entities, notably thrush and glossitis, may be encountered in chronically ill patients who have been receiving prolonged antimicrobial therapy. The precise relationship of the chemotherapy to the furtherance of the monilia infection in such situations has not been established.

Bronchitis, both the acute and chronic varieties, results from bronchial infections. The symptoms resemble those of bacterial bronchitis, but the sputum usually is mucoid or gelatinous.

Pneumonitis occurs as an acute or subacute process. The lungs may show massive patchy consolidation in one or more lobes. There is cough, malaise, fever and leukocytosis, but usually the patients are less toxic than with bacterial infections. The sputum is mucoid or mucopurulent and may contain blood.

Diagnosis. The diagnosis is established by cultivating and identifying the potentially pathogenic *Candida* (*Monilia*) *albicans.* *Candida* is frequently a secondary invader in tuberculosis, pulmonary abscess, bronchiectasis, neoplasm and even other types of mycoses.

Prognosis. The pulmonary and septicemic forms may be fatal. The bronchial and localized infections are often chronic and resist treatment, but rarely kill the patient.

Treatment. Bronchial and pulmonary moniliasis should be treated with potassium iodide as outlined in the chapter on Blastomycosis. In some cases the patients have positive skin tests to *Monilia* vaccines and may not respond to the iodides until partial desensitization with vaccine has been effected. Intravenous gentian violet in doses of 5 mg. per kilogram of body weight each day, or every other day, for four to six doses sometimes cures massive pulmonary infections.

The acute oral lesions usually respond to alkaline washes or to gargles with 1:10,000 gentian violet. Recently a jelly-like preparation of sodium propionate has been found very effective in curing *Monilia* vaginitis.

DAVID T. SMITH

References

Alter, R. L., Jones, C. P., and Carter, B.: The Treatment of Mycotic Vulvovaginitis with Propionate Vaginal Jelly. Am. J. Obst. & Gynec., 53:241, 1947.

Benham, R. W.: Certain Monilias Parasitic on Man. J. Infect. Dis., *49*:183, 1931.

Conant, N. F., and others: Manual of Clinical My-
    cology. 2nd ed. Philadelphia, W. B. Saunders
    Company, 1954.
Craig, W. McK., and Gates, E. M.: Metastatic My-
    cotic Abscesses of the Brain. Arch. Neurol. & Psy-
    chiat., 62:314, 1949.
Hauser, F. V., and Rothman, S.: Monilial Granu-
    loma. Report of a Case and Review of the Litera-
    ture. Arch. Dermat. & Syph., 61:297, 1950.
Hopkins, J. G.: Moniliasis and Monilids. Arch. Der-
    mat. & Syph., 25:599, 1932.
Hurwitz, A. H., and Yesner, R.: Report of a Case of
    Localized Bronchopulmonary Moniliasis Success-
    fully Treated by Surgery. J. Thoracic Surg., 17:
    826, 1948.
Kunstadter, R. H., McLean, H., and Greengard, J.:
    Mycotic Endocarditis Due to Candida albicans.
    J.A.M.A., 149:829, 1952.
Oblath, R. W., and others: Pulmonary Moniliasis.
    Ann. Int. Med., 35:97, 1951.
Smith, D. T.: The Disturbance of the Normal Bac-
    terial Ecology by the Administration of Antibi-
    otics with the Development of New Clinical Syn-
    dromes. Ann. Int. Med., 37:1135, 1952.

SPOROTRICHOSIS

Definition. Sporotrichosis is a chronic infection characterized by the formation of
gumma-like nodules, abscesses and ulcers.
The lesions usually are confined to the skin
and superficial lymph nodes.

History. Schenck in 1896 isolated a fungus, later
identified as Sporotrichum by E. F. Smith, from a
patient in Johns Hopkins Hospital. The second case
was described by Hektoen and Perkins in 1900, who
named the fungus Sporotrichum schenckii. The disease was recognized in France in 1903 by de Beurmann and Raymond, and their organism was named
Sporotrichum beurmanni by Matruchot and Raymond.

Etiology. The disease occurs throughout
the world, but most often in males, especially
farmers, laborers and horticulturists. The
primary lesion was on some part of the upper
extremities in 90 of 102 cases. Sporotrichosis
occurs spontaneously in horses, dogs and rats;
Meyer infected himself while working with
an equine strain. Plants may be the primary
host.

Mycology. The yeastlike tissue form of
the organisms will grow on Francis' glucose
cystine blood agar at 37° C. in five to ten
days. The white moldlike form grows on
Sabouraud's medium at room or incubator
temperature after five to ten days and slowly
becomes brown or black on further incubation.

Immunology. Agglutinins and complement-fixing antibodies may appear in the
serum, and occasionally a tuberculin-like sensitivity develops in the patient.

Pathology. The gumma-like nodules usually consist of a central abscess surrounded
by granulation tissue with giant and epithelioid cells and a peripheral zone of connective
tissue, histologically resembling syphilitic, tuberculous or other chronic inflammations.
In the living tissue Sporotrichum occurs as
oval bodies of fairly uniform size, 2 to 3
microns broad and 3 to 5 microns long.

Clinical Manifestations. The primary lesion usually is in the skin and may appear
as early as twenty days or as long as three
months after the initial infection. The primary lesion is a hard, spherical, elastic, movable, subcutaneous nodule, not adherent to
the overlying skin. It becomes attached to the
skin, which first becomes pink and then
purplish and finally black and necrotic. This
lesion (sporothrix chancre) may persist for
months. Usually after a few days or weeks
multiple subcutaneous nodules appear along
the course of the lymphatic drainage. These
nodules are at first freely movable, but later
adhere to the overlying skin, become reddened and ulcerate through to the surface,
discharging a small amount of thin pus. The
lymph vessels between the nodes may become
so thickened they can be felt as hard cords.

De Beurmann and Gougerot classified the
clinical types of the disease as (1) lymphatic,
(2) disseminated, (3) epidermal, (4) sporotrichosis of the mucous membranes, (5)
skeletal sporotrichosis and (6) visceral sporotrichosis. In the rare disseminated gummatous form single or successive crops of
nodes develop at intervals. Pulmonary sporotrichosis is rare.

Diagnosis. The diagnosis is established by
cultivating the organisms from the discharges
or from material removed at biopsy. The disease may simulate syphilis, tuberculosis, blastomycosis, cryptococcosis, glanders, tularemia, leprosy or pyogenic infections.

Prognosis. Uncomplicated sporotrichosis
is rarely fatal; when untreated, it persists for
months or years, but appropriate treatment
usually is followed by rapid healing.

Treatment. Potassium iodide should be
given in slowly increasing doses up to 4 to 6
gm. or more daily. If absorption of closed
abscesses is slow, they may be punctured,
aspirated and injected with a weak solution
of iodide. Incision and curettage are to be
avoided. Ulcerated lesions may be painted
with tincture of iodine and dressed with a

solution containing water, 500 cc., potassium iodide, 10 gm., and iodine, 1 gm. The treatment should be continued for at least a month after apparent recovery.

DAVID T. SMITH

References

Benham, R. W., and Kesten, B.: Transmission of Sporotrichosis to Plants and Animals. J. Infect. Dis., 50:437, 1932.

Campbell, C. C.: Use of Francis' Glucose Cystine Blood Agar in the Isolation and Cultivation of Sporotrichum Schenckii. J. Bact., 50:233, 1945.

Cawley, E. P.: Sporotrichosis, a Protein Disease: With Report of a Disseminated Subcutaneous Gummatous Case of the Disease. Ann. Int. Med., 30:1287, 1949.

Conant, N. F., and others: Manual of Clinical Mycology. 2nd ed. Philadelphia, W. B. Saunders Company, 1954.

de Beurmann, L., and Gougerot, H.: Les Sporotrichoses. Paris, Libraire Felix Alcan, 1912.

Foerster, H. R.: Sporotrichosis an Occupational Dermatosis. J.A.M.A., 87:1605, 1926.

Meyer, K.: The Relation of Animal to Human Sporotrichosis. J.A.M.A., 65:579, 1915.

Norden, A.: Sporotrichosis. Clinical and Laboratory Features and Serologic Study in Experimental Animals and Humans. Acta Path. et Microbiol. Scand. suppl., 89:3, 1951.

Robinson, H. M.: Industrial Sporotrichosis. South. M. J., 42:343, 1949.

Schenck, B. R.: On Refractory Subcutaneous Abscesses Caused by a Fungus Possibly Related to the Sporotrichia. Bull. Johns Hopkins Hosp., 9:286, 1898.

Singer, J. I., and Muncie, J. E.: Sporotrichosis. Etiologic Considerations and Report of Additional Cases from New York. N. Y. State J. Med., 52:2147, 1952.

Smith, L. M.: Sporotrichosis; Report of 4 Clinically Atypical Cases. South. M. J., 38:505, 1945.

Symposium: Sporotrichosis Infection on Mines of the Witwaterstrand Transvaal Chamber of Mines, Johannesburg, 1947.

MADUROMYCOSIS

(Madura Foot)

Maduromycosis, or mycetoma, is a chronic infection affecting principally the foot, but in rare instances other parts of the body. It is characterized by multiple abscesses and sinuses and the development of granulation and connective tissues.

Mycology. Carter, in 1860, proved that the disease was a mycosis and introduced the term "mycetoma" or fungous tumor. The disease may be caused by any one of thirteen species of the genus *Actinomyces* or any one of nineteen species of molds belonging to two classes and eight genera (Gammel).

Etiology. The specific cause is contained in the white, yellow, deep brown or black granules which appear in the discharges from the affected region. The disease is most common in males and in farmers or other persons who come directly in contact with the soil.

Pathology. The pathologic reaction is essentially the same regardless of the type of invading fungus. There is local and general swelling of the parts affected with a corresponding degree of deformity. In old chronic cases the skin is darkened and the surface studded with pitted scars, open sinuses and nodular fungating elevations. Dense masses of scar tissue are found in the healing lesions. The abscesses connected with the sinuses are filled with mucoid fluid in which the characteritic granules are floating.

Prognosis and Treatment. Sulfonamide therapy may cure the type of maduromycosis which is caused by *Actinomyces* or *Nocardia*. The disease does not heal spontaneously, and the patients eventually die of secondary infection unless the infected limb is amputated.

DAVID T. SMITH

References

Ajello, L.: The Isolation of *Allescheria boydii* Shear, an Etiologic Agent of Mycetomas, from Soil. Am. J. Trop. Med. & Hyg., 1:227, 1952.

Benham, R. W., and Georg, L. K.: *Allescheria boydii,* Causative Agent in a Case of Meningitis. J. Invest. Dermat., 10:99, 1948.

Burns, E. L., Moss, E. S., and Brueck, J. W.: Mycetoma Pedis in the United States and Canada. Am. J. Clin. Path., 15:35, 1945.

Conant, N. F., and others: Manual of Clinical Mycology. 2nd ed. Philadelphia, W. B. Saunders Company, 1954.

Emmons, C. W.: *Allescheria boydii* and *Monosporium apiospermum.* Mycologia, 36:188, 1944.

Gammel, J. A.: The Etiology of Maduromycosis. Arch. Dermat. & Syph., 15:241, 1927.

CHROMOBLASTOMYCOSIS

Chromoblastomycosis, or verrucous dermatitis, is characterized by the formation of warty cutaneous nodules which, through slow progressive growth, become transformed into prominent papillomatous vegetations which may or may not ulcerate. Usually the lesions are confined to the feet and legs, but may be limited to the hands and arms.

In 1911 Pedroso, of São Paulo, Brazil, isolated a pigmented organism from patients with verrucous lesions of the skin which was later named *Hormodendrum pedrosoi*. Large spherical bodies, dark brown in color, are present in abundance in the verrucous lesions and grow readily on Sabouraud's medium.

Pathology. The disease is chronic and may last for years. With the development of extensive fibrosis in the deeper dermal lesions, the lymphatics are blocked and the patient suffers an elephantiasis of the extremity.

Treatment. Complete destruction of the lesion by surgical excision or electrotherapeutic methods would seem to be logical when the disease is diagnosed in its incipient stage. Surgical amputation is not justifiable, because the lesions rarely become severely infected and usually make sufficient response to medical treatment to leave the patient with a useful limb. The internal treatment consists of large doses of potassium iodide, up to as much as 1 to 9 gm. per day. Iontophoresis with copper sulfate was used with considerable success in the case reported by Martin, Baker and Conant.

DAVID T. SMITH

References

Auzlay, R. D.: Experimental Chromoblastomycosis in Man. J. Invest. Dermat., *19*:307, 1952.
Carrión, A. L.: Yeastlike Dematiaceous Fungi Infecting the Human Skin. Arch. Dermat. & Syph., *61*:996, 1950.
Conant, N. F., and Martin, D. S.: The Morphologic and Serologic Relationships of the Various Fungi Causing Dermatitis Verrucosa (Chromoblastomycosis). Am. J. Trop. Med., *17*:553, 1937.
——, and others: Manual of Clinical Mycology, 2nd ed. Philadelphia, W. B. Saunders Company, 1954.
Martin, D. S., Baker, R. D., and Conant, N. F.: A Case of Verrucous Dermatitis Caused by Hormodendrum Pedrosoi (Chromoblastomycosis) in North Carolina. Am. J. Trop. Med., *16*:593, 1936.
Powell, R. E.: A Survey of Chromoblastomycosis in Queensland. Australian J. Dermat., *1*:214, 1952.

ASPERGILLOSIS

Certain species of Aspergillus, especially *Aspergillus fumigatus,* produce inflammatory granulomatous lesions in the skin, external ear, vagina, nasal sinuses, orbit, bronchi, lungs and occasionally bones and meninges.

The disease was first recognized by Bennett in 1842, and the first careful necropsy of pulmonary aspergillosis in man was by Virchow in 1856. Renon's monograph, published in 1897, established the frequency and importance of aspergillosis in France.

Extensive pulmonary lesions may occur in instances in which there are overwhelming exposures to the spores, as in pigeon feeders, hair cleaners and certain agricultural workers. Aspergilli grow readily on dextrose agar or Sabouraud's medium at either room temperature or at 37° C. Infection may be suspected from the greenish or brown color of the discharges. Aspergilli are frequently secondary invaders or accidental contaminants, and the diagnosis should not be made exclusively on the appearance of the organism on culture. One should demonstrate the mycelial forms directly in the discharges before the material is planted.

The standard treatment is with potassium iodide. If hypersensitiveness to an autogenous aspergillus vaccine can be demonstrated, then vaccine therapy is also indicated. For superficial lesions thymol iodide dusting powders or 2 per cent thymol in 70 to 95 per cent alcohol may be used.

DAVID T. SMITH

References

Hertzog, A. J., Smith, T. S., and Giblin, M.: Acute Pulmonary Aspergillosis. Report of a Case. Pediatrics, *4*:331, 1949.
Ross, C. F.: A Case of Pulmonary Aspergillosis. J. Path. & Bact., *63*:409, 1951.
Virchow, R.: Beiträge zur Lehre von den beim Menschen vorkommenden pflanzlichen Parasiten. Arch. f. path. Anat. u. Physiol., *9*:557, 1856.
Weed, L. A., Baggenstoss, A. H., and Baugher, L.: Some Problems in the Diagnosis of Actinomycosis. Proc. Staff Meet., Mayo Clinic, *24*:463, 1949.

PENICILLIOSIS

Several species of the genus *Penicillium* are capable of producing lesions in the ear and skin and occasionally in the lungs. Clinically the infections resemble those caused by the *Aspergillus,* and the same care has to be exercised in establishing the etiologic relationship between the culture and the disease. The treatment is the same as for aspergillosis.

DAVID T. SMITH

References

Aimé, P., Crewzé, P., and Kresser, H.: Mycosis of Lungs Due to Penicillin Crustaceum; Case with Clinical and Roentgen Aspects of Abscess. Presse méd., *41:*761, 1933.

Conant, N. F., and others: Manual of Clinical Mycology. 2nd ed. Philadelphia, W. B. Saunders Company, 1954.

Gilliam, J. S., Jr., and Vest, S. A.: *Penicillium* Infection of the Urinary Tract. J. Urol., *65:*484, 1951.

Raper, K. B., and Thom, C.: A Manual of the Penicillia. Baltimore, Williams and Wilkins Co., 1949.

MUCORMYCOSIS

Mucormycosis is a rare disease with clinical characteristics resembling those of aspergillosis. Several cases of pulmonary mucormycosis have been reported. The first authentic case in man was studied by Paltauf in 1885. The initial infection was in the lungs, but metastatic abscesses developed in various organs before death. The treatment is the same as for aspergillosis.

DAVID T. SMITH

References

Baker, R. D., and Severance, A. O.: Mucormycosis with Report of Acute Mycotic Pneumonia. Am. J. Path., *24:*716, 1948.

Conant, N. F., and others: Manual of Clinical Mycology. 2nd ed. Philadelphia, W. B. Saunders Company, 1954.

Gregory, J. E., Golden, A., and Haymaker, W.: Mucormycosis of the Central Nervous System. A Report of Three Cases. Bull. Johns Hopkins Hosp., *73:*405, 1943.

Paltauf, A.: Mycosis mucorina. Virchows Arch. f. path. Anat., *102:*543, 1885.

Wadsworth, J. A. C.: Ocular Mucormycosis; Report of a Case. Am. J. Ophth., *34:*405, 1951.

RHINOSPORIDIOSIS

Rhinosporidiosis, caused by *Rhinosporidium seeberi,* is characterized by the development of pedunculated or sessile polyps in the nose and conjunctivas. The disease is prevalent in India and Ceylon, but occurs in temperate regions. More than 15 cases have been recognized in the United States.

The diagnosis is established by demonstrating the sporangia and spores in the tumor tissue. Surgical excision cures the early cases.

DAVID T. SMITH

References

Andleigh, H. S.: Rhinosporidiosis in Rajasthan. Report of Three Cases. Indian J. M. Sc., *6:*16, 1952.

Arnold, R., and Whildin, J.: Rhinosporidiosis of Conjunctiva: Case Report. Am. J. Ophth., *25:* 1227, 1942.

Conant, N. F., and others: Manual of Clinical Mycology. 2nd ed. Philadelphia, W. B. Saunders Company, 1954.

Seale, W. H., Flinn, C. B., and Britt, E. C.: Rhinosporidiosis. Arch. Otolaryng., *40:*203, 1944.

SPIROCHETAL INFECTIONS

SYPHILIS

Definition. Syphilis is an infectious disease, generalized at first, subsequently localized and dispersed, which may involve many organs of the body. It is caused by a spirochete, *Treponema pallidum*. The infection is unique in the benign character of the illness produced during the period of blood stream invasion, and in the infrequency of late metastases and remarkably slow progression once localization has occurred. The characteristic histologic lesion is a vasculitis of the smaller vessels. This is surrounded by areas of cellular reaction and tissue destruction which are conditioned in extent by the stage of the disease and the nature of the underlying tissue. Despite the slow tempo, the untreated infection eventually cripples or kills approximately one quarter of the persons afflicted.

Etiology. *Treponema pallidum* is the cause of syphilis. It is an actively motile, thin, spiral organism which varies from 6 to 14 microns in length and divides by transverse fission. *T. pallidum* is morphologically indistinguishable from several other varieties of spirochetes, and adsorbs most stains poorly. The characteristic motility pattern which this organism displays in a wet preparation, when observed through the darkfield microscope, is an essential criterion for its identification. The identity of spiral organisms which are demonstrated by stain or silver impregnation in fixed tissue specimens can be established only by inference.

Transmission of Syphilis. *T. pallidum* cannot withstand drying, and even in a liquid environment the organisms do not survive outside the host for more than a few hours. Thus, in order to produce infection the organisms must be transferred directly, in a liquid vehicle, from host to host. Coitus provides the necessary conditions for such transfer of liquid infectious material. The genitals are not uniquely susceptible to infection, however, and any form of intimate bodily contact (such as kissing), if it happens to involve the transfer of liquid infectious material, may result in the production of syphilis. Indirect transmission of the in-fection occurs only rarely and requires a rapid contact between host, object and susceptible, such as might develop from the handling of recently contaminated surgical instruments. The fetus of a syphilitic woman can be infected *in utero,* presumably through the placenta. There is no evidence to support the notion that a syphilitic father can transmit the infection to his offspring in the absence of syphilis in the mother.

Host-Parasite Reactions in Syphilitic Infection. Once the micro-organisms have traversed the epithelium at the site of deposition, multiplication and local extension occur. The treponemes enter the lymphatics almost immediately and are carried to the regional nodes. Through the lymphatic system, and perhaps by direct invasion of venules in the region of the initial lesion, the organisms are carried to the venous blood stream, traverse the pulmonary circulation, and are transported in the arterial blood to all the tissues of the body. As is the case with other bacteria, it is probable that *T. pallidum* does not multiply in the circulating blood. During passage through the smaller vessels, the organisms leave or are removed from the circulating blood and initiate metastatic lesions in and around the vessels of many tissues. These lesions may eventually become demonstrable in the tissues of ectodermal origin, i.e., skin, mucous membranes, central nervous system and eye. Presumably, similar but less easily demonstrable lesions also develop in the small vessels of other organ such as the liver and aorta.

The generalization of the treponemes from the site of original implantation occurs within a period of a few days to a week and conceivably may begin in less than 24 hours. Thus, long before any lesion of syphilis becomes evident, the infection is established in the form of (*a*) a focus near the site of implantation; (*b*) innumerable metastatic foci throughout the body; and (*c*) a spirochetemia which is continuously or intermittently augmented from either source. Multiplication of treponemes with resulting tissue reaction proceeds simultaneously in all of the foci. The focus near the site of initial infection because of its seniority is usually the first to progress to the point where it is recognized externally as the primary chancre. In an appreciable number of infected persons, however, either the initial or the secondary foci may fail to progress sufficiently to attain recognition.

Host Resistance. Virtually nothing is known concerning the precise mechanisms by which the treponemes are destroyed within the body. There is no clear-cut evidence that living treponemes are phagocytized. Indeed, darkfield microscopy of material obtained at intervals from a healing lesion suggests that *T. pallidum* is killed extracellularly and rapidly autolyzes.

Humoral immunity appears early in the infection and can be detected by animal protection tests (Turner) or by the *in vitro* treponemal immobilization test of Nelson. (This antibody is distinct from the antibody *syphilis reagin* which is revealed by the diagnostic tests.) Whether the "immobilizing" antibody plays a role in the destruction of *T. pallidum in vivo* is not known. It is conceivable that it might play such a role and even, through this or other mechanisms, might play an important part in maintaining the steady equilibrium of latent syphilis.

Whatever may be the character of the defenses mobilized by the host against *T. pallidum,* it is clear that they are impressive. The influence of this resistance may be seen in: (1) the enormous numbers of treponemes which are eventually destroyed with the spontaneous healing of the surface lesions; (2) the control of the spirochetemia and the prevention of its subsequent reappearance; (3) the phenomenon that the tissue reaction to reinoculation with *T. pallidum* immediately assumes the character of the particular stage of evolution of the original infection, i.e., chancre, secondary papule or gumma.

After a period which may vary from a few weeks to many months, *T. pallidum* disappears from the circulating blood and from most of the lesions, including all of the visible ones. The inflammation then resolves, usually without leaving residual traces. In some instances, this process of generalization followed by extensive resolution does not occur all in one cycle, but rather as repeated episodes of spirochetemia and metastases, each one of which is less extensive than its predecessor. Regardless of whether the spirochetemia and surface lesions appear in one or in several waves, they no longer occur once the immune forces of the host have attained maximum effectiveness. The period of time required for the development of this state of relative immunity varies in individual infections from a few months to several years. *Thus the development of the infectious state or the appearance of new lesions in previously uninvolved areas is not to be anticipated subsequent to the first few years after the initial infection.*

The development of refractoriness to the redissemination of the organisms can apparently be prevented by the administration of subcurative antimicrobial therapy. In such instances a reappearance of the manifestations of the acute phase of the infection is not uncommon. Moreover, the fully acquired resistance can be overcome by some influences which are operative during pregnancy. In the latter instance, however, the breakdown in the forces of immunity is limited, as the development of new lesions on the body surfaces or in the nervous system does not occur. Aside from pregnancy, no conditions are known which will diminish this state of resistance to spirochetemia once the state has become fully established. Even in the presence of extreme debilitation caused by starvation or a wasting disease, the spirochetes apparently do not spread from their sites of localization to invade other areas of the body. This serves to emphasize the unique character of the host-parasite relationship in syphilis.

Course of Syphilitic Infection. After a variable period of generalization, the spirochetes disappear from the blood stream and the surface lesions, and the latter completely resolve. Presumably at the same time, destruction of spirochetes and healing of lesions are taking place in other tissues of the body. It is not established whether the process of resolution ever goes on to completion at this time with a resulting eradication or "biologic cure" of the infection. Certainly in most syphilitic infections a complete eradication of the organisms does not occur and one or more foci persist in various locations. If the presence of these foci is hidden beyond diagnostic reach, the state of the infection is designated as *latent*. The presence of persistent foci in the central nervous system is not hidden beyond diagnostic reach, as they are detectable by examination of the cerebrospinal fluid. *Therefore, unless it can be demonstrated that the fluid is normal, a patient cannot be regarded as having inapparent or latent syphilis.* If evidence of infection is present in the cerebrospinal fluid (in the absence of clinical signs of infection), the stage of the disease is designated as *asymptomatic neurosyphilis.* Although the presence of neurosyphilis may not become clinically evident until many years after the initial infection, the process originates during the period of spirochetemia. The persons with asymptomatic neurosyphilis represent a minority in whom the metastatic lesions of the early invasion fail to disappear from the central nervous system at the time of resolution of the generalized infections.

The term *latent syphilis* is thus limited to those instances in which the presence, but not the location, of syphilitic foci is evident.

As surface lesions are not present, the person with latent syphilis cannot transmit the infection. Nevertheless, such a person is at risk from the development of infections or other metastatic lesions until acquired resistance has been fully attained. Thus, until the possibility of redissemination has become remote, the prognosis and the principles of therapy of latent and of infectious syphilis are identical. It has been found convenient, therefore, to subdivide the term, *latent syphilis,* into early or late, at a point four years after the onset of infection. The line of division is arbitrary, and is based on the assumption, true in virtually all instances, that after four years the reappearance of the generalized stage of the infection is no longer to be anticipated.

Early latent syphilis thus may return to the metastatic or infectious variety. Once the focalization of the process becomes stabilized, the disease enters into the stage either of *asymptomatic neurosyphilis* or of *late latent syphilis.*

Late Latent Syphilis. After the stage of late latency has been reached, the infection may pursue any one of three possible courses: (1) The foci still present after resolution of the infectious lesions may heal slowly over a period of years with complete eradication of the infecting organisms (biologic cure). The incidence of this phenomenon is not known, but it probably occurs in approximately 25 per cent of those infected (Brunsgaard). (2) The foci of infection may persist throughout the life of the host but evoke such a minimal or fortuitously located tissue reaction that the health of the infectious person is unimpaired. This course, which is analogous to the "healthy carrier" state in other infections, undoubtedly occurs with frequency. (3) The foci may progress at a slow and inconstant rate until sufficient tissue reaction has occurred to produce clinical evidences of disease. This occurs in approximately 25 per cent of the persons with late latent syphilis. The resulting clinical disease may be fatal or benign depending upon the amount of damage and the importance of the structure affected. Although there is virtually no prospect that a person with late latent syphilis (cerebrospinal fluid normal) will subsequently develop neurosyphilis, the person with neurosyphilis may eventually develop clinically demonstrable lesions in other areas of the body in the same manner as occurs in late latent syphilis.

Location and Character of the Lesions of Late Syphilis. Syphilis may attack virtually any organ or tissue of the body. In the past this fact has been grossly overemphasized, for almost without exception

serious or fatal syphilis in adults is limited to involvement of the aorta, the central nervous system or the eye. Less frequently the infection becomes evident as the localized single or multiple granulomas which are designated as gummas. The fundamental histopathologic lesion of the late forms of syphilis is essentially the same as that of the early lesions and consists of vascular and perivascular cellular infiltration associated with tissue necrosis and ultimate fibrosis. The chief features which distinguish early from late lesions are that in the latter the amount of necrosis is greater and the cellular reaction less intense. Moreover, the treponemes are present in the late lesions only in small numbers and are difficult to demonstrate. Gummas increase in size at an inconstant rate and the destruction of tissue is accompanied by partial healing and fibrosis.

Prenatal Syphilis. The lesions of prenatal syphilis resemble in general the lesions of acquired syphilis of comparable duration. However, in infants who fail to survive for more than a few weeks (or in stillborn infants) the syphilitic process is unusually acute and is characterized by massive spirochetal invasion of all tissues including the lung (*pneumonia alba*). Aortic syphilis, which is so common in the infection acquired by adults, occurs only rarely in those who survive a prenatal infection.

Serologic Response to Syphilitic Infection. Shortly after infection with *T. pallidum* two distinct antibodies become detectable in the serum of the host. One of these, designated *syphilis reagin,* exists in close association with the gamma globulin fraction of the plasma; the other, known as *treponemal immobilizing antibody* (T.P.I.), can be detected by an *in vitro* test originated by Nelson.

Only the first named antibody, *syphilis reagin,* can be detected by the various serologic tests for syphilis (hereinafter designated S.T.S.). As with serologic tests in other infections, the amount of syphilis reagin present in a specimen of serum can be crudely quantitated by repetition of the test with serial dilutions of the unknown serum. The highest dilution of serum which contains detectable reagin is designated as the titer of the reaction.

The interval between the onset of infection and the appearance of detectable reagin in the serum is dependent upon the sensitivity of the technique employed and varies among individual infections. Usually the

S.T.S. becomes positive between the third and the sixth weeks after the disease has been contracted. In a minority of instances, however, the process requires more time, and the serologic tests may not become positive until approximately three months after the onset of infection. With modern techniques, the S.T.S. is invariably positive when the dissemination of the infection has become sufficiently intense to result in metastatic lesions in the skin and mucosa.

Less precise knowledge is available concerning the length of time during which detectable reagin will persist in the serum of persons who receive no treatment. It is probable that the serologic tests for syphilis, once positive, do not spontaneously revert to negative for at least ten years. Whether spontaneous serologic reversal occurs in a significant number of patients (exclusive of tabetics) after the first decade of the disease has not been established; but this probably occurs in some persons.

The antibody detected by the treponemal immobilization test, once present, apparently persists for life. The appearance of this antibody can be prevented, however, by appropriate treatment very early in the course of syphilitic infection.

CLINICAL PICTURE OF SYPHILIS

Acquired Syphilis of Adults. *Early Syphilis (Infectious or Early Latent).* Infectious syphilis is the generalized form of the disease in which one or more lesions, rich in *T. pallidum,* are present on the exterior of the body. The lesions may appear at any time from a week to several years after onset of infection. In an appreciable number of instances (females 50 per cent, males 30 per cent), the lesions either fail to appear at any time or remain unrecognized by the infected person. Infectious lesions vary in character and extent from a solitary primary or metastatic lesion to a generalized involvement of the skin and mucous membranes. The initial or primary lesion serves as an historic landmark of the portal of entry of the infection but is otherwise intrinsically the same as the metastatic lesions. Even the value of the primary lesion as a landmark is modified by the fact that solitary metastatic lesions occur and may be erroneously identified as primary. Frequently when the patient is first observed by the physician, both primary and metastatic lesions are present.

SYMPTOMS OF INFECTIOUS SYPHILIS. A unique feature of the early syphilitic infection is the fact that it usually produces virtually no symptoms of systemic disease despite the presence of spirochetemia and widespread metastatic lesions. A possible exception is headache, which may occur as a manifestation of the generalization of the infection, but more often is a reflection of metastatic involvement of the central nervous system or skull. Fever occurs only rarely, and seldom rises higher than 100.2° F. (38° C.). The urine is normal. There is no anemia or leukocytosis of the peripheral blood.

Because of the virtual absence of systemic symptoms, the patient with syphilis may not seek medical care during the period of infectiousness unless local lesions give rise to symptoms or awaken a suspicion of disease. Thus the physician is usually faced with the problem of identifying a serious generalized infection from a clinical manifestation which appears to be purely local and trivial in nature.

The *initial lesion* (primary chancre) may appear at any time between the tenth and the ninetieth day after infection but usually is evident within two or three weeks. *There is nothing fundamentally characteristic about the appearance of a chancre.* The diagnosis can be established only by the demonstration of the presence of the organisms in the lesion even though the syphilitic etiology may be suspected from clinical examination. Because of the subacute nature of the inflammatory process with the extensive occlusion of small vessels, the chancre tends to be indurated, circumscribed, relatively avascular and painless. Any or all of these characteristics may be so modified by the location of the lesion, and the presence of other infectious processes, that no typical picture is consistently produced.

As would be anticipated from the epidemiology of syphilis, the initial lesion usually occurs on the skin or mucous membranes of the genitalia, the perianal region, the lips or the oral cavity. Less frequently the finger or the female breast is the site of implantation of the organisms. An ulcerative lesion of these or other areas, particularly one which persists for several weeks, may represent the initial lesion of syphilis and can be identified as such only by the proper use and interpretation of laboratory examinations.

Regardless of the site of infection, the appearance of the chancre is usually accompanied by a moderate enlargement of the regional lymph nodes. The nodes are firm, discrete, movable and are not usually tender. Syphilitic infection does not lead to suppuration of lymph nodes, but occasionally a purulent process may develop in inguinal nodes which are involved simultaneously by syphilis and another infection.

On the genitalia, multiple infectious lesions of syphilis are common, particularly in the female. In the latter instance the lesions

extent from one or several lesions in a single area to widespread involvement of skin and mucosa. Although the cutaneous and mucosal lesions frequently coexist, it is important to realize that they may occur independently of each other. The character of the cutaneous lesions is protean. With the exception of a vesicular eruption, which is never produced by acquired syphilis, virtually any type of rash may develop. The forms which are most

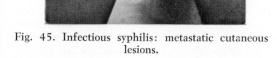

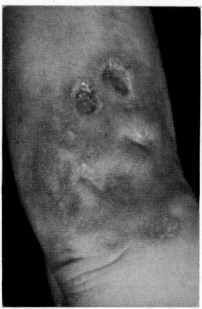

Fig. 45. Infectious syphilis: metastatic cutaneous lesions.

Fig. 46. Late syphilis: cutaneous gumma of elbow before treatment.

are usually metastatic. In the male, multiple chancres of the penis are by no means rare.

The primary lesion of syphilis is frequently, but by no means invariably, accompanied or followed by the development of metastatic lesions of the skin and mucous membranes. Regardless of whether secondary lesions occur, the initial lesion slowly heals usually in a two- to six-week period, and may or may not leave a thin atrophic scar. The regional lymphadenopathy subsides less rapidly and may be present in some degree for several or more months. The generalized enlargement of the lymph nodes may resolve or may persist and become more prominent if widespread metastatic lesions develop.

Metastatic Lesions (Secondary Syphilis). The visible manifestations of the generalization of the syphilitic infection are encountered chiefly in the skin and mucous membranes. The surface involvement varies in

frequently encountered are a faint red macule (1 to 3 mm. in diameter), a reddish brown papule or a folliculopapule. Although the pigmentation of the papule is presumably caused by the extravasation of blood, the process never becomes sufficiently acute to give rise to hemorrhagic lesions. Less frequently the infection produces an annulopapular, pustular, rupial (ulcerated) or psoriasiform eruption. The annulopapular, pustular and folliculopapular varieties are encountered more frequently in Negroes.

The distribution of the cutaneous lesions may be of more value than the morphology in directing the suspicion of the clinician toward the possibility of the presence of syphilis. As the infection is blood-borne, the lesions are generalized and may develop on the palms, soles and face in addition to, or independently of, involvement of the skin of the trunk and extremities. In infections other than syphilis (meningococcemia, staphylococcemia, the rickettsial and viral diseases) in which skin lesions appear in the characteristic blood-borne distribution, the patient usually presents obvious evidence of acute systemic disease. Syphilitic lesions of the palms or soles usually appear as dark reddish brown macules or papules. Occasionally on the hands and feet the infection may produce a superficial scaling eruption which simulates a fungal infection.

INVOLVEMENT OF MUCOUS MEMBRANES. Metastatic (secondary) syphilitic involvement of the mucous membranes may appear as a simple erosion, a papulo-erosion, or as a hypertrophic, papular or symmetrically spread lesion which is designated by the term *condyloma latum**. The simple erosive and papulo-erosive lesions occur in the buccal mucosa or on the genitalia. The erosion is usually covered by a thin, silvery gray membrane (*mucous patch*) and is surrounded by little inflammatory reaction. Multiple lesions are common, particularly in the oral cavity. The erosions do not usually produce any symptoms unless they are located on the tonsillar pillar or tonsil, where they may cause moderately severe symptoms of a tonsillitis or pharyngitis.

Condyloma latum occurs most frequently in moist areas such as the lips, the female genitalia, and in the perianal region of both sexes. On the labia majora the lesions are usually multiple and consist of flat raised nodules which are approximately a centimeter in diameter. In the other areas, particularly around the anal orifice, the condyloma may appear as an indurated slightly raised, purple-brown lesion which extends symmetrically over the surrounding skin for an area of 2 or 3 cm. Unless traumatized or secondarily infected, condylomas are not usually ulcerated. A perianal condyloma, like any lesion close to the anal sphincter, may cause considerable pain on defecation. In the presence of this symptom the highly infectious condyloma is frequently mistakenly identified as a "fissure" or a "thrombosed hemorrhoid."

A mucocutaneous lesion of syphilis which is deserving of special mention is the so-called *"split papule."* The lesion consists of a tiny moist papule which develops at the angle of the mouth where it becomes split in one or more places. A papule in this location may

* Not to be confused with *condyloma acuminatum,* the venereal or genital wart which has the characteristic appearance of warts occurring elsewhere.

represent the sole demonstrable lesion of a syphilitic infection yet may easily be overlooked because of the frequent occurrences of innocuous traumatic fissures at the corners of the mouth.

INFECTIVITY OF CUTANEOUS AND MUCOSAL LESIONS. All of the cutaneous and mucosal lesions of early syphilis contain *T. pallidum* in considerable numbers and hence are potentially infectious for others. The most dangerous lesions from the standpoint of transmissibility are the innocuous appearing ulcerated lesions about the lips or in the mouth.

EARLY NEUROSYPHILIS. Involvement of the central nervous system during the course of infectious syphilis is demonstrable in an appreciable number of patients by examination of the cerebrospinal fluid. Usually this inflammatory process is not sufficiently intense to produce symptoms other than a mild or moderately severe headache. Occasionally, however, the presence of the infection in the central nervous system becomes clinically evident. *This early symptomatic neurosyphilis is an extremely rare occurrence among patients with untreated infectious syphilis but develops not infrequently in patients who have received subcurative therapy.* The presenting clinical picture of early symptomatic neurosyphilis is characterized by evidence of disease of the meninges or of the arteries of the brain and is discussed in a subsequent chapter (p. 364).

OTHER METASTATIC LESIONS OF EARLY SYPHILIS. The metastatic lesions of early syphilis which may occur in addition to those already described are: a generalized enlargement of lymph nodes only rarely accompanied by splenic enlargement; alopecia of an irregular, "moth-eaten" type distinct from the completely hairless areas of alopecia areata; and three types of ocular disease, *iritis, neuritis* or *retinitis*. For a detailed presentation of the ocular involvements which may occur during the course of infectious syphilis, the authoritative review of Woods should be consulted.

It is reasonable to assume that the development of metastatic lesions during the course of infectious syphilis is not limited to those structures in which the presence of infection is so easily demonstrated. Nevertheless, the development of clinically detectable disease of other organs or structures is remarkably infrequent.

Diagnosis of Infectious Syphilis. No

matter how experienced the clinician or how "characteristic" the lesions, the diagnosis of infectious syphilis cannot be established with certainty except by darkfield microscopy. Less certain but generally acceptable evidence of the presence of the infectious state is the finding of consistently positive S.T.S. in a patient who presents lesions which have the appearance of syphilis and which respond promptly to antisyphilitic therapy. Although patients who present this combination of findings are usually syphilitic, there is no proof that the infection is recent, and the presumed infectious lesions may represent manifestations of a coincidental disease. Despite the fact that the proof of the diagnosis of infectious syphilis rests entirely on laboratory procedures, it is essential that the physician be alert for possible clinical evidences of syphilis in order that the laboratory tests may be properly employed.

The finding of a genital lesion, no matter how nondescript or apparently benign, should immediately arouse a suspicion of syphilis. The possibility of syphilis should also be suggested by the presence of a lesion, particularly one which persists for several weeks, anywhere on the body. Moreover, a cutaneous eruption of blood-borne distribution in a patient who shows no evidence of acute systemic infection is highly suggestive of infectious syphilis. In the presence of these frank manifestations of syphilitic infection, the physician is usually prompt in obtaining the necessary diagnostic laboratory tests. In an impressive number of instances, however, the presence of syphilis is by no means so readily apparent. The greatest opportunity for error does not arise from the presence of a genital lesion or a generalized eruption, but from the apparently solitary lesions in other areas. The tendency is strong for the physician, or the regional specialist, to regard a particular abnormality as a localized and trivial disease, and to fail to ascertain that similar abnormalities are present in other regions of the body.

Exclusion of the Presence of Infectious Syphilis. Not infrequently the physician is confronted by a patient who fears that he has contracted syphilis from a particular exposure and who presents cutaneous or mucosal lesions, genital or otherwise, in which T. *pallidum* cannot be found. The question immediately arises as to whether the eruption or ulceration is a manifestation of infectious syphilis. In the case of a generalized cuta-

neous eruption the problem may be solved immediately by the performance of an S.T.S. If the test is negative, syphilis can be excluded from consideration, for the serologic tests attain virtually 100 per cent sensitivity in the presence of a generalized eruption. The problem is not so easily solved if the lesion is solitary. The proper procedure is to examine material from the suspected lesion under the darkfield microscope for three successive days and to obtain blood for serologic testing. If no spirochetes are found, and the lesion heals, S.T.S. should be obtained at four- or five-day intervals during the first two weeks and at two-week intervals thereafter. The serologic follow-up should be continued for ninety days after the suspected exposure, or after the appearance of the lesion if multiple exposures had previously occurred. The physician should emphasize the fact that the negative S.T.S. obtained during the course of the period of observation do not exclude the presence of early syphilis. To be sure, as the follow-up continues from week to week, the significance of negative tests is steadily increased and the chances that the person is developing syphilis become increasingly remote.

Early Latent Syphilis. The term *early latent syphilis* merely designates those patients who fail to present any lesions of infectious syphilis at the time of examination. As mentioned previously, the patients with early latent and with overt infectious syphilis present essentially the same problem in management. The diagnosis of early latent syphilis is made from (*a*) a history of a recent diagnosis of infectious syphilis; (*b*) serologic evidence of syphilis in a person with a history suggestive of a recently acquired infection; (*c*) discovery of serologic evidence of syphilis in a person known to have been free from infection in the recent past.

LATE SYPHILIS

Late Latent Syphilis. An understanding of the clinical entity of *late latent syphilis* is essential, for approximately 80 per cent of the syphilitic patients seen by the practitioner are in this stage of the disease. Many patients with late latent syphilis are either grossly overtreated or sadly neglected. Once true latency has been established, the subsequent course of the infection is usually benign. It is important, therefore, that this relatively benign and frequently encountered form of syphilis be clearly distinguished from the potentially serious types of infection which may require different therapy.

As defined previously, *late latent syphilis* is the term which designates those patients with serologic or historical evidence of syphilis of more than four years' duration, but in whom no evidence of syphilitic disease is detectable by (*a*) complete physical and neurologic examination; (*b*) an examination of the cerebrospinal fluid; (*c*) roentgenographic examination of the heart and aorta.

Unless these criteria are met it is possible to overlook detectable and potentially serious syphilitic infection. Therefore, the physician should obtain the information made available by these three procedures as quickly as possible. Although the problem of establishing the latency of a syphilitic infection presents no difficulties, it may be difficult to prove that the infection is of more than four years in duration. Frequently the patient will relate a history of the previous discovery of a positive serologic test or of some lesion which was diagnosed and treated as syphilis. In the absence of such a history, the physician must exercise his own judgment as to whether the undoubtedly latent infection is recent or old. As with other chronic infections such as tuberculosis, it is advisable to regard syphilis of unknown duration in a young person as a recently acquired infection.

Syphilis of the Cardiovascular and Central Nervous Systems. Virtually all of the fatalities from syphilis arise from involvement of either the cardiovascular or central nervous systems. It is not generally appreciated that aortic and neurosyphilis frequently occur together. These two most serious forms of syphilis are discussed in following chapters.

Ocular Involvement in Late Syphilis. The most frequently encountered and serious forms of ocular syphilis, optic neuritis, optic atrophy and interstitial keratitis are discussed below and in the chapter on Neurosyphilis. In addition, iritis, chorioretinitis, and rarely a gumma of the orbit or eye, may develop as late manifestations of the infection. Both iritis and chorioretinitis occur in association with many diseases other than syphilis, and the syphilitic form of these ophthalmic disorders is in no way distinctive.

Gummas. Although the development of a gumma has been observed at one time or another in virtually every organ of the body, these focal lesions of late syphilis seldom occur in tissues other than those of the skin,

bones, liver, testes or larynx. It must be appreciated that it is not usually possible to establish with certainty that a particular lesion is a gumma either by the examination of biopsy specimens or by the demonstration of *T. pallidum* in the affected tissue. *T. pallidum* is notoriously difficult to demonstrate in most lesions of late syphilis, and the histopathologic picture of a gumma, while characteristic of syphilis, may also be simulated by a number of other chronic granulomas. From the standpoint of diagnosis, therefore, a gumma is a chronic granulomatous lesion, reasonably "characteristic" in appearance, which develops in a person with syphilis and which resolves with residual fibrosis within a few weeks of the institution of antisyphilitic therapy. The results of the S.T.S. are of great value in the diagnosis of a gumma; with modern techniques, the tests are almost invariably positive in high titer. Conversely, the finding of a negative S.T.S. (with no history of previous antisyphilitic therapy) constitutes strong evidence against the possibility that a particular granuloma is syphilitic in origin.

Skin. In contrast to the multiple lesions of the skin which may appear during the course of infectious syphilis, cutaneous gummas are usually localized to a single area. The skin of the face, neck and extremities is most frequently involved, presumably because of the influence of trauma. The lesion arises in or under the skin as a nodule which enlarges at so slow a rate that it produces no pain or tenderness. The nodule may eventually break down, forming a symmetrically rounded ulceration with an indurated base which is covered with a small amount of exudate. Although the individual intact nodules are reddish brown, there is a gray-blue coloration along the periphery of the gumma which is sufficiently characteristic to be helpful in diagnosis. The ulcerated or indurated lesions heal slowly and are replaced by a thin smooth scar which retains the configuration of the active process, and is surrounded by a pigmented border. If untreated, a cutaneous gumma may persist in varying stages of activity for a period of months or even for several years. Gummas of the skin may simulate a number of diseases, and are frequently mistaken for varicose ulcers of the legs or for lupus erythematosus (discoid type) of the face.

Juxta-articular nodules are firm subcutaneous gummas which may develop on the extensor aspects of the elbows or knees, close to the insertion of the muscle. The nodules seldom enlarge to more than 1 or 2 cm. in diameter and rarely ulcerate.

Skeletal System. Gummatous lesions of the skeletal system develop in approximately 5 to 10 per cent of patients with late syphilis, more commonly in Negroes than in whites. The process may involve the periosteum, the cortex or the medullary cavity. The periostitis is primarily proliferative, but in osteitis and osteomyelitis both destructive and proliferative processes are present together. In syphilitic involvement of the skull, the lesions are predominantly destructive in character.

Syphilitic disease of bone is often mistaken for sarcoma, tuberculosis or metastatic carcinoma. Gummas may be differentiated from these other diseases by: (*a*) the S.T.S., which is almost invariably positive in high titer in the presence of syphilis of bone; (*b*) the appearance of the lesion in the roentgenogram; (*c*) biopsy; and (*d*) the response to antisyphilitic therapy.

The finding of a negative S.T.S. constitutes strong evidence against the diagnosis of osseous syphilis. Moreover, it is essential to realize that if a suspected lesion is an active gumma, it will show evidence of healing within a few weeks of the institution of therapy. Unless definite symptomatic improvement appears within a four-week period, therapeutic trial should be discontinued and a biopsy performed because of the possibility of neoplastic disease.

Syphilis of the Liver. Syphilis is a rare cause of clinically detectable disease of the liver and is discussed in the chapter on Diseases of the Liver.

Gumma of the larynx develops occasionally in persons with late syphilis. The chief clinical manifestation of this form of syphilis is the development of severe and persistent hoarseness in a person who is otherwise completely asymptomatic. Gummas may closely simulate tuberculous or neoplastic disease of the larynx. Therefore, a therapeutic test should not be attempted until an effort has been made to exclude the presence of these more serious diseases.

Gumma of the testicle or epididymis occurs rarely and is characterized by the development of a firm, smooth, occasionally nodular mass which slowly enlarges in size. Testicular gummas seldom produce symptoms other than a dragging sensation caused by the weight of the mass. As neoplasms arising from the testicle may grow and metastasize with great rapidity, the physician must be unusually wary in order to avoid the serious error of performing a "therapeutic test" for syphilis in a patient with a malignant neoplasm.

Gummatous Formation on Other Structures. As mentioned previously, the development of the localized gummatous lesion of late syphilis has been observed in virtually every tissue of the body. Because of the rarity with which gummas appear in structures other than those noted above, no attempt will be made to catalogue all the possible sites of involvement. Nevertheless, certain points should be emphasized.

Gummas usually produce clinical manifestations similar to those caused by chronic infectious or neoplastic disease of a particular structure. Therefore, even in a patient known to have syphilis, the physician should be slow to accept the diagnosis of gumma in a site of infrequent involvement until the possibility of neoplasm has been excluded (by biopsy or surgical exploration if necessary). Moreover, even in patients who have been infected with syphilis the presence of a gumma is distinctly unlikely if the S.T.S. is negative.

SYPHILIS IN PREGNANCY

A woman infected with syphilis can transmit the disease to a fetus for an undetermined period of years after she has contracted the infection. As would be anticipated, the chance of intrauterine transmission of syphilis is greatest when the infection has been recently acquired, and diminishes throughout successive pregnancies. Infection of the fetus usually occurs after the fifth month of pregnancy and may result in spontaneous abortion, miscarriage, a stillborn fetus or a fatally ill infant.

Prenatal Syphilis. The clinical manifestations, course, and diagnostic problems presented by syphilitic infection in infancy and early childhood are beyond the scope of the present article. The clinical manifestations and the course of prenatally acquired syphilis in *adults* are with few exceptions essentially the same as in acquired infections of comparable duration. The unique features of the prenatal variety are the frequency of *interstitial keratitis* and the virtual absence of aortic involvement. Ophthalmalogic texts should be consulted for a discussion of interstitial keratitis. Localized gummatous lesions occur in prenatally acquired syphilis and are identical in every respect with the gummas of late syphilis acquired in adult life. Skeletal involvement is not uncommon, and in the form of osteitis or periostitis may produce "saddle nose" or "sabre shins." A nongummatous form of skeletal involvement which is unique to prenatally acquired syphilis is the characteristic malformation of the teeth described originally by Hutchinson. The changes are most conspicuous in the central incisors, which are unusually small, widely spaced, notched and less broad at the cutting edge than at the gum margin. A rarely encountered syndrome of *Hutchinsonian teeth, interstitial keratitis* and *eighth nerve deafness* (caused by meningeal involvement) is known as *Hutchinson's triad* and is considered to be unequivocal evidence of the presence of prenatal syphilis.

Pregnancy. Adult women with prenatally acquired syphilis may transmit the infection to their offspring during pregnancy. Such "third generation" syphilis is extremely rare but seemingly indisputable instances of its occurrence have been reported. More often, an apparent instance of this phenomenon is the result of syphilitic infections contracted independently by a mother and her daughter and the subsequent intrauterine transmission of the disease by the latter.

SEROLOGIC DIAGNOSIS OF SYPHILIS

The serologic tests for the presence of *syphilis reagin* (S.T.S.) assume a greater or lesser importance in diagnosis depending upon the type of syphilitic infection which is under consideration. In infectious syphilis the serologic tests are distinctly secondary in importance to the demonstration of *T. pallidum* by darkfield microscopy. In certain varieties of cardiovascular and neurosyphilis the serologic tests are chiefly of value as an additional confirmation of the clinical diagnosis. In the great bulk of infections observed by the practitioner, however, the diagnosis of syphilis can be established only by serologic testing. It is essential, therefore, that an S.T.S. be obtained as part of the routine of the initial examination of every patient. It is equally important that the results of such tests be subjected to proper interpretation.

The Wassermann test and the other tests designated by proper names are all based on the same immunologic phenomena and all detect the same substance, *syphilis reagin*. In a very real sense all of these tests are nonspecific. This fact presents no difficulties when the S.T.S. is employed to *confirm* a diagnosis of syphilis made by clinical examination or from the patient's history. The nonspecificity becomes of the greatest importance, however, *when a positive S.T.S. represents the sole indication that a patient might have syphilis.* For, in addition to syphilis and the other treponemal infections (yaws, pinta, bejel), there are other states not necessarily infectious, which may give rise on occasion to a positive S.T.S. Such results of serologic testing are designated *biologic false positive reactions* or B.F.P. The incidence of these reactions has not yet been defined, but it has been credibly estimated (Moore) that in certain highly selected populations in the U.S. the incidence may approach 50 per cent.

The finding of a positive S.T.S. in a person with absolutely no clinical or historical evidence of syphilis is thus to be regarded as a highly significant lead but it does not certainly establish the presence of syphilis.

Situations in which it is well for the physician to be particularly wary of the diagnosis of syphilis solely on serologic evidence are: (*a*) the presence of a positive S.T.S. in a patient who is suffering or convalescing from an acute infection; (*b*) the finding of a positive S.T.S. in a patient who has had a recent negative test and whose sexual partners are nonsyphilitic; and (*c*) the finding of a series of doubtful (i.e., "one to three plus") S.T.S., possibly punctuated by an occasional positive in a person who credibly denies having experienced any previous manifestations of syphilis or antisyphilitic therapy.

The problem of the person with the recent acute infection is relatively simple, as the false positive S.T.S. which occur in this setting are usually transient. The treponemal immobilization reaction of Nelson can be of immense help and it is current practice to regard all S.T.S. reactors whose serum is negative by the immobilization test as being truly nonsyphilitic. Unfortunately, however, relatively few laboratories are presently able to perform the treponemal immobilization test on a service basis. Hence, in most circumstances, the problem must be managed by the exercise of arbitrary judgment.

Accordingly, whenever the standard S.T.S. are repeatedly positive in a person with no clinical or historical evidence of syphilis or the other states mentioned above, it is advisable to treat the patient as if early latent syphilis were present (see below). For a detailed discussion of this question of the significance of serologic tests for syphilis the reader should consult the reports by Moore and Mohr and by Davis.

TREATMENT

Early Syphilis. The goal of antimicrobial therapy in syphilis is to effect a drastic reduction of the population of *T. pallidum* to a census readily manageable by the host. In early syphilis (infectious and early latent) attainment of this goal by penicillin is followed in 85 to 90 per cent of infected persons by an apparently complete disappearance of *T. pallidum* from the body. In the remainder, after disappearance of the acute manifestations, the infection survives into the late latent stage or reappears as an infectious or neurologic relapse. The possibility of such relapse can be minimized by continuation of the antimicrobial therapy for a matter of months. In such circumstances it is highly unlikely that the continued therapy *per se* eradicates the persisting *T. pallidum*. On the contrary, eradication during prolonged therapy is presumably accomplished either by the defenses of the host or more probably by the "natural" death of the parasites after their prolonged physiologic confinement.

As the incidence of relapse after short-term therapy is so relatively low, it seems impracticable and indeed inadvisable to subject all patients with early syphilis to the months of treatment necessary for only a few. Accordingly, an acceptable procedure is to treat all patients with early syphilis with only a single large dose of one of the "long-lasting" preparations of penicillin.

A satisfactory regimen for this purpose consists of the intramuscular injection at multiple sites of a total dose of 2.4 million units of one of the "long-lasting" penicillins. The entire dose may be administered at one visit or may be divided over two successive days. The most satisfactory preparation is *benzathine penicillin G fortified with procaine penicillin G,* which is available under a variety of proprietary names. Procaine penicillin in oil containing 2 per cent aluminum monostearate can be substituted in the same dosage.

In the relatively remote event that relapse or other failure of treatment should be detected on subsequent observation, the patient could either be retreated with the above described regimen or could be given 900,000 units of procaine penicillin per day on eight successive days, excluding Sundays. In situations in which it is desired to reduce the chance of relapse to a minimum, it is advisable to prolong therapy for a six-month period by the addition of 300,000 units of procaine penicillin once or twice weekly to either of the two short-term regimens.

A number of other drugs, notably chloramphenicol and the tetracyclines, represent relatively imperfect substitutes for penicillin in the treatment of syphilis. Regimens for the use of these other drugs have not been clearly defined. Hence when penicillin cannot be used, it would seem advisable to administer chloramphenicol or a tetracycline drug orally for a two-week period in a total daily dose of 2 gm. with unusually meticulous clinical and serologic follow-up observations thereafter.

Course of Early Syphilis Under Treatment. In early syphilis an acute exacerbation of any visible lesions may become evident within six to ten hours of the initiation of treatment. This exacerbation soon after the institution of antimicrobial therapy is designated the *Herxheimer reaction,* and occurs to some degree in the majority of patients with early syphilis. It is seldom sufficiently emphasized that the intensity of a Herxheimer reaction reflects the intensity of the syphilitic inflammation before treatment. Thus lesions which are poor in *T. pallidum* are less likely to develop an acute exacerbation following the start of therapy than the infectious lesions of early syphilis. The duration of the reaction is short (two to four hours), and in early syphilis the phenomenon is in no way harmful.

The rate of disappearance of *T. pallidum* and the healing of the external lesions are modified by their number and size. In general, within 24 hours of the start of therapy, *T. pallidum* is no longer demonstrable in the lesions and the latter show evidence of the onset of resolution. During the succeeding week, healing proceeds rapidly. All but the most unusually extensive processes are completely healed, save for residual pigmentation or scarring, within seven to ten days after the start of therapy.

At this point, the patient presents little or no clinical evidence of syphilitic infection, but unless treatment was started before the development of seropositivity, the serologic tests are still positive.

During the first six months after the start of treatment, the patient should be seen at two-weekly intervals and questioned for symptoms suggestive of mucocutaneous, ocular or neurologic relapse. Moreover, the questioning should be supplemented by a complete examination of the skin, oral cavity, genital and perianal regions, superficial lymph nodes, anterior eye and fundus, cranial nerves and the tendon reflexes of the extremities. Material from a lesion which makes its appearance should be examined by darkfield microscopy. At the same two-week interval, a specimen of blood should be obtained for serologic testing. When facilities are available, the blood specimens obtained before, during and after treatment should be tested in serial dilution, if the usual qualitative test is positive (i.e., "four plus"). A pronounced fall in titer (e.g., positive when diluted 1 to 128, changed to positive when diluted 1 to 4 and negative on further dilution) may be detectable at a time when the usual qualitative test would be reported simply as *positive* (i.e., "four plus"). Even with the aid of quantitative tests, a change in the S.T.S. may not become evident until the third or fourth month after the start of treatment. Between the third and the sixth month after the institution of therapy, the serologic reactions gradually become negative in the majority (approximately 80 per cent) of treated cases. In a small number of patients (5 or 10 per cent) the reaction may not be consistently negative at six months, but the titer will have fallen considerably and the reaction will become completely negative by the ninth or twelfth month after the start of treatment. In the remaining group of infected persons (5 or 10 per cent), despite some fall in titer during and after treatment, the serologic tests for syphilis will be repeatedly positive (i.e., "four plus") one year after the institution of therapy. Some of this latter group may attain seronegativity during the second post-treatment year.

In a small proportion of treated infections persistently positive serologic reactions may show a steady increase in titer or the reaction once negative will again become positive. In evaluating such serorelapse, it is essential that the physician realize that minor fluctuations below the range of complete positivity (i.e., so-called "one plus to three plus reactions") are merely a reflection of the day-to-day variation in the sensitivity of the serologic test in the laboratory, and have no significance in respect to a change in the serologic status of the patient. Only a change from complete negativity to complete posi-

tivity or a two-fold change in titer can be considered as definite evidence of serologic relapse. Although clinical relapse does not invariably accompany or follow serologic relapse, a correlation between the two phenomena is so frequent that they have an identical significance in terms of therapy.

A satisfactory serologic response to treatment in early syphilis may thus be defined as complete or virtually complete seronegativity, six months after treatment was started. It is probable that many persons who fail to show such prompt serologic reversal require no further therapy. In the present state of knowledge, however, it is advisable to regard all such cases as therapeutic failures and to reinstitute therapy.

Six months after the start of therapy, it is essential to determine the total cell count, total protein, colloidal gold and S.T.S. of the *cerebrospinal fluid*. In the event that abnormalities are present, treatment for early neurosyphilis should be instituted according to the principles discussed in a following chapter. If the cerebrospinal fluid is normal at this time, it is necessary to examine it on one more occasion after an interval of one year, i.e., eighteen months after therapy.

If at six months after the start of therapy for early syphilis the patient presents no evidence of relapse on clinical or cerebrospinal fluid examination and the blood serologic tests have shown a satisfactory response, the interval between examinations (clinical and serologic) may be extended to one month. The procedure at the time of each visit should be exactly the same as when the patient was examined at fortnightly intervals, and the monthly examination should be continued for one year. The clinical and serologic follow-up should be continued for a total period of five years, but the interval between examinations may be gradually lengthened to three to six months after the first eighteen months of observation have been completed.

Prognosis of Early Syphilis Following Peni- may be expected following the use of present-logic cure (i.e., complete eradication of *T. pallidum*) or of permanent latency which may be expected following the use of present-day methods for the penicillin treatment of early syphilis cannot yet be stated with precision. In broad terms it can be said that biologic cure is apparently attained in 85 to 90 per cent of the persons who receive one course of treatment and in a substantial proportion of those who require retreatment.

The ultimate outcome of the infection among patients with apparent biologic cure two or three years after treatment is almost uniformly excellent. A few patients with early syphilis will fail to become serologically negative. If they have been adequately treated including a second course of penicillin treatment for the seroresistance, and have no evidence of syphilis other than a low titer on quantitative serologic test, they may be safely followed without further treatment.

Relapse and Reinfection in Early Syphilis. Post-treatment relapse of early syphilis is a phenomenon which if unrecognized has serious implications. The incidence of complicating lesions in the eye or nervous system is appreciably higher in the case of relapsing infections than in the course of untreated syphilis. Moreover, opportunity for transmission of the infection is enhanced, as the person may not appreciate that the cutaneous or mucosal lesions of relapse are related to the treated "venereal" infection of several months previously.

Reinfection probably accounts for a considerable number of the treatment failures. The patient is cured of his infection before he has mobilized resistance to *T. pallidum* and hence can become reinfected. With the old long-term arsenical and bismuth therapy the patient was protected from reinfection while he was under treatment and presumably also had developed considerable immunity by the time therapy was completed.

Late Latent Syphilis. It is probable that once true latency (*vide supra*) has been established there is no need for the administration of antisyphilitic therapy. Moreover, the possibility exists that the organisms which persist within the host after the development of true latency are not particularly susceptible to antimicrobial therapy. Unfortunately there is no way by which apparently latent syphilis can be distinguished from active disease of the aorta or other viscera which has not progressed to the point of clinical recognition. Thus, the physician has no choice other than to treat all persons with late latent syphilis.

From the preliminary experience in the treatment of early syphilis with penicillin and from the available knowledge of the course of the infection once late latency has been established, it would seem that regimens which constituted adequate therapy for early syphilis would be at least equally effective in the treatment of late latent syphilis. Because the problem with late latent syphilis is

less urgent, however, it is permissible to use a regimen of 600,000 units of procaine penicillin administered twice weekly for a four-week period.

Course Under Therapy and Prognosis. As by definition, persons with late latent syphilis exhibit no clinical evidences of infection, they will show no change in clinical status as a result of successful therapy. In an individual patient with late latent syphilis, a precise evaluation of the result attained by therapy or natural immunity can only be made by following the patient throughout his entire lifetime. Until sufficient time has elapsed to permit a long-term evaluation of the results of the penicillin therapy of late latent syphilis, therefore, the expected outcome of the infection in a person treated with penicillin can only be surmised from the results of penicillin therapy in other forms of syphilis. A reasonable prediction would be that less than 2 per cent of patients with late latent syphilis who are properly treated will subsequently develop a serious manifestation of late syphilis. The few who do exhibit evidence of progression despite theoretically "adequate" treatment will be chiefly those in the older age groups who had well established but clinically unrecognizable aortitis at the time of the treatment of the apparently latent syphilis.

Serologic Reversal in Late Latent Syphilis. In late syphilis (including the latent variety), the serologic tests do not reverse to normal after treatment so readily and uniformly as they do following the therapy of recently acquired infections. This frequent failure of the serologic tests to become normal is designated *seroresistance*. There are two important facts concerning seroresistance which must be fully appreciated by the physician. (1) There is no reason to believe that the phenomenon of seroresistance alters the outcome of the treated infection in any way. (2) Seroresistance cannot be influenced by additional therapy. Once it is established that a patient with late latent syphilis has received a proper regimen of therapy, it is as irrational to continue therapy because of a persistently positive S.T.S. as it would be to persist with antituberculous chemotherapy merely because of the continued presence of a positive tuberculin reaction. The physician should realize that the laity, almost without exception, hold the erroneous notion that a positive S.T.S. signifies the actual presence of *T. pallidum* in the particular specimen of blood which was tested. Therefore, it is important to explain in understandable terms the true significance of serologic tests to each patient who is infected with syphilis. It must be appreciated that seroresistance, by definition, is the phenomenon observed only in *latent* syphilitic infections. The persistently positive serologic tests in persons with obvious progressive lesions of the aorta or nervous system are not to be considered as examples of seroresistance.

Examination of the Cerebrospinal Fluid in Late Latent Syphilis. In contrast to the situation which exists in early syphilis, the cerebrospinal fluid is examined *before* the institution of therapy in late latent syphilis, for a normal fluid is one of the prerequisites for the diagnosis of latency. In the event that a latent infection has been proved to be really late, i.e., of more than four years' duration, subsequent examinations of the cerebrospinal fluid are not necessary. In those instances in which it is impossible to determine the duration of the infection, and hence the possibility of early latent syphilis cannot be excluded, the cerebrospinal fluid should be reexamined eighteen months after the institution of therapy.

Treatment of Gummas. The penicillin regimens appropriate for late latent or for early syphilis are entirely adequate for the treatment of a gumma. If aortic or neurosyphilis is also present it should receive precedence in the choice of therapy, and a penicillin regimen appropriate for aortic or neurosyphilis would also be appropriate for a gumma. When a gumma is strategically located, as in the larynx, it is advisable to administer only two 25,000 unit doses of penicillin on the first day of treatment. In this way, the intensity of a Herxheimer reaction might be modified even though its occurrence cannot be completely prevented. The complete regimen can then be started on the following day. Within the first week of treatment, there will usually be subjective and objective evidence of improvement in the status of the lesion. Resolution of the lesion or lesions is steadily progressive, but the time required for complete healing will vary from several weeks to several months depending upon the original size of the gumma. Once the lesions are completely healed, the subsequent course and the management of the patients are the same as in late latent syphilis.

Treatment of Syphilis in Pregnancy. An S.T.S. should be obtained on every pregnant woman during the first and last trimesters of pregnancy, and any woman who has had syphilis should be evaluated as to the need for antisyphilitic treatment with each pregnancy. Formerly, treatment was repeated with each pregnancy. This is no longer deemed necessary and the present practice is to allow a pregnant woman to reach term untreated provided that she has received theoretically adequate therapy in the past, shows no clinical evidence of active syphilis and is seronegative.

Early syphilis in the pregnant woman carries the greatest risk of infection of the fetus. Nevertheless, with penicillin, a normal infant can be expected even if the disease is discovered late in pregnancy. The penicillin regimens recommended for early syphilis are satisfactory for the treatment of syphilis in pregnancy. If the infection is not discovered until after the thirty-second week of pregnancy, however, it is advisable to administer 300,000 units of procaine penicillin three times daily for at least eight days.

Treatment of Prenatally Acquired Syphilis. Except for interstitial keratitis, the treatment of the various manifestations of prenatally acquired syphilis which are first recognized during adult life is the same as in the corresponding situations with syphilis contracted during adult life. *Interstitial keratitis* is a potentially serious complication which should be treated promptly and intensively with penicillin and cortisone or corticotropin. Procaine penicillin, 300,000 units intramuscularly, should be administered each day for a two-week period. Preliminary observations indicate that cortisone and corticotropin systemically are equally effective but apparently no more so than cortisone when used locally. Whenever possible, interstitial keratitis and the other ocular manifestations of syphilis should be treated in consultation with an ophthalmologist.

INDIVIDUAL PROPHYLAXIS AND THE PREVENTION OF SYPHILIS

The most effective prophylaxis against syphilis is the use of a condom during sexual intercourse and a thorough cleansing of the genitalia and adjacent areas with soap and water immediately thereafter. These measures afford an appreciable amount of protection to either sex against the direct genital transmission of the infection. There is no efficacious method of protection against transmission by other bodily contacts. The most practicable method for the *prevention* of syphilis among a civilian population is to effect a reduction in the *prevalence of infectious syphilis* by the prompt recognition and proper therapy of all persons with recent infections. In this way the incidence of new contact infections can be sharply reduced.

PSYCHOLOGIC AND SOCIAL ASPECTS OF SYPHILITIC INFECTION

The mechanics of the diagnosis and treatment of syphilis are simple and require but little of the physician's time. Not infrequently, however, the patient's discovery that he or she has syphilis immediately gives rise to problems which occasion considerable mental distress. Although these problems appear uniquely insolvable to the person concerned, they can usually be settled satisfactorily by the physician who is willing to devote the time. It is not sufficient for the physician merely to "answer any questions." Frequently, a reticent patient will cherish all manner of unwarranted fears about the effects of the infection on himself or his intimates without betraying such fears to his physician. Therefore, at the same visit at which the diagnosis of syphilis is announced, it is essential that the physician undertake an active discrediting of the folklore of syphilis and an honest presentation of the facts and potentialities of syphilitic infection. The questions of transmissibility to others, the risk of neurosyphilis, the chances of having nonsyphilitic children, and the significance and expected course of the serologic tests should be discussed in detail. The circumstances under which it would be proper for the patient to marry depend upon the stage of the infection. In general, it is not advisable for the patient to marry a nonsyphilitic person until the danger of infectious relapse is minimal, i.e., one year after an adequate course of penicillin therapy. An infection of more than four years' duration should not constitute a barrier to marriage from the standpoint of transmission of infection to the spouse. The presence of neurosyphilis, however, constitutes a certain economic liability and, in decisions on the advisability of marriage, should receive exactly the same consideration as any other physical handicap. Obviously, if the physician knows or suspects that a patient has paresis, every effort should be made to prevent marriage.

In marital and premarital problems the physician should exert all his influence to have the patient inform spouse or fiancée of the diagnosis of syphilis. Although the patient (and some physicians) frequently believe that the announcement to the marital partner that the patient has syphilis will "break up the marriage," such fears are almost invariably unwarranted. In the unusual event that a patient with *potentially infectious* syphilis refuses to inform the marital partner, the physician should undertake to do so.

Walsh McDermott

References

Moore, J. E.: The Modern Treatment of Syphilis. 2nd ed. Springfield, Charles C Thomas, 1941.
———, and Mohr, C. F.: Biologically False Positive Serologic Tests for Syphilis. J.A.M.A., *150*:467, 1952.
Nelson, R. A., Jr., and Mayer, M. M.: Immobilization of *Treponema pallidum in vitro* by Antibody Produced in Syphilitic Infection. J. Exper. Med., *89*:369, 1948.
Turner, T. B.: Protective Antibodies in the Serum of Syphilitic Rabbits. J. Exper. Med., *69*:867, 1939.
———, Fleming, W. L., and Brayton, N. L.: Protective Antibodies in the Serum of Human Syphilitics (abstract). Proc. 31st Annual Meeting Am. Soc. Clin. Investigation. J. Clin. Investigation, *18*: 471, 1939.
Woods, A. C.: Syphilis of the Eye. Am. J. Syph., Gonor. & Ven. Dis., 27:133, 1943.

SYPHILITIC AORTITIS AND ANEURYSM

History. In the latter half of the sixteenth century Ambroise Paré remarked upon the frequent occurrence of aortic disease (aneurysm) in "those who have often had the unction and sweat for the cure of the French disease." The writings of Lancisi of Rome (1654–1720) and Morgagni of Padua (1761) indicate their recognition of syphilis as an etiologic factor in aortic aneurysm. Erichson credits Donald Monro, 1760, with the first reference in English to syphilis as a causative factor: "sometimes a scorbutic or venereal taint . . . has been accused." Welch in 1875 presented data proving syphilis to be the cause of aortic aneurysm in 66 per cent of 53 cases of aneurysm found at autopsy. Heller and subsequently Döhle (1895) published a description of the gross and microscopic lesions. *Treponema pallidum* was demonstrated in lymph nodes in syphilis by Schaudinn and Hoffmann in 1905 and in the wall of the aorta in syphilitic aortitis by both Reuter and Schmorl in 1907.

Prevalence. A quarter century has passed since a conservative estimate indicated that syphilitic aortitis and its complications constituted from 8 to 18 per cent of all heart disease; that it accounted for from 20 to 40 per cent of organic heart disease in Negroes and from 4 to 10 per cent among whites. There is every reason to believe that the incidence of cardiovascular syphilis is being sharply reduced in the United States by prompt recognition and effective modern treatment of early syphilis, and that the figures cited from the pre-penicillin literature are now much too high.

While the figures furnished by pathologists indicate that aortitis is a common visceral manifestation of acquired syphilis, indeed the commonest recognized at necropsy, they do not supply the clinician with reliable information concerning the incidence of aortitis in living persons who have been infected with syphilis. It should be remembered that, even when acute syphilis is untreated, many subjects reach the pathologist without gross changes indicative of the infection. Such cases are not detectable at autopsy and their occurrence obviously distorts inferences with respect to the prevalence of aortic syphilis. It is probable that the incidence of aortitis in syphilis does not exceed 10 to 12 per cent.

Morbid Anatomy. Syphilitic aortitis constitutes the basic pathologic lesion—the foundation pathology—of syphilitic cardiovascular disease. The changes occur most commonly in the root and arch of the aorta.

The route traversed by *T. pallidum* in its invasion of the aorta is not known. The location and extent of the resulting pathologic changes are of the greatest importance, for they determine the clinical manifestations of aortitis in the individual case. Thus, as commonly happens, involvement at the level of the sinuses of Valsalva carries the threat of dilatation of the aortic ring or extension of the inflammatory reaction to the aortic valve with resulting incompetency, or of narrowing of the orifices of the coronary arteries with embarrassment of the myocardial blood supply. If the predominant involvement is considerably distal to both the coronary ostia and the valvular insertions, the only important lesion which can develop is an aneurysm.

The histologic changes are those of a destructive mesaortitis. Fibrosis converts the media "into merely a débris of patches of distorted muscle and elastic tissue separated by scars" (MacCallum). The intima is irregularly thickened and is frequently hyalinized and exhibits irregular sunken areas beneath which the wall of the aorta is actually thinner

than elsewhere. If the syphilitic process is fairly evenly distributed, only elongation and dilatation of the arch of the aorta may result. Focal weakness of the wall may lead to aneurysm formation. If the root of the aorta is involved, dilatation of the aortic ring, widening and sagging of the commissures with separation of the leaflets of the aortic valve, or syphilitic changes in the leaflets themselves may occur and result in aortic valve incompetency. Finally, narrowing of the orifices of the coronary arteries, resulting in interference with blood flow to the myocardium, may take place.

CLINICAL AND SUBCLINICAL FORMS OF AORTIC SYPHILIS

Because of the nature of the pathologic change in syphilitic aortitis the manifestations of the disease fall naturally into several groups: (*a*) uncomplicated syphilitic aortitis; (*b*) syphilitic aortic insufficiency and congestive heart failure; (*c*) syphilitic atresia of the coronary ostia; and (*d*) aortic aneurysm. Combinations of *b, c* and *d* are frequent.

Uncomplicated Syphilitic Aortitis. The term uncomplicated syphilitic aortitis describes a lesion in which syphilitic changes are present in the aorta, but the process has not extended sufficiently to produce an aneurysm or detectable involvement of the valves or coronary ostia. As would be anticipated from its nature, uncomplicated syphilitic aortitis presents no consistent clinical manifestations and hence cannot be convincingly diagnosed during life. At one time, various phenomena such as dilatation of the ascending aorta or the quality of the aortic second sound were thought to be sufficiently distinctive to permit detection of uncomplicated aortic syphilis. Continued experience, however, revealed that the auscultatory phenomena were untrustworthy and the roentgenographic findings in question were not uncommon in diseases other than syphilis. For example, hypertension, arteriosclerosis, and perhaps even a loss of aortic elasticity with age, all produce an aortic dilatation indistinguishable from that caused by syphilis. Conversely, in the presence of clinically demonstrable aortic syphilis such as aortic valvular insufficiency, the aorta is dilated in only about one-half the cases. Irrespective of width, syphilis is the most frequent cause of calcification of the ascending aorta. Hence when calcification permits clear visualization of the supervalvular and ascending portions of the aorta on a roentgenogram, syphilis is almost invariably present. In such an extensive type of involvement, however, the process usually involves the aortic valve as well, so that even this roentgenographic finding is of no real value in the diagnosis of *uncomplicated* syphilitic aortitis.

To all intents and purposes, therefore, during the very phase of aortic syphilis in which it should be most amenable to treatment, namely uncomplicated aortitis, it is a subclinical entity. As a consequence, the only way in which aortic syphilis can be treated, while still uncomplicated, is by the careful identification and treatment of all persons with latent syphilis (see section on Latent Syphilis). When this is done, clinically overt cardiovascular syphilis rarely develops.

Syphilitic Aortic Insufficiency. As the root of the aorta at the level of the sinuses of Valsalva is the commonest location for syphilitic aortitis, one would predict that involvement of the aortic valve and the coronary orifices would be the commonest complication. Such is the case. Aortic valve incompetency is present in approximately 30 per cent of all cases of syphilitic aortitis at necropsy (24 per cent of the Vanderbilt University Hospital series) and in about 60 per cent of the cases recognized during life. Patches of aortitis above the commissures of the valves lead to widening of the commissures with separation of the valve leaflets; extension of the process along the free border of the cusp produces thickening and contraction; penetration of the cusp along the attachment to the aorta results in thickening and contraction. All lead eventually to incompetency of the valve. Aortic regurgitation results in cardiac enlargement and, eventually, congestive heart failure, conditions not encountered in uncomplicated aortitis or aneurysm unaccompanied by aortic insufficiency.

Clinical Manifestations and Course of Aortic Insufficiency With or Without Coronary Ostial Atresia. The clinical manifestations of syphilitic aortic insufficiency and its attending cardiac embarrassment, which help to differentiate it from other forms of aortic valvular disease, are: (1) the eventual development of cardiac failure after an asymptomatic phase of greater or lesser duration; (2) the simultaneous presence of coronary arterial insufficiency and aortic insufficiency in the absence of aortic stenosis; and (3) collateral neurologic or serologic evidences of syphilis.

The eventual development of frank cardiac insufficiency is an important difference between the aortic valvular insufficiency produced by syphilis and that caused by rheumatic fever. With the latter disease, when the sole valvular defect is an aortic insufficiency, cardiac failure seldom if ever develops (Grant). In contrast, with syphilitic aortic insufficiency, the patient may remain asymptomatic for five to twenty years after the diagnosis is established, but cardiac failure develops sooner or later in almost virtually all instances. In a joint study at the Johns Hopkins and New York Hospitals, the natural history of aortic insufficiency was tabulated for 1020 patients. It was found that the long-term prognosis for the entire group was not so poor as had at one time been believed. Between 33 and 43 per cent of the patients survived ten years and some 20 to 30 per cent survived fifteen years after the diagnosis was made at one or the other of these hospitals. Nevertheless, of the patients who died, 75 per cent died with predominant symptoms of cardiovascular disease.

The presence and association of aortic regurgitation and coronary arterial insufficiency is of considerable help in distinguishing between syphilitic and rheumatic aortic valvular disease. To be sure, coronary arterial insufficiency may occur as a part of rheumatic valvular disease, but only with severe aortic *stenosis,* a condition which is easily differentiated by clinical examination from the aortic regurgitation of syphilis. Indeed, as described above, the nature of the syphilitic process is such that it cannot produce *stenosis* of the aortic valve. Nevertheless, two points should be stressed in this connection. First, a loud systolic murmur and even a systolic thrill may be present over the aortic area in certain advanced cases of syphilitic aortic valvular regurgitation. No real problem is thus presented, for the diastolic murmur in such cases has the greater prominence and, together with the very low diastolic pressure, clearly indicates the absence of significant aortic stenosis. Second, calcific disease of the aortic valve has been observed to develop in certain patients who have received many years of chemotherapy for presumed aortic syphilis. It is not yet established whether such cases represent medical curiosities with the coincidence of two independent processes or are a late result of an artificially influenced syphilitic lesion.

Even in the late nineteenth century before it was realized that either tabes dorsalis or aortic insufficiency could be caused by syphilis, astute clinicians had noted that the two conditions tended to occur together as a clinical syndrome. As the syphilitic nature of other forms of neurosyphilis was subsequently established, it became evident that they too were frequently associated with aortic regurgitation and the other manifestations of aortic syphilis. With respect to serologic evidence in the differentiation of syphilitic aortic insufficiency from that due to other causes, the situation has been somewhat clouded by the widespread use of penicillin for a variety of illnesses. In the era immediately before the introduction of penicillin into the therapy of syphilis, the serologic techniques in use for the diagnosis of syphilis were highly sensitive. As a consequence, untreated aortic syphilis was almost invariably associated with a positive serologic test for syphilis. Although serologic reversal is not to be anticipated in the large majority of persons with aortic syphilis who have received penicillin intentionally or for another disease, such therapy would presumably have some influence in some cases. Hence it is not possible to rely on a negative serologic test for excluding the presence of syphilis in a patient with aortic insufficiency or aneurysm with quite the same confidence as was the case in the early days of World War II. As antisyphilitic therapy for late syphilis does not influence the treponemal immobilization test, however, the result of this reaction should provide strong collateral evidence of the presence or absence of syphilis in a patient with aortic insufficiency. (See section on Serologic Diagnosis in preceding chapter on Syphilis.)

Once cardiac failure does appear in syphilitic aortic insufficiency, left ventricular enlargement and failure may develop rapidly. As this enlargement may be out of proportion to the changes in size and function of the right heart, *paroxysmal dyspnea* is an impressive early symptom of failure. A *sensation of sternal pressure* is commonly complained of and frank *angina pectoris* occurs not infrequently. Death often occurs suddenly. It results usually from congestive heart failure, coronary ostial atresia, ventricular fibrillation or intercurrent bronchopneumonia.

Syphilis of the Ostia of Coronary Arteries. Narrowing of the orifice of one or both coronary arteries is present in syphilitic aortitis in 10 to 20 per cent of the cases at necropsy (approximately 10 per cent of the Vanderbilt University Hospital series), and is due to localization of the syphilitic process in the sinuses of Valsalva or to the abnormally high origin of the arteries at or above the upper level of the sinuses (von Glahn) where syphilitic involvement of the aorta is common. Syphilitic endarteritis in the course of the vessels is rare, though the writer has seen it in association with a gumma of the myocardium. The occlusive lesion of the orifice is of slow development and may lead to complete stenosis without producing symptoms of myocardial ischemia.

The *angina pectoris* may be identical with that seen with atherosclerosis of the coronary arteries or it may occur in relatively bizarre patterns. For example, the attacks of pain may not be directly attributable to either exercise or rest, may persist for twenty to thirty minutes before relief by nitrites, and may occur even in bed patients as often as ten to twenty times a day.

Syphilitic involvement of the orifice of one or both coronary vessels may also occur in the absence of involvement of the aortic valve. It is of interest, however, that such isolated stenosis of a coronary orifice by syphilis is seldom if ever recognizable ante mortem by the clinician. In recent years it has become evident that, almost without exception, the instances of "isolated stenosis" observed post mortem are in medical examiners' material and not in the autopsy material of the general hospitals. A reasonable inference from this fact is that isolated syphilitic involvement of coronary ostia is a totally asymptomatic condition either up to a few moments before death or *until the development of aortic regurgitation.* Presumably when the process results in death before the development of aortic insufficiency, the patient has so little warning that he neither consults a physician nor is admitted to a general hospital. Hence the old concept of a clinical entity of "syphilitic angina" *in the absence of aortic regurgitation* has no solid basis in clinical experience. To all intents and purposes the clinical manifestations of the coronary arterial insufficiency of aortic syphilis are an additional clinical manifestation of syphilitic aortic regurgitation. From the standpoint of therapy, both entities may be considered together.

Treatment. The nonspecific treatment of syphilitic aortic insufficiency does not differ from that of other forms of aortic insufficiency in congestive heart failure. The reader is referred to the chapters on Chronic Valvular Disease and Diseases of the Myocardium. The symptomatic and supportive treatment of coronary disease is considered in the chapters of this book dealing with Diseases of the Coronary Arteries.

The principal agent for use in the chemotherapy of aortic syphilis is penicillin. Nevertheless, previous experience indicated that bismuth and the iodides were probably beneficial when used with the arsenicals in the treatment of chronic syphilis. It seems reasonable to allow for this possibility, therefore, and to employ these slowly acting remedies before and after the administration of penicillin. The use of them before penicillin is given in syphilitic cardiovascular disease provides, in addition, the possible advantage of "preparing" the patient for the rapid powerful action of penicillin. It must be recognized, however, that the concept that the Herxheimer reaction, which occurs in the acute inflammatory lesions of syphilis, is of any significance in aortic syphilis has been challenged in recent years.

The penicillin may be administered in single daily injections of 600,000 units of procaine penicillin or in six or eight injections daily of aqueous penicillin. In either case therapy should be continued for eight to ten days or until 4.8 to 6 million units have been given. Doses two and three times as large have been employed. Another plan of treatment providing slowly absorbed penicillin over a prolonged period is the injection of 600,000 units of penicillin intramuscularly twice a week for six weeks (for dosage forms see Treatment of Early Syphilis in preceding chapter).

Systematic follow-up examinations with annual or biannual courses of antisyphilitic treatment are in order. The serologic reaction is not usually reversible in aortic syphilis and especially is this true when neurosyphilis is also present.

The evaluation of the usefulness of penicillin in syphilitic aortitis with aortic insufficiency must await the passage of time. As it is clear, however, that the long-term prognosis of the natural course of this condition is by no means discouraging, it seems reasonable to provide penicillin therapy for every patient with aortic syphilis.

It cannot be stated as yet whether a surgical approach will prove to have as much usefulness in the treatment of syphilitic aortic insufficiency as has been the case with other forms of valvular heart disease. Nevertheless, Hufnagel has already been successful in instituting a functionally competent valvular mechanism in patients with aortic regurgitation due to syphilis.

Aneurysms of the Thoracic Aorta. Arteriosclerosis and hypertension in the absence of syphilis commonly produce diffuse dilatation of the aorta, but rarely, if ever produce a saccular dilatation of the thoracic aorta. Pathologists agree that definite, saccular aneurysms of the aorta almost invariably represent complications of syphilitic aortitis. When the destructive changes in the elastic and muscle layers of the aorta, which are characteristic of syphilis, are more excessive at one area of the vessel than elsewhere, the blood pressure tends to balloon out the wall at that point and sacculation occurs. This complication is present at necropsy in 10 to 30 per cent of all cases of syphilitic aortitis (11 per cent of the Vanderbilt University Hospital cases). Multiple sacs may develop, though this is rare. Because syphilitic aortitis develops, in the vast majority of instances, in the thoracic rather than the abdominal portions of the vessel, thoracic aortic aneurysms are over ten times as frequent as abdominal aortic aneurysms; and, since the segments which constitute the ascending, transverse and descending arch of the aorta are the ones principally affected by syphilis, aneurysms occur here almost ten times as commonly as below the arch (Kampmeier). The condition is most frequently encountered in Negro males and in the second or third decade of syphilitic infection.

Pathology. Little can be added to the following graphic description by MacCallum: "the sac most commonly springs from the convexity of the arch and . . . intense sclerotic alterations of the aorta surround its mouth. The orifice is round or irregular in outline, and the edge is rolled over into it somewhat, so as almost to overhang its cavity. The cavity itself may reach a very great size, the sac thus formed pushing aside the surrounding organs or embedding itself in them in the most remarkable way. Mechanical effects produced in this way are of great variety, depending largely upon the point of origin and size of the sac. Pressure on the recurrent laryngeal nerve produces an alteration of the voice from spasm or paralysis of the vocal cord, coughing, dyspnea, etc. Pressure on the trachea flattens it and causes dyspnea. Later the aneurysm may rupture into it after eroding its wall. The lungs yield and collapse before the aneurysm. Pressure on a bronchus narrows it and behind the obstruction bronchiectasis arises. When the sac reaches the bony structures of the thorax, which do not yield, it hammers its way through them, appearing under the skin through a hole in the ribs or sternum. If it extends backward to the spine, it destroys the centra of the vertebrae even down to the spinal canal leaving the yielding intervertebral discs standing almost unaltered; in the same way it may break through the ribs in the back and appear under the skin there. Then it is not long before the skin becomes thinned out and bluish, and finally the sac ruptures, so that death follows at once. Often it ruptures, long before reaching the skin, into the pleura or pericardium, trachea or esophagus, or even into the superior or inferior vena cava." MacCallum states further that "such a sac which can produce a huge and destructive tumor, which destroys itself as soon as it completes its advance . . . is not really composed of the stretched-out walls of the vessels . . . but [of] connective tissue, and that essentially new formed . . . the current of blood eddies about in the cavity, and its pulsation gives the sac its power of breaking down the resistance of the tissues. But the endothelial lining is imperfect and thrombosis occurs . . . layer after layer of compact thrombus material may be hammered down on the wall of the sac. . . . Occasionally, the aneurysm may be completely obliterated in this way. . . ."

Symptoms, Physical Signs. The symptoms of thoracic aneurysm are produced by pressure of the sac upon neighboring structures, thus producing interference with their function, or upon the bony framework of the thoracic cage. Thus a small aneurysm, arising from the sinus of Valsalva, may remain "silent" until rupture occurs in the pericardial sac with resulting hemopericardium and cardiac tamponade; or, if the sac points anteriorly, it may rupture into the pulmonary artery. Aneurysms arising from the aorta in the region between the aortic valve and the innominate artery (the ascending arch) may attain great size without producing symptoms. Here the sac tends to point upward, forward and to the right. Physical signs may be abundant ("the aneurysm of signs"). Proximity to the anterior chest wall results in visible pulsations in the suprasternal notch and pulsations of the upper sternum and upper right interspaces, with or without an actual expansile bulging in these regions. The heart may be displaced downward and to the left and substernal dullness increased to the right over the region of the sac. Compression or traction on the innominate artery results in a demonstrable diminution in the size of the pulse in the right carotid, subclavian, brachial and radial arteries and lowering of the blood

pressure in the right arm. A systolic thrill and diastolic shock are usually palpable over such aneurysms, and on auscultation a rough, systolic murmur followed by a snapping sound coincident with closure of the aortic valve (if not incompetent) may be heard. Aneurysms rising from this region may point posteriorly or attain enormous size and compress the right bronchus or lung (resulting in atelectasis), compress and deflect the trachea (dyspnea, tracheal tug), compress the superior vena cava (venous stasis, cyanosis), recurrent laryngeal nerve (hoarseness, "brassy cough"), esophagus (dysphagia) and sympathetic ganglia (anisocoria, unilateral sweating). These manifestations, however, are much more likely to develop when the sac arises from the transverse portions of the arch (Broadbent's "aneurysm of symptoms"). Aneurysms below the arch, in that part of the aorta extending from the level of the sixth to the twelfth dorsal vertebrae, are rare, frequently nonproductive of either symptoms (unless spinal nerve roots are compressed) or physical signs, and are usually discovered only by roentgenographic examination or at necropsy. In large aneurysms of the transverse and descending portions of the arch, pulsations may be visible in the left interscapular region.

Aneurysms rarely develop in patients with syphilitic aortitis already complicated by the presence of syphilitic aortic insufficiency. Whether this is due to the shortening of life of patients with the latter complication or to the protection afforded the weakened aortic wall by the low diastolic blood pressure which is associated with aortic regurgitation is not clear. The presence of aneurysm, however, is no protection against the subsequent development of syphilitic aortic insufficiency. Narrowing of the orifices of the coronary arteries occurs in about one fifth of the cases, and coronary sclerosis unrelated to syphilis may be present. Syphilitic aortitis with aneurysm uncomplicated by aortic valve or coronary orifice involvement does not produce cardiac enlargement or congestive heart failure.

Pain, dyspnea and cough are the commonest symptoms of thoracic aneurysm. The former occurred in 65 per cent of Kampmeier's series of 596 cases. It may consist merely of a persistent sense of subternal discomfort. The latter may be referred to the neck, shoulder or back and sometimes undergoes periodic intensification of great severity. Bone erosion may produce boring, agonizing pain which is almost intolerable, or may be painless. A striking feature is that certain positions assumed by the patient may cause intensification of pain or afford relief. True angina pectoris, occurring either at rest or after exertion and relieved by nitroglycerin, occurs with approximately the same frequency as involvement of the coronary ostia and aortic valves is encountered at autopsy. *Dyspnea* is complained of almost as commonly as pain. When bronchial or tracheal compression is present, it may be continuous and associated with inspiratory stridor. In the absence of pressure on the air passages and aortic insufficiency, dyspnea is rarely present. When aortic insufficiency complicates the condition, paroxysmal dyspnea and frank attacks of acute pulmonary edema are not uncommon. *Cough,* often of a "brassy" character, is an important symptom in almost half of the cases. It is the result of either recurrent laryngeal nerve, tracheal or bronchial pressure or, in patients with aortic insufficiency, congestive heart failure.

Prognosis. The average time which elapsed from onset of symptoms to death in Kampmeier's series was seven to eight months. Extremely rare cases are recorded in which the aneurysmal sacs became obliterated by laminated clots which subsequently organized. Even calcification may occur. Such patients may live many years. The increasingly rapid developments in vascular surgery provide hope of satisfactory treatment for some patients with thoracic aneurysms. Each patient with this condition presents a special problem, however, so that no generalizations are possible concerning the over-all results to be expected from surgery.

Diagnosis. "Silent" aneurysms are discovcovered usually by roentgenographic examination of the chest or at necropsy. When productive of either symptoms or physical signs, the condition must be differentiated from other mediastinal or thoracic tumors. Neoplasms are not apt to erode bone and may be associated with superficial lymphadenopathy, cachexia and anemia. The following points may be emphasized in the differentiation of aneurysm from mediastinal neoplasm: (1) the history of syphilis or serologic or physical evidence of its presence (aortic regurgitation, Argyll Robertson pupils, absent knee or ankle jerks, superficial gummas or scars, gumma of liver, and so forth); (2) the presence of a mediastinal tumor which, regardless of the "neighborhood" pressure symptoms and signs, is demonstrably expansile by physical examination (pulsations in chest walls, systolic thrill and murmur, diastolic shock and accentuated second sound or tracheal tug); (3) expert roentgenographic examination, including angiocardiography, if necessary. Tuberculosis may be suggested by the pulmonary signs resulting from bronchial or lung compression. Fever, and tubercle bacilli in the sputum, are absent, and roentgenographic examination usually dispels all doubt as to the true nature of the condition.

Roentgenographic Examination. Except in infrequent, small sacculations of the aorta which are situated in such positions that they cannot be brought into profile and made a part of the aortic silhouette, ordinary roentgenography is of inestimable diagnostic value. Moreover, even the less easily detected aneurysms can usually be detected by angiocardiography.

Treatment. The treatment of thoracic aneurysms is directed to: relief of symptoms; the arrest of the syphilitic process by chemotherapy; and, in certain cases, the employment of vascular surgery. Complete bed rest often affords great relief from pain, dyspnea and cough. The iodides have a strikingly beneficial effect upon the pain of aneurysms. Fifteen to 20 drops of the saturated solution of potassium iodide thrice daily is sufficient. Nitroglycerin or amyl nitrite is indicated for angina pectoris. In the late stages of the illness, morphine should be used freely for its analgesic and soporific effects.

Antisyphilitic therapy should be instituted in the same way as described above for the treatment of aortic insufficiency. If the patient's general condition makes it at all reasonable, he should be seen in consultation with a vascular surgeon for consideration of some type of surgical therapy.

Abdominal Aneurysms. Abdominal aneurysms due to syphilis are rare. In asthenic patients with thin abdominal walls the normal aorta can be palpated readily. A definitely expansile tumor along the course of the aorta, the upper and lower limits of which are clearly definable by palpation, is rarely encountered. Syphilis is the major cause of aneurysms of the *upper* abdominal aorta. Aneurysms of the *lower abdominal aorta and its branches* are usually arteriosclerotic. Excruciating, boring abdominal pain is the characteristic manifestation of abdominal aneurysms, and this is usually due to erosion of the bodies of the lumbar vertebrae. The blood pressure in the legs may be reduced to a figure equal to or lower than in the arms. In three fourths of the cases roentgenographic demonstrations of eroded bodies of lumbar vertebrae is possible and is of great diagnostic assistance. Rupture of the aneurysm may occur into the peritoneal cavity or retroperitoneal spaces and, less frequently, into the gastro-intestinal tract. The attending shock and abdominal rigidity may result in a condition suggesting perforation of a hollow viscus.

Dissecting Aneurysms. These are discussed in the chapter on Arteriosclerosis.

HUGH J. MORGAN

References

Allen, E. V., Barker, N. W., and Hines, E. A., Jr.: Peripheral Vascular Diseases. 2nd ed. Philadelphia, W. B. Saunders Company, 1955.

Blitch, C. G., Morgan, H. J., and Hillstrom, H. T.: Early (Subclinical) Syphilitic Aortitis. South. M. J., 25:709, 1932.

DeBakey, M. E., and Cooley, D. A. Successful Resection of Aneurysm of Thoracic Aorta and Replacement by Graft. J.A.M.A., 152:673, 1953.

————: Surgical Treatment of Aneurysms of Abdominal Aorta by Resection and Restoration of Continuity with Homograft. Surg., Gynec. & Obst., 97:257, 1953.

Grant, R. T.: After Histories for Ten Years of a Thousand Men Suffering from Heart Disease. Heart, 16:275, 1933.

Hufnagel, C. A.: Surgical Correction of Aortic Regurgitation. Bull. Georgetown Univ. M. Center, 6:60, 1953.

Ivins, J. C., and others: Symposium on Recent Advances in the Surgical Treatment of Aneurysms. Proc. Staff Meet., Mayo Clin., 28:705, 1953.

Kampmeier, R. H.: Saccular Aneurysm of the Thoracic Aorta: A Clinical Study of 633 Cases. Ann. Int. Med., 12:624, 1938.

————, and Morgan, H. J.: The Specific Treatment of Syphilitic Aortitis. Circulation, 5:771, 1952.

MacCallum, G. W.: Textbook of Pathology. 7th ed. Philadelphia, W. B. Saunders Company, 1940.

McDermott, W., Tompsett, R., and Webster, B.: Syphilitic Aortic Insufficiency: The Asymptomatic Phase. Am. J. M. Sc., 203:202, 1942.

Morgan, H. J.: The Prognosis of Syphilis. J.A.M.A., 112:311, 1939.

Scott, V.: Abdominal Aneurysms. Am. J. Syph., Gon. & Ven. Dis., 21:682, 1944.

Webster, B., and others: Studies in Cardiovascular Syphilis. III. The Natural History of Syphilitic Aortic Insufficiency. Am. Heart Journal, 46:117, 1953.

SYPHILIS OF THE CENTRAL NERVOUS SYSTEM

(Meningovascular Tabetic and Paretic Neurosyphilis, Congenital Neurosyphilis)

"Neurosyphilis" is a general term which includes all those disorders of the nervous structures, the envelopes surrounding them, and the blood vessels traversing them, which are caused by the *Treponema pallidum*. The organism usually invades the nervous system early in the course of syphilis, although symptoms may not appear for many years. The symptoms may be of almost any variety, but may logically be considered variations of a common disease caused by a single type of organism. The clinical manifestations depend on the localization of the organism and the pathologic changes, which, in turn, depend on the inherent reaction of the tissue invaded. From the viewpoint of morbid anatomy and clinical symptomatology it is convenient to think of neurosyphilis as predominantly meningeal, vascular or parenchymatous. Such is the basis of the following discussion.

Etiology. *Treponema pallidum* is the cause of all neurosyphilis. In most instances, invasion of the central nervous system occurs early in syphilitic infection, but demonstrable neurosyphilis becomes evident eventually in only 30 to 40 per cent of those infected. This subject is discussed in a previous chapter.

Morbid Anatomy. In the vast majority of cases the primary pathologic changes occur in the meninges and blood vessels and are, therefore, similar to the syphilitic lesions in other mesenchymal tissues. The reaction in the meninges is of an exudative nature, and the tissue is invaded by inflammatory cells, for the most part by small lymphocytes, but also by a few large lymphocytes and endothelial cells and an occasional plasma cell. The lesion is chiefly confined to the pia mater, although at times the arachnoid and dura are involved. The meningitis may be relatively localized, or so diffuse as to affect all the cerebrospinal meninges, brain and the thoracic portion of the spinal cord. Gummatous lesions which may develop are similar to the gummatous tumors seen in other parts of the body.

The cranial and spinal nerves are frequently involved in the inflammatory process.

Direct invasion of the optic nerves and optic chiasm from the meningeal covering is the most widely accepted cause of *syphilitic optic neuritis* and *primary optic atrophy,* although some believe primary optic atrophy is a degenerative process similar to tabes dorsalis. The specific lesion of *tabes dorsalis* is degeneration of the posterior spinal nerve roots, posterior columns of the spinal cord, and, to some extent, of the posterior root ganglia. Meningitis, generally of a mild chronic type, is also usually present. In *general paresis* the pia arachnoid is thickened and considerable central atrophy may be present, especially over the frontal region and about the lips of the sylvian fissures. The ventricles may be enlarged. The architecture of the frontal cortex is often greatly disturbed by degeneration of ganglion cells, gliosis, perivascular cuffing and round cell infiltration.

Involvement of the small blood vessels, and rarely of the larger ones, is common in all types of neurosyphilis. There is some question whether the process starts in the intima, media or adventitia, but it is probable that the media undergoes the first change. The relation of the coats becomes altered, and because the elastica splits and the intimal lining is broken, thrombi frequently form. Occasionally hemorrhages occur from the weakened vessels.

Symptoms. In the earliest phase of central nervous system invasion by *T. pallidum,* the symptoms are generally mild and frequently pass in a short time without their importance and significance being recognized. They usually consist of headache, general malaise, blurring vision and dizziness. Later, after the invading organisms have become well established within the tissues, symptoms are more persistent and their character is dependent upon the location and extent of the pathologic change. In the first several years symptoms result primarily from meningeal inflammation, whether diffuse or relatively localized, mild or severe. Later, symptoms of vascular disease with or without chronic meningitis may appear and, still later, symptoms of neuron degeneration develop. It is well to keep in mind that neurosyphilis is a progressive disease potentially affecting the entire central nervous system, and although symptoms may wax and wane, with or without treatment, irreparable and disabling damage may occur almost at any time as long as activity of the syphilitic process is present.

ASYMPTOMATIC NEUROSYPHILIS

Neurosyphilis of all types in which there are symptoms or signs is preceded by a period without symptoms. This asymptomatic phase may vary in length from a few weeks to forty or more years, apparently dependent upon the success or failure of the body's defense mechanisms for eradicating or holding the infection in check. During this time the location and character of the disease which is to follow is established. It is during this time, prior to the appearance of symptoms or signs, that the greatest success in therapy can be obtained. Examination of the cerebrospinal fluid is the only means of detecting asymptomatic neurosyphilis, and this examination, together with the knowledge of the approximate duration of the infection, is the only means of estimating the character and prognosis of the disease. A strong spinal fluid reaction of a high cell count, considerable increase in the total protein and a positive Wassermann reaction in high dilution portend the early appearance of symptoms. A near normal spinal fluid, however, gives no assurance that symptoms will not develop. The earliest change in the spinal fluid is usually a pleocytosis of slight to moderate degree with a rise in protein content as the next change. The Wassermann reaction occasionally becomes positive very early, but is almost always positive a year or two after the central nervous system invasion.

MENINGOVASCULAR NEUROSYPHILIS
(Cerebral Syphilis, Spinal Syphilis, Cerebrospinal Syphilis, Syphilitic Meningitis, Cerebral Gumma)

Definition. Meningovascular neurosyphilis is an involvement of the membranes and vessels of the nervous system by *T. pallidum,* with or without secondary involvement of the nervous parenchyma. Although it is usual for both meninges and blood vessels to be involved, there are many instances in which one or the other is predominantly affected, but only rarely is there almost exclusive involvement of either structure.

Incidence. The condition is said to develop usually within the first five or six years after infection, but is not rare many years later, and is associated with prenatal as well as with acquired syphilis. No very definite statements can be made about the incidence of the various types of meningovascular neurosyphilis, but it may be stated that in approximately 20 to 30 per cent of all patients with syphilis meningovascular symptoms develop.

Symptoms. The symptoms of meningovascular neurosyphilis vary greatly according to the location and extent of the lesion, the relative severity of the meningeal and vascular changes, and the extent of the pathologic process.

Although symptoms may develop within the very earliest period of the syphilitic infection or not appear until forty years or more after the primary stage, certain manifestations have come to be associated with the different stages of the disease. In the first weeks of the syphilitic infection the symptoms of cerebrospinal involvement are usually mild and consist chiefly of headache (probably due to meningeal irritation), tinnitus aurium, vertigo and blurring of vision. At times, pains may be caused throughout the body by irritation of the spinal nerves. Opthalmoscopic examination frequently reveals papillitis. During this period, however, there may be symptoms of a severe cerebrospinal meningitis, with intense headache, rigidity of the neck, Kernig's signs and complete prostration. Such a syndrome requires prompt and vigorous antisyphilitic treatment.

In the period beginning six months to a year after the primary stage, severe meningovascular disasters, including meningo-encephalitis, occur with relative frequency. The meningitis may be either cerebral or spinal. A palsy of one or more of the cerebral nerves may develop, which is fleeting and disappears within a few days or may be more permanent. When it is of short duration, recurrences are frequent. Headache, dizziness and visual and auditory symptoms are often noted. Spinal cord symptoms are less frequent, but may develop as "rheumatic" pains in any part of the body, and occasionally as disturbances of the sphincters. Marked spinal meningitis at the dorsal level sometimes leads to compression of the cord, or to so-called "transverse myelitis" with resulting spastic paraplegia. Erb considered the syphilitic spastic paraplegia which bears his name as a primary degeneration of the corticospinal tracts. Gummas are infrequent in the first year.

The *vascular* disorders are the most dreaded complication of the early period. Thrombosis of one of the large meningeal or cerebral vessels is not infrequent. The sylvian and lenticulostriate arteries are particularly susceptible to this lesion which results in hemiplegia. These apoplectic conditions often come on without warning, or, on the contrary, the patient may awake after a few days of headache and dizziness to find himself paralyzed. The paralysis is the result of destruction of brain tissue, due to the shutting off of the blood supply. Although this condition usually develops during the first five to seven years after infection, the syphilitic patient is liable to such manifestations of meningovascular syphilis throughout life.

Cerebrospinal Fluid. During the primary and early secondary period of mild neurosyphilis the changes in the spinal fluid are relatively insignificant. Occasionally the Wassermann reaction is positive, but more frequently there is slight pleocytosis (10 to 25 cells per cubic millimeter). A little globulin may be present, and there may be a weak gold-sol reaction. The serologic tests for syphilis (S.T.S.) of the blood are negative during the early part and positive during the latter part of the primary period. In the early secondary period of mild cases the spinal fluid is similar to that found during the primary stage, while the S.T.S. of the blood are usually positive.

In patients with symptoms the reactions of the spinal fluid are likely to be rather strong after a few months. In most instances the Wassermann reaction is positive with 1 cc. of fluid. The cell count may be high (20 to 200 cells per cubic millimeter) and, when the meningitic symptoms are relatively severe, may run up into the thousands. The fluid nearly always contains globulin and an increased quantity of albumin. The gold reaction usually follows the so-called "luetic curve." At times the spinal fluid reactions may be strongly positive and resemble those of paretic neurosyphilis.

If the lesions are chiefly vascular the spinal fluid findings may be the same as those of the meningeal form, but often they approach normal.

Prognosis. The outlook for patients with meningeal lesions, whether early or advanced, is usually excellent if treatment is properly administered. Of the strictly vascular conditions there are two types: one which becomes manifest at an early period and may be so arrested by suitable treatment that there are no further vascular changes; and another which appears at a later stage and responds to therapy less satisfactorily because the vascular lesions are more generalized and irreparable damage has occurred.

TABETIC NEUROSYPHILIS

(Tabes Dorsalis, Locomotor Ataxia, Syphilitic Posterior Spinal Sclerosis)

Definition. Tabetic neurosyphilis is a condition characterized by visceral crises, and symptoms referable to the afferent spinal nerves and the nerves of special sense. The kinesthetic and pain fibers are, as a rule, first affected; this leads to progressive loss of position sense and to lancinating pains. Trophic disturbances and disorders of the cerebral nerves are also frequently associated with the condition.

Symptoms and Signs. Most of the typical signs and symptoms of tabetic neurosyphilis appear only after the disease has persisted for some time, and relatively few develop during the very early stages. In the early stages tabes may be of two types: in one the symptoms develop before the neurologic signs; in the other the signs are the first to appear. In fact, in one group of patients the neurologic findings may be nearly normal, while there are such typical symptoms as lancinating pains, gastric and other visceral crises. The diagnosis is confirmed by the spinal fluid findings. In another group, Argyll Robertson pupils and the absence of the tendon reflexes may be obvious before any symptoms develop.

Of the characteristic *symptoms,* the most common are related to the sensory system and are apparently caused by pathologic change in the posterior roots. These symptoms are of the type of painful sensations or kinesthetic abnormalities, the latter of which lead to motor incoordination. The cerebral nerves of special sense, especially the optic, are often involved with subsequent symptoms, such as blindness and deafness. Visceral symptoms such as gastric, rectal and laryngeal crises, probably depend on disorders of the sympathetic and autonomic fibers. Trophic changes (perforating ulcer and Charcot joint) also occur.

Pain, which is the most common of the early symptoms, usually begins in the legs, and sooner or later becomes severe. It is often described as a burning, gnawing or lancinating sensation, such as might be produced if a hot knife were stuck into the flesh and twisted. The attacks often last for hours and may recur throughout many years. In some instances there is a sensation of constriction about the waist or chest (girdle sensation), which follows involvement of the radicular nerves. Associated with the attacks are all sorts of abnormal sensory phenomena, such as paresthesia, numbness, and sensations of cold, warmth or tingling. When the pain is severe, pressure on the skin may give relief, or be intolerable because of the exquisite sensitiveness. Occasionally ecchymoses appear on the skin in the region where the pain is felt.

Ataxia (incoordination), the result of loss of the fibers of the posterior roots and posterior columns, often appears after the onset of the pain, although it may be the earliest symptom and be unassociated with any other disorder of sensation. It usually involves the lower extremities, but occasionally affects the hands when the spinal lesions are cervical. The change of gait, which usually develops slowly, is ordinarily first noticed when the patient is walking in the dark. Once in a while the change comes suddenly. The abnormality varies from a slight unsteadiness in the early stages to a marked change of gait in the late stages in which the foot is thrown into the air and brought down unsteadily as if being slapped on the floor. This latter condition is characteristically tabetic.

During the early stages there is little if any loss of the tactile, pain or temperature *senses.* Hypesthesia and hypalgesia develop later. Hyperesthesia, especially of radicular distribution, is common. Rarely, in the late stages, complete anesthesia develops and is followed by disappearance of the pain, which may have been severe. The loss of kinesthetic sense, as shown by inability to feel passive movements of the toes or fingers, may be noted early. Loss of pain sense about the tendo achilles is an early finding.

The *visceral crises* are relatively common manifestations. That most frequently met is the *gastric crisis,* characterized by recurrent abdominal distress and vomiting, often associated with considerable pain in the abdomen. The attacks come on without relation to food, and may persist for hours or days at a time. After the crisis has passed, the patient feels well and has no gastrointestinal symptoms. The attack may be extremely severe and controlled only by large doses of morphine. The character of the crises varies greatly. Some patients have mild nausea and distress, while others vomit almost continuously. This manifestation is not related to the general function of the gastrointestinal tract, and gastric analyses and roentgenographic studies are entirely negative in the typical uncomplicated case. Since, in some patients, gastric crises are accompanied by no other

troublesome tabetic symptoms and the reflexes may be normal, some authorities consider the gastric crises a separate syndrome.

Crises of other organs also occur. Those in
the rectum are characterized by diarrhea or
tenesmus; those in the larynx by local spasm.

Disorders of the sphincters are at times
the first symptoms. Incontinence of urine,
usually beginning as "dribbling," with great
difficulty in starting the stream and inability
to completely empty the bladder, is a common
symptom. The bladder has reduced tone, dependent on loss of sensation, and is readily
recognized on cystoscopy as a "spinal cord
bladder." In relatively few cases there is also
loss of control of the rectal sphincter. Loss of
sexual power is a frequent and often an early
symptom.

Atrophy of the Nerves of Special Sense.
Mild *optic atrophy* occurs in many cases of
tabes; that leading to marked diminution of
vision or complete blindness, however, develops in about 10 per cent of all tabetic patients, and may be an early or almost isolated
symptom. Like gastric tabes, it may occur
without the usual cord signs and symptoms,
and is often designated as "optic tabes." The
auditory nerve is sometimes similarly involved, but marked degeneration is less frequent. Symptoms depending upon atrophy of
the *other nerves of special sense* are rare.

Although *trophic disturbances* usually appear during the late stages, *Charcot joints*
may develop at any period, occurring most
often in weight-bearing joints, e.g., hip, knee,
ankle and spine. The lesion is to be looked
upon as the result of repeated trauma to the
joint surface because of lack of sufficient
joint sensation and consequent deficient
muscular protection. *Perforating ulcers,*
which were formerly seen frequently, are
now extremely rare, possibly because of modern methods of treatment.

The most important *neurologic* signs are
(1) absence of the knee jerks and ankle jerks,
and less frequently of the tendon jerks of the
upper extremities; (2) the Romberg sign;
(3) ataxia of the legs and less often of the
hands; (4) pupillary changes: irregularity,
inequality, sluggishness, and the typical
Argyll Robertson condition; (5) loss of control of the sphincters, and sexual impotence;
(6) sensory disturbances such as hypesthesia
and even anesthesia.

The *tendon reflexes* are typically lost early,
frequently before the appearance of any
symptoms. Their absence is caused by interruption of the reflex arc when the fibers of
the posterior roots are destroyed. Those of the
lower extremities often disappear while the
reflexes of the upper extremities are retained,
although, when the upper part of the cord is
involved, the reverse is true. The ankle jerks
are frequently lost before the knee jerks. In
many cases of tabes the reflexes are retained,
especially when there is evidence of gastric
crises or optic tabes. The *skin reflexes* may be
present or absent. The *abdominal reflexes* are
likely to be absent, as they are in other forms
of syphilis, probably also because of interruption of the reflex arc in the posterior roots.
The *cremasteric reflexes* persist, except in unusual or advanced conditions.

The noteworthy *Romberg sign* (inability to
maintain equilibrium with eyes closed and
feet placed close together) may be observed
before the patient has noticed any difficulty in
walking, because of the reduction of the normal flow of impulses from tendons and joints
which are essential for reflex standing.

Pupillary Signs. As in other types of neurosyphilis, irregularity and inequality of the
pupils are common early signs. The pupils
are almost always unequal, and their early
sluggishness of response usually increases
until they are of the typical Argyll Robertson
type, i.e., respond in accommodation but not
to light. This type of reaction is seen more
commonly in tabes than in any other form of
neurosyphilis. The pupils may be so contracted that their diameter is less than
that of a small pin head, but they may
also be large. In not a few cases they
become fixed and react to neither light nor
accommodation.

Motor Palsies. Paralyses of the extrinsic
eye muscles, especially the levator palpebrae
and the external or internal recti, may be the
first manifestation of tabetic neurosyphilis to
attract the patient's attention. Such palsies
may occur years before any of the other characteristic symptoms of tabes. They are usually
temporary, lasting for a few days or weeks,
but are sometimes permanent. As a rule, they
are accompanied by reflex anomalies in other
parts of the body which are revealed by examination. Lid drop or diplopia often precedes by several years the symptoms of which
a tabetic patient complains, but, since these
conditions right themselves rather promptly,
they are often not seriously considered. Muscle tone is generally decreased in the extremities affected, because of the reduction of afferent impulses to the cord. Joint capsules

are relaxed, and increased mobility of the joints can be demonstrated.

In the late stages of the disease the intrinsic muscles of the hand or foot may become wasted and also, although more rarely, the larger muscles. This may result from degeneration of the anterior horn cells, pinching of the anterior root by the meninges, or, as Richter suggests, from degeneration of the anterior root caused by treponemal action at the junction of the anterior and posterior roots.

Cerebrospinal Fluid. Probably in the tabetic type, as well as in the other forms of neurosyphilis, changes take place in the spinal fluid before either signs or symptoms of the disease become manifest. The reactions of the blood and spinal fluid in tabetic neurosyphilis are similar to those in the meningovascular type. Not infrequently the spinal fluid resembles that recovered from paretic patients; occasionally it is entirely negative, apparently because of spontaneous arrest, a condition which leads to the concept of a burned-out process.

Diagnosis. Blood and spinal fluid tests usually permit recognition of tabetic neurosyphilis before the appearance of marked symptoms and signs. Consequently, when laboratory methods of diagnosis are used and modern treatment is promptly instituted, fewer cases are allowed to assume the typical characteristics. It is well to bear in mind that a typical case is relatively far advanced and is past the stage in which the clinician can take pride in making a diagnosis.

Prognosis. Without treatment the symptoms usually increase slowly for many years until the patient finally becomes bedridden. Frequently, however, the progress is so slow that the change from year to year is only slight. On the other hand, symptoms may develop rapidly. Under treatment, improvement is the rule, and occasionally arrest of the progress occurs spontaneously.

PARETIC NEUROSYPHILIS
(*General Paresis, General Paralysis, General Paralysis of the Insane, Dementia Paralytica*)

Definition. Paretic neurosyphilis is a chronic syphilitic meningo-encephalitis, characterized by progressive dementia and a diffuse, generalized paralysis which terminates in death.

Incidence. About 3 per cent of syphilitic patients exhibit symptoms of paresis. They occur approximately three to five times as frequently in men as in women, although the incidence of syphilis is not greatly different in the two sexes.

Symptoms. The symptoms of paretic neurosyphilis are protean in character and form almost any syndrome. The onset is at times insidious, at other times sudden. For systematic discussion the mental symptoms may be divided into three stages: (1) those of the period of onset, often spoken of as the "medico-legal state"; (2) those of the period of full development of the disease; and (3) those of the terminal period, in which the patient is bedridden. Such a division is entirely arbitrary and in many cases impracticable. A galloping form of the disease is described which progresses rapidly and leads to death within a short period.

1. *The Early Stage.* Any *change in the personality of an adult* should arouse suspicion of paretic neurosyphilis. The first changes in character may be slight and of brief duration, a slight change in manner, for instance, greater irritability, carelessness about the clothes and person, lack of judgment, absent-mindedness, inabilty to concentrate, increased fatigability, hypersuggestibility and slowness of comprehension. These symptoms may develop early and be of little apparent significance in themselves. They may, however, lead to such disasters as heavy losses in business, alcoholism, and loss of reputation because of various excesses. Frequently *neurasthenic symptoms* develop into mild depression or, on the other hand, into euphoria and elation. These symptoms may become much more marked after a period of days, weeks, months or even years, and lead to symptoms characteristic of the well established phase of the disease.

The early physical signs and symptoms include headache, visual disorders and loss of weight. Often there is a slight disturbance of manual dexterity, i.e., tremors of the outstretched hands and inability to make coordinated movements. The frequent decrease of muscle tone, especially in the face, results in flattening of the nasolabial folds which reduces the facial expression and markings and often makes the patient appear younger than he is. Another characteristic symptom is a speech defect which causes poor enunciation of such test phrases as "Methodist Episcopal," "third riding artillery brigade," and so on.

The *pupillary changes* of neurosyphilis appear in the paretic form as in all others. The typical Argyll Robertson pupil can only infrequently be seen. In the early stage the reaction of the pupils may be normal, or the dilated pupil may respond poorly to light. Later there is no reaction to light, but there is response to accommodation, and finally both types of reaction are lost.

Changes in the *tendon reflexes* are common. Atrophy of the efferent or afferent pathways may be so balanced as not to alter the reflexes, or may increase, diminish or destroy them. As a rule, the changes of the tendon reflexes are relatively late manifestations, although they may take place before the onset of any other recognizable symptoms. An extensor plantar response (Babinski sign), ankle clonus and other pathologic reflexes are to be observed in the early stage, but are usually associated with atypical conditions or vascular complications; late in the disease they are common. In the early stages the sphincters are rarely involved, and there is often increased sexual potency.

Sometimes the period of onset is short, and the disease attains the full developed stage with great rapidity; in fact, a seizure may occur in a person in apparently good mental and physical condition and be followed by well developed symptoms of the established stage. The progress may, however, be so slow that a year or more elapses between the onset of mental symptoms and the development of the characteristic syndrome.

2. The *stage of full development* is characterized by varied symptoms which may mimic any type of mental disease. Sometimes there is *euphoria,* and the patient is grandiose, elated with delusions of wealth and great prowess, and feels better than ever before. This classic syndrome appears in only 10 to 20 per cent of cases. Another type is that of *depression,* with anxiety, fear of impending danger and self-accusation. A third well recognized syndrome is that of a *simple dementia,* in which, without excitement, depression or delusion formation, the mind of the patient deteriorates. In a fourth form, *paranoid ideas* predominate. There are many other variations.

Common to all the forms and of the greatest importance is the *progressive dementia.* Loss of memory, especially for recent events, later for past events as well, difficulty in calculation and writing and defects of judgment are sooner or later apparent.

Paretic seizures of either the epileptiform or apoplectiform type, which are frequently accompanied by transient paralyses, are characteristic of this stage. The defect of speech is more marked, and the disorders of the reflexes become prominent.

3. *Terminal Stage.* In the third stage physical weakness becomes great. The patient becomes bedridden and finally reaches the condition of a vegetative organism. There is emaciation, bed sores develop, and generalized paralysis of all the muscles of the body ensues. If death is not caused by a seizure or by intercurrent disease, it finally results from paralysis of the respiratory muscles.

Prognosis. Paretic neurosyphilis has in the past been considered invariably fatal, but at the present time the prognosis is more hopeful because of the newer forms of therapy. Untreated patients live on the average two and one-half to three years after the onset of definite symptoms. Some patients, however, die in a seizure at the very onset of the disease; others linger for five to six years; exceptionally, a patient lives as long as nine or ten years.

Spontaneous remissions are characterized by improvement of both the mentality and the physical condition of the patient. This may be so great as to allow the patient to return to his former occupation. These remissions usually last no longer than six months; rarely they continue for a year. In a few cases they have been reported to persist for a period of years. Spontaneous remissions occur in 2 to 10 per cent of patients.

Syphilitic epilepsy is not a well defined syndrome, and there is much discussion concerning its existence. Three types are described: in the first, though there is no pathologic or serologic evidence of neurosyphilis, epileptic seizures develop some time after the syphilitic infection of a person supposedly without hereditary epileptic taint who has never had previous convulsions; the second type is supposed to be related to meningovascular neurosyphilis and is apparently the result of irritation of the brain; in the third type there is a parenchymatous disorder of syphilitic origin. In the two latter there is the suggestion of an etiologic connection between the convulsions and syphilis; in the first, such a hypothesis has little foundation. It is true that epileptiform seizures are not rare in all types of cerebral neurosyphilis, but the recurrence of convulsions over a period of years is uncommon.

Syphilis of the peripheral nerves may be secondary to disease of such nearby struc-

Table 1. Cerebrospinal Fluid Formulas in Meningovascular and Tabetic Neurosyphilis

WASSERMANN REACTION	CELLS	TOTAL PROTEIN	GLOBULIN	GOLD SOL.
Positive in 0.05 to 1 cc.; 40 per cent negative with 0.2 cc. Pure vascular neurosyphilis usually negative with 1 cc.	Tabes 0 to 200+ Average 25 to 50	17 to 150 mg. per 100 cc. Average 78.	0 to ++++	0122100000 0134431000 3332100000 4443210000 5555431000
	Meningovascular and acute meningitis 200 to 2000	Average 99 mg. per 100 cc.		
	Chronic 0 to 200+	Average 73 mg. per 100 cc.		
	Vascular, often no increase	Average 50 mg. per 100 cc.		

Table 2. Varieties of Cerebrospinal Fluid Formulas in Meningovascular Neurosyphilis

WASSERMANN REACTION	CELLS	TOTAL PROTEIN	GLOBULIN	GOLD SOL	REMARKS
1. Positive 0.6 cc.	90	70	++	0244310000	Average
2. Positive 0.4 cc.	1200	118	++++	4432100000	Acute meningitis
3. Positive 1 cc.	2	45	+	0122100000	Pure vascular
4. Positive 0.05 cc.	40	130	+++	5555431000	Paresis sine paresi asymptomatic
5. Positive 1 cc.	10	30	+	1233210000	Mild
6. Negative	35	35	+	Negative	Mild meningitis
7. Negative	75	50	++	4443100000	Infrequent

Table 3. Variations of Cerebrospinal Fluid Formulas in Tabetic Neurosyphilis

WASSERMANN REACTION	CELLS	TOTAL PROTEIN	GLOBULIN	GOLD SOL	REMARKS
1. Positive 0.66 cc.	25	70	++	0244310000	Average
2. Positive 0.05 cc.	75	95	+++	5555421000	Not rare
3. Positive 1 cc.	40	30	+	Negative	Relatively inactive
4. Negative	50	50	++	0244310000	Infrequent
5. Positive 0.4 cc.	4	25	+	Negative	Infrequent
6. Negative	30	35	+	Negative	Infrequent
7. Negative	3	17	0	Negative	Burned out or stationary

Table 4. Cerebrospinal Fluid Formulas in Paretic Neurosyphilis

WASSERMANN REACTION	CELLS	TOTAL PROTEIN	GLOBULIN	GOLD SOL	REMARKS
Positive in 0.05 to 0.2 cc. in 95 per cent; slightly weaker reaction rarely found	0 to 200 Average 25 to 50	50 to 150 mg. per 100 cc. Average 89	+++	5432100000 5554321000 5555555555	Unusually weak Average Unusually strong

tures as bones, fasciae and muscles. Gummas may encroach upon and implicate the nerves. The peripheral nerves may, however, be affected by a direct extension of the inflammatory reaction along the lymph channels and perivascular spaces. Such neuritis is said to cause palsy of motor nerves or, in the case of the sensory nerves, neuritic pains.

Prenatal neurosyphilis closely simulates all the syndromes of acquired neurosyphilis. About 20 per cent of the patients with prenatal syphilis show clinical or serologic evidence of neurosyphilis. Symptoms may make their appearance in the first years of life, or may be delayed until adolescence, when they suggest meningovascular, tabetic or paretic neurosyphilis.

Juvenile tabetic neurosyphilis is unusual.

The symptoms are similar to those of the acquired form, except that pains are perhaps less frequent.

Juvenile paresis is relatively frequent as compared with juvenile tabes (50:1 in the author's series). The usual age of onset is between 8 and 18 years. The patient may have appeared normal before the paretic symptoms developed, showing few, if any, stigmata of prenatal syphilis. The characteristic clinical manifestation is usually dementia, which progresses rather rapidly. Occasionally the symptoms are those of grandiosity. In other instances the child fails to develop mentally and is considered feebleminded. The duration of life without treatment is usually from three to five years after the onset of mental symptoms.

Syphilitic feeblemindedness is described in many textbooks, but the author has not recognized such an entity. Unless there is definite syphilitic involvement of the brain, the juvenile syphilitic usually has the mentality characteristic of his family.

Diagnosis. As the various syndromes of neurosyphilis simulate almost any organic or functional disease of the nervous system, it is necessary to consider the possibility of the disease whenever neuropsychiatric signs or symptoms develop. The history of syphilis and examination of the blood and spinal fluid usually suffice for diagnosis of neurosyphilis. It is unusual and rare for the S.T.S. to be negative. Frequently it is only by examination of the spinal fluid that diagnosis is possible. When the serologic tests are negative, the diagnosis of neurosyphilis is hardly ever permissible, since experience has shown that such conditions are usually nonsyphilitic. It is nearly always advisable to confirm the clinical diagnosis by examination of the spinal fluid.

Differentiation of the various forms of neurosyphilis is made by the symptoms and to some extent by the condition of the cerebrospinal fluid. Even pathologically, however, it is not possible to distinguish all types. Thus syphilitic meningitis may simulate the tabetic condition in spite of a quite different course; it is then known as "syphilitic pseudotabes." Likewise, the meningovascular type may be erroneously diagnosed as paresis, and vice versa.

Tables 1 to 4 outline the changes usually found in the spinal fluid in the different types of neurosyphilis and offer some possible aids to differentiation.

TREATMENT

Penicillin has proved to be an adequate drug for the control and arrest of most forms of neurosyphilis. General paresis, which has been one of the most recalcitrant forms of neurosyphilis, responds excellently to this form of treatment as indicated by continued life and, in most instances, alleviation of symptoms, a lack of progress of the disease and improvement or reversal of abnormalities in the cerebrospinal fluid.

An adequate dosage for most cases is 12 to 15 million units of penicillin given over a period of fifteen days. This may be given satisfactorily either in aqueous solution every 3 to 4 hours or in a slowly absorbed form given once or twice per day.

Reduction in the cell count and the total protein of the cerebrospinal fluid usually begins before the treatment is ended or shortly thereafter. In most instances the cell count will become normal and the total protein will be greatly reduced within two to three months. The serologic tests and colloidal tests are usually much slower in response, and indeed in not a few cases will remain positive for many years. Therefore, they are not the best indicators of the success of treatment, whereas the cell count and total protein generally reflect the activity of the infection. If there is lack of satisfactory response in these tests or an increase of cells and total protein after a preliminary diminution, it suggests that the infection is reactivated and a repetition of treatment is indicated. These elements of the spinal fluid examination almost always indicate probable relapse and precede the appearance of other symptoms. Relapses after the first course of 15 million units of penicillin in a two-week period are quite exceptional, and failure to respond to a second course is indeed rare. If failure of response is evident, a combination of fever treatment with the penicillin is probably indicated.

The final mental state of the patient is apparently dependent upon the amount of brain damage that has occurred before the treatment was instituted and on the type of symptoms and the personality structure of the individual. Symptoms simulating those of schizophrenia are often continued even after the original disease process seems to have been arrested. Such cases require psychiatric treatment and, in some instances, electric shock therapy may be advisable.

The tabetic syndromes usually respond to

somewhat smaller doses of penicillin, but it is wise to treat such cases with at least 10 million units over a ten-day span. Arrest is to be expected in almost all cases of tabetic neurosyphilis. However, symptoms such as lancinating pains, gastric crises and ataxia may persist and must be treated symptomatically. The cerebrospinal fluid may be expected to become normal in nearly all cases within six months to a year or, at the most, two years after cessation of treatment. Most cases of meningeal vascular neurosyphilis, meningeal neurosyphilis and asymptomatic neurosyphilis respond to relatively smaller doses of penicillin. However, it would seem that conservative treatment would be advisable, and 10 million units over a ten-day period is good treatment.

Optic atrophy is a form of neurosyphilis which responds less satisfactorily to chemotherapy or to chemotherapy in conjunction with fever. Nevertheless, this serious condition should be treated intensively with both penicillin and fever therapy. The spinal fluid usually becomes normal after treatment as in other forms of neurosyphilis. However, when optic atrophy is reasonably advanced, the continuance to blindness is highly probable. In cases in which only one optic nerve is involved, there is good probability of retention of vision in the other eye if treatment is given.

Other drugs such as the tetracyclines also have considerable effectiveness in the treatment of neurosyphilis but, on the basis of present-day experience, penicillin is the drug of choice.

The present reliance on penicillin in the treatment of neurosyphilis is based on the experience and extensive studies carried on by many clinics in the United States since the drug has been available. The exigencies of World War II brought about a coordination of investigative efforts which permitted a gain of maximal information in a relatively short period of time. The greatest amount of experience has been with aqueous crude penicillin and crystalline penicillin G given intramuscularly at three- to six-hourly intervals over periods of from one to three weeks' time. Experience with slowly absorbed penicillin preparations (see Treatment of Early Syphilis) which may be given intramuscularly once a day, is rapidly accumulating, and these may well replace the aqueous variety.

Experimental evidence in neurosyphilis indicates that a relatively small total dose of penicillin given over a period of two weeks or more is more effective than a relatively large dose given over a period of one week or less. Intravenous or intrathecal administration of penicillin is unnecessary, and the latter route carries certain risks which should be avoided.

After the administration of penicillin, patients with any form of active neurosyphilis commonly experience a reaction of temperature elevation and a slight to moderate shortlasting period of intensification of symptoms (*Herxheimer reaction*). Thereafter many symptoms quickly subside, weight is gained, and often a sense of well-being develops, even in cases classified as asymptomatic. The most striking improvement appears in patients with symptoms of meningeal inflammation, and reversal of some neurologic signs frequently occurs in patients with early neurosyphilis. However, improvement in symptoms in general paresis, meningovascular neurosyphilis and tabes occurs within a few weeks and often continues gradually for several months. Arrest in the progression of visual or auditory loss, ataxia or intellectual deterioration frequently appears promptly, though full recovery of these functions may not be possible because of permanent damage to nervous tissue. Lightning pains, which accompany meningeal inflammation, subside promptly after treatment. But in those cases of tabes without evidence of active inflammation, pains may persist unabated.

The Herxheimer reaction, which occurs in active neurosyphilis with penicillin, has not been found to be of sufficient danger, even when cardiovascular syphilis is present, to justify withholding treatment.

The spinal fluid should be examined before and at regular intervals after treatment of all types of cases. The cell count and total protein determinations are the most reliable guides to activity of the syphilitic process within the nervous system. Following penicillin treatment, changes in the spinal fluid abnormalities in a high percentage of cases are to be found. The cell count may be expected to return to normal or near normal at the end of three months. Total proteins fall more slowly, but usually reach approximately normal levels by the end of nine to twelve months and considerably ahead of the gold sol curve and titrated Wassermann reaction. Spinal fluid abnormalities in early neurosyphilis may reverse to normal within a year or two after penicillin treatment, but in the majority of late cases, regardless of clinical type, the gold sol and Wassermann reaction remain abnormal from three to five years or more. If spinal fluid is carefully examined every four to six months, a good estimate of the course of the disease can be obtained. When the cell count and/or total protein remain abnormal for several months without showing a steady decline, or when one or both of these determinations return to abnormal levels after once showing improvement, clinical progression or relapse of the disease may be expected. The cell count and total protein therefore are to be considered the best guides to the need for more therapy.

In cases of primary optic atrophy with continuing loss of vision, and in cases of unquestionable general paresis, it is important to risk no further progression once the diagnosis has been established. In these, fever therapy in addition to penicillin is strongly indicated. In other types of cases, if the patient can be kept under close observation, penicillin as the only treatment may be safely utilized.

HARRY C. SOLOMON

References

Dattner, B., and others: Management of Neurosyphilis. New York, Grune & Stratton, 1945.

Merritt, H. H., Adams, R. D., and Solomon, H. C.: Neurosyphilis. New York, Oxford University Press, 1946.

Moore, J. B., and others: Modern Treatment of Syphilis. 2d ed. Springfield, Ill., Charles C Thomas, 1943.

Stokes, J. H., Beerman, H., and Ingraham, N. R.: Modern Clinical Syphilology: Diagnosis, Treatment, Case Study. 3rd ed. Philadelphia, W. B. Saunders Company, 1944.

NONSYPHILITIC TREPONEMATOSES

For many years it has been recognized that there are a number of disease syndromes, occurring principally among the more backward peoples of warm countries, that are syphilislike in their general course and symptomatology. These syndromes have both clinical and epidemiologic features which still make it useful to give them distinguishing names, such as *yaws, bejel, pinta* and *endemic syphilis*.

It is now known that the etiologic agent of each of these disease syndromes is a spiral micro-organism which is indistinguishable morphologically from the treponeme of syphilis, *Treponema pallidum*. Moreover, infected persons develop serum antibodies—Wassermann antibody and treponemal immobilizing antibody—just as do persons with syphilis; significant degrees of cross-immunity can be demonstrated experimentally; and each disease responds well to the usual antisyphilitic drugs, such as penicillin and the arsenicals.

On the basis of the foregoing considerations, it is becoming common practice to refer to this group of diseases, including syphilis, as the *treponematoses*. Nevertheless, real clinical and biologic differences do exist among the various diseases belonging to this general group, differences which bear on problems of diagnosis, treatment, prevention and community control. From a more academic standpoint the relationship of these diseases one to another presents absorbing problems to the medical biologist interested in microbial variation and mutation as influenced by climate, race and other ecologic factors.

It is clear from clinical, epidemiologic and laboratory investigations that these are not simply different manifestations of the same disease, for each disease will reproduce itself under controlled experimental conditions. Laboratory experiments suggest, however, that long-continued exposure of infected hosts to different environmental conditions eventually results in modification of certain biologic characteristics of the particular treponemes. To what extent this same phenomenon may occur in nature is still only a matter for speculation.

Finally, to complete and at the same time confuse the picture of this group of diseases, there is a naturally occurring disease of domestic rabbits, designated venereal spirochetosis, caused by a treponeme (*T. cuniculi*) which is morphologically indistinguishable from the human pathogenic treponemes. The disease is likewise characterized by the development of Wassermann and treponemal immobilizing antibodies, ready response to antisyphilitic drugs, and some degree of reciprocal immunity to syphilis and yaws. No human infection with this treponeme has been recorded.

THOMAS B. TURNER

YAWS

Definition. Yaws is a specific disease caused by a spirochetal organism, *Treponema pertenue*. It is largely limited to tropical countries and is characterized by an initial cutaneous lesion, followed by a multiple papular, granulomatous skin eruption, and in some instances by late destructive lesions of the skin and bones. Lesions of the soles of the feet are especially common. Among synonyms for the disease are frambesia tropica, pian (French), bouba (Spanish-American) and parangi (Ceylon). Many others are listed by Hermans (1931).

History. The earliest reliable accounts of yaws now available date to the seventeenth century. Since Negroes were brought from Africa to the West Indies as early as 1510, it cannot be determined whether yaws was introduced into the Americas through this means, or whether the disease already existed among the native tribes. Undoubtedly it was prevalent among slaves imported from Africa, and by the eighteenth century yaws had become a serious problem on plantations in the West Indies.

Etiology. The spirochete of yaws (*T. pertenue*) was first described by Castellani in 1905, soon after the discovery of *T. pallidum* by Schaudinn. The organism measures from 8 to 20 microns in length and about 0.2 micron in diameter. It has six to fourteen closely placed spirals and morphologically is indistinguishable from the spirochete of syphilis. It is best seen in the fresh state by darkfield illumination. The organism stains with difficulty.

Among laboratory animals *T. pertenue* is pathogenic for monkeys, rabbits and hamsters; subclinical infection only is produced in mice, rats and guinea pigs. At ordinary temperatures the organism survives for only a few hours when removed from a living host; in special media it will survive for several days but multiplication does not occur. It remains virulent for years when stored at $-70°$ C. in 15 per cent glycerin.

Epidemiology. *Distribution and Prevalence.* Yaws as an endemic disease is practically limited to the tropics. It is particularly common in equatorial Africa, the West Indies, parts of India, Ceylon, the Philippines, the Netherlands East Indies, and throughout the entire group of Southern Pacific Islands. Endemic foci occur in parts of Brazil and Colombia in South America, and in several countries of Central America. Only sporadic cases have been reported from North America and Europe. The disease is not distributed uniformly, however, even within the tropics. The situation as found by the epidemiologic studies of the Jamaica Yaws Commission (Turner, Saunders, Kumm and others, 1935–1937) is interesting and may be representative of that in other countries. In that country the distribution of yaws is uneven. Areas of high prevalence lie within a few miles of communities in which it is rarely encountered, and there is a close correlation between its prevalence and certain environmental factors. Where yaws is common there is practically always a heavy rainfall, and a fertile moisture-holding soil supporting an abundant vegetation.

It is principally a disease of rural peoples, the lowest social and economic groups showing the highest attack rate. There is no clear evidence of racial immunity.

Yaws is usually acquired in childhood, but no age is free from the risk of infection. In one community in Jamaica (Bath) prevalence rates rose from 26 per cent among all children under 5 years of age, to 75 per cent among those 10 to 14 years of age. Approximately 90 per cent of all persons found to have infectious lesions were under 20 years of age.

Transmission. Yaws can be transmitted by direct person-to-person contact, but it is probable that nonbiting insects also play a role in the spread of the disease. There is no evidence for the existence of an animal or avian reservoir. The initial yaws lesions, which develops at the point of implantation of the spirochete, is frequently observed at the site of a previous injury, and is located on the lower extremity in the majority of cases. Sexual transmission rarely occurs. Transmission from mother to child in *utero* has not been established.

Since earliest times the possibility of transmission by insects has been recognized. Studies in Jamaica (Kumm and others, 1935–1936) indicate that in this country a small gnat, *Hippelates pallipes,* is a likely mechanical vector.

Pathology. Histologically, the cutaneous papule or frambesioma shows marked epithelial hyperplasia, elongation of the papillae, exudation of leukocytes on or near the surface, with many lymphocytes and plasma cells in the dermis. Silver stains show spirochetes in large numbers in the epidermis and more superficial dermis. The late ulcerative lesions of yaws are histologically similar to syphilitic gummas. On the whole, the histologic criteria for the differentiation of the cutaneous and subcutaneous lesions of yaws and syphilis are unreliable (Ferris and Turner, 1937). The occurrence of visceral

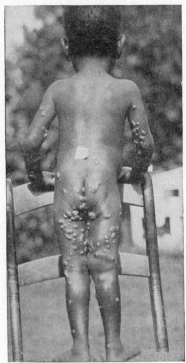

Fig. 47. Yaws in a child, showing generalized frambesiform lesions.

lesions in yaws is still debated. Evidence is accumulating that the aorta is sometimes involved (Choisser, 1929; Chambers, 1936; Weller, 1937). With possibly rare exceptions, the central nervous system is not affected.

Clinical Manifestations. *Skin.* Within two to eight weeks after infection the initial or primary lesion appears at the point of implantation of yaws spirochetes. This lesion is a granuloma and may develop into a large cauliflower-like growth from which *T. pertenue* can be recovered. There is accompanying enlargement of the regional lymph nodes. The initial lesion usually persists for several months and heals with scar formation.

During the first weeks of the disease *T. pertenue* gains access to the blood stream, and symptoms attributable to generalization of the organism soon become manifest. These consist of widely distributed skin lesions, often enlargement of the superficial lymph nodes, bone and joint pains and in some cases clinically recognizable lesions of these structures. Mild constitutional symptoms, such as low grade fever, loss of appetite and slight loss of weight, may occur, but in many cases the general health of the person is not materially affected. Within one or two weeks after development of the initial lesion blood serologic tests similar to those used in the diagnosis of syphilis (Wassermann, Kahn, Eagle, Hinton) become positive, increase rapidly in titer, and remain positive for many years unless rendered negative by specific therapy. The treponemal immobilization test and the treponemal agglutination test also become positive and remain so for many years in untreated patients.

The generalized rash may comprise at first only scaly macular lesions. More commonly, however, from the beginning the rash is polymorphous, comprising scaly macules, folliculopapules, papules and, most prominent of all, large granulomas—the yaw or frambesioma, which is characteristic of this disease. As the disease progresses, the frambesiform lesions become more numerous and larger; the patient with a fully developed generalized frambesiform rash presents an arresting picture, one which can scarcely be confused with any other disease (Fig. 47). The individual lesion stands out from the skin level like a giant wart, measuring 0.5 to 4 cm. in diameter. The surface of the lesion, which may be covered by a crust, is granular, like the surface of a raspberry—hence the name "frambesia." Serum from the lesion yields large numbers of motile *T. pertenue*.

After several months, retrogression of the generalized lesions may begin. The smaller lesions heal and the large frambesiform lesions tend to become smaller and less numerous, but it may be many months before they have entirely disappeared .Even then relapses are not uncommon, so that infectious types of lesions may be present off and on for several years after the onset of the disease. Eventually a stage of latency is usually reached, but this stage may likewise be interrupted, at intervals, by the occurrence of more bizarre types of lesions in which *T. pertenue* cannot be readily demonstrated.

After several years have elapsed, skin lesions similar to the syphilitic gumma may occur. These so-called "late-lesions" are characterized by tissue destruction and ulceration often involving large areas of skin and subcutaneous tissue. *Treponema pertenue* cannot be found, but other types of spirochetes, notably *Borrelia refringens,* may be present. Healing often leads to extensive scarring, which, if located in the region of a joint, may lead to contractures.

Lesions of the soles of the feet are common and account for a good deal of the disability from the disease. Two types, which may occur alone or together, are recognized. One type consists of one or more eroded papules somewhat analogous to the frambesiform lesion of the skin. Instead of protruding above the plantar surface, however, the papule lies at the base of a small opening in the sole, and is exquisitely tender. Serum from these lesions is usually rich in *T. pertenue.* Like other infectious lesions, plantar papules are observed most commonly in the first years of the disease.

The other type of plantar lesions consists of widespread hypertrophy, stripping or fissuring of the superficial layers of the sole, and less frequently of the palms, giving rise to a curious mottled pattern characteristic of yaws. There is usually no ulceration, and *T. pertenue* cannot ordinarily be demonstrated. Plantar hyperkeratosis, the so-called "crab yaws," may occur at almost any period during the course of yaws; it has been observed in patients soon after development of the generalized rash as well as twenty years or more after infection.

Bones. In the Jamaica series bone lesions were observed in about 15 per cent of all patients showing active manifestations. On the basis of roentgenographic changes two types are recognized, although not infrequently both types are present simultaneously. In the one type periosteal proliferation, similar to that seen in syphilis, is the most prominent feature. In the other type areas of rarefaction or destruction in the shafts of the long bones are observed. These areas are round or oval and usually multiple, with a surrounding zone of increased density. Clinically, the patient complains of pain in the affected region, and there may be tenderness and swelling of the overlying soft parts (Goldman and Smith, 1943; Helfet, 1944). The bones of the forearms, legs and hands seem most often to be affected; involvement of the skull, pelvis and spine is rare. Both periostitis and osteitis may occur either in association with infectious skin lesions, or in later years after the generalized skin lesions have healed.

Other Yaws Lesions. Among the less common but more spectacular lesions of yaws are gangosa, goundou and juxta-articular nodules. In *gangosa* the cartilaginous and bony structures of the nose are partially or completely destroyed by a late ulcerative process. Cutaneous leishmaniasis may cause somewhat the same picture. *Goundou* is an egg-shaped paranasal enlargement arising from the superior maxillary bone. The tumors may be sufficiently large to interfere with vision (Strong and Shattuck, 1930). *Juxta-articular nodules* are firm, freely movable, painless, subcutaneous fibroid tumors situated in proximity to a joint.

Differential Diagnosis. A case of yaws with typical generalized lesions cannot easily be confused with any other disease. Individual lesions may resemble those of secondary syphilis or cutaneous leishmaniasis, but, when the case as a whole is considered, little difficulty should be experienced. Demonstration of the treponeme in skin lesions serves to differentiate yaws from all conditions except those of the syphilis group. Late ulcerative lesions of yaws are often indistinguishable from the tertiary lesions of syphilis. The late effects of yaws, ulcerative lesions, contractures, partial amputation of digits, may resemble the lesions of leprosy. In areas where yaws is common, serologic tests for syphilis are of limited value in differential diagnosis.

Prognosis. The disease is rarely directly fatal except in young infants. Without treatment the disease leads to months of partial incapacity, with the possibility of relapses over a period of many years. A not inconsiderable proportion of infected persons apparently go on, after many years, to spontaneous clinical and serologic cure. The indirect mortality from the disease, because of secondary infection of cutaneous ulcers or bone lesions, is probably higher than is commonly supposed. In areas of high yaws endemicity, a substantial proportion of the beds in chronic disease hospitals and poorhouses are occupied by patients whose disability stems primarily from yaws. With early treatment the prognosis is entirely favorable.

Prophylaxis. No methods of artificial immunization are available. In regions where yaws is prevalent the chances of infection can be reduced by avoiding minor injuries to the skin, and by protecting all open wounds and abrasions from contamination by flies. Children with infectious lesions should be excluded from school until rendered noninfectious by treatment. Efforts to control insect vectors are not practicable at the present time.

Treatment. Yaws responds to the same therapeutic agents that are effective in syphilis, but smaller amounts of drug are required for yaws. Penicillin is the drug of choice; other drugs tested have been much less effective. Use of the arsenical drugs or bismuth is not recommended.

For the treatment of the usual case of yaws, procaine penicillin in 2 per cent aluminum monostearate and oil is recommended in doses of 1,200,000 units (4 cc.) for adults and children 10 years of age and older, and 600,000 units (2 cc.) per injection for younger children. Two injections a week for a total of four doses should be given. Injections should be made intramuscularly in the buttocks. The more recently developed long-lasting penicillin preparations (see Treatment of Early Syphilis) could presumably be substituted in the same dosage. Oral penicillin has not had an adequate clinical trial.

For mass treatment campaigns the Expert Committee of the World Health Organization has recommended one intramuscular injection of 1,200,000 units, because of the impracticability of administering multiple injections.

The response to penicillin is dramatic. Initial and generalized lesions commonly become darkfield negative for *T. pertenue* within forty-eight hours, and healing is complete within one week. Serologic titers decline rapidly, but a substantial proportion of patients may still show a low titer serologic test after six months.

Late skin lesions as a rule respond promptly to antiyaws drugs, but the more chronic lesions of the skin and bones may require local surgical treatment in addition to chemotherapy.

Prevention. In areas of high prevalence, effective control of yaws depends upon reducing the attack rate by measures directed to the source of infection, i.e., the infectious cases, in the community. The control program instituted by the Jamaica Yaws Commission comprised the following: (1) survey of a given area by sanitary inspectors for the purpose of detecting all infectious cases; (2) rendering these patients noninfectious through treatment; (3) close observation of the community by sanitary inspectors in order that patients with new infections may be

promptly treated. Since over 90 per cent of the infectious cases occurred among persons under twenty years of age, it was to this portion of the population that control measures were directed. By these methods the attack rate in the control areas was reduced by 80 per cent (Turner, Saunders and Johnston, 1935; Saunders, 1937).

THOMAS B. TURNER

References

Ash, J. E., and Spitz, Sophie: Pathology of Tropical Diseases; An Atlas. Philadelphia, W. B. Saunders Company, 1945.
Helft, A. J.: Acute Manifestations of Yaws of Bone and Joint. J. Bone & Joint Surg., 26:672, 1944.
Hermans, E. H.: Framboesia Tropica, Acta Leidensia. Vol. VI, 1931 (English translation). Many references.
Mackie, T. T., Hunter, G. W., and Worth, C. B.: Manual of Tropical Medicine. 2nd ed. Philadelphia, W. B. Saunders Company, 1954.
Rein, C. R., and Kitchen, D. K.: Time-dosage Relation in Penicillin Therapy with Special Reference to Yaws. 2. Clinical Basis for Effective Therapy. Bull. World Health Org., 8:91, 1953.
Turner, T. B., Hollander, D. H., and Schaeffer, K.: Biological Investigations on Treponemes. Bull. World Health Org., 8:7, 1953.

BEJEL

Bejel is a chronic infectious disease of the treponematosis group occurring principally among seminomadic inhabitants of the Arabian Peninsula, Asia Minor and the Middle East. It is a family disease, the infection being acquired usually in childhood with subsequent transmission to adults living in the same tent, unless these have been protected by previous infection. Drinking utensils often constitute the vehicle of transmission and initial lesions are particularly common about the lips and within the oral cavity. Serologic surveys indicate that as high as 90 per cent of the inhabitants of some villages are affected.

The evolution of the disease follows much the same pattern as that in syphilis and yaws. Generalized lesions tend to be confined to the oral cavity and the mucocutaneous borders of the lips, genitalia and anal regions. The bejel treponeme, which is morphologically indistinguishable from *T. pallidum,* can be readily demonstrated in early lesions by darkfield examination. Bone lesions are common in both the early and late stages; roentgenographic examination shows the changes to be similar to those observed in yaws. Late lesions of the skin, and gummatous involvement of the palate and nasal septum, are also common in untreated cases. No definitive data are available on the occurrence of visceral lesions.

Bejel is an important cause of chronic illness in endemic areas, but penicillin is as effective in bejel as in the other treponematoses. In the control campaign initiated by the World Health Organization in Iraq, good clinical results were obtained with penicillin in aluminum monostearate and oil in one dose of 1,200,000 units given intramuscularly. A second dose at an interval of three to seven days was given to those with osseous involvement. While the immediate results were good, it is not known what proportion of infected persons was cured by this treatment.

THOMAS B. TURNER

PINTA

(Mal del Pinto, Carate)

Definition. Pinta is a chronic endemic infectious disease, characterized by dyschromic papular skin lesions, which eventually become depigmented splotches.

Etiology. The disease is caused by a spirochete, *Treponema carateum* (also *T. herrejoni*), which is morphologically indistinguishable from *T. pallidum*. This spirochete can be demonstrated in the initial and generalized papular lesions by darkfield examination, but not in the depigmented spots. It has not been successfully propagated in laboratory animals or cultivated *in vitro*.

Epidemiology. Pinta is endemic in localized areas in Central America and the tropical portions of South America. It has also been reported from the West Indies, tropical Africa and various islands and countries of the South Pacific. Pinta is biologically closely related to syphilis, yaws and other members of the treponematosis group of diseases, and in these areas certain diagnostic confusion between pinta and yaws is encountered.

There is no racial immunity. Transmission is usually by direct person-to-person contact. Intrauterine transmission is believed not to occur. Pinta is acquired mostly by children and young adults, but because of its chronic nature many older persons exhibit signs of the disease.

Pathology. Active lesions appear to be confined to the skin and lymph nodes. The initial and generalized papular lesions are similar histologically, being characterized by thickening of the epidermis, dense infiltration of lymphocytes and plasma cells into the dermis, with foci of intracellular edema. Perivascular infiltration is usually present. The wide variation in the color of the lesions is a reflection of the degree of vascularity, migration of the chromatophores into the more superficial layers of the skin, and natural racial variation in skin pigmentation. As lesions grow older, there is a progressive decrease in vascularity, cellular infiltrate and pigment.

Symptomatology. In a series of 28 purposeful inoculations of volunteers Leon-Blanco found the usual incubation period to be fourteen to twenty days. The initial or primary lesion is papular, and enlarges slowly, often becoming psoriasiform in appearance, with smaller satellite papules. When present alone, it may be mistaken for psoriasis or lichenified eczema, and its true nature can be established with certainty only by demonstration of *T. carateum*. The regional lymph node is usually enlarged, and *T. carateum* can be recovered by aspiration.

The secondary stage, which develops in five to twelve months after infection, is characterized by a generalized eruption of macules or miliary papules, called pintids, which are often pinkish or violaceous and slightly scaly. Most of these lesions heal, but some enlarge and coalesce to form patches resembling psoriasis or lichenoid eczema. They are particularly common on the face and other exposed parts of the body. These lesions are exceedingly chronic and may last for years, often remaining darkfield positive for *T. carateum* all the while. Itching is not a prominent symptom. Hyperkeratosis of the soles and palms also occasionally occurs.

It is this tertiary or dyschromic stage in which the characteristic symptomatology of pinta is observed. When the low grade inflammatory process is still present, the lesions usually exhibit some color, sometimes a dull red or violet, but more often a leaden or slate blue. As time goes on, the active process subsides, the skin becoming atrophic and white because of the loss of pigment. In some patients considerable disfigurement occurs from the extensive areas of vitiligo.

Standard serologic tests for syphilis are usually negative during the primary stage of the disease, but become positive soon after the appearance of generalized lesions. In the later stages of the disease the serum of nearly all patients gives a positive test, often in high titer. Immobilizing antibody to T. *pallidum* is also present. The only constitutional symptoms are those attributable to a mild chronic infection. Reports of examination of the cerebrospinal fluid have yielded conflicting results, a few observers reporting an increase in cell count in some cases. Likewise, the occurrence of enlargement of the aorta believed to be due to pinta has been reported, but the occurrence of such lesions has not been definitely established.

Prognosis. Pinta rarely causes disabling illness or death. Aside from the mild symptoms of a chronic infection, the disfigurement due to the dyschromic and achromic lesions with accompanying abnormal psychic reactions is the most serious feature of the disease. The results of penicillin therapy are excellent.

Treatment. Penicillin is specific. In a series of 700 cases, Rein and his associates observed a dramatic response to one intramuscular injection of 1,200,000 units (4 cc.) of penicillin in 2 per cent aluminum monostearate and oil. Other long-lasting penicillin preparations (in Treatment of Early Syphilis) may be used in the same dosage. Both early papular and late pigmented lesions healed promptly, and even the vitiligoid spots, if present less than five years, often regained pigment. After one year serologic tests were negative in about half the patients. When practicable, a second injection of the same amount of penicillin should be given one week after the first injection.

THOMAS B. TURNER

References

Ash, J. E., and Spitz, S.: Pathology of Tropical Diseases. Philadelphia, W. B. Saunders Company, 1945.

Fox, H.: Cutaneous Manifestations of Some Tropical Diseases. Arch. Dermat. & Syph., 59:127, 1949.

Leon-Blanco, F., and de Laosa, O.: The Primary Lesion of Pinta. Am. J. Syph., Gonor. & Ven. Dis., 31:600, 1947.

Stokes, J. H., Beerman, H., and Ingraham, N. R.: Pinta: A Review of Recent Etiologic and Clinical Studies. Am. J. M. Sc., 205:611, 1943.

RELAPSING FEVER

(Febris Recurrens, Spirillum Fever, Famine Fever, Mianeh Fever, Carapata Disease, Tick Fever, Kimputu)

Definition. The term "relapsing fever" is applied to a large group of acute infectious diseases, clinically similar but etiologically distinct, which are prevalent in many parts of the world. These diseases are characterized by an initial febrile period lasting three to ten days, which usually begins and ends abruptly and is followed after several days of apparent recovery by one or more relapses. If untreated, the total course of the infection may last six to eight weeks. The relapsing fevers are caused by various closely related species of spirochetes of the genus *Borrelia,* which are demonstrable in the patient's blood during the febrile attacks. The infections may be divided into two large groups: namely, the louse-borne and the tick-borne relapsing fevers.

History. The first known description of relapsing fever was afforded by Rutty, who in 1739 reported an epidemic at Dublin. The name "relapsing fever" was proposed by Henderson, who, in 1843, described an epidemic in Edinburgh and differentiated the disease from typhus fever. In 1869 Obermeier (1873) discovered the causative spirochete in the blood of relapsing fever patients whom he studied during an epidemic in Berlin. This observation was confirmed by Munch, who, in 1874, inoculated himself with blood containing motile relapsing fever spirochetes and subsequently acquired the disease; also by Motschutkoffsky (1876), who proved the infectivity of the spirochete by inoculating the blood of patients into healthy persons.

In 1891 Flügge suggested that the human body louse might act as a vector, and Mackie (1907) in India reached a similar conclusion. This belief was later confirmed by the inoculation into monkeys of crushed lice taken from relapsing fever patients. In 1904 Ross and Milne, in Uganda, showed that the "tick fever," mentioned by Livingston in 1857, was caused by a spirochete which invaded the peripheral blood stream. These observations were confirmed in the Congo by Dutton and Todd (1905), who reported the mechanism of infection in the tick *Ornithodoros moubata* and the hereditary transmission of the spirochetes through the egg to succeeding generations of ticks.

Geographic Distribution. Relapsing fevers occur in many parts of the world, as is indicated graphically in the accompanying map (Fig. 48), and the distribution is influenced by various factors, including the distribution of the arthropod vectors.

The *louse-borne* relapsing fevers have been reported as endemic in the following regions: (1) Europe, including the British Isles, Denmark, Germany, Poland, Russia, the Balkans and Turkey; (2) Asia, including India, China, Japan, Manchuria, Iran and Siberia; (3) Africa, especially in northern Africa, including Egypt, Algeria, Ethiopia and Sudan, and in western Africa, including the Gold Coast, Nigeria, Senegal and the French Sudan; and (4) on many occasions during the past the disease has been imported from Europe to the United States and has caused epidemics in cities along the Atlantic Coast. In 1869–71 there was a

regions. *B. recurrentis* (European), *B. duttonii* (West African), *B. kochii* (East African), *B. berbera* (North African), *B. carteri* (Indian) and *B. novyi* (American), *B. hermsi* and *B. parkeri* (western United States), *B. turicatae* (Mexican) and *B. venezuelensis* (South American).

BACTERIOLOGY. *Morphologically,* these spirochetes are indistinguishable, and in general they conform to the description of

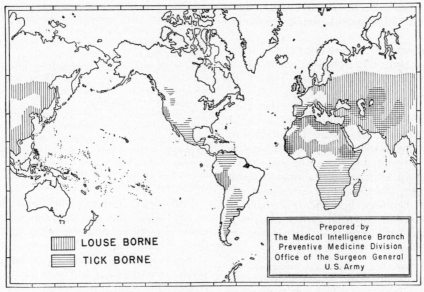

LOUSE BORNE
TICK BORNE

Prepared by
The Medical Intelligence Branch
Preventive Medicine Division
Office of the Surgeon General
U.S. Army

Fig. 48. Geographic distribution of relapsing fever.

widespread American epidemic which affected New York City, Philadelphia, Washington, D. C., and many other cities.

The *tick-borne* relapsing fevers are endemic in (1) Africa, especially tropical Africa and north Africa; (2) Asia, including Arabia, Persia, India and other parts of central Asia; (3) Europe, including Spain; (4) North America, including Canada, the United States and Mexico; (5) Central America; and (6) South America, including Colombia, Venezuela, Peru, Uruguay and the Argentine Republic. In the United States the disease has been reported in California, Colorado, Arizona, Texas and Kansas. Because of the manner of their transmission the tick-borne fevers rarely become epidemic.

Etiology. *The Spirochetes.* The relapsing fevers are caused by spirochetes, similar to the *Spirochaeta recurrentis* discovered by Obermeier in 1868, which are demonstrable in the blood of patients during the febrile periods. According to Bergey's Manual of Determinative Bacteriology, 1948, the genus *Borrelia swellengrebel* includes ten species which cause relapsing fevers in the following

Borrelia recurrentis. This is a delicate spiral threadlike organism 8 to 30 microns long and 0.3 to 0.5 micron thick, with pointed ends, and from four to ten large wavy irregular coils. There is a springlike axial filament on which there is a layer of contractile protoplasm enveloped in a delicate periplast, also fine terminal filaments, but no flagella. The organism can move in either direction. The spirochetes may be stained with the ordinary aniline dyes and preferably by methods commonly used for staining blood films. They can be destroyed by exposure to 10 per cent saponin or 10 per cent bile salts.

According to Geiman no one has produced quantitative information to support claims of multiplication *in vitro.*

Certain lower animals are susceptible to experimental infection, and, according to Novy and Knapp, *B. recurrentis, B. novyi* and *B. duttonii* have been differentiated according to their infectivity for monkeys, mice and rats. It is claimed that rabbits and guinea pigs are relatively unsusceptible, although they may be infected with *B. carteri,* and guinea pigs have been infected with some American strains. It is of interest to note that spirochetes resembling those of relapsing fever, but producing different symptoms, have been found in various natural infections of lower animals and birds.

In man and in animals, recovery from the infection is followed by a transient immunity and the appearance in the serum of agglutinating and complement fixing antibodies (Stein).

Transmission. Relapsing fever can be transferred by the injection of blood containing the spirochetes into normal persons. The organisms are able to penetrate the mucous membranes of the eye and possibly of other parts of the body; they can also cause infection when rubbed into the apparently intact skin. It appears that under natural conditions the disease is spread by blood-sucking arthropods, which may act either as contaminated mechanical carriers of infection or as biologic vectors. Fleas, bedbugs, lice and ticks have all been suspected as potential carriers, but most of the infections appear to be spread by either lice or ticks.

LICE. Human lice (*Pediculus humanus,* var. *corporis* and *capitis*) have long been accepted as vectors of *B. recurrentis* (synonym *S. recurrentis*), the cause of European typhus fever. Manson-Bahr believes that *B. novyi, B. carteri* and *B. berbera* are similar to *B. recurrentis* and that the fevers which they cause in Europe, Asia and North America are conveyed by lice. Strong states that European, Indian, Chinese, West African and some of the North African infections are transmitted by the louse, *P. humanus.*

Lice feeding on patients during febrile periods may ingest spirochetes, some of which survive the louse's gastric juice, quickly enter the hemocele, and are distributed throughout the entire body cavity. After four to six days the organisms become abundant in the hemocele and the louse contains infective spirochetes for several weeks and possibly during the rest of its life. The organisms do not pass through the egg to the louse's offspring. Apparently the infection is transmitted to man, not by the bite of the louse or through contamination with the feces, but by crushing the infected louse on the human skin. The released spirochetes may then enter the skin, or contaminate the fingers and thus reach the mucous membranes of the eye.

TICKS. The tick-borne relapsing fevers caused by *B. duttonii* and other species or varieties of spirochetes are transmitted by ticks of the family *Argasidae,* especially of the genus *Ornithodorus.* The following species have been suspectde or shown to be vectors: *O. moubata* in southeast and central Africa; *O. erraticus* in Tunis; *O. papillipes* and *O. tholozani* in central Africa and Palestine; *O. marocanus* in Spain and Morocco; *O. venezuelensis* and *O. talaje* in northern South America, Central America and Mexico; *O. turicata* in Texas and Kansas; and *O. hermsi* in California.

Available experimental data indicate that within a few days after the tick ingests infected human blood, the spirochetes disappear from the digestive tract; but within several days they multiply in the malpighian tubules and other organs, including the coxal glands, salivary glands and legs. It appears probable that the tick does not transmit the organisms through its proboscis while biting, but that infection occurs by contamination of the skin-puncture wound with the spirochete-containing fecal fluid excreted by the tick. The spirochetes are transmitted from adult female ticks through the eggs to their offspring for at least three generations. Ticks of the species *O. turicata* have remained infected for at least six and one half years. There appears to be no specific relationship between the kind of tick and the species of spirochete.

It is now believed that ticks normally become infected by feeding on infected lower animals. Such animal reservoirs are probably afforded in West Africa by a shrew mouse, in Panama by a monkey, *Leontocebus geoffroyi,* in Texas by armadillos and opossums, and in California by squirrels and chipmunks and probably other animals.

Pathology. The spirochetes may be found in the blood and the internal organs, especially the spleen and the brain, but the autopsy findings are not diagnostic. Often the skin is jaundiced, and there may be numerous small subcutaneous or submucous hemorrhages. The spleen is enlarged, and histologically it shows simple hyperplasia. The liver is slightly enlarged. Hemorrhagic meningitis has been reported. It appears likely that death is rarely caused by the relapsing fever, but can be attributed to complicating conditions and infections.

Clinical Manifestations. The many types of relapsing fevers described in various parts of the world naturally differ considerably in their clinical characteristics. Wide variations also occur in the symptoms observed in a single epidemic. Manson-Bahr has described five clinical types as follows: (1) a cosmopolitan type due to *B. recurrentis;* (2) an Iranian type due to *B. persica;* (3) a Central African type caused by *B. duttonii;* (4) a Spanish type due to *B. hispanica;* and (5) a Central and South American type produced by *B. venezuelensis.* Strong has discussed the symptomatology of the relapsing fevers of Africa, North Africa, Europe, India, China, Persia, Panama and North America.

The more important characteristics of these different types may be briefly summarized as follows:

The *incubation period* is estimated at from two to fifteen days, the average being about seven days.

The *initial attack* may last two to seven or more days. It usually starts abruptly with chilliness or a chill followed by a high fever, intense headache, pains in the muscles and joints, nausea, vomiting, photophobia, dizziness and sometimes epistaxis. The temperature rises quickly to 104° or 105° F. or higher, and except for slight morning remissions it remains elevated throughout the initial febrile period, at the end of which it falls to normal by crisis. The pulse also rises quickly and soon reaches 110 to 140 beats per minute. Periods of sweating may occur during the first day, but thereafter the skin is hot and dry, and the face is flushed. Jaundice may occur, but is more likely to appear later. An erythematous rash is common during this period, and later rose-colored spots may occur on the trunk and limbs. According to Manson-Bahr, "the rash generally is most marked in the region around the neck, spreading in a semicircular fashion from the tips of the mastoid processes; thence it ranges in a symmetrical manner round the shoulders, down the sides of the chest and abdomen to the inner aspects of the thighs, and to the extensor and flexor aspects of the forearms. The individual petechiae may be as large as a three penny bit, and need to be carefully differentiated from the exanthemata of typhus and hemorrhagic smallpox." Labial herpes may occur.

Frequently the patient complains of severe headaches and of muscular and joint pains. In case of high fever there may be delirium. Insomnia may be an important symptom, and hyperesthesias of the taste and tactile senses may occur. It has been suggested that the spirochetes of relapsing fever are neurotropic. They may persist in the brains of experimental animals for periods of more than a year. In the tick-borne central African type, severe nervous lesions have been noted. On rare occasions, optic atrophy has occurred immediately after the fever or several months later. At times, hemiplegia, aphasia or other nervous symptoms may occur suddenly during the disease. In such instances the spirochetes may be demonstrable in the cerebrospinal fluid, which also contains an excess of lymphocytes and is under increased pressure. Cases have also been reported with symptoms sembling those of encephalitis and meningitis.

The tongue is usually coated and moist, but in severe cases it may be dry and brown. Nausea and vomiting are common and may persist even during the apyrexial period. The vomitus may contain bile or may resemble the black vomit of yellow fever. Anorexia is common, and the patient usually is constipated; however, diarrhea has been associated with severe types of the disease. Abdominal pain is a common symptom, and gastric or intestinal hemorrhages have been reported. The liver may be enlarged and tender; and jaundice may be severe. The spleen is usually large and tender.

Pulmonary symptoms, including bronchitis, frequently occur during the initial febrile period. In some epidemics, pneumonia occurs in 5 per cent of the patients and is a serious complication.

Urine collected during the paroxysm may contain albumin, less frequently casts and rarely blood. Spirochetes have been found at times in the urine and prostatic fluid.

Blood collected during the febrile attack usually contains spirochetes. There is a polymorphonuclear leukocytosis of 15,000 to 26,000 per cubic millimeter, and the Arneth count is deflected to the left. In about 20 per cent of cases serologic tests for syphilis are positive during the period of infection.

The period of the initial attack usually ends abruptly with profuse sweating and a rapid fall of the temperature to normal or below. This may be accompanied by diarrhea. In elderly or weak patients a dangerous state of collapse may occur.

The *first period of apyrexia* which follows the crisis of the initial attack lasts three to ten days. The fever and all other symptoms subside. The spirochetes disappear from the peripheral blood stream. The skin becomes cool and pale, and the pulse falls to the normal rate and is of poor quality. The prostration is great at first, but in a few days the appetite and strength return and the patient feels so well that he considers himself completely recovered.

The *first relapse* follows this symptomless interval. It is characterized by a repetition of the more important symptoms of the initial attack. It may be more severe, but, as a rule, it is milder. Jaundice is more common. Conjunctivitis may occur, and iritis is not rare. Transient cranial nerve defects may occur, and there may be uterine hemorrhages or abortion. The relapse seldom lasts as long as the first attack, and it also ends by crisis.

Subsequent Relapses. The end of the first

relapse is often coincident with convalescence, but in many instances additional relapses occur. Frequently these are shorter and milder than the previous febrile periods. In the louse-borne relapsing fever of Europe and Asia there are rarely more than two, three or four relapses. This is also true of the tick-borne infections of North America. The tick-borne infections of Persia and central Africa usually have four or five relapses, and the latter may have as many as eleven relapses.

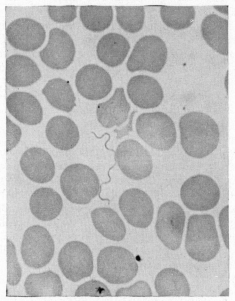

Fig. 49. *Borrelia recurrentis* in blood smear. (Photograph courtesy of Colonel J. E. Ash, M. C., Director, U. S. Army Medical Museum.)

Convalescence may be protracted, and there may be various sequelae, including iritis, otitis, parotitis, adenitis, neuritis, polyarthritis, nephritis and pneumonitis.

Diagnosis. The relapsing fevers may be confused with various other diseases, including malaria, dengue, yellow fever, Weil's disease, enteric fever, typhus, influenza, pneumonia and early smallpox. They may be differentiated from these diseases on the basis of clinical differences. However, the specific diagnosis depends on the demonstration of typical relapsing fever spirochetes in the patient's blood. This is commonly done by the microscopic examination of blood as follows: (1) fresh preparations examined by dark-field illumination, (2) thin films prepared with Wright's stain, (3) thick films stained with Wright's or Giemsa's stains. Care is required to avoid mistaking artefacts for

spirochetes. The spirochetes are usually found during the febrile attacks, being more numerous early. Rarely they may be present in the afebrile period. If spirochetes are not demonstrable microscopically, specimens of blood should be injected into white rats or white mice. The blood of these animals should then be examined for spirochetes daily for several days.

Prognosis. The reported mortality has usually been low, 2 to 6 per cent, but in certain epidemics in West Africa the death rates have exceeded 50 per cent. The deaths usually occur among weak, poorly nourished persons, especially young children and the aged. Untreated cases may last as long as six to eight weeks. However, the disease can be cured in a short time by specific treatment.

Immunity. Recovery from an attack of relapsing fever confers a transient immunity, at least to the same type of spirochete. It also produces specific antibodies in the serum, which, according to Stein, can be detected as long as thirty-six years after the initial infection. Possibly the relapses are usually less severe than the initial attack because the immunity increases with each relapse until the infection is overcome. It has been reported that reinfection can occur in man within two months.

Prevention. The prevention of relapsing fever naturally depends on the protection of susceptible persons from the arthropod vectors. The louse-borne fevers can be prevented by taking all the precautions necessary to avoid exposure to body or head lice. These measures include the maintenance of good personal hygiene and cleanliness, and the disinfestation of lousy persons and clothing. Military experience in World War II shows that the 10 per cent DDT louse powder used by the U. S. Army is the most satisfactory agent available for delousing either individuals or large groups of infested persons.

The tick-borne infections are more difficult to control, since these arthropods do not live on the victim, but as a rule live in the floor or walls of native houses, in the earth of old camp sites, in cracks in the floors and walls of caves and in the burrows of various small animals. Infested places should not be selected as camp sites, and care should be taken to avoid exposure to ticks, which usually come out of their hiding places at night and feed on their hosts.

According to Manson-Bahr, a prophylactic vaccine made of killed cultures of B. *recur-*

entis has been used by Russian workers and found to produce specific spirochetolysins in the serum. However, attempts to protect animals with killed vaccines have failed.

Treatment. The patient should be kept in bed, on a liquid diet. The treatment previously recommended consisted of a single intravenous injection of one of the arsenical compounds. According to Manson-Bahr (1940), who preferred novarsenobillon, the arsenical should be given when the temperature is on the rise and not when it is declining or during the apyrexial period. If treatment is not begun during the initial attack, one should wait until the first relapse and then give it as the temperature rises. If given toward the end of the attack, just before the crisis, a severe reaction may occur, presumably because of the liberation of toxic substances from the destroyed spirochetes. In such circumstances fatal complications may result. Albuminuria is not considered a contraindication.

Previously, neoarsphenamine was commonly used in a single intravenous dose of 0.01 gm. per kilogram of body weight, followed, if necessary, by a second or possibly a third dose. Arsenoxide was preferred by some because of its low toxicity and ease of administration. It is used in doses of 0.045 gm. Larger doses may cause toxic reactions. In some cases it may be desirable to give two doses of 0.03 and 0.045 gm., respectively, with one day intervening. When intravenous injections cannot be given, Stovarsol may be used by mouth in doses of six tablets (0.25 gm. each) daily.

The antibiotics have been studied intensively since 1943, and a review by Schuhardt in 1952 indicates that many workers have found penicillin to be effective using 1,000,000 units or more in divided doses at intervals of 3 hours for at least four days of treatment. Narain and Kalra in 1950 reported the cure of tick-borne relapsing fever in Kashmir using streptomycin 1 gm. daily in divided doses at 3- to 4-hour intervals on two consecutive days. Aureomycin has been used successfully by others (Mazzotti; Gilchrist; Yeo; Innerfield). The clinical studies with these and other antimicrobial drugs now being conducted in various parts of the world undoubtedly will provide a number of excellent new chemotherapies in the near future.

JAMES STEVENS SIMMONS†

† Deceased.

References

Ash, J. E., and Spitz, Sophie: Pathology of Tropical Disease: An Atlas. Philadelphia, W. B. Saunders Company, 1945.

Augustine, D., Weinman, D., and McAllister, J.: Rapid and Sterilising Effect of Penicillin Sodium in Experimental Relapsing Fever Infections and Its Ineffectiveness in Treatment of Trypanosomiasis and Toxoplasmosis. Science, 99:19, 1944.

Eagle, H., and Magnuson, H. J.: The Therapeutic Efficacy of Penicillin in Relapsing Fever Infections in Mice and Rats. Pub. Health Rep., 59:583, 1944.

Gaud, M., and Morgan, M. T.: Epidemiological Studies of Relapsing Fever in North Africa (1943–1945). Bull. World Health Organization, 1947, Vol. 1, No. 1, p. 69.

Geiman, Q. M.: Metabolism of Spirochetes. Ann. Rev. Microbiol., 6:300, 1952.

Manson-Bahr, P. H.: Manson's Tropical Diseases. Baltimore, Williams and Wilkins Company, 1942.

Moursund, W. H.: Historical Introduction to the Symposium on Relapsing Fever, A Symposium on Relapsing Fever in the Americas. Publication 18, AAAS, Washington, Chap. 1, 1942.

Nicolle, C., Blagiot, L., and Consil, E.: Etiologie de la fièvre recurrente. Ann. Pasteur Inst., 27:204, 1913.

Obermeier, Otto H. F.: Vorkommen feinster eine Eigenbewegung zeigender Fäden im Blute von Rekurrenskranken. Zentralbl. f. d. Med. Wissenschr., 11:145, 1873.

Schuhardt, V. T. Treatment of Relapsing Fever with Antibiotics. Ann. N. Y. Acad. Sci., 55:967, 1952.

Stein, G. J.: The Serological Diagnosis of Relapsing Fever. J. Exp. Med., 79:115, 1944.

Strong, R. P.: Stitt's Diagnosis, Prevention and Treatment of Tropical Diseases. 7th ed., Philadelphia, Blakiston Company, 1944, Vol. 1.

RAT-BITE FEVER

Two etiologic and clinical entities are included in the medical literature under the term rat-bite fever, the only important factor common to both being the usual mode of transmission to man indicated by the name. The two diseases will be designated, respectively, *spirillary rat-bite fever* and *streptobacillary fever* in accordance with the nature of the etiologic agent of each (Watkins).

History. Transmission of a febrile disease to man by the bite of a rat has been known for centuries. The first clinical description of the disease was by Wilcox in 1840, and a monograph by Miyaka in 1900 awakened interest in the disease. In 1914 Schottmüller isolated a streptobacillus from a case of rat-bite fever, and in 1916 Futaki and his associates demonstrated a spirillum. Cases have been reported from many parts of the world. Watkins collected 184 cases reported in the United States, up to 1946; of these a streptobacillus was demonstrated in 39 and a spirillum in 41. Since 1946 most of the cases reported have been of the streptobacillary type. No case has been reported in which both etiologic agents were demonstrated to be present simultaneously, although such cases may plausibly occur.

SPIRILLARY RAT-BITE FEVER
(Sodoku)

Definition. The disease caused by *Spirillum minus* is characterized by an indurated ulcer at the site of inoculation, regional lymphadenitis, relapsing type of fever, skin rash and often false positive serologic tests for syphilis.

Etiology. Of 39 proved cases recorded by Watkins, 37 followed the bite of a rat, one the bite of a weasel, and one simple trauma with no known animal contact. This is in contrast to Weil's disease which is rarely transmitted by actual rat bite. The source of the spirilla at the time of rat bite is believed to be the eye discharge produced by keratoconjunctivitis of the infected rat; this discharge, in which spirilla have been demonstrated, drains into the oral cavity of the rat.

Spirillum minus is a short, thick, spiral organism 2 to 5 microns in length, with one to three angular curves, and polar flagellae. It moves with a rapid darting motion which can best be seen by darkfield microscopic examination. It cannot be cultivated in artificial media, but upon intraperitoneal inoculation of laboratory animals (guinea pigs, rats, mice) blood stream invasion and peritoneal involvement occurs. In guinea pigs intradermal inoculation often gives rise to a local lesion in which the spirillum can be demonstrated.

Clinical Manifestations. Unless complicated by secondary infection, the rat-bite wound heals promptly. After an incubation period of five to twenty-eight days there is sudden onset with flare-up of the rat-bite wound, regional lymphangitis and lymphadenitis, chills, fever, malaise and headache.

The site of inoculation becomes swollen, indurated, painful, with an angry purplish hue, and may subsequently ulcerate. After several days both local and generalized symptoms subside, only to reappear again in a few days. Periods of fever may then alternate with afebrile periods, the temperature rising abruptly and remaining elevated for 24 to 48 hours, then falling rapidly to normal.

This relapsing type of fever is typical and may continue for weeks in untreated cases. The first few relapses are usually accompanied by an exacerbation of the inflammation in the wound and the appearance of a rash. The eruption is of a dusky red macular or maculopapular character and is sparsely distributed over the trunk and extremities. The spleen is often palpable. Arthritis is not a common or prominent symptom, in contrast to streptobacillary fever, although arthralgia and muscle pains may occur. A leukocytosis is often but not invariably present, and may reach 20,000 or more per cubic millimeter. False positive serologic tests for syphilis occur in a high proportion of cases. The fatality rate as recorded has been about 10 per cent, but this should be reduced by modern therapy.

Diagnosis. Confirmation of the diagnosis is made by demonstration of *Spirillum minus*. Exudates from the local lesion and material aspirated from the enlarged regional lymph node should be examined by darkfield microscopy, inoculated into the scrotal skin of guinea pigs, and intraperitoneally in mice. Darkfield examination of blood is unrewarding, but freshly drawn blood plasma should be inoculated intraperitoneally in guinea pigs and mice. Spirilla may be demonstrated by darkfield examination of the animal's blood and peritoneal exudates five to fourteen days after inoculation. As both mice and guinea pigs occasionally carry spirilla as a natural infection, an effort should be made to demonstrate the organism in more than one inoculated animal.

Treatment. In the pre-penicillin era the response to one of the arsenical drugs, such as neoarsphenamine, was usually prompt. Both penicillin and the tetracyclines have been shown to be effective. Crystalline penicillin in doses of 30,000 to 40,000 units every 6 hours for a period of seven days has proved to be satisfactory. Penicillin in aluminum monostearate in doses of 600,000 units twice daily, continued for three to four days after the temperature has returned to normal, should likewise be adequate.

Chlortetracycline (aureomycin) in an initial dosage of 10 mg. per kilogram body weight with daily maintenance doses of 30 mg. per kilogram given orally has also been recommended. No reports on the use of other antimicrobials have been made.

STREPTOBACILLARY FEVER
(Haverhill Fever; Erythema Arthriticum Epidemicum)

Definition. Streptobacillary fever is an acute infection acquired often but not exclusively by rat-bite, and characterized by acute onset, intermittent fever, erythematous rash and polyarthritis.

Etiology. *Streptobacillus moniliformis* is a gram-negative, pleomorphic organism 2 to 15 microns in length, which grows in chains, interspersed with swollen bodies among the bacillary forms. It is a common inhabitant of the nasopharynx of wild and laboratory rats, and most cases of this disease have followed the bite of a rat. However, one epidemic originally described as haverhill fever (Place and Sutton) was milk-borne, and there have been a number of sporadic cases reported in which no direct contact with rats could be established.

Clinical Manifestations. The incubation period is usually one to five days, thus tending to be shorter than in spirillary rat-bite fever. If the disease follows rat-bite, the local wound ordinarily heals without incident but occasionally an abscess develops in the wound. Regional lymphadenitis is not a prominent feature. The onset of the disease is abrupt with chills, fever, vomiting, headache and rather severe pains in the back and joints. A maculopapular rash develops early, usually within the first 48 hours, and at this stage the disease is dengue-like in its manifestation. Often there is a remission of the fever after 48 to 72 hours. Within the first five days, however, one or more joints usually become swollen, red and painful, with recurrence of the septic type of fever. The acute arthritis is one of the most prominent and persistent symptoms in streptobacillary fever. Subcutaneous abscesses, from which the infecting organism has been recovered, have been observed. Bronchopneumonia also occurs in a small proportion of cases. There is a leukocytosis of 10,000 to 20,000 cells per cubic millimeter with a relative increase in neutrophils. False positive serologic tests for syphilis occur only rarely, in contrast to spirillary rat-bite fever.

Relapse is rare, but in the absence of specific therapy convalescence may be prolonged because of the affected joints. About 7 per cent of reported cases have been fatal, but this proportion can probably be substantially reduced by modern therapy. Ulcerative endocarditis and myocardial abscesses have been found post mortem.

Diagnosis. Even without a history of rat-bite, an acute febrile illness accompanied by nonmigratory polyarthritis and skin rash is highly suggestive of streptobacillary fever.

Serum agglutinins for *Streptobacillus moniliformis* develop within ten days and reach a maximum in three to four weeks. An agglutination titer of 1:80 or higher is regarded as diagnostic; demonstration of a four-fold or greater rise in titer is especially significant. *Streptobacillus moniliformis* may be recovered from the patient's blood or more readily from fluid aspirated from an affected joint or abscess. Isolation is accomplished by implantation in special media containing serum or ascitic fluid, or by intraperitoneal inoculation of mice. Infection is usually fatal to mice in six to twelve days, and the organism can in turn be demonstrated in their blood. In liquid or semisolid media colonies develop well below the surface of the medium and have a characteristic fluffy, cotton-ball appearance. Mice which survive the infection frequently develop joint lesions from which the organism can be isolated.

Treatment. Penicillin appears to be specific for this disease, although relatively few cases have been reported since this drug has been available. In the absence of more definitive information, large doses of penicillin, 1,200,000 units per day of the aqueous form for adults and older children and one-half this amount for young children, should be given daily for at least seven days. Further experience may show smaller doses to be effective.

Streptomycin in a dose of 1 to 2 gm. daily until the patient has been asymptomatic for two to three days has also been found to be effective. No data are available on the efficacy of the other antimicrobial drugs. In contrast to spirillary rat-bite fever, the arsenical drugs are not effective in the streptobacillary disease.

Thomas B. Turner

References

Bayne-Jones, S.: Rat-bite Fever in the United States. Internat. Clin. (41st series), 3:235, 1931.

Brown, T. McP., and Nunemaker, J. C.: Rat-bite Fever: a Review of the American Cases with Reevaluation of Etiology; Report of Cases. Bull. Johns Hopkins Hosp., 70:201, 1942.

Lominski, I. R. W., Henderson, A. S., and McNee, J. W.: Rat-bite Fever due to *Streptobacillus moniliformis*. Brit. M. J., 2:510, 1948.

Place, E. H., and Sutton, L. E.: Erythema Arthriticum Epidemicum (Haverhill Fever). Arch. Int. Med., 54:659, 1934.

Watkins, C. G.: Ratbite Fever. J. Pediat., 28:429, 1946.

THE LEPTOSPIROSES

Definition. The leptospiral infections of man comprise a group of syndromes, including Weil's disease, pretibial fever, meningitis, nephritis, arthritis, iridocyclitis and a mild grippe-like illness.

More than twenty different strains of leptospirae have been recognized by serologic methods. The strains known to be associated with human infection in the United States include *L. icterohemorrhagiae, L. canicola, L. pomona, L. autumnalis* and *L. grippotyphosa.*

Epidemiology. A variety of wild and domestic animals, including rats, mice, dogs, cattle and swine, may become infected by leptospirae, and the infection is usually a chronic one, characterized by excretion of living organisms in the urine for long periods of time. Humans may become infected by contact with materials contaminated by such urine; for this reason certain occupations carry a special hazard of leptospiral infection. These include sewer work, ditch digging, fish cutting, farming and slaughterhouse work. Infection has also been acquired from swimming in contaminated pools of water.

Pathogenesis and Pathology. The portal of entry is believed to be either the respiratory or the gastrointestinal tract, although conceivably leptospirae can gain access through cuts or abrasions of the skin. Once the organisms have penetrated the mucosal or skin barrier, the type of clinical disease produced will depend upon the strain of infecting organism as well as on the host's response. In young persons the *mild grippe-like* and *meningeal* forms of disease are more likely to develop, whereas in persons past the age of 30 the more severe *Weil's disease* is commonest. This form is most frequently associated with infection by *L. icterohemorrhagiae,* although it is occasionally produced by *L. canicola.*

Presumably in all forms of infection there is an initial leptospiremia. This can be demonstrated in the great majority of cases of Weil's disease any time during the first three to five days of illness. Circulating antibodies usually make their appearance during the second week of illness and organisms can seldom be demonstrated in the blood after that time. Leptospirae may appear transiently in the urine during the latter part of the second or the third week. A chronic urinary carrier state does not become established in the human, as it so frequently does in animals.

The cellular response to acute inflammation produced by leptospirae varies. The muscle lesions of Weil's disease are principally those of acute localized degenerative changes in muscle fibers with little inflammatory reaction about them. In the liver the microscopic evidence of disease is often surprisingly meager, even in deeply jaundiced patients. There may be minimal evidences of cytoplasmic degeneration, some active hepatocellular regeneration and bile stasis. In the most severe cases areas of focal necrosis may be observed. In the kidney the pathologic changes may be more obvious; here one finds degeneration and necrosis of convoluted tubules, diffuse interstitial inflammation and numerous granular casts and cellular debris in the collecting tubules. The cellular response in meningitis is principally lymphocytic. The circulating leukocytes of the blood vary in number according to the disease picture: in the grippe-like, meningeal and pretibial fever syndromes, the leukocyte count is usually in the normal range, whereas in Weil's disease a well marked leukocytosis is the usual finding.

WEIL'S DISEASE

Clinical Manifestations. The incubation period is usually eight to twelve days. The onset is abrupt, often with one or more chills, followed by fever varying from 102° to 104° F. Headache and photophobia are prominent symptoms, and the patient complains of severe muscular pains in the lumbar region and calves. There may be nausea, vomiting or diarrhea. Sore throat and cough are less common. The conjunctivas are conspicuously injected. Herpes simplex may develop about the mouth. The spleen seldom becomes palpably enlarged.

Fever usually lasts four to seven days, then terminates by rapid lysis. There may, however, be no real improvement in the clinical state, since it is at about the fifth or sixth day that hepatitis and nephritis are likely to become obvious. About 60 to 70 per cent of cases recognized as having Weil's disease show *hepatitis,* with icterus and enlarged tender liver. Jaundice deepens during the next few days, then usually begins to subside by the twelfth or fourteenth day. In cases terminating fatally there may be increasing cholemia until death. *Nephritis* is somewhat less frequent, being evident in less than half of the recognized cases. It is manifested by albuminuria and hematuria and, in severest cases, by oliguria and azotemia. Renal involvement is rare without evidence of liver disease. In about 10 per cent of cases there is clinical evidence of meningeal inflammation, i.e., pain and stiffness of the neck, with Kernig's and Brudzinski's signs. Other unusual manifestations include *petechial and purpuric lesions* of the skin, and *iridocyclitis* or *optic neuritis.*

Relapse, with fever and muscle pain, occurs in about 20 per cent of all cases, during the third or fourth week. The symptoms are usually milder than in the original attack.

Diagnosis. Leptospirae have been identified in the blood by darkfield microscopy during the first five to seven days of illness. This procedure is reliable only in the hands of an experienced observer, since it is easy to mistake strands of fibrin moved about by brownion motion for leptospirae. A preferable procedure is to inoculate young guinea pigs intraperitoneally with the patient's blood. These animals show signs of infection (fever and jaundice) three to fifteen days later, and the organisms can be recovered from their tissues. After the first week of illness it is rarely possible to demonstrate leptospirae in the blood, but during the second or third week they may be recovered from the urine, by animal inoculation, in perhaps 20 per cent of cases. Occasionally leptospirae can be recovered from the blood or urine of human beings by cultural methods.

Antibodies usually appear in the blood during the second week of illness and reach peak levels by the third or fourth week. Agglutinin titers of 10,000 to 100,000 are not uncommon. For best results the antigen should be freshly prepared from cultures.

In the *blood* a polymorphonuclear *leukocytosis,* from 10,000 to 30,000 per cubic millimeter, is the rule. This is of considerable value in differential diagnosis. There may be a moderate reduction in blood *platelets,* although not usually sufficient to account for the hemorrhagic tendency sometimes manifested. Examination of the *cerebrospinal fluid* is a useful guide to diagnosis of Weil's disease. In 80 to 90 per cent of all cases, regardless of the presence of clinical signs of meningitis, there is a pleocytosis, varying from 10 to several hundred cells per cubic millimeter, the majority being lymphocytes.

In patients with jaundice the cerebrospinal fluid also becomes xanthochromic. The *urine* may show no abnormality during the first few days, but with the development of hepatitis, bilirubin may appear. Nephritis is evidenced by hematuria, cylindruria and proteinuria.

Muscle biopsy can also provide an early presumptive diagnosis of Weil's disease, for the tissue obtained may reveal a characteristic picture, consisting of areas of focal necrosis in a segment of muscle fiber, with little vascular change or infiltration by inflammatory cells.

Differential Diagnosis. During the first few days of illness the picture is that of an acute systemic infectious disease which can hardly be differentiated from a variety of other processes, including acute pyogenic infections, influenza and typhus fever. Severe muscle pain, suffusion of the conjunctivas, leukocytosis and pleocytosis in the cerebrospinal fluid are features which should suggest leptospiral infection. After the first week there may be little or no fever, but jaundice is likely to appear. At this stage the principal problem is differentiation from viral hepatitis. Again the presence of conjunctival suffusion, leukocytosis and cerebrospinal fluid abnormalities are helpful. In acute hemolytic jaundice, reticulocytosis is likely to be present, and bile may not be found in the urine.

Prognosis. The fatality rate is approximately 5 per cent in recognized cases of Weil's disease. As many mild forms of the disease probably go unrecognized, the actual death rate is doubtless considerably lower. The prognosis is grave if there is severe hepatic and renal involvement, with deep jaundice, azotemia, oliguria or circulatory impairment.

Treatment. General supportive measures to be used in acutely ill patients are the same as for any acute infectious disease.

It has been difficult to evaluate different kinds of specific therapy in Weil's disease, because of its variable severity and natural early subsidence of fever. In view of good results in the treatment of experimental infection with antiserum, a few attempts have been made in humans to give serum therapy or transfusions of blood from patients who have recovered from the infection. The results have not been clear-cut, and neither procedure has been widely accepted.

Penicillin is effective in therapy of experimental infections, if given early in the course of the disease but not after the infection has become well established. The drug has been administered more or less routinely to patients with Weil's disease since 1944, but its value still remains questionable. Deaths have occurred despite administration of moderately large doses of the drug. Very large doses, 5,000,000 units or more a day, may be tried. The tetracyclines (Aureomycin, Terramycin) and chloramphenicol are also effective in experimental infections but their usefulness in treatment of human disease has not been clearly demonstrated. In a study of various antimicrobial drugs alone and in combination, carried out in Puerto Rico, there was no definite benefit demonstrable with any.

PRETIBIAL FEVER
(Fort Bragg Fever)

An acute infectious disease which was observed among soldiers stationed at Ft. Bragg, North Carolina, during the period 1942–44, was given the names pretibial fever and Fort Bragg fever. An agent, probably responsible for the disease, was isolated from the blood of a patient in 1944, and maintained by animal passage in laboratories for some years thereafter. Originally assumed to be a filterable virus, this agent was shown in 1952, by Gochenour and associates, to be L. autumnalis. The serums saved from patients convalescent from pretibial fever were found to contain specific agglutinins for this agent. Sporadic cases of the syndrome are still observed occasionally in North Carolina and in Georgia, and it is to be presumed that the disease still occurs in those regions.

The clinical manifestations are those of an acute, self-limited, exanthematous infectious disease. There is an abrupt onset with chilliness, or chills, malaise, headache and photophobia. Some patients have cough and coryza, some have nausea and vomiting. On examination the distinctive physical findings are splenomegaly and a cutaneous eruption. The rash appears about the fourth day of illness. It is most often located only on the anterior aspects of the legs (hence the name "pretibial"), but is occasionally generalized, even to the face. The lesions consist of irregular, slightly raised areas of erythema, varying in size and shape, occasionally being 5 cm. in diameter.

The course of illness is brief, fever subsiding in four to eight days, and there are no residual defects.

The distinctive laboratory finding is leukopenia in the early stages, with return to normal levels in convalescence.

Definitive diagnosis can be made by isolating L. autumnalis from the blood during the early stage of illness, or by demonstrating the appearance of specific antibodies for that organism during convalescence.

LEPTOSPIRAL MENINGITIS
(Swineherd's Disease)

This form of leptospirosis is most commonly observed in young persons and there is a peak incidence in the latter part of the summer. It was first described in Europe, where it was called swineherd's disease. For a time it was thought to be due to a virus similar to that of lymphocytic choriomeningitis, but the leptospiral etiology has since been established beyond doubt. Cases have been shown to be caused by L. icterohemorrhagiae, L. canicola and L. pomona. The clinical picture is indistinguishable from that of other nonpurulent meningitides caused by viruses such as lymphocytic choriomeningitis, mumps and nonparalytic poliomyelitis. There is usually an abrupt onset of illness with headache, fever, pains in the muscles, some stiffness of the back and neck. The temperature may go as high as 103° or 104° F. The cerebrospinal fluid may be normal during the first two or three days; later a mononuclear pleocytosis develops, the cell count usually being between 50 and 300 with occasionally as many as 50 per cent being polymorphonuclears. Dextrose content of the cerebrospinal fluid is normal and the protein is moderately elevated, usually being 50 to 100 mg. per 100 ml. The peripheral leukocyte count is normal. Symptoms of headache and malaise persist for two to ten days, then subside, and complete recovery ensues. Diagnosis can be made only by isolation of leptospirae from the blood or cerebrospinal fluid or by serologic tests.

GRIPPE-LIKE ILLNESS AND OTHER FORMS OF LEPTOSPIRAL INFECTION

Grippe-like Illness. In many parts of the world leptospiral infection is commonly observed in the form of a brief febrile disease without localizing manifestations pointing either to hepatic or to meningeal involvement. These infections are usually caused by strains of leptospirae other than L. icterohemorrhagiae, such as L. canicola, L. pomona and L. grippotyphosa. According to the occupational factors these diseases are designated variously as *rice-field fever, mud fever, cane fever* and so forth. There are no distinctive manifestations and diagnosis can only be made by demonstration of the agent in the blood or urine or by serologic methods. In a case recently reported from Tennessee, in addition to the above symptoms of fever and malaise there was an acute polyarthritis with a clinical picture somewhat suggestive of acute rheumatic fever.

Iridocyclitis. Acute inflammation of the iris and uveal tract may occur as a late complication of Weil's disease, usually coming on in the third or fourth week, but sometimes as an isolated entity several months after recovery from generalized leptospiral infection. Such cases may come under the care of ophthalmologists, and the relationship to the preceding leptospiral infection may not be recognized because of the long latent period which has occurred. The outcome is usually satisfactory, with subsidence after two or three weeks, leaving no permanent damage to the eye.

Nephritis. In rare instances leptospiral infection is principally manifested by involvement of the kidney with hematuria, pro-

teinuria, cylindruria and oliguria. Such a picture can easily be confused with that of acute glomerulonephritis. The eventual outcome is complete recovery.

PAUL B. BEESON

References

Beeson, P. B., Hankey, D. D., and Cooper, C. F., Jr.: Leptospiral Iridocyclitis; Evidence of Human Infection with Leptospira pomona in the United States. J.A.M.A., *145*:229, 1951.

Beeson, P. B., and Hankey, D. D.: Leptospiral Meningitis. Arch. Int. Med., *89*:575, 1952.

Daniels, W. B., and Grennan, H. A.: Pretibial Fever, an Obscure Disease. J.A.M.A., *122*:361, 1943.

Gochenour, W. S., Jr., Smadel, J. E., Jackson, E. B., Evans, L. B., and Yager, R. H.: Leptospiral Etiology of Fort Bragg Fever. Pub. Health Rep., *67*:811, 1952.

Gsell, O.: Leptospirosen. Bern, Switzerland, Medizinischer Verlag Hans Huber, 1952.

Hall, H. E., and others: Evaluation of Antibiotic Therapy in Human Leptospirosis. Ann. Int. Med., *35*:981, 1951.

Stiles, W. W.,Goldstein, J. D., and McCann, W. S.: Leptospiral Nephritis. J.A.M.A., *131*:1271, 1946.

Sutliff, W. D., Shepard, R., and Dunham, W. B.: Acute Leptospira pomona Arthritis and Myocarditis. Ann. Int. Med., *39*:134, 1953.

PROTOZOAN INFECTIONS

AMEBIASIS

Definition. Amebiasis is the disease caused by infection with the protozoan, *Endamoeba histolytica*. It affects the colon primarily, and other organs secondarily, especially the liver. Amebiasis is characterized by gastrointestinal and constitutional symptoms, and almost always runs a chronic course, which is subject to acute exacerbations. The term, *amebic dysentery,* is properly applied only to the severe cases in which there is diarrhea with blood and mucus in the stools. The term, *acute amebic dysentery,* is often applied to the acute exacerbations, but truly acute cases are probably rare. They are the result of heavy infections such as may occur in epidemics due to contamination of water supplies with sewage.

Etiology and Pathogenesis. The parasite has two phases, trophozoite and cyst. The active trophozoites, which are present in infected tissues, cause the pathologic changes, and the cysts, which develop from trophozoites on the surface of the mucosa of the colon, are responsible for the transmission of the disease. The trophozoites are 10 to 40 microns in diameter. They exhibit progressive, flowing motility, and have a nucleus with uniform distribution of peripheral chromatin and a delicate, usually centrally placed nucleolus. Some show ingested erythrocytes. Cysts are from 5 to 20 microns in diameter and contain one to four nuclei similar to those of the trophozoites, as well as chromatoid bodies with blunt rounded ends. They have a well-defined wall, and are resistant to freezing and partial drying, but not to boiling or complete drying.

When cysts are swallowed, they pass to the cecum. There, by a process called excystation, several trophozoites emerge from each cyst and attack and invade the tissues of the colon. It is evident that intestinal bacteria aid in the production of the intestinal lesions, for the administration of antimicrobial drugs which are inactive against amebas will produce improvement and evidence of healing in many cases of amebiasis. This does not necessarily imply bacterial invasion of the tissues. *E. histolytica* does not grow in culture in the absence of other micro-organisms; evidently it depends on bacteria for some metabolic product or products. Antibacterial agents may interfere with the multiplication of the amebas by decreasing the numbers of bacteria or their output of certain metabolites.

Incidence and Epidemiology. Amebiasis is by no means limited to the tropics but is world-wide in distribution and is found as far north as the Arctic Circle. Amebiasis is more prevalent and more severe in the tropics; however, it may produce severe and even fatal illness in persons who have lived only in the temperate zones. It is more prevalent in areas where sanitation is poor. In areas devoid of any sanitary facilities, rates of infection are often more than 50 per cent. In the United States as a whole, Craig has estimated that 10 per cent of the population is infected. The writer found an infection rate of 16 per cent in a group of food handlers in New York City. Some published studies have shown comparable infection rates in similar population groups in other temperate zone cities. It is evident that infection with *Endamoeba histolytica* may be of frequent occurrence even in areas where sanitation is good.

Amebiasis may occur at any age. In unsanitary areas, children tend to show the same rates as adults, once they have passed the age of 5 years. In areas of good sanitation, children show a much lower incidence than adults. Infection rates are little influenced by sex, but 85 per cent to 90 per cent of amebic liver abscesses occur in adult males. Children rarely, if ever, develop this complication.

Infection takes place when the cysts are ingested. This usually results from fecal contamination of food or drink. Water is contaminated by sewage. Food may be contaminated by being fertilized with human excreta, by flies exposed to previously infected excrement, or by food handlers who are careless in their habits. The last method is responsible for the endemicity of amebiasis in places with well protected water and food supplies. Children may infect themselves when playing in soil contaminated with feces. Infection by close personal contact occurs in institutions for mental illness when fecal contamination of the environment plus uncontrollable personal habits are combined.

Epidemics of amebiasis occur occasionally. Perhaps the most famous is that which occurred in Chicago in 1933, when there were more than 1400 cases and more than 100 deaths. Epidemics are usually the result of direct contamination of the water supply with sewage, due to faulty plumbing.

Morbid Anatomy. Amebiasis is characterized by ulceration of the colon which varies greatly in extent and intensity. In patients who die of the disease, ulcers are most often present throughout the colon and occasionally extend to the terminal ileum. In 30 to 40 per cent of cases, however, the process is focal and the lesions tend to concentrate in the region of the cecum and ascending colon, and to a lesser degree in the rectosigmoid area. In patients in whom amebiasis is an incidental finding at death, the tendency of the lesions to concentrate in the upper colon is even more striking. The ulcers vary in size. The larger ulcers penetrate to the submucosa and extend laterally, assuming a flask shape. The mucous membrane between the ulcers is usually normal.

In the liver there is focal necrosis. In some patients the process goes no further, resulting in low grade hepatitis. In others, the necrotic areas coalesce to form an abscess which has a ragged wall and contains necrotic material, usually of a brown color. The same liquefaction necrosis characterizes lesions of the lung and brain. Histologic examination usually shows little cellular reaction to invasion by *E. histolytica.*

Clinical Manifestations. The symptoms of amebiasis vary greatly from patient to patient, both with respect to severity and to the presence or absence of specific complaints. They may also vary in severity in the same patient, and there may be intervals of relatively good health. The classic dysenteric form with cramps, diarrhea and bloody, mucoid stools is seen in only a small proportion of cases, at least in the temperate zones. Patients with severe dysentery usually have a history of preceding milder gastrointestinal disturbances, although this may be brought out only on careful questioning.

Many infected persons have no complaints. They may be called "carriers" in the sense that they constitute a source of infection for others. In the biologic sense, however, the term "carrier" does not apply, since they often have pathologic changes in the colon and may develop clinical manifestations, including liver abscess, at any time. In any case, these asymptomatic infections should always be treated. Sometimes, following treatment, the so-called carrier will recognize that he has really been having symptoms, which were so mild that he was not aware of them. The insidious character of mild amebiasis is striking. The symptoms are often vague and difficult to describe; they may be peculiarly described by the patient. Consequently, a functional disturbance may be suspected, especially since the blood count, erythrocyte sedimentation rate and other routine studies are usually normal in mild infections. Patients with amebiasis are not infrequently treated for spastic colon or referred for psychiatric advice.

Diarrhea is a common, but by no means constant symptom. About one third of patients do not have it. The diarrhea may be persistent or intermittent, mild or severe. In some instances it is so mild that it is not noticed by the patient. It may alternate with constipation and, in some instances, the latter is the more prominent symptom. When there is diarrhea, stools vary from slightly loose to watery. They sometimes contain mucus and less frequently blood. Other common gastrointestinal symptoms are abdominal distress, distention, abdominal pain and tenesmus. *Vomiting* is unusual but nausea occurs in some cases. *Abdominal pain* may be generalized or localized. When it is localized, it is often felt in the right lower quadrant, owing to involvement of the cecum. In such instances appendicitis may be suspected, and a normal appendix is sometimes removed before the correct diagnosis is made. True amebic appendicitis occurs, but it is rare.

Constitutional symptoms often accompany the gastrointestinal manifestations and may overshadow them. They include undue fatigue, fever, which is most often not high, vague somatic aching, backache and arthralgias. Rarely actual arthritis suggesting the rheumatoid form is seen. There may also be nervousness, irritability or dizziness, suggesting a neuropsychiatric disorder. Weight loss is not characteristic. It may occur in relatively severe cases but is rare in mild cases. Patients with pronounced diarrhea may maintain a normal weight and are sometimes actually obese. Anemia is rare in mild cases, but frequent when manifestations are severe.

Patients with uncomplicated amebic colitis may have tenderness over the cecum or other portions of the colon. Otherwise, physical signs are usually absent unless a very severe dysentery occurs. In such cases, the patient shows varying degrees of emaciation and dehydration.

Sigmoidoscopic examination is most often negative in amebiasis. In hospital practice it is not unusual to find ulcerations or other abnormalities in one third or more of cases; in office practice, however, at least in the temperate zone, less than 5 per cent of those infected show visible changes. The most typical finding is the presence of ulcers of an irregular shape set in an otherwise normal mucosa. In some cases, there is a friable, hemorrhagic mucosa suggesting nonspecific ulcerative colitis; it is probably due to secondary bacterial infection.

Roentgenographic examination of the colon is usually negative, but a substantial minority of cases do have abnormal findings. Most often these are observed in the cecum, which is irregular, narrowed and altered in shape due to edema and spasm. Spasm may occur in other portions of the colon.

Both sigmoidoscopic and roentgenographic examinations are desirable in amebiasis. They give some indication as to the extent of the disease, and if abnormalities are found, their reversion to normal following treatment can be utilized as an indication of cure. The examination will also detect coexisting but unrelated conditions such as neoplastic disease.

Complications. *Abscess of the liver* is the most common serious complication of amebiasis. It may occur in patients with no previous history of intestinal disorder. There is usually only one abscess and in a large majority of cases it occurs in the right lobe. While the onset of symptoms may be acute, it is usually insidious and the diagnosis is frequently difficult. The initial symptom may be *unexplained fever*. *Pain* over the liver may not occur until several weeks have passed. The pain may be felt in the upper abdomen or right lower chest and may be referred to the right shoulder or scapular area. Anorexia and weight loss are frequent. Nausea may occur but vomiting is rare. The fever is usually moderate in degree; it may be associated with sweats.

The physical signs depend on the direction in which the liver enlarges. When the enlargement is chiefly upward, dullness and diminished breath sounds may be noted at the right lung base, simulating pneumonia. If the enlargement is downward, it can be detected by palpation. In either case, there is tenderness over the liver edge and pain on percussion over the liver area. Roentgenographic examination of the chest may show elevation and fixation of the right diaphragm, or merely impairment of its excursion. In some cases, there is a localized bulge in its contour. Pleural effusion is present in some instances. The blood shows a moderate increase in the leukocyte count, most often not exceeding 20,000 per cubic millimeter, with a moderate increase in the percentage of neutrophils, usually only to 75 or 80 per cent. Anemia is frequent. Marked leukocytosis and high fever are usually associated either with a perforated abscess or with secondary bacterial infection. Perforation is not unusual, since the diagnosis may be overlooked for weeks or months. Most often the abscess perforates into the subphrenic space, right pleural cavity or right lung. Less often perforation occurs into other organs adjacent to the liver, or into the peritoneal cavity.

There may be less profound involvement of the liver with manifestations indicating recurrent *acute hepatitis* or low grade *chronic hepatitis*. In these cases jaundice is rare, but one or more of the tests of liver function frequently show an abnormal result. The liver may or may not be enlarged to palpation. Tenderness over the liver is often but not invariably present. Symptoms suggesting chronic hepatitis are right upper quadrant pain, nausea, variable appetite and intolerance to alcoholic beverages.

Pulmonary abscess is usually the result of extension from a liver abscess; occasionally it occurs independently as an isolated phenomenon. Other rare complications are brain abscess, and involvement of the skin, usually in contiguity with internal infection, that is, adjacent to the rectum, a colostomy or the drainage tract of a liver abscess. In the colon, major complications are very unusual. They include perforation, stenosis, and a localized productive inflammation called ameboma, which produces the clinical manifestations of a tumor.

Diagnosis. The laboratory plays a major role in the diagnosis of amebiasis. The infection should be suspected in patients with ill defined gastrointestinal complaints as well as those with diarrhea, in patients with unexplained constitutional symptoms, and in patients with anicteric hepatitis. Periodic routine examination of the stools for *E. histolytica* is advisable in persons exposed to unsanitary conditions.

The diagnosis of intestinal amebiasis is only exceptionally justified without the demonstration of *E. histolytica* in the stools. The parasite is most readily found in diarrheal stools, so that, if diarrhea is not present, it should be produced by the administration of a saline cathartic. These diarrheal stools must be examined promptly, using warm slides and saline, in order that the characteristic motility of the trophozoites may be observed. Some workers prefer to fix such specimens and stain them with iron-hematoxylin so that permanent preparations are available for study. Specimens obtained through the sigmoidoscope are useful in diagnosis when there are visible lesions. However, since the lesions are more common in the upper colon and frequently limited thereto, purged stool specimens are more likely to yield positive results than material obtained through the sigmoidoscope.

In diarrheal stools it is usual to find only trophozoites. Cysts may occur but are more frequently found in formed stools. In many patients, cyst formation is a variable process, so that for periods as long as several weeks, it may be impossible to detect them. Hence, reliance on casual specimens greatly reduces the likelihood of a positive finding.

Cultures have only a limited value in the diagnosis of ambiasis for, in many cases, the amebas do not grow readily. In selected cases, the method is a useful adjunct to the direct examination of fresh stools.

The administration of antimicrobials such as the sulfonamides, the tetracyclines, or even penicillin by injection, before the stool specimens are obtained greatly increases the difficulty of finding E. histolytica. Hence, the empiric treatment of diarrheas with these agents is not advisable. The presence of mineral oil and barium in the intestinal tract temporarily interferes with the detection of amebas.

When there are manifestations suggestive of amebic abscess of the liver, the demonstration of E. histolytica in the stools helps to confirm the diagnosis. In some cases, it is not possible to find the parasite. This is true especially if antimicrobials have been given empirically because the patient has had an unexplained fever. The specific complement fixation reaction is of considerable value, since it appears to be positive in all cases of liver abscess due to E. histolytica. In patients with hepatitis but no abscess the reaction may be either positive or negative. With the technique currently used in most laboratories, the test is negative in the large majority of cases of uncomplicated intestinal amebiasis. In cases in which the reaction is positive, it may remain so for many months after cure.

Further corroborative evidence for the diagnosis of amebic abscess is the response to specific therapy. In uncomplicated amebic abscess, there is almost always prompt and dramatic abatement of symptoms within 24 to 48 hours after emetine is started. The response to chloroquine is less dramatic.

Some patients are so seriously ill that there may not be time to carry out proper stool examinations and therapeutic tests. In these cases, it may be necessary to perform an exploratory laparotomy because the diagnosis is obscure and an acute surgical condition is suspected. If, in the course of such an operation, an abscess of the liver is encountered, it should be aspirated and specific therapy for amebiasis instituted immediately, pending laboratory examination of the material obtained. In the absence of some other obvious infection, liver abscess is almost always amebic. If the aspirated material is brown in color, one can be almost certain of the diagnosis even though it does not usually contain demonstrable E. histolytica. However, if open drainage has been instituted and, inadvertently, no emetine or chloroquine has been given, the parasites can sometimes be found in the discharge after several days, since the material now comes from the ameba-containing abscess wall.

The aspirate should be cultured for bacteria. A negative result supports the diagnosis of amebic abscess. A positive result indicates either secondary infection of such an abscess, or a nonamebic abscess.

Prognosis. Many cases of mild amebic colitis respond rapidly and completely to a single course of an oral amebacide. A few prove more resistant. In general, the more severe the manifestations, the more likely the case is to be resistant to cure. In acute hepatitis and liver abscess, the prognosis as to cure is excellent. Low grade hepatitis often requires prolonged treatment and may be difficult to clear up permanently and completely. Death from amebiasis occurs only when the disease goes unrecognized or, occasionally, in patients weakened by other illness or subjected to massive amebic infection. A fatal outcome is most often due to liver abscess or its complications.

In those cases of amebiasis in which cure is not accomplished, the patient can be kept in reasonably good health with periodic specific treatment. Reasonable criteria of cure are freedom from clinical manifestations for one year together with post-cathartic stool specimens which are repeatedly negative for E. histolytica. Stool specimens should be examined on approximately six different occasions at increasing intervals over the period of one year following the completion of therapy.

Treatment. The therapy of amebiasis depends upon the character and the severity of the clinical manifestations. In asymptomatic amebiasis, and in mild, uncomplicated amebic colitis, a single treatment with an effective oral amebacide will result in cure in about 90 per cent of the cases. The amebacides in general use in the United States, and their doses, are as follows:

Iodine-quinoline compounds
    Diodoquin   0.65 gm. 3 or 4 times a day for 20 days
    Vioform   0.5 gm. 3 times a day for 10 days
    Chiniofon   1.0 gm. 3 times a day for 10 days
    (Anayodin, Yatren)
Arsenical compounds
    Carbarsone   0.25 gm. 3 times a day for 10 days
    Milibis   0.5 gm. 3 times a day for 8 days

Some of the oral antimicrobials, notably the tetracyclines, are capable of eradicating amebic infections. They may not have a direct amebacidal action, but may produce their effects by suppressing intestinal bacteria. Chloramphenicol rarely produces satisfactory results. The drugs which have been shown to be reasonably effective, and their doses, are as follows:

Chlortetracycline   0.5 gm. 4 times a day for 2 days or more, followed by 0.25 gm. 4 times a day for the balance of 7 days

Oxytetracycline   0.5 gm. 4 times a day for 7 days

Bacitracin   20,000 units 4 times a day for 10 days

Owing to its relative freedom from untoward effects, *Diodoquin* is the most generally useful drug. *Carbarsone* is equally effective, but somewhat more likely to produce side effects, especially diarrhea. *Chiniofon* is frequently not tolerated in adequate doses because it produces marked diarrhea. *Vioform* is slightly more prone to produce side effects than *Diodoquin,* but is approximately as effective if used in twice the dose usually recommended, that is, 0.5 gm. rather than 0.25 gm. three times a day. In adults, *Milibis* seems to have about the same effectiveness as *carbarsone,* but in children, with the appropriate reduction in dose, it is distinctly less effective. *Chlortetracycline* (Aureomycin) and oxytetracycline (Terramycin) are about equally effective. In adequate doses, they cure 85 to 90 per cent of mild cases of amebiasis. However, they are apt to produce marked gastrointestinal symptoms which may be more pronounced than the symptoms of the disease. *Bacitracin* rarely produces important gastrointestinal disturb-

ances, but it is effective in only 70 per cent to 80 per cent of mild cases.

Fumagillin, a drug which has a high amebacidal activity in the test tube, and no significant antibacterial activity, has recently been made available. It appears to rank with Diodoquin and carbarsone in effectiveness in mild amebiasis, but it has not yet been fully evaluated. The dose is 10 mg. three times a day for ten days.

Because there is no evidence that the cure rate of oral amebacides is enhanced by the concurrent administration of *emetine,* this drug should not be used in mild or asymptomatic amebic colitis. In more severe cases of amebic colitis, treatment should be started with emetine hydrochloride, 1 mg. per kilogram of body weight, administered daily by deep subcutaneous injection. On the first day it should be divided into two doses in order to observe the patient for possible idiosyncrasy. Thereafter it is given in a single dose until severe symptoms are controlled. Frequently this is accomplished after two or three days. It is advisable to limit emetine treatment to a maximum of five days, in order to avoid the serious toxic effects which it may produce. Emetine is remarkably effective in controlling diarrhea and other acute symptoms but it is essentially symptomatic therapy. Even with a total dose of 10 mg. per kilogram of body weight, cure will result in only 15 to 20 per cent of cases of intestinal amebiasis if no other specific is used.

Emetine should be followed by antibacterial therapy. This may consist of a tetracycline drug, 1 gm. per day in divided doses, or a combination of sulfasuxidine, 1 gm. four times a day, and penicillin, 500,000 units intramuscularly once a day. After five days of antibacterial therapy, Diodoquin, 0.65 gm. four times a day for twenty days, or one of the other oral amebacides should be prescribed. A second oral amebacide of different chemical character from the first should be administered one or two weeks after the first course is completed. If Diodoquin is used first, it may be followed either with carbarsone or with Milibis.

For *amebic infection of the liver* there are two effective drugs, *emetine hydrochloride* and *chloroquine diphosphate* (Aralen). The latter is as effective as the former but considerably less toxic. In the case of emetine, the margin between the effective dose and the toxic dose is small. The most important toxic effects occur in the heart. Chloroquine is not free of toxic effects. It frequently produces visual disturbances and nausea as well as insomnia. Occasionally other forms of psychic disturbance appear, such as nightmares or manic tendencies. However, all of these are promptly relieved when the drug is discontinued.

For acute amebic hepatitis or liver abscess, chloroquine should be prescribed in a dose of 0.25 gm. three times a day for two weeks. If there is marked nausea or mental aberration, the dose is reduced to 0.25 gm. twice daily and it is continued, if possible, to a total dose of 10 gm. If emetine is used, the dose is 10 mg. per kilogram of body weight in a period of ten days. The pulse and blood pressure should be checked before each injection. If there is a pronounced fall of blood pressure or rise in pulse rate, the treatment should be stopped. The patient's activity should be markedly restricted not only during therapy but for four weeks thereafter, since emetine is slowly excreted.

Specific therapy will cure a majority of cases of liver abscess. If there is persistent fever or other evidence of incomplete resolution of the abscess, drainage by aspiration or open operation is indicated.

In *chronic amebic hepatitis,* the dose of chloroquine should be 0.25 gm. twice a day, since these patients seem to tolerate it less well than those with acute involvement. A total dose of 10 gm. should be used, unless here is marked intolerance. In addition, the general measures used in other chronic hepatic disease are indicated. All cases of amebic liver disease should be treated for intestinal involvement as well, even if there are no symptoms of colitis. Neither emetine nor chloroquine can be relied upon to clear up the intestinal infection.

Emetine bismuth iodide is frequently used by British physicians. It has not found favor in this country because of its toxicity. Thioarsenites have been tried recently because they seem effective against both liver and intestinal infections. Since they are prone to produce vomiting and other signs of gastrointestinal irritation, they have not had wide acceptance.

Prevention. Preventive measures consist essentially of protection of food and water supplies from contamination. This is accomplished in part by: sanitary disposal of feces; filtration plus chlorination of water supplies; and periodic examination for cross-communication between water supply and sewage system. Chlorination alone, as ordinarily used, cannot be relied on to kill cysts and indeed may serve to mask the evidence of fecal contamination by keeping the bacterial counts at a satisfactory level. Individual chlorination (Halazone tablets) is likewise of only limited effectiveness, for the amebic cysts can resist the concentrations of chlorine attainable within the limits of palatability. A tablet containing tetraglycine hydroperiodide effective against common water-borne bacteria and amebic cysts has recently been developed. It is marketed under the designation "Iodine Water Purification Tablet." Measures to reduce fly breeding are helpful. Detection and treatment of mild or asymptomatic infections, especially in food handlers, are important.

HOWARD B. SHOOKHOFF

References

Conan, N. J., Jr.: The Treatment of Hepatic Amebiasis with Chloroquine. Am. J. Med., 6:309, 1949.
Craig, C. F.: The Etiology, Diagnosis and Treatment of Amebiasis. Baltimore, Williams and Wilkins Company, 1944.
Golden, R., and Ducharme, P.: The Clinical Significance of Deformity of the Cecum in Amebiasis. Radiology, 45:565, 1945.
Hussey, K. L., and Brown, H. W.: The Complement Fixation Test for Hepatic Amebiasis. Am. J. Trop. Med., 30:147, 1950.
Klatskin, G.: Observations on Amebiasis in American Troops Stationed in India. Ann. Int. Med., 25:773, 1946.
Loesch, F.: Massenhafte Entwickelung von Amoeben im Dickdarm. Virchows Arch. f. path. Anat., 65:196, 1875.
Ochsner, A., and DeBakey, M.: Surgical Consideration of Amebiasis. Internat. Abstr. Surg., 69:392, 1939.
Walker, E. L., and Sellards, A. W.: Experimental Entamoebic Dysentery. Philippine J. Science, 8:253, 1913.
Weingarten, M., and Herzig, W. F.: The Clinical Manifestations of Chronic Amebiasis. Rev. Gastroenterol., 20:667, 1953.

SPOROZOAN INFECTIONS

Sporozoan infections are produced by the one-celled animals belonging to the Class SPOROZOA. All members of this class are parasitic, and all require an alternation of asexual reproduction (*schizogony*) and sexual reproduction (*sporogony*) to complete a life cycle. The two important groups of Sporozoa which parasitize man are the HEMOSPORIDIA (i.e., malaria parasites) and the COCCIDIA.

In the HEMOSPORIDIA of man, all or part of the asexual stage and the mother sex cells develop in the human body, while maturation of the sex cells, fertilization and sporozoite production take place in the *Anopheles* mosquito.

In the COCCIDIA only a single host is required. In the host not only asexual propagation but maturation and fertilization of the sex cells are carried out, with a brief extrinsic phase for the production and ripening of the sporozoites.

COCCIDIOSIS
(*Coccidiasis*)

Etiology. Coccidiosis is an infection caused by sporozoan parasites belonging to the genera *Isospora* and *Eimeria*. Several species of these organisms have been reported from man, but all except two (*Isospora belli* and *I. hominis*) have, on careful scrutiny, been found to be "spurious parasites," taken into the human digestive tract in infected fish.

Isospora belli and *I. hominis* have been inadequately studied, owing for the most part to their relatively uncommon occurrence in areas where modern medical examination is available, in part to the moderate symptoms usually associated with their presence, and finally to the fact that no postmortem data are available. During the period 1943–45 many cases of coccidiosis were diagnosed in American military personnel stationed in the Southwest Pacific including the Philippines.

History. More recently Meira and Corrêa (1950), in São Paulo, Brazil, and Elsdon-Dew and Freedman (1953), in Durban, Natal, have found both *I. hominis and I. belli* in their patients, while Matsubayashi and Nozawa (1948), in Japan, have experimentally infected two human volunteers with *I. belli*.

Morbid Anatomy. The schizogonic phase of the cycle in man is believed to occur in the villi of the lower portion of the ileum. The encysted fertilized ova (*oocysts*) pass down the bowel and out in feces. They are delicate, slightly irregular elongate-ovoidal objects measuring 20 to 33 by 10 to 19 microns for *I. belli* and 16 by 10.5 microns for *I. hominis,* and contain a single spherical cell. In fecal samples at warm room temperatures the single cell soon matures to provide two internal cells, each containing four crescentic *sporozoites*. The *sporocyst* with its eight sporozoites is now infective for man and, if

taken into the mouth in feces-contaminated food or drink, will hatch in the small bowel and initiate a new infection.

Clinical History. The infected patients have a history of watery mucous diarrhea of several days' standing and moderate to extreme weakness. If they are put to bed and placed on a bland diet, they usually recover in a week to ten days and the infection is spontaneously evacuated; but if they disregard the debilitated condition, the infection may become chronic and persist for years. There is no known chemotherapy for this infection.

Although many species of *Isospora* have been described from domestic and wild animals, none is morphologically similar to *I. belli* or *I. hominis*.

Prevention consists of ensuring a water supply free of living spores of the two species of *Isospora* infective for man. This may be accomplished by boiling for 10 minutes at 212 degrees F. or by passage through diatomaceous filters. Cold food contaminated by carriers should likewise be avoided.

ERNEST CARROLL FAUST

Reference

Elsdon-Dew, R., and Freedman, L.: Coccidiosis in Man: Experiences in Natal. Trans. R. Soc. Trop. Med. & Hyg., *47*:209, 1953.

MALARIA

Definition. Malaria is an infectious febrile disease produced by several species of protozoa belonging to the single genus *Plasmodium*. It is transmitted naturally from host to host only by the bite of an infected anopheline mosquito. In the mosquito the development of the parasite is observed on the stomach wall and in the salivary glands, while in man it is continued in the erythrocytes. Clinically, the disease is characterized by paroxysms of severe chills, fever and sweating. These paroxysms may occur daily (quotidian), on alternate days (tertian) or with an interval of three days between chills (quartan). After recovery from the acute attack the disease has a tendency to become chronic with occasional relapses.

History. Some of the earliest records of man show that malaria was recognized as a definite clinical entity. In the fifth century B.C. Hippocrates differentiated the fever into quotidian, tertian and quartan types. In 1880 a French army surgeon by the name of Laveran recognized the pigmented parasites in the erythrocytes of a soldier in Algiers and was convinced that they were the cause of malaria. Soon all the different asexual stages of the parasites were recognized in the erythrocytes. In 1897 MacCallum saw the fertilization of a female gametocyte following the exflagellation of a male parasite and correctly assumed that the malaria parasite had a sexual and an asexual cycle. The incrimination of the mosquito as the vector for malaria followed the work of Theobald Smith, who was the first to discover the arthropod transmission of disease, when the tick was shown to be the essential intermediate host in Texas cattle fever. English and Italian workers quickly applied the same principle to malaria and found that certain anopheline mosquitoes were infected and responsible for the transmission in man. By 1900 the details of the cycle in man and mosquito were known, and the highly specialized manner by which this disease propagates itself was understood. This complete information, in addition to the long-known efficacy of quinine as a treatment, led many to believe that malaria would soon be eradicated, but fifty years later this belief remains far from realization.

Epidemiology. Malaria at the present time is one of humanity's chief scourges, and there are many fertile areas that remain uninhabitable because of its influence. It is probable that the combined number of deaths in all parts of the world where malaria exists amount to almost 2,000,000 annually. In India the figures of the annual malaria survey show that there are approximately 100,000,000 cases with 1,000,000 deaths. In the United States indigenous malaria has practically disappeared.

Malaria in World War II. The introduction of American troops in World War II into South Pacific areas, Africa, Middle East, China, Burma and India resulted in thousands of malarial infections. Malaria soon became the outstanding medical problem of the war, not from the standpoint of mortality, because there were relatively few deaths, but because of the high degree of morbidity. The most disturbing feature was the great number of *vivax* relapses, which occurred at periodic intervals, usually every four to six weeks. For several years after World War II and the Korean conflict there was a considerable residue of men with relapsing infections. Some of these patients experienced as many as forty or more distinct episodes.

The malaria acquired overseas was both the *falciparum* and the *vivax* variety. As the former has an extremely low relapse rate, practically all malaria seen in the United States is the less severe and more persistent *vivax* form. A noticeable feature of the malaria seen in the returning serviceman is the absence of malarial cachexia so prevalent in populations native to endemic areas. Enlarged spleens, anemia and other commonly associated debilities are not frequently encountered even in servicemen with a long history of malaria. This suggests that cachexia develops only when malaria is associated with other infections or poor nutritional states.

Etiology. The specific etiologic agent of malaria is a unicellular organism which lives at the expense of the erythrocytes in certain reptiles, birds and mammals and belongs to the order of *Hemosporidia,* class *Sporozoa,* and the single genus *Plasmodium.* The species within the genus are not numerous, and they are capable of producing infections only in hosts that are closely related. In man malaria is produced by four specific parasites known as *Plasmodium vivax, P. malariae, P. falciparum* and *P. ovale.* There are certain similarities among these parasites, but each has a distinct morphology and definite pathogenicity, and none of them has been found infectious for any of the lower animals. Unlike viral or bacterial diseases, the etiologic agent of malaria has not been successfully cultivated on an artificial medium or in the presence of living cells outside its respective host. The only means of transmission in nature is by anopheline mosquitoes, although different species act as vectors in different parts of the world. The anopheline mosquito does not act as a mere mechanical transmitter of the pathogen from man to man, but serves as a haven where the parasite undergoes a definite development necessary for the perpetuation of the organism. An artificial method of transmission is the hypodermic syringe commonly used by drug addicts, which results in the actual transfer of infected blood from a carrier to a susceptible person. This type, which occurs more often in the larger cities, is responsible for many deaths, since it is usually the highly virulent falciparum malaria. Less frequently malaria is acquired in nonendemic areas after transfusions from an infected donor. There are many authenticated reports of children becoming infected from parent donors who last had symptoms twenty or more years previously. It is interesting to note that in practically all such instances the causative agent has been *P. malariae.*

The Mosquito Host. Many different species of anopheline mosquitoes have been described from various parts of the world. Although most of them can transmit malaria, they vary enormously in their susceptibility. In North America *Anopheles quadrimaculatus* has been shown to be the only important vector. The habitat of this mosquito extends to the southern border of Canada, but the severe winters, in addition to agricultural drainage and clearing, have largely limited its activity as a disease carrier to the southern states. The adult anopheline mosquito is identified by its spotted wings and its habit of resting at an angle. Only the female mosquito can become infected, since she requires a blood meal to produce fertile eggs. The male is not blood-sucking. Anopheline mosquitoes lay their eggs in swamps, ponds and streams; and the larvae lie and feed horizontally on the surface of the water, a characteristic which makes them more liable to destruction by floating larvicides, particularly oils and Paris green. The common pest mosquito, *Culex,* lays its eggs in eaves, tin cans, cisterns or any container of water in and about houses. The larvae hang head downward with an air siphon sticking above the surface of the water, and the body of the adult is parallel to the surface of its resting place. It is not concerned with the transmission of malaria and is definitely a domestic mosquito, while the anopheline prefers a wilder environment.

Development of the Malaria Parasite in the Mosquito. In order to become infected, a female mosquito must first bite a person who has male and female malaria parasites in the circulating blood, since the asexual parasites cannot survive in the mosquito's stomach. The sexual forms, known as gametocytes, initiate the cycle of development within the stomach of the mosquito, where they undergo fertilization. This is accomplished by the male parasite pushing out several flagella, which break loose and come into contact with the female form. Many attempt to penetrate, but when one succeeds, the foiled ones depart for other quarry. (This also can be observed readily under the darkfield microscope.) The fertilized forms then push their way out between the stomach cells and form cysts on its outer wall. These cysts, known as oöcysts, gradually enlarge so that by the eighth or tenth day they are mature and measure about 75 microns in diameter. If examined under the microscope, the oocysts will be seen to be distended with spindle-shaped sporozoites. At this time they rupture into the body cavity of the mosquito, and the liberated sporozoites make their way to the salivary glands, where they lie and await an opportunity to enter the blood stream of a susceptible person. The sporozoites escape from the salivary glands as the infected mosquito bites a person, thus initiating the cycle of development in the human host. At this step there is a missing link in the life history of the malaria parasite; it was last seen as a spindle-shaped sporozoite in the salivary gland of the mosquito and next observed about ten days later as a "ring-shaped" parasite in the human erythrocytes. No one has recognized an intermediary form or understood the exact manner in which it attacks the erythrocytes.

Malaria Parasites in Man. The most common variety is *Plasmodium vivax.* About ten days after an infection has been acquired through the bite of an infected anopheline, the first parasites are observed in the erythrocytes as circles of cytoplasm with a mass of red chromatin. This stage is commonly referred to as the "ring form." There follows a progressive growth of the parasite into an ameboid stage characterized by irregular arrangement of the cytoplasm, appearance of pigment granules and enlargement of the chromatin. The infected erythrocyte becomes somewhat larger and paler than normal and contains numerous reddish granules known as Schüffner's dots, which occur only with this species of parasite. As the parasite continues to enlarge, the amount of pigment increases and the nucleus starts to divide. At the end of 48 hours the erythrocyte is a mere membrane; all hemoglobin has been devoured or replaced by the parasite. The nuclear fragments have assumed a "rosette" form with each unit known as a merozoite, which is a daughter parasite. As the erythrocyte ruptures, the cluster of merozoites, usually sixteen in number, are released, and each attaches itself to a new cell. The cycle is then repeated every 48 hours, but, fortunately for man, not every merozoite that is released finds its way unhindered to reproduce its full quota of progeny. Fully 90 per cent of the merozoites are destroyed by the macrophages located chiefly in the spleen, liver and bone marrow. For some unknown reason there is a tendency for the *vivax* merozoite to prefer a reticulocyte to a mature erythrocyte for initiating its development.

The asexual reproduction of the parasite continues for several days, when new forms appear, the sexual ones (gametocytes). They fill the entire erythrocyte. Their pigment is scattered, and chromatin is diffuse. The male parasite may be differentiated from the female by its pale-staining cytoplasm with Giemsa or other Romanowsky stains. The gametocytes are concerned only with infection in the mosquito, have no clinical importance, and usually persist in the blood in limited numbers for two or three weeks. The characteristics which differentiate *P. vivax* from other parasites are a 48-hour cycle, sixteen merozoites in the mature parasite at time of segmentation, and an enlarged, pale, parasitized erythrocyte usually stippled with red-staining granules.

Plasmodium malariae, which produces quartan malaria in man, requires 72 hours to complete each asexual cycle in the erythrocyte. Except for its slower metabolic activity, this parasite bears a close similarity to the behavior of *P. vivax*. Morphologically, the young parasite is frequently observed as a "band" form across the cell. The parasitized erythrocyte seems to have a greater concentration of hemoglobin and is somewhat reduced in size. There are usually only eight merozoites in the mature parasite, and after segmentation they prefer to attach themselves to mature erythrocytes rather than the younger reticulocytes.

The asexual cycle of *Plasmodium falciparum* is first recognized as an extremely small "signet ring" in the erythrocyte approximately one-half the size of a *P. vivax* ring. Only in the severest cases are the more mature stages of the parasite seen in the erythrocyte. The reason for this seems to be that early in the acute infection there is a tendency for the ring forms to aggregate in the capillaries throughout the body, where they undergo their usual development. The required time for one cycle is not definitely known, but is probably between 24 and 48 hours. The gametocytes are crescent-shaped, a definite diagnostic finding, since no other known malaria parasite has this morphology. The parasite seems to attack young and old erythrocytes indiscriminately.

Plasmodium ovale, first described in 1923 by Stephens and now generally accepted as a definite species, derived its name from the fact that the infected erythrocyte always assumes an oval shape. Otherwise, its morphology and behavior are practically identical with those of *P. vivax.*

Morbid Anatomy. Patients with tertian or quartan malaria rarely come to autopsy except when the malaria is a contributory cause of death. The pathologic lesions in these instances are, in the main, due to the disintegration of parasitized erythrocytes and the accumulation of pigment. In the spleen one finds the maximum evidence of an active or latent malaria infection, and because of the collection of pigment no other disease presents a more pronounced pathognomonic picture, either macroscopically or microscopically. The spleen is usually markedly enlarged, slate gray in color, and of soft consistency during the acute disease. The capsule is smooth and tense, and may even rupture spontaneously. The cut surface exudes a brownish pulp, and the malpighian bodies stand out. Microscopically, the sinuses are distended with parasitized and normal erythrocytes. The macrophages are laden with parasitic debris which is mostly pigment. The liver is usually somewhat enlarged and slightly darker than normal. Microscopic examination reveals that the Kupffer cells are engorged with parasites in various stages of disintegration. There is little or no evidence of toxic degeneration in the parenchymal cells. The heart, lungs, kidneys and pancreas have a normal cellular structure, and the only finding of interest is again the presence of pigment in the active macrophages.

Falciparum malaria is responsible for the majority of deaths due to uncomplicated malaria, and likewise presents some pathologic lesions not present in *vivax* or quartan malaria. Fatal cases are usually associated with an overwhelming infection and cerebral involvement. The brain shows a gross brownish discoloration of the gray matter with macroscopic punctuate hemorrhages in the white matter. Stained sections reveal the capillaries filled with parasites in various stages of development. The cerebral capillary occlusion which is characteristic of *falciparum* malaria may also frequently be generalized and present a pathologic picture of congestion. A pathologist is frequently able to make the correct diagnosis of this disease from a glance at the exposed tissues because of the slate gray tinge due to capillary engorgement with pigmented parasites.

Symptoms. The symptoms of malaria vary according to the type of parasite producing the disease. Each of the four parasites has a characteristic behavior and time of sporulation which give rise to different clinical pictures. Symptoms also vary according to host resistance or immunity. For example, in areas of high malaria endemicity, people may go about their work with no apparent difficulty, despite the presence of a considerable number of circulating parasites in their blood stream. Less intense infections, gauged by the number of circulating parasites, will completely prostrate a nonimmune person coming into the same area. There is evidence to show that strains of the same species of parasite may also have different virulence. However, the initial infections in susceptible persons have certain classic features according to the species involved.

Vivax or Tertian Malaria. This is by far the most common, the mildest and most likely to recur. Because large numbers of persons have received the beneficial effects of *vivax* malaria in the treatment of neurosyphilis, excellent opportunities have been afforded for observing the symptoms of vivax infections in great detail. The most thoroughly studied malaria infections were induced by the bite of infected mosquitoes, and once established, they were allowed to run their full course in order to obtain greatest therapeutic results. In a typical infection, about six days after the bite of the mosquito, the patient has a mild backache, muscle soreness and a low grade fever with-

of intense heat with a hot, dry skin. This portion of the paroxysm lasts about two hours.

SWEATING STAGE. The sweating stage is ushered in with an abrupt onset, and the patient breaks out into a profuse perspiration. Temperature drops to normal, the headache disappears, and a feeling of well-being comes over the patient. Although somewhat drowsy and weak, he feels able to resume work.

Quartan Malaria. This parasite produces an infection (after a prolonged incubation period) which may vary from eighteen to forty days. The onset is similar to that of

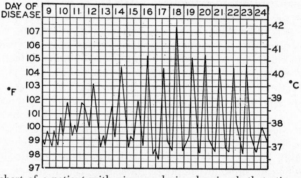

Fig. 50. Temperature chart of a patient with *vivax* malaria, showing both tertian and quotidian types of fever. (Photograph by J. B. Haulenbeek.)

out chills. Febrile paroxysms appear about the fourteenth day. Usually these paroxysms occur on alternate days and coincide with the segmentation of the mature parasite. They may occur daily (quotidian), however, which means that there are two broods of the same parasite, one segmenting on even days and the other on odd days of the disease, or the two types may occur during the course of the one infection as shown in Figure 50. A typical paroxysm for *vivax* malaria consists of a "cold," "hot" and "sweating" stage.

COLD STAGE. The patient has a chilly sensation over the entire body which gradually increases in intensity, the teeth chatter, the skin becomes blue and cold, and there is an uncontrollable shaking. In spite of heat pads and blankets, it is impossible to keep the patient warm. The pulse is rapid and weak, and occasionally there is nausea and vomiting. The cold stage lasts on the average of one hour, and subsides as the body temperature rises.

HOT STAGE. In this stage the patient has a flushed face and severe headache, and may be partially delirious with a temperature often as high as 107° F. There is a sensation

vivax malaria, being initiated by a low grade remittent fever lasting three to five days without chills. The paroxysms usually occur every 72 hours, the time required for the complete development of the asexual cycle in the blood. However, the total period from the beginning of the day of one chill to the end of the day of the next paroxysm is four days (Fig. 51), which accounts for the unfortunate name quartan malaria. A double quartan infection produces a chill on two consecutive days with an intervening day of normal temperature. Rarely does one encounter daily chills with quartan malaria. When compared with *vivax* malaria, the paroxysm lasts longer, is slightly more severe, and the patient feels less like leaving his bed between chills.

Falciparum Malaria. Falciparum or estivo-autumnal malaria is a more severe disease than the others and as such is responsible for the origin of the purely descriptive terms of the disease as cerebral, algid, hemorrhagic, pernicious and many others. The latter refer to symptoms which depend largely upon the localization of the parasites. The incubation period is commonly twelve days; the fever is irregular and not characteristic. The paroxysms are similar to those accompanying other malarias, although of longer duration and occurring at more irregular intervals. The temperature is usually high. If there is a cerebral localization of the parasites, the onset is rapid with delirium or coma, and death frequently ensues without a return to consciousness. The disease may present a gastrointestinal syndrome with abdominal cramps, diarrhea, vomiting and only a few parasites in the peripheral blood. The patient is markedly dehydrated and may have a high or low grade fever. Stools may contain blood result-

mortality being approximately 50 per cent. The only known treatment is absolute rest. The body fluid should be restored as rapidly as possible, preserving normal concentrations of protein and salt. Excessive blood transfusions should be avoided since cardiac failure often results.

Diagnosis. An absolute diagnosis of malaria depends upon the recognition of the parasite in stained thin or thick blood smears. Ordinary thin smears should be made on slides that have been thoroughly cleaned to ensure even spacing of the erythrocytes. They

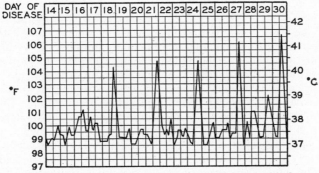

Fig. 51. Temperature chart of a patient with quartan malaria.

ing from intestinal capillary thrombosis and ulceration.

Blackwater Fever. Blackwater fever, sometimes called hemoglobinuria, is the most serious and frequent complication of malaria, but occurs almost entirely in the falciparum variety. The etiology of blackwater fever is not understood. At one time this complication was very prevalent in the United States but it is no longer present there and occurs only in certain of the more heavily endemic areas of Africa and the Orient. Blackwater fever does not appear until the patient has had repeated attacks of malaria. The first sign is a pronounced darkening of the urine produced by the hemoglobin released during extensive intravascular hemolysis. The blood pigments very rapidly increase in amount in the urine until there is a copious amorphous deposit. The pulse becomes very rapid; the fever is high, 105° F. or more, and, curiously enough, parasites are usually absent at this stage. The erythrocyte count drops to two million cells per cubic millimeter or lower within 24 or 48 hours, while vomiting and jaundice are likewise early symptoms. The appearance of blackwater fever is associated with a very poor prognosis, the

can be stained with Giemsa's, Wright's or Hastings' stain. For the uninitiated the thin smear method is preferred because there is less opportunity to be confused by artefacts. It is easy to overlook parasites by this method, however, although they may be present in sufficient numbers to produce clinical activity. The thick smear method is advantageous because it affords a means of concentrating the blood. The thick film should be about the size of a dime on a very clean slide. The two preferred methods of staining are with Giemsa's or Field's. The former is satisfactory and is accomplished by adding one drop of Giemsa to 1 cc. of distilled water and staining for 30 minutes. Field's method has many advantages: long drying of the film is unnecessary, the entire staining takes less than 10 seconds and there are fewer artefacts. (Consult J. W. Field, *Trans. Roy. Soc. Trop. Med.,* 35:35, 1941.) The greatest number of parasites appears in the blood stream immediately after the chill and for the following 6 hours. The inability to find parasites in blood films does not exclude the presence of malaria, particularly in a subsiding or chronic infection. Splenic puncture for diagnostic purposes is unwarranted and dangerous, since it may lead to the rupture of an enlarged tense spleen.

The chief complaint of the patient is usually a severe chill, high fever and sweating. In the history there also is usually information showing that malaria is endemic where the patient resides or that he has traveled in infected areas; for example, campers and hunters frequently acquire malaria in this manner.

There are few physical signs. The patient appears anemic, the degree varying according to the duration and severity of the disease. The spleen, if sufficiently enlarged to be palpated, is soft in the acute disease and firm in chronic cases.

A therapeutic diagnostic test is useful if correctly interpreted. If a potent antimalarial drug fails to reduce a patient's fever, it is strong evidence that the fever is not caused by malaria. Likewise, it is extremely important that the physician ascertain whether the patient has taken some remedy on his own initiative before seeking medical aid. This self-medication is a common practice and accounts for a temporary cessation of symptoms and disappearance of parasites from the blood stream.

In addition to the diagnosis of the individual case the physician is frequently called upon to determine the prevalence of malaria in a community. The established routine procedure is to determine the incidence of parasitemia (by blood smear examination) in as large a group of persons as is feasible. At the same time a determination of the number of enlarged spleens and the degree of splenomegaly furnishes additional information. Personal history about malaria infections in previous years is also included. Such a survey will give data permitting the quantitative expression of the amount of malaria in a community and, if continued, will furnish a guide to yearly endemicity of the disease.

Prognosis. Patients with *vivax* or quartan malaria rarely, if ever, succumb unless the malaria is complicated with other diseases, malnutrition or exposure. Even in endemic areas where many infections are self-treated, deaths are few. Moreover, in paretics in whom malaria has been induced for therapeutic purposes and allowed to run a full course without intervention, the death rate is almost nil. *Vivax* and quartan malaria are diseases of high morbidity and low mortality.

Falciparum malaria is the cause of practically all deaths due to malaria, but, if rec-

ognized early, usually responds to therapy. A guarded prognosis must be held for patients with the cerebral type in coma or stupor. Malaria with hemoglobinuria always presents a grave prognosis.

Relapses are to be expected with all types of malaria. These may occur at any time, but are most likely to occur after exposure, change of climate, hemorrhage, or when body resistance is lowered from any cause.

Immunity. A malaria infection confers a low grade but specific immunity upon its host after the acute attack has subsided. This acquired immunity in man is of short duration, and a person may have repeated attacks produced by the same organism within a relatively short space of time. In experimental animals the residual immunity following complete eradication of the infection persists only a few weeks. Many believe that a host is immune to malaria only in the presence of infection. There is no cross-immunity in human malaria, since it is frequently observed that a person may have a simultaneous infection with two or more types of plasmodia. It is highly probable that a person is resistant only to the malaria in his particular locality; for example, it has been shown that a person immune to a strain of *vivax* malaria in Florida behaves as a normal when exposed to infection from a *vivax* parasite from Cuba.

The mechanism of immunity in malaria is not clearly understood, but it is possible to demonstrate specific protective and complement-fixing antibodies and agglutinins in the serum of experimental animals after recovery from the acute attack. The chief defense of the body against an acute malaria infection or recovery from a relapse probably depends upon a greatly accelerated rate of phagocytosis by the individual macrophages of the reticuloendothelial system.

Treatment. The accepted treatment for malaria is the administration of certain chemotherapeutic drugs. Specific antiserum prepared from animals or serum from convalescent patients has not proved beneficial in the prevention or treatment of the disease.

It now seems possible for the first time to state that satisfactory suppressive and curative compounds for *vivax* and *falciparum* malaria are available. There have been insufficient tests of these recently introduced compounds in quartan malaria. Moreover, preliminary studies indicate that certain of the new compounds are probably true prophylactic agents. This would be in contrast to the previously available "prophylactic" drugs which did not actually prevent infection but suppressed evidence of disease so long as "prophylaxis" was continued. These goals, visualized and sought by malariologists for centuries, now seem at hand.

It is now possible to make these statements because of the results of a research program initiated at the beginning of World War II and continued until the present. Nevertheless, it would be incorrect to assume that no problems continue to exist, for evaluation must continue for years; no disease as formidable as malaria is easily conquered.

Suppression. For the suppression of malaria, two compounds, *chloroquine* (Aralen) and *amodiaquine* (Camoquin), have had wide laboratory, experimental and field trials and thus far have proved to be eminently satisfactory. The use of chloroquine was compulsory among the troops in the endemic areas of Korea. Malaria, although acquired, remained at subclinical levels and no problem was recognized until infections appeared in this country among those exposed and who had discontinued the drug. The suppression of malaria is indicated in personal traveling or living in endemic areas of malaria such as soldiers, laborers, and others. Thus far neither chloroquine nor amodiaquine has been used on a large scale in native populations. Both of these drugs require only one dose weekly, are readily absorbed, and have not been observed to produce any untoward or disagreeable side effects.

The dosage of chloroquine diphosphate (Aralen) is 0.25 gm. (two tablets) weekly taken the same day each week. For heavily endemic areas the dose can be increased by one to two tablets for adults. Amodiaquine (Camoquin), 4-[7-chloro-4-quinolylamino] -a-diethylamino-o-cresol, is also equally effective at two or three tablets (0.4 to 0.6 gm.) once weekly.

Mention should also be made of two other drugs. The first, *chlorguanide* (proguanil, Paludrine), is an inexpensive compound to make and effective as a suppressant. Unfortunately, when used in minimal doses in many areas for the suppression of malaria it has resulted in a high degree of drug resistance by the indigenous strains of parasites. The second drug is *pyrimethamine* (Daraprim). Promising but meager trials as compared with those made with other drugs

do not permit the recommendation of pyrimethamine at this time.

Because of availability and long usage, *quinine* and *quinacrine* (Atabrine) will be used for many years to come. If quinine is to be used for suppression, 0.3 gm. daily is usually sufficient. The dosage of quinacrine, a synthetic drug used since 1930, is 0.1 gm. once daily for six days, with one day without therapy each week. Although very useful, neither of these two drugs is recommended if the newer compounds are available.

Therapy for the Acute Attack. Either chloroquine or amodiaquine is recommended for an acute attack of malaria, either for the first illness or a relapse. The therapeutic action of these drugs is exceedingly prompt without toxic reactions. Neither of these compounds will result in an eradication of infection for *vivax* malaria, but will do so for *falciparum*.

The usual chloroquine regimen consists of an initial dose of 1.0 gm. (four tablets) followed by 0.5 gm. (two tablets) after 6 hours. On the second and third day, 0.25 gm. (two tablets) is given.

The treatment of the acute attack of malaria with quinine or quinacrine will continue to be the practice of many physicians since both drugs are effective, although somewhat less so than the newer compounds. The dosage of quinine sulfate is 1.0 gm. every 6 hours in capsule form, for three doses, followed by 0.6 gm. two to three times daily for seven to ten days. If the patient is unable to tolerate medication by mouth, quinine dihydrochloride should be given intravenously in 10 cc. of sterile water every 6 hours until the oral route of administration can be used. The dosage of quinacrine is 0.3 gm. every 6 hours for five doses, then 0.1 gm. three times daily for six days.

Radical Cure. Vivax malaria has a constant tendency to relapse in spite of maximum tolerated amounts of antimalarial drugs or their administration over an extended period. The only drugs thus far shown to be effective in the complete eradication of a chronic *vivax* malaria are the 8-aminoquinoline compounds. Pamoquine (Plasmochin) was the first to be recommended but has now been discarded in favor of *primaquine,* a more effective and less toxic derivative. Primaquine has been tested in many thousand whites and nonwhites and found to be a safe compound when given in the recommended dosage. When tested for its curative value in several hundred experimental and naturally acquired infections, it was demonstrated to be of considerable value. Primaquine, in doses of 15 mg. (base) daily for fourteen days, has reduced the relapse rates in Korean *vivax* malaria to less than 1 per cent by destroying the tissue stages of the parasite. Since primaquine is relatively ineffective against the asexual blood stages, it should be used in combination with chloroquine. The recommended double therapy regimen for radical cure consists of 0.3 gm. (base) of chloroquine during the first 24 hours followed by 0.3 gm. daily on each of the two succeeding days, accompanied by primaquine started simultaneously at 15 mg. doses daily and continued for a total period of fourteen days. Although as mentioned above the toxic properties are not severe, the possibility of hemolytic reactions should be borne in mind. Frequent blood and urine examinations should be made.

The general treatment consists of simple measures aimed at keeping the patient comfortable, especially during the acute paroxysms. In infections complicated by vomiting or diarrhea special effort should be made to maintain the normal fluid level. It is advisable that convalescent patients receive iron in any of the available forms, since it is extremely beneficial in the restoration of hemoglobin deficiency. Many favorable reports have followed the use of liver therapy. There are occasional reports advising splenectomy in chronic cases with gross enlargement of the spleen, but this practice is to avoided at all costs because it removes the body's chief organ of defense.

L. T. COGGESHALL

References

American Association for the Advancement of Science: Human Malaria. Lancaster, Pa., The Science Press, 1941.

Ash, J. E., and Spitz, Sophie: Pathology of Tropical Diseases; An Atlas. Philadelphia, W. B. Saunders Company, 1945.

Bispham, W. N.: Malaria—Diagnosis, Treatment and Prophylaxis. Baltimore, Williams and Wilkins Co., 1944.

Coggeshall, L. T.: Malaria and Filariasis in the Returning Serviceman. Am. J. Trop. Med., 25:177, 1945.

Mackie, T. T., Hunter, G. W., and Worth, C. B.: Manual of Tropical Medicine. 2nd ed. Philadelphia, W. B. Saunders Company, 1954.

Russell, P. F., West, L. S., and Manwell, R.: Practical Malariology. Philadelphia, W. B. Saunders Company, 1946.

Strong, R. P.: Stitt's Diagnosis, Prevention and Treatment of Tropical Diseases. 7th ed. Philadelphia, The Blakiston Company, 1944.

TRYPANOSOMIASIS

AFRICAN TRYPANOSOMIASIS
(Sleeping Sickness)

Two varieties of trypanosomiasis occur in tropical Africa. The Gambian type is irregularly distributed over an enormous area. It is found on the west coast from Senegal southward to Angola, and extends eastward from Bahr el Ghazal, Lake Albert and Lake Victoria on the north to Lake Banguelo in the south. The Rhodesian type is limited to a much smaller area, occurring only in parts of Nyasaland, Rhodesia, Tanganyika Territory and Portuguese East Africa.

Gambian Sleeping Sickness. The causative agent, *Trypanosoma gambiense,* is a typical polymorphic mammalian trypanosome which varies in length from 10 to 39 microns. It reproduces by longitudinal fission and, as far as is known, retains its trypaniform structure in man. Transmission from man to man is effected chiefly by the tsetse fly, *Glossina palpalis.* A related species, *G. tachinoides,* is important in certain areas of the Gold Coast and Nigeria. The parasites undergo a developmental cycle in the fly which lasts twenty days or more. Eventually they invade the salivary glands, where, once established, they constitute a constant source of infection when the fly bites uninfected persons. Occasionally transmission may take place mechanically by means of *Glossina* or other biting insects, or by coitus.

In man, the trypanosomes are found in the blood, lymph and cerebrospinal fluid and may invade the parenchyma of various organs. Pathologic lesions are found chiefly in the lymph nodes of the neck, submaxillary region and mesentery and in the central nervous system.

Clinical Course. The incubation period may be as short as fourteen days. It is usually followed by two ill defined and overlapping clinical stages: (1) the *trypanosome fever stage* and (2) the *sleeping sickness stage,* or stage of central nervous system involvement. "The first is characterized principally by irregular attacks of fever, chronic polyadenitis, exanthemata, frequency of the pulse and respiration, and asthenia; the second, by exaggeration of the symptoms of the first stage, marked emaciation, and by the appearance of nervous symptoms, tremors, incoordination of movements, paralyses, mental disturbances, apathy, somnolence, coma and death" (Blacklock and Yorke).

Rhodesian sleeping sickness is caused by *Trypanosoma rhodesiense*. In man its morphology is identical with that of *T. gambiense*. The disease is similar to the Gambian type except that it may run such a rapid course that patients may succumb before the typical sleeping sickness stage develops, and it is more difficult to treat. *Trypanosoma rhodesiense* is transmitted chiefly by *G. morsitans* and may be a human-adapted strain of *T. brucei* of animals. Development in the fly may be completed within fourteen days after ingestion of infected material.

Diagnosis. Although certain clinical symptoms arouse suspicion, trypanosomiasis can be diagnosed only by demonstrating parasites in the blood, enlarged lymph nodes or spinal fluid.

Microscopic examination of the blood is difficult, especially in the Gambian type, because of the usual scarcity of parasites in the peripheral blood. Stained thin films are of little value, but some workers use stained thick films. Fresh preparations are preferable because trypanosomes agitate the blood cells in a characteristic fashion. If parasites cannot be found in a small drop of blood, they may be concentrated in 10 to 20 cc. of blood. The blood is first citrated and then centrifuged at a low speed (1000 to 1500 r.p.m.) for 10 minutes to throw down the erythrocytes. The supernatant and leukocytic cream are then recentrifuged at a higher speed (2000 r.p.m.) for 15 minutes and the sediment examined for parasites. When autoagglutination of erythrocytes is observed, further search is advisable.

Lymph Node Puncture. Tissue fluid from lymph nodes that are soft and enlarged (particularly those of the posterior triangle of the neck) almost invariably contains trypanosomes. A small quantity of this may be sucked out with a sterile, dry hypodermic needle for diagnostic purposes. Sclerosed nodes in chronic or treated cases do not contain parasites.

Lumbar puncture is of value in the second stage of nervous involvement because the sediment from centrifuged spinal fluid often contains trypanosomes. Since the cells and protein content of the spinal fluid increase with cerebrospinal involvement, they may furnish a rough index of the extent of cerebrospinal invasion.

Inoculation into Susceptible Animals. Laboratory animals, such as rats, mice, guinea pigs, rabbits and monkeys (*Macacus* and *Cercopithecus*), may be inoculated subcutaneously or intraperitoneally with suspected blood, lymph node juice or spinal fluid, and their blood examined for trypanosomes.

Treatment of the diseases has greatly advanced since 1920, when tryparsamide and Bayer 205 were introduced. Of the drugs now in clinical use, especial mention should be made of the following: (1) the arsenicals, tryparsamide and the Melarsen group; (2) suramin sodium which is also known as Naphuride, Antrypol, Germanin or Bayer 205; and (3) the aromatic diamidines, pentamidine and propamidine.

The efficacy of *tryparsamide* in the treatment of trypanosomiasis probably lies to a large extent in the ease with which it penetrates the central nervous system. In first stage cases, according to Chesterman, six to eight weekly injections should be given. The dose per kilogram of body weight in children should be 0.07 gm.; for young adults, 0.055 gm.; and for adults, 0.045 gm. Second courses are not advised. In second stage conditions the doses per kilogram of body weight should be increased to 0.09 gm. for children, 0.07 gm. for young adults and 0.06 gm. for adults. In advanced second stage cases two or three large doses should be given at five-day intervals, followed by a rest of ten to fourteen days. The maximum dose for adults should be 4 gm. The drug may be given intravenously or intramuscularly. The severe toxic reaction is optic atrophy.

Great promise is shown by the melarsen group: Melarsen, Melarsen oxide and Mel B. There is still question as to which is the best drug for general use. A typical treatment consists of two series of four daily intravenous doses of 0.0036 gm. Mel B per kilogram of body weight, separated by a week. The drug is especially indicated in tryparsamide-resistant cases. Close supervision of patients with cerebrospinal involvement is necessary because the toxicity of Mel B appears to increase with the severity of the disease.

Suramin or *Bayer 205* is of great value in the early stages of the disease. Its ineffectiveness later may be due to the fact that it does not readily penetrate into the central nervous system. The relatively few toxic reactions include transient edema, skin rashes, pruritus, purulent conjunctivitis, stomatitis, skin rashes and mild peripheral neuritis. The drug should be given cautiously to patients with impaired kidney function. Suramin may be given intravenously or intramuscularly. Various investigators have reported cures after administering a total of about 10 gm. of the drug. The exact course of treatment varies with different authorities. The usual single intravenous dose for an adult is 1 gm. dissolved in 10 cc. of water given weekly for a course of five treatments.

Excellent results in the lymphohematogenous stage and after moderate cerebrospinal fluid change are reported after seven daily intramuscular injections of 0.3 gm. pentamidine di-isethionate. Some workers have increased the amount to 0.005 gm. per kilogram body weight daily for ten days without evidences of serious toxicity. Many patients, especially after the first few injections, show transient symptoms, such as flushing of the face, indefinite epigastric sensations, headache, rapid pulse, sweating, retching and occasional vomiting. The drug is contraindicated in renal disease.

A combination of two drugs may reduce the development of drug-resistant strains and may be more efficient chemotherapeutically. Pentamidine may be combined with suramin or tryparsamide. The older combination of suramin and tryparsamide is considered too toxic.

SOUTH AMERICAN TRYPANOSOMIASIS
(*Chagas' Disease*)

South American trypanosomiasis, or Chagas' disease, has been found from Chile and Argentina to Mexico. It is confined to rural areas where infection rates may be as high as 10 to 20 per cent. Many mammals, including dogs, cats and rodents, act as reservoirs of infection. The parasite occurs in reduviid bugs and rodents in Arizona, California, New Mexico and, in addition, in armadillos and opossums in Texas.

Etiology. The causative agent, *Trypanosoma cruzi,* occurs in the blood as a trypanosome and in the tissues as a leishmania stage. Each stage can change into the other. Reproduction occurs only in the tissue stages. The infection is transmitted from man to man or from animal to man chiefly by *Panstrongylus megista, Triatoma infestans* and *Rhodnius prolixus.* The bug receives its infection by ingesting infected blood, and its feces are later infective to man. It lives in cracks in the walls of houses and feeds at night.

Clinical Course. The disease can generally be divided into two stages—acute and chronic. The *acute stage* generally lasts twenty to thirty days and is usually characterized by edematous swelling of one eyelid, inflammation of the lacrimal gland and swelling of the preauricular node (Romaña's sign). These may be the only symptoms associated with mild fever in adults, but in children there may also be generalized edema, high fever, cardiac and nervous symptoms. During the acute stage, trypanosomes are present in the blood and leishmaniform bodies in the tissues. If the patient survives this stage, the disease becomes chronic and may persist for many years. During the *chronic stage,* which can occur as the initial form in adults, trypanosomes are extremely rare in the blood, but leishmaniform bodies occur in the tissues. Heart involvement is the chief manifestation of the chronic stage. Its intensity and symptomatology are variable, and arrhythmias and heart block are frequent. Sudden death is common with or without heart symptoms. Mild or asymptomatic infections often occur in nontropical countries.

Diagnosis. Diagnosis can be definitely made only by finding parasites. Trypanosomes may be found in the blood during the acute stage, but they are seldom numerous. Their presence can be demonstrated by microscopic examination or injection into susceptible laboratory animals such as the guinea pig. They are occasionally found in small numbers during the chronic stage, but whether this is due to the chronic infection or to reinfection is not known. In endemic regions they are sometimes accidentally discovered in thick blood films prepared for malarial surveys. *Xenodiagnosis* often discloses an infection when other methods fail. By this method, laboratory-raised uninfected reduviid bugs are fed on suspected patients and their hind gut content examined for parasites about two weeks later. Lumbar puncture sometimes yields parasites during cerebrospinal involvement. Biopsy examination of excised tissue from the preauricular lymph node and the conjunctiva on the affected side have occasionally revealed leishmania stages. Complement fixation using Davis' antigen made from cultures preserved with merthiolate is the serologic method of choice.

Treatment. The usual trypanocides are not effective. The most effective drug is the quinaldine derivative, Bayer 7602 Ac, but relapses invariably occur. In experimental animals, pentaquine, isopentaquine and especially primaquine are markedly suppressive. A number of patients apparently recover spontaneously.

Prophylaxis consists in constructing houses so as to avoid cracks in the walls, etc., and in using insecticides, such as Gammexane.

W. H. TALIAFERRO

References

Belding, D. L.: Textbook of Clinical Parasitology. 2nd ed. Appleton-Century-Crofts, Inc., 1952.
Mackie, T. T., Hunter, G. W., and Worth, C. B.: Manual of Tropical Medicine. 2nd ed. Philadelphia, W. B. Saunders Company, 1954.
Manson-Bahr, P, H.: Manson's Tropical Diseases. 13th ed. Baltimore, Williams and Wilkins Co., 1950.
Mazza, S.: Chagas' Disease. In Gradwohl, R. B. H., Benétez Soto, L., and Felsenfeld, O.: Clinical Tropical Medicine. St. Louis, C. V. Mosby Co., 1951, pp. 127–155.
Strong, R. P.: Stitt's Diagnosis, Prevention and Treatment of Tropical Diseases. 7th ed. Philadelphia, Blakiston Co., 1944.
Tropical Diseases Bulletin. Bureau of Hygiene and Tropical Diseases, London. (Abstracts of current literature.)

LEISHMANIASIS

The diseases described under this title are all caused by infection with parasites of the protozoon genus *Leishmania.* A number of specific names have been given to parasites recovered from patients with differing clinical conditions in various parts of the world and, in addition, from dogs. Such species, however, have not so far been satisfactorily distinguished. At present three species are generally recognized, corresponding to the three diseases described below: namely, kala-azar, oriental sore or cutaneous leishmaniasis as seen in Mediterranean and Asiatic areas, and American or mucocutaneous leishmaniasis as seen in South and Central America. It should be noted that in certain circumstances cutaneous and mucocutaneous lesions occur in kala-azar. The separation of these diseases and of the parasites associated with them rests on epidemiologic, clinical and immunologic grounds. Kirk has suggested that the clinical conditions encountered may represent stages in the course of infection with the same parasite, the appearance of which is greatly influenced by differences in parasite strains, by the previous life history of the infecting strain in a particular insect vector (and in a particular animal reservoir), and by the dietary habits and nutritional state of the patient. The following account, however, conforms to the views generally accepted.

KALA-AZAR
(Visceral Leishmaniasis)

Definition. Kala-azar is a chronic infection caused by *Leishmania donovani* with its principal seat in the reticuloendothelial system. It may affect all the parts of the body and should be regarded as a general disease. The outstanding characteristics are fever, enlargement of spleen and liver, leukopenia, anemia and hyperglobulinemia.

Etiologic Agent. The discovery of the causative agent was reported in 1903 by Leishman and Donovan independently. *Leishmania donovani* is a parasitic protozoon which is found in two forms during its life cycle. In man and other susceptible vertebrates the parasites have roughly oval shapes, are about 3 microns long, and have no flagella ("Leishman-Donovan bodies"). With Wright or Giemsa stains, L-D bodies have pale blue cytoplasm and bright red nuclei, the presence of a kinetoplast which appears as a purplish dot is important. In appropriate insects and in cultures the organisms have spindle-like shapes, are 14 to 20 microns long, and have prominent flagella (leptomonad forms). Neither form has been found outside animal hosts. Both forms succumb rapidly in water or soil. A number of animals are susceptible to artificial infection with either of these forms, certain hamsters being the most useful. Cultures are readily made, starting with either form of the parasite.

Epidemiology. Kala-azar is widespread, but the areas in which its existence is well known are discontinuous, and the importance of the disease varies greatly in localities relatively near one another. The incidence is especially high in parts of China north of the Yangtse River and of eastern India, particularly in Bihar, Bengal and Assam. The disease is endemic in the region about Tashkent in southern Asiatic Russia, and occurs in Mesopotamia, Arabia and Turkey. It is present in areas scattered all around the Mediterranean Sea and in a belt across Africa from Eritrea and Kenya through Abyssinia and French Equatorial Africa to Nigeria. Cases have been reported from Argentina, Paraguay, Bolivia, Brazil,

Venezuela and Colombia, but so far the disease does not seem to be very important in South America. Autochthonous cases have not been found in the United States, but many imported cases have been reported, especially in soldiers previously stationed in endemic areas. Kala-azar is predominantly a disease of childhood and youth, but cases occur at all ages. There is no evidence of any variation in susceptibility between the sexes or among races. Multiple cases have a tendency to occur in small foci and even in particular houses. Occasionally the disease appears in epidemic form.

Sandflies of the genus *Phlebotomus* have been shown to be important vectors of kala-azar in India and China. Since various species of *Phlebotomus* exist wherever the disease occurs, these insects may be vectors in other areas. In China and elsewhere a natural reservoir host for *Leishmania* has been found in dogs, in addition to that in infected human beings. In endemic areas in India, however, dogs apparently rarely if ever harbor the infection. It is generally assumed that in India kala-azar is transmitted by sandflies directly from patient to patient. This may be one of the methods of infection in all endemic areas. Although parasites are present in the stools, urine and nasopharyngeal secretions of patients, there is no evidence that infection arises from these sources. The disease has been inadvertently transmitted by blood transfusion.

Morbid Anatomy. The principal reaction of the tissues is marked proliferation of the cells of the reticuloendothelial system. Leishman-Donovan bodies may be found in all parts of the body, but they are overwhelmingly localized in the cells of this system. Intracellular parasites grow and multiply, while the host cells gradually swell and finally disintegrate. The reticuloendothelial proliferation is often so great that other cells are encroached upon or crowded out. The process is most severe in the spleen, liver and bone marrow. In the spleen and liver, marked congestion develops, with enlargement which may be enormous. Capsular thickening causes these organs to become firm. Groups of lymph nodes are often enlarged. Subcutaneous nodules composed chiefly of macrophages may appear.

Pathologic Physiology and Chemistry. The most important abnormalities are found in the blood. About 90 per cent of patients have leukopenia which is largely due to reduction in the number of granulocytes. Leukopenia usually develops early. After the disease is established, counts of 3000 or less per cubic millimeter are common. In rare instances agranulocytosis is seen. A normal leukocyte count or a moderate elevation is sometimes associated with another infection. The differential formula shows a shift to the left. There is usually a relative lymphocytosis; sometimes an absolute increase is seen. The same changes occur in the mononuclears. Occasionally (but usually with difficulty), parasitized macrophages or mononuclears are seen in blood smears. Anemia is also characteristic. It develops more slowly than leukopenia and may be absent or trivial in early cases. As a rule after the first month, hemoglobin values are 40 to 60 per cent of normal and erythrocyte counts are from 2 to 4 million per cubic millimeter. The icterus index is normal. Thrombocytopenia is regularly present; bleeding times and clotting times are in the upper range of normal or somewhat elevated, and clot retraction may be defective, but these changes are seldom extreme. Serum proteins show an increase in globulin (chiefly in the gamma component), which may be so marked that total globulin amounts to 8 or 9 gm. per 100 cc. Serum albumin is usually decreased, especially in longstanding cases. A cold-precipitable protein has been found in some serums. Bromsulfalein tests give normal results, while cephalin flocculation and thymol turbidity tests are strongly positive. The latter must be interpreted in the light of the marked hyperglobulinemia. The urine shows nothing remarkable.

Patients with kala-azar have a decided lack of resistance to other infections. It is usually considered that those who have recovered are immune to further infection with kala-azar, but not to other forms of leishmaniasis.

Symptoms. In the proper sense of the term, the incubation period is not definitely known. Symptoms have appeared from three weeks to nearly three years after exposure, but the long silent periods should be attributed in part to latent disease. The onset is often sudden, with fever and chills, but it may be insidious, with no striking symptoms. The diagnosis is occasionally made by accident in asymptomatic patients. Symptoms may be apparently precipitated by unusual exertion or stress. The temperature chart usually shows remittent or intermittent fever. There may be wide daily swings, but sustained elevation occurs in some cases. Double or triple temperature peaks in 24 hours are not infrequently seen. Chills, sweats, dizziness and headache are common. Other symptoms include malaise, vague pains in muscles, bones or joints, conjunctivitis, coryza, cough, bleeding from the nose or gums, abdominal distention or the presence of an abdominal mass, occasionally nausea and vomiting. Mental changes are rare, except that young children may show clouding or, rarely, convulsions. In many cases symptoms are strikingly vague or few. On examination patients often appear remarkably well in spite of fever. Pallor accompanies anemia. Purpura is occasionally present. Petechiae are unusual findings. Rose spots do not occur. Jaundice is rare. In late cases the skin may become dark, the hair may fall, and there is often much loss of weight. Some patients show painless enlargement of groups of lymph nodes. Subcutaneous nodules are found in a few cases. The pulse rate is increased with fever. Rales may be heard in the lungs. In the great majority of cases the outstanding physical signs are splenomegaly and hepatomegaly. Both organs may enlarge rapidly, but the diagnosis has been made when enlargement was not detectable. These organs are not usually tender, but occasionally a new infarct produces splenic tenderness. Ascites and edema are rare.

In the Sudan some patients with general manifestations of kala-azar have cutaneous and mucocutaneous lesions containing L-D bodies. In this area and in central Asia, a primary cutaneous lesion has been described in some cases.

Course and Complications. In the absence of treatment the course is usually prolonged, often as much as two or three years. Remissions and relapses are common. Fulminating cases are occasionally seen. The commonest complications are bronchitis and pneumonia. The rare development of agranulocytosis has already been noted. Stomatitis and noma may appear in children with advanced disease. Nephritis is an occasional complication. An interesting sequel to kala-azar, postkala-azar dermal leishmaniasis, has been seen especially in India. This condition develops a year or more after recovery from the generalized disease. The lesions, which take various forms and are considered to be distinct from those of oriental sore, contain *Leishmania,* but are not accompanied by any evidence of visceral infection. The commonest types are hypopigmented macules, a butterfly erythema on the face and, relatively later, nodules which resemble those of leprosy. The nodules may persist for years.

Diagnosis. A sojourn or residence in an endemic area, fever, splenomegaly, granulocytopenia and hyperglobulinemia should suggest the possibility of kala-azar. Double daily temperature peaks should bring the disease

to mind, but they are not pathognomonic. The formol-gel test and the antimony test, which depend upon the presence of hyperglobulinemia and hypoalbuminemia, are helpful in the Far East. These tests, however, may be negative in the first few weeks of the disease and are positive in certain other dis-

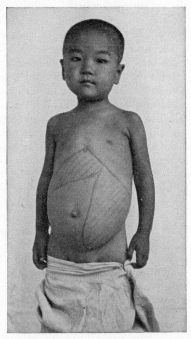

Fig. 52. Kala-azar in a Chinese child. Note protuberant abdomen with enlargement of liver and spleen. (Photograph by E. B. Struthers.)

eases, though rarely to the degree commonly seen in kala-azar. Actual measurement of serum globulin and albumin supplies data useful both in diagnosis and in following the course of treatment.

The *formol-gel test* is done by adding 1 or 2 drops of formalin to 1 cc. of clear serum. Complete opacity within 24 hours constitutes a positive result. Partial opacity is a doubtful result, and a persistently clear serum is negative, even though it gels.

The *antimony test* consists in diluting serum ten times with distilled water and adding to 2 cc. of diluted serum the same amount of 4 per cent solution of ethylstibamine (Neostibosan) in distilled water. The materials are mixed by rotating the test tube between the palms. A positive result is indicated by a heavy flocculent precipitate, a doubtful one by mere clouding, and a negative one by complete absence of precipitation.

The diagnosis should always be confirmed

by demonstration of the parasite. Although L-D bodies are probably always present in the blood of active cases, they are usually so difficult to find that reliance should not be placed on blood smears. A small amount of tissue for examination should be obtained from one of the sites in which parasites are normally plentiful, which include spleen, liver, sternal bone marrow, lymph nodes and skin lesions. The simpler procedures for obtaining the necessary material are aspiration of sternal bone marrow or enlarged lymph nodes and excision of lymph nodes or nodules. The spleen has been shown, however, to be the most reliable source of diagnostic material. Spleen puncture is commonly regarded as presenting serious danger, although it has been done in thousands of cases in the Far East with only rare accidents. The procedure is not free from risk, but experience amply justifies its use with proper precautions when bone marrow or lymph node material is negative in a case in which kala-azar is a reasonable possibility. It is important that the spleen extend well below the costal margin and that the bleeding and clotting times be within normal limits. The technique is described in detail by Most.

The tissue obtained should be prepared with a Giemsa or Wright stain. The parasites probably live mostly within other cells, but since macrophages are often ruptured in making smears, extracellular Leishman-Donovan bodies are common in such preparations. They should not be confused with platelets. Several preparations should be persistently searched for parasites conforming to the description given previously.

When prolonged study of smears is fruitless, one can rely on cultures or, if a suitable species is available, on animal inoculation. Both methods are highly successful. The material used is generally the same as that for smears; the leukocyte layer of 10 cc. of centrifuged citrated blood may also be tried. Cultures are made on rabbits' blood-agar medium (Nicolle, Novy, McNeal, N.N.N.), and are incubated at 22° C. Special care must be taken throughout to maintain aseptic technique. In one to four weeks actively motile leptomonad forms may be found on high power search of a sample mixed with a little saline solution on a slide. The organisms are sometimes best found in the water of condensation. Details should be studied in stained smears. The usual laboratory animals are refractory to infection with *Leishmania,*

but several species of hamster are highly susceptible. Intratesticular inoculation of rabbits has been successfully used for diagnostic purposes. Complement fixation, agglutination and skin sensitivity tests have been used, but their practical value is uncertain and the necessary materials are not generally available.

Differential Diagnosis. In differential diagnosis, various forms of leukemia have been the most frequent cause of confusion in the United States. Hodgkin's disease and infectious mononucleosis have also been diagnosed here instead of kala-azar. Histoplasmosis, which closely resembles kala-azar, in some instances can be separated only by close attention to the comparative characteristics of the parasites. Many other diseases may superficially resemble kala-azar, including especially malaria; also brucellosis, typhoid fever, bacterial endocarditis, disseminated lupus, tuberculosis, Weil's disease, relapsing fever and schistosomiasis. In all these instances the separation must be made by close study of the history and clinical picture and by use of applicable laboratory tests.

Prognosis. In the absence of treatment about 75 per cent of patients die, often with an intercurrent infection and usually within two or three years. Spontaneous recovery has been observed in rare proved cases. Good treatment ultimately cures about 98 per cent of patients (including relapsing patients who are retreated), with the exception that this high cure rate has not been attained in the Sudan, where fulminating and drug-resistant cases are apparently numerous.

Treatment. When fever, severe anemia or leukopenia, or serious complications are present, patients should be kept in bed. Special care should be given to the mouth. Blood transfusions are indicated for severe anemia, leukopenia or bleeding tendency. An antimicrobial drug may be given for an intercurrent infection at the same time as treatment for kala-azar. Patients with noma should receive penicillin. Chemotherapy should be started as soon as the diagnosis of kala-azar is established, unless agranulocytosis is present. Therapeutic tests and "tinkering" treatment are especially unwise. If it is considered necessary to begin treatment without demonstration of the parasite, a full course of the drug in adequate dosage should be given.

Effective therapy of kala-azar began with the use of antimony and potassium tartrate, but this drug was superseded long ago by pentavalent antimony compounds. More recently a new type of drug has been introduced.

The use of ethylstibamine (Neostibosan) has been highly successful, except in the Sudan. This drug is recommended for first courses in general. It should be given slowly by vein as a 5 per cent solution in sterile distilled water. The solution is relatively unstable and must be freshly prepared for each injection. It should be used as soon as possible, without boiling or heating. The first dose for adults is 0.2 gm., and subsequent doses are 0.3 gm. Unless untoward effects appear, doses should be given daily until a total of 3 to 5 gm. has been administered. Nausea and vomiting are the commonest side effects. Dizziness, cough, abdominal and muscular pain, diarrhea, renal disturbances, urticaria and increased bleeding are unusual toxic effects. Increased fever is usually the result of the presence of pyrogens in the distilled water. Anaphylactic shock has been reported in rare instances. If agranulocytosis develops, as it may rarely, treatment should be interrupted until this condition has improved, but should be resumed as soon as possible. Otherwise it should rarely be necessary to interrupt chemotherapy completely, though it is not infrequently wise to restrict drug administration to alternate days or to reduce the dosage when untoward effects appear. Pentavalent antimony compounds which may be used instead of ethylstibamine include sodium antimony gluconate (Pentostam, formerly designated Solustibosan) and stibamine glucoside (Neostam). These drugs are said to be both less toxic and less effective than ethylstibamine, but they possess the advantage that they can be given intramuscularly.

Patients under treatment should be followed closely, with special attention to the leukocyte count. The response to therapy is sometimes dramatic, sometimes slow. Fever is usually absent after the first two weeks, but may persist briefly after completion of treatment. The leukocyte count is generally normal in three or four weeks. Improvement in the erythrocyte count is heralded by a marked increase in reticulocytes. It may take many weeks for erythrocytes and hemoglobin to become wholly normal. Serum proteins take three to six months to reach normal values. The spleen and liver often recede rapidly, but in longstanding cases the spleen may remain large for months. Cure may follow a single course of therapy, even though progress is slow. The treatment outlined rarely fails entirely, but 5 to 10 per cent of patients relapse. Most relapses occur within two months, but the interval is sometimes four or five months. Patients should be followed for six months before being declared cured. Relapses are usually marked by the return of fever, followed by the characteristic picture. The continued presence for a few weeks of *Leishmania* alone does not necessarily indicate that a relapse will occur, but clinical suggestions of a relapse should be confirmed by demonstration of the parasite. When the occurrence of a relapse is established, another course of treatment should be given. This may again consist of ethylstibamine, in which case larger doses are desirable (up to 0.5 gm. a day for twenty days). Such second courses have cured many patients. Or recourse may be had to one of the newer drugs.

Certain aromatic diamidines have given better results than pentavalent antimonials in the treatment of kala-azar in the Sudan and in some resistant cases elsewhere, although they have not been found more satisfactory in general. These drugs have potentially great toxicity which calls for special care in their use. In most areas they are best held in reserve for cases resistant to pentavalent antimonials. The most extensively tested of these drugs are stilbamidine isethionate and pentamidine isethionate. The former is both the more efficacious and the more toxic. It is essential that these drugs be used in freshly prepared solutions. The action of light on solutions produces dangerous hepatotoxic compounds. A number of immediate reactions to intravenous injection, including circulatory collapse, may occur, especially with stilbamidine and particularly with rapid injection. After a course of stilbamidine (sometimes months later), a peculiar neuropathy, usually having a trigeminal distribution, appears in some cases. Stilbamidine must be given intravenously, the daily dose being dissolved in 200 cc. of sterile fluid. For adults, the first dose is 25 mg. In the absence of untoward effects, the dose is increased each day by 10 to 20 mg. until the dose of 150 mg. is reached. The total amount in a course varies, usually falling between 2 and 4 gm. Pentamidine can be given intravenously in doses of 2 to 4 mg. per kilogram of body weight dissolved in

200 cc. of sterile fluid; or it can be given intramuscularly in similar doses dissolved in 5 cc. of sterile fluid. The total dose for a course is from 2 to 4 gm.

In rare cases several courses of treatment with proper doses of antimonial and diamidine drugs are unsuccessful. In a few such instances in which the spleen remained large and firm, splenectomy has been quickly followed by apparent cure. This operation should be considered in such cases, but it should not be done unless the patient has had more than one course of chemotherapy and it should also be followed by a full course of chemotherapy.

Postkala-azar dermal leishmaniasis is relatively refractory, but the best available treatment is a full course of ethylstibamine as outlined for the visceral stage.

Prevention. The source of the infection should be attacked by treatment of patients and, in areas where dogs are infected, by suitable steps against such animals. The sandfly vector should be attacked by removing the conditions in which they abound. Cracks and dark corners in walls and floors, rubbish and vegetation in and around houses should be eliminated. DDT residual spray is effective. Ordinary screens and sleeping nets do not exclude sandflies, but, sprayed thoroughly with DDT or impregnated with repellent, they do constitute a barrier. Sandflies bite mostly after sunset. Clothing is protective, except near openings. A repellent, such as dimethylphthalate, applied to exposed skin keeps sandflies off for four to five hours.

ORIENTAL CUTANEOUS LEISHMANIASIS
(Oriental Sore)

Definition and Incidence. This name is given to an infection with *Leishmania tropica* which is characterized by cutaneous granulomas with a strong tendency to ulceration. The disease is limited to the skin, there being no evidence of involvement of other parts of the body. It was formerly known by many local names, such as Aleppo boil. Its distribution is focal, but widespread, with centers in western India, southwestern Asiatic Russia, Iran, Iraq, Turkey, Arabia, all countries bordering on the Mediterranean Sea, Abyssinia, the Sudan, French Congo and Nigeria. In spite of the broad coincidence of its distribution with that of kala-azar, the two diseases are not closely associated in most

areas. A number of imported cases have been seen in the United States.

Etiology and Pathology. The disease is caused by protozoa of the genus *Leishmania,* which are known as *Leishmania tropica,* although many parasitologists agree that this parasite cannot be reliably distinguished from *Leishmania donovani,* the characteristics of which were previously described. Sandflies of the genus *Phlebotomus* have been shown to transmit the disease from person to person, and this is believed to be the common method of transmission. Animal reservoirs, however, are probably important. They exist in the dog in many areas and in the gerbil (a small rodent) in Asiatic Russia. The evidence indicates that this form of cutaneous leishmaniasis is transmitted by other species of sandflies than those responsible for the spread of kala-azar. Direct inoculation from a sore sometimes occurs, but is rare. The pathology is that of the local lesion. The basic change is an infiltration of all the layers of the skin, mainly by reticuloendothelial cells (macrophages), which behave as they do in kala-azar. The circulation is interfered with and necrosis occurs, followed by ulceration, granulation and, with healing, the proliferation of fibrous tissue. The infection is usually followed by immunity, at least to the same strain of *Leishmania tropica,* but apparently not to kala-azar.

Symptoms. The period from infection to manifest disease extends from a few weeks to two or three years. Systemic symptoms are rare and consist only of transient slight fever and malaise. The lesions are usually multiple, sometimes solitary. They are commonly located on exposed surfaces, especially the face, ears, neck, backs of the hands, and forearms. The scalp, palms and soles escape. In its earliest stages the lesion takes the form of a small red papule which often itches. A slight exudate gives rise to fine adherent scales. The papule enlarges slowly until in the course of a month or two it is 1 to 3 cm. in diameter. A thick rupia-like scab usually forms. Necrosis ordinarily takes place in the center of this lesion, resulting in the formation of a roughly circular ulcer with clear-cut margins, which bleeds easily. Pyogenic infection is common at this stage. The surrounding area is somewhat swollen and indurated. In addition to this typical evolution, the lesion may take various other forms. The infection is characteristically indolent, usually lasting a year or more, but occasionally sores follow an abortive course. Fairly large lesions heal slowly with the formation of a contracted scar which is often disfiguring.

Diagnosis. In endemic areas the diagnosis is often based on the clinical picture, but the lesions may be confused with those of many other diseases, including syphilis, yaws, tuberculosis, leprosy and various mycoses. The diagnois should alway be confirmed by the demonstration of *Leishmania tropica,* which can usually be found without difficulty in stained smears or N.N.N. cultures of material from early lesions. In large lesions material for examination should be obtained by puncturing or scraping the cleaned edges. It is useless to study the central exudate. Skin sensitivity tests have been used, but their value is uncertain.

Treatment. This form of leishmaniasis responds less satisfactorily to chemotherapy than kala-azar. Cure and healing often require several weeks. Numerous agents have been used, but there is no general agreement as to the best method of treatment. On account of the relatively benign nature of the disease, treatment is usually given by local applications or injections. Among the agents so used with success are superficial radiation, solid carbon dioxide and, by local injection, berberine sulfate (2 per cent solution), quinacrine hydrochloride (10 per cent), stibamine glucoside (Neostam) and other pentavalent antimony preparations (2 per cent). Local injections should consist of about 2 cc. given in various points on the periphery of the lesion at weekly intervals. Judicious débridement of large ulcers is recommended. Secondary infection should be treated by the systemic administration of an appropriate antimicrobial drug. The pentavalent antimony compounds used for kala-azar are sometimes given intravenously for oriental sore, but the results are not clearly superior to those following local treatment. A somewhat less intensive course of one of these drugs than that recommended for kala-azar is advisable when the lesions of oriental sore are numerous.

Efforts to prevent this form of leishmaniasis should follow the lines laid down for kala-azar. In addition, lesions should be protected so that sandflies and other insects do not have access to them. In highly endemic areas, advantage is taken of the immunity which usually follows infection to protect selected persons against disfigurement by artificial inoculation of living parasites in inconspicuous areas.

AMERICAN MUCOCUTANEOUS LEISHMANIASIS
(*Espundia and Other Local Names*)

Definition and Incidence. This form of leishmaniasis, which is attributed to *Leishmania brasiliensis,* resembles the oriental cutaneous type in that it is characterized by skin granulomas, but in addition many cases show ulcerative lesions of the nose, mouth and pharynx. The infection is endemic in most if not all Central and South American countries and in the Yucatan peninsula (Mexico). It is especially common in forested areas. It is considered to be distinct from kala-azar, which also occurs in certain parts of South America.

Etiology and Pathology. The disease is caused by *Leishmania* assigned to the genus *L. brasiliensis,* although the organisms cannot be reliably separated from those responsible for the other forms of human leishmaniasis. Sandflies are capable of transmitting the infection. The parasite has been recovered from dogs, but dogs do not seem to be an important source of human disease. The basic pathologic changes are similar to those in oriental cutaneous leishmaniasis, but in many cases the infection spreads regionally through local lymphatic or blood channels, producing involvement of the naso-oral mucosa and neighboring lymph nodes. Systemic disease does not result. Little is known about immunity in connection with this infection.

Symptoms. There are usually three or four skin lesions, but often only one and rarely a large number, located on exposed parts of the body. In form the lesions often resemble those of oriental sore. Ulceration may not appear for months or even years and sometimes does not occur. In the absence of ulcer formation the lesion may acquire a verrucose form. In a few cases, nodules are formed along lymphatics and regional lymph nodes are enlarged. The incidence of mucosal lesions is variable in different areas, but reaches 20 per cent in Brazil. These lesions usually appear about a year after the skin lesions, occasionally only many years later. They begin as swellings which ulcerate and slowly spread so that they may become extensive and cause serious destruction anywhere in the nose, mouth or pharynx. The infection is persistent, often lasting for many years if not for life in the absence of treatment. Secondary infection of ulcerated areas is common and may be fatal.

Diagnosis. The diagnosis should always be based on the demonstration of the parasite, which is recoverable from the more recently invaded tissue of skin and mucosal lesions. In many cases the organism can be found in material from regional lymph nodes and from the nasal mucosa even in the absense of mucosal lesions. Appropriate methods were described for kala-azar.

Treatment. No standard plan is generally recognized, but the use of both local and systemic therapy is recommended for most cases. Local treatment of skin lesions should follow the lines suggested for oriental cutaneous leishmaniasis. For systemic treatment the standard intravenous course of a pentavalent antimonial used against kala-azar deserves careful trial, which it has not yet had. Snapper has described the successful treatment of a patient with mucosal lesions by the use of a stilbamidine derivative. The parenteral therapy most frequently used has consisted either of antimony and potassium tartrate or of stibophen (Fuadin), both given intravenously. Extensive mucosal lesions require much attention. The persistence and pains used to secure and maintain cleanliness are more important than the particular drug applied locally. Sodium perborate or boric acid solution may be used. Systemic treatment with a suitable antimicrobial drug should be given for concurrent infections. Patients should be followed for a year to see that mucosal lesions do not develop or recur. The prevention of this disease follows the recommendations given for kala-azar and oriental cutaneous leishmaniasis.

FRANCIS R. DIEUAIDE

References

Ash, J. E., and Spitz, Sophie: Pathology of Tropical Diseases; An Atlas. Philadelphia, W. B. Saunders Company, 1945.

Conrad, A. H. Jr., and others: Cutaneous Leishmaniasis. Report of Cases Occurring in Great Britain and the United States. Arch. Dermat. & Syph., 62: 502, 1950.

Kirk, R.: Differentiation and Nomenclature of Leishmania. Parasitol., 39:263, 1949.

Most, H., and Lavietes, P. H.: Kala-azar in American Military Personnel. Medicine, 26:221, 1947.

Napier, L. E.: Principles and Practice of Tropical Medicine. New York, The Macmillan Company, 1946.

Schoenbach, E. B., and Greenspan, E. M.: Pharmacology, Mode of Action and Therapeutic Potentialities of Stilbamidine, Pentamidine, Propamidine, and Other Aromatic Diamidines. Medicine, 27: 327, 1948.

Shortt, H. L.: Diagnosis of Kala-azar. Trop. Dis. Bull., 44:145, 1947.

Snapper, I.: American Mucocutaneous Leishmaniasis Successfully Treated with 2-Hydroxystilbamidine. Am. J. Med., 13:655, 1952.

Snow, J. S., and others: American Cutaneous Leishmaniasis. Arch. Dermat. & Syph., 57:90, 1948.

Stone, H. H., and others: Kala-azar (Visceral Leishmaniasis): Report of Case with 34-Month Incubation Period. Ann. Int. Med., 36:686, 1952.

Tuckman, E.: Treatment of Chinese Kala-azar with Sodium Antimony Gluconate. J. Trop. Med., 52: 199, 1949.

TOXOPLASMOSIS

Etiology. Until recently toxoplasmosis was poorly understood and poorly defined. The infection is produced by species of *Toxoplasma,* protozoa which have been recovered from body fluids and exudates, but typically reside intracellularly in mononuclear and epithelioid cells, nerve cells, muscle fibers, endothelial cells of capillaries, and polymorphonuclear and eosinophilic leukocytes. They are minute (2 to 6 by 1.5 to 2 microns), distinct, oval, pyriform, rounded, crescentic or elongated protoplasmic masses, each with a more or less central nucleus. They occur singly or in clusters in the host cell and multiply by repeated binary fission, at times suggesting a primitive type of schizogony.

As a result of clinical and postmortem studies, demonstration of the organism in experimental animals inoculated with material from human sources, protection tests and other evidence of *Toxoplasma* antibodies, toxoplasmosis has been found to be rather widely distributed in the United States, Europe, South America, and possibly in other areas.

Morbid Anatomy. Toxoplasmosis may develop as an intrauterine disease, as an early postnatal infection or in older children and adults (Zuelzer, 1944). Although the portal of entry is unknown, the toxoplasmas first typically involve the blood vessels, with an acute vasculitis which leads to rapid necrosis of the vessels and perivascular tissues. This is followed by an inflammatory infiltration by plasma cells, large monocytes and some eosinophils. Thus granulomas develop, usu-

several species nan
in reptiles, birds a
sheep, cattle, hors
species, *Sarcocysti*
1878, has been re
from man.

The Organism.
muscles and conn
unstriated muscles
elongated spindle-sl
sules having rounde
The exact manner i
fected is unknown,
ripe spores are ac
food or drink and
ferment (*sarcocystin*
culature via the inte

ally terminating in calcification of the involved areas. In the intrauterine variety the disease may develop to the granuloma-calcification stage at birth, with evidence of advanced encephalitis and hydrocephalus. In cases with evidence of postuterine exposure the symptoms indicate involvement of the lungs, with diffuse pneumonitis; of the kidneys, with necrotic glomerulitis; and of the superficial blood vessels, with exanthem.

Symptoms. Congenital encephalitis patients exhibit fever, inanition and opisthotonos and usually die of the disease during the first few weeks of life. In the infantile variety there are early convulsions and other neurologic symptoms, including the relatively pathognomonic triad of internal hydrocephalus, chorioretinitis and eventually evidence of intracerebral calcifications. There may be an enlargement of the liver and spleen with elevated icteric index. The cerebrospinal fluid is exanthochromic and has an increased cell count and protein content. Survivors have impaired vision and retarded mental development. In older children and adults the involvement is mostly extraneural, with acute exanthem and interstitial pneumonia, but may have associated chorioretinitis (Wilder).

It is possible that inapparent toxoplasmosis may be relatively common in human beings and in various animals, which then may serve as carriers, although the method of transmission is unknown. Warren and Sabin (1943) developed a complement fixation test for the rapid diagnosis of the disease, and more recently Sabin and Feldman (1948) have described a dye test which is much simpler and equally accurate in the diagnosis of this infection. In clinically active infections the **prognosis** is almost invariably grave. There is no **specific treatment,** although sulfonamides and other antimicrobials have been shown to be toxoplasmostatic in experimental animals. Protection tests in laboratory animals suggest the possible development of protective vaccines. Mothers who give birth to a *Toxoplasma*-infected baby are not in danger of having subsequent children similarly afflicted.

ERNEST CARROLL FAUST

References

Feldman, H. A.: The Clinical Manifestations and Laboratory Diagnosis of Toxoplasmosis. Am. J. Trop. Med. & Hyg., 2:420, 1953.

Jacobs, L.: The Biology of Toxoplasma. Am. J. Trop. Med. & Hyg., 2:365, 1953.
Wilder, H. C.: Toxoplasma Chorioretinitis in Adults. Arch. Ophth., 48:127, 1952.
Wolf, A., Cowen, D., and Paige, B. H.: Human Toxoplasmosis: Occurrence in Infants in Encephalomyelitis: Verification by Transmission to Animals. Am. J. Path., 15:657, 1939.

CILIATE INFECTIONS
BALANTIDIASIS
(*Balantidiosis*)

The Ciliata, a distinct class group of the Protozoa, are unicellular organisms which have numerous rows of relatively short threadlike extensions of their cytoplasm, the *cilia,* which are used in locomotion. Ciliates multiply by transverse binary fission. Some species encyst when environmental conditions are unfavorable to growth and propagation. The great majority of ciliates are free-living forms, but a few are obligatory parasites. Only *Balantidium coli* is medically important.

In reservoir hosts (hogs and monkeys) this parasite has an extensive distribution in warm and temperate climates. Human infection is more prevalent in tropical countries.

Etiology. *Balantidium coli* is the largest of the protozoan parasites of man, ranging in length from 50 to 100 microns and in breadth from 40 to 70 microns. The living organism is a sturdy, ovoidal, glassy-green object, covered with many rows of cilia arranged in a slightly oblique pattern. A cell mouth lies somewhat to one side of the anterior extremity. Within the cytoplasm there are a large, slightly curved *macronucleus,* and near the center of its concave margin a minute *micronucleus.* Numerous food and contractile vacuoles may also be observed. By means of its cilia *B. coli* progresses in a slightly spiral path. It may be observed under the microscope to "plough" through a semiliquid film of feces, then become relatively quiescent, round up, partially retract its cilia and secrete a tough cyst wall around itself. It does not multiply during the cystic stage.

Morbid Anatomy. As a parasite of man, *B. coli* invades the wall of the large bowel, especially in the region of the cecum. Its entry into the tissues is primarily mechanical, although it probably has some lytic properties. In uncomplicated infections the lesion produced is cuplike or flasklike, but, because of its relatively larger size, the opening is

larger than tha
tolytica. At tir
or burrows
cularis mucos;
not invade th
organs. In un
evidence of l
lar reaction to
fibroblastic re
the lesion is f
terial invaders
leukocytes and
diate vicinity.
Clinical M
tient harboring
ciation with
reservoir. Most
parent infectic
a moderate to ;
usually withou
tion may altern
has seen these
in China, Pan;
Orleans and
United States.
fection is mor
than has been
balantidial dys
charge of bloo
the characteris
in Venezuela.
variety results
sion of a strain
come adapted
even if there i;
colon and no
dence of invasi
hyperemic, wi
hemorrhage.
In most pat
dysentery is ac
tenesmus, naus
tite, headache,
and loss of we
poor digestion ;
is at times a p
membranes and
physical examir
over the colon.
ing watery diar
Diagnosis o
demonstration
zoites or cysts
are readily seen
scope in uncon
essential featur
fresh films stai

METAZOAN INFECTIONS

The Metazoa are animals made up of many cells, which in aggregates are usually specialized into tissues and organs performing particular but coordinated functions of the entire organism. In this respect the Metazoa differ from the Protozoa, the one-celled organisms, in which all the functions are performed by specialized parts of the protoplasm within a single cell unit. The parasitic Metazoa are found primarily within the following invertebrate groups: the PLATYHELMINTHES, or flatworms; the NEMATODA, or roundworms; the HIRUDINEA, or leeches; and the ARTHROPODA, comprising the insects and their allies.

ERNEST CARROLL FAUST

THE PLATYHELMINTHES

(Flatworms)

Members of this group are invertebrates which have a longitudinal axis, with anterior and posterior ends, and are bilaterally symmetrical. With few exceptions they have either an incomplete digestive tract or none at all. There is no body cavity. Most of the flatworms are hermaphroditic; thus each individual is a complete reproductive unit. Among the flatworms there are two classes containing important human parasites: the TREMATODA, or flukes, and the CESTOIDEA, or tapeworms.

TREMATODE OR FLUKE INFECTIONS

(Trematodiasis)

Trematodiasis is an infection with species of Trematoda (flukes), in which the ciliated epithelium is confined to the larva (*miracidium*) hatched from the egg; typically with a mouth, surrounded by a muscular sucker, a pharynx, esophagus and a pair of intestinal ceca which end blindly in the subdistal part of the body. All flukes parasitizing man have a complicated life cycle involving a minimum of three generations and obligatory utilization of certain species of snails (or other molluscs) as intermediate hosts. The larval stage hatched from the egg (*miracidium*) actively invades the appropriate snail, in which two (or at times three or more) generations develop, each with production of progeny. The tailed larva emerging from the snail (*cercaria*) becomes a free-living aquatic form and has one of three recourses, depending on the species of fluke. It may directly infect man by the skin route (blood flukes); it may crawl onto aquatic vegetation, drop its tail and encyst on the surface of the plant (sheep liver fluke); it may penetrate into the soft tissues of certain animals, where it encysts (Chinese liver fluke). In the latter two groups, man acquires the infection by ingesting raw or inadequately cooked plant or animal food infected with the respective cysts.

Most flukes infecting man are hermaphroditic and have two distinct suckers, one surrounding the mouth and a blind acetabulum on the ventral side of the body. These species are referred to as *distomes,* and their infection is properly designated as *distomiasis.* Important exceptions are the blood flukes, or *schistosomes,* which are unisexual (i.e., dieccious); the infection is designated as *schistosomiasis.*

INTESTINAL DISTOMIASIS

Etiology. Several species of flukes parasitize the digestive tract of man, in most instances the small bowel, where the worms are attached to the mucosa by means of their suckers.

FASCIOLOPSIS BUSKI

The large fleshy fluke, *Fasciolopsis buski,* is an important parasite of man (and the pig) in the neighborhood of the China Sea, the southern Pacific Ocean, Burma and eastern India. It lives primarily at the levels of the duodenum and jejunum. These fleshy flukes lay large, colorless, transparent, thin-shelled ovoidal eggs which have a minute, inconspicuous operculum. They mature only after they have been evacuated in feces into fresh water. After several days a miracidium hatches from each egg, penetrates into its appropriate snail host, and undergoes multiplication within the snail. The cercariae which are shed from the snail a few weeks later crawl onto and encyst upon certain water plants, which constitute the source of human infection.

Symptoms. Wherever the adult worm is attached to the intestinal mucosa there is first a focus of inflammation, and later a necrotic center, with hemorrhage and frequently abscess formation. Many worms attached near one another at one level of the bowel may produce an acute obstruction. Towards the end of the incubation period of about ninety days there is a toxic diarrhea, with hunger pains. Heavy infections may simulate peptic ulcer and the patient may become asthenic. Generalized toxemia is usually manifested in the form of edema, particularly of the face, abdominal wall and lower extremities. Ascites develops in severe infections, especially in children. Generalized abdominal pain is frequent. The diarrhea continues, and the stool becomes foul-smelling and contains much undigested food. Anorexia, nausea and vomiting are characteristic. Death is commonly due to anasarca. Most of the patients have a marked leukocytosis with absolute eosinophilia, but some chronic cases have a relative lymphocytosis. There is no significant anemia.

Diagnosis is based on the history of the patient, his residence in endemic foci and the recovery of the characteristic eggs in the feces. These eggs require differentiation from those of the sheep liver fluke (*Fasciola hepatica*) and some of the larger species of echinostomes.

Prognosis is fair to good in properly treated cases.

Treatment. The treatment of choice consists in the administration of hexylresorcinol crystoids (Crystoids anthelmintic) in amounts of 0.4 to 1 gm., depending on the age of the patient. The drug is administered in 0.2 gm. hard gelatin capsules on an empty stomach, and is followed in two hours with sodium sulfate (Glauber salts) purgation (30 cc. or 30 gm. dissolved in a glass of water). Food must not be taken until four hours after the anthelmintic has been administered. In severe infections supportive treatment for the circulation (e.g., norepinephrine) may be needed during and immediately after specific therapy. Treatment with hexylresorcinol has a 75 to 100 per cent worm-removal value for *F. buski* and may be repeated safely within one week. Carbon tetrachloride (adult dose, 3 cc.), preceded and followed by sodium sulfate purgation, is equally specific, but is relatively dangerous in this infection.

Prevention can be provided by immersing raw vegetables in boiling water for a few seconds. The "seedbeds" of the infection may be eradicated by mass treatment of the infected population, together with destruction of the snails by the use of copper sulfate solution (1:50,000) or calcium cyanide as fertilizer in submerged fields where the infected water plants are grown.

OTHER INTESTINAL FLUKES

Several species of flukes, small to large and fleshy in character, are provided with an incomplete circlet of hooks on the cervical region of their body and are designated as echinostomes.

Species belonging to the genera *Echinostoma, Himasthla, Paryphostomum* and *Echinochasmus* have been reported as parasites of the human bowel, particularly in the Far East, as well as in Rumania and elsewhere.

Infection results from eating a variety of raw animal products, including snails, limpets, tadpoles, fresh-water fish, and so on, in which the cercariae have encysted. The smaller species produce only minor intestinal symptoms, but the larger species cause grave symptoms comparable to those of *Fasciolopsis* infection.

Treatment should be carried out along lines indicated for *F. buski*.

Prevention consists in the thorough cooking of all animal foods.

Another type of intestinal distomiasis is produced by many flukes belonging to the family Heterophyidae, and represented by the species *Heterophyes heterophyes, Metagonimus yokogawai* and their kin, which have an extensive distribution in the Far East, Egypt and Southeastern Europe. These worms are minute forms, at times barely visible to the naked eye, are ovoidal, pyriform or nearly cylindrical, and have a peculiar union of their ventral and genital suckers. They lay minute ovoidal eggs (measuring 26 to 30 by 15 to 17 microns) with a distinct operculum at one end. The encysted cercariae are found in the tissues of many species of fresh-water and some brackish-water fishes.

Morbid Anatomy. When various mammals (and frequently birds) eat the infected fish, either raw or inadequately cooked, the worms gain entrance to the small bowel, excyst and attach themselves directly to the lining cells of the glandular crypts or become buried in the cells, at times even reaching the stroma of the villi. They produce an inflammation of the contiguous or invaded cells, with excessive mucous secretion and erosion of cell membranes. Worms which have entered the mucous membrane remain there until they die. If the number of worms is large and the involved areas of mucosa are considerable, a mucous diarrhea may result. Africa and his colleagues (1935 *et seq.*) in the Philippines have demonstrated that in man the minute eggs of some heterophyid species not infrequently get into the mesenteric lymphatics or venules and are carried to many sites in the body, including the myocardium, brain, spinal cord, kidneys, and elsewhere, setting up trains of symptoms dependent on the organs and tissues involved.

Treatment should be instituted, if possible, before the worms burrow into the intestinal mucosa. Hexylresorcinol crystoids, as recommended in *Fasciolopsis buski* infection, may be undertaken, but tetrachlorethylene (C_2Cl_4) is believed to be more specific. The adult dosage is 3 cc., given in the morning on an empty stomach, preceded the night before and followed two hours after treatment by sodium sulfate purgation (30 cc. or 30 gm. dissolved in a glass of water). No food should be permitted until a copious posttreatment bowel movement has been obtained. Tetrachlorethylene is safe in the absence of alcohol and absorbable fats and should remove all heterophyid worms except those which are deeply imbedded in the bowel wall.

Prevention consists in the thorough cooking of all fish in endemic areas.

AMPHISTOMES

Two other large intestinal flukes, referred to as amphistomes because their suckers are at opposite ends of their body, have been reported from man, *Watsonius watsoni* in West Africa and *Gastrodiscoides hominis* in India, Indo-China and occasionally among East Indian immigrants in British Guiana. Practically nothing is known of the life cycles or epidemiology of these flukes, although there is suggestive evidence that exposure results from ingesting and swallowing vegetation on which the encysted larvae have become attached. They produce severe diarrhea, indigestion and generalized toxemia with anasarca. Hexylresorcinol crystoids, as for *F. buski*, is likely to prove efficacious for their removal.

HEPATIC DISTOMIASIS

Etiology. Hepatic distomiasis is produced by the sheep liver fluke (*Fasciola hepatica*) and its relatives, the Chinese liver fluke (*Clonorchis sinensis*) and its relatives (*Opisthorchis felineus* and *O. viverrini*), and by the lancet fluke (*Dicrocoelium dendriticum*).

FASCIOLA

Fasciola hepatica and its kin, *F. gigantica,* are the largest hepatic flukes, measuring about 30 by 13 mm.

Life History. As adults they live in the more proximal bile ducts and gallbladder, where they lay large, colorless, transparent, thin-shelled, unembryonated, ovoidal eggs with a minute operculum. The eggs, hardly distinguishable from those of *Fasciolopsis buski,* pass down into the lumen of the bowel and are evacuated in feces. They mature in fresh water and undergo an extrinsic life history paralleling that of *F. buski.* Herbivorous animals grazing on infected swampy pastures are commonly exposed to infection. After the cysts are swallowed with grass and excyst in the duodenum, the larvae bore through the intestinal wall into the peritoneal cavity, then bore through Glisson's capsule into the liver, burrowing through the parenchyma and liver cells until they reach the larger bile ducts. Here they grow into adults. Sheep liver fluke infection is cosmopolitan wherever sheep are raised. In recent years human infections have been repeatedly reported from Cuba, several other countries in Latin America, Hawaii, southern France and Algeria. The commonest source of human fascioliasis in Europe and the Western Hemisphere is water cress used as salad greens.

Morbid Anatomy. Heavy invasion of the liver by *F. hepatica* results in extensive necrosis of the parenchyma ("liver rot" of sheep). After the worms reach the bile ducts they provoke a hyperplasia of the biliary epithelium with a circumscribing fibrous encapsulation, resulting in pressure necrosis of the parenchyma and eventual periportal cirrhosis. Symptoms and signs in human infections are hepatic colic, cholecystitis, cholelithiasis, generalized abdominal rigidity and pain on pressure, irregular fever, more or less persistent diarrhea, leukocytosis and eosinophilia, marked anemia, anasarca, and rarely hemoglobinuria. At times these worms become located in ectopic foci, such as the abdominal wall, the muscles of the neck or, rarely, the brain and eyeball.

Diagnosis consists in recovering the characteristic eggs in the feces of persons outside Fasciolopsis-endemic areas, or from biliary drainage. False distomiasis, resulting from the consumption of infected sheep or cattle liver, must be excluded.

Prognosis is fair to poor, depending on the degree of involvement.

Treatment, as outlined by Kourí (1932), consists in the intramuscular administration of emetine hydrochloride (0.03 gm. daily for seventeen to eighteen days) and has been demonstrated to be quite effective in killing the adult worms in the bile tracts. Surgical intervention is required when the worms migrate to ectopic foci and develop in these locations.

Prevention consists in meticulous care not to eat raw water cress or other water plants in endemic foci.

OTHER HEPATIC FLUKES

Clonorchis sinensis, Opisthorchis species and *Dicrocoelium dendriticum* are delicate, transparent, narrowly oval flukes which parasitize the distal bile ducts, especially near the margins of the liver. *Clonorchis sinensis* has a wide distribution in the Far East; *Opisthorchis felineus* is prevalent in Siberia, east Prussia, southeastern Europe and French Indo-China. *Opisthorchis viverrini* has been found only in northern Siam. *Dicrocoelium dendriticum* has been reported as a human parasite from Europe, Africa and Asia. *Clonorchis* and *Opisthorchis* are contracted from eating raw fish containing the encysted larvae; *Dicrocoelium* infection results from accidentally swallowing certain ants, which live in contaminated pastures and are hosts for the advanced larval stage of the worm.

Life History. The excysted larvae crawl up the ampulla of Vater to the distal bile ducts and develop into adult worms. Here they may live for fifteen to twenty-five years, producing hyperplasia of the biliary epithelium, a circumscribing fibrosis of the ducts, pressure necrosis of the parenchyma and, in heavy infections, periportal cirrhosis and ascites. Light infections are essentially symptomless; moderate infections produce progressive hepatic dysfunction, with loss of appetite, a feeling of fullness of the abdomen, diarrhea, indigestion, edema and hepatomegaly. Heavily infected persons suffer from cholangitis, anasarca, tachycardia, vertigo, tremors, abdominal cramps and mental depression.

Diagnosis is based on recovery of the characteristic operculate eggs in feces or by duodenal drainage (*Clonorchis,* 28 by 16 microns; *O. felineus,* 30 by 11 microns; *O.*

viverrini, 26 by 13 microns; *Dicrocoelium,* 38 to 45 by 22 to 30 microns). Care must be exercised not to diagnose as "positive" persons who have eaten sheep livers infected with *Dicrocoelium.*

Prognosis is good in early light infections, poor in heavy or chronic infections.

Treatment. There is no eminently satisfactory anthelmintic for any of these infections. However, in recently acquired *Clonorchis* infection the administration of gentian violet or tartar emetic will prove clinically beneficial and may kill most of the worms. The gentian violet may be administered in 1½-hr. Seal-Ins enteric coating (0.06 gm. three times daily for sixteen days). The tartar emetic, as 0.5 per cent solution, should be administered intravenously on alternate days, beginning with 8 cc. and increasing the dose gradually to 24 cc. until 320 cc. (containing 0.576 gm. of antimony) has been given.

Prevention consists in thoroughly cooking all fresh-water fish (*Clonorchis, Opisthorchis*) and greens obtained from moist meadows (*Dicrocoelium*) in endemic foci.

PULMONARY DISTOMIASIS
(*Paragonimus Infection*)

Etiology. Pulmonary distomiasis is produced by the lung fluke, *Paragonimus westermani,* a moderately small (7.5 to 12 by 4 to 6 by 3.5 to 5 mm.), thick, ovoidal worm, which most typically lives in little encapsulated pockets that open into the bronchioles and are almost invariably provided with small blood vessels. The infection has a wide distribution in the Far East, New Guinea, Java, Sumatra, parts of Africa, and has been found in native populations in Peru, Ecuador and Colombia.

Life History. Eggs (golden brown in color, operculate, measuring 80 to 118 by 48 to 60 microns) are laid by the parent worms into the adventitious capsular pockets and are usually discharged into the bronchiole, frequently with flecks of hemorrhaged blood and cellular debris. They are coughed up and discharged in sputum, or swallowed and evacuated with the feces. They embryonate and hatch in fresh water, and the miracidial larvae enter appropriate snails. After sojourn and multiplication through two complete generations in the snail, the emerging cercariae enter the soft tissues of fresh-water crabs or crayfishes, and encyst. Man and other mammals acquire infection from eating uncooked crab or crayfish meat.

Morbid Anatomy. The excysted larvae in the small bowel bore through the intestinal wall, traverse the peritoneal cavity, bore

424

through the diaphragm and enter the lungs, eventually reaching sites near the smaller air passages where they settle down and develop into adults. Some of the migrating larvae get sidetracked in the abdomen, others in the thorax; still others get into the cranium and may wander into the brain or its envelopes. The lesions produced (Musgrave, 1907) consist of (1) abscesses around eggs infiltrated in host tissue; (2) pseudotubercles developed around eggs; (3) suppurative, and (4) ulcerative processes. In the lungs the pathologic picture may consist of generalized or localized diffuse fibrosis, cystic dilatation of the bronchi, pneumonitis and tubercle-like abscesses, with accompanying painful cough and hemoptysis. Physical signs may suggest bronchopneumonia or pleural effusion. The abdominal implantation may slough into the intestine or through the somatic tissues. Lymph node involvement may be accompanied by fever. Brain tumors, the size of a hazelnut or larger, may produce a jacksonian type of epilepsy. Cerebral lesions may suggest epilepsy of other etiology, or encephalitis. In Japan and Korea, pulmonary distomiasis is common in children.

Diagnosis is based on finding the characteristic eggs in sputum, which is usually blood-tinged, or in the feces. Because of the macroscopic resemblance of the eggs to minute iron filings, there is no serious likelihood of confusing the discharge of pulmonary distomiasis with that of pulmonary tuberculosis or bronchial spirochetosis.

Prognosis is usually good unless the worms become lodged in foci such as the brain.

Treatment. There is no eminently satisfactory treatment. The intramuscular administration of 60 mg. of emetine hydrochloride daily for not more than twelve days is at times temporarily helpful in inhibiting egg production and thus alleviating bronchial irritation. Unless reinfected, the average patient eventually overcomes the parasites and the lesions heal without dysfunctioning fibrosis.

Prevention consists in care not to eat raw or pickled crab or crayfish meat in endemic areas.

ERNEST CARROLL FAUST

References

Africa, C. M., Garcia, E. Y., and De Leon, W.: Intestinal Heterophyidiasis with Cardiac Involvement. A Contribution to the Etiology of Heart Failure. Philippine J. Pub. Health, 2:1, 1935.

Alicata, J. E.: Human Fascioliasis in the Hawaiian Islands. Hawaii M. J., 12:196, 1953.

Faust, E. C.: Human Helminthology. 3rd ed. Philadelphia, Lea & Febiger, 1949.

———, and Khaw, O. K.: Studies on Clonorchis sinensis (Cobbold). Am. J. Hyg., Monogr. Ser., No. 8, 1927.

Komiya, Y., Yokogawa, M., and others: Studies on Paragonimiasis in Shizuoka Prefecture. II. Studies on the Treatment of Paragonimiasis. Japan. J. M. Sc. & Biol., 5:433, 1952.

Krull, W. H., and Mapes, C. R.: The Second Intermediate Host of Dicrocoelium Dendriticum. Cornell Veterinarian, 42:2, 1952.

SCHISTOSOMIASIS

(Bilharziasis)

Etiology. Schistosomiasis is produced by the schistosomes, or blood flukes, of which there are three important species of the genus Schistosoma parasitizing man over extensive areas of the globe. These worms are delicate elongate organisms which live in the portal circulation and collateral venous circulation. They are unisexual (i.e., diecious). During insemination and the long period of oviposition the female lies within the ventral trough of the male (the gynecophoral canal). Pairs of the adult worms typically reside in the smaller venules of the bowel wall (Schistosoma japonicum and S. mansoni), or of the vesical and pelvic plexuses (S. haematobium).

Life History. At the time of oviposition the female extends her threadlike anterior extremity as far as she can up into the lessening diameter of the venule, then deposits an egg. She then contracts a little and lays a second egg just behind the first, and another and another, until the entire venule is filled with the eggs. The pair then back out, enter another venule and repeat the process. This continues until the entire venous radicle is packed with eggs. Soon after the eggs are laid the larvae (miracidia) within the eggs are fully embryonated and secrete lytic ferments that ooze out through submicroscopic pores in the eggshell into the venule in which the eggs are trapped. The digestive action of this ferment, together with the pressure within the venule occasioned by the presence of the eggs, weakens and soon ruptures the wall of the venule, causing the discharge of the eggs into the perivascular tissues of the bowel or bladder wall. Some of these eggs in the mucous or submucous membranes soon effect a passage to the lumen of the respective organ, are carried down the bowel or urethra, and are evacuated with feces or urine. Hemorrhage from the wall of the organ at the time the eggs escape is characteristic of the discharge. Thus in the intestinal types there is dysentery; in the vesical type, hematuria.

When the schistosome eggs come in contact with fresh water, they hatch, and the miracidia swim about and seek out appropriate snails, which they enter. After two generations of development and multiplication within the snails the fork-tailed cercarial progeny emerge. When the skin of human beings swimming, wading, bathing or washing clothes comes in contact with infested water (i.e., containing the fork-tailed cercariae), the cercariae become attached, and burrow down to the peripheral capillary beds as the surface film of water drains off. The cercariae are then transported through the afferent blood to the right heart and lungs. They slowly squeeze through the pulmonary capillaries, and are carried through the left chambers of the heart and out into the aorta. Only those which get into the mesenteric arteries and pass through to the portal vessels survive. Within the intrahepatic portion of the portal blood the successful blood fluke larvae begin to feed and grow rapidly. Approximately twenty days after skin exposure the adolescent worms migrate against portal blood out to the mesenteric and vesical venules. *Schistosoma japonicum* typically migrates to the superior mesenteric venules draining the small bowel; *S. mansoni* migrates to the venules draining the large bowel (i.e., colic branch of the superior mesenteric vein and the inferior mesenteric vein); *S. haematobium,* through the inferior mesenteric vessels and via the hemorrhoidals or pudendals into the vesical or pelvic veins. The incubation periods are: in *S. japonicum,* four to five weeks; in *S. mansoni,* six to seven weeks; in *S. haematobium,* ten to twelve weeks. However *S. haematobium* may mature and oviposit in the rectal venules at a somewhat earlier period.

Endemic Regions. Schistosomiasis japonica, produced by *S. japonicum,* has a widespread distribution in the Orient, including Japan, extensive areas throughout Central and South China, several foci in the Philippines and one in Celebes. Although this species occurs in Formosa, it infects only domestic and wild mammals, and not man. Tens of millions of people in these countries are yearly exposed to infection. Schistosomiasis mansoni, produced by *S. mansoni,* has an extensive distribution in Egypt, East, Central and West Africa, and in many countries of the West Indies and northern South America. Schistosomiasis haematobia (vesical schistosomiasis, bilharziasis), produced by *S. haematobium,* is common throughout the continent of Africa and on the island of Madagascar, has been reported from the southern tip of Portugal, and is prevalent in areas of the Near East and Middle East. An endemic focus has recently been found in India, not far from Bombay.

INTESTINAL AND VISCERAL SCHISTOSOMIASIS

These types of schistosomiasis are due to *Schistosoma japonicum* and *S. mansoni,* and on occasion constitute a part of the clinical picture produced by *S. haematobium.*

Clinical Course. The disease may be divided into three stages: (1) incubation, (2) acute, (3) chronic. The *incubation period* is initiated by the boring of the cercariae into the skin. This rarely causes any considerable degree of trauma or cellular infiltration, but at times produces a needle-like pricking pain at each site of entry. While the larvae are

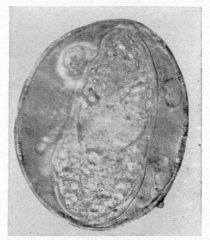

Fig. 53. Mature egg of *Schistosoma japonicum* with motile larva (miracidium). × 680. (Photomicrograph after Faust and Meleney in Studies on Schistosomiasis Japonica, courtesy of Am. J. Hyg.)

squeezing their way through the pulmonary capillaries, they frequently rupture the delicate blood vessels and set up an acute cellular reaction at each site, with a characteristic infiltration of neutrophils and eosinophils, occasionally epithelioid and giant cells. Several days later, after the larvae have reached the portal blood and have begun to feed, or have filtered out elsewhere as foreign proteins, there is typically a giant urticaria (especially in white patients) attributed to allergic reaction to the parasites. Towards the end of the incubation period the liver becomes acutely inflamed and intensely painful, and there is generalized abdominal discomfort and evidences of generalized intoxication, late afternoon fever and night sweats. The final prodromal symptom is a toxic diarrhea.

With the initiation of egg laying the *acute stage* is ushered in. The eggs work their way through the intestinal wall and escape with blood and necrotic tissue cells in the dysenteric discharge. In schistosomiasis japonica the small bowel is at first primarily involved, later the colon; in schistosomiasis mansoni the large bowel bears the brunt of the damage. Soon many of the eggs freed into the perivascular tissues become the centers for intense cellular infiltration, leading to miliary abscesses. The deeper ones usually become transformed by invasion of epithelioid cells, giant cells and fibroblasts into pseudotubercles. Gradually the acute period is transformed into the *chronic stage*. There is increased difficulty in the digestion and absorption of food, and more extensive open ulceration of the bowel occurs. In addition, eggs in constantly increasing numbers are carried into the liver, where they initiate miliary abscesses which later transform into pseudotubercles. Meanwhile the passage of portal blood through the liver becomes increasingly embarrassed, with compensatory passive congestion of the spleen, which may lead to tremendous splenomegaly. Some eggs get into the peripheral venous circulation and reach the lungs, where multiple pseudotubercles are formed in the pulmonary parenchyma. Occasionally eggs may pass into the systemic circulation, possibly via the vertebral venous circulation, and are then filtered out in the central nervous system, or the skin of the abdomen, chest or extremities.

Symptoms. There is recurrent daily fever, epigastric pain with acute tenderness of the abdominal viscera, enlarged tender liver and spleen, loss of appetite and weight, and profound malaise. Such an acute episode may terminate in a few weeks, but is exacerbated with exercise. The blood picture at the initiation of the acute stage is one of leukocytosis with intense eosinophilia; later it gradually changes to a leukopenia, with anemia, although the eosinophilia remains a prominent feature. As the chronic stage supersedes the acute period, weakness, skin pallor and dyspnea on slight exertion become conspicuous. Digestion is poor, emaciation is evident, and the superficial veins of the abdomen and thorax become dilated. Ascites may be a prominent feature. Digestion of food now becomes negligible. This stage may be prolonged for years, or the patient may die of pneumonia or other supervening infectious diseases. Lesions in the lungs resulting from pseudotubercle formation may suggest pulmonary tuberculosis, while neurologic manifestations, such as hemiplegia or jacksonian type of epilepsy, indicate involvement of the central nervous system by infiltration of eggs of the parasite.

On the whole, schistosomiasis japonica is a more rapidly developing and fatally terminating infection than schistosomiasis mansoni, because of the larger number of eggs laid per female per day, the greater percentage of eggs which reaches the liver and sets up tissue changes, and the more intense systemic intoxication produced by the worms and their eggs. Ileitis is more conspicuous in the former infection; colitis, in the latter. In both infections, however, the average case seen by the physician presents a complex picture of early and late stages, owing to repeated exposure.

Diagnosis in these infections is based specifically on the recovery of the eggs of the respective species in feces. In the acute stage these appear in the dysenteric exudate or in flecks of blood and mucus attached to formed or semiformed feces. In the chronic stage fewer eggs are discharged and require concentration of the stool for their recovery. Repeated sedimentation of the stool after dilution in ten to twenty-five parts of 0.5 per cent glycerin in water allows the eggs to settle to the bottom of a large urinalysis glass so that they may be picked up with a pipet. Eggs of *S. japonicum* are broadly ovoidal, and measure 70 to 100 by 50 to 65 microns. Those of *S. mansoni* are elongated-ovoidal with a conspicuous lateral spine, and measure 114 to 175 by 45 to 68 microns. In both types of intestinal schistosomiasis proctoscopic examination may reveal small granulomatous nodules in the lower sigmoid colon or upper rectum. Scraping or biopsy of these nodules will provide material for the demonstration of nests of eggs of the parasite. The history of intestinal and visceral involvement, together with splenomegaly, hepatic cirrhosis with ascites, and eosinophilia is suggestive of schistosomiasis, although Banti's syndrome must be excluded.

Prognosis. In overwhelming exposures the prognosis is almost invariably grave. With good management and specific therapy the outlook for persons in the acute and early chronic stage of the disease is good. In the late chronic stage, with advanced hepatic cirrhosis, the prognosis is relatively poor.

Treatment. Antimony compounds are indicated for specific therapy, but tolerance of these drugs is at times relatively low because of their high residual concentration in a liver which is already seriously damaged by the parasites. Tartar emetic (potassium antimony tartrate) has been used since 1918 in the treatment of schistosomiasis. In more recent years Fuadin and Anthiomaline have frequently replaced tartar emetic. There is evidence, however, that when comparable amounts (in terms of metallic antimony) are administered, relapses are much more frequent with Fuadin and Anthiomaline than with tartar emetic. During 1945 a new, well tolerated regimen with tartar emetic was developed for the treatment of schistosomiasis japonica among American Army personnel. This consists of the intravenous administration of a 0.5 per cent solution of the drug as follows: first day, 8 cc.; third day, 12 cc.; fifth day, 16 cc.; seventh day, 20 cc.; ninth day and on alternate days through the twenty-ninth day, 24 cc. (total, 320 cc., containing 0.576 gm. of antimony). A relapse rate of about 16 per cent may be expected following one course of treatment, compared with approximately 70 per cent with a course of Fuadin (65 cc. of a 6.3 per cent solution) containing the same amount of antimony. Miracil D, administered orally, is ineffective for these types of schistosomiasis.

Prevention consists in avoiding contact with infested water. For drinking purposes, water may be treated with chlorine (one part per million residual after 30 minutes guarantees death of the infective cercariae). Populations must be educated to avoid contact with infested water and to defecate in sanitary locations. Facilities for the safe washing of clothes must be provided. In localized endemic foci, bodies of water may be treated with copper sulfate (1:50,000) in order to kill the molluscan intermediate hosts (*Schistosoma mansoni*), or banks of canals and ditches may be sprayed with dinitro-cyclohexylphenol (Dow) in the amount of 100 gm. per 100 linear feet (schistosomiasis japonica). Flowing water (streams, canals, irrigation ditches) may be treated with sodium pentachlorophenate (schistosomiasis mansoni and schistosomiasis haematobia). Ultimately, control will require that feces of infected persons be mechanically or chemically sterilized with respect to the schistosome eggs before the excreta are discharged into bodies of water in which the appropriate snails develop. In areas of schistosomiasis japonica the control problem is complicated by the fact that several domestic mammals are natural reservoirs of the infection.

VESICAL SCHISTOSOMIASIS
(*Bilharziasis*)

This type of schistosomiasis is commonly due to S. *haematobium,* rarely to S. *mansoni.*

The pathology and the symptomatology are confined primarily to the bladder and pelvic organs, but there may be considerable pulmonary disease resulting from infiltration of eggs via the caval system into the perivascular tissues of the lungs.

Clinical Course. The *incubation period* resembles that of intestinal schistosomiasis except that it is more prolonged and never has toxic diarrhea at its termination. The *acute stage* is usually ushered in with the painless passage of blood in the urine about three months or more after exposure. In some patients there may be an earlier or an associated involvement of the rectum, due to maturing of the worms and oviposition in the rectal venules en route to the vesical venules. This may produce temporary dysentery, with recovery of eggs in flecks of blood and mucus evacuated per rectum. On the other hand, for months or years there may be no subjective evidence of the disease, but sooner or later there is a burning sensation at the time of micturition and increased desire to urinate, together with bladder colic and dull pains in the loins and suprapubic region. Cystoscopic examination will reveal an inflammatory hyperplasia of the urethra and lower level of the bladder, incipient papillomata, and concretions of uric acid and oxalates around eggs in the bladder lumen. Eggs which have infiltrated into the prostate cause inflammation and fibrosis of this organ.

The *chronic stage* of vesical schistosomiasis, with tissue proliferation and repair, begins while egg deposition and extrusion is under way. It is characterized by increasing lodgment of the eggs in nearby tissues, with multiple abscess and pseudotubercle formation, leading to hyperplasia and fibrosis of the entire bladder wall. Cystoscopic examination now become difficult, bladder calculi develop, the urethra may become occluded, and an intermittent, frequently uncontrolled, discharge of urine, blood, pus and eggs ensues. Pyogenic invaders may extend the lesions to the periurethral or perivascular areas, or fistulas may extend into the rectum or scrotum. The patient becomes incontinent and usually succumbs to extensive dysfunction of the genitourinary system. Neoplastic disease of the involved tissues is a not infrequent occurrence.

Diagnosis consists in the recovery of eggs from the sediment which settles out at the bottom of a urinalysis glass into which the patient has passed a specimen. If there is rectal involvement the eggs may be passed in the stool. Biopsied specimens of the bladder or rectum may contain eggs of the worms when urine and stool examinations are negative. The eggs of S. *haematobium* are elongated-ovoidal, with a distinct terminal spine, measure 112 to 170 by 40 to 70 microns, are pale yellow, with a moderately thick wall, house a fully developed motile larva, and frequently have cellular debris adherent to the shell.

Prognosis is relatively good except in the terminal stage, provided specific treatment is administered.

Treatment consists in the administration of antimony as recommended for intestinal schistosomiasis. However, since there is relatively slight involvement of the liver in vesical schistosomiasis, the patient is usually able to tolerate tartar emetic by vein in 2 per cent and at times even 6 per cent solution. In vesical schistosomiasis due to S. *haematobium*, miracil D, administered by mouth three times daily for three to five days, appears to be relatively specific. This drug is particularly valuable for treatment of small children in whom intravenous therapy is difficult.

Prevention is similar to that of the intestinal types, except that urine is the source for infection of the appropriate snails. Moreover, there are no important reservoirs of S. *haematobium*, so that the control problem is much simpler than in schistosomiasis japonica.

SCHISTOSOME DERMATITIS

Etiology. The fork-tailed larvae (cercariae) of several species of nonhuman blood flukes have been found capable of penetrating the skin of persons wading or bathing in infested fresh and salt water, with resulting *schistosome dermatitis*.

Symptoms. As the infected water drains off or evaporates from the victim's skin, the cercariae penetrate below the epidermis and for a week or more may remain alive in the deeper skin layers. At the time of skin penetration there is a prickling sensation with macule formation, followed by urticarial wheals and modification of the macule into a papule. Within a few hours to two to three days, intense pruritus of the involved areas is experienced, with a marked edema and transformation of the papule into a pustule. Palliatives, such as calamine lotion, should be applied, and attempts should be made to prevent secondary bacterial invasion.

Control. Schistosome dermatitis is relatively prevalent in some of the glacier lakes of Michigan, Wisconsin and northern Minnesota. Similar reports have come from the state of Washington, El Salvador in Central America, Germany, France, Wales and the Federated Malay States. Moreover, infection has occurred on the bathing beaches of New England, Florida, California and Hawaii. Summer guests in endemic foci, especially children, should be warned concerning the dangers of exposure. Copper carbonate in the amount of $\frac{3}{10,000}$ pound per calculated cubic foot of infested water should be distributed in fresh water along the shore every two weeks during the guest season to kill the snails in which the cercariae develop.

ERNEST CARROLL FAUST

References

Cort, W. W.: Studies on Schistosome Dermatitis. XI. Status of Knowledge after More Than Twenty Years. Am. J. Hyg., 52:251, 1950.
Expert Committee on Bilharziasis: First Report. World Health Org., Tech. Ser. No. 65, Geneva, 1953, 45 pp.
McMullen, D. B.: Schistosomiasis and Molluscacides. Am. J. Trop. Med. & Hyg., 1:671, 1952.
Wright, W. H., and Dobrovolny, C. G.: Experiments in the Control of Schistosomiasis in Brazil. Pub. Health Rep., 68:1156, 1953.

CESTODE OR TAPEWORM INFECTIONS

(*Cestodiasis*)

Cestodiasis is an infection with species of *Cestoidea* (tapeworms). The mature worm (*strobila*) consists of a "head" (*scolex*), the organ of attachment, which is provided with suckers and usually with anterior hooklets; the "neck," situated immediately behind the head, which constitutes the region of growth of the tapeworm; and a chain of successive "segments" (*proglottids*), which arise from the distal end of the "neck" and become larger and more mature sexually as their distance from the "neck" increases. Each mature proglottid is a complete hermaphroditic reproductive unit, sexually comparable to a complete trematode. The mature egg of human tapeworms contains an *oncosphere* or *hexacanth embryo*. After the oncosphere stage there are one or more larval stages before the worm is ready to mature. Most tapeworms require two or three hosts for the completion of their life cycles.

Human tapeworm infections are of two types: (1) those in which the mature worm is attached to the bowel wall (i.e., *intestinal cestodiasis*), and (2) those for which man is an acceptable larval or intermediate host (*visceral* and *somatic cestodiasis*).

INTESTINAL CESTODIASIS

Etiology. Thirty or more distinct species of tapeworms produce intestinal infection in man. Only six of these are common as human parasites. They are as follows: *Taenia saginata* (beef tapeworm); *T. solium* (pork tapeworm); *Diphyllobothrium latum* (fish tapeworm); *Hymenolepis nana* (dwarf tapeworm); *H. diminuta* (rat tapeworm); and *Dipylidium caninum* (dog tapeworm).

Taenia saginata (Beef Tapeworm). This worm measures 12 to 15 feet or more in length, and consists of about one thousand to two thousand proglottids. The "head" is small, quadrate-rhomboidal, has four deeply excavated suckers, but lacks an anterior circlet of hooklets. The "neck" region is delicate and narrow, and measures a centimeter or more in length. Immature and mature proglottids constitute approximately the proximal half of the strobila, while the gravid ones make up the distal half. The uterus of the gravid proglottid consists of a long, median longitudinal sac with fifteen to twenty-one (usually eighteen) main lateral rami on each side of the main stem. Each uterus contains myriads of characteristic eggs, each consisting of a walnut-colored, hull-like, spherical shell, 31 to 43 microns in diameter, and, inside, the six-hooked embryo. Though eggs of this worm are at times shed inside the human bowel, usually the distalmost gravid proglottids, singly or in chains, break off from the parent worm and are passed in feces or actively migrate out the bowel. Cattle, the only known intermediate host, pick up the eggs when grazing on moist pastureland contaminated with human sewage. The embryos hatch in the ox's small bowel, migrate to striated muscle and in three months metamorphose into the mature bladder worm larvae (*Cysticercus bovis*). When man consumes this infected meat inadequately cooked, he acquires the infection, which requires about three months for incubation. This infection is prevalent throughout countries where people eat essentially raw beef, including the United States.

Taenia solium (Pork Tapeworm). This tapeworm seldom reaches 10 feet in length and consists of less than one thousand proglottids. The "head" is armed with a circlet of hooklets anterior to the suckers; the "neck" is relatively short and stout; the gravid proglottids have a uterus with only seven to thirteen (usually nine) main lateral rami on each side of the main stem. The eggs are indistinguishable from those of *T. saginata,* and usually escape from the human body in unbroken gravid proglottids. Hogs which feed on human feces become infected, and within three months the bladder worm larva or pork

"measle" (*Cysticercus cellulosae*) is fully developed in their striated muscle. Man becomes infected from eating inadequately cooked pork. This infection is uncommon in the United States, but is prevalent in eastern and southeastern Europe, in many countries of Asia and in Latin America, especially Mexico.

Diphyllobothrium latum (Fish Tapeworm). This tapeworm is unlike any other common tapeworm of man in many respects. It has a narrow, spatulate "head," which is provided only with a pair of longitudinal grooves or sulci for purpose of attachment. The strobila may reach several feet in length, but never develops strictly gravid proglottids. In each mature proglottid there is a uterine pore, through which immature eggs are discharged soon after they are produced. They are broadly ovoidal, measure about 70 to 45 microns, are straw-colored and have an operculum at one end. When infected human stools are discharged into fresh water, the eggs mature, the operculum of each egg opens, and ciliated six-hooked embryos escape into the water. If these swimming embryos are eaten by "water fleas" (*Diaptomus* or *Cyclops*), they develop to the first larval stage. When fresh-water fishes eat the infected fleas, they become infected with the second larval stage, which matures in the flesh of the fish. The infection is now ready for man, if he eats infected raw fish. However, the fishes which commonly ingest "water fleas" are usually too small for human food, but when these smaller fishes are eaten by larger, game fish, the flesh of the latter constitutes the source of human infection. *Diphyllobothrium latum* infection is mostly confined to the North Temperate Zone. It is common in Europe, the U. S. S. R., Japan, central south Canada and the northern parts of Minnesota and Michigan. A small endemic focus has been described from northern Florida, and other endemic areas have been noted in fresh-water lakes of Chile and Argentina. In the Western Hemisphere it is particularly prevalent in Scandinavian peoples and in Polish Jews. Iced fish shipped from endemic foci to many urban centers in the United States has provided the source for numerous infections.

Hymenolepis nana (Dwarf Tapeworm). This is a minute worm only a few centimeters long and is correspondingly small in other dimensions. Its "head" is provided with four suckers and an anterior circlet of hooklets. The distalmost proglottid disintegrates in the small bowel, setting the characteristic eggs free. These eggs are nearly spherical, measure 30 to 47 microns in diameter, and have a hyaline outer shell and an inner shell provided with a pair of polar thickenings and polar filaments. The presence of these filaments is species-diagnostic. The eggs, when evacuated in human stools, require no intermediate host. If they are accidentally taken into the mouth of the same or another person and swallowed, they hatch and develop to the mature worms. However, a brief sojourn in the stroma of the intestinal villi is required for the transformation of the six-hooked embryo into a larval stage. This infection is much more prevalent in children than in adults and tends to be familial or institutional in its distribution. Worms morphologically indistinguishable from *H. nana* are common parasites of rats and mice, but are physiologically distinct. Hence human infection is of human origin. The infection is cosmopolitan, but is especially common in the southern Appalachian area of the United States, in Latin America and in Mediterranean countries.

Hymenolepis diminuta (*Rat Tapeworm*) *and Dipylidium caninum* (*Dog Tapeworm*). These tapeworms are relatively uncommon in man, although at least 200 authentic cases of the former and several dozen cases of the latter have been reported from the human host, including several cases diagnosed in children in the southern United States. The intermediate hosts for these species are insects, frequently fleas ectoparasitic, respectively, on rats or mice and dogs or cats. Human infection results from accidentally ingesting infected intermediate insect hosts.

Symptoms. The pathogenicity and symptomatology of tapeworm infections probably do not differ with the species of tapeworms involved, but depend on several factors, including the number and mass of the worms, trauma and ulceration produced at the sites of attachment to the wall of the small intestine, host reaction to the metabolites of the worms, and probably consitutional reactions of the host. Except for *H. nana* and *D. latum,* it is common to have only a single tapeworm present in the small bowel. However, although a 15-foot *T. saginata* may fill a 2-liter container, many adult patients who harbor such a parasite have no subjective symptoms resulting from the infection. On the other hand, some persons are extremely sensitive to the presence of a single *H. nana.*

Clinical Course. An average history of a patient harboring *T. saginata* or *T. solium* or *Diphyllobothrium latum* is as follows. Towards the end of the three-month incubation period following the consumption of essentially raw beef, pork or fresh-water fish there is a toxic diarrhea and false hunger pains, and at times a systemic toxemia. During the early acute stage there is a moderate leukocytosis, with an eosinophilia usually not in excess of 13 per cent. There may be diarrhea alternating with constipation. After several weeks the average patient will have no apparent evidence of the infection except, in the *Taenia* infections, the almost daily annoyance of proglottids crawling out of the anus and frequently down the leg. There may be a mild microcytic or normocytic anemia, later a moderate leukopenia. In other patients parasitized by *T. saginata* or other intestinal tapeworms there may be abdominal colic, with or without diarrhea; anorexia, loss of appetite and weight; insomnia; extreme weakness, nervousness, convulsions in children; pronounced anemia of a normocytic or macrocytic type (especially in *D. latum* infection).

Diagnosis consists in recovery of the characteristic gravid proglottids in the feces or migrating out the anus, less commonly eggs in the feces (*T. saginata, T. solium, D. caninum*); recovery of the eggs consistently in the feces (*D. latum, H. nana, H. diminuta*). **Prognosis** is usually good, especially with specific treatment.

Treatment. Several anthelmintics have been used with success for the evacuation of intestinal tapeworms. The writer's recent experience favors the use of *quinacrine* (Atabrine). Routine treatment involves semistarvation the day before treatment, and before going to bed that night taking 30 cc. (30 gm.) of sodium sulfate dissolved in a glass of water. On the morning of treatment the patient remains in bed, takes no food or drink except water or black coffee. At 7 A.M., 0.5 gram of quinacrine (Atabrine hydrochloride, five 0.1 gm. tablets) is administered in a glass of water containing one or two teaspoonfuls of baking soda ($NaHCO_3$). Two hours later post-treatment with sodium sulfate is carried out. The worm is usually passed soon thereafter, intact with the "head" attached, stained a bright saffron yellow. For children the amount of quinacrine prescribed should be reduced according to apparent (not chronologic) age. Although vomiting may possibly follow administration of the drug, usually a sufficient amount reaches the worm to penetrate its tissues, cause it to release its attachment and to be evacuated. Only in constipated patients is this method of treatment likely to be unsuccessful.

For children harboring the dwarf tapeworm (*Hymenolepis nana*), it may be advisable to try hexylresorcinol crystoids (Crystoids anthelmintic) before utilizing the more toxic specifics. Pretreatment sodium sulfate purgation is indicated the night before treatment. In the morning in a single dose, on an empty stomach, the hexylresorcinol is administered in hard gelatin capsules, as follows: for children of preschool age, 0.4 gm.; for children 6 to 10 years, 0.6 to 0.8 gm.; for those over 10 years, the adult dosage of 1 gm. Sodium sulfate purgation is recommended 2 hours later, and food is proscribed for 4 to 5 hours.

Hernández Morales and Santiago Stevenson (1949) have reported considerable success in eradicating taenias after transduodenal intubation of crystalline hexylresorcinol in an emulsion.

Prevention consists in abstinence from

eating raw or rare beef (*T. saginata*), pork (*T. solium*) or fresh-water fish (*D. latum*), together with sanitary disposal of human excreta; more careful personal and group hygiene (*H. nana*), campaigns against domestic rats and mice (*H. diminuta*) and frequent disinfestation (by dusting with DDT) and de-worming (with arecoline hydrobromide) of dogs and cats, especially house pets (*D. caninum*).

ERNEST CARROLL FAUST

References

von Bonsdorff, B.: *Diphyllobothrium Latum* and Pernicious Anemia. Acta Med. Scandinav., 129, 142 and 213, 1947.

Dixon, H. B. F., and Smithers, D. W.: Epilepsy in Cysticercosis (*Taenia solium*). A Study of Seventy-one Cases. Quart. J. Med., 3:603, 1934.

Faust, E. C.: Human Helminthology. 3rd ed. Philadelphia, Lea & Febiger, 1949.

Hernández Morales, F.: The Treatment of Taenia Saginata with Atabrine. Puerto Rico J. Pub. Health & Trop. Med., 25:78, 1949.

Magath, T. B.: Factors Influencing the Geographical Distribution of *Diphyllobothrium latum*. Skrjabin Anniversary vol. (Moscow), 1937, p. 366.

Sodeman, W. A., and Jung, R. C.: Treatment of Teniases with Quinacrine Hydrochloride. J.A.M.A., *148*:285, 1952.

Wardle, R. A., and Green, N. K.: Tapeworm Anemia: The Influence of Tapeworm Fatty Acid Ingestion upon the Host Blood Picture. Tr. Roy. Soc. Canada, 3d Ser., Sec. V, 35:85, 1941.

VISCERAL AND SOMATIC CESTODIASIS

Under this group of diseases are included cysticercosis, cenurosis, echinococcosis (hydatid disease) and sparganosis.

CYSTICERCOSIS

Etiology. Cysticercosis is infection with the larval or bladder-worm stage of a species of *Taenia*. There are on record only 3 cases of cysticercosis of man referable to the beef tapeworm, *T. saginata;* in contrast, there are thousands of published clinical and necropsy reports of human cysticercosis cellulosae, due to the pork tapeworm, *T. solium*.

Life History. Man is an acceptable intermediate host of *T. solium*, as well as the only known definitive host of this worm. There are three possible methods by which man may acquire cysticercosis: (1) he may accidentally take into his mouth and swallow the eggs of *T. solium* passed in the stools of someone else harboring the intestinal worm; (2) he himself may harbor the intestinal worm and by anus-to-mouth contamination may ingest the eggs; (3) he himself may harbor the intestinal worm, and, by regurgitation, eggs discharged from gravid proglottids may be carried up into his stomach, then returned to his duodenum. Whatever the method by which the eggs reach the upper levels of the human small bowel, they may hatch and the embryos migrate through the bowel wall into the mesenteric venules or lymphatics. They are then carried to all tissues of the body, where they lodge and develop into cysticerci within three months. In man the cysticerci can develop in any soft body tissue, including muscle, subcutaneous layers, the heart valves, the orbit, and the ventricles, tissues or envelopes of the brain.

Symptoms and Morbid Anatomy. The presence of a few to hundreds of cysticerci in the subcutaneous tissues and somatic muscle produces only slight inconvenience and is essentially painless. On the heart valves, in the orbit or in the tissues of the brain or its envelopes, cysticerci provoke lesions which interfere with important functional processes. Possibly little damage may result in these foci until the larvae begin to die, whereupon there is an intense cellular infiltration in the area, at first inflammatory, later fibroblastic, in an attempt to wall off the irritating process. The most common site for these damaging lesions is within the eyeball or within the brain tissues, where it may provoke a jacksonian type of epilepsy. Approximately 10 per cent of patients who require brain surgery in Mexico are afflicted with cerebral cysticercosis (Mazzotti, 1944). Persons with subcutaneous or muscular cysticercosis usually develop epileptiform seizures as a result of concomitant cerebral cysticercosis.

Treatment and Prevention. There is no satisfactory treatment for most of these brain or eye cases, although occasionally it is possible to remove the intracranial tumor or intraocular parasite. Meticulous personal hygiene is indicated in areas where *Taenia solium* is prevalent.

Cenurosis. Related to cysticercosis is the rather rare condition of cenurosis, infection with the larval stage of certain tapeworms of the genus *Multiceps*. Usually the larvae develop in sheep, hogs, or rabbits, occasionally in man. One species, *Coenurus cerebralis,* localizes in the brain, with an invariably fatal outcome.

ECHINOCOCCOSIS
(*Hydatid Disease*)

Etiology. Echinococcosis, or hydatid disease, is caused by the larval stage (i.e., hydatid cyst) of the tapeworm *Echinococcus granulosus,* of which the dog is the common definitive host, and sheep, hogs, cattle and man the most usual intermediate hosts.

Life History. The mature worm is a minute organism which lives attached to villi or in the glandular crypts of the dog's small intestine. The gravid proglottid disintegrates, setting *Taenia*-like eggs free in the bowel lumen, so that they are evacuated in feces. Whenever these eggs contaminate food or drink, or otherwise get into the mouth of a susceptible mammal and are swallowed, they hatch in the duodenum and the six-hooked embryos gain entrance to the bowel wall. They reach the mesenteric venules or lymphatics and are filtered out in various foci.

Morbid Anatomy. In man 50 to 70 per cent of the organisms usually lodge in the liver, increasingly smaller percentages in the lungs, osseous tissues, brain and other tissues of the body. In Peru and Chile, however, the lungs and liver are equally involved. On reaching the site where the organisms are filtered out, the embryos transform slowly into minute vacuolated cysts; then, as they gradually increase in size, they are found to have an inner germinative membrane, an outer laminated layer, and usually a fibrous adventitious capsule. The cystic cavity is filled with hydatid fluid. The size of the cyst is limited only by its physical and mechanical confines. Thus, in five years or more a hepatic hydatid cyst may average from 5 to 25 cm. in diameter. From the germinative membrane multiple scolices or "heads" (*hydatid sand*) are produced and set free into the fluid-filled cavity. These scolices vacuolate and develop into daughter cysts. Such a mother cyst is viable and is termed "*unilocular.*"

At times the original implantation of the embryo is in a site mechanically incompatible with unilocular growth. Scolices from the germinative membrane then migrate through the laminated layer and reach the unconfined host tissue, through which they multiply and metastasize as *alveolar hydatids*. If the scolices reach the spongy tissue of bones, the organism develops as a syncytium, eroding its way as an *osseous hydatid*.

Endemic Regions. Echinococcosis is widely distributed over the face of the earth, but is particularly prevalent in sheep-raising countries. Human infection has an extensive distribution in Europe, the Near East, the U. S. S. R., China and Japan, the north coast of Africa, and South Africa. The disease is of greatest human importance in Argentina and Uruguay, in which countries it is a major public health problem. In the United States there were previously many case reports of hydatid cyst, mostly from immigrants from eastern Europe. Today the number is diminished, but several native-born patients are diagnosed each year and provide evidence of rather widespread endemic areas in the South, Middle West, Mountain States and California. Dogs usually become infected from eating the carcasses of sheep and hogs having the cystic stage.

Symptoms. If a unilocular hydatid cyst has become well walled off in an organ or tissue of the abdominal cavity, there is characteristically no train of symptoms for several years after exposure. Five years or more after implantation the growth of the cystic mass begins to cause pressure on the surrounding organs. Pulmonary echinococcosis may also produce a similar history and is almost invariably well encapsulated. Rupture of the cyst from pressure or a blow will spill the cyst contents into the patient's body cavities, possibly produce anaphylactic shock, and will usually allow scolices to become implanted on the nearby membranes. Osseous hydatid is commonest in long bones and the pelvis, proceeds as a protoplasmic stream, and invariably causes erosion and eventual fracture of the bone. Original cardiac or brain implantations may produce relatively early, frequently fatal episodes.

Diagnosis may be suggested by eosinophilia in patients with large tumor masses, especially of the abdomen. If intracystic "thrill" can be demonstrated, the evidence is more convincing. However, preoperative diagnosis is dependent on an immunologic reaction to specific antigen, as complement fixation, precipitin reaction or intracutaneous test. The Casoni skin test, using sterile hydatid fluid from human or sheep cysts, or the Dennis powdered concentrate, is the most practical method.

Prognosis depends on the site where the hydatid originally became implanted, the amount of its growth, its type, whether unilocular, alveolar or osseous, and the experience of the physician and surgeon. Alveolar hydatid invariably has a fatal termination, and repair of bone invaded by hydatid usually is unsatisfactory.

Treatment. There is no thoroughly tested nonsurgical method for reducing the lesion. Unilocular cysts are usually operable, even though 50 per cent recur. After the surgeon has incised the overlying tissues down to the site of the cyst, before the cyst wall is opened aspiration of the fluid contents and scolices is attempted through a trocar, and caution must be exercised not to spill the contents on the adjacent membranes. Then the cyst is opened and, if possible, completely enucleated. Failing this, its wall is scraped as thoroughly as possible, sterilized with several cubic centimeters of 10 per cent formalin, then washed out with physiologic salt solution, collapsed, and the operative cavity preferably closed, since open drainage prolongs recovery.

In the heavy endemic-enzootic areas of hydatid disease in Argentina, Uruguay, Chile and southern Brazil, *biotherapy* is being employed in cases with multiple or inoperable cysts. The method consists in using hydatid antigen in small but increasing amounts to desensitize the tissues and kill the parasite. This technique provides considerable promise for patients who otherwise have a very unfavorable outlook.

Prevention consists in keeping dogs from eating carcasses of sheep, hogs and other intermediate hosts (i.e., deep burying of dead animals); in keeping children away from dogs in endemic foci; in periodic deworming of dogs with arecoline hydrobromide; and in scrupulous care not to contaminate food, drink, or mess kits with dog's feces.

ERNEST CARROLL FAUST

References

Asenjo, A., and Bustamente, E.: Die neurochirurgische Behandlung der Cysticerkose. Deutsche med. Wchnschr., 75:1180, 1950.
Belleville, G. I.: Terapéutica Biológica de la Hidatidosis. Bol. Acad. Argent. Ciruj., 34:244, 1950.
Dixon, H. B. F., and Hargreaves, W. H.: Cysticercosis (*Taenia Solium*). A Further Ten Years'

Clinical Study Covering 284 Cases. Quart. J. Med., 13:107, 1944.
Johnstone, H. G., and Jones, O. W., Jr.: Cerebral Coenurosis in an Infant. Am. J. Trop. Med., 30:431, 1950.
Leche, Junior: Ocular Cysticercosis. Am. J. Ophthalm., 32:523, 1949.

SPARGANOSIS
(Sparganiasis)

Etiology. Sparganosis is due to infection with the second larval stage (*sparganum*) of certain species of *Diphyllobothrium* (not *D. latum*). Infection may be acquired from ingesting raw drinking water containing species of water "fleas" (*Cyclops*) harboring the first larval stage, but is more commonly contracted from eating raw, infected flesh of frogs, snakes, birds or mammals or application of the parasitized tissues to an injured, inflamed or ulcerated site. This disease is prevalent throughout many countries of the Far East, but has been described occasionally from other parts of the world, including the United States. Ocular sparganosis is a common affliction in the Orient. Surgical removal of the larva is the indicated treatment. In endemic foci, boiled or filtered drinking water will preclude ingestion of infected *Cyclops*. Native peoples should be taught the dangers of applying fresh flesh poultices to injured members of their bodies.

ERNEST CARROLL FAUST

References

Faust, E. C.: Human Helminthology. 3rd ed., Philadelphia, Lea & Febiger, 1949.
Weinstein, P. O., Krawzyk, H. J., and Peers, J. H.: Sparganosis in Korea. Am. J. Trop. Med. & Hyg., 3:112, 1954.

THE NEMATODA
(Roundworms)

NEMATODA (true roundworms or nematodes) are unsegmented, frequently cylindroidal invertebrates, with a cuticle which may be smooth, but is at times provided with spines or hooklets, particularly around the mouth. There is a complete digestive tract. The sex organs are greatly elaborated and occupy the major part of the body cavity. Most nematodes are oviparous, but a few are larviparous. Some eggs are fully embryonated when laid; others require a period of incubation outside

the human body. Some eggs hatch in the soil, grow and metamorphose into infective-stage larvae. Some nematodes require an intermediate host for completion of their larval development. Man acquires most nematode infections by the oral route, but hookworm and *Strongyloides* larvae actively invade the skin, and filaria larvae gain entrance into the skin after escape from their blood-sucking insect hosts.

The following important nematode infections of man will be considered here: trichinosis, trichocephaliasis, strongyloidiasis, creeping eruption, ascariasis, oxyuriasis, filariasis, dracunculosis and hookworm disease.

ERNEST CARROLL FAUST

TRICHINOSIS

(Trichiniasis, Trichinelliasis)

Definition. Trichinosis is an infestation of striated muscle by the larvae of the roundworm, *Trichinella spiralis*. It is transmitted by inadequately cooked food and represents the greatest uncontrolled public health problem in this country.

Etiology. Live, encysted larvae of the parasite are ingested in meat. After being liberated by protein digestion they anchor themselves to the mucosa of the duodenum and jejunum, from which they extract oxygen and liquid food. Within the next two days they develop into sexually mature adults— the males 1.5 mm. and the females 3 to 4 mm. in length. After copulation the male may die, but the female burrows deeper into the mucosa. The eggs develop and hatch *in utero*. About 1500 larvae (which are 100 microns in length) are discharged through the vulva in the anterior fifth of the body into the lymphatics and lacteals of the host's small intestine, at the rate of one each half hour over a period of approximately six weeks; the female then dies.

Epidemiology and Prevention. The parasite exhibits no specificity for species and can infect a wide variety of carnivorous and herbivorous animals. The chief reservoir for human infection is swine. The incidence of infestation in hogs fed on grain or allowed to root in the field is about 0.5 per cent, but in those fed on uncooked garbage it is in the range of 5 per cent. The meat becomes infectious within seventeen days after the pig ingests the parasite.

The epidemics which occur are small and are usually confined to a family or group which has held a picnic or barbecue. Infection may follow the tasting of raw pork, as in the preparation of sausage. In meat products prepared commercially from the pooled muscles of many hogs the infected sample is so diluted that the infestation in any given person is light, though it may be spread among many people. Only about 70 per cent

of the pork raised in this country is processed in plants which are under close supervision; hence a large part of the country's total supply of pork products may carry live parasites. As much as 10 per cent of the sausage in large city markets has been found infected. It has been estimated that each American consumes three servings of trichinous pork in a year. The cysts do not calcify in pork and are almost invisible to the naked eye; hence they are not looked for in the government inspection of meat. No economically feasible technique for detecting trichinella infection in hogs by anatomic or immunologic methods has been developed.

Autopsy studies indicate that approximately 16 per cent of the human population is infected; this incidence is the same in both sexes. The fact that the number and density of infections are greater in older patients suggests many separate invasions of the body by a small number of parasites. The greater prevalence of the disease in the Midwest and other areas where Germans and Italians have settled reflects local customs in the preparation of food.

All the basic scientific facts necessary for complete prevention of the disease in human beings have been known for years. Trichinae can be killed by cooking or irradiation. Smoking, pickling and other methods of processing or preserving meat do not kill the parasite. Pork should be cooked at a minimum temperature of 140° F. for at least thirty minutes per pound; otherwise large roasts may not be completely done in the center. Freezing of meat at 0° F. (−18° C.) for at least 24 hours, or at 5° F. (−15° C.) for twenty days, will usually kill all trichinae. These preventive measures are effective and their general use has been shown by autopsy studies to reduce the incidence of human infection.

Pathogenesis and Morbid Anatomy. Invasion of the intestine by the adult parasite produces little local reaction. About the seventh day the larvae enter the general circulation and are widely distributed to all tissues; they then break out of capillaries between muscle fibers and penetrate into serous cavities and even into the cerebrospinal fluid. In initial infections, invasion of striated muscle fibers produces necrosis, hyaline degeneration and an inflammatory response consisting of polymorphonuclear neutrophils, lymphocytes and variable numbers of eosinophils. The reaction of the body produces around the coiled trichina a cyst which begins to calcify between six and eighteen months after invasion, and in which the larvae may live for ten years or more.

The heaviest infestation occurs near the tendinous portion of the diaphragm, of the gluteus, pectoral, deltoid, gastrocnemius or intercostal muscles, in that order of frequency. The extraocular muscles, the masseters and the muscles of the larynx may also be involved. The heart is invaded, but the parasite seems unable to establish itself in cardiac or smooth muscle.

In approximately four fifths of the human infections proved at autopsy, less than ten trichinae per gram of muscle are present— a degree of infection which probably produces few symptoms. In some cases, however, as many as 1000 trichinae per gram of muscle may be found.

In reinfections the muscle walls of arterioles may show degenerative and inflammatory changes similar to those seen in serum sickness and periarteritis nodosa—a finding which suggests an allergic or immune reaction. The fatty change found in the liver in fatal cases probably results from inadequate intake of protective foods. The renal tubules occasionally show degenerative changes which are reflected clinically by albuminuria. The bone marrow shows hyperplasia, chiefly in eosinophilic myelocytes.

Pathologic Physiology and Chemistry. The mechanism responsible for the development of edema is obscure. The number of capillaries mechanically ruptured is inadequate to explain it, and production of a toxin by the parasite or by the destruction of muscle has never been demonstrated. Measurements of the fluid space in animals indicate that the increased permeability of capillary walls and of cells may result from an immune reaction.

In some instances the blood chlorides and total serum proteins (particularly the albumin fraction) are decreased and the nonprotein nitrogen is elevated.

In cases with neurologic involvement, the cerebrospinal fluid may contain erythrocytes and increased amounts of protein.

Symptoms. The symptoms are highly variable and depend largely upon the degree of infection. If the meat is heavily infected, the *invasion* of the intestinal mucosa one to four days after ingestion may cause local irritation, producing symptoms of nausea, vomiting and diarrhea which resemble those of "food poisoning." In other cases these symptoms may be entirely absent.

Beginning on the seventh day, the *migration* of the larvae usually produces muscular weakness, stiffness or pain, accompanied by remittent fever which may reach 104° F. (40° C.)—a rare finding in disease caused by larger parasites. The fever may persist for several weeks and usually drops by lysis. The elevation of temperature, as well as occasional transient skin rashes, probably results from the liberation of foreign protein, since a large number of larvae are destroyed during their migration. Depending upon the muscles invaded, the patient may note backache which resembles that of influenza, or pain on chewing, swallowing, breathing, or moving the eyes or limbs.

Next to the muscular symptoms edema is the most common finding; it may appear at any time after invasion. Edema is most frequently manifested as puffiness around the eyes involving the upper lids, though it may be generalized. Many of the protean manifestations of the disease result from the involvement of arterioles and from the edema. Symptoms in the central nervous system, such as headache, delirium and psychic or visual disturbances suggest encephalitis, but are usually transient. Hemiplegia or localized paralysis occasionally occurs and may be permanent. Dyspnea may result from the edema and from invasion of the muscles of respiration. The great variety of symptoms, the variation in their intensity, and the lack of regularity in the course are characteristic of trichinosis.

After *encystment* the only symptom may be vague aching in the muscles.

Diagnosis. A *clinical* diagnosis is extremely difficult to make except in cases of heavy infection. The early gastroenteritis is nonspecific. The most useful physical signs are tenderness to pressure on the muscles; edema, especially about the eyes; the splinter hemorrhages under the nails or in the conjunctivas. Only a fraction of the cases are recognized and reported.

Laboratory methods are helpful for confirmation of the diagnosis, but are of little aid in therapy. If a portion of the suspected meat can be obtained, it should be ground in a household meat chopper and digested in hydrochloric acid and pepsin. After the suspension has been digested for an hour, several portions are examined for larvae by means of a dissecting microscope.

Examination of the stools for adult worms is useless. During the stage of migration, larvae can occasionally be found in the centrifuged blood.

Beginning ten days after infection, the larvae may be found in biopsy specimens removed from the tendinous insertion of the deltoid or gastrocnemius muscle. One gram of the unfixed muscle should be spread between two pieces of plate glass measuring roughly 18 by 12 by 0.6 cm., compressed with screw clamps, and examined under the low power microscope. During the second or third week the larvae may be parallel to muscle fibers and are sometimes difficult to recognize. After encystment they can hardly be confused with anything else. The samples removed at biopsy are usually too small to examine by the digestion technique. Routine methods of cutting and staining microscopic preparations rarely detect the parasite and show only a myositis.

The simplest diagnostic procedure is the intradermal skin test, performed by injecting 0.1 cc. of a 1:10,000 dilution of dried, powdered trichinae dissolved in saline. A positive reaction is usually not obtained before the end of the third week of the infection. The skin reaction may be immediate (wheal) or delayed (tuberculin) in type. Many false positive tests are obtained; some are group cross reactions due to infestations with closely related parasites (such as *Trichuris,* the whipworm), but the significance of most is unknown. The skin test usually remains positive for about seven years.

Immunologic tests made on the patient's serum after the third week of the disease, and utilizing the precipitin, complement fixation or flocculation techniques, are more specific, but may not be positive in an overwhelming infection. Involvement of the reticuloendothelial system, particularly with Hodgkin's disease, may give rise to false positive reactions. The most accurate serologic reaction uses living trichinella larvae suspended in the patient's serum; a highly refractive precipitate forms around the worm. This mechanism probably explains how most of the ingested living larvae are prevented from penetrating the intestinal mucosa in reinfections. The serologic tests revert to negative after a year.

In acute infections caused by a moderate number of parasites the eosinophils in the peripheral blood will begin to increase ten days after infection, reaching a peak in the third or fourth week. The proportion of eosinophils may vary from 5 to 70 per cent, and the total leukocyte count is usually between 10,000 and 20,000 per cubic millimeter. The eosinophilia precedes the development of positive skin or serologic reactions, but may be present in severe infections or suppressed by a simultaneous bacterial infection. In subclinical or very mild cases the eosinophil count is of no diagnostic value. Eosinophilia may persist for five to seven years.

Reversible changes in the T waves may be detected by electrocardiograms after the second week of the disease.

Prognosis. In subclinical or mild infections the prognosis is excellent; in small epidemics the mortality may vary from 5 to 30 per cent. The over-all mortality must be low, since few patients in whom the infestation is detected at autopsy have had clinical symptoms suggestive of the disease. In individual cases the ultimate prognosis is poor if symptoms, particularly pronounced diarrhea, develop within two day of exposure or if little evidence of immune response can be detected by eosinophil counts, skin tests or serologic reactions. Most patients who die succumb to pneumonia or cachexia between the fourth and sixth weeks.

Treatment. No specific treatment is known. If the parasite can be demonstrated in the suspected meat while the patient is still having gastrointestinal symptoms, administration of an anthelmintic such as three gelatin capsules containing 1 cc. of tetrachlorethylene (which is also effective in related parasitic infestations), followed in four hours by a saline purge, may remove some of the adult worms.

No drug has been found effective against the larvae. After encystment of the parasite has begun, the damage is done.

In human cases and in experimental animals, the administration of corticotropin (ACTH) or cortisone has reduced the acute manifestations of the disease. The benefit probably results from suppression of host response to the presence of the parasite or its products. The dose and duration of hormone therapy must be carefully adjusted to the individual case.

Because of the tendency to hypoproteinemia, a high protein diet is probably of some value in supportive therapy. In very heavy infections, with severe symptoms and marked edema, caution should be exercised in the administration of crystalloids such as glucose and saline. Infusions may be necessary to overcome dehydration, but unless the intravascular osmotic pressure is maintained with plasma or human serum albumin, circulatory collapse may be produced by fluid replacement therapy.

The muscular aching may require the intermittent administration of analgesics such as salicylates. It is possible that the administration of antihistamine drugs from the second to the fifth week might reduce the allergic manifestations of the disease.

GEORGE T. HARRELL

References

Beard, R. R.: Incidence of Trichinella Infections in San Francisco, 1950. J.A.M.A., *146*:331, 1951.

Gomberg, H. J., and Gould, S. E.: Effect of Irradiation with Cobalt-60 on Trichina Larvae. Science, *118*:75, 1953.

Gould, S. E.: Trichinosis. Springfield, Illinois, Charles C Thomas, 1945.

Harrell, G. T., and Horne, S. F.: Trichinella Skin Tests in Tuberculosis Sanatoriums, Hospitals for Mental Diseases, and General Hospitals. Am. J. Trop. Med., 25:51, 1945.

Luongo, M. A., Reid, D. H., and Weiss, W. W.: The Effect of ACTH in Trichinosis. New England J. Med., *245*:757, 1951.

Skinner, J. C.: Neurologic Complications of Trichinosis. Report of Two Cases. New England J. Med., 238:317, 1948.

Southam, C. M., Thomason, A. E., and Burchenal, J. H.: False Positive Trichina Precipitin Reactions in Neoplastic Disease. Pro. Soc. Exper. Biol. & Med., 72:354, 1949.

Spink, W. W.: Cardiovascular Complications of Trichinosis. Arch. Int. Med., 56:238, 1935.

TRICHOCEPHALIASIS

(Trichuriasis, Whipworm Infection)

Etiology. This is an infection with the whipworm, *Trichocephalus trichiurus* (synonym, *Trichuris trichiura*), and involves primarily the cecum and appendix.

Life History. The adult worms have a delicate threadlike anterior half and a fleshy posterior half. The females have a club-shaped posterior extremity, the males a flatly spiralled posterior end. The anterior end of the worm is inserted or basted into the mucous membrane of the parasitized level of the bowel wall. In light infections the worms are characteristically confined to the level of the cecum and appendix; in heavy infections (i.e., several hundred worms) they extend throughout the colon and at times into the rectum. The female lays daily a few thousand radially symmetrical, barrel-shaped eggs,

which are usually bile stained and have a blister-like "plug" at each pole. These eggs are unembryonated when evacuated in feces. On moist, shaded, warm earth they develop in ten to fourteen days or more to the infective stage. Upon being swallowed they hatch in the duodenum. The emerging larvae slowly migrate down to the cecum or appendix, become attached, and in about three months after ingestion develop to the adult stage. The infection is relatively cosmopolitan in all except cold climates, but is dependent on moist, shaded earth for the extrinsic incu-

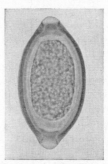

Fig. 54. Egg of *Trichocephalus trichiurus*. × 666. (Photomicrograph after Faust in Brennemann's Practice of Pediatrics, courtesy of W. F. Prior Co.)

bation of the eggs. Heavy infections are most frequent in the moist tropics, but are not infrequent in the coastal areas of the southern United States. Children are more commonly exposed than are adults.

Symptoms. Mild infections (i.e., with low worm burden) seldom produce a distinct train of symptoms. Nevertheless, children are occasionally intolerant of whipworms even in small numbers, as indicated by an eosinophilia of 8 to 25 per cent, loss of appetite, insomnia, nervousness, loss of weight, urticaria and, rarely, convulsions. The entire colon may be raw and inflamed, irritable, and the surface covered with excess mucus, blood and necrotic epithelial cells. In patients who have several worms attached to the rectum there is frequently a prolapse. At times, in heavy infections (i.e., several hundred worms) the clinical picture simulates that of severe hookworm disease.

Diagnosis of trichocephaliasis depends on the recovery of the characteristic eggs in the feces of the patient. Concentration techniques, as with brine or zinc sulfate centrifugal flotation, may be required to apprehend eggs in mild infections. Prognosis is good, except in heavy infections or those to which children show marked intolerance to the parasite.

Treatment. Probably the most efficient available treatment consists in the administration of 2.7 cc. of tetrachlorethylene combined with 0.3 cc. of oil of chenopodium (adult dose). The medication should be preceded by sodium sulfate purgation and a high retention enema of tepid physiologic salt solution, followed by sodium sulfate purgation.

In case there is extensive involvement of the colon and rectum the worms at the lower levels of the large bowel may be removed by several retention enemas of hexylresorcinol (1 gm. in 300 cc. of a 10 per cent mucilage of acacia), using 500 to 1000 cc. for each administration. With removal of these worms the tone of the bowel wall greatly improves and prolapse of the rectum can usually be corrected. Should the enema produce intense colonic cramps, the enema should be rapidly evacuated and the colon washed out with tepid water or physiologic salt solution.

Prevention consists in care not to contaminate food, drink or fingers with soil containing embryonated eggs.

ERNEST CARROLL FAUST

References

Basnuevo, J.: Recientes Adquisiciones en la Clínica y en la Terapéutica de la Tricocefaliasis Infantil. Rev. Kuba, 8:4, 1952.
Faust, E. C.: Human Helminthology. 3rd ed. Philadelphia, Lea & Febiger, 1949.
Jung, R. C., and Beaver, P. C.: Clinical Observations on *Trichocephalus Trichiurus* (Whipworm) Infestation in Children. Pediatrics, 8:548, 1952.

STRONGYLOIDIASIS

(Strongyloidosis)

Etiology. Strongyloidiasis is produced by *Strongyloides stercoralis,* a delicate threadworm which exhibits capacities for complete parasitic existence on the one hand and complete free-living existence on the other.

Life History. The adult parasitic worms are primarily parasites of the intestinal tract. The parasitic male, when found, is tenuously attached to the mucous membrane of the bowel, predominantly at the level of the duodenum. The delicate threadlike female is typically buried in the mucosa of the bowel wall, most commonly at the level of the duodenum, but heavy infections may extend from the pyloric wall of the stomach to the anus. Within the mucous membrane these worms lay partially embryonated eggs resembling those of the hookworms. Embryonation is completed in the glands and villi of the bowel,

and hatching takes place here. The escaping first-stage (i.e., rhabditoid) larvae burrow out to the lumen of the bowel, and are passed down and evacuated in feces. If the feces are deposited on wet, shaded, sandy humus in a favorably warm climate, the rhabditoid larvae feed, grow, and metamorphose into postfeeding *filariform larvae,* which are the infective stage.

Endemic Regions. Strongyloidiasis is apparently coincident with hookworm infection over the face of the globe, being most prevalent in the moist tropics. Strongyloidiasis is rather widely prevalent throughout rural areas in the southern United States, and autochthonous cases have been sporadically reported from regions as far north as central New York State and southern Canada. There are no important reservoirs of this infection.

Morbid Anatomy. On contact with exposed human skin, the larvae penetrate under the epidermis and down to the cutaneous blood capillaries. On gaining entry to the afferent blood vessels, the organisms are carried through the chambers of the right heart to the lungs. They burrow out of the pulmonary capillaries into the air sacs, slowly migrate up the respiratory tree, crawl over the epiglottis and are swallowed. Meanwhile they have grown in size, have become adolescent and, by the time they have reached the level of the duodenum, have become sexually differentiated. Within twenty-eight days after skin exposure, egg laying begins. Should larvae be blocked in the air sacs or bronchioles by cellular infiltration, the worms continue to grow in these sites, and the females may burrow into the bronchial epithelium and establish foci of infection there. This type of life cycle is referred to as the *direct mode of development.*

In favorable warm climates, however, the rhabditoid larvae evacuated in human stools onto moist ground develop into free-living rhabditoid adults, which mate, lay eggs and continue through one or more free-living generations. Eventually, however, filariform larvae are produced and the parasitic phase is again established. This alternation of parasitic and free-living cycles is the *indirect mode of development.*

A third type of development is *auto-infection.* In some patients, usually chronically infected with *Strongyloides,* rhabditoid larvae in transit down the bowel, or lodged in moist feces on the perianal skin, become transformed into filariform larvae and are enabled to penetrate the mucous membrane of the intestine or the perianal skin, and thus initiate superinfection without having left the host. Moreover, at times rhabditoid larvae metamorphose into filariform larvae without leaving the intestinal mucosa. However, all larvae must make a "lung journey" before they can mature in the intestinal wall.

Pathology. The characteristic pathology produced by *Strongyloides stercoralis* consists of trauma due to the slow migration of the parasitic female in the intestinal mucosa, the escape of eggs into the glands and stroma and the burrowing of hatched rhabditoid larvae. The usual cellular reaction is an infiltration of polymorphonuclear and eosinophilic leukocytes around the worms. Irritation of the mucosal cells causes a mucositis, and from time to time little patches of necrotic mucosa are sloughed off, leaving denuded areas. If the infection is extensive, a mucous, watery diarrhea may alternate with constipation and be reactivated at times of dietary indiscretions or overexertion. In heavy infections dehydration may be extreme.

Symptoms. Epigastric pain is the most common subjective symptom. There is a hypereosinophilia (up to 40 per cent or more) with leukocytosis during the acute stage, followed by a leukopenia with a somewhat reduced eosinophilia. As the chronic stage develops, larvae are fewer in the stools and more difficult to discover. Meanwhile the patient tends to become toxic, and suffers dull headaches and periods of despondency. Although the parasitic females presumably live for only a year or two, patients who have been studied by the writer over more than 25 years have had persistent infection in spite of the impossibility of a new external source of inoculation.

In addition to the intestinal lesions there are those due to lodgment of larvae and their development in the bronchial epithelium. This results in bronchial irritation, production of bronchial mucus containing necrotic tissue cells and polymorphonuclear leukocytes, and paroxysmal, relatively nonproductive cough, with blood-tinged sputum.

Diagnosis consists in the discovery of typical rhabditoid larvae, occasionally filariform larvae, usually in loose or diarrheic stools, in duodenal drainage, or at times in sputum. These must be differentiated from similar stages of hookworm, which may develop in feces left standing in the diagnostic laboratory. The **prognosis** is fair to good in mild early cases given the benefit of specific therapy; poor to grave in severe cases left untreated. Absence of eosinophilia is a poor prognostic sign.

Treatment consists in the adequate administration of gentian violet medicinal, first advocated in the United States by the author in 1930. For the average adult case 0.06 gm. is given with meals three times daily (two 0.03 gm. Seal-Ins, 1½-hr. coating) until 3.0 gm. have been taken. One or two such courses of treatment produce cure in about 90 per cent of *Strongyloides* patients who have recently acquired the infection. For refractive cases and those which develop intestinal colic from taking the enteric-coated tablets, transduodenal intubation of 25 cc. of a 1 per cent solution of the drug is effective. The rationale of treatment consists in the deep staining of the mucous membrane of the intestine, particularly that of the duodenum (hence 1½-hr. coating), down to the muscularis mucosae, to reach all the worms. Sometime during the administration of the enteric-coated tablets and after transduodenal intubation, nausea and vomiting may be expected. If pulmonary strongyloidiasis occurs, intravenous injection of 0.5 per cent solution of filtered gentian violet medicinal may be given to hospitalized patients in amounts not to exceed 20 cc. each every alternate day for one month. Even when the drug is introduced slowly into the vein, one may expect a temporary increase in temperature and palpitation of the heart. As a precaution against hyperinfection, constipation should be combated by adequate catharsis.

Prevention consists in care not to walk barefooted or otherwise expose the skin to polluted soil; in the sanitary disposal of human feces; and in adequate treatment of detected cases until they have been cured.

ERNEST CARROLL FAUST

References

Faust, E. C.: Human Helminthology. 3rd ed. Philadelphia, Lea & Febiger, 1949.
Jones, C. A.: Clinical Studies in Human Strongyloidiasis. I. Semeiology. Gastroenterology, *16:* 743, 1950.
Napier, L. E.: *Strongyloides Stercoralis* Infection. Part II. Strongyloidiasis Among Ex-Prisoners-of-War. J. Trop. Med. & Hyg., 52:46, 1949.
Palmer, E. D.: A Note on the Treatment of Strongyloidiasis with Gentian Violet. Am. J. Trop. Med., 30:91, 1950.

CREEPING ERUPTION

(Cutaneous Larva Migrans)

Etiology. Creeping eruption is a dermatitis produced by invasion into the deeper layers of the skin by nematode or fly larvae, which continue to migrate for weeks or months through serpiginous tunnels in the stratum germinativum. Among the nematode larvae the hookworm *Ancylostoma braziliense* is most commonly incriminated, but those of other species of hookworms and of *Strongyloides stercoralis* at times produce similar lesions. Filariform larvae of canine and feline strains of *A. braziliense,* on contact with human skin, are unable to negotiate an entry into the cutaneous blood vessels, but progress intracutaneously at the rate of several millimeters to a few centimeters a day, producing an inflamed, elevated tunnel which becomes vesicular and frequently is complicated by invasion of pathogenic bacteria. There is an intense pruritus of the involved area, almost invariably provoking scratching and allowing bacterial and mycotic invasion of the scarified skin as well as the tunnels. This infection is distributed throughout the coastal areas of the southeastern and Gulf States, especially in Florida, but occurs elsewhere in warm climates. The foot is most frequently involved, but any other area which comes in contact with moist sandy soil where *A. braziliense*-infected dogs or cats have previously defecated is readily subject to infection.

Another nematode whose larvae cause creeping eruption is *Gnathostoma spinigerum,* with a distribution in the Orient. The lesions of gnathostomiasis may be similar to those described for *A. braziliense* or may be more like cutaneous abscesses.

Creeping eruption produced by fly larvae (i.e., *maggots*) is a dermal myiasis due primarily to skin invasion by maggots of the horse bot, *Gasterophilus.* Other species of maggots, such as *Hypoderma bovis, H. lineatum* and *Dermatobia hominis,* are more likely to bore down more deeply into the subcutaneous tissues. Eggs are laid on the human skin, hatch, and the maggots penetrate down to the stratum germinativum or corium, then travel in this layer for weeks or months like *A. braziliense* larvae. Differential diagnosis can readily be made by massaging the involved site with clear machine oil. If numerous black bands (of spines) are seen with a hand lens, the agent is *Gasterophilus;* otherwise most likely it is *A. braziliense.* Prognosis is good if secondary infection with bacteremia is avoided.

Treatment. Recommended treatment for *A. braziliense* creeping eruption is the application of ethyl chloride spray to freeze the site at the inner end of the tunnel where the larva resides, or combining this topical therapy with systemic medication. For *Gasterophilus,* the treatment consists in removing the larva with a sterile sharp needle and dressing the wound with mild antiseptic bandages; for *Gnathostoma,* radical enucleation. Where pyogenic infection of the wound has developed, topical application of an appropriate antimicrobial ointment or powder might be useful.

Prevention. Control of creeping eruption of hookworm origin consists in avoiding skin contact with sites where dogs or cats have defecated. For *Gasterophilus,* intensive campaigns to eliminate horse flies should be instituted. Human infection with *Gnathostoma* is due primarily to eating raw fish or other flesh containing the larval stage of this worm.

ERNEST CARROLL FAUST

References

Caplan, J. P.: Creeping Eruption and Intestinal Strongyloidiasis. Brit. Med. J., *1*:396, 1949.
Daengsvang, S.: Human Gnathostomiasis in Siam with Reference to the Method of Prevention. J. Parasitol., 35:116, 1949.
Hitch, J. M.: Systemic Treatment of Creeping Eruption. Arch. Dermat. & Syph., *55*:664, 1947.
Kirby-Smith, J. L.: The Treatment of Creeping Eruption. South. M. J., *28*:999, 1935.

ASCARIASIS

Etiology. Ascariasis is produced by the giant intestinal roundworm, *Ascaris lumbricoides,* which inhabits the lumen of the small bowel. The worm is elongate and cylindroidal, and tapers bluntly at the anterior end and to a moderately sharp point posteriorly. The males average 15 to 31 cm. in length by 2 to 4 mm. in diameter; the females, 20 to 35 cm. by 3 to 6 mm. The male is curved ventrally at the posterior extremity.

Life History. Each female lays up to 200,000 eggs a day. These may be infertile or fertile. The former are more elongated and have a disorganized mass of granules and globules completely filling the inner shell. The fertile eggs are broadly ovoidal, and have a spherical, heavily granular, unsegmented egg cell, a thick, hyaline inner shell and a thick, mammillated, usually bile-stained outer shell. When evacuated in human feces onto the ground, they proceed to embryonate and in nine days or more will contain a motile rhabditoid larva coiled inside. In another week this unhatched larva sheds its cuticle and now becomes infective but does not hatch. It remains infective for months and possibly years within its shell. Only direct sun's rays or heat will kill the embryonating or infective-stage egg. When human beings pick up these mature eggs on their fingers or otherwise get them into their mouths and swallow them, the eggs hatch in the duodenum or jejunum, and the emergent larvae enter the intestinal wall and make their way to the lungs via the mesenteric lymphatics or venules, vena cava, right heart and pulmonary arteries. They break out of the pulmonary capillaries into the air sacs, migrate up the respiratory tree, crawl over the epiglottis, are swallowed and in sixty to seventy-five days after exposure become adult worms in the lumen of the small intestine.

Endemic Regions. Ascariasis is cosmopolitan in its distribution, but is more prevalent in warm than in cold climates. Its epidemiology differs materially from that of hookworm disease or oxyuriasis. The soil is "seeded" with *Ascaris* eggs passed in feces of infected persons. Primarily this is the result of promiscuous defecation by small children in and around the home (Cort). These same children and their associates later on become exposed to new infections when they pick up eggs that have become fully embryonated. Thus infection in an environment tends to become endemic, and infected persons may harbor adult egg-laying *Ascaris* and young worms in the intestine, as well as larvae en route through the lungs.

Morbid Anatomy. The first important lesions produced in ascariasis are in the lungs, because of the breaking out of the migrating larvae from the pulmonary capillaries into the air sacs. These rhabditoid larvae are considerably more robust than migrating larvae of hookworms and *Strongyloides,* and produce more trauma and hemorrhage, at times resulting in an atypical pneumonia, especially in small children. During the lung migration the larvae also produce host sensitization, and this commonly results in allergic manifestations such as bronchial asthma, which differs from Loeffler's syndrome and tropical eosinophilia. In the small bowel, adolescent and adult ascarids may produce no apparent

disturbance, even when present in moderate numbers. The worms will be passed spontaneously or die within the bowel in approximately a year's time. Digestive upsets or other abnormal conditions within the bowel frequently irritate these worms and provoke activities hazardous to the patient. They may be regurgitated and vomited, escape through the external nares, or rarely be inhaled into a bronchus; they may block the common bile duct or the appendiceal lumen, setting up acute inflammatory processes, or may perforate the intestinal wall and initiate peritonitis. They may cause acute abdominal symptoms, intussusception or paralytic ileus. The most common complaint in *Ascaris* patients is intestinal colic. Rarely the worms have been found in the parenchyma of the liver and in the pleural cavity. Not infrequently in small children knotted masses of worms produce acute obstruction of the bowel and require immediate surgical intervention. Even when the worms cause little or no traumatic damage, the by-products of living or dead worms may produce marked "toxic" manifestations, such as edema of the face and giant urticaria, accompanied by insomnia, loss of appetite and weight, extreme nervousness and, in extreme cases, cachexia. Moreover, it has been convincingly demonstrated that *Ascaris*-children, like hookworm-children, are mentally retarded. A moderate eosinophilia may be expected; otherwise the blood picture is not materially altered.

Diagnosis is made by the recovery of the eggs of *Ascaris lumbricoides* in human feces. Usually fertile eggs will be found along with some infertile ones, but when female worms alone are present only infertile eggs will be found. In about 5 per cent of infections only males are present, and diagnosis must be tentatively based on symptoms until a therapeutic test has been made. The spontaneous passage of one or more worms by anus or mouth does not necessarily mean that additional worms are present. This can be verified by stool examination two or three days after the worms have been evacuated.

Prognosis is good except in patients in whom obstruction or grave traumatic injury has been produced by the worms.

Treatment is best accomplished by the administration of hexylresorcinol crystoids (Crystoids anthelmintic), which has a 90 to 95 per cent worm removal rate for *Ascaris.*

After pretreatment purgation the night before with 30 gm. of sodium sulfate dissolved in a glass of water, the drug is administered in one dose in the morning on an empty stomach, in hard gelatin capsules of 0.1 or 0.2 gm. size. For children of preschool age the dosage is 0.4 to 0.6 gm.; for children from 6 to 10 years, 0.8 gm.; for older children and adults, 1 gm. The patient is required to swallow the capsules without chewing them, to prevent superficial irritation of the buccal mucosa. Food is proscribed for 4 to 5 hours, and a post-treatment purge of sodium sulfate is given 2 hours after the drug, to evacuate dead and dying worms as soon as possible and thus prevent absorption of their "toxic" products. In patients suffering from diarrhea the pretreatment and post-treatment purges should be omitted. An alternative prescription, which is valuable in combined infections of Ascaris with hookworms or Trichocephalus, is the following: tetrachlorethylene, 2.7 cc.; oleum chenopodii, 0.3 cc. in 0.5 cc. capsules or on a teaspoon with sugar. Pretreatment sodium sulfate purgation the night before, administration of the anthelmintic on an empty stomach, and post-treatment sodium sulfate purgation are indicated. For children, the dosage is 0.18 cc. per year of age up to 15 years.

These prescriptions are eminently satisfactory for intestinal ascariasis. During migration of Ascaris larvae through the lungs and for ectopic infections there is no specific chemotherapeutic procedure. Physicians are requested to be "Ascaris-conscious" in cases of atypical pneumonias, especially in children in Ascaris communities.

Prevention constitutes an integral part of the protection of human beings against the possible dangers of Ascaris infection, since successful treatment of individual cases does not prevent reinfection from the same "seed beds" where infective-stage eggs are planted. Children must be taught to use sanitary toilets or privies on all occasions, and must be warned of the dangers of contaminating fingers, candy or play objects with soil. Heavily infested ground around the house should either be treated with live steam (70° C. for 5 minutes is lethal for Ascaris eggs) or spaded up and the top soil turned under. Ascariasis in hogs is not a source of human infection, since human and porcine strains are physiologically distinct.

ERNEST CARROLL FAUST

References

Beaver, P. C.: The Detection and Identification of Some Common Nematode Parasites of Man. Am. J. Clin. Path., 22:481, 1952.
Cort, W. W.: Recent Investigations on the Epidemiology of Ascariasis. J. Parasitol., 17:121, 1931.
Headlee, W. H.: The Epidemiology of Human Ascariasis in the Metropolitan Area of New Orleans, Louisiana Am. J. Hyg., 24:479, 1936.
Lamson, P. D., Brown, W. H., and Ward, C. B.: Anthelmintics; Some Therapeutic and Practical Considerations of Their Use. J.A.M.A., 99:295, 1932.
Milwidsky, H.: The Surgical Complications of Ascariasis. Acta Med. Orient., 4:370, 1945.

VISCERAL LARVA MIGRANS

Only during recent years has this clinical entity become recognized and the *etiology* confirmed by biopsy and at necropsy. The causative agents are nematode larvae poorly adapted to development in the human body. The most common of these is the dog ascarid, *Toxocara canis,* but the cat ascarid, *T. felis,* may also be involved and possibly other roundworms which have a required migration through the lungs. When human beings, usually dirt-eating small children, ingest infective-stage eggs of these nematodes, hatching occurs in the duodenum and the freed larvae proceed to burrow into the intestinal wall enroute to the lungs. Almost invariably they are trapped in the liver or other viscera by host-cell infiltration, with the development of a granuloma around each larva. Clinical manifestations consist of hepatitis, eosinophilia for several months, and fever. Similar lesions around larval nematodes have been found in the eyeball and rarely in the brain. Hepatic larval granulomas usually have a favorable prognosis. Ophthalmic involvement requires removal of the eye. Cerebral infection has a relatively poor prognosis. *Diagnosis* is made presumptively on the symptoms, confirmed by biopsy or at autopsy. *Treatment* is nonspecific. *Control* consists in the teaching of better personal hygiene in small children and periodic deworming of dogs and cats.

ERNEST CARROLL FAUST

References

Milburn, C. L., and Ernst, K. F.: Eosinophilia-Hepatomegaly Syndrome of Infants and Young Children. Pediatrics, 11:358, 1953.
Parsons, H. E.: Nematode Chorioretinitis. A.M.A. Arch. Ophth., 47:799, 1952.
Wilder, H. C.: Nematode Endophthalmitis. Tr. Am. Acad. Ophth., Nov.-Dec., 99, 1950.

ENTEROBIASIS

(Oxyuriasis, Pinworm Infection)

Etiology. Enterobiasis, familiar to most clinicians as oxyuriasis, is infection with the pinworm or seatworm, *Enterobius vermicularis*. The adult worms are small, delicate objects. The male has a ventrally curved posterior end, the female a sharply pointed tail.

Life History. These worms live as young adults typically in the cecum and appendix, with their heads attached to the mucosa. Gravid females become free and migrate in the bowel, usually down and out the anus, especially at night when the patient retires. The worms crawl in a sinuous path on the perianal and perineal skin, discharging several thousand eggs en route. They seldom, if ever, return to the bowel. In female patients the worms may enter the genital tract. Eggs are laid within the bowel only in about 5 per cent of positive cases, and such eggs are usually nonviable. Those deposited outside the anus are practically mature when deposited. They are hyaline, colorless, ovoidal objects, with a relatively thick shell, usually flattened on one side, and contain a coiled, frequently motile larva.

They may produce infection by direct anus-to-mouth contamination, the common method of reinfection; by contaminating fingers with objects in a bedroom or elsewhere on which eggs have settled from the air; by breathing in and swallowing eggs carried in air currents; or occasionally by the hatching of eggs on the moist anal surface and the migration of the hatched larvae retrograde up the bowel to the cecal area. Infection is commonest in children, especially in large families or in institutions. Enterobiasis is also common in mental hospitals. The highest incidences of infection occur in large dormitory groups, the lowest in families where each person has his own bedroom. The mature eggs, upon being swallowed, hatch in the small bowel, and the emerging larvae migrate slowly down to the levels of the cecum and appendix, where they become attached and develop into adults in two months or possibly less.

Morbid Anatomy. Pathologic processes at times develop at the sites where the adult worms reside, especially in the tip of the appendix. Considerable hemorrhage may occur at the points of attachment, while pyogenic organisms invade the abandoned sites and may initiate inflammatory reactions, at times leading to submucosal abscess formation. The clinical picture is that of acute or subacute appendicitis. Eosinophilia and leukocytosis may or may not be produced. The principal difficulty in enterobiasis is associated with the migration of the gravid females out of the anus and on the perianal and perineal skin, at times causing almost insufferable pruritus. This leads to scratching of the area and con-

sequent contamination of fingers. Frequently the itching skin becomes inflamed or raw and may require treatment with antiseptic ointment, such as yellow oxide of mercury, penicillin or sulfonamide. Chronic pruritus leads to insomnia, nervousness, at times hysteria, rarely convulsions in small children. Nocturia in boys and heightened excitability of the genitalia in adolescent girls are complicating states not infrequently observed.

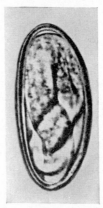

Fig. 55. Photomicrograph of fully embryonated egg of *Enterobius vermicularis* obtained by perianal swabbing. × 800. (From Cram in Introduction to Nematology, Washington, D. C.)

Diagnosis based on recovery of eggs of *Enterobius* in feces, even by concentration techniques, is hopelessly inadequate. Swab examinations of the perianal and perineal skin, preferably in the morning before the patient bathes or defecates, is the ideal method for determining if a suspected person is infected. Several types of swabs are available, but the most practical and efficient one consists of a 2-inch length of Scotch cellulose tape held sticky-side-out over the end of a tongue depressor. The moist anal mucosa and surrounding skin folds are firmly blotted with the tape, which is then placed, sticky-side-down, in a drop of toluene on a microscopic slide and examined. Eggs of other helminths, including *Ascaris, Trichocephalus,* tapeworms and intestinal schistosomes, are at times also demonstrated by this technique.

Prognosis is almost always good, especially with adequate treatment.

Treatment consists preferably in the administration of gentian violet medicinal, in the form of four-hour Seal-Ins or Enseals coated tablets of 0.012 or 0.03 gm. size. For adults, a course of treatment consists of 0.06 gm. three times daily with meals for 8 days; rest one week, then repeat treatment. For children, the dose is 0.01 gm. daily for each year of apparent, not actual, age. This treatment should be given to all infected persons in the family or other environmental group; otherwise there will be repeated reinfection. With mass therapy as recommended 90 per cent cures may be expected, but permanent eradication may require several courses of treatment. Phenothiazine is also efficient in eradicating pinworms, but is much too toxic for routine use. Oxytetracycline (Terramycin) and piperazine have recently been given clinical trial and are promising as alternatives for children intolerant of gentian violet.

Prevention has not been successful where only hygienic measures have been carried out. On the other hand, mass therapy with gentian violet has proved successful in most groups. Occasional refractory cases suggest need for temporarily moving to an uninfested location, for it is unlikely that the eggs remain viable for more than a few weeks. Only by persistent efforts can eradication be affected.

ERNEST CARROLL FAUST

References

Beaver, P. C.: Methods of Pinworm Diagnosis. Am. J. Trop. Med., 29:577, 1949.

Brown, H. W.: Use of Antibiotics in the Treatment of Helminthic Infections. Ann. N. Y. Acad. Sci., 55:1133, 1952.

Kuitunen-Ekbaum, E.: Phenothiazine in the Treatment of Enterobiasis. Canad. J. Pub. Health, 37:103, 1946.

White, R. H. R., and Standen, O. D.: Piperazine in the Treatment of Threadworms in Children. Report on a Clinical Trial. Brit. M. J., 2:755, 1953.

FILARIASIS

Etiology. Filariasis is an infection with one or more of several true filaria worms, which are threadlike and have the following general characteristics and life cycle.

Life History. The female worms in their natural habitats in the human body give birth to delicate, elongate embryos known as *microfilariae*. If the old egg shell remains around the microfilaria, it is said to be "sheathed"; if the microfilaria is naked, it is "unsheathed." These microfilariae periodically or constantly migrate through peripheral blood vessels (or through cutaneous tissues), from which they are taken up by appropriate species of blood-sucking flies. Within the fly the microfilariae migrate from the lumen of the "stomach" to the thoracic muscles, where they metamorphose into sausage-shaped first-stage larvae. These larvae grow, metamorphose through several stages and in approximately two weeks or less become motile filariform larvae. They now migrate down the proboscis-sheath of the fly and at the time of the fly's next blood meal are introduced into or nearby the puncture wound which they make in the human skin. These infective-stage larvae then penetrate more deeply into the skin, migrate through lymphatic or blood vessels and eventually come to rest in sites where the adult worms will mature. The biologic incubation period is usually one year or less, after which the females of this new generation give birth to a brood of microfilariae.

BANCROFT'S FILARIASIS

This filarial infection is produced by *Wuchereria bancrofti,* a delicate, threadlike worm which lives in lymph vessels and lymphoid tissues, particularly in the groin and the lymphoid tissues associated with the external genitalia.

Life History. Infection is initiated when the filariform larvae are introduced onto or into the skin by infected mosquitoes, especially *Culex fatigans,* the tropical house mosquito. Little is known of the subsequent history of these larvae until they mature into adult worms and the fertilized females begin discharging microfilariae. This *incubation period* requires about one year or less and may or may not be symptomless. This may be succeeded by a *latent symptomless period,* which continues for months or even years. The microfilariae pass from the immediate vicinity of the parent worms into lymph vessels and thence into visceral blood vessels. Typically at night (especially between midnight and 2 A.M.), when the patient relaxes, the microfilariae surge through the peripheral circulation, but return to the viscera during daytime when the patient is active.

Symptoms. In native populations in endemic areas, exposure to bites of infected flies begins early in childhood. In adults new to the area there may be episodes of lymphangitis and lymphadenitis during the biologic incubation period, owing to adolescent worms becoming temporarily lodged immediately retrograde to lymph nodes. The worms may even become strangulated and die without maturing. At other times the incubation period may be symptomless. Sooner or later, however, the patient usually becomes "toxic," with frontal headache and a feeling of depression. These prodromes are followed by the *acute period,* with inflammation of the involved superficial lymph vessels, which become raised and exquisitely painful, and an associated lymphatic fever. After ten days to two weeks the lymphangitis disappears, and temporarily the patient returns to a state of well-being. Recurrence of the inflammatory process may be anticipated, usually at periodic intervals, and eventually the *chronic period* gradually replaces the acute stage. Repeated infection tends to produce sensitization to the foreign body and is probably responsible for the more pronounced types of elephantiasis and varicose lymphatic vessels.

Morbid Anatomy. The pathologic basis for the acute and chronic stages consists fundamentally in cellular infiltration around the adult worms. The acute reaction is inflammatory, consisting of a hyperplasia of the endothelium of lymphatic vessels together with endolymphatic and perilymphatic infiltration, with eosinophils, histiocytes, epithelioid and occasionally giant cells. The process is followed by extensive fibrous encapsulation of the vessels in the locations where the worms have lodged. Fibrosis extends retrograde along these channels until elephantiasis with nonpitting edema of the member develops, or lymph varix is produced. The lower extremities, male genitalia and lymph nodes of the groin are most frequently involved, but the processes may extend into the peritoneal cavity (with chylous ascites) or into the bladder (with chyluria). It is inevitable that, with the almost complete loss of cutaneous blood circulation in the involved member and the consequent cracking of the skin, pathogenic bacteria and fungi enter and complicate the picture; they may, in fact, be responsible for initiating recurrent acute attacks of lymphatic fever.

Several thousand American troops were exposed to Bancroft's filariasis in a hyperendemic area in the South Pacific during the earlier years of World War II. About 25 per cent of the exposed troops had acute lymphangitis and lymphadenitis during the biologic incubation period (i.e., before the worms had matured). Many had localized funiculitis, with or without epididymitis, orchitis or hydrocele, but relatively few manifested an elevation of temperature or constitutional symptoms. After removal to a nonendemic area the symptoms subsided; very few troops had chronic sequelae. However, six years after the symptoms had disappeared, the return of some of these troops to a nonfilarious tropical location has served to resensitize them to the lymphangitic syndrome.

Diagnosis may be accomplished during the patent symptomless period and the acute stage by the recovery at night of the characteristic microfilariae in thick-drop blood films stained with Giemsa stain. Before the worms mature, diagnosis depends on history of exposure in an endemic area, the symptom complex and at times the demonstration of immature worms in biopsied specimens of involved lymph nodes. When the adult worms die, the production of microfilariae ceases, so that dependence must be placed on gross pathology and roentgenographic evidence of calcified worms in the midst of the lesions.

Prognosis. Prognosis is relatively good if the disease is apprehended early and people are removed from areas of exposure. On the other hand, prognosis is relatively poor for native populations in hyperendemic areas who are subject to repeated exposure and tend to have permanent lymphatic obstruction.

Treatment. Until recently, chemotherapy in filariasis has been distinctly discouraging. Even the antimonials and arsenicals tested intensively by Brown and co-workers and by Culbertson and associates left much to be desired. One arsenical, an arsenamide, may prove to be a valuable filaricidal drug (Otto et al.). However, the use of Suramin sodium (Naphuride sodium, Bayer 205, Germanin) and of diethylcarbamazine (Hetrazan) suggests that drugs are now available which are effective for Bancroft's filaria. *Hetrazan* (1-diethyl carbamyl-4-methyl piperazine HCl) is particularly promising, since it is administered orally and in well-tolerated amounts rapidly inhibits production of microfilariae and then causes death of the parent worms. Kenney and Hewitt treated 239 controlled cases of this infection in British Guiana (118 asymptomatic with circulating microfilariae and 121 symptomatic, of whom 101 had demonstrable microfilariae). The drug was administered three times daily in doses of 0.2 to 2 mg. each per kilogram of body weight for periods up to thirty-five days. When the amount was 0.5 mg. or more, the microfilariae usually disappeared within a week from the blood, which remained negative. Clinical improvement occurred in most of the symptomatic cases, including 50 per cent of those with advanced lesions. Penicillin should be used for streptococcal and staphylococcal invaders. Surgical procedures include radical operations to remove elephantoid tissues, and a modified Kondolean operation for the lower extremity. Knott (1938) used tight Turkish-towel bandaging of the involved lower extremity and reported marked success in reestablishing drainage through collateral lymph channels, reduction of the elephantoid tissues and reestablishment of blood circulation in the skin.

Prevention of Bancroft's filariasis is a difficult problem. It involves fundamentally the clearance of mosquito-breeding sites around endemic foci, particularly with DDT spraying of breeding places, while considerable protection may be temporarily afforded by screening, together with the use of pyrethrum sprays, and repellents against adult mosquitoes.

FILARIASIS MALAYI

Filariasis malayi is produced by *Wuchereria malayi,* which is closely related to, but specifically different from, *W. bancrofti.* The development in the mosquito (*Mansonioides, Anopheles,* and so on), method of inoculation of the human victim, incubation period, latent symptomless period, and the development of the acute and chronic states are much the same as in Bancroft's filariasis, except that the lesions occur preponderantly in the upper trunk and upper extremities. **Diagnosis** is made in a similar manner. The **prognosis** is usually much better, even without surgical intervention. The *clinical aspects* of filariasis malayi have been little studied. In Travancore, India, new infections have been greatly reduced by removing the water plants on which the larval stages of the mosquito, *Mansoniodes annulifera,* live (Sweet and Pillai, 1937), while in Ceylon the use of 2-4-D (Weedone) to kill these plants has provided a considerable degree of control.

OTHER FILARIAL INFECTIONS

Filaria infections due to *Acanthocheilonema perstans* and *Mansonella ozzardi* have a widespread distribution, but produce few pathologic effects or symptoms of clinical grade. It is important to recognize the diagnostic characters of their microfilariae so that infections with these worms will not be confused with pathogenic filariae of man.

ONCHOCERCOSIS

Onchocercosis is produced by *Onchocerca volvulus,* which is transmitted by the biting gnat, *Simulium.* In Africa it has an extensive distribution; in the Western Hemisphere its distribution is limited to a narrow strip of coffee-growing uplands on the Pacific slope of Guatemala and adjacent Mexico, and to a newly discovered focus in eastern Venezuela. The adult worms live tightly coiled, usually in pairs, in fibrous subcutaneous tumors,

which become palpable within a year or less after exposure to the infection. They vary in size from a pea to a small orange. The tumors may be located on any part of the body. In Africa they are found conspicuously at the junctions of long bones; in Guatemala and Mexico most of the tumors are on the head, especially in the temporal areas and occiput. The "unsheathed" microfilariae escape from the parent tumors and migrate through the skin and subcutaneous tissues, frequently accumulating in the corneal conjunctiva, tissues of the eyeball or in the optic nerve. The parent lesion is usually painless, seldom abscesses, and causes little functional damage. On the other hand, invasion of the microfilariae into the tissues of the eye provokes damaging changes leading to photophobia and diminished vision. Involvement of the optic nerve leads to complete blindness. Moreover, inflammation of the tissues in the temporal area may produce an erysipelatoid appearance especially around the ear and on the ear lobes.

Diagnosis of onchocercosis may be suspected in patients living in endemic areas or previously exposed there, who have one or more characteristic parent tumors, especially with evidence of diminished vision. Specific diagnosis requires the demonstration of the microfilaria of *O. volvulus,* obtained from biopsied skin near the tumor or from biopsied corneal conjunctiva, or in the aspirate of the tumor after puncture.

Treatment. Both suramin sodium and Hetrazan have been given clinical trial in onchocercosis. Both appear to be effective in inhibiting microfilarial production, while the former drug also kills the parent worms. However, tolerance to these drugs, particularly Hetrazan, is very low compared with their tolerance in Bancroft's filariasis. This is interpreted as hypersensitization to the catabolic by-products of the onchocercas following drug administration rather than to the direct effect of the drug on the patient. Thus these drugs must be administered in comparatively small amounts, requiring much longer treatment periods. Even with adequate chemotherapy, in order to reduce the indirect toxic effect of the drug on the patient and to guard against unnecessary damage to the eyes by microfilarial invasion, the onchocercomas should be excised as rapidly as they develop.

Prevention might be accomplished by cleaning out breeding places of the *Simulium* intermediate hosts, but since these locations are usually under stones in mountain streams, no practical control has been developed. Larvicidal use of DDT at times of the pool stage of mountain streams in which the *Simulium* breed, has been suggested as a simple practical means of control of the flies and the infection which they transmit. Relatively good results have been demonstrated in endemic foci by enucleation of the parent tumors in patients as soon as they appear.

LOAIASIS

Etiology. Loaiasis is produced by *Loa loa,* the "eyeworm," so called because of its propensity to wander across the front of the cornea during its continual migrations through the peripheral tissues of the body. This threadlike nematode lives as a mature organism in the subcutaneous tissues, but is not immobilized within a fibrous tumor as is *Onchocerca volvulus.* It characteristically advances a few centimeters a day in a raised serpentine track, and during its wanderings typically reaches the temporal region and passes under the corneal epithelium across the front of one eye, the bridge of the nose, then the other eye, and finally out to the other temple and down the neck to the trunk. In its migrations the worm sets up a temporary inflammatory reaction referred to as a "fugitive swelling." There is no permanent impairment of tissues or organs—only the inconvenience and nervous reaction from constant slight irritation, and at times giant urticaria and other allergic reactions. The microfilariae are diurnal in their appearance in the peripheral blood stream. They are picked up by the mango fly, *Chrysops,* in which they are transformed into infective-stage larvae and are then inoculated again into man. The disease is confined to tropical Africa, but in the United States occasional patients are seen with a history of having lived in endemic foci.

Diagnosis is frequently provided by patients who know of the migrations of the parent worms in their peripheral tissues. The lesions must not be confused with those of creeping eruption (*vide supra,* p. 440). The characteristic sheathed microfilariae present in peripheral blood in the daytime provide specific diagnosis.

Prognosis is always good.

Treatment consists in the skillful extraction with a sharp hooked needle of the parent worm as it migrates under the epithelial layer of the cornea. Procaine anesthesia is not advised, since it drives the worm back into inaccessible tissues. Hetrazan has recently been found to have specific effects on this filaria.

Prevention. Avoid water courses around which mango flies breed and hover.

DIROFILARIASIS

A number of cases of human filariasis have been reported from the Mediterranean area, the Near East, Middle East, South America and the southern United States, in which the parasite has been identified as a species of *Dirofilaria.* In two instances a single adult worm was found, once in the left ventricle (Brazil) and once in the inferior vena cava (Louisiana). In the remaining cases only immature worms were discovered in subcutaneous nodules. Three of these were obtained from patients in Florida. It is most likely that all of these infections have been due to a filaria which is poorly adapted to man but is a relatively common parasite of a host closely associated with man. The filaria which conforms to this requirement is the dog heart worm, *Dirofilaria immitis* (Faust et al.). No serious symptoms have developed in these atypical human infections.

ERNEST CARROLL FAUST

References

Beye, H. K., and others: Preliminary Observations on the Prevalence, Clinical Manifestations and Control of Filariasis in the Society Islands. Am. J. Trop. Med. & Hyg., 1:637, 1952.

Burch, T. A., and Ashburn, L. L.: Experimental Therapy of Onchocerciasis with Suramin and Hetrazan; Results of a Three-Year Study. Am. J. Trop. Med., 31:617, 1951.

Culbertson, J. T., and others: Experimental Chemotherapy of Filariasis. Tr. Roy. Soc. Trop. Med. & Hyg., 41:18, 1947.

Faust, E. C., and others: Unusual Findings of Filarial Infections in Man. Am. J. Trop. Med. & Hyg., 1:239, 1952.

Goldman, L., and Ortiz, L. F.: Types of Dermatitis in American Onchocerciasis. Arch. Dermat. & Syph., 53:79, 1946.

Kenney, M., and Hewitt, R.: Treatment of Bancroftian Filariasis with Hetrazan in British Guiana. Am. J. Trop. Med., 29:89, 1949.

Knott, J.: The Treatment of Filarial Elephantiasis of the Leg by Bandaging. Tr. Roy. Soc. Trop. Med. & Hyg., 32:243, 1938.

Michael, P.: Filariasis among Navy and Marine Personnel. U. S. Nav. Med. Bull., 42:1059, 1944.

O'Connor, R. W.: The Etiology of the Disease Syndrome in *Wuchereria bancrofti.* Tr. Roy. Soc. Trop. Med. & Hyg., 26:13, 1932.

Otto, G. F., and others: Arsenamide in the Treatment of Infections with the Periodic Form of

Filaria, *Wuchereria Bancrofti.* Am. J. Trop. Med. & Hyg., *1:*470, 1952.

Strong, R. P.: Onchocerciasis in Africa and Central America. Am. J. Trop. Med., Suppl., *18:*1, 1938.

Vargas, L.: Consideraciones sobre Una Campaña contra la Oncocerciasis. Medicine (México), 32: 189, 1952.

Woodruff, A. W.: Destruction of Microfilariae of *Loa Loa* in the Liver in Loaiasis Treated with Banocide (Hetrazan). Tr. Roy. Soc. Trop. Med. & Hyg., *44:*479, 1951.

DRACUNCULOSIS

(*Dracontiasis*)

Etiology. Dracunculosis is produced by *Dracunculus medinensis,* referred to as the dragon worm, Medina worm or Guinea worm. This worm superficially resembles the true filaria worms, but in structure and life cycle is quite different. The male worm is a small thread, while the female more nearly resembles a length of grocer's twine and may be a meter long.

Life History. The mature worms live in the viscera or deeper somatic tissues of man and several species of mammals. The gravid female migrates to the skin and on arrival produces a cutaneous blister over her anterior extremity. When this area comes in contact with fresh water, or a goat-skin water bag seeps water onto the skin of the carrier's back, the blister bursts and the dragon worm discharges a brood of rhabditoid larvae into the water. These larvae are picked up by little "water fleas" of the genus *Cyclops,* migrate to the hemocelic cavity of the *Cyclops* and mature. When man or other susceptible host then swallows raw water containing the infected fleas, he acquires the infection, which requires about one year for incubation. After this the gravid female migrates to the skin to shed her progeny.

Endemic Regions. This infection is highly endemic in extensive areas of India, Arabia, Iran, Afghanistan, Turkestan, the southeastern states of the U. S. S. R., and Africa.

Symptoms. During the migration of gravid female dragon worms from the deeper tissues of the body to the skin there is typically a pronounced histamine-like symptom complex, which is readily amenable to epinephrine therapy. The subsequent period of weeks during which the female is discharging larvae through the skin opening is subject to invasion of pyogenic bacteria, which constitute the greatest hazard of the infection. Since time immemorial infected natives have pulled out the worm a centimeter or two a day by coiling it around a small stick which is bound to the site between manipulations. Attempts to pull the worm out rapidly invariably causes it to break off in its tunnel, with suppuration.

Diagnosis is usually self-made by infected patients, who regard the infection as a "God-sent" affliction.

Prognosis is good except when serious bacterial infection develops.

Treatment. Until recently there was no satisfactory anthelmintic treatment. Elliott found that an emulsion, consisting of 2 gm. of finely powdered phenothiazine, 0.35 gm. of lanolin and 35 cc. of sterile olive oil in 5 cc. of sterile water, when introduced under local procaine anesthesia along the path of the worm, soon causes complete relaxation of the parasite so that it may be removed intact by gentle traction. Probably the most practical *control measure* consists in placing small fishes in all bodies of fresh water, such as ponds, wells, and so forth, in endemic areas, to eat the infected *Cyclops,* and thus break the cycle of the parasite.

The GORDIACEA, or "hair worms" ("hair snakes"), have from time to time been reported as parasites of the digestive tract of man. All cases investigated have proved to be ones of temporary parasitism, due most likely to ingestion of raw water containing the immature or maturing worms, which are temporarily free-living after a parasitic phase in grasshoppers and other insects.

ERNEST CARROLL FAUST

References

Elliott, M.: A New Treatment for Dracontiasis. Tr. Roy. Soc. Trop. Med. & Hyg., 35:291, 1942.

Faust, E. C.: Human Helminthology. 3rd ed. Philadelphia, Lea & Febiger, 1949.

HOOKWORM DISEASE

(*Ancylostomiasis, Uncinariasis, Tropical Chlorosis, Miner's Anemia*)

Definition. Hookworm *disease* is a clinical syndrome caused by infection with *Ancylostoma duodenale* or *Necator americanus.* Hookworm *infection* implies the harboring of hookworms in the intestine, with or without symptoms.

History. *Ancylostoma duodenale* was discovered by Dubini in Italy in 1843. *Nector americanus* was discovered by Allen J. Smith in Texas and by Ashford in Puerto Rico and was named by Stiles in 1902. Clinical hookworm disease was first recognized as such by Perroncito in 1880 in laborers who were constructing the Saint Gotthard tunnel through the Alps. Looss in Egypt discovered that the larvae penetrate the skin and in 1904 demonstrated the route of migration of the larvae through the blood and respiratory tract to the intestines.

Distribution and Incidence. Hookworm infection is endemic in many parts of the world between 36 degrees north latitude and 30 degrees south latitude. Light infections are found in hot, dry climates and moist, cooler climates where environmental conditions are favorable. Moisture, warmth, sandy or loose soil and promiscuous defecation are the chief factors responsible for heavy infections. A mean monthly temperature of 50° F. is necessary for the development of the larvae in the soil. Regions having less than 40 inches of rainfall a year may show a high incidence of light infections, but rarely have heavy infections. The disease is almost entirely rural except for mines where excreta disposal is unsanitary. The occupations, in addition to farming and mining, most often associated with hookworm disease are coffee, tea, sugar, cacao, banana and sweet potato raising, and mulberry growing for silkworm cultivation, in all of which people work barefoot in contaminated soil. Loughlin and Stoll (1947) also showed that infection could be acquired by contact with moist contaminated clothing or bedding. The two species of hookworms originally had separate areas of distribution, both being limited to the Old World, *Ancylostoma* north of the twentieth parallel of north latitude, *Necator* south of this parallel. The present distribution is due to the migration of people from the original areas. *Ancylostoma* is present alone in the Mediterranean area, parts of India, northern China and Japan, and in most mines; *Necator* in Central and South Africa, and in North and South America. The two worms are found together in parts of India, southern Asia and parts of Central and South America. The hookworm belt in the United States is principally along the Atlantic and Gulf seaboards from North Carolina to eastern Texas. The other important area is the southern Appalachian region, including southwestern Virginia, western North Carolina, eastern Kentucky and eastern Tennessee. In some tropical areas where hookworm campaigns have not been conducted, practically 100 per cent of the rural population are infected. Where such campaigns have been conducted and where sanitary disposal of excreta has been introduced, a considerable reduction has taken place. Studies by Keller and Leathers from 1930 to 1938 in six southern states showed that there had been a reduction in incidence of hookworm infection in the rural white population of these states from 39 per cent to 18 per cent since 1910–1914, when the original survey was made by the Rockefeller Sanitary Commission. Hood showed that by 1947 the incidence and intensity of infection in Florida had dropped still further. Examination of returned American military personnel after overseas service, especially in the Far East, revealed many light infections with *Ancylostoma*. Loughlin and Stoll and others have warned of the possibility that this may lead to the establishment of endemic foci of this worm in the southern United States.

White and Oriental peoples are more susceptible than the Negro. In infected families the larger the number of infected persons, the greater is the average intensity of infection. Incidence and intensity increase with age up to the 15 to 19 year group, after which there is a gradual decline. Males show a higher incidence and intensity than females, and the peak comes a little later in life. This is undoubtedly due to greater exposure.

Etiology. The human hookworms are nematodes (round worms) measuring about 1 cm. in length, the female being slightly larger than the male. *Ancylostoma* is slightly larger than *Necator*. The anterior end is curved dorsally. The buccal cavity is armed with ventral teeth (*Ancylostoma*) or cutting plates (*Necator*). The male has a copulatory bursa at the posterior end consisting of finger-like rays.

The worms inhabit the small intestine, mainly the jejunum. They attach themselves to villi which are sucked into the buccal cavity, and they secrete toxic fluid which causes dilatation and rupture of the capillaries and prevents coagulation of the blood. The worms feed mainly on blood and lymph pumped into the intestine of the worm by the muscular esophagus. The worms are wasteful of this food, only fluid constituents being absorbed. Most of the ingested material is rapidly excreted through the anus. Wells showed that a single dog hookworm could ingest 0.8 cc. of blood daily if it fed continuously. Although a hemolytic toxin has been demonstrated in extracts of hookworms, it has not been shown that such a toxin contributes directly to the anemia or other symptoms. The life span of the hookworm may be several years;

the heavier the infection, the shorter the average life span of individual worms.

A female hookworm lays between 6000 and 15,000 eggs a day, *Ancylostoma* more than *Necator*. The larva develops rapidly in the egg and hatches under favorable conditions of moisture and temperature in about three days. The rhabditiform larva ruptures the egg shell and after two moltings within a few days becomes an infective filariform larva enclosed in a transparent sheath. This larva may travel upward or downward in the soil for a few inches as changes in moisture require. Its life span may be several weeks in moist soil, although it does not feed as long as it retains its sheath. When the skin of man is exposed to infected soil, the larva penetrates rapidly, enters a blood vessel and is carried to the lungs, where it breaks out into an alveolus. It then makes its way up the bronchi and trachea into the pharynx and is swallowed and passes into the small intestine, where it develops into an adult. About six weeks are required from the time of penetration of the skin until eggs appear in the stools.

Clinical symptoms depend mainly upon the chronic loss of blood, producing a secondary anemia. A diet low in iron content, as is found among the rural people in many parts of the world, prevents recuperation from the loss of blood, sometimes even after the worms have been expelled. A vicious cycle consisting of poor nutrition, inability to work and poverty is established in heavy infections and contributes largely to the problem of the disease.

Morbid Anatomy. The *blood* in heavily infected persons presents a picture of microcytic hypochromic anemia. In extreme cases a picture of macrocytic hyperchromic anemia may be present. There is usually an eosinophilia ranging from 5 to 25 per cent. The *bone marrow* shows an increase of erythropoietic cells. The *liver* may show marked fatty infiltration. In fatal cases the *small intestine* usually shows some atrophy of the epithelium and increase in the connective tissue elements of the mucosa. Petechial hemorrhages are found at the site of attachment of the worms. The *heart* is dilated and its muscle flabby. There is often edema of the subcutaneous tissues, and sometimes even of the brain, and free fluid in the serous cavities.

Symptoms. *Stage of Invasion.* The larvae, in penetrating the skin, produce lesions which are called "ground itch." They consist of maculopapules which become small vesicles. These are often confluent and rupture, discharging serous fluid. They are surrounded by local erythema and swelling. Itching is severe. The commonest site is on the feet, particularly between the toes, but in miners may be on the arms, legs or but-tocks. Regional lymph nodes are often enlarged, especially if secondary infection takes place.

The larvae, in passing through the lungs, may produce bronchitis if a heavy infection occurs at one time. It may be accompanied by fever. It has been noted particularly among miners.

Symptoms Produced by Adult Worms. Very light infections usually produce no recognized symptoms, but elimination of the worms sometimes increases the vigor or accelerates normal development in children. *Mild cases* show slight pallor of the skin with a yellow tinge, dryness of the skin with decreased perspiration, sometimes slight discomfort in the abdomen, slight palpitation of the heart on exertion, slight weakness of the muscles, and distaste for work. The appetite may be increased. Bowel movements are usually normal. Such cases usually show 4,000,000 to 5,000,000 erythrocytes per cubic millimeter, a hemoglobin concentration between 9 and 12 grams per 100 ml., and slight or marked eosinophilia.

Moderately severe cases show an exaggeration of these symptoms. The hair is dry and lusterless, the expression of the face is dull, there may be general itching of the skin, the appetite may be voracious, and the eating of earth or other mineral material may be indulged in, although it is rarely admitted. The tongue shares in the general pallor and may show atrophy of the papillae. The bowels are usually constipated, but there may be irregular intervals of diarrhea. The heart shows slight hypertrophy, the pulse is rapid and often weak, and a hemic systolic murmur is usually heard over the precordium. There is usually dyspnea on exertion. There may be dizziness, tinnitus and *headache*. Weakness is marked, fatigue is rapid, and movements are slow. There may be a slight amount of albumin in the urine, with or without a few casts. There may be edema of the feet. The blood picture shows from 3,000,000 to 4,000,000 erythrocytes per cubic millimeter. The hemoglobin is between 4 and 9 grams, and eosinophilia is usually present.

Severe cases show further intensification of the anemia and cardiac dilatation. Weakness and stupor are apparent. Edema may involve the entire body, including the face and the serous cavities, and cardiac insufficiency may be present. Slight exertion causes severe dyspnea. The reflexes may be abolished, and paresthesias are present. The skin is very dry. The appetite may be enormous or poor. The stomach may become dilated, and nausea and vomiting are frequent. Diarrhea may predominate over constipation. The stools do not contain gross blood, but occult blood is readily found. The urine may show more albumin and casts. These patients show between 2,000,000 and 3,000,000 erythrocytes per cubic millimeter and 2 to 4 grams of hemoglobin. The color index sometimes exceeds 1. Eosinophilia is usually absent.

In addition to these symptoms, hookworm disease retards general development. Puberty is often delayed, and, if it occurred before infection took place, sexual development may recede. The age of the patient may appear five to ten years younger than it actually is. Mental development is proportionately retarded. In adults, impotence may occur in men and menstruation cease in women.

Diagnosis. The final diagnosis of hookworm infection is based entirely upon the demonstration of ova in the stools. The simplest method is by a slide-cover slip preparation of an emulsion of stool in water or saline. A rough estimate of the intensity of infection may be gained from such a preparation, but light infections may be missed. The salt flotation method, in which an emulsion of about 1 cc. of feces is made in 10 cc. of a saturated solution of sodium chloride and allowed to stand for half an hour, brings the eggs to the surface and permits the finding of light infections. Various methods developed for estimating the number of worms in the intestine are valuable in surveys of population groups in order to determine the clinical importance of the disease in such groups. These methods, however, are not necessary in clinical practice, since all persons harboring hookworms, no matter how few in number, should be treated. The most important element in diagnosis is to keep the disease in mind in the presence of symptoms, and to examine routinely the feces of every patient in areas where the disease might be present.

Prognosis. Unless the patient is in the last stages of the clinical disease, elimination of the worms should be followed by ultimate cure in the absence of reinfection. Even the most severe cases may show dramatic improvement when the worms are eliminated and iron is administered. Studies by Rhoads, Castle and their associates have shown, however, that, in Puerto Rico at least, chronic cases in which the anemia is pronounced do not improve rapidly after removal of the worms unless iron is given in large doses, and that almost the same improvement in the blood picture can be obtained by the administration of iron without removal of the worms. This emphasizes the importance of stimulating blood formation in hastening recovery from the disease.

Treatment. Preparation for anthelmintic treatment is important, but can be overdone. The patient should have a light evening meal without fats and should receive the drug in the morning before breakfast. A preliminary purge is not necessary unless constipation is present. Food should be omitted for a few hours and alcohol for 24 hours after treatment. A purge is usually advisable four hours after treatment in order to eliminate the worms and the drug. Sodium sulfate is preferable to magnesium sulfate, because the latter sometimes acts as a depressant.

Oil of chenopodium in three doses of 0.5 cc. each in hard gelatin capsules at intervals of a half hour removes 70 to 90 per cent of the worms. Children may be given 0.03 cc. per year of age up to age 15. A considerable number of deaths from this drug have been reported, apparently due to idiosyncrasy or to excessive absorption. The toxic symptoms of oil of chenopodium usually appear 2 to 24 hours after treatment. They consist of nausea, vomiting, dizziness, stupor and coma. They should be treated as early as possible by purging, preferably with sodium sulfate, and by general supportive measures.

Hexylresorcinol in crystalline form in specially prepared hard gelatin capsules will remove 50 to 60 per cent of hookworms. The adult dose is 1 gm. The dose for children is 0.1 gm. for each year of age up to age 10. The advantage of this drug is that it is entirely nontoxic. The crystals, however, will burn the mouth if the capsules are crushed, and the drug combines quickly with organic matter, so that food must be strictly avoided for 12 hours before and 4 hours after treatment.

Tetrachlorethylene is probably the drug of choice because of its relative efficiency and lack of fatal toxicity. The only reported death was in an emaciated beggar in India (Chaudhuri and Mukerji). Dizziness sometimes occurs. The dose is 3 cc. in hard gelatin capsules or in skimmed milk given at one time. Children may be given 0.2 cc. for each year of age up to age 15. This treatment will re- move from 60 to 80 per cent of *Necator,* but only about 40 per cent of *Ancylostoma* worms. If a heavy Ascaris infection is present with the hookworms, Ascaris should be re- moved by hexylresorcinol before treatment for hookworms is given, because tetrachlor- ethylene only stimulates Ascaris to activity and a large number of these worms might produce intestinal obstruction.

Carbon tetrachloride should not be used as an anthelmintic because it may cause fatally toxic necrosis of the liver and is but little more effective than tetrachlorethylene.

Since one treatment with an anthelmintic rarely removes all the worms, the stools should be carefully examined for eggs five or six days after treatment; if eggs are found, the treatment should be repeated at weekly intervals until the stools become negative.

Iron should be given in large amounts. The recommended daily dosage is 1 gm. of ferrous sulfate (exsiccated) in capsules or 6 gm. of ferric ammonium citrate in a 50 per cent solution. These preparations should be given in three divided doses after meals. It is best to start with smaller doses in order to avoid intolerance. Children should receive doses in proportion to their weight. This treatment produces rapid stimulation of reticulocytes and increase of hemoglobin and erythrocytes with rapid general improvement of the pa- tient. Liver extract is of no value except for its iron content. The diet should be abundant and well balanced, but this alone will not cause rapid improvement unless it has a high iron content.

Prophylaxis. There are three important elements in prevention: treatment, the wear- ing of shoes and sanitary disposal of excreta. Treatment is only of temporary value if rein- fection can take place. The wearing of shoes is dependent upon local customs and educa- tion. The only effective method of prevention is sanitary disposal of excreta. This must be adapted to the individual and community involved. Since the larvae cannot climb up a vertical surface to any height, the deposi- tion of excreta anywhere except on the ground is sufficient for prevention. The bored hole latrine in many parts of the tropics and the pit privy in the rural parts of the United States are sufficient to insure prevention if they are properly used. Hookworm is still an important public health and clinical problem in many parts of the world, including certain areas in the United States, and will continue to be until sanitary disposal of excreta becomes universal.

HENRY E. MELENEY

References

Ash, J. E., and Spitz, Sophie: Pathology of Tropical Disease; An Atlas. Philadelphia, W. B. Saunders Company, 1945.

Ashford, B. K., and Igaravidez, P. G.: Uncinariasis (Hookworm Disease) in Porto Rico. 61st Con- gress, 3rd Session, Senate Document No. 808. Washington, Government Printing Office, 1911.

Carr, H. P., Pichardo Sardá, M. E. and Nuñez, N. A.: Anthelmintic Treatment of Uncinariasis. Am. J. Trop. Med. Hyg., 3:495, 1954.

Chang, K., and co-workers: Studies on Hookworm Disease in Szechwan Province, West China. Am. J. Hyg. Monographic Series, No. 19, 1949.

Chaudhuri, R. N., and Mukerji, A. K.: Death Fol- lowing Administration of Tetrachlorethylene. In- dian M. Gaz., 82:115, 1947.

Dubini, A.: Nuovo verme intestinale umano (Agchy- lostoma duodenale) constituente un sesto genere dei nematoidei proprii dell'uomo. Ann. univ. di med. e. chir., Milan, 106:5, 1843.

Hood, M.: The Present Status of Hookworm Infec- tion in Florida. Am. J. Trop. Med., 27:505, 1947.

Leathers, W. S., and Keller, A. E.: Investigations Concerning Hookworm Disease in Southern States with Suggestions for Continued Control. South. M. J., 29:172, 1936.

Looss, A.: Die Wanderung der Ankylostomum- und Strongyloides-Larven von der Haut nach dem Darm. Compt-rend. 6 Cong. internat. de zool., Geneva, 225–233, 1905.

Loughlin, E. H., and Stoll, N. R.: Fomite-borne An- cylostomiasis. Am. J. Hyg., 45:191, 1947.

———, and Stoll, N. R.: Hookworm Infections in American Servicemen with Reference to the Es- tablishment of *Ancylostoma duodenale* in the Southern United States. J.A.M.A., 136:157, 1948.

Mackie, T. T., Hunter, G. W., and Worth, C. B.: 2nd ed. Manual of Tropical Medicine. Philadel- phia, W. B. Saunders Company, 1954.

Rhoads, C. P., Castle, W. B., Payne, G. C., and Law- son, H. A.: Observations on the Etiology and Treatment of Anemia Associated with Hookworm Infection in Puerto Rico. Medicine, 13:317, 1934.

Stiles, C. W.: A New Species of Hookworm (*Un- cinaria americana*) Parasitic in Man. Am. Med., 3:777, 1902.

———: Report upon the Prevalence and Geographic Distribution of Hookworm Disease in the United States. U. S. Pub. Health and Marine Hosp. Serv- ice, Hyg. Lab. Bull. No. 10, 1903.

Strong, R. P.: Stitt's Diagnosis, Prevention and Treatment of Tropical Diseases. 7th ed. Philadel- phia, Blakiston Co., 1944.

Wells, H. S.: Observations on the Blood-Sucking Activities of the Hookworm, *Ancylostoma cani- num.* J. Parasitol., 17:167, 1931.

ARTHROPODS AND HUMAN DISEASE

Arthropods, which comprise the insects and their relatives (crustaceans, centipedes, scorpions, spiders, ticks and mites), constitute the largest single group in the animal kingdom. They are medically important in three capacities: (1) as causative agents of disease; (2) as mechanical carriers of pathogenic micro-organisms; and (3) as necessary hosts (or incubators) and transmitters of pathogens to man. In the first category are all the blood-sucking species, those which venenate, and those which actually parasitize the human body. In the second group are those species, especially flies, which come in contact with disease-producing organisms through their filthy feeding and breeding habits, and then pass on the pathogens to man. In the third group are the obligatory arthropod hosts of such agents of disease as the malaria parasites, the filaria worms, the rickettsiae, the relapsing fever spirochetes, plague bacilli and others.

ERNEST CARROLL FAUST

ARTHROPODS AS CAUSATIVE AGENTS OF DISEASE

All blood-sucking arthropods, i.e., ticks, many species of mites, lice, blood-sucking bugs, blood-sucking flies and fleas, puncture the skin and introduce minute amounts of saliva into the puncture wound before taking a blood meal. If the puncture wound is small, as from mosquitoes and other blood-sucking gnats, the trauma is slight, but the protein in the introduced saliva may lead to allergic reactions, with local or generalized edema and inflammation, accompanied by fever. In the case of ticks, the wound is moderately large and may become ragged if attempts are made to remove the tick with its mouth parts unrelaxed. Moreover, red mites ("chiggers") usually bury their heads in the skin of their victim, so that removal is difficult. The sarcoptic mite (*Sarcoptes scabiei*) actually tunnels in the skin and multiplies there, and the follicular mite (*Demodex folliculorum*) utilizes the hair follicles for similar purposes. The female chigoe flea (*Tunga penetrans*) burrows into the skin to obtain food to develop her eggs.

SARCOPTIC ITCH
(*Scabies*)

The sarcoptic or itch mite is widely prevalent in groups of the population with low personal hygiene. The disease is also known as *sarcoptic mange*. The female, which measures 330 to 450 microns in length by 150 to 200 microns in breadth, burrows into the skin via hair follicles and develops a somewhat tortuous tunnel several millimeters to a few centimeters in length and nearly parallel to the skin surface. At the inner end of the tunnel she lays about forty ovoidal eggs over a period of four to five weeks. Within three to five days after oviposition a larva hatches from each egg. The larvae develop lateral burrows or come out of the tunnel and produce new burrows. Four to ten days later they have moulted and become sexually mature. New sites of infestation develop in this way in the skin of the same person, or his clothing or bed linen serves to infest his associates.

Morbid Anatomy. The *lesions* develop rapidly as raised red linear channels in the epidermis, and are most common between the fingers, on the backs of the hands, elbows, axillae, groin, breasts, umbilicus, penis, shoulder blades and the small of the back. Deposition of little fecal pellets by the mites in their burrows produces vesiculation with itching, which is intensified by warmth and moisture. Scratching produces an open weeping lesion which frequently becomes infected with pyogenic bacteria.

Diagnosis is based technically on the recovery of the mites from the inner ends of the tunnels, but the lesions are so characteristic that clinical diagnosis is relatively satisfactory.

Prognosis is good with persistent treatment.

Treatment. Cannon and McRae, also Wooldridge, have reported excellent results from the topical application of a bland ointment containing 0.5 per cent lindane (Gammexane) (gamma isomer of benzene hexachloride), which produces no skin sensitivity. Clinical cures were obtained by the former workers in 100 per cent of their patients (61 per cent with one application, 36 per cent with two treatments, and the remaining 3 per cent with three). Lindane ointment lends itself to mass treatment of large groups of ambulatory patients, institutional inmates or prisoners of war.

Sulfur ointment (5 per cent flowers of sulfur in lanolin) has been commonly used, and some physicians prefer the more complicated Danish treatment. After all suspected lesions have been scrubbed with green soap and soaked in warm water, the ointment is rubbed in before the patient retires. The next day fresh clothing is put on and all soiled clothing and bed linen are sterilized by boiling. This is repeated the second night and at least once again between the sixth and tenth nights to kill larvae freshly hatched from eggs. For patients sensitive to sulfur, pyrethrum ointment (0.75 per cent pyrethrins one part, lanolin 2 parts and petrolatum one part) or 2 per cent rotenone in petrolatum may be substituted.

PEDICULOSIS

Pediculosis is a louse infestation and may refer to head lice (pediculosis capitis), body lice (pediculosis corporis) or pubic lice (pediculosis pubis). Head lice (*Pediculus humanus* var. *capitis*) infest the head and attach their eggs near the base of the hair shafts; body lice (*P. humanus* var. *corporis*) feed on the skin, but usually attach their eggs to the fibers of body clothing; pubic lice (*Phthirus pubis*) live closely appressed to the skin, usually in areas of the pubic, axillary and breast hairs, occasionally in the eyebrows and eyelashes, attaching their eggs to these hairs. They all produce an irritating roseate, papular dermatitis.

Treatment. For *head lice,* the hair should be cut short and the head skin thoroughly rubbed with lindane ointment (0.5 per cent pure benzene hexachloride in a vanishing cream), which kills both the active stages and the eggs ("nits"). This same treatment is equally effective for *pubic lice* when the ointment is massaged into the skin of infested areas. For *body lice* dusting of the body and infested clothing with 4 per cent DDT (U.S.P.) in an inert (pyrophyllite) powder is effective in all localities except Korea, Manchuria and Japan, where the lice have become resistant. In these regions chlordane is substituted for DDT.

BITES

For treatment of *dermatitis* due to "bites" of flies, fleas, mites and other arthropods, application locally of phenolated camphor in pure mineral oil ("Campho-phenique") is a satisfactory, well tolerated palliative, and will usually prevent secondary bacterial infection.

MYIASIS
(*Maggot Infestation*)

The largest group of tissue invaders among the arthropods is that of fly larvae (i.e., mag-

gots), producing myiasis. The mother fly may lay eggs on food or in drink which is accidentally taken into the digestive tract and produces temporary *intestinal myiasis;* or may by design deposit eggs or young maggots in or nearby a wound, or on the unbroken skin. The maggots hatching from eggs or those already hatched invade the whole or damaged skin or mucous membranes and cause *cutaneous, ophthalmic, rhinal, aural* or *urethral myiasis.* The myiasis-producing flies frequently cause permanent disfigurement of the invaded skin and underlying tissues and may be responsible for death of the victim, especially in small children. Moreover, wounds infected secondarily with pyogenic bacteria are much more difficult to handle than uncomplicated ones. *Surgical removal* of these maggots should be accomplished as soon as diagnosis has been made, to forestall further damage and possibly fatal injury.

VENENATING ARTHROPODS

The venenating arthropods include centipedes, scorpions, spiders, some ticks, bees, wasps and ants, blister beetles and the caterpillar of several moths and one family of butterflies.

Centipedes have a pair of hollow oral "fangs" through which venom is introduced into the victim when they penetrate the skin. This produces local and at times general inflammation, but probably never has a fatal termination.

True scorpions have a single curved, hollow caudal fang, through which the venom elaborated in a pair of basal glands is emptied into the skin. This venom contains neurotoxins, hemolysins and endotheliolysins. In many warm countries, including the southwestern United States, species of scorpions frequently venenate human beings whose skin accidentally contacts the scorpion, as the unprotected surface of the foot or arm. In the southwestern United States, Durango State, Mexico, Trinidad and in parts of India and Africa, death, especially in small children, is not uncommon as a result of scorpion sting, with ascending motor paralysis, at times accompanied by acute pancreatitis. Local application of an icepack or freezing with ethyl chloride is recommended to prevent systemic dissemination of the venom. Specific antivenins can be prepared, but are not generally available. Caution should be exercised to prevent direct skin contact with these creatures. Residual spraying of DDT emulsion within and around homes in areas where these dangerous scorpions are present is effective in reducing their number.

Spiders. All spiders are venomous, but only a few species are able to penetrate human skin with their pair of oral "fangs," through which the venom is discharged. The most notorious spider is the "black widow" (*Latrodectus mactans*), which has a wide distribution from Canada to Chile. Its venom is a toxalbumin, containing fractions which produce both an ascending motor paralysis and destruction of peripheral nerve endings. There is sharp pain, swelling and reddening at the site of the "bite," dizziness and weakness, tremor of the legs, and abdominal cramps after lymphatic absorption of the venom. Boardlike ridigity and spasm of the abdominal muscles may simulate acute appendicitis or tetanus. More advanced symptoms include urinary retention, reduced heart beat and feeble pulse, labored breathing and speech, light stupor, convulsions in small children and delirium.

Treatment. With a history of black widow spider "bite" (*arachnidism*), the patient should be placed in bed, given 10 cc. of a 10 per cent solution of calcium gluconate intravenously to reduce pain and protect peripheral nerve endings, and then given immune serum (Antivenin *Latrodectus mactans,* Mulford's). Care must be exercised not to disturb "black widow" or other dangerous spiders lurking in their webs in caves, under rocks, around the base of posts or lumber piles, or on the under side of the seats of outdoor privies. Dusting of DDT in and around the webs of these spiders is lethal to them and affords considerable protection.

Ticks. The Rocky Mountain wood tick (*Dermacentor andersoni*), the eastern dog tick (*D. variabilis*) and some other species of hard-bodied ticks introduce a poison into the skin along with their saliva, causing an ascending motor paralysis. This is not due to a neurotoxic virus. It is most concentrated in adult females which have not previously fed and most dangerous when the tick "bites" at the base of the medulla. No specific relief has been developed. Abbott has provided a comprehensive review of the epidemiology and clinical aspects of tick paralysis.

Bees and **wasps** have a posterior sting apparatus, the modified ovipositor, through which venom is introduced into human skin. The venom consists of acid and alkaline fractions and a histamine-like fraction. Honey

bees deposit the entire sting apparatus in the wound. For most persons the wound is painful and may produce mild systemic reaction. Some sensitized persons die as a result of repeated stinging, unless treated with epinephrine. They should then be desensitized with whole bee venom made up in Coca's solution. **Blister beetles** contain a vesicant which produces blisters when the coxal or body fluid of the beetle is discharged on the

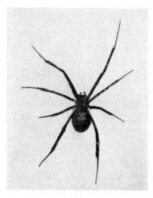

Fig. 56. Ventral view of the female "black widow" spider, *Latrodectus mactans,* showing characteristic scarlet hour-glass pattern. × ½. (Modified by Faust from Strong: Stitt's Diagnosis, Prevention and Treatment, in Craig and Faust: Clinical Parasitology, courtesy of Lea and Febiger.)

skin. Mild applications, such as damp baking soda, should be applied topically. Many types of *moth larvae* (i.e., **caterpillars**) have hollow poison hairs, at times concealed by tufts of nonpoisonous hairs. In contact with human skin the poison hairs discharge minute amounts of an urticating substance, which behaves like a chemical burn and heals with difficulty. Palliative treatment consists in the application of calamine lotion.

ERNEST CARROLL FAUST

ARTHROPODS AS MECHANICAL CARRIERS OR ESSENTIAL HOSTS

As Mechanical Carriers of Pathogenic Micro-organisms. Because of their filthy feeding and breeding habits, many of the common flies serve as mechanical vectors of several pathogenic organisms affecting man. These flies (common house fly, lesser house fly, biting and nonbiting stable flies, green bottles, blue bottles, blow flies, flesh flies, fruit flies, and so on) commonly feed on garbage and the dung of man and domestic animals. Usually they oviposit or larviposit on such decaying organic material, and the larvae (i.e., maggots) feed and grow in these media. After a pupal stage, during which the apparently resting organism undergoes a profound internal reorganization, the adult fly emerges from the pupal case, dries its wings and flies about to take food. It feeds on dissolved and finely particulate material which it sucks up into its proboscis. After ravenously feeding, it defecates and vomits. If the feeding ground is an open privy or other deposit of human feces and the fly next alights on human food or utensils in the kitchen or on the dining table, not only are pathogenic micro-organisms likely to be transferred in vomit drops or fecal pellets to food, drink or containers, but moist feces temporarily lodged on the outside of the fly's body (i.e., proboscis, trunk and legs) may be a source of contamination.

Role in Epidemics. Substantial proof has been furnished that filth flies have been responsible for epidemics of several enteric diseases, including typhoid fever, bacillary dysentery, cholera and amebic enteritis. Moreover, suspicion has been directed to filth flies in the transmission of infantile paralysis, and it is epidemiologically possible that trachoma may be mechanically contracted from flies which breed in profusion in regions such as India and Egypt. Likewise, it is possible that infectious hepatitis may be transmitted by filth-breeding flies. Biting stable flies, contaminated with horse manure, may introduce tetanus and anthrax spores into the skin. Eye gnats (*Hippelates* species) have been incriminated in epidemics of acute conjunctivitis ("pink eye") and are potential vectors of the spirochete of yaws.

Control of Epidemics of several of these diseases at times depends primarily on *control of fly breeding*. Homes should be adequately screened; garbage cans should be tightly covered, the garbage collected daily and completely incinerated; outdoor privies should be soundly constructed and screened and the pit kept clean with generous, frequent applications of quick-lime, crude oil or preferably a 5 to 10 per cent solution of DDT in kerosene. Barnyard manure should be adequately treated and drained to prevent the breeding of stable flies. In cities where

screening and sanitary disposal of garbage are carried out, the dangers of fly convection of pathogenic micro-organisms have been greatly reduced. But in rural areas, particularly on large farms, flies are still a menace to human health. Area spraying of DDT emulsion by airplane is helpful in reducing or terminating epidemics of enteric diseases which are mechanically transmitted by filth flies. Nevertheless this measure cannot be depended on for long-term control, for the flies rather rapidly develop resistance to this toxicant.

As Essential Hosts (or Incubators) of Pathogenic Micro-organisms. The disease entities for which arthropods play an essential role in development or multiplication and transmission to man are considered in other chapters of this book. Hence it is necessary here only to direct the reader's attention to these important diseases for which arthropods serve as necessary vectors.

ERNEST CARROLL FAUST

References

Abbott, K. H.: Tick Paralysis: A Review. Proc. Staff Meet., Mayo Clin., *18*:39, 59, 1943.
Barnett, H. C., and Knoblock, E. C.: Chemical and Biological Studies on DDT Resistance of Lice. U.S. Armed Forces M. J., 3:297, 1952.
Bogen, E.: Arachnidism. Arch. Int. Med., 38:623, 1926.
Cannon, A. B., and McRae: Treatment of Scabies. J.A.M.A., *138*:557, 1948.
Craig, C. F., and Faust, E. C.: Clinical Parasitology. 5th ed. Philadelphia, Lea & Febiger, 1951.
Efrati, P.: Poisoning by Scorpion Sting in Israeli. Am. J. Trop. Med., 29:249, 1949
Hawley, J. E., Penner, L. R., Wedberg, W. E., and Kulp, W. L.: The Role of the House-fly, *Musca Domestica*, in the Multiplication of Certain Enteric Bacteria. Am. J. Trop. Med., 31:572, 1951.
Herms, W. B.: Non-Bloodsucking Flies as Vectors of Pathogenic Micro-organisms. Ann. Entomol. Soc. America, 25:623, 1932.
James, M. T.: The Flies that Cause Myiasis in Man. U. S. Dept. Agr. Misc. Publ. No. 631, Washington, D. C., 1947, 175 pp.
Rockwell, E. M., and Johnson, P.: The Insect Bite Reaction. II. Evaluation of the Allergic Reaction. J. Invest. Dermat. 19:137, 1952.
Stahnke, H. L.: The L-C Treatment of Venomous Bites or Stings. Am. J. Trop. Med. & Hyg., 2:142, 1953.
Waterman, J. A.: Some Notes on Scorpion Poisoning in Trinidad. Tr. Roy. Soc. Trop. Med. & Hyg., 31:607, 1938.

DISEASES OF UNPROVED ETIOLOGY

SARCOIDOSIS

*(Boeck's Sarcoid, Lupus Pernio, Be-
nignes Miliär-lupoi, Benign Lymphogranulomatosis, Osteitis Tuberculosa
Multiplex Cystoides, Mortimer's Malady, Hutchinson-Boeck's Disease, Maladie de Besnier-Boeck, Besnier-Tenne-
son's Disease, Schaumann's Disease,
Uveoparotid Fever or Heerfordt's Disease)*

Definition. Sarcoidosis is a chronic indolent and benign infectious disease of unknown
cause, involving the skin, lymph nodes, eyes,
salivary glands, lungs, and bones of the hands
and feet especially. In addition to these conspicuous lesions, disseminated systemic manifestations bespeak widespread pathologic
changes. The predominance of certain lesions
has perpetuated as clinical entities such groupings of clinical details as *uveoparotid fever*.

Etiology. Most observers have cited tuberculosis as the underlying cause of sarcoidosis.
Acid-fast organisms have at times been seen
in the lesions, but Koch's postulates have not
been fulfilled in any further detail. Furthermore, the reactions to large doses of old tuberculin are conspicuously feeble or negative.
Singularly, the lesions of sarcoidosis disappear
upon the development of active tuberculosis.
Some maintain that the products of the *Mycobacterium tuberculosis* rather than the organism itself may be responsible for the disease.
Mycobacterium leprae has received some
attention in this connection. The difficulty in
cultivating the acid-fast bacilli from the sarcoid lesions and in reproducing the disease
might well raise this question; but with certain similarities in the cutaneous and bony
manifestations of the two diseases the clinical
resemblance ceases. The intracutaneous injection of an emulsion of a sarcoid nodule into an
affected subject has induced an apparently
specific cytologic reaction (Kveim reaction).
This result, however, can scarcely be admitted as conclusive evidence of a viral etiology.

Sarcoidosis may occur at any period of life,
but usually is found in patients between 15
and 40 years old. The rare occurrence of this

disease in siblings does not favor a familial or
communicable basis. Sex exerts no influence.
In this country there is an apparent predilection for the Negro. Confirmed statistics for
the United States Army in World War II give
a ratio of sixteen Negro soldiers to one white
soldier with sarcoidosis. Moreover, the greater
portion of the military cases occurred in men
from the southeastern states. No race is exempt from its inroads. Sarcoidosis appears
more commonly in rural than in urban dwellers. Most instances have been reported from
the North Temperate zone, especially in
Scandinavia, northern Europe, England and
North America.

Morbid Anatomy. The fundamental lesion
is granulomatous. Large pale epithelioid cells
are collected in isolated nests or well defined
nodules. As a rule, these areas are not sharply
demarcated from normal tissue. Occasional
pale multinucleated giant cells complete the
picture. Frequently, laminated or doubly refractile bodies (Schaumann) are observed in
these giant cells. Their optical characteristics
suggest calcification. Neither necrosis nor caseation is observed. In the natural evolution
of sarcoidosis, fibrosis may be anticipated.
These lesions have been found in the skin,
breast, mucous membrane, salivary gland,
lachrymal gland, lymph node, tonsil, eye,
nervous system, pituitary body, thyroid gland,
heart, lung, serous membrane, liver, intestine,
spleen, kidney, endometrium, prostate, testis,
epididymis, voluntary muscle, tendon sheath,
bone and marrow.

Pathologic Physiology. The manifestations of disturbed function may be as widespread as the lesions of sarcoidosis. Xerostomia
may attend the active phase of the uveoparotid syndrome, but permanent alteration
of salivary function is rare. Visual disorders in
this syndrome may be persistent, and occasionally permanent difficulties, even as serious as blindness, may result. Invasion of the
pituitary body has given rise to diabetes insipidus. Myxedema may arise from thyroid
involvement. Extensive pulmonary sarcoidosis
may lead to polycythemia, right heart strain
and overstrain (chronic cor pulmonale).
Tachycardia, arrhythmia and heart failure

have been attributed to cardiac invasion by this process. The hyperglobulinemia may reflect the hepatic phase of the disease. Renal involvement rarely advances to the degree of frank uremia, but altered glomerular function is indicated by occasional albuminuria and hematuria. Eunuchoidism may attend testicular encroachment. Hypersplenism may lead to thrombocytopenia with purpura.

Symptoms. The patient suffering from sarcoidosis experiences slight constitutional reaction as a rule. Fever is unusual. Even major degrees of pulmonary involvement may occur without any increase in temperature. Mild malaise and indisposition may appear. Distaste for food, vague gastric symptoms and diarrhea occasionally supervene. Night sweats and arthralgia have been noted. So insidious may be the onset that only the cutaneous eruption or the lymphadenopathy arouses clinical suspicion as to the true state of affairs. The skin lesions appear in about 50 per cent of patients with sarcoidosis. Boeck's description of three characteristic eruptions still obtains: (1) Small firm cutaneous nodules (*kleinknotige*) may be noted in the butterfly area of the face, on the arms and back. These nodules are sharply demarcated, smooth, brown or blue. (2) Similar but larger nodules (*grossknotige*) may appear. (3) The skin may be diffusely infiltrated and thickened (lupus pernio) over the nose, face and ears. The tense skin over the affected area may be bluish, but tiny yellow granules appear at the margins. This eruption is not painful nor attended by pruritus. Having reached its peak, there may be no change for months. Atrophic scars may mark the sites of earlier lesions, but ulceration never occurs. Erythema nodosum may occur in sarcoidosis. The mucosa of the nose and oropharynx may be reddened and nodular.

The *involvement* of the *hands* serves as a clue to the diagnosis. Firm nodules appear at the interphalangeal joints. These may present a remarkable symmetry. A knotty appearance may be imparted to the affected fingers and hands. Scaling of the skin occurs over these projections. The subject complains of tightness or stiffness of the fingers, but they are not painful or tender. General lymphadenopathy may early attract the attention. Pre- and postauricular involvement is particularly significant. The cervical, submaxillary, axillary, epitrochlear and inguinal nodes may be involved. As a rule the individual nodes are not especially large, but there are exceptions.

These nodes are firm in consistency, discrete and nontender. Pressure symptoms rarely arise from them. Cough, dyspnea and remittent low grade fever may attend mediastinal or pulmonary involvement; but extensive intrathoracic invasion may occur without significant subjective or objective evidence. Interscapular dullness and bronchial breath sounds are occasionally elicited. At times the pulmonary process may be so extensive as to lead to right heart embarrassment. Hepatomegaly and splenomegaly may arise from sarcoid involvement of these organs.

Uveoparotid fever constitutes an expression of sarcoidosis requiring especial attention. Insidiously, as in the commoner forms of sarcoidosis, the picture is evolved after nonspecific prodromes of lassitude, drowsiness, malaise and indefinite gastrointestinal symptoms. Intermittent pyrexia of moderate degree may attend. Firm, painless swelling of the parotid glands usually precedes ocular involvement. Although bilateral in a vast majority, the invasion of the parotid glands is not simultaneous. Dryness of the mouth may be a distressing symptom. Mastication is not embarrassed by the parotid swelling. The induration of the glands may be permanent.

Occasionally the ophthalmic symptoms anticipate the parotitis. Uveitis is the most common detail of this picture, but there have also occurred conjunctivitis, corneal herpes, keratitis, corneal opacities, vitreous hemorrhage, optic neuritis, neuroretinitis, chorioretinitis, glaucoma, aqueous turbidity and cataract. Relapses are not infrequent.

The third component in the uveoparotid syndrome is the cranial nerve involvement. A majority of these patients have seventh nerve paralysis, unilateral or bilateral, suddenly a few days to a few months after the onset of the parotitis. The lower facial distribution is more involved than the upper. Usually the facial palsy subsides *pari passu* with the parotitis, but it may appear after its subsidence. Occasional neurologic involvement of different orders may be observed, such as paralysis of the soft palate, dysphagia, intercostal neuralgia, paralysis of the vocal cords, deafness, ptosis of the eyelid, wasting of the muscles of the hand, loss of vibratory perception in the legs, and polyneuritis.

The *sarcoid of Darier-Roussy* (*sarcoïdes noueuses et nodulaires des membres*) represents an artificial segmentation of the general reaction. Under this designation in the past have been grouped sarcoid lesions with a subcutaneous distribution. Histologically, the individual nodules are comprised of giant and epithelioid cells and lymphocytes with a fibrous capsule. Caseation, liquefaction and ulceration do not occur. The tuberculous etiology has been postulated; but in common with other forms of sarcoidosis neither cultivation of *Mycobacterium tuberculosis* nor transmission of the disease to experimental animals has been accomplished.

The lesions of Darier-Roussy sarcoid are usually limited to the trunk with especial predilection for the sides of the abdomen and the lower back. Imperfect symmetry has been described. These deeply seated nodules vary in size from a few millimeters to a few centimeters. They are discretely rounded or oval and insensitive to palpation. At times they form chains which follow the course of blood vessels. Devoid of constitutional or local reaction as a rule, with more extensive involvement the overlying skin may become adherent, irregular and reddish or violaceous. The progression of these sarcoid lesions is self-limited, and after an indeterminate course spontaneous arrest of further development occurs. Singularly, it is a disease of adults.

A slight hypochromic, microcytic anemia may be anticipated in sarcoidosis. The leukocytes are normal in number, or there may be a slight leukopenia. Monocytosis prevails. Eosinophilia of a slight to moderate degree (up to 35 per cent) may occur in a minority. Increased sedimentation speed is the rule. Serologic tests for syphilis are negative. The blood calcium and alkaline phosphatase are regularly increased, and the blood phosphorus and cholesterol normal. The total plasma proteins are increased largely by reason of the increase in the plasma globulin. The albumin:globulin ratio is frequently reversed. In the uveoparotid syndrome there may be added pleocytosis and increased protein in the cerebrospinal fluid.

Roentgenograms of the chest may disclose two fundamental types of intrathoracic involvement. Tracheobronchial and mediastinal lymphadenopathy may assume varying proportions. From the hilum there may occur an extension along the peribronchial structures to involve the lung in an advancing process of fibrosis that fades centrifugally. Patches of fibrous density may be scattered irregularly through the lung. These changes are most marked at the bases. In the second type of pulmonary sarcoidosis a reticular appearance is lent to the whole lung field and tiny densities stud it to indicate a miliary distribution of the pathologic process.

Particularly significant is the roentgenographic appearance of the shafts of the phalanges and metacarpal bones. Without periosteal involvement or thickening, rarefaction of the medullary portion of these bones takes place. Eventually small punched-out areas appear in the small bones of the hands and feet (osteitis tuberculosa multiplex cystoides). Less commonly the long bones of the arms and legs are involved. Sarcoidosis of the skull has been reported. The bony changes are more extensive than are disclosed by the roentgenogram. Biopsies of the sarcoid lesions of the skin, parotid, tonsil and bone marrow are recommended in a diagnostic survey, but the tonsil is not so regularly the seat of the pathologic changes as was once thought. More recently the study of the liver and spleen by biopsy has disclosed an unusually high incidence of positive returns.

Diagnosis. The diagnosis of sarcoidosis is usually made from the nature of the cutaneous eruption and the lymphadenopathy with or without the support of roentgenograms of the thorax and hands. Hutchinson's description of the skin lesions is significant in this relation: "The disease is characterized by the formation of multiple, raised, dusky-red patches which have no tendency to inflame or ulcerate. They are very persistent, and extend but slowly. They occur in groups, their bilateral symmetry, and the absence of all tendency to ulcerate or form crusts, are features which separate the malady from lupus vulgaris. To none of the other forms of lupus has the malady any resemblance."

The uveoparotid syndrome adds the parotid tumor, uveal tract involvement and facial palsy. Invasion of the lachrymal and salivary glands may satisfy the diagnostic criteria of *Mikulicz's syndrome*. Only blood studies and biopsy of the affected structures will properly catalogue its several origins. General lymphadenopathy and splenomegaly may lead to the suspicion of Hodgkin's disease or hyperplastic tuberculosis. The singular absence of constitutional symptoms and the sluggish course in sarcoidosis contrast to the rule in Hodgkin's disease and tuberculosis. The degree and order of the pulmonary involvement upon roentgenographic study contrast strikingly with the clinical well-being of the patient with sarcoidosis. This circumstance alone militates against the diagnosis of Hodgkin's disease and tuberculosis. The negative Mantoux reaction and persistently negative sputum would be further evidence against a tuberculous explanation. It should be noted that the negative cutaneous reaction to tuberculoprotein characteristically shown by the sarcoid patient is "nonspecific" in the sense that cutaneous reactivity to a number of other substances is reduced or abolished in sarcoidosis. A roentgenogram of the hands and feet should give the clue in a considerable proportion of doubtful diagnoses. Absence of periosteal change would tend to exclude syphilis as well as tuberculosis, but a negative Wassermann reaction would be helpful. The virtual absence of constitutional symptoms and the benign course exclude leprosy.

The industrial history might afford the answer to a possible confusion with silicosis and *berylliosis*. Conspicuous lags between the exposures to beryllium and the development of pulmonary fibrosis may render judgment difficult, and this represents the major diagnostic problem with respect to intrathoracic sarcoidosis. It is important to attempt to differentiate the two conditions because the response to steroid (e.g., cortisone) therapy is considerably more marked in sarcoidosis. The principal ways by which this can be done consist of rather elaborate studies of pulmonary physiology (McClement et al.) or by both histopathologic and chemical observations on a piece of lung tissue obtained by wedge resection. The demonstration of beryllium in the urine signifies only the fact of beryllium exposure and is not sufficient evidence to establish the diagnosis in a case of pulmonary disease. Examination of biopsy material from accessible lesions would arbitrarily exclude Hodgkin's disease and lymphosarcoma; but there might be raised the question of tuberculosis, which may be met as stated. Although the differences between tuberculous or syphilitic iridocyclitis and uveitis of uveoparotid fever may be finely drawn, parotitis and facial palsy are peculiar to the latter. Furthermore, a positive Mantoux reaction on one hand or a positive Wassermann reaction on the other would establish the respective etiologies. The geographic distribution of coccidioidomycosis together with appropriate laboratory studies should serve to differentiate it from sarcoidosis. The coccidioidin test and the isolation of *Coccidioides immitis* would confirm the diagnosis. Histoplasmosis and toxoplasmosis should also be considered but could be identified by appropriate laboratory procedures.

As the diagnostic horizon is lifted, an extension of sarcoidosis to include a number of systemic disorders, such as regional ileitis, may increase the problem. Early attempts to establish a diagnostic test for sarcoidosis using the Frei technique failed because the nonspecificity of the prompt reaction (24 to 36 hours) was not appreciated. However, with appropriate antigens, specific reactions have been obtained in patients with sarcoidosis one to two weeks after the intracutaneous injection. The delay in the reaction may be up to 200 days. The antigenic property of the extracts bears no direct relationship to the degree of the pathologic change in the tissue extracted. In general, antigens prepared from cutaneous nodules have proved more effective than those from affected lymph nodes. The cytologic reaction to such emulsions is analogous to the sarcoid lesion (Kveim). Since a sluggish ulcer may persist at the site of the reactive nodule, resection has been advised. This test has not been widely employed in this country, perhaps by reason of the reliance upon the biopsy and other diagnostic measures.

Prognosis. Although interrupted by relapses, the course of sarcoidosis is singularly benign and free from grave constitutional symptoms. Spontaneous recovery may be anticipated in a majority of patients. The pathologic lesions tend to heal by fibrosis. Atrophic scars may mark obsolete cutaneous eruptions. The lymph nodes become more dense. Although the symptoms of the uveoparotid syndrome usually disappear entirely, some induration of the parotid gland and more or less serious visual disturbances may persist. The pulmonary changes may lead to chronic cor pulmonale with congestive failure. Approximately 10 per cent of these patients acquire clinical tuberculosis. Clinical abatement of cutaneous sarcoidosis has attended activation of pulmonary tuberculosis. In the occasional instance of invasion of some important structure, such as the pituitary body, thyroid gland or heart, by the granulomatous process, replacement of essential parenchyma may determine serious collateral effects. Myocardial sarcoidosis may prove particularly dangerous. Tachycardia may be the first and most significant warning of myocardial involvement. On the other hand, cardiac enlargment, abnormal rhythm or electrocardiographic evidence of faulty conduction may be present. With or without such warning, myocardial failure may supervene.

The mortality from all forms of sarcoidosis does not exceed 5 per cent.

Treatment. The therapy of a disease with such a natural history is difficult to evaluate. No specific treatment has been reported.

Nitrogen mustard has failed of its early promise. Corticotropin and cortisone have been extensively studied in sarcoidosis. The immediate results have commonly been spectacular, but relapses have frequently occurred. Profound influences upon the ocular changes, pulmonary physiology and hypercalcemia justify continued close study under controlled conditions. Topical applications of cortisone or hydrocortisone in uveal tract involvement are especially promising.

Phospholipid compounds are responsible for certain epithelioid reactions in lupus vulgaris. By analogy this principle has been carried into the therapy of sarcoidosis. To favor the excretion of phosphorus and to interrupt this cytologic response, calciferol, 150,000 to 900,000 units, with or without calcium, or dihydrotachysterol, 3.75 mg. reduced to 1.2 mg., is administered daily by mouth. These doses are large, and toxic evidence of hypercalcemia must be anticipated and met. The cutaneous, lymphoid and pulmonary lesions of sarcoidosis have apparently responded favorably to this therapy. Splenectomy has resulted in relief of thrombocytopenic purpura in sarcoidosis. Since neither infectivity nor, for that matter, tuberculous etiology has been established, sanatorium treatment should be discouraged.

WILLIAM S. MIDDLETON

References

Bernstein, S. S., and Sussman, M. L.: Thoracic Manifestations of Sarcoidosis. Radiology, *44*:37, 1945.

Boeck, C.: Multiple Benign Sarkoid of the Skin. J. Cutan. & Genito-Urin. Dis., *17*:543, 1899.

Curtis, A. C., Taylor, H. J., and Grekin, R. H.: Sarcoidosis. I. Results of Treatment with Varying Amounts of Calciferol and Dihydrotachysterol. J. Invest. Dermat., *9*:131, 1947.

Fisher, A. M., and Davis, B. D.: The Serum Proteins in Sarcoidosis: Electrophoretic Studies. Bull. Johns Hopkins Hosp., *71*:364, 1942.

Heerfordt, C. F.: Ueber eine Febris uveo-parotidea subchronica an der Glandula parotis und der Uvea des Auges lokalisiert und häufig mit Paresen cere-brospinalen Nerven kompliciert. Arch. f. Ophthal., *70*:254, 1909.

Kveim, A.: Preliminary Report on New and Specific Cutaneous Reaction in Boeck's Sarcoid. Nord. Med., *9*:169, 1941.

Longcope, W. T.: Sarcoidosis, or Besnier-Boeck-Schaumann Disease. J.A.M.A., *117*:1321, 1941.

————, and Fisher, A. M.: The Effect of Schaumann's Disease upon the Heart and its Mechanism. Acta Med. Scandinav., *108*:529, 1941.

McClement, J. H., Renzetti, A. D., Himmelstein, A. and Cournand, A.: Cardiopulmonary Function in the Pulmonary Form of Boeck's Sarcoid and Its Modification by Cortisone Therapy. Am. Rev. Tuberc., *67*:154, 1953.

Mylius, K., and Schürmann, P.: Universelle Sklerosierende tuberkulöse grosszellige Hyperplasie, eine besondere Form atypischer Tuberkulose. Beitr. z. Klin. d. Tuber., *73*:166, 1930.

Pautrier, L. M.: La Maladie de Besnier- Boeck, Presse méd., No. 8, 146, 1935. Une nouvelle grande réticulo-endothéliose maladie de Besnier-Boeck-Schaumann. Paris, Masson et Cie, 1940.

Pohle, E. A., Paul, L. W., and Clark, E. A.: Roentgen Therapy of Boeck's Sarcoid. Am. J. M. Sc., *209*:503, 1945.

Putkonen, J.: Über die infrakutanreaktion von Kveim (KR) bei Lymphogranulomatosis benigna. Acta Derm.-Vener., 23:(Suppl. K), 1, 1943.

Sands, J. H.: Personal Communication regarding experience at Fitzsimmons Army Hospital.

Schaumann, J.: Lymphogranulomatosis Benigna in the Light of Prolonged Clinical Observations and Autopsy Findings. Brit. J. Dermat. & Syph., *48*:399, 1936.

Shulman, L. E., Schoenrich, E. H., and Harvey, A. M.: The Effects of Adrenocorticotropin (ACTH) and Cortisone on Sarcoidosis. Bull. Johns Hopkins Hosp., *91*:371, 1952.

Van Beek, C., and Haex, A. J. C.: Aspiration-Biopsy of the Liver in Mononucleosis Infectiosa and in Besnier-Boeck-Schaumann's Disease. Acta med. Scandinav., *113*:125, 1943.

MILIARY FEVER

Definition. Miliary fever is an acute infectious disease which occurs in epidemic form and is characterized by abrupt onset of fever, excessive sweating, prostration and erythematous rash.

Incidence. Most of the epidemics have occurred in Europe, and the "sweating sickness" which swept over England during the fifteenth and sixteenth centuries was probably miliary fever. An epidemic occurred in France in 1907. Zeiss made an epidemiologic study of the disease in Russia in 1932. So far as is known, the disease has never occurred in the United States.

Etiology. The cause of miliary fever is not

known, nor is its mode of transmission understood. The epidemics which have been studied have occurred most frequently in the spring and summer months. Persons of all ages are susceptible. The mode of spread is rapid, in this respect resembling that of epidemic influenza.

Symptoms. The most striking feature of miliary fever is the profuse perspiration. It begins with the onset of fever, which continues throughout the course of the disease. The eruption, which appears on the third or fourth day, is usually of the papulovesicular type, occurring first on the neck, back and chest, and later in the axillae and between the thighs. Occasionally a purpuric form of the disease with other manifestations of hemorrhage is noted. As the rash appears, there is gradual diminution in the intensity of the symptoms and, after two or three days, desquamation occurs. Convalescence is characterized by weakness, loss of weight and slow recovery.

Prognosis. The prognosis is usually favorable, but occasionally a high fever, dyspnea and rapid pulse develop, followed by delirium and death.

Treatment. Treatment is symptomatic.

RUSSELL L. CECIL

References

Beckman, H.: Treatment in General Practice. 6th ed. Philadelphia, W. B. Saunders Company, 1948.

von Lemser, H.: Der englische Schweisz in seiner Abhängigheit von Rasse, Boden und Klima. Ztschr. f. Hyg. u. Infektionskrankh., p. 476, April, 1937.

Wallis, Conrado. Exantema febrile vesiculoso, miliar, de caracter epidemico. Medicina, México, 27:94, 1947.

Zeiss, H.: Über englischen Schweiss und Schweissfriesel in Russland. Arch. f. Hyg., 107:243, 1932.

AINHUM

(Dactylolysis Spontanea)

Definition. Ainhum is a chronic disease of unknown cause usually affecting the little toe and characterized by the formation of a furrow at the digitoplantar fold, which deepens and extends until the toe is encircled and eventually separated from the foot.

Incidence. Ainhum has been observed chiefly on the west coast of Africa and in Brazil. Cases have been reported also from the West Indies, Panama, and rarely from the southern part of the United States. Apparently, white people are not susceptible; nearly all the cases reported have been observed among nonwhites. There is some evidence that ainhum is a familial disease, since it may occur in several members of the same family or in repeated generations of the same family. It occurs chiefly in male adults between 25 and 30 years of age.

Etiology. There have been various theories as to etiology. Some have claimed that ainhum was related to leprosy. This seems, however, most unlikely; it is much more probable that the disease is a trophoneurosis secondary to some local trauma. Kean and Tucker reviewed 45 cases from the Isthmus of Panama in 1946 and concluded that the cause of ainhum is still unknown and its pathogenesis not clear.

Morbid Anatomy. In a typical case a fibrous cord replaces the bony structures normally attaching the bone to the foot. The skin becomes thickened, and the walls of the blood vessels show an endarteritis with a secondary rarefying osteitis.

Symptoms. According to Still, the little toe is the one affected in 90 per cent of the cases; more rarely, the fourth toe and very rarely both the fourth and the little toe are implicated. Both little toes may be attacked at the same time, but the condition usually starts in one toe. The initial appearance is featured by a crack in the digitoplantar fold of the little toe. This extends laterally and finally appears on the dorsum of the toe. The distal portion of the toe enlarges and becomes bulbous. In the final stages the connection between the foot and the little toe is a slender fibrous cord which permits the toe to wobble in various directions and to interfere greatly with walking.

The course of the disease extends over several years if the toe does not undergo spontaneous amputation as a result of injury to the pedicle. The disease is practically painless.

Treatment. Ainhum is best treated in the early stages by longitudinal incision into the grooved furrow. In the later stages amputation is usually necessary.

RUSSELL L. CECIL

References

Ash, J. A., and Spitz, Sophie: Pathology of Tropical Diseases; An Atlas. Philadelphia W. B. Saunders Company, 1945.

Jacobs, E. C., Butz, W. C., and Felts, J. H.: Ainhum (Dactylolysis spontanea). Am. J. Clin. Path., 21: 56, 1951.

de Jimenez, J.: Ainhum in Dominican Republic, with Report of 5 Cases. Bol. Asoc. med. Santiago, 4:55, 1946.

Kean, B. H., and Tucker, H. A.: Ainhum; Etiologic Concepts and Pathologic Aspects. Arch. Path., 41: 639, 1946.

Strong, R. P.: Stitt's Diagnosis, Prevention, and Treatment of Tropical Diseases. 7th ed. Philadelphia, Blakiston Co., 1944.

MILK SICKNESS

(Trembles)

Milk sickness, better known as the trembles, is an afebrile disease due to the ingestion of milk, milk products, or the flesh of animals suffering from the disease.

Milk sickness is now more or less of a medical curiosity, but in the first half of the nineteenth century it constituted a major problem on the western frontier of the United States.

History. Nicolay and Hay, in their "History of Abraham Lincoln," claim that Nancy Hanks, the mother of Lincoln, died of milk sickness. "In the autumn of 1818 the little community of Pigeon Creek was almost exterminated by a frightful pestilence called the 'milk-sickness.'" Nancy Hanks was one of the victims.

Incidence. At the present time milk sickness is a rare disease, but a century ago the condition was common in various parts of the United States. It was quite prevalent throughout the Mississippi Valley, particularly in Ohio, Indiana, Illinois and Michigan. There is no record of milk sickness having ever occurred outside the United States.

Etiology. The evidence seems to be fairly conclusive that milk sickness is caused in the majority of cases by a plant known as white snakeroot, *Eupatorium urticaefolium*. In New Mexico and Arizona this plant has not been observed, but what is apparently the same disease also occurs in these states and is due to another herb, the rayless goldenrod, *Aplopappus heterophyllus*, which probably

contains the same toxic agent found in white snakeroot. In man the disease results from eating butter or drinking the milk from cattle which have ingested the weed. It is also possible for the human being to be poisoned by the beef of cattle that have eaten of this plant. When extract of white snakeroot is fed to laboratory animals, they become ill, refuse food and develop a generalized tremor. Couch, who was one of the first to isolate a toxin from white snakeroot, named it *trematol* which, according to Couch, exists in the plant partly in ester combination with a resinous acid.

Symptoms. Milk sickness is characterized by a gradual onset of weakness, loss of appetite and vomiting. These early symptoms are followed by constipation and abdominal distress. There is no fever, but marked thirst is usually noted. The mind is clear, but in fatal cases, coma may precede death by several hours. The average duration of the disease is seven to nine days, although symptoms may continue much longer.

Prognosis. The prognosis is grave in both acute and subacute cases. Moseley states that the death rate is about 25 per cent.

Treatment. The treatment is purely symptomatic. Prophylaxis consists of avoiding meat and milk products of animals with trembles, and in pasturing cattle on cleared or plowed land.

RUSSELL L. CECIL

References

Couch, J. F.: The Toxic Constituent of Richweed or White Snakeroot. Report from J. Agr. Research, 35:547, Washington (Sept. 15) 1927.

Doyle, J. T.: Milk Sickness. North Carolina M. J., 8:404, 1947.

Jordan, E. O., and Harris, N. M.: Milk Sickness. J. Infect. Dis., 6:401 (Sept. 20) 1909.

Jordon, P. D.: Milk Sickness in the Western Country Together with an Account of the Death of Lincoln's Mother. Ohio State M. J., 40:848, 1944.

Moseley, E. L.: Milk Sickness Caused by White Snakeroot. Pub. jointly by The Ohio Acad. Sci. and author, Bowling Green, Ohio, 1941.

Sackett, W. G.: The Connection of Milk Sickness with the Poisonous Qualities of White Snakeroot, *Eupatorium Urticaefolium*. J. Infect. Dis., 24: 231 (Mar.) 1919.

Steun, Fred: The Pioneer History of Milk Sickness. Amer. Med. Hist., 9:23, 1937.

Diseases of Allergy

INTRODUCTION

RELATION OF ANTIGEN-ANTIBODY REACTIONS TO ALLERGIC DISEASES

The clinical manifestations of allergic reactions result from the combination of an antigen with an antibody which has been formed by the host, generally in response to prior contact with the antigen. Hay fever, asthma, food and drug allergy, and allergic dermatitis usually are caused by noninfectious antigens of environmental or extrinsic origin. However, the pathologic changes of chronic infection often may be caused, in large part, by an allergic response of the host to the invading micro-organism. Furthermore, the morphologic and physiologic changes which characterize the so-called "collagen diseases," glomerulonephritis, rheumatic fever and encephalomyelitis, are thought by some to result from autoantibody production to antigens present in the individual's own tissues. In erythroblastosis fetalis, antibodies derived from the mother pass through the placenta to combine with antigens on the erythrocytes of the fetus. The degeneration of homologous skin and other tissue grafts may be also attributed to the formation by the recipient of antibodies to the grafted tissues. From the immunologic standpoint, therefore, allergy is an ever-broadening field with a profoundly important relation to pathology and clinical medicine.

Allergic reactions to extrinsic antigens may be separated broadly into two groups. One of these is associated with the presence of circulating antibody in the serum of affected individuals, and includes anaphylaxis, Arthus reactions, serum sickness, allergies involving the characteristic wheal and erythema reaction, hay fever, urticarias, angioedema, asthma and certain gastrointestinal allergies. In the other, an antibody having a high affinity for tissue cells has been demonstrated and circulating antibody is thought not to be involved. This latter group includes contact dermatitis (e.g., poison ivy sensitivity), drug allergies (sulfonamides, penicillin) and certain allergies of infection. The allergic reactions observed in these two groups are frequently referred to as "immediate" and "delayed," respectively. These terms are sometimes useful in distinguishing anaphylaxis and urticarial reactions from contact dermatitis and tuberculin sensitivity, but are ambiguous as applied to the Arthus and tuberculin reactions, as well as drug sensitivities, in which microscopic evidence of reaction occurs early but in which several hours are required before they become visible grossly.

Since allergic diseases are a manifestation of the response of tissues to an antigen-antibody reaction, an understanding of their mechanism depends largely upon a knowledge of: (1) the nature of the inciting antigens; (2) the ways in which sensitization can take place; (3) the nature of any predisposing or hereditary factors; (4) the properties of the antibodies involved; (5) the relationship of the reacting quantities of antigen and antibody to the severity of the allergic reaction; (6) the mechanisms by which the combination of antigen and antibody causes the various manifestations of allergic reactions, both local and systemic; and (7) factors affecting antibody formation and the allergic response. None of these problems have been completely solved, but a substantial body of information has been accumulated from studies on human allergy and from animal experimentation.

1. The Nature of the Inciting Antigen(s). Proteins and polysaccharides are capable of stimulating antibody formation in animals and in man, and these comprise most of the allergenic substances. Both are widely distributed throughout the animal and plant world, and almost any protein constituent (and some polypeptides) can, under suitable experimental circumstances, be shown to elicit an antibody response. In sensitivities caused by low molecular weight substances, such as common drugs, it is generally believed from the work of Landsteiner and co-workers that these substances are in some way coupled to protein in the animal and in this way induce the formation of antibody. To be antigenic, proteins must be foreign to the circulation of the host, e.g., antibodies are not produced by the injection of human serum proteins from man to man. In hemolytic anemias, the production of autoantibodies to erythrocyte antigens may occur but the mechanism of this sensitization is unknown; a recent case was shown to be due to production of antibodies to one of the rare Rh factors, e or Hr″, by an individual whose erythrocytes contained this antigen.

Purified polysaccharides are antigenic in certain species but not in others. The type-specific pneumococcal polysaccharides and dextrans, for example, are antigenic in man and give rise on injection to precipitins and to wheal and erythema sensitivity. Antibodies and skin sensitivity to certain polysaccharides occur in a considerable proportion of humans, sensitization probably resulting from micro-organisms in the nasopharynx and the gastrointestinal tract which produce these polysaccharides. Indeed, the infusion of certain dextrans into such sensitized individuals has produced urticarial and other anaphylactic symptoms. In other species, such as the rabbit and guinea pig, these polysaccharides are antigenic only when combined with protein or in the intact micro-organism.

In experimental animals, using well defined or purified proteins, the sensitivities produced are most frequently associated with circulating antibody, and are similar to the allergies encountered in the administration of foreign proteins (e.g., horse antitoxins) to man as typified by serum sickness and anaphylactic reactions. The high proportion of allergic sensitizations affected by contact with such foreign proteins in man necessitates the use of a preliminary intracutaneous test prior to parenteral administration of even small amounts of an antitoxin or other foreign protein. This may be performed with about 0.01 to 0.02 cc. of 1:10 diluted serum; a positive wheal and erythema reaction after about 20 minutes indicates sensitivity.

Delayed type allergic reactions are less amenable to study, since they are generally the result of infections with intact micro-organisms which are extremely complex mixtures of antigens (e.g., tuberculin, mallein) and thus are far more complicated from the immunologic standpoint. Drug sensitivities and poison ivy sensitivity are also of this delayed type; the experimental production of drug sensitivities in animals provides instances of less complicated antigenic systems.

The factors determining whether a substance will be antigenic and whether allergic sensitization will or will not be associated with circulating antibody are completely obscure, and our present knowledge is entirely empiric.

2. Ways in Which Sensitization Can Take Place. Sensitization to various antigens may occur following introduction of antigen by parenteral, respiratory, oral or other routes. In experimental animals and man, sensitization to serum proteins of another species can be induced in almost all instances. Serum sickness has occurred in over 90 per cent of individuals treated with large amounts of horse antipneumococcal serum. Similarly, the development of skin sensitivity to tuberculin may be produced in tuberculin-negative individuals by vaccination with BCG. On the other hand, only a relatively small proportion of the population develop the usual allergic diseases produced by grass and tree pollens, danders and certain foods. Efforts to induce skin sensitivity, hay fever, asthma or other manifestations of allergy with these antigens in man have been generally unsuccessful, although anaphylactic sensitivity may be produced in guinea pigs fairly readily. Naturally occurring human allergies are sometimes termed spontaneous allergies to distinguish them from induced allergies.

3. Predisposing or Hereditary Factors. Studies in various experimental animals have shown that by inbreeding and selection it is possible to establish strains differing widely in susceptibility to certain bacterial infections, capacity to produce antibody and ability to become sensitized to certain simple chemical compounds. Such data indicate that heredity influences these phenomena. Evidence that similar genetic factors affect the development of the spontaneously occurring allergies in man is far more difficult to obtain. Suggestions that these allergies are inherited on a Mendelian basis have been based on the occurrence of families with a large proportion of allergic individuals. A recent critical reexamination of such family studies established that in about 40 per cent of the families only a single individual was allergic and that in an additional 25 per cent only one other member had allergy; only a small fraction of the families had many allergic members. With only such data the existence of genetic determinants in these human allergies must be considered as unproved.

4. Properties of the Antibodies Involved. A number of antibodies have been recognized in both experimental animals and man which differ in their capacities to induce allergic sensitivities. These antibodies may vary in their ability to react with antigen, to sensitize a heterologous species passively, to elicit a wheal and erythema reaction, or in their affinity for tissue cells. To a limited extent certain of these properties have been related to certain types of allergic response.

The usual type of precipitin produced after the injection into a rabbit of a foreign protein such as egg albumin can passively sensitize the guinea pig or rabbit for anaphylactic shock or the Arthus reaction. However, the antibodies produced by the rabbit to such an antigen are not all identical but are thought to represent a spectrum of antibodies differing in reactivity. Certain of the antibody molecules in such an antiserum do not by themselves precipitate with antigen. They precipitate with other antibody molecules if sufficient antigen is added at one time, but remain in the supernatant serum if precipitation is carried out fractionally by successive serial addition of small amounts of antigen. This type of antibody is termed nonprecipitable since it cannot precipitate with antigen by itself, but can only attach itself to a specific precipitate formed in the presence of precipitable antibody. Precipitable and nonprecipitable rabbit antibodies to egg albumin have been shown to be equally effective in inducing passive anaphylactic sensitization in the guinea pig; the nonprecipitable antibody, however, was incapable of inducing an Arthus type of sensitization passively. Conversely, certain types of horse antibody such as horse antibody to the pneumococcal polysaccharides are, for unknown reasons, incapable of inducing passive anaphylactic sensitization of the guinea pig. However, they precipitate with the pneumococcal polysaccharides and have been shown to induce a passive Arthus reaction in the guinea pig. From this and other evidence, the Arthus reaction may best be interpreted as due to mechanical damage to blood vessels resulting from precipitation of antigen and antibody, while anaphylaxis is a consequence of the combination of antigen with antibody and is largely independent of precipitation. Some individuals have been shown to produce a nonprecipitating variety of diphtheria antitoxin which was also capable of passive anaphylactic sensitization of the guinea pig. Precipitating antibodies have been found in hu-

mans who have developed serum sickness. Since horse serum is a complex mixture of antigens, the relation of the clinical manifestations to the disappearance of antigen and the appearance of antibody is difficult to determine. However, in studying serum sickness following the administration of crystalline bovine albumin, Kendall was able to demonstrate that the clinical manifestations coincided with accelerated disappearance of antigen from the circulation and that circulating antibody appeared shortly after symptoms subsided.

It is of importance to remember that individuals who have experienced serum sickness or formed antibody to such foreign protein may be thrown into anaphylactic shock. Furthermore, lesions wholly similar to those of periarteritis nodosa have been found in animals and in man following administration of large amounts of foreign serum. Rare instances have also been recorded in which an acute demyelinating disseminated encephalomyelitis followed the administration of pertussis vaccine.

The spontaneous allergies of the wheal and erythema type have been shown frequently to be associated with antibody in the circulating blood. The antigen or antigens responsible for such sensitivity may be identified by skin testing with a variety of extracts from trees, grasses and pollens. Because of the danger of inducing severe systemic reactions, minute doses of such extracts are employed. Extracts are standardized on the basis of their protein nitrogen content and their potency is frequently expressed in units; one unit is 0.01 microgram protein nitrogen. Two techniques are generally used—the scratch test and the intracutaneous test. The former is considered to be somewhat safer, but the latter is more sensitive. Skin tests are generally performed on the arm or forearm, a location which offers the opportunity for controlling development of any systemic reaction from the test by application of a tourniquet. The scratch test is usually performed by making a small scratch with a hypodermic needle, gently rubbing a drop of the allergenic substance into the skin over the scratch. The intracutaneous test is carried out by the injection into the most superficial layers of the skin of about 0.01 cc. of the allergen solution; this quantity is usually the minimum amount producing a detectable bleb. Control tests with diluent alone are always carried out. The appearance after 15 to 30 minutes of a wheal with surrounding erythema which is absent in the control is taken as a positive test. In carrying out such tests, it is essential to start with extremely dilute solutions (10 to 100 units per cubic centimeter) to avoid severe constitutional reactions. If negative results are obtained, further tests may be made with increasing concentrations, usually tenfold increments.

Antibodies in the serum of individuals showing such skin sensitivity may be identified by passive transfer of such serum into the skin of nonsensitive individuals (Prausnitz-Küstner reaction). After from 6 hours to five or ten or even more days, antigen is injected into the same site and the occurrence of a wheal and erythema reaction noted.

While allergic individuals generally show skin sensitivity of the wheal and erythema type to one or more of the offending antigens, it is not uncommon to find skin sensitivity in individuals who do not show clinical manifestations of disease on exposure to this allergen. A substantial proportion of individuals with skin sensitivity to a given antigen have antibodies in their serum capable of giving a Prausnitz-Küstner reaction. Despite extensive study no unequivocal *in vitro* manifestation of the presence of these skin sensitizing antibodies has been demonstrated. Recent attempts to associate them with a nonprecipitating antibody are open to considerable question in view of the failure to employ serums shown to be free from precipitating antibodies to other antigenic impurities.

Another type of antibody in human serum to antigens associated with the wheal and erythema types of allergy has been demonstrated by Cooke and co-workers, by Harley and subsequently by others. This antibody is formed in response to the parenteral injection of antigen. It may be formed in sensitive individuals receiving injections of antigens such as ragweed extracts for therapeutic purposes, and is also formed when nonallergic individuals receive similar injections. These antibodies do not sensitize human skin but combine with their homologous antigen so that the antigen cannot react with the skin-sensitizing antibody to give a wheal and erythema response. These antibodies, which have been termed *blocking antibodies,* differ in several respects from skin-sensitizing anti-bodies. They are stable to heating at 56° C. for 4 hours, a procedure which destroys the activity of the skin-sensitizing antibody. Unlike the skin-sensitizing antibody they diffuse away from the site of injection and also are able to pass the placenta. Finally, recent studies have shown that serums with high titers of blocking antibody to ragweed extract not only combine with antigen to prevent a skin reaction, but can also bind antigen so that the antigen is unable to combine and fix complement with rabbit antibody to ragweed extracts; this latter capacity is measured by a "complement fixation inhibition" or "indirect complement fixation" test. Blocking antibody may eventually be shown to be a classic type of precipitating antibody if obtainable in adequate quantities. The major unsolved problems in wheal and erythema allergy are the nature of the skin-sensitizing antibody, the manner in which it is produced, how it is able to attach itself to skin and whether or not it would behave as a precipitating antibody if obtained in sufficient quantities.

The antibody associated with allergies of the delayed type appears to be different from these other antibodies. Individuals and animals showing delayed or tuberculin type sensitivities do not appear to have antibodies which can passively transfer this type of sensitivity in their serum. Studies of Landsteiner and Chase, however, have shown that skin sensitivity of the delayed type in guinea pigs may be transferred passively to nonsensitive animals of the same species by the administration of cell exudates. Subsequent studies in man have also successfully demonstrated passive transfer of sensitivity to tuberculin by injecting leukocytes from tuberculin-positive into tuberculin-negative subjects. To elicit such effects the cells must be living. The sensitivity does not make its appearance for two to three days after the cells are introduced, and a probable explanation is that these cells continue to elaborate antibody during this period. With larger amounts of washed cell exudates, Chase has also been able to transfer anaphylactic sensitivity and antitoxic immunity. Since all kinds of antibodies must of necessity have been elaborated by cells, further progress may make it possible to account more clearly for these diverse types of antibody activity.

5. Quantitative Relationships between Antibody and Antigen and the Allergic

Responses. An important consideration in the understanding of the mechanisms of allergy is a knowledge of the amounts of antibody required to bring about allergic reactions. Passive sensitization may be affected by injecting measured volumes of rabbit or guinea pig antiserum to purified antigens of known antibody content into guinea pigs, and then after a suitable interval injecting antigen. With this technique, it has been shown that only 30 micrograms of rabbit or guinea pig antibody nitrogen need be present in a 250 gm. guinea pig for uniformly fatal anaphylactic shock to occur; with human diphtheria antitoxin about 100 micrograms was needed. Uterine strips from a guinea pig passively sensitized to egg albumin might be expected to contain about 0.01 microgram of antibody N; such uterine strips show maximal contraction when exposed to antigen in a Dale bath. Ovary has shown that injection into guinea pig skin of but 0.003 microgram antibody N was sufficient to cause a wheal and erythema type of reaction on contact with antigen. The latent period in passive anaphylaxis, e.g., the time interval between the sensitizing dose of antibody and the shocking dose of antigen, has been shown both in systemic anaphylaxis and with isolated uterine strips to be a function of the quantity of antibody used for sensitization; with large amounts of antibody N fatal anaphylaxis could be obtained with no latent period but as the quantity of antibody N used for sensitization decreased, the latent period increased.

The passive Arthus reaction, however, requires far larger quantities of antibody N. To produce a minimal Arthus reaction, 25 micrograms of antibody N in the rabbit and about 10 micrograms in the guinea pig must be injected into a skin site. These quantities of antibody are of the order of 1000 to 2500 times larger than that estimated to be present in a contracting uterine strip, or 3000 to 10,000 times greater than that responsible for a wheal and erythema reaction in guinea pig skin.

The very minute amounts of antibody required to elicit wheal and erythema and anaphylactic reactions suggest the possibility that the failure to detect *in vitro* manifestations of skin-sensitizing and blocking antibodies may be due to the small quantities involved; it cannot be excluded, however, that certain of these antibodies may possibly prove to be of the nonprecipitable variety which,

as described above, can produce anaphylactic sensitivity.

6. The Mechanisms by Which Combination of Antigen and Antibody Causes An Allergic Response. A number of the physiologic and pathologic manifestations of immediate type anaphylactic reactions, notably the patterns in anaphylactic shock, the wheal and erythema reaction in human skin, and the contraction of smooth muscle, may be produced by the injection of histamine, and these findings have led to the belief that the antigen-antibody combination liberates histamine or some pharmacologically similar H substance (or possibly acetylcholine) which is responsible for these manifestations. Further evidence that histamine is liberated in allergic reactions rests on the similarity of the effects produced in various animal species, notably in the guinea pig by certain diamines, and mono- or diamidines, a group of substances termed histamine liberators. For instance, if a sensitized guinea pig which has also received an injection of pontamine sky blue is thrown into anaphylactic shock, the localization of the blue dye in certain characteristic areas is very similar to that produced in a guinea pig injected with a histamine liberator. Furthermore, the areas of skin selectively colored by the blue dye in both instances are those which contain the highest concentrations of histamine. On the other hand, it has not been established that histamine or acetylcholine liberation can explain all of the manifestations in these reactions. For instance, the uterine muscle of a sensitized guinea pig, placed in a Dale bath and repeatedly exposed to histamine until it no longer contracts, will nevertheless respond by contraction when antigen is introduced into the bath; similarly sensitized uterine muscle will contract when exposed to antigen even when acetylcholine action is counteracted by atropine. The failure of both atropine and antihistaminics to alleviate symptoms in asthma also requires clarification. It is possible, however, that the histamine or other substances released from within cells may act differently than when introduced from outside the cell. Little is known of the mechanisms by which antigen-antibody combination brings about other allergic manifestations.

7. Factors Affecting Antibody Formation and the Allergic Response. Roentgen irradiation has been shown to reduce or inhibit antibody formation if administered prior to the injection of antigen. Several substances, notably the nitrogen mustards and ACTH and cortisone, have also been shown to suppress but not completely abolish antibody formation and to have a suppressive effect on the specific anamnestic response. As a consequence, in actively sensitized animals receiving these drugs, the Arthus reaction which requires fairly substantial antibody levels has been reduced in severity. However, anaphylactic reactions in actively sensitized animals which require relatively minute quantities of antibody are not affected by these substances. Cortisone and ACTH have been shown not to influence the combination of preformed antigen and antibody in that both passive anaphylaxis and the passive Arthus reaction are unaffected. Cortisone has been found useful in the treatment of certain allergies, notably serum sickness, hay fever, asthma, contact dermatitis, infantile eczema and drug allergies, and less effective in urticarias and angioedema; it also reduces the intensity of the tuberculin reaction. These effects may also result from an effect on inflammation rather than from suppression of antibody formation, since the cortisone frequently acts more rapidly than an effect on antibody would be expected.

ELVIN A. KABAT

References

Chase, M. W.: In Dubos, R. J.: Bacterial and Mycotic Infections of Man. 2nd ed. Philadelphia, J. B. Lippincott Co., 1952, Chap. 8.

Cooke, R. A.: Allergy in Theory and Practice. Philadelphia, W. B. Saunders Co., 1946.

Fischel, E. E.: The Role of Allergy in the Pathogenesis of Rheumatic Fever. Am. J. Med., 7:772, 1949.

Kabat, E. A., and Mayer, M. M.: Experimental Immunochemistry. Springfield, Ill., Charles C Thomas, 1948.

Landsteiner, K.: The Specificity of Serological Reactions. Revised edition. Cambridge, Mass., Harvard University Press, 1945.

Pappenheimer, A. M., Jr., Editor: The Nature and Significance of the Antibody Response. New York, Columbia University Press, 1953.

von Pirquet, C., and Schick, B.: Serum Sickness (translated by B. Schick). Baltimore, Williams and Wilkins Co., 1905, 1951.

Ratner, B., and Silberman, D. C.: Critical Analysis of the Hereditary Concept of Allergy. J. Allergy, 24:371, 1953.

Symposium on Allergy: Am. J. Med., 3:509, 1947.

Combined Staff Clinics, College of Physicians and Surgeons: Antigen-Antibody Reactions. Am. J. Med., 13:352, 1952.

HAY FEVER

Definition. *Allergic rhinitis* is a reaction of the nasal mucosa manifested by edema, itching and increased mucous secretion, and is the result of allergy to a specific antigen. When caused by allergy to pollens it is called *hay fever* or pollenosis, and is characterized by seasonal recurrence during the period of pollination of the causative plants. In present usage, the term hay fever is not limited to allergy of grass pollens but is applied also to that due to tree and weed pollens. Allergic rhinitis due to antigens other than pollens is called *nonseasonal* or *perennial allergic rhinitis*. The term *vasomotor rhinitis* is applied both to perennial allergic rhinitis and to morphologically similar chronic edema of the nasal mucosa due to nonantigenic irritants, or probably in some cases to neurogenic and psychosomatic causes.

Etiology. The occurrence of symptoms of hay fever depends upon the development of allergy of the "wheal and erythema type" for pollen and subsequent inhalation of the specific pollen in adequate quantity to elicit the allergic reaction. The allergic sensitization producing hay fever is the same type associated with infantile eczema, atopic dermatitis, bronchial asthma and certain forms of food allergy, so that persons manifesting one of these diseases frequently develop others of the group. While diseases of this group tend to occur in certain families, neither the particular disease manifestation nor allergy to a specific antigen is inherited, only a tendency to become allergic to antigens to which the individual is exposed.

In general, only those plants depending on the wind for cross-pollination and producing an abundance of buoyant, windborne pollen are important factors in the causation of hay fever. These include grasses, many families of weeds, and most of the trees of temperate climates. Plants with showy and odoriferous blossoms, including roses and goldenrod, which are adapted to insect pollination and produce relatively small amounts of heavy, sticky pollen, rarely cause hay fever. Allergy to tree and weed pollens is specific for the genus rather than the species of plant, so that the use of pollen of one species of a genus in testing and treatment suffices. In the case of the grasses, the pollens of all the common genera are antigenically quite similar, so that for practical purposes a mixture of the pollens of three or four of the grasses most common in a given area may be used as if a single antigen.

Specific diagnosis of hay fever requires a knowledge of the flora of the patient's locality and the seasons of pollination of the plants. Throughout the greater portion of the United States and southern Canada, spring hay fever (April and May) is due to tree pollens, early summer hay fever (June and July) to grass pollens, with plantain and sorrel also important in some areas, and late hay fever (August and September) to weed pollens. The important trees vary considerably in different areas; ash, beech, birch, cedar, hickory, maple, oak, sycamore and poplar produce an abundance of antigenic windborne pollen and may be presumed important where they grow commonly. The pollens of the pines and other conifers are relatively less antigenic and less often cause hay fever even where abundant. The grass pollens are everywhere important, their season being prolonged through much of the year in the extreme south. In the East and Middle West ragweed is by far the most important weed pollen; it also occurs in most of the Far West, except for the North Pacific coast, but its importance in the mountain and coast areas is less than that of sage, amaranth and Russian thistle. For detailed accounts of the windborne pollens causing hay fever in various areas of the United States and southern Canada, reference to the works of Wodehouse and of Durham is suggested. The tree and grass hay fever seasons in northern Europe correspond closely to those of the United States; the weed pollens are relatively much less important, ragweed not being indigenous to the area.

Incidence. It has been estimated that 8 to 10 per cent of the population of the United States is affected by hay fever, but a large proportion of these cases are not severe enough to require medical treatment. The white, Negro and yellow races are susceptible. Both sexes are equally affected. In areas where ragweed is abundant, approximately 75 per cent of hay fever sufferers are affected by this pollen; in 50 per cent it is the only significant cause. About 50 per cent are affected by grass pollens alone or in combination with other pollens. Tree hay fever is statistically less important and usually occurs in patients also affected by grass or weed pollens.

Pathology and Physiology. Since one of the chief functions of the nose is to warm and purify the inhaled air, a large proportion of suspended dust particles are deposited on its mucosa, which is therefore peculiarly exposed to inhaled allergens. As has been described in the introductory section on allergy, sensitization of the type causing hay fever consists in the development of sensitizing antibodies present in the conjunctiva, nasal mucosa, skin and blood plasma. Contact of the allergenic pollen with the sensitized mucosa elicits an antigen-antibody reaction which is manifested by engorgement of the blood vessels, edema, increased secretion of watery mucus, and itching which gives rise to sneezing. The physiologic effects of the antigen-antibody reaction are believed to result from the release of histamine, which acts locally. There is little evidence that the central nervous system is involved.

While the symptoms produced by inhalation of pollen are localized to the mucosae with which it comes in contact, the sensitization is systemic. Injection of too large a quantity of antigen into a highly allergic patient in a diagnostic skin test or in treatment, may elicit a *constitutional reaction* similar to experimental anaphylactic shock. It is manifested within 20 minutes or less, by coughing, sneezing, asthma, urticaria or general flushing and itching of the skin and, in severe cases, collapse. Such reactions may be serious or even fatal if not promptly treated.

Repeated injections of the antigen, for the specific treatment of hay fever, stimulate the formation of blocking antibody, distinct from the preexisting sensitizing antibody. This blocking antibody appears to be responsible for the increase of tolerance for injected antigen, and may be responsible for the clinical benefits of treatment, although evidence of the latter is still inconclusive.

Symptoms. The symptoms of hay fever characteristically recur each year at the same season with the beginning of pollination of the causative plant, the date of onset in a given locality rarely varying by more than a week or so, although the amount of pollen produced and hence the severity of symptoms varies considerably from year to year depending on the weather. During the season, symptoms are worse on dry, windy days and decrease during heavy rain. They usually tend to be worse in the morning. The termination of symptoms at the end of the pollen season is less abrupt than the onset, owing to the persistence of pollen in the air and, in many cases, to the complicating effects of nonseasonal allergens and superimposed respiratory infections.

The most characteristic symptom is sneezing, usually in paroxysms of several sneezes in rapid succession. The nasal mucosa is congested and there is an increased flow of watery mucoid secretion. The conjunctivas are red and itchy with increased lacrimation. Itching of the soft palate and pharynx is usual, and in severe cases the ears may also itch severely. Cough, wheezing and dyspnea are commonly present but are actually indicative of pollen asthma rather than hay fever itself.

Diagnosis. When the pattern of seasonal recurrence has become established, the diagnosis of hay fever is easy and the causative pollen is usually apparent to the physician acquainted with the pollen seasons of the area. During the first season, differentiation from infective rhinitis may be difficult, although the paroxysmal sneezing, the itching of the eyes and pharynx, the watery nasal discharge, the normal temperature, the absence of sore throat and of general malaise are helpful, as is a personal or family history of allergies of the wheal and erythema type. In doubtful cases, smears of the nasal secretion may be stained with Wright's stain; an abundance of eosinophils is characteristic of allergic rhinitis.

Allergic rhinitis due to antigens other than pollens, particularly airborne molds, such as Alternaria and Hormodendrum, may have a seasonal exacerbation during warm weather, but lacks the precise onset and cessation characteristic of pollen allergy. Occasional cases of allergic rhinitis due to fruits or vegetables eaten at certain seasons may be confusing but can be distinguished by skin tests.

The diagnosis of hay fever is established, and the specific cause demonstrated, by eliciting the wheal and erythema reaction in skin tests with the antigen, performed with the technique and precautions outlined in the introductory section on allergy. Both the *scratch test* and the *intracutaneous test* are useful; the former is simpler and involves less danger of a general constitutional reaction, the latter is more sensitive and more useful in estimating the degree of sensitization. For the typical case of seasonal hay fever, a few tests with pollens appropriate to the season and locality suffice. If the season is prolonged, additional tests with mold spores and other inhalants may be added. (See section on Nonseasonal Allergic Rhinitis.)

Reactions are read after 10 to 15 minutes. A slight but definite wheal is considered one plus; a moderate reaction (wheal 6 to 10 mm., without pseudopods) two plus; a wheal of 10 to 15 mm. with pseudopod formation marked or three plus; and wheals larger than 15 mm., four plus.

The initial intracutaneous tests with pollens should be made with solutions of antigen containing no more than 10 protein nitrogen units per cubic centimeter (0.0001 mg. of protein nitrogen per cubic centimeter) and not more than six tests done at one time. If little or no reaction is obtained, subsequent tests may be made with solutions containing 100 units and then 1000 units per cubic centimeter, until a two or three plus reaction is elicited. If pollen extracts not standardized on the basis of protein content are used, one must be guided by the recommendations of the manufacturer.

The degree of sensitivity is roughly indicated by the highest dilution producing a marked (three plus) skin reaction in the intracutaneous test: Class A, highly sensitive, 10 units per cubic centimeter, Class B, average, 100 units, and Class C, less sensitive, 1000 units. A moderate (two plus) reaction to the 1000 unit strength is evidence of sensitivity if consistent with the seasonal incidence of symptoms. Many patients with definite allergy to one pollen show slight or moderate reactions to many other pollens. These are not to be considered significant unless confirmed by the history.

Prognosis. Hay fever is essentially a permanent idiosyncrasy, more troublesome than disabling, and without danger to life. Variations in severity may occur spontaneously or as a result of a change of residence or habits which alters the intensity of exposure to pollen. Since hay fever is a manifestation of allergy of the wheal and erythema type, patients affected by it often develop other diseases of this type, particularly asthma. This complication eventually occurs in approximately 30 per cent of untreated cases, but the incidence is greatly reduced by specific treatment. Patients with hay fever are unusually susceptible to upper respiratory infection and the development of sinusitis is a common complication, especially of the fall type, which persists until the cold weather when respiratory infections are prevalent.

Treatment. The treatment of hay fever consists of: (1) avoidance of the causative pollen; (2) palliative drug therapy; (3) lessening of sensitivity by injections of the specific antigen. When treatment is started during the season of symptoms, the first two methods produce the most immediate relief, but the most satisfactory results over the long term are achieved by antigen injections started at least two months before the season.

Avoidance. When the severity of symptoms warrants it, relief may be obtained by a trip to an area known to be free of the causative pollen, or by a sea voyage. Exposure to pollen may also be lessened by air-condi-

Dosage in Protein Nitrogen Units for Treatment of Hay Fever

DOSE	CLASS A (HIGHLY SENSITIVE)	CLASS B (AVERAGE CASE)	CLASS C (LESS SENSITIVE)
1	2	10	20
2	5	20	40
3	10	40	80
4	20	80	150
5	35	140	250
6	50	200	400
7	75	300	600
8	110	400	850
9	150	600	1200
10	200	800	1800
11	300	1000	2500
12	400	1500	3500
13	600	2000	5000
14	800	3000	6500
15	1000	4000	8000
16	1000	5000	10000

If the allergens used are not standardized on the basis of protein content, the advice of the manufacturer should be followed.

tioning or the use of suitable pollen filters in the window of the bedroom or other rooms, to a lesser degree by simply remaining indoors with windows and doors closed.

Palliative Treatment. The most useful drugs are the antihistaminics, which produce satisfactory relief in a majority of cases. Tripelennamine (Pyribenzamine) 50 mg., chlorprophenpyridamine (Chlor-trimeton) 4 mg., and chlorcyclizine (Perazil or Di-Paralene) 25 mg., are examples of the many suitable drugs of the group. They may be taken after each meal and if necessary every 4 hours at night. Phenergan (12.5 to 25 mg.) has a more potent and lasting antihistaminic action and is useful at bedtime but is too sedative for general use during the day.

Patients with severe symptoms or with coexisting pollen asthma, not relieved by the antihistaminics, may be given cortisone 25 mg., every 6 to 8 hours, or corticotropin in a slowly absorbed vehicle 40 units intramuscularly daily. The dose of either drug should be reduced by 25 to 50 per cent as soon as relief is obtained and is generally continued only for seven to ten days at the height of the pollen season.

For relief of the conjunctival symptoms, eye drops containing cocaine hydrochloride 0.3 per cent, epinephrine hydrochloride 0.025 per cent and boric acid 3 per cent, in rose water, are useful, one drop in each eye two or three times a day if necessary.

Specific Treatment. Treatment with specific pollen antigen consists of a series of twelve to sixteen subcutaneous injections of gradually increasing doses of antigen, given at intervals of three to seven days, starting in time to reach the top dose before the onset of the pollen season. The doses are planned on the basis of the degree of sensitivity as indicated by the skin test, but often must be modified subsequently in accordance with the tolerance of the individual patient. The following schedules will serve as a guide:

The injections are given on the lateral aspect of the upper arm or the thigh, with a rubber tourniquet and epinephrine 1:1000 at hand for use in case of a constitutional reaction. The patient is kept under observation for 20 minutes after the injection.

Normally the injections produce a slight local swelling which subsides within 24 hours. If the local reaction is troublesome or lasts longer than 36 hours, the same dose is repeated after the usual interval, then increased or again repeated as indicated by the resulting reaction.

If a constitutional reaction follows the injection, a rubber tourniquet is applied promptly proximal to the site of the injection and epinephrine 1:1000, 0.4 to 0.6 cc., injected every 10 minutes until relief is obtained. Mild constitutional reactions may be relieved by tripelennamine (Pyribenzamine) 50 to 100 mg. orally or 25 mg. subcutaneously, but since they may rapidly become more serious, the inexperienced physician is wise to use epinephrine. When a constitutional reaction has occurred, the dosage should be dropped back two steps on the schedule and then increased more gradually. If a second constitutional reaction occurs at the same dosage, the subsequent dosage should be kept below that level.

The dose which has been reached at the beginning of the season is repeated weekly during the period of active pollination, without further increase. Suitable injection treatment produces satisfactory results in at least 75 per cent of cases but may be supplemented with drug treatment if necessary. If the results of injection treatment are not satisfactory and no undue reactions have occurred, the following season one may plan to reach a dose two or three times as great.

If treatment is to be repeated the following year, more satisfactory results may be expected with no greater total number of injections, by the perennial method of treatment. After the end of the season, the same dose is repeated every four weeks until the following spring. When a fresh supply of extract is obtained, the dose must be reduced 50 to 60 per cent to allow for the deterioration of the year-old antigen; it can then be increased to the previous or a somewhat higher dose by giving injections every two weeks and progressing in accordance with the above schedules.

If injections of antigen have not been given before onset of symptoms, attempts to start specific treatment during the season are rarely effective, and palliative treatment is more satisfactory.

NONSEASONAL ALLERGIC RHINITIS, VASOMOTOR RHINITIS

Allergic rhinitis due to nonseasonal antigens is essentially similar to hay fever and often affects the same individuals, but if exposure to the antigen is persistent, it assumes a chronic form. Perennial allergic rhinitis may be due to inhaled antigens (inhalants), or to allergic reactions to the bacteria of the nose and paranasal sinuses, and rarely to foods or ingested drugs. Ordinary house dust contains antigens distinct from the known substances contributing to its formation, but possibly resulting from their deterioration, and is one of the most important inhalant antigens.

Vasomotor rhinitis, practically indistinguishable from chronic allergic rhinitis, may result from prolonged exposure to nonantigenic irritants, of which the most frequently encountered are vasoconstricting nose drops such as ephedrine, Privine and Neo-Synephrine. When these drugs have been used persistently, they frequently prove to be the principal cause of prolonged rhinitis and marked improvement results within a week after their discontinuation. A similar edema of the nasal mucosa can also result from psychosomatic factors which may occasionally be the sole cause, but more often are a contributory cause in allergic cases.

In rhinitis due to any of these causes, the nasal mucosa is markedly swollen and presents a pale grayish appearance. In chronic cases there are often mucous polyps, particularly in the ethmoid region. The nasal secretion is increased in amount and mucoid in character, with an abundance of eosinophils in the stained smear.

To evaluate the importance of extrinsic allergens, skin tests with eighteen or twenty of the principal inhalants should be done as outlined in the section on asthma. Tests with food antigens are indicated only if the history is suggestive or if the inhalant tests give negative results. Skin tests are not satisfactory for determining the existence of bacterial allergy in the causation of vasomotor rhinitis. It may be suspected in the presence of associated chronic sinusitis, particularly hyperplastic sinusitis, and is strongly suggested by the coexistence of nasal polyps. If the patient has been using vasoconstricting nose drops persistently, their use should be discontinued before the importance of other factors is estimated. The importance of psychogenic factors in certain cases of vasomotor rhinitis, either as the principal cause or as a contributory factor in allergic patients, must be judged by the history, by the careful elimination of allergic and infective causes, and by observation over a period of time.

Treatment is best directed to the cause. In cases due to specific inhalant antigens such as feathers or animal danders, elimination of contact is far more effective than injection treatment. Allergy to inhalants with which contact is unavoidable, such as house dust and airborne mold spores, is treated by injection of antigens in progressive dosage similar to that advised for pollen antigens. For symptomatic treatment, the antihistaminic drugs in the doses advised for hay fever are useful, but are somewhat less effective in chronic than in acute cases. Cortisone and corticotropin are highly effective in severe cases but the relief is only temporary and prolonged use involves risk of undesirable side effects.

Perennial allergic rhinitis, like hay fever, is not dangerous to life, but if specific treatment is neglected, is often followed by asthma. Susceptibility to nasal and sinus infection is also greatly increased.

WILLIAM B. SHERMAN

References

Blackley, C. H.: Experimental Researches on the
Cause and Nature of Catarrhus Aestivus, London,
1873.

Coca, A. F., Walzer, M., and Thommen, A. A.:
Asthma and Hay Fever in Theory and Practice,
Springfield and Baltimore, Charles C Thomas,
1931.

Cooke, R. A., and Vander Veer, A.: Human Sensitization. J. Immunol., *1*:201, 1916.

———: Allergy in Theory and Practice, Philadelphia, W. B. Saunders Co., 1947.

Durham, O. C., in Feinberg, S. M.: Allergy in Practice. Chicago, Year Book Publishers, 1944, p.
125.

Wodehouse, R. P.: Hay Fever Plants. Waltham,
Mass., Chronica Botanica Co., 1945.

ASTHMA

Definition. Bronchial asthma is a chronic disease, manifested by a characteristic form of wheezing, dyspnea and expectoration of thick tenacious sputum. Typically it occurs in paroxysmal recurrences with intervals of relative comfort, but may also assume a mild continuous form with exacerbations; or the acute attack may persist for days or weeks as *status asthmaticus.*

Etiology. Approximately half of the cases of bronchial asthma result from allergy to external antigens, most often dusts suspended in the inhaled air, but occasionally ingested foods or drugs. This type of asthma is usually classed as *extrinsic asthma.* The remainder, in which no evidence of hypersensitivity to specific allergens is found by skin tests, is classed as *intrinsic asthma.* Most of the cases in the latter category can be shown to result from infections of the respiratory system.

Asthma of the extrinsic type results from the same "wheal and erythema" type of hypersensitivity as hay fever, differing only in the site of the allergic reaction, and the two conditions frequently coexist in the same person. The reasons for localization of the allergic reaction in the bronchi rather than the nasal mucosa are not established, although it has been suggested that inflammation of the bronchial mucosa by intercurrent infections, such as acute bronchitis or pertussis, or by nonspecific chemical irritants, may play a part in some cases.

The allergens causing extrinsic asthma are the same as those causing allergic rhinitis. By far the most important are inhaled organic dusts, such as pollens, mold spores, animal danders, feathers, insecticides, glue and lint from fabrics. Ordinary house dust, in addition to the substances obviously contributing to its formation, contains additional antigens apparently arising from the disintegration of fibers or from contamination with molds and bacteria. Although house dust is a complex and variable mixture, for most practical purposes an extract of a mixture of dusts from several houses may be used as if a single antigen. Grain dust, flour, spices and such vegetable seeds as cottonseed, flaxseed and castor bean, are important causes in persons exposed as a result of their occupations and occasionally affect those with only casual contact. The proportion of cases due to foods is not large, but practically any food may occasionally be a cause. Among those most active as antigens are eggs, fish, shellfish, nuts, spices and chocolate. In general, the antigens are proteins or similar compounds of somewhat lower molecular weight, but certain synthetic drugs, such as aspirin, may cause severe asthma, presumably through acting as haptenes.

The infections of the respiratory system causing asthma are recurrent or chronic infections of the bronchi, often secondary to chronic infections of the paranasal sinuses, tonsils or adenoids. The sinusitis is usually of the chronic hyperplastic type, with purulent secretions only during the more acute phases, and is often accompanied by mucous polyps in the nasal cavity or within the sinuses. Cultures of the secretions of the respiratory system in such cases usually show a mixed growth, with pneumococcus, *Streptococcus viridans* and *hemolyticus, Neisseria catarrhalis, Klebsiella pneumoniae* and *Hemophilus influenzae* the most common organisms. Only occasionally can the etiologic importance of a single organism be clearly established.

The role of allergy in asthma due to respiratory infection is less obvious than in extrinsic asthma, but there is considerable evidence that infective asthma results from specific hypersensitivity to the bacteria present. The asthma may continue severe at times when the infection is in a relatively quiescent chronic stage. The symptoms and clinical findings are similar in infective and extrinsic asthma, including the abundance of eosinophils in blood and sputum. The personal or family history of other diseases due to extrinsic allergy is almost as frequent in infective asthma as in the extrinsic type. Skin tests with the available bacterial antigens rarely give immediate urticarial reactions comparable to those produced by pollens and other extrinsic antigens, but confirmatory evidence of hypersensitivity is occasionally furnished by the occurrence of an asthmatic attack after the injection of bacterial antigens (usually those derived from cultures of the patient's own secretions), either intracutaneously for skin tests or subcutaneously in attempts at immunization.

Although the distinction between extrinsic and infective asthma is useful in the discussion of diagnosis and treatment, it is important to remember that many, if not most, asthmatic patients are affected both by extrinsic allergens and by infective factors. Studies of the etiology of a case of asthma should attempt an evaluation of the importance of both extrinsic and infective causes, rather than simply classification in one group or the other.

Once the asthmatic pattern of reaction has developed through allergy to extrinsic agents or infection, paroxysms of asthma may be precipitated by many factors unrelated to the original causes. Such secondary factors include emotional stress, changes of temperature and humidity, irritating fumes or smoke, strong odors and physical exertion. These factors may be the obvious precipitating causes of individual attacks. Their recognition and control play an important part in therapy and, in occasional cases in which the underlying allergic or infective basis is obscure or resistant to treatment, may constitute the main approach. However, there is little evidence that true bronchial asthma arises purely from them, and when the allergic or infective factors are determined, the most satisfactory results usually come from treatment directed at the primary causes. In asthma primarily due to extrinsic allergens, acute respiratory infections may be a secondary factor precipitating attacks. Here also, the best results are obtained by treatment directed at the underlying primary cause.

Incidence. Asthma is a common disease ranking high among the causes of disability in America and Europe. Apparently all races are susceptible. The incidence in the two sexes is essentially equal, and it may occur at any age from early infancy to old age. The onset of extrinsic asthma usually occurs in the first four decades of life; infective asthma may begin at any age, but more often begins in middle age.

Morbid Anatomy. The lungs of patients dying during asthmatic attacks are voluminous, distended and less elastic than normal. The lumina of many of the smaller bronchi are occluded by thick, tenacious, mucoid secretions. The bronchial mucosa and submucosa are thickened. Microscopic sections show the alveoli of the lungs to be irregularly distended, with thinning and rupture of septums. Isolated areas of atelectasis may be present. The bronchial epithelium usually shows many goblet cells, and a thickened hyaline basement membrane. The submucosa is thickened and infiltrated with wandering cells, the mucous glands are generally large and active. Evidence of spasm of the bronchial muscle is rarely seen in autopsy material.

Pathologic Physiology. In extrinsic asthma, the hypersensitivity is mediated by the skin-sensitizing antibody demonstrable in the blood serum by the Prausnitz-Küstner reaction and also present in the bronchial tissues and skin. Contact of the sensitized mucosa with the antigen, which is direct in the case of inhaled allergens, and through the blood stream in the case of ingested antigens, elicits an antigen-antibody reaction in the tissues. The exact immunologic mechanism of infective asthma has not been established but, for the reasons mentioned previously, an antigen-antibody reaction is believed to be involved.

The immunologic reaction gives rise to a physiologic reaction in the bronchi similar to the nasal reaction in hay fever. The lumina of the smaller bronchi are greatly narrowed by swelling of the mucosa and submucosa. It is widely believed that spasm of the bronchial muscle also contributes to the constriction of the air passages, but conclusive proof of smooth muscle contraction is lacking. The narrowed lumina are further obstructed by the secretion of thick tenacious sputum from the bronchial glands.

The physiologic changes resulting from the antigen-antibody reaction have been attributed to release of histamine, acetylcholine or similar metabolites. In patients subject to asthma, attacks may be induced by the administration of either histamine or Mecholyl. This experimental asthma in general resembles that occurring spontaneously, except that attacks produced with histamine are readily controlled by antihistamine drugs and those produced with Mecholyl by atropine, while these agents, separately or in combination, are not particularly effective in spontaneous asthma. Thus the precise mechanism remains in doubt.

The extent to which asthmatic attacks are influenced by nervous control is not clear. Many authors have suggested that reflexes stimulated by irritation of the nasal passages may produce asthma, and the influence of psychogenic factors in producing certain attacks in susceptible persons appears to be well established. However, surgical procedures attempting to prevent asthma by excision of the autonomic nerve fibers supplying the bronchi have not been successful, indicating that the asthmatic reaction may occur independently of nervous control. It has been suggested that psychogenic factors may produce asthmatic attacks through causing hyperventilation, which in itself may precipitate an attack in a susceptible person.

The narrowing of the bronchial air passages and further obstruction by mucoid sputum greatly hamper the ventilation of the lungs in both the inspiratory and expiratory phases. Increased respiratory effort, with utilization of the accessory muscles of respiration, tends to increase the efficiency of inspiration more than that of expiration, so that the lungs tend to become progressively distended with air as the attack progresses, producing an acute emphysema. Spirometric tracings made during even mild asthma show a decrease of the vital capacity, with the reserve air component greatly decreased or absent after a forced inspiration. The maximum breathing capacity is markedly reduced, attempts at increased ventilation rapidly increasing the residual air. Aeration of the blood is obviously impaired by the ventilatory difficulty and in severe attacks cyanosis may be apparent. The heart is relatively little affected, except as preexisting cardiac disease is aggravated by anoxemia.

Subsidence of the attack follows widening of the constricted bronchi, permitting expectoration of mucous plugs. With the obstruction relieved, the lungs rapidly return to normal after an acute attack. However, persistence of even mild asthma over a long period of time may lead to progressive emphysema which is only partially reversible.

Symptoms. In its most typical form asthma occurs in sporadic paroxysms, with respiratory function essentially normal during the intervening intervals. Attacks often occur at night but may also follow exposure to a specific allergen, unusual exertion, a sudden change of temperature, onset of a respiratory infection or excitement. The onset is marked by a sense of suffocation and pressure in the chest, often with a nonproductive cough. Respiration is marked by a wheeze which is often audible to the patient and bystanders. The respiratory rate is little changed, expiration is often prolonged, but the respiratory effort is greatly increased. The patient sits upright or leans forward to secure maximum use of the accessory muscles of respiration. The chest rapidly becomes distended with air and remains in a relatively expanded state at the end of expiration, the following inspiratory effort producing little further expansion. Termination of the attack is usually marked by cough productive of a considerable quantity of thick, stringy, mucoid sputum. Attacks are often followed by pains in the lower chest, apparently resulting from muscle soreness induced by the violent respiratory efforts.

Most attacks subside spontaneously in a half hour to several hours. In certain cases, particularly those in which the asthma follows respiratory infection, the acute attack may persist for days or weeks and recur promptly even if temporary relief has been obtained with suitable medications. Such persistently severe asthma (status asthmaticus) through fatigue, loss of sleep and inadequate nutrition rapidly debilitates the patient.

A considerable proportion of patients remain in a chronic state of mild asthma with the symptoms barely noticeable at rest, but with dyspnea and wheezing apparent after any exertion, a hearty meal, laughing, singing or emotional excitements. Usually these are patients who have had severe acute attacks, but occasionally the onset of the disease is marked by this chronic state, with no severe attacks for months or years.

Physical signs of asthma are quite characteristic. The wheezing may be audible with the unaided ear and is very apparent through the stethoscope, with sonorous and sibilant rales heard in all portions of the lung fields, usually during both inspiratory and expiratory phases. Cyanosis is rarely present in mild cases, but may be marked in the more severe attacks. The chest shows signs of acute emphysema, with a low, relatively immobile diaphragm and decreased cardiac dullness.

When examined a few hours after cessation of an acute attack, the chest may be amazingly normal. However, in many other cases, the persistence of mild chronic asthma may be manifested by sibilant or sonorous rales heard chiefly at the lung bases and brought out by cough or forced expiration.

Diagnosis. The diagnosis of bronchial asthma consists of two steps: first, the differentiation of asthma from other diseases causing dyspnea, and second, the determination of the causative agents producing asthma in the particular patient.

The differential diagnosis is rarely difficult if the patient is seen during an acute attack. The dyspnea, the presence of sonorous and sibilant rales throughout the chest, the thick, tenacious, mucoid sputum and the history of periodic attacks are very characteristic. A history of asthma and other allergic diseases in the family or of previous allergic disease in the patient is valuable contributory evidence.

Laboratory examination of the sputum shows distinctive features which are confirmatory evidence. The gelatinous globules, when smeared on a slide, are found to be elongated spiral casts of the smaller bronchi (Curschmann's spirals). Also visible with the microscope are Charcot-Leyden crystals, elongated, pointed octahedral crystals varying in length from 20 to 40 microns. Streaks of blood may be visible in the sputum during severe asthma, but the occurrence of real hemoptysis is rare and suggests the possibility of some other disease. In stained smear, a large proportion of the cell are seen to be eosinophils. When asthma is associated with acute respiratory infection, the sputum is intermediate in character between that of simple asthma and the purulent sputum of bronchitis, and some of the typical features may be lacking.

Examination of the blood usually shows a moderate increase in the proportion of eosinophils, ordinarily 5 to 8 per cent, but occasionally 30 per cent or higher in severe infective asthma.

Roentgenograms of the chest show no features characteristic of asthma. There may be a moderate increase of the bronchovascular markings, and in advanced cases, some degree of emphysema is usually apparent. They are valuable, however, to rule out diseases of the lung parenchyma, cardiac hypertrophy and tumors causing pressure on the trachea or bronchi.

The wheezing rales of asthma are usually present throughout the chest during the attack, although the sounds may be temporarily suppressed in one area if plugging of a bronchus with mucus has produced atelectasis. The persistence of sonorous or sibilant rales limited to one portion of the lungs is suggestive of bronchial obstruction by a tumor, foreign body, or endobronchial tuberculosis. In such cases, roentgenograms are of great value, but when the differentiation between bronchial asthma and a local obstruction of the air passages is difficult, bronchoscopy is indicated.

Sonorous and sibilant rales are often heard in patients with acute bronchitis; in such cases dyspnea is not a significant symptom and the sputum does not show the characteristic features of asthma. Differentiation during the first attack is not always easy, and it is important to remember that recurrent attacks of acute bronchitis, with increasingly severe dyspnea, often mark the development of true bronchial asthma. A sharp distinction between chronic bronchitis and mild chronic asthma also is often not possible. Many patients with chronic bronchitis show a degree of wheezing dyspnea, with typical physical signs of asthma, and are benefited by therapy appropriate for asthma; such a condition is justifiably described as asthmatic bronchitis.

Dyspnea due to heart disease only occasionally has the wheezing character of bronchial asthma, and sonorous and sibilant rales, if present, are usually overshadowed by moist or crepitant sounds. When severe attacks of cardiac dyspnea occur at rest, other evidences of heart disease are usually apparent. Since both asthma and hypertensive or arteriosclerotic heart disease are common in elderly persons, the coexistence of the two conditions is not unusual and the symptoms may be intermingled to a confusing degree.

When the diagnosis of bronchial asthma has been established, determination of the etiologic factors is essential for rational long-term management. This requires meticulous inquiry as to the time, place and circumstances in which attacks have occurred, and the potential allergens to which the patient is exposed. Asthma during the spring and summer months suggests pollens or mold spores and a precisely dated season may indicate one particular pollen. (See section on Hay Fever for discussion of pollen seasons.) Attacks limited to the winter months obviously suggest an infective cause, although bedding, such as a down quilt, used only during the cold weather may be the cause. Persistence throughout the year suggests household contacts, pets or bedding, but may also be due to chronic respiratory infection. An observed relationship to certain foods or drugs or to acute respiratory infection is important. Certain occupations involve exposure to distinctive antigens; the farmer to animal danders, feeds and fertilizers, the baker to flour, and so forth. Attacks occurring in certain houses may be due to pets, to bedding or upholstered furniture or the molds and fungi they harbor. In evaluating the history, one should remember that a majority of patients with asthma are affected by more than one factor, a large number by both extrinsic and infective factors.

The properly taken history usually calls attention to possible antigens, but, except in cases of pollen asthma, only occasionally completely establishes the cause. Sensitivity is demonstrated by testing the skin with the possible allergens suggested by the history. These skin tests may be carried out by either the scratch or intracutaneous method, as described in the two preceding sections.

The dilutions of some of the common antigens considered safe for intracutaneous tests on the average case of asthma are shown in the following table, expressed in protein nitrogen units per cubic centimeter. If the history suggests *violent* sensitivity to one or more antigens, these are tested first in a concentration one tenth of that shown in the table. If the allergens used are not standardized on the basis of protein content, the advice of the manufacturer must be followed. Not more than six intracutaneous tests are done at one time, but if no undue reaction is noted after 10 minutes, further groups of six may be done to a total of eighteen or twenty-four at one sitting. Antigens which give doubtful, one plus or two plus reactions when tested in dilutions of 10 or 100 units per cubic centimeter should be retested with successive tenfold increases of concentration until three plus reactions are obtained or until a concentration of 1000 units per cubic centimeter is reached.

INHALANTS

Grass pollen 100	Cottonseed 10
Ragweed pollen 100	Flaxseed 10
House dust 1000	Kapok 100
Alternaria 1000	Fish glue 10
Hormodendrum 1000	Silk 1000
Cat 100	Wool 1000
Dog 100	Feathers 1000
Horse 100	Tobacco 1000
Orris 100	Pyrethrum 1000

FOODS

Cow's milk 10,000	Banana 5000
Egg white 100	Orange 5000
Egg yolk 100	Peach 5000
Wheat 1000	Carrot 5000
Corn 1000	Peas 5000
Rice 1000	Potato 5000
Beef 1000	Tomato 5000
Chicken 1000	Mustard 100
Lamb 1000	Flounder 1000
Pork 1000	Salmon 1000
Chocolate 1000	Oyster 1000
Peanut 1000	Shrimp 1000

If skin tests are properly performed and read, the positive reactions indicate sensitization of the skin to the antigens tested. The importance of these substances in the actual production of clinical asthma must be judged from correlation of the skin reactions with the history of the case. A one plus or two plus reaction which explains the observed time and circumstances of attacks is of value, while a strong reaction to a substance with which the patient has little or no contact is of limited significance. In general, skin reactions to inhaled antigens, which come into direct contact with the sensitized mucosa, are of greater significance than skin reactions to foods, which are greatly altered by cooking, digestion and metabolism before reaching the bronchi through the blood stream. Positive skin reactions to foods are regarded as suggestive evidence of their etiologic importance in asthma, and the final evaluation is by clinical judgment based either on the past history or the observed results of eliminating the foods from the diet. Not only may foods giving positive skin reactions prove innocuous when eaten, but occasionally foods showing negative skin reactions cause asthmatic attacks, usually delayed several hours after ingestion and presumably due to the production by digestion of an antigen not present in the original material. This situation, while rare, obviously calls for careful observation rather than acceptance of skin tests as the final criterion.

Evaluation of infective factors in the causation of asthma is not always easy. Attention may be directed to this possibility by the absence of skin reactions to all probable extrinsic allergens, but in many cases both extrinsic allergens and infection are important. As previously noted, the onset of asthma after the age of 40 years is statistically suggestive of infective asthma, and at any age, the coexistence of chronic sinusitis, particularly of the hyperplastic type, or of nasal polyps, indicates a potential infective factor. Skin tests with bacterial antigens have not proved a reliable criterion, except in those cases in which an exacerbation of constitutional symptoms is inadvertently produced. In patients requiring hospitalization, the persistence of asthma after three or four days in an environment which eliminates, insofar as possible, contact with inhalant allergens usually indicates the presence of endogenous, usually infective, factors.

As previously mentioned, asthmatic patients are often made worse by nonspecific secondary factors, such as changes of temperature and humidity, irritating fumes and odors, acute infections, exertion, excitement and emotional stress. These conditions, rather than changes in exposure to antigens, may be the actual precipitating causes of individual attacks. Their importance, which can only be judged by careful inquiry into the circumstances of occurrence of exacerbations, must be evaluated if treatment is to be successful. However, obvious as their relationship may be, they should be recognized as secondary influences and not confused with the fundamental allergic or infective causes of the asthmatic state.

Prognosis. Asthma is a chronic disease with a marked tendency to periodic recurrence over a period of many years, unless the causative factors are recognized and satisfactorily handled. Present methods of treatment do not afford the prospect of actual cure. Approximately 25 to 30 per cent of the cases beginning in early childhood undergo spontaneous recovery during adolescence, but since an essentially equal number become worse during the same period, withholding treatment in hope that the condition will be outgrown is not justified. During adult life, the tendency to spontaneous recovery is much less marked, and there is a greater probability of the attacks becoming progressively more frequent and prolonged, with the remission less complete and with nonspecific factors playing an increasing part in the causation. With repeated attacks over a period of years, asthma originating as a strictly seasonal reaction to a specific pollen may be prolonged progressively beyond the pollen season, and gradually enter into a chronic state lasting throughout much of the year. Infective asthma in elderly patients is particularly apt to become chronic. Persistent asthma from any cause is apt to produce pul-

monary emphysema and permanent ventilatory disability.

The danger to life in the average attack is slight, although death occasionally occurs in acute attacks caused by allergy to rapidly absorbed drugs such as aspirin, or in attacks resulting from injection of an overdose of antigen in testing or treatment. However, in severe status asthmaticus with persistent cyanosis, failing to respond to corticotropin or cortisone, the mortality is considerable. Some deaths are attributable to depression of respiration and cough by injudicious use of sedatives, but many are entirely uninfluenced by attempts at therapy.

Treatment. Therapy of asthma comprises three types of efforts: (1) symptomatic relief of the attack; (2) control of specific causative factors; (3) general care of the patient.

Symptomatic Relief. During the acute attack, relief may usually be attained with epinephrine 1:1000 injected subcutaneously or intramuscularly. Since patients vary both in tolerance and response, best results are obtained with 0.3 to 0.5 cc. (0.1 to 0.2 cc. for infants or small children), repeated if necessary every 5 or 10 minutes for two or three doses. This treatment will terminate mild attacks, but in more persistent cases may be required every two or three hours. Frequent repetition may be avoided by the use of a slowly absorbed form of epinephrine, such as epinephrine in oil 1:500, 1 cc. intramuscularly every 6 to 12 hours. For the ambulatory treatment of patients with frequent mild attacks, inhalation of an aerosol of epinephrine 1:100 or isopropylarterenol (Isuprel) 1:200 from a suitable nebulizer is a convenient measure often producing prompt relief. Also effective in mild attacks, and having the advantage of oral administration, is ephedrine 25 mg. every 4 hours if necessary. The stimulating effects of ephedrine may be minimized by combination with a mild sedative such as phenobarbital 15 mg. All drugs of the epinephrine group should be used cautiously in patients with coexisting hypertension, heart disease or hyperthyroidism.

In acute attacks not relieved by epinephrine, aminophylline 0.25 to 0.5 gm. injected slowly intravenously is often effective and may be repeated after 2 to 3 hours if necessary. A slower but more prolonged effect may be obtained by administering aminophylline 0.5 gm. (0.25 for children) by rectum every

8 to 12 hours if needed, either as a suppository or dissolved in 20 to 30 cc. of water. Oral use of aminophylline in asthma is limited by the tendency of adequate doses to produce nausea. However, a combination of aminophylline 120 mg., ephedrine 25 mg. and phenobarbital 15 mg., every 4 hours if necessary, is useful for mild attacks.

Sedatives are useful adjuncts in the relief of severe asthma but the danger of depressing respiratory function precludes their employment as the principal therapy. Demerol is preferable to morphine and may be used in doses of 50 mg. every 4 hours if necessary. The barbiturates, such as phenobarbital 30 mg. every 4 hours for daytime use and pentobarbital 100 mg. at night, are valuable. If strong sedation is needed, ether, 60 cc. in 120 cc. of oil by rectum, is relatively safe. Codeine 15 mg. or elixir of terpene hydrate with codeine, 5 cc. every 4 hours, may be used to control excessive cough.

In persistent asthma, expectorants are often valuable to facilitate discharge of tenacious mucoid sputum. The most effective is potassium iodide, 0.6 gm. three times a day after meals. Ammonium chloride in the same doses may be tried by patients who do not tolerate iodide.

In severe asthma which is not readily controlled by medications, oxygen administered by tent, nasal catheter or mask is a useful supportive measure. Positive pressure is of value only in the inspiratory phase; the ordinary masks applying pressure during the expiratory phase are not helpful.

If acute asthma persists for several days or fails to respond to the medications previously mentioned, the use of corticotropin or cortisone is of great value for temporary relief. In the most severe cases, corticotropin 15 to 20 mg. is given in an intravenous drip of 1 liter of 5 per cent glucose solution over a period of 8 hours, repeated daily if necessary. In less urgent situations, corticotropin 40 mg. in gelatin is injected intramuscularly daily, or cortisone 50 mg. given by mouth every 6 hours. As soon as relief is obtained, the dose is reduced by 25 to 50 per cent and then rapidly tapered off over a period of four to five days. Both drugs must be used with caution in patients with heart disease, diabetes or mental disease, and are generally contraindicated in patients with pulmonary tuberculosis or pregnancy. Careful observation for evidence of fluid retention is essential, particularly if the treatment is continued for more than a week. Salt intake should be restricted and potassium chloride given in 1 gm. doses three to five times daily.

In severe chronic asthma which cannot be controlled by other symptomatic or specific treatment, the use of small maintenance doses of cortisone over a prolonged period may be considered, if the disability caused by the asthma outweighs the potential risks of a prolonged hyperadrenal state. After the symptoms have been controlled by the usual doses of cortisone, the dose is reduced to the minimum which will maintain a satisfactory degree of relief, usually not exceeding 25 mg. every 8 to 12 hours. Patients receiving such treatment should be kept under close supervision and intercurrent infections treated promptly.

Numerous other measures are of some value in various phases of asthma. In persistent severe asthma with retention of thick sputum, bronchoscopic aspiration is sometimes effective. Fever therapy, usually produced with intravenous typhoid vaccine, has been used in status asthmaticus, but is rarely as effective as cortisone or corticotropin. For the relief of mild attacks, inhalation of the fumes of burning stramonium leaves is reasonably effective. The antihistamine drugs are also mildly efficacious but offer no advantage over ephedrine and aminophylline.

Specific Treatment. Satisfactory handling of asthma over the long term requires the control of the causative factors. Asthma due to extrinsic antigens is best treated by the avoidance of contact with the antigen when possible. Elimination of household pets, feather pillows, and so forth, generally produces more satisfactory relief than any attempt at immunization. In the case of occupational allergens, such as flour in baker's asthma, a trial of injection treatment may be warranted but usually a change of occupation eventually proves necessary. Avoidance of windborne pollen is possible as a temporary measure, either by a trip to a location free of the offending plant or by air filtration, but continuation of the patient's usual residence and activities requires injection treatment. Contact with house dust may be minimized by stripping the bedroom of carpeting, drapes and heavy furniture, and by careful cleaning, but coincident injection treatment is usually needed.

Treatment by injections of antigen, variously described as immunization, desensitization or hyposensitization, is generally indicated in asthma due to house dust, mold spores or pollens, and may be desirable in the cases due to other protein antigens, with which the patient cannot completely avoid contact. The general principle is to begin treatment with an injection of no more than twice the actual amount of antigen injected in the intracutaneous test giving a moderate (two plus) or marked (three plus) skin reaction, and to proceed with injections once or twice a week, gradually increasing the dose, aiming to reach a dose approximately 500 times the initial one after about sixteen injections. The schedules included in the section on Hay Fever, in which allowance is made for the variations in degree of sensitivity as indicated by the skin tests, are generally applicable to the treatment of asthma, but in patients highly sensitive to nonseasonal allergens, it may be necessary to proceed somewhat more slowly if the patient is constantly exposed to the antigen while treatment is progressing. In the case of house dust allergen, the strengths of available solutions may not permit as great a range of dosage as with pollens. Usually a top dose of 0.5 to 0.8 cc. of the strongest available dust extract is adequate.

The injections are given subcutaneously on the lateral aspect of the upper arm or thigh, with a rubber tourniquet and epinephrine hydrochloride 1:1000 solution at hand in case of an excessive reaction. After the injection, the patient should be kept under observation for 20 minutes to observe the local reaction and to treat any constitutional symptoms that may develop. (See section on Hay Fever.)

While the antigen dosage schedules serve as a guide, they must be modified in accordance with the individual patient's reaction. As the dosage progresses, a local reaction, manifested by redness and swelling 2 to 4 cm. in diameter, usually occurs at the site of injection, and need not cause a change in the program of doses. If the local reaction is uncomfortably large or persists for more than 36 hours, the same dose should be repeated at the next injection rather than progressing according to the schedule. When this dose no longer produces an excessive reaction, one may increase as indicated in the schedule or somewhat more cautiously. If an injection produces a constitutional reaction, the following dose should not exceed one-half the dose producing the reaction and should not be given sooner than one week later.

Subsequent increases should be about one-half as large as those listed in the schedules, with careful observation of the local reaction each time. If it becomes apparent that the patient cannot tolerate a larger dose, the schedule is abandoned and treatment continued with a dose one-quarter to one-third less than that which produces an excessive reaction.

The maintenance dose, either the top dose indicated in the schedule or that comfortably tolerated by the patient, is repeated every two weeks. If the symptoms are completely controlled, the interval between injections may be increased to three or four weeks, the individual doses remaining the same. Treatment may be expected to be necessary for several years or indefinitely. Once a year the skin tests with antigens used in treatment are repeated and if some have become essentially negative, those antigens may be discontinued while carefully observing the patient for recurrence of symptoms.

Treatment of Infective Asthma. Infections of the respiratory system believed to be causative factors in asthma should be treated vigorously with available medical and surgical measures. During the more acute stages the antibiotics, penicillin, chlortetracycline (Aureomycin), tetracycline (Achromycin) and oxytetracycline (Terramycin), are often effective. Adequate drainage of infected paranasal sinuses should be maintained by local treatment, with excision of nasal polyps if necessary. If recurrences of infection are very frequent, prophylactic doses of a sulfonamide, such as sulfisoxazole (Gantrisin) 0.5 to 1.0 gm. twice a day, may be given during the fall and winter months.

Injections of bacterial vaccines or filtrates are often of value in recurrent infective asthma, but must be given cautiously in patients highly allergic to bacterial products. General reactions with exacerbations of asthma, often delayed one or two days after the injection and lasting several days, are easily provoked by excessive doses. If the concentrated vaccine is 1 per cent by volume or approximately 5 billion organisms per cubic centimeter, the first dose should not exceed 0.1 cc of a 1:1000 dilution, and subsequent doses at weekly intervals may be gradually increased up to 0.1 to 0.2 cc. of the concentrated material in a manner similar to that employed for pollen antigens.

If the sinuses show evidence of chronic disease and conservative measures are not effective, consideration may be given to surgical measures. Since the thickened membrane of the sinuses is the site of infection, satisfactory surgical treatment requires widely opening all the sinuses shown by roentgenograms to be involved and complete removal of the hyperplastic or polypoid membrane. When such operations are thoroughly performed, the results are favorable in a sufficient proportion of cases to warrant their employment in cases not otherwise relieved.

General Measures. The general care of the asthmatic patient involves chiefly the avoidance of those secondary factors which are apt to aggravate asthma regardless of the primary cause. Extremes of cold and humidity should be avoided, particularly outdoor exertion in cold, damp weather. Exposure to respiratory infections should be avoided as far as reasonably possible. For these purposes, spending the winter in a warm, dry climate may be helpful. Smoking should be avoided or restricted to a minimum. Physical exercise should be limited to the tolerance of the patient, with the more violent forms of exertion avoided. Causes of emotional stress should be eliminated when possible; psychotherapy is only occasionally needed.

In patients with chronic asthma who are developing emphysema, breathing exercises which stress complete expiration rather than deep inspiration are helpful both to increase ventilatory efficiency and to lessen the development of chest deformity. Manual pressure on the lower ribs and diaphragm during expiration is helpful in emptying the chest.

Maintenance of an optimistic mental state is important. Needless to say, few things will contribute more to this attitude than the combination of effective and readily available symptomatic relief with a logical plan for determining and coping with the causative factors.

WILLIAM B. SHERMAN

References

Cooke, R. A.: Infective Asthma, Indication of its Allergic Nature. Am. J. M. Sc., *183*:309, 1932.
————: Allergy in Theory and Practice. Philadelphia, W. B. Saunders Co., 1947.
Feinberg, S. M.: Allergy in Practice. Chicago, Year Book Publishers, 1944.
Gay, L. N.: The Diagnosis and Treatment of Bronchial Asthma. Baltimore, Williams and Wilkins Co., 1946.
Salter, H. H.: Asthma, Its Pathology and Treatment. 2nd ed. London, J. & A. Churchill, 1868.
Sherman, W. B.: Cortisone, ACTH, and the Allergic Reaction. Practitioner, *170*:347, 1953.

DRUG ALLERGY

Definition. Drug allergy is a general, often loosely used term for a multiplicity of sensitivity reactions, including skin eruptions, edema, arthritis, lymphadenopathy, hematologic abnormalities, fever and periarteritis, which occur during or following the administration of a variety of therapeutic agents. The symptoms bear no relation to the primary pharmacologic properties of the drug concerned, and resemble in important respects the manifestations of serum sickness. It is generally assumed that the reactions are due to the presence of antibody against the drug itself, or against an antigenic conjugate between the drug and a protein in the blood or tissues. This assumption is based in part on experimental studies, by Landsteiner and his associates, of the antigenicity of simple chemicals, and there is some evidence to support it in several types of reaction in human beings. However, in actual practice, the majority of reactions cannot be proven to involve an antigen-antibody mechanism. Some of the manifestations attributed to allergy, such as agranulocytosis, hemolytic anemia and hepatitis, cannot be reproduced in experimental animals, nor can the presence of antibody be demonstrated in patients. The designation of such reactions as drug allergy should therefore be regarded as tentative.

Incidence. Although allergic reactions have been reported to occur with almost every medication in common use, there are large differences in the capacity of different drugs to produce reactions. Important differences also exist in the susceptibility of different persons; patients with a history of other allergic diseases are more apt to develop drug reactions. As an example, aspirin rarely causes sensitization in normal individuals, while patients with bronchial asthma are remarkably prone to exhibit asthma or urticaria after taking the drug. The incidence of penicillin reactions has been stated to be as high as 10 or 15 per cent, but there is a great variation in different reports, depending on the degree of purity of the penicillin, the presence of other substances in the vehicle employed, the route of injection, the duration of treatment and the amount administered. At the University of Minnesota Hospitals, 2.5 per cent of a recent series of 562 patients developed reactions to penicillin, consisting of skin eruptions and mild fever; no severe reactions occurred.

Certain drugs, such as phenylethylhydantoin (Nirvanol), arsphenamine and thiouracil, are known to produce sensitivity reactions in a high proportion of patients. "Nirvanol sickness," a syndrome closely resembling serum sickness, has been reported to occur in all patients given large doses of the drug.

The incidence of drug allergy depends to some extent on prior exposure to the drug, although this seems to be much less important than in serum sickness. Reactions to the sulfonamides and penicillin are more likely to occur in previously treated patients, but many occur at the first contact with the agents.

Pathogenesis. Landsteiner and his associates made a series of important experimental observations which have led to an interesting concept of the mechanism of drug allergy. It was shown that animals could be specifically sensitized to simple chemical compounds, such as picric acid or dinitrochlorobenzene, by repeated exposure to the substances or by the injection of conjugates of the chemicals with protein. Sensitization with chemical alone was found to involve a union *in vivo* with body protein, yielding antigenic complexes whose immunologic specificity was determined by the chemical hapten. Antibody formed against such complexes was capable of reacting either with the chemical alone, or with the chemical-protein conjugate, but not with the protein.

It has been postulated that a similar mechanism may account for drug allergy in man. The administration of a drug would, under this theory, be followed by the formation of a union between tissue or blood proteins, and the drug or a breakdown product of the drug. Antibody produced against the conjugate would subsequently react with the drug itself (or with the breakdown product), and also with protein-drug conjugate formed after readministration of the drug. Moreover, since specificity of the antibody is determined by the structure of the chemical hapten, it is possible that sensitization would also occur to closely related substances.

If this concept is correct, the mechanism of drug allergy would involve several variable factors which might affect the incidence of reactions and also the tissue sites involved.

The capacity of a drug to unite with body protein, and differences in the degree of union in different individuals, would be of much importance. If the complex of drug and body protein were soluble and rapidly absorbed, the sensitivity would probably be of the immediate, anaphylactic type. If the protein constituent of the complex were confined to a particular tissue or cell, and not removed or absorbed, reactions of the local, delayed type would occur. Furthermore, if the haptene were not the drug itself but a metabolic breakdown product, individual variations in the metabolism of the substance would play a role in the incidence of drug allergy.

Further investigation of the problem in man has been delayed because of the absence of satisfactory methods for detecting the presence of antibody in almost all types of drug allergy. Ackroyd has described a complement fixation reaction with the serums of patients with thrombocytopenia due to Sedormid sensitivity, in which the "antigen" consists of a mixture of Sedormid and platelets; no fixation of complement occurred with Sedormid alone, or with platelets alone. Leftwich reported that sulfonamide sensitivity could be detected by an intradermal injection of serum containing the sulfonamide, but not with solutions of sulfonamide alone, implying that a protein-sulfonamide complex was necessary for the production of a skin reaction. However, a large number of investigators have been unable to demonstrate antibody in various types of drug allergy by any of the available methods.

Pathology. Death is a rare event in drug allergy, and there is little information concerning the pathology of the disease. Rich and his associates found typical vascular lesions of periarteritis nodosa similar to the changes in experimental serum sickness, in several patients with severe reactions to sulfonamides. Similar lesions have been described in patients dying with hypersensitivity reactions to penicillin, iodine, thiourea and Dilantin.

Symptoms. The most common type of drug reaction is a mild systemic illness with the clinical features of typical serum sickness, including erythematous and urticarial *skin eruptions, arthralgia* or *arthritis, lymphadenopathy* and *fever*. Such reactions may occur during treatment with penicillin, the sulfonamides, chlortetracycline, streptomycin, aspirin, barbiturates, Dilantin, thiouracil, iodides and many other drugs. The disease usually begins between six and twelve days after the start of medication, and lasts two or three days. More prolonged reactions may occur if the drug is not withdrawn promptly.

Immediate anaphylactic type reactions to drugs are uncommon but occasionally occur in patients with extreme degrees of sensitization; persons with other allergic diseases are more susceptible to such reactions. The symptoms, which are similar to those of an acute serum accident, may appear within a few minutes after injection of certain drugs. Some of the acute, fatal reactions to penicillin are of this type. Procaine produces a similar reaction in susceptible individuals; it is not known whether this is based on allergy or a pharmacologic idiosyncracy.

Isolated symptoms are common in drug allergy. Patients may develop only fever, without other allergic manifestations, usually during the second week of treatment with penicillin, sulfonamides, arsphenamine, iodides and barbiturates. The fever continues until the drug is discontinued, and will usually reappear with a second administration. Other isolated signs of drug allergy may be skin eruption, conjunctivitis, lymphadenopathy, abdominal pain and vomiting, and pharyngitis. Proctitis and diarrhea are frequent complications of treatment with chlortetracycline, oxytetracycline and chloramphenicol, but there is no evidence that this represents an allergic reaction.

Other forms of skin eruption, differing from the erythema and urticaria of serum sickness, occur as reactions to certain drugs. *Exfoliative dermatitis* is a complication of treatment with gold, arsphenamine, penicillin, iodide, quinine, Dilantin and the sulfonamides. *Fixed eruptions,* which recur in the same skin area on readministration of the drug, are caused by numerous drugs, including barbiturates, phenolphthalein, bromide, iodide, sulfonamides and Bromsulphalein. *Erythema nodosum, photosensitization* and *contact dermatitis* have occurred as reactions to various drugs.

The hematologic reactions to drugs are of major importance. The most frequent and serious of these is *agranulocytosis,* which may occur during treatment with the sulfonamides, thiouracil, aminopyrine, arsphenamine, Butazolidin and gold. Agranulocytosis usually appears during or after the fourth week of continuous treatment; the onset may be earlier in previously sensitized patients. *Thrombocytopenic purpura* has been associated with Sedormid, quinine, quinidine,

thiouracil, Mesantoin, and the sulfonamides. *Hemolytic anemia* was a frequent complication of treatment with the older sulfonamide preparations, particularly sulfapyridine and sulfanilamide; hemolysis usually occurred within the first five days of treatment, and was not proved to be due to allergy. *Aplastic anemia* is an infrequent event during therapy with chloramphenicol, gold, trimethadione and the sulfonamides; the allergic basis for this complication is also open to question.

Periarteritis nodosa has occurred during treatment with the sulfonamides, penicillin, iodine, thiourea and Dilantin. The studies of Rich and his associates indicate that this disease may represent a basic type of hypersensitivity reaction to many antigenic substances.

Severe *liver damage* is sometimes produced by arsphenamine, cinchophen and the sulfonamides. There is no direct evidence to indicate an allergic basis for such reactions. The same is true for *peripheral neuritis* and *hemorrhagic encephalitis,* which are rare complications of drug therapy. It is possible that the latter diseases may occur as manifestations of periarteritis nodosa.

Longcope has emphasized the importance of renal involvement in drug allergy. Acute *hemorrhagic nephritis* has appeared during reactions to Nirvanol, arsphenamine and the sulfonamides.

A syndrome resembling *lupus erythematosus,* with arthritis, fever, polyserositis and hyperglobulinemia, has been described in patients receiving prolonged therapy with hydralazine (Apresoline) for hypertension. The plasma of these patients produced the characteristic alteration of leukocytes which occurs in lupus (the "L.E. phenomenon"), which has also been observed in allergic reactions to penicillin.

Diagnosis. Discontinuation of the drug in question is the safest and most reliable diagnostic measure, and the prompt disappearance of symptoms permits a presumptive diagnosis of drug allergy. There are no specific diagnostic tests of proven value. If symptoms recur when the drug is administered a second time the diagnosis becomes more certain, but this procedure is rarely justified. Skin tests, and attempts to demonstrate antibody by test tube or passive transfer, are negative in most instances. Eosinophilia may occur in patients with skin eruptions, and the "L.E. phenomenon" may be present in severe, systemic drug reactions.

Treatment. In most cases, the symptoms are completely relieved when the medication is stopped, and no other treatment is required. In mild reactions, and when the therapeutic agent is of vital importance, the medication may be continued under close observation, but if another drug can be substituted this should always be done. Agranulocytosis should be treated with appropriate antibiotic therapy to control infection. Benadryl or pyribenzamine, in a dose of 50 mg. every 4 hours, may relieve the itching and discomfort of skin eruptions. Epinephrine should be given for immediate anaphylactic reactions, in a dose of 0.5 to 1.0 cc. of the 1:1000 dilution by subcutaneous injection; it is also useful for temporary relief of urticaria.

ACTH and cortisone may be of great value in the treatment of severe reactions. Either of these hormones, in a dose of approximately 100 mg. daily, should be used in cases of exfoliative dermatitis, prostrating or extremely painful systemic reactions, and inflammatory reactions involving the eye. Considerably larger doses of cortisone or hydrocortisone may be required for a short period of time in severe cases.

LEWIS THOMAS

References

Ackroyd, J. F.: Sedormid Purpura: An Immunological Study of a Form of Drug Hypersensitivity. In Kallós, Paul: Progress in Allergy. Vol. 3, New York, Interscience Publishers, 1952, p. 531.

Chase, M. W.: The Allergic State. In Dubos, R. J.: Bacterial and Mycotic Infections of Man. Philadelphia, J. B. Lippincott Co., 1952, Chap. 6.

Feinberg, S. M.: Drug Allergy—Some Clinical and Immunological Aspects. Ann. Allergy, 10:260, 1950.

Harvey, A. M., and others: Series of Papers on ACTH and Cortisone. Bull. Johns Hopkins Hospital (Special Issue), 87:349, 1950.

Landsteiner, K.: The Specificity of Serological Reactions. Springfield, Ill., Charles C Thomas, 1936.

Longcope, W. T.: Serum Sickness and Analogous Reactions from Certain Drugs Particularly the Sulfonamides. Medicine, 22:251, 1943.

Rich, A. R.: Hypersensitivity in Disease. Harvey Lectures, 42:106, 1946.

SERUM SICKNESS

Definition. Serum sickness is the systemic reaction which follows an injection of foreign serum, and is the result of interaction between specific antibody and an antigenic protein or proteins contained in the injected serum. In its fully developed form, the illness is characterized by skin eruptions, fever, lymphadenopathy, arthralgia, abdominal pain, nausea and vomiting. It may occur at any time within two weeks after the injection of serum. In individuals previously sensitized to the foreign protein the antibody response is accelerated, and the incubation period is several days shorter than in normal persons. With sufficiently high degrees of preexisting sensitization an extremely severe and sometimes fatal reaction may occur immediately after injection; such reactions are commonly referred to as *serum accidents*.

Incidence. The introduction of prophylactic toxoids and specific antibacterial therapeutic agents has greatly reduced the use of serum therapy and therefore the incidence of serum sickness. The disease now occurs as an occasional complication of the management of diphtheria, tetanus, clostridial infections, botulism and snake venom poisoning. The incidence of reactions is greater after injections of whole horse serum than when highly purified antiserums are employed, presumably because of the reduced number of different antigens in the latter preparations.

Neither age, sex, state of health nor route of injection appears to influence the incidence of serum sickness. There is some evidence that Negroes and American Indians are less susceptible than white persons. The major factors which determine the incidence as well as the severity of the disease are (1) the amount of serum injected, and (2) the previous immunological status of the patient.

When the amount of serum is 10 cc. or less, serum sickness occurs in approximately 10 per cent of patients. The incidence rises to 90 per cent when 100 cc. or more is injected. Patients with a history of previous injections of the same foreign serum may be expected to develop serum sickness more frequently and in greater severity than normal persons.

Instances of serum sickness have occurred following transfusion with human whole blood. Some of these are due to passive transfer of antibody against antigens to which the recipient of the transfusion is exposed; others have been shown to be caused by the presence of antigens in the transfused blood to which the recipient is hypersensitive.

A syndrome which is indistinguishable from serum sickness is known to occur during the course of treatment with certain drugs, and it is possible that a similar immunologic disturbance is involved. This type of reaction is discussed in the section on Drug Allergy.

Pathogenesis. The basic mechanisms which are responsible for serum sickness have received much investigation, in man and in experimental animals. It is known that within six to twelve days after an injection of foreign protein in the rabbit, precipitating antibody appears in the blood. In subjects previously exposed to the same antigen, antibody may appear within the first two or three days. Simultaneously with the appearance of antibody, the foreign protein, which has been detectable in the blood until this time, disappears completely. It has been suggested that a precipitation reaction between antigen and antibody, followed by clearance of the conjugate from the blood, may be occurring during this period. The mechanism of removal and destruction of the antigen is not understood. The level of serum complement undergoes a sharp reduction during the time of appearance of antibody and disappearance of antigen from the blood; perhaps this is a manifestation of fixation of complement *in vivo.*

Comparable events have been observed in human serum sickness, and it is generally accepted that a causal relationship exists between the antigen-antibody interaction and the symptoms of the disease. A correlation has been shown to exist between the occurrence of serum sickness and the degree of antibody formation, although the antibody is usually not demonstrable until late in the course of the illness. Patients who do not develop serum sickness have little or no demonstrable antibody, and the antigen is demonstrable in the circulating blood for much longer periods of time. As to the actual events which lead to tissue damage in serum sickness, there is very little information. It has been suggested that injury to endothelial and smooth muscle cells may be caused by the local release of histamine, acetylcholine or proteolytic enzymes; direct proof for these hypotheses is lacking.

Recurrences of symptoms sometimes occur after apparent recovery from serum sickness. These relapses, which are usually seen in patients given whole horse serum, probably represent successive, independent episodes of antigen-antibody interaction involving different antigenic proteins in the serum.

Pathology. Serum sickness is almost always a relatively benign, brief illness, and very few deaths resulting from the disease itself have been recorded. The most important information concerning the pathologic alterations in tissues has been contributed by Rich and his associates, who described vascular lesions indistinguishable from those of periarteritis nodosa in patients with serum sickness. Similar arterial lesions have been shown to occur frequently in experimental animals following the intravenous injection of large amounts of foreign protein. On the basis of these observations, it has been suggested that periarteritis nodosa, and related "collagen" diseases such as rheumatic fever and disseminated lupus erythematosus, may be based on an immunologic disturbance analogous to serum sickness.

Symptoms. The incubation period is usually between six and twelve days after the injection of serum, but may be much shorter in previously sensitized persons. The illness begins with a *skin eruption,* which may take the form of urticaria, patches of erythema, or a diffuse morbilliform rash, or combinations of these. Such skin manifestations are the most conspicuous and constant feature of the disease, and occur in over 90 per cent of patients. Occasionally, petechiae or purpuric skin lesions are encountered. *Itching* occurs shortly before the skin eruption is obvious, and usually persists throughout the illness; it is most bothersome in patients with extensive urticarial lesions. A generalized *lymphadenopathy* is present in most patients at the time of or just prior to the appearance of the skin eruption. *Edema* of the face, eyelids, hands and feet occurs in approximately 30 per cent of cases; it is more frequent and severe in children than in adults. Edema of the glottis is in rare instances sufficiently intense to require tracheotomy. Some patients without obvious edema undergo a rapid gain in weight during the period of the disease, owing to retention of water. The renal excretion of sodium chloride and water is markedly reduced at this time.

In many patients, the disease is limited to the above-mentioned manifestations, and these disappear within two to three days. In more severely ill patients, the skin eruption lasts for a week or longer and, on the third or fourth day after onset, *fever* appears, with daily elevations of temperature to 101 or 102° F. During the febrile period, constitutional symptoms such as *malaise, headache, abdominal pain, nausea* and *vomiting* are often present.

Involvement of the joints occurs in approximately 50 per cent of patients with serum sickness, usually beginning two to three days after the appearance of skin eruption. There may be mild *arthralgia* and some stiffness on movement or, less commonly, there may be outright *polyarthritis* resembling the joint symptoms of acute rheumatic fever. Swift and Boots found the joint fluid to be an inflammatory exudate containing numerous polymorphonuclear leukocytes. The earliest joint to be involved is usually the temporomandibular; pain and limitation of motion in this joint may be misinterpreted as early tetanus in patients treated with antitetanus serum.

Neurologic manifestations sometimes occur in severe serum sickness. *Stupor, coma* and transient *hemiplegia,* associated with an increase in cerebrospinal fluid pressure, have been observed. *Optic neuritis* may occur as a complication of serum sickness. *Peripheral* neuritis, usually involving the cervicobrachial plexus, may cause severe root pains in the shoulder girdle and upper extremities, with temporary weakness or paralysis of arm muscles.

Diagnosis. Laboratory studies provide little if any assistance. Patients with serum sickness following injections of horse serum may exhibit elevated titers of heterophile antibody for sheep erythrocytes. Leukocytosis and eosinophilia are uncommon but may occur late in the course of illness. The urine may show slight albuminuria and a few casts, but there are no significant evidences of renal impairment. The erythrocyte sedimentation rate is usually normal.

The disease may be mistaken for rheumatic fever, if a history of serum administration is unobtainable. In cases with inconspicuous or absent skin eruptions, the symptoms may resemble those of complications of the disease for which serum was administered, for example, tetanus. In general, however, the typical syndrome of serum sickness is unmistakably recognizable.

Serum Accidents. The acute, immediate, shock-like reactions which follow an injection of foreign serum in previously sensitized individuals are in all probability based on the same immunologic disturbance as that involved in serum sickness. The early onset and severity of symptoms are due to the existence of antibody at the time of injection of antigen, and the situation is quite similar to anaphylactic shock in animals. Within a few seconds after injection the patient may exhibit extreme apprehension, violent itching, sneezing and coughing, and asthmatic breathing. Generalized urticaria may appear within minutes. The blood pressure falls, and the pulse becomes weak or imperceptible. There may be sudden loss of consciousness, accompanied by generalized convulsive seizures. The temperature is usually elevated shortly after the beginning of symptoms. Death can occur within less than 10 minutes, or after several hours. Patients who survive such episodes usually exhibit other evidences of typical serum sickness during the next few days.

The pathologic findings in fatal serum accidents include extensive acute emphysema of the lungs, dilatation of the right ventricle, and multiple small hemorrhages in the heart, lungs, kidneys and adrenal glands.

Treatment. Recognition of hypersensitivity in patients prior to the administration of foreign serum is of the first importance in avoiding serum reactions. All patients should be carefully questioned concerning previous injections of serum. A history of asthma, hay fever or other allergic reactions is an indication for special caution in the administration of serum. *All* patients, regardless of history, should be tested for cutaneous and conjunctival sensitivity before undertaking serum treatment. The intracutaneous test may be performed with 0.02 cc. of a 1:10 dilution of the serum to be used; for the conjunctival test a drop of 1:100 dilution is employed. If either test is positive, the use of serum treatment should be reconsidered in the light of the potential danger involved. If it is imperative that serum be administered, an attempt should be made to desensitize the patient. This may be done by giving repeated injections of small amounts every 15 minutes, starting with 0.1 cc. of a 1:100 dilution subcutaneously and doubling the amount with each dose until 1 cc. has been given by this route. Intravenous injections are then begun in the same fashion, beginning with 0.1 cc. and doubling the dose every 15 minutes until the required amount has been administered.

Serum reactions of the immediate, anaphylactic variety are treated with epinephrine, which should be available in a syringe whenever serum is injected. A dose of 0.5 to 1.0 cc. of a 1:1000 dilution should be given subcutaneously at the first sign of an acute serum reaction, and repeated after a few minutes if indicated.

The usual case of serum sickness is a mild, self-limited disease presenting few problems of therapy. The itching discomfort associated with urticaria may be temporarily relieved by subcutaneous injections of epinephrine, or by the oral administration of pyribenzamine in a dosage of 50 mg. every 4 hours. Cortisone and ACTH have been used with success in the treatment of allergic reactions to drugs, and may be useful in controlling the discomfort in severe or prolonged attacks of serum sickness; most cases, however, are so mild that such treatment is unnecessary.

LEWIS THOMAS

References

Chase, M. W.: The Allergic State. In Dubos, R. J.: Bacterial and Mycotic Infections of Man. Philadelphia, J. B. Lippincott Co., 1952, Chap. 6.

Kojis, F. G.: Serum Sickness and Anaphylaxis. Am. J. Dis. Child., 64:93, 313, 1942.

Longcope, W. T.: Serum Sickness and Analogous Reactions from Certain Drugs Particularly the Sulfonamides. Medicine, 22:251, 1943.

Rich, A. R.: Hypersensitivity in Disease. Harvey Lectures, 42:106, 1946.

CONTACT DERMATITIS

Definition. Contact dermatitis is a common expression of allergy wherein an eczematous lesion of the skin appears after repeated contact with specific agents.

Etiology. The two factors responsible for the production of contact dermatitis are (*a*) the nature of the offending agent (contactant) and (*b*) the responsiveness of the skin.

Contactants. These vary from simple chemical substances to complex biological products. Although strong chemicals applied to the skin may cause irritation, the specific agents responsible for contact dermatitis are usually not irritating when first applied to normal skin. Those which penetrate the horny layer of the skin most readily to reach the underlying epidermis are, as a rule, encountered most frequently. Thus, common contactants are plant oils, such as that from poison ivy, which are easily dissolved in the fatty substances of the skin surface, dyes which become fixed in the horny layer and

come in close contact with the epidermis, and local anesthetics such as procaine which have an affinity for epidermal structures. Thousands of contactants have been identified as responsible for dermatitis. They are associated for the most part with industry and trades. The disease occurs frequently in bakers, beauty parlor operators, chemists, furriers, gardeners, jewelers, munition workers, nurses, painters, photographers, printers, tanners, and so on. Sulfonamide compounds, penicillin, streptomycin and other drugs of more recent origin have accounted for many cases from incorporation in ointments or by direct handling.

Skin Responsiveness. Although, quantitatively, there is a wide variation in the capacity of the skin of different persons to react, no one is considered immune, provided the epidermis is exposed sufficiently to repeated application of a known contactant. The mechanism by which the skin becomes sensitized is apparently by an attachment of the contactant to proteins of the epidermal cells, and the combined molecule acts as an antigen. Antibodies to the contactant (haptene) then are produced and the lesion represents a specific antigen-antibody reaction.

Morbid Anatomy. The essential lesion is epidermal edema. This occurs, apparently, as the result of an escape of fluid from dilated blood and lymph capillaries at the site of irritation. As fluid continues to accumulate, vesicles are formed within the epidermis and appear on the surface of the skin as small blisters. In the more chronic stages, prolonged irritation may lead to hyperkeratosis and lichenification.

Symptoms. The only symptom is pruritus, felt as itching and burning at the site of the lesion. In the acute cases there appears first an erythema with superimposed papules, and then vesicles. The time of appearance of the eruption following contact is extremely variable. Once hypersensitiveness is established, however, the lesion usually appears within 24 hours after the last exposure. In some instances in which the lesion is very acute, a generalized eruption may appear as the process spreads, presumably via the lymphatics. When there is continual contact, as in certain industries, the vesicular eruption is replaced by thickened, fissured, dry dermatitis. Secondary infection is common.

Differential Diagnosis. This concerns (*a*) the distinction from other types of eczema and (*b*) the detection of the specific contactants.

Contact dermatitis may resemble the lesions of other types of eczema, such as those from fungus infections, seborrheic dermatitis, chemical dermatitis and particularly atopic dermatitis. This lesion, however, is frequently associated with other atopic disorders, as asthma and hay fever, and this type of allergy is hereditary. It occurs most frequently in infants and children, and sites of predilection are the face, neck, and folds of the elbows and knees. Contact dermatitis occurs most frequently in adults. The distribution of the lesion frequently indicates the diagnosis and may even suggest the contactant at fault. Thus, an eczematous eruption limited to the skin about the eyes strongly suggests a cosmetic such as mascara; that which occurs only on the neck is frequently caused by fur dyes; and that beneath the arms from dress shield material. Other eczemas rarely have such a distribution.

Detection of the offending contactant is made from the case history and from patch tests. The site of the localized lesion and meticulous questioning will frequently elicit a clue. The possible contactants are then applied to uninvolved skin. Unlike intradermal tests, the patch test material is gently rubbed onto the skin, moistened if necessary, covered with cellophane and held in place with adhesive material for 24 to 48 hours, or less if intense itching occurs at the site of the test. A positive reaction is an eczematous dermatitis at the patch site. The contactant at fault will be revealed in the majority of the cases tested. Precautions to be carefully observed are the removal of the patch if itching becomes marked, and limitation of the number of tests at one time to twenty or less. Necrosis of the skin and marked exacerbation of symptoms may occur if the application is too intense.

Prognosis. All patients eventually recover, sometimes quickly after the offending substance is removed.

Treatment. It is a moot question whether the injection of extracts of at least some of the contactants will build up a resistance to them. This is particularly important in poison ivy. Although, experimentally, such prophylactic or phylactic treatment does not seem valid, clinically there are favorable reports. The only certain cure is the discovery of the offending allergen and its avoidance.

The principles of local treatment are important, since drugs applied repeatedly to excoriated skin may cause a superimposed contact dermatitis on one for which treatment is sought. Wet dressings of saturated solution of boric acid or 5 per cent aluminum acetate for the acute stage followed by a bland grease such as 3 per cent boric acid in nonallergic cold cream will often allay itching, provided the contactant has been removed. There is always danger of overtreatment, and in severe, stubborn cases, hospitalization, so that the patient can be protected and nursed, is recommended. In the acute and subacute forms, hydrocortisone ointment in 1 and 2.5 per cent concentrations may be very effective.

HARRY L. ALEXANDER

References

Eisen, H. N., Orris, N., and Belman, S.: Elicitation of Delayed Skin Reactions with Haptens. The Dependence of Elicitation on Hapten Combination with Protein. J. Exper. Med., 95:573, 1952.

Rauchwerger, S. M., Erskine, F. A., and Nalls, W. I.: Streptomycin Sensitivity. Development of Sensitivity in Nursing Personnel through Contact during Administration of the Drug to Patients. J.A.M.A., 136:614, 1948.

Rostenberg, A., Jr., and Kanof, N. P.: Eczematous Sensitizations. The Specificity of the Sensitization from the Viewpoint of Chemical Configuration. J. Invest. Dermat., 6:201, 1945.

Schwartz, L.: Industrial Dermatosis. U. S. Pub. Health Rep., 1935.

———, and Peck, S. M.: Cosmetics and Dermatitis. New York, Paul B. Hoeber, Inc., 1946.

Sulzberger, M. B.: Dermatologic Allergy. Springfield, Ill., Charles C Thomas, 1940.

———: Hydrocortone (Compound F) Acetate Ointment in Dermatologic Therapy. J.A.M.A., 151: 468, 1953.

ANGIONEUROTIC EDEMA

(Angioedema)

Definition. Angioneurotic edema is characterized by transient, circumscribed, edematous swellings of the skin or mucous membrane, occasionally of the viscera. One form is hereditary and is frequently terminated by a fatal edema of the glottis; another form is relatively benign, and in some cases is dependent upon a demonstrable food allergy. Urticaria and angioneurotic edema are frequently associated.

History. Quincke in 1882 described the nonhereditary form. Priority has usually been assigned to him, although Milton in 1876 described the same condition under the title of "Giant Urticaria." The first descriptions in American literature were from

Osler, in 1888; he reported a remarkable family history in which the disease was transmitted for five generations.

Incidence. The condition is not rare. Bulloch in 1909 collected 170 cases of the hereditary form from the literature. The nonhereditary type is seen with some frequency.

Etiology. From Quincke's time, belief in an angioneurosis as the important pathogenetic factor has persisted, and certainly in many of these patients psychologic difficulties appear to participate in the etiology. Recent evidence makes it probable that in some of the *nonhereditary* cases the condition is due to *food allergy*. The offending food, however, can be discovered only exceptionally from skin reactions; these usually yield no helpful information. This form is frequently associated with urticaria. Focal infection, drugs and endocrine disturbances have been thought to be etiologic factors in some cases, but critical scrutiny of the evidence in any series of these cases leaves a large percentage in which the etiology must be said to be undetermined. The *sexes* are about equally affected. The appearance of the lesion in childhood is unusual, but the onset at puberty has been noted in numerous cases. The majority of instances appear in adults. The *hereditary form* of the disease may be transmitted through several generations by both affected and unaffected persons without sex linkage. The families studied do not show transmission according to the theoretical expectations of a mendelian dominant. It has been suggested that urticaria and angioneurotic edema are dependent on the same mechanism; that in the former the vessels of the skin affected are more superficial than in the latter form. The mechanism which produces both these cutaneous reactions seems to consist in vasodilation and transudation; the vasodilator substance is probably histamine—free or in loose combination—or a histamine-like substance. The mechanisms involved in wheal formation have been thoroughly studied by Lewis. Recently Rose has reported a marked diminution of the histamine content of the blood when acute symptoms of angioneurotic edema were present. In recent years several cases of angioneurotic edema and urticaria due to penicillin have been reported.

Symptoms. The swellings appear, as it were, spontaneously. An itching, prickly or burning sensation may precede the appearance of a smooth, rounded elevation varying in size from a few millimeters up to large areas covering nearly the entire back. The swellings may be tense and elastic or rarely soft and pitting. The skin may not change in color over the swellings, or may become pink or dusky red. Areas commonly involved are the lips, the skin about the eyes, chin, hands, feet and tongue, but any part of the body surface may be affected. A swelling may persist several days, but more frequently disappears after 24 to 36 hours. There may be years between attacks, or edematous areas may appear almost daily for years. In rare cases there is a periodic recurrence of attacks. Involvement of the genitals has caused urethral occlusion. Visceral involvement, much more common in the hereditary form, may cause death by edema of the glottis. Gastro-intestinal crises with vomiting and abdominal pain have occurred in many familial cases. Cases simulating acute ileus, ruptured tubal pregnancy, appendicitis, acute cholecystitis, renal colic and intussusception are on record. Kennedy has described cases of angioneurotic edema of the brain. Fever may occur, but from available reports leukocytosis seems to be rare.

Associated skin lesions not infrequently observed are urticaria, erythema multiforme and purpura.

Prognosis. In the hereditary form the danger of death from edema of the glottis is serious. Of the 170 patients cited by Bulloch, 21.1 per cent died in this way, and 67.9 per cent of all the deaths were due to this lesion. In the nonhereditary form the prognosis is much better. Spontaneous cessation after a few months or years is to be expected. Edema of the glottis is rare in this group.

Treatment. In a small percentage of cases a specific allergen is found to be responsible for the occurrence of the swellings. In such patients, elimination of the offending substance from the diet may prevent recurrences. The procedure in this regard which is sometimes effective is to restrict the diet to one or two simple foods, such as rice and milk, for ten days or two weeks. The swellings may cease when the number of foods is thus limited. If one article of food is then added at intervals of three or four days, it may be possible to observe that when a certain food is given the swellings reappear, and that when it is withdrawn the swellings disappear. In some patients it is possible to discover by this method the offending food and to prevent recurrence of the swellings by its elimination from the diet. Such treatment is, however, rarely successful. Nonspecific measures consist first of drug therapy. Ephedrine (0.025 to 0.05 gm. three times a day by mouth), antihistamine drugs such as Benadryl and Pyribenzamine in doses of 50 mg. every 6 hours, and epinephrine subcutaneously (0.3 to 0.5 cc.) may all have some temporary ameliorating effect. Cortisone, as in urticaria, is by far the best symptomatic remedy. Initial daily doses should be sufficient to overcome the lesion; and 200 to 300 mg. or more may be required. Usually the amount may soon be reduced to much smaller maintenance levels. The beneficial effect of injections of histamine in cases of long standing is doubtful. Cold local applications are comforting. A concurrent acute infection may cause a temporary disappearance of the lesion. Persons who have the hereditary form should carry with them at all times a nebulizer containing epinephrine hydrochloride, 1:100, or a hypodermic syringe containing epinephrine, 1:1000, for self-administration. A quick tracheotomy may be lifesaving.

GEORGE M. MACKENZIE

Revised by Harry L. Alexander

References

Bulloch, W.: Angioneurotic Edema. The Treasury of Human Inheritance (Eugenics Laboratory Memoirs, IX). London, Dulan & Co., 1909, Part III, 38.
Crowder, J. R., and Crowder, T. R.: Five Generations of Angioneurotic Edema. Arch. Int. Med., 20:840, 1917.
Dunlap, H. F., and Lemon, W. S.: The Hereditary Type of Angioneurotic Edema. Am. J. M. Sc., 177:259, 1929.
Lewis, T.: The Blood Vessels of the Human Skin and Their Responses. London, Shaw and Sons, Ltd., 1927.
Osler, W.: Hereditary Angioneurotic Edema. Am. J. M. Sc., 95:362, 1888.
———: On the Visceral Manifestations of the Erythema Group of Skin Diseases. Am. J. M. Sc., 127:1, 1904.
Quincke, H.: Ueber akutes umschriebenes Hautödem. Monatschr. f. prak. Dermat., 1:129, 1882.
Rose, B.: Studies on Blood Histamine in Patients with Allergy. J. Clin. Investigation, 20:419, 1941.
Schulman, L. E., Schoenrich, E. H., and Harvey, A. M.: Allergic Reactions to Therapeutic Agents: Treatment with Adrenocorticotropic Hormone (ACTH) or Cortisone. Bull. Johns Hopkins Hosp., 92:196, 1953.

URTICARIA

Definition. Urticaria is an expression of several allergic disorders. It is characterized by multiple, circumscribed, red, raised, pruritic wheals. These, like angioneurotic edema, are caused by dilatation of capillaries with transudation of plasma and some cellular elements through their walls. This is essentially an inflammatory process. The lesions, regardless of their intensity or duration, are reversible and leave no visible trace.

Etiology. As with angioneurotic edema, there is evidence that a histamine-like substance is released in the skin at the sites of the wheal. This process may be brought about in a number of circumstances, including antigen-antibody mechanisms that mediate allergic responses. One characteristic example is urticaria following ingestion of shell fish in a person hypersensitive to this allergen. Another is its appearance in those allergic to drugs such as acetylsalicylic acid or penicillin. It occurs as a cardinal sign of serum sickness and after the injection of an excessive amount of antigen, as in the treatment of hay fever with pollen extract. These are acute episodes. Chronic urticaria appears not infrequently with localized infection, and it is presumed that this represents bacterial allergy. The lesion may be induced in certain persons by physical agents such as exposure to but moderate degrees of cold or heat or sunlight or on stroking the skin (dermatographism). The term "physical allergy" has been applied to such cases; this is not allergy in its true sense, but evidently a histamine-like substance is released by some other mechanism. In a substantial number of patients with chronic urticaria no etiology is detectable, although, in some of these, emotional situations may exaggerate the eruption.

Treatment. As in all allergic situations, if the allergen at fault can be avoided, the eruption disappears thereafter. Skin tests are usually unrevealing in detecting the offending substance. Hence indirect methods such as careful history evaluation, elimination diets and drug exclusion are used. In chronic urticaria, search for a focus of infection and appropriate treatment of it may cure the eruption. When it is due to heat, daily tub baths beginning at temperatures just below those that cause whealing, and increasing by increments of 1 or 2 degrees F., will usually within a few weeks greatly enhance the patient's tolerance. The same process in reverse order applies to those sensitive to cold. Cortisone is, by far, the most effective drug for symptomatic relief. In severe cases, substantial doses may be required initially such as 200 mg. or more for the first day or two, with subsequent reduction as the eruption comes under control. This form of therapy is feasible for acute cases since these usually are not of long duration. Antihistamine drugs bring symptomatic relief in many cases of urticaria, presumably by blocking the formation of histamine in the skin. Side effects are frequent, although with newer preparations these are less prominent.

HARRY L. ALEXANDER

PURPURA

Allergic purpura (anaphylactic purpura) is encountered in patients with drug sensitivity, serum sickness and other allergic disorders. It usually appears without a depression of blood platelets, and it discussed in other chapters of this section.

HARRY L. ALEXANDER

ERYTHEMAS

The term "erythema," which indicates redness, has application to an extensive variety of eruptions. In several instances erythema is accompanied by exudation and inflammatory changes as in urticaria and erythema multiforme. In these two eruptions the pathologic pictures of transudation of plasma and inflammatory cells through the capillaries resemble each other. Moreover, each may occur as a dermatologic expression of the same underlying disorder, such as rheumatic fever or serum sickness. In this connection, purpura in which there may be no changes in blood elements, but extravasation of red cells through the capillaries, also appears at times interchangeably with urticaria and erythema multiforme, so that all three have been linked together by the designation "the erythema group." Osler used this expression to apply to certain cases in which there were associated visceral lesions such as arthritis, abdominal pain, nephritis and signs referable to other organs. Henoch's purpura is one representation of this syndrome. Many of

these patients have been found to be allergic to foods, inhalants and bacterial products.

Of the several types of erythematous lesions, some are linked to allergy, others not.

ERYTHEMA MULTIFORME

Definition. This is an acute process characterized by bright or dark red macules, papules, vesicles, and bullae. The lesions have multiform shapes and sizes, and occur particularly on the face, neck and dorsal surfaces of the extremities and on the mucous membranes. The eruption is an acute process lasting at most but a few weeks and, like urticaria, disappears completely unless the vesicles become secondarily infected. The eruption is a common manifestation of hypersensitivity to drugs.

Systemic manifestations per se are few. Very occasionally, erythema multiforme is associated with an acute, febrile, sometimes fulminating systemic disorder (Stevens-Johnson syndrome). The mucous membranes of the gastrointestinal canal may be involved, and bronchitis, pneumonitis and various ocular disturbances are part of the picture. Loss of vision has occurred and there have been fatalities.

Treatment. In several instances in which allergy has been demonstrated a given food was at fault. As in urticaria, skin tests are usually not revealing, and elimination diets are used. In some instances, as in rheumatic fever, hypersensitiveness to bacterial products is presumed to be the cause, and in these, eradication of infected foci may bring relief. Recently, improvement with antihistamine drugs has been described, and cortisone has been beneficial according to some reports.

ERYTHEMA NODOSUM

Definition. Unlike erythema multiforme, erythema nodosum is usually limited to comparatively few red, oval, tender lesions several centimeters in length, deeply embedded in the skin. They appear most frequently on the extensor surfaces of the legs and arms, but may be more widespread. There is intense infiltration of the corium with tightly packed red and white blood cells which have extravasated through the capillaries.

Etiology. In view of recent observations the older conventional concept that erythema nodosum is a common expression of tuberculosis and rheumatic fever is no longer tenable. It appears to be part of a systemic infection in many cases, since it is usually preceded by upper respiratory symptoms in which the beta hemolytic streptococcus is often isolated. Moreover, a polyarthritis commonly precedes or follows the skin manifestations. In a reported series positive skin tests with beta hemolytic streptococcus antigen far exceeded controls and even reactivated the disease. Although the incidence of associated tuberculosis is not remarkable, it is of interest that erythema nodosum has been found to appear at the time of the development of a positive tuberculin test. There are other instances in which the eruption is definitely associated with hypersensitiveness to drugs such as iodides. Again, erythema nodosum has been found to be interchangeable with erythema multiforme, and has appeared simultaneously with evident allergic purpura. The eruption occurs with other infections such as coccidioidomycosis and ulcerative colitis. The lesion is now generally considered to be an expression of hypersensitiveness to infectious agents, drugs and probably to other allergens.

Treatment. There is no specific treatment. Chemotherapy and antibiotics have had no notable effect. Salicylates are recommended. Cortisone or ACTH gives symptomatic relief but should not be employed if the cause is believed to be tuberculosis. The lesion is self-limited and disappears usually within one month.

Other erythemas which may be identified with allergy are the diffuse morbilliform eruption of *"erythema of the ninth day,"* which occasionally follows injections of arsphenamine or neoarsphenamine. A few cases have been attributed to bismuth, and the lesion is considered an expression of drug hypersensitiveness. Other drugs such as quinine, atropine and the barbiturates may produce a diffuse erythematous eruption in those hypersensitive to these agents.

The erythema of scarlet fever is probably due to an erythrotoxin rather than to bacterial allergy, as claimed by some.

Other erythemas such as *induratum,* in which the tubercle bacillus is usually recovered from the lesion, and *infectiosum,* which occurs in epidemics and is presumably due to an unknown infectious agent, have no apparent allergic implication.

Harry L. Alexander

References

Agostas, W. N., Reeves, N., Shanks, E. D. and Sydenstricker, V. P.: Erythema Multiforme Bullosum (Stevens-Johnson Syndrome). New England J. Med., *246:*217, 1952.

Crawford, G. M., and Luikart, R. H.: Severe Erythema Multiforme with Intestinal Involvement. J.A.M.A., *140:*780, 1949.

Favour, C. B., and Sosman, M. C.: Erythema Nodosum. Arch. Int. Med., *80:*435, 1947.

Feinberg, S. M.: Histamine Antagonists. J. Allergy, *17:*217, 1946.

Finland, M., Joliffe, L. S., and Parker, F. J.: Pneumonia and Erythema Multiforme Exudativum. Am. J. Med., *4:*473, 1948.

Lever, W. F.: Severe Erythema Multiforme. Arch. Dermat. & Syph., *49:*47, 1944.

Montgomery, H., O'Leary, P. A., and Barker, N. W.: Nodular Vascular Diseases of the Legs. J.A.M.A., *128:*335, 1945.

Waldbott, G. L.: An Etiological Survey of Chronic Urticaria. Progress in Allergy. New York, S. Karger, 1949, p. 236.

Collagen Diseases

INTRODUCTION

The term, "collagen disease," is not a diagnostic symbol which identifies a specific morbid entity, well defined by characteristic clinical features or postmortem tissue alterations. It rather refers to a concept founded upon pathologic-anatomic observations which suggests that clinically heterogeneous maladies have a common denominator in generalized alterations of the connective tissue, specifically of its intercellular components. The meaning of the concept will best be illustrated by a review of its evolution.

Schade, in the first decades of the century, called attention to the loose connective tissue, particularly to its extracellular components as a widely distributed colloidal system of importance for physiology. He called it the "connective tissue organ." The pathologic significance of systemic alterations of the intermediary substances of the collagenous tissue was first recognized by Klinge. He correlated fibrinoid connective tissue damage, previously established as a characteristic microscopic feature of rheumatic fever and rheumatoid arthritis, with morphologically similar alterations in experimental animals provoked by protein hypersensitivity. He regarded fibrinoid connective tissue damage as a microscopic lesion specific to tissue allergy. Consequently, he adopted the sweeping generalization that the presence of this type of connective tissue damage in human diseases was adequate evidence of a hypersensitivity background. Thus, he collected into a group with common pathogenesis several maladies which hitherto had not been considered as related, such as the rheumatic diseases, polyarteritis nodosa, dermatomyositis, thromboangiitis obliterans, malignant nephrosclerosis, subacute bacterial endocarditis and certain nephritides. Subsequently, generalized scleroderma was included when Masugi and Yä-Shu observed fibrinoid arteriolar damage in the kidneys.

In the aforementioned diseases vascular involvement was a conspicuous feature, with the walls of small arteries frequently showing fibrinoid degeneration, as well as necrosing inflammation. This vascular implication seemed to be a conspicuous histopathologic feature of systemic diseases with allergic etiology. Microscopic studies of the organs of patients dying of systemic (acute disseminated) lupus erythematosus revealed the presence of widespread and most intensive fibrinoid connective tissue damage in significant frequency. It was tempting to apply the same pathogenetic interpretation and to classify systemic lupus erythematosus with the diseases of hypersensitivity. However, it had become evident that Klinge's original generalization deserved critical reexamination. *Local* fibrinoid connective tissue changes are observed in a variety of morbid situations in which allergy can be excluded as a pathogenetic factor, such as the base of the peptic ulcer, the vicinity of pancreatic necrosis or acute bacterial infections. It is widespread and conspicuous in the vasculature of animals made hypertensive by the Goldblatt mechanism or by desoxycorticosterone, and of dogs treated with repeated epinephrine injections. The diversity of human pathologic and experimental conditions in which fibrinoid tissue damage was observed challenged Klinge's pathogenetic generalization applied to human disease. Moreover, while it could not be denied that fibrinoid connective tissue damage occurred in experimental and human hypersensitivity, it was obvious that the correlation was purely empiric; the mechanism by which the hypersensitivity state provokes connective tissue changes was, and still is, entirely obscure. Pathogenetic research cannot be advanced if one remains satisfied with interpreting ill defined histologic structural alterations in terms of poorly understood experimental phenomena.

These were reasons which made the allergic theory in its universal scope untenable. Yet Klinge's basic premise that the widespread fibrinoid tissue alteration observed in a great variety of etiologically obscure human disease is of great significance was, and still is, fully acceptable. It seemed, however, that comprehension of this ill defined area of human pathology could be advanced only by unbiased investigation of all factors which might be responsible for the fundamental connective tissue alteration. Klinge's definition based on the specific allergic etiology therefore had to be abandoned. In its place the noncontroversial descriptive criterion of structural alteration of the intermediate substances of the connective tissue was chosen as the principle of a tentative classification. Since the collagen fibers seemed to be prominently affected in the morbid process, the term "collagen disease" was proposed for the group of diseases so characterized. This cautious nosologic formulation was to serve as temporary foundation until the pathogenesis of the basic tissue changes was established by further investigations. It was realized that a rational inquiry into the cause of the pathologic states identified by alterations of the intercellular substances of the connective tissue must rest upon comprehension of their normal constitution and biology.

It was fortunate that during the years when these studies in pathology were slowly advancing, studies of the biology of connective tissue became the focal point for investigations in chemistry, physiology and histology to clarify the nature of the intercellular material, its origin and its role in the economy of life. The many aspects of these recent studies have concerned themselves with the fundamental constitution of the intercellular substances, their plasticity as influenced by enzymes and hormones, and their mode of formation. Most of these investigations have not yet been advanced far enough to clarify the clinical manifestations of the diseases defined so far only by their morphology. However, recent pathologic-anatomic studies suggest that the fibrinoid connective tissue damage is the result of precipitation of abnormal proteins within the amorphous ground substance. These abnormal proteins are circulating within the blood plasma and reach the ground substance by transudation. It is probable that the intermediate substances of the connective tissue under normal conditions are in intimate genetic relationship with the plasma proteins, and that a disturbance of this relationship is one of the factors in the pathogenesis of diseases characterized by systemic implication of the intermediate substances of the connective tissue. The concept of collagen disease applies not only to the rheumatic maladies, hypersensitivity angiitis, systemic lupus erythematosus, generalized scleroderma and, possibly, dermatomyositis,

but might well be considered in investigations of the pathogenesis of vascular diseases including arteriosclerosis. It is, however, of heuristic value only, and will have served its purpose when the abnormalities of the intercellular substances have been fully appreciated and comprehended.

PAUL KLEMPERER

References

Duran-Reynals, F.: Introduction to Symposium on The Ground Substance of the Mesenchyme and Hyaluronidase. Ann. N. Y. Acad. Sci., 52:943, 1950.

Klemperer, P.: The Significance of the Intermediate Substances of the Connective Tissue in Human Disease. Harvey Lectures, 1954.

———, Pollack, A. D., and Baehr, G.: Pathology of Disseminated Lupus Erythematosus. Arch. Path., 32:569, 1941.

———, Pollack, A. D., and Baehr, G.: Diffuse Collagen Disease. J.A.M.A., 119:331, 1942.

Klinge, F.: Der Rheumatismus. Ergebn. d. allg. Path. und path. Anat., 27:1, 1933.

Masugi, M., and Yä-Shu: Die diffuse Sklerodermie und ihre Gefässveränderung. Virchows Arch. f. path. Anat., 302:39, 1938.

Schade, H.: Die physikalische Chemie in der inneren Medizin. Dresden und Leipzig, T. Steinkopff, 1923.

Zeek, P. M.: Periarteritis Nodosa: A Critical Review. Am. J. Clin. Path., 22:777, 1952.

DISSEMINATED LUPUS ERYTHEMATOSUS

Definition. Among the heterogeneous groups of so-called rheumatoid diseases, disseminated lupus erythematosus constitutes a disease entity, distinguished by a prolonged clinical course which usually terminates fatally, by a striking predilection for young females and by characteristic pathologic changes in the collagenous tissues which especially affect the vascular system and the serous and synovial membranes. Because in many instances an erythematous rash is apt to appear on the face and other parts of the body at some stage of the disease, the condition was first described about the middle of the nineteenth century by dermatologists (Hebra, Casenave, Kaposi), who named it lupus erythematodes or erythematosus. In spite of its name this disease bears no relationship whatever to tuberculosis and lupus vulgaris, or to that benign indolent skin lesion known to dermatologists as discoid lupus.

Unlike discoid lupus, erythematous lupus is not a primary disease of the skin. It is a disease of the body as a whole and is usually fatal.

In recent years it has been recognized that the skin rash is not invariably present, and that when it appears it is a superficial manifestation of a widespread injury to the collagen, which serves as a matrix and binding substance for capillaries and other small blood vessels in various parts of the body. The appearance of an erythema spreading in a butterfly pattern across the bridge of the nose and the malar eminences in a patient suffering from fever and the other systemic manifestations of this disease greatly facilitates the diagnosis. But even in the absence of the rash the characteristic combination of other clinical manifestations should be adequate for the diagnosis. On the other hand, an erythema on the bridge of the nose and the malar eminences may be due to a variety of other causes, and it alone does not warrant a diagnosis of disseminated lupus erythematosus if fever and the other clinical features of this disease are absent.

Incidence. In its milder and clinically atypical forms, the disease is often unsuspected by clinicians unfamiliar with its protean symptomatology. In recent years, as physicians have become increasingly aware of its frequently atypical features, it has gradually come to be recognized as a rather common disease, especially among young females. Using the L.E. cell test of Hargraves as a sensitive diagnostic aid, 44 cases were recognized in the Los Angeles County Hospital during 1950 and 1951, compared with 18 cases of Hodgkin's disease and 88 cases of acute rheumatic fever.

One of the most remarkable characteristics of the disease is its sex linkage. About 85 per cent of all clinically recognizable cases are in females. The disease occurs in childhood but is most common during adolescence and early adult life. It is rare after the menopause.

Etiology. Bacteriologic studies have revealed no clue concerning the cause of this disease. The cultivation of a virus was recently reported by Moolten but his work has not been confirmed. Blood cultures are negative, unless there is an intercurrent pneumonia or a terminal streptococcal or staphyloccal blood infection. There are as a rule no clinical or other evidences of allergy.

In spite of the fact that more than 85 per cent of the patients are females, no endocrine disorder can be recognized, nor do the few young males with the disease show any endocrine abnormalities. The predominant predisposition of females indicates that, whatever the exact nature of the primary cause, the disease must be conditioned upon a peculiarity in the constitution of the host. This is supported by the observation that this relatively uncommon disease may occur in siblings. The effects of the unknown agent are manifested by a change in the chemistry of mesenchymal tissues, chiefly the subendothelial connective tissue of capillaries and small arteries, the endocardium, and various serous and synovial surfaces.

Morbid Anatomy. At the autopsy table the frequent paucity of severe gross anatomic changes and the absence of a distinctive lethal lesion is in striking contrast to the profound toxemia and the train of clinical events leading to the death of the patient. The widespread and heterogeneous visceral lesions usually revealed by microscopic study can be ascribed to alteration in the ground substance and collagen fibrils of the connective tissues of the body.

Pericardial involvement occurs frequently and in its severest form appears as a thick, gelatinous, connective tissue completely obliterating the pericardial space. This appearance is due to a series of proliferative and degenerative changes of the collagenous tissue underneath the mesothelium. A similar type of pleuritis, perisplenitis and perihepatitis is also exceedingly common.

In about 30 per cent of the cases examined grossly the *endocardium* of one or more valves exhibits a pathognomonic lesion first described by Libman and Sacks as indeterminate endocarditis to distinguish it from vegetations due to known bacteria. The endocardial vegetations may be small and verrucous or large, broad and flat. They may occur on either side of the valvular leaflets, sometimes also on the chordae tendineae or the mural endocardium of the ventricle. Microscopically, the lesion begins as a fibrinoid degeneration or necrosis of the connective tissue fibrils and a swelling of the ground substance immediately beneath the endocardium. A subendothelial accumulation of collagenous material develops, which protrudes as an excrescence on the surface of the endocardium. In the terminal period of the disease such advanced endocardial vegetations may occasionally become infected secondarily with bacteria.

Focal lesions of the interstitial collagenous tissue of the myocardium morphologically identical with those seen in the endocardium and pericardium are present in about 35 per cent of cases. Aschoff bodies are not found.

The small arteries and arterioles of various viscera and especially of the kidneys may show fibrinoid degeneration and necrosis of the connective tissue matrix of the vessel wall. This may lead to a reactive proliferation of the lining endothelium and to a thrombotic occlusion of the affected arterioles. The renal glomeruli may show focal necroses of occasional loops, or the walls of some glomerular capillaries may be thick, rigid, deeply eosinophilic, the so-called "wire loop" lesion. These alterations are merely another expression of the widespread damage to subendothelial collagen.

The spleen is usually not enlarged significantly unless there is an intercurrent secondary bacteremia. Microscopically, the central arteries of the malpighian lymph follicles are surrounded characteristically by conspicuous concentric rings of connective tissue.

Erythematous areas of skin may show few microscopic changes except capillary dilatation, small red cell extravasations, edema, and some swelling of the ground substance between connective tissue fibrils. Older lesions may show fibrinoid degeneration of the collagenous tissues of the upper corium and of small blood vessels, but microscopic examination of a small biopsy specimen is often disappointing.

The regional lymph nodes are usually enlarged during periods of exacerbation and, on biopsy, sometimes show areas of necrosis. Bronchopneumonia is a frequent terminal complication.

Pathologic Chemistry. The histologic changes observed in this disease are the expression of fundamental disturbances in cellular chemistry. In some of the affected areas of connective tissue this is revealed by the increase and deep metachromatic staining of the intercellular ground substance, which consists of mucoprotein, and by the swelling and fibrinoid degeneration of collagen fibrils which may melt together into more or less homogeneous eosinophilic masses of collagenous substance. Klemperer has made the important observation that another deep purplish-staining material may be found in some of the affected areas of connective tissue, which he has identified histochemically as consisting largely of desoxyribonucleic acid and which must therefore be derived from the enzymatic disintegration of nuclear ma-

terial. This is apparently the same abnormal chromatin material observed in the so-called "L.E. cells" of the blood and bone marrow in this disease by Hargraves, Richmont and Morton.

These indications of a disturbance in cellular enzyme chemistry, especially of connective tissues, suggest that the efficacy of cortisone (and of ACTH) in arresting the disease process in rheumatoid arthritis and in disseminated lupus erythematosus may depend upon the ability of these hormonal agents to reverse the destructive enzymatic processes in the affected cells rather than upon a direct influence upon the unknown cause of the disease. This hypothesis is supported by the prompt effect of the therapy and, in most instances, the equally prompt recurrence of illness upon its discontinuance.

Symptoms. The salient clinical manifestations are (1) a prolonged irregular fever with a tendency to remissions of variable duration (weeks, months or even years); (2) a tendency to recurrent involvement of synovial and serous membranes (polyarthritis, pleuritis, pericarditis); (3) depression of bone marrow function (leukopenia, moderate hypochromic anemia, moderate thrombopenia); and (4) in advanced stages, clinical evidences of vascular alterations in the skin, retina, kidneys and other viscera.

In the absence of the rash the condition may resemble an infectious polyarthritis. The pain and sometimes swelling of various joints may at first make it difficult to distinguish the condition from rheumatic fever or from rheumatoid arthritis. Suspicion may first be directed to its true nature by finding a leukopenia, the white blood cell count usually ranging between 3500 and 6000, while the polymorphonuclear leukocytes are proportionately reduced. The characteristic leukopenia may be replaced by leukocytosis whenever secondary intercurrent infections occur, such as bronchopneumonia. As the disease progresses, the hemoglobin falls more rapidly than the red cell count, but rarely below 60 per cent. In the more advanced stages the blood platelet count is apt to be depressed to about 100,000, occasionally below 40,000. Patients with lower platelet counts during exacerbations may have generalized purpuric manifestations resembling those of primary thrombocytopenia, for which splenectomy has in a few instances been mistakenly performed.

The so-called L.E. cells of Hargraves are

found in stained blood and bone marrow smears, especially in those made from clotted blood or from the buffy layer of heparinized blood. They consist of phagocytes, usually neutrophilic polymorphonuclear leukocytes, containing masses of chromatin material which take a deep purplish color with Wright's or Giemsa's stain. The phagocytized material is apparently derived from the products of nuclear disintegration, for

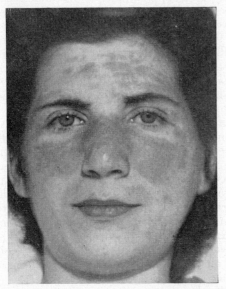

Fig. 57. Typical butterfly lesion of lupus erythematosus on the bridge of the nose and on the cheeks.

Klemperer has demonstrated that it contains desoxyribonucleic acid. Although the finding of L.E. cells in blood or bone marrow is diagnostically specific, they are not invariably demonstrable at all stages of the disease.

During exacerbations of the disease the percentage of total plasma proteins and of serum albumin declines out of proportion to the albuminuria. Coincidentally, the percentage of globulin rises and may exceed the serum albumin, both the α and β globulin fractions usually being conspicuously increased (Coburn and Moore, and Reiner). Although usually negative, a falsely positive Wassermann test is not infrequent and may antedate by years other manifestations of the disease.

Suspicion that the illness is not rheumatic fever or rheumatoid arthritis is warranted when red blood cells are found in the microscopic examination of the urine. The presence of red blood cells in the urine is due to the development of renal vascular lesions, a

pathologic alteration which does not commonly occur in rheumatic fever without heart failure or in rheumatoid arthritis. Small amounts of albumin are also usually to be found. The appearance of large amounts of albumin, red blood cells and casts, resembling the urinary findings of an acute glomerulonephritis, signifies the development of extensive vascular changes and of glomerular damage. It occurs in the advanced stage of the disease and completely eliminates the diagnosis of rheumatic fever.

In addition to arthralgia and arthritis, attacks of pleurisy or of pericarditis may occur at any time during the disease. Probably because of peritoneal serositis, some patients may at times complain of abdominal pain and present abdominal distention and diffuse tenderness.

When the fever is high and the patient's state is unusually toxic, the heart is apt to have a gallop rhythm. Unless pericarditis is present, the electrocardiogram reveals no characteristic changes as a rule except low voltage. In some patients a soft systolic murmur is audible at the apex of the heart or to the left of the sternum. In most instances it is not to be regarded as evidence of endocarditis, since it may be due to the effect of fever or anemia. If it becomes unusually conspicuous, it may indicate the peculiar type of endocarditis (Libman-Sacks) which develops in the advanced stage of the illness in about 30 per cent of the cases.

Either at the onset or sometimes at a later stage, vascular lesions become visible on the skin as erythematous macules or patches which tend to become confluent. The rash first appears as a rule upon the more exposed parts of the face, the bridge of the nose and the cheeks, above the eyebrows, on the upper lip, the prominence of the chin and the edges of the pinna. It is also commonly found on the V-shaped exposed area of the upper chest. It may at times be characteristically located on the tips of the fingers and around the nail beds or as erythematous macules on the thenar and hypothenar eminences, the palms, occasionally on the ends of the toes and the balls of the feet. Areas of skin on parts of the body which are subject to rubbing or other mechanical trauma may become erythematous, such as the elbows and knees, the shoulders, the malleoli, the buttocks and the dorsal aspects of the forearms.

If the rash has existed for some time, minute telangiectases may be scattered in the midst of the erythema as evidence of more permanent vascular changes. At times the intensely erythematous areas may present a purplish blush, especially on the face, fingers, elbows and chest, owing to diffuse extravasations of red cells and plasma. Small groups of purpuric or petechial hemorrhages are sometimes seen on the skin and mucous membranes at the height of the disease. During periods of remission the erythema tends to disappear, but macules of brown pigmentation will then persist in the previously affected areas.

marked, both in the skin and mucous membranes, owing to the intense vascular injury and perhaps in part to a tendency to thrombopenia. In a few instances hemorrhagic vesicles or even small hemorrhagic necroses develop on the intensely erythematous areas of of the face or hands.

Aside from the skin and mucous membrane lesions, the progressive injury to the peripheral vascular system results in microscopic hematuria and albuminuria which, when marked, may give rise to a suspicion of glomerulonephritis. Severe examples of renal

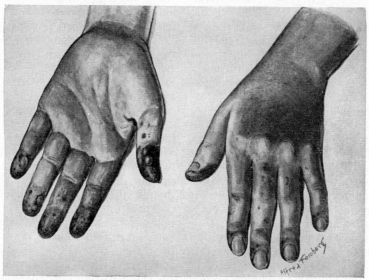

Fig. 58. The skin lesions of lupus erythematosus may also occur on the hands and feet. When present, the erythema commonly involves the palmar surface of the terminal phalanges and area of skin around the nail beds on the sides and dorsum of the fingers. In the midst of the erythema are petechial hemorrhages and telangiectases. The blebs occur only rarely and in cases with the most intense skin lesions. Scattered erythematous macules are sometimes observed on the palms and on the thenar and hypothenar eminences.

Some patients give a history of exposure to the sun immediately before the onset of the disease or of an exacerbation. Others, who have suffered mildly for weeks or months with a low grade fever and migrating arthralgia, expose themselves to sunlight during convalescence and only then have the facial rash followed by an exacerbation of the illness. In other cases no history of exposure to sunlight is given.

At the height of the disease erythematous or petechial macules may appear on the mucous membranes, especially of the mouth, which soon develop into shallow ulcers surrounded by an erythematous or hemorrhagic areola. These lesions tend to heal. In some patients the tendency to purpura may become

damage may be associated with fixation of specific gravity of the urine and, sometimes in the terminal stages of the disease, azotemia. In spite of severe vascular injury and renal damage, the blood pressure is usually normal, sometimes moderately elevated. Moderate edema of the face and extremities occurs at times, due either to the diffuse vascular disturbance in the skin or to hypoproteinuria. If prolonged albuminuria results in profound hypoproteinuria, general anasarca may develop. A complicating clinical picture resembling nephrosis is especially apt to occur in young children.

Some discrete enlargement of regional lymph nodes is common, especially when the skin and mucous membrane manifestations are conspicuous. The spleen may be palpable, but is usually not. Ophthalmologic examination in advanced cases reveals characteristic evidences of vascular injury, perivascular hemorrhages, segmentation of arteries, scattered fluffy exudates and at times circumpapillary edema and even flame-shaped hemorrhages.

Prognosis. The fever and other manifestations of the disease may continue for many months, with long alternating periods of exacerbation and remission. In some cases complete remissions may last for years, but the ultimate prognosis is grave. Occasionally a patient who has been critically ill for months may improve slowly and recover clinically. However, most sufferers from this disease ultimately die. Death is due to the toxemia of the disease, to renal insufficiency (azotemia) or to an intercurrent pneumococcal, streptococcal or staphylococcal infection. Unless renal damage and insufficiency have developed, prompt remission of the clinical manifestations of the disease may usually be induced by therapy with appropriate doses of cortisone administered either orally or parenterally, or by the parenteral or intravenous administration of the adrenocorticotropic hormone of the pituitary (ACTH). Although they do not cure the disease, both hormonal substances are capable of altering its course and of prolonging life. However, they do not affect irreversible morphologic alterations in the kidneys and other organs nor the resulting disturbances in their physiologic function, such as renal azotemia.

Treatment. No form of specific therapy is available. Gold chloride has long been the favorite remedy of dermatologists. There is no reason to believe that it has any genuinely favorable influence upon the disease. It is to be avoided because it may further depress bone marrow function, it may increase the severity of the vascular lesions, and it is certainly capable of increasing the severity of renal damage. In spite of some favorable reports, therapy with bismuth and with paraaminobenzoic acid has also proved disappointing. The erythema may be improved by daily oral administration of small doses of chloroquine.

Remissions in the disease have occurred in patients treated in a variety of ways. Confinement to a darkened room or one in which the windows are covered with red cellophane seems to be helpful. Although a vitamin deficiency is not responsible for the condition, nutritional deficiencies of various kinds may appear as in any prolonged wasting disease, especially when painful mouth lesions interfere with the ingestion of food. A high calorie diet is therefore indicated with generous vitamin supplementation, orally or parenterally. Most patients have a low blood level and a low excretion rate for ascorbic acid, but the prolonged administration of generous amounts of this vitamin to the point of complete saturation does not affect the progress of the disease or prevent the petechial lesions.

Because of the susceptibility of girls and young women, estrogens as well as androgens have been administered, and even castration has been performed, with doubtful effects. Remissions have sometimes coincided with the administration of large doses of testosterone propionate over prolonged periods. Such irregular therapeutic results are difficult to evaluate because of the tendency of the disease to spontaneous remissions.

During active febrile periods the prophylactic use of sulfadiazine (0.5 to 1 gm. twice a day) or of procaine penicillin (600,000 units intramuscularly twice a week) may prevent intercurrent bacterial infections. Although they have no influence upon the course of the primary disease, full therapeutic doses of the appropriate antibiotics are indicated for the control of such secondary infections.

As in rheumatoid arthritis, cortisone and ACTH have proved effective in inducing prompt clinical remissions which may persist as long as these precious therapeutic agents are continued. Adequate therapy with ACTH (0.025 gm. every 6 hours intramuscularly) is promptly effective as a rule, the temperature falling to normal within 24 hours and other clinical manifestations subsiding during the succeeding days. The oral administration of cortisone or the intramuscular injection of hydrocortisone is as a rule equally effective in comparable amounts (0.15 to 0.30 gm. daily in four divided doses). After a week or ten days on maximum therapy, the drugs should be slowly reduced by gradually diminishing the daily dose every two or three days until a minimum maintenance level is ultimately reached below which fever, arthritis and other evidences of clinical activity are observed to recur. After another two or three weeks an attempt may again be made to reduce the daily maintenance dose, again by *very* slow downward gradations in the daily dosage, a small reduction being made only at intervals of a few days. In this manner the patient may gradually be weaned from ACTH or cortisone therapy, or at least reduced to minimal doses which will not induce distressing hormonal effects. In the minority of cases a remission in the disease, not a cure, is achieved by such progressive reduction of the daily dose until the injections can finally be discontinued. In most instances the patients continue to require a small maintenance dose for an indefinite period, sometimes as little as 0.025 to 0.050 gm. of cortisone once a day or every second day, or 0.01 gm. of ACTH (Acthar Gel) once a day or every other day.

To prevent hypochloremic alkalosis and hypokalemia while the patient is receiving large doses of ACTH or cortisone, it is advisable to give large amounts of potassium chloride daily. This is especially necessary when mercurial diuretics are being administered to control water retention and edema.

As the cardiovascular apparatus is severely impaired during acute exacerbations of disseminated lupus erythematosus, the therapy is more likely to precipitate acute congestive circulatory failure and pulmonary edema in this disease than in other collagen diseases. This complication is the result of the changes in blood and tissue electrolytes and the associated increase in body water which often follow the administration of large doses of these hormones. It can be prevented in part by keeping the patient on a minimum salt diet (less than 0.2 gm. of sodium daily) during the early weeks of treatment. Other possible complications of the therapy include Cushing's syndrome, diabetes, hypertension, hypochloremia, alkalosis, hypokalemia, epileptiform convulsions and transitory psychotic states. Cortisone or ACTH therapy of patients with this disease should therefore be initiated in a hospital where the daily fluctuations in body weight can be carefully watched and accurate clinical and physiologic observations can be made.

GEORGE BAEHR

References

Baehr, G.: Disseminated Lupus Erythematosus and Diffuse Scleroderma. J.A.M.A., *134:*1169, 1947.
———, Klemperer, P., and Schifrin, A.: A Diffuse Disease of the Peripheral Circulation (Usually Associated with Lupus Erythematosus and Endocarditis). Tr. A. Am. Physicians, 50:139, 1935.
———, and Pollack, A. D.: Diffuse Vascular Diseases. Modern Concepts of Cardiovascular Diseases. Am. Heart A., *15:*12, 1946.
———, and others: Influence of Cortisone and Adrenocorticotropin in Disseminated Lupus Erythematosus. Tr. A. Am. Physicians, 63:89, 1950.
———, and Soffer, L. J.: Treatment of Disseminated Lupus Erythematosus with Cortisone and Adrenocorticotropin. Bull. New York Acad. Med., 26:229, 1950.
Coburn, A. F., and Moore, D. H.: Plasma Proteins in Disseminated Lupus Erythematosus. Bull. Johns Hopkins Hosp., 73:196, 1943.
Dubois, E. L.: The Effect of the L.E. Cell Test on the Clinical Picture of Systemic Lupus Erythematosus. Ann. Int. Med., 38:1265, 1953.
Ginzler, J. M., and Fox, T. T.: Disseminated Lupus Erythematosus. Arch. Int. Med., 65:26, 1940.
Hargraves, M. M., Richmond, H., and Morton, R.: Presentation of Two Bone Marrow Elements: the "Tart" Cell and the "L.E." Cell. Proc. Staff Meet. Mayo Clin., 23:25, 1948.
Haserick, J. R.: Plasma L.E. Test in Systemic Lupus Erythematosus. J.A.M.A., *145:*16, 1951.
Kaposi, M.: Neuer Beitrag zur Kenntniss des Lupus erythematosus. Arch. f. Derm. u. Syph., 4:36, 1872.
Klemperer, P.: Diseases of the Collagen System. Bull. New York Acad. Med., 23:581, 1947.
———: The Pathogenesis of Lupus Erythematosus and Allied Conditions. Ann. Int. Med., 28:1, 1948.
Soffer, L. J., and Bader, R. B.: Corticotropin and Cortisone in Acute Disseminated Lupus Erythematosus. J.A.M.A., *149:*1002, 1952.
———, Levitt, W. F., and Baehr, G.: Use of Cortisone and Adrenocorticotropic Hormone in Acute Disseminated Lupus Erythematosus. Arch. Int. Med., 86:558, 1950.
Wagener, H. P.: Retinal Lesions in Acute Disseminated Lupus Erythematosus. Am. J. M. Sc., *211:* 240, 1946.

DERMATOMYOSITIS

(Neuromyositis, Polymyositis, Dermatomucosomyositis, Poikilodermatomyositis)

Definition. There has been no more satisfactory definition of this disease in its classic form than that proposed by Steiner: "An acute, subacute or chronic disease of unknown origin characterized by a gradual onset with vague and indefinite prodromata followed by edema, dermatitis, and multiple muscle inflammation." The common denominator of this syndrome is the acute or subacute degeneration of skeletal muscles, and the descriptive terms are utilized to indicate the combination of tissues involved in the individual case.

Etiology and Incidence. The etiology is unknown. Many cases have had their onset during or after some type of infection but no causative relationship has been established. Other observers have suggested an allergic background, a disturbance in vitamin E metabolism or an endocrine factor, but no conclusions can be reached from the information available. In the past few years an increasing number of cases have been reported in which there was an associated neoplasm of some type, such as carcinoma of the breast, stomach, ovary or kidney. No conclusions can be drawn as to any part these tumors may play in the pathogenesis of the disease, although it has been suggested that the relationship is more than a coincidental one.

As evidence of the rarity of this syndrome, only 31 proven cases have been observed in the Johns Hopkins Hospital since 1933. The youngest patient was 2 and the oldest 76 at the time of onset, the largest incidence being in the fifth decade. There was no sex predominance, and 3 of the patients were Negroes.

Pathology. Histologically the skin may reveal vacuolation of the epithelium, perivascular lymphocytic infiltrations, atrophy of the epidermis, flattening of the rete pegs and edema or fibrosis of the cutis. These changes are not specific for this disease. The affected muscles may appear swollen and pale in color, and have a firm consistency. The primary process is one of degeneration of muscle fibers, but there may be a variable degree of inflammatory reaction. The sarcolemmal nuclei of altered fibers may be increased, and vacuolization, granular degeneration and fragmentation can be seen in many fibers. In the acute stage there is active phagocytosis of involved fibers, and hemorrhages may occur, leading to the use of the term "hemorrhagic myositis." In the chronic form one sees vacuolated fibers which contain shrunken sarcolemmal nuclei, and there is an increase in the endomysial collagen.

Clinical Features and Natural History of the Syndrome. Some observers have differentiated cases into two clinical types: (1) acute dermatomyositis which is more commonly seen in children and is characterized by an erythematous eruption, edema, tenderness, swelling and weakness of the proximal muscles of the extremities, fever and leukocytosis. Involvement of the respiratory muscles may lead to a fatal termination, but the process may have a self-limited course; (2) chronic polymyositis which runs a more chronic course, begins in the peripheral limb muscles and is not associated with dermal involvement. However, there are all gradations between these two extremes, and cases which begin acutely with erythema and edema of the skin and extensive muscle involvement may pass into the chronic stage with atrophy and fibrosis. The dermal and muscular involvement do not always parallel one another, and there may be an interval of many months between the appearance of the cutaneous lesions and the evidence of muscle dysfunction.

The disease often begins with muscle tenderness, followed by weakness, and the appearance of cutaneous signs. Raynaud's phenomenon may be an early manifestation. The muscular involvement is not constant in its distribution and may be limited to one group such as the shoulder or pelvic girdle or may be generalized from the onset, in which event the course is usually a fulminating one. The element of pain and tenderness seems to depend on the degree of edematous change and may be very intense, slight or even absent. The muscles may at first feel doughy, later become firm, and finally show extensive wasting. Stiffness and weakness are usually complained of early and are often symmetrical in distribution. When muscle involvement is extensive the patient may be bedridden. Later there is marked atrophy and fixation of joints may occur. Striated muscles in areas other than the limbs and trunk may be involved, giving rise to such symptoms as diplopia, dysphagia, difficulty in respiration, facial weakness and impairment of sphincter control. Heart failure may occasionally be present owing to similar changes in the cardiac muscle.

The areas most frequently involved by the mucocutaneous lesions are the face, eyelids, ears, buccal mucosa, V area of the neck, and the skin overlying articulations. The eyelids may be swollen and have a characteristic heliotrope coloration due to the presence of small telangiectases. Important are the symmetrical cutaneous lesions overlying the small joints of the hands which may show edema, a violaceous hue and telangiectasia. Similar changes may be seen about the larger joints and, when scaling is prominent, may resemble psoriasis. As the lesions regress pigmentation may develop; in some cases this may be so widespread as to resemble Addisonian discoloration. Cutaneous alterations may be present which resemble the changes seen in scleroderma. When there is extensive involvement, lesions in various stages of development, from acute erythema and edema to atrophy and pigmentation, may be observed. Subjective symptoms such as pruritus are usually absent. As in lupus erythematosus there may be a relation between the appearance or intensity of the cutaneous manifestations and exposure to sunlight. In some cases there is extensive calcification in the subcutaneous tissues.

An intermittent fever may be present. Malaise, anorexia and loss of weight are common. Involvement of the joints is rarely seen, although pain in periarticular areas often results from lesions of the soft tissues and tendons. Alopecia of varying degree may develop, and hyperhidrosis is occasionally noted. Occasionally present are lymphadenopathy, splenomegaly, paresthesias and hemorrhagic phenomena. Polymyositis haemorrhagica differs from the usual acute form in that there are hemorrhages in the skin and muscle.

A mild anemia is often recorded. Leukocytosis is infrequent, but in some cases there may be an increase in eosinophils, lymphocytes or monocytes. Creatinuria is a constant finding when there is · moderate or severe muscle involvement. Other laboratory abnormalities which have been recorded include increase in serum globulin, proteinuria, hematuria and reduction in serum albumin.

The *course* is a progressive one to death in about half of the cases. However, there may be remissions and exacerbations of activity of the disease. The terminal event may be respiratory insufficiency, cardiac failure or a complicating infection. It would appear that the majority of the patients who survive the first year may enter a very long period in which the process may become quiescent or remain mildly active.

Diagnosis. When the classic features described are present, they are usually sufficient when combined with muscle biopsy to make the diagnosis with certainty. Early in the course it may be difficult to distinguish this disease from the edematous stage of scleroderma or scleredema. Periorbital edema and muscle tenderness may mimic trichinosis, and in other cases there may be a resemblance to polyneuritis, myasthenia gravis, muscular dystrophy, pseudobulbar palsy, thyrotoxic myopathy, Addison's disease and periarteritis nodosa. In the acute form there may be symptoms similar to those of systemic lupus erythematosus, such as facial erythema, vague arthralgias, fever and weakness, and sensitivity to sunlight. However, there are usually distinguishing features. As noted by Banks, there are transitional cases in which the clinical picture has seemed to fit one disease well, only to have at a later stage the typical histologic picture of the other. For example, the atrophic dermal changes of scleroderma may be seen in patients with systemic lupus erythematosus or dermatomyositis, and in advanced scleroderma there may be extensive muscular involvement. However, the associated findings, the laboratory examinations and the histologic picture usually serve to make the diagnosis clear.

Treatment. Symptomatic treatment should include rest in bed, suitable physiotherapeutic measures and special exercises to minimize contractures. Salicylates may be helpful in the relief of pain and tenderness, but in the acute phase more potent analgesics may be necessary. In the early stages when activity of the process is evident, adrenocorticotropic hormone and cortisone may produce dramatic relief but large doses may be necessary over a period of several weeks. Striking objective improvement in muscle power may be brought about and sustained with maintenance therapy. A few patients have remained in remission when the dose of hormone was gradually reduced and then treatment discontinued after a period of several months. When advanced atrophy and fibrosis have developed, there is no return of function after hormone administration.

A. McGehee Harvey

References

Adams, R. D., Denny-Brown, D., and Pearson, C. M.: Diseases of Muscle: A Study in Pathology. New York, Paul B. Hoeber, Inc., 1953, p. 309.

Banks, B. M.: Is There a Common Denominator in Scleroderma, Dermatomyositis, Disseminated Lupus Erythematosus, Libman-Sacks Syndrome and Polyarteritis Nodosa? New England J. Med., 225:433, 1941.

Keil, H.: The Manifestation in the Skin and Mucous Membranes in Dermatomyositis with Special Reference to the Differential Diagnosis from Systemic Lupus Erythematosus. Ann. Int. Med., 16:828, 1942.

O'Leary, P. A.: Dermatomyositis. M. Clin. North Amer., 33:21, 1949.

Sheard, C., Jr.: Dermatomyositis. Arch. Int. Med., 88:640, 1951.

Steiner, W. R.: Dermatomyositis with Report of a Case which Presented a Rare Muscle Anomaly but Once Described in Man. J. Exper. Med., 6:407, 1901–05.

POLYARTERITIS

(Periarteritis Nodosa, Polyarteritis Nodosa, Necrotizing Angiitis)

Definition. Kussmaul and Maier introduced the term periarteritis nodosa in 1866 to describe a systemic disease which was characterized by visible nodules along the course of the medium-sized muscular arteries. The lesions are segmental in their distribution and involve arteries throughout most of the body in varying degree, so that the resulting clinical picture is one of polymorphic manifestations which may seem unrelated. Some observers have placed all of the pathologic conditions of the vascular system characterized by inflammation and fibrinoid necrosis in the category of periarteritis nodosa, including the angiitis which follows an allergic reaction to a drug or foreign protein. Others have suggested "necrotizing angiitis" as a better term to use collectively for all vascular lesions showing this type of histologic picture.

Etiology and Incidence. During the past few decades numerous observers have recorded vascular phenomena in association with allergic reactions of various types, and new ideas concerning the pathogenesis of necrotizing inflammatory lesions in blood vessels have been advanced. Longcope demonstrated that when foreign protein was administered to an animal and sufficient time allowed for the formation of antibodies, areas of degeneration with extensive inflammatory reaction were produced in the myocardium, liver and kidneys. Gruber first suggested that periarteritis nodosa might be a general hyperergic reaction to infectious or toxic agents to which the vessel walls had previously been exposed. In 1937 Clark and Kaplan described necrotizing vascular lesions accompanying serum sickness. The clinical and experimental studies of Rich and Rich and Gregory helped to clarify these relationships. They found lesions similar to those seen in periarteritis nodosa in patients dying from serum sickness and allergic reactions to sulfonamides and iodine. These workers produced the lesions of periarteritis nodosa experimentally, sometimes accompanied by glomerulonephritis, in rabbits by the establishment of an anaphylactic state analogous to human serum sickness. Hawn and Janeway, using bovine serum, produced segmental arterial lesions in the rabbit which were similar to those which followed the injection of horse serum. Of interest was the production by the albumin fraction of lesions confined almost exclusively to arteries, and by gamma globulin of lesions principally in the glomeruli and in a lesser degree in the heart. However, in most cases of periarteritis nodosa there is no history of any type of allergic reaction either to drugs or foreign proteins. It has been suggested that various infectious agents may be etiologic factors but no substantiating evidence exists.

Zeek and her co-workers believe that drug-induced lesions are different morphologically and in distribution from those seen in human periarteritis nodosa, and state that vascular changes like those described by Kussmaul and Maier have been produced experimentally by procedures that usually resulted in severe hypertension but did not cause hypersensitivity. They prefer the term necrotizing angiitis for this entire group of arterial diseases and believe that five types may be differentiated: (1) periarteritis nodosa; (2) hypersensitivity angiitis; (3) rheumatic arteritis; (4) allergic granulomatous angiitis; and (5) temporal or cranial arteritis.

The nature of so-called fibrinoid necrosis is fundamental to study of the pathogenesis of these various vascular lesions. It is generally believed that this type of reaction in connective tissue is not pathognomonic of allergy but is merely a nonspecific response to injury. Altshuler and Angevine have produced evidence that it represents the precipitation of acid mucopolysaccharides in the ground substance of connective tissue.

Pathology. In periarteritis nodosa the arterial lesions consist of necrosis, fibrinoid alteration and hyalinization of the media, with a marked perivascular infiltration of mononuclear and polymorphonuclear cells but without foreign body giant cells. The affected vessels may show intimal proliferation leading to thrombosis and arterial obstruction with infarct formation. The artery may become distended into an aneurysmal saccule and even rupture. In some instances the vascular changes may be limited to the vessels of one system or to a few isolated organs with the result that no single clinical finding is invariably present. It is stated that lesions are not found in the pulmonary circulation unless there is pulmonary hypertension, although the bronchial arteries may be affected. Repair and fibrosis of the adventitial lesions may produce characteristic nodules which on occasion can be felt along the course of the artery. The lesions in this disease may be seen in all stages in any given case from acute ones to those which are completely healed. The process apparently spreads through the wall of the vessel, the intima being the last coat involved. Similar lesions have been described in patients with typical rheumatoid arthritis and also in individuals dying with systemic lupus erythematosus.

In contrast, in hypersensitivity angiitis, according to Zeek, the smallest branches of intrinsic blood vessels, both arterial and venous, are involved, the lesions probably begin in the intima, and the intense cellular reaction contains many eosinophils. In the kidney a necrotizing glomerulitis is often found and the vessels of the pulmonary tree are frequently affected. The lesions in the individual case are of the same age and no chronic or healed lesions are noted.

In so-called allergic granulomatous angiitis small nodules usually related to blood vessels are found predominantly in the heart. These consist of eosinophils undergoing necrosis, fibrinoid change and granulomatous proliferation of epitheloid cells with the formation of giant cells. In temporal arteritis, or cranial arteritis, differentiation from periarteritis nodosa cannot be made on the basis of the histologic changes. These changes, however, are limited to the vessels of the lower half of the head.

Clinical Features and Natural History of the Syndrome. The widespread nature of the vascular lesions reflects itself in symptoms and signs so variable, and so often superficially unrelated, that no standard clinical description can amply relate the polymorphic manifestations of these illnesses. In cases of periarteritis nodosa the general clinical picture presented may be that of (1) a nonspecific subacute or chronic pyrexial illness, (2) an atypical abdominal illness, (3) a primary renal disease or (4) a combination of polyneuritis and polymyositic manifestations. In the accompanying table are listed the principal signs and symptoms as recorded in several hundred reported cases. Fever occurs at some time during the course of the disease in almost every case. Approximately half of the patients describe a sudden onset accompanied by fever. The kidneys are frequently involved, albuminuria and hematuria being common findings. Hypertension occurs in over half the cases, and the association of

Symptoms and Signs of Periarteritis Nodosa With Frequency of Occurrence in 300 Cases

	%		%
Fever	85	Jaundice	10
Abdominal pain	65	Convulsions	10
Hypertension	60	Eruptions	10
Edema	50	Diarrhea	10
Neuritis	50	Muscle soreness	10
Weakness	45	Leukocytosis	80
Weight loss	45	Albuminuria	60
Cough and dyspnea	40	Hematuria	40
Vomiting	30	Eosinophilia	25
Headache	30	Uremia	15
Precordial pain	25		

this finding with continued pyrexia of unknown origin is a particularly significant combination.

The frequency with which the characteristic arterial lesions of periarteritis nodosa are found in one or more of the abdominal viscera or the intestinal tract accounts for the common occurrence of abdominal pain, which is often violent and maximal in the umbilical region or in the gallbladder area. Anorexia, nausea, vomiting and bloody diarrhea have been observed, and thrombosis of mesenteric arteries may lead to infarction of the bowel. Such arteritic lesions may involve the appendiceal, pancreatic and hepatic vessels as well, resulting in a clinical picture simulating appendicitis, hemorrhagic pancreatitis or hepatic necrosis. Mucosal ulceration with hemorrhage and perforation has been reported frequently.

A painful peripheral neuritis, usually bilateral and often asymmetrical, is a common finding, particularly in the lower limbs. Many other signs and symptoms due to arteritic lesions in the nervous system have been noted, including meningeal irritation due to subarachnoid hemorrhage, facial palsy, hemiplegia, cerebellar signs, visual disturbances, headache, vertigo and convulsions.

The vessels supplying the myocardium may be involved with the production of a large myocardial infarct or multiple small areas of necrosis. Frequent attacks of precordial pain may be noted, and the picture of congestive heart failure may ensue. In hypersensitivity angiitis heart failure has been associated with miliary myocardial infarcts. Heart failure may also be associated with the severe hypertension which is often present. Pericardial tamponade may follow rupture of an aneurysm along a superficial coronary vessel.

Pain in the chest may be due to pleural vasculitis, and a hemorrhagic effusion may result. Pulmonary vascular thrombosis leading to hemoptysis and excavation may simulate pulmonary tuberculosis. An "anaphylactoid pneumonia" has been described in cases which follow drug reactions. The association of asthma together with paresthesias of the extremities and eosinophilia was noted by Rackemann and Greene. More recently, Churg and Strauss have described a syndrome characterized by severe asthma, fever and hypereosinophilia, together with manifestations of vascular involvement in other organ systems, which they have called allergic granulomatosis. They feel that this is an entity apart from classic periarteritis nodosa and suggest that other allergic syndromes such as that of Loeffler may represent benign forms of allergic granulomatosis.

Joint pains and myalgia have been frequently noted in periarteritis nodosa. Muscle pain and soreness may be so prominent that when eosinophilia is also present, trichinosis is suspected. Joint swelling is rarely seen and often the tenderness or pain is associated with peripheral neuritis.

In periarteritis nodosa the ovaries, testes and epididymes are frequently involved. Extensive vasculitis of the bladder may lead to gross hematuria and dysuria as an early manifestation of the disease.

A variety of cutaneous lesions may be seen in periarteritis nodosa as well as in hypersensitivity angiitis. These include scarlatiniform eruptions, urticaria, angioneurotic edema, vesicular and bullous lesions. The latter may become necrotic and ulcerate, involving large areas of skin.

Leukocytosis is often a prominent feature, and in some cases a conspicious eosinophilia is present. A severe anemia may develop and marked elevation of the sedimentation rate is common.

The *course* of periarteritis nodosa is variable. The onset may be insidious or sudden due to a vascular thrombotic lesion. The disease is usually fatal but cases have been reported which were characterized by remissions, long intermissions and exacerbations. Complete recovery may take place from hypersensitivity angiitis. In both situations healing may occur clinically as well as histologically, but when there is extensive involvement of the pulmonary, cardiac, renal or intraabdominal arteries, recovery is rare.

Knowles, Zeek and Blankenhorn have divided cases of periarteritis nodosa into two groups on the basis of the clinical findings. In the first group the nodular vascular lesions were unassociated with any other major disease process and the illness had progressed to fatal termination in periods up to twelve months. In the second group the lesions developed shortly before death in patients with severe renal disease and/or hypertension. In the first group renal infarcts were common, being produced by vascular lesions which were limited in extent so that renal insufficiency did not develop. In the second group malignant nephrosclerosis was the most frequent type of renal disease. The high incidence of gross hematuria in this group was considered to be of diagnostic significance.

In their cases designated as primary periarteritis nodosa there was a long clinical course characterized by gastroenteric symptoms, peripheral neuropathy, hypertension usually, and eosinophilia occasionally. In contrast, the clinical features of hypersensitivity angiitis were fever, skin rash, nephritis and myocarditis.

Diagnosis. The diagnosis may be difficult as proof is dependent on histologic evidence. As the disease progresses many regions of the body may be involved, and the multiplicity of signs and symptoms may suggest the correct diagnosis. From the diversified symptomatology which has been described, it is evident that periarteritis may simulate a great many other diseases. When a biopsy is taken, the skin and subcutaneous tissues, as well as the muscle, should be sent for microscopic section. As the lesions in the vessels are segmental in distribution, many sections must be made. In a recent case in which serial sections were made of a muscle biopsy, the first classic lesion was found on the fiftieth slide.

Treatment. Treatment in the past has been for the most part symptomatic. In view of recent work every effort should be made to exclude any antigens that might be responsible. Care should be taken in following the course of any patient receiving a drug to which manifestations of hypersensitivity may develop. Immediate relief of many of the manifestations of periarteritis are noted after the administration of adrenocorticotropic hormone and the adrenal hormones. All histologic signs of inflammation may disappear within a few weeks. In the process of healing fibrous obliteration of the lumina of vessels may occur with resulting infarction, particularly in the kidneys, heart and intestinal tract. Occasional cases have been reported in which complete spontaneous remission took place, and the only difference in these cases and those treated with the hormones is the rapidity and extent of the healing. There is not yet sufficient information available as to whether these hormones will influence the over-all course of the various types of angiitis. However, in view of the rapid development of new therapeutic agents it is of importance that further information be obtained concerning the pathogenesis of periarteritis nodosa and so-called hypersensitivity angiitis, and whether there is any fundamental difference between them that cannot be explained by the nature and time-course of the antigen-antibody reaction.

A. McGehee Harvey

References

Baggenstoss, A. H.: Effect of Cortisone on Lesions of Periarteritis Nodosa. Am. J. Path., 27:537, 1951.

Churg, J., and Strauss, L.: Allergic Granulomatosis, Allergic Angiitis, and Periarteritis Nodosa. Am. J. Path., 27:277, 1951.

Grant, R. T.: Observations on Periarteritis Nodosa. Clin. Sc., 4:245, 1940.

Hawn, C. V., and Janeway, C. A.: Histological and Serological Sequences in Experimental Hypersensitivity. J. Exper. Med., 85:571, 1947.

Kilbourne, E. D., and Wolff, H. G.: Cranial Arteritis: Critical Evaluation of Syndrome of "Temporal Arteritis", with report of a case. Ann. Int. Med., 24:1, 1946.

King, F. H.: Protracted Course of Periarteritis Nodosa. J. Mt. Sinai Hosp., 15:97, 1948–49.

Miller, H. G., and Daley, R.: Clinical Aspects of Polyarteritis Nodosa. Quart. J. Med. (New Series), 15:255, 1946.

Rich, A. R., and Gregory, J. E.: The Experimental Demonstration that Periarteritis Nodosa is a Manifestation of Hypersensitivity. Bull. Johns Hopkins Hosp., 72:65, 1943.

Spiegel, R.: Clinical Aspects of Periarteritis Nodosa. Arch. Int. Med., 58:993, 1936.

Zeek, P. M.: Periarteritis Nodosa and Other Forms of Necrotizing Angiitis. New England J. Med., 248:764, 1953.

PROGRESSIVE SYSTEMIC SCLEROSIS

(Scleroderma, Sclerema Adultorum, Dermatosclerosis)

Definition. Progressive systemic sclerosis is a disease involving the collagenous connective tissue which may cause widespread, symmetrical, leathery induration of the skin followed by atrophy and pigmentation. The cutaneous lesions are merely the external manifestation of a systemic disease, and the muscles, bones, mucous membranes, heart, lungs, intestinal tract and other internal organs may be involved by the same process, resulting in functional impairment such as heart failure or pulmonary insufficiency.

Etiology and Incidence. The specific etiology of scleroderma is unknown. Similar changes in collagen tissue may occur in disseminated lupus erythematosus, rheumatic fever, rheumatoid arthritis and serum sickness; but the pathologic process is not of sufficient specificity to serve as a common denominator for the classification of these diseases. The possible role of infections and of abnormalities of certain endocrine glands has been postulated, but no consistent relationships have been noted.

Both the localized form, known as *morphea,* and the generalized disease are relatively uncommon. Scleroderma appears most frequently in the middle period of life, and females are more frequently affected than males.

Pathology. Histologic studies show that scleroderma is primarily a collagenous tissue alteration, thus accounting for the stiffness and hardness of the affected structures. There is at first swelling of collagenous intercellular substance which later becomes dense and sclerotic. The vascular lesions show thickening of the intima, often with fibrinoid degeneration and occlusion resembling those seen in disseminated lupus erythematosus, and are thought by some to have a relationship to the sclerodermatous alterations in the skin. Later, there is atrophy of the epidermis including the appended structures. Calcification develops in some cases. Similar changes occur in collagen tissue in other organs including the heart, lungs and gastrointestinal tract.

Symptoms and Signs. The focal form of the disease, known as *morphea,* is characterized by indurated lesions found on the trunk, extremities or neck which may follow the distribution of the peripheral nerves. This is a benign process which only rarely may precede the development of diffuse cutaneous or visceral involvement. In the linear form firm irregular bands several centimeters in width may be distributed over the skin of the extremities, forehead and scalp, but seldom the trunk. There may be involvement of underlying muscle and the development of contractures.

In the diffuse or systemic disease the cutaneous changes pass through several stages, the first of which is a brawny edema which commonly starts on the hands and feet, and later involves the face, neck and often the trunk. The nonpitting edema gives the skin a puffy white appearance with smoothing of the normal folds. In the second or indurative stage the skin becomes smooth, waxy, leathery and tight so that it cannot be lifted from the deeper structures. This may be most prominent on the fingers, dorsum of the hands, and the ankles. The face becomes mask-like with the expression fixed. Constitutional manifestations such as weakness and loss of weight are common, and joint pains and fever are prodromal symptoms in many cases. Raynaud's phenomenon and sclerodactyly, often associated with dysphagia due to esophageal involvement, may be present for years before cutaneous thickening in other areas is noticed. This has been referred to as the acrosclerotic form.

As the disease advances to the atrophic stage the skin becomes thinner, smoother and completely adherent to the shrunken muscles. The movement of joints is progressively restricted until the patient resembles a living mummy. There may be extensive brownish pigmentation of the skin, and in some cases calcium is deposited in the diseased portions. Other developments include anhidrosis, coldness of the digits, loss of hair, telangiectasia, and the appearance of indolent, painful ulcers. Lesions may also be noted in the mucous membranes with painful induration of the tongue as well as the gums. In some cases dyspnea, cyanosis and edema are attributable to involvement of the heart muscle by this peculiar type of fibrosis, and diffuse pulmonary scleroderma may result in severe functional impairment. Disturbances in thyroid, pancreatic, pituitary and adrenal function have been described by various observers, although these organs may show no histologic lesions characteristic of this disease. The difficulty in swallowing is the result of atrophy and sclerosis of the esophagus leading first to dilatation and loss of normal peristaltic movements. Later, there may be partial obstruction with the development of a chronic esophagitis. When there is diffuse involvement of the intestinal tract, pain, nausea, vomiting, diarrhea or constipation may develop.

In contrast to other connective tissue diseases such as disseminated lupus erythematosus, hematologic and biochemical alterations are not regularly present. There may be a mild anemia, and increase in the sedimentation rate. Serum albumin may be below normal levels, and occasionally some elevation in serum globulin is noted. The urine may contain albumin, red cells, white cells and casts. Roentgenograms may reveal diffuse osteoporosis, and destructive lesions of bone have been described. Involvement of the heart, lungs and intestinal tract may be recorded also by radiologic and electrocardiographic studies. The roentgenographic appearance of the lungs is usually a diffuse linear infiltration which may be more prominent in the lower half of the lungs. These changes interfere with diffusion of oxygen across the alveolo-capillary membrane, and the physiologic and clinical disturbance resembles that of "diffusion fibrosis" seen also in sarcoidosis and beryllium intoxication. The electrocardiogram may show change in rhythm, T wave alteration and other evidence indicative of myocardial involvement. These changes are not specific or diagnostic of scleroderma.

Diagnosis. The typical case presents no difficulties in diagnosis, but sclerodactyly in the early phases may be diagnosed as Raynaud's disease, or the joint pains as some type of arthritis. Fever, arthralgia and erythema of the skin may suggest disseminated lupus erythematosus, and the distinction from dermatomyositis is at times difficult. In the stage characterized by edema, differentiation must be made from scleredema which is a relatively benign condition. Probably the majority of cases of scleredema are diagnosed as scleroderma, and this may account for many of the instances in which dramatic improvement in scleroderma is believed to have occurred. The hands which are so uniformly involved in scleroderma are almost always spared in scleredema. Scleredema does not progress to atrophy, contractures or pigmentary changes, and spontaneous remission is the rule. There may be pleural or pericardial effusion in scleredema but serious involvement of the heart, lungs, esophagus or intestinal tract is not characteristic, as in scleroderma.

Other conditions which may be characterized by some type of cutaneous edema are in most instances easily differentiated. These include trichinosis, myxedema and edema of cardiac or renal origin.

Prognosis. In the localized type (morphea) healing takes place, leaving a smooth depressed area in the skin. Scleroderma of the slowly advancing generalized type may pass through periods of activity and remission, during which extension to a new area may be accompanied by remission in areas involved earlier. Disability may finally be extreme, and death in the chronic form often results from some intercurrent infection or from specific involvement of such areas as the heart or lungs.

Treatment. The long list of therapeutic agents tried in this condition, including various metals, hormone preparations and peripheral vasodilators, makes it obvious that no specific treatment has been discovered. Local heat, massage, hydrotherapy and softening ointments may be beneficial. In the vascular form, with vasospasm and a formal vasodilatory response, protection from cold, vasodilator drugs and sympathetic ganglionectomy may be recommended according to the principles, and with the limitations, followed in the treatment of Raynaud's disease. A number of cases have now been treated with pituitary corticotropin or cortisone. With aggressive therapy temporary beneficial effects may be obtained in the early phases, but treatment after the development of atrophy and contractures has not been helpful. More experience is needed before any final evaluation is possible. No improvement in pulmonary function has been observed to follow hormonal therapy.

Most important is the intelligent utilization of physiotherapy to prevent deformities resulting from contracture and to maintain muscle function to the greatest possible extent.

A. McGehee Harvey

References

Baehr, G., and Pollack, A. D.: Disseminated Lupus Erythematosus and Diffuse Scleroderma. J.A.M.A., *134*:1169, 1947.

Beerman, H.: The Visceral Manifestations of Scleroderma. A Review of the Recent Literature. Am. J. M. Sc., *216*:415, 1948.

Beigelman, P. M., Goldner, F., Jr., and Bayles, T. B.: Progressive Systemic Sclerosis (Scleroderma). New England J. Med., *249*:45, 1953.

Hale, C. H., and Schatski, R.: Roentgenological Appearance of the Gastrointestinal Tract in Scleroderma. Am. J. Roentgenol., *51*:407, 1944.

Longcope, W. T.: Scleroderma. In Oxford Loose-Leaf Medicine, Vol. 6. New York, Oxford University Press, 1945, p. 828.

Mayo, W. J., and Adson, A. W.: Raynaud's Disease, Thrombo-angiitis Obliterans and Scleroderma; Selection of Cases for and Results of Sympathetic Ganglionectomy and Trunk Reaction. Ann. Surg., *96*:771, 1932.

Shuford, W. H., Seaman, W. B., and Goldman, A.: Pulmonary Manifestations of Scleroderma. Arch. Int. Med., *92*:85, 1953.

Weiss, S., Stead, E. A., Jr., Warren, J. V., and Bailey, O. T.: Scleroderma Heart Disease with Consideration of Certain Other Visceral Manifestations of Scleroderma. Arch. Int. Med., *71*:749, 1943.

SCLEREDEMA

(Scleredema Adultorum of Buschke, Scleriasis)

Definition. This rare condition, which usually follows an acute infection and has a benign course, is characterized by a brawny edema of the skin which may resemble closely the early stage of scleroderma.

Pathology. The dermis is thickened and there is a moderate perivascular cuffing with mononuclear cells. In the deeper layers the collagen fibers are hypertrophied and swollen. A mucin-like material which stains with cresyl violet may separate these enlarged collagen bundles producing a fenestrated appearance. Similar changes have been described in other organs.

Etiology. Scleredema has been considered to be a diffuse disease of collagen. It usually develops one to six weeks after an infection which is most frequently of streptococcal origin. The disease is predominantly one of females. Selye has reported that the topical application of estrogens in mice produces a pathologic picture resembling scleredema, but at present there is insufficient knowledge upon which to base a sound opinion as to etiology. The majority of cases develop in childhood and early adult life, but the diagnosis has been made in the neonatal period and as late as the seventh decade.

Symptoms and Signs. The characteristic waxy, brawny edema of the skin usually appears abruptly although a brief prodromal period with slight fever, malaise and myalgia has been described. In the majority of cases the neck is involved first, but within one to two weeks there is spread to the face, chest, abdomen and extremities. The hands and feet are almost always spared. There may be an erythematous blush to the involved skin, but pigmentation and atrophy do not develop. There is no pitting on pressure and the skin is difficult to pick up. There is a sense of being "hidebound," and when the chest is involved dyspnea may result from the restriction of thoracic movement. Involvement of the tongue and pharyngeal tissues results in dysphagia and dysarthria. Parotid swelling has been described, and the occasional development of hydrarthrosis, pleural effusion and hydropericardium is cited as evidence of the systemic nature of this disease.

Diagnosis. Scleredema and the early stage of scleroderma may be easily confused. The onset of scleroderma may also follow an infection, and the histologic changes seen at this stage may not be distinctive. In scleredema the induration is more prominent in the superficial layers of the cutis, and atrophy, pigmentation and telangiectasia do not develop. In contrast to scleroderma involvement of the hands and feet is rare. The early phases of dermatomyositis may resemble scleredema so closely that a final diagnosis must be delayed until the more distinctive features appear. Other conditions such as trichinosis, myxedema, and edema of cardiac and renal origin are easily distinguished by the associated manifestations.

Prognosis. There is resolution of the edema in from six to eighteen months in most of the cases. However, the disease may remain essentially static for years or regress in certain areas leaving islands of edema which slowly resolve.

Treatment. As in scleroderma, many forms of treatment including artificial heat, hormonal substances, vasodilators and antihistaminics have been tried, but thus far none may be considered specific. The general tendency to spontaneous recovery makes evaluation of therapy difficult. In cases treated intensively with pituitary corticotropin there may be partial clearing of the edema, but the response is usually not dramatic.

A. McGEHEE HARVEY

References

Buschke, A.: Vorstellung eines Falles von Skleroedem vor der Berliner Gesellschaft für Dermatologie. Arch. f. Derm. u. Syph., 53:383, 1900.
Leinwand, I.: Generalized Scleredema: Report with Autopsy Findings. Ann. Int. Med., 34:226, 1951.
Madison, L. L.: Scleredema. Am. J. Med., 9:707, 1950.
Vallee, B. L.: Scleredema: A Systemic Disease. New England J. Med., 235:207, 1946.

Diseases Due to Physical Agents

AVIATION MEDICINE

The human factor is an important aspect of nearly all aviational activities and these in turn have important influences on man and on mankind. Aviation medicine, broadly defined, is concerned with all of these aspects. So defined, it is to be regarded as a special area of interest rather than a specialty *per se,* embracing as it does many disciplines both within and without the field of medicine.

Even with regard to the clinical aspects of aviation medicine there is a sharp separation of interests between flight surgeons in the military and those associated with the commercial air lines. Flight surgeons in military service try to protect the aviator from the stresses associated with the ever-increasing flight performance of airplanes. Flight surgeons for the air lines are mainly interested in the state of health of the pilot and the comfort of the passenger.

The well-being of the passenger is of chief concern to the physician acting as medical advisor to persons contemplating travel by air. To discharge this responsibility satisfactorily requires a knowledge of the travel stresses to be encountered and the probable effects of such stresses on the individual. The problem is that of passenger comfort except in the case of patients who are suffering either from severe illness or from some disability which renders them peculiarly susceptible to flying stresses.

What follows is divided into three main parts. The first is concerned with the principal causes of flying stresses, the estimation of their magnitude, the symptoms they cause, and suggestions for their prevention or relief. The second part has to do with the medical appraisal and contains a listing of diseases and conditions which increase susceptibility to flying stresses. The third part deals with the final evaluation of fitness for air travel together with logical recommendations based on this evaluation.

FLYING STRESS

The principal stresses encountered in flying are related to (1) reduced atmospheric pressure, (2) danger, (3) accelerations, (4) noise and vibration.

Reduced Atmospheric Pressure. The extent and speed of reduction are the two basic variables which determine the physiologic effects of a fall in atmospheric pressure. The relationship between altitude and barometric pressure is shown in Figure 59. The relation is nearly linear at low but not at high altitudes; thus, the pressure is reduced approximately one-quarter at 8000 feet, one-half at 18,000 feet, but only three-quarters at 42,000 feet. Paul Bert demonstrated that the important factor in the production of physiologic effects is the diminished partial pressure of oxygen; the decrease parallels the fall in barometric pressure, though the percentage of oxygen remains the same. In regard to the effects of exposure to hypoxia, the longer the exposure the greater the effects due to hypoxia, whereas the shorter the decompression time the greater the likelihood of biologic effects due to expansion of free gas and release of dissolved gas.

Thus, the air traveler exposed to ambient atmospheric pressures is affected by the rate of ascent, the altitude reached and the length of time aloft. These may give rise to three specific stresses within the body, namely, free gas expansion, release of gases in solution and hypoxia. These same stresses may be present even in a pressurized-cabin type of plane but are normally under greater control.

Hypoxia. The relationship between altitude, on the one hand, and the alveolar oxygen pressure and the arterial oxygen saturation, on the other, is approximately as shown in Figure 60. It should be noted that the relation is not linear in either case. The fall in partial pressure of oxygen is less than might be expected, because of a compensatory increase in pulmonary ventilation which becomes a considerable factor above 10,000 feet. Much more remarkable, however, is the fact that the fall in arterial oxygen saturation is far less than the fall in oxygen pressure. This is due to the characteristic manner in which oxygen and hemoglobin combine. At 8000 feet the fall in saturation is so small as to be almost negligible. Even at 12,000 feet the fall is not great, but thereafter the fall is precipitous. In other words, a healthy person at rest just begins to notice the effects of oxygen lack at 8000 feet and may complain only of slight dyspnea and after-fatigue at 12,000 feet. However, patients with severe anemia, with cyanosis of central origin, or with greatly decreased cardiopulmonary re-

masks made of plastic are comfortable and efficient.

Expansion of Bodily Gases. Free gases in the body expand and contract as a function of the changing pressure of the ambient air. The volume is doubled at approximately 18,000 and tripled at 28,000 feet. The biologic effects are produced mainly during pe-

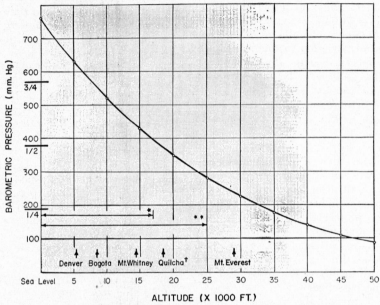

Fig. 59. Relationship between atmospheric pressure and altitude.

    * Extreme range for nonpressurized cabin airplanes.
  ** Usual range for pressurized cabin airplane.
    † Aucanquilcha, Chile, highest permanent habitation.

serve from any cause may derive benefit from supplemental oxygen at altitudes of 5000 feet and above.

The problem of hypoxia is met by limiting the maximum altitude of flight operations, by cabin pressurization and by providing supplemental oxygen. Scheduled air carriers (nonpressurized) under the Civil Aeronautics Board (CAB) are not permitted to fly above 17,000 feet. Their regulations further state that supplemental oxygen shall be provided on each air carrier for flights of more than 30 minutes' duration above 8000 feet and that progressively larger amounts shall be carried at progressively higher altitudes. Similar safeguards are also provided in pressurized-cabin airplanes for operations at flight altitudes above 8000 feet. In cases in which the slight effect of moderate altitude is undesirable, it is usually possible to arrange for supplemental oxygen administration throughout the flight. The new disposable oxygen

riods of change in pressure because either the body accommodates to it or the excess is released or absorbed. From a practical standpoint we are interested in the free gas in middle ear, paranasal sinuses and gastrointestinal tract.

MIDDLE EAR. The middle ear cavity is normally "ventilated" by the eustachian tube which becomes slit-like near the pharyngeal end. Here the walls are in apposition, and they act like a flutter valve, opening readily when air pressure increases from within the middle ear but closing more tightly when pressure is increased from without. The "valve," however, normally opens during such acts as swallowing, chewing and yawning. Armstrong states that during ascent air escapes unaided with every rise of about 400 feet, but that during descent voluntary efforts are required. Indeed, if a pressure differential of 80 or 90 mm. Hg (3000 feet to sea level) is allowed to develop, the tensor and levator muscles can no longer open the lips of the tube, which becomes "locked." Pressure differentials equivalent to descents of from 7000 to 15,000 feet lead to damage and even rupture of the drum membrane.

Aerotitis media is the term coined by Armstrong and Heim to describe the inflammation caused by barotrauma. In commercial planes sudden changes in pressure are deliberately avoided by limiting the rate of descent for nonpressurized aircraft, and by control of cabin pressure in pressurized planes. Despite these efforts to limit the stress, earache is still a frequent complaint among air travelers, and the following suggestions may prove helpful. Persons with acute sinusitis, common cold or sore throat should avoid flying if there is obstruction of the eustachian tube. A simple test for patency is to swallow while holding the nostrils closed; a feeling of pressure in the ears indicates that the tubes are patent. The use of amphetamine or other agents designed to shrink the mucous membranes of the nasopharynx may be of benefit. Anyone anticipating difficulty should instruct the flight attendant to ensure his being awake prior to let-down. If frequent swallowing does not suffice during descent, relief may be obtained by holding the nostrils closed while attempting forcibly to exhale

through them. In case of air lock immediate relief can be obtained only by reascent or intubation.

SINUS OBSTRUCTION. Symptoms due to inability to ventilate the nasal sinuses are infrequent and rarely severe. Anyone with acute sinusitis should avoid, if possible, traveling by air. Inhalations and sprays designed to shrink congested membranes may be successful in temporarily relieving obstruction.

GASTROINTESTINAL TRACT. Abdominal distention during ascent is usually relieved by passage of gas but occasionally may produce pain and other distressing symptoms. Patients with colostomies, herniation, peptic ulcer with complications, and recent abdominal wounds may experience difficulty. If allowed to fly, they should be properly advised with regard to their particular problems and should avoid eating gas-forming foods prior to flight.

Bends. Decompression sickness or bends, caused by a rapid decrease of atmospheric pressure which releases nitrogen normally held in solution, is not a problem in flights below 25,000 feet. Hence, it is not encountered in commercial aviation except in the rare event of explosive decompression in pressurized aircraft flying above this altitude.

Fear. Many persons are fearful of flying,

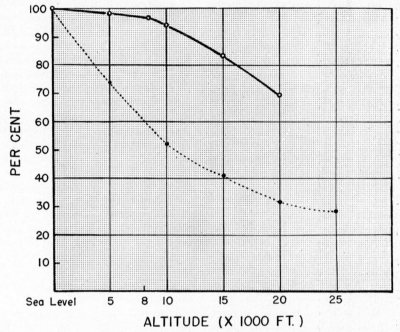

Fig. 60. Approximate fall in arterial oxygen saturation (solid line) and alveolar oxygen pressure (dotted line) as a function of altitude. Values for both are expressed as per cent of normal.

and passengers often become frightened during flight. Although fear is not listed as an important complaint in passenger comfort surveys, it is perhaps the most important problem in the passenger-carrier relationship. The ostensible reason for fear is the anticipation of danger to life and limb, although some passengers are fearful of developing earache, becoming air sick or developing claustrophobia. Actually, the danger to life while traveling on scheduled airliners is less than that while traveling by automobile*; hence, the reasons for fear probably lie not so much in the fatality rates as in circumstances which are regarded as frightening, such as poor visibility, "pancaking," stormy weather and oil streaks on the fuselage. The things which frighten the passenger rarely alarm the pilot, partly because of his greater familiarity with flying and partly because of the up-to-the-minute information on which his actions are based.

The prevention of anxiety begins with the recognition that it is an important problem. Lack of familiarity with flying is overcome through explanation and experience; one or two short "familiarity flights" might be helpful in certain instances. Travelers should be urged to express their anxieties to the flight attendant, who may be able to reassure them. Moderate sedation is effective, but soporific drugs may be given only on the recommendation of a physician.

Accelerations. The air traveler is subjected to two types of accelerative forces. The first, angular acceleration, is generated during rotations of the plane about one or more of its principal axes (pitch, roll and yaw) and is the physiologic stimulus for the semicircular canals. Coriolis acceleration is the term applied when the acceleration involves more than one axis, thus stimulating more than one pair of canals. This condition is experienced not only in association with simultaneous rotations of the plane about two of its axes, but, more frequently, in association with combined movements of head and plane. Coriolis accelerations are a principal factor in causing motion sickness.

The second type of accelerative force is generated during a change in speed or direction of the plane and forms a resultant vector with the force of gravity. In commercial aviation the flight patterns do not permit the

---

* However, the fatality rate for the air carriers is somewhat higher than that of the bus lines and railroads.

development of large G forces, and the problem of "grayout" or "blackout" does not arise. In turbulent air, however, linear accelerations resembling those experienced in elevators may, through their effects on the otolith organs and abdominal contents, contribute to motion sickness. Short-lived linear accelerations may also contribute to these effects and, in addition, cause buffeting.

Motion sickness is a more frequent complaint among air travelers than all others combined. Although the most important etiologic factor is the pattern of movement through space, others include basic individual susceptibility, anxiety, illness, lack of fitness and other unfavorable or unpleasant factors in the environment. Motion produces its principal effects through the labyrinthine, visual and kinesthetic pathways, and motion sickness may be the result of disharmony among the cues they provide. With few exceptions, flyers become less liable to motion sickness with experience just as do sailors on ships. However, this increased tolerance may be lost; indeed, following unpleasant experiences, tolerance may fall below the initial level. For further information see Chapter on Motion Sickness.

Vibration and Noise. Vibration and noise are important principally because they contribute to fatigue. The problem they present is rapidly disappearing, and large airliners compare favorably with any other form of transportation in this regard.

The Estimation of Travel Stress. In attempting to estimate travel stress it is necessary to consider all steps of the proposed journey from point of origin to final destination. These include (1) the trip to and from the airport, (2) the length and inclination of the ramps, (3) the climb getting aboard the plane, (4) the number of transfers and (5) the flight itself. The most important factors which modify the specific stresses during flight are (1) weather conditions; (2) type of plane; and (3) the flight plan, which includes (a) duration of flight, (b) estimated altitude and (c) number of stops en route. Unfavorable weather may cause anxiety, motion sickness and delays. Unfortunately, it is not always possible accurately to predict weather conditions; hence, weather is an uncertain variable. Planes having four engines, a large cruising range and pressurized cabins with adequate space and toilet facilities have important advantages over planes without these features. The superior plane may be able to fly above or around bad weather and maintain low pressure altitudes. The four engines afford a measure of safety which is reassuring to many passengers. The duration of the flight, altitude reached and the number of let-downs are variables the importance of which is obvious. It is only after a careful consideration of all of these factors that a valid estimation of travel stress can be made.

FITNESS FOR FLIGHT

The fitness of the individual to travel by air depends on what might be termed his basic susceptibility to flying stresses and the possible presence of some defect, disorder, disease or other condition which acts adversely either by increasing susceptibility to a factor already present or by introducing a new one.

Individual Susceptibility. Just as there are great variations in flying stress, so are there great variations in individual susceptibility to such stress. For the healthy adult this susceptibility is estimated in terms of his tendency to develop anxiety, motion sickness, fatigue, and symptoms due to hypoxia and obstruction of middle ear or sinus.

In the case of the experienced traveler this evaluation may be easy, but, even in the case of a "neophyte," much useful information may be obtained by a little inqury. In general, persons who readily become nervous are more likely to develop symptoms of anxiety aloft than are those who do not, though there are exceptions to this rule. Similarly, persons who tend to develop motion sickness in swings, cars, trains and ships are more prone to develop motion sickness in flight. It is even possible to estimate the probability with which earache may develop on the basis of past experience when traveling over hills and mountains or riding in elevators. Examination of the ears and throat and a test for patency of the eustachian tubes also provide much information in this regard.

Medical Evaluation. The following is a list of diseases and other conditions which render the passenger less fit or even unfit for travel by air:

Acute illness. This and convalescence from recent illness are the most common known causes of "incidents of unconsciousness" during flights.

Alcoholism. Excessive consumption of alcohol increases susceptibility to hypoxia and motion sickness.

Anemia. Susceptibility to hypoxia increases rapidly as hemoglobin levels fall below 11 gm.; severely anemic passengers should receive supplementary oxygen at altitudes over 5000 feet.

Angina pectoris. Patients with a history of attacks precipitated by anxiety or by slight physical effort should not fly at all or only after anticipatory precautions have been taken.

Asthma. This is a serious hazard only if attacks are severe or controlled with difficulty.

Cardiopulmonary failure. Patients who are cyanotic or who have greatly reduced vital capacity or poor exercise tolerance require special attention and should receive supplemental oxygen at altitudes over 5000 feet.

Common cold. Obstruction of ear or sinus causes pain but other complications are rare. Postponement of trip may be advisable.

Congestive failure. Flying is contraindicated if congestion is severe; even if slight, the possibility of aggravation by hypoxia, anxiety and physical effort must be carefully considered; supplemental oxygen should be given at altitudes above 5000 feet.

Diaphragmatic hernia. Expansion of gases may produce symptoms.

Head injury. Changes in barometric pressure are poorly tolerated.

Heart disease. In general, great cardiac enlargement, congestive failure, and inability to climb stairs are contraindications to flying under usual conditions. For details see recent review by the writer.

Hemorrhagic tendency. Recent history of hemorrhage from lung or gastrointestinal tract is a contraindication to travel by air.

Hypertension. In itself this is not a contraindication to flying; complications and the possibility of their aggravation by excitement or exercise require individual consideration.

Infancy. During the first ten days of infancy air travel is poorly tolerated.

Menière's disease. Two factors require consideration, namely, the possibility of turbulence inducing an attack and the limited facilities for care and treatment should an attack occur.

Myocardial infarction. Recent or resolving infarction is a contraindication to air travel. Healed infarction with major residua may impose a risk, and careful evaluation is required.

Pneumothorax. Careful evaluation is required; flying is contraindicated except under urgent circumstances if more than a small amount of air is present.

Postoperative convalescence. In general, air travel should be avoided during the first ten days; following chest and abdominal surgery longer avoidance may be needed.

Pregnancy. Prolonged hypoxia may cause miscarriage, and pregnant passengers may have an increased susceptibility to motion sickness. A history of repeated abortion or other serious complications is a contraindication to air travel except under urgent circumstances. Air lines differ in their regulations regarding travel during the ninth month of pregnancy; some will not accept passengers, and others require a statement from the attending obstetrician to the effect that the delivery date is at least three days beyond the time of arrival at destination.

Sinusitis. Patients with acute sinusitis and obstruction should avoid flying if possible.

Tuberculosis. Flying may be contraindicated in case of pulmonary cavitation and pneumothorax.

Valvular heart disease. Patients with severe mitral stenosis, especially if there is a history of attacks characterized by collapse, should not fly except in urgent circumstances. Even in mitral insufficiency, diffusion is impaired and supplemental oxygen should be given at altitudes over 8000 feet.

In summary, then, to estimate susceptibility to flying stress first determine the individual's basic tendency to develop symptoms in flight, particularly in regard to anxiety, fatigue, motion sickness and obstruction to middle ear. Then determine whether there exists some disease or other condition which may affect fitness for air travel.

THE FINAL EVALUATION

In making the final appraisal two approaches should be kept in mind. One might be called the "limiting factor concept," in which a particular stress such as hypoxia or a clearly defined disability such as pneumothorax is the only important factor requiring consideration. The other is a general approach made necessary either by the multiplicity of factors present or the inability to define them clearly.

From a practical standpoint one of three opinions can be reached with respect to the health hazard involved: first, that there is no hazard and that the problem, if one exists at all, is a matter of passenger comfort; second, that a significant hazard exists which must be accepted as a calculable risk if the flight is made; third, that the hazard is so great that the flight should not be made.

If there is a considerable hazard involved, the question of postponing the trip should be raised. If the trip is urgent, alternate modes of travel should be considered. Flying may still be the preferred means of travel. The advantages of short travel time, the services of a flight attendant and the availability of supplemental oxygen may outweigh the advantages of any other means of transportation. Air ambulance is also a possibility; the splendid record in the military services suggests that this is often preferable to any other mode of conveyance.

The attitude of the domestic air lines toward carrying patients is best expressed in the following regulation passed by the Air Transport Association of America:

"Participating carriers will refuse to carry or will remove en route any person whose status, age, physical or mental condition is such, in the opinion of the participating carrier, as to render him incapable of caring for himself without assistance, contributing to the discomfort of or making himself objectionable to the other passengers or involve any hazard or risk to himself, to other persons, or property."

ASHTON GRAYBIEL

References

Armstrong, H. G.: Principles and Practice of Aviation Medicine. 3rd ed. Baltimore, Williams & Wilkins Co., 1952.
——, and Heim, J. W.: The Effect of Flight on the Middle Ear. J.A.M.A., 109:417, 1937.
Chinn, H. I., Gammon, W. R., and Frantz, M. E.: Prevention of Airsickness among Airborne Troops. J. Appl. Psychol., 5:599, 1953.
——, and Milch, L. J.: Comparison of Airsickness Preventives. J. Appl. Psychol., 5:162, 1952.
Graybiel, A. G.: Air Travel and Heart Disease. Mod. Concepts Cardiovas. Dis., 23:217, 1954.
Johnson, W. H., and Mayne, J. W.: Stimulus Required to Produce Motion Sickness. Restriction of Head Movement as a Preventive of Airsickness— Field Studies on Airborne Troops. J. Aviation Med., 24:400, 1953.
——, Stubbs, R. A., Kelk, G. F., and Franks, W. R.: Stimulus Required to Produce Motion Sickness. 1. Preliminary Report Dealing with Importance of Head Movements. J. Aviation Med., 22: 365, 1951.
King, B. G.: Cases of In-flight Unconsciousness and/ or Death of Passenger. Dept. of Comm., CAA, Med. Div., Personal Communication. 31 October 1952.
McFarland, R. A.: Human Factors in Air Transportation. New York, McGraw-Hill Book Co., 1953.
Smedal, H. A.: Air Transportation of Persons with Cardio-Respiratory Disease and/or Injury. J. Aviation Med., 23:33, 1952.
Strickland, B. A., Jr., and Rafferty, J. A.: Effects of Air Transportation on Clinical Conditions. J.A.M.A., 145:129, 1951.
U. S. Civil Aeronautics Board. Civil Air Regulations. Part 61. Scheduled air carrier rules. As amended to Sepetmber 1, 1949.

MOTION SICKNESS

(Air Sickness, Sea Sickness)

Air sickness and sea sickness may be defined as conditions due to frequently repeated oscillatory movements of the body in a ship or airplane, and characterized by dizziness, nausea, vomiting, pallor and sweating.

Etiology. In a ship the pitching, see-saw movement on a transverse axis through the center of the ship, the rolling movement on its long axis and the movement of the entire ship up and down constitute the usual motions to which a person is subjected. In airplane travel, vertical accelerations and excessive rotary motions bring on the disturbance. Recent evidence indicates that the basic cause of air sickness is violent head motion which affects the fluid in the labyrinthine channels of the inner ear. Visual, psychogenic and kinesthetic factors play a subsidiary role, varying with the person.

Symptoms. The symptoms may come on without warning. A man who was previously in good spirits may suddenly become quiet and subdued. He feels nauseated and is aware of excessive salivation. Mental depression is almost constantly present. Vomiting may then take place with mild headache. Pallor and cold sweats are common; true vertigo is rare. There are no characteristic objective signs, although a drop in systolic blood pressure has been reported accompanied by tachycardia or a slow pulse rate. The nervous component in both air and seasickness is at times important.

Treatment. Fixing the eye on a definite object in space undoubtedly is of real help in both air sickness and sea sickness. The eye should not be allowed to shift with the position of the airplane, for the earth or sky will swim past the eyes and produce dizziness or nausea in a manner comparable to the development of this condition when one whirls rapidly on a piano stool. Head rests in airplanes have significantly decreased motion sickness. When possible, travelers should place their heads firmly against the back of the seat, lessening forward and backward movements.

Many drugs have been advocated which either act as sedatives to the entire organism or effectively suppress the parasympathetic nervous system. Dramamine, 50 to 100 mg., has been preferred to hyoscine, 0.6 to 1.0 mg. by some. The initial dose should be taken about one-half hour before expected exposure to motion sickness and at about 4- to 6-hour intervals thereafter as needed. The long-lasting antihistamine, Bonamine, administered as a 25 mg. tablet once daily, effectively prevents motion sickness for 12 hours; drowsiness is noted in a small percentage of cases.

ALVAN L. BARACH

References

Chinn, H. I., and others: Evaluation of Some Drugs in Seasickness. J. Pharmacol. & Exper. Therap., *108:*69, 1953.

Gay, L. N., and Carliner, P. E.: The Prevention and Treatment of Motion Sickness. I. Seasickness. Bull. Johns Hopkins Hosp., 84:470, 1949.

Johnson, W. H., and Wayne, J. W.: Stimulus Required to Produce Motion Sickness. Restriction of Head Movement as a Preventive of Air Sickness— Field Studies on Airborne Troops. J. Aviation Med., 24:400, 1953.

Morren, H., Trolin, S., Denayer, R., Grivsky, E., and Marioq, J.: New Prolonged-Action Antihistaminic Substances. Bull. Soc. Chim. Belg., 60:282, 1951.

HEAT EXHAUSTION, HEAT STROKE AND HEAT CRAMPS

Heat exhaustion is a physiologic breakdown following exposure to heat and is characterized principally by peripheral vasomotor collapse. *Heat stroke,* on the other hand, has for its distinguishing manifestation an extreme elevation of body temperature. *Heat cramps* are muscular cramps due to excessive salt loss. Although manifestations of two or even all three of these conditions may coexist, the mechanisms by which they are produced are quite different.

Heat exhaustion results usually from physical exertion in a hot environment, when vasomotor control and cardiac output are inadequate to meet the needs of increased skin circulation in addition to muscle and cerebral circulation. It may be precipitated in even the most fit man by heavy enough work or a severe enough environment. The severity of the environmental heat stress is determined by temperature, humidity and wind velocity. The wet bulb temperature is probably the best single index paralleling physiologic stress.

Heat exhaustion is a nonfatal physiologic disturbance unless complicated by coexisting disease. The factors in normal adaptation are important in understanding the morbid physiology. When a man is exposed to a hot environment, a considerable part of his circulation must be directed into the blood vessels of the skin in order to radiate heat from the surface and to support activity of the sweat glands. The ease of these adaptations is rapidly enhanced by repeated exposures to work in the heat, a process known as acclimatization, caused, at least in part, by increased adrenocortical activity and manifested by increased blood volume, better vasomotor control and more efficient sweating. Obviously, even a minor degree of dehydration will prevent maximum cardiovascular adaptation and so predispose to heat exhaustion.

Salt deficiency from any of several causes predisposes to heat exhaustion. Restricted salt intake or lack of supplemental salt during very heavy sweating is a common cause of salt deficiency. Recently described excessive salt concentrations in the sweat of patients with fibrocystic disease of the pancreas and in some normal members of their families illustrate another rather special mechanism of salt depletion.

Faintness, usually with subjective sense of palpitation, is the predominant symptom. Nausea, vomiting, syncope, headache and restlessness are common. Other symptoms may appear from underlying cardiac or other disease.

The patient who has collapsed in the heat and is perspiring freely almost surely has heat exhaustion and not heat stroke, even though his temperature is somewhat elevated. Under general supportive treatment he will usually recover consciousness promptly unless dehydration, salt deficiency, cardiovascular disease or some other complicating condition is important in the picture. In older patients a cardiovascular complication should be suspected if the symptoms persist.

The *prognosis* of simple heat exhaustion is invariably good, and the *treatment* is simple. Rest in a comfortable environment and mildly salted fluids by mouth as tolerated will usually suffice. Occasionally, when vomiting is severe and cardiac disease is absent, intravenous injection of 1000 ml. of 5 per cent glucose in physiologic saline may hasten recovery. The most important phase of treatment is that related to cardiac or vascular disease, which may manifest itself.

Heat stroke is a failure of adequate heat elimination almost always related to a breakdown of the sweating mechanism; it may occur whenever heat regulation is dependent on sweating for long periods of time. Experimentally, the rate of sweating in normal individuals has been found to decrease progressively during work in the heat and finally to lead toward real deficiency of sweating. In heat stroke this process has apparently gone on to complete breakdown of the mechanisms of temperature regulation, to

complete cessation of sweating and extreme elevation of body temperature.

At autopsy the important and primary tissue damage is in the central nervous system, consisting in edema and, in severely involved areas, destruction of nerve cells, chiefly in the cerebral cortex. Other changes are probably related to the secondary vasomotor shock which occurs in severe cases: congestion, edema and hemorrhages in various organs.

Although the exact mechanisms of maintenance of sweating are not known, it is clear that they fail in incipient heat stroke and the process behaves like a local fatigue of the glands. Heat stroke rarely occurs if relief from sweating is afforded during a part of the day, such as in desert areas with cool nights or where air-conditioned sleeping quarters are available. In extremely hot environments the development of full-blown stroke may be a matter of a few minutes after cessation of sweating, since all the normal heat loss under these conditions may be by evaporation of sweat. Dehydration is not a factor; in fact, superhydration has been reported. Leukocytosis is the rule, often above 20,000 per cubic millimeter; diminution of platelets is common in severe cases.

The patient may occasionally be aware of cessation of sweating, but often he is not. Sensation of extreme heat is the rule. The first overt symptoms are often those referable to the central nervous system: mental confusion, staggering gait, headache, delirium or coma. In the early phases the circulation is maintained (rapid, full pulse), but soon a stage of vasomotor collapse supervenes with low blood pressure and rapid, weak pulse.

The *diagnosis* of heat stroke is no problem in the classic instance with warm dry skin, temperature of 105° F. or higher, history of long exposure to heat, lack of evidence of other cause, and coma or near-coma. The chief confusion is with other diseases of the central nervous system causing coma and hyperpyrexia, and occasionally with overwhelming sepsis without external manifestations, or terminal liver disease. In some instances therapy to lower the temperature should be given before a sure diagnosis is made.

True heat stroke calls for heroic measures and is one of the few true medical emergencies. The aim of *treatment* is to reduce the body temperature to a safe range (102° F. or lower) as rapidly as possible, since brain damage is a function of both temperature and time. Total immersion in an ice bath or in water as cold as possible is probably the most efficient method of cooling. The alleged danger of heat retention from peripheral vasoconstriction and of increased shock has not been supported experimentally or clinically. Evaporative cooling by sprays and fans is effective, provided the environment is cool and dry enough to allow rapid evaporation. An important adjunct, often neglected, is vigorous massage of the extremities during the cooling, to overcome the peripheral stagnation regularly seen and to allow the more rapid transfer of heat. Vigorous cooling should be stopped when the rectal temperature reaches 102° F., but may need to be reinstituted if the temperature rises again. Intravenous fluids should be given with care and only with definite indications, because of the dangers of pulmonary edema. Persistence of coma and shock after cooling probably means severe brain damage, and therapy is often disappointing. Irregularity of temperature regulation is to be expected for several days in those who recover.

Prognosis is wholly a function of the promptness of treatment. All untreated patients will die. Probably all would recover if heat stroke were detected early and treated vigorously. Most of those who have recovered retain some intolerance to heat. Late effects of brain damage are possible, but have not been reported frequently.

Heat cramps are painful contractions of various skeletal muscles, a symptom most commonly seen among manual workers in hot environments whose body fluids have been depleted of sodium chloride by unreplaced heavy losses (up to 20 gm. a day) in sweat. Occasionally a similar condition is observed in patients with chronic cardiac or hepatic disease on prolonged salt restriction. Lowering of the plasma chloride concentration (often to 90 mEq. per liter) is a regular and diagnostic finding, but many questions concerning individual susceptibility and mechanism of cramp causation remain poorly answered. Once established, the symptoms are specifically relieved by the replacement of salt (and water). The intravenous administration of 600 to 1000 cc. of normal saline may be necessary to start relief of acute symptoms. More important is prevention, which is most surely achieved by adding 0.1 per cent sodium chloride to drinking water. Heavy salting of food and the use of salt tablets are effective, but more difficult to enforce.

ROBERT C. DARLING

References

Borden, D. L., Waddill, J. F., and Grier, G. S., III: Statistical Study of 265 Cases of Heat Disease. J.A.M.A., *128*:1200, 1945.

Daily, W. M., and Harrison, T. R.: A Study of the Mechanism and Treatment of Experimental Heat Pyrexia. Am. J. M. Sc., *215*:42, 1948.

di Sant'Agnese, P. A., Darling, R. C., Perera, G. A., and Shea, E.: Sweat Electrolyte Disturbances Associated with Childhood Pancreatic Disease. Am. J. Med., *15*:777, 1953.

Ferris, E. B., Jr., Blankenhorn, M. A., Robinson, H. W., and Cullen, G. E.: Heat Stroke: Clinical and Chemical Observations on 44 Cases. J. Clin. Investigation, *17*:249, 1938.

Ladell, W. S. S., Waterlow, J. C., and Hudson, M. F.: Desert Climate: Physiologic and Clinical Observations. Lancet, *2*:491, 527, 1944.

Malamud, N., Haymaker, W., and Custer, R. P.: Heat Stroke. Clinicopathological Study of 125 Fatal Cases. Mil. Surgeon, *99*:397, 1946.

Robinson, S., and Gerking, S. D.: Thermal Balance of Men Working in Severe Heat. Am. J. Physiol., *149*:476, 1947.

Talbott, J. H.: Heat Cramps. Medicine, *14*:323, 1935.

DECOMPRESSION ILLNESS

(*Caisson Disease*)

This term refers to the group of symptoms produced by the sudden reduction in pressure of the atmosphere. It is seen (1) among workers in compressed air after return to atmospheric pressure (caisson workers, tunnel workers and deep-sea divers) or (2) on rapid ascent in open airplanes to heights usually above 25,000 feet. It should be noted that in both instances the symptoms occur during or after an abrupt drop in atmospheric pressure, always to at least one half of the initial pressure and usually to one third or less. Various terms have been applied to the separate symptoms seen in this illness, such as "bends" for pains in muscles and joints, "staggers" for vestibular involvement, and "the itch" for skin manifestations.

Etiology. All the manifestations except an occasional symptom are clearly due to the evolution of bubbles of nitrogen in the tissues and blood stream. The nitrogen, in solution at the higher pressure, is freed by the lowering of pressure. Nitrogen is the gas chiefly concerned, because the pressure change of this gas is greatest and because oxygen and carbon dioxide diffuse rapidly and chemically combine more readily, although the latter gases do diffuse into nitrogen bubbles when once formed. Bubbles cause symptoms by plugging small vessels and by the pressure of their expansion, particularly in confined regions.

Morbid Anatomy. Actual bubbles have been demonstrated only rarely. The usual cause of death is damage to the central nervous system, most severe in the spinal cord, especially the lower thoracic region. In the early stages there are areas of nonspecific softening, later replaced by gliosis. Frequently the pathologic changes are more widespread than suspected from clinical findings.

Bone changes are those of small sterile infarcts. In sudden deaths there is frequently intense congestion of all the internal organs.

Pathologic Physiology. The amount of nitrogen dissolved in the tissues of the body at any pressure is considerably more than would be dissolved in a similar volume of water. This results from the greater solubility (five times as great) of the gas in fat than in water. The high lipoid content of the central nervous system is the chief factor causing the vulnerability of that tissue.

Gradual reduction in the pressure of nitrogen will result in harmless diffusion of dissolved nitrogen from the tissues into the blood stream and elimination by the lungs. It is only by marked reduction in pressure (to one half or greater) that bubbles may form. Even then, a solution (or the tissues) may remain supersaturated unless disturbed. Thus, trauma and exercise predispose to bubble formation (and symptoms) and often determine the site. The circulation of the tissues is another important factor; relatively ischemic tissues will retain nitrogen longer.

Nitrogen may be removed prophylactically from the tissues by reducing the nitrogen content of the gas breathed, without danger of bubble formation. Thus, breathing 100 per cent oxygen for 3 hours before high altitude ascent will practically eliminate the incidence of symptoms. At pressures above two atmospheres, however, oxygen is highly toxic, and therefore its use in compressed air work must be limited to an aid in the later stages of gradual decompression. Helium, chiefly because of its rapid diffusion, has become an important replacement for nitrogen in work at very high pressures, such as in deep-sea diving.

Symptoms. The onset of symptoms occurs usually from a few minutes after decompression to three hours later. By far the most common manifestation is pain in joints, muscles or periarticular tissue coming on usually suddenly in one or several joint regions, and varying in intensity from a mild ache to a tearing, excruciating pain. Mild pains may disappear with rubbing. Very severe pain may lead rapidly to collapse.

Manifestations in the skin, considered among the mild forms of the disease, consist in itching, either mild or severe, usually with blotchy purplish erythema, sometimes with a mild degree of edema and occasionally with palpable crepitation.

Neurologic symptoms are of grave importance. The lower extremities are the chief site. They may vary from mild paresthesia and weakness to total paralysis. Loss of control of bladder and rectal sphincters is almost invariable, even with little other paralysis. Symptoms from higher cord lesions are much less common, and rare from brain damage.

Symptoms from bubbles in the lung capillaries (the "chokes") are often indicative of a severe form of the disease. The patient complains of inability to take a satisfactory deep breath, constriction of the chest, and a dry cough. Severe symptoms may progress rapidly to general collapse resembling asphyxia.

In severe forms of the disease resulting from accidents and sudden escape from high pressures, rapid collapse and sudden death may occur without premonitory symptoms.

This description is more strictly that of decompression after work in compressed air. In decompression to high altitude, involvement of the nervous system is much less frequent; otherwise the symptoms are quite similar.

Diagnosis. Correct diagnosis depends entirely on a history of recent exposure to compressed air. The high altitude syndrome will be met only *during* high altitude flight. Without adequate history the condition cannot be surely distinguished from other conditions causing muscle and joint pain or spinal cord disease. Occasionally abdominal pain due to decompression might be confused with acute peritonitis.

It is well to distinguish carefully the symptoms of decompression illness from other symptoms due to pressure change. Painful ears and sinuses occur chiefly on *increase* in pressure. Nitrogen at high pressures has a narcotic effect seen again on *increase,* not decrease, in pressure. Intestinal gases may cause pain by simple expansion *during decompression.*

Treatment and Prognosis. The sole effective treatment is recompression and gradual decompression. At high altitudes, descent to 20,000 feet will usually suffice. The syndrome after compressed air requires a compressed air chamber in which the patient should be recompressed to his original working pressure. Except in some instances of cord damage, symptoms will usually disappear, provided treatment is prompt enough.

Decompression after relief or control of symptoms should be gradual, usually lasting 2 to 3 hours, and recompression again is indicated by any recurrence of symptoms. Details of management may vary markedly. Breathing oxygen during the later stages of decompression helps to remove nitrogen.

Prognosis in invariably good if there is no cord damage. Even then, prompt recompression is often successful. Recovery of cord function after more than transient damage is variable; some patients with complete physiologic cord transection make a gradual complete recovery; others are permanent paraplegics. Other residual defects are related to the bones, which may show permanent radiographic change of "aseptic infarction" at the ends of long bones and be the site of secondary hypertrophic changes.

Medical management of the workers by elimination of elderly, obese and particularly susceptible men and by well controlled slow decompression after work periods, has reduced and can continue to reduce both the incidence and severity.

ROBERT C. DARLING

References

Behnke, A. R., Jr.: Effects of High Pressure; Prevention and Treatment of Compressed Air Illness. M. Clin. North America, 26:1213, 1942.
Bridge, E. V., and others: Decompression Sickness—Nature and Incidence of Symptoms during and after Decompression to 38,000 Feet for 90 Minutes with Exercise during Exposure. J. Aviation Med., 15:316, 1944.
Harvey, E. N.: Decompression Sickness and Bubble Formation in Blood and Tissues. Bull. New York Acad. Med., 21:505, 1945.
Hoff, E. C.: A Bibliographical Sourcebook of Compressed Air, Diving and Submarine Medicine. Bureau of Medicine and Surgery, Navy Department, Washington, D. C., 1948.
Taylor, H. K.: Aseptic Necrosis in Adults; Caisson Workers and Others. Radiology, 42:550, 1944.
Thorne, I. J.: Caisson Disease Study Based on 300 Cases Observed at Queens-Midtown Tunnel Project. J.A.M.A., 117:585, 1941.

BLAST INJURY

Blast injury is the term applied to the physiologic disturbances and internal structural damage caused by the pressure wave from an explosion. The blast injury itself is not characterized by evidence of injury on the body surface, but it frequently occurs concomitantly with other forms of trauma. In this discussion, we are not concerned with the purely psychiatric syndrome which also has been labeled "blast injury."

The rapidly expanding gases from an explosion generate a sharp rise in pressure in the surrounding zone of air or water; this pressure wave is then propagated in a manner analogous to the transmission of a single sound wave. When this pressure wave meets a human body it has little effect on solid organs and tissues, but may cause rapid and damaging distortion of those tissues containing air, such as the eardrums, the lungs and the intestinal walls. The amount of damage is related fairly closely to the maximum pressure of the wave; pressures between 3 and 15 atmospheres cause detectable, but not necessarily fatal, injuries to the lungs in animals.

Minimum trauma in the lungs consists of petechial hemorrhages, mostly on the lung surfaces between ribs. If the hemorrhages are at all extensive, secondary edema occurs in the hour or two after injury, and local areas of emphysema are common. In more intense blasts, the hemorrhages occur more widely in the lung, and involve larger vessels so that gross blood may escape into bronchi and trachea. In the intestines, trauma consists similarly in mild cases of intramural hemorrhages; in severe cases, of rupture. The colon and lower small intestine are most often involved. Lung injuries are predominant in air explosions; in water, the incidence of intestinal injuries is considerably increased. Hemorrhages in the brain are caused occasionally; apparently, the pressure is transmitted from the great vessels in the thorax to the cerebral vessels.

The person suffering blast injury in air will usually be bowled over by the explosion and most likely rendered temporarily unconscious. When conscious, he may be dazed; almost surely he will have ear pain and partial or complete deafness, but otherwise he may have no symptoms. If the lungs are injured, he will soon complain of dyspnea and chest pain which may progress rapidly. If the damage is severe, cyanosis will become apparent and blood may appear in the sputum. Severe blood loss into the lungs not infrequently leads to shock. Abdominal symptoms are rare in blast injury and when present are found usually in association with severe lung injury. In immersion blast injury, the abdominal symptoms often predominate and vary from the mild pain of a few petechial hemorrhages to the acute abdominal catastrophe of intestinal rupture.

The primary point of **diagnosis** lies in the recognition that internal injuries may exist without external evidence of trauma. Even if burn, fractures or lacerations are present, the possibility of blast injury should be kept in mind. The presence of damage to eardrums adds greatly to the suspicion of internal blast injury. Bradycardia, often extreme, has been frequently noted and may be a useful diagnostic sign.

Prognosis in air blast injury depends almost entirely on the extent of pulmonary damage. Grossly bloody sputum is a dire prognostic sign as is intense cyanosis or shock.

Treatment is primarily aimed at the relief of dyspnea and anoxia by the use of inhalation oxygen, tracheal aspiration and rest. Since shock, if present, is associated with internal blood loss, whole blood transfusion is the treatment of choice. Treatment of the rarer manifestations in other organs is that of internal trauma to these organs from other cause.

ROBERT C. DARLING

References

Clemedson, C.-J.: An Experimental Study on Air Blast Injuries. Acta physiol. Scandinav., *18,* Supplement 61, 1949.

Hooker, D. R.: Physiological Effects of Air Concussion. Am. J. Physiol., 67:219, 1924.

Tunbridge, R. E.: Cause, Effect and Treatment of Air Blast Injuries. War Med., 7:3, 1945.

Wakeley, C. P. G.: Effect of Underwater Explosion on the Human Body. Lancet, 1:715, 1945.

MOUNTAIN SICKNESS

The ascent to high altitudes of persons accustomed to life under the pressure of practically one atmosphere (760 mm. of mercury) may produce distressing and possibly serious consequences. The effects of diminished pressure may be manifested quickly if the ascent is rapid, as in airplanes or balloons, or more gradually during mountain climbing. These are not produced by the reduction of mechanical pressure, but result from the diminished partial pressure of oxygen. In persons permanently resident in rarefied air there are structural and functional adaptive changes. Few persons escape slight discomfort, at least, on ascending more than 12,000 feet above sea level, corresponding to a reduction of oxygen pressure of about one third.

The principal factors, in acclimatization are (*a*) increased volume of air breathed; (*b*) increased alveolar oxygen pressure; (*c*) increase in red cells in proportion to the increase in hemoglobin; (*d*) increase in size of red cells; (*e*) increase in viscosity of the blood and in resistance to hemolysis; (*f*) increase in serum proteins; (*g*) diminution in available alkali; (*h*) decreased alveolar carbon dioxide; (*i*) decrease in arterial oxygen saturation. At high altitudes new formation of red cells has been indicated by the large percentage of reticulated cells in the blood. Hurtado found an increase in the midcapacity of the lungs, a true physiologic emphysema and augmented vital capacity.

Symptoms of mountain sickness differ in kind and severity in different persons and at different altitudes. In mountain climbing the effects of diminished pressure may be observed at much lower altitudes than in aviation because of the association of rarefied air, and more or less severe physical exertion. Patients suffering from cardiovascular disease are, of course, at a peculiar disadvantage, and in them the effects of a rarefied atmosphere are correspondingly intensified. Frontal headache, vertigo, malaise, mental dullness, abnormalities of vision and hearing, epistaxis, nausea, vomiting, thirst, cyanosis, dyspnea, palpitation and muscular weakness are commonly noted. Baker reports a much higher incidence of allergic manifestations. There may be slight fever. The pulse is accelerated and the systolic blood pressure moderately raised. With rest, some degree of accommodation is ordinarily acquired within a few days. Oxygen affords prompt relief.

Treatment. To relieve oxygen want in mountain sickness, oxygen should be given. Discussions on methods of protection of flying personnel against the many hazards that are encountered, and the treatment of affections following exposure to these hazards, can be found in the chapter on Aviation Medicine (p. 511).

W. J. McCONNELL

References

Aste-Salazar, H., and Hurtado, A.: The Affinity of Hemoglobin for Oxygen at Sea Level and at High Altitudes. Am. J. Physiol., *142*:733, 1944.

Baker, Julia: A Note on a Possible Allergic Factor in Altitude Sickness. J. Lab. & Clin. Med., *29*:831, 1944.

Clinton, M., Jr., Thorn, G. W., and Davenport, V. D.: Studies on Altitude Tolerance. Bull. Johns Hopkins Hosp., *79*:70, 1946.

Houston, C. S., and Riley, R. L.: Respiratory and Circulatory Changes during Acclimatization to High Altitude. Am. J. Physiol., *149*:562, 1947.

Hurtado, A.: Chronic Mountain Sickness. J.A.M.A., *120*:1278, 1942.

Kerwin, A. J.: Heart Size of Natives Living at High Altitudes. Am. Heart J., *28*:69, 1944.

ELECTRIC SHOCK

Electric shock may result when the body becomes part of the path of flow of current between poles of different potential. Broadly speaking, alternating currents are considered much more dangerous than direct currents. Fatal shock seldom results from contact with a direct current of less than 300 volts, but the danger increases as higher voltages are attained. Alternating currents, if of few cycles (15 to 60), may cause death in well grounded subjects, even at the 110 to 115 volts commonly used for home lighting, but alternating currents of high voltage, if of very high frequency, may be handled with relative safety. Maclachlan concluded, from an analysis of 479 cases of electric shock, that the severity of shock decreased or the success of resuscitative efforts increased as the potential of the circuit involved increased. The resistance offered by the body, as a conductor, is a factor determining the severity of shock. The resistance of dry skin is about 50,000 ohms per square centimeter, varying in different parts of the body. Moisture from sweating or wet clothing may lower the resistance to 1200 or 1500 ohms. If skin resistance reaches 1200 ohms, an alternating current of 110 volts may prove fatal. The nature of the "ground" may determine the seriousness of shock. A subject immersed in a water-filled bath might be killed by a current which could be tolerated under other circumstances. The duration of contact is also of great importance, since the severity of shock increases with an increase in the duration of contact. Prolonged contact with low voltages is more likely than with high voltages, for in the latter case the victim often "falls clear," aided by violent muscular contractions.

Etiology. The tendency of currents of low voltage is to arrest the heart without affecting the respiration. Alternating currents of low tension throw the heart in fibrillation. High-tension currents affect the central nervous system, causing inhibition of respiration. In one, the result is heart death; in the other, respiratory paralysis. It is inadvisable to generalize regarding the action of currents of moderate tension, since many variable factors such as skin resistance, grounding, source voltage, amperage, duration of contact and kind of current determine the severity of the shock. Much remains unknown concerning the mechanism and the effects of electric shock, although the studies of Urquhart, Hoff and Nahum, Maclachlan, and their associates, have contributed greatly to knowledge in this field.

Morbid Anatomy. Postmortem evidences of electrocution are variable. Extensive charring may mark the points of entrance and exit of the current, or the burns may be slight or absent. The superficial destructive effects of direct currents are usually more extensive than those of alternating currents. The blood is often dark and is rarely coagulated. Minute hemorrhages and areas of destruction may be found in the brain and cord. Reference should be made to the detailed reports of studies of the effects of electric shock upon the nervous system published by Kouwenhoven and by Morrison, Weeks and Cobb.

Symptoms. Loss of consciousness, momentary or prolonged, and burns of varying degree usually accompany severe electric shock. Death may be instantaneous or result after some moments or hours. Convulsions and priapism are common. Those who recover from shock may suffer various after-effects, such as persistent muscular pain, fatigue, headache and nervous irritability. Progressive loss of vision with opacity of the lens has been reported. There are usually no permanent effects in those recovering from shock. Because of the tendency to electrolysis of deep tissues and to the destruction of vessel walls, the possibility of delayed hemorrhage must be kept in mind in the treatment of cases involving extensive burns.

Prognosis. In cases of cardiac failure due to ventricular fibrillation, death must be expected. Respiratory paralysis often responds to artificial respiration. (In experimental animals, however, cardiac function has been restored after induced ventricular fibrillation: Wiggers.) Jex-Blake considered death due to (1) prolonged muscular tetany resulting in asphyxia; (2) ventricular fibrillation; (3) respiratory failure through effects on the nervous system; or (4) delayed effects of burns. To these causes Kouwenhoven would add the more immediate effects of heat production and tissue coagulation.

Treatment. When the victim is freed from the current, artificial respiration is the first measure necessary in the treatment of electric shock. It should be instituted at once, since a delay of even moments may result in death. Although the "back pressure-arm lift" method is rapidly replacing the "prone pressure" method, either may be used and should be continued until rigor mortis sets in. One patient, at least, was revived after 8 hours of effort. There is some evidence that the return of normal respiration is hastened by the supplementary use of oxygen inhalations. "Countershock," or stimulation by mechanical means, has been advocated, but there is little or no reason to believe that it is of value. Different authors, following the experimental work of Levy, who showed that ventricular arrhythmias leading to ventricular fibrillation and death could be induced by conditions which stimulated the heart and by equivalent conditions which removed or reduced depressing influences, have called attention to the often fatal consequences of administering epinephrine and other stimulating drugs in electric shock. Hoff and Nahum discovered that acetylcholine given to experimental animals protects them from ventricular fibrillation and death when they receive an electric shock of the strength which normally causes fibrillation of the ventricles. The important clinical application which is suggested by these findings is obvious. Spinal punctures as a hospital procedure in the after-treatment for persistent headache or signs of cerebral pressure are of some value.

W. J. McCONNELL

References

Brown, H. S.: Treatment of Low-Voltage Injuries. National Safety News, 67:6, 1953.

Dickson, W. E.: Accidental Electrocution: with Direct Shock to the Brain Itself. J. Path. & Bact., 59:359, 1947.

Hoff, H. E., and Nahum, L. H.: Nature of Ventricular Fibrillation Following Electric Shock and Its Prevention by Acetyl β-Methyl Choline Chloride. Am. J. Physiol., 110:675, 1935.

Jex-Blake, A. J.: The Goulstonian Lectures on Death by Electric Currents. Brit. Med. J., 1:425, 1913.

Kouwenhoven, W. B.: Electricity and the Human Body. Safety Rev., (U. S. Navy), 8, 4–9:3, 1951.

Levy, R. L.: Disorders of the Heart and Circulation. New York, Thomas Nelson and Sons, 1951.

Maclachlan, W.: Electrical Injuries. J. Indust. Hyg., 16:1, 1934.

Morrison, L. R., Weeks, A., and Cobb, S.: Histopathology of Different Types of Electric Shock on Mammalian Brains. J. Indust. Hyg., 11:324, 1930.

Urquhart, R. W. I.: Experimental Electric Shock. J. Indust. Hyg., 9:140, 1927; also with Noble, E. C.: J. Indust. Hyg., 11:154, 1929.

Wiggers, C. J.: Physiologic Basis for Cardiac Resuscitation from Ventricular Fibrillation: Methods for Serial Defibrillation. Am. Heart. J., 20:413, 1940.

Diseases Due to Chemical Agents

CARBON MONOXIDE POISONING

Carbon monoxide is a gas produced by the imperfect oxidation of carboniferous material and is probably the most widely distributed of toxic agents. It is slightly lighter than air, nonirritating, colorless, tasteless and, in moderate concentrations, odorless. Ordinarily, carbon monoxide does not appear in nature, but may be encountered in the home through accidental leakage of manufactured gas from open burners and defective appliances, and from incomplete combustion of various commercial gas products. It is also encountered in many industries, particularly in coal mining, in the steel industry, in gas manufacturing, in processes utilizing gas heat, and in connection with the use of explosives in confined spaces. It is found in smoke, in compartments which have been painted with oil paints and sealed, and in the exhaust of internal combustion engines. Many deaths have occurred in closed garages from motor exhaust gas, and manufactured gas long has been used in suicide. Coal gas contains about 16 per cent carbon monoxide; blast furnace stack gas, 28 per cent; mine air after dust explosions, 1 to 8 per cent; and the exhaust from automobile motors, about 7 per cent.

Incidence. Without doubt, countless persons are daily affected to some degree by carbon monoxide. There is a striking variation in individual susceptibility, but no evident racial or sex predisposition. Children are believed to be more susceptible than adults, probably because of their relatively greater respiratory exchange, body weight considered. Persons with cardiorespiratory disease are handicapped when exposed to carbon monoxide, and the preexistence of certain nervous disorders may, in persons poisoned, result in aggravation of the nervous manifestations. Some degree of acclimatization to carbon monoxide develops among those continually or frequently exposed to the gas and is shown in the lessening of symptoms during successive exposures to the same concentrations. The possible explanation of this acclimatization is suggested by Killick as due to (1) a selective activity of the alveolar membrane producing either a secretion of oxygen from the alveoli into the blood, or an excretion of carbon monoxide from the blood into the alveoli; or (2) removal of carbon monoxide from the blood by oxidative or other processes in the tissues.

Etiology. Carbon monoxide has an affinity for hemoglobin two hundred to three hundred times that of oxygen. The reaction, however, is reversible and depends upon the relative tensions of carbon monoxide and oxygen in the alveolar air. The gas is harmful in that it produces anoxemia. Death is due to respiratory failure. Though the problem has occasioned much study, it has not been demonstrated that carbon monoxide is, of itself, specifically toxic. Haldane suggested that it may poison a catalyst of oxidation.

Poisoning depends, not only upon the carbon monoxide content of inspired air, but also upon the duration of exposure to the gas. Particularly when exposed to moderate concentrations, the blood does not attain the full saturation theoretically possible. The maximum allowable concentration of carbon monoxide recommended by the American Standards Association is 100 parts per 1,000,000 parts of air by volume with atmospheric oxygen not below 19 per cent by volume for exposures not exceeding a total of eight hours daily, and 400 parts per 1,000,000 parts of air by volume for exposures not exceeding a total of one hour daily.

Morbid Anatomy. In the postmortem examination of victims of carbon monoxide poisoning there is often noted a bright, cherry color of the blood. Lining membranes are exceptionally red or show ecchymoses. Particularly important are pathologic changes in the brain, characterized by hyperemia, edema, hemorrhage and diffuse degeneration. Softening in the lenticular nucleus is regarded as the most typical lesion in carbon monoxide poisoning. Yant and others found, in dogs, that the cells of the cortex, the corpus striatum, the dorsal motor nucleus of the vagus, and the dorsal sensory areas of the medulla were especially involved. Neurons were severely damaged, showing disruption, marked chromatolysis and other degenerative effects. Though still a matter of some dispute, the effects of carbon monoxide upon the nervous system are generally considered to be due, essentially, to asphyxia and not to immediate toxic action. There have been reports of the disappearance of chromatin from adrenal cortical cells and of colloidal material from the thyroid in cases of acute poisoning.

Symptoms. It has been observed by Sayers and others that the character and severity of symptoms under any degree of blood saturation depended largely upon the duration of exposure and the accompanying muscular activity; and, further, that with a blood concentration resulting from long exposure to a low atmospheric concentration there were noted more severe symptoms and after-effects than with a similar blood concentration resulting from a short exposure to a richer carbon monoxide mixture. In general, a concentration of 0.06 per cent, or 6 parts of carbon monoxide in 10,000 parts of air, produces headache within an hour, and unconsciousness in 2 hours, while 0.1 per cent carbon monoxide, or 10 parts in 10,000, produces unconsciousness in a little more than an hour and may prove fatal in 4 hours.

Carbon monoxide may kill with great suddenness. Victims of mine dust explosions have been found in attitudes indicating that there was no warning of impending danger. Though headache is usually the first symptom, the onset may be insidious. There have been many cases displaying a progressive muscular weakness without loss of consciousness, but with disturbances of memory, the victim passing into a rather insouciant oblivion, from which he may emerge promptly or from which he may pass into full coma.

The after-effects in those recovering from acute poisoning are extremely varied. Headache, vertigo, muscular weakness and nausea are common. More rarely encountered are serious disturbances of memory, vision, hearing and speech; or psychoses, neuritis and paralysis. Cerebral hemorrhage has been observed some days after apparent recovery. A moderate polycythemia may persist for some time after all carbon monoxide has disappeared from the blood.

Chronic poisoning by carbon monoxide is believed by many authors to be a clinical entity. The alleged effects produced by repeated exposures to low concentrations of carbon monoxide are headache, malaise and an ill defined debility. However, carbon monoxide is neither cumulative nor proved to be toxic, and other causes should be sought for these and other subjective symptoms which persist long after the exposures to carbon monoxide have ceased.

Diagnosis. Absolute diagnosis is dependent upon the identification of carbon monoxide hemoglobin. The pyrotannic acid method affords a reasonably accurate quantitative estimation of carbon monoxide in blood or air. Of the laboratory methods, the iodine pentoxide method, though time-consuming, is now the generally accepted standard method for carbon monoxide analysis. Carbon monoxide indicators are now available on the market which indicate by direct reading of a meter the percentage of carbon monoxide present. One of these is said to be sensitive down to 0.005 per cent.

Treatment. Emergency treatment requires immediate artificial respiration if breathing has ceased, preferably by the back-pressure arm-lift method. It may be used advantageously for a short while, even though the victim is breathing, if asphyxia is marked. The use when possible of an inhalator for the administration of oxygen is most desirable. The inhalation of pure oxygen greatly accelerates the release of carbon monoxide, freeing it about four or five times as rapidly as does air.

Patients should not be permitted to make any physical exertion and should be kept warm. Seriously poisoned patients, after receiving emergency treatment, may well be placed under observation in a hospital. Medication and blood transfusions are rarely if ever indicated.

W. J. McConnell

References

Drinker, C. K.: Carbon Monoxide Asphyxia. New York, Oxford University Press, 1938.

Haldane, J. B. S.: Carbon Monoxide as a Tissue Poison. Biochem. J., 21:1068, 1927.

Killick, E. M.: Acclimatization of the Human Subject to Atmospheres Containing Low Concentrations of Carbon Monoxide. J. Physiol., 87:41, 1936.

Meigs, J. Wister: Acute Carbon Monoxide Poisoning, An Analysis of One Hundred Five Cases. A. M. A. Arch. Indust. Hyg. and Occ. Med., 6:344, 1952.

von Oettingen, W. F.: Poisoning: A Guide to Clinical Diagnosis and Treatment. New York, Paul B. Hoeber, 1952, p. 524.

Sayers, R. R., Yant, W. P., Levy, Edward, and Fulton, W. B.: Effect of Repeated Daily Exposure of Several Hours to Small Amounts of Automobile

Exhaust Gas. Public Health Bull. No. 186, March 1929.

Sendroy, Julius: Hazards from Thermal Decomposition of Motor-Insulating Materials. A. M. A. Arch. Indust. Hyg. and Occ. Med., 5:330, 1952.

Sievers, R. F., Edwards, T. I., Murray, A. L., and Schrenk, H. H.: Effect of Exposure to Known Concentrations of Carbon Monoxide. J.A.M.A., 118:585, 1942.

Yant, W. P., Chornyak, J., Schrenk, H. H., Patty, F. A., and Sayers, R. R.: Studies in Asphyxia. Public Health Bull. No. 211, Aug. 1934.

CARBON TETRACHLORIDE POISONING

Definition. Carbon tetrachloride (tetrachloromethane) poisoning may be defined as an acute, subacute or chronic intoxication caused by carbon tetrachloride or its vapor. It is characterized clinically by acute abdominal symptoms or pulmonary involvement as well as by serious injury to the liver and kidneys. The clinical picture in some instances is dominated by pulmonary and renal injury, either alone or combined, with hepatic effects not evident; in others, signs of liver damage with evident jaundice and hepatic tenderness are outstanding. In some persons gastrointestinal symptoms may be so severe as to lead to an early diagnosis of food poisoning or even of acute perforative appendicitis. A defatting of the skin with a resulting dermatitis may follow contact with carbon tetrachloride.

Etiology. Carbon tetrachloride is the most widely used of the halogenated hydrocarbon group of organic solvents. It is encountered industrially as an extractant for fats and oils, as a solvent in rubber cements, textile soaps and other combinations, and as a cleaning fluid and in fire extinguishers. It is used in offices and homes as a dry-cleaning and degreasing agent. Medicinally it is occasionally used as a vermifuge.

Carbon tetrachloride, alone or mixed with other solvents, has been sold under many trade names, such as Carbona, Asordin, Chlorasol (25 per cent carbon tetrachloride, 75 per cent ethylene dichloride), Phoenipine, Katarine, Pyrene, Spectral, Tetra, Tetracol, Tetraform and no doubt, under other names.

Like other volatile solvents, carbon tetrachloride exercises its effects only after absorption into the body. The severity of the effects is generally proportional to the quantity absorbed. Absorption may take place by inhalation of the vapor, ingestion of the liquid, or through prolonged or repeated contact of the liquid with the skin and mucous membranes. The mode of entrance appears to have little or no influence on the results produced, except that acute poisoning almost always follows exposure to an atmosphere highly contaminated with vapor or to mistaken drinking of the liquid carbon tetrachloride. Elimination takes place primarily through the lungs.

The threshold limit value for 1954 adopted by the American Conference of Governmental Industrial Hygienists is 25 parts carbon tetrachloride per million parts of air for an 8-hour working day. Quantities in excess of 3 to 4 cc. orally may cause death. Individual susceptibility varies and is probably enhanced by the use of alcohol.

Pathology. In fatal poisoning, which may follow a single exposure to a high concentration of the vapor, damage to the liver, kidneys, heart, adrenal glands and nervous system, as well as a cerebral hemorrhage and bronchopneumonia with pulmonary edema, may result. Liver sections show a disseminated central necrosis with degenerative changes in the peripheral cells. Petechial hemorrhages may be found on the surfaces of the lungs. Some areas of consolidation are not unusual. The kidneys may reveal a lower nephron nephrosis in which the distal convoluted tubules disclose a severe grade of degeneration with little change in the proximal tubules. Mallory describes the changes as like those in a kidney injured by transfusion, crush or sulfonamides.

Symptomatology. There is considerable variation in the signs and symptoms of carbon tetrachloride poisoning, depending upon the nature of exposure. Acute intoxication results when an excessive amount of the vapor or liquid is absorbed into the body within a short period of time. The first acute reaction is similar to that to chloroform—dizziness, nausea, vomiting, backache, malaise, headache, giddiness and unconsciousness—but is more toxic. The narcotic effects are less marked than those of chloroform, but the effects on the liver, kidneys and heart are much more rapid. The effects on the heart are important in acute poisoning, because, in addition to acting as a heart depressant, there is a tendency to cause fibrillation. Death may occur from circulatory or respiratory failure, or the patient may recover within one or two days without any apparent after-effects.

Subacute poisoning, usually resulting from

prolonged or repeated exposure to an atmosphere containing a high concentration of the vapor, but insufficient to cause loss of consciousness, may cause headache, nausea, fatigue, vomiting, dizziness, visual disturbances, subconjunctival hemorrhage, coughing, and bleeding from the mucous membranes. Some cases present hypertension. Acute renal damage with albumin and casts in the urine or anuria may develop early, and toxic hepatitis with a moderate degree of jaundice frequently occurs, particularly in subjects who have ingested rather than inhaled carbon tetrachloride. Pulmonary complications and coma may follow within a week after exposure and in some cases end fatally in one to two weeks.

Chronic poisoning, which is the result of daily exposures, each small in itself, over a longer period of time, may be recognized by local symptoms of irritation of the mucous membrane of the eyes, nose and upper respiratory tract. The patient invariably complains of headache, sleepiness, fatigue, and, in more advanced stages, abdominal pain, edema and oliguria or anuria. Jaundice may or may not be present. Affections of the central nervous system have been observed.

Diagnosis. There may be confusion in the diagnosis of carbon tetrachloride poisoning because of the variability in its manifestations. A history of absorption of an adequate quantity of carbon tetrachloride, irrespective of the portal of entrance, together with the symptoms and signs of the intoxication, should make the diagnosis reasonably certain. In general medical or hospital practice, carbon tetrachloride poisoning is encountered most frequently after inhalation or skin contact with cleaning fluids in a closed room or after ingestion by alcoholics.

Liver function tests, kidney function tests, roentgen findings in the chest and electrocardiograms should be carefully evaluated. Laboratory procedures offer greater value in confirming an obvious intoxication than in prognosticating the final outcome. Laboratory findings may show an increase in serum bilirubin and nonprotein nitrogen. Albumin and casts in the urine are found in renal involvement. There may be changes in the blood in the direction of a leukocytosis, but these do not dominate the picture as they do in poisoning by hydrocarbons of the benzene ring group of solvents.

Roentgen findings in the lungs may vary from a mild prominence of linear markings to complete consolidation of one or more lobes of the lungs.

Prognosis. Although the fatality rate from carbon tetrachloride poisoning is low compared with the number of cases of intoxication reported, there are a sufficient number of deaths to emphasize the need for precaution against carelessness in its use and inadequate safety measures. In fatal cases, nearly all deaths result from kidney and liver damage, and occur three to ten days after exposure. Most patients who survive the acute illness recover completely.

Treatment. Most important in the case of any poisoning is the prompt separation of the victim from the offending substance. In instances in which the victim is overcome from inhalation of carbon tetrachloride vapors, immediate removal to an uncontaminated area where he can rest quietly and be kept warm is imperative. If breathing has stopped, artificial respiration and the administration of oxygen are indicated. Hot tea or coffee may be given as a stimulant if the patient is conscious, but alcoholic stimulant or epinephrine is contraindicated in all stages of carbon tetrachloride poisoning. When carbon tetrachloride is swallowed, absorption from the stomach and intestines is rapid, but early lavage or induced vomiting may be helpful. This may be followed with Epsom salt (1 tablespoon) in water. All contaminated clothing should be removed and affected skin areas should be washed thoroughly with a mild soap and warm water. A mild ointment containing petrolatum or lanolin may be applied to the affected skin areas. Any of the liquid carbon tetrachloride entering the eyes should be flushed out with copious quantities of water at room temperature.

In the absence of specific therapy, further treatment must be largely symptomatic, varying with the individual symptoms and signs. When kidney function is impaired, the treatment is that of acute urinary suppression as outlined in the section on Diseases of the Kidneys. In anticipation of liver damage, glucose is of value. When the patient is able to tolerate food orally, the diet commonly used today is a high protein, high carbohydrate, low fat diet, which may be supplemented with vitamins in the form of brewers' yeast, thiamine and ascorbic acid. The amino acid, methionine, is said to have been used successfully in the treatment of several cases of carbon tetrachloride poisoning.

Prevention. The measures at our disposal

for the control of harmful concentrations of carbon tetrachloride, as well as other solvent vapors, in the plant atmosphere fall within three special fields, safety, engineering and medical. Safety measures must be used against accidents or irregularities in operation. Labels on cans and drums should indicate the hazardous nature of the substance, and workmen should be instructed as to the dangers. Personal protective devices, such as protective clothing, goggles and respirators— the latter are only for short exposures— should be provided when necessary. Good housekeeping and sanitary facilities are essential and include segregation of processes, care of spilled solutions, receptacles for soaked rags, and ample general ventilation.

W. J. McCONNELL

References

Abbott, G. A., and Miller, M. J.: Carbon Tetrachloride Poisoning; Report on Ten Cases. Pub. Health Rep., 63:1619, 1948.
Allebach, H. K. B., and McPhee, W. R.: Carbon Tetrachloride Poisoning. Missouri Med., 50:106, 1953.
Harris, F. H.: Acute Carbon Tetrachloride Poisoning. U. S. Armed Forces Med. J., 3:1023, 1952.
Mallory, T. B.: Case Records of the Massachusetts General Hospital. New England J. Med., 238:776, 1948.
Miller, L. L.: Nutritional Factors Affecting the Toxicity of Halogenated Hydrocarbons. Occup. Med., 5:194, 1948.
Myatt, A. V., and Salmons, J. A.: Carbon Tetrachloride Poisoning. A.M.A. Arch. Indust. Hyg. and Occ. Med., 6:74, 1952.

BENZENE POISONING

Benzene (benzol, C_6H_6, to be distinguished from petroleum benzine) is, with disturbing frequency, the cause of serious and even fatal poisoning. Benzene is obtained by the distillation of coal and the cracking of certain grades of petroleum. It is used widely in the manufacture of rubber goods and artificial and patent leather; in lacquers, paints, printing processes; as a solvent for fats and greases, and motor fuels; and for a great variety of other purposes. Commercial benzene contains a number of impurities such as thiophene and various homologues of benzene, particularly xylene and toluene. Extended investigation of the toxicity of such impurities has produced conflicting evidence, but the preponderance of opinion favors the belief that they are not responsible for the effects generally attributed to benzene.

Etiology. Benzene poisoning is usually caused by inhalation of its vapor, though it can be produced by skin absorption. Although individual susceptibility to benzene varies greatly for reasons not determined, the American Conference of Governmental Industrial Hygienists (1954) has adopted the threshold limit value of 35 parts benzene per million parts of air for the maximum average atmospheric concentration to which workers may be exposed for an 8-hour working day without injury to health.

Morbid Anatomy. Most striking among postmortem findings are multiple hemorrhages throughout the body; uncoagulated blood; abnormalities of the bone marrow, spleen and lymph nodes; and evidences of secondary infection.

Symptoms. *Acute poisoning* may take place with great rapidity and death may ensue in a few minutes. Beginning with sudden dizziness, the victim may quickly show great muscular weakness and lapse through drowsiness into coma. Tremors, delirium or convulsions are more infrequent. There is often marked dyspnea with, possibly, a sense of constriction of the chest, which may proceed to death from respiratory failure. The pulse is small and rapid, the skin pallid or cyanotic, occasionally showing ecchymoses.

Chronic poisoning or subacute poisoning is much more frequent and is manifested usually after days or months of exposure to benzene. The early evidences of disease are commonly rather vague, such as loss of appetite and weight, headache, vertigo and muscular weakness. As the condition progresses, pallor is marked and is associated with a true anemia. Dyspnea and air hunger may be striking. Convulsions and delirium are rare. Abdominal pain and gastrointestinal irritation with nausea and vomiting are common. Hemorrhages from the nose, gums, bowels, kidneys and vagina, as well as into the skin and mucous membranes, are typical. The urine often shows evidences of nephritis, with casts, albumin and blood. Furunculosis may be encountered, and possibly dermatitis related to skin contact with benzene.

The blood picture may vary considerably from the so-called classical changes. Leukopenia, neutropenia, thrombocytopenia, hypochromia, eosinophilia and anemia may or may not be present. The bone marrow may not be affected, or it may be aplastic, hyperplastic or leukemic. Resistance to infection is low-ered.

Diagnosis. The use of arbitrary criteria for diagnosis is not advocated. The diagnosis cannot be made upon blood findings alone, since these may simulate various blood dys-crasias. The blood picture of agranulocytosis may be similar to that produced by benzene and the other well known causes of leuko-penia. A history of exposure to benzol should be the determining factor in the diagnosis of benzene poisoning.

Prognosis. Many seriously poisoned pa-tients have died after several days or weeks; others have recovered after prolonged illness. The mortality among severe cases has in the past been about 50 per cent.

Treatment. Acute poisoning requires re-peated washing of the stomach, followed by the administration of 2 to 3 tablespoons of magnesium sulfate in 250 cc. of water. In instances of respiratory failure prompt arti-ficial respiration is indicated. The use of oxygen, administered with an inhalator, is advised. Serious blood destruction and hemor-rhage are best treated by blood transfusion, possibly repeated many times. The blood pic-ture should be observed frequently. Prepara-tions of liver have been used to advantage. Lane reports that ACTH has been used suc-cessfully in some cases of aplastic anemia due to benzene. Other treatment is symptomatic. Because of lowered resistance to infection, complications may appear, such as pneu-monia, bronchitis and cystitis.

Prophylaxis involves careful control of in-dustrial processes in which benzene is used, adequate ventilation, the selection of healthy persons as workers with benzene, and the periodic examination of persons exposed, to the end that those even slightly affected may be removed.

W. J. McCONNELL

References

Bowers, V. H.: Reaction of Human Blood-Forming Tissues to Chronic Benzene Exposure. Brit. J. Indust. Med., 4:87, 1947.
Browning, E.: Benzene as Hazard in Industry. Brit. J. Phys. Med., 7:122, 1944.
Dinberg, M. C.: Benzol Poisoning. Canad. M. A. J., 52:176, 1945.
Hunter, F. T.: Chronic Exposure to Benzene. II. Clinical Effects. J. Indust. Hyg. & Toxicol., 21: 331, 1939.
Lane, R. E.: Blood Changes in Industrial Diseases. Brit. J. Indust. Med., 9:245, 1952.
Mallory, T. B., and others: Chronic Exposure to Ben-zene. III. Pathologic Results. J. Indust. Hyg. & Toxicol., 21:355, 1939.
Sacca, J. D.: Myelogenous Leukemia Resulting from Benzol Poisoning. New York State J. Med., 48: 1619, 1948.
Sroka, K. H.: Occupational Poisoning Caused by Benzene and Its Homologues. Deutsche med. Wchnschr., 77:959, 1952. Abst. in A.M.A. Arch. Indust. Hyg. and Occ. Med., Dec. 1952, p. 546.

CHRONIC BROMIDE POISONING

(Bromism)

Bromide therapy, first introduced in 1857, has been widely used on account of its seda-tive action in the treatment of nervous dis-orders, in idiopathic epilepsy and in kindred states. Self-medication with proprietary bro-mide preparations, which are extensively ad-vertised to the public and readily available without prescription, is common, and it is important, therefore, that the physician as-certain the extent of previous or simultaneous consumption of these preparations by the pa-tient when prescribing bromides.

The bromides are readily absorbed from the stomach when given by mouth and exert a depressing effect on the central nervous sys-tem, especially on the brain and medulla. Their prolonged and indiscriminate use, how-ever, may cause an intoxication, often accom-panied with a transitory delirium, due to ac-cumulation of bromides in the blood and other body fluids. This accumulation is at the expense of the body chlorides, which fall in the same proportion and are excreted by the kidney in preference to bromides.

Symptoms. The clinical features, particu-larly in the milder forms of bromide intoxica-tion, may be somewhat masked by the under-lying disturbance or disease for which the bromide was administered, and the only clue may be an apparent exaggeration of the pre-existing illness. The patient may complain of headache and dryness of the mouth and show evidence of weakness. In the more severe bro-mide intoxications the symptoms and signs of toxic delirium predominate and are mani-fested by fear, delusions, hallucinations, dis-orientation, visual disturbances and disturb-ances of memory and equilibrium.

Skin rash, usually acneiform or maculo-papular, is a characteristic manifestation of bromism, but is absent in many instances.

Diagnosis. Though the symptoms may be sufficiently suggestive to permit clinical recog-nition in a number of cases, a laboratory de-termination of bromide in the blood should always be made. Although a variety of methods for determining bromide concentration has been suggested, Wuth's modification of the Walter-Hauptmann method is popularly used. A blood bromide level averaging 200 mg. per 100 cc. of serum is apt to produce intoxication, although susceptible persons may show symptoms with a much lower level; conversely, others more resistant may tolerate higher levels with impunity.

While admitting the adequacy of the gold chloride method for the initial diagnosis of bromide intoxications, Gray and Moore point out certain inaccuracies in the method and suggest that the determination of urine and blood chlorides, along with bromides, is a far better indication of the progress of treatment or of the validity of a diagnosis.

Treatment. Treatment consists in discontinuing the bromides plus the administration of sodium chloride in doses of 2 to 4 gm. three times daily in addition to that contained in the diet. Salt can be pleasantly administered in the form of 1 gm. enteric-coated tablets of sodium chloride. Fluids should be moderately forced, and the patient should be given a high caloric diet rich in vitamins. Spinal puncture and withdrawal of up to 20 cc. of spinal fluid has been found helpful in some cases of severe bromide poisoning.

W. J. McCONNELL

References

Craven, E. B., Jr.: Clinical Picture of Bromide Poisoning. Am. J. M. Sc., *186:*525, 1933.
Dax, E. C.: Overdosage with Bromides. Brit. M. J., 2:226, 1946.
Gray, M. G., and Moore, M.: Blood Bromide Determinations: Their Use and Interpretation. J. Lab. & Clin. Med., 27:680, 1942.
Levin, M.: Transitory Schizophrenias Produced by Bromide Intoxication. Am. J. Psychiat., *103:*229, 1946.
Logan, W. P.: Bromide Intoxication. Florida Med. Assoc. J., 34:123, 1947.
von Oettingen, W. F.: Poisoning. New York, Paul B. Hoeber, 1952, p. 285.

ENTEROGENOUS CYANOSIS

(Methemoglobinemia, Sulfhemoglobinemia, Parhemoglobinemia)

Definition. Enterogenous cyanosis connotes methemoglobinemia or sulfhemoglobinemia. The original entity, described by Stokvis and by Talma in 1902, consisted of attacks of cyanosis associated with bowel dysfunction. Today the term embraces various forms of cyanosis due to increased amounts of abnormal hemoglobin (parhemoglobinemia) in contrast to cyanosis due to reduced hemoglobin.

Pathologic Biochemistry and Physiology. Methemoglobin differs from hemoglobin in that its iron is ferric, not ferrous; in this form it does not combine with oxygen and cannot participate in oxygen transport. In plasma, hemoglobin becomes oxidized slowly to methemoglobin, reaching equilibrium at about 50 per cent conversion; within the normal erythrocyte the equilibrium is maintained at less than 1 per cent methemoglobin, perhaps largely by systems involved in the oxidation of glucose and lactate.

The mechanism which maintains normal concentrations of methemoglobin may be impaired (a) by inactivity or suppression of the necessary reducing system, or (b) by exposure of intracellular hemoglobin to various oxidants which produce methemoglobin at a rate which overwhelms the capacity of the erythrocyte to reduce it to hemoglobin.

The conversion of hemoglobin to methemoglobin imposes two different stresses on the oxygen transport mechanism. First, inactivation of part of the normal respiratory pigment reduces the total oxygen transport capacity, as in anemia. Second, the presence of methemoglobin alters unfavorably the oxygen-dissociation characteristics of the remaining normal hemoglobin so that unloading of oxygen at the tissues is restricted, as in carbon monoxide poisoning. In acute forms of methemoglobinemia these effects sum to produce hypoxemic symptoms when as little as 20 per cent of circulating hemoglobin has been converted. In chronic methemoglobinemia, due, for example, to congenital inactivity of the specific reducing system, symptoms are strikingly absent despite concentrations of methemoglobin which range from 40 to 50 per cent of the total pigment.

The structure of sulfhemoglobin is unknown; it has been surmised that sulfur replaces nitrogen in the constituent pyrrole rings of hemoglobin. In contrast to methemoglobin, this change is irreversible. The functional deficit imposed by the accumulation of sulfhemoglobin is qualitatively similar to that of methemoglobin, but details have not been studied.

Etiology. The cause of the original cases of enterogenous cyanosis remains obscure. Instances of this syndrome are distinguished by episodic constipation and diarrhea. The suggestion has been advanced that the abnormality of the bowel permits growth of nitrite-producing micro-organisms and enhances the absorption of nitrites which, as oxidizing agents, are notoriously capable of producing methemoglobin and sulfhemoglobin.

The commonest cause of parhemoglobinemia is ingestion of one of a large, diverse series of compounds which have nitro (NO_2) and amino (NH_2) groups in common. Relatively common examples are sulfonamides (sulfanilamide, sulfathiazole and sulfapyridine), nitrates (especially bismuth subnitrate and contaminated well water) and a host of aromatic compounds, including aniline and its industrial congeners. The aniline derivatives of medicinal importance are acetophenetidin (Phenacetin) and acetanilid (Antifebrin). Indeed, an appreciable number of persons with enterogenous cyanosis associated with constipation were habitual users of aniline analgesics.

The third form of methemoglobinemia occurs as a congenital and familial defect in an intra-erythrocytic reducing system ordinarily active in reverting methemoglobin (see Congenital Methemoglobinemia, p. 634).

Symptoms. Acute methemoglobinemia, induced, for example, by ingestion of nitrates, produces a clinical picture similar in most respects to that encountered in acute hypoxemia: headache, mild confusion, dizziness, dyspnea on exertion, and cyanosis. The train of symptoms accompanying the rare instance of true enterogenous cyanosis is complicated by episodes of constipation during which the cyanosis becomes intense.

Diagnosis. Detectable cyanosis in the absence of an adequate cardiovascular or respiratory basis should awaken suspicion of the presence of abnormal hemoglobin, and the suspicion will deepen if the mucous membranes display a brownish hue. Shed venous blood containing abnormal hemoglobin may be recognized by its chocolate or deep terracotta hue. If venous blood is then shaken with air, the familiar scarlet of oxygenated hemoglobin fails to develop or appears muddy.

Advantage may be taken of certain characteristics of various forms of enterogenous cyanosis to make an approximate differentiation. If the brown hue disappears from blood after standing several hours, the methemoglobinemia results from a chemical agent; if the color remains, it indicates either sulfhemoglobinemia or congenital methemoglobinemia. There are more precise physical and chemical means for spectroscopic and gasometric identification and estimation of the amount and form of the abnormal hemoglobin.

Treatment. Many reducing agents will revert or reduce methemoglobin (ferric) to hemoglobin (ferrous). A commonly used agent is methylene blue (methylthionine chloride). It may be administered *slowly* as a 1 per cent solution intravenously in doses of 1 (adults) to 2 mg. (children) per kilogram of body weight. Maximum conversion occurs within 30 minutes, and the same dose may be repeated several times at 60-minute intervals if the cyanosis has not receded. Slower but more prolonged effect is obtained by peroral administration in doses of 3 to 10 mg. per kilogram of body weight. Patients who present a combination of recurrent cyanosis with disordered bowel function may respond to correction of constipation or repair of a structural defect.

Sulfhemoglobin cannot be reverted chemically, but, if the causal agent is removed, will disappear at a rate equivalent to the rate of formation of new erythrocytes. In a severe instance, exchange transfusions of red blood cells may be indicated.

Joseph L. Lilienthal, Jr.

References

Barcroft, H., Gibson, Q. H., and Harrison, D. C.: Methaemoglobinemia. In Roughton, F. J. W., and Kendrew, J. C.: Hemoglobin. New York, Interscience Publishers, 1949.

van den Bergh, A. A. H.: Enterogene Cyanose. Deutsches Arch. f. klin. Med., 83:86, 1905.

Bodansky, O.: Methemoglobinemia and Methemoglobin-Producing Compounds. Pharmacol. Rev., 3:144, 1951.

Darling, R. C., and Roughton, F. J. W.: Effect of Methemoglobin on Equilibrium between Oxygen and Hemoglobin. Am. J. Physiol., 137:56, 1942.

Finch, C. A.: Methemoglobinemia and Sulfhemoglobinemia. New England J. Med., 239:470, 1948.

Graybiel, A., Lilienthal, J. L., Jr., and Riley, R. L.: Idiopathic Congenital (Familial) Methemoglobinemia. Bull. Johns Hopkins Hosp., 76:155, 1945.

Lemberg, R., and Legge, J. W.: Hematin Compounds and Bile Pigments. New York, Interscience Publishers, 1949.

Rieders, F., and Brieger, H.: Mechanism of Poisoning from Wax Crayons. J.A.M.A., 151:1490, 1953.

Wendel, W. B.: Control of Methemoglobinemia with Methylene Blue. J. Clin. Investigation, 18:179, 1939.

ARSENIC POISONING

Arsenic poisoning is usually the result of exposure to one of the oxides of arsenic, such as arsenious acid (As_2O_3), or to arsenical salts, such as emerald green (aceto-arsenite of copper) or lead arsenate. Arseniuretted hydrogen (arsine AsH_3) is highly toxic, but produces effects different from those of arsenic salts.

Incidence. Most industrial arsenic poisoning is seen in workmen engaged in extracting white arsenic (As_2O_3) from cobalt and arsenical pyrites; in chemical works, glass making and cadmium plating; in agricultural spraying and dusting; in the use of sheep dip; or in handling skins treated with arsenic. Poisoning has been reported from the use of the organic arsenic compounds, from fruit sprayed with arsenic and from certain cosmetics and proprietary remedies.

Arsine is produced when an acid and a metal, either or both containing arsenic, are brought into contact, with a resulting liberation of nascent hydrogen which combines with arsenic to form the toxic gas. Poisoning has occurred in chemical and galvanizing works; in submarines, because of arsenic in storage battery plates or acid; on ships carrying ferrosilicon, which in contact with air and moisture tends to decompose and liberate arsine; and in the preparation of hydrogen for balloon inflation.

Etiology. Arsenic oxide and the salts are local irritants to the skin and the mucous membranes of the mouth and respiratory passages; inhalation or ingestion of them produces local and systemic changes. Acute poisoning is usually due to the use of arsenic with suicidal intent. One grain (65 mg.) of white arsenic has proved fatal. Though the normal therapeutic dose of this substance is 2 mg., the "arsenic eaters" of Styria can safely take over 400 mg. twice a week.

Arsine is primarily a hemolytic agent. The inhalation of the gas, over a period of several hours, in a concentration of 30 parts per 1,000,000 will produce poisoning and the lethal dose, as variously stated, ranges from 100 mg. to over 500 mg. There is apparently marked individual susceptibility.

Morbid Anatomy. Delepine reported that after poisoning by arsenic trichloride there is found granulofatty degeneration of the heart, liver, kidneys, pancreas and gastric and duodenal glands. After death from poisoning by arsine the liver has been found to be large and edematous, with some evidence of fatty degeneration; the kidneys large, and the renal epithelium degenerated and necrotic. Ecker found significant alterations in the nervous system, marked by alterations in the ganglion cells and by regions of perivascular necrosis.

Symptoms. Arsenic oxides or salts, as dusts, produce superficially a dermatitis or even ulceration about folds of skin, as in the axillae or about the scrotum. Increased pigmentation may be noted about the axillae, the nipples, the eyelids and on the neck. Keratosis of the palms and soles may develop after prolonged ingestion of arsenic, and skin cancer has been reported to follow the use of the drug. The causal relation of arsenic to skin cancer is much disputed. The septum of the nose in some cases is perforated. Other symptoms are edema of the lids, coryza, pharyngitis and laryngitis. With more serious poisoning, vomiting, abdominal pain and diarrhea may be marked. A peripheral neuritis with pronounced paresthesia is moderately common. Paralysis similar to that produced by lead may result from the absorption of arsenic, the legs being more notably affected than the arms. Tendon reflexes are diminished or lost. Diffuse cerebral symptoms such as headache, vertigo, fatigue, drowsiness and impairment of mental activity may result from chronic absorption.

Poisoning by arsine is manifested, usually 3 to 6 hours after the gas is inhaled, by malaise, vertigo, weakness, headache, nausea and vomiting. There may be abdominal pain and diarrhea. A few hours later hemoglobinuria or hematuria and albuminuria are noted. The pulse may become rapid and feeble and the respiration increased. Within a day or two jaundice and a coppery cyanosis may be observed. Oliguria may develop. The red blood cells and hemoglobin are much reduced. In very severe cases there is a high color index and evidence of extreme blood destruction as well as of regeneration. The leukocytes are ordinarily not involved, though in some cases there is a slight leukocytosis. There develops, rarely, after several weeks, a transitory toxic polyneuritis with pain or anesthesia, but no motor involvement.

Diagnosis of arsenic poisoning is facilitated by careful inquiry into the nature of the patient's work and by chemical analysis of the urine, hair and nails. In connection with such analyses it should be noted that "normal" arsenic frequently has been found in the hair, nails and excreta of persons not known to be exposed to arsenic.

Prognosis. Industrial poisoning by arsenical oxides or salts is rarely fatal. Manifestations of the disease may persist for weeks or months. Poisoning by arsine, if severe, is usually fatal within about a week, death being due essentially to blood destruction. The mortality is approximately 30 per cent. Serious damage to the kidneys is almost inevitable, and impaired renal function complicates recovery. Convalescence is slow.

Treatment of chronic arsenic poisoning is largely by the promotion of elimination through the kidneys and bowels. During World War II, 2,3-dimercaptopropanol (BAL or Dimercaprol) was developed as an antidote to the arsenical blister gases. This agent appears promising as a treatment for systemic arsenical poisoning. It is recommended that 3 mg. per kilogram of Dimercaprol (10 per cent in oil) be given intramuscularly every 4 hours for the first two days, four injections on the third day, and injections twice daily thereafter for ten days or until complete recovery. In milder cases the dosage per injection may be reduced to 2.5 mg. per kilogram, and only four injections need be given on each of the first two days, two on the third day, and a single injection daily for ten days or until complete recovery.

In poisoning by arsine, oxygen should be promptly administered and the inhalations prolonged. Transfusion may be necessary. In the few cases of arsine poisoning in which BAL was given the results proved generally unsatisfactory. Pinto and others found that it neither stopped nor prevented the destruction of red cells.

W. J. McCONNELL

References

Council on Pharmacy and Chemistry: "BAL" (British Anti-Lewisite) in the Treatment of Arsenic and Mercury Poisoning. J.A.M.A., *131*:824, 1946.

Currie, A. N.: The Role of Arsenic in Carcinogenesis. Brit. M. Bull., *4*:402, 1947.

Fairhall, Lawrence T.: Toxicology. Ann. Rev. Med., *3*:265, 1952.

Goldwater, L. J.: Physiology of the Bone Marrow in Relation to Industrial Intoxication. Occup. Med., *4*:439, 1947.

Pinto, S. S., Petronella, S. J., Johns, D. R., and Arnold, M. F.: Arsine Poisoning. A.M.A. Arch. Indust. Hyg. and Occ. Med., *1*:437, 1950.

Steel, M., and Feltham, D. V. C.: Arsine Poisoning in Industry. Lancet, *258*:108, 1950.

Talbott, J. H.: Untoward Effects of the Newer Drugs. New York State J. Med., *48*:280, 1948.

MERCURY POISONING

Mercury has long been used in the arts and in medicine. Paracelsus (1493–1541) advocated its use for the treatment of syphilis.

ACUTE POISONING

Etiology. Acute poisoning is usually caused by ingestion of bichloride of mercury, accidentally or with suicidal intent. The absorption of mercury administered therapeutically by mouth, injection, inunction or in vaginal douches may produce a mild acute or subacute poisoning, as does, rarely, an industrial exposure to massive doses of mercury vapor. Ingestion of 0.1 gm. of mercuric chloride may result in acute poisoning, although usually 1 gm. or more is required to render the condition serious. Mercury is quickly absorbed from the stomach and, after brief storage in the liver, is widely distributed.

Morbid Anatomy. In patients dying within 24 hours after ingestion of mercury, there is observed marked gastritis and possibly some nephritis. Patients dying within two to seven days after ingestion show a necrotic nephrosis and marked colitis. Those dying after one week show a tendency toward healing of the gastric and renal lesions, but a severe gangrenous colitis.

Symptoms. The onset is usually rapid; within a few minutes after ingestion abdominal pain develops, especially in the epigastrium. This is, fortunately, in most cases associated with vomiting and rejection of part of the ingested poison. There is a metallic taste and often a marked stomatitis and congestion, or even ulceration, of the pharynx and esophagus. The vomitus may early contain blood-streaked mucus. Stools are loose and bloody. There may be prompt collapse and, in exceptional cases, delirium and convulsions. Examination of the blood during the first few days shows blood nitrogen increased, the blood chlorides reduced, and the alkali reserve lowered. When the intoxication is not promptly fatal, signs of gastrointestinal inflammation and striking evidence of injury to the kidneys usually continue. Albumin, casts and blood appear in the urine a few hours after ingestion of the poison, and gradual suppression of the urine and anuria may be noted.

Diagnosis. It is important to ascertain with certainty that mercury has been ingested. Some of the new methods for the determination of mercury are the electrolytic, dithizone, selenium sulfide, spectographic and photoelectric. Spectro-analysis has become a valuable diagnostic aid. Small amounts of mercury have been found in the urine and stools of apparently normal, healthy persons.

Prognosis. If mercurial salts are vomited within 15 minutes of ingestion, the patient usually recovers. The frequent estimation of blood nonprotein nitrogen is of aid in prognosis. The majority of deaths occur within the first two or three days. The mortality among proved cases may run over 40 per cent, though with prompt and thorough treatment in hospital it should be less than 10 per cent. If death is not caused by shock or severe gastroenteritis, it is usually attributable to kidney damage.

Treatment. Emergency treatment may include induced emesis and gastric lavage or treatment of shock. The treatment described by Weiss is devised to overcome the effects produced by the poison rather than to provide an antidote to mercury. It may be outlined as follows:

The stomach is immediately washed with a saturated solution of sodium bicarbonate, the operation being continued until the washings are clear. At least 2 liters of the solution should be used.

Lavage with 250 cc. of a 5 per cent solution of sodium formaldehyde sulfoxylate has been recommended, particularly in cases seen early. Before withdrawing the stomach tube 6 ounces of a saturated solution of magnesium sulfate are administered. A soapsuds enema is then given.

From the onset, a beverage made by dissolving 4 gm. (1 teaspoonful) of potassium bitartrate and 2 gm. (½ teaspoonful) of sodium citrate in a glass of water, orangeade or lemonade is to be administered six to eight times daily. Weiss has seldom used rectal irrigation or hot packs. He permits a liberal diet after diarrhea ceases.

Dimercaprol (BAL) has also been used with success in mercury poisoning. The initial dose should be 5 mg. per kilogram (approximately 300 mg.), intramuscularly, followed in one or two hours by a dose of 2.5 mg. per kilogram. After a lapse of 2 to 4 hours a second dose of 2.5 mg. per kilogram should be given within the first 12 hours of therapy. On the second day, two 2.5 mg. per kilogram doses may be administered. It should be emphasized that the successful treatment of arsenic or mercury poisoning with Dimercaprol depends on the institution of treatment at the earliest possible moment before irreparable tissue damage has occurred, and on the use of adequate amounts of Dimercaprol at frequent intervals.

Renal damage with suppression of urine is usually a major problem in acute mercury poisoning. For management of urinary suppression, see page 1088.

SUBACUTE POISONING

Subacute poisoning is ordinarily caused by the excessive therapeutic use of mercury. The common symptoms—salivation, gingivitis and diarrhea—subside upon withdrawal of the drug.

INDUSTRIAL POISONING

Industrial mercury poisoning is almost invariably a chronic intoxication resulting from the inhalation of volatilized mercury for a long period. One milligram of mercury per 10 cubic meters of air has been accepted by the American Standards Association as the maximum allowable concentration for work places. The most hazardous trades are the production of mercury and its derivatives, the manufacture of scientific apparatus (thermometers and barometers), the preparation of hatters' fur and felt hat making, the extraction of gold and silver by amalgamation, the application of antifouling plastic paint for the protection of hulls of warships against the growth of aquatic life, and the preparation and handling of the fulminate of mercury as a detonator of explosives. Since the recent discovery of a substitute for mercury in the treatment of fur, certain states, by agreement with the manufacturers of felt hats, have issued regulations prohibiting the use of mercurial carrot in the preparation of hatters' fur, or the use of mercurial carroted hatters' fur in the manufacture of hats.

Symptoms. Chronic mercurialism has various manifestations, not all of which may be observed in any one case. The most typical symptoms are included in the first three of the following groups:

1. *Stomatitis,* salivation, a metallic taste, reddish-brown discoloration of the buccal mucosa, gingivitis, loosening of the teeth, and occasionally a marking of the gums similar to the lead line.

2. *Erethismus mercurialis,* a peculiar psychic disturbance characterized by ready excitability and a strange shyness in the presence of strangers, a symptom of great interest and

importance; insomnia; headache; vertigo; mental depression and dullness; and, rarely, hallucinations.

3. *Tremors* of the orbit, lips, tongue, fingers and limbs. These are usually moderately fine at first, but at intervals become a coarse jerking. They may become severe and in rare instances involve contractions of the limbs of such volence as to require restraint. The tremor is intentional and subsides during rest. Under observation it may increase and diminish, rhythmically recurring. When it is marked, the patient may require assistance in eating and in other activities. Weakness of both the flexor and extensor muscles of the hand and forearm has been reported, but marked paresis is rarely, if indeed ever, caused by mercury. Polyneuritis is said to result occasionally from exposure to mercury. No ataxia occurs, and reflexes are not notably affected.

4. *Albuminuria and High Blood Pressure.* While the severe nephritis associated with acute mercurial poisoning is not associated with the chronic type, these symptoms appear with such frequency as to warrant the belief that the kidneys are usually involved in chronic poisoning.

5. *Loss of appetite, indigestion, and diarrhea* are occasionally observed. There is loss of weight in severe cases. The blood is normal except for a moderate secondary anemia.

6. *Dermatitis* characterized by erythema and desquamation is not uncommonly produced by contact with mercuric chloride or even by ingestion of mercury. In susceptible persons fulminate of mercury produces severe dermatitis. Punched-out and penetrating ulcers may develop about the fingernails and knuckles. The conjunctivas and the mucous membranes of the mouth, nose and larynx are often affected.

Prognosis. There is apparently no acquired immunity to mercury. The severity of symptoms is usually determined by the length and degree of exposure to the poison. Though most severe symptoms tend to decrease when the subject is removed from contact with mercury, such manifestations as erethism and tremor may persist for a long time.

Treatment should eliminate the metal through the bowels, kidneys and skin. In acute mercury poisoning, BAL has been effective. For the dosage of BAL, the reader is referred to the chapter on Arsenic Poisoning.

Mercury dermatitis may be prevented and to some degree relieved by application of a 10 per cent solution of sodium hyposulfite. A 2 per cent solution may be used as a wash for conjunctivitis.

W. J. McCONNELL

References

Batson, R., and Peterson, J. C.: Acute Mercury Poisoning: Treatment with BAL and, in Anuric States, with Continuous Peritoneal Lavage. Ann. Int. Med., 29:278, 1948.

Bidstrup, P. L., Bonnell, J. A., Harvey, D. G., and Locket, S.: Chronic Mercury Poisoning in Men Repairing Direct-Current Meters. Lancet, 2:856, 1951.

Lawrence, J. B.: How Poisonous is Mercury? Chem. & Eng. News, 29:3529, 1951.

Locket, S., and Nazroo, I. A.: Eye Changes Following Exposure to Metallic Mercury. Lancet, 1:528, 1952.

Longcope, W. T.: Value of BAL in the Treatment of Poisoning by Mercury Bichloride. Bull. Ayer Clin. Lab., 4:61, 1952.

Mayers, M. R.: Mercury Poisoning. Industrial Hygiene Newsletter, U.S.P.H.S., Federal Security Agency, 9:7, 1949.

Williams, C. R., Eisenbud, M., and Pihl, S. E.: Mercury Exposures in Dry Battery Manufacture. J. Indust. Hyg. & Toxicol., 29:378, 1947.

LEAD POISONING

(Plumbism)

Definition. Lead poisoning is a toxic state which results when the levels of lead absorption exceed those of excretion. Considerable amounts of toxic lead compounds may be absorbed, stored and excreted without producing intoxication. Depending on the exposure, acute or chronic poisoning with variation in the clinical picture may result. Lead poisoning in children differs strikingly from that in adults.

Etiology. Lead may be absorbed through the lungs as vapor or dust, through the gastrointestinal tract following ingestion of the metal or its compounds, or through the unbroken skin. In adults the inhalation of toxic lead compounds is the chief means of intoxication. The majority of infants become intoxicated by ingesting lead-containing paint, either by picking up flakes which are peeled off old woodwork or by chewing on painted surfaces. This habit, called pica, is often the result of mental deficiency but is also seen in children of adequate endowment, possibly because of emotional factors. Certain organic lead compounds such as tetraethyl lead are absorbed through the unbroken skin.

Dangerous paint usually contains 5 to 50 per cent lead by weight and is easily analyzed for this content, the flake eaters being poisoned by lower concentrations. Amounts of lead under 1 per cent by weight are found in many paints and are probably unimportant since the small amount of lead ingested is readily excreted. Because of its cost, lead paint is seldom used inside new buildings today, but in older houses and tenements the original paint or trim frequently contains chrome green or chrome yellow, both lead pigments. Outside white paint often contains white lead and should not be applied where children can chew it, either on porch railings, or in repainting furniture or toys at home. In sampling paint for analysis it is obviously important to include all the layers, down to the wood. Unusual sources of lead are water pipes, cisterns, lead nipple shields, or lead-containing ointments used by nursing mothers, and in the Orient, face powders containing white lead, which may contaminate the mother's skin and possibly her milk.

The solubility of a given lead compound in body fluids and the quantity in the breathing zone determine the degree of its hazard. The U.S. Public Health Service sets 0.1 mg. per liter as the limit of safety for lead in drinking water. Adults are commonly poisoned industrially by inhaling dust or fumes which contain lead compounds. Since the manufacture of lead storage batteries accounts for about one third of the industrial use of lead, lead poisoning is a prevalent hazard in this industry. Any process in which lead compounds are reduced to a fine dry dust or are volatilized by heat should be carried on only with proper safeguards. The upper limit of safety of air contamination is considered 1.5 mg. per 10 liters of air. Good hygiene throughout the work place and clean work clothes are essential in order to emphasize the toxicity of lead and prevent excess contamination.

In determining the degree of hazardous lead exposure some knowledge of common industrial usage is helpful in history-taking. Paint spraying such as is done on structural steel in highway building and paint sanding and scraping, widely practiced, are highly dangerous operations involving intense exposure to toxic white and red lead. As pointed out, modern indoor paint seldom contains lead but white lead paint is a not infrequent source of poisoning in sanding and scraping antique furniture and surfaces in old houses. Burning of lead in salvage operations, and oxy-gas cutting of red lead painted steel in dismantling elevated railways or ships, are sources of in-

toxication. Smoothing of lead surfaces with mechanical devices in automobile manufacture, a practice recently growing, is a danger. Because lead is combined with iron, copper and zinc to make bronze, with tin to make solder, with tin and antimony to make type metal, the pouring and grinding of these materials are a potential source of excessive lead exposure. Paint mixing if soluble lead compounds are used can be very hazardous. In modern industrial practice, enameling and glass manufacture are done without danger of lead exposure. Because of the great toxicity of tetraethyl lead, its use in gasoline manufacture is surrounded with elaborate safeguards in spite of which there are occasional cases of lead poisoning in this industry.

Pathology. After absorption lead is deposited at first in all the viscera but chiefly in the liver. It is soon transferred for storage to the skeleton. There it exists in the following equilibrium: $3\ PbHPO_4 \rightleftharpoons Pb_3(PO_4)_2 + H_3PO_4$. At pH 7.45 virtually all the lead is in the form of trilead phosphate which is soluble at a rate of 0.13 mg. per liter; but as the pH moves toward the acid side more and more of the dilead phosphate, which has a solubility of 12.6 mg. per liter, is formed. This salt can be redistributed by the blood stream to the liver, lungs and nervous system. Since homeostasis is relatively weak in children as compared to adults, significant changes in pH with consequent redistribution of and poisoning by lead stores in the skeleton occur in the former with relatively great frequency.

Lead may affect a wide variety of organs. In the lead poisoning of childhood both the peripheral and central nervous systems are implicated. Occasionally the spinal cord shows loss of anterior horn cells. The brain shows flattening of convolutions due to edema, increase in weight and circulatory changes secondary to thrombosis and compression of vessels and necrosis of capillaries. Herniation of the medulla through the foramen magnum is common. The cerebral hemispheres are most involved, but the cerebellum and brain stem are also affected.

During the years of rapid growth the zones of provisional calcification at the metaphysial ends of the shafts of the long bones show on microscopic examination abnormally thick and numerous trabeculae of calcification in the intercellular substance, with giant cells and abnormal osteoclasts and osteoblasts. The renal tubular cells and less frequently the hepatic cells show rather characteristic acidophilic intranuclear inclusion bodies, which are diagnostically important at autopsy, especially when combined with skeletal changes.

Symptoms and Clinical Pathology. The clinical manifestations of lead poisoning may be grouped under six physiologic systems: gastrointestinal, hematopoietic, renal, skeletal, nervous and probably general metabolic.

Gastrointestinal symptoms include colic, constipation and vomiting. Colic is severe in adults, often simulating the pain of intestinal obstruction. It is seen more strikingly in adults than children. Vomiting often occurs before breakfast and may be related to encephalitis. A flat roentgenogram of the abdomen in children who have ingested paint may show flecks of radiopaque material and may confirm pica previously unobserved by parents. The examination must be made before evacuation of the contaminated feces in the hospital.

Black deposits are frequently seen in the gum margins about pyorrheic teeth in adults and are evidences of ingestion or inhalation of lead or bismuth. Since children rarely have pyorrhea, this sign is unusual in childhood. A bit of white paper slipped between the gum and tooth makes the deposits more apparent. These deposits constitute the so-called *"lead line."*

A *hypochromic anemia* with basophilic stippling of the red cells is usual, though normochromic anemia is sometimes encountered. Pallor is usually out of proportion to the hemoglobin level and is in part the result of vasospasm. With overwhelming intoxication acholuric jaundice or even hemoglobinuria is seen. The number of stippled cells seen in any smear depends so much on the staining technique employed that no absolute figure for stippled cells is possible, but often 0.01 to 0.1 per cent of the cells show this abnormality. Stippled cells are rarely found in blood smears of normal children.

In children injury of the *renal tubules* is shown by mild glycosuria, never of great degree, in the presence of normal blood sugar levels. With Benedict's qualitative reagent green to brown precipitates are frequently encountered in children.

Coproporphyrinuria commonly accompanies lead poisoning and is presumably an evidence of the metabolic disturbance caused by the metal. It may well be the most delicate clinical indicator of the toxic action of lead. Once present it ordinarily persists for months. It is readily demonstrated by acidifying 5 cc. of urine, adding two drops of hydrogen peroxide, shaking with 5 cc. of ether and allowing 10 minutes to pass. When held under an ultraviolet light a cherry red fluorescence of the ether layer shows the presence of coproporphyrin.

The *skeletal changes* in children who have ingested toxic lead compounds are demonstrable as dense radiopaque bands at the growing ends of the shafts of the long bones and the margins of the flat bones. These are most marked at the faster growing epiphyses, such as those at the knee joint. They are usual in infants and young children with plumbism and increasingly uncommon in school age children and are not seen in adults. Withdrawal of lead is followed by their disappearance often long before the skeletal stores of lead have been excreted. Many circumstances other than lead poisoning produce densities in the roentgenogram indistinguishable from those caused by lead.

Peripheral neuritis and acute and chronic *encephalitis* are the usual neurologic manifestations of plumbism. The neuritis tends to affect the most used muscle groups rather than the muscles supplied by any one nerve, the extensors of the wrist in painters, and the dorsiflexors of the feet in children. In children, especially, the weakness may become profound and generalized. Tendon reflexes are lost in the affected muscle group, but except for some suggestions of peripheral type of ataxia, sensation remains intact.

Acute encephalopathy in adults and children usually is manifested by loss of memory, headaches, irritability and sleeplessness. In severe cases convulsions, mania and coma may finally occur. Early tendon reflexes are increased, but with severe collapse they may be lost. The spinal fluid protein content is usually increased to levels between 50 and 200 mg. per 100 cc., and occasionally lymphocytes up to 200 per cubic millimeter may be found. Total protein increase may often be found prior to the onset of acute cerebral symptoms.

Chronic encephalitis of children is characterized essentially by a failure of cerebral maturation, which may appear in the absence of preceding acute encephalitis and results in defects in attention, judgment, self-control and visual learning. Many of the young victims of plumbism may be verbally facile, but unable to master the basic school techniques of reading, writing and arithmetic in spite of fairly adequate I.Q.'s. Those who were defective prior to plumbism show the type of amentia well described by the I.Q., whereas those previously adequate often show the so-called brain injury type of psychologic impairment which may be missed by the usual I.Q. type of examination.

Diagnosis. Since none of these symptoms or signs is pathognomonic of lead poisoning, a constellation of at least one item from each of three classes is necessary to sustain a purely

lead poisoning concentrations of 0.25 mg. or more are sometimes found. In children, because of the wide fluctuations of urine volume, the measurement of the 24-hour excretion of lead should be estimated. More than 0.08 mg. per 24 hours has regularly been associated with lead poisoning (Fairhall technique of analysis), though lead poison-

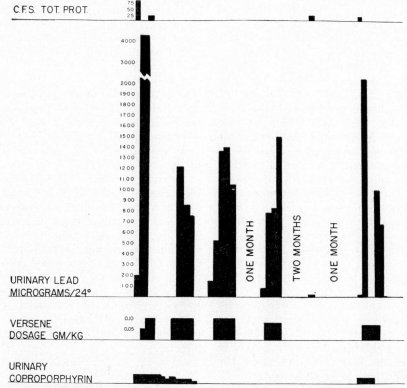

Fig. 61. Urinary output of lead in micrograms per 24 hours before and during Versene treatment, correlated with total protein in spinal fluid and urinary coproporphyrin. Recurrence of coproporphyrinuria with acute cervical adenitis four months after treatment. (Each column represents one day.)

clinical diagnosis of plumbism. When an adequate source of lead can be chemically demonstrated, symptoms from two groups are adequate to prove poisoning and from one group to indicate its probability. In the final analysis, poisoning as opposed to absorption implies some disability as the result of the chemical action of lead. From the compensation point of view the distinction between lead absorption, present in everyone, and lead poisoning is important.

The *chemical recognition* of lead poisoning, apparently so logical, is beset with difficulties. In suitably collected urine samples of about a liter amounts of lead over 0.1 mg. suggest dangerous levels of lead absorption, though in adults with no known evidence of

ing may exist in the presence of outputs of one-fourth this amount. Blood levels of lead over 0.07 mg. per 100 cc. suggest intoxication, but occasional levels up to 0.12 mg. per 100 cc. have been found in control adults with no known exposure or intoxication. Fecal excretion of over 0.5 mg. per gram of dry ash indicates a dangerous level of lead intake.

Prevention. The prevention of industrial lead poisoning is a complicated matter beyond the scope of this article. It combines regular medical examination of personnel, chemical examination of urine, engineering safety measures and personal hygiene of the workers.

Treatment. The treatment of lead poisoning depends on removal of lead from the body, relief of symptoms and prevention of after-effects.

Calcium disodium versenate given intravenously in amounts of 1 gm. per 15 kg. of body weight per day offers a safe and effective method of removing lead from the soft tissues and causing its excretion in the urine. One-half the 24-hour dose is given at intervals of 12 hours in approximately 250 to 300 cc. of 5 to 10 per cent glucose solution, an hour or so being used for each dose. A test dose of one-tenth this amount is a good precaution, but in critical situations such as acute encephalopathy should be omitted. Treatment should be continued three to five days, followed by an interval of three days, and a total of at least three or four courses should be given. Symptoms of lead poisoning usually subside in three or four days, spinal fluid total proteins return to normal in a few days, coproporphyrinuria usually disappears in ten days to two weeks and recent neuritis begins to improve in about a week.

A large fraction of the stored lead in the skeleton remains after treatment as a threat to children who may apparently without further lead exposure develop recurrences of lead poisoning over periods of at least a year and probably longer. Attacks of fever or vomiting in such children should for the present be regarded as emergencies requiring prompt investigation by tests for coproporphyrinuria and blood smears, and retreatment with Versene in hopes of preventing the chronic encephalopathy of childhood.

The recent development of an oral preparation of Versene may make it possible to continue treatment for long periods in these chronic cases. Its applicability to acute cases is still under investigation. Oral Versene is definitely dangerous if lead is being ingested.

Acute encephalopathy with evidence of medullary compression requires immediate and very extensive surgical decompression of the skull.

Acute colic is virtually instantly relieved by the intravenous administration of 10 cc. of 20 per cent calcium gluconate in adults and proportionately smaller doses in children. This measure often clarifies the differential diagnosis between lead colic and a surgical abdominal disease.

Lead neuritis requires the usual orthopedic protection of the weakened muscles and overstretched ligaments.

Patients with chronic lead poisoning should avoid excessive use of alcohol. A high calcium diet should be recommended and this should be supplemented by sunshine and vitamin B_1, but these may be dangerous if lead is still being ingested.

Following recovery from lead poisoning children must be protected against a recurrence of lead ingestion, and in most instances this means chemical recognition and removal of the offending paint from the child's environment. If this is not possible (as when paint is chewed at a neighbor's house), removal of the family to a new environment may be necessary.

Psychologic supervision is usually important in developing understanding by parents, school and social agencies of the mental and emotional consequences of lead poisoning on the growing nervous system of children. This may ameliorate social and educational difficulties.

Industrial workers should be excluded from exposure to lead unless proper precautions are observed. There is no good evidence that workers who have had lead poisoning are any more susceptible to new lead absorption than normal individuals.

An adult worker recovered from lead intoxication needs the benefit of adequate protective devices and medical control if for economic reasons he returns to a potential lead exposure. Obviously, repeated attacks mean he must find work in a lead-free atmosphere.

RANDOLPH K. BYERS

References

Aub, J. S., Fairhall, L. T., Minot, A. S., and Resnikoff, P.: Lead Poisoning. Medicine, 4:1, 1925.

Byers, R. K., Maloof, C. C., DeSimone, A., and Morrell, M. E.: The Use of Calcium Disodium Versenate in The Treatment of Lead Poisoning in Children. Am. J. Dis. Children, 87:559, 1954.

Hamilton, Alice, and Hardy, Harriet: Industrial Toxicology. New York, Paul B. Hoeber, 1949.

Ingraham, F., and Matson, D. D.: Neurosurgery of Infancy and Childhood. Springfield, Illniois, Charles C Thomas, 1953.

Karpinski, F. E., Jr., Rieders, F., and Girsh, L. S.: Calcium Disodium Versenate in The Therapy of Lead Encephalopathy. J. Pediat., 42:687, 1953.

Maloof, C. C.: Role of Porphyrins in Occupational Disease. 1. Significance of Coproporphyrins in Lead Workers. Arch. Indust. Hyg., 1:296, 1950.

Mayers, M. R.: Lead Poisoning. Oxford Loose-Leaf Medicine Vol. 4. New York, Oxford University Press, 1951, p. 662.

Occupational Lead Exposure and Lead Poisoning. Report of Committee on Lead Poisoning. New York, Am. Pub. Health Association, 1943.

BERYLLIUM POISONING
(Berylliosis)

Definition. Beryllium poisoning, or beryl-liosis, is a general term which includes all those acute and chronic manifestations resulting from exposure to the fumes and dusts of beryllium salts and alloys. In human beings the major clinical forms have been characterized chiefly by acute pneumonitis and chronic pulmonary granulomatosis. Surface contact with the material may cause lesions such as conjunctivitis, corneal ulcer, dermatitis on the hands, arms, face, and neck, skin ulcer or granuloma, and subcutaneous granuloma.

Pathology. In the acute form of the disease the lungs present a picture of bilateral diffuse pneumonitis with pronounced intra-alveolar and interstitial exudates. The air spaces are filled with plasma cells, lymphocytes and mononuclear phagocytes, attended occasionally with edema and hemorrhagic extravasation. These may infiltrate the smaller blood vessels and bronchioles. There is an early proliferation of fibroblasts. Unlike cases of acute chemical pneumonitis from other causes, the polymorphonuclear leukocytes are relatively absent.

The chronic form of the disease is characterized by marked emphysema and a bilateral diffuse granular or nodular infiltration scattered through the lung fields. The normal structure of the lungs may be altered and is often obliterated by these changes.

The nodular granulomatous lesions are located in the thickened walls of the alveoli and in the fibrous tissue around the bronchi and blood vessels. The central core of the lesions consists of fibrinoid material, lymphocytes, plasma cells, large mononuclear phagocytes and giant cells of the Langhans type. The peripheral zone consists of fibrous tissue infiltrated with small round cells. Giant cells may or may not be present. Conchoidal bodies are present in most cases.

The mediastinal and axillary lymph nodes are infiltrated in some instances by a similar granulomatous process. Liver involvement also has been observed. The skin and subcutaneous tissues may be the sites of granulomas following accidental introduction of beryllium compounds.

Morbid Physiology. The extensive changes in the parenchymal lung tissue and associated thickening of the walls of the alveoli interfere seriously with cell metabolism and the exchange of gases in the lungs. Occasional deaths from failure of the right side of the heart occur.

Symptoms. The acute form of the disease develops usually after a relatively short period of exposure. The symptoms may appear insidiously or suddenly, beginning with an acute irritation of the upper respiratory tract; cough which is often nonproductive; dyspnea; substernal discomfort or pain; anorexia; weakness; and weight loss. The objective signs reveal a thin anxious person with little or no elevation in body temperature. There is usually some swelling and redness of the mucous membranes of the nose and throat. Cyanosis is evident in severe cases. Rales may be detected in both lung fields. Vital capacity is diminished. The illness may subside within a few weeks or extend into several months.

The symptoms and signs in chronic cases appear insidiously and include exertional dyspnea, weakness, irritative cough and weight loss. The onset of symptoms may be delayed for periods of several weeks to five or six years following termination of exposure. As the disease progresses, the symptoms become more localized and intense. There is a progressive loss in weight and variable degrees of respiratory distress. The patient appears nervous and complains of pain in the chest and abdomen, weakness and fatigability. Cyanosis and clubbing of the nails may be present. The pulse rate is usually increased, and definitely accelerated in cases of cyanosis. The blood pressure usually drops during the course of the disease. Rales and loss of resonance have been observed. Reduction in vital capacity may become marked as the disease progresses. The duration of the disease is prolonged usually for a period of several months.

Diagnosis. The diagnosis is made after a careful evaluation of the occupational history, type of onset and clinical manifestations, roentgenographic characteristics, and chemical findings of beryllium in tissues obtained by skin biopsy or in the urine.

The occupational history should include all occupations in which the patient has been engaged and the duration of employment in each, as well as all obtainable information on the amount and kind of dust and fumes to which he has been exposed and the extent to which protective devices were used. The inhalation of beryllium dust after breaking fluorescent lamps may occur, and this possibility should be inquired into when taking the history.

In roentgenographs of the lungs in acute pneumonitis a diffuse haziness may be noted two to three weeks after the early symptoms of the disease. There is usually prominence of the peribronchial markings and irregular opaque shadows suggestive of pulmonary edema, followed by discrete small or large conglomerate nodules scattered throughout both lung fields. Clearing of lung fields occurs usually after one to four months.

The roentgenographic changes in the chronic disease are characterized by small discrete stippling and fine nodulation scattered throughout both lung fields, resembling the shadows cast in miliary tuberculosis, in sarcoidosis and in early, uncomplicated silicosis. As the disease progresses, confluent nodular shadows with emphysematous spaces between appear throughout both lung fields. There may be an accompanying enlargement of the hilar lymph nodes.

Prognosis. The course and prognosis of beryllium poisoning depend largely upon the form of the disease. The mortality rate is low in the acute form. Only occasionally has death occurred early in its course. The transition from acute pneumonitis to chronic pulmonary granulomatosis has so far rarely been observed. Machle and his co-workers, however, report that an attack of acute disease has been followed two years later by the onset of chronic berylliosis, and gradations of intermediate degree occur.

The chronic course of the disease is one of protracted convalescence in a few, and gradual progression and eventually death in many. Machle reports a fatality rate of 20 per cent in his series of cases. Cutaneous lesions do not readily heal unless all particles of the beryllium material are removed and granulomas of the skin are excised.

Treatment. In the absence of specific therapy in the acute and chronic pulmonary forms of the disease, the treatment must be largely supportive. Enforced bed rest in early and severe cases is indicated. Oxygen therapy is required to overcome cyanosis and dyspnea, and to prolong life. Cortisone and ACTH have been shown to induce striking improvement in pulmonary function with marked clinical improvement in a number of patients with pulmonary granulomatosis. Antibiotics may be of value in preventing secondary infections.

Dermatitis and conjunctivitis, although severe at times, tend to clear up after removal from work. The application of a mild antipruritic or antihistaminic ointment may aid in the treatment of affected skin areas, and a soothing antibiotic ophthalmic ointment may be applied in cases of conjunctivitis. Cutaneous ulcers are best treated by scraping away the base of the ulcer with a curet. Cutaneous and subcutaneous granulomas should be widely excised.

Prevention. Prevention consists in both medical and engineering control. A periodic checking of workers possibly exposed to beryllium-containing fumes and dusts is a valuable health measure in detecting early cases. A monthly check of each worker's body weight for evidence of persistent loss, and interrogation as to symptoms, such as cough, anorexia and fatigue, is desirable. When suspicion points to possible disease of the respiratory system, a roentgenogram of the chest should be made. All workers incurring breaks in the skin should be required to seek immediate treatment so that the medical attendant can remove all particles of beryllium compounds in the wound.

Good engineering practice consists in meticulous housekeeping and systematic determinations of the beryllium content of air at breathing levels of the workers. Until safe limits of concentrations are determined, every effort should be made through engineering control methods to prevent beryllium-containing fumes or dusts from escaping into the atmosphere.

W. J. McConnell

References

DeNardi, Joseph M., Van Ordstrand, H. S., Curtis, George H., and Zielinski, John: Berylliosis. A.M.A. Arch. Indust. Hyg. and Occ. Med., 8:1, 1953.

Hardy, H. L., and Tabershaw, I. R.: Delayed Chemical Pneumonitis Occurring in Workers Exposed to Beryllium Compounds. J. Indust. Hyg. & Toxicol., 28:197, 1946.

Machle, W., Beyer, E., and Gregorius, F.: Berylliosis. Occup. Med., 5:671, 1948.

Symposium on the Treatment of Chronic Beryllium Poisoning with ACTH and Cortisone. A.M.A. Arch. Indust. Hyg. and Occ. Med., 3:543, 1951.

U. S. Atomic Energy Commission Symposium on Beryllium. AECD-1803. Obtainable from Technical Information Division, Oak Ridge, Tenn.

Vorwald, A. J.: Pathologic Aspects of Acute Pneumonitis and Pulmonary Granulomatosis in Beryllium Workers. Occup. Med. 5:684, 1948.

RADIATION INJURY

Definition. The term "radiation injury" describes a number of clinical syndromes which have exposure to ionizing radiation as a common etiology. The term "radiation sickness" has generally been used to designate the nausea and loss of appetite which follow exposure to penetrating radiations used for therapeutic purposes. Radiation injury in a less restrictive sense is reserved to indicate those clinical and subclinical manifestations which result from toxic local or general exposure to penetrating radiations originating from an external source or from the presence of radio-elements within the body itself. For practical purposes, the agents capable of producing injury to the body are x-rays, gamma rays, fast and slow neutrons, beta and alpha particles. Radiation which arises from sources outside the body is conventionally referred to as external radiation, while radiation arising from radio-elements within the body is referred to as internal radiation.

Etiology. Beta particles are energetic electrons which travel several millimeters in tissues; ordinary alpha particles are helium nuclei which travel a maximum of about 40 microns in tissue; whereas energetic x-rays, gamma rays or fast neutrons are many times more penetrating than either. X-rays and gamma rays expend their energy and produce biologic effects in cells and tissues by the acceleration of electrons; fast neutrons by acceleration of protons (hydrogen nuclei), and slow neutrons by the release of gamma rays or fast atomic nuclei when they are captured by the atomic nuclei of the chemical elements present in the tissue. Thus the significant sources of external radiation include all those mentioned except alpha particles. Internal radiation involves alpha and beta particles and gamma rays.

The clinical manifestations of exposure to radiation vary because the injury sustained depends on the type and energy of the radiation, the area of the body exposed, and the dose and the length of time over which a given dose is sustained. The biologic effects of penetrating ionizing radiation delivered to the whole body within a few milliseconds or minutes will differ remarkably from the effects resulting if this same amount of radiation is sustained over a period of weeks, months or years. The degree of selective localization of radio-elements within the body and the half life of the isotope are additional factors to be taken into consideration.

Radiation exposure until 1934 was largely confined to professional and technical personnel involved in the preparation of radium and its by-products, to persons employed in the manufacture of x-ray tubes and equipment or engaged in the diagnostic and therapeutic use of x-rays and gamma rays, and to a lesser extent to persons using these radiations as tools of physical research. The invention of the cyclotron by Lawrence in 1934 brought the added hazard of the fast neutron and gamma rays and artificial radioelements. In 1942 the first chain-reacting uranium pile was placed in operation by Enrico Fermi, adding as a consequence a radiation hazard several thousand times greater than that which had existed theretofore. Thus the uranium pile, the processing of the many radio-elements produced in the fission reaction and the increased medical and research uses of radiation and radio-elements and the eventuality of atomic warfare make the prevention, diagnosis and treatment of acute and incipient radiation injury a public health problem of growing national importance.

The entry of radioactive elements into the body may occur as a result of ingestion (deliberate or accidental), inhalation, introduction through penetrating wounds, absorption through the skin or deliberate intravenous administration, as in the use of these materials for therapeutic purposes.

Measurement of Radiations and "Tolerance" or "Permissible Exposure." In 1931 a committee of the Bureau of Standards set 0.1 roentgen per day of x-rays or gamma rays as the "tolerance" or permissible dose to which the human body could be exposed indefinitely without the production of harmful effects. More recently the permissible dose has been reduced to 0.3 roentgen per week. The maximum permissible dose of certain radio-elements with long half lives that may be accumulated in the body has also been established.

The unit of measurement of ionizing radiations for medical and biological purposes is the roentgen. A roentgen designates that amount of radiation which corresponds to an energy absorption of about 83 ergs per gram of tissue.

Experimental Radiation Injury. Experiments on animals have been performed to give baseline information and to supplement the very limited data that are available on the effects of ionizing radiations in human beings. The reader is referred to papers by Prosser, Lorenz, Friedman, Dunlap, and Jacobson, since only a brief summary of these studies is presented here.

Single Exposure (Whole Body) to Dosages in the Midlethal Range. The dosages of x radiation required to kill half of irradiated groups of animals (within thirty days) of the species commonly used in laboratories are:

Guinea pig . . . . 250 roentgens
Dog . . . . 325 roentgens
Goat . . . . 350 roentgens
Mouse . . . . 550 roentgens
Rat . . . . 650 roentgens
Rabbit . . . . 800 roentgens

In all these species death usually occurs between the sixth and the fourteenth days. The chief pathologic findings are confined largely to the hematopoietic system, the gastrointestinal tract and the gonads. Doses below the midlethal point produce progressively less damage in these species. Single doses below 25 roentgens produce neither hematologic nor histopathologic evidence of effect.

Repeated Exposure (Whole Body) to Relatively Low Dosages in the Permissible Range. Experiments on mice, guinea pigs and rabbits indicate that a dosage of 0.1 roentgen per day (radium-gamma rays) is tolerated throughout the normal life span of the animal (more than three years) without the appearance of recognizable evidence of damage, except for an increased incidence of ovarian tumors in female mice. With dosages of 1, 2, 4 or 8 roentgens per day, the hematopoietic depression, shortening of the life span, and the incidence of sterility and of benign and malignant tumors becomes increasingly more significant.

Morbid Anatomy. The pathologic changes associated with whole body exposure to lethal or semilethal doses of penetrating radiations (400 to 600 roentgens) as described by Warren are essentially limited to the findings of an aplastic marrow, depletion of lymphatic tissue, destruction and atrophy of gonadal tissue, edema, mucosal sloughing and hemorrhage in the gastrointestinal tract, multiple pyogenic abscesses or other infection, hemorrhages in the skin, subcutaneous tissue, muscle and viscera, and an increase in tissue mast cells. Erythema, edema, loss of skin surface with delayed healing, and epilation are common after exposure to doses of about 600

roentgens or more. Doses below the lethal range produce correspondingly less pathologic change.

Acute or chronic exposure to whole or partial body radiation below the lethal but above the permissible range may produce no demonstrable pathologic effects, or the effects may be confined to degenerative changes in the hematopoietic system, gonads, skin, and eyes and to the induction of neoplasms.

The pathologic changes associated with radioactive elements such as radium, strontium and plutonium which are deposited largely in bone are a hyperplastic immature or aplastic type of marrow, rarefaction of bone, fracture and incomplete healing, irregularities of the epiphysis, and growth arrest. As described by Martland, sarcomas of bone are complications of these long-lived "bone seekers."

Pathologic Physiology and Chemistry. Absorption of radiation in cells and fluids of the body is attended by release of energy. This release of energy is considered by many authorities to consist of transient ionization of water molecules followed by the formation of hydrogen peroxide and chemical radicals which in turn inhibit or denature the sensitive enzymes or enzyme systems. There is a great difference in the radiosensitivity of cell types within the body. The radiosensitivity of the same cell type differs from person to person and from species to species. Rapidly proliferating cells such as lymphocytes and spermatogonia are more radiosensitive than the cells of the brain or the kidney. Cells in mitosis, especially in prophase, are more susceptible to radiation injury than cells in the resting phase. It is also apparent that a latent period varying from minutes to years may be interposed between the initial effect of irradiation on cells and their death or functional derangement.

In acute lethal or midlethal radiation injury, regeneration and repair proceed too slowly to overcome the overwhelming pathologic alteration induced by the widespread death of cells. In chronic radiation exposure, regeneration and repair may so closely parallel injury that pathologic alteration does not become manifest for long periods of time, if at all.

No single organ system or tissue appears to be universally critical in producing death after lethal or midlethal whole body exposure to single doses of external radiation. Death appears to occur usually as a result of a combination of pathologic processes which include plasma and electrolyte loss, destruction of hematopoietic tissue, infection, hemorrhage and nonspecific toxemia.

The functional effects of acute or chronic external exposure, such as temporary or permanent sterility and amenorrhea, can usually be correlated directly with pathologic changes in the ovary or testes. On the other hand, the altered capillary physiology, the role of histamine release, the loss of adrenal lipid, the increased incidence of neoplasia and accelerated aging process are as yet poorly understood from the standpoint of the mechanism of the acute or chronic radiation injury syndrome.

Symptoms and Signs. Injury from overwhelming doses to the whole body is followed within minutes to hours by severe nausea, vomiting and diarrhea, erythema and edema of the skin, severe prostration, circulatory collapse, coma and death within 48 hours.

Lethal or near-lethal doses (400 to 600 roentgens) produce severe weakness, malaise and prostration, nausea and vomiting and diarrhea within a few hours after exposure. Fever appears within the first 24 hours. Infections such as painful ulcerations in the throat or about the teeth, skin abscesses or evidence of other local or more general infection appear after two to four days. Bleeding from the gums and bloody diarrhea usually appear at the end of the first week after exposure and may increase in extent and severity through the third week or more unless recovery or death occurs. Disorientation may appear early and progress to coma. If patients survive infection, hemorrhage and shock resulting from plasma and electrolyte imbalance in the first three to four weeks, anemia may be sufficiently severe as a result of hemorrhage and failure of marrow recovery to produce death. Temporary or permanent sterility, amenorrhea and an increased incidence of acute and chronic leukemia are observed in survivors.

Whole body exposure to single doses of 200 to 400 roentgens of penetrating radiation can be expected to produce marked weakness, malaise, nausea, vomiting and diarrhea. Individual susceptibility will dictate the outcome of persons in the group in the absence of supportive treatment. All will have leukopenia and thrombocytopenia, but the seriousness of infection, anemia, hemorrhage and electrolyte imbalance will vary from mild to severe. Death can be expected to occur in less than 50 per cent of this group from circulatory collapse, infection, hemorrhage or combinations thereof. Temporary sterility and epilation will occur in an unpredictable number of the persons thus exposed.

Single doses of 100 to 200 roentgens can be expected to produce nausea, vomiting, anorexia, malaise, fever and diarrhea. These symptoms would appear early, but would be transient. Leukopenia and thrombocytopenia would occur, but variability in the severity should be expected. Hemorrhagic manifestations would be moderate or absent, an anemia would be unlikely. Recovery could be expected in all persons so exposed.

Single doses of 50 to 100 roentgens produce no symptoms, or only a mild nausea and malaise. Reduction in leukocyte and platelet values of the peripheral blood may occur in an occasional person, but will be transient. No symptoms or signs occur from whole body exposure to 25 roentgens or less.

Injury from chronic exposure to radiation of external origin produces local or general symptoms and signs, depending on whether whole or partial body exposure was sustained. Delayed healing of abrasions or the development of painful benign or malignant ulceration in the friable, atrophic skin of the hands may be distressing. Weakness and fatigue are associated with the onset of a leukemia or the presence of an anemia and may also occur in circumstances in which only a leukopenia is demonstrable. Premature menopause with its attending symptoms in the female and sterility in the male with aspermia or morphologically abnormal sperm may occur. The development of lens opacities is attended with a gradual loss of vision.

The clinical picture produced by lethal amounts of radioactive elements such as radiophosphorus (P^{32}) or radiostrontium (Sr^{89}) is similar in most respects to that observed after lethal doses of whole body radiation from an external source, except that the onset of symptoms is delayed. The symptoms preceding death are chiefly due to severe anemia, leukopenia and thrombocytopenia with widespread hemorrhage or infection, or both, since these radioactive elements seriously affect the hematopoietic system. Lesser amounts of these and other radioisotopes produce signs and symptoms dependent on the degree of localization. For example, after the administration of radioiodine (I^{131}) in single or divided doses sufficient to produce a remission in hyperthyroidism, hypothyroidism may insidiously supervene as a result of thyroid destruction.

Since, in therapeutic radiology, every effort is made to minimize discomfort to the patient or damage to normal tissue, complications are relatively rare. Nausea, anorexia and malaise are frequently associated with therapeutic radiation involving abdominal viscera; diarrhea may supervene in some instances. Leukopenia, thrombocytopenia and anemia occasionally complicate therapeutic irradiation when the portals involve hematopoietic tissue.

Diagnosis. The diagnosis of radiation injury after whole body exposure to a single burst of penetrating radiation in or near the lethal range as a result of accidents involving cyclotrons, betatrons, large gamma ray sources, and nuclear reactors will offer no problem; the difficulty will be found in establishing the exact or approximate dose received and thus the probable prognosis or, in the case of an atomic bomb, attempting to distinguish radiation injury from thermal and blast injury. With doses below the lethal range, but above 100 roentgens, the characteristic symptoms of nausea, vomiting, diarrhea, anorexia and malaise are likely to appear within hours of the exposure, while the leukopenia and thrombocytopenia follow within a week, and anemia even later. Temporary, complete or partial epilation, temporary sterility in both males and females and temporary amenorrhea in women should always be looked for after exposures in this range. The diagnosis of radiation injury after accidental or therapeutic exposure of a part of the body to single or divided doses of penetrating external radiation may rest on the history, since the local findings, the symptoms and hematologic picture will depend to a large extent on the size of the area irradiated and the total dose sustained.

The diagnosis of radiation injury from chronic exposure to external radiation above the permissible range is based on the history of exposure plus such findings as dermatitis, atrophy or distortion of the epidermal ridges of the fingers, hyperkeratosis, epilation, indolent skin ulcers, neoplasia, sterility, amenorrhea, lens opacities and hematologic abnormalities.

Even in the presence of suggestive clinical or laboratory evidence of radiation injury from internal emitters such as radium and plutonium, the diagnosis must be confirmed on the basis of the demonstration of evidence of actual deposition within the body. This may be done by survey of the body with a modified Geiger counter, or isolation and identification of the radio-element in the urine.

Prophylaxis. Prevention of radiation injury involves the maintenance of conditions which reduce the hazard of exposure to external and internal radiation to the permissible dose level or below. The techniques involved in working with radiations require special experience and knowledge if chronic overexposure and disastrous accidents are to be avoided. Orientation of personnel should precede work with penetrating radiations or radioactive elements. Such orientation should embrace: (1) understanding of "permissible exposure" and basic knowledge of the biologic effects and physical properties of radiation; (2) understanding of the principles of radiation protection from the various radiations; (3) ability to utilize existing instruments for determining a given radiation hazard; (4) familiarity with the techniques and procedures basic to work with these physical agents.

The supervisor must assume the responsibility for his professional and technical staff and demand and enforce observation of accepted standards of operation. One careless person working with radioactive elements can hopelessly contaminate a laboratory and jeopardize the health of his colleagues.

Even when the most stringent precautions are enforced to minimize radiation exposure, such as education of personnel, shielding of radiation sources and effective ventilation, the following additional precautions must be observed: (1) periodic medical examination, which should include a general physical examination with special reference to evidence of atrophic changes in the skin or of dermatitis; (2) periodic hematologic studies to detect leukopenia, thrombocytopenia or anemia; (3) daily monitoring of skin and clothing of personnel for contamination with radioactive elements; (4) periodic examination of urine, sputum, feces and exhaled air from personnel to detect actual presence of radio-elements in the body; (5) continuous monitoring of personnel during working hours in order to measure dose received (film badge, pocket electroscope, and so on); (6) periodic monitoring of laboratory facilities or radiation source installation for evidence of radioactive contamination or unsuspected faulty shielding. This involves analysis of air samples in certain circumstances.

Evidence of actual overexposure of a person (physical measurements) or clinical or laboratory evidence of radiation injury should be followed by immediate removal of the person from all sources of further exposure until the situation can be properly assessed and remedial measures instituted if necessary. The decision whether a person once or repeatedly overexposed to radiation, with or without evidence of radiation injury, may or may not be allowed to continue work with radiation will be difficult to make with certainty.

Treatment. In general, there is no specific treatment for radiation injury. Treatment of radiation injury from single doses in the lethal range consists largely in symptomatic, supportive and prophylactic measures. Maintenance of fluid and electrolyte balance with physiologic saline and other necessary aids, combating protein deficiency and vascular collapse by the liberal administration of plasma and whole blood, parenteral feeding with glucose and protein digests, prevention or management of infection with antibiotics, management of blood loss with whole blood transfusion, compression bandages for severe surface burns, and liberal use of sedation such as morphine for pain and restlessness are the major steps to be taken. In the event of an atomic bomb the treatment would be essentially similar, except that the flash burns and penetrating wounds would require immediate attention. The severe nausea, vomiting and diarrhea which attend serious radiation injury respond poorly to any attempt at specific management. Persons exposed to doses of whole body radiation below the mid-lethal range, but from which gastrointestinal symptoms, infection and hemorrhage of unpredictable seriousness may arise, should be managed in accordance with the clinical and laboratory evidence of involvement.

The treatment of accidental or deliberate exposure of limited areas of the body to external radiation with injury to vital internal organs or tissues or damage to the skin (erythema) will depend on the area involved and the severity of the pathologic process.

Treatment of evidence of radiation injury resulting from chronic exposure to penetrating external radiation should begin by removal of the person from further exposure or reducing the exposure to permissible or negligible levels. Such manifestations as radiation dermatitis, atrophy of the skin, indolent ulcers, carcinoma of the skin, leukopenia, leukemia and lens opacities will require specific symptomatic, supportive treatment or corrective surgery.

The treatment of radiation injury following the entrance of massive doses of radio-elements into the body is essentially similar to the treatment of massive exposure to penetrating external radiation. No effective methods are available which materially hasten the excretion of radio-elements fixed in the body. The treatment of the anemia, leukopenia, thrombocytopenia and hemorrhagic manifestations which follow therapeutic administration of radiophosphorus (P^{32}), radiosodium (Na^{24}) and radiostrontium (Sr^{89}) is largely confined to blood transfusion and the use of antibiotics as indicated if local or general infection occurs.

LEON O. JACOBSON

References

Dunlap, C. E.: Effects of Radiation on the Blood and the Hemopoietic Tissues, Including the Spleen, the Thymus, and the Lymph Nodes. Arch. Path., 34:562, 1942.

Folley, J. H., Borges, W., and Yamawaki, T.: Incidence of Leukemia in Survivors of the Atomic Bomb in Hiroshima and Nagasaki. Japan. Am. J. Med. 13:311, 1952.

Friedman, N. B.: Effects of Radiation on the Gastrointestinal Tract, Including the Salivary Glands, the Liver, and the Pancreas. Arch. Path., 34:749, 1942.

Hamilton, J. G.: The Metabolism of the Fission Products and the Heaviest Elements. Radiology, 49:325, 1947.

Hollaender, A., Ed.: Radiation Biology. New York, McGraw-Hill Co., 1954.

Jacobson, L. O., and Marks, E. K.: The Hematological Effects of Ionizing Radiations in the Tolerance Range. Radiology, 49:286, 1947.

Jacobson, L. O., Stone, R. S., and Allen, J. G.: Physicians in an Atomic War. J.A.M.A., 139:138, 1949.

Lorenz, E., Heston, W. E., Eschenbrenner, A. B., and Deringer, M. K.: Biological Studies in the Tolerance Range. Radiology, 49:274, 1947.

Martland, H. S.: The Occurrence of Malignancy in Radioactive Persons. Am. J. Cancer, 15:2435, 1931.

Prosser, C. L., and others: The Clinical Sequence of Physiological Effects of Ionizing Radiation in Animals. Radiology, 49:299, 1947.

Warren, S.: The Pathologic Effects of an Instantaneous Dose of Radiation. Cancer Research, 6:449, 1946.

WAR GASES

Certain war gases, notably the nerve gases and mustard gas, are capable of inflicting heavy casualties on an unprepared civilian population. The nerve gases are extremely toxic and are suitable for long-range air attack. For shorter-range attacks, mustard gas is effective in inflicting large numbers of burns and in denying the use of important facilities by hazardous contamination. This presentation is limited to these two types. The reader is referred to the armed services manual "Treatment of Chemical Warfare Casualties" for more comprehensive discussion.

THE NERVE GASES

Properties. The nerve gases are a family of colorless, essentially odorless, liquid, organic phosphorus compounds. They are extremely toxic on inhalation of the vapors or by absorption of the liquids through the skin or mucous membranes. *Sarin* is largely vaporized by explosive munitions into a highly lethal, but nonpersistent, gas cloud. Others vaporize slowly and are more persistent.

Mechanism of Action. Nerve gases inhibit cholinesterase irreversibly, causing the accumulation of acetylcholine in the central and peripheral nervous systems. Parasympathomimetic effects predominate, and uncontrolled potentiation of synaptic and myoneural transmission and grand mal convulsions, followed by synaptic and myoneural depression and generalized flaccid paralysis, occur.

Morbid Anatomy. Lesions characterizing asphyxial death are typical and the pharynx and larger air passages may contain much fluid and ropy mucus. The constricted pupils dilate terminally.

Symptoms. Traces of vapor induce miosis, mild intermittent bronchoconstriction and watery nasal discharge. Slightly greater exposure increases bronchoconstriction and causes ciliary spasm, with pain in or back of the globes, headache and photophobia. One or a few breaths of a high concentration of vapor cause the rapid development of most of the classic symptoms of both muscarine and nicotine poisonings. Tightness in the chest and beginning muscular incoordination are noted in a few seconds, and marked miosis, collapse and unconsciousness develop within a minute. Massive salivation, increased mucoid secretions in the upper respiratory tract, labored and stertorous respiration, falling pulse rate and blood pressure, muscular twitching and jerking, clonic and tonic convulsions, followed in severe cases by flaccid paralysis and respiratory failure, all occur in the next 2 to 4 minutes. Without treatment, asphyxia, cyanosis, circulatory collapse and cardiac arrest may lead to fatal termination in 5 to 10 minutes.

Liquid nerve gas absorbed through the eye or digestive tract produces similar symptoms with equal rapidity. Absorption through the skin is slower and symptoms may not occur for 5 to 40 minutes. Sweating, persistent for days, and muscular twitching at the site of skin contamination may occur. Temporary mental depression and irritability sometimes follow nerve gas poisoning.

Diagnosis. Timely diagnosis depends upon recognition of anticholinesterase poisoning, plus knowledge of an enemy attack resulting in numerous similar casualties. Diagnosis can be confirmed by measuring the cholinesterase activity of the erythrocytes, which may be below 25 per cent of normal in severe cases.

Prognosis. Prompt treatment can save victims of several lethal doses of nerve gas, but under war conditions most apneic cases may die. Victims who escape respiratory paralysis usually recover, though occasional deaths from vascular collapse may occur. Survivors have shown no sequelae, but hypoxic cerebral damage is possible in apneic cases. Symptomatic recovery usually is complete in one to two weeks, but normal cholinesterase levels are not restored for two to three months.

Treatment. The basic treatment consists in *large* doses of atropine, plus artificial respiration for apneic cases. Mild symptoms, except ocular, are relieved by oral doses of 1 mg. of atropine sulfate every 4 to 8 hours, as required for mild atropinization (dry mouth), for 12 to 48 hours. More severe ambulatory cases require intramuscular injections of 2 mg. of atropine sulfate every 30 minutes for mild atropinization, and maintenance of atropinization thereafter, as required for relief of symptoms, by 1 mg. oral doses for one to three days.

Miosis, ciliary spasm and headache are relieved by ocular instillations of 2 per cent homatropine hydrobromide or 1 per cent atropine sulfate solutions until mydriasis is obtained and repeated as often as miosis returns.

Severe cases usually collapse in the contaminated area, which the physician cannot enter without a military-type gas mask. If he has none, others who have must rescue and transfer the victim to clean air. If this cannot be done in seconds, the victim must be protected with a gas mask from additional exposure. If rescue requires several minutes, the rescuers must initiate treatment, or the patient may reach the physician too late to revive.

If the patient is breathing but is unconscious or in convulsions, 6 mg. of atropine sulfate* should be injected intravenously or intramuscularly immediately. The physician should continue injections of 2 mg. of atropine sulfate, intravenously if possible, every 15 minutes until atropinization is achieved (increased pulse rate, decreased salivation). Atropinization should be maintained with intramuscular injections of 2 mg. until consciousness returns, and then with oral doses of 1 mg., for one to two days. One milligram oral doses thereafter should be employed every 4 to 8 hours, as long as needed to control symptoms.

If convulsions are exhausting or cause cyanosis, they should be controlled symptomatically, with ether anesthesia or intravenous thiopental sodium, until they cease to threaten life, but depression of respiration should be avoided by using minimal dosage. Muscular fasciculations are not dangerous and their control with intramuscular magnesium sulfate is too hazardous to justify its use. If the patient is unduly apprehensive, mild sedatives may be administered.

The apneic victim requires removal of massive secretions by improvised prone postural drainage and wiping the pharynx, or by aspiration through a large bore (quarter-inch internal diameter) catheter, followed at once by artificial respiration. A mechanical resuscitator, if immediately available, may be tried, using intermittent positive pressure in preference to "suck-and-blow." If not available, the arm lift-back pressure manual (modified Holger-Nielsen) method of artificial respiration should be used and an oropharyngeal airway should be inserted if available. As necessary, artificial respiration should be interrupted *briefly* for administra-

* Atropine Ampins (Strong, Cobb & Co., Cleveland, Ohio) or Atropine Syrettes (E. R. Squibb & Sons, New York City) each contain the equivalent of 2 mg. of atropine sulfate, ready for immediate injection, and are convenient for this purpose.

tion of the required atropine, using dosages described above. If possible the patient should be transferred to a body respirator, because several hours of artificial respiration may be required. Convulsions are absent, since these patients are paralyzed, and convulsions do not recur with return of muscular function. Consciousness and muscular control return soon after spontaneous respiration begins.

Liquid contaminations are highly dangerous and must be removed *quickly*. Contaminated clothing should be removed and *left outdoors*. Contaminated skin should be flooded with water and then washed gently with soap and rinsed. The skin must not be rubbed with dry materials, for this increases absorption. Swabbing with 5 per cent sodium carbonate solution is best, if it is immediately available. A patient should never be brought indoors until all liquid contamination is removed, for the vapors endanger other patients and attendants.

MUSTARD GAS

Properties. Mustard gas, bis-(beta-chloroethyl) sulfide, $S\text{-}(CH_2CH_2Cl)_2$, is a colorless to brown oily liquid, heavier than water, with an odor like horseradish or garlic. It is soluble in fats, oils and organic solvents, but only slightly in water. It vaporizes slowly to yield toxic, highly vesicant vapors. Its principal use is to contaminate facilities and terrain. This is accomplished from the air by bombs or spray, and on the ground by chemical mortar and artillery shells and land mines. Hazardous contamination persists for days to weeks.

Mechanism of Action. Mustard gas is a general cytotoxic poison, which inhibits or destroys many enzymes, notably hexokinase. It produces necrotizing lesions of the skin and mucous membranes. Rarely, systemic absorption of liquid mustard injures hematopoietic tissues, producing leukopenia and thrombocytopenia, and depresses cholinesterase activity, giving moderate parasympathomimetic effects. Extensive, severe mustard burns may cause shock and derangements of fluid and electrolyte balances, similar to those seen in thermal burns. Its cytotoxic effects are highly cumulative and irreversible.

Morbid Anatomy. Hyperemia and edema of the conjunctivas and necrosis of corneal tissue external to Bowman's membrane are the common eye changes, though occasionally iritis and deep corneal ulcerations and vascularization occur.

Hyperemia and patchy necrosis of the lining epithelium of the upper respiratory tract occur with moderate exposures. With severe exposure, exudation below the larynx produces a pseudomembrane which may form a cast of the tracheobronchial tree, and there is congestion, scattered edema, moderate emphysema and focal atelectasis of the lung parenchyma. Secondary infection, with development of bronchitis or bronchopneumonia, is common. Chronic bronchitis, bronchiectasis and pulmonary fibrosis are found in chronic exposure cases.

Hyperemia in the corium, and dermal edema, followed by liquefaction necrosis of the lower epidermal cells, lead to blister formation. The gray centers of doughnut-shaped blisters show coagulation necrosis of the full thickness of the dermis.

Symptoms. Most victims are unaware of exposure to mustard. Its insidious action gives no warning until a latent period of one hour, in the case of liquid mustard in the eye, to five days, in the case of mild vapor exposure of the skin in cool weather, has elapsed. The eyes are extremely sensitive. Exposure for one hour to a concentration of only 0.001 mg. per liter of air produces conjunctivitis, while this exposure has no significant effect on the respiratory tract or skin.

Following a latent period, usually 2 to 6 hours, lacrimation and a sensation of grit in the eyes develop. The conjunctivas and lids become red and often so edematous that the eyes cannot be opened voluntarily. In World War I, 75 per cent of patients suffered only conjunctivitis and recovered in one to two weeks. Fifteen per cent had blepharospasm, photophobia and orange-peel roughening of the cornea, requiring two to six weeks for recovery. Ten per cent had iritis and superficial corneal erosions, followed by some corneal scarring and vascularization. Relapses were common during healing, and hospital convalescences lasted two to three months. With liquid contamination, ischemic necrosis of the conjunctivas and dense corneal opacification, with deep ulceration and vascularization, were rarely encountered. Vision was permanently impaired and recurrences of corneal ulceration were common. Chronic exposure to traces of vapor induces a punctate keratitis which clears slowly on termination of exposure.

Inhalation of mustard vapor affects primarily the mucosa of the nose, pharynx, larynx, trachea and larger bronchi. Erythema, edema and superficial necrosis develop slowly and do not reach maximum for several days. Symptoms begin with hoarseness and may progress to aphonia. A dry cough, worse at night, later becomes productive. Nasal and pharyngeal hyperemia and tenderness may be prominent. In severe cases, fever, dyspnea and moist rales develop and the incidence of bronchopneumonia is high. Hoarseness clears and the nasal and pharyngeal mucosa heal in two to three weeks, but nocturnal cough persists a month or longer.

The action of mustard on the skin is influenced strikingly by temperature. Warm, moist skin is injured much more rapidly and severely than cool, dry skin. The burns, largely first and second degree, give symptoms and run clinical courses like those of thermal burns of like severity, except that initial pain is usually less, and itching, nausea and vomiting are more common with mustard burns.

Moderate vapor exposure produces erythema which has the same appearance, symptoms and clinical course as sunburn of equal severity. It terminates with tan pigmentation and desquamation, like sunburn. Greater exposure produces edema, stiffness and tenderness of the skin and multiple pinpoint vesication. In severe cases, the blisters coalesce into large, thin-walled bullae, filled with clear fluid and surrounded by erythema. The fluid clots in two or three days and is resorbed in about a week, leaving thin crusts under which new epithelium grows. However, accidental rupture of the thin-walled bullae is common, leaving painful denuded surfaces. The scrotal skin seldom vesicates, but develops marked edema and painful fissures. Liquid mustard contamination of the skin or clothing may result in such intense local exposure that isolated, doughnut-shaped blisters are produced with gray, nonvesicated, third-degree, coagulated centers, each surrounded by a ring of bullae and erythema.

Diagnosis. Diagnosis depends upon history of exposure to mustard gas. Several plants cause vesication like that due to mustard, but these rarely involve the eyes and respiratory tract. Unprotected individuals rarely develop mustard blisters without involvement of the eyes and respiratory tract.

Prognosis. The mustard gas fatality rate in World War I was 2 per cent due almost entirely to bronchopneumonia. This should be lowered by chemotherapy, not available then. Ninety per cent of eye lesions heal without sequelae within six weeks and permanent impairment of vision is rare. Convalescence from acute respiratory injury is slow, taking one or more months, but permanent disability is rare. However, chronic exposure to traces of mustard vapor may initiate chronic bronchitis and progressive pulmonary fibrosis within a year and eventuate in bronchiectasis, low vital capacity and permanent disability. The average healing times for mustard blisters are: one week on the face; two to four weeks on the neck, trunk, arms and anterior surfaces of the thighs; three to six weeks on the legs, buttocks and posterior surfaces of the thighs; one to two months on the feet, genitalia and scrotum. The centers of doughnut-shaped blisters do not heal until the necrotic coagulum has sloughed, and this may require six to eight weeks. Without skin grafts, these centers heal leaving thin, readily traumatized scars. Otherwise, in the absence of active infection, scarring from mustard burns is insignificant. Unless liquid mustard is ingested in food or water, systemic poisoning is rare.

Treatment. Mustard gas injuries are irreversible and there are no known means to neutralize or modify the effects of mustard absorbed into tissues. Hence, every effort must be made to minimize exposure. Escape from mustard vapor within 5 minutes in hot weather to 15 minutes in cool weather, and removal of liquid mustard from the skin within 30 seconds in hot weather to 2 minutes in cool weather, are essential to avoidance of more than moderate injury. No method of decontamination will prevent severe blistering if liquid mustard remains on the skin for 2 minutes in hot weather and 5 minutes in cool weather. Heavily contaminated clothing must be removed in a few minutes and left outdoors. Injury is inevitable if liquid mustard contacts the eye, but thorough irrigation with water within one minute may save vision.

Decontamination is worthless for vapor exposure, but vapor exposed clothing should be discarded within an hour and aerated outdoors for several days. In the removal of liquid mustard, time is more important than correct materials. Whatever is immediately available should be used. Contaminated hair should be shorn off. Excess liquid should be blotted off with any dry absorbent material,

but smearing should be avoided. The contaminated skin should be flooded with water, then soaped and rinsed. If immediately available, a slurry of bleaching powder (hypochlorite), or household chlorinated laundry bleach, will do a better job. Bleaches should be rinsed off the skin within 5 minutes. A patient should never be taken indoors until all liquid contamination is removed, because mustard vapors will endanger other patients and attendants.

Mild conjunctivitis requires no treatment. For severe conjunctivitis, with blepharospasm and photophobia, one drop of 1 per cent atropine sulfate solution may be instilled and also penicillin or chlortetracycline (Aureomycin) opthalmic ointment, every 8 hours. The patient should be kept in a darkened room for a few days. If pain is severe, 10 mg. of morphine sulfate should be given subcutaneously. Local anesthetics, compresses, accumulated secretions and pressure on the lids predispose to corneal ulceration. Secretions should be removed by gentle irrigation with the minimum of 1 per cent sterile saline. When edema subsides, so that the lids can be opened without trauma to the cornea, a drop of 2 per cent fluorescein in saline should be instilled and the eyes rinsed with a few drops of saline. If the cornea stains, or if severe photophobia persists, an ophthalmologist should treat the patient.

Rhinitis and pharyngitis are treated symptomatically, as for acute respiratory infections. Steam inhalations give some relief of the laryngitis and tracheitis. Codeine cough syrups help control the sleep-wrecking nocturnal cough. If evidences of bronchitis or parenchymal involvement of the lungs appear, penicillin should be given prophylactically. If bronchopneumonia develops, it should be treated like any other bronchopneumonia.

Mustard erythema requires no treatment, unless itching is annoying. Itching may be controlled and tenderness soothed by local applications of calamine lotion containing 1 per cent each of phenol and menthol. Blisters must be protected from rupture and should not be aspirated. Burns of the genitalia and scrotum require light petrolatum gauze dressings and suspensory bandage. Otherwise, techniques for the treatment of mustard burns are identical with those for thermal burns of like severity.

JOHN R. WOOD

References

Departments of the Army, Navy and Air Force: Technical Manual 8-285, Treatment of Chemical Warfare Casualties, August 1951.

Freedman, A. M., Willis, A., and Himwich, H. E.: Correlation Between Signs of Toxicity and Cholinesterase Level of Brain and Blood During Recovery from Di-isopropyl Fluorophosphate (DFP) Poisoning. Am. J. Physiol., *157*:80, 1949.

Gordon, A. S., Raymon, F., Sandov, M., and Ivy, A. C.: Manual Artificial Respiration: Comparison of the Effectiveness of Various Methods on Apneic Normal Adults. J.A.M.A., *144*:1447, 1950.

Grob, D., and Harvey, A. M.: Observations on the Effects of Tetraethyl Pyrophosphate (TEPP) in Man, and on Its Use in the Treatment of Myasthenia Gravis. Bull. Johns Hopkins Hosp., *84:* 532, 1949

————, Harvey, A. M., Langworthy, O. R., and Lilienthal, J. L.: The Administration of Di-isopropyl Fluorophosphate (DFP) to Man: III. Effect on the Central Nervous System With Special Reference to the Electrical Activity of the Brain. Bull. Johns Hopkins Hosp., *81*:257, 1947.

Riker, W. F., and Wescoe, W. C.: The Relationship Between Cholinesterase Inhibition and Function in a Neuro-effector System. J. Pharmacol. & Exper. Therap., *95*:515, 1949.

Wood, J. R.: Chemical Warfare: A Chemical and Toxicological Review. Am. J. Pub. Health, *34:* 455, 1944.

————: Medical Problems in Chemical Warfare. J.A.M.A., *144*:606, 1950.

————: Chemical Defense. J.A.M.A., *145*:1264, 1951.

————, Dickens, P. F., Jr., Rizzolo, J., and Bayliss, M. W.: Treatment of Nerve-Gas Casualties. U. S. Armed Forces M. J., *11*:1609, 1951.

HYPERVITAMINOSIS

History. Since vitamins were first used as therapeutic agents, there have been sporadic reports of ill effects following their administration. Despite the size of the therapeutic dose, however, the administration of most of the vitamins is not followed by any untoward effects. The water-soluble vitamins tend to reach a certain concentration in the blood and are then quickly excreted. Undoubtedly cases of individual idiosyncrasy may produce unpleasant reactions to these substances even when taken in small amounts. Such symptoms are not those of hypervitaminosis. There is considerable evidence that repeated massive doses of the fat-soluble vitamins A and D sometimes produce so-called hypervitaminosis. This discussion will be limited to the hypervitaminosis caused by vitamin A and by vitamin D.

Hypervitaminosis A is a term which is used for a varied and sometimes bizarre condition arising from the administration of massive doses of vitamin A. Numerous investigators have reported injurious effects following the administration of large doses of vitamin A to rats. The coats of the animals become rough, and they develop cachexia, conjunctivitis and diarrhea, striations in the muscle fibers of the heart, degeneration of the testes and changes in the liver. The excessive administration of vitamin A to young rats and guinea pigs has been associated also with bone fragility and fractures.

Although in the human being the administration of up to 300,000 U.S.P. units of vitamin A daily for a number of months has not produced detectable harmful effects, some persons have developed sensitivity to cod liver oil. It is of interest that the ingestion of polar bear liver results in serious illness, which is due to the large amount of vitamin A in polar bear liver at certain times of the year. Analysis of polar bear liver shows that it may contain as much as 18,000 I.U. of vitamin A per gram of wet material. Affected persons develop severe headaches and vomiting. While some investigators have not accepted the idea that it is vitamin A which causes toxicity of polar bear liver, the author sees no reason to look beyond this. Hypervitaminosis A, in its chronic form, is characterized by anorexia, loss of weight, sparsity of hair, hepatomegaly and tenderness over the long bones, which show characteristic roentgeographic changes occurring most frequently in the ulna and tibia.

It is important to emphasize that the physician should not discontinue vitamin A therapy until he is certain that it is vitamin A which is producing the undesirable symptoms.

Hypervitaminosis D. In 1928 and 1929 considerable interest was centered on the effect of administering repeated, massive doses of vitamin D to experimental animals. In a study on normal animals, Kreitmair and Moll found that the administration of massive doses of irradiated ergosterol was followed by calcium deposition in some of the tissues. In a study of the effect of repeated large doses of irradiated ergosterol to experimental animals with either acute or chronic tuberculosis, Spies found extensive deposition of calcium salts within the caseous lesions. He also corroborated the findings of other workers who reported that massive and repeated dosage of vitamin D was followed by loss of weight, cachexia and calcification of many of the tissues. In addition he observed an even more widespread calcification than had been reported previously and a retention of nitrogenous products in the blood which was associated with marked kidney lesions. When such toxic manifestations occurred in animals, the possible danger of giving repeated large doses in clinical practice was obvious.

In human beings, hypercalcemia follows the repeated administration of large doses of vitamin D. Reed believes, however, that the toxic effects of vitamin D are independent of its action in raising the calcium and inorganic phosphorus concentration in the blood serum. Although persons treated for a prolonged period of time with massive doses of vitamin may exhibit calcification of the soft tissues, Spies and Hanzal showed that the oral administration of massive doses of irradiated ergosterol to young adults over a few days produced an elevation of blood calcium and phosphorus without histopathologic calcification of the tissues.

Frequently it is difficult to obtain a history of excessive vitamin D therapy, but in all cases of unexplained hypercalcemia the patient should be carefully questioned in regard to vitamin D therapy. This is particularly important should an operation for adenoma of the parathyroid gland be considered. According to Park, early symptoms of overdosage are nausea, headache, diarrhea, loss of appetite, frequent micturition, nocturia and lassitude. Examination of the urine may reveal evidence of overdosage. Albright and his collaborators noted that, after enormous doses of vitamin D in a child with intractable rickets, the urine was loaded with calcium and contained many calcium casts such as have been observed in cases of hyperparathyroidism.

Two cases of hypercalcemia with calcification of soft tissues and renal damage have been reported by Danowski, Winkler and Peters. Bauer and Freyberg have reported a fatal case of vitamin D intoxication in an adult woman who received massive doses of vitamin D for over one year. At autopsy white chalky deposits of calcium salt were found in the myocardium, kidneys and arteriovascular system.

Therapy with massive doses of vitamin D for very long periods of time demands careful supervision by the physician. Serum calcium should be determined frequently, and at the first suggestion of hypercalcemia the dosage should be reduced. The patient should never be allowed to continue treatment on his own initiative. The greatest danger of all, perhaps, comes in taking doses of vitamin D large enough to produce cumulative effects over a very long period of time. Once the diagnosis of hypervitaminosis D is made, the patient should be prohibited everything which tends to increase the blood calcium.

TOM D. SPIES

References

Albright, F., Butler, A. M., and Bloomberg, Esther: Rickets Resistant to Vitamin D Therapy. Am. J. Dis. Child., 54:529, 1937.
Bauer, J. M., and Freyberg, R. H.: Vitamin D Intoxication. J.A.M.A. 130:1208, 1946.
Danowski, T. S., Winkler, A. W., and Peters, J. P.: Tissue Calcification and Renal Failure Produced by Massive Dose Vitamin D Therapy of Arthritis. Ann. Int. Med., 23:22, 1945.
Kreitmair, H., and Moll, T.: Hypervitaminosis through Large Doses of Vitamin D. München. med. Wchnschr., 75:637, 1928.
Park, E. A.: The Therapy of Rickets. J.A.M.A., 115: 370, 1940.
Reed, C. I., Dellman, L. M., Thacker, E. A., and Klein, R. L.: The Calcification of Tissues by Excessive Doses of Irradiated Ergosterol. J. Nutrition, 6:371, 1933.
Wolbach, S. B.: Pathology in Relation to Nutritional Research. Nutrition Rev., 3:193, 1945.

BARBITURATE POISONING

Definition. Barbiturate poisoning refers to the physiologic and psychologic changes produced by the ingestion of amounts of barbiturate drugs in excess of those used therapeutically. The drugs most commonly involved in the United States are pentobarbital (Nembutal), secobarbital (Seconal), amobarbital (Amytal), phenobarbital and barbital. Poisoning with these substances may be acute or chronic.

ACUTE BARBITURATE POISONING

Incidence. Acute barbiturate poisoning is the most common type of poisoning with solids and causes approximately 1500 deaths yearly in the United States. It is more common in women than in men; occurs more frequently in urban centers than in rural; is most frequent among persons between the ages of 30 and 50 years; and the incidence is high among individuals who have easy access to these drugs (physicians, pharmacists, nurses and members of their families).

Etiology. Poisoning from barbiturates may

result from unusual sensitivity to the drug, may be accidental, but most frequently results from suicidal attempts.

Morbid Anatomy. Characteristic histopathologic changes do not occur in acute barbiturate intoxication. Changes that are seen are related to asphyxia and to the development of pulmonary complications.

Pathologic Physiology. The effects of the barbiturates are due to depression of all types of cells in the central nervous system. According to Echols, barbiturates stabilize the soma of neurons and make depolarization more difficult. Biochemically, barbiturate depression may be based on inhibition of transformation of diphosphopyridine to triphosphopyridine nucleotide. Small doses of barbiturates induce drowsiness by an effect on the reticular activating system in the midbrain and diencephalon. As the dose is increased the cells of the cerebral cortex are affected, leading to difficulty in thinking and impairment of judgment. The basal ganglia, cerebellum and spinal cord are involved next, resulting in incoordination, ataxia and depression of spinal reflexes. As the degree of intoxication increases, sleep passes into coma, the deep tendon reflexes disappear, and respiration becomes depressed. Respiration, finally, may be carried on through the anoxic drive from the carotid and aortic chemoreceptors. This latter fact is important since, in severe poisoning, the administration of oxygen alone may remove the stimulus to respiration and cause cessation of breathing. Eventually, the vasomotor center may become involved, resulting in vasomotor collapse.

Signs and Symptoms. The signs and symptoms of acute barbiturate poisoning vary in general with the amount and type of drug and the length of time after ingestion. The rapidly acting drugs, such as pentobarbital and secobarbital, produce coma quickly, but recovery is relatively rapid. Barbital and phenobarbital produce coma slowly, but recovery is rather slow. These differences are due in part to variations in the speed of detoxification of the different barbiturates and their storage in fat depots. Within limits, the longer the time which has elapsed between ingestion of the drugs and examination of the patient, the greater is the degree of depression.

Acute barbiturate poisoning resembles alcoholic intoxication except that the face is not flushed, the conjunctivas are not suffused and there is no odor of alcohol present on the breath. Mental symptoms in order of their appearance include impairment of mental ability and judgment, emotional instability (easy laughing or crying), garrulousness, confusion, drowsiness, sleep and coma. A group of neurologic signs, including those suggestive of cerebellar disease, is present. These include in rough order of appearance: absence of superficial skin reflexes, dysarthria, transient nystagmus on lateral gaze, ataxia in gait and station, constant nystagmus, adiadochokinesis, positive Babinski signs, depression or absence of tendon reflexes, constricted pupils (dilatation occurs if anoxia becomes severe), and absent corneal and pharyngeal reflexes. Respiratory rate and volume are reduced but adequate in mild and moderate degrees of poisoning. In severe grades respiration is very slow, shallow, and frequently periodic. Pulse rate and blood pressure are little affected in mild poisoning but in severe intoxication peripheral circulatory collapse is present.

Cases of barbiturate poisoning may be classified as mild, moderate or severe dependent upon the degree of depression. Differentiation of these grades is important in planning treatment. *Mild poisoning* is characterized by the following: (1) Mental ability and judgment are impaired; (2) the patient is readily roused; (3) nystagmus is transient, not constant; (4) reflexes, other than the superficial skin twitches, are not depressed; (5) respiration and blood pressure are not significantly depressed.

Moderate intoxication is characterized by the following: (1) Sleep or light coma—the patient can be aroused by vigorous manual stimulation, by cerebral electrostimulation or by Metrazol; (2) nystagmus is constant; (3) dysarthria is marked and patient cannot answer questions; (4) tendon reflexes are depressed but corneal and gag reflexes are active; (5) respiration is slow and shallow but usually not periodic; (6) blood pressure is not depressed. *Severe intoxication* is characterized by: (1) coma from which the patient cannot be roused by manual or electrostimulation or by Metrazol; (2) marked depression or absence of tendon reflexes; (3) absent corneal and pharyngeal reflexes; (4) markedly depressed respiration, frequently periodic; (5) shock.

Laboratory Findings. Methods are available for the detection of barbiturates in blood and urine. These techniques are complicated, however, and require a great deal of time. In mild and moderate grades of barbiturate poisoning the electroencephalogram presents a very characteristic fast-slow pattern. In severe barbiturate poisoning, the electroencephalogram shows only slow waves.

Diagnosis. The diagnosis of barbiturate poisoning should be considered in any patient who presents signs and symptoms resembling those of alcoholic intoxication, but who has no odor of alcohol detectable on the breath. In cases of coma with quiet or depressed respiration, the diagnosis is always likely. A positive history of ingestion of large amounts of barbiturates obtained from the patient, friends or relatives is of great importance. The patient and his living quarters should be carefully searched for bottles, boxes, capsules or tablets. Frequently, remains of the characteristic colored capsules can be found in the mouth or in gastric washings.

Acute barbiturate poisoning must be differentiated from all other conditions which cause clouding of the sensorium and coma. Head injuries, cerebrovascular accidents, brain tumors, meningitis, encephalitis, diabetic and uremic and hepatic coma, coma due to hypoglycemia, cardiovascular disturbances and poisoning with alcohol, morphine, bromides and chloral must be considered. Complete physical and laboratory examination usually suffices for the differentiation. One must keep in mind that head injuries are a frequent complication of barbiturate intoxication, and that barbiturate poisoning is frequently complicated by the use of other intoxicants, especially alcohol.

Prognosis. The mortality rate in all grades of acute barbiturate poisoning is only 8 per cent. The outlook in mild and moderate cases is excellent. Danger of death is great only in severe poisoning. The larger the dose of barbiturate ingested, and the longer the time since the drug was taken, the more serious is the prognosis. The outlook is worse in individuals intoxicated with barbital or phenobarbital than in patients who have ingested pentobarbital or secobarbital. The deeper the coma and the longer coma has been present, the worse is the outlook. Mortality is higher in elderly people and in patients who are in poor physical condition. Severe intoxication with a mixture of alcohol and barbiturates is more serious than severe intoxication with either drug alone. The presence of pneumonia, massive aspiration of gastrointestinal contents, pulmonary edema and shock are of serious import.

Treatment. The treatment of acute barbiturate poisoning is dependent upon the grade of intoxication. It is important to remember that the mortality rate in barbiturate poisoning is low (about 8 per cent), and that most patients will recover without any treatment whatever. Only patients falling in the severe category are in grave danger. The use of the powerful analeptic drugs is contraindicated in noncomatose patients.

In mild and moderate cases, if ingestion of barbiturates has been recent, gastric lavage should be performed. The stomach should be emptied completely in order to avoid aspiration of stomach contents into the lungs. The patient should not be allowed to go to sleep, but should be kept awake by talking and by manual stimulation. Mild analeptics, such as coffee, caffeine sodium benzoate and amphetamine, may be used if desired.

Comatose patients who can be aroused with vigorous manual stimulation or by electrostimulation with the Reiter apparatus (moderate poisoning) should also be treated conservatively. The patient should be under constant observation for signs of respiratory depression. Caffeine sodium benzoate (0.5 gm.) may be given intramuscularly. Ten to 40 mg. of amphetamine sulfate orally or intramuscularly may be of value. If coma deepens, or if serious respiratory depression appears, more vigorous treatment should be instituted.

The treatment of patients with severe barbiturate poisoning constitutes a medical emergency. Symptomatic treatment is more important than analeptic therapy, and the greatest attention must be paid to maintaining a sufficient degree of pulmonary ventilation. The services of an expert anesthesiologist are of greatest value. The foot of the bed should be elevated, mucus aspirated from the mouth and pharynx, an airway inserted, if necessary, and artificial respiration begun, preferably using an approved type of automatic positive-pressure respirator. Manual artificial respiration must be used if a respirator is not available.

As soon as an adequate degree of pulmonary ventilation is obtained, the patient should be examined thoroughly and blood, spinal fluid and urine obtained for laboratory tests. If the patient is in shock, a plasma expander or whole blood should be administered at once. Because of the danger of aspiration pneumonia, lavage should be avoided in seriously depressed patients.

After the measures designed to remedy respiratory depression and circulatory collapse have been instituted, one must consider analeptic therapy. Application of the modulated unidirectional periodic electrocerebral stimulation (Reiter apparatus) may make analeptic therapy unnecessary, and should always be tried first. If electrostimulation is not effective, one should inject 5 cc. of a 10 per cent solution of Metrazol slowly, intravenously. If twitching and grimacing occur and corneal and deep tendon reflexes return, Metrazol is the analeptic of choice, and the drug should be repeated every 15 minutes until the patient is out of danger. If there is no response to the initial "orientation" dose of Metrazol, a second dose of 8 cc. of Metrazol may be given 15 minutes after the first. If this dose does not produce definite analeptic effects, the administration of picrotoxin may be necessary. Within 10 to 15 minutes after the last dose of Metrazol, 2 cc. of a solution of picrotoxin containing 3 mg. per cubic centimeter should be injected intravenously at the rate of 1 cc. (3 mg.) per minute. The patient should be observed for muscular twitching and the return of corneal reflexes as the picrotoxin is injected. The injection should be stopped if either of these analeptic effects appear. If the initial dose of picrotoxin does not produced the desired effects, it should be followed in 15 minutes by a second dose of 3 cc. If a definite analeptic effect is not obtained with this amount, the dose should be increased in steps of 1 cc. until 5 cc. (15 mg.) is being given every 15 minutes.

The administration of picrotoxin should be continued until definite improvement in the patient's condition is evident. After the depth of coma lessens, the dose of picrotoxin may be decreased and intramuscular administration begun. One should attempt to keep the patient constantly restless and active, but stop short of a convulsive dose. Neither Metrazol nor picrotoxin should be used unless a rapidly acting anticonvulsive agent, preferably Pentothal sodium, is at hand. If convulsions do occur, 2.5 per cent Pentothal sodium should be administered intravenously until they are controlled. For this purpose, minimal doses of 2 to 3 cc. repeated as required should be employed.

If the desired effects are obtained with the analeptic drugs, artificial respiration may be discontinued and the patient maintained on analeptic therapy until partial consciousness has returned. Antibiotics should be administered in an effort to prevent the development of hypostatic pneumonia. Careful nursing is necessary; the patient must be turned frequently, and attention given to the skin over the bony prominences.

If the degree of depression does not lessen under analeptic therapy, supportive measures must be continued. It may be advisable to transfer the patient to a Drinker respirator for ease of handling. Fluid intake should be maintained at a level of at least 3000 cc. daily by hypodermoclysis or by slow intravenous infusion. If evidence of atelectasis or aspiration of gastric contents appears, bronchoscopy should be done at once, or mechanical devices for inducing artificial cough should be employed.

Following recovery from coma, the patient will be confused and will require continued protection and nursing. Toxic psychoses are quite common at this time, and small amounts of paraldehyde may be given to induce sleep and prevent exhaustion.

After the patient has fully recovered, complete psychiatric evaluation followed by appropriate treatment is necessary for patients who ingested the drugs with suicidal intent.

Complications. The most common complications of acute barbiturate poisoning are pulmonary. Atelectasis and bronchopneumonia due to decreased pulmonary ventilation, aspiration of vomitus, and so on often occur. Ulcers may develop over bony prominences and may require extensive dermatologic treatment. It is not unusual for acute barbiturate poisoning to be superimposed on chronic barbiturate poisoning. After the patient has recovered from coma, one should therefore ascertain whether he has been ingesting the drugs chronically. If this is true, severe withdrawal signs may appear and these are best prevented by replacing the patient on barbiturates and then slowly withdrawing the drugs, as prescribed in the section on Chronic Barbiturate Poisoning.

HARRIS ISBELL

References

Kappanyi, T., and Fazekas, J. F.: Acute Barbiturate Poisoning. Am. J. Med. Sci., 220:559, 1950.
Mayer, L. D., and Greenfield, I.: Barbiturate Poison-

ing. Report of Thirty-Three Cases. Arch. Int. Med., *84*:379, 1949.

Nilsson, Eric: On Treatment of Barbiturate Poisoning. Acta med. Scandinav., Supplement 253, Accompanies Vol. *139*, 1951.

Robie, T. R.: Treatment of Acute Barbiturate Poisoning by Nonconvulsive Electrostimulation. Postgrad. Med., *9*:253, 1951.

CHRONIC BARBITURATE INTOXICATION (BARBITURATE ADDICTION)

Incidence. The incidence of chronic barbiturate poisoning is unknown and, although it is probably more common than is usually believed, the incidence is low when the huge consumption of these drugs is considered. Barbiturate addiction complicates about 1 out of 5 cases of morphine addiction.

Etiology. The etiology of chronic barbiturate poisoning, like that of other addictions, is multifactorial. The pharmacologic effects of barbiturates play a definite role since these drugs diminish anxiety and ego controls, and permit the patient to act out a solution for, or to satisfy directly, basic psychic drives. Chronic barbiturate intoxication is always associated with some psychiatric disorder, usually a psychoneurosis or a character disorder. Neuroses associated with anxiety and insomnia are particularly important in the genesis of this condition. Other addictions, particularly addiction to alcohol or opiates, predispose to barbiturate addiction.

Patterns of Abuse. These resemble patterns of abuse of alcohol. Barbiturates may be used for short sprees of less than 24-hours' duration, for debauches lasting a few days to several weeks, or they may be ingested in large amounts daily for months or years. Generally, barbiturate addicts prefer the rapidly acting drugs of short duration of action, such as pentobarbital and secobarbital, to the drugs with slow onset but long duration of action (barbital and phenobarbital). The drugs are usually taken orally but some morphine addicts may attempt to inject them. Neurotic patients ordinarily do not elevate their doses rapidly, but gradually increase the amount taken over a relatively long period of time. Psychopaths, on the other hand, take the barbiturates for the purpose of becoming intoxicated rather than to relieve anxiety and induce sleep. Such persons usually elevate their dosage quite rapidly and may be taking very large amounts after only a week or two of chronic intoxication. Concomitant use of barbiturates and alcohol is very common in this latter group, as is the combined abuse of barbiturates and sympathomimetic amines.

As is the case in alcoholism, it is difficult to define the point at which proper use of the barbiturates ceases and abuse begins. Clinical data suggest that most persons can ingest 0.2 gm. or less of any of the barbiturates daily for months or years without incurring any definite harm. The ability and efficiency of the individual who takes as much as 0.8 gm. of a potent barbiturate daily is greatly impaired and, if this amount is ingested for as long as six weeks to two months, severe symptoms will appear on abrupt withdrawal. Patients who have been ingesting 0.3 to 0.7 gm. of barbiturate daily fall into an intermediate class. Practically all of these patients will show some impairment of mental ability on close examination, and mild withdrawal symptoms are the rule after abrupt discontinuation of barbiturates. Occasionally, convulsions and mild delirium are observed.

Morbid Anatomy. Increases in the number of corpora amylacea have been observed in the central nervous system of animals chronically poisoned with barbiturates. Whether similar changes occur in man is unknown, but if any anatomic changes are produced, they must be relatively minor in extent or reversible since clinical recovery appears to be complete.

Pathologic Physiology. The mechanisms underlying tolerance to and physical dependence on barbiturates are not understood.

Signs and Symptoms. Signs and symptoms of chronic barbiturate poisoning are identical with those of mild to moderate acute intoxication. Mental symptoms include difficulty in thinking, confusion, increased emotional instability and, occasionally, a toxic psychosis. Neurologic signs are quite characteristic and include nystagmus, dysarthria, dysmetria, hypotonia, ataxia in gait and station, decreased superficial skin reflexes and normal tendon and pupillary reflexes. No abnormal sensory findings are present. The symptoms fluctuate in intensity greatly in the same individual from time to time. The variation is related in part to the variation in food intake.

Abstinence Syndrome. If a person who has been taking 0.8 gm. or more of one of the potent barbiturates daily discontinues use of these drugs, a stereotyped train of symptoms resembling alcoholic delirium tremens ensues. In the first 8 hours following withdrawal of the drug the degree of intoxication declines, confusion lessens and the patient appears to be improving. Soon thereafter, increasing anxiety, tremor and marked weakness upon standing appear. Twenty-four hours after barbiturates have been discontinued, twitching of various muscle groups and uncontrollable bouts of shaking of the extremities without loss of consciousness may ensue. In 75 per cent of the cases one or more typical grand mal convulsions occurs, usually during the second day of abstinence, but occasionally as late as the seventh day. The number of seizures varies greatly from patient to patient. After the convulsive phase is over, the patient usually improves and may recover without further incident. In about 60 per cent of cases anxiety reappears and insomnia becomes complete. Finally, between the third and the seventh day of abstinence a psychosis appears which is characterized by vivid hallucinations and delusions. The hallucinations are predominantly visual but auditory hallucinations occur. The delirium is apt to begin and be worse at night; it fluctuates in intensity from moment to moment. The patient usually becomes disorientated in time and place but not in person. Recovery usually occurs in three to five days. The illness terminates suddenly as a rule with an 8- to 12-hour period of sleep. Partial memory of the hallucinatory experiences is usually retained. During the delirium body temperature is usually elevated from 1.8 to 3.6° F. A rapidly rising temperature is an ominous sign and may indicate a fatal termination.

Laboratory Findings. The ordinary laboratory findings are negative in maintained barbiturate addiction. Tests for barbiturates in blood and urine may be positive. The electroencephalogram shows the characteristic fast pattern superimposed on random slow waves. During withdrawal of barbiturates, the fast activity disappears in the first 24 hours and the electroencephalogram becomes generally slowed. During the second and subsequent days, paroxysmal bursts of high voltage slow waves, or of spike and dome complexes, may occur.

Diagnosis. The diagnosis of barbiturate addiction is usually made by a history of chronic ingestion of large amounts of barbiturates obtained from either the patient or his relatives. Frequently, patients give histories of taking 1 to 5 gm. of barbiturates daily. The diagnosis should always be considered when slightly confused, mildly intoxicated individuals present themselves with complaints of insomnia and request prescriptions for barbiturates. It must be differentiated from morphine addiction, bromide intoxication, cerebral arteriosclerosis, parkinsonism, encephalitis, multiple sclerosis and brain tumor.

Barbiturate withdrawal convulsions must be differentiated from all other causes of seizures. The combination of seizures followed by a typical delirium is usually characteristic of either abstinence from barbiturates or alcoholic delirium tremens. Barbiturate delirium must be differentiated from toxic psychoses due to infections, from bromide psychoses, from uremia, from manic depressive and schizophrenic psychoses and from alcoholic delirium tremens.

Complications. The most common complications of barbiturate addiction are injuries resulting from a fall while intoxicated or from a convulsion during withdrawal. Exhaustion and bronchopneumonia constitute the chief dangers during withdrawal.

Prognosis. The immediate prognosis with respect to chronic barbiturate intoxication is good. If delirium has developed during withdrawal of barbiturates, prognosis should be guarded since this condition occasionally is fatal. Prognosis with respect to continued abstinence from barbiturates or other intoxicants must be guarded since, as is the case in alcohol and morphine addictions, relapse is very common.

Treatment. Abrupt withdrawal of barbiturates from addicted persons is absolutely contraindicated. Treatment should always be carried out in a hospital where absolute control of the patient's environment can be achieved. If the diagnosis of barbiturate addiction is made before objective signs of abstinence have appeared, the patient should be given pentobarbital in amounts sufficient to maintain a state of mild barbiturate intoxication. Usually 0.2 to 0.3 gm. of pentobarbital orally every 6 hours will suffice for this purpose. The patient's barbiturate intake should be maintained at this level until all necessary examinations have been completed. Careful gradual withdrawal of barbiturates is then begun. The dosage should not be reduced more than 0.1 gm. daily. When the daily dosage has been reduced to half of the stabilization dose, reduction should be stopped for two or three days and then resumed. If anxiety, insomnia, tremor, weakness or paroxysmal slow activity appears in the electroencephalogram, withdrawal should be stopped and the dosage of barbiturates held at whatever level has been reached until these symptoms have disappeared. Withdrawal of barbiturates can usually be accomplished in fourteen to twenty-one days. There is no contraindication of concomitant withdrawal of opiates or other drugs.

Individuals undergoing withdrawal of barbiturates should be kept under close observation. They should not go to the bathroom unattended and their beds should be provided with sideboards. Usually, no special dietary or other therapy is required. Precautions must be taken to prevent smuggling of barbiturates to these patients.

If a diagnosis of barbiturate addiction is made after a major convulsion has occurred or after delirium has appeared, the patient should immediately be given 0.3 to 0.5 gm. of pentobarbital or amobarbital either orally or parenterally. He should then receive barbiturates every 4 to 6 hours in amounts sufficient to induce mild intoxication. After reintoxication with barbiturates has been achieved, gradual withdrawal is conducted as described above.

After withdrawal of barbiturates has been completed, full psychiatric evaluation followed by appropriate psychotherapy should be instituted.

HARRIS ISBELL

References

Isbell, H., and others: Chronic Barbiturate Intoxication. An Experimental Study. Arch. Neurol. & Psychiat., 64:1, 1950.

Kalinowsky, L. B.: Convulsions in Non-epileptic Patients on Withdrawal of Barbiturates, Alcohol and Other Drugs. Arch. Neurol. & Psychiat., 48:946, 1942.

Pohlisch, K., and Panse, F.: Schlafmittelmissbrauch. Leipzig, George Thieme, 1934.

ALCOHOLISM

Clinical Definition. The various syndromes resulting from the ingestion of alcohol (C_2H_5OH) are usually grouped together under the general term "alcoholism." These effects are far from negligible, in spite of the widespread social use of alcohol and the casual attitude most people show toward it. The drinking of alcohol is an ancient custom related intimately to religion, social mores, law and medicine.

Medically, alcohol has little value other than as a tissue preservative, a hardener and cleanser of the skin, a reducer of fever by cooling of the skin, an anesthetic in nerve blocks, and as an antiseptic. It is generally used, otherwise, for purposes of relaxation, relief from tension, as a stimulant to the appetite, and as an almost universal means of promoting a sense of social ease. The dangers of alcohol far outweigh its advantages. The toll exacted in human misery as a result of acute alcoholism, delirium tremens, chronic alcoholism and alcoholic psychoses is enormous. Between 10 and 25 per cent of all patients admitted to state hospitals suffer from alcoholic conditions. There are a million known chronic alcoholics in this country. Traffic accidents show 5 to 50 per cent of the fatalities to be due to alcohol.

Alcoholism is one of the great unsolved public health problems of America. There are few facilities for the treatment of alcoholics. Few people recognize that chronic alcoholism is an illness, not a weakness of character. Most alcoholic patients land in jail or correctional institutions instead of in the hands of the medical profession. In one year Bellevue Hospital in New York City admitted 12,000 alcoholics. Most of these stayed in the hospital less than 72 hours and were turned back into the community. Only a minute percentage get more than emergency therapy.

Physiology and Chemistry. Alcohol is usually ingested, but it can be absorbed through the lungs by inhalation. After ingestion, absorption of alcohol takes place rapidly from the stomach and intestines in an unchanged stage. About 20 per cent is absorbed in the stomach, the rest in the intestine, especially in the jejunum. The speed of absorption varies directly with the concentration. Food slows absorption, especially fatty foods. The effects of alcohol, therefore, are much less marked when it is taken during meals than on an empty stomach.

Alcohol is distributed throughout all organs and fluids of the body fairly uniformly except in the brain and spinal fluid, where the concentration is slower in rising and falling. Ninety to 95 per cent of alcohol is oxidized almost completely within the body. Available energy is released and carbon dioxide and water produced. Man oxidizes approximately 10 cc. of alcohol per hour. Alcohol therefore is of little value for energy, since its rate of oxidation cannot be increased to meet body needs. Its incapacity to be stored in the body tissues also decreases its value as a food. Initial oxidation takes place in the liver, and insulin is required for this function. There seems also to be a definite relation between the oxidation of alcohol and the oxidation of glucose. This fact points to the importance of glucose and insulin as therapy in the rapid reduction of blood alcohol levels. In addition, there is some evidence which suggests that the oxidation of alcohol is related to the presence of thiamine. Both thiamine and nicotinic acid may be necessary for the rapid oxidation of alcohol.

Alcohol which escapes oxidation is excreted primarily in the urine and through the lungs. The concentration in the urine varies with the concentration in the blood. The usual amount of excretion, however, rarely exceeds 3 per cent of that ingested.

Alcohol is detectable in the blood within 5 minutes of ingestion. The blood level rises rapidly in the first and second hours, and then begins to fall. This peak is reached more quickly in habitual drinkers, in whom the curve descends rapidly in 2 hours. It is believed that blood alcohol concentrations of 0.2 per cent are usually associated with mild or moderate intoxication. Concentrations beyond 0.3 per cent usually indicate marked intoxication. The fatal concentration of alcohol in the blood ranges between 0.5 and 0.8 per cent. There is an individual variation in the reaction to blood alcohol concentrations and in the amount of alcohol which must be ingested to reach any given blood level.

Definite tolerance to alcohol usually develops in repeated users. This is variously ascribed as being due to decreased absorption, increased oxidation, increased cell tolerance or increased excretion. It is well known also that serious addiction occurs. The true mechanism of addiction is not known, but addiction is more likely in persons whose tolerance is great than in those who tolerate little alcohol. Other factors contributing to addiction are idiosyncrasy and need for the sedative effect. A strong addiction to alcohol, once acquired, is difficult to break.

Physiologic Action of Alcohol. Alcohol affects all the tissues of the body, and notably the central nervous system, upon which it acts as a depressant or inhibitor. What the average person assumes to be stimulation is really the depressant effects upon the inhibitory cortical controls of behavior. In this respect alcohol is like a general anesthetic. The effect on the central nervous system is that of any irregularly descending depressant. Respiratory depression may occur late in alcoholic intoxication. The pulse rate usually increases, though cardiac effects are inconstant. Vasodilatation occurs, especially at the cutaneous vessels. Dilatation of coronary arteries may occur from moderate doses of alcohol. The body temperature is reduced because of increased cutaneous blood flow. As a result, heat loss increases. With the ingestion of large quantities of alcohol there is a further loss of heat by disturbance of the heat-regulating center. Where conservation of body heat is important, as in cold climates, alcohol is contraindicated.

The effects on the alimentary tract are usually those of increased salivary secretion, increased gastric secretion of high acidity and low pepsin. For this reason alcohol is frequently used to determine the ability of the gastric glands to secrete hydrochloric acid. With higher concentrations of alcohol, gastric secretion may be inhibited. The long-continued use of alcohol almost invariably results in some degree of gastritis. Urine flow is increased by alcohol, which acts as a powerful diuretic. Alcohol may increase sexual desire because of the abolition of inhibitions, but usually decreases sexual potency. By impairment of the general health, excessive alcohol may reduce the resistance to infection, but in moderate amounts there is little evidence that it directly affects susceptibility or resistance. Moderate drinking of alcohol appears to have little effect upon longevity, but life insurance statistics show that heavy drinkers have a shorter life span.

People who drink regularly or too much usually eat inadequately and thereby suffer a vitamin lack. It is likely that many of the chronic effects of alcohol upon the nervous system are primarily the results of vitamin deficiency. Because of increased vomiting, voiding or diarrhea, drinkers suffer from loss of water and salt.

Pathologic Effects. The nervous system and digestive system are most markedly affected. The wet brain or edema seen in death from acute alcoholism is the most striking finding. Edema may be present in the pia-arachnoid and the parenchymous tissues of the brain and lungs. Only after the prolonged use of large amounts of alcohol are pathologic findings characteristic, and even in such instances the results may well be those of food and vitamin deficiency rather than a direct result of the alcohol. In persons who have died in acute alcoholism no specific gross or microscopic lesions are detectable. The usual finding is lividity of the extremities and congestion of the mucous membranes of the stomach, with frequent punctiform hemorrhages and superficial erosions. The right chamber of the heart may be distended. In chronic alcoholism peripheral neuropathies are frequent. It has been estimated that 50 per cent of all chronic users of alcohol suffer some peripheral neuritis, but few if any specific characteristic lesions are defined. In some cases a Laënnec's cirrhosis or fatty infiltration of the liver is present. The role of alcohol in the etiology of hepatic cirrhosis is still not clear, since similar cirrhosis is seen in abstainers. Other findings which have been described, but which have been poorly defined, are fatty infiltration and degeneration of cardiac muscle (myocardium), fibrosis of the spleen depending on the degree of liver fibrosis, and, occasionally, degenerative changes in the optic and peripheral nerves. Little is known about the respective roles of alcohol and the accompanying dietary difficulties in the production of these histopathologic changes.

Contraindications. Alcohol is contraindicated in patients with hepatic and renal disease, hyperacidity, gastric or duodenal ulcer, infections of the urinary tract, epilepsy, in all persons who give history of addiction, intolerance, or dependence, and in those persons of unstable personality who use alcohol to escape from the stresses and strains of daily life.

Principles of Treatment. Whereas most people consume alcohol in moderation and for many the drug is an aid to relaxation and stimulates appetite, many people insist on drinking too much and thereby run the risk of developing some of the disorders which have been described. Such people need therapy, the crux of which is psychiatric understanding, guidance and treatment. The entire problem is essentially a psychiatric one. The person with an alcoholic problem is not a weakling, but must be thought of as a sick patient who first needs help to get over the effects of alcohol, and secondly instruction in how to live without the need for alcohol as a conscious or subconscious escape. The most urgent need is for a program of public education toward the prevention of alcoholism. Although the problem is now generally recognized as essentially medical, there has been no systematic attack upon it on nation-wide

basis. Nor are the medical profession and the public fully aware of its serious importance. Many people find it difficult to realize that alcoholism is actually symptomatic of underlying psychiatric disorders which require medical and psychiatric aid.

From a consideration of the physiologic metabolic data, it is evident that the main principles of medical treatment as well as prevention include the restoration of adequate nutrition and an appropriate vitamin intake. Since alcohol oxidation involves glucose and insulin metabolism in addition to nicotinic acid and thiamine, these substances are important in therapy.

ACUTE ALCOHOLISM

Acute intoxication with alcohol results in a characteristic progression of symptoms. These begin with a mild tingling of the mucous membranes of the mouth and throat, increasing sense of warmth and general feeling of well being, loquaciousness, sense of relaxation, mild dizziness, increasing euphoria with unnatural optimism, abandonment of worry, and subjective awareness of increased energy and strength. Speech becomes loud and boisterous. There may be tremulousness and increasing clumsiness of movements. As real intoxication occurs, all normal inhibitions are removed, and verbosity, inordinate sense of power, staggering, clumsiness, dysarthria, elation or sadness appears. Thereafter the person may become increasingly drowsy, pugnacious, argumentative, angry, weeping or shouting. Nausea and vomiting may occur with poor control of sphincters. Diplopia, tinnitus and numbness gradually appear. The pupils are dilated, the face is flushed, the pulse is full, the heart rate is rapid. In extreme degrees of intoxication the end result is usually stupor, with heavy breathing, a deep degree of anesthesia, and sometimes death. Circulatory collapse and disturbance of heat regulation may develop. Death may occur rapidly or after hours of deep coma.

Instead of coma, automatic behavior may occur (alcoholic trance or automatism). Upon recovery, amnesia of the entire event is frequent.

After the acute alcoholic episode there is usually severe headache, lassitude and dehydration. Vomiting may be persistent. During coma, pneumonia may result either from exposure or from aspiration of food material. During acute intoxication fundamental personality traits and conflicts are released. Because of poor judgment, sexual encounters are common. Venereal disease may result from exposure, and misdemeanors and criminal acts may ensue.

Diagnosis. Diagnosis is facilitated by the odor of alcohol, a history of alcoholic consumption, the determination of the blood level of alcohol or the alcohol content of the urine. The skin is cold and clammy, body temperature is low, respiration is slow and noisy, pupils are dilated and tachycardia is present. Death is rare unless coma is protracted over many hours, or trauma or infection complicates the picture. Any such comatose patient must be carefully examined, for evidence of injury, fracture of the skull, intracranial hemorrhages or cerebrovascular accident. Uremia and diabetes must be excluded. A complete physical examination is imperative in all cases to rule out accidental injuries.

Prognosis. Acute alcoholic intoxication without coma usually disappears spontaneously. The presence of coma renders the prognosis more serious.

Treatment. The majority of patients suffering from acute alcoholism require little in the way of special treatment and usually sleep off the intoxication. Patients in coma, however, require emergency medical care. The patient must be kept warm. Posture should be changed frequently. The stomach should be washed out through a tube. Inhalation of a mixture of 5 to 10 per cent carbon dioxide and 90 to 95 per cent oxygen is effective if the respiration is appreciably depressed. The use of stimulants may be necessary and may be administered in the form of 0.75 to 1 gm. of caffeine sodium benzoate orally or hypodermically. Benzedrine sulfate is an extremely efficient stimulant in oral doses of 5 to 10 mg. For rapid oxidation of blood alcohol it is wise to give 100 cc. of 50 per cent glucose solution combined with 20 units of insulin and thiamine chloride in doses of 50 to 100 mg. ACTH (see discussion of Chronic Alcoholism) may be tried. When dehydration is present, ample fluids containing sodium chloride should be administered. In case of circulatory collapse, other usual stimulants, such as ephedrine sulfate intramuscularly (0.3 gm.) every 2 hours, can be tried. Postalcoholic headache and gastritis call for immediate cessation of continued alcohol, sodium chloride and ample fluids, preferably milk, accompanied by a full and liberal diet.

CHRONIC ALCOHOLISM

Definition. The chronic alcoholic is one who habitually relies on alcohol, who is unable to abstain from alcohol, who finds it impossible to start the next day's work without a drink. In contrast, the moderate drinker is one who limits his consumption, who does not become regularly intoxicated, whose judgment is never blurred by his drinking, who never becomes physically unsteady or tremulous from it, who never lets it interfere with his work, and who is not dependent on alcohol for escape or for relief of uncomfortable anxiety. The physician must also recognize the heavy social drinker (one who drinks heavily during social occasions but whose drinking is not a serious handicap) and the excessive drinker (one who uses alcohol frequently in such quantity that he may behave in pathologic ways but who is capable of stopping when necessity warrants).

Chronic alcoholics fall into two main groups: the spree drinker and the steady drinker. The spree drinker is a person who may not drink for days, weeks or months at a time, but at intervals finds himself driven to alcohol, usually in large amounts. He is often a solitary drinker, and he may stay on his spree for days at a time, unable to stop his drinking. A steady drinker consumes too much alcohol regularly and daily. Chronic alcoholism is a disease. The alcoholic almost invariably is seeking escape from worries and anxieties or from unconscious conflicts within his own personality which he does not recognize. In general, the alcoholic falls into several categories.

1. *Reactive Alcoholics.* These are the persons who seek to escape from intolerable environmental circumstances which may lie in difficulties of adjustment to their vocational, marital, sexual, economic or physical status. They find reality too difficult to face and know that alcohol will substitute an unrealistic phantasy for their monotonous or overdemanding lives.

2. *Symptomatic Alcoholics.* In these people alcoholism develops as a more or less prominent symptom of more widesweeping personality disorders or psychotic conditions. Thus a person who is consistently depressed may seek relief in alcohol. A self-assertive, extravagant manic may celebrate with alcohol. The feeble-minded may be inadequately protected and imitate others. Persistent alcoholism may mask schizophrenia. Persons of constitutional psychopathic make-

up drink as part of their general instability, inadequacy and unreliability.

3. *The Psychoneurotic Drinker.* These people use alcohol as a relief from their anxiety. Here we find a maladjusted person seeking escape from his intolerable inner conflicts. He finds in alcohol a socially acceptable way of covering his timidity, fears and sensitiveness.

4. *Persistent chronic drinkers* who drink primarily because they like the taste and effect of alcohol.

Many attempts have been made to define a specific personality type, among alcoholics, without much success. In general the alcoholic is insecure, self-centered, narcissistic, immature, rigid, compulsive and often driven by unrecognized sexual conflicts. The majority of patients have clear-cut psychoneurotic reactions or psychopathic personalities. He commonly presents a family history of alcoholism, and often comes from families in which there is an aggressive, successful father and a spoiling indulgent mother. Excessive drinking usually begins early in life and is used to bolster sexual insecurities and to provide security in marriage. Sexual maladjustment is common, and divorce frequently follows.

Diagnosis. Diagnosis is best made by the history of chronic continued use of alcohol, by the presence of anorexia, nausea, vomiting, diarrhea, abdominal pain, loss of weight, malnutrition and dilatation of skin capillaries. The changes in personality as reported by relatives are usually striking in the direction of irritability, lowering of moral standards, inability to work and general deterioration of habits. There may also be present enlargement of the liver, polyneuritis, persistent tremors of the face and hands, and evidences of avitaminosis. The mental processes become dulled. There may be irritability, temper outbursts, emotional lability. Psychiatric evaluation will elicit characteristic personality difficulties and conflicts.

Diagnosis is not always easy, particularly when a patient denies the use of alcohol. Many such patients recognize their difficulties but deny their inability to solve the problem, and refuse therapy.

Treatment. Psychiatric hospitalization is the most effective method of treatment. The patient must first recognize that he has a problem, that he is unable to solve it alone and that the time has come when he must seek medical help. Throughout the difficult days of withdrawal and the attendant anxiety and discomfort, the patient is best in a psychiatric hospital where he has the advantages of hydrotherapy, occupational therapy, sedation and psychotherapy. In most cases hospitalization of three to six months is indicated. Few patients are willing to stay this long and are apt to leave the hospital during the period of euphoria which characteristically occurs several weeks after the cessation of alcohol intake. Commitment, either voluntary or forced, is sometimes necessary to keep the patient under therapy during this period. In general, psychiatric treatment aims first at getting the patient to accept the fact that he has an illness, that he cannot afford to be casual about it, that he is genuinely sick, that he must avoid all the usual cliches of blandness and rationalization, and that he must finally relinquish his problem to the physician. The hospital environment permits a full study of the personality make-up and the basic pathology and allows the physician to study the many factors at work in the 24-hour living, particularly the individual's adjustment to a group environment. Anxiety can be analyzed as it emerges. Once the initial psychiatric study is well under way, the patient can be permitted to test out his reactions to reality by increasing visits outside of the hospital until the time when he can become an ambulatory patient. Long-term psychiatric treatment is indicated in most cases, i.e., one year or longer. Only when the patient becomes fully aware of the multiple factors at work, often unrecognized and unconscious, is he able to combat the addiction.

The results of therapy at best are poor. Many patients relapse. This factor has led to considerable discouragement among the medical profession. Hospital facilities are limited. There are few hospitals specifically for the treatment of alcoholism. Most private psychiatric hospitals are reluctant to admit such patients. Only a few state hospitals in this country have specific services devoted to the treatment of alcoholics. Several states have recently passed legislation to expand their treatment facilities for this group, notably Connecticut and Virginia. Most alcoholics go untreated. There is urgent need for vast expansion of facilities for the care of such patients.

Other factors enter into the effectiveness of cure, aside from the physician's skill and the patient's willingness. It is difficult for the average nondrinker to find a social group in which alcohol is not the common medium of social exchange. The most effective organization to meet this need for companionship, understanding, sharing and self-help is the organization known as "Alcoholics Anonymous." This is a society of ex-alcoholics— started 20 years ago, now numbering over 100,000 members in over 6000 chapters throughout the major cities and towns of America and in thirty-four other countries. This organization provides opportunities for the alcoholic to be accepted by others in the same dilemma, all with the same common desire to remain abstainers. It provides social life and companionship, frequently obtains employment and cooperates with hospitals and physicians in the treatment of individual members. This society has been uniquely effective. One fifth of the arrested alcoholics at a large private psychiatric hospital achieved recovery through affiliation with Alcoholics Anonymous.

No specific medication of importance is known at present, although striking therapeutic results have been claimed for the method of conditioned reflex therapy. The method is not new. It consists in the injection of 0.25 to 1 cc. subcutaneously of a mixture containing emetine, 3.3 gm., pilocarpine, 1.5 gm., and ephedrine, 11.5 gm., in 40 cc. of water. Injection is given at the same time the patient is offered alcohol. Violent nausea and vomiting results. Theoretically, a conditioned response of vomiting to alcohol is set up. Treatments are given once a day for three to seven days. Reinforcement single treatments are given at the end of one month, two months, and after that at three month intervals for one year. The procedure should be combined with psychotherapy.

Antabuse (tetraethylthiuram disulfide), first described by Hald, Jacobsen and Larsen in Denmark in 1948, is of definite value as long as patients persevere in taking the drug. When taken by mouth it renders the patient unable to tolerate alcohol in any form because of the formation of acetaldehyde which causes severe nausea, vomiting, flushing, increased cardiac rate and decreased blood pressure. The earlier claims that this drug is chemically inert are not sustained. During early weeks on the drug many patients experienced drowsiness, fatigue, headache and gastrointestinal disturbances. Such symptoms are usually mild and disappear as the dosage continues. The drug level is usually built up at the rate of 1 to 3 gm. per day, reducing the dosage to 125 mg. daily for maintenance. Some workers use a test dose of one ounce of alcohol on the fifth day (when the drug level is achieved) so that the patient may experience a severe effect from drinking. Several deaths have resulted. The danger probably does not justify the use of the test dose. The probable contraindications to its use are cardiovascular disease, liver damage, diabetes and epilepsy. Reports on the use of Antabuse therapy indicate 50 to 60 per cent of cases remain sober for a year or more. There are more and more reports on relapse and of the development of serious mental illness. Unstable and poorly organized patients rarely remain in therapy. Antabuse is, however, a useful adjunct to general psychiatric therapy.

ACTH and cortisone have been tried in the treatment of cases of acute alcohol intoxication, delirium tremens, alcoholic hallucinosis and Korsakoff's psychosis. The effects of this therapy however are usually not striking, and may be actually harmful.

Roger Williams believes that nutritional defect is etiologically significant in chronic alcoholism. He found that distinctive metabolic patterns occur which give the total picture of metabolism of any given individual and he believes there are hereditary differences. He postulates that individuals with a strong tendency to become alcoholic possess distinctive metabolic features and that the appetite for alcohol arises as a result of a deficiency of the B vitamins.

Diethelm and co-workers, through biologic assay of chemical substances in the blood of alcoholic patients, have found that the prevailing emotions, in chronic alcoholic patients, of anxiety, tension and resentment are regularly accompanied by the appearance of a substance in the blood resembling epinephrine (in anxiety), of a cholinergic substance (with tension) and of an unknown substance accompanying resentment. This latter substance in the blood of alcoholic patients repeatedly disappears when alcohol is ingested. Similarly, the anxiety substance disappears with the administration of dibenamine and the tension substance with barbiturates. These findings offer valuable leads for possible therapeutic application in the future.

A chronic alcoholic must be prepared to abstain totally and permanently. He cannot rationalize with himself that he can tolerate beer or wine. This rarely if ever succeeds.

Religion and other suggestive influences

and group psychotherapy may be used. The patient's entire way of life needs to be reorganized. Families and relatives need education in the fundamental nature of the disease, and their cooperation is important in the therapeutic process. Social service is often of extreme importance in reorienting the patient and his family.

The National Research Council, Medical Science Division, has established a Committee on Problems of Alcohol to advise and support research in the field. Help and advice can also be obtained through the National Committee for Education on Alcoholism in New York City.

Alcoholism as a broad medical problem is equally a public health and community responsibility. Planning in the United States lags far behind that of Switzerland and Sweden. In Sweden there is a local official temperance board in every community which possesses broad power and is said to obtain 30 to 40 per cent cures. In our country there is a great lack of organization in plans and not enough recognition of the need for diagnostic centers and clinical research. General hospitals are the logical point of attack, but most general hospitals refuse to admit alcoholic patients.

DELIRIUM TREMENS

Delirium tremens is an acute, serious and sometimes fatal syndrome seen usually in chronic alcoholics, characteristically during periods of withdrawal or after particularly heavy bouts of drinking. It constitutes an acute psychotic episode, characterized especially by disorientation as to time, place and person, marked fear, and hallucinations, particularly of the visual type, which are usually terrifying (snakes, bats, other animals). The episode is usually transient, lasting three to seven days, and recovery is the rule. However, delirium tremens after an operation or after an accident can be extremely dangerous to life. The illness, coming on after prolonged drinking, lack of food and sleeplessness, is generally ushered in by restlessness, insomnia and the development of increasingly severe tremors of the entire body. During the delirium the patient may be excited, overactive, attempting frantically to escape from his hallucinatory fears. In his confusion he may mistake a window for a door and inadvertently injure himself. He should always be considered a potential suicidal risk. The delirium is characteristically like an active, vivid, terrifying dream. Paranoid suspicion and distrust may color the picture. The condition is usually worse at night or in dimly lighted rooms where the patient cannot visually orient himself. Infectious diseases, such as pneumonia, or a severe injury may precipitate the condition.

Diagnosis. Diagnosis is made from the characteristic delirious picture, history of abrupt cessation of alcoholic intake, flushing or pallor, profuse perspiration and tachycardia. Pneumonia and circulatory collapse are the usual immediate causes of death, which may supervene with great rapidity.

Treatment. Delirium tremens is an acute, self-limiting disorder which requires emergency care. Hospitalization is imperative, and competent, wise nursing care is the best single aid to therapy. Sedation is always indicated, and paraldehyde is preeminently the drug of choice—10 to 20 cc. by mouth, or 15 to 25 cc. by rectum. Immediate cessation of alcohol is indicated. There is little justification for gradual withdrawal. If paraldehyde is refused, chloral hydrate may be given in doses of 1 to 2 gm. Barbiturates also have value; Sodium Amytal in doses of 0.5 gm. is preferred because of its fairly rapid action. The main effort is to secure relaxation, freedom from fear, and sustained sleep. Hydrotherapy in the form of prolonged baths is helpful. Restraint should never be used, since it increases the patient's fearfulness. The patient must be protected against accidentally harming himself through panic. Suicidal precautions are necessary.

Immediate therapy should also include the use of ample fluids and the combination of 100 cc. of 50 per cent glucose solution intravenously with 20 units of insulin, intramuscularly. Thiamine chloride (50 to 100 mg.) and nicotinic acid (10 mg.) should be given immediately and repeated three times daily. Some therapists have recommended massive vitamin medication as high as 1500 mg. of nicotinic acid and 500 mg. of thiamine chloride as an emergency procedure. The enthusiasm for lumbar puncture has waned. It is doubtful if the procedure has great value. Hypertonic glucose solution should be injected intravenously to reduce cerebral edema. Magnesium sulfate by mouth may also be effective. The patient should be digitalized only if signs of congestive cardiac failure develop. As stated above, ACTH in doses of 25 mg. every 6 hours, may be a specific and its trial is justified.

The main effort should be toward supportive treatment. The patient should be kept warm in bed, but permitted freedom of movement. The diet should be liquid or soft, and high in carbohydrate, electrolytes and vitamins. Constant reassurance is necessary. The patient is best kept either in a brightly lighted room or in total darkness, since shadows tend to increase visual misinterpretations. Complete recovery is the rule, although death occurs in approximately 5 to 15 per cent of the cases.

CLINICAL DISORDERS RELATED TO CHRONIC ALCOHOLISM

The long-continued use of alcohol can result in the following varieties of disturbances: (1) acute alcoholic excitement, (2) pathologic intoxication with epileptoid complications, (3) alcoholic hallucinosis (acute or chronic), (4) Korsakoff's psychosis, (5) alcoholic deterioration, (6) paranoid disorders and jealousy reactions, (7) neuritis, (8) Wernicke's syndrome—mistakenly related to alcoholism, actually the result of vitamin deficiency. These will be briefly defined.

1. **Acute Alcoholic Excitement.** In susceptible persons alcohol can result in an acute, brief, self-limiting psychotic episode of great excitement and combativeness, with or without hallucinations.

2. **Pathologic Intoxication with Epileptoid Complications.** In any history of epilepsy or epileptoid behavior it is necessary to rule out alcoholism as the major factor, since it can produce atypical epileptic pictures in susceptible persons.

3. **Alcoholic Hallucinosis (Acute or Chronic).** In this condition the main picture is one of auditory hallucinations in the presence of otherwise clear mental processes. Coupled with this is commonly a paranoid reaction of suspicion, distrust and ideas of persecution. Jealousy is common. The person remains well oriented and in grasp of himself and his situation, but complains primarily of disturbing auditory hallucinations. The disorder may be short or last for weeks or months.

4. **Korsakoff's Psychosis.** This type of psychosis may develop in persistent alcoholics and is characterized by marked and obvious difficulties in memory and by the presence of confabulation (filling in of imaginary details to cover up the memory deficit). The psychosis may start with delirium or may be insidious, as a memory deficit disorder. Usually associated with the psychosis there are manifestations of polyneuritis and at times pellagra-like skin lesions. Though nutritional deficiency (particularly of vitamin B) commonly plays a role, the prognosis is usually serious and the damage is apt to be irreversible in spite of vitamin replacement therapy.

5. **Alcoholic Deterioration.** This is a slowly evolving deterioration of the whole personality resulting in a loss of mature standards of behavior and in the development of an irresponsible, jovial and carefree outlook upon life, or impulsive behavior leading to serious breaking of the social and moral codes, particularly in the realm of sexual behavior.

6. **Paranoid Disorders and Jealousy Reactions.** Persistent drinkers are particularly prone to the development of marked jealousy reactions mainly directed at their spouses or members of their families and, in full-fledged reactions, with the development of outstanding systematized or poorly systematized delusional syndromes of a paranoid nature.

7. **Neuritis.** The polyneuritis associated with alcoholism is in all likelihood due to a vitamin B deficiency. It is relatively uncommon when nutrition is well maintained and vitamin replacement therapy is carried out. The onset may be gradual with paresthesias of the hands and feet, increasing pain in muscle groups or motor manifestations in the form of paralysis involving the feet, legs and arms. The extensor muscles of the feet are commonly affected, giving rise to a characteristic gait. The patient complains of persistent burning sensations or severe pain in the extremities. Sphincter disturbances may also occur. Tachycardia is a frequent manifestation. The condition may persist for weeks or months, but usually responds to massive doses of vitamin B preparations. The picture may also be complicated by manifestations of pellagra, including glossitis, achlorhydria, diarrhea, nutritional edema or cardiac decompensation.

8. **Wernicke's Syndrome.** The usual clinical picture is that of ophthalmoplegia, pupillary disturbances, clouding of consciousness and ataxia. The lesion is a midbrain syndrome with marked deterioration of parenchyma, blood vessel proliferation and hemorrhage. This is a nutritional deficiency

which results principally from a lack of thiamine and possibly other vitamins of the B complex group.

Treatment of Neurologic and Psychiatric Disorders Associated with Continued Use of Alcohol. Mention has already been made of the common sequelae that attend the continued use of alcohol and the dietary deficiency that almost invariably attends it. The prognosis for these conditions is often grave. Treatment is preeminently vitamin replacement therapy, particularly with thiamine and nicotinic acid, but also with all the other fractions of the B complex group. Daily replacement doses should be administered orally, and in cases of doubtful absorption the material should be given parenterally. Emphasis upon full dietary intake is important. A diet rich in carbohydrate and protein is indicated. Small doses of insulin, 5 to 15 units, one-half to one hour before meals, can be given to promote appetite in patients unable to eat adequately.

Nursing care and hospitalization may be indicated when defective judgment or personality deterioration renders the patient subject to impulsive antisocial acts. If advanced avitaminosis is present, treatment should be similar to that for pellagra. Physiotherapy, massage and reeducation may be effective in neuritic states.

THOMAS A. C. RENNIE

References

Diethelm, O., Fleetwood, M. F., and Milhorat, A. T.: The Predictable Association of Certain Emotions and Biochemical Changes in the Blood. Life Stress and Body Disease. Baltimore, Williams and Wilkins Co., 1950, Chapter XVI.

Emerson, H.: Alcohol and Man. New York, The Macmillan Company, 1932.

Goldfarb, W., Bowman, K. M., and Parker, S.: The Treatment of Acute Alcoholism with Glucose and Insulin. J. Clin. Investigation, 18:581, 1939.

Haggard, H. W.: The Physician and the Problem of Alcoholism. Bull. New York Acad. Med., 21: 451, 1945.

Hald, J., Jacobsen, E., and Larsen, V.: The Sensitizing Effect of Tetraethylthiuramdisulphide (Antabuse) to Ethyl Alcohol. Acta pharmacol., 4:285, 1948.

Lemere, F., and others: Conditioned Reflex Treatment of Chronic Alcoholism: VII. Technic. Dis. Nerv. System, 3:243, 1942.

Piker, P.: Clinical Evaluation of Use of Fluids in Treatment of Delirium Tremens. Arch. Neurol. & Psychiat., 39:62, 1939.

Rotman, D. B.: Alcoholism, A Social Disease. J.A.M.A., 127:564, 1945.

Smith, J. J.: A Medical Approach to Problem Drinking. Quart. J. Stud. on Alcohol, 10:251–257, 1949.

————: The Treatment of Acute Alcoholic States with ACTH and Adrenocortical Hormones. Quart. J. Stud. on Alcohol., 11:190–198, 1950.

Strecker, E. A., and Chambers, F. T.: Alcohol, One Man's Meat. New York, The Macmillan Company, 1943.

Tintera, J. W., and Lovell, H. W.: Endocrine Treatment of Alcoholism. Geriatrics, 4:274–280, 1949.

METHYL ALCOHOL POISONING

Methyl alcohol (CH_3OH: wood alcohol, Columbian spirit) has no medicinal uses. Serious poisoning leading to death can occur from its ingestion or from exposure in industry. It is used as a solvent in industry and formerly as an adulterant in ethyl alcohol. The main toxic results arise from its oxidation in the body into formaldehyde and formic acid, both of which are exceedingly toxic. The effects of methyl alcohol are due to depression of the central nervous system, the state of acidosis created, cerebral edema and a specific toxic effect upon the optic nerve, respiratory center and vagus nerve. The amount of methyl alcohol necessary to cause blindness or death varies from 10 cc. upwards, the lethal dose being usually 100 to 250 cc. In the absence of a history of ingestion the diagnosis of an individual case may be difficult. Most cases occur because of the inadequate labelling of methyl alcohol as a poison.

Symptoms. The common symptoms of poisoning, which occur within a few hours after drinking, are prolonged inebriation, drowsiness, general weakness, headache, photophobia, blurring of vision, nausea, vomiting, abdominal pain, dyspnea and cyanosis. Coma, delirium and unconsciousness may ensue. Blindness may occur in a few hours or be delayed several days. The impaired vision is usually but not necessarily irreversible. The patient may die in one to three days. Coma caused by methyl alcohol may last three or four days.

Diagnosis. Diagnosis is facilitated by the history of ingestion when available, the odor of methyl alcohol on the breath, and the presence of flushed face, cyanosis, rapid pulse, labored and elevated respiration, various degrees of drowsiness, confusion or delirium, ocular abnormalities consisting in loss of vision, supraorbital or retro-orbital pain, dilated and sluggish pupils, mild hyperemia of the disk and retina, haziness of disk margins and engorgement of the blood vessels, and difficulties of memory. The urine may contain traces of albumin and ketones, and numerous hyaline and granular casts. The urine may be strongly acid and show the presence of abnormally large amounts of formic acid. The presence of methyl alcohol in the blood may be demonstrated.

Pathologic Findings. Postmortem examination findings reveal moderate to severe cyanosis, lividity, emphysema, edema of the lungs, hemorrhages into the subpleural and subpericardial tissues and the mucosa of the stomach. An outstanding feature is the edema and swelling of the brain and brain stem.

Treatment. Treatment should include enforced complete bed rest, warmth and adequate nutrition. Even though the patient is not in immediate distress, collapse may occur suddenly. Routine measures include a gastric lavage, a high saline enema, 45 cc., magnesium sulfate orally or through a stomach tube, repeated intravenous infusions of 15 gm. of sodium bicarbonate or sodium lactate dissolved in 1000 cc. of 5 per cent dextrose in saline. This should be repeated every six hours or more frequently until the urine pH reaches 7.0. In addition, 6 gm. doses of sodium bicarbonate should be given orally at 4-hour intervals. If pain is severe or delirium ensues, morphine, scopolamine or barbiturates may be used in the usual dosage, provided that no respiratory depression is evident. Cerebral edema can be combated by intravenous hypertonic glucose solution (50 to 100 cc. of 50 per cent solution) and 30 to 60 gm. of magnesium sulfate orally. Oxygen therapy may be necessary in some cases, and hypodermic stimulants of 1 gm. of caffeine sodium benzoate, ephedrine (10 to 30 mg. intramuscularly), coramine (2 to 4 cc. intravenously), or artificial respiration may be needed as respiratory stimulants. The eyes should be protected from exposure to strong light. The administration of vitamins—thiamine, nicotinic acid and specifically vitamin K—is indicated. The patient should receive a transfusion of whole blood or plasma.

In two reports from the U. S. Navy the importance of correcting acidosis by intravenous sodium bicarbonate or lactate therapy is emphasized.

Reiner, also of the U. S. Navy, reviews evidence for the existence of cerebral edema and recommends the therapeutic value of drainage of the cerebrospinal fluid in acute methyl alcohol poisoning. Abnormal elevation of spinal fluid pressure occurs frequently during the week following ingestion. Repeated lumbar puncture is recommended until spinal fluid pressure returns to normal. Death and blindness may thereby be prevented.

Thomas A. C. Rennie

References

Buller, F., and Wood, C. A.: Poisoning by Wood Alcohol: Cases of Death and Blindness from Columbian Spirits and Other Methylated Preparations. J.A.M.A., 43:1213, 1904.

Harrop, G. A., Jr., and Benedict, E. M.: Acute Methyl Alcohol Poisoning Associated with Acidosis. J.A.M.A., 74:25, 1920.

Jacobson, B. M., Russell, H. K., Grimm, J. J., and Fox, E. C.: Acute Methyl Alcohol Poisoning. U. S. Nav. M. Bull., 44:5, 1945.

Kaplan, A., and Levreault, G. V.: Methyl Alcohol Poisoning (Report of 42 Cases). U. S. Nav. M. Bull., 44:5, 1945.

Reiner, E. R.: The Cerebrospinal Fluid in Methyl Alcohol Poisoning. Arch. Neurol. & Psychiat., 64:528, 1950.

Voegtlin, W. L., and Watts, C. D.: Acute Methyl Alcohol (Methanol) Poisoning. Synopsis of Subject with Case Report. U. S. Nav. M. Bull., 41:1715, 1943.

MARIHUANA INTOXICATION

(Cannabis)

The term "marihuana" (hemp) refers to any part of the hemp plant or extract therefrom which induces somatic and psychic changes in man. From the flowering tops of the hemp plant, which grows wild in many parts of the world, including the United States, there is obtained an intoxicating principle which has been known since 1500 B.C. Variously prepared, the active principle can be inhaled or ingested in the form of a candy or liquid preparation. In America it is most commonly used as cigarettes called "reefers." The drug is habitually used for its psychic effects and is unique in the reactions it produces. Its physiologic effects have been likened to those of atropine and the psychic effects of those of alcohol.

Chemistry. The chemistry of marihuana is complicated and confusing. By synthesis, it has been proved that the formula for one of two active substances contained is 1-methyl-3-n-amyl-6,6,9-trimethyl-6-dibenzo-pyran (cannabinol). Marihuana belongs botannically to the genus *Cannabis,* of which *Cannabis indica* is one of the few varieties.

Symptoms. The effects are mainly those of acute intoxication, containing sensory, motor and subjective elements lasting several hours to several days. Toxic psychoses as a direct result, and atypical psychoses initiated or colored by marihuana, have been described.

The effects manifest themselves almost entirely on the central nervous system. There are several successive phases to intoxication. The subject first feels strong, agile and capable of extraordinary feats of prowess, the state of being "high." This phase is characterized by sensations of floating in the air, lightness or dizziness in the head, ringing in the ears and heaviness of the limbs. The euphoria is manifested in volubility and increased psychomotor activity, and later in a subjective feeling of pleasant lassitude. Distance and time intervals appear elastic: time seems infinitely slow and spatial conceptions are impaired. Sight and hearing are extremely acute, but the perceptions are distorted sometimes to the degree of illusions or hallucinations. Succeeding this is a phase of fatigue and sleepiness, which may last 1 to 6 hours. When the subject awakes, he feels "down," although the clinical phenomena may linger for another few hours. Throughout the period of intoxication the subject may appear apprehensive, loquacious and somewhat suspicious. His talk may be circumstantial. Attention, concentration and comprehension may be impaired. The subject, upon awakening, usually remembers what he had experienced during the period of intoxication.

Disagreeable symptoms may occur, especially with overdosage. These include pains in the head and neck, feelings of apprehension and anxiety and even panic, and the development of suspicions which may flare into hatred resulting in fits of terror and assaultiveness. In unstable, poorly organized personalities the administration of large amounts of marihuana may precipitate psychoses which last for weeks or months. During acute psychotic reactions the physiologic and psychic manifestations become quantitatively greater. Respirations become labored, and pallor, perspiration, tachycardia and an irregularity of the pulse may occur, together with urinary urgency, diarrhea, nausea and vomiting. Pathologic emotional reactions may include negativism, catalepsy, pseudohallucinations, micropsia and macropsia.

The prolonged effects of the drug consist in increased fatigability and vague generalized aches and pains. The aftermath is like that of an alcoholic hangover.

While all substances derived from cannabis are narcotic drugs, by act of Congress, marihuana does not give rise to biologic or physiologic addiction, for discontinuance of the drug after prolonged use does not result in withdrawal symptoms. However, habituation or dependence can occur. Increasingly larger doses are not necessary in order to continue the original degree of pleasure. No permanent effect results from acute intoxication. It is doubtful that prolonged use leads to physical, mental or moral deterioration or to any degenerative brain disease. While the drug acts primarily by lowering inhibitions, thereby accentuating the fundamental traits of personality, it does not of itself impel to violent action or crime, but may permit the release of antisocial tendencies formerly repressed. Marihuana as a direct cause of criminal acts has been overstressed. The drug has no proved therapeutic value in modern medicine.

Treatment. A drug having such properties is, of course, dangerous. As with alcohol, the addict needs medical and psychiatric care, preferably in a psychiatric hospital. Under such a regimen immediate withdrawal of marihuana is indicated. There are no known hazards from immediate withdrawal. Treatment must include primary attention to the personality make-up and emotional problems of the patient, and psychotherapy is the main tool in rendering the patient free of his dependence and need for stimulation by marihuana. In this respect the treatment aims are the same as those applied to the addicts of alcohol (see discussion under Alcoholism).

THOMAS A. C. RENNIE

References

Adams, R.: Marihuana. Science, 92:2380, 1940.
Allentuck, S., and Bowman, K. M.: The Psychiatric Aspects of Marihuana Intoxication. Am. J. Psychiat., 99:1942–43.

Bromberg, W.: Marihuana. J.A.M.A., *113*:1, 1939.

Walton, R. P.: Marihuana: America's New Drug Problem. Philadelphia, J. B. Lippincott Company, 1938.

Yawger, N. S.: Marihuana, Our New Addiction. Am. J. M. Sc., *195*:3, 1938.

OPIUM POISONING

Definition. Opium poisoning refers to the intoxication produced by opium, any of its preparations or alkaloids (morphine, heroin, Dilaudid, codeine and the like), and to intoxication by synthetic drugs with morphine-like action (meperidine and methadone). Poisoning with any of these drugs may be acute or chronic.

ACUTE OPIUM POISONING

Etiology. Acute opium poisoning sometimes occurs because of ingestion of the drugs in suicidal attempts, but usually results from an accidental overdose. Occasionally it may be due to an abnormal sensitivity to opiates. Narcotic drug addicts with active habits are seldom acutely poisoned because of the high degree of tolerance they have developed to opiates. Occasionally, addicts, after having been withdrawn from drugs, may mistakenly take the same dose of the drug which they were using when addicted and become acutely poisoned. Fatal doses vary greatly and are affected by the particular drug or preparation taken, the route of administration, the age, sex and physical condition of the patient. In general, the ingestion of 60 mg. of morphine, or an equivalent dose of any of the other drugs, is dangerous to an adult. Doses of 240 mg. or more may be fatal unless treatment is begun promptly. Both infants and elderly people are more sensitive to morphine than are young adults. Women are more sensitive than men. The toxicity of these drugs is increased in any condition associated with diminished vital capacity, such as bronchial asthma, pulmonary fibrosis and emphysema. Patients suffering with hypothyroidism are also very sensitive to the toxic effects of morphine.

Pathology. There are no specific anatomic changes due to acute intoxication with drugs of this type. The pathologic findings are those associated with asphyxia and peripheral vascular collapse, and include petechial hemorrhages beneath serous membranes, pooling of the blood in the great veins, and pulmonary and cerebral edema.

Pathologic Physiology. The symptoms of acute opium poisoning are due to depression of the cerebral cortex and the respiratory center, and to the development of abnormalities of cardiovascular function, which are caused by direct peripheral vasodilatation and by depression of the vasomotor center and the carotid bodies.

Symptoms. The symptoms of poisoning with all the derivatives of opium or with methadone are identical, but the symptoms of poisoning by meperidine are somewhat different. After the ingestion of toxic amounts of any opiate, or methadone, symptoms usually appear within 30 minutes and consist in flushing of the face and the upper part of the body, giddiness, nausea, vomiting and itching of the skin. Patients become drowsy, sleep, and finally slip into coma, which is characteristically light in proportion to the degree of respiratory depression. Patients breathing only three or four times a minute can frequently be aroused by mild reflex stimulation, such as slapping or pinching. The pupils are constricted, and the temperature is depressed about 1 degree C. Respiratory rate and minute volume are decreased, and Cheyne-Stokes respiration is frequently seen. Systolic blood pressure falls slightly, the pulse rate is slowed, and a tendency to postural hypotension is present. Signs of severe poisoning include dilatation of the pupils, severe respiratory depression, cyanosis, marked depression of blood pressure, tachycardia and pulmonary edema. Convulsions rarely occur.

Poisoning due to meperidine is characterized by respiratory depression, dilatation of the pupils, dryness of the mouth and mucous membranes, and by muscular tremors and convulsions.

Diagnosis. The triad of miosis, coma and marked respiratory depression should always suggest the diagnosis of acute opium intoxication. A history of the ingestion of opiates obtained from friends or relatives, the presence of needlemarks on the skin, or the finding of boxes or bottles which have contained the drug may be helpful. A therapeutic test with N-allylnormorphine should distinguish between opiate poisoning and all other causes of coma with respiratory depression. If spectacular respiratory stimulation does not follow the intravenous administration of 10 mg. of this drug (see below), it is unlikely that one is dealing with opiate poisoning.

Prognosis. The availability of N-allylnormorphine has greatly altered the prognosis of opiate poisoning. If the diagnosis is made before shock, pulmonary edema and pneumonia are present, treatment is almost invariably successful.

Treatment. The treatment of acute opiate poisoning consists of specific antidotal therapy with N-allylnormorphine combined with symptomatic and supportive measures. Whenever the diagnosis of acute opium poisoning is suspected, the patient should be given as soon as possible 5 to 10 mg. of N-allylnormorphine intravenously or subcutaneously. This compound, though chemically related to morphine, specifically reverses the respiratory depressant, sedative and circulatory depressant effects of morphine, methadone, meperidine and related drugs. Following the administration of N-allylnormorphine to a person severely poisoned with any of the drugs mentioned above, dramatic respiratory stimulation will occur. This effect is so marked and consistent that failure to obtain it weighs heavily against the diagnosis of opiate poisoning. Concomitantly, coma lightens and the patient can be aroused. The effect of N-allylnormorphine on consciousness is, however, less than on the respiratory depression. If the blood pressure has been depressed by the opiate, N-allylnormorphine will elevate it into the normal range. Since the length of action of N-allylnormorphine is shorter than that of some of the opiates, patients may slowly become depressed after being aroused with the drug. Repetition of the dose of N-allylnormorphine will promptly revive the patient. Not more than 40 mg. of N-allylnormorphine in divided doses should be given in a 12-hour period.

Symptomatic treatment includes maintenance of an open airway. The nasopharynx should be kept clear by suction. Continuous reflex stimulation should be applied using light pinching, slapping and talking. The patient should not be walked since postural hypotension is a feature of acute opium poisoning. If the breathing is greatly depressed and N-allylnormorphine is not available, artificial respiration should be instituted, preferably using an automatic positive pressure device or a Drinker respirator. Oxygen should be administered by mask or catheter. Periodic stimulation of respiration with 5 per cent carbon dioxide and 95 per cent oxygen is of value. Until N-allylnormorphine can be obtained, injections of 0.5 gm. of caffeine sodium benzoate, 10 to 20 mg. of amphetamine sulfate and 5 cc. of 25 per cent solution of

nikethamide may be tried. The patient should be turned in bed periodically and fluid intake maintained. Antibiotics should be given in an attempt to prevent the development of hypostatic pneumonia.

CHRONIC OPIUM POISONING
(Narcotic Addiction)

Definition. Chronic opium poisoning, or narcotic drug addiction, is a condition in which a person compulsively uses opium, or any equivalent drug, to such an extent that he becomes emotionally and physically dependent upon it. Narcotic drug addiction is usually described as embracing three intimately related phenomena: (a) *tolerance*—a decrease in the effects of the same dose of a drug on repeated administration; (b) *physical dependence*—the development of an altered physiologic state brought about by the repeated administration of a drug, which results in the development of a characteristic train of symptoms called an abstinence syndrome when the drug is withheld; and (c) *habituation*—emotional dependence upon the use of a drug.

Incidence. Since 1950 an increased incidence of addiction to heroin among adolescents and young adults has occurred in some of the large cities of the eastern seaboard and Great Lakes region. Despite this, the number of addicts in the United States is estimated to have fallen from 150,000 to 200,000 in 1916 to not more than 60,000 in 1952. Narcotic addiction is more common among males than females, occurs more often among residents of large cities and is more frequent in persons who engage in underworld activities. Physicians and nurses are especially likely to become addicts—particularly to meperidine—probably because of the ease of access to drugs.

Drugs Used. The drugs most popular with addicts are the more potent ones—heroin, Dilaudid, morphine and methadone. Meperidine, being less potent, is less frequently used, and addiction to codeine is fairly rare.

Most addicts inject their drugs, and usually prefer the intravenous route. Use of the drugs orally or as a snuff is now uncommon. Opium smoking remains the preferred method among Asiatics. Addicts obtain the greater part of their supply of drugs by purchase from persons engaged in illegal trafficking in drugs. The drugs available in the illegal market are usually impure, diluted with other substances, and frequently contaminated with fungi and bacteria.

Etiology. The etiology of drug addiction is multifactorial, involving sociologic, pharmacologic and psychologic factors. The important sociologic factors include association with criminals, slum-living, minority group pressures and membership in gangs. The pharmacologic factors are the effects of opiates which fulfill certain of the potential addict's psychologic needs. The most important effects are the reductions in "primary" needs or motivations, particularly hunger, pain and sexual urges. Though these are primary, "secondary" gains may be important. The use of drugs may provide a means of expressing hostility towards individuals, or society or a way of self-punishment. Psychiatric factors are of prime importance, and all addicts can be shown to have a personality defect, which, so far as can be judged from the history, antedates the addiction. There is nothing specific about the personality defects found in addiction. Most addicts suffer from a character disorder (constitutional psychopathic inferiority), a psychoneurosis or, most frequently, a mixture of the two. Reactive depressions appear to play a role in some cases. Schizophrenia and manic-depressive psychoses are of no importance in the etiology of addiction. If one excludes persons who must have opiates over a long period of time for relief of pain due to a chronic incurable disease, the number of persons who become addicted as a result of medical administration of analgesics accounts for less than 5 per cent of the total number of addicts. Moreover, patients who do become addicted as a result of medical contact usually have deep-seated personality problems.

Morbid Anatomy. No specific pathologic changes are directly attributable to the chronic use of opiates. Such changes as do occur are probably attributable to malnutrition, abscess formations in the injection sites and to diseases not related to the addiction.

Pathologic Physiology. Addicts take narcotic drugs because they regard the effects of the drug as pleasurable. These effects are described as including a sense of "pep" or "drive" followed by a pleasurable sense of warmth and muscular relaxation which is associated with the development of a dreamy, semisomnolent state in which all worries vanish and all problems can be deferred.

When morphine is taken intravenously a tingling sensation, which has been likened to a sexual orgasm, spreads over the body. This sensation is extremely attractive to psychopaths. In all probability, these effects, which are readily described by addicts, are of lesser importance than reduction in pain, anxiety, hunger and sexual urges. The sensations produced by morphine and allied drugs are, of course, due to the effects of the drug on the cells of the central nervous system, the most important of which may be the reduction of reflexes mediated through multineuron arcs.

Although addicts originally take the drug to enjoy the pleasurable effects, they find that, as the experience is repeated, larger and larger doses are required to produce the desired results. This phenomenon is spoken of as tolerance. Its mechanism is as yet unknown, but it is believed to represent in part the development of physiologic counter-responses within the nervous system which antagonize some of the actions of morphine. Nearly complete tolerance develops to the toxic, euphoric, emetic and analgesic effects of morphine, but no tolerance to the constipating action, and only partial tolerance to the cardiovascular, respiratory and miotic actions. The amount of drug a tolerant addict can take appears to be limited only by the available supply and by the mechanical difficulty of preparing and injecting the solution. Patients observed under carefully controlled conditions have injected as much as 5 gm. of morphine intravenously in 16 hours without any serious toxic symptoms.

As the addict becomes tolerant, he finds that, if he discontinues his drug, he suffers a characteristic illness (abstinence syndrome) which is immediately abolished by another injection of the drug. Physical dependence has frequently been attributed to psychologic mechanisms, but this view is no longer tenable. Abstinence symptoms occur in the paralyzed extremities of dogs whose spinal cords have been severed and in dogs without cerebral cortex. The mechanism of abstinence is probably closely related to the mechanism of tolerance, appears to be diffuse throughout the central nervous system, and may represent a release from the check imposed by the drug on the counter-responses developed against the actions of morphine.

Psychopathology. Although morphine addiction is nearly always based on a preexisting psychiatric disorder, continued use of opium or an equivalent drug always produces still more emotional damage and leads to a lower level of social adjustment. Although the ability of addicts to perform work is not greatly impaired by the drug, they are content to sit and dream. Their will to work and to produce is markedly impaired. This reduced social productivity represents the real loss from narcotic addiction. The use of the drug comes to represent the answer to all of life's problems, and obtaining the drug replaces all other drives and motives. The necessity for secrecy in using the drug, difficulties with the law, and the high cost of the drug, all contribute to social and moral regression.

Although many criminals are drug addicts, the use of morphine does not release or increase tendencies to commit violent crime. Because of the high cost of the drugs, many addicts who are not basically criminal must engage in minor thievery or in confidence games in order to obtain funds to support their addiction.

Symptoms. Prior to development of tolerance, the symptoms of addiction are chiefly those of mild to moderate opium intoxication and include miosis, nausea, vomiting, itching of the skin, scratching, and the development of semisomnolent state characterized by periods of alternating sleep and wakefulness. The pulse is slightly slowed, systolic blood pressure is reduced, and body temperature is at first somewhat depressed. After tolerance has developed there are practically no pathognomonic signs of morphine addiction. Partial tolerance to the miotic action of morphine develops so that too great reliance cannot be placed on the presence or absence of constricted pupils. Behavior of tolerant addicts is not strikingly different from that of unaddicted persons. Patients are usually pale and malnourished as a result of neglect of their diet in favor of drugs. They do not show ataxia, are able to carry out skilled movements, can converse normally and can work. The presence of scars, abscess and needlemarks, particularly in the form of linear tattoos over the veins, is the most constant finding, but does not indicate whether the patient is taking the drugs at the time of the examination. Patients using methadone have marked thickening, induration and inflammation of the skin over the injection sites. Addicts chronically intoxicated with meperidine may, if they are using as much as 1 or 2 gm. of the drug daily, have muscular tremors, twitching, marked dilatation of the pupils, and possibly convulsions.

Abstinence Syndrome. The clinical course of abstinence from morphine is one of the most characteristic and stereotyped syndromes seen in clinical medicine. If patients become tolerant to 24 mg. or morphine or more daily, and medication is abruptly stopped, no signs are noted during the first 8 to 14 hours of abstinence. Patients then become somewhat restless and nervous. Despite the restlessness, they are sleepy and drift into a restless, tossing slumber which may last several hours. On awakening from this abnormal sleep, patients start to yawn and begin to exhibit rhinorrhea, lacrimation and slight perspiration. As time goes on, they become more restless. Twenty-four to 36 hours after the last dose is given, they are unable to remain still, turn and toss from side to side, change from one position to another, constantly twitch their legs and arms, and complain of alternating sensations of warmth and chilliness, of cramps in the legs and back. Waves of gooseflesh and dilatation of the pupils are seen. Yawning, lacrimation, rhinorrhea and perspiration are present continuously, appetite is decreased, and patients at this state usually take only liquids. They may have frequent spells of vomiting. Diarrhea develops. Slight fever, hyperpnea, elevation of systolic blood pressure, leukocytosis and mild hyperglycemia are present. The peak intensity of symptoms is reached at the forty-eighth hour and maintained until the seventy-second hour. After the third day the symptoms decline, and after five to seven days no acute symptoms are detectable, although patients are still weak, have poor appetites, and sleep poorly. After fourteen days the only remaining symptoms are nervousness and insomnia, which may persist for two to four months.

The course of abstinence from other morphine-like drugs differs from abstinence from morphine chiefly in time of onset, and intensity and duration of symptoms. Abstinence from heroin, Dilaudid, dihydrocodeinone and ketobemidone (a derivative of meperidine) is characterized by a rapid onset of signs, great intensity and a rapid decline of the acute symptoms. Signs of abstinence from meperidine appear sooner than signs of abstinence from morphine, are not as severe, and decline more rapidly than do signs of abstinence from morphine. Signs of abstinence from codeine are quite mild, appear more slowly, and decline at approximately the same rate as abstinence from morphine. Signs of abstinence from methadone are mild, usually are not detectable until the third or fourth day of abstinence, and very few signs of disturbed autonomic function are present. Changes in blood pressure, body temperature, pulse and respiratory rates during abstinence from methadone, while definite, are small. The abstinence syndrome from methadone is, however, prolonged and is characterized by weakness and slow recovery as compared to morphine.

The intensity of abstinence symptoms from morphine is conditioned more by the dose which the addict is taking than by any other single factor. Mild grades of symptoms can be produced in either nonaddicts or former morphine addicts by the administration of as little as 10 to 20 mg. of morphine four to six times daily for twenty-one to thirty days. Moderate to severe abstinence syndrome is seen after administration of as much as 240 mg. or morphine daily for thirty days. The maximum grade of abstinence syndrome appears after the use of 480 mg. or more of morphine daily for thirty days or longer.

Diagnosis. The diagnosis of drug addiction usually presents no great difficulties, since most patients readily admit their addiction. Some addicts, however, are quite clever in concealing their addiction and in obtaining drugs from physicians. The possibility of addiction should immediately come to mind when a strange persons presents himself with a glib, smooth story of some organic disease for which little physical evidence can be found. The presence of needlemarks and abscess scars is helpful. In doubtful cases the only way in which the diagnosis can be made is by isolation of the patient and observation for the characteristic signs or by precipitating abstinence with N-allylnormorphine. The latter procedure should not be carried out without obtaining the written permission of the patient or his guardian. The technique consists of injecting 3 mg. of N-allylnormorphine subcutaneously; if the patient has been using 60 mg. or more of morphine daily (or an equivalent amount of dihydromorphinone, Dromoran, heroin or methadone), definite abstinence will appear in less than 20 minutes; if the reaction to the first injection is

negative, a second dose of 5 mg. may be given 30 minutes after the first; and if the test is still negative, a third dose of 8 mg. 30 minutes after the second dose; if the test is still negative and if typical signs of *direct* effects of N-allylnormorphine have appeared (dizziness, pseudoptosis, mild drunkenness, miosis, slowing of respiratory rate), one may safely conclude that the patient is not addicted *at the time the test is done.* A negative test does not preclude the possibility that the patient is taking scattered doses of analgesics or that he was actively addicted the week before the test was made. The procedure is also not reliable in meperidine addiction. The test is contraindicated in persons with serious organic disease of any kind.

Complications. The most important complication of drug addiction is the presence of concomitant addiction to barbiturates, which is best managed by slow reduction of barbiturates at the same time reduction of morphine is carried out. Other complications include the development of multiple abscesses at the injection sites, and bacterial endocarditis, which results from unsterile intravenous injections.

Prognosis. The prognosis of drug addiction must always be guarded, since the tendency to relapse is always great. The prognosis is better in patients who have been addicted for a comparatively short time than in patients who have been addicted for a long time, and is better in persons who have been addicted only once than in persons who have been addicted repeatedly. At least 15 to 20 per cent of addicts remain abstinent for five years or more after one adequate period of treatment. Others may remain abstinent for years before relapsing, and such periods of abstinence represent a considerable gain.

Treatment. One should not attempt to treat narcotic addiction on an outpatient basis. The patient should be referred to a private institution devoted to the treatment of narcotic addiction or, if he is unable to pay for treatment, to a government institution. *Addicts should never be given a prescription for narcotics for self-administration.* Also, physicians are not legally allowed to prescribe opiates merely for relief of withdrawal symptoms. Only after the addict has agreed to go to an institution and has taken definite steps to obtain admission, may the physician administer narcotics and then only in the minimal amounts necessary (usually

15 to 60 mg.). The patient should not be allowed to procrastinate and administration should not be continued unless the addict promptly obtains admission to an institution. Information concerning admission to the U. S. Public Health Service Hospital at Lexington, Kentucky, or Fort Worth, Texas, can be obtained by writing either to the Surgeon General, U. S. Public Health Service, Washington, D.C., or directly to the hospitals.

Treatment can be divided into two phases: withdrawal and rehabilitation.

Withdrawal. When a patient is first admitted, methadone should be substituted for whatever drug the patient has been using. This scheme of treatment is based on the fact that, while methadone is a completely adequate substitute for morphine, abstinence from methadone is milder than abstinence from morphine. Methadone has a very long duration of action and is effective orally so that two oral doses daily will effectively suppress abstinence symptoms from withdrawal of whatever drug the patient has been using. During the first two or three days of treatment the least amount of methadone which will just prevent the appearance of signs of abstinence is determined (stabilization dosage). Generally, 10 to 90 mg. of methadone orally at 12-hour intervals will suffice. If signs of abstinence appear, 10 to 20 mg. of methadone may be given hypodermically and the oral dosage increased in steps of 10 per cent until signs of abstinence disappear. During the stabilization period, physical and laboratory examinations can be completed and preliminary psychiatric assessment made. After these data have been obtained, reduction of methadone is begun. On the first day of reduction, the total dose of methadone is cut 50 per cent. The patient is maintained on this level for two days and then reduced to about one third of the original substitution dose of methadone. Thereafter, the dosage is reduced according to the needs of the individual patient. In the ordinary case, withdrawal should be completed within ten days after reduction is begun. Minor signs of abstinence are to be expected near the end of the withdrawal period. Importunities by the patient to increase the dose or to change the withdrawal schedule must be resisted kindly but firmly.

In cases complicated by severe organic disease the length of the withdrawal period is increased in accordance with the needs of the patient. Even patients with cardiac decompensation can be subjected to withdrawal without danger, if the reduction is carried out slowly enough.

The emotional reaction to withdrawal is frequently more difficult to handle than is physical reaction. All sorts of hysterical and anxiety reactions may occur, and a great deal of malingering and complaining is to be expected. The physician must maintain a sympathetic but firm attitude toward such manifestations and, in general, should follow his prearranged plan of reduction as closely as possible despite the patient's complaints.

Warm flow baths help ease the nervousness and muscular cramping associated with withdrawal. The patient's fluid intake should be maintained. No special dietary measures are required if reduction of methadone is the withdrawal treatment used. Sedatives are generally not required during the first half of the reduction schedule. Thereafter, 0.2 gm. of pentobarbital or 1.3 gm. of chloral hydrate may be administered at bedtime. One must be cautious in the use of sedatives and should permit no more than are necessary to obtain 4 or 5 hours' sleep nightly. The use of sedatives should be discontinued as soon as possible.

Methods of treatment which involve the use of hyoscine, atropine, insulin, heavy sedation with barbiturates, intravenous alcohol, adrenocorticotropin, cortisone or electroconvulsive therapy are not only irrational but are also harmful and should not be used.

Rehabilitative Treatment. After withdrawal has been completed any physical defects or diseases which the patient may have should be treated and corrected, if possible. If the patient is suffering from an incurable chronic disease, such as asthma, arthritis, migraine, treatment should be aimed at producing the greatest degree of improvement possible and at educating the patient to manage his disease without the aid of narcotics.

If the addiction is due to the presence of severe, chronic pain caused by some irremediable disease, appropriate surgical methods such as rhizotomy, prefrontal lobotomy or chordotomy should be instituted.

All patients should engage in a program of individual occupational and recreational therapy which should provide them with an opportunity to carry out at least 8 hours of useful, productive work daily, preferably of the type which maintains and improves any special skills they may have, or which adds new skills to those they already possess. Recreational therapy should include an organized athletic program, ample reading matter, opportunity to see movies, hear music and pursue hobbies.

As far as possible, individual psychotherapy aimed at helping the patient to understand his fundamental problems should be administered. Unfortunately, a large proportion of addicts is resistant to any type of psychotherapy; also, a sufficient number of therapists is not available to give individual attention to all who need it. This deficiency in facilities can partially be bridged by organizing group psychotherapeutic sessions. If possible, the addict should be encouraged to join with the groups known as Alcoholics Anonymous or Addicts Anonymous and to participate in their activities.

HARRIS ISBELL

References

Council on Pharmacy and Chemistry, American Medical Association: What To Do With A Drug Addict. J.A.M.A., *149*:1220, 1952.
Fraser, H. F., and Grider, J. A.: Treatment of Drug Addiction. Am. J. Med., *14*:571, 1953.
Isbell, H.: Nalline—A Specific Narcotic Antagonist. Clinical and Pharmacologic Observations. Merck Report, 62:23, 1953.
———, and White, W. M.: Clinical Characteristics of Addictions. Am. J. Med., *14*:558, 1953.
Kolb, L.: Drug Addiction: A Study of Some Medical Cases. Arch. Neurol. & Psychiat., 20:171, 1928.
Vogel, V. H., Isbell, H., and Chapman, K. W.: Present Status of Narcotic Addiction, with Particular Reference to Medical Indications and Comparative Addiction Liabilities of the Newer and Older Analgesic Drugs. J.A.M.A., 138:1019, 1948.
Wikler, A.: Opiate Addiction. Psychological and Neurophysiological Aspects in Relation to Clinical Problems. Springfield, Illinois, Charles C Thomas, 1953.

COCAINE POISONING

Definition. Cocaine poisoning refers to the pathologic changes in physiology produced by that drug. Cocaine poisoning may be either acute or chronic.

ACUTE COCAINE POISONING

Etiology. Acute cocaine poisoning may result from an accidental overdose, from mistaking cocaine for another drug, or may be due to an idiosyncrasy to the drug. Cocaine is practically never used in suicidal attempts. The fatal dose of cocaine is extremely variable. The average fatal dose is usually said to be 1.2 gm., but fatal poisoning due to idiosyncrasy has occurred after as little as 20 mg. of cocaine. Because of the great variation in the toxicity of cocaine, the drug is no longer used hypodermically for the induction of local analgesia, but it still remains the most effective and favored agent for inducing anesthesia by topical application.

Morbid Anatomy. No specific changes are found after death from acute cocaine intoxication.

Pathologic Physiology. The effects of cocaine are due to direct stimulation of the cerebral cortex, to stimulation of centers in the midbrain, and to sympathomimetic effects. The pathologic physiology of death due to cocaine idiosyncrasy is not understood.

Symptoms and Signs. Mild intoxication with cocaine is characterized by garrulousness, easy laughter, lack of appetite, anxiety and confusion. Hallucinations and delusions may develop with larger doses. Signs referable to peripheral stimulation of the sympathetic nervous system are usually present and include tachycardia, elevation of systolic blood pressure, dilatation of the pupils and increased sweating. With larger doses, dyspnea, Cheyne-Stokes respiration and tremors appear. In severe intoxication, convulsions may occur and death result from apnea. Poisoning associated with idiosyncrasy to cocaine is manifested by sudden cardiovascular collapse.

Treatment. The best treatment is prophylactic. Cocaine should be used only for inducing topical anesthesia and should never be injected. A preliminary dose of 0.2 gm. of Sodium Amytal or 0.1 gm. of pentobarbital should be given before the administration of cocaine.

The treatment of acute cocaine intoxication consists primarily in the administration of cortical depressants. In mild or moderate intoxication, 0.25 gm. of Sodium Amytal should be administered intramuscularly. In more severe poisoning, rapid treatment may be necessary, and 0.5 gm. of Sodium Amytal or sodium pentobarbital should be injected intravenously at a rate of 0.1 gm. per minute.

Symptoms of intoxication due to idiosyncrasy to the drug usually occur so rapidly that treatment is ineffective. Patients should be placed in the shock position, and given artificial respiration and intravenous injections of nikethamide.

CHRONIC COCAINE POISONING
(Cocaine Addiction)

Definition. Chronic cocaine poisoning, or cocaine addiction, refers to a condition in which a person willfully uses cocaine to such an extent that the individual or society, or both, are harmed.

Etiology. The chewing of coca leaves is culturally accepted among certain South American Indians, and does not have as great psychopathologic significance as does cocaine addiction in other parts of the world. In the United States, chronic cocainism is always based on some personality defect. Psychoneurotic persons do not like the effects of cocaine and usually try it only once or twice. Persons with psychopathic personalities, however, obtain intense pleasure from cocaine and begin and continue the use of the drug in order to experience its exhilarating effects. Contact with the drug is always made because of association with persons who are already taking the drug, and almost never as a result of medical usage.

Routes of Administration. In the United States cocaine was formerly used as a snuff, but this practice has almost completely been replaced by intravenous injection. Pure cocaine addiction is rare in this country, but mixed addiction to cocaine and opiates is fairly common. North American addicts seldom take the drug continuously, but prefer to use it for short debauches. The compulsion to repeat the dose at frequent intervals appears to be great, and ordinarily users exhaust their supply rapidly, or else stop taking the drug temporarily because of the appearance of disagreeable symptoms.

Morbid Anatomy. There is no clear-cut evidence to show that chronic cocaine addiction produces any anatomic changes directly attributable to the drug itself. Chronic use leads to emaciation and malnutrition because of the great depression of appetite which the drug produces. Subcutaneous injection causes marked abscess and scar formation.

Pathologic Physiology. Like acute intoxication, the pathologic physiology of chronic cocaine intoxication is closely related to the pharmacologic actions of the drug. The drug is taken primarily to enjoy the transient feelings of ecstasy which are due to cortical stimulation. North American habitues describe this sensation as being similar to sexual orgasm. The sense of ecstasy after cocaine is fleeting, and in order to recapture it the cocainist repeatedly injects the drug at intervals of 15 to 30 minutes. After a sufficient number of injections, signs due to excessive stimulation of the cerebral cortex and the sympathetic nervous system appear.

Symptoms and Signs. Persons who have been using cocaine are nervous, apprehensive, tremulous and easily startled, and speak in soft tones and may complain of formication. Tachycardia, hypertension and mydriasis are usually seen. Patients who have been using as much as 1 to 2 gm. of cocaine a day may have a toxic psychosis manifested by visual and auditory hallucinations and delusions. In this state, cocainists are dangerous and may assault and even kill harmless people. When a cocaine addict becomes excessively apprehensive or begins to experience hallucinations, he discontinues taking cocaine or takes an injection of morphine as an antidote to the effect of the cocaine.

Concomitant use of any of the potent opiate drugs increases the addict's tolerance for cocaine, so that larger amounts of it may be used over longer periods of time.

Unlike opium addiction, the use of cocaine increases the propensity of people with psychopathic personalities to commit violent crime.

Diagnosis. Diagnosis is based on the history and on the signs of nervousness and tremulousness, mydriasis, tachycardia, mild hypertension, and the presence of needle-marks in the skin or over the veins. Amphetamine intoxication, anxiety states and, at times, the psychoses must be differentiated.

Prognosis. Prognosis is guarded, since relapse frequently occurs. Prognosis in addiction to both cocaine and opium is worse than that for addiction to either drug alone.

Treatment. If the patient is excessively nervous or if he is experiencing hallucinations or delusions, he should be given one of the rapidly acting barbiturates. As much as 0.5 gm. of sodium pentobarbital may have to be injected intravenously to produce the desired degree of sedation. Morphine, in doses of 20 to 30 mg., is an effective antidote and is the one generally desired by the cocaine addict.

No conclusive evidence has been brought forward to show that tolerance develops during chronic administration of cocaine or that any physiologic dependence is present. For this reason, no treatment, other than mild sedation until the acute effects of the cocaine have subsided, is necessary. Rehabilitative and psychiatric therapy is identical with that of chronic opium poisoning.

HARRIS ISBELL

References

Kolb, L.: Drug Addiction in Its Relation to Crime. Ment. Hyg., 9:74, 1925.

Tatum, A. L., and Seevers, M. H.: Experimental Cocaine Addiction. J. Pharmacol. & Exper. Therap., 36:401, 1929.

Wolff, P. O.: The Treatment of Drug Addicts. Bull. Health Organ., League of Nations, 12:656, 1945–6.

CHRONIC POISONING WITH SYMPATHOMIMETIC AMINES

Definition. Chronic poisoning with sympathomimetic amines refers to the state brought about by continued consumption of excessive amounts of sympathomimetic amines over long periods. The drugs most commonly abused are amphetamine (Benzedrine), methamphetamine (desoxyephedrine, Desoxyn) and dextro-amphetamine (Dexedrine). These drugs all have powerful cortical excitant actions in addition to their sympathomimetic actions. Their effects are similar to those of cocaine but are milder and do not develop as rapidly. True incidence of chronic poisoning with these drugs is unknown. Their abuse is common among alcoholics and barbiturate addicts. They are popular among thrill-seeking adolescents and inmates of penal institutions.

Route of Administration. These drugs are almost always taken orally as tablets. Occasionally, they may be injected subcutaneously or intravenously by morphine and barbiturate addicts. Amphetamine inhalers are no longer available and do not constitute a problem. Dosages taken may be enormous. Some users may take as much as 250 mg. of amphetamine at a dose and may ingest 1 to 1.5 gm. daily. Concomitant use of barbiturates increases tolerance for these drugs.

Symptoms. The symptoms are similar to those of mild to moderate intoxication with cocaine. The patients are nervous, apprehensive, jerky and tremulous, and have tachycardia, hypertension, mydriasis, insomnia and anorexia. A toxic psychosis, characterized by the development of hallucinations and delusions of a paranoid character, may appear.

Treatment. Treatment consists of sedation, abrupt withdrawal of the sympathomimetic amines, and a program of psychotherapy similar to that used in the treatment of morphine addiction.

HARRIS ISBELL

Reference

Monroe, R. R., and Drell, H. J.: Oral Use of Stimulants Obtained from Inhalers. J.A.M.A., 135:909, 1947.

SNAKE VENOM POISONING

Venomous serpents are particularly abundant in those tropical and subtropical countries which are under intensive agricultural cultivation. The normal ophidian population of those places is always stimulated as a result of the increase in the number of rats, mice and other rodents, which accompanies the production of crops. India, Java, Malay, southeastern Brazil, southwestern United States, eastern Mexico and the Central American republics since the advent of widespread cultivation may be cited among the highly snake-infested regions of the world.

Venomous snakes feeding on rodents are rather rare in forests or in wooded districts even in the tropics, because, in order to survive, they must resist active competition on the part of many species of predatory and stronger animals, both birds and mammals, which also feed on rodents and live in woody sections.

Etiology. The introduction of toxic principles actually occurs when some type of snake bears sufficient secretion in its supralabial glands at the moment it bites a victim. From a purely biologic point of view, most serpents must be considered *venomous*, for on each side of the head they have a gland that yields a viscous secretion capable of producing toxic or destructive effects on the animal tissues. From a medical standpoint, however, only those ophidians are considered *veneniferous* which, upon biting or stabbing, are able to inject the secretion of their supralabial glands more or less deeply into the tissues of their prey or potential enemy.

These snakes are all included in two groups or series which in ophiology are called PROTEROGLYPHA and SOLENOGLYPHA. The PROTEROGLYPHA bear small fangs, longitudinally grooved, one on each side of the anterior upper jaw; each fang is firmly implanted in the maxilla, which is articulated with other skull bones. The coral snakes are the only representatives of this group in America.

The SOLENOGLYPHA bear rather large

fangs, hollow like a hypodermic needle, in a series on each anterior aspect of their upper jaw; of each series the foremost fang is the acting one, the others being suppletory. The ophidians of this group are the vipers, which are of two kinds, the more important being the pit vipers, named after the hole or pit on each side of the head between the nostril and the eye. Among the true pit-less vipers the most dreaded species is the Gaboon viper which is provided with very voluminous venom glands and large fangs. The pit vipers are found in the United States, where they are represented by the copperhead, the water moccasin and the rattlers, of which there are some twelve species. Of the rattlers the most dreadful and venomous ones are the Florida rattler, the Texas rattler, the prairie rattler and the black-tailed rattler. In Latin America the most important pit vipers are the fer-de-lance or barba-amarilla, the cascabel or cascavel, the surucucú or bushmaster, the jararaca, the jararacuçú and the urutú.

The venom apparatus is made up of a gland, a duct and an active fang on each side. Physiologically, the venom acts as a sort of saliva and serves both to facilitate the swallowing of the prey and to initiate the digestion of the prey's tissues through enzymic action. The amount of venom a serpent can eject varies from a few drops to 2 cc.; the active constituents may weigh as much as 650 mg. (exceptionally, 1 gm.).

Chemistry of Snake Venoms. Venoms are composed chiefly of proteins, including toxins and enzymes, which are responsible for their toxicity. The toxicity of a venom may be lost if it is treated by chemicals or exposed to both light and heat. However, venoms are little modified by glycerin, which serves as the best means for their preservation in the field. In the laboratory full stability can be achieved only when the venom is frozen and desiccated under high vacuum immediately after being obtained from the snake and is subsequently kept in the dark and at low temperature.*

For many years little was known of the chemical composition and the real na-

* From a biochemical standpoint the following powerful enzymes have already been recognized by electrophoresis in snake venoms, serving both to complicate the action of the poison toxins and to induce harmful progressive chain-effects on the tissue constituents: proteases (including nucleotidase), λ amino-acid oxidase, hyaluronidase ("spreading factor"), phosphatases (including phospholipase A) and acetylcholesterinase.

ture of the toxic principles of venom. Professor Karl Slotta and his associates, working at the Instituto Butantan, under my direction, have confirmed the findings of Micheel and Jung as to the chemical nature of the venom active principles and are inclined to ascribe to the presence of 5 to 7 atoms of sulfur (bound to cystine) an important binding role in the large protein molecule of the neurotoxin, giving it a peculiar specificity. Moreover, they have succeeded in isolating from the South American rattler's venom a pure principle, "crotoxin," the formula of which is $C_{1386}H_{2086}O_{470}N_{372}S_{41}$. Crotoxin, which is the first crystallized substance ever isolated from snake venoms or from any animal protein venin and which contains 18 amino acids at least, has a molecular weight of about 30,500 according to Svedberg's ultracentrifugal investigations. Crotoxin, which is also a homogenous substance, has proved, in the course of electrophoresis experiments, to have the value of $d\mu/dpH_0$ as its isoelectric point. Crotoxin exerts both neurotoxic and hemolytic actions in the body. From the venom of the India cobra a purified enzyme, different from the neurotoxin, has been obtained in crystalline form; it represents the hemolytic principle of this venom, being about 33 times more potent than the latter.

According to Singer and Kearney, the yellow color found in most venoms, particularly those of the Nearctic rattlers and the Neotropical species of *Bothrops,* seems to be due to riboflavin, the action of which is correlated with the presence of an enzyme, the l-amino-acid oxidase.

Pathologic Physiology. Every venom appears to have unique properties. The individual physiologic peculiarities are due to the variations in composition which are found among even the species of the same genus. Thus the venom of the South American rattler *Crotalus terrificus* acts very slowly upon the organism and produces nervous symptoms (blindness, local paralyses, and so forth) only after an incubation period of a few hours and never causes even local pain. The venom of nearly all the North American rattlers (*Crotalus atrox, adamanteus, ruber, molossus* and others) acts rather rapidly upon the body and causes marked swelling and other local symptoms in the virtual absence of any sign of nervous disturbances.

The active constituents of snake venoms are usually classified as neurocytolysins, hemolysins and hemocoagulins, proteolysins and cytolysins.

Neurocytolysins have a systemic effect, are slow to act, and affect the respiration and circulation, or the vision and other specialized functions. They are prevalent in the venom of the South American rattler and all the Western World coral snakes, the Indian cobras, the African mamba, and others.

Hemolysins, acting on both the red cells and the leukocytes, complicate the local symptoms produced by proteolysins and cytolysins which act in the earlier stages of the poisoning, and are responsible for the respiratory disturbances which sometimes appear during the later phases of the venenation. By altering the blood composition through the lysis of red cells, hemolysins contribute to the reduction of the oxygen intake of the tissues. They are particularly prevalent in the venom of the Indian cobra and daboia, the Texas rattler, the South American urutú and fer-de-lance.

Hemocoagulins act both on the coagulating and the anticoagulating mechanism of the blood. Some venoms have trypsin-like enzymes and react with prothrombin to form thrombin, while others bear papain-like enzymes and react with fibrogen to precipitate fibrin, the result in both cases being blood coagulation. In the former group may be included the venoms of the South American jararaca and fer-de-lance and some coral snakes; in the latter group are the venoms, not only of the Florida rattler and the South American cascavel, but also of the South American jararaca and fer-de-lance. Finally, those venoms that prevent blood coagulation appear to destroy either prothrombin or fibrinogen, or else they neutralize thrombin itself, thus acting in the same manner as heparin. This type of venin is secreted by such snakes as the American water moccasin, the African puff adder, the Texas rattler, the Indian daboia and the European sand viper while heparin-like action is caused by the Indian cobra venom.

Proteolysins and *cytolysins* are the typical phlogogenous substances responsible for the local symptoms, such as pain, swelling, discoloration, necrosis and mutilation, which follow the stab of certain vipers and pit vipers. They are particularly noticeable in the secretion of such snakes as most North American rattlers, the Latin American fer-de-lance, jararaca, jararacuçú and urutú, the Japanese habú, the Asiatic and Mayalan green pit viper and the Indian daboia. By

dissolving the tissue proteins, proteolysins open the way for cytolysins, which in turn are responsible for the destruction of the cell structure.

Symptomatology. The symptoms of venenation vary widely according to the chemical composition of the poison. They may be briefly summarized as follows, according to the species or groups of snakes:

1. *Coral snakes:* salivation and lacrimation; depression and somnolence; trembling and convulsions—all resulting from the action of the chemical constituents of the venom on the autonomic nervous system. The poisoning may result in death.

2. *South American rattler:* impairment of vision or complete blindness; paralysis of both eyelids and eyeballs; paralysis of peripheral muscles (especially about the neck, which acts as though it were broken)—all caused by the action of the chemical principles on the neuromuscular apparatus; finally, lesion of the lower nephron with occasional hematuria. Death is usually the outcome.

3. *Spectacled cobra:* salivation and vomiting; hemorrhages and fall of blood pressure; prostration and somnolence; dyspnea, apnea and death—all caused by the effect of the venom on the blood and the autonomic nervous system.

4. *King cobra:* dyspnea, polypnea, profuse sweating and death, resulting from the direct action of the venom on the central nervous system and the phrenic nerve endings.

5. *North American rattlers:* local pain, edema and discoloration, followed by ecchymoses and phlyctenules; blood destruction all through the affected tissues; prostration, nausea, vomiting or diarrhea, following absorption of residues of both tissue and blood; collapse and sometimes death.

6. *Indian daboia:* strong local swelling and tissue destruction; profuse hemorrhages because of the lack of blood clotting; fall of blood pressure and collapse; hematuria, albuminuria, anemia and emaciation sometimes resulting in death.

7. *Latin American pit vipers,* excluding the cascabel and the bushmaster; extensive local reaction, with edema, ecchymosis and adenitis; thirst and diarrhea, hemorrhages through the eyes, ears, mouth, intestines or kidneys; prostration, exhaustion, followed sometimes by death. The symptoms following the stab by the Japanese habú and most of the Asiatic and Malayan pit vipers are more or less comparable to these.

Diagnosis. The diagnosis of a case of venenation is based primarily on the capture or examination of the snake that caused the bite and secondarily on the description of its characteristics by the victim. Failing this, the physician, being acquainted with the local ophiologic fauna, must examine the patient thoroughly in order to establish his diagnostic conclusion. In this connection his judgment must be extremely sound, since the specificity of the treatment to be applied depends on the correctness of his findings. Final diagnosis will be based chiefly on the discovery of puncture marks at the site of the alleged "bite."

Prognosis and Death Rate. The prognosis of snake poisoning is contingent upon the seriousness of the particular case. This is always grave when the patient is small or young, when the amount of venom injected by the bite is large or when the snake fang happens to enter a vein, thus forcing the poison directly into the circulation.

It may happen that a serpent has recently eaten or bitten an animal before biting a human being. In this instance little venom may be present in the glands and the accident will be mild. In contrast, the serpent may be fullgrown or may have been quiet for a long time; in such circumstances its glands will contain a large amount of secretion. For this reason snake poisoning is usually more severe in early spring, when the reptiles start crawling out from their winter retreats.

In the event that symptoms develop rapidly, and the patient loses sight, becomes unconscious or experiences a rapid fall in blood pressure, the accident must be considered serious, and the prognosis bad.

The death rate depends directly upon the types of snakes prevailing in any region. With species like the Latin American cascabel, the Indian cobras and daboia, and the African mamba, whose venoms are extremely powerful, or secreted in amounts too great for human resistance, the death rate will be relatively high. An average of 25,000 deaths occur annually in India from ophidic accidents, the majority of which are due to the spectacled cobra alone. In contrast there were but 14 fatal cases of poisoning in Europe, all caused by local vipers, from 1883 to 1892. In the Okinawa islands an annual average of about 225 persons used to be poisoned by the habú with a death rate of about 15 per cent.

In this country, statistics prepared by the Antivenin Institute of America seem to indicate that the yearly number of cases of snake bites may amount to 2000 to 3000, the death rate varying from 10 to 35 per cent.

Prophylaxis. The dreadful consequences of the venenation may be prevented in two ways: first, by avoiding snake bites; second, by properly treating the accident.

The prevention of snake bites may be achieved by wearing heavy shoes and leather leggings whenever one goes into a snake-infested district, and by avoiding the use of the bare hands in climbing a rock or a ledge where snakes may be encountered.

Treatment. The treatment of snake poisoning consists in the application of specific antivenins followed by additional measures when necessary; if antivenins are unavailable, local therapy should be applied.

Antivenins are the only known agents capable of neutralizing venoms and arresting their harmful effects on the body. Injections of these specific serums may be made hypodermically, intramuscularly or intravenously (the patient being properly prepared against allergic reactions) according to the seriousness of every case.

If the antivenin can be given at once or within the first 2 hours after the bite, about half the dose should be injected immediately around the wound in order to prevent local destruction of the tissues by venom of the phlogogenic type, such as that of the American and Oriental pit vipers and the daboia. In late treated cases, however, this local application is not indicated. In such cases, and always in those in which the symptoms are severe, intravenous injection of the specific antivenin is strongly advised.

As to dosage, the physician must remember that the age or weight of the victim of the bite is an important factor. Its relation to the amount of serum is just the reverse of the usual rules for dosage. In the case of ophiotoxosis the concentration of venom per kilogram of body weight is relatively greater in young or light persons (or animals) than in adult or heavy persons. Therefore, the smaller or lighter the person the greater and the more urgent the need of the antivenin. When there is reason to believe that the venin inoculated by the serpent was of unusually large quantity or whenever the symptoms develop quickly and in severe form, as, for instance, in children, it is advisable to start with a double dose and repeat it, at short intervals, if the previous dose has not caused an amelioration of the symptoms. For adults or heavy patients the usual dose is one to three syringes or ampules of 10 cc. each. The serum to be given may be either of the liquid type, kept in the icebox for preservation of its potency, or of the lyophilized type, in which case the powder is previously dissolved in the usual way.

In all cases the victim should be watched for 3 to 5 hours after every injection, and, if his condition has not markedly improved within that time, an additional injection should be made.*

The special procedure to be carried out whenever specific serum or antivenin is *not* available may be summarized:

1. Apply a ligature or tourniquet above the bite site. This should be applied tightly at first, but must be partially released for a few seconds at 5- to 10-minute intervals so as to maintain the necessary circulation in the limb. There is no particular advantage in making an incision, or in applying permanganate of potassium in solution or crystals or any of the other chemical agents empirically recommended for this purpose. In fact, it is advisable to avoid any further mutilation or injury that might facilitate the development of tetanus, gas gangrene or secondary infection and thus complicate the patient's condition. Exception to this rule may be made only in those cases with large swelling and discoloration, followed by severe general symptoms, such as result from a bite by the Indian daboia or the majority of the North American rattlers. The venoms of these serpents are both hemolytic and noncoagulant, and cause intense edema and extravasations of blood. The toxins absorbed by the lymph vessels and at the site of their inoculation form a poisonous substance (*lysocythin* due to the splitting action of phospholipase A on lecithin) from the extravasated blood. For this reason it is advisable, in these particular instances, to make a series of incisions around the puncture marks left by the snake and to apply strong suction by means of a

* Since some venoms, particularly those causing local hard edema and late tissue destruction, appear to act also through the so-called "anti-spreading factor" (hyaluronic acid) which hinders the absorption of the antivenin given around the site of the "bite," it is advisable, previous to injecting the specific serum, to mix with its dose a certain amount (about 1 to 2 mg.) of hyaluronidase and administer the mixture subcutaneously. In this case, in order to prevent the rapid dissemination throughout the system of the toxic derivatives of the venom held up by the swollen tissues, it is necessary to take special precautions with the patient, by giving him an extra dose of antivenin with ephedrine intravenously and by watching his heart and kidney functions.

hydraulic pump (a good vacuum rubber bulb pump may be used), attempting to extract the lysocythin together with the residues of destruction of both blood and tissues.

2. Strychnine, caffeine, black coffee or strong tea may be given to the patient if symptoms of weakness and giddiness develop.

3. It is important to bear in mind that in late and severe cases, complicated by profuse bleeding, symptoms of liver injury, low blood pressure or dehydration, instant relief may sometimes be obtained from the intravenous administration of saline, followed by glucose solution or Ringer-sodium lactate solution.

AFRÂNIO DO AMARAL

References

Amaral, A. do: Thesis, Harvard Univ. School of Public Health, 73 p., 1924; Contrib. II. Harvard Inst. f. Trop. Biol. & Medicine (Harvard Univ. Press). 64 p., 16 pl., 1925; Bull. Antivenin Inst. of America, 1:61, 77, 1927; *loc. cit.*, 1:103, 1928; Chapter in Brennemann's Practice of Pediatrics, 2(37), 1942; Animais Veneniferos, Venenos e Antivenenos (Edit. Caça e Pesca Ltda. S. Paulo), 169 p., 61 figs., 1945.
Ditmars, R. L.: Snakes of the World. New York, The Macmillan Company, 1943.
Githens, T. S.: Antivenin: Its Preparation and Standardization, Bull. Antivenin Inst. of America, 4:81, 1931.
Gralén, N., and Svedberg, T.: The Molecular Weight of Crotoxin, Biochem. J., 32:1375, 1938.
Klauber, L. M.: Bull. Antivenin Inst. of America, 1: 27, 1927; Transact. San Diego Soc. Nat. Hist., 6: 95, 1930; Bull. Zool. Soc., San Diego, 6:72, 1930.
Li, C. H., and Fraenkel-Conrat, H. L.: J. Am. Chem. Soc., 64:1586, 1942.
Micheel, F., and Jung, F.: Ztschr. f. Physiol. Chem., 239:217, 1936.
Singer, T. P., and Kearney, E. B.: Arch. Biochem., 27:348, 1950.
Slotta, K. H., and Forster, W.: Mem. Inst. Butantan, 12:513, 1938.
———, and Fraenkel-Conrat, H. L.: Mem. Inst. Butantan, 11:121, 1937; 12:505, 1938.
Strong, R. A.: Intern. M. Dig., 12:233, 1928.
Wieland, H., and Konz, W.: Sitz.-Ber. math.-nat. Abt. bayr. Akad. Wiss., 177, 1936.

FOOD POISONING

INTRODUCTION

Food poisoning may occur from the ingestion of a diverse group of inciting agents. The literature contains records of many outbreaks of gastrointestinal illnesses in which the inciting agent given is in error. Some of the errors in the earlier reports were due to lack of knowledge concerning the inciting agents. For example: Salmonella organisms have been assigned as the cause of several outbreaks of food poisoning which were obviously due to staphylococci. The term "ptomaine poisoning" is still used in newspaper reports of outbreaks of food poisoning and, unfortunately, is occasionally used by the medical profession. This term came into use soon after the word was coined by the Italian toxicologist Selmi in 1870. Much work has been done with toxic products extracted from foods and tested by parenteral injection into animals. Animals receiving injections of these materials frequently manifested shock and developed diarrhea and labored respiration preceding death. Many filtrates prepared from broth cultures of Salmonella bacilli are toxic when injected intravenously into rabbits and other experimental animals. The peculiar feature of this toxicity is that it is limited to *parenteral* injections—the same material often is without any effect when given by *mouth*. This situation also applies to the products of putrefaction, among which are the amines. The "ptomaine" theory would never have gained prominence if experimental animals had reacted similarly to man when fed foods implicated in outbreaks of food poisoning. Perhaps the majority of so-called "ptomaine food poisoning" outbreaks may be attributed to staphylococci. There is abundant evidence to indicate that putrefied foods in the absence of food-poisoning agents are without ill effect when ingested. It is well known, for example, that the Eskimo considers putrefied seal meat a delicacy. Others races similarly prefer putrefied protein foods. In the United States, perhaps the best example of a putrefied food is Limburger cheese. In some of the earlier outbreaks of food poisoning in which Cheddar cheese was found responsible, Limburger cheese was singularly mentioned as not being involved. It is, therefore, evident that putrefaction in a food does not implicate it as a cause of food poisoning in the absence of specific food-poisoning agents.

Some persons are allergic to certain items of food, which, though wholesome to most people, may act as poisons to those who are sensitized to them. One example is the case of the *Vicia fava* bean, which is cultivated extensively in New York, New Jersey, Illinois and California and is a staple article of diet, particularly with people of Italian extraction. Sensitization to the bean appears to be on a hereditary basis, since in certain families every member for generations has been reported severely affected. Therefore, susceptibility varies, and certain persons, after years of eating the beans with impunity, may suffer a single, severe attack and none subsequently. Illness may follow inhalation of pollen from the blossoming plant or within an hour after eating the beans. The illness is characterized by acute febrile anemia with jaundice, hematuria and hemoglobinuria.

A number of *chemicals* have been taken by mistake or accident and thus have been implicated in food poisoning. Usually illnesses from chemical poisoning occur within a few minutes to an hour or two after ingesting the chemical. The poisons include antimony, arsenic, barium carbonate, cadmium, sodium fluoride, lead, methyl chloride, mercury, nitrates and zinc. Of this list, *cadmium* and sodium fluoride have been most commonly involved. If acid foods are placed in cadmium-plated utensils, such as pitchers or ice trays in mechanical refrigerators, sufficient cadmium is dissolved to cause abdominal cramping, severe diarrhea and vomiting within 15 to 30 minutes after eating or drinking the foods or beverages. *Sodium fluoride* is widely used to exterminate cockroaches from food establishments. Since it is a white powder, it has frequently been mistaken for baking powder, soda or flour. Illness usually follows within a few minutes to two hours and is characterized by an acute poisoning—vomiting (often hemorrhagic), diffuse abdominal pains, and diarrhea occur with great constancy; convulsions, toxic or clonic spasms of certain muscle groups, paresis of certain groups of muscles (eye muscles, facial muscles, hand extensors and those of lower extremities), hiccup and contraction of pupils. Paresthesia occasionally is present in extremities and has led to confusion with botulism. Arsenic, lead and mercury poisoning are discussed at length elsewhere in this book under their respective titles.

Of the *animal poisons,* perhaps one of the best recognized is *shellfish* or *mussel poisoning.* It has occurred along the West Coast, in central California, with a sprinkling of severe outbreaks from Juneau, Alaska, to southern California, the Gulf of California and Mexico. In the eastern part of North America it has been found due to shellfish from the Bay of Fundy. The illnesses have been traced to the food of the shellfish, *Gonyaulax;* in the cases on the West Coast, to *Gonyaulax catanella.* Chemical studies have been made of the poison, and some preparations have been made which have a toxicity greater than 1

MU per microgram. The MU is the amount of mussel poison which, when dissolved in 1 cc. of water and injected intraperitoneally into a 20 gm. white mouse, will cause death in 15 minutes. Shellfish poisoning is characterized by respiratory paralysis. Symptoms vary from trembling about the lips to complete loss of power in the muscles of the neck. The illness develops within 5 to 30 minutes and longer after eating the poisoned mussels.

Of the more common *plant poisons,* snakeroot poisoning, mushroom poisoning, ergotism and water hemlock poisoning may be mentioned. The most poisonous of the mushrooms is *Amanita phalloides.* It has been reported that two or three of these mushrooms may be sufficient to cause illness and death in the adult. A patient with mushroom poisoning has hypoglycemia which may be accompanied by convulsions, severe abdominal pain, intense thirst, nausea, retching, vomiting and profuse watery evacuations. The illness occurs within 6 to 15 hours after ingestion of the poisonous mushrooms. *Ergot poisoning* has occurred from eating rye meal or rye bread prepared from diseased rye containing a fungus, *Claviceps purpurea,* and may develop after several meals of diseased rye. The symptoms are drowsiness, headache, giddiness, painful cramps of the limbs and itching of the skin. In the more severe cases, gangrene may occur, involving especially the fingers and toes and occasionally the ears and nose. *Water hemlock poisoning* occurs when the leaves and roots of the water hemlock are eaten. The onset of illness comes one to two hours after ingestion and is characterized by nausea, vomiting and convulsions.

In all instances of poisoning it is important to recognize the type in order to prevent the occurrence of further cases. Often there is no specific treatment; the vomiting and diarrhea serve the useful purpose of eliminating the poison which is not already absorbed. Symptomatic treatment should be given, and, with the types of poisoning characterized by severe vomiting and diarrhea, parenteral fluids should be administered if dehydration and loss of electrolytes in the body have been excessive.

BACTERIAL FOOD POISONING

Food poisoning from bacteria may be divided into two general categories: first, when toxins are preformed in the food by the growth of micro-organisms and the illnesses are due to the *toxins* and not to the ingested *organisms;* in the other category the living *organisms* alone are responsible for the illnesses, filtrates or heated dead cultures being without effect.

PREFORMED TOXINS
BOTULISM

Today most outbreaks of botulism occur from the use of home-canned foods. In the United States ten to fifteen outbreaks occur annually. The term "botulism" originated from the word "botulismus," meaning a sausage, and was coined by physicians in southern Germany in the beginning of the nineteenth century. The causative agent, *Clostridium botulinum,* is a large, gram-positive, rod-shaped organism which is an anaerobic spore-former. The organism is a natural saprophyte and is commonly found in the soil. The spores are very heat resistant, and in foods that are not properly processed they may germinate and produce toxin. There are five toxigenic types: A, B, C, D and E. Of these five, three have been found to cause food poisoning in man: namely, types A, B and rarely E. The symptoms produced by all types of toxin are the same, but the antitoxin differs for each type.

Symptoms. In some, but not all, persons the central nervous system symptoms characteristic of botulism are preceded by an active digestive disturbance and vomiting. In general, nausea and vomiting occur in less than 24 hours and appear to bear some relation to the degree of spoilage and to the amount of incriminated food consumed. Although dehydration may develop early in some cases, constipation is present in the later stages of the disease. Typical symptoms usually appear in 12 to 36 hours. In many instances the earliest symptom is a peculiar lassitude or fatigue, sometimes associated with dizziness or headache and attributed to constipation. Double vision or diplopia may occur early. The difficulty with vision is usually due to involvement of the extraocular muscles. Photophobia, nystagmus and vertigo are occasionally recorded. Difficulty in swallowing and in speech is observed later in the disease. A sense of constriction of the throat is described occasionally. Usually the tongue is coated and swollen. Paralysis of the pharyngeal muscles occurs in fatal cases, and it is not uncommon for fluids to be regurgitated through the nose and mouth. The muscles in the neck are often weakened, and there may be muscular incoordination. There is no retention of urine, although the amount secreted may be small, since patients cannot swallow, and proper fluid balance is not maintained. The temperature is usually normal or subnormal. Bronchopneumonia may develop because of aspiration of mouth contents. The pulse may be normal, but often becomes rapid in the later stages, even though the temperature remains normal. The respiration occasionally becomes irregular, and Cheyne-Stokes breathing has been observed just before death. The blood pressure is usually normal, and no abnormalities in type or number of blood cells have been found. Death results from respiratory failure. Life has often been sustained for several hours by artificial respiration. The Drinker respirator has been used in several cases, but without success. The duration of illness in fatal cases is usually three to six days after ingestion of the poisonous food.

Diagnosis. The diagnosis of botulism can usually be made from the symptoms. Confusion has sometimes occurred in cases of chemical poisoning involving methyl chloride and sodium fluoride. In acute sodium fluoride poisoning, vomiting, abdominal pains and diarrhea are marked. The paralysis of certain groups of muscles (eye muscles, facial muscles, hand extensors and those of the lower extremities), contraction of the pupils, and paresthesia in the extremities have led to confusion with botulism. In botulism the gastrointestinal symptoms are mild, if present, and the diplopia, aphonia and labored breathing are pronounced. Methyl chloride poisoning is characterized by progressive drowsiness, mental confusion, stupor, nausea, pain in the abdomen and vomiting. In severe cases, convulsions and cyanosis alternating with coma have led to confusion with botulism. In botulism the sensorium is usually clear up to the time of death. In the majority of cases there is a history of ingestion of home-canned foods which frequently may have had a rancid or slightly putrefactive odor or taste. In the laboratory diagnosis, blood taken from patients occasionally may contain sufficient toxin to cause the death of mice into which 1 cc. of serum has been injected intraperitoneally. If the food has been discarded and fed to chickens, limberneck may develop in the chickens, causing death. Suspected items of food should be sent to the laboratory and examined for toxin and/or the presence of C. *botulinum.* The toxin can be typed in the laboratory using the specific antitoxins.

Prognosis. The mortality from botulism in the United States is approximately 65 per cent, but in Europe it is much lower. When a large dose of toxin is ingested, symptoms occur within a short time, usually less than 24 hours. In nonfatal cases the symptoms subside slowly, and usually several weeks elapse before all residual signs of the disease have disappeared and recovery is complete.

Treatment. The treatment of botulism is unsatisfactory. The sooner the disease is recognized, the better the opportunity for the physician to treat those more fortunate persons who have eaten less of the poisonous food and have not manifested symptoms early. Since the majority of cases are due to type A or B, it is advisable to give polyvalent antitoxin for these two types. In the presence of symptoms, antitoxin is frequently given too late, for it cannot repair the damage already done to the patient by the toxin. Antitoxin should be given, even though the disease is advanced, in the hope of neutralizing any toxin which is not already fixed in the tissues. At least 50,000 units of antitoxin should be given intramuscularly after the patient has been tested for serum hypersensitivity and, if necessary, desensitized.

It is important that other measures be taken in addition to specific treatment with antitoxin. The fluid balance of the body should be maintained, and, in the presence of pharyngeal paralysis, which occurs early, fluids should be administered parenterally. The taking of fluids or food by mouth should be discouraged when pharyngeal paralysis is marked, in order to avoid the danger of aspiration pneumonia. Saliva should be expectorated or aspirated from the throat in such cases. The patient should be kept quiet in restful surroundings and encouraged to avoid even the slightest unnecessary movement. In outbreaks of botulism involving several persons, those who have only tasted the food or eaten sparingly of it usually do not exhibit symptoms until some time after those who have eaten generously of the poisonous food. In such cases antitoxin should prove of great prophylactic value.

STAPHYLOCOCCAL FOOD POISONING

Definition. Staphylococcal food poisoning also is caused by a toxin formed in the food before ingestion. In the United States it is probably the most common of all food poisonings. Since it is not a reportable disease, the number of cases occurring annually is unknown. It is an ailment which involves most persons at one time or another during their lives, and no great attention is paid to it unless large groups of people are attacked, such as at banquets, encampments or in public institutions.

Etiology. Although the relation of staphylococci to foods implicated in this type of food poisoning has been known since 1884, staphylococcal food poisoning was not generally recognized until 1930. This failure to recognize the disease was due to the fact that, when implicated foods and cultures made from them were fed to experimental animals, no illness followed. Unfortunately, man appears to be peculiarly susceptible to the poison, although extremely potent preparations cause vomiting and diarrhea when fed to kittens and monkeys (*Macaca mulatta*). However, portions of enterotoxin-containing food which cause serious illness in man may be fed to these animals without ill effect. Not all strains of staphylococci produce enterotoxin, and it is probable that only a few of the total strains in nature have this property. The enterotoxin has been shown to develop within as short a period as 4 to 5 hours when food is kept at 86° F. Unlike diphtheria, botulinum and tetanus toxins, it is relatively heat-stable and has caused illness in a human volunteer after having been boiled for 30 minutes. A wide variety of foods have been implicated, including milk, Cheddar cheese, ice cream, cream-filled bakery goods, rapid-cured hams, potato salad, dried beef, sausage, chicken gravy, tongue sandwiches, hollandaise sauce, liver sausage, pressed pickled beef, bread pudding and chicken salad.

Symptoms. Symptoms of staphylococcal food poisoning usually appear within about 3 hours, although occasionally they develop 1 to 6 hours after ingestion of food containing enterotoxin. The incubation period is influenced by the amount of enterotoxin consumed and the susceptibility of the person. The first symptom observed is salivation, which is subsequently followed by nausea, vomiting, retching, abdominal cramps, prostration and diarrhea. In severe cases blood and mucus have been observed in the stools and vomitus. In mild cases nausea and vomiting without diarrhea may occur, or there may be cramps and diarrhea without vomiting. Muscular cramps, headache and sweating often occur when symptoms are moderately severe. In severe poisoning marked prostration accompanies the vomiting and diarrhea, and symptoms of shock have been observed. A few fatal cases have occurred, usually in the very young, the aged or the debilitated. As a rule the acute symptoms are of short duration and generally subside after 5 or 6 hours.

Diagnosis. The short interval of time between the eating of the incriminated food and the onset of symptoms is one of the most characteristic features of staphylococcal food poisoning. If a list of foods served at the previous meal is available, the various food items can be tabulated for those made ill as well as those who were not ill. With such a list it is often possible to implicate one item of food as a common denominator. The suspected food should be sent to the laboratory for a bacteriologic examination. Usually, implicated foods contain enormous numbers of staphylococci. However, it must be remembered that the enterotoxin is not destroyed by boiling. In some outbreaks the food item has been bacteriologically sterile, although enterotoxin was present. In such instances, if the food is smeared on slides, stained and examined microscopically, large numbers of the heat-killed cocci are observed. Usually, there is a history of the food having been kept at a warm temperature for a period of several hours before being cooked and served.

When individuals rather than groups of people are taken ill with symptoms resembling those of staphylococcal food poisoning, it is important first to eliminate other possible causes of the illness, such as gallbladder disease, appendicitis, certain forms of intestinal allergy, onset of infectious diseases and functional bowel distress associated with emotional upsets. The diagnosis of staphylococcal food poisoning must be seriously considered when several members of a family or a group suddenly become ill with symptoms of vomiting, diarrhea, abdominal cramps and prostration coming on within two and one-hour to three hours after a meal. Enteric infections caused by bacteria or viruses are not of the explosive nature characterizing staphylococcal food poisoning, and the illnesses appear over a longer period of time.

Prognosis. In general, the acute illness in staphylococcal food poisoning usually does not persist longer than 5 hours, although anorexia and diarrhea may continue for several days after the acute attack. Fatalities are rare. A death occurred in one member of a family made ill by contaminated beef, and in one outbreak two children, 3 and 4 years old, died within 24 hours after each drank 250 cc. of milk from a goat suffering from acute suppurative mastitis. Other deaths have been reported in young children, aged or debilitated persons.

Treatment. Vomiting and diarrhea are

usually severe; therefore it is not necessary to empty the stomach with a stomach pump or to give cathartics to free the gastrointestinal tract of enterotoxin. Prostration occurs in severe cases, and the blood pressure may fall precipitously. The symptoms of shock are due to loss of body fluids and electrolytes, resulting in decreased circulating blood volume, and should be corrected immediately by the administration of saline solutions parenterally. The amount of fluid to be given should be governed by the age of the patient and the severity of the vomiting and diarrhea. There is no specific drug or serum therapy.

Prevention. Since staphylococci are abundant in nature and commonly present in the secretions of the nose and throat and in purulent lesions of the skin, it is impossible to exclude them from foods exposed to the air. Staphylococci will grow in the presence of amounts of salt and sugars which are inhibitory to the common enteric bacilli. Because of this fact, many foods which the housewife would regard as preserved might provide a good medium for staphylococci. When staphylococci grow in food, there is no perceptible off-flavor or taste to indicate their presence. It has been shown experimentally that enterotoxin is not formed in periods up to four weeks at temperatures maintained by the ordinary mechanical refrigerators, even though other conditions necessary for enterotoxin production are fulfilled. Therefore, at the present time, the best control of staphylococcal food poisoning consists in adequate refrigeration of perishable foods.

LIVING ORGANISMS
SALMONELLA FOOD POISONING

Since Salmonella infections are discussed elsewhere in this book, only brief reference will be made here to the role of Salmonella in food poisoning. Strains of Salmonella have long been associated with food poisoning, and many theories have been proposed to implicate them as causative agents when bacteriologic studies have been negative or inconclusive. An attempt has been made to explain some outbreaks on the basis that these organisms produce endotoxins which survive heat treatments that would destroy the living Salmonella. Most of the work with endotoxins involved *parenteral* injections into experimental animals. Human volunteers *fed* filtrates and heat-killed cultures of Salmonella, which are toxic by parenteral injections into animals, have not become ill—only *living organisms* have caused illness in man. If symptoms are caused by endotoxins, the living organisms undoubtedly must invade the tissue to by-pass the natural barrier of the gastrointestinal tract. In Salmonella infections characterized by acute gastrointestinal disturbances, the onset of symptoms may vary from 7 to 72 hours after eating contaminated food.

ENTEROCOCCI IN RELATION TO FOOD POISONING

Although the role of enterococci in food poisoning has not been clearly established, a number of food-poisoning outbreaks have been described involving specific items of food which contained per gram hundreds of millions of *Streptococcus faecalis,* a normal inhabitant of the human intestine. Human volunteers fed either the item of food or cultures prepared from the food have, in many instances, had symptoms similar to those involved in the outbreaks. Filtrates or heat-killed cultures have failed to produce symptoms when fed to human volunteers. Many volunteers fed cultures which were under laboratory cultivation for long periods of time also have failed to become ill. Since *S. faecalis* has been shown to decarboxylate tyrosine, leaving an appreciable amount of tyramine in the food, it was postulated that perhaps the tyramine was responsible for the symptoms. However, human volunteers fed tyramine in amounts as large as 1 gm. have remained well. The symptoms of this type of food poisoning are generally mild and are characterized by nausea, sometimes vomiting, colicky pains and diarrhea, developing within 2 to 18 hours after eating the incriminated food and usually subsiding within a few hours, thus requiring no specific treatment. In these outbreaks a number of different types of foods have been involved, such as Vienna sausage, beef croquettes, turkey dressing, evaporated milk, dried eggs, charlotte russe, roast beef and ham bologna.

G. M. DACK

References

Dack, G. M.: Food Poisoning. Chicago, The University of Chicago Press, 1949.
——, Niven, C. F., Jr., Kirsner, J. B., and Marshall, H.: Feeding Tests on Human Volunteers with Enterococci and Tyramine. J. Infect. Dis., 85:131, 1949.
Edwards, P. R., Bruner, D. W., and Moran, A. B.: The Genus Salmonella: Its Occurrence and Distribution in the United States. Kentucky Agricultural Experiment Station Bulletin 525, 1948.
Meyer, K. F.: Botulismus. Handb. d. Pathogenen Mikroorg., 4:1261, 1928.

Deficiency Diseases

INTRODUCTION

The nutritional deficiency diseases are a group of diseases caused by an inadequate intake or absorption of essential food factors. Intake may be insufficient for the usual or normal requirements, or only relatively insufficient, that is, inadequate for abnormally increased needs or abnormal destruction. The essential food factors include, not only the vitamins, but the energy principle (calories), protein and certain amino acids, some minerals, possibly some fatty acids, and water. In medical practice, deficiencies are usually multiple, although the signs and symptoms of one or two predominate. Curiously, complete starvation is not accompanied by evidence of deficiencies other than of calories.

Although the effects of many of the deficiencies are represented by long-recognized syndromes, such as beriberi and scurvy, the modern concept of deficiency disease really begins with the discovery of the vitamins. These substances were hinted at by Lind's classic observations on lime juice and scurvy, but had their real beginning in the search for the substance in rice bran that cured polyneuritis in pigeons, an unknown substance to which Funk gave the name "vitamine." From these studies came the impetus for the discovery of not only thiamine (vitamin B_1), but nearly a dozen other vitamins now believed to be essential for man.* The names and structural formulas of these are shown in Figure 62. More recently, increasing interest has developed in the deficiencies of calories, proteins and minerals.

In the beginning, medical interest and knowledge were confined to the gross manifestations of severe deficiencies represented by well known diseases whose etiology and pathogenesis had long been obscure—scurvy, beriberi, pellagra, hunger edema, keratomalacia and others. As further progress was made, new essential nutrients and the syndromes due to their deficiency were discovered—vitamin K and the hemorrhagic states related to it, for example. New and hither-

* Other vitamins are necessary nutrients for other species of animal life or plants.

to unrecognized results of deficiencies of previously known factors were found. Finally, it was realized that, besides the severe and advanced deficiencies hitherto recognized, there are many instances of deficiencies so slight that they either cause no recognizable symptoms or produce symptoms too mild and nonspecific to constitute reliable diagnostic evidence of the deficiency. To detect such deficiencies, objective laboratory tests and special procedures are required.

The various nutritive factors and the diseases associated with them have many characteristics which serve to distinguish them as a group. Except for the energy principle (calories) and protein, the various nutrients are needed in very small amounts, much as catalysts. This is true even of certain minerals, the nutritive requirements of which are many times smaller than the pharmacologic doses. Even for protein the required amounts of the essential amino acids are relatively small.

None of the truly essential dietary factors can be formed or synthesized by the body; they must be obtained in a preformed state in the diet. This characteristic, which is relative and shows considerable species variation, is well expressed in man. He can complete the synthesis of vitamin A from carotene, can obtain vitamin K and perhaps certain newly recognized vitamins from the action of bacteria in his intestine, and can form vitamin D from the action of ultraviolet light on his integument. Except for these limited abilities, he is dependent upon preformed substances from outside sources.

Another characteristic of the various nutritive factors is their relative lack of toxicity or potentiality for harm. Excessive amounts are in general excreted without untoward effect, even of such minerals as iodine, if the amounts are at all near the range of nutritional requirements. This lack of untoward effect, however, is concerned with a direct toxic action and not with possible ill effects of a nutritional nature caused by an imbalance of nutritive factors. Little is known of possible disturbances of this kind, but such disturbances can occur. A simple example is the increased requirement for thiamine

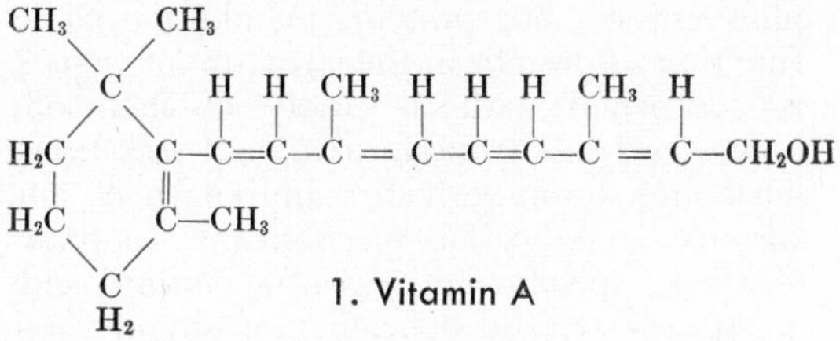

1. Vitamin A

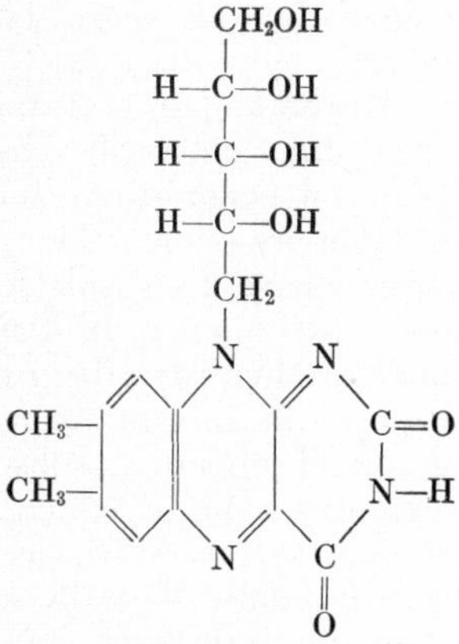

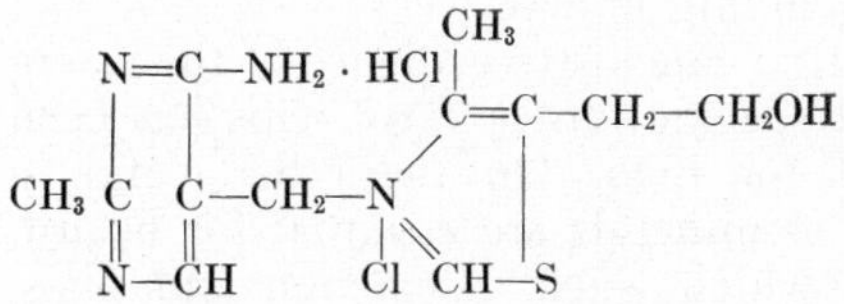

2. Thiamine hydrochloride

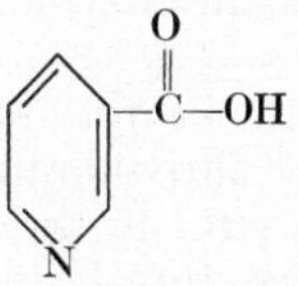

3. Riboflavin

4. Niacin ((Nicotinic acid)
(Pyridine—3—carboxylic acid)

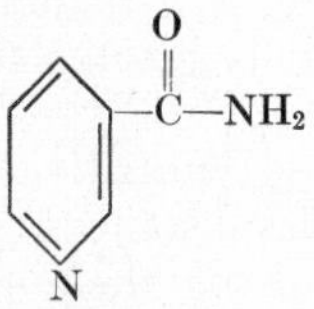

5. Niacinamide

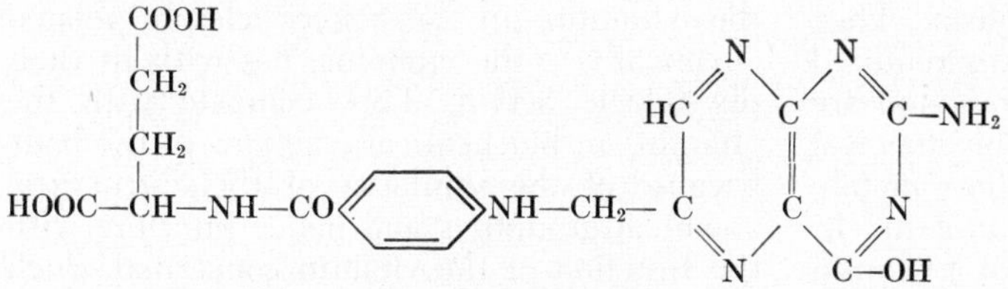

6. Pteroylglutamic acid

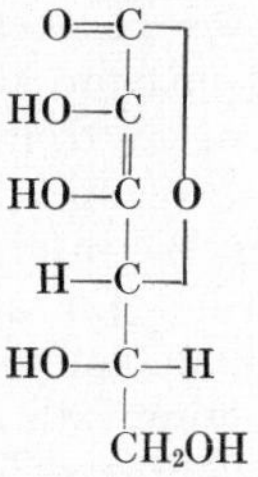

7. L-Ascorbic acid

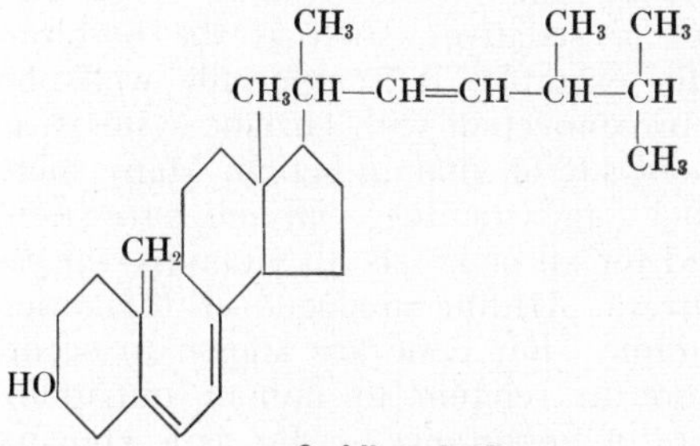

8. Vitamin D_2

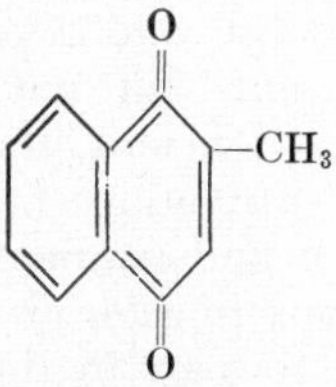

9. Menadione ($C_{11}H_8O_2$)
2-methyl-1, 4-naphthoquinone

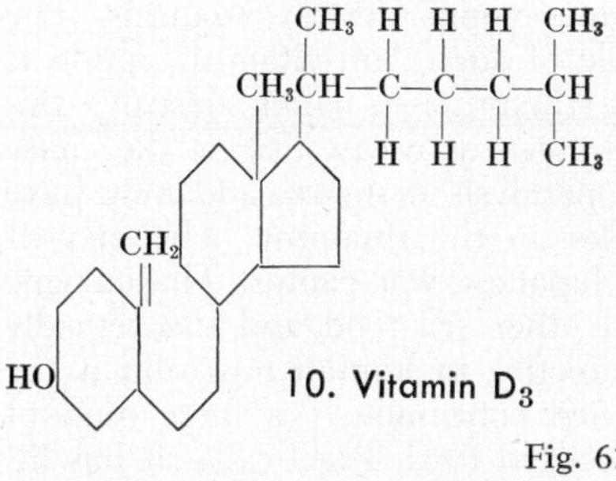

10. Vitamin D_3

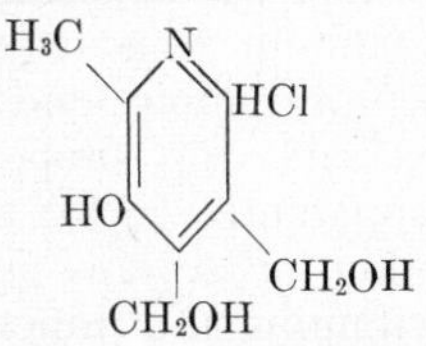

11. Pyridoxine hydrochloride

Fig. 62. Structural formulas of vitamins.

caused by an increased carbohydrate intake.

All the known essential nutritive products are distinct chemical substances. The nature, chemical composition and structure of most of them are known. Many of the organic substances have been isolated and synthesized— one of the most brilliant achievements of modern chemistry. In a number of instances the specific factors are members of a related group of chemical substances, natural and artificial, some of which may have an effect similar to, or serve as precursors of the actual vitamin. Usually such substances have a less marked effect than that of the natural vitamin; occasionally (vitamin K, for example) the potency of a related, even an artificial, compound is greater than that of the natural vitamin.

Because these nutritive essentials are known chemical substances, we have considerable knowledge of their physical characteristics and chemical reactions. For example, most members of the so-called B complex of vitamins are concerned in the intimate biochemical processes of metabolism. They constitute a part of enzyme systems required for the release of energy from foods and are concerned with highly specific biochemical reactions involved in the intermediary metabolism of carbohydrate, fat and protein. In the absence of adequate amounts of a vitamin the biochemical reaction fails or is imperfect. For example, in thiamine deficiency there is an imperfect oxidation of glucose and abnormal quantities of a metabolite (pyruvic acid) accumulate. When ascorbic acid, another water-soluble vitamin and a powerful oxidation-reduction agent, but not a member of the B complex, is deficient, there is a failure of the proper formation of intercellular ground substance and connective tissue. Although the actions *in vivo* of vitamin A are in part obscure, its part in the formation of visual purple and its breakdown and regeneration necessary for the visual function of the cones of the retina is well established. Vitamin D controls in part the adsorption and perhaps the deposition (in bone) of calcium; vitamin K is required for the formation of prothrombin, and pteroylglutamic acid is necessary for proper hematopoiesis as well, apparently, as for the normal intestinal absorption of several substances, including some vitamins and minerals and even such a simple substance as glucose.

Combustion of fat and carbohydrate supplies energy, but protein, in addition to its function as protein in the structure of tissues, is concerned with a variety of metabolic processes, such as the formation of secretions, hormones, immune bodies and enzymes, and various detoxification mechanisms. In many of these, specific and essential amino acids are necessary, and deficiency of any of these leads to a failure of normal physiologic processes, including growth.

As yet no conclusive evidence of the essentiality of specific fats or fatty acids has been obtained for man. On the other hand, a number of minerals are essential for health, some of which, such as calcium and phosphorus, are used for body structure, others in various biochemical actions as in enzymes. Many are necessary for both.

Recently, interest has arisen in the so-called *antivitamins*. The term "antivitamin" has been rather loosely used to refer to three kinds of actions or substances interfering with the availability or utilization of vitamins. These are as follows:

1. The action of structural analogues of the vitamins in substances closely related chemically to the vitamins, but without their physiologic action. They compete with the vitamins in biochemical reactions in the body because of the similarity of their structural chemical groupings and hence interfere with the function of the vitamin concerned. Such substances are sometimes called vitamers. Basically, the action is similar to that which accounts for much of the action of drugs, anesthetics or sedatives, such as the barbiturates, for example. It is especially well observed in connection with enzyme systems, a prominent site of vitamin action. Many such analogues (antivitamins) can and have been prepared for all or nearly all vitamins—pyrithiamine, a pyridine analogue of thiamine, for example—but none are known to occur in nature in relation to human nutrition. They are of importance, as far as is known, only experimentally.

2. Enzymes which destroy vitamins. The best example of such "antivitamin" action is the enzyme thiaminase, which destroys thiamine. It is formed in raw fish, is the cause of Chastek paralysis in foxes, and may have been a factor in the thiamine deficiency of inmates of Japanese war camps. The enzyme is found in other sea food and theoretically might be effective in human nutrition if the diet contained continuously a large amount of such uncooked food. Practically, it has lit-

tle significance as far as is known. A some-what related process is the oxidative destruction of vitamin A, against which the tocopherols (vitamin E) may be protective.

3. The action of chemical substances in "binding" a vitamin and rendering it unabsorbable or ineffective. An example is the avidin in raw egg white which reacts with and binds biotin. Such instances must be rare, however, because of the peculiar circumstances necessary to produce such an effect.

A final example of possible "antivitamin" activity should be given. The competition between para-aminobenzoic acid and the sulfa drugs in the nutrition of bacteria is often used as a good illustration of antivitamin activity. Para-aminobenzoic acid is used in the synthesis of pteroylglutamic acid (folic acid). Since the production of pteroylglutamic acid by bacteria in the gut may play some part in human nutrition, another possible antivitamin action in man may be envisioned. Recently, more subtle functions and reactions, such as those concerned with detoxification mechanisms, immune body production and the like, disclose new fields of study and development.

As a group, the nutritional deficiencies, that is, the diseases resulting from a lack of the specific nutrients, have many characteristics in common, as do the nutritive factors themselves. Clinically, these deficiency diseases appear in epidemic as well as in endemic and sporadic form. The sporadic cases are of more immediate interest to practicing physicians, but existing endemic deficiencies provide a large backlog of nutritional illness which may complicate all manner of other disease and, under conditions of stress, may often develop into a major problem by itself. Simple, idiopathic deficiencies are those which are the result simply of failure to consume enough of one or more nutrients. Conditioned deficiencies are brought about by the influence of some other disease on the intake, absorption or utilization of food. They constitute the largest group of deficiencies seen in medical practice and are found in all specialties and types of practice.

The importance of the nutritional factor in injury and disease has been greatly emphasized by the recent discovery and recognition of the influence of negative nitrogen balance, calorie deficiency and certain vitamin disturbances occurring in injury, shock and in certain infectious diseases. The proper management of these factors has resulted in a reduction in morbidity, mortality and the period of convalescence in such conditions as serious fractures, major operations, burns, infectious hepatitis, meningitis and typhoid fever. In this direction lies much of the future development in the field of nutrition.

So far the goal of clinical medicine in the prevention and control of nutritional deficiencies has been the "absence of disease." Little is known of optimum nutrition or even of optimum amounts of single factors. The problem is exceedingly complex, concerned as it is with the interaction of a large number of independent major nutritive factors, besides many lesser influences. Yet in the direction of such optimum nutrition lies a potentially tremendous advance in public and individual health.

JOHN B. YOUMANS

References

Funk, C.: The Etiology of the Deficiency Diseases. Beriberi, Polyserositis in Birds, Epidemic Dropsy, Scurvy, Experimental Scurvy in Animals, Infantile Scurvy, Ship Beriberi, Pellagra. J. State Medicine, London, 20:341, 1912.

Hawk, P. B., Oser, B. L., and Summerson, W. H.: Practical Physiological Chemistry. 12th ed. Philadelphia, The Blakiston Co., 1947, p. 1212.

Lind, J.: A Treatis of the Scurvy. 3rd ed. London, 1772.

Malnutrition during Convalescence. Prepared under Direction of the Committee on Convalescence and Rehabilitation of the National Research Council. War Medicine, 6:1, 1944.

Sydenstricker, V. P., and others: Preliminary Observations on "Egg White Injury" in Man and Its Cure with a Biotin Concentrate. Science, 95:176, 1942.

UNDERNUTRITION

Definition. As used here, the term *undernutrition* means a state of nutritional deficiency predominantly of calories and protein. There may or may not be a deficiency of other nutrients. The term is not a fortunate one, lacking specificity as to nutrient and degree of nutritional deficiency. Nevertheless, the term has come to have rather wide acceptance as meaning calorie and protein deficiency disease primarily.

Although it is customary to distinguish between calorie deficiency and protein deficiency, calorie deficiency disease is in effect protein deficiency. Experimentally, protein deficiency can be produced by feeding either a protein-deficient diet or a diet inadequate in calories. In the latter case the calorie deficiency leads to the burning of protein for fuel (energy), and, even though the amount of protein is adequate as such, the protein is diverted to combustion and becomes insufficient for the body's needs as protein. A deficiency of calories in the diet causes disease only when it causes too much body protein to be burned for energy. This occurs only after the fat stores have been consumed or nearly consumed. In a person of normal weight these stores will not be large and may be soon exhausted, depending on the extent of calorie deficiency. In obese subjects the process is much longer (it is the basis of weight reduction). When fat is gone, protein is next consumed. Injury and deficiency disease may be said to exist when more than the small reserve of body protein has been burned. Thus calorie deficiency disease becomes in effect protein deficiency disease. In practice, the deficiency is usually mixed from the beginning.

Etiology. Deficiencies of protein and calories result from an inadequate intake, absorption and utilization of food and are common in many diseases, ranging from the psychoneuroses to gastrointestinal obstruction. Simple, idiopathic starvation is only occasionally encountered.

However, deficiencies in the *intake* of protein and calories, though common enough in disease and injury, are not the only cause of actual protein deficiency disease or undernutrition. Many kinds of injury and disease are accompanied by a spontaneous, idiopathic, negative nitrogen balance. This is occasioned by an excess urinary excretion of nitrogen, apparently mediated by the action of adrenal cortical hormones. This excess secretion of nitrogen is independent of intake, which is often reduced in disease and injury, and is apparently the result of tissue breakdown. In fact, it may be impossible to match the excretion by increasing the intake, i.e., to bring about nitrogen balance, even when the intake is increased by artificial means to high levels. This fact has led some persons to conclude that the negative nitrogen balance is a beneficial or protective reaction to injury despite the untoward effects it causes. This is possibly true. Nevertheless, there are many examples of reaction to disease, primarily beneficial, which, when excessive, become harmful and retard recovery.

The phenomenon just described is sometimes spoken of as the *catabolic* phase of reaction to injury or disease. It persists for a variable length of time and exists to a variable degree, depending on a variety of factors. Even so simple a restriction as confinement to bed may produce this effect. The most striking and uncomplicated examples are seen in fractures of the long bones in previously healthy and well nourished persons, or in severe burns. In these circumstances the negative nitrogen balance stands out as a sharply defined abnormality, clearly related to the acute injury and without any background of disease or other apparent cause.

The reaction occurs in a variety of injuries and diseases: in severe burns; after major surgical operations, especially those in which the peritoneum is opened; with infections such as osteomyelitis, empyema and abscesses; and with some infectious diseases such as typhoid fever and meningitis. In addition to the original reaction, similar, though usually less severe, reactions may occur as the result of complications during the course of an illness. The changing of casts, secondary operations, the opening of abscesses and the occurrence of secondary or complicating infections or infectious disease, all may be accompanied by a return, or exaggeration and prolongation, of the nitrogen deficit and hence a delay in the onset of the anabolic or recovery phase.

It is clear that in many instances the nitrogen deficit will be aggravated and increased by a diminished intake of proteins and calories. A number of factors are responsible for this diminished intake. After injury and in many diseases there is often a loss of appetite and hence a lessened intake of food. With this specific loss of appetite there are often the factors of unappetizing meals, poorly prepared and served; weakness; difficulties of recumbency and apparatus; nausea, vomiting, and the mental changes of illness. Unfortunately, to these are often added indifference to nutritional problems on the part of the physician and nurse, and even misconception and ignorance regarding the proper diet and nutrient requirements. In some cases the nitrogen (protein) deficit is still further increased by loss of nitrogen from hemorrhage, exudates, transudates, and discharge from wounds and burned surfaces, from diarrhea and vomiting, even from albuminuria when this is present.

The catabolic phase, just described is followed by an *anabolic* phase during which the nitrogen balance becomes positive (provided intake is adequate), nitrogen is retained and protein formed, the tissues are restored and weight is regained. It corresponds to the period of convalescence and recovery and is deficient or lacking in unfavorable circumstances.

Morbid Anatomy and Physiology. The effect of this negative nitrogen (and calorie) balance depends on its severity and duration and on the nutritional state of the patient. As has already been stated, it is ordinarily most severe in a previously healthy and well nourished person (for a given grade of injury), and, curiously, slight or absent in those already ill and poorly nourished, as though the body lacked the ability to respond normally (and defensively?) to injury. It should be remembered, however, that the latter group are already in a state comparable to the end stage of an initially well nourished group which has suffered from the full and severe effects of such a reaction. The restorative, if not the preventive, treatment is therefore the same in both.

The spontaneous result of the reaction, therefore, represents a balance between the severity and duration of the reaction and the resistance (nutrition) of the patient. If the process is mild and of short duration in a well nourished patient, little harm is done. Such would be the effect from a mild burn or minor fracture. The body has a sufficient reserve of protein and calories (fat) to tide it over. To say in such cases that nutritional deficiency disease is present would be incorrect. However, if the reaction is severe and prolonged, is not limited by treatment, and consumes the reserve resources of the body, actual deficiency disease does occur. Primarily, it is a protein deficiency, although other nutrients, as will be shown later, may be involved.

Keys and his associates have well demonstrated experimentally the effects of this deficiency without the complications of accompanying disease. They may be described as illustrating the basic harmful results of such a deficiency. These may be aggravated or complicated by the effects of the primary injury or illness.

The principal outward manifestation of this undernutrition is loss of body weight, at first slight and representing mostly loss of fat. When it is more severe and of longer duration, there is a loss of tissue protein, revealed externally by atrophy of muscles. There is, however, a concomitant loss of native protein from parenchymatous organs and the blood plasma. This is easily demonstrable by measurements of heart size and is also clearly evident in the liver and other parenchymatous organs. There are accompanying physiologic changes such as weakness, hypothermia, bradycardia and lowered basal metabolism, together with significant mental changes of a character resembling those of the psychoneuroses. With the hypoproteinemia there may be edema, which, if severe, is not necessarily confined to the legs. Decubital ulcers are a common complication.

There is evidence also that more subtle changes of a harmful nature may accompany this undernutrition, such as interference with immune body formation, and hence with resistance to infection (a notorious complication of debility), and with production of secretions and enzymes. Besides interference with such specific defenses against infection, there may be secondary infection and impaired healing of wounds, related to impaired health of tissues resulting from edema.

In the presence of disease many of these abnormalities that are clearly evidenced in uncomplicated experimental undernutrition are aggravated or modified. Fever and infection may prevent bradycardia and elevate the metabolism. The weakened heart may be enlarged instead of smaller. Edema may be massive, with effusions into the serous sacs, and weight may fail to decrease or may even increase because of the dropsy.

So far, little has been said of a deficiency of other nutrients, such as vitamins and minerals. Deficiencies of these are relatively uncommon in the condition described here, particularly in those who were in good health and nutrition before the onset of the particular disease or injury. The reduction in calorie consumption and slowing of metabolic processes accompanying many disease states themselves tend to reduce requirements, particularly of the vitamins concerned with enzymatic processes. Body reserves protect in the case of those nutrients for which there is a large storage capacity—vitamin A, for example. Forced feeding to prevent or minimize the colorie and protein deficit will, of course, expose the patient to deficiencies of those vitamins, such as the B complex, concerned with metabolic oxidative mechanisms, unless natural vitamin-carrying foods are supplied. A good example of the need for supplement is parenteral feeding with glucose after operations.

One important exception to the general lack of vitamin and mineral deficiencies in undernutrition should be made, namely, that relating to calcium. In a variety of traumas, excessive calcium excretion, mainly urinary, accompanies the excess secretion of nitrogen. If it is continued and sufficiently severe, there occurs an actual calcium deficiency represented by demineralization of the skeleton in varying degree, sometimes sufficient to result in pathologic fractures. This loss, like that of nitrogen, can often be minimized, but not always overcome, by an increased intake of calcium. There is the added complication of urinary calculi, formed because of the high concentration of calcium in the urine, combined in some cases with relative immobility (confinement to bed). There is insufficient evidence, however, that added calcium in reasonable amounts in the diet increases to any significant degree the likelihood of stone formation.

Diagnosis. The diagnosis of undernutrition is, on the whole, easy; in fact, the condition can in many instances be anticipated and prevented—true preventive medicine.

A patient, when seen by the physician, should have an appraisal of the state of nutrition, the probable effects of the disease on his nutrition and what is needed for the prevention or treatment of nutritional disease. Often this will require only the usual history, physical examination and routine laboratory work, but special laboratory tests may be needed. For the patient who is injured or acquires an illness while in a normal state of nutrition the need can be determined in general from the nature of the illness and its severity and probable duration, but complications and variations in the response of the patient and his cooperation may require modification from time to time. For instance, in fractures of the large bones, or severe trauma, in serious burns and in most major surgical operations for acute diseases, an immediate negative nitrogen balance and calorie deficit can be anticipated. This should be met by nitrogen and calorie intakes to overcome or minimize these deficiencies.

Weight is, of course, the earliest and at the same time simplest guide to undernutrition unless it is masked by edema. Losses below 10 per cent of calculated ideal body weight may in general be considered evidence of actual protein deficiency. However, in some circumstances obese persons may have protein deficiency without calorie deficiency or reduc-

tion of weight below the ideal level. Hypoproteinemia can be detected by determining the concentration of and total circulating plasma proteins. Ordinarily the determination of the total serum proteins by the simple specific gravity methods suffices as a general diagnostic test and guide, but the greater significance of the albumin fraction and the possibility that albumin is depressed while total proteins remain normal or near normal make it desirable to determine serum protein fractions when such a situation is suspected. Accurate nitrogen balance studies are not often needed in these patients. Edema, except in patients with complicating renal or cardiac disease, is nearly always related to the hypoproteinemia and is in itself a strong indication of protein deficiency. It should indicate the need for a serum protein determination. It must be emphasized that edema may mask actual loss of tissue. Retention of 10 pounds of water can occur without visible edema.

The diagnosis of other possible nutritional deficiencies is made in the usual manner. Knowledge of the situation should lead one to anticipate such possible deficiencies and be on the watch for them.

Treatment. In practice, two stages of the reaction to injury or disease can be rather sharply differentiated and differ in their practical management. The first is the initial period when only the metabolic disturbance is present and no nutritional deficiency disease has occurred. In this stage there is the possibility of preventing or minimizing serious effects. The second stage is that in which a greater or lesser deficiency has developed.

The prevention and treatment of undernutrition are simple and easy in principle. No difficult, highly specialized or expensive techniques are necessary. With occasional exceptions, inexpensive materials may be used. But they do require close attention and supervision on the part of the physician, the nurse and other personnel, as well as the wholehearted cooperation of the patient. Much help can be derived from the use of standardized procedures or "routines," particularly in a hospital. However, as always, each patient will present an individual problem, his requirements will differ as will his response, and he will need individual attention. Routines can provide only the basic framework of the procedure, within which adjustments must be made for each patient. Standardized regimens will indicate the amount and kind of food and route of administration. They will not assure its consumption. Finally, it is to be remembered that too much food in early realimentation of the severely undernourished may be harmful.

A number of excellent diets for this purpose have recently been published. In general, 3000 to 5000 calories and 120 to 150 gm. of protein are necessary and advisable in the types of injury and disease in which possible undernutrition may develop. Experience has shown that in many cases it is not necessary or desirable and may be harmful to secure complete nitrogen equilibrium during the early and more marked stage of the catabolic reaction, the disadvantages and difficulties of attempting to supply huge amounts of protein outweighing the advantages. However, sufficient protein and calories should be administered to provide a high intake of nitrogen, overcome the calorie deficit, and take full advantage of the beginning of the anabolic period, which will probably be hastened by this treatment.

When possible, this nourishment should be provided as ordinary food, supplemented when necessary by special feedings. In general, an attempt should be made to secure an intake of around 2500 calories and 90 to 100 gm. of protein by ordinary meals. The additional requirements are met by supplements. These are most satisfactorily furnished as milk drinks, composed of milk with added skim-milk powder, or prepared casein, and glucose. A variety of satisfactory formulas have been devised. A typical one provides 28 gm. of protein and 343 calories for each 240 cc. Therefore, three such feedings will add 84 gm. of protein and 1029 calories, or a total of 160 to 180 gm. of protein and 3500 calories if the regular meals are consumed.

A careful record of intake—calories and nitrogen—should be maintained in such patients, and it can be assumed that, if intakes of around 3500 to 4000 calories and 120 to 150 gm. of protein are secured, the nitrogen deficit will be abolished or minimized in most cases. Losses beyond about 10 per cent of calculated ideal body weight should be avoided; if losses exceed this figure, a more careful determination of the nitrogen balance should be made. In burned patients, particularly, and in those with exudates, draining sinuses, dysentery and other causes of abnormal loss of protein, a careful check of the probable balance must be made to determine the necessary intake, which in some cases may be unusually large. For instance, it has been calculated that an average-sized man with a third degree burn of 50 per cent of his body surface may lose as much as 19.9 gm. of nitrogen in 24 hours from the burned surface, equivalent to 124 gm. of protein.

With patients who are already in a state of nutritional deficiency disease, more strenuous treatment is necessary because the problem is one of replacement rather than prevention —the replacement of losses rather than maintenance of reserves. Furthermore, speed is highly desirable, and delay merely prolongs recovery and convalescence. Weight and muscle atrophy, with due consideration for edema, are again the best general evidence of the state of protein nutrition. Hypoproteinemia indicates the cause of edema and gives a rough index of the degree of protein loss from other body tissues and organs. Intakes graduated up to as high as 5000 to 6000 calories or higher and 200 to 300 gm. of protein may be required and be very effective in severe deficiencies.

In patients with nutritional disease already established, and in some other circumstances, the ordinary intake of food by mouth may be inadequate and tube or parenteral feeding may be necessary. It may also be necessary in delirious or mentally ill patients, in those with disease of the gastrointestinal tract, especially as a preoperative procedure, when haste is necessary or desirable, and for those who do not cooperate by ingesting adequate amounts of food. Often such feeding is best accomplished by stomach or duodenal tube, which can be used intermittently or for a continuous drip. For this purpose a variety of formulas for liquid foods are available, most of them similar to those used for supplemental feeding by mouth. In some cases it may be necessary to use intravenous feeding, alone or in combination with gastric or duodenal gavage. Ordinarily, such intravenous feeding is only for replacement of nutrients lost acutely, such as in operations or trauma, and includes red blood cells, plasma, fluid and electrolytes. It is assumed in this discussion that such replacement of acute losses has been made. Occasionally, however, intravenous feeding is necessary for the maintenance or restoration of nutrition. For this purpose plasma or a solution of amino acids is used for nitrogen, and glucose for fuel. Except for replacement of acute losses, plasma is relatively ineffective. Nitrogen and calorie balance can be maintained by these means, though usually only with difficulty, and ordinarily only a portion of the nutritive requirements can be supplied in this manner. The development of preparations of fat with their high caloric value, suitable for intravenous injection, will make complete intravenous alimentation possible. Such preparations are not yet generally available.

There are numerous drawbacks to intravenous feeding, however. One is the amount of fluid necessary, which may overtax a weak heart, cause circulatory failure, induce or exaggerate edema, and even provoke pulmonary edema and secondary pneumonia. The salt in solutions of amino acids may be undesirable. Thrombosis of the veins used for injection occurs and may interfere with prolonged feeding. Febrile reactions may occur. The psychologic influence of eating is lacking. Therefore intravenous feeding, particularly by itself, should be used only after careful consideration of the need and suitability, and for no longer than necessary. Supplements of other nutrient such as vitamins and minerals should be given when necessary.

Except perhaps in burned patients, vitamins and minerals present little difficulty in previously healthy persons unless the illness is severe and prolonged and has resulted in severe undernutrition. Adequate amounts for maintenance should be assured; if these amounts are not available in the food, they should be provided as supplements. In particular, provision should be made for adequate amounts of those vitamins directly concerned with cellular oxidations—thiamine, riboflavin and niacin—when patients are maintained on large intakes of pure carbohydrates such as glucose, that carry with them no complementary vitamins. In parenteral administration, somewhat larger doses of these vitamins should be given than are normally required, because of greater excretion. In previously ill patients, or those seen for the first time with nutritional deficiency disease, an appraisal should be made of their status in respect to vitamins and minerals, and adequate restorative and maintenance treatment should be instituted.

JOHN B. YOUMANS

References

Bontwell, R. K., Brush, M. K., and Rusch, H. P.: Some Physiological Aspects Associated with Chronic Caloric Restriction. Am. J. Physiol., 154: 517, 1948.

Cuthbertson, D. P.: Post-shock Metabolic Response. Lancet, 1:433, 1942.

Howard, J. E., and others: Studies on Fracture Convalescence. I. Nitrogen Metabolism after Fracture and Skeletal Operations in Healthy Males. Bull. Johns Hopkins Hosp., 75:156, 1944. II. The Influence of Diet on Post-traumatic Nitrogen Deficit Exhibited by Fracture Patients. Ibid., 75: 209, 1944.

Keys, A.: Caloric Undernutrition and Starvation, with Notes on Protein Deficiency. J.A.M.A., 138: 500, 1948.

———, and others: The Biology of Human Starvation. Minneapolis, University of Minnesota Press, 1950.

Kimbrough, J. C., and Denslow, J. C.: Urinary Tract Calculi in Recumbent Patients. J. Urol., 61:837, 1949.

Koop, C. E., Drew, J. H., Riegel, C., and Rhoads, J. E.: Studies on Nutrition. The Effect of Preoperative Forced Feeding on Surgical Patients. Ann. Surg., 124:1165, 1946.

Lund, C. C., and others: Ascorbic Acid, Thiamine, Riboflavin and Nicotinic Acid in Relation to Acute Burns in Man. Arch. Surg., 55:557, 1947.

Minutes of the Fifth Conference on Metabolic Aspects of Convalescence. Josiah Macy Jr. Foundation, 1943.

Plasma Proteins: Symposia on Nutrition of the Robert Gould Research Foundation, Inc. Vol. II. John B. Youmans, Ed. Springfield, Ill., Charles C Thomas, 1950.

Schiele, B. C., and Brozek, J.: 'Experimental Neurosis' Resulting from Semistarvation in Man. Psychosomat. Med., 10:31, 1948.

Stewart, J. D., Hale, H. W., and Schaer, S. M.: Management of Protein Deficiency in Surgical Patients. Intravenous and Intrajejunal Injections. J.A.M.A., 136:1017, 1948.

Varco, R. L.: Preoperative Dietary Management for Surgical Patients, with Special Reference to Lesions of Stomach and Duodenum. Surgery, 19: 303, 1946.

VITAMIN A DEFICIENCY

Vitamin A is a pale yellow substance soluble in fat solvents. It is an unsaturated cyclic alcohol.

As far as is known, the original source for all the vitamin A in all species of fish, birds and mammals is the carotenes and related carotenoids. Vitamin A occurs only in the animal kingdom and is present chiefly in the liver, although the kidney, lungs and fat droplets may contain some. For many years vitamin A_1 has been known to occur in sea fish oils, and more recently vitamin A_2 has been found in the oils of certain fresh-water fish. The provitamins A are not ordinarily found in large quantities in the healthy person, since they are transformed into vitamin

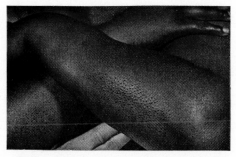

Fig. 63. Follicular hyperkeratosis of vitamin
A deficiency.

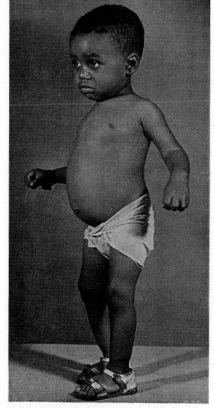

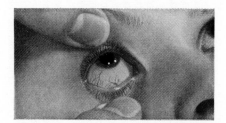

Fig. 64. Hemorrhagic jaundice of vitamin
K deficiency.

Fig. 65. Rickets due to vitamin D deficiency.

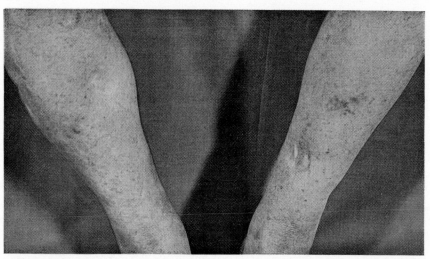

Fig. 66. Pitting edema of legs ("wet beriberi") and peripheral neuritis of vitamin B
deficiency.

Food and Nutrition Board, National Research Council Recommended Daily Dietary Allowances[1], Revised 1953

Designed for the Maintenance of Good Nutrition of Healthy Persons in the U.S.A.

(Allowances are considered to apply to persons normally vigorous and living in temperate climate)

	AGE YEARS	WEIGHT KG. (LB.)	HEIGHT CM. (IN.)	CALORIES	PROTEIN GM.	CALCIUM GM.	IRON MG.	VITAMIN A I.U.	THIAMINE MG.	RIBO-FLAVIN MG.	NIACIN MG.	ASCORBIC ACID MG.	VITAMIN D I.U.
Men.....	25	65 (143)	170 (67)	3200[2]	65	0.8	12	5000	1.6	1.6	16	75	
	45	65 (143)	170 (67)	2900	65	0.8	12	5000	1.5	1.6	15	75	
	65	65 (143)	170 (67)	2600	65	0.8	12	5000	1.3	1.6	13	75	
Women....	25	55 (121)	157 (62)	2300[2]	55	0.8	12	5000	1.2	1.4	12	70	
	45	55 (121)	157 (62)	2100	55	0.8	12	5000	1.1	1.4	11	70	
	65	55 (121)	157 (62)	1800	55	0.8	12	5000	1.0	1.4	10	70	
	Pregnant (3rd trimester)			Add 400	80	1.5	15	6000	1.5	2.0	15	100	400
	Lactating (850 ml. daily)			Add 1000	100	2.0	15	8000	1.5	2.5	15	150	400
Infants[3]...	0-1/12[4]												
	1/12-3/12	6 (13)	60 (24)	kg.x120	kg.x3.5[3]	0.6	6	1500	0.3	0.4	3	30	400
	4/12-9/12	9 (20)	70 (28)	kg.x110	kg.x3.5[3]	0.8	6	1500	0.4	0.7	4	30	400
	10/12-1	10 (22)	75 (30)	kg.x100	kg.x3.5[3]	1.0	6	1500	0.5	0.9	5	30	400
Children...	1-3	12 (27)	87 (34)	1200	40	1.0	7	2000	0.6	1.0	6	35	400
	4-6	18 (40)	109 (43)	1600	50	1.0	8	2500	0.8	1.2	8	50	400
	7-9	27 (59)	129 (51)	2000	60	1.0	10	3500	1.0	1.5	10	60	400
Boys......	10-12	35 (78)	144 (57)	2500	70	1.2	12	4500	1.3	1.8	13	75	400
	13-15	49 (108)	163 (64)	3200	85	1.4	15	5000	1.6	2.1	16	90	400
	16-20	63 (139)	175 (69)	3800	100	1.4	15	5000	1.9	2.5	19	100	400
Girls.....	10-12	36 (79)	144 (57)	2300	70	1.2	12	4500	1.2	1.8	12	75	400
	13-15	49 (108)	160 (63)	2500	80	1.3	15	5000	1.3	2.0	13	80	400
	16-20	54 (120)	162 (64)	2400	75	1.3	15	5000	1.2	1.9	12	80	400

[1] In planning practical dietaries, the recommended allowances can be attained with a variety of common foods which will also provide other nutrient requirements less well known; the allowance levels are considered to cover individual variations among normal persons as they live in the United States subjected to ordinary environmental stresses.

[2] These calorie recommendations apply to the degree of activity for the average active man and woman. For the urban "white-collar" worker they are probably excessive. In any case, the calorie allowance must be adjusted to the actual needs of the individual as required to achieve and maintain his desirable weight.

[3] The recommendations for infants pertain to nutrients derived primarily from cow's milk. If the milk from which the protein is derived is human milk or has been treated to render it more digestible, the allowance may be in the range of 2-3 gms. per kg. There should be no question that human milk is a desirable source of nutrients for infants even though it may not provide the levels recommended for certain nutrients. (See discussion in text.)

[4] During the first month of life, desirable allowances for many nutrients are dependent upon maturation of excretory and endocrine functions. Therefore no specific recommendations are given.

A and utilized in that form. A low plasma vitamin A and a high plasma carotene content suggest a failure in liver function.

One of the chief functions of vitamin A in the body is the maintenance of epithelial tissues. In the absence of vitamin A over a sufficient period of time, the cells atrophy and some of the basic cells proliferate. This produces a picture of keratinized epithelium. This type of epithelium is susceptible to bacterial invasion. In the late stages, severe infections of the eye, respiratory organs, genitourinary tract and mouth are likely to occur. Another function of vitamin A is its participation in the so-called "visual cycle." After prolonged deprivation of vitamin A, impairment of vision may occur, giving rise to a form of night blindness. Wolbach has brilliantly demonstrated that the skeletal growth of young rats is retarded by vitamin A deficiency. He showed that mechanical damage of the brain and spinal cord results from the continual growth of the central nervous system within its skeletal framework.

A deficiency of vitamin A can sometimes be detected by dark-adaptation tests or by an examination of scrapings from the eye or from the vagina. There is no absolute correlation between the vitamin A content of the blood and biophotometer readings, or examination of the scrapings from the epithelial surfaces, or the general physical examination. The first symptom referable to the eyes is loss of visual acuity in dim light. This symptom occurs in various diseases affecting the eye and is not pathognomonic. It should be seriously considered, however, in a person whose diet has been deficient in vitamin A or in a patient who has cirrhosis of the liver, any generalized alimentary tract disease, or nutritive failure. In the late stages the ocular disease is termed *xerophthalmia*.

Within the past few years cutaneous lesions caused by a deficiency of vitamin A have been described. The earliest clinical skin change is simple dryness. The most characteristic skin lesions are the plugs which form in the hair follicles, resulting in a rough dry skin known as hyperkeratosis (see Fig. 65).

Treatment. Green leafy vegetables, all yellow vegetables and fruits supply provitamin A in the human diet. Vitamin A proper is supplied by milk, liver and, to a lesser extent, by kidneys and animal fats. A liberal supply of these foods in the diet is excellent prophylactic therapy. Persons with night blindness, xerophthalmia or keratomalacia can usually be relieved by ingestion of 5000 to 50,000 units of vitamin A daily in the form of synthetic vitamin A, a potent fish liver oil or carotene. The skin lesions may require doses of 50,000 units of vitamin A daily. They respond slowly; as a rule, three to four months of therapy elapse before beneficial results are observed.

Tom D. Spies

References

Harris, P. L., Hickman, K. C. D., Jensen, J. L., and Spies, T. D.: Survey of the Blood Plasma Levels of Vitamin A, Carotene, Ascorbic Acid, and Tocopherols of Persons in an Area of Endemic Malnutrition. Am. J. Pub. Health, 36:155, 1946.

Moore, T.: Vitamin A and Carotene. XIII. The Vitamin A Reserve of the Adult Human Being in Health and Disease. Biochem. J., 31:155, 1937.

The Vitamins, published by the American Medical Association, under the auspices of the Council on Pharmacy and Chemistry and the Council on Foods, 1939.

Wolbach, S. B.: The Pathologic Changes Resulting from Vitamin Deficiency. J.A.M.A., 108:7, 1937.

VITAMIN B DEFICIENCIES

BERIBERI

Definition. Beriberi is a clinical syndrome associated etiologically with a faulty food supply or an alteration of metabolism associated with thiamine deficiency. It is characterized clinically by multiple neuritis, serous effusions, edema, muscular atrophy and cardiovascular changes. It occurs sporadically and endemically and passes in great waves over the Oriental countries. The disease is associated with ignorance and poverty and may appear in any race and at any age. It is prevalent among infants whose mothers have beriberi.

History. Though the precise origin of the word "beriberi" is unknown, the term undoubtedly arose from an Oriental language many centuries ago. There is good reason to believe that the disease was described in the Niching (2697 B.C.). In 1642, Jacobus Bontius, the first Occidental physician to describe the disease, pointed out that the natives of Java called it beriberi. During the nineteenth and twentieth centuries great interest arose in the recognition and prevention of beriberi and closely related diseases. During this period of renewed clinical interest, investigators applied dietary methods of prevention to special groups of the population with great success.

Incidence. Beriberi occurs sporadically

throughout the world. It is prevalent both among infants and adults in the endemic areas of China, Japan, the Netherlands East Indies, Brazil, India, the Malay Peninsula and the Philippine Islands. At times, sudden outbreaks of the disease occur in these countries and in prisons and asylums of the Western World.

For many years it was believed that beriberi seldom occurred in the Western Hemisphere. Recent studies show, however, that beriberi (nutritional peripheral neuritis) is much more prevalent than is commonly supposed. Its incidence is high among pellagrins, alcohol addicts and pregnant women. It is frequently associated with organic disease and often coexists with other nutritional deficiencies.

Etiology. The results of clinical and experimental studies point to a definite relationship between an unbalanced diet, abundant in decorticated cereals, and the development of beriberi. Such diets are known to be deficient in thiamine (Vitamin B_1). Although it has not been proved that one specific factor is the sole cause of the disease, clinical and experimental studies leave no doubt that persons with beriberi are greatly benefited by vitamin B_1 therapy.

It appears that man cannot synthesize thiamine, nor can he store it to any great extent. The length of time or the degree to which a deficiency must be present before clinical evidence of the disease appears is not known. Clinical studies show that the depletion period is extremely variable, ranging from a few weeks to months or years. They show, also, that certain factors predispose to, and precipitate the development of, the disease. Prominent among these are: increased physical exercise, fevers, hyperthyroidism and other conditions which are accompanied by an increased metabolic rate; pregnancy and lactation; digestive disturbances and chronic debilitating diseases which cause improper ingestion, assimilation or utilization of food.

At the present time the precise manner in which a deficiency of thiamine operates to produce the symptoms of beriberi is not understood. It has been shown, however, that cocarboxylase (thiamine pyrophosphate) has antineuritic properties and that it is a fundamental enzyme which plays a prominent role in oxidation and reduction.

There is considerable evidence that other nutritional diseases often coexist with beriberi. Persons with beriberi frequently have

a deficiency of nicotinic acid and riboflavin, and symptoms which arise from these deficiencies are benefited by the administration of these synthetic chemical substances. The number of factors involved in the development of the disease is not known, and knowledge concerning the physiologic mechanism is incomplete. Nevertheless, the synthesis of thiamine, nicotinic acid and riboflavin has stimulated investigation, and during the next few years much of the confusion over the relationship between the various symptoms of beriberi, and between beriberi and other diseases, should be eliminated.

Morbid Anatomy. Postmortem examinations are of little value in making a diagnosis or in explaining the pathologic physiology of the disease. The findings are not constant, but the process, in general, is one of degeneration, affecting especially the myocardium, the gastrointestinal tract and the nervous system. The most common gross findings are emaciation of the body and atrophy of the muscles, particularly in the legs. The body is often edematous, the heart is dilated and hypertrophied, and serous effusions and chronic passive congestion of the viscera are commonly observed. Microscopic studies show diffuse edema in various tissues and degeneration of the involved nerves, muscles and myocardium. Degeneration of the nerves varies from slight alteration to complete degeneration of the myelin and axis cylinder. The affected muscles show a diffuse parenchymatous degeneration with loss of striations, and hyaline and fatty changes. The cardiac muscle fibers are often fragmented and contain hyaline and fatty material. Postmortem findings in infants dying of beriberi are practically identical with those found in the adult. The degenerative changes in the nerves are, however, less striking in the infant.

Symptoms. Beriberi may be an acute or chronic disease. In the infant it is nearly always acute; in the adult it is nearly always chronic. The symptoms of infantile beriberi appear identical with those of the fulminating type in the adult. Infantile beriberi is characterized by a rapid onset with diminished urinary secretion, constipation, rigidity of the body and cyanosis. The child has a peculiar whine and cries most of the time. He is weak, has a rapid, irregular pulse, edema of the legs, and usually dies suddenly or is rapidly and completely cured by treatment.

In contrast, the onset in the adult is usually insidious and the prodromata are vague and general. Lassitude, general itching, dyspepsia, tachycardia, fatigue on exertion, and tenderness of the muscles occur early. After a variable period of time the symptoms can be associated with degeneration of the nervous system, alteration of the gastrointestinal tract, the presence of edema and serous effusions, or enlargement and dilatation of the heart. When the disease affects chiefly the peripheral nerves, it is commonly called the "dry type"; when it is especially characterized by acute cardiac symptoms, it is known as the "fulminating type"; and when it is associated primarily with edema and serous effusions, it is referred to as the "wet type" (Fig. 66). Beriberi strikingly selects the vagi, the peripheral nerves of the extremities and the vasomotor system.

Not all symptoms are necessarily present in a given patient, and the order of their appearance may vary. A patient with predominating cardiac symptoms may suddenly exhibit gastrointestinal symptoms such as a distaste for food, vomiting or diarrhea; the patient with gastrointestinal distress may suddenly display such myocardial symptoms as dyspnea, precordial pain and circulatory failure. Either or both of the foregoing types may have, or may develop, peripheral neuritis; conversely, a patient with peripheral neuritis may have cardiorespiratory or gastrointestinal symptoms. Serous effusions and edema may precede, accompany or follow the cardiac, gastrointestinal or nervous symptoms.

The symptoms subside slowly in the adults who recover; many months may pass before there is a restoration of function, if, indeed, complete restoration ever does take place. Often, after the active phase of the disease disappears, residual paralysis, muscular atrophy and cardiac enlargement remain for a long time.

Nervous Symptoms. The chronic cases have involvement of the nervous system. The early course is characterized by tingling of the hands and feet and by weakness of the legs. The clinical manifestations are caused by an ascending, symmetrical, peripheral neuritis. The deep reflexes of the extremities at first increase, later diminish and finally are absent. Tenderness in the calf muscles and sharply defined patches of anesthesia and numbness often appear early. This process affects particularly the extremities and sometimes the diaphragm, producing wasting of the muscles, contractures, ataxia, lack of co-ordination and dyspnea. Sensations of touch, pain and temperature are usually decreased, but at times may be increased. Anxiety states and mental confusion are common manifestations.

Cardiorespiratory Symptoms. When the disease is characterized especially by cardiac

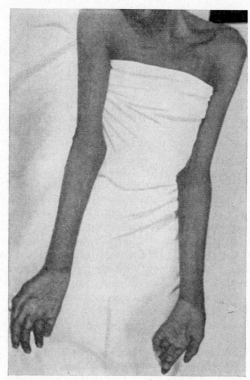

Fig. 67. Muscular atrophy of the upper extremities in a beriberi patient with severe peripheral neuritis. Compare the wasting of all muscle groups in the arms with fairly normal muscles of the shoulder girdle and neck.

symptoms (fulminating type), the adult patient usually dies suddenly and without a history of prodromal symptoms. Occasionally, however, a person with gastrointestinal and neurologic symptoms suddenly suffers the fulminating type of the disease. The cardiac symptoms are always striking. The most common ones are palpitation, tachycardia, dyspnea, lowered blood pressure, cardiac murmurs, changes in the electrocardiogram and paralysis of the diaphragm, associated with "high output" failure. Before death there is nearly always cardiac enlargement and dilatation, pulmonary congestion, edema, cyanosis and vasomotor collapse.

Digestive Symptoms. Frequently there is nausea, vomiting and epigastric distress.

These symptoms are especially prominent in the acute fulminating type and are often found with cardiac decompensation.

Other Symptoms. Edema is the most striking feature in many cases. It usually begins in the legs and may progress until the whole body becomes involved. Sometimes a typical case, with the body bloated from anasarca, appears emaciated after diuresis. Hydropericardium and effusions into various serous cavities are common, and a low serum protein can be demonstrated frequently. At times the organs of taste, smell, hearing and sight are involved. Libido decreases. Anemia may appear in the later stages of the disease.

Diagnosis. The typical case can be readily diagnosed by means of a reliable dietary history and by the presence of certain characteristic physical findings. Almost without exception, the history reveals that adults who have beriberi have subsisted on a monotonous diet abundant in carbohydrates (chiefly milled rice, wheat or corn). The physical findings are an enlarged heart, peripheral neuritis, edema, and tenderness and atrophy of the muscles. Infants who are restricted to the milk of women with beriberi usually acquire the disease during the first three months of life. The diagnosis is made on the following objective findings: constipation, diminution in the volume of urine, rigidity of the body, irritability, a rapid and irregular pulse, weakness, edema, cyanosis and a peculiar whine.

Though the atypical or mild cases occurring in infancy or later are probably more common than the typical ones, the manifestations in such cases vary greatly and the disease is not easily recognized. Since there is no specific laboratory test for beriberi, it is often necessary to exclude the possibility of various types of heart disease, diphtheria, nephritis, tabes, alcoholism, lead and arsenic poisoning, pellagra, scurvy and sprue before a positive diagnosis of beriberi can be made.

Prognosis. No disease requires more conservatism in making a favorable prognosis than does beriberi, for a patient who seems to be recovering may suddenly exhibit cardiac symptoms and die. The mortality rate is variable, being around 5 per cent in the mild cases and reaching well over 50 per cent in the more severe ones. The ultimate prognosis is dependent upon the age and general condition of the patient and upon the severity and duration of the disease. In general, patients with acute cardiac symptoms are least likely to survive. If the adult is left untreated, eventually incapacitation or even death is to be expected. If, however, the disease is recognized and treated early, the outlook is good, provided the patient can and will follow recommendations. Recovery is rapid and complete in infants who are given early and persistent treatment.

Prevention. Prevention in the adult or infant is dependent upon the ingestion, assimilation and utilization of sufficient quantities of a well balanced diet. Beriberi would practically disappear if it were possible to make proper diets available to all. We cannot hope, however, to achieve this ideal in the immediate future, since its fulfillment is dependent upon educating the masses and raising their economic level. The most logical means of ending beriberi as a world problem in the near future would be to pass and enforce a law preventing the overmilling of rice, wheat and corn. Grain products have long been the principal component of the poor man's diet. Overmilling of the cereals has deprived the finished product of much of its natural mineral and vitamin content. Consequently, the foods which may constitute the major part of the diet of persons most in need of improvement in their nutritional status are nutritionally inferior. The enrichment of flour and bread in this country is a step forward in improving the diets of these persons. Until such time as proper diets are available to all people, or until a law prohibiting the sale of overmilled cereals is passed and enforced, the incidence of beriberi can be greatly decreased by the application of the following recommendations:

1. Whole grain or enriched flour and bread should be substituted for the highly milled products.

2. Foods must not be overcooked, since excessive heat destroys vitamin B_1. The common habit of adding soda during the cooking process is detrimental and should be discontinued. Foods should be cooked in as little water as possible, and the water in which they are cooked should be used in soups or broths rather than discarded.

3. Lean meat, milk, eggs, fresh vegetables, dried vegetables and nuts should make up at least 50 per cent of the daily diet.

4. Any one of the following relatively inexpensive supplements is helpful in preventing beriberi and should be added to the daily diet whenever possible: dried brewers' yeast (1 ounce), wheat germ (2 ounces) or

tikitiki (1 ounce). Infants are given indirect protection by preventing the disease in mothers and can be given additional protection by supplementing their daily diet with an alcoholic extract of 40 gm. of rice polishings (tikitiki).

It is of great significance to note that in recent years in Alabama the author has not been able to find any cases of nutritional neuritis due to lack of vitamin B_1. This is due to the so-called "enrichment program," to better food habits on the part of the people, and to the interest of the medical profession in protecting the population against these disorders.

Treatment. Crystalline vitamin B_1 (thiamine hydrochloride) is recommended for every case in which the diagnosis of beriberi is established. It may be administered intravenously, intramuscularly or orally. Parenteral administration is recommended in severely ill cases, especially when thiamine deficiency is associated with severe gastroenteric disturbances or with cardiac failure. In such cases 30 to 50 mg. should be given intravenously in sterile physiologic saline twice daily. For the average cases the parenteral administration of 10 mg. twice daily is adequate. Oral administration of 5 to 10 mg. twice daily is sufficient for the mild case. Brewers' yeast, wheat germ and tikitiki (an alcoholic extract of rice polishings) are effective therapeutic agents in the average case of thiamine deficiency. The usual dose of brewers' yeast and wheat germ is 6 ounces, and of tikitiki, 3 ounces. The yeast and wheat germ are best tolerated if given in iced milk or eggnog at frequent intervals. All persons who have a thiamine deficiency should be given a well balanced, high caloric diet, including foods rich in vitamin B_1. These foods are whole grain bread and cereals, legumes, lean pork, liver, heart, kidney and milk. All patients, whether the disease is mild or severe, should be kept at complete rest until convalesence is well established.

For infants with beriberi the parenteral administration of 5 to 10 mg. of crystalline vitamin B_1 is recommended. After convalescence is established the same amount may be administered orally. If crystalline vitamin B_1 cannot be procured, an alcoholic extract of 100 gm. of rice polishings (tikitiki) may be given daily. If the child's mother has latent or manifest beriberi, cow's milk should replace breast milk.

Tom D. Spies

References

Blankenhorn, M. A., and Spies, T. D.: Prevention, Treatment and Possible Nature of the Peripheral Neuritis Associated with Pellagra and Chronic Alcoholism. Tr. A. Am. Physicians, 1:164, 1935.

Cowgill, G. R.: The Vitamin B Requirement of Man. New Haven, Yale University Press, 1934.

Jolliffe, N., and Jaffe, P. M.: Relation of Vitamin B (B_1) Intake to Neurological Changes in the Alcoholic Addict. Proc. Soc. Exper. Biol. & Med., 32: 1161, 1935.

Spies, T. D., and Aring, C. D.: The Effect of Vitamin B_1 on Peripheral Neuritis in Pellagra. J. A. M. A., 110:1081, 1938.

————, Vilter, R. W., and Ashe, W. F.: Pellagra, Beriberi, and Riboflavin Deficiency in Human Beings; Diagnosis and Treatment. J.A.M.A., 113: 931, 1939.

Strauss, M. B.: The Etiology of "Alcoholic" Polyneuritis. Am. J. M. Sc., 189:378, 1935.

Vedder, E. B.: Beriberi. New York, Wm. Wood and Co., 1913.

Wenckebach, K. F.: Das Beriberi-Herz. Pathologie und Klinik in Einzeldarstellungen. Berlin and Vienna, Julius Springer, 1934.

Williams, R. R., and Spies, T. D.: Vitamin B_1 and Its Use in Medicine. New York, The Macmillan Company, 1938.

PELLAGRA

Definition. Pellagra is a noncontagious, nonhereditary clinical syndrome affecting the skin, alimentary tract and nervous system. It is characterized by seasonal recurrences and relapses, may occur in any race and at any age, and is associated with deficiency in niacin and other factors in nutrition.

History. The term "pellagra," from the Italian "pelle agra," meaning rough skin, was first used in medical literature in 1771 by the Italian physician Frapolli, who found the word in common use among the peasant population of Lombardy. The authentic history of the disease begins somewhat earlier in northern Spain. In 1735 Gaspar Casal, physician to King Philip V, recorded his observations on "mal de la rosa," a malady prevalent among the peasantry in the province of Asturias. Twenty years later, Antonio Pujati reported its presence in northern Italy, and in 1784 a special hospital for the treatment of pellagrins was established at Legano by warrant of Joseph II of Austria. During the nineteenth century the disease was observed in many other countries, chiefly in France, Egypt and Rumania. In the United States, sporadic cases had been reported as early as 1864 from New York and Massachusetts, but it was not until 1907, when Searcy called attention to the presence of a large number of cases of endemic pellagra in an asylum in Alabama, that the seriousness of the situation in the southern part of the United States was appreciated. Within the next few years many cases were reported from practically all southern and from many northern States.

Incidence. Pellagra formerly was prevalent in many countries. The incidence was high in Egypt, United States, Rumania, Serbia, Bulgaria, Russia, Italy and Spain. Wilson stated that 30 per cent of the population of Egypt was affected with pellagra, and the United States Public Health Service estimated that there were 400,000 cases annually in the United States. It was believed that at least 10 per cent of the inmates of the insane asylums in the southern part of the United States were admitted because of pellagra. Owing to the use of nicotinic acid, pellagra has virtually been eradicated from the United States and greatly decreased in other countries.

Etiology. For many years opinion in regard to the cause of pellagra was divided. The two prevailing theories were (1) that it was a dietary deficiency disease, and (2) that it was an infection in which diet played a more or less important role. The spectacular improvement in so many pellagrins who receive intensive dietary treatment leaves no doubt that the disease may be explained on the basis of a dietary deficiency. At the present time the opinion is accepted that pellagra is a clinical syndrome caused primarily by a nutritional deficiency which may arise in one or more of the following ways: (1) The person's diet may be inadequate in the antipellagric foods. (2) His absorption may be impaired because of altered gastrointestinal function. (3) His requirement for the antipellagric substances may be in excess of the amount supplied by a liberal well balanced diet.

Goldberger advanced the theory that the pellagra-preventive factor is a single substance, vitamin B_2 (G), the thermostable portion of the vitamin B complex, and until recently many students of nutrition accepted this theory. It is now known that vitamin B_2 is not a single substance, but is composed of a number of active principles. Three of these, namely, niacin, riboflavin and pyridoxine, have been synthesized and, thus far, are the only ones which have been found to play a role in human nutrition. It has been shown that niacin is a specific curative agent for the mucous membrane lesions, for many of the symptoms arising from the alimentary tract and for the mental symptoms of human pellagra, and that it aids in preventing recurrences of these symptoms. Its relationship to the dermatitis of pellagra has not been fully established. After the administration of nicotinic acid, the concentration of coenzymes I and II in the blood and urine of pellagrins is increased from subnormal to normal values. The increase in concentration of these coenzymes, which are fundamental to cell respiration, parallels the clinical improvement of the patient. Recent work has shown that tryptophan when given in large amounts promotes relief of symptoms in pellagrins.

Certain predisposing and precipitating factors often play a role in the pathogenesis of the disease. Important among these are fatigue, insomnia, loss of teeth, infections, food idiosyncrasies, chronic alcoholism and diseases which cause improper ingestion, assimilation or utilization of food. Failure to consider all these conditions as underlying factors in the cause of pellagra has led to the designation of certain cases as "pseudopellagra," "pellagra sine pellagra," "postalcoholic dermatitis," "alcoholic pellagra" and "secondary pellagra." Such terms are confusing and should be abandoned; the disease is or is not pellagra.

During the past twelve years, from the study of over 10,000 pellagrins, we have found that the inadequate diets of these persons predispose them simultaneously to a number of nutritional deficiencies and that pellagra frequently coexists with beriberi and riboflavin deficiency. The diagnosis of pellagra, therefore, necessitates a thorough search for evidence of other deficiency syndromes, and the institution of therapy specific for each deficiency.

Morbid Anatomy. The most common gross findings are generalized emaciation of the body and atrophy of various organs. Pellagra can be diagnosed at the postmortem table only when the characteristic oral and skin lesions persist. In some cases the walls of the gastrointestinal tract may show swelling, reddening and ulceration of any portion; in other cases the walls may be thin and atrophic. The liver occasionally contains abnormal amounts of fat. Histologically, the skin lesions vary from atrophy to an intensive inflammatory reaction. Similarly, the microscopic picture of the intestinal lesions varies from atrophy to acute inflammation characterized by fibrin formation and collections of inflammatory cells. When changes in the nervous system are demonstrable, they are characterized by irregular areas of degeneration, often involving the posterior and lateral columns of the spinal cord, the posterior spinal ganglia, and the Betz and Purkinje cells.

Symptoms. These arise chiefly from the skin, gastrointestinal tract and nervous system. They vary greatly with each patient, arising in some from only one of the systems, and in others, from two or more.

Prodomal Symptoms. The onset of pellagra is often so gradual that the earliest symptoms may not be noticed by the patient. Early in the disease there is a loss of strength, particularly in the legs, a change in appetite, and usually, though not always, a decrease in body weight. There may be, also, a change in mood or personality. Pellagra, in the early stages of the disease, is often incorrectly diagnosed as neurasthenia.

Skin. Pellagra dermatitis is not always present, but, when observed, may be readily diagnosed by its appearance, symmetry, location and course. Symmetric lesions may appear on any part of the body, but are most common over sites of irritation, such as the hands, wrists, elbows, neck, under the breasts, knees, feet, and in the perineal region. A sharp line of demarcation at the periphery of the lesion separates the affected area from the healthy skin. In the majority of cases, pellagrous dermatitis is restricted to the exposed parts of the body, and the dermal lesions of pellagra often appear after exposure to sunlight. The dermatitis begins as an erythema resembling sunburn. As the disease progresses, the area becomes reddish-brown, roughened, scaly and keratotic; vesicles and bullae may form. Desquamation usually begins at the center of the lesion, and the underlying skin appears red and thickened. The intensity of the pigmentation and the thickening of the skin tend to increase with each recurrence of the disease; after repeated recurrences, the skin may become either permanently pigmented, thick and roughened, or thin and atrophic (see Figs. 71, 72, 73, 74).

Alimentary Tract. Both glossitis and stomatitis are early and common symptoms and are usually such as to be diagnostic of the disease. In the beginning only the tip and lateral margins of the tongue are swollen and reddened (Fig. 70). If treatment is not given, the swelling increases, the red discoloration becomes more intense, and deeply penetrating ulcers may appear along the sides and tip—rarely on top. Frequently a thick, gray membrane filled with debris and Vincent's organisms covers the surface. The tongue is usually hypesthetic, though it may be hypersensitive. The buccal membranes, the mucocutaneous surface of the lips, the gums and the palate may likewise be affected. The course of the stomatitis is similar to that of the glossitis. A burning sensation of the tongue and of the mucous membranes of the pharynx, esophagus and stomach is not uncommon; this is often aggravated by hot or acid foods. Ptyalism, nausea and vomiting may occur early, but as a rule these are advanced symptoms of the disease. About 50 per cent of pellagrins have no free hydrochloric acid even after histamine stimulation; rennin and pepsinogen are likewise absent. This achylia gastrica tends to persist during remissions. The stools may be hard, soft or watery, but the odor is invariably foul. Contrary to what is generally taught, the bowels in the majority of mild cases act normally or are constipated. Severe, persistent diarrhea, with several watery stools each hour, tends to appear only in the more acute cases. Abdominal distention, discomfort and pain may be present at any time during the course of the disease, but are more severe after a large meal.

Nervous System. Nervous symptoms are common, but at the onset of the disease are often vague and ill defined. The patient may complain of nervousness, insomnia, headaches, dizziness, muscular weakness, and a bilateral burning of the hands, feet and other parts of the body. The tendon reflexes are frequently altered. At first they may be exaggerated, later decreased; finally they may be absent. The extremities, particularly the legs, may "feel numb" or become paralyzed. Typical subacute combined degeneration of the spinal cord with spasticity and ataxia is found. Tremor and a spastic or ataxic gait are often associated with peripheral neuritis in the advanced cases.

Mental Changes. Pellagrins are subject to periods of depression and apprehension, and unless treatment is administered, hallucinations, confusion, delirium and complete disorientation may develop. Tremor, jerky movements and rigidity of the body frequently accompany these mental symptoms. If such cases are given early and intensive treatment, the mental symptoms seldom persist, but in the absence of treatment the patient is likely to become insane.

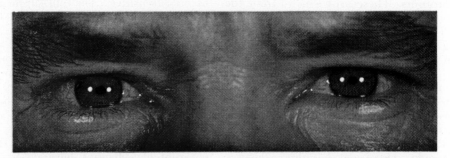

Fig. 68. Photophobia, epiphora and scleral injection in riboflavin deficiency.

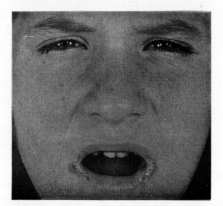

Fig. 69. Cheilitis and photophobia in riboflavin deficiency.

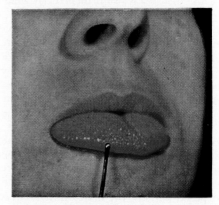

Fig. 70. Glossitis of nicotinic acid deficiency.

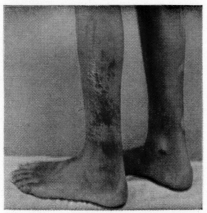

Fig. 71. Pellagrous dermatitis of nicotinic acid deficiency.

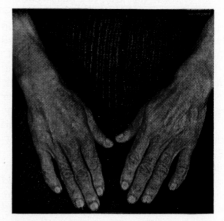

Fig. 72. Pellagrous dermatitis of hands in nicotinic acid deficiency.

Organs of Special Sense. Any of the organs of special sense may be affected; loss of taste and smell is common.

Genitourinary System. Burning on urination occurs frequently. Libido is often decreased; sterility is unlikely. In the female, acute pellagrous vaginitis with Vincent's infection is a usual finding. Menstruation may be scanty or absent.

Circulatory System. In the mild case a slightly subnormal blood pressure is often noted. In the severe case there is an increased pulse rate, lowered blood pressure and vasomotor collapse. Syncope and sudden death frequently occur.

Blood. The hemoglobin is less than 70 per cent in the majority of patients with severe pellagra. The anemia is either macrocytic or microcytic in type.

Temperature. The temperature of the mild, uncomplicated case is usually normal; an elevation of several degrees is serious, since it denotes the presence of an infection or a severe type of the disease.

Diagnosis. The typical case is easily diagnosed on the basis of a reliable history and careful physical examination. The history is usually one of an inadequate or unbalanced diet, high in carbohydrate and fat content. Physical examination reveals the characteristic dermal and lingual lesions. Atypical cases are many and can be recognized only by careful clinical study, since there is no specific laboratory test for pellagra. Were it not for the skin and oral changes characteristic of pellagra, neither the typical nor the borderline cases could be distinguished from cases of chronic alcoholism, beriberi, pernicious anemia or sprue.

Prognosis. Pellagra is always a serious disease. A favorable course depends on an early diagnosis followed immediately by intensive and persistent treatment. If untreated or incompletely treated, it usually becomes chronic and continues through remissions and recurrences until either the pellagra itself or a coexistent or resultant secondary disease produces incapacitation or death. The disease tends to increase in severity with each attack, but the author has observed recovery after thirteen distinct relapses. Even in cases with rare recurrences, the daily life of the patient must be properly regulated, or he will fail to make satisfactory progress. Without special treatment the death rate is more than 50 per cent in the severe cases. Once the disease, mild or severe, has remitted, the

prognosis is good if no other predisposing condition or organic disease is present and provided the patient is cooperative and has perseverance and the capacity to continue treatment.

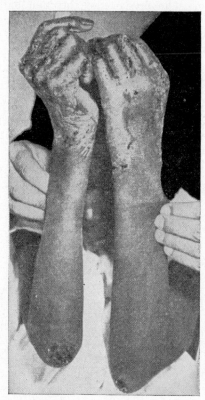

Fig. 73. Symmetric exfoliating lesions on elbows and dorsal surface of the hands of a pellagrin in relapse. Multiple areas of ulceration and a few large bullae can be seen.

Pellagrins who seem to be making satisfactory progress often become suddenly worse and die. No single manifestation can be used as the sole indicator of the prognosis. In each case the immediate outlook is contingent upon the general condition of the pellagrin and upon the presence or absence of other diseases.

The outlook is most grave when severe mental symptoms, hallucinations, violent motor excitement, opisthotonos, delirium, rigidity, tremors, ankle clonus, Babinski's sign or convulsions are present. Extensive and severe gastrointestinal symptoms such as intractable diarrhea and vomiting, severe glossitis, stomatitis and cachexia may also have an unfavorable effect on the course of the disease. Refusal of food, long-continued abdominal distention and marked anemia should be regarded as ominous signs. Pellagra is not usually accompanied by fever; a temperature of 103° F. makes for an unfavorable prognosis. The danger is increased if chronic addiction to alcohol, fatigue or surgical operations intervene. The presence of infection darkens the outlook, for, just as infectious diseases predispose to pellagra, so are pellagrins unusually susceptible to infections.

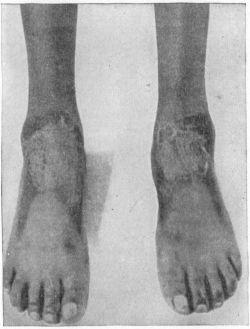

Fig. 74. Photograph showing symmetric dry, scaly pellagrous dermatitis on the feet of a Negro. Note the sharply demarcated borders and the hyperpigmentation at the periphery of the lesions.

Prevention. Pellagra can be prevented by the intelligent application of medical knowledge. In order to eradicate pellagra, persons with organic disease, those who are poor, chronic alcohol addicts, food faddists and those with improper dietary habits must receive special attention.

Organic Disease. Organic disease often predisposes to pellagra by affecting the general nutrition and probably by increasing susceptibility. Particular attention to the diet, while the disease is being treated, prevents the development of pellagra. The incidence of pellagra is abnormally high among people having metabolic diseases, chronic infections and diseases of the gastrointestinal tract.

Poverty. Although pellagra often develops as the result of financial inability to buy proper food, lack of knowledge in regard to diet is an important contributing factor. If sufficient amounts of a well balanced diet are eaten regularly, pellagra will not develop. Education of the poor in correct dietary habits is indicated, so that those who can, but do not, may buy the inexpensive protective foods and those who cannot afford them may obtain protective substances, such as yeast and wheat germ, through relief agencies.

Chronic Alcoholism. Chronic alcohol addicts who do not eat adequate amounts of a well balanced diet acquire pellagra. Alcohol alone does not cause the disease, but it often decreases the patient's appetite and diminishes his food intake. This is easily understood when we consider that often the heavy drinker receives from 3000 to 4000 calories per day from the alcohol alone. When alcoholic pellagrins are induced to stop drinking, their appetites return, they eat more food, and the disease is arrested and is not likely to recur. Likewise, alcoholic pellagrins who can be persuaded to eat large amounts of food do not have recurrences.

Improper Dietary Habits. It is a popular fallacy to believe that our customary diets are adequate. Many people live on a diet of narrow range, too high in fats and carbohydrates, because of custom, preconceived ideas as to what foods are good for one, and dependence upon the appetite as the guide in the proper selection of foods. Education of the masses in the essential dietary requirements is imperative.

The pellagrin develops this disease because for one reason or another he does not get in his tissues sufficient niacin or materials which act similarly. Large amounts of tryptophan can be converted into niacin. Corn and corn products tend to be low in both salts of niacin and the amino acid tryptophan; hence, the association between the endemic pellagrin who eats a great deal of maize and maize products and his disease. For over five years the author has not seen a case of endemic pellagra in the southern part of the United States. The disappearance of this disease which was so debilitating and rampant a few years ago has been due to the "enrichment program," to better dietary habits and to general interest on the part of the medical profession.

Treatment. Pellagra is a systemic disease and must be treated as such, early, promptly, intensively and persistently. The essence of successful treatment is improved nutrition, adequate rest and good medical and nursing care. The methods must be adapted to the special needs of each patient and can be carried out most effectively if the patient is hospitalized and placed under the direct supervision of a physician, assisted by a nurse and a dietitian.

Treatment of the Mild Case. Every adult with mild pellagra must ingest and retain a well balanced, high protein diet of at least 4000 calories per day; the diet should include 1500 cc. of sweet milk, ½ pound of lean meat or liver, and eight eggs. Additional milk should be given instead of water, except in very dehydrated cases. Water tends to decrease the amount of food ingested; the milk will not only supply fluid, but will also be an additional source of nourishment. Diets abnormally high in carbohydrate or fat content are contraindicated. The diet should be supplemented, especially at night, by large amounts of a potent, specific therapeutic agent, prepared by a reputable concern. When administered by mouth, dry powdered brewers' yeast (30 gm. three times daily), wheat germ (60 gm. three times daily), crude liver extract (30 gm. three times daily), or niacin or niacinamide (10 doses, 50 mg. each daily) is effective. The amide is preferable to niacin when one wishes to avoid vasodilating reactions.

Treatment of the Severe Case. The severe case, that is, one with central nervous system involvement, intractable diarrhea, persistent vomiting, marked anemia, a pulse rate exceeding 120, or a temperature of 103° F., must have immediate supportive as well as antipellagric therapy. As in the mild case, success of treatment depends upon improved nutrition, adequate rest and appropriate medical and nursing care. The food intake must be increased to at least 4500 calories per day. The specific therapeutic agent must be administered in amounts three times as large as those used for the mild case. Absolute rest in bed is imperative. Parenteral liver extract (probably the crude preparation is more efficacious that the refined), given intramuscularly in doses of 20 cc. three to five times daily, in addition to the wheat germ, yeast or liver extract by mouth, is often beneficial, especially to patients with persistent vomiting or diarrhea. Niacin orally (50 mg., ten times daily) or niacinamide parenterally (50 mg. in physiologic solution of sodium chloride, two or three times daily) is astoundingly effective. Healing of the oral and dermal lesions, even in the most severe cases, usually

begins within 72 hours after treatment is begun, and the relief of the psychoses of pellagra is spectacular.

Special Treatment of Symptoms. Symptomatic treatment often aids in remitting the disease. Exacerbation of the stomatitis, vomiting, diarrhea and abdominal pain must not deter the physician from continuing the administration of proper diets, specific therapeutic agents and indicated symptomatic therapy.

ORAL LESIONS. The use of a mouth wash is beneficial. The teeth should be brushed gently to avoid severe hemorrhages.

SKIN LESIONS. Potassium permanganate solution (1:5000), used as soaks, offers some relief and in the moist type of lesion diminishes the possibility of secondary infection.

DIARRHEA. Tincture of opium, 2 cc., can be given every 4 hours unless symptoms of overdosage appear. This is sometimes beneficial and is particularly indicated whenever an analgesic is required. The severe case should receive fluids by a parenteral route. The administration of niacin is effective.

VOMITING. Absolute rest in bed and feedings of an iced fluid such as eggnog, ginger ale or malted milk in small quantities (10 to 15 cc.) at intervals of 10 to 15 minutes are necessary, and should be continued until the patient has not vomited for 12 hours. Yeast, wheat germ or liver extract should be added to these feedings in amounts of 4 to 5 gm. until the daily requirement has been given. In the more severe case, parenteral liver extract must be given immediately and continued until the patient is able to retain the required amount of the recommended diet together with any one of the potent, specific therapeutic materials.

ABDOMINAL PAIN. The pain is often increased after meals, thus discouraging the patient from eating. Codeine will relieve this and should be used generously.

ANEMIA. If the hemoglobin is below 50 per cent, blood transfusions should be given. After recovery has started, large doses of iron or folic acid and sometimes vitamin B_{12} should be administered.

FEVER. Alcohol sponges are indicated when the temperature is more than 103° F.

TACHYCARDIA. Patients with tachycardia must have constant rest.

MENTAL SYMPTOMS. Large doses of niacin or niacinamide result in spectacular relief of the mental symptoms, and their use is indicated instead of sedatives.

PERIPHERAL NEURITIS. Ice-bags and local medications containing phenol (1 per cent) and menthol afford temporary relief. Physical therapy and splints are often beneficial. For use of vitamin B_1, see Beriberi.

TOM D. SPIES

References

Goldberger, J.: Pellagra—Its Nature and Prevention. United States Pub. Health Rep. No. 1174, 1927.

Harris, S.: Clinical Pellagra. St. Louis, C. V. Mosby Company, 1941.

Jolliffe, N., McLester, J. S., and Sherman, H. C.: The Prevalence of Malnutrition. J.A.M.A., 118:944, 1942.

Mulholland, H. B., and King, R. L.: Pellagra. Review of Cases, with Special Reference to the Gastric Secretions. J.A.M.A., 101:576, 1933.

Ruffin, J. M., and Smith, D. T.: The Treatment of Pellagra with Certain Preparations of Liver. Am. J. M. Sc., 187:512, 1934.

Sebrell, W. H.: Table Showing the Pellagra-Preventive Value of Various Foods. United States Pub. Health Rep. No. 1632, 1934.

Spies, T. D.: The Treatment of Pellagra. J.A.M.A., 104:1377, 1935; 111:584, 1938.

———, and Aring, C. D.: The Effect of Vitamin B_1 on the Peripheral Neuritis of Pellagra. J.A.M.A., 110:1081, 1938.

———, and Butt, H. R.: Vitamins and Avitaminoses. In Duncan, G. G.: Diseases of Metabolism. 3rd ed. Philadelphia, W. B. Saunders Company, 1952.

———, and DeWolf, H. F.: Observations on the Etiological Relationship of Severe Alcoholism to Pellagra. Am. J. M. Sc., 186:521, 1933.

———, Grant, J. M., Stone, R. E., and McLester, J. B.: Recent Observations on the Treatment of Six Hundred Pellagrins with Special Emphasis on the Use of Nicotinic Acid in Prophylaxis. South. M. J., 31:1231, 1938.

Sydenstricker, V. P.: The Clinical Manifestations of Nicotinic Acid and Riboflavin Deficiency (Pellagra). Ann. Int. Med., 14:1499, 1941.

Turner, R.: Pellagra Associated with Organic Disease of the Gastro-intestinal Tract. Am. J. Trop. Med., 9:129,1929.

Youmans, J. B.: Nutritional Deficiencies. Philadelphia, J. B. Lippincott Co., 1941.

RIBOFLAVIN DEFICIENCY

The importance of riboflavin in human nutrition was observed independently by Sebrell and Butler, and Vilter, Vilter and Spies. Riboflavin deficiency occurs in either sex, at any age, and is common in persons who subsist, over a considerable period of time, on a grossly inadequate diet. It tends to occur in the spring and to disappear during the summer months. It is probably the most common clinically recognized deficiency disease in the United States.

Diagnosis depends upon the recognition of characteristic angular stomatitis associated with transverse fissures in the corners of the mouth. Another lesion, occurring less frequently, is the accumulation of greasy seborrheic material around the alae nasae and occasionally around the eyes and on the ears. In the Nutrition Clinic of the Hillman Hospital, Birmingham, Alabama, we have observed over 5000 persons with riboflavin deficiency. In our experience we have found that diagnosis depends upon the recognition of certain symptoms and their response to the administration of synthetic riboflavin or substances containing riboflavin. The symptoms characteristic of riboflavin deficiency are angular stomatitis associated with transverse fissures in the corners of the mouth and lips and an abnormal shiny redness of the mucous membranes of the lips; a "sharkskin" appearance of the skin around the alae nasae and eyes, and occasionally over the ears and malar prominences; ocular symptoms characterized by bulbar conjunctivitis, lacrimation, burning of the eyes and failing vision, and invasion of vessels of the cornea (Figs. 68, 69). These symptoms disappear within four to six days after the administration of adequate amounts of riboflavin.

Treatment. In the average case the administration of 5 mg. of synthetic riboflavin three times a day was followed by the disappearance of the lesions within three to six days. Two patients who were given 2 mg. of synthetic phosphoric acid ester of riboflavin three times a day showed similar improvement within six to eight days. In these cases Ashe and Spies found that the daily excretion of flavin (determined as riboflavin) was 18 per cent below normal. Diminished output of flavin has been observed in other patients who have not had the typical lesions described. After the administration of riboflavin the level in the urine rises. These studies suggest that in persons subsisting on inadequate diets riboflavin deficiency is not uncommon. Our figures indicate that the riboflavin requirement for an adult is approximately 3.5 mg. daily.

Comprehensive reviews of the physiology and pathology of riboflavin deficiency and of the chemical nature of riboflavin have been published, and its importance in human nutrition has been established, but at the present time the exact mechanism of its action is not understood. Nevertheless, it is known that the lesions of riboflavin deficiency disappear and the patient has an increased feeling of well being after the ingestion of an adequate, well balanced diet, the administration of brewers' yeast or synthetic riboflavin.

Tom D. Spies

References

Hogan, A. G.: Riboflavin: Physiology and Pathology. J.A.M.A., *110*:1188, 1938.
Sebrell, W. H., and Butler, R. E.: Riboflavin Deficiency in Man, A Preliminary Note. Pub. Health Rep., *53*:2282, 1938.
Spies, T. D., Bean, W. B., and Ashe, W. F.: Recent Advances in the Treatment of Pellagra and Associated Deficiencies. Ann. Int. Med., *12*:1130, 1939.
Sydenstricker, V. P., Sebrell, W. H., Cleckley, H. M., and Kruse, H. D.: The Ocular Manifestations of Ariboflavinosis. J.A.M.A., *114*:2437, 1940.
Vilter, R. W., Vilter, S. P., and Spies, T. D.: Relationship between Nicotinic Acid and a Codehydrogenase (Cozymase) in Blood of Pellagrins and Normal Persons. J.A.M.A., *112*:420, 1939.

ACRODYNIA
(Pink Disease)

Definition. Acrodynia, or "pink disease," is primarily a disease of infancy and early childhood, characterized by painful, red, swollen hands and feet, tachycardia, hypertension, hypomotility, mental apathy, anorexia and photophobia. The onset is insidious, and the disease may persist for months. The outcome is favorable unless terminated by intercurrent infection.

History. The term "acrodynia" was used in describing an outbreak of disease in Paris in 1828. It was attributed to arsenic poisoning and was confined largely to adults, and, therefore, had little to do with the syndrome as we now know it in children. The first series of cases to receive prominence in medical literature were reported by Swift in Australia in 1914. A number of descriptions of the disease were published in the United States about 1920, and a few years later it was described in Europe.

Etiology and Morbid Anatomy. The disease is of unknown etiology. It is impossible to trace familial incidence. It usually occurs between the ages of four months and three years. Transmission of the disease to other members of the family rarely occurs. One theory is that it is the result of a dietary deficiency, but it does not appear to be a deficiency of any of the known vitamins. Another theory is that it is caused by a filterable virus, but no virus has been isolated. Histologic studies show a degenerative process which affects both the central and peripheral nervous systems. There is widespread peripheral nerve degeneration with demyelinization of the nerve sheaths. The anterior horn cells and the cells of the posterior root ganglia often show chromatolysis. It is possible that acrodynia includes a number of disease entities. Among them may be included the "burning feet" syndrome, which some believe to result from a pyridoxine deficiency.

Symptoms. Because of the insidious onset the mother frequently cannot state (with any degree of accuracy) when the disease began. In some instances the onset is associated with an upper respiratory infection or is manifested by cessation of growth and progressive loss of weight, followed by fretfulness, sleeplessness and refusal of food. The child is excessively irritable and usually lies curled up in a knee-elbow position with his face buried in a pillow. He constantly rubs together his reddened, desquamating hands, and when exposed to light, he rubs his eyes. He cries frequently, especially when disturbed. The cheeks are bluish-red, and in many cases the tip of the nose is red. Areas of hyperemia alternating with ischemia appear on the skin of the hands and feet. Papular rashes may appear over the whole body.

Diagnosis. The diagnosis is based on the presence of painful red hands and feet, peeling of the skin, prostration, perspiration and photophobia, accompanied by tachycardia and hypertension. The most constant features of the disease are photophobia, hypotonia and cutaneous rash. The mild or borderline cases are not so clearly defined, and in such instances diagnosis is more difficult. The erythema in acrodynia, however, is readily distinguished from that of pellagra or the erythema caused by heat or cold.

Prognosis. Generally speaking, the mortality rate is low. When death occurs, it is usually the result of an intercurrent infection.

Treatment. Ignorance of the true nature of the disease prohibits specific therapy. In our Nutrition Clinic, where several of these patients are treated each year, we use two principles. First, we attempt the judicious use of barbiturates or other sedatives, and we do everything possible to ensure the ingestion of a high-vitamin, high-caloric diet. Secondly, we give a mixed vitamin preparation containing 50 mg. of niacinamide, 5 mg. of thiamine, 5 mg. of riboflavin and 50 mg. of ascorbic acid in the baby's milk three times a day. At times we have given parenteral liver extract. The mixed vitamin preparation and liver extract both seem to give considerable symptomatic relief. It has recently been reported that infusions of saline and the administration of desoxycorticosterone acetate in debilitated infants with pink disease afford prompt improvement. This is based on the presumed presence of adrenal insufficiency.

TOM D. SPIES

References

Blackfan, K. D., and McKhann, C. F.: Oxford Medicine, 4:272, Part II.

Chaudhuri, K. C.: Pink Disease or Acrodynia. Indian J. Pediat., 10:70, 1943.

Hay, J. D.: Intramuscular Vitamin B$_1$; 8 Cases. Practitioner, 146:264, 1941.

Swift, H.: Erythroedema. Australian Med. Congress. Child. Dis. Sect., Lancet, 1914.

Vijnovsky, B.: Acrodynia and Pellagra as Disease Entity. Día Méd., 15:331, 1943.

BURNING FEET SYNDROME

This disabling disease of nutritional origin was little known to American physicians prior to World War II. It has been described under various names but has been noted in the Orient among underfed people for more than one hundred years. Painful burning feet were so common among the prisoners of war in the Orient that sleep was practically impossible and walking difficult. The patients improved slowly with general dietary improvement, and to this day the patients who have had that trouble complain "that the doctors did not understand their condition." At best, malnutrition and undernutrition are associated with this syndrome because it appears only among groups on very restricted diets. The incidence of endemic nutritive failure among the population of the southeastern United States where the author has worked so long has decreased greatly in the past eighteen years. When the incidence was high, burning feet was a common presenting symptoms of the patients. Many, but not all of them, could be relieved by the administration of thiamine. In recent years the general nutrition of the population has improved, and the physician rarely sees persons who complain of burning feet arising from general dietary failure.

TOM D. SPIES

PYRIDOXINE (VITAMIN B$_6$) DEFICIENCY

Between 1951 and 1953 many physicians throughout the United States observed that artificially fed young infants taking a pyridoxine (vitamin B$_6$)-deficient formula developed hyperirritability and convulsive seizures. These clinical observations provided much important information. It was soon recognized that in each case there was a uniform pattern of symptoms varying in degree of severity. The convulsions were unassociated with any other signs of illness, and there were no physical findings or laboratory abnormalities indicative of any etiologic factor. The infants had normal birth histories and had grown and developed normally until they were at least eighteen weeks of age. The onset of the convulsions was sudden. All the physicians reporting their occurrence found that the infants invariably had been fed on a liquid SMA formula, which consisted of defatted cows' milk, vegetable and animal fats, vitamins and iron. No cases were encountered in which the infants received the powdered SMA formula which contained pyridoxine. When the infants were fed a formula other than liquid SMA or when they were given supplementary foods such as cereals, meats, fruits and vegetables, or when they were given pyridoxine either orally or by injection, the convulsions disappeared and did not recur if a supplement of pyridoxine was continued. The Wyeth Company, which makes both the liquid and powdered SMA formula, was most energetic and cooperative in taking the deficient material from the market and in adding a thermostable form of pyridoxine to their liquid product.

Although far too little is known regarding the function of pyridoxine in human beings, its essential function had been demonstrated previously. Many years ago an etiologic relationship was established between pyridoxine deficiency and convulsive seizures in rats, chicks and pigs. Synthetic pyridoxine was first administered to human beings in 1939 by Spies, Bean and Ashe, who published their observations that patients on inadequate diets who developed deficiencies of niacin, riboflavin and thiamine also were likely to be somewhat deficient in pyridoxine. Specifically, they stressed that after the deficiencies of niacin, riboflavin and thiamine were corrected, and if the patients remained on their deficient diets, pyridoxine would produce an additional improvement. Snyderman and associates and Stokes and associates (quoted by Coursin) have made interesting observations on single patients suggesting a relationship between pyridoxine deficiency and convulsive seizures.

In discussing this work and particularly the work of Spies, Bean and Ashe, Elvehjem in 1952 stated that dogs on a diet which produced a niacin deficiency responded well to niacin therapy, unless the treatment were repeated too many times. He and his associates learned that tryptophan could replace niacin in correcting these deficiencies. From these observations and from the fact that tryptophan metabolism is associated with pyridoxine, it was concluded that there is an interrelationship between these substances and that a pyridoxine deficiency reduced the conversion of tryptophan to niacin and its derivatives.

TOM D. SPIES

References

Chick, H., El Sadr, M. M., and Worden, A. N.: Occurrence of Fits of Epileptiform Nature in Rats Maintained for Long Periods on Diet Deprived of Vitamin B$_6$. Biochem. J., 34:595, 1940.

Coursin, D. B.: Convulsive Seizures in Infants with Pyridoxine-Deficient Diet. J.A.M.A., 154:406, 1954.

Daniel, E. P., Kline, O. L., and Tolle, C. D.: A Convulsive Syndrome in Young Rats Associated with Pyridoxine Deficiency. J. Nutrition, 23:205, 1942.

Elvehjem, C. A.: Nutritional Interrelationships. Internat. Ztschr. f. Vitaminforsch., 23:299, 1952.

Hughes, E. H., and Squibb, R. L.: Vitamin B$_6$ (Pyridoxine) in the Nutrition of the Pig. J. Animal Sc., 1:320, 1942.

Lerkovsky, S., and Kratzer, F. H.: Pyridoxine Deficiency in Chicks. J. Nutrition, 24:515, 1942.

Molony, C. J., and Parmelee, A. H.: Convulsions in Young Infants as a Result of Pyridoxine (Vitamin B$_6$) Deficiency. J.A.M.A., 154:405, 1954.

Ruegamer, W. R., Brickson, W. L., Torbet, N. J., and Elvehjem, C. A.: Response of Dogs to Liver Extracts Containing Pernicious Anemia Factor. J. Nutrition, 36:425, 1948.

Snyderman, S. E., Carretero, R., and Holt, L. E., Jr.: Pyridoxine Deficiency in the Human Being. Fed. Proc., 9:371, 1950.

———, Holt, L. E., Jr., Carretero, R., and Jacobs, J.: Pyridoxine Deficiency in the Human Infant. J. Clin. Nutrition, 1:200, 1953.

Spies, T. D., Bean, W. B., and Ashe, W. F.: A Note on the Use of Vitamin B$_6$ in Human Nutrition. J.A.M.A., 112:2414, 1939.

Williams, J. N., Jr., and Elvehjem, C. A.: The Effects of Tryptophan Deficiency upon Enzyme Activity in the Rat. J. Biol. Chem., 183:539, 1950.

VITAMINS (FOLIC ACID AND VITAMIN B$_{12}$) AND BLOOD REGENERATION

A number of years ago when Spies and associates showed that folic acid, a single synthetic compound of known molecular structure, was capable of producing hemopoiesis in persons with certain types of macrocytic anemia, the chemical era of vitamins and blood regeneration was initiated. Folic acid was the first of many synthetic chemical substances shown to produce blood regeneration in persons with pernicious anemia, nutritional macrocytic anemia, macrocytic anemia of pregnancy, macrocytic anemia of sprue and megaloblastic anemia of infancy. Soon it was demonstrated that folic acid failed to protect against or to prevent the symptoms arising from acute degeneration of the spinal cord so frequently associated with pernicious anemia, and it became clear that folic acid was not a complete therapeutic agent for the treatment of pernicious anemia, but that it is an essential therapeutic agent for the treatment of the average case of macrocytic anemia of pregnancy and megaloblastic anemia of infancy. It is a most useful therapeutic agent in the treatment of sprue and nutritional macrocytic anemia.

Folic acid is an important member of the vitamin B complex. The administration of folic acid, or foods which contain it, to expectant mothers whose diets are low in folic acid is mandatory. In this way the macrocytic anemia of pregnancy, infancy and early childhood can be prevented. It is recommended that at least 2 mg. per day be administered in the last third of pregnancy, if the diet is deficient in folic acid. It is interesting to note that the mother can concentrate folic acid and transmit it through her milk to the infant so as to produce a therapeutic response in the infant with megaloblastic arrest.

During the past eight years, by administering folic acid as a supplement to the diet, we have enabled numerous patients to continue working. These patients had tropical sprue or nutritional macrocytic anemia, were totally incapacitated, and probably would have died if specific therapy had not been administered either orally or parenterally. The precise dose of folic acid varies from patient to patient, but in the average case 5 to 10 mg. per day, and usually much less, produces a prompt hemopoietic response which is paralleled by a striking clinical response. The glossitis heals, the patient's appetite increases and his strength rapidly increases.

Like vitamin B_{12}, which will be discussed later, folic acid is composed of a family of substances. Its chief factors are what are called "pteroyl glutamates." These substances differ from each other in the number of glutamic radicals in the side chain. Folic acid is essential in some form or other for all forms of life.

Vitamin B_{12} is the newest of the family of B vitamins to be isolated. It was first crystallized from liver by Rickes and others, and independently by E. Lester Smith. Soon it was found in streptomycin residues, and at the present time the material available for the physician comes from streptomycin cultures. The vitamin B_{12} of course is identical, whether isolated from liver or from streptomycin, and has similar chemical and physiologic properties.

Pernicious anemia has been recognized as a definite clinical entity for more than one-hundred years. Very recently we have come to realize that it can be controlled by maintaining an adequate amount of vitamin B_{12} in the tissues. Substances with vitamin B_{12} activity are widely scattered in nature. They exist in such small quantities, however, that the ingestion of them does not produce beneficial effects in persons with pernicious anemia. The active principle of liver extract is vitamin B_{12}, but in refined liver extract it exists in rather small amounts.

All members of the vitamin B_{12} family are of great interest, and it is possible that not all of them have as yet been identified. We summarize a few pertinent points as follows:

1. Vitamin B_{12a} and vitamin B_{12b} are identical.

2. Vitamin B_{12} contains a cyano group which is not present in vitamin B_{12a}.

3. The cyano group is present in the vitamin B_{12} cobalt coordination complex.

4. Cobalamin designates all the vitamin B_{12} molecules except the cyano group. Vitamin B_{12} can then be termed cyano-cobalamin and vitamin B_{12a} termed hydroxo-cobalamin.

5. Both have been found active by parenteral injection in producing clinical and hemopoietic improvement in persons with pernicious anemia, nutritional macrocytic anemia and tropical sprue.

Vitamin B_{12} contains 4 per cent cobalt and phosphorus and is easily destroyed by excessive light.

The bone marrow biopsy and peripheral blood findings in pernicious anemia are indistinguishable from those found in nutritional macrocytic anemia, tropical sprue and nontropical sprue in relapse, and the administration of vitamin B_{12} is effective in each of these conditions. A number of types of steatorrhea, which sometimes are associated and confused with endemic sprue, as a rule are not relieved by this material. It should be emphasized that the average patient who receives vitamin B_{12} should receive it parenterally, or orally in association with an active intrinsic factor. Parenteral therapy is effective in a higher percentage of cases. When given in small doses by mouth, vitamin B_{12} does not usually benefit persons with pernicious anemia in relapse unless an intrinsic factor is added. It seems that in working with a very concentrated intrinsic factor material, we are dealing with a protein, the chemical nature of which is not known.

Neither vitamin B_{12} nor folic acid should be considered as a universal blood regenerating therapeutic agent. Individual cases vary a great deal when there is an inadequate amount of vitamin B_{12} in the nervous tissues. Pain, tingling, numbness and stiffness of the extremities develop, and this condition may advance to complete or partial paralysis. It is now accepted that the symptoms arising in the nervous system can be ameliorated when treated promptly by injections of vitamin B_{12}. The chronic phase of the disease does not respond well to treatment and changes are irreversible. The essence of the best treatment for pernicious anemia depends on an early and precise diagnosis.

The mechanism concerning vitamin B_{12} is delicately balanced, and if too much vitamin B_{12} is administered, the excess is excreted in the urine. It is the most potent therapeutic substance per unit of weight known to man; about one microgram of vitamin B_{12} per day has a detectable effect. It is arbitrarily accepted that one microgram of vitamin B_{12} is approximately equivalent to one U.S.P. unit of liver extract, which in itself is an arbitrary standard. The striking clinical response which parallels the hemopoietic response is rarely fully appreciated. When glossitis is present, it heals spectacularly; when the appetite has failed, there is a voracious desire for food. Vitamin B_{12} is innocuous at the dose level effective for human beings.

It is interesting that many compounds with entirely different chemical structures can induce blood regeneration in the same patient with macrocytic anemia in relapse.

Tom D. Spies

References

Hartman, A. M., Dryden, L. P., and Cary, C. A.: The Role and Sources of Vitamin B_{12}. J. Am. Dietet. A., 25:929, 1949.

Kaczka, E., Wolf, D. E., and Folkers, K.: Vitamin B_{12}. V. Identification of Crystalline Vitamin B_{12a}. J. Am. Chem. Soc., 71:1514, 1949.

Pierce, J. V., Page, A. C., Jr., Stokstad, E. L. R., and Jukes, T. H.: Crystallization of Vitamin B_{12b}. J. Am. Chem. Soc., 71:2952, 1949.

Smith, E. L.: Purification of Anti-pernicious Anemia Factors from Liver. Nature, 161:638, 1948.

Spies, T. D.: Experiences with Folic Acid. Chicago, Year Book Publishers, Inc., 1947.

———, and Stone, R. E.: Some Recent Experiences with Vitamins and Vitamin Deficiencies. South. M. J., 40:46, 1947.

———, Stone, R. E., and Aramburu, T.: Observations on the Antianemic Properties of Vitamin B_{12}. South. M. J., 41:522, 1948.

———, Stone, R. E., Kartus, S., and Aramburu, T.: The Treatment of Subacute Combined Degeneration of the Spinal Cord with Vitamin B_{12}. South M. J., 41:1030, 1948.

———, and others: Antianemic Properties of Reaction Products of Vitamin B_{12} and the Intrinsic Factor. J.A.M.A., 151:1264, 1943.

———, and others: Thymine, Folic Acid and Vitamin B_{12} in Nutritional Macrocytic Anemia, Tropical Sprue and Pernicious Anemia. Lancet, 2:519, 1948.

Vilter, C. F., Vilter, R. W., and Spies, T. D.: The Treatment of Pernicious and Related Anemias with Synthetic Folic Acid. J. Lab. & Clin. Med., 32:262, 1947.

West, R.: Activity of Vitamin B_{12} in Addisonian Pernicious Anemia. Science, 107:398, 1948.

VITAMIN C DEFICIENCY

(Scurvy)

Definition. Scurvy is a nutritional disorder caused by prolonged inadequacy of the supply of ascorbic acid. In its mild forms it gives rise to apathy, anorexia, fatigability and loss of strength, with tenderness of the extremities; to these symptoms is added, in more severe cases, a striking tendency to hemorrhage. The manifestations of the disease depend on the age of the patient. Infantile scurvy (Barlow's disease or Moeller-Barlow disease) differs from adult scurvy principally in the extent to which the growing bones are involved.

History. The name "scurvy" appeared first in the Middle Ages as a folk word, having various forms phonetically allied in several European tongues. Its origin is therefore obscure. The Latinized "scorbutus" is an artificial implant.

Possibly the earliest clear-cut description of the disease was made by de Joinville, whose account of its appearance among the Crusaders of the thirteenth century leaves no room for doubting its identity. To Joseph Lind, an officer of the British navy, belongs the credit of amassing convincing evidence, first, that scurvy is a disorder of nutrition and not a contagion or strictly an occupational disease, and, second, that it results, not from excessive consumption of certain articles of diet, but from insufficient intake of others. His "Treatise on the Scurvy," published in 1753, was ultimately responsible for the introduction of lemon juice into the seaman's ration. Sharp as was the decline in the general morbidity of scurvy after the widespread adoption of effective preventive measures, the disease nevertheless continues to appear in circumstances of stress.

Scurvy was produced in laboratory animals by Theobald Smith in 1895, but the discovery was not followed up. The experimental period began with the work of Holst and Frölich, which was published in 1907.

In 1928, Szent-Györgyi isolated from the suprarenal glands of oxen and from various plant sources a crystalline compound of formula $C_6H_8O_6$ which he named "hexuronic acid." The wide distribution of this compound in animal tissues and in growing plants was soon appreciated, as were also its strong reducing properties, but it was not until 1932 that Szent-Györgyi determined by appropriate feeding experiments that he had been dealing with the specific antiscorbutic factor, vitamin C. Simultaneously and independently, King and Waugh isolated a highly active antiscorbutic compound from lemon juice and showed that it was identical with "hexuronic acid." By common agreement the latter term was abandoned in favor of "ascorbic acid."

Etiology. Ascorbic acid is essential for the proper formation of collagen by fibroblasts, and there is evidence that it participates in the production of intercellular material in other tissues, such as the cement substance of vascular endothelium and the attachment of striated muscle cells to tendon. Because of its strong reducing property, ascorbic acid has been assumed to play an important role in biochemical oxidations, but the actual mechanisms involved have thus far largely escaped elucidation. In the absence of adequate ascorbic acid the oxidation of tyrosine is incomplete, phenyl ketone and hydroxyacids appearing in the urine. The body's requirement of folic acid is elevated when the intake of ascorbic acid is restricted.

Fresh fruits, vegetables and raw meats contain ascorbic acid in sufficient quantity to prevent the appearance of scurvy if the diet is composed largely of uncooked or freshly cooked natural products. The juice of ripe oranges has a fairly constant content of ascorbic acid at about 0.5 mg. per cubic centimeter. Other citrus fruits, though showing greater variation under market conditions, contain similar quantities. In general, there is a fairly close parallelism between the ascorbic acid content of plant tissues and their store of carotenoids or chlorophyl; green leaves and shoots of all kinds, as well as tubers, whether edible or those generally regarded as inedible, are sources of vitamin C.

In animal tissues the concentration of ascorbic acid is highest in adrenal cortex, hypophysis, corpus luteum, lens and aqueous humor, and somewhat less in brain, pancreas, liver, spleen and kidney; it is considerably lower in muscle tissue, distinctly low (about 0.5 to 1.5 mg. per cent) in blood plasma, and virtually absent from fat. Cow's milk as processed for urban consumption does not provide a reliable dietary quota of vitamin C. Chemical synthesis of ascorbic acid from sorbitol is now more economical than is its extraction from natural sources.

The human organism, being unable to synthesize ascorbic acid, depends on extraneous sources for its essential requirements. If the supply is cut off for a sufficiently long time, a matter of months, clinical scurvy supervenes. The minimal daily requirement has not been accurately determined. A group of British volunteers remained in good health when on a daily intake of as little as 10 mg. for nine months, and as a result British nutritionists commonly cite 30 mg. as the minimal daily intake needed. American authorities, on the other hand, usually quote a higher figure, of the order of 1 mg. per kilogram or, for an average adult, 75 mg. per day. Even on a daily intake of this size there is no assurance that the body's capacity to utilize ascorbic acid has been exceeded, for with additional dietary load retention continues for a time until loss through urinary excretion takes place above a threshold level of approximately 1.5 mg. per 100 cc. of plasma. On an average diet the normal adult excretes from 5 to 50 mg. of ascorbic acid in the urine in 24 hours. An increase in the intake augments this output, though not immediately and not quantitatively. If to an average diet one adds a daily supplement of 500 mg. of ascorbic acid, equivalent to about 1 liter of orange juice, the urinary excretion of the vitamin will rise significantly within the first or second 24-hour period and will level off at about 80 per cent of the intake. After this equilibrium has been established, withdrawal of the supplement results in a similarly steep falling off of the excretion, so that within three or four days the output has returned to the starting level. It would seem, in other words, that the organism has a limited capacity for storing vitamin C, that on an average diet the stores are not filled to the saturation point, and that, after saturation, the major portion of the intake spills over into the urine.

Infections and other forms of "stress," rheumatic activity and hyperthyroidism accelerate vitamin depletion. Withdrawal of vitamin C from the diet of a normal subject for a period of one or two weeks causes a clearly detectable change in the economy of the vitamin when a supplement is subsequently added; the daily administration of a liberal quantity of ascorbic acid after such a vitamin-free period may fail to produce an increased output in the urine for four days or even longer.

In scurvy the body stores of ascorbic acid are significantly depleted; the plasma concentration is zero or nearly so, and the small quantities reported present in urine may well reflect merely the error of analysis. In the depletion process the white blood cells and platelets, which normally contain ascorbic acid at a concentration some thirty times as great as that of cell-free plasma, retain their stores with relative avidity; yet they likewise lose their ascorbic acid by the time symptoms appear. On administration of the vitamin, relief of symptoms and signs of scurvy precedes the restoration of a normal urinary output of ascorbic acid or the establishment of a stable plasma concentration at a normal level.

The time required to bring out symptoms of scurvy on a deficient diet varies greatly in ordinary clinical circumstances, since complete deprivation is seldom encountered except under experimental conditions and since the intake of even a small quantity of the vitamin tends to delay the onset of symptoms. In a notable human experiment carried out by Crandon under controlled conditions of strict dietary deficiency, the subject's plasma level of ascorbic acid fell to zero by the forty-first day, the white blood cells and platelets became depleted after four months, yet objective signs of scurvy in the form of cutaneous hemorrhages were not evident until the 161st day of the experimental diet. These intervals presumably represent approximately minimal values. Subjective symptoms of a less specific nature—languor, fatigability and anorexia—preceded the appearance of objective signs.

Most cases of scurvy seen in infancy develop six months or so after the institution of artificial feeding. A few examples have been reported in infants considerably younger, but in these instances the mother could invariably be shown to have subsisted on an inadequate diet during pregnancy; and since the concentration of ascorbic acid in fetal tissues is directly influenced by the mother's diet, the period of vitamin deprivation as it affected such a mother's infant obviously commenced before birth. The concentration of ascorbic acid in human milk, while invariably higher than that in maternal plasma, closely reflects the adequacy of the mother's intake.

Pathology. In fatal cases of scurvy in adults, hemorrhages into the skin are found as a rule; in only one of the 23 cases reported by Aschoff and Koch were superficial hemorrhages absent. They may vary from petechiae to large ecchymoses. The larger spots are apt to be found on the trunk, the smaller ones on the extremities. Almost invariably the lower extremities are more markedly involved than the upper; the face, palms, soles, lateral aspects of the thigh and region of the knee joint tend to be spared. Many of the hemorrhages involve hair follicles, or at least begin there; follicular keratosis frequently occurs in association with the disease.

Edema and accumulation of fluid in body cavities are characteristic of scurvy, the transudates remaining strikingly uncontaminated with blood. Localized areas of superficial edema are apt to overlie deep hemorrhages, which occur most frequently in the lower extremities both because of their increased liability to trauma and because of the greater hydrostatic pressure to which their blood vessels are normally subjected. Such hemorrhages appear to arise from capillary oozing rather than from macroscopic rupture of a

larger vessel, but they may attain almost any size. Intramuscular hemorrhages are common at sites of particular mechanical stress. Subperiosteal hemorrhages are relatively uncommon in adult scurvy, but invariably accompany severe cases of infantile scurvy; owing to loosening of the periosteal attachment, which is a primary feature of the functional pathology of the disease, capillary bleeding may dissect the periosteum free over a large area. Most commonly these subperiosteal hemorrhages are found at the lower end of the femur, the upper end of the humerus, both ends of the tibia, and at the costochondral junction of the middle ribs, but they may be found in almost any location in severe cases, as over the skull, the clavicles or the scapulas.

The lesions of the gums will be described among the clinical signs. Scurvy causes striking changes in the teeth: separation of the odontoblast layer from the dentin and development of hemorrhages within the pulp cavity. Although the teeth are capable of functional recovery, the healing process is never anatomically complete, so that histologic identification of an antecedent attack is possible throughout life.

The suppression of collagen formation, which is an essential feature of scurvy, may not produce a striking morphologic picture. Its effects become evident in experimental studies of wound healing, such as those which Crandon added to his self-imposed nutritional privations. By the time hemorrhagic manifestations of scurvy had appeared, a little more than five months after initiation of the C-free diet, a freshly inflicted surgical incision showed no evidence of organization for some days, until the administration of ascorbic acid started the healing process on its normal course. Similarly, the degradation of intercellular cement substance which accompanies scurvy is less evident morphologically than are its results in the form of hemorrhages or detachment of periosteum.

Symptoms. The symptoms of the disease begin, as a rule, insidiously with a feeling of general weakness and inadequacy, negativism, depression or even melancholia. The normal degree of alertness is replaced by a disposition to inactivity. Appetite fails, and the taking of food is additionally hampered by painful gums, which are disposed to bleed easily. The skin is dry and rough, with prominent, gritty follicles. In areas in which capillary pressure is high, as in the lower extremities or in regions distal to constricting bands of clothing, minute hemorrhages are to be seen in the hair follicles.

Increasing mental depression accompanies progressive loss of muscle power. The lips become cyanotic, and the gums begin to show erosion of the mucous membrane at their margins, with formation of friable clots adherent to the teeth; almost invariably these are accompanied by fetid breath. The lower extremities develop swellings in the muscle masses, particularly in the extensors and adductors of the thighs and in the calves, and the knees are held in partial flexion; efforts toward full extension are accompanied by great pain. There is increased swelling of the subcutaneous tissue of the feet, particularly between the Achilles tendon and the tibia. Tenderness on deep pressure may be elicited in any part of the limb. Finally, ecchymoses appear, especially over the lower third of the thigh, above the malleoli, or on the dorsa of the feet. Hemorrhage into the muscle masses or beneath the periosteum is generally accompanied by induration. There may be either microscopic or gross hematuria. Not all the symptoms mentioned are necessarily of simultaneous occurrence. Mental depression is rarely absent, but ecchymoses may occur in the absence of stomatitis, and the disease may be clinically recognizable before extensive intramuscular or subperiosteal hemorrhages have taken place.

With healing, recovery occurs in more or less the following order: stomatitis, mental depression, induration, cutaneous hemorrhages and, last, follicular keratosis.

In particularly severe cases the course is progressively downhill. The necrotic changes in the gums involve the alveolar process; the teeth loosen and fall out, often with uncontrollable hemorrhage. There may be hemorrhage from the nose, stomach or intestines, or an extravasation of blood may suddenly appear without provocation at some bizarre site, as in the orbit, causing proptosis and ecchymosis of the eyelids. The pulse becomes rapid and weak, and the patient may suddenly die from relatively mild physical exertion, or may expire from progressive prostration or intercurrent infection.

In infants, apathy and irritability alternate, but anorexia is the rule. In contrast to the afebrile state of older patients, elevation of temperature is almost always present. Petechial hemorrhages are generally less conspicuous than in the adult. The tenderness of the involved extremities and the changes in contour brought about by subperiosteal hemorrhages and epiphyseal infraction are often extreme. On the other hand, the oral signs are usually limited to swelling and purple discoloration of the gums around deciduous teeth which have already erupted or are about to erupt, while the formation of large vegetations is rare and fetor exceptional. Anemia of some degree is almost always found. The leukocyte pattern is not affected in uncomplicated cases.

Scurvy often goes hand in hand with other deficiency diseases.

Diagnosis. The diagnosis of scurvy is generally made on the history of an inadequate diet combined with the detection of some of the more obvious physical manifestations of the disease. Subperiosteal hemorrhage supervening on mild or insignificant trauma is always suggestive; in fact, any bleeding which does not depend on some demonstrable cause must give rise to a suspicion of scurvy. Tenderness may be confined to the region of the long bones of the lower extremities or may at times be so capricious in its orientation as to bring the patient under suspicion of neurosis or even malingering. The changes in the gums produced by scurvy may be simulated in thrombocytopenic purpura, leukemia or mercurial poisoning. In infants the roentgen picture in the long bones is pathognomonic, but in children and especially in young adults this diagnostic aid is less helpful. Subperiosteal hemorrhage is not ordinarily recognizable in roentgenograms until some days after the institution of effective therapy, and until the formation of new bone has been resumed in the elevated periosteum. Demonstration of capillary fragility is suggestive, but must be supported by more specific evidence.

Biochemical assay of the ascorbic acid stores plays a salient part in diagnosis. A plasma level close to zero accompanies all cases of untreated scurvy, but identical values may be found in many subjects who are symptom-free and who in consequence cannot be described as scorbutic. The same may be said of low urinary concentrations. Accurate evaluation of the degree of depletion may be achieved in any of three ways: (1) simultaneous determination of the concentration of ascorbic acid in the patient's plasma and in the white cell and platelet layer of centrifuged blood; (2) measurement of the plasma level in the fasting state and after intravenous or intramuscular administration of a test load of ascorbic acid; (3) daily estimation of the total urinary excretion of ascorbic acid for several days after liberal dosage of the vitamin (of the order of 500 mg. daily). Depleted stores are indicated in (1) by low values in both determinations; in (2) by a low, flat 4-hour curve; in (3) by a delay of two days or more in the rise of urinary excretion.

Since the response of a scorbutic patient to specific antiscorbutic therapy is usually prompt and dramatic, a simple therapeutic diagnostic test is rational and often decisive.

Prognosis. Scurvy is readily amenable to treatment, provided it is recognized in time. Convalescence prolonged more than a month after the institution of adequate antiscorbutic therapy usually reflects the presence of some additional dietary deficiency, e.g., protein, thiamine, riboflavin or niacin. Conspicuous as is the tendency to hemorrhage in the symptomatology of the disease, fatal bleeding is rare except as a result of surgical intervention when the presence of scurvy has not been recognized. Under ordinary conditions of civil life, deaths from uncomplicated scurvy are almost unknown.

Treatment. The optimal intake of vitamin C for the normal subject has yet to be determined; dietitians argue that anything less than a state of repletion of the stores compromises the body's economy, but historical and general clinical evidence suggests that moderate unsaturation is not inconsistent with physiologic efficiency. In a therapeutic test for diagnostic purposes the daily administration of 250 mg. of ascorbic acid, or about 16 ounces of fresh orange juice, may be expected to dispel anorexia, relieve mental depression to a considerable degree, eliminate tenderness of the extremities, and obviate the appearance of fresh capillary hemorrhages within two days to a week, provided these symptoms have their origin in a deficiency of vitamin C. The total quantity of ascorbic acid required to resaturate a scorbutic patient varies from about 2 gm. up to ten times that amount. Absorption of orally administered ascorbic acid is usually complete or nearly so, appreciable reduction in absorption occurring only in the presence of diarrhea or chronic disease of the intestinal tract. Solutions of ascorbic acid are well tolerated in the blood stream, as much as 6 gm. having been given in a single dose without adverse effect. In spite of its acidity, a 1 or 2 per cent solution of ascorbic acid in normal saline need not be buffered or neutralized for intravenous injection.

RUSTIN MCINTOSH

References

Accessory Food Factors Committee, Medical Research Council: Vitamin-C Requirement of Human Adults; Experimental Study of Vitamin C Deprivation in Man. A Preliminary Report. Lancet, 1:853, 1948.

Aschoff, L., and Koch, W.: Skorbut. Veröffentl. aus d. Geb. d. Kriegs- u. Konstitutions-pathol., 1:1, 1919.

Crandon, J. H., Lund, C. C., and Dill, D. D.: Experimental Human Scurvy. New England J. Med., 223:353, 1940.

Follis, R. H., Jr.: The Pathology of Nutritional Diseases. Springfield, Illinois, Charles C Thomas, 1948.

Holst, A., and Frölich, T.: Experimental Studies Relating to "Ship Beriberi" and Scurvy. J. Hyg., 7: 634, 1907.

Lind, J.: A Treatise of the Scurvy, etc. Edinburgh, Sands, Murray and Cochran, 1753.

McMillan, R. B., and Inglis, J. C.: Scurvy: Survey of 53 Cases. Brit. M. J., 2:233, 1944.

Ralli, E. P., and Sherry, S.: Adult Scurvy and the Metabolism of Vitamin C. Medicine, 20:251, 1941.

Westin, G.: Ueber Zahnveränderungen in Fällen von Skorbut bei Homo. Stockholm, Fahlkrantz, 1931.

VITAMIN D DEFICIENCY

(Privational Rickets)

Definition. Privational rickets is a disease characterized chiefly by clinical and roentgenologic abnormalities of the skeleton which result from deficient deposition of lime salts in growing cartilage and in newly formed bone. It is a deficiency disease caused by insufficient vitamin D during the age when growth is rapid. Since the human organism is able to supply its need for the vitamin either by ingestion or by autosynthesis in the presence of sunlight, rickets is an expression of the combined absence of two factors, one dietetic and the other environmental.

Incidence. The disease primarily affects infants at the age when rapid growth is taking place. Several months must usually elapse before the manifestations are perceptible clinically; the disease is, therefore, extremely rare in the early weeks of life, and the majority of cases are diagnosed between the ages of 4 months and 2 years. Formerly the incidence was exceedingly high. Observations in different places indicate that from 50 to 98 per cent of the infant population was affected. Today in the United States the widespread use in infant feeding of milks fortified with vitamin D has had an amazing effect in lowering the incidence. In most areas severe rickets is a rare disease. It is observed more commonly in breast-fed than in artificially fed infants.

The premature infant is particularly susceptible to rickets. The susceptibility is so extreme that one is almost justified is saying that moderate or severe rickets will develop in all premature infants unless preventive measures are instituted. Twins belong in the same category.

Rickets is predominantly a disorder of the Temperate Zone. It is rare in the Far North, where fish constitute the chief source of food; the influence of sunlight prevents its occurrence in the Tropics. There is a seasonal incidence; in the Northern Hemisphere the peak occurs during the winter and spring months when the rays of sun from the south are slanting. Environmental variations in the amount of exposure to the sun also account for a greater prevalence in urban than in rural communities. The Negroes and Italians who dwell in the cities of the United States are unusually susceptible to rickets; the susceptibility is accounted for, at least in part, by the dark pigmentation of the skin, which offers a barrier to the penetration of radiant energy.

Pathology. Distinctive findings are limited to the skeleton and result chiefly from the failure of deposition of lime salts in growing cartilage and in newly formed bone. The uncalcified bone or osteoid tissue is morphologically similar to normal bone, but, because it lacks the elements essential for rigidity, it is soft and easily distorted. In health the formation of new bone is greatest at the ends of the long bones and at the costochondral junctions; in these places rickets produces the greatest change. Calcification fails in the zone of proliferating cartilage cells, which then persist in scattered tonguelike aggregations. Capillaries from the shaft invade the region between cartilage cells and carry with them an envelope of connective tissue. Thus the regular "epiphyseal line" of health disappears, and in its place there develops a zone composed of osteoid and connective tissues, blood vessels and cartilage cells. This is the "rachitic metaphysis." It is soft, and in response to external stress the bone will bend

in this region. The constant pull of muscles and tendons tends to mushroom the firm epiphyseal cartilage into the metaphysis. The resulting increase in circumference is the epiphyseal enlargement of rickets.

Evidence of the disorder is also found in the shafts. In healthy bone the process of destruction by osteoclasts and replacement by osteoblasts is continuous; in rickets the process is similar except that replacement is by osteoid rather than by osseous tissue. Trabeculae of bone come to be enveloped by a mantle of osteoid tissue. Fractures are frequently found. In health the production of cortical bone is a function of the periosteum. In rickets the periosteum is sometimes excessively active in laying down concentric layers of lime-deficient bone so that the shaft becomes considerably increased in thickness.

When rickets begins to heal, the first change results from calcification of the matrix about the more recently differentiated cartilage cells. The new epiphyseal line which is formed is demonstrable by roentgenogram and demarcates the distal end of the rachitic metaphysis. The hiatus which remains between the new line and the shaft is obliterated more slowly.

Etiology. *Metabolic and Chemical Aspects.* Vitamin D has a profound effect both on the absorption of calcium and phosphorus from the intestine and on the reabsorption of phosphorus by the renal tubules. During rickets large amounts of ingested calcium and phosphorus are excreted in the stools. With healing a strongly positive balance is established until the skeleton has been replenished. Thereafter the larger part of the excess phosphorus over that required for growth is excreted in the urine, while the bowel continues to be the principal route for eliminating calcium.

The serum of healthy infants normally contains, per 100 cc., 10 to 11 mg. of calcium and 4.5 to 5.5 mg. of inorganic phosphorus. According to Howland and Kramer the product of the calcium and phosphorus, when both are expressed in milligrams per 100 cc., furnishes an index of the presence or absence of rickets. A product less than 30 indicates the presence of rickets; a product between 30 and 40 may or may not be associated with rickets; a product greater than 40 indicates either that rickets is absent or that the disease is undergoing healing. In most cases of rickets the low product results from a deficit in inorganic phosphorus. When tetany complicates rickets, the calcium level is affected chiefly.

Symptoms and Physical Signs. The accuracy which the roentgenogram has contributed to the diagnosis of rickets has made it clear that the only characteristic signs are those which pertain to the skeleton. Other manifestations, such as irritability, excessive sweating or muscular hypotonia, are either difficult to evaluate or common to so many disorders as to be of no aid in recognizing the disease. As a single exception, the manifestations of tetany during infancy strongly suggest the presence of rickets. Tetany, however, is a complex of symptoms which accompanies only a small fraction of all cases of rickets and which may occur from causes other than those responsible for rickets. The skeletal signs of rickets are the combined result of the softened state of bone in the regions where growth is occurring and of the external stresses to which these regions are exposed. Since age is a factor in determining the sites of rapid growth and since new stresses come into play when the child learns to sit and to stand, it is apparent that the manifestations of rickets must vary in relation to the age at which they develop. Long after the disease has ceased to be active, the residual deformities are evidence of the age at which the process was most intense.

Craniotabes may be the earliest demonstrable sign of rickets; it is rare after the eighth or ninth month of life. It develops in the occipital or parietal bones in one or more areas removed from the lambdoidal suture and invariably on that side of the head upon which the infant has habitually lain. It is usually associated with softening along the suture line. Craniotabes is often overlooked on routine physical examination; its presence is detected by pressure with the finger over the probable sites of involvement and the finding of relatively soft areas where the skull buckles and snaps back when the pressure is released. The sensation is much the same as one experiences when pressing on a celluloid ping pong ball. As the infant approaches the end of the first year of life, craniotabes generally disappears, even though the rickets continues to be active. By this time, however, the skull may present other evidence of the disease. The eminences of the frontal and parietal bones become unusually prominent, and later are thickened into actual bosses which produce a square head (*caput quadratum*). Sometimes the eminences stand out as

four rounded elevations separated by depressions which mark the lines of sutures (*hot cross bun* head; *caput natiforme*). Rickets also results in delayed closure of the fontanels. In severe cases the anterior fontanel may still be membranous at the age of three or four years.

Thoracic deformities belong among the early signs of rickets. Rapid growth of the ribs during infancy renders the costochondral junctions, particularly the sixth and seventh, unusually susceptible. Here rounded enlargements make their appearance and can be palpated along a line which extends downward and laterally on either side of the chest. This is the *rachitic rosary*. As the disease progresses, the weakened metaphyses of the ribs yield to the force of negative pressure in the thorax and bend inward. When the enlargements at the rib-cartilage junctions are palpable externally, they are even more prominent on the inner wall of the thorax. Finally an external groove or depression develops along the line of the rosary. At its lower end the groove merges with a girdle-like depression (*Harrison's groove*) which appears when the ribs have bent inward along the attachments of the diaphragm. Harrison's groove is generally accentuated by flaring of the lower ribs and distention of the abdomen. Park and Howland have pointed out that the functional embarrassment which attends severe rickets of the thorax may actually endanger life. The thoracic cage, instead of expanding with each downward excursion of the diaphragm, may even become more constricted; pulmonary ventilation is further reduced by wide areas of atelectasis; respiration is rapid and difficult; and a relatively mild infection may have a fatal termination.

Enlargements at other epiphyses develop more slowly than at the costochondral junctions, but are often well developed before the end of the first year of life. They are recognized most easily at the wrists and ankles where the subcutaneous tissue is relatively thin. When the swelling is slight, it is difficult to be sure that one is not dealing with the normal protuberances of the malleoli or styloid processes. In examining the wrist the writer has made it a practice to palpate the dorsal as well as the lateral aspects, since an abnormal swelling at the former surface is less liable to be confused with normal styloid processes. Another type of bony enlargement may result from excessive production of subperiosteal bone. In the hands it leads to fusiform enlargement of the proximal and middle phalanges (*string of pearls* deformity).

Most conspicuous among the permanent malformations caused by rickets are the *bending* deformities. To a large extent they originate when the disease continues to be active after the child has learned to sit. The rachitic child shows little inclination to engage in the incessant activity which characterizes his healthy peers; a posture, once chosen, becomes habitual, and he sits for hours in essentially the same position. The resulting stress on the skeleton leads to deformity, not only because the bones are unusually yielding, but also because the direction of application is unusually constant. Commonly the child sits with thighs slightly spread apart and with one lower leg crossed over the other; the hands are placed on the floor or on the thighs to assist the spine in holding the trunk erect. The pull of gravity on the foot is augmented by that of the Achilles tendon, so that the lower epiphyses of the tibia and fibula are displaced backward, producing an angular deformity (*saber shin*). At the time of its origin the maximal convexity is just above the ankle. With increasing age the bones grow in length beyond this site, and ultimately the greatest bend is about one third the way up the shaft of the tibia. Stress on the femur from the same posture leads to lateral and forward bowing, and the femoral head is bent forward toward the shaft (*coxa vara*). That portion of the spine which is unsupported by the thorax is unusually vulnerable, and marked lumbar kyphosis is not uncommon. The combined deformities of lumbar kyphosis, pot belly and flattened thorax produce a striking picture when the child is viewed in profile; the outline is that of an erect, truncated cone with the base at the level of the navel. Less conspicuous bending deformities may develop in the upper extremities. The humerus bows outward, and the lower epiphyses of the radius and ulna may be bent to one side or the other, depending upon the direction in which the hands are habitually turned. When the child with rickets has learned to stand, the stresses are altered. Kyphosis is replaced by lumbar lordosis, coxa vara is increased, and bowlegs or knock knees make their appearance. The significant rachitic flattening of the pelvis probably begins during infancy from the force of gravity and is increased by the stresses applied during sitting and standing.

Diagnosis by Roentgenogram. The roentgenographic changes characteristic of rickets are most easily recognized in pictures of the lower ends of the radius and ulna. The earliest changes are seen almost exclusively at the cartilage-shaft junction. The normally sharp termination of the shaft becomes blurred and finely irregular (*fraying*); the line of termination tends to become concave (*cupping*); the end of the bone is widened (*spreading*); and in some instances *cortical spurs* may be present at the lateral margins where lime salts have been deposited in the perichondrium, which is adjacent to the periosteum. As the disease progresses to the moderate and more severe stages, the alterations become unmistakable. The spreading increases, the end of the shaft is hollowed out into a crater, and the fraying widens into a fringe which may be 1 cm. or more in width. Severe rickets is also attended by distinctive roentgenographic findings in the shaft. These include marked osteoporosis, either thinning or sometimes a lamellated type of thickening of the cortex, and cloaking of the shaft with rarefied subperiosteal bone. Change in the shaft, however, is rarely useful in establishing an early diagnosis and is a less sensitive index of the progress of successful therapy than is the cartilage-shaft junction.

The beginning of healing is heralded in roentgenograms by the appearance of new deposits of lime salts in the zone between bone and cartilage. Particularly prominent is the reappearance of an epiphyseal line at the proximal boundary of the cartilage. At this stage the end of the bone is marked by two horizontal lines between which the area of greatest disorder is isolated. The final obliteration of signs of the disease in x-ray films may require many months.

Prophylaxis and Treatment. The Food and Nutrition Board of the National Research Council has recommended that normal infants receive a daily dosage of 400 to 800 international units of vitamin D. Vitamin D milks, either fresh or reconstituted from the evaporated state, furnish about 400 units per quart. Full-term infants reared from birth on formulas made from vitamin D milk do not acquire clinically detectable rickets; mild roentgenologic rickets, if it develops, disappears as growth continues. Since young infants ingest less than a quart of milk a day and because the deleterious effect of slight vitamin overdosage is unimportant, most physicians prescribe a small supplement.

Cod liver oil, to be acceptable by the

U.S.P., must contain 85 units of vitamin D per gram (400 units per teaspoon); the products of the better pharmaceutical houses are generally more potent. Concentrates contain from 50 to 300 units per drop. The physician should be aware of these variations in prescribing dosage. Infants on formulas made from vitamin D milk do not derive benefit from a supplement of more than one teaspoon per day of cod liver oil of minimum U.S.P. strength; for infants on nonenriched formulas two teaspoons are ample. When concentrates are used, the dose must be measured in drops.

When active rickets must be treated or when the disease is to be prevented in premature infants, one of the many available concentrates should be prescribed. Dosage in the neighborhood of 5000 units daily is satisfactory.

A. ASHLEY WEECH

References

Bills, C. E.: Physiology of the Sterols Including Vitamin D. Physiol. Rev., 15:1, 1935.

Eliot, M. M., and Park, E. A.: Rickets, in Brennemann's Practice of Pediatrics. Hagerstown, Md., W. F. Prior Company, 1936, Vol. I, Chap. 36.

Hess, A. F.: Rickets, Including Osteomalacia and Tetany. Philadelphia, Lea & Febiger, 1929.

Howland, J.: Etiology and Pathogenesis of Rickets. Medicine, 2:349, 1923.

Park, E. A.: Some Aspects of Rickets. Canad. M. A. J., 26:3, 1932.

VITAMIN E DEFICIENCY

In 1922 Evans and Bishop first demonstrated the existence of this vitamin. Five years later Evans and Burr wrote a monograph on the subject which is the foundation of our knowledge today.

The term "vitamin E" has been applied to alpha tocopherol and, to a lesser extent, to the other tocopherols and certain synthetic substances which restore fertility to the vitamin E-depleted rat. Vitamin E is synthesized in plants. The vegetable seed oils such as wheat germ oil and cotton seed oil contain tocopherols. In 1936 Evans, Emerson and Emerson isolated three tocopherols: alpha, beta and gamma. Each of these has been artificially synthesized.

Experimental studies on animals, carried out under standardized conditions, have produced distinct results. Symptoms of vitamin E deficiency appear earlier in the male than in the female rat. The weight of the testes decreases, and spermatozoa become nonmotile. In the female the fetuses die young if the deficiency is mild; if it is greatly advanced, absolute sterility occurs. In rats and rabbits on a vitamin E-deficient diet, one of the earlier signs is a dystrophy of the striated muscles and greatly increased urinary creatine. After the administration of vitamin E the creatine content of the urine decreases promptly. No such definite changes have been found in the urine of man with any neuromuscular disturbance. Vitamin E has a remarkable influence on the storage of vitamin A in experimental animals and is often considered an antioxidant.

Experimental studies on human beings have not yet demonstrated sufficient usefulness of vitamin E to warrant making definite claims as to its role in human nutrition. It is claimed that it has a beneficial effect in habitual abortion, and it has been reported to be beneficial in primary fibrositis. These claims have not been substantiated, however. Harris, Hickman, Jensen and Spies have shown that the plasma level of tocopherols is lower in persons with nutritional deficiency diseases than in well nourished persons. That the administration of vitamin E produces no harmful effects has been observed by the writer, who administered 100 mg. daily to patients for three months without untoward symptoms.

Much work on the action of vitamin E has been carried out, but its fundamental action in the human body remains obscure. We know practically nothing of either man's requirement for it or its biologic action in human beings. Many of the studies reported have been poorly controlled, and their evaluation has been uncritical.

TOM D. SPIES

References

Evans, H. M., and Bishop, K. S.: On the Existence of a Hitherto Unrecognized Dietary Factor Essential for Reproduction. Science, 56:650, 1922.

———, and Burr, G. O.: The Antisterility Vitamin. Fat Soluble E. Mem. Univ. Calif., No. 28, 1927.

———, Emerson, D. H., and Emerson, G. A.: The Isolation from Wheat Germ Oil of an Alcohol Alpha Tocopherol Having the Properties of Vitamin E. J. Biol. Chem., 113:319, 1936; Science, 83:422, 1936.

Harris, P. L., Hickman, K. C. D., Jensen, J. L., and Spies, T. D.: Survey of the Blood Plasma Levels of Vitamin A, Carotene, Ascorbic Acid, and Tocopherols of Persons in an Area of Endemic Malnutrition. Am. J. Pub. Health, 36:155, 1946.

Spies, T. D., and Butt, H.: Vitamin E, in Duncan, G. G.: Diseases of Metabolism. 3rd ed. Philadelphia, W. B. Saunders Company, 1952, Chap. 7, p. 426.

Steinberg, C. L.: Vitamin E in the Treatment of Fibrositis. Am. J. M. Sc., 3:347, 1941.

VITAMIN K DEFICIENCY

Definition. Deficiency of vitamin K is characterized by a hemorrhagic diathesis caused by a lowered blood prothrombin level which is detectable as an increase in the prothrombin clotting time. The disease occurs primarily in patients with jaundice or certain intestinal disorders, and in the newborn infant. It is not a true primary dietary deficiency disease, but rather a nutritional deficiency in the sense that more factors than vitamin K deficiency alone are necessary for its production. In the absence of complicating factors, however, vitamin K therapy results in the relief of all signs of the disease.

History. For generations physicians and surgeons observed many jaundiced patients bleed to death in spite of all forms of treatment. Fatal hemorrhage occurred frequently in jaundiced persons after surgical operation and was also common in the newborn infant and in patients with various intestinal disorders. As the cause of these deaths was unknown, no satisfactory form of therapy was available.

During the past few years many of these perplexing problems have been solved. Dam and his associates in Copenhagen produced a disease in chicks by feeding them a diet washed in ether, and observed that a widely distributed antihemorrhagic substance was curative. Dam proposed a term, "vitamin K," for this. Quick, in America, then suggested that a deficiency of vitamin K was present in patients who had obstructive jaundice. Butt and his associates showed that such patients had a deficiency of prothrombin.

Maccorquodale, McKee, Doisy, Almquist, Klose, Fieser and many other investigators made possible the final isolation and synthesis of vitamin K.

A number of compounds have been tested for vitamin K activity, and many have been found active; the two most important at the present time are vitamin K_1 and vitamin K_2. These are fat-soluble and at low temperatures form yellow crystals.

Etiology. The importance of prothrombin for hemorrhage lies in its relationship to blood coagulation; for coagulation is thought to involve a reaction between prothrombin, platelets and calcium to form thrombin, which, in turn, combines with fibrinogen to produce fibrin. Hemorrhage may occur when the concentration of blood prothrombin is sufficiently reduced; and this deficiency can be corrected by vitamin K in all cases except those in which there is severe hepatic damage.

Because of this relationship to prothrombin, vitamin K appears to be necessary for normal physiologic function of the liver and for blood coagulation.

In man an inadequate intake of vitamin K is seldom, if ever, responsible for prothrombin deficiency. The vitamin is widely distributed in chlorophyll-containing plants such as green leaves, alfalfa, spinach and cabbage. As it is fat-soluble, it is not absorbed from the upper intestine unless conditions are favorable for the absorption of fat. An intact hepatic parenchyma is essential if vitamin K is to enter into prothrombin formation. The vitamin is said to be stored in only small amounts in the body. Many chronically debilitated persons have moderate hypoprothrombinemia, which apparently is not directly attributable to primary vitamin K deficiency.

Diagnosis. Blood coagulation time and bleeding time have been found unsatisfactory indices of the potential danger of hemorrhage because abnormal values do not appear until hemorrhage is imminent. The measurement of the prothrombin concentration or prothrombin clotting time is a more accurate measure of the tendency to bleed.

The decrease in concentration of prothrombin is a phenomenon in which numerous factors are involved. Bleeding because of prothrombin deficiency may be anticipated in any disease state which results in inadequate intestinal absorption or hepatic utilization of vitamin K. Hemorrhage may result when bile is excluded from the gastrointestinal tract, by obstruction due to pancreatic neoplasm, postoperative stricture of the common duct, intermittent obstruction by stones, or hepatic injury from chronic cholecystic disease or hepatotoxins. The bleeding may manifest itself as a slow oozing of blood from the gums, nose or gastrointestinal tract, or more frequently from the incisional site. The hemorrhage occurs most frequently on the first to fourth postoperative days, but may occur later. Severe melena or hematemesis may occur, though uncommonly, and may even be uncontrollable with repeated transfusions. Invariably a prolonged "prothrombin clotting time" will be found. According to Smith, postoperative bleeding occurs if the prothrombin concentration is less than 20 per cent of normal. A multiplicity of factors may produce this situation: loss of blood, trauma, anesthesia and an already depleted prothrombin.

Hemorrhage in patients with various intestinal disorders, such as sprue, celiac disease, chronic ulcerative colitis, intestinal obstruction with intubation, external biliary fistulas, ileac stomas with profuse discharge, short-circuiting operations and ileitis, should lead the physician to suspect prothrombin deficiency. In such conditions it is of utmost importance to follow the prothrombin level. A special problem is encountered in infants who manifest a deficiency of prothrombin at birth. This is attributed to the absence from the intestinal tract of bacterial flora which have some relationship to the synthesis of vitamin K, to the limited absorption of fat, to the insufficiency of bile and to the usually hypermotile gut during the first few days of life. The deficiency of prothrombin in infants is often spontaneously remedied within three or four days after birth. If a surgical procedure is contemplated in the newborn infant, one should follow the prothrombin level with particular caution.

In order to use vitamin K effectively the physician must have a satisfactory method of measuring the level of prothrombin in the circulating blood. Two methods are available, both of them indirect and not entirely satisfactory on physiologic grounds. The first, described by Quick, Stanley-Brown and Bancroft, is well adapted for the usual clinical laboratory. The second method, that of Warner, Brinkhous and Smith, measures the concentration of prothrombin quantitatively and requires a large laboratory with specially trained technicians.

Treatment. In most instances vitamin K_1 or K_2 or related compounds are effective in the prevention and control of bleeding due to a lowered prothrombin level. The tendency of a patient to bleed is not always accurately indicated by the prothrombin measurement. Thus, when prothrombin deficiency is suspected, therapy should be instituted before bleeding starts. The water-soluble preparations (menadione bisulfite) may be given parenterally when intestinal absorption is poor, but adequate functioning liver parenchyma is necessary in any circumstance.

Minimal requirements for the infant, child, mother or adult are not known, but a dose of 1 to 2 mg. per day of menadione usually corrects the deficiency usless there is in-adequate absorption or an increased need because of diarrhea or sprue. The development of untoward reactions from the oral or parenteral administration of preparations of vitamin K need not be feared. Amounts far above the therapeutic dose have been given to adults (50 mg. orally, 10 mg. intravenously) without the appearance of any signs of toxicity. The oral administration of larger amounts (180 mg. of menadione) to human beings has been followed by vomiting and porphyrinuria.

Bleeding may occur with little warning. It is the writer's practice to determine the prothrombin clotting time of every patient with jaundice or other conditions which may lead to hypoprothrombinemia and to administer vitamin K (2 mg. of menadione) with bile salts orally, or water-soluble synthetic progenitors (menadione bisulfite, 4.8 mg.) parenterally if the prothrombin clotting time is prolonged. One to 2 mg. of a synthetic compound with vitamin K activity, together with 1 to 3 gm. of animal bile salts, given orally, usually suffices. This dosage should be repeated as indicated.

Preoperative and postoperative care in the jaundiced patient is of utmost importance. After an operation the prothrombin clotting time usually increases to some extent for three or four days, but may increase rapidly days later. In such patients the prothrombin concentration should be determined daily for at least four days and then every other day for another ten days. Some think it is best to administer vitamin K regardless of the postoperative prothrombin clotting time.

The problem of treating patients who are actively bleeding is difficult. The alimentary tract is often filled with blood and the patient frequently is dehydrated and in shock. Such cases usually require a transfusion of blood, which provides a temporary store of prothrombin for about 8 hours. In cases in which severe bleeding into the alimentary tract is associated with low prothrombin, 25 mg. of a water-soluble vitamin K (menadione bisulfite) can be given either orally or parenterally. Absorption is more certain when the parenteral route is used.

In cases of severe hepatic damage 3 to 5 mg. of substances with vitamin K activity should be administered daily, even though the prothrombin clotting time response is slight. Death from hemorrhagic diathesis rarely occurs when such therapy is applied. Should the usual dose be tripled without effect, no additional amount will be effective. When hepatic damage is severe, utilization of vitamin K substances may prove inadequate.

The newborn infant may be treated by giving 1.5 mg. of menadione at birth, which prevents transitory hypoprothrombinemia and hemorrhagic disease. Many obstetricians advocate giving vitamin K to the mother 12 to 24 hours before parturition, since it has been found that the infant has a higher prothrombin level when the mother has received vitamin K prior to delivery. The author prefers to give a pregnant woman 2 mg. daily for one week preceding delivery, and during labor if necessary.

TOM D. SPIES

References

Barr, D. P.: Modern Medical Therapy in General Practice. Baltimore, Williams & Wilkins Co., 1940, Vol. II, p. 2401.
Brinkhouse, K. M.: Plasma Prothrombin—Vitamin K. Medicine, 19:329, 1940.
Butt, H. R., and Snell, A. M.: Vitamin K. Philadelphia, W. B. Saunders Company, 1941.
Quick, A. J., Stanley-Brown, Margaret, and Bancroft, F. W.: A Study of the Coagulation Defect in Hemophilia and Jaundice. Am. J. M. Sc., 190:501, 1935.
Warner, E. D., Brinkhous, K. M., and Smith, H. P.: A Quantitative Study on Blood Clotting: Prothrombin Fluctuations under Experimental Conditions. Am. J. Physiol., 114:667, 1936.
———, Spies, T. D., and Owen, C. A.: Hypoprothrombinemia and Vitamin K in Nutritional Deficiency States. South. M. J., 34:161, 1941.

MIXED DEFICIENCY DISEASES

Diets that fail to supply one nutrient in adequate amounts are deficient in others and every method of study has indicated the predominance of mixed rather than single deficiencies. Accordingly, a person may have a number of diseases simultaneously, although diagnostic evidence of only one may be apparent at the time he is examined by the physician. The basis of treatment of all patients with deficiency diseases is a diet that supplies liberal amounts of all the essential nutrients. In many instances, however, food cannot be consumed in sufficiently large amounts to supply the patient with the quantities of nutrients needed to restore him to health. Too often it is forgotten that we must treat the patient rather than his disease, and

that treatment must be adapted to the individual case. Even a liberal well balanced diet should be supplemented with all the vitamins known to be essential for human nutrition. They may be given as crystalline vitamins, as concentrates, or in the form of therapeutic materials such as dried brewers' yeast or liver extract.

In treating the clinical syndromes of beriberi, pellagra, riboflavin deficiency and scurvy, we give a basic formula consisting of 10 mg. of thiamine, 50 mg. of niacin, 5 mg. of riboflavin, 75 mg. of ascorbic acid and 5 mg. of folic acid. When we find that the symptoms of one deficiency disease predominate, we add to this formula more of the vitamin specific for the predominating deficiency. In beriberi, 10 mg. of thiamine is added daily; in riboflavin deficiency, 5 mg. of riboflavin twice daily; in scurvy, 100 mg. of ascorbic acid three times a day; and in mild pellagra, 50 mg. of niacinamide three times a day. If the pellagra is severe, the patient is given 150 mg. of niacinamide three times a day in addition to the basic formula. When the patient is moribund, it may be necessary to resort to parenteral injections in order to prolong and indeed even to save life. When large amounts of glucose are injected daily, we recommend the inclusion of 20 mg. of niacinamide, 7.5 mg. of riboflavin and 5 mg. of thiamine. In a few instances we have found it desirable to inject 50 mg. of ascorbic acid in physiologic solution of sodium chloride.

When there is any tendency to bone marrow failure in patients with definite deficiency disease states, we proceed to make a precise diagnosis. On many occasions it is found that the patients have evidence of nutritional macrocytic anemia or iron deficiency anemia.

Deficiency diseases frequently occur in patients with true pernicious anemia or in women who are pregnant; thus a group of diseases may be operating simultaneously in the patient who may have physiologic stress, such as pregnancy or lactation, or who may have organic and primary disturbances, such as failure of the intrinsic factor of the stomach.

The four principles used in treating mixed deficiency diseases are:

1. DIET. 4000 calories, 120 to 150 gm. protein, rich in vitamins and minerals.

2. BASIC THERAPY. Thiamine, riboflavin, niacinamide, ascorbic acid, orally.

3. ADDITIONAL MEDICATION. Synthetic vitamins as indicated, orally or parenterally.

4. NATURAL B COMPLEX. Brewers' yeast or extract, or rice bran extract, and/or liver extract orally or parenterally.

One of the basic formulas employed is:

	Daily
Folic acid	5 mg.
Thiamine	10 mg.
Niacinamide	150 mg.
Riboflavin	10 mg.
Ascorbic acid	150 mg.
Vitamin B_{12} and "Activator"*	10 mcg. vitamin B_{12}

KWASHIORKOR
(Malignant Malnutrition)

Kwashiorkor, an African term meaning "red boy," is the name given a disease associated with characteristic skin and hair discoloration. It was described for the first time eighteen years ago by Cecily Williams who observed it in a children's hospital on the African Gold Coast. There is general agreement that the term has been applied to dietary deficiency conditions which arise from various causes in different parts of the world. Many investigators believe that kwashiorkor develops as a result of varying mixtures of protein deficiency, undernutrition and hunger edema, but the precise cause remains obscure.

The disease occurs in infants and adults living in certain tropical and subtropical countries (we have not found a true case of kwashiorkor in Cuba, Puerto Rico or the southern part of the United States). It apparently is related to fatty infiltration of the liver. In children the disease is fairly distinctive. The child is seriously ill, his height and weight are subnormal, there is diarrhea, the abdomen is distended, and there is edema involving the feet and face, which later tends to become generalized. The hair shows some changes; in the African it becomes soft and straight. Whatever the original color of the hair, depigmentation tends to occur. Perhaps, as in other deficiency states, the advanced cases are likely to be typical but the less common, mild case is difficult to define precisely. The clinical picture may be distinctive, but it is doubtful that all signs are invariably present or that they occur only in this order. For example, a patient may be typical in all other respects but may show

* Equivalent to 10 micrograms of vitamin B_{12} and intrinsic factor adequate to form its conjugate.

no depigmentation of the hair; other patients may have little or no edema.

There are no biochemical findings which definitely characterize the disease, although in the acute stages there is hypoalbuminemia.

The diets eaten by persons who develop kwashiorkor are low in protein, and the best treatment is a diet high in protein. Concentrated milk proteins give good results, and plant proteins also are effective. We have learned that when a diet is grossly deficient in proteins and calories it likewise is deficient in all the other essential nutrients and, consequently, there are many nutritional complications including electrolyte disturbances.

TOM D. SPIES

References

Dean, R. F. A.: The Treatment of Kwashiorkor with Milk and Vegetable Proteins. Brit. M. J., 2:791, 1952.
———, and Schwartz, R.: The Serum Chemistry in Uncomplicated Kwashiorkor. Brit. J. Nutr., 7: 131, 1953.
Spies, T. D.: Symposium on Nutrition. M. Clin. North America, 27:1943.
———, and Butt, H. R.: Vitamins and Avitaminoses, in Duncan, G. G.: Diseases of Metabolism. 3rd ed. Philadelphia, W. B. Saunders Co., 1952.
Trowell, H. C., Davies, J. N. P., and Dean, R. F. A.: Kwashiorkor: Clinical Picture, Pathology and Differential Diagnosis. Brit. M. J., 2:798, 1952.
Waterlow, J. C.: Fatty Liver Disease in Infants in the British West Indies. Special Report Series, Medical Research Council, London, No. 263, 1948.
———: Liver Choline-Esterase in Malnourished Infants. Lancet, 258:908, 1950.

SPRUE
(Psilosis)

Definition. Sprue, or psilosis, is a chronic, afebrile disease with marked tendency to remissions and relapses. It is characterized by recurrent glossitis, aphthous stomatitis, flatulent indigestion, diarrhea, general weakness and anemia. The full-blown cases show marked loss of weight, signs of premature aging, abdominal distention, intractable diarrhea accompanied by the passage of voluminous, often fatty and frothy, foul-smelling stools, and a severe macrocytic anemia with a megaloblastic bone marrow.

History. The term "sprue" was first used by a Dutchman, V. Katelaer (1669), who applied the term to the aphthous stomatitis, accompanied by the passage of voluminous stools that occurred among the Belgians. An Englishman, Hillary (1766), is credited with the first clear description of the disease, his observations having been based on clinical experience during a six-year residence in the Barbadoes (1753–1759). Real scientific interest in this disease may be said to date from the writings of the Scotsman, Sir Patrick Manson (1880), in China, and of another Dutchman, Van Der Burg (1880), in Batavia. Van Der Burg's contribution was based on the study of 1407 cases during his thirty years' experience in Java. Manson was probably the first to suggest that "bad or insufficient food" was of major importance in the causation of sprue. In more recent years, especially in America, a renewed interest in the disease was undoubtedly brought about by the studies, observations and contributions of Ashford in Puerto Rico.

Incidence. For many years sprue was supposed to be limited to tropical and subtropical latitudes. In 1932 Thaysen reported the first cases of the so-called "nontropical" sprue in northern Europe. Shortly afterwards many such cases were being reported from the United States of America, not only from the southern, but also from the northern states. Snell (1936) reported many instances in the northwestern states, while Hanes and his collaborators from the Duke Hospital Clinic in Durham, North Carolina (1943), had observed 66 cases of indigenous sprue in a period of eight years. There is no doubt that tropical and nontropical sprue are the same disease.

No less than 500 cases of sprue have been studied in Puerto Rico during the last 30 years, though the incidence of sprue in Puerto Rico and elsewhere has diminished in frequency and severity during recent years. A more adequate diet through better education, improvement in the economic status of the people, and the more liberal use of the various antianemic substances probably account for the present lower incidence of the disease.

Etiology. The etiology of sprue remains unknown, but the concept of a deficiency state is one of the theories that have been able to withstand prolonged investigation. In favor of this theory is the fact that cases of sprue have been successfully treated in the past with different diets: marmite soup, meat diet, milk and strawberry diet, and others. The remarkable effect produced by the administration of liver extract, folic acid or vitamin B_{12} seems to give additional support to the view that sprue is a deficiency disease.

A suggestive link in the chain of evidence of the relation between food deficiency and sprue has been supplied by Miller and Rhoads, who by feeding a deficient diet produced a disorder in hogs which they believe is closely analogous to the human sprue syndrome.

While working in Puerto Rico, Castle and Rhoads and their collaborators confirmed the belief that a deficient diet frequently antedates the onset of clinical sprue. They demonstrated that feeding vitamin B complex in the form of autolyzed yeast produces reticulocyte crises and improvement of the blood picture in certain cases. The intrinsic factor was found lacking in other instances, and some of the more severe or advanced cases showed an apparent defect in absorption from the intestinal canal.

Many theories have been offered from time to time to explain the etiology of sprue. Most of them have been discarded. Ashford attributed the onset of the disease to an unbalanced diet made up largely of carbohydrates and fatty foods with little protein of good biologic value, a view that has been widely accepted. He thought, however, that the nutritional *imbalance* led to gastrointestinal conditions favorable to the growth of a yeastlike fungus, *Monilia psilosis,* which, in turn, aided in producing the clinical picture known as sprue. His writings made a deep impression on the opinion of the medical profession in America. The studies on sprue in Puerto Rico by Castle and Rhoads, and of several English and Indian investigators in the Orient, did not substantiate the theory of the pathogenic action of Monilia.

The theory of infection, which has had ardent advocates, has also been practically abandoned. The afebrile course of the disease, the absence of leukocytosis and of anatomico-pathologic evidences of bacterial invasion, point against the theory of an infectious disease. There is no doubt that infectious diseases, debilitating influences, pregnancy and many conditions that are associated with disorders of digestion or assimilation of food may serve as contributory or conditioning factors.

The part played by a constitutional or inherited defect is difficult to evaluate. It is impossible, however, to escape the conviction that the constitution of the patient plays a role in the development of the disease. It is also an accepted fact that there is a definite racial predisposition.

Epidemiology. Sprue is a regional rather than a climatic disease; according to most authors, it preeminently attacks Europeans. Dark-skinned people are less liable to acquire the disease, though it is occasionally seen in the Mongolian race, in Malayans, and in Indians. In a study of 150 patients, 121 were white, 26 mulattoes, and only 3 Negroes. The ages ranged from 9 to 84 years. The majority of the patients were middle-aged, and one third were less than 40, a point of difference from true Addisonian anemia.

The disease is apt to occur in one or more members of the same family. A history of sprue or pernicious anemia in one of the patient's parents can often be elicited. In rare instances, sprue develops in husband and wife. Women appear more liable to have the disease than are men. Atmospheric temperature does not seem to influence the incidence of the disease, for it originates at high altitudes in Ceylon and in the Himalayas, where the climate resembles that of Europe.

Sprue and pernicious anemia have so many features in common that it has been repeatedly suggested that the former may constitute a geographical variant of the latter.

Morbid Anatomy. All storehouses of fat are found depleted, and the internal organs are small. The weight of the liver varies from 720 to 1620 gm., with an average of 1060 gm.; the heart from 140 to 270 gm., with an average of 230 gm.; and the spleen from 5 to 140 gm., with an average of 74.9 gm. The lingual mucosa shows atrophy or zones of atrophy alternating with hyperplasia. The gastric mucosa is moderately atrophied in half the cases, while chronic gastritis is a frequent finding. Distinct shortening and blunting of the villi of the small intestine are noted in half the cases (not attributable to postmortem changes). The colon is occasionally found normal, but mild acute colitis and a few nonspecific ulcers are often seen.

Symptoms. The chief complaints are usually a persistent diarrhea and general weakness. There is also flatulent dyspepsia, anorexia, and a sense of fullness in the epigastrium. On questioning, one finds that the illness dates back several months or years and that it has been progressive in character.

Physical examination usually reveals a white, pale, weak and emaciated young or middle-aged person, showing no fever, with a normal pulse and respiration, while lying comfortably in bed. The skin is dry and wrinkled, occasionally hyperpigmented, and rarely shows purpuric spots on the forearms and external ears. A slight subicteric tint may be observed in the conjunctivas. The tongue is inflamed, with crops of minute, whitish, painful ulcerations with fiery red borders in

the early stages, or complete and total atrophy of both the filiform and the fungiform papillae in the more advanced cases. The heart and lungs are not abnormal, but the abdomen is distended, with dilated intestinal loops that are clearly visible. The liver and spleen are not palpable; the endocrine glands are normal, and, in the majority of cases, there is no evidence of central nervous system involvement, although many patients complain of cramps in the legs, paresthesia and emotional instability. Subacute combined degeneration of the spinal cord has been observed in only 2 per cent of the patients, some of them showing free hydrochloric acid in their gastric secretion.

Stools are frequent, copious, frothy and foul-smelling; from three to twenty bowel movements a day are common. The diarrhea may cause severe electrolyte depletion, particularly of sodium and potassium.

The onset of the disease is usually insidious, but the course may be subacute or chronic. Subacute forms may last for one or two years, the chronic cases for ten or fifteen years.

At the time the sprue patient applies for medical treatment, the laboratory test usually reveals the presence of a macrocytic hyperchromic anemia, a megaloblastic bone marrow, a flat, oral glucose tolerance curve, and either a hypochlorhydria or a histamine-resistant achlorhydria.

Patients who have received inadequate doses of liver extract are likely to show a normal tongue and mouth in the presence of a persistent and, at times, troublesome diarrhea.

Diagnosis. The typical case is usually a white, young or middle-aged person who complains of general weakness, diarrhea and glossitis that has persisted, off and on, for months or years. On examination there is evident weight loss, premature aging, and some abdominal distention. The laboratory will establish the diagnosis with the following findings: a macrocytic hyperchromic anemia, megaloblastic bone marrow, flat, oral glucose tolerance curve, low or absent free hydrochloric acid in the gastric secretion, increase of fat content in the stools, and roentgenologic evidences of a deficiency state.

A diagnosis based exclusively on clinical grounds is prone to error. A combination of glossitis, anemia, loss of weight and diarrhea, with or without steatorrhea, may be observed in various conditions unrelated to sprue. To the superficial observers, simple achlorhydric anemia may be confused clinically with sprue, as well as some cases of hookworm anemia, syphilitic glossitis, intestinal and peritoneal tuberculosis, chronic enteritis and colitis, Hodgkin's disease and other neoplastic diseases of the intestine, and Addisonian pernicious anemia.

Differential Diagnosis. Both sprue and *pernicious anemia* present glossitis, a macrocytic anemia and a megaloblastic bone marrow. Both diseases may show neurologic signs and symptoms, sprue in only 2 per cent of the cases, and pernicious anemia in 60 per cent. Histamine-resistant achlorhydria may be found in both, in 100 per cent of the cases of pernicious anemia, but in only 20 to 30 per cent of sprue patients. Both conditions may show a subicteric tint to the sclerae, and loss of weight. However, progressive emaciation is an outstanding sign of sprue, whereas the loss of weight in pernicious anemia, if it does occur, is minimal. The blood sugar curve is normal in pernicious anemia, but low in sprue. The spleen is frequently enlarged or palpable in the first and smaller or normal in the last.

Pellagra and *Addison's disease* bear only a superficial resemblance to sprue and should cause no real diagnostic difficulties. Pancreatic steatorrhea, unlike the diarrhea of sprue, is characterized by great loss of nitrogen in the feces (azotorrhea), which can be demonstrated microscopically in the form of undigested striated muscle fibers; the blood sugar curve may be diabetic in type.

In *intestinal* and *mesenteric tuberculosis* there may be steatorrhea due to obstruction to the lacteal flow of chyle, but the blood glucose curve is not low, the anemia is hypochromic, and the finding of tuberculosis elsewhere in the body clarifies the diagnosis.

Simmonds' disease and *anorexia nervosa* may resemble sprue only superficially, but the severe cachexia and anorexia are the only features common to these three conditions.

Gastrocolic and other fistulous connections between the stomach and intestines will sometimes give rise to steatorrhea and azotorrhea, as well as to a pernicious type of anemia. Roentgenographic investigation will establish the diagnosis.

Fecal Fat Determinations. In determinations of the fat content of the dried stools of sprue patients receiving their usual inadequate diet, it was observed that only one third showed values above 30 per cent. In other words, only 33 per cent apparently showed steatorrhea. In a more recent study, in which the sprue patients were on a controlled diet of known fat content, the stools were collected every 24 hours, and determinations of fat output and fat absorption were made, using the wet method developed by Dr. C. F. Asenjo. Five of 7 patients showed definite evidences of steatorrhea.

Gastroscopic Findings. Nine of 10 full-blown cases in Rodriquez-Olleros' series, and 55 per cent of the cases studied by Hernandez-Morales, showed atrophic gastritis. After treatment, the gastric mucosa of 62 per cent of the cases returned to normal.

Rectosigmoidoscopic examinations during the acute diarrheal stage revealed several types of lesions, such as patches of atrophy, edema, friability, purpuric spots and superficial inflammation.

Roentgen Studies of the Intestinal Tract. Seventy per cent of the acute cases studied showed the so-called "deficiency pattern:" segmentation or "moulage" sign of the small intestine. Most of the roentgenologic evidence of the disease is found in the jejunum.

Prognosis. Sprue may be considered a curable disease only in the young and in those receiving early treatment. Most of the patients will require a maintenance dose of antianemic substance, and a special diet, probably for the rest of their lives, at least while living in the tropics. Even severe and advanced cases often respond dramatically to adequate treatment. Relapse of gastrointestinal manifestations is occasionally observed, in the presence of a satisfactory blood picture, in patients who have discontinued therapy or have been unable to follow the recommended diet. At present, death from uncomplicated sprue is rare.

Treatment. The best therapy for sprue consists of an adequate diet rich in animal proteins, rich in vitamins and low in fats, carbohydrates and roughage, plus the parenteral administration of liver extract or vitamin B_{12}, or parenteral or oral administration of folic acid. Blood transfusion is occasionally life-saving. Such drugs as hydrochloric acid, calcium, vitamin D, phosphorus, pancreatin, cholagogues and glandular extracts are of little if any value. Iron in large doses is sometimes necessary during the course of treatment. Its use during the acute stage of the disease is not only ineffective, but may be detrimental.

Liver Extract. From a historical point of

view, it is interesting to recall that liver therapy was first used by Chinese physicians in the treatment of sprue, hundreds of years before the epoch-making discovery of Minot and Murphy.

When used parenterally, either the crude or concentrated liver extracts produce satisfactory response, the former in doses of 6 cc. (1 cc. $=$ 1 to 2 units), intramuscularly and daily for a week or ten days, and then at biweekly intervals for several months. The maintenance dose of the diluted preparation is usually 6 cc. every three to seven days. Concentrated liver extract (1 cc. $=$ 10 to 15 units) is also administered intramuscularly in doses of 1 cc. daily for three consecutive days; then 1 cc. every third day for the first month, and 1 cc. every five days during the second month of treatment. The maintenance dose is 1 cc. every five to seven days.

The sprue patient, as a rule, improves dramatically for the first ten days to a month or a month and a half under appropriate diet and parenteral liver therapy. However, in spite of large doses of liver extract and the addition of iron, progress from then on is slow and tedious, so much so that only few cases reach an absolutely normal blood picture at the end of two months. The same holds true for folic acid.

Folic Acid. Spies and his collaborators have proved conclusively that sprue patients can be adequately treated with folic acid (pteroylglutamic acid) both by the parenteral and by the oral routes. The oral dose varies from 10 to 20 mg. daily for the acute cases, and the maintenance dose, from 2.5 to 5 mg. The response to oral administration of folic acid compares favorably with that obtained by the parenteral administration of a potent liver extract, and is far superior to the response induced by oral administration of liver extract.

Patients showing the slightest manifestations of neurologic involvement should not be given folic acid, unless supplemented by the administration of parenteral vitamin B_{12}.

Citrovorum Factor (Leucovorin or Folinic Acid). This has proved effective in intramuscular doses of 3 mg. daily (20,000,-000 units) for one week and the subsequent administration of the same dose at weekly intervals. Orally administered in combination with *calcium, leucovorin* is also effective when given in doses of 15 to 20 mg. daily.

Vitamin B_{12}. This substance administered parenterally induces striking hematologic and clinical response in sprue, as well as in pernicious anemia. It is, per unit of weight, the most effective antianemic substance known. As little as 4 micrograms has induced a slight reticulocytosis. Spies and his collaborators are correct in stating that probably 100 micrograms or less will induce a maximal response. A number of sprue patients have been maintained in perfect clinical and hematologic remission for over four years with the administration of only 15 micrograms every ten days. The rare sprue patient showing spinal cord involvement responds to the administration of vitamin B_{12}.

ACTH and Cortisone. Although optimistic reports on the use of ACTH and cortisone in sprue have appeared in the literature, we do not recommend these hormones for the routine treatment of the disease. Both substances may induce a sense of well being and euphoria but no significant hematologic improvement, although a slight increase in the reticulocytes and improvement in the intestinal absorption of glucose and fats have been observed following ACTH administration.

Authenticated and uncomplicated sprue rarely needs any other therapy than oral folic acid and/or parenteral vitamin B_{12}.

RAMON M. SUAREZ

References

Castle, W. B., Rhoads, C. P., Lawson, H. A., and Payne, G. C.: Etiology and Treatment of Sprue. Observations on Patients in Puerto Rico and Subsequent Experiments on Animals. Arch. Int. Med., 56:628, 1935.

Hanes, F. M., and McBryde, A.: Identity of Tropical Sprue, Non-tropical and Celiac Disease. Arch. Int. Med., 58:1, 1936.

Hernandez-Morales, F.: Gastroscopic and Rectosigmoidoscopic Observations in Tropical Sprue. Puerto Rico J. Pub. Health & Trop. Med., 20:257, 1944.

Manson-Bahr, P. H.: Manson's Tropical Diseases. Baltimore, Williams and Wilkins Co., 1940.

Spies, T. D., and others: Tentative Appraisal of Vitamin B_{12} as a Therapeutic Agent. J.A.M.A., 139:521, 1949.

Strong, R. P.: Stitt's Diagnosis and Treatment of Tropical Diseases. Philadelphia, The Blakiston Co., 1945.

Suarez, R. M., Spies, T. D., and Suarez, R. M., Jr.: The Use of Folic Acid in Sprue. Ann. Int. Med., 26:643, 1947.

———, Suarez, R. M., Jr., Busó, R., and Sabater, J.: The Effect of Orally Administered Folinic Acid in the Treatment of Tropical Sprue. Blood, 9:489, 1954.

Diseases of Metabolism

INBORN ERRORS OF METABOLISM

Garrod characterized the inborn errors of metabolism as "metabolic sports, the chemical analogues of structural malformations"— anomalies in metabolic pathways which are presumably present from birth. They show "no tendency to become aggravated as time goes on, and they are little likely to be influenced by any therapeutic measures at our disposal." On these grounds Garrod drew a distinction between such metabolic diseases as diabetes and the true inborn errors of metabolism, which he listed in 1923 as including albinism, alkaptonuria, cystinuria, congenital porphyrinuria, congenital steatorrhea and pentosuria. Subsequent experience has greatly expanded the list.

Included among the inborn errors of metabolism now are gout, some of the lipoidoses and essential hypercholesterolemias, the glycogen storage diseases, congenital galactosemia, fructosuria, phenylpyruvic oligophrenia, tyrosinosis, Wilson's disease, the Fanconi syndrome and related disorders, congenital methemoglobinemia, sicklemia and other hemoglobin anomalies responsible for hemolytic anemias, familial periodic paralysis, and some of the progressive muscle dystrophies and myotonias. Doubtless more remain to be uncovered.

In certain respects the criteria set up by Garrod no longer apply. Some inborn errors of metabolism are not as innocuous as initially supposed. Some are now known to become aggravated with age, while others are apt to recede. In some instances appropriate therapy for complete or partial control of manifestations has been devised in consequence of clarification of basic mechanisms; others remain resistant.

The inborn errors of metabolism have acquired a significance altogether out of proportion to their rarity and practical clinical importance. Their study has clarified important problems of intermediary metabolism, even to the identification of specific enzyme deficiencies. Moreover, the genetic implications of the inborn errors have thrown new light upon the relation of genes to the chemical and enzymatic constitution of cells.

ALEXANDER B. GUTMAN

References

Garrod, A. E.: Inborn Errors of Metabolism. 2d ed. London, Henry Frowde, 1923.
Inborn Errors of Metabolism (Combined Staff Clinic). Am. J. Med., 8:90, 1950.

THE GLYCOGEN STORAGE DISEASES
(Glycogenosis, von Gierke's Disease)

Definition. Glycogen storage disease is a composite term referring to a group of distinct inborn errors of carbohydrate metabolism characterized by excessive deposition of glycogen in tissues, usually associated with an anomaly of one or another enzyme system concerned with glycogen degradation or synthesis. In the hepatorenal form, *von Gierke's disease,* glycogen storage occurs chiefly in the liver and kidney. In *generalized glycogenosis* the distribution of excessive glycogen is more diffuse but is preponderantly in cardiac and skeletal muscle; this rare disorder is often referred to as the cardiac form of glycogen storage disease. A possibly related form of glycogen disease, a myopathy due to inability of the skeletal musculature to utilize muscle glycogen properly, has recently been described by McArdle as another probable inborn error of carbohydrate metabolism (*McArdle syndrome*).

Etiology. Cori has shown that in most cases of the hepatorenal type the excessive liver glycogen is of normal molecular structure but there is a deficiency of the liver enzyme, glucose-6-phosphatase, which specifically accelerates the formation of glucose from glucose-6-phosphate. Hence glycogen can be formed from glucose but glucose-6-phosphate derived from liver glycogen, or from ingested glucose through the action of hexokinase, cannot be broken down again to regenerate glucose when required. In occasional cases of von Gierke's disease there is no deficiency of glucose-6-phosphatase, but the metabolic error appears to be a lack of branching enzyme (1,4→ 1,6 transglucosidase) or of debranching enzyme (amylo-1, 6-glucosidase). These deficiencies are associated with abnormal molecular structure of glycogen and inadequate utilization for glucose formation because of inaccessibility of the major part of the glycogen molecule to the action of phosphorylase. In generalized glycogenosis the metabolic error has not yet been identified—there appears to be neither abnormal glycogen synthesis nor an absence of specific glucose-6-phosphatase. In the McArdle syndrome there would seem to be a deficiency of 1, 3-diphosphoglyceraldehyde dehydrogenase in skeletal muscle.

Symptoms and Signs. Von Gierke's disease usually becomes manifest in infancy or early childhood as a problem in feeding or because of undue prominence of the abdomen or delayed growth. The most characteristic physical finding, usually present in infancy, is marked hepatomegaly due to the excessive deposits of glycogen, often associated with a considerable increase in neutral fat. Jaundice may appear. The spleen ordinarily is not enlarged.

Because of the limited availability of glucose upon demand, hypoglycemia and ketosis develop, particularly in the fasting state. The symptoms of hypoglycemia may dominate the picture, shock or generalized convulsions occurring typically in the early morning hours. The realization that frequent feedings allay these symptoms may later result in obesity. There is usually delay in growth and development of afflicted children.

Generalized glycogenosis is characterized by very marked globular enlargement of the heart in infants, with progressive and refractory cardiac failure leading to death in the early weeks or months of life. This is due to massive glycogen infiltration of the ventricular musculature, giving a "lacework" appearance to the myocardium. There is associated cyanosis, dyspnea and malnutrition. Macroglossia due to glycogen storage in the musculature of the tongue may be striking. Metabolic indications of impaired glycogenolysis have not been marked.

In the *McArdle syndrome* no abnormality is apparent other than a myopathy characterized by pain, stiffness and weakness, with prolonged contracture of the skeletal muscles, upon moderate exercise. There is no demonstrable disability of the muscles at rest.

Diagnosis. Liver puncture biopsy offers the most direct method of diagnosis in the hepatorenal form of glycogen storage disease. The liver cells, engorged with glycogen, present a characteristic plant cell appearance and give the typical staining reactions for glycogen; a deficiency of glucose-6-phosphatase may be inferred if the glycogen disappears at a normal rate upon incubation with normal liver homogenate. The presence of excessive neutral fat may lead to confusion with hypertrophic steatosis or fatty liver associated with diabetes mellitus.

Von Gierke's disease should be suspected in infants or children who have marked enlargement of the liver, hypoglycemia and ketosis or rapid development of these manifestations when food is withheld, and subnormal or no response of the blood sugar to injection of epinephrine (due to unavailability of liver glycogen stores). Additional findings are low serum carbon dioxide combining power, ketonuria, increased serum glycogen, delayed rise in blood sugar after glucose tolerance tests, and low curves with rapid fall in levulose and galactose tolerance tests. Hyperlipemia and hypercholesterolemia may be so marked as to cause diagnostic difficulties.

The cardiomegaly of generalized glycogenosis in infants may simulate subendocardial fibroelastosis and multiple rhabdomyomas of the heart, the latter usually associated with tuberous sclerosis of the brain. Definitive diagnosis can be made only at necropsy by histochemical or chemical demonstration of glycogen in the tissues.

Treatment. Treatment in the hepatorenal form of glycogen storage disease is directed toward improvement of nutrition and correction of hypoglycemia and acidosis. This is accomplished by frequent feedings, including night feedings, and the use of glucose or Dexin between meals. Bridge and Holt recommend an extra high protein meal of ground beef and bread late at night. Ulstrom et al. found corticotropin useful for this purpose. Gradual symptomatic improvement as the children grow older is the rule, although hepatomegaly usually persists.

ALEXANDER B. GUTMAN

References

Bridge, E. M., and Holt, L. E., Jr.: Glycogen Storage Disease. J. Pediat., 27:299, 1945.
Cori, G. T.: Glycogen Structure and Enzyme Deficiencies in Glycogen Storage Disease. Harvey Lect., 48:145, 1952–53.

Di Sant'Agnese, P. A., Andersen, D. H., and Mason, H. H.: Glycogen Storage Disease of the Heart. II. Critical Review of the Literature. Pediatrics, 6:607, 1950.

Mason, H. H., and Andersen, D. H.: Glycogen Disease. Am. J. Dis. Children, 61:795, 1941.

McArdle, B.: Myopathy Due to a Defect in Muscle Glycogen Breakdown. Clin. Sc., 10:13, 1951.

Ulstrom, R. A., Ziegler, M. R., Doeden, D., and McQuarrie, I.: Metabolic and Clinical Effects of Corticotropin (ACTH) on Essential Glycogenosis (von Gierke's Disease). Metabolism, 1:291, 1952.

Van Creveld, S.: Glycogen Disease. Medicine, 18:1, 1939.

CONGENITAL GALACTOSEMIA
(Galactemia, Galactose Diabetes)

Congenital galactosemia is an inborn error of metabolism characterized by a defect in enzymes concerned with utilization of galactose. Large amounts of galactose therefore appear in the blood and urine after feedings of milk or other lactose- or galactose-containing foods.

The children from birth are feeding problems, refusing their bottles, vomiting, failing to show normal weight gain and growth, and exhibiting prominence of the abdomen because of distention and marked hepatomegaly. Jaundice and abnormal glycogen storage in the liver, with cirrhosis, may occur. Mental retardation is a common accompaniment. Bilateral cataracts develop early, as in experimental animals on a high galactose diet.

The fasting blood sugar and glucose and fructose tolerance curves are normal, but lactose and galactose tolerance tests show a marked and sustained rise in nonfermentable sugar. The urine contains large amounts of galactose for several hours after a lactose-containing meal. A trace of albumin is usually present.

All symptoms and signs disappear when milk and other foods containing lactose or galactose are excluded from the diet.

ALEXANDER B. GUTMAN

References

Bell, L. S., Blair, W. C., Lindsay, S., and Watson, S. J.: Galactose Diabetes (Galactosemia). J. Pediat., 36:427, 1950.

Townsend, E. H., Jr., Mason, H. H., and Strong, P. S.: Galactosemia and Its Relation to Laennec's Cirrhosis. Pediatrics, 7:760, 1951.

FRUCTOSURIA

After ingestion or intravenous infusion of fructose, appreciable amounts may appear in the urine of normal persons ("alimentary fructosuria"), larger quantities in the presence of severe liver damage. Because fructose reduces the reagents ordinarily employed in testing urine for sugar, fructosuria is often mistaken for glycosuria.

In essential fructosuria, an inborn error of metabolism, blood fructose levels are excessive and renal tubular reabsorption of fructose is inadequate to remove fructose altogether from the glomerular filtrate. The principal defect may be a deficiency of fructokinase.

The experience of Silver and Reiner indicates that fructosuria may not be as rare as is generally supposed. The disorder involves no disability, although a considerable proportion of ingested carbohydrate may be lost from diets rich in fruits or sucrose.

ALEXANDER B. GUTMAN

References

Peters, J. P., and Van Slyke, D. D.: Quantitative Clinical Chemistry. 2nd ed. Baltimore, Williams and Wilkins, 1946, Vol. I, p. 213.

Silver, S., and Reiner, M.: Essential Fructosuria. Arch. Int. Med., 54:412, 1934.

PENTOSURIA

Pentosuria is a rare inborn error of metabolism characterized by the excretion of pentose, usually of d-xyloketose, occasionally of l-xyloketose or d-ribose. Essential pentosuria is to be distinguished from alimentary pentosuria, which may occur in normal persons after the ingestion of large amounts of vegetable gums, fruits or berries rich in pentosans. The condition involves no disabilities, but may be confused with glycosuria because of the reducing properties of the pentoses in question. The distinction may be made by means of the orcinol reaction, lack of fermentation with yeast, and preparation of the phenylosazone derivative.

ALEXANDER B. GUTMAN

Reference

Peters, J. P., and Van Slyke, D. D.: Quantitative Clinical Chemistry. 2d ed. Baltimore, Williams and Wilkins, 1946, Vol. I, p. 212.

CONGENITAL METHEMOGLOBINEMIA

Definition. Congenital methemoglobinemia is a disorder characterized by an inborn specific enzyme deficiency in erythrocytes leading to accumulation of methemoglobin and consequent inadequate oxygen transport.

Etiology. Unlike the acquired form resulting from ingestion of acetanilid and other aniline derivatives, nitrites, chlorates or sulfanilamide, there is no history of exposure to toxic agents in congenital methemoglobinemia. The conversion of methemoglobin, containing hemoglobin iron in the ferric state and therefore incapable of carrying oxygen, to hemoglobin, containing ferrous iron, is inherently deficient. As a result, methemoglobin may comprise 30 to 40 per cent of the total pigment as compared with the normal of approximately 0.4 per cent.

This conversion, a reduction, has been shown by Gibson to involve a complex series of enzyme reactions within the red cell, the pathway of electron transport being glucose or lactate → coenzyme I → coenzyme factor I (diaphorase, a flavoprotein) → methemoglobin. Gibson's work indicates that in congenital methemoglobinemia this transfer is interrupted because of a specific deficiency in erythrocyte coenzyme factor.

Symptoms and Signs. Congenital methemoglobinemia becomes manifest early in life as a diffuse, persistent, gray or slate-blue cyanosis, simulating in appearance that of the "blue babies" associated with congenital heart lesions of the cyanotic type. Cardiac or respiratory distress is notably absent, although exertion often elicits dyspnea, palpitation, fatigability and severe headache. Cardiac murmurs are uncommon, and clubbing of the fingers does not occur. The conjunctivas are injected. The retinal veins appear dark and congested. In severe cases marked compensatory polycythemia develops, with associated reticulocytosis.

The blood has a chocolate hue and, when oxygenated, fails to recover its normal red color. The pigment is identified as methemoglobin spectroscopically by its absorption band.

Treatment. Recognition of congenital methemoglobinemia is important because confusion with surgically amenable congenital heart disease may lead to needless exploration and because effective treatment is available once the proper diagnosis has been established. Continued administration of methylene blue by mouth will restore the oxygen capacity of the blood and maintain the patient free of cyanosis, headache and associated symptoms. Eder and his co-workers found that daily doses of 240 mg. in enteric-coated tablets alleviated all signs and symptoms, including polycythemia and reticulocytosis, and were well tolerated. Excessive amounts should not be used because methylene blue in massive dosage causes methemoglobin formation. Ascorbic acid in daily oral doses of 300 to 500 mg. is also efficacious, probably exerting a direct reducing action on methemoglobin.

The prognosis as to life is good.

ALEXANDER B. GUTMAN

References

Codounis, A.: Hereditary Methaemoglobinaemic Cyanosis. Brit. M. J., 2:368, 1952.

Eder, H. A., Finch, C., and McKee, R. W.: Congenital Methemoglobinemia. A Clinical and Biochemical Study of a Case. J. Clin. Investigation, 28: 265, 1949.

Gibson, Q. H.: The Reduction of Methaemoglobin in Red Blood Cells and Studies on the Cause of Idiopathic Methaemoglobinaemia. Biochem. J., 42: 13, 1948.

Taggart, J. V.: Congenital Methemoglobinemia, in Combined Staff Clinic on Inborn Errors of Metabolism. Am. J. Med., 8:102, 1950.

FANCONI SYNDROME

Definition. The term "Fanconi syndrome" is used to describe a somewhat variable complex of metabolic errors deriving from congenitally defective renal tubular reabsorptive and secretory mechanisms, usually without glomerular insufficiency, at least of proportionate degree. As originally described by Fanconi in children, the symptom complex of stunted growth and hypophosphatemic rickets with acidosis, renal glycosuria and amino-aciduria but (in contrast to hyperphosphatemic "renal rickets") without azotemia, has come to be classified as the more severe *juvenile* form. In *adults* the renal tubular deficiencies are apt to be less severe, although not different in essentials, and osteomalacia is the presenting skeletal disorder. Closely related is the more or less distinct symptom complex designated *renal tubular acidosis*.

Etiology. Microdissection of nephrons in two cases of Fanconi syndrome by Clay and associates revealed essentially normal appearing glomeruli, but there was a congenital anomaly of the proximal convoluted tubules, which were much shorter than the normal and joined to the glomerulus by an elongated, narrow "swan neck." The abnormal structural configuration of the first convolution implies functional deficiency, which is further indicated by histochemical evidence of absence of alkaline phosphatase in its usual location there. Some thinness and atrophy of the epithelium of the distal tubule were also noted.

These findings are, on the whole, in accord with renal function studies in Fanconi syndrome which suggest marked deficiencies in the reabsorptive capacities of the proximal convoluted tubule and relatively minor impairment of distal tubular function, usually with substantial preservation of the glomerular filtration rate. Thus there is excessive urinary loss of metabolites believed normally to be reabsorbed largely in the proximal convoluted tubule: glucose, phosphate, bicarbonate, amino acids, uric acid, acetoacetic acid and acetone; and with these a loss of fixed base, notably of potassium, and of ammonia. The characteristic systemic hyperchloremic acidosis may be attributed chiefly to inadequate tubular conservation of bicarbonate, and its consequences; this presumably also is responsible in part for frequent failure of the urine to show the low pH appropriate to the degree of systemic acidosis. Urinary losses account for the characteristically low serum bicarbonate, phosphate, potassium, uric acid and low normal or low glucose. The prolonged hypophosphatemia is probably the chief cause of the development of rickets in children and of osteomalacia in adults, although acidosis and possibly also parathyroid overactivity may play a role.

Symptoms and Signs. Severely afflicted children are malnourished and dehydrated, there is marked polyuria with isosthenuria and excessive thirst. Characteristic are acidosis without hyperglycemia or azotemia (other than due to dehydration), renal glycosuria and marked urinary excretion of organic acids, chiefly amino acids in wide variety and acetoacetic acid. Weakness may be pronounced, typical hypokalemic episodes may occur. Growth and development are delayed and the characteristic deformities of low-phosphorus rickets, relatively resistant to vitamin D, are present.

In the adult, weakness and marked weight loss may supervene, and one must be alert to the development of hypokalemic periodic paralyses, but the clinical picture is apt to be ushered in and dominated by the manifestations of osteomalacia. These include bone pain and tenderness, waddling gait, pathologic fractures and eventual incapacitation. Chemical studies reveal hypophosphatemia, normal calcium, elevated alkaline phosphatase, low bicarbonate, hypophosphatemia and the other findings already mentioned in the blood and urine, notably renal glycosuria and amino-aciduria. Roentgenograms show the typical pseudofractures of Milkman's syndrome, symmetrical infractions of bone particularly in the ribs, pubic bones, scapulas and femurs. Nephrocalcinosis does not occur. Progressive glomerular insufficiency is a common late sequel.

Renal tubular acidosis resembles the Fanconi syndrome in many of its clinical manifestations but is likely to be less severe and more amenable to management. In the adult, females are more commonly affected. Skeletal indications of progressive osteomalacia usually predominate. Nephrocalcinosis or renal calculi (with intermittent colic) are the rule. Polyuria, polydipsia and signs of urinary tract infection usually appear in the course of the disorder. Low serum bicarbonate, with hyperchloremic acidosis, is a regular finding, as well as hypophosphatemia and hypokalemia, occasionally sufficiently pronounced to cause marked muscle weakness and periodic paralysis. These are all attributable to excessive urinary excretion of these electrolytes. Renal glycosuria and distinct amino-aciduria, in contrast to the Fanconi syndrome, are absent. The urine is usually conspicuously alkaline or neutral in reaction, despite the marked systemic acidosis. Ammonia production and acidification of the urine are more consistently impaired than in the Fanconi syndrome, suggesting more extensive distal tubule involvement.

Treatment. Replacement of lost base by daily oral administration of 5 to 10 gm. of sodium bicarbonate or the equivalent of an alkalinizing mixture of citrates effectively relieves the acidosis and restores electrolyte balance in most cases. The manifestations of osteomalacia or rickets respond gratifyingly to vitamin D in doses of 50,000 units a day and calcium salts by mouth; to avoid further renal damage, however, these should not be pushed to hypercalcemia and should be discontinued upon healing of the skeletal lesions. Hypokalemic episodes require administration of potassium salts.

ALEXANDER B. GUTMAN

References

Albright, F., and Reifenstein, E. C., Jr.: The Parathyroid Glands and Metabolic Bone Disease. Baltimore, Williams and Wilkins Co., 1948.

Clay, R. D., Darmady, E. M., and Hawkins, M.: The Nature of the Renal Lesion in the Fanconi Syndrome. J. Path. & Bact., 65:551, 1953.

Dent, C. E.: Amino-Aciduria in Fanconi Syndrome. Biochem. J., 41:240, 1947.

Fanconi, G.: Der frühinfantile nephrotisch-glykosurische Zwergwuchs mit hypophosphatämischer Rachitis. Jahrb. f. Kinderh., 147:299, 1936.

McCune, D. J., Mason, H. H., and Clarke, H. T.: Intractable Hypophosphatemic Rickets with Renal Glycosuria and Acidosis (the Fanconi Syndrome). Am. J. Dis. Children, 65:81, 1943.

Milne, M. D., Stanbury, S. W., and Thomson, A. E.: Observations on the Fanconi Syndrome and Renal Hyperchloraemic Acidosis in the Adult. Quart. J. Med. 21:61, 1952.

Pines, K. L., and Mudge, G. H.: Renal Tubular Acidosis with Osteomalacia. Am. J. Med., 11:302, 1951.

Sirota, J. H., and Hamerman, D.: Renal Function Studies in an Adult Subject with the Fanconi Syndrome. Am. J. Med., 16:138, 1954.

CYSTINURIA AND CYSTINOSIS

Excessive urinary excretion of cystine has long been recognized as a rare familial metabolic error. Recent investigation by Dent and others indicates that lysine and arginine are also excreted in large amounts and that there may not be a sharp distinction from the amino-aciduria of the Fanconi syndrome. It has also been found that cystinurics can readily oxidize administered cystine, the cystine excreted in the urine arising largely from the methionine of ingested proteins, by way of cysteine.

The chief hazard of cystinuria is the formation of cystine calculi in the urinary tract. This may be minimized by maintaining an alkaline and copious urine.

Cystinosis is an inborn error of metabolism characterized by deposition of cystine throughout the reticuloendothelial system and in various organs, notably the kidneys. Renal insufficiency, renal rickets and dwarfism result. No treatment is known, and death in childhood is the rule.

ALEXANDER B. GUTMAN

References

Dent, C. E., and Rose, G. A.: Amino Acid Metabolism in Cystinuria. Quart. J. Med., 20:205, 1951.

Eberlein, W. R.: Aminoaciduria in Childhood: Cystinuria and Cystinosis. Am. J. M. Sc., 225:676, 1953.

Freudenberg, E.: Cystinosis: Cystine Disease (Lignac's Disease) in Children. In Advances in Pediatrics, Vol. 4, Chicago, Year Book Publishers, 1949, p. 265.

ALKAPTONURIA AND OCHRONOSIS*

Definition. Alkaptonuria is a rare disorder of the metabolism of the amino acids, tyrosine and phenylalanine, characterized by the excretion of homogentisic acid in the urine.

Pathogenesis. It occurs most commonly in males and is believed to be transmitted as a recessive trait. More than 200 cases have been described. It is now believed that homogentisic acid appears in the normal catabolism of tyrosine and phenylalanine and that these individuals have a deficiency of an enzyme system essential for its oxidation. Homogentisic acid is the only abnormal substance excreted in the urine. The metabolic disturbance is complete and the amount of homogentisic acid excreted is proportional to the amount of protein catabolized.

Diagnosis. The diagnosis is often suggested early in life by diapers or linen stained black or brown by urine and by a family history of alkaptonuria.

Urine. The color of the urine is normal when acid and freshly excreted; when alkaline, it may be dark. When alkali is added, it turns black. It reduces Benedict's solution, imparting a brown or black color to the supernatant fluid. This appearance should suggest the presence of an abnormal reducing substance other than glucose. Further identification can be made by more specific chemical tests, and if the diagnosis still remains in doubt, isolation of homogentisic acid from the urine will establish the diagnosis with certainty.

Ochronosis. Ochronosis is a clinical state characterized by the deposition of bluish black pigment in the cartilages, tendons and other types of connective tissue. The term ochronosis was derived from the ochre-like color of the pigment on histologic examination. In time, probably all alkaptonuric individuals develop some degree of pigmentation, but the intensity and distribution as seen clinically varies considerably. In its fully developed form, as seen in older alkaptonurics, it is manifested by a patch of light brown or slate gray pigment in the scleras on

* The author wishes to express his deep appreciation to Dr. Morton Galdston for his valuable assistance in the revision of this article.

either side of the corneal limbus, by a bluish discoloration of the external ears, nasal cartilage and superficial tendons of the hands, and brown pigmentation in the skin, cerumen, sweat and the nails. The pigmented ears are opaque to the transmission of light.

The term ochronosis also applies to similar pigmentation associated with clinical conditions other than alkaptonuria. It was formerly seen after long-continued application of phenol dressings to leg ulcers and it may occur in association with melanuria. The pigmentation observed after the use of phenol gradually recedes after the causative agent is discontinued. In contrast, the pigmentation associated with alkaptonuria, by virtue of the permanence of the metabolic disturbance, is persistent and progressive.

In spite of the similarity in distribution and appearance of the ochronotic pigments, their origin is distinct. Alkaptonuric pigment is a derivative of homogentisic acid, whereas melanotic pigment is derived from 3,4 dihydroxyphenylalanine ("dopa"). The enzyme tyrosinase catalyzes the oxidation of "dopa" to melanin, but there is no reason to believe it is also involved in the polymerization of homogentisic acid to the ochronotic pigment. The pathway by which phenol is converted to ochronotic pigment is unknown.

Arthritis. Pigment deposition in joint cartilages is accompanied by degenerative changes and arthritis. The severity of the arthritis is not necessarily proportional to the degree of joint pigmentation, but arthritis may be the chief complaint of middle-aged alkaptonurics and it is a prominent feature of the condition. The joints usually affected are the hip, knee, shoulder and the spine. The rate of progression of the arthritis and the intensity of symptoms vary widely among different patients.

Roentgenographic Findings. Roentgenographic examination of the spine may show the presence of intense calcification of the intervertebral disks which is characteristic of the disease. In addition, degenerative osteoarthritic changes are generally apparent in the involved joints. Calcific deposits are commonly seen in muscle tendons about the large joints. Stones may be demonstrated in the urinary bladder, prostate gland and the urethra.

Prognosis. The disease does not apparently decreased life expectancy. Except for the passage of black urine and the appearance of pigmentation in the second and third decades,

as described under Ochronosis, patients are relatively free of symptoms until the onset of arthritis in middle age.

Treatment. No specific treatment is available for alkaptonuria or for ochronosis associated with it. Scorbutic guinea pigs fed phenylalanine or tyrosine excrete homogentisic acid in the urine and this defect is corrected by vitamin C. In contrast, clinical alkaptonuria is not due to a vitamin C deficiency and this vitamin has no effect on the metabolic defect. The only effect of vitamin C in clinical alkaptonuria is that it delays to some degree the darkening of the urine because of its strong reducing properties. A restriction of dietary protein has been advocated, since this decreases the amount of homogentisic acid excreted per day and might theoretically decrease the rate of development of ochronosis. The arthritis resembles osteoarthritis and should be treated similarly. It does not respond favorably to agents found effective in rheumatoid arthritis, such as ACTH, cortisone and phenylbutazone.

J. MURRAY STEELE

References

Duncan, G. G.: Diseases of Metabolism. 3rd ed. Philadelphia, W. B. Saunders Company, 1952, pp. 168 and 675.

Galdston, M., Steele, J. M., and Dobriner, K.: Alcaptonuria and Ochronosis. With a Report of Three Patients and Metabolic Studies in Two. Am. J. Med., *13:*432, 1952.

Garrod, A. E.: Inborn Errors of Metabolism. 2nd ed. London, Henry Frowde, 1923.

Kohlmann: Alkaptonurie mit Ochronosis im Röntgenbilde. Verhandl. d. deutsch. Roentgengesel., 20:88, 1929.

Lerner, A. B.: Metabolism of Phenylalanine and Tyrosine. In Advances in Enzymology, Vol. 14. New York, Interscience Press, 1953, pp. 73–128.

Neubauer, O.: Handbuch der normalen und pathologischen Physiologie. Vol. 5. Berlin, Julius Springer, 1928, p. 851.

Oppenheimer, B. S., and Kline, B. S.: Ochronosis, with a Study of an Additional Case. Arch. Int. Med., 29:732, 1922.

HEPATOLENTICULAR DEGENERATION
(Wilson's Disease)

The disorder known as Wilson's disease is a familial, coarsely nodular cirrhosis of the liver, which in some patients is associated with progressive damage to the nervous system, resulting in the appearance of tremor and rigidity. There are two chief types of the disease. One is a more rapidly progressive disorder appearing in late childhood or early adolescence, with parkinsonian rigidity and pseudobulbar symptoms in addition to tremor, and is the "progressive lenticular degeneration" of Wilson. The other is a slowly progressive disorder characterized chiefly by tremor and titubation, appearing in the third or fourth decade, and running a course of many years ("pseudosclerosis"). Intermediate, mixed types are more common than these extremes.

Pathology. Some degree of coarsely nodular cirrhosis of the liver is found in all cases, with variable extent of recent degeneration of some lobules, of the type seen in acute yellow atrophy. Regenerative activity is intense. In a few cases portal obstruction and its effects are obvious, but in most this is minimal.

The nervous system may appear normal to the naked eye except for some shrinkage of the basal ganglia, and brownish pigmentation of the putamen (the outer segment of the lenticular nucleus). Throughout the central nervous system, but most evident in the cerebral cortex, basal ganglia, thalamus and dentate nuclei, there is a great increase in number of the large astrocyte nuclei. These astrocytes are sometimes present in lobulated or even giant cell forms, with light brown pigment in the cytoplasm. In the more rapidly progressive forms of the disease edematous areas in the glia appear in the frontal cortex, lenticular and dentate nuclei. When intense this process leads to the appearance of cavitation in these situations, as originally described by Wilson.

The pigmentation of the cornea is present in fine granules in Descemet's membrane, and has been shown chemically and spectroscopically to contain chiefly copper, with traces of zinc and other metals. The pigment in the cerebral glia, the liver and occasionally the skin appears to be identical. The copper content of the liver and of the brain, especially the basal ganglia, is greatly increased. There is no evident renal lesion, and in distinction from the Fanconi syndrome the first collecting tubule is reported to be of normal length.

Symptoms and Signs. In some families the cirrhosis is a prominent feature, and episodes of ascites or hematemesis are frequent. More commonly, symptoms of liver damage are entirely absent, though cirrhosis is invariably present in some degree. Jaundice is not a symptom, and tests of liver function are usually not helpful unless there has been clinical evidence of a recent hepatic embarrassment. Cephalin and thymol flocculation have been the most frequently positive liver function tests.

A consistently high output of urinary amino acids and high urinary copper content are the most constant findings. Normally all copper is excreted in the bile, but in Wilson's disease 200 to 700 micrograms is excreted in the urine in 24 hours. This copper is derived from the diet. The characteristic copper-containing protein in blood plasma, ceruloplasmin, is greatly reduced in amount, and more loosely bound copper is also reduced. Administration of amino acids increases the output of copper in the urine, presumably bound to amino acids. Similar amino-aciduria has been found with uranium and lead poisoning. The significance of low blood ceruloplasmin is uncertain, but it is possibly primarily related to the overabsorption of copper from the gut, its abnormal accumulation in the tissues and abnormal excretion.

The patient may succumb to the effects of hepatic cirrhosis without developing neurologic symptoms other than terminal coma. More commonly tremor and dystonia with pseudobulbar phenomena in the form of dysarthria and fixed smiling expression appear. In the more rapidly progressive forms of the disease dystonic attitudes such as overpronated postures of the arms, choreic movements, inversion of the feet, open-mouthed fixed smile and difficulty in mental concentration first appear between the ages of 14 and 18, the earliest age reported being 8 years. In a few months the limbs may become greatly distorted by dystonic rigidity, and slow rhythmical tremors appear, leading to a termination in one to three years. If the onset occurs after the age of 18 to 20 the course is slower and the characteristic tremor is prominent. When the neurologic disorder appears after the age of 30, tremor and dysarthria may be the only signs, associated with slow mental deterioration. The tremor is a flapping of the hands at the wrist, as in waving good-by, and is present when the hands are outstretched. It is then accompanied by alternating adduction-abduction at the shoulder. Titubation of the head and dysarthria are common, indicating that the essential tremor is cerebellar in type. In more progressive types of the disease a plastic rigidity of the limbs and set expression of the face appear, and in time the pill-rolling tremor of the fingers of parkinsonian type is added. The lower limbs then also become affected.

Pigmentation of the outer margin of the cornea in the form of a smoky brownish ring (the Kayser-Fleischer ring), seen best by oblique lighting, is absolutely characteristic of this disease. It is constant in the more chronic forms, but may be absent in the more rapidly progressive forms of the disease.

Treatment. Treatment by diets designed to favor liver function has not had any lasting effect on the neurologic symptoms. Improvement, sometimes striking in degree, has followed the periodic mobilization of copper deposits by courses of BAL (2,3-dimercaptopropanol), 1 to 1.5 cc. of 10 per cent solution in peanut oil, once daily for twenty days repeated at intervals of two to six months. Calcium disodium versenate, a chelating agent, given by mouth in the form of 250 mg. tablet before each meal, lessens absorption of copper and delays the intervals before symptoms again worsen and BAL is again required. Sulfite and amino acids have been used for the same purpose. No satisfactory way of eliminating copper from the diet has been found. Stramonium somewhat lessens the rigidity. General anesthetics and barbiturates are very poorly tolerated.

D. DENNY-BROWN

References

Cummings, J. N.: The Copper and Iron Content of Brain and Liver in the Normal and in Hepatolenticular Degeneration. Brain, 71:410, 1948.

Denny-Brown, D.: Diseases of the Basal Ganglia and Subthalamic Nuclei. In Christian, H., Ed.: Oxford System of Medicine, Vol. 6, New York, Oxford University Press, 1945, Chap. 11.

———, and Porter, H.: The Effect of BAL (2,3,-Dimercaptopropanol) on Hepatolenticular Degeneration (Wilson's Disease). New England J. Med., 245:917, 1951.

Hall, H. C.: La Dégénérescence Hépato-lenticulaire. Paris, Masson et Cie, 1921.

Matthews, W. B., Milne, M. D., and Bell, M.: The Metabolic Disorder in Hepato-lenticular Degeneration. Quart. J. Med. 21:245, 1952.

Scheinberg, I. H., and Gitlin, D.: Deficiency of Ceruloplasmin in Patients with Hepatolenticular Degeneration (Wilson's Disease). Science, 116:484, 1952.

Uzman, L., and Denny-Brown, D.: Amino-aciduria in Hepatolenticular Degeneration (Wilson's Disease). Am. J. M. Sc., 215:599, 1948.

———, and Hood, B.: The Familial Nature of the Amino-aciduria of Wilson's Disease (Hepatolenticular Degeneration). Am. J. Med. Sc., 223:392, 1952.

Zimdahl, W. T., Hyman, I., and Cook, E. D.: Metabolism of Copper in Hepatolenticular Degeneration. Neurology, 3:569, 1953.

FAMILIAL PERIODIC PARALYSIS

This syndrome is characterized by periodic attacks of flaccid paralysis usually involving the muscles of all four extremities and the trunk, but occasionally affecting only the arms or legs. The condition is hereditary, has its onset during the first or second decade of life, and persists for a number of years. The attacks usually develop during the night and, if untreated, last for a few hours to a few days. The tendon reflexes are abolished; the muscles can be completely refractory to all types of stimulation, and during particularly severe attacks cardiac and respiratory involvement can occur. Sensation and mental faculties are not impaired. During periods between attacks the findings are normal. The attacks are associated with low levels of serum potassium and can be terminated by the oral administration of potassium chloride (5 to 10 gm.). Recurrences can be prevented by doses of potassium chloride daily (2 or more gm. before retiring) and the avoidance of measures that significantly lower the serum potassium, such as the ingestion of large amounts of carbohydrates.

A. T. MILHORAT

References

Gass, H., Cherkasky, M. and Savitsky, N.: Potassium and Periodic Paralysis. A Metabolic Study and Physiological Considerations. Medicine, 27:105, 1948.

Stewart, H. J., Smith, J. J., and Milhorat, A. T.: Electrocardiographic and Serum Potassium Changes in Familial Periodic Paralysis. Am. J. M. Sc., 199:789, 1940.

Talbott, J. H.: Periodic Paralysis. A Clinical Syndrome. Medicine, 20:85, 1941.

PHENYLPYRUVIC OLIGOPHRENIA
(Phenylpyruvic Amentia, Phenylketonuria)

Definition and Genetics. Phenylpyruvic oligophrenia, first described by Fölling in 1934, is a hereditary disease characterized by severe mental deficiency and by a metabolic aberration manifested by the urinary excretion of phenylpyruvic acid ($C_6H_5CH_2CO$

COOH). Genetic studies of families have proved that the condition is transmitted as a simple mendelian recessive trait. Jervis, in a study of 125 families, found 52 in which more than one sibling was affected. In England, Penrose studied the families of 203 initial cases and found that 129 of 638 siblings were affected; in 30 of the 203 families the parents were first cousins. Evidence of other etiologic factors, such as maternal toxemia, birth injury, infectious disease or endocrine disorder, is lacking.

Incidence. The reported incidence of the disease varies in different countries and probably depends to some extent on the awareness of investigators. In the United States and Great Britain, where extensive genetic, clinical and metabolic studies have been conducted, the incidence in the total population seems to be about 1:25,000 and 1:50,000 respectively; in institutions for the feebleminded, 0.3 to 0.8 per cent of inmates of all ages. In Norway, Fölling and his associates discovered 34 cases, or 1.4 per cent of about 2400 mental defectives tested. Swiss investigators found only 3 cases, or about 0.1 per cent, in tests on about 2500 mental defectives. Apparently no search has been made in Germany. The disease has not to date been reported in Negroes; only one case has been described in a Jewish child.

Clinical Findings. The most striking and consistent clinical finding is mental deficiency, generally of severe degree. Psychometric tests of institutionalized phenylketonurics place about 60 to 65 per cent in the idiot range (I.Q. below 20) and 30 to 35 per cent in the imbecile range (I.Q., 20 to 50). Their responses to standard intelligence tests are more characteristic of failure of development than of deterioration of previously developed mentality. The mental retardation is commonly recognized at an early age. As infants, they display lack of interest in their surroundings and are slow to walk and talk. Many also have convulsions. The patients usually continue apathetic and good-natured in later life; however, they often exhibit transient restlessness and noisy irritability when disturbed, as by examination procedures.

The physical appearance of these patients is usually characteristic and quite distinctive from that of patients with other specific and nonspecific forms of mental deficiency. More than 85 per cent of phenylketonurics have blond hair and fair complexion, some even approaching albinism. Their coloring is often lighter than that of their parents and normal siblings. They have attractive facies, and a slightly small or average-sized head and stature. A number of pregnancies are recorded in phenylketonuric patients, some resulting in normal infants; in one family in which the mother was affected there were two normal and two phenylketonuric children.

The frequency and variety of skin manifestations are probably related to the low content of skin pigment. They range from dermatographia, photosensitivity, and increased sweating, to eczema which may be patchy and transient or extensive and intractable. Eczema was prominent in three patients under three years of age admitted to The New York Hospital. In Jervis' survey of 213 cases from several American institutions, at least 50 per cent had an eczematoid eruption; on the other hand, in some smaller American series it was not noted or was specifically stated to be absent, and it does not appear to be a conspicuous finding in the British accounts.

Besides the skin manifestations, another prominent clinical feature involves the nervous system. Neurologic signs vary greatly in individual patients. Clumsiness and hyperactive reflexes are almost universally present; the patients learn to walk late (two and one-half to eight years), and many have a stiff, jerky, short-stepped gait often associated with kyphotic posture or a semirigid forward bending at the hips. Stereotyped repetitive motions, including head-nodding and so-called "digital mannerisms," sometimes described as athetoid, are common; fine tremors are less common. Recurrent daily epileptiform seizures are seen in some patients. Higher grade phenylketonurics may exhibit normal posture and gait and none of the neurologic stigmata except hyperactive tendon reflexes and occasional tremors. Many investigators consider these symptoms part of an extrapyramidal syndrome; most are of the opinion that the varied neurologic pictures are nonspecific.

Metabolic Aberration. Diagnosis is established by a simple qualitative chemical test of freshly voided urine for phenylpyruvic acid, which is constantly excreted in amounts ranging from about 0.5 to 2 gm. daily. To about 5 cc. of urine, acidified with dilute sulfuric acid, a few drops of fresh 5 per cent ferric chloride solution are added; if phenylpyruvic acid is present, a deep bluish green color appears immediately.

Phenylketonemia is as characteristic of the disease as phenylketonuria; Jervis found blood levels of phenylpyruvic acid from 0.31 to 1.78 mg. per 100 cc. in 39 patients aged 4 to 68 years. Blood phenylalanine is also abnormally high.

The primary metabolic defect is not a failure of the tissues to break down phenylpyruvic acid, but an inability to handle phenylalanine through one of its normal metabolic channels: hydroxylation in the para position to tyrosine. A part of the unconverted phenylalanine is deaminated; in the light of Jervis' recent studies it appears that this takes place both in the kidneys and in extrarenal tissue. Either d-, or d,l-phenylalanine ingested by one of these patients causes a rise in the blood level. Dann et al. showed a dose of d,l-phenylalanine to be quantitatively accounted for: within 48 hours it was excreted, about 50 per cent as phenylpyruvic acid and the rest as phenyllactic acid and phenylalanine in d- and l- forms, the extra-urinary output of the amino acid and these intermediates equaling the test dose. At the same time, ingestion of this amino acid did not raise the urinary output of tyrosine and its derivatives. The metabolic breakdown of ingested tyrosine was complete, just as in normal persons.

It is presumed that an enzymatic lack underlies the metabolic defect; Jervis demonstrated, in extracts of liver obtained at autopsy from two of these patients, the absence of a factor capable, in controls, of catalyzing the conversion of phenylalanine to tyrosine. However, doubt has been cast on the completely quantitative nature of the defect, and therefore on the theory of a simple enzyme deficit as its cause, by Udenfriend and Bessman, who reported recovery as tyrosine of a small but measurable fraction of C^{14}-labeled d,l-phenylalanine fed to two patients with the disease.

The relationship between this innate metabolic aberration and albinism, alkaptonuria, tyrosinosis and the experimental defect in aromatic amino acid metabolism induced in some animals and premature infants in the absence of ascorbic acid is a fascinating subject that deserves exploration. It is also of interest that temporary phenylketonuria has been produced in normal adults and in albino rats by oral d-phenylalanine intakes.

There is no real evidence to indicate that the intrinsic failure to convert phenylalanine to tyrosine is causally related to the mental defect or to the skin manifestations of phenylketonurics. Fölling suggested that the metabolic defect may be primary, and diminished mental capacity secondary. However, Jervis did not find a positive correlation between degree of mental deficiency and phenylpyruvic acid levels in the blood, as might have been expected if the metabolic defect were a cause of the mental one; instead, there appeared to be a positive relation between food intake and blood level of the keto acid. Since in none of the many published reports have phenylketonuria and normal mentality been associated, and, conversely, since relatives of affected persons whose urine is negative show no higher incidence of mental disease than the population as a whole, it seems reasonable to infer that the metabolic and mental defects are inseparably associated because they are inherent in the same gene. With respect to the skin manifestations, one could conjecture that the low content of melanin in these subjects might stem from their inability to convert phenylalanine into tyrosine, the precursor of melanin. Experimental evidence for this concept is still lacking.

Pathologic Findings. There is no consistent pathologic picture. In the few reported autopsies a variety of abnormalities of the central nervous system has been described in isolated cases: edema of the brain, cord and optic nerves; gliosis; degeneration of myelin; multiple nerve tumors, and hypoplasia of the hypophysis. Other cases have shown only a diminished size of the brain. None of these findings is specific.

Prognosis. The prognosis for normal or even fair mental development is unqualifiedly bad; that for life, in a sheltered environment, is apparently good, though in the low grade patients there is the same liability to succumb to intercurrent infection found in other idiots. No specific treatment is of any value; administration of ascorbic acid or thiamine has no influence on the metabolic error.

The importance of prompt diagnosis, despite the discouraging prospect, is not to be discounted. It enables the physician to give a definitive prognosis, to prepare for institutionalization in those cases (the great majority) in which it is desirable, to rule out the disease in siblings whose urine gives a negative ferric chloride test, to warn against consanguineous marriages in relatives of patients, and to prevent "shopping around" for ineffectual attempts at treatment.

S. Z. Levine
Margaret Dann

References

Dann, M., Marples, E., and Levine, S. Z.: Phenylpyruvic Oligophrenia. Report of a Case in an Infant with Quantitative Chemical Studies of the Urine. J. Clin. Investigation, 22:87, 1943.

Fölling, A.: Ueber Ausscheidung von Phenylbrenztraubensäure in den Harn als Stoffwechselanomalie in Verbindung mit Imbezillität. Ztschr. f. physiol. Chem., 227:169, 1934.

———, Mohr, O. L., and Ruud, L.: Oligophrenia Phenylpyrouvica. A Recessive Syndrome in Man. Dybwad. Oslo, 1945.

Jervis, G. A.: The Genetics of Phenylpyruvic Oligophrenia. J. Ment. Sc., 85:719, 1939.

———: Studies on Phenylpyruvic Oligophrenia. Phenylpyruvic Acid Content of Blood. Proc. Soc. Exper. Biol. & Med., 81:715, 1952.

———: Phenylpyruvic Oligophrenia. Deficiency of Phenylalanine-oxidizing System. Proc. Soc. Exper. Biol. & Med., 82:514, 1953.

Penrose, L. S.: Phenylketonuria, a Problem in Eugenics. Lancet, 1:949, 1946.

Udenfriend, S., and Bessman, S. P.: The Hydroxylation of Phenylalanine and Antipyrine in Phenylpyruvic Oligophrenia. J. Biol. Chem., 203:961, 1953.

GOUT AND GOUTY ARTHRITIS

Gout is a disease of unknown origin characterized by: (1) acute recurrent arthritis, sometimes chronic arthritis later, (2) slow accumulation of sodium biurate, manifested by hyperuricemia and tophi, and (3) sometimes terminal lesions affecting the kidneys, or blood vessels of the heart or brain. "Acute gout" is a misnomer; gout *per se* is always chronic.

Gout is seen commonly by those looking for it. It is not the disease but an awareness thereof which "disappears" from time to time.

Predisposing Factors. About 95 per cent of patients are males. If a writer states that many more than 5 or 10 per cent of his gouty patients are females, his diagnostic criteria are open to question. The reported incidence of active familial gout has been low (7 to 18 per cent) among American patients, much higher (22 to 80 per cent) among British patients. Heredity is more apparent among juveniles than adults with gout. Gout occurs mostly in temperate zones. It is common in England and France, less common in North America, uncommon in Scandinavia, Poland and Russia, and almost unknown in the Orient and tropics. Negroes are rarely affected. Habitual or episodic excesses of food and drink probably do not predispose to gout *per se,* but they may incite acute gouty arthritis. They are provocative, not predisposing factors. Gout can occur in vegetarians and teetotalers. Commonly affected are those in occupations favored by the well-to-do or those exposed to gastronomic indulgence. Although the incidence of gout is higher among patients with blood dyscrasias (myeloid metaplasia, polycythemia, leukemia), most patients so afflicted do not develop gout.

Morbid Anatomy. In gout, urates tend to deposit in cartilage (ears, joints, rarely the nose), epiphysial bone, other articular structures, and kidneys, rarely elsewhere. Crystalline urates produce local necrosis and (unless tissue is avascular) an ensuing foreign body reaction with proliferation of fibrous tissue, the "gouty granuloma." Cartilaginous degeneration, synovial proliferation, destruction of subchondral bone ("destructive arthritis"), proliferation of marginal bone ("hypertrophic arthritis"), often synovial pannus, and sometimes fibrous or bony ankylosis may slowly develop. In the kidneys one finds gross and microscopic urate deposits in tubules, medulla and interstitial tissues, linear streaks in the pyramids, and uratic gravel or calculi. Secondary destructive and inflammatory reactions develop. Urate deposits have reportedly been found in heart valves.

Nonspecific lesions include: in the kidneys—glomerular fibrosis and hyalinization, nephrosclerosis, sometimes focal areas of pyelonephritis; elsewhere—nonurate degenerative lesions which may affect blood vessels of the heart and brain.

Evolution of Symptoms: Clinical Stages of Gout. The chief features (arthritis, hyperuricemia, tophi, late renal and cardiovascular complications) are the outward signs of a fundamental disturbance of which little is known. This disturbance ("gouty diathesis"; "gout *per se*") is in operation long before it first manifests itself as *clinical gout.* Developing fully, gout passes through successive stages: a larval, prearthritic stage; next, a stage of acute recurring gouty arthritis; and later, in some instances, a stage of chronic gouty arthritis.

Larval Stage. During this stage, which is generally symptomless or subclinical, the body is being unobtrusively conditioned for subsequent events. Asymptomatic "genetic" or "essential hyperuricemia" may or may not become manifest. Rarely, tophi or renal colic from urate gravel develops in this prearticular stage; their presence or significance is commonly overlooked. Gout and gouty arthritis are not synonymous; the latter is merely the dominant *symptom* of gout.

Stage of Chronic Gouty Arthritis. From five to forty (average twelve) years after the first attack, an important change may become apparent: the onset of chronic gouty arthritis, the second form of articular gout. Sometimes, when first discovered, it appears to be the residue of an acute attack; a joint no longer recovers completely. But it may develop insidiously, *without* immediate reference to any (previous) attack.

Chronically affected joints may be subject to superimposed acute attacks (phase 3, Fig. 75). But sometimes acute attacks (or "ex-

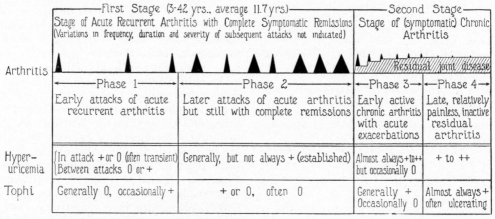

First Stage (3-42 yrs., average 11.7 yrs.)		Second Stage	
Stage of Acute Recurrent Arthritis with Complete Symptomatic Remissions (Variations in frequency, duration and severity of subsequent attacks not indicated)		Stage of (symptomatic) Chronic Arthritis	
Arthritis		Residual joint disease	
Phase 1	Phase 2	Phase 3	Phase 4
Early attacks of acute recurrent arthritis	Later attacks of acute arthritis but still with complete remissions	Early active chronic arthritis with acute exacerbations	Late, relatively painless, inactive residual arthritis
Hyperuricemia {In attack + or 0 (often transient) {Between attacks 0 or +	Generally, but not always + (established)	Almost always +to++ but occasionally 0	+ to ++
Tophi Generally 0, occasionally +	+ or 0, often 0	Generally + Occasionally 0	Almost always + often ulcerating

Fig. 75. The basic pattern of gout and gouty arthritis (untreated). (P. S. Hench; J. Lab. & Clin. Med., Vol. 22.)

Stage of Acute Recurrent Arthritis With Complete Remissions. The first attack of acute arthritis usually occurs suddenly, lasts several (perhaps three to fourteen) days, then disappears completely. It affects a great toe or, with almost equal frequency, ankle, instep, knee. Sooner or later (a few months, a year or longer) there is another attack, perhaps more severe or longer; it also disappears completely. Then attacks commonly increase in severity and frequency, coming semiannually or oftener.

Early attacks are generally monarticular, afebrile and short (phase 1, Fig. 75). Later attacks are often polyarticular, longer and perhaps febrile (phase 2). Permanent roentgenologic changes may slowly develop, despite which, in this stage of the disease, joints recover full, symptomless function.

During phases 1 and 2, attacks of acute olecranon bursitis may develop, also with complete remissions; in early attacks thereof there may be no palpable bursal tophi. Acute bursitis may develop with or without acute arthritis.

acerbations") cease to recur (phase 4). Chronic gouty arthritis usually become polyarticular; hands and feet may be misshapen by tophaceous deposits and deformities. Tophi are usually present on the ears. By now olecranon or prepatellar bursal walls may be chronically thickened from urate deposits and the tissue reactions thereto. Chronic tophaceous "bursitis" may be painless or mildly painful, a process apparently independent of the acute attacks of bursitis which may or may not continue to recur.

Thus the pattern of classic gouty arthritis can be divided *clinically* into two great stages comprising four phases (Fig. 75). Although the stage of chronic gouty arthritis (or chronic bursitis) *always* appears after that of acute recurrent gouty arthritis, these two clinical stages are not completely or necessarily interdependent; indeed from the etiologic or pathogenetic standpoint acute gouty arthritis and chronic gouty arthritis may be independent, unrelated developments.

Patients whose first attack develops in middle or later life may never reach stage 2 or develop notable tophaceous deposits, chronic gouty arthritis or significant renal involvement.

Acute Gouty Arthritis. *Typical Attack.* Some patients recognize prodromes: irritability, melancholia, nocturia, polyuria, vague muscular symptoms, nausea, dyspepsia, or sometimes euphoria and a ravenous appetite. Attacks begin any time, day or night. Those beginning at night, if severe, may awaken the patient in the early morning hours; if

ing subsides there may be itching and desquamation. Spontaneous recovery is sometimes slow, but often rapid—within a few or several days. In articular stage 1, clinical recovery is complete whether or not there are roentgenographic residues—a point of diagnostic importance. "A person subject to gout has won the race at the Olympiac games during the interval of the disease" (Aretaeus).

Predisposing and Provocative Factors. PREDISPOSING FACTORS. Among men over 35

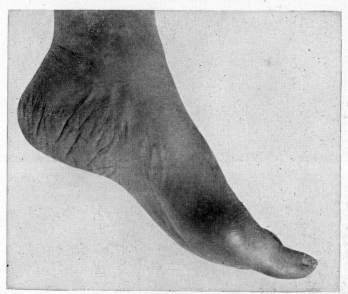

Fig. 76. Acute gouty arthritis of great toe.

mild, they do not awaken the patient but are noted first when, on awakening, he puts his foot to the floor.

In gout there is a gradient of articular vulnerability whereby distal joints—feet, ankles, hands, wrists—are most commonly affected. Knees and elbows are less vulnerable. Shoulders and hips are rarely affected *clinically* except in severe or late gout. Although the spinal column may be affected by urates, it practically always escapes attacks. Olecranon bursitis and tendinitis, especially of Achilles' tendon, often occur.

Attacks generally develop rapidly, sometimes slowly. Maximal disability may appear within 12 to 36 hours. Pain may be mild or moderate, but is often severe—so excruciating that the weight of bedclothes or vibration of the bed is unbearable. It is not always worse at night.

The affected part is swollen and tender, sometimes exquisitely so. The skin may be bright or deep red, sometimes dusky. Inflammatory, pitting edema may develop. As swell-

years of age gouty arthritis is the commonest form of acute arthritis. It should always be suspected when acute trauma and gonorrhea are excluded. Attacks come any time, commonly in spring and fall. Habitual (in contrast with acute) excesses of "rich" or purine-rich food and drink may condition patients to frequent attacks.

Precipitating Factors. There are many provocatives of acute gouty arthritis: trauma, acute indiscretions as to food or alcoholic drinks, psychic upsets, chilling and hemorrhage; certain therapeutic agents or procedures—liver extract, mercurial diuretics, ergotamine tartrate, testosterone propionate, roentgen therapy, probenecid (Benemid), thiamine chloride (vitamin B_1), dehydrocholic acid (Decholin), high-fat or ketogenic diets, penicillin, sulfathiazole, transfusion, purging, bleeding, possibly injections of pollen extract, and also corticotropin (ACTH) under certain circumstances. Contact with provocatives must be sought; patients rarely recognize them.

Attacks may be precipitated by minor trauma, as from excessive walking, long motoring (pedaling) and sports. True traumatic arthritis begins immediately after trauma; the reaction is proportionate to the severity trips with their trauma and indiscretions around the camp fire (meats, venison, liquor). The hunter may return home with game, gun and gout. Episodic excesses of food and alcohol do not cause the gout *per se* any more

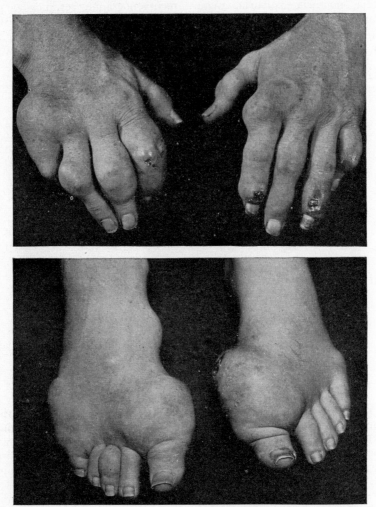

Fig. 77. Severe chronic gouty arthritis with ulcerating tophi.

of trauma, is confined to the traumatized region and is not relieved by colchicine; characteristics of gout (history, hyperuricemia, tophi) are absent. In post-traumatic gouty arthritis the reaction is often delayed some hours, is disproportionately severe after trivial trauma, often progresses to other joints, and is relieved by colchicine; other characteristics of gout may be discoverable.

Gouty arthritis is often provoked by acute dietary excesses associated with birthdays, weddings, Thanksgiving, New Year's Day, conventions, vacations and lodge night. Potent provocatives are hunting and fishing than sugar causes diabetes, but they may provoke quiescent gout and cause acute gouty arthritis. Some attacks seem to be provoked by foods, such as asparagus, which are not rich in purines but contain "allergens."

Surgical procedures commonly provoke acute gouty arthritis within the first seven postoperative days. "In a case of acute postoperative arthritis, suspect gout."

Accumulation of Urates. The following data refer mainly to untreated gout. Estimations of urates in *serum* are preferable to those made on whole blood. The upper limits of normal values for males are 6 or 6.5 mg.; for females, 5 or 5.5 mg. per 100 cc. of serum. According to certain writers, once arthritis occurs, hyperuricemia is present and persistent unless uricosuric agents are used. But many observers have found *normal* urate concentrations in serum or whole blood in 15 to 20 per cent of gouty patients at various

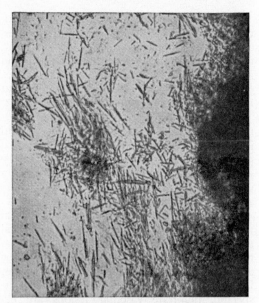

Fig. 79. Urate crystals from gouty tophus (× 435).

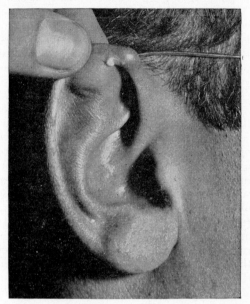

Fig. 78. Two tophi on ear.

stages of the disease, and increased values in 80 to 85 per cent (Hench; Mason). The blood urate levels of normal and gouty patients fluctuate considerably from day to day. In some gouty patients they fluctuate above and below the upper limit of normal, at least early in the disease; in others, concentrations remain above normal but fluctuate without regard to attacks or to the use of nonuricosuric agents, such as colchicine. In summary, hyperuricemia may or may not be present in phase 1 (Fig. 75), is generally present in phase 2, and is almost always present in phases 3 and 4.

Urinary concentrations of urate (during periods without treatment) fluctuate considerably even on a fixed diet. Estimations are not diagnostic.

Visible or palpable *subcutaneous tophi* may develop at any stage, occurring in about 40 to 50 per cent of cases. They are rare in the prearthritic stage, uncommon in phase 1, more frequent in phase 2, and almost always present in phases 3 and 4, when they may be multiple and ulcerating. They occur

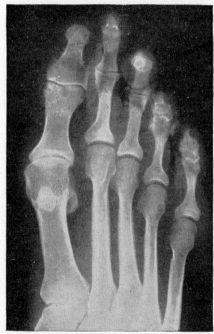

Fig. 80. Area of erosion (tophus), distal end of proximal phalanx of great toe.

usually on the ears (Fig. 78), and about olecranon bursae and peripheral joints. A "tophus" is not a proved tophus until urate crystals have been recovered therefrom (Fig. 79). Sometimes its identity should be certified by the murexide test or histologic study.

Areas of erosion of articular *bone* in gout represent replacement of bone by urates (Fig. 80). Osseous tophi are uncommon in phase

1, fairly common in phase 2, and more numerous and larger in phases 3 and 4. Areas of erosion (replacement of bone by nonurate debris) may occur in rheumatoid arthritis, osteoarthritis or lupus pernio. Hence erosions are not pathognomonic for gout, but if large or numerous they are usually gouty.

Sooner or later urate depositions affect certain renal tissues and constitute microtophi in the kidneys. On the distal side of the renal pelvic membrane, urates may precipitate, especially in acid urine, coalesce and form urogenital gravel or stones. Urate deposits may affect tendons but not muscular tissues *per se.*

Except for exceedingly rare endocardial urate deposits, the only examples of visceral gout are the urate accumulations, degenerative and inflammatory lesions in the kidney and the late, degenerative vascular changes in the kidneys, heart and brain. The nonspecific, nonurate vascular lesions are believed to be more than coincidental in gout —probably true complications.

About 10 to 20 per cent of gouty patients develop gouty nephritis or renal colic or both. Hence "suspect gout in cases of acute or chronic arthritis with renal colic or nephritis." Ulcerating tophi may complicate late gout and lead to amputation of digits.

Additional Laboratory Data. Erythrocyte sedimentation rates may be normal between attacks and in mild attacks, but elevated, sometimes markedly, in severe acute attacks and in chronic gouty arthritis. Serum concentrations of total cholesterol and esters are usually normal between attacks, sometimes subnormal during attacks (Wolfson and co-workers, 1949). Concentrations of urinary 17-ketosteroids are reported as being subnormal (average 3 mg. daily) by some, but as normal (average 9.5 mg. daily) by others who used a different method.

Cause of Death. Patients with mild gout and those responsive to prolonged therapy commonly live their full span of years and die from something coincidental to their gout. But there are many exceptions. Common causes of death are uremia from "gouty nephritis," myocardial infarction and apoplexy, recalling the old aphorism that "gout is to the arteries what rheumatic fever is to the heart."

Roentgenographic Appearance. The development of radiologically visible osseous tophi appears to be governed more by the gradient of articular vulnerability than by the general intensity of urate accumulation or the number and severity of attacks in any given joint. Even in severe gout when many proximal or less distal joints are extensively affected by urates (as shown later by necropsy), areas of erosion rarely become *apparent* roentgenographically except in the feet and hands. Such erosions appear occasionally in phase 1 (Fig. 75), but commonly in phase 2 and thereafter. Because the appearance of erosions is often delayed, roentgenograms of joints are of limited diagnostic usefulness. Periarticular thickening and nonspecific hypertrophic and destructive changes may involve joints, sometimes in phase 1 but generally not until phase 2 and thereafter.

Roentgenograms of the kidneys are also of limited value—urate stones cast no shadow.

Etiology and Pathogenesis. *Dissociation of Clinical Features.* It is impossible to regard a single factor, either an hereditary abnormality such as a "gouty gene" or one chemical substance such as urate, as the prime cause of all features of gout. The dominant clinical features are (1) the acute articular attacks and (2) the accumulation of urate (with the renal and *chronic* articular consequences thereof). But temporal relationships between the two are far from close, and their pathogenetic relationships are quite uncertain. Thus, although the patterns of acute gouty arthritis and of urate accumulation often, or commonly, develop together at what might be called the same *general* rate, the evolution of the one does not necessarily parallel that of the other or depend on it; the two patterns are often dissociated. If so, the proximate causes of gout's two main features may be quite separate, and one is obliged to study separately the pathogenesis of each feature of the disease.

Urate Accumulation: Etiology and Pathogenesis, Nature and Extent. Isotopic techniques now permit more accurate measurement of urate accumulations by estimation of the "miscible pool" of urate (Stetten; Talbott). When a small, measured amount of isotopically labelled uric acid of known concentration or "isotopic abundance" is injected intravenously into man, it mixes freely with the body's natural urates, the degree of dilution depending chiefly on the total amount of urates momentarily present in the body. Calculation of this dilution measures the "miscible pool," which is that quantity of urates in the body capable of mixing promptly with the injected urates and consequently of diluting the isotope (Stetten; Benedict and co-workers; Talbott). Among normals the miscible pool varies between 700 and 1400 mg. (average about 1 gm.), and about 500 to 850 mg. of old uric acid is replaced daily by newly formed (unlabelled) urate, a turn-over rate of 50 to 75 per cent. Among the few gouty patients studied to date the pool has always been increased, ranging between 1900 and 3400 mg. in mild or moderate gout, and 31,000 mg. in old, severe, un-treated, tophaceous gout. The peripheral, most recently precipitated, microcrystalline layers of tophi still in contact with body water are capable of either prompt resolution (under the influence of uricosuric agents) or reprecipitation, but the more central and solid urates are more resistant.

In a patient with severe tophaceous gout the miscible urate pool after irregular treat-ment was 18,450 mg. (15 times normal), rose after 4.5 months without treatment to 31,000 mg., then fell to 2084 mg. after the use of aspirin (2 to 4 gm. daily) for three or four months. But the serum urate re-mained practically constant (Benedict and co-workers). ACTH, cortisone or probenecid, given for short periods, reduced pools about 30 to 50 per cent and doubled the turnover rates by increasing renal clearance of urates and mobilizing the solid phase of miscible urates (Stetten). Such studies have been few and have utilized mathematical calculations, the accuracy of which has been questioned (Thannhauser, 1950).

Hereditary Factor in Hyperuricemia. LA-TENT GENETIC HYPERURICEMIA. Of 449 members of 87 gouty families, 21 per cent had clinical gout (arthritis and hyperuricemia or tophi), 15 per cent had symptomless hy-peruricemia with no (other) signs of gout, and 64 per cent had neither hyperuricemia nor active gout. The conclusion is that in-herent susceptibility to gout is transmitted by a single autosomal (that is, not sex-linked) dominant (gouty or "hyperuricemic") gene with a low penetrance in both sexes. (Talbott, 1940; Smyth and co-workers, 1948; Stecher and co-workers, 1949.) Most nonhyperuri-cemic relatives do not develop hyperuricemia in later life. Although hyperuricemia was present in certain relatives by the time they were examined, it was rarely present in boys or premenopausal women. In other words, about 20 to 25 per cent of members of gouty

families are born, not with actual hyperuri-cemia (postnatal, infantile or even juvenile), but as *carriers* of (latent) gouty hyperuri-cemia.

FRANK SYMPTOMLESS GENETIC HYPER-URICEMIA. Latent genetic hyperuricemia does not develop into hyperuricemia until after puberty in males or near the menopause in females. Nonhereditary factors related to sex, renal function and normal androgenic activity are considered responsible for this change. This inherited or "pregouty hyper-uricemia" is symptomless; it represents, not clinical gout, but susceptibility to clinical gout.

Regardless of its ultimate cause, by what mechanism does symptomless hyperuricemia develop? Three mechanisms have been con-sidered.

1. Diminished Destruction of Urates. Are gouty patients deficient in purinolytic fer-ment (for example, uricase), hence do not destroy urate adequately? Studies with iso-topically labelled uric acid suggest that in-testinal bacteria normally destroy small amounts of urate in the gut, and that the tis-sues of gouty patients (but not of normals) also destroy some urate (Benedict and co-workers).

2. Deficient Excretion. It was formerly be-lieved that urinary urate excretion was often subnormal in gouty patients, especially before acute attacks. But some gouty patients during and between attacks excrete more urate than nongouty controls. This does not necessarily indicate that the kidneys of gouty patients excrete urate in a normal manner (Berliner, 1940).

3. Increased Production: Biosynthesis of Uric Acid. Formerly the idea of overproduc-tion of urate in gout seemed untenable, since gouty hyperuricemia is not accompanied by increased excretion or accumulation of phos-phates as would be expected if destruction of nuclear protein were increased. But a differ-ent mechanism for urate production has been discovered.

Feeding experiments with glycine-N[15] reveal that uric acid in man is not solely de-rived from ingested purines, or nucleopro-teins, but can be synthesized from simple carbon and nitrogen compounds present in carbohydrate, protein and fat. Whether gouty patients differ from normals is not yet known. The mechanism responsible for urate ac-cumulation in gout is still unknown, but these newer data suggest overproduction of urate, at least in some cases.

Pathogenesis of Acute Gouty Arthritis. It is often assumed that there is a direct connection between hyperuricemia, urate deposits and acute articular attacks. Just before an articular attack, it is supposed, urinary urate excretion decreases, blood urate increases, and then irritating urate crystals are precipitated within articular tissues and cause the acute inflammatory reaction which constitutes the attack. Some time during the attack the mechanism is presumed to reverse: sudden urate diuresis promotes decrease in the blood urate level and articular healing. Actually, it is not known when urates are deposited, whether long before, just before, during or between attacks. According to some writers, an acute attack develops either when urate crystals are suddenly precipitated *de novo* (from supersaturated blood or extravascular fluid) into previously uncontaminated articular tissues, or when urates already present in articular cartilage suddenly burst into the joint space. But acute gouty arthritis is not a disease of the joint *space;* it is an intense inflammation of various articular and periarticular *tissues.*

Massive infiltration of articular tissues by urate can be long present and painless. Why would articular tissues remain long tolerant of their (sometimes extensive) urate infiltration and then suddenly react *acutely* either when some of this old urate is extruded into the joint *space,* or when a new crop of crystals is precipitated in the articular tissues?

In considering what relationship (if any) exists between urates and acute gouty arthritis, this summary should be noted: 1. In gout the evolution of *hyperuricemia* does not necessarily parallel that of acute gouty arthritis. 2. The pattern of acute gouty arthritis does not necessarily parallel that of subcutaneous or intra-articular urate deposition. Thus, (*a*) one patient with a few attacks develops extensive tophaceous gout and chronic gouty arthritis, whereas another with many attacks develops few tophi and no chronic arthritis; (*b*) joints never affected acutely or chronically have been found at necropsy to be "whitewashed" with urates; spinal joints do not escape urate deposition but acute gouty spondylitis almost never occurs; and (*c*) *per contra,* certain joints repeatedly attacked acutely have shown no *gross* urate deposits. 3. Acute attacks are unrelated to any consistent change in the urate concentration of

blood or urine; serum and urinary urate do not change in any characteristic way just before or during attacks. 4. The anti-inflammatory and uricosuric effects of drugs useful in gout can be dissociated. Thus, (*a*) acute attacks are relieved by certain antiphlogistic agents (for example, colchicine) which have no proved effect on urate metabolism or at least on urate excretion; (*b*) acute attacks are *not* relieved by large, uricosuric doses of probenecid; and (*c*) the comparative effectiveness of cortisone, corticotropin and salicylates on attacks is *not* based on their relative uricosuric activity. 5. The hyperuricemia of leukemia, polycythemia, and so forth, usually remains symptomless. 6. Urates *per se* are relatively innocuous. Thus, (*a*) peripheral tophi are usually painless, (*b*) acute arthritis is not provoked when urates are injected intravenously into nongouty persons or into gouty patients during or between attacks, and (*c*) urates injected subcutaneously are painless (Brown, 1938) or are no more painful in the gouty than the nongouty (von Muller, 1927). 7. Certain provocatives of acute gouty arthritis (purine-free liver extracts, wine, Salyrgan, Gynergen, surgical operations) have little or no obvious connection with urates or with marked changes in urate metabolism.

All these data suggest strongly that acute gouty arthritis bears little or no (direct) relationship to urates. But some precursor of urate might be responsible (Gutman).

Pathogenesis of Chronic Gouty Arthritis. Tissue reactions to foreign matter (tophaceous deposits) in and around joints are considered responsible for the slow development of chronic gouty arthritis.

From the foregoing, it would appear that urates may have little or nothing to do with acute gouty arthritis but "everything" (more or less) to do with chronic gouty arthritis, and that chronic gouty arthritis is not merely the end result of acute gouty arthritis or the sum total of acute attacks, but that acute and chronic gouty arthritis may be quite unrelated to each other, each having a different immediate cause and an independent (though sometimes parallel) evolution. The same can be said for the relationship between acute gouty bursitis (for example, olecranon) and chronic tophaceous bursal thickenings, painless or painful.

Pathogenesis of Gouty Nephritis. Renal dysfunction is considered the cause of gout by some, the result of gout by others. Whether or not the undefined "primary renal dysfunction" in the minds of the former is purely hypothetical or will some day be demonstrated, it is not to be confused with the secondary renal dysfunction of gouty nephritis—a late characteristic of gout. Intrarenal urate deposits presumably elicit a foreign body tissue reaction. Varying degrees of dysfunction and destruction of renal units result; superimposed thereon may be secondary infection.

Pathogenesis of Vascular Complications. The vascular lesions which may complicate severe or late gout bear no direct or obvious histopathologic relationship to urate; at least urate is practically never found therein. The mechanism of their production is unknown.

Adrenocortical, Anterior Pituitary or Hypothalamic Dysfunction. Recently the hypothesis has been advanced that gout is an endocrine disease characterized by deficiency of 11-oxysteroids. Presumably, chronic, *relative* lack of 11-oxysteroids is characteristic of symptomless, interval gout, and an even greater acute deficiency is related to acute attacks (Robinson and co-workers; Wolfson and co-workers). Since the adrenal cortices appear to be normally responsive in gout, at least to exogenous ACTH, the hypothetical dysfunction involves either the anterior pituitary or, more likely, the hypothalamus, with sluggishness in providing enough endogenous ACTH to satisfy the 11-oxysteroid requirements put upon the gouty patients by various stresses.

Space does not permit elaboration of the pros and cons of this hypothesis, but no adrenocortical dysfunction during or between attacks has been found by other workers. Colchicine does not increase adrenocortical activity. Clinically recognized disorders of the anterior pituitary or adrenals either with hypofunction or hyperfunction are not associated with gout. There is as yet no convincing evidence that pituitary or adrenocortical dysfunction plays a *primary* role in the etiology or pathogenesis of either gout or acute gouty arthritis.

Diagnosis. The presence of any characteristic feature (podagra, hyperuricemia, peripheral tophi, erosions) is of great diagnostic significance, but the appearance of any one is often delayed until rather late in the disease. The metatarsophalangeal joint of a great toe is affected early or repeatedly in some cases, rarely or never in others. Also hyperuricemia is usually present, but one must not insist on its presence or that of podagra before diagnosing gout. Usually a long, rather than a short, time elapses between "toe and tophus." If other features are present, a diagnosis of pretophaceous gout is appropriate without tophi. The pattern of recurrent arthritis with complete remissions is of itself so distinctive as to be almost pathognomonic, although episodic rheumatoid arthritis and palindromic rheumatism must be excluded. If diagnosis of any single attack is not helped by the history of previous attacks or if the initial attack is under consideration, diagnosis is based on the characteristics of an attack as described, including predisposing and provocative factors. If an attack promptly responds to treatment (especially to colchicine, specific for gout) and if the disease subsequently is largely controlled by a gout regimen, the diagnosis of gout is justified even before the development of tophi. Provocative tests are of uncertain diagnostic value; no provocative is consistently effective, probably because of the variable "goutiness" of patients.

Prognosis. Prognosis is best for those who first manifest gout late in life, poorest for those whose symptoms begin before the age of 20 or 25 years. But estimation of prognosis is difficult. The frequency of attacks and the rate of urate accumulation may change capriciously. "The disease sticks to him till death," so wrote Aretaeus about 1600 years ago. This is still true, but thanks to recent developments patients now have better means of controlling their disease. Therapeutic results depend largely on the patient's self-discipline and ability to follow throughout life an individualized, sometimes changeable regimen. He must understand the nature of gout, and realize that his acute attacks are merely the episodic, surface explosions of an underlying disease which is always present even when symptomless, and that he has a lifelong campaign to conduct, not just the next short-lived acute skirmish to control. More patients fail from ignorance or lack of will power than from unresponsiveness to treatment. Optimism is justified: irreversible gout is now less common than ever before.

Prophylaxis and Treatment. Although one could prescribe measures to slow the progress of symptomless, genetic or "pregouty" hyperuricemia among relatives of gouty patients, as a rule none is advocated; few gouty candidates would accept them. If a person, usually a male, is found, perhaps accidentally, to have hyperuricemia and either a small tophus or renal colic from urate, he has definite clinical gout even though acute gouty arthritis has not yet developed. Such (rare) patients should consider seriously the regimen for interval gout.

Each phase and feature of classic gout requires its own treatment. Measures for acute gouty arthritis are chiefly anti-inflammatory; those for symptomless interval gout are uricosuric and prophylactic; those for chronic gouty arthritis are uricosuric and anti-inflammatory; and those for gouty nephritis, renal colic or tophaceous ulcers are of a special nature.

Acute Gouty Arthritis. Most important for the treatment of acute gouty arthritis is its recognition; few conditions respond more promptly to appropriate measures.

For suspected attacks: Patients who recognize some characteristic *non*articular prodrome or wonder whether mild articular twinges represent an impending attack may abort it by taking orally a few doses of colchicine (0.65 mg. every 1 to 2 hours). It is wiser to do this for a possible false alarm than to let an attack become established.

For recognized attacks: Affected parts should be completely rested, preferably in bed, sometimes in a light splint. Lower extremities should be protected from bedclothes by a light wooden or metal cradle. Activity or weight-bearing should be curtailed until pain and tenderness are gone; otherwise an exacerbation may result. Hot water or ice-cold compresses (every 2 to 3 hours) are often preferable to dry heat; compresses of magnesium sulfate or lead lotion are sometimes prescribed.

Colchicine, given orally, is generally the treatment of choice. But it is commonly misapplied. Necessary for success are: (1) prompt administration, (2) proper total dosage and (3) proper rate of dosage, so as to provide a maximal antiarthritic effect with minimal gastrointestinal irritation. If individual doses are too large or too closely spaced, gastrointestinal irritation may develop before articular relief is obtained. If doses are too small or too widely spaced, effective blood concentrations are not obtained. The sooner colchicine is given the smaller is the total dose required and the better the chance for relief without significant gastrointestinal irritation.

Colchicine tablets, each containing 0.53 or 0.65 mg., are prescribed thus: two tablets initially and one tablet usually every 2 (waking) hours, sometimes every hour or every 3 hours, depending on individual responsiveness, severity of attacks and probable "nearness" to toxicity. Colchicine is given until gastrointestinal symptoms (diarrhea, sometimes nausea or vomiting) appear. If a second course is required, two or three days should intervene between courses, or until diarrhea subsides. Some patients, having learned their toxic or "diarrheal dose" (usually about six to fourteen tablets), may be able in subsequent attacks to obtain a therapeutic, without a toxic, effect by taking one or two less tablets to a course. If not, and if troublesome diarrhea impends or develops, codeine or paregoric may prevent or control it. Patients should always keep colchicine tablets handy at home, at the place of business, and especially in the suitcase for travel emergencies. If attacks are treated promptly, relief may begin within a few (12 to 24) hours, and be more or less complete within about 24 to 72 hours. But in severe attacks or in patients less responsive to colchicine, symptoms may persist for days or even weeks.

Colchicine given intravenously usually produces quicker results, often without toxicity. This is indicated (1) whenever rapid relief is particularly desirable, (2) when good results from colchicine given orally are complicated by marked gastrointestinal irritation, (3) for acute postoperative attacks, (4) for attacks unresponsive to colchicine given orally, perhaps belatedly. Individual doses have varied from 0.65 mg. one to three times daily to 3 mg. once daily; the latter is the most effective (Graham and Roberts; Ward). Patients often require only one or two injections, occasionally more. Relief may begin within an hour or two of the first injection, is often notable within 6 to 12 hours and is more or less complete within 18 to 36 hours (Ward). Gastrointestinal irritation rarely develops from one or two injections (1.5 to 3 mg. each, 8 to 24 hours apart), but may be mild or moderate if several injections are required.

Colchicine is very irritating if injected outside the vein.

Corticotropin (ACTH) (aqueous) in sufficient doses rapidly controls most acute attacks, even those unresponsive to colchicine. If enough ACTH or cortisone is given long enough, attacks are usually controlled without relapses. Misnamed "withdrawal flares" are simply relapses of attacks caused by premature discontinuance of temporarily adequate treatment, or discontinuance of doses which were never adequate, and are not due to ACTH-induced pituitary-adrenocortical insufficiency, as has been stated.

If aqueous ACTH is used alone (that is, without colchicine), recommended doses are: for the first day, 100 to 200 mg. (in divided doses) depending on the attack's severity; for the next three days or so, 80 to 120 mg. daily. Thereafter, *even though symptoms are more or less completely controlled,* use of ACTH should be continued, though in progressively smaller daily doses, for four to eight more days, total treatment lasting about a week or two. Colchicine-resistant attacks, or attacks which develop despite prophylactic use of colchicine between attacks, often require larger doses of ACTH than otherwise. From adequate doses relief begins often within 4 hours of the first dose, may be marked (75 to 90 per cent relief) within 24 hours and complete within 24 to 72 hours. Even so, the attack, though symptomatically suppressed, has generally not run its full course until a week or two have passed.

Attacks are controlled with long-acting ACTH gels given intramuscularly once daily (total doses comparable to those of aqueous ACTH), or with ACTH given by *intravenous* infusion (20 to 30 U.S.P. units in 500 ml. of fluid over a period of 6 to 8 hours).

The combined use of ACTH and colchicine is generally but not always effective. According to one plan, aqueous or long-acting ACTH is given on the first day or two of an attack; concurrently colchicine is given in the usual way (0.65 mg. three or four times a day) to the point of gastrointestinal irritation; then after a 24-hour pause colchicine is given again in smaller doses. But prompt relief without gastrointestinal irritation may be obtained by another scheme: for one or two days the patient is given long-acting ACTH (100 mg. or more, once daily) or aqueous ACTH (40 mg. two or three times daily for a total of 80 or 120 mg. daily); also from the onset, colchicine in *submaximal* doses (1 or 2 mg. daily) for several days.

According to some writers, *cortisone* is inferior to ACTH—indeed, relatively useless. Consequently, relatively few patients have been treated with cortisone given intramuscularly, and even fewer with cortisone or hydrocortisone tablets given orally despite great practical advantages. But critical review indicates that unsatisfactory results have been largely from underdosage or pre-

mature discontinuance, and that if enough cortisone is given long enough most attacks are controlled promptly. Rapid relief without relapses has resulted from cortisone, given occasionally for only three to four days, but generally for one to three weeks. Successful doses have been: either 200 to 300 mg. daily (intramuscularly) for the first three to four days, then progressively smaller doses for one to two weeks more; or 100 mg. daily for about two to three weeks.

The combined use of cortisone and colchicine has been effective, for example, in daily amounts of 100 mg. of cortisone and 2 mg. of colchicine (0.65 mg. three times daily) for a week or more. Relapses due to premature discontinuance of cortisone (used alone) have been controlled either by giving cortisone a few more days or by giving cortisone plus colchicine.

Attacks have been controlled promptly by injections (often one only) of 25 to 50 mg. of *hydrocortisone acetate* into gouty joints or bursae (Hollander).

Phenylbutazone (Butazolidin) is also effective. It has been used in the following doses: intramuscularly, 0.6 to 1.0 gm. (generally the latter) once daily; or orally, 100 to 800 (generally 400 to 600) mg. daily, in four divided doses. The oral preparation is effective and convenient; intramuscular use is preferred by some. (Gutman and Yü; Kidd and co-workers; Kuzell and co-workers.) Serum concentrations of urate are reduced; urinary excretion of urate is increased only by large doses.

Chief limitations are the frequent toxic reactions, which increase with length of treatment. The more severe reactions usually occur early. Toxic reactions affected 13 per cent of patients treated briefly for acute gouty arthritis, and 32 per cent of those treated longer for chronic gouty arthritis; reactions necessitated cessation of treatment in 4 and 8 per cent respectively. Reactions include edema, nausea, epigastric pain, morbilliform rash, granulocytopenia and activation of peptic ulcer. The drug is contraindicated whenever edema from cardiac, renal or hepatic disease might develop. Probenecid counteracts the therapeutic effects of phenylbutazone (Kidd and co-workers).

The old concept that attacks are related to urate retention and precipitation led to the use of uricosuric agents in acute gouty arthritis, the rationale of which is by no means established. Except for cortisone and

ACTH (which appear to control attacks by anti-inflammatory rather than by uricosuric action), uricosuric agents do not certainly prevent or control acute gouty arthritis. Indeed, acute attacks are sometimes precipitated by diuretic or uricosuric agents (salicylates, cinchophen, mersalyl [Salyrgen], probenecid). Despite its uricosuric effect probenecid (Benemid) is of no value for acute attacks; indeed, their incidence may increase during the early weeks of such therapy.

DIET. The diet currently recommended for acute gouty arthritis is one adequate in proteins, low in purines and fats, and rich in carbohydrates and purine-free proteins. This diet (the same as for interval gout) minimizes formation of exogenous urates. Its rationale may be questioned because many patients during attacks excrete urate normally or even excessively; furthermore, attacks bear no proved relation to urate levels or to any precursor thereof. Future work must determine how necessary dietary restrictions are *during* attacks. But then, of all times, patients are receptive to instruction in those dietary measures which the interval treatment of gout seems to require. Intake of fluids should be large. Complete avoidance of alcohol is advisable.

Interval Treatment of Symptomless Gout. Interval treatment aims to reduce the number and severity of attacks, to retard or even reverse the process of urate accumulation, and to prevent or postpone the late, sometimes critical vascular and renal "complications." These intentions require the use, not of a single remedy, but of several measures combined.

Preventive measures include the prophylactic use of colchicine, and the avoidance, reduction or control of the psychic, medicinal, alcoholic, dietary, traumatic and surgical provocatives of acute gouty arthritis. Contrary to older opinions it is now believed that the more or less continuous use of *colchicine* in nonirritating doses is of prophylactic value (Cohen, 1936). In mild cases (less than one attack yearly) one pill (0.53 mg.) is given two or three times daily for one week each month, or for two or three days each week. In moderate cases (more than one attack yearly) at least one tablet daily is given. In severe cases a tablet is given two or three times daily more or less continuously if well tolerated. Gutman and Yü (1952) prescribed 0.5 to 1.0 mg. every

night or two in most cases, and 1.5 to 2.0 mg. nightly in more refractory cases. Sometimes this made the difference between virtual incapacitation and relatively normal activity. Patients have taken colchicine daily for 5 to 10 years without discomfort or drug tolerance (Kersley and co-workers, 1950; Talbott, 1942, 1953). Most patients continue to tolerate about 1.3 to 2.6 mg. colchicine daily, occasionally less.

Dietary management aims chiefly to control, not acute attacks, but accumulation of urate. But any food that seems repeatedly to provoke attacks should be avoided. Some veterans of gout insist that they can consistently tolerate certain alcoholic drinks, but not others; since they (and their physicians) cannot agree on which are harmless, gouty patients should avoid alcohol unless they are prepared to pay the price of personal experimentation.

Postoperative gouty attacks can generally be prevented by use of either a high-carbohydrate, purine-free diet and salicylates for five days before and five days after operation (Hench), or colchicine (0.5 mg. three times a day if given orally, or 1.5 mg. once a day if given intravenously) for at least three days before operation (Kersley and co-workers, 1950; Talbott), or ACTH (with or without colchicine orally) for two to three days before and after operation (Coste and co-workers).

Some control or even reversibility of urate accumulation can be accomplished by diet and uricosuric drugs. This is important for the prevention of tophaceous gout, chronic gouty arthritis, gouty nephritis and renal colic.

Dietary management aimed at preventing formation of tophi is in a period of transition. If urates are synthesized not only from purines but from carbohydrates, fats and purine-free proteins, restriction of purines alone is of limited value. There are limits to restrictions which patients with a lifetime disease will accept. Each patient must be treated individually, as his disease and temperament dictate. It is still logical to decrease the purine load by avoiding purine-rich foods, excesses of fats which decrease urate excretion, and excesses of carbohydrates which produce obesity. A basic diet low in purines, poor in fat and limited in proteins (50 to 75 gm. daily) is recommended empirically; this consists chiefly of cereals, grain products, eggs, cheese, milk, fruits and nonleguminous vegetables (Gutman and Yü; Hench). When gout is mild or well controlled, the diet can

Purine Content of Certain Foods*†

LIST 1. Foods which contain very large amounts (150–1000 mg.) of purine bodies in 100 gm.:

Heart, sheep	174 mg.	Mussels	154
Herring	172	Sardines	234
Herring roe	484	Smelts	168
Meat extracts	236–356	Sweetbreads	426
		Yeast	570–990

LIST 2. Foods which contain a large amount (75–150 mg.) of purine bodies in 100 gm.:
Anchovies, bacon, codfish, goose, grouse, haddock, liver, kidneys, mackerel, mutton leg, partridge, pheasant, pigeon, salmon, scallops, trout, turkey, veal, venison

LIST 3. Foods which contain a moderate amount (up to 75 mg.) of purine bodies in 100 gm.:
Asparagus, bass, beef, bouillon, brains, chicken, crab, duck, eel, halibut, ham, kidney beans, lentils, lima beans, liverwurst, lobster, mushrooms, mutton chop, navy beans, oysters, peas, plaice, pork, rabbit, roe, shrimp, spinach, tongue, tripe

LIST 4. Foods which contain an insignificant amount of purine or no purine:
   1. Beverages
        Carbonated
        Chocolate
        Cocoa
        Coffee
        Fruit juices
        Postum
        Tea
   2. Butter‡
   3. Breads and breadstuffs (refined and whole grain)
   4. Caviar
   5. Cereals (refined and whole grain)
   6. Miscellaneous cereal products
        Arrowroot
        Hominy
        Macaroni
        Noodles
        Sago
        Spaghetti
        Tapioca
        Vermicelli
   7. Cheese of all kinds‡
   8. Eggs
   9. Fats of all kinds (but eat in moderation)‡
   10. Fruits of all kinds
   11. Gelatin
   12. Milk
        Buttermilk
        Condensed milk
        Malted milk
   13. Nuts of all kinds
        Peanut butter
   14. Pies (except mincemeat)‡
   15. Sugar and sweets
   16. Vegetables (except those in list 3)
   17. Vegetable and cream soups (to be made with allowed vegetables and without meat stock)
   18. Vitamin concentrates
        Cod liver oil
        Halibut oil

---

* Bridges, M. A.: Food and Beverage Analyses. Ed. 3, Philadelphia, Lea & Febiger, 1950, pp. 188–192.
Dirr, K., and Decker, P.: Über den Nichteiweiss-Stickstoff der Hefe. Biochem. Ztschr., *316:*239, 1944.
   † To calculate the purine or "purine bodies" in a given food, the purine nitrogen is multiplied by 3; for example, 200 mg. of purine nitrogen equals 600 mg. of purine bodies.
   ‡ These foods are high in fat.

be liberalized to include one serving of meat, fish or fowl five days a week.

Until isotopic techniques become practical, the rate of urate accumulation must be gauged by the degree of hyperuricemia, tophaceousness (number and size of tophi), chronic arthritis or renal insufficiency. If the accumulation is adjudged to be mild, avoidance of foods in list 1 (table) and prolonged use of a uricosuric agent may suffice. Other patients require greater purine restriction. Normal diets contain 600 to 1000 mg. of purines daily; a low-purine diet contains 100 to 150 mg. and can be attained roughly by allowing one food from list 2 one or two days a week, and one from list 3 four days a week, besides whatever is desired from list 4. Coffee and tea are permissible. Deficiencies in protein, iron and vitamin B must be avoided; generally, gout diets should be reinforced with an approved vitamin preparation, for example, one hexavitamin capsule U.S.P. every one to two days. Normal weight should be maintained and obesity avoided or corrected.

As to the use of uricosuric agents in interval treatment of symptomless gout, *probenecid,* a benzoic acid derivative, is probably the best agent for prolonged use (Gutman and Yü; Talbott). Serum urate is decreased, and excretion of urinary urate is notably increased by suppression of tubular resorption. For uricosuria, probenecid (Benemid) (2 gm. daily) is much more effective than neocinchophen (3 gm. daily) or aspirin in small doses (2 to 3 gm. daily), and more effective than aspirin, 5 gm. daily, but less effective than aspirin plus sodium bicarbonate, 5 gm. of each daily (Gutman and Yü).

Doses of probenecid are 0.5 to 2 gm. or more daily. The incidence of toxicity is proportional to dosage. Most toxic reactions are minor; they include nausea, anorexia, constipation and rash. Allergic reactions sometimes develop. One severe reaction (headache, muscular aching, pruritus, dyspnea, nausea, vomiting, chill, fever) developed after ten days of therapy (2.0 gm. daily) and recurred later after a single test dose of 0.125 gm. (Kloempken and Montgomery, 1952). Doses now recommended are: 0.25 gm. twice daily the first week, thereafter 0.5 gm. twice daily taken with food. Larger doses (2.0 gm. daily) are rarely needed unless renal insufficiency or extensive tophaceous deposits are present. Patients should receive also a liberal fluid intake and sodium bicar-

bonate (about 2 to 5 gm. daily) to prevent renal gravel. Probenecid and salicylates should not be given concurrently: each counteracts the uricosuric effect of the other (Gutman and Yü, 1951; Pascale and co-workers). ACTH does not interfere with probenecid.

Probenecid tends to provoke gouty arthritis during the first weeks of treatment (in 18 per cent of cases); thereafter attacks may become fewer than before treatment. Vigorous uricosuria from overzealous dosage together with insufficient fluids and alkalis may produce a momentary "flash colic," a true renal colic or urate crystalluria and hematuria.

Marked uricosuria is produced by *aspirin* or *sodium salicylate* in daily (divided) doses of 4 to 6 gm. or more but not by daily doses of less than 3 or 4 gm. (Hanzlik, 1927; Graham, 1920, 1933). Salicylates inhibit tubular resorption of urate. The uricosuric effect of salicylates may be enhanced by the concurrent use of sodium bicarbonate (Gutman, 1950). Prolonged use of aspirin or sodium salicylate (1 to 1.3 gm. or 15 to 20 grains four times a day) and sodium bicarbonate (1.3 gm. four times a day) may be recommended for those few who tolerate such amounts without salicylism; thus salicylates are an alternate for probenecid to reduce the miscible pool of urate (Benedict and co-workers; Stetten).

The prolonged use of the cortisones, corticotropins, cinchopens and phenylbutazone as uricosuric agents is not recommended.

Sodium bicarbonate is given (1) to increase the solubility of urinary urates so as to prevent the spontaneous or therapeutically induced formation of uratic calculi or (2) to enhance salicylate uricosuria. Gouty patients, whether or not they are taking urate eliminants, are commonly advised to take enough sodium bicarbonate to alkalinize their urine, for example, 2 to 5 gm. daily in divided doses (Gutman, 1951) or 0.5 gm. with each dose of probenecid or salicylate (Talbott). They should be taught to test urine with litmus papers. Sodium bicarbonate occasionally produces gastrointestinal symptoms erroneously ascribed to the uricosuric agent. Then an alternate method of urinary alkalinization is necessary.

Chronic Gouty Arthritis. Joints "whitewashed" with urates can be symptomless. Apparently, chronic gouty arthritis requires for its production, not just urates, but a sufficient inflammatory reaction thereto. Hence treat-

early age, they now live to become vi
of the arteriosclerotic period of life.

Age. Diabetes may develop at any ag
the curve of incidence reaches its peak i
fifth and sixth decades. According to J
approximately 50 per cent of all dia
occurs between the ages of 40 and 60
Only 5 per cent occurs in the first d
and 3 per cent in the eighth.

Sex. Between the ages of 40 and 70
diabetes is significantly more commo
women than in men, the ratio being ap
imately 3 to 2. In earlier life there ap
to be a slight preponderance in males.
possible that the high incidence in w
more than 40 is related to the high inci
of obesity in this group.

Etiology. It must be emphasized a
outset that the etiology of diabetes melli
undetermined in the vast majority of pat
However, it is apparent from experim
studies and clinical observation that a
ber of factors may disturb the normal in
mechanism and thereby induce the hyp
cemia and glycosuria typical of diabetes
this reason it might be more accurate to
sider "the etiologies" of diabetes.

The capacity to metabolize carbohy
as well as other substances, must be co
ered a fundamental process inherent in
if not all, tissue cells. This property pro
constitutes a heritage from our unice
ancestors. What part primary disturban
the intrinsic enzyme systems concerned
these oxidative processes may play in dia
mellitus is still obscure. It is known, how
that certain endocrine glands, through
elaboration of their respective hormone:
able to influence profoundly the metab
of various foodstuffs; therefore the rela
of these glands to the origin of diabetes
be considered.

The Pancreas. Insulin is elaborated b
beta cells of the islands of Langerhans i
pancreas. It is therefore to be expected
total pancreatectomy will terminate in
production, thus giving rise to severe
rapidly fatal diabetes. This is true i
dog, but in other species the diabetes inc
by pancreatectomy is much less intense.

Total pancreatectomy in man has been
formed on a number of occasions. Dia
appears promptly after this procedure,
in contrast to that in the dog, is not of
severity. Patients may require 25 to 50
of insulin daily with a liberal ingestic
carbohydrate. This dosage of insulin,

ment must combat the chief factor, the sec-
onary *inflammation,* as well as urate deposition. But perhaps still another factor intrudes.

The effects of *colchicine* on *chronic* gouty
arthritis are inconstant—sometimes satisfactory, often not. The nature of the "acute
exacerbations" of chronic gouty arthritis is
not precisely known. Since colchicine appears
to relieve some exacerbations but not others,
they may be of different types. Perhaps those
responsive to colchicine are analogous to the
early, discrete attacks of acute arthritic non-
uratic inflammation, whereas exacerbations
unresponsive to colchicine may represent a
flare of the posturatic inflammation. If such
be true, individualized care of each patient
with chronic gouty arthritis and its exacerbations is required.

Uricosuric agents (probenecid; salicylates) constitute the *long-term* remedies for
chronic gouty arthritis; their prolonged use
reduces the size of periarticular tophi and
fosters resorption of urate from osseous tophi
and the sclerotic repair thereof (Gutman
and Yü, 1952). But as *short-term* remedies
for painful chronic gouty arthritis and its
exacerbations, uricosuric agents are inadequate. Some prompt-acting antiphlogistic
agent is required. Colchicine should be tried
first, in full therapeutic, not prophylactic,
doses (oral or intravenous). When it fails,
one has the choice of short-term systemic
usage of phenylbutazone, ACTH or cortisone,
of hydrocortisone given intra-articularly, or
of a combination thereof (Coste and co-
workers; Engleman and co-workers; Kuzell
and co-workers).

*Gouty Nephritis: Prevention and Treat-
ment.* Prolonged administration of a uricosuric agent is useful for the prevention and
treatment of renal lesions, as are also abundant intake of fluids, especially water, and
constant alkalinization of the urine. Special
measures are required for pyelonephritis,
renal insufficiency or uremia.

*Vascular Accidents: Prevention and Treat-
ment.* One can only speculate on the mechanism or agent responsible for vascular
complications. For their prevention the physician must rely on the general regimen already
outlined.

Treatment of Gross or Ulcerating Tophi.
Special treatment is required for some tophi
such as painful ones on weight-bearing surfaces, large ones which prevent use of regular
shoes or gloves, or those in which fistulous
ulcers are present or impending. Prolonged

therapeutic uricosuria may heal draining
sinuses. If tophi remain troublesome they
should be excised. The removal of a small
tophus under local anesthesia can be done
usually without a postoperative flare. But
when one or more large tophi are to be excised and if general anesthesia is used, one
should institute, prior to tophectomy, a regimen to prevent acute postoperative (that is,
post-tophectomy) gouty arthritis.

PHILIP S. HENCH

References

Benedict, Jean D., Forsham, P. H., Roche, Marcel, Soloway, Sidney, and Stetten, DeWitt, Jr.: The Effect of Salicylates and Adrenocorticotropic Hormone Upon the Miscible Pool of Uric Acid in Gout. J. Clin. Investigation, 29:1104, 1950.

Graham, Wallace, and Roberts, J. B.: Intravenous Colchicine in the Management of Gouty Arthritis. Ann. Rheumat. Dis., 12:16, 1953.

Gutman, A. B., and Yü, T. F.: Benemid (p-[di-n-propylsulfamyl]-benzoid Acid) as Uricosuric Agent in Chronic Gouty Arthritis. Tr. A. Am. Physicians, 64:279, 1951.

———, and Yü, T. F.: Current Principles of Management in Gout. Am. J. Med., 13:744, 1952.

Hench, P. S.: Diagnosis and Treatment of Gout and Gouty Arthritis. J.A.M.A., 116:453, 1941.

Hollander, J. L.: Intra-articular Hydrocortisone in the Treatment of Arthritis. Ann. Int. Med., 39:735, 1953.

Mason, R. M.: Some Observations on the Blood Uric Acid Levels in Gout. Proc. Roy. Soc. Med., 44:289, 1951.

Pascale, L. R., Dubin, Alvin, and Hoffman, W. S.: Therapeutic Value of Probenecid (Benemid) in Gout. J.A.M.A., 149:1188, 1952.

Robinson, W. D., Conn, J. W., Block, W. D., and Louis, L. H.: Role of the Adrenal Cortex in Urate Metabolism and in Gout. J. Lab. & Clin. Med., 33:1473, 1948.

Smyth, C. J., Stecher, R. M., and Wolfson, W. Q.: Genetic and Endocrine Determinants of the Plasma Urate Level. Science, 108:514, 1948.

Stetten, DeWitt, Jr.: The Pool of Miscible Uric Acid in Normal and Gouty Man, Studied With the Aid of Isotopic Nitrogen. J. Mt. Sinai Hosp., 17:149, 1950.

Talbott, J. H.: Gout and Gouty Arthritis. Modern Medical Monographs. New York, Grune and Stratton, 1953, 92 pp.

Wolfson, W. Q., and others: Physiologic and Clinical Studies With Long-acting Preparations of Pituitary Adrenocorticotrophic Hormone. Univ. Michigan M. Bull., 16:152, 1950.

Wolfson, W. Q., Hunt, H. D., Cohn, Clarence, Robinson, W. D., and Duff, I. F.: ACTH and Colchicine in the Clinical Treatment of Acute Gouty Arthritis: Physiological Considerations and Review of Therapeutic Results in Fifty-one Attacks. J. Michigan M. Soc., 49:1058, 1950.

DIABETES MELLITU[S]

Definition. The disease known [as diabetes]
mellitus is a disorder of carbohyd[rate metab-]
olism characterized by hypergly[cemia and]
glycosuria. This disorder is associ[ated with a]
disturbance of the normal insuli[n mechan-]
ism. When the carbohydrate met[abolism be-]
comes seriously deranged, there [are also]
demonstrable abnormalities of p[rotein and]
fat metabolism. The latter may g[ive rise to]
ketosis, acidosis, coma and death[. The dis-]
turbance in the insulin mechanism [appears]
to be due in most cases to a decr[eased]
elaboration of insulin by the panc[reas; how-]
ever, in certain cases it probably r[esults from]
an increase in insulin requireme[nts of the]
tissue cells to maintain normal ca[rbohydrate]
metabolism.

History. The growth of our knowledg[e of diabetes]
mellitus demonstrates admirably a patt[ern of scien-]
tific development which has led repea[tedly to sig-]
nificant medical progress. Clinical descr[iption of the]
disease came first. Aretaeus appropriate[ly described]
a "melting down of the flesh and limbs t[o urine." The]
first and crude demonstration of the c[hemical na-]
ture of the disorder is ascribed to Suśrut[a, who in the]
fifth century described "honey urine," [followed]
by Thomas Willis 1200 years later, an[d by Dobson]
who in the eighteenth century demo[nstrated the]
presence of sugar in the urine. The thir[d important]
step was the physiologic demonstration [by von Mer-]
ing and Minkowski, in 1889, that extir[pation of a]
dog's pancreas was followed by the deve[lopment of a]
condition strikingly similar to diabet[es in man.]
Hyperglycemia, glycosuria and ketonu[ria resulted]
and, when glucose was fed, it was exc[reted quanti-]
tatively in the urine. After this, his[tologic]
studies in man by Opie, in 1900, show[ed some de-]
gree of correlation between degeneratio[n of islet tis-]
sue in the pancreas and the presence [of diabetes.]
This supported the experiments of Sobo[lev, who in]
the same year demonstrated that degene[ration of the]
tryptic portion of the pancreas did n[ot produce]
diabetes.

The final step which appeared to c[omplete the]
proof that diabetes mellitus arises fr[om primary]
disease of the pancreas was accompli[shed by the]
classic studies of Banting, a surgeon, an[d Best,]
a medical student, in 1921. They prep[ared an ex-]
tract of the islet tissue of the pancre[as whose]
tryptic portion had degenerated after li[gation of the]
pancreatic ducts. This extract depresse[d the blood]
sugar of the diabetic dog as had extracts [prepared by]
Zuelzer in 1907, and others at later [dates from]
whole pancreatic tissue. These extracts [were unpre-]
dictable in terms of toxicity, but prepa[rations suitable]
for clinical use were soon prepared by [the ex-]
traction procedures developed by J. B. C[ollip, a mem-]
ber of Banting's group. With the dev[elopment of]
insulin which corrected the disturbance[s of carbohy-]
drate metabolism in diabetic dogs and [man, there]

---

were not accompanied by any histologic
change in the pancreas. Haist and Best inferred from their studies that "resting" the
pancreas relieved the "strain" imposed by
hyperglycemia and is beneficial. The observations of Haist and Best showing a decrease
in insulin content of the pancreas with rest
furnish at least a partial explanation for what
is termed *"starvation diabetes"* encountered
in man and certain animals. It has been repeatedly observed that, after starvation or a
low carbohydrate diet, the administration of
glucose is followed temporarily by hyperglycemia of an abnormal degree and duration,
often associated with glycosuria. Transient
diabetes has also been observed following the
surgical relief of recurrent hypoglycemia due
to islet cell tumors. In this case, also, it appears that time is required for the islet
cells to regain their normal function after
prolonged relative inactivity. Mirsky has indicated that prolonged "rest" of the beta cells
resulting from long-continued hypoglycemia
leads in time to atrophy of these insulin-pro-
ducing cells. These observations await confirmation.

Diabetes in man occasionally occurs in association with a variety of diseases of the
pancreas. In *hemochromatosis* it is not unusual to have associated diabetes, which
some believe to be due to extensive siderosis
and fibrosis of islet tissue. Mild diabetes appears in a few patients with *carcinoma* of the
pancreas and may result from destruction of
islet tissue, as may also be true in the case
of large pancreatic *cysts.* Acute *hemorrhagic
pancreatitis* is not infrequently associated
with hyperglycemia and glycosuria, and permanent diabetes has been reported following
recovery from pancreatitis. *Trauma* of the
pancreas has been purported to be a cause of
diabetes, but this view is not established on
firm grounds.

The Pituitary. It has long been known
that diabetes mellitus is frequently found in
association with acromegaly. It was therefore
natural to suspect that hormones of the anterior lobe of the pituitary gland were in
some way capable of disturbing carbohydrate
metabolism. Evans, Houssay, Lassen and
others subsequently established the fact that
the intensity of diabetes could be enhanced
by the parenteral administration of anterior
pituitary extract and that, in normal animals,
transient hyperglycemia and glycosuria could
be induced by this procedure. It remained,
however, for Young (1937) to demonstrate

---

that typical diabetes could be permanently
established in dogs by the administration of a
potent extract of the anterior lobe of the pituitary (APE) when injections were continued daily for about four weeks. Histological
study of the pancreas of these animals showed
lesions characteristically found in many patients with diabetes.

These important studies of Young left in
doubt the question whether anterior pituitary
extract exerted a direct effect upon beta cells
of the islets similar to that observed following
alloxan. Best, Haist and Campbell showed
that the administration of a diet low in carbohydrate or the administration of insulin
inhibited the diabetogenic effect of anterior
pituitary extract, as well as the development
of histologic changes in the pancreas. The
basis for the development of "Young's diabetes" was finally established through the
ingenious experiments of Lukens and Dohan.
They induced "Young's diabetes" in partially
pancreatectomized cats in which hydropic
degeneration of beta cells persists for some
months before fibrosis occurs. These investigators found that, after the injections of
anterior pituitary extract were discontinued
and before fibrosis of islet tissue occurred, the
diabetes which had been established was
curable. Cure could be effected in any one of
three ways, each of which abolished hyperglycemia: first, by reduction in carbohydrate
intake; second, by the administration of insulin; and third, by the administration of
phlorizin. In other words, the permanent
diabetes induced by APE appears to result in
the main from exhaustion of the beta cells
by interference with carbohydrate utilization
and long-continued hyperglycemia. Young
and others believe it also acts through stimulation of glucagon and possibly insulin. Of
importance is the further observation of Lukens and Dohan, who have shown that permanent diabetes with characteristic pancreatic
changes can also be induced in normal cats
through the maintenance of hyperglycemia
for a period of ten days by the intraperitoneal
injection of glucose alone.

How many fractions of anterior pituitary
extract may play a part in the genesis of diabetes is not yet established. "Pure" growth
hormone or somatotropin (STH) unquestionably has the capacity to induce permanent
diabetes in dogs and cats, but only in partially pancreatectomized rats. Also, Cori and
Bornstein have found a lipoprotein in beef
pituitary which inhibits the glucokinase re-

action and thus may prove to be diabetogenic. The observations of Ladd and of White concerning the onset of diabetes in children suggest that, among others, the growth hormone may be implicated. Thus Ladd found that 30 out of 34 children carefully studied were overgrown or overweight, or both, at the onset of their disease. White reports that 86 per cent of children with diabetes were definitely overheight within three months prior to the onset of their disease. Obesity was not a significant factor in White's patients. Furthermore, there are numerous reports of women who have given birth to oversized infants some months before the onset of diabetes in themselves, suggesting hypersecretion of growth hormone in the mother during pregnancy. The role of ACTH in the genesis of human diabetes appears to be a minor one, since a vast number of individuals have been given this hormone in amounts sufficient to induce prolonged and intense hypercorticism with only infrequent initiation of transient diabetes. However, the enhancement of diabetes by ACTH is not to be questioned.

The Adrenal Glands. Lukens and Long first showed that extirpation of the adrenal glands ameliorated pancreatic diabetes in dogs and cats, just as Houssay found a beneficial effect from hypophysectomy. With these observations the importance of the adrenal cortex in the genesis of disturbances of carbohydrate metabolism became firmly established. Ingle has been able to induce heavy glycosuria in intact rats by intensive administration of 17-hydroxycorticosterone or 17-hydroxy-11-dehydrocorticosterone, cortisone, thus further emphasizing the importance of certain adrenal steroids in their capacity to act either directly or indirectly as an "anti-insulin." The increase in glycosuria induced by 11-oxysteroids in the rat is ascribed by Stetten and Ingle to an increase in gluconeogenesis.

Himsworth points out that patients with diabetes (and probably nondiabetic persons) can be divided into insulin-resistant and insulin-susceptible groups. The whole implication of this generalization is not known, but it is probable that either pituitary or adrenal cortical hormones, or both, are significantly concerned with at least some of the variations in insulin resistance. In support of this view is the fact that the diabetes occurring with acromegaly or Cushing's syndrome may be mild, as judged by the degree of glycosuria and hyperglycemia, but the dosage of insulin required to relieve it is reputed to be inordinately great. On the other hand, in the absence of adrenal cortical hormones, or in pituitary insufficiency, even intense diabetes may be incredibly sensitive to minute amounts of insulin.

It remains to be determined how frequently excessive secretion of anterior pituitary extract or certain adrenal cortical steroids with their antagonistic behavior toward insulin activity may be of importance in the development of diabetes in man.

Whereas *epinephrine* is responsible for transient hyperglycemia as a result of increased glycogenolysis, there is no convincing evidence suggesting that the adrenal medulla plays any part in the initiation of diabetes mellitus.

The Thyroid Gland. Wilder reported an incidence of 3.2 per cent of frank diabetes mellitus in a series of patients with hyperthyroidism. Diabetes occurred more than three times as often in Wilder's patients with toxic nodular goiter as in patients with exophthalmic goiter, probably because of the higher incidence of nodular goiter in older age groups in whom diabetes is most prevalent. Experience dictates that overactivity of the thyroid gland should always be suspected in diabetics who are difficult to regulate and require large doses of insulin, since it is well established that hyperthyroidism intensifies diabetes mellitus. However, it has not been possible to establish permanent diabetes in animals by thyroid administration, in contrast to the effect of the administration of anterior pituitary extract. Consequently it is probable that hyperthyroidism merely intensifies latent diabetes and does not induce the disease.

Obesity. Among 1000 diabetics reported by Joslin, 77 per cent were definitely overweight and only 8 per cent were below the normal zone. Among 252 diabetics between the ages of 51 and 60, only 2 were below normal weight prior to the onset of their disease. It is a striking fact that the correlation between obesity and diabetes occurs only in the adult group and particularly among older adults.

A majority of older obese diabetic patients lose evidence of a disturbance in carbohydrate metabolism with reduction in weight. Thus it appears that the capacity of these patients to metabolize carbohydrate tends to be impaired only in association with a carbohydrate intake sufficiently in excess of normal to establish obesity. When their caloric intake is reduced to a level commensurate with the maintenance of normal weight, diabetes tends to disappear.

It seems possible that the "strain" on the pancreas to elaborate insulin essential for oxidation of excessive carbohydrate or possibly for fat storage may lead in time to diabetes in those people with a genic predisposition to the disease. In this connection it is of interest to note that diabetes appears in mice exhibiting hereditary obesity. Also, Long and his co-workers have shown that rats rendered obese by hyperalimentation after hypothalamic injury may in time develop diabetes. From a practical standpoint the essential fact is that a relationship between obesity and diabetes is found in more than 50 per cent of persons with diabetes.

Heredity. A family history of diabetes can be obtained in at least 25 per cent of patients. Furthermore, the incidence of diabetes in both of identical twins is approximately 70 per cent in contrast to less than 10 per cent in twins derived from separate ova. These facts, in addition to studies of White and Pincus and also of Wilder, indicate that the predisposition to diabetes is inherited as a Mendelian recessive which is not sex-linked. *It is not known whether the genic defect finds its expression at the hormonal level in the form of "imbalances" or at a more fundamental level involving defects in enzymatic processes.* Be that as it may, the implication of White's and Pincus' studies is that 100 per cent of the offspring of two diabetic parents will develop the disease—assuming the etiology of diabetes in both parents is the same.

There is a mass of evidence offered in support of different etiologies for juvenile diabetes and the diabetes of older obese persons. To be mentioned are the acute onset in the juveniles and typically mild symptoms in the obese; the lack of fat in the liver in juvenile diabetics and classic fatty liver of the obese; the relative insulin sensitivity in the juveniles and comparative resistance in the obese; also the possible overactivity of the pituitary gland in juvenile diabetics as suggested by their oversize. *Nevertheless, it must be remembered that persons who develop their diabetes when they are fat and elderly may have children who develop classic juvenile diabetes.* This fact suggests strongly a single basis for both types.

Infection. One of the most characteristic features of diabetes is the fact that infection intensifies the disease process and may increase enormously the demand for insulin.

This is particularly true of febrile diseases, but is also true of infections as trivial as the common cold. The mechanism by which activation of diabetes takes place is wholly obscure. It is not known whether infectious processes decrease the formation of insulin. They do, however, stimulate liberation of ACTH with increased secretion of steroids of the adrenal gland.

Diabetes often develops after an acute infectious disease, but it seems improbable that the infection initiates diabetes in these patients. More probable is the explanation that these patients are potential diabetics and that infection merely brings the latent disease to light.

Race. It is a generally accepted fact that diabetes is more common among Jews than among other people. This high incidence is almost entirely limited to elderly Jews and is in all likelihood associated with a high incidence of obesity.

Disturbances of the Nervous System. Certain authors have emphasized that the incidence of diabetes is highest among persons whose occupations are associated with "nerve strain" and great responsibility, but it must be recognized that a sedentary existence associated with consequent obesity in this group is probably of greater significance. The appearance of glycosuria following sudden emotional upsets or cerebral trauma is well established and was commented upon by Willis in 1679, but this is transitory in nature and is probably dependent upon sympathetic discharge of epinephrine. It seems certain that "psychic trauma" can temporarily increase the severity of established diabetes and consequently increase insulin requirements. This becomes a point of practical importance in the management of the disease. It is conceivable that continued outpouring of epinephrine in patients with inherited susceptibility to diabetes might, through pituitary stimulation, induce excessive secretion of ACTH, which in turn might induce glycosuria by the liberation of adrenal steroids. This is not established, but is suggested by the fact that certain patients with a pheochromocytoma exhibit diabetes mellitus.

Whatever the etiology of diabetes, the disease can be looked upon from a standpoint of practical management as a disorder in which the amount of endogenous insulin available is inadequate to meet the metabolic demands.

Physiology. The ability of a physician to understand the disturbances responsible for the clinical picture of diabetes mellitus and likewise his ability to treat the disease intelligently and successfully are dependent upon knowledge of the metabolic processes involved. It is essential in gaining this background of information to contrast certain aspects of normal metabolism with the deviations encountered in diabetes.

Carbohydrate Metabolism. Normal carbohydrate metabolism proceeds along a number of pathways as indicated in Figure 81. A portion of the glucose, from which carbohydrate metabolism originates, is converted into glycogen in the liver and muscles. The remaining glucose is broken down by means of anaerobic glycolysis to lactate and pyruvate and possibly to other 3-carbon fragments without the interposition of glycogen formation, likewise shown in Figure 81. The phosphorylation of glucose to glucose 6-phosphate is the first and essential step both for its conversion to glycogen and its degradation to smaller fragments. The 3-carbon fragments, lactate and pyruvate, are decarboxylated to form acetyl coenzyme A (acetyl coA). The condensation of two molecules of acetyl coenzyme A yields acetoacetyl coenzyme A which may give rise to acetoacetic acid as an end product. However, normally, most of the acetoacetyl coenzyme A enters the cycle of Lynen and of Green and upon further condensation with acetyl coenzyme A it ultimately forms the longer chain fatty acids. Thus, in 8 turns about the cycle, the chain is lengthened to form stearic acid. The major portion of acetyl coA combines under normal circumstances with oxaloacetate to be oxidized to CO_2 and water via the tricarboxylic acid cycle.

Essentially all carbohydrate is broken down in the gut into the three hexoses, glucose, fructose, and galactose, before being absorbed. It is generally believed that these sugars are phosphorylated in their passage through the gut wall and that they do not traverse the mucosa of the small intestine by simple diffusion alone. This viewpoint is borne out by the fact that the rates of absorption of these hexoses are unequal; e.g., galactose and glucose are absorbed rapidly, whereas fructose enters the portal blood much more slowly. Furthermore, these hexoses are absorbed from the gut even when their concentrations are lower than that in the blood.

Three Sources of Body Glucose. Obviously the largest amount normally comes from the food; a second source is liver glycogen; and a third source is that derived from gluconeogenesis.

Liver glycogen is derived from glucose, either ingested or synthesized in the body, and from lactic or pyruvic acid, elaborated to a large extent in the muscles. It turns out from studies on the rat by Stetten that the total amount of glycogen stored in the normally fed animal in 24 hours is equivalent to only about 3 per cent of the total glucose metabolized. Hence stored glycogen appears to be almost insignificant as a source of glucose for metabolic requirements in the normal animal. This statement does not detract,

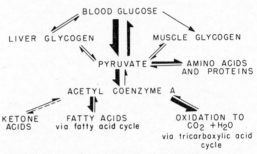

Fig. 81. Diagram of normal carbohydrate metabolism. (Thickness of arrows indicates possible magnitude of the reactions.)

however, from the vital importance of liver glycogen as an emergency stabilizing factor for the blood sugar level. The glycogen of the liver, as well as that in the muscles, derived from glucose, appears as a product elaborated by a series of reactions involving the phosphorylation of glucose. These reactions are reversible except for the initial phosphorylation of glucose, but it is worthy of note that the final step in the degradation of liver glycogen to glucose is accomplished by a specific phosphatase present in the liver, but not in muscles; consequently no free glucose can be formed from muscle glycogen.

In addition to glucose absorbed from the gut and to that derived from liver glycogen, glucose may be synthesized from a variety of building blocks within the body. This synthesis is termed *gluconeogenesis.* Gluconeogenesis appears to take place primarily in the liver from 2- or 3-carbon fragments which appear in the course of the metabolism of protein, fat and carbohydrate. Included in these are certain amino acids from protein (e.g., alanine), glycerol from fat, lactate and pyruvate from glucose, and probably many other substances. The amount of glucose made available by gluconeogenesis in the normal rat, according to Stetten, is approximately tenfold that derived from glycogen. The importance of this process in body economy is apparent.

The Normal Fate of Glucose in the Body. As stated before, only about 3 per cent of the glucose metabolized by the normal rat is to be accounted for by glycogen formation. Of the remaining 97 per cent, Stetten has shown that 30 per cent, i.e., ten times as much as goes to glycogen, is converted to fatty acids after breakdown to acetyl coenzyme A. The portion of glucose not con-

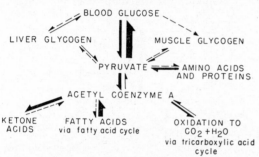

Fig. 82. Diagram of carbohydrate metabolism in diabetes mellitus. (Thickness of arrows indicates possible magnitude of the reactions.)

verted to glycogen or fatty acid (about 70 per cent of the total), after being split to lactate, pyruvate and other 3-carbon fragments, is either oxidized (chiefly in the muscles) by means of the tricarboxylic and succinic acid cycles to carbon dioxide and water, or is made available for amino acid and ultimately protein synthesis.

Carbohydrate Metabolism in Diabetes. The major defect in carbohydrate metabolism in diabetes mellitus is due to a decrease in the utilization of glucose. Actual increase in glucose production from fatty acids is not quantitatively significant. It seems probable that gluconeogenesis from protein is significantly increased by 11-oxysteroids of adrenal origin. Studies of Stetten have demonstrated conclusively that the amount of extra glucose found (gluconeogenesis) in phlorizin diabetes, in which the loss of sugar is dependent solely upon a renal lesion, is just as great as it is in the truly diabetic animal (alloxan-poisoned) in which the loss of glucose is due to a disturbance in the insulin mechanism. In other words, *there is no more "overproduction" of glucose in alloxan diabetes than in renal glycosuria induced with phlorizin.* It appears at the present time that "underutilization" of glucose results from the summation of three

defects (*vide* Figs. 81 and 82); first, a decrease in oxidation of glucose and a decrease in its utilization in amino acid and protein synthesis and some increase in gluconeogenesis; second, a decrease in fatty acid formation from glucose to about one twentieth of the normal, thus making this nonmetabolized glucose also available for urinary excretion; and third, a decrease in glycogen storage in the liver and muscles, which, however, contributes only slightly to the total amount of glucose excreted over any considerable period of time.

It must be emphasized that, whereas the capacity to oxidize glucose and the ability to convert glucose to glycogen may be seriously impaired in diabetes, these functions, contrary to earlier thought, are not completely interrupted. It may well be that the oxidation of glucose, which does continue in the brain and probably in other tissues in diabetes, is independent of insulin action and is akin to that in unicellular organisms, which utilize carbohydrate without a pancreas. This is also suggested by the fact that the depancreatized animal is capable of increasing the utilization of glucose in response to muscular work.

Glucose may be oxidized after phosphorylation by a pathway known as the "hexose monophosphate shunt." This pathway, still not wholly understood, does not follow the steps of the conventional Embden-Meyerhof anaerobic glycolysis. Its importance has not been entirely clarified, but it appears to be involved, at least, in the formation of ribose for nucleic acid synthesis.

Insulin. This hormone of the islands of Langerhans is a single protein, the biologic activity of which is dependent upon the integrity of the disulfide bridges between cysteine residues in adjacent polypeptide chains. The monomeric insulin molecule has a molecular weight of about 12,000 or perhaps 6000 and it exists in micelles of molecular weight of about 36,000.

The mechanism of action of insulin is not firmly established, and two views continue to prevail. Levine and Park and also Martin have presented impressive evidence favoring the idea that insulin acts by enhancing the passage of glucose and of galactose through cell membranes, and that in the diabetic animal glucose fails to be utilized because it is incapable of entering the cells where it is normally phosphorylated and then utilized. Cori and Cori, on the other hand, maintain that the defect in diabetes results from an inhibition of phosphorylation of glucose to glucose-6-phosphate by a factor in the pituitary gland. This may be growth hormone or a lipoprotein. They believe that insulin counteracts this pituitary inhibition of glucokinase. Stadie has shown that the insulin "sticks" onto the normal rat diaphragm which has been briefly immersed in a solution containing insulin, and that it does not stick onto the diaphragm of the diabetic rat or on one treated with pituitary extract. The utilization of glucose appears to be dependent upon this adherence of insulin to the muscle. Stadie's observations can be harmonized with either viewpoint concerning insulin action. Chaikoff has shown, as has Miller, that, *in vitro* or *in vivo*, fructose in contrast to glucose is utilized normally by tissues of the diabetic organism. Levine suggests that this is because insulin is not needed for the penetration of fructose into cells. With the alternative hypothesis it would be assumed that the fructokinase reaction is intact whereas the glucokinase reaction is disturbed in the diabetic. The balance of evidence at present favors the view of Levine.

Regardless of the mechanism of action of insulin, its over-all effects are readily demonstrable in the diabetic animal. The reactions which appear to benefit at least indirectly from the administration of insulin are indicated in Figure 83. Here it will be seen that insulin enhances the normal breakdown of glucose to pyruvate which is ultimately oxidized to carbon dioxide and water, and which also serves as a "steppingstone" in the conversion of glucose to fatty acids. Furthermore, insulin appears to aid indirectly in the synthesis of certain amino acids and their incorporation into body protein. By virtue of increasing glucose oxidation, insulin decreases gluconeogenesis in the diabetic and thereby decreases the loss of nitrogen from the body. The increase in glucose utilization following insulin injection similarly decreases the need for mobilization and oxidation of fat in the diabetic. It appears that both fat storage and protein synthesis are dependent upon the oxidation of glucose. In the absence of insulin, protein synthesis induced by growth hormone is minimal. Insulin also greatly increases glycogen storage in the liver and to a less extent in striated muscle in diabetes. It actually decreases glycogen storage in cardiac muscle and kidney.

In the normal animal, insulin tends to decrease glycogen storage in the liver. This appears to result from an increase in glycogen storage or glucose utilization in striated muscle, which results in a decrease in the blood sugar level. This in turn results in glycolysis in the liver to reestablish the level. The action of insulin at the periphery was demonstrated by its augmentation of the arteriovenous difference in blood sugar in an extremity, in the early studies of Cori and Cori.

A number of *types of insulin* are now available for clinical use. All are derived from either hog or beef pancreas and all have the same basic actions on carbohydrate metabolism. The preparations of insulin in use include *regular insulin, crystalline insulin,*

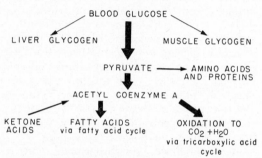

Fig. 83. Diagram of processes apparently enhanced by insulin in the diabetic.

globin insulin, protamine zinc insulin, NPH insulin and *zinc insulin mixtures.* The chief difference in these modifications of insulin is in the time of action. Thus, in the fasting diabetic, regular and crystalline insulin exert their effect on blood sugar for about 6 to 8 hours with a peak effect at about 3 to 4 hours. Globin insulin is active for about 20 to 24 hours with maximal action at 8 hours. NPH or isophane insulin, about equivalent to 2:1 mixture of regular and protamine zinc insulin, exerts action for 24 to 28 hours with maximal action also at about 8 hours. Protamine zinc insulin (PZI) may have activity persisting in excess of 30 hours with a peak effect between 12 and 24 hours. The Danish zinc and insulin mixtures (insulin lenta) vary in their duration of action from 18 to 30 hours. The duration of action of any insulin varies in different persons depending on rates of absorption and other unknown factors.

The *adrenal glands* exert important influences on carbohydrate metabolism. *Epinephrine,* the product of the medullary portion of the gland, when administered to the well nourished animal, characteristically raises the blood sugar as a result of increasing the breakdown of liver glycogen to glucose. When liver glycogen stores are depleted, epinephrine appears to decrease muscle glycogen similarly with the liberation of lactic acid, which is transported to the liver and resynthesized to glycogen or glucose. Epinephrine may also stimulate liberation of ACTH by the pituitary gland with secondary liberation of adrenal cortical hormones. The *adrenal cortex,* as mentioned under Etiology, is capable of causing profound changes in carbohydrate metabolism. The steroids with an oxygen atom in the 11-position, e.g., corticosterone or 17-hydroxycorticosterone, induce glycosuria and an increase in nitrogen excretion in normal animals, and they intensify already-existing diabetes. The mechanism of action of these steroids has not been established, but the site of action appears to be in the liver. Cori and his associates suggest that these adrenal steroids exert their "anti-insulin" effect primarily by intensifying the inhibitory action of anterior pituitary extract upon hexokinase, the enzyme responsible for the phosphorylation of glucose to glucose-6-phosphate.

As stated above, growth hormone, particularly in association with insulin, is effective in increasing nitrogen storage by augmenting protein synthesis. It is also diabetogenic as discussed elsewhere.

The effect of the *thyroid* hormone, as mentioned before, intensifies glycosuria in the diabetic and causes transient glycosuria in normal persons. This effect appears to result primarily from the fact that thyroid substance increases the rate of absorption of glucose so that the threshold for excretion is readily exceeded. It also increases glycogen breakdown.

Blood Sugar. The concentration of glucose in the blood at any given time is the resultant of forces tending to remove glucose to the tissues for utilization and forces leading to the synthesis of glucose or to an increase in its flow to the blood stream, as indicated by the arrows in Figure 81. The most important factor quantitatively determining the height of the blood glucose level is obviously the glucose absorbed from the gut. The normal fasting blood sugar level is 80 to 120 mg. per 100 cc., of which about 20 mg. is not glucose and is accounted for by other reducing substances. After the ingestion of a liberal amount of carbohydrate the level rises normally to about 150 mg. per 100 cc. in 30 to 60 minutes and returns to the fasting level or lower in the course of 2 hours.

In order to maintain the normal fasting blood sugar level, the pancreas must liberate the proper amount of insulin. This control mechanism is generally believed to be regulated by vagal stimulation and the concentration of glucose in the blood. Thus, when the blood sugar level begins to rise, the islet cells are stimulated to elaborate more insulin. When the level tends to fall, insulin formation is diminished and the liberation of epinephrine is believed to stimulate glycogenolysis in the liver which restores the blood sugar level. The part played by anterior pituitary extract and certain adrenal cortical steroids in the maintenance of the normal blood sugar level is undoubtedly also of great importance and may, under conditions of stress, result indirectly from the liberation of epinephrine, which causes release of ACTH by the hypophysis. The role of glucagon in regulating the normal blood sugar level has not been fully determined.

When the blood sugar level is in excess of about 170 mg. per 100 cc., glycosuria appears. Under these conditions the renal tubules are unable to reabsorb all the glucose present in glomerular filtrate. In a number of older diabetics the normal renal threshold is raised and the urine remains sugar-free even when the blood glucose level is greater than 300 mg. per 100 cc. Possibly this elevation of threshold can in some way be correlated with capillary glomerulosclerosis which is common in this group of patients and results from a decrease in filtration and in some instances an increase in tubular reabsorption.

Fat Metabolism. The storage of neutral fat occurs chiefly in the subcutaneous depots. This fat is derived normally from that ingested and from fatty acids derived from glucose, as described under Carbohydrate Metabolism. The liver, which is intimately involved in fat metabolism as well as in carbohydrate metabolism, normally contains 2 to 4 per cent of fat. Concentration of fat in excess of 10 per cent may appear in the liver, however, under a great array of circumstances, including obesity, pregnancy, starvation, phlorizin diabetes and in elderly obese but not in juvenile diabetics. Diets containing large amounts of fat, biotin or cystine, or diets deficient in methionine, choline or betaine, also give rise to an increase in the fat content of the liver, as do chloroform and other liver poisons.

The mechanisms by which *fat is mobilized* from the peripheral tissues to the liver are not understood. However, a substance in the anterior pituitary, "adipokinin," is capable of inducing this "migration" of fat. The importance of this pituitary stimulus for fat mobilization in the variety of conditions under which liver fat is increased is not known, and the way in which it affects mobilization is also obscure.

The total lipid concentration of the normal plasma is from 500 to 600 mg. per 100 cc. Approximately one half of this is in the form of neutral fat and fatty acid, and the remainder is composed of cholesterol and its esters, and phospholipid. When the rate of mobilization is greatly increased, as in uncontrolled diabetes complicated with severe ketosis, the concentration of blood lipid may be enormously increased; in one of the writer's patients it reached 25 per cent.

The *oxidation of fat* begins in the liver (except for a small increment in the kidneys and other tissues) and proceeds, as originally postulated by Knoop and by Dakin, by stepwise oxidation of the long-chained fatty acids occurring normally in nature which contain an even number of carbon atoms.

The oxidation takes place in the beta position and yields at each step a fatty acid chain shortened by 2 carbon atoms and a 2 carbon fragment, acetyl coenzyme A. This process of degradation of fatty acids takes place in the fatty acid cycle of Lynen and of Green and the events are the exact reverse of those described for the formation of fatty acids in the section on Carbohydrate Metabolism. In the complete degradation of fatty acid, acetyl coA enters the tricarboxylic acid cycle and is ultimately oxidized to CO_2 and H_2O. Acetoacetic acid results from the condensation of two molecules of acetyl coA. Beta-hydroxybuteric acid and acetone, the other "ketone bodies," are elaborated from acetoacetate.

The ketone bodies and acetic acid are rapidly transported from the liver to other tissues, notably the muscles, where they serve, both in the normal and the diabetic, as a source of energy and are ultimately oxidized to carbon dioxide and water. This utilization is so complete that under normal conditions only traces of ketone bodies appear in the blood and urine.

Ketosis and Acidosis. In the course of uncontrolled diabetes, glycosuria increases in intensity and is accompanied by a large rise in the urinary excretion of nitrogen due to an increase in gluconeogenesis (the gluconeogenesis appears to be, at least in part, due to the inability to store protein normally in the absence of insulin). Soon there follows a great increase in the catabolism of fat. The rate of breakdown of fat to ketone bodies, in itself a normal process, is far in excess of the rate at which acetoacetic and beta-hydroxybutyric acids can be utilized by muscles and other tissues. Consequently, the ketone bodies increase in the blood, at times reaching levels of 200 mg. per 100 cc. or more. This ketonemia is associated with the excretion of both ketone acids and acetone in the urine in amounts which may exceed 60 gm. a day.

Ketosis develops also in other disorders in which adequate amounts of glucose are not available, as in the course of starvation or in phlorizin poisoning. It also appears when the diet contains fat in excess of about 4 gm. for each gram of glucose available as such, or that derived from protein (about 58 per cent). The nature of the stimulus for unusually great catabolism of fat and its ensuing ketosis has not been ascertained with certainty. However, it seems certain that glucose oxidation is essential both for the storage of fat and the synthesis of body protein. When oxidation of glucose is sharply reduced in diabetes as a result of an inadequate supply of insulin or in starvation because of an inadequate supply of glucose, then mobilization and breakdown of fat with varying degrees of ketone formation transpire by the routes indicated above. Also in the absence of glucose oxidation negative nitrogen balance ensues because of failure of protein synthesis and because of gluconeogenesis from amino acids.

One of the many unresolved problems concerning the mechanism of ketosis is the unpredictability with which it appears. For example, one of two wholly similar diabetics may, in the course of 24 hours after the withdrawal of insulin, exhibit serious ketosis in association with heavy glycosuria. The other under apparently identical circumstances and with the same glycosuria will develop essentially no ketonemia or ketonuria despite persisting glycosuria and nitrogen loss.

Because two of the three ketone bodies are acids, their continued elaboration leads to *disturbances of acid-base equilibrium.* Their accumulation in the blood plasma reduces the bicarbonate content and ultimately causes severe acidosis. Both acetoacetic and beta-hydroxybutyric acids are relatively strong acids, and, whereas they are in part excreted as such, a much larger part calls upon base for elimination. Some of this is furnished by the ammonia and phosphate mechanisms, but there is also serious depletion of fixed cation, including sodium, potassium and calcium as acidosis progresses. Moreover, Atchley, Richards and the writer showed that the loss of inorganic base in severe diabetes actually begins coincidentally with the development of heavy glycosuria and before ketosis occurs. This loss of base is associated with the loss of intracellular and extracellular water as well as with the breakdown of cells, as judged by nitrogen loss. The general problem of acidosis is dealt with elsewhere in this volume.

The accumulation of beta-hydroxybutyric acid in the body is relatively harmless except for its effect upon acid-base equilibrium. On the other hand, acetoacetic acid and acetone are distinctly toxic, and their accumulation depresses the central nervous system. It seems probable that a considerable part of the picture of diabetic coma may properly be ascribed to intoxication by these ketone bodies. Kety has demonstrated a 40 per cent reduction in cerebral utilization of oxygen in diabetic coma and ascribes it, in part, to the acidosis and more significantly to the ketosis and possibly other factors.

Caloric Requirements. Age, sex, surface area, physical activity, state of nutrition, fever, thyroid activity and probably many other factors influence energy requirements. Consequently, to attempt to set down the number of calories required by any person to maintain a given weight is not, in most instances, helpful. In general, sedentary adults require in the neighborhood of 30 calories per kilogram; the requirements of children are greater, and those of the aged tend to be less. The deviations from these generalizations are, however, great, and the only practical procedure to be followed in establishing caloric requirements is that of trial and error, using body weight as an index. It should be noted that the caloric requirements of the diabetic do not differ from those of the normal.

The protein requirements are also variable and are governed more or less by the same factors which influence the total caloric needs. The amount of carbohydrate in the diet, however, has a significant effect upon the protein intake essential to maintain nitrogen equilibrium. An intake of 100 to 150 gm. of carbohydrate daily cuts down nitrogen loss in starvation appreciably. With increase in carbohydrate beyond this amount, Butler has shown that additional "nitrogen-sparing action" of carbohydrate is inappreciable, at least in normal young adults.

Morbid Anatomy. The commonest histologic lesions in diabetes mellitus are found in the pancreas. It is interesting to note, however, that in the meticulous studies of postmortem material by Cecil and others, more than 10 per cent of the cases failed to reveal any pancreatic lesions. In the cases in which changes are encountered in the pancreas, no one distinctive lesion is uniformly present in the islets. In some cases there appears to be a reduction in the total number of islets without other lesions demonstrable. In others, hydropic degeneration of the beta cells has been noted. The most frequently encountered lesions are hyaline degeneration and sclerosis of the islands of Langerhans. The lesions observed may be secondary to an abnormality of carbohydrate metabolism originating outside the pancreas, as in "Young's diabetes," or as in cats maintained hyperglycemic by the prolonged administration of glucose intraperitoneally. Local destructive disease of the pancreas including diffuse pancreatitis, extensive tumors and large cysts may be the cause of diabetes. Also hemochromatosis with intensive infiltration of the pancreas with hemosiderin and ceroid is often associated with diabetes.

The kidney is frequently the site of a variety of lesions in diabetes mellitus. Commonest is pyelonephritis, infection in the kidneys perhaps being enhanced by high concentrations of glucose. Capillary glomerulosclerosis characterized by hyaline globules in the walls of the capillary loops is present in about 20 per cent of patients. When the lesions are marked, as is the case in 5 to 10 per cent, they may be associated with albuminuria, hypoalbuminemia, hypercholesterolemia and arterial hypertension, i.e., the Kimmelstiel-Wilson syndrome. Glomerulosclerosis, retinopathy and neuropathy frequently occur in the same patient and this combination has been termed the "diabetic triopathy." There are those who believe that patients exhibiting this syndrome have a special form of diabetes, though the evidence for this is not convincing. Necrotizing papillitis occurs occasionally, and most frequently in patients with severe acidosis and hypotensive shock. Deposition of glycogen in the loops of Henle, as in cardiac muscle, is present in severe diabetes.

Sherlock has demonstrated, by liver biopsy,

striking increase in deposition of fat in the older, relatively resistant obese diabetics in contrast to juvenile diabetics in whom there is no increase in liver fat.

Arteriosclerotic lesions are extraordinarily prevalent in patients with diabetes. This is discussed more fully in the section on Complications.

Clinical Symptoms and Signs. In children and young adults an abrupt onset or one which can be dated within a two months' period is encountered in about 65 per cent of patients, according to Joslin. In the older age groups the onset is usually so insidious that it cannot be established. Among these patients the disease is often discovered only in the course of routine examination of the urine, because, if symptoms do exist, they are not sufficiently severe to cause the patient to seek medical attention. Other patients more than 40 years old first see the physician when a complication arises, suggesting that diabetes may have been present but unrecognized for years.

The most common and characteristic symptom of diabetes, and the one from which it derives its name, is *polyuria*. Patients not infrequently pass large amounts of urine day and night, and the volume is often in excess of 3 or 4 liters. Inordinate thirst, *polydipsia*, may torment the patient and lead him to seek medical advice. Less frequent, but not uncommon, is a striking increase in appetite, *polyphagia*. This is particularly true in children who are brought to the physician by parents because, despite a great "improvement" in appetite, the children fail to gain weight or strength. Many patients complain of *loss of weight* or *loss of strength*, or both, losses of 20 to 40 pounds in the course of a few weeks or months being not unusual. The symptoms of polyuria, polydipsia, polyphagia, loss of weight and loss of strength are generally associated with the more acute and severe forms of the disease. Among older patients there may be an abnormal tendency to postprandial *drowsiness*, not related to ketosis; at times there are vague aches in the legs or other symptoms, as already mentioned, referable to some complication.

In uncomplicated diabetes there are but few *physical signs* which alone would lead one to suspect the disease. Possibly marked emaciation and dryness of the skin and mucous membranes without obvious cause might be considered evidence. In uncon-

trolled diabetes in children, hepatomegaly is common and is at times associated with splenomegaly.

The characteristic feature of the *urine* in diabetes is obviously the presence of glucose. The concentration of sugar may vary from mere traces to as much as 10 per cent, and the total excreted in 24 hours varies from insignificant amounts to several hundred grams. In general, the amounts excreted are indicative of the intensity of the disorder at the time. The specific gravity of the urine may naturally be much higher than the pale-colored urine would suggest. In the presence of ketosis the urine usually contains large quantities of ketone bodies which can be detected by the nitroprusside and ferric chloride reactions. Proteinuria and numerous casts are often present in ketosis. The *blood sugar* level may be normal or markedly elevated, depending upon the circumstances of the test and the severity of the disease; in severe uncontrolled diabetes it may exceed concentrations of 1000 mg. per 100 cc. It has already been mentioned that blood lipids are often increased in diabetes, particularly when ketosis is present. When emaciation is marked, hypoproteinemia may be extreme and there is a sharp reduction in the serum albumin fraction. It is rare, at the present time, to find cases which have reached this stage of protein depletion. In uncomplicated diabetes there is no reduction in the *erythrocyte count* except in the presence of marked malnutrition, when mild secondary anemia may be present. With severe dehydration in ketosis, hemoconcentration may be moderate. The *leukocyte count* is normal except in severe ketosis and acidosis, when it usually rises to 20,000 or 30,000 per cubic millimeter. The *sedimentation rate* of the red cells is essentially normal except in the presence of acidosis or complications of infectious origin.

Complications. With the increasing span of life of patients with diabetes, complications may be expected to increase; consequently they deserve particular consideration in management of the disease.

Acidosis and Coma. In days before the advent of insulin, approximately 50 per cent of diabetics died from these complications. Today, death in coma is a rare occurrence in well organized clinics, and a case terminating fatally deserves critical review to determine the reasons for coma and for failure of therapy. Analysis of 7 patients in diabetic coma admitted to the Presbyterian Hospital and dying thereafter reveals that 5 of these arrived at the hospital in this stage of the disease without the diagnosis of their underlying diabetes ever having been established prior to admission.

Whereas deaths from acidosis have become a rare occurrence, it must be emphasized that any diabetic may succumb in two or three days if control of his disease is not rigidly exercised. Ketosis with its sequelae, acidosis and coma, is usually precipitated by one of the following disorders: (1) infections of the respiratory, genitourinary or gastrointestinal tract, or pyogenic infections; (2) surgical procedures or trauma; (3) gastrointestinal disturbances with reduction of food intake or vomiting. *The commonest contributing factor to ketosis in these conditions is the ill advised reduction or omission of insulin by the patient because of a decrease in food intake. In reality, all these disturbances effect an increase in the insulin requirement!* It should be emphasized that in many instances emotional disturbances are the basis for increases in glycosuria, ketonuria, "digestive disturbances" and the subconscious or conscious rationalization for the withdrawal of insulin.

The development of acidosis is usually associated with *symptoms* of increasing weakness, weariness, dull headache and general malaise. The onset may be abrupt or insidious. Insatiable thirst soon becomes a prominent feature, and, as acidosis progresses, hyperpnea or the "air-hunger" of Kussmaul appears with little if any subjective distress. Epigastric aching pain adds to the discomfort of the patient and is associated with increasing nausea and vomiting and persistent thirst. The abdominal symptoms, in association with the striking leukocytosis, usually present in severe ketosis, often arouse suspicion of acute inflammation in the peritoneal cavity. The patient becomes more and more listless and may sink into coma quietly and die, or coma may be preceded by a period of great restlessness, irritability and confusion.

On *physical examination* the patient in severe diabetic acidosis shows marked dehydration of the mucous membranes and loss of turgor of the skin. The eyes are sunken, the lips and tongue red and parched, and the cheeks either flushed or else very pale. The breath has the characteristic "fruity" odor of acetone, and hyperpnea is apparent. These signs are accompanied by a rapid, feeble pulse, a temperature which may either be elevated or subnormal, and by arterial hypotension. The blood pressure may fall to 60 to 70 mm. of mercury as coma deepens and anuria supervenes, together with progression of peripheral circulatory collapse. In older patients this state of shock, if allowed to continue, gives rise to myocardial insufficiency, probably because of decreased blood flow in the coronary arteries.

The *severity* of diabetic acidosis may be arbitrarily but conveniently classified in relation to the bicarbonate-combining power of the blood serum. When the serum carbon dioxide falls below 25 volumes per 100 cc., severe acidosis may be said to be present. A carbon dioxide of 25 to 40 volumes per 100 cc. may be considered indicative of moderately severe acidosis, and values between 40 and 50 volumes are consistent with mild acidosis. This is a purely clinical classification and is not correlated with actual shift of the pH from normal, which is obviously more significant than is the CO_2 level. Deep coma due to ketosis and acidosis rarely if ever develops with a blood carbon dioxide above 25 volumes per 100 cc. When the carbon dioxide is higher, it is particularly important to exclude other causes of coma. The other typical blood and urine findings have been described. It should be added for emphasis that loss of bicarbonate and also of chloride results from their replacement by ketone acids and from a loss of sodium from the blood and intercellular fluids by renal excretion. *In the presence of renal failure, occurring in the course of peripheral circulatory collapse, ketone bodies may virtually disappear from the urine. Failure to appreciate this fact may result in failure to recognize severe diabetic acidosis.* In these patients large quantities of acetone can be demonstrated in the blood plasma with the simple nitroprusside reaction. Patients exhibiting renal insufficiency may also have retention of nonprotein nitrogen in excess of 200 mg. per 100 cc.

Arteriosclerosis. Because about 50 per cent of diabetes occurs in the fifth and sixth decades, it is to be expected that arteriosclerosis in its various forms will appear concurrently. It seems, however, that the two disorders are more intimately related, since 50 per cent of White's children who had diabetes for more than fifteen years had calcification of leg vessels. How much metabolic factors, such as long-continued hyperglycemia and hypercholesterolemia, contribute to the arteriosclerotic process is not known. It is of interest that Mendlowitz has demonstrated decreases in digital blood flow in young diabetics and that this change is largely independent of intensity and duration of the diabetes and the age of onset. This suggests the possibility that the vascular lesions may be at least in part unrelated in their genesis to the intensity and duration of overt disturbances in carbohydrate metabolism. Decrease in circulation in the legs gives rise to *trophic ulcers* in the soles of the feet and also serves as a basis for *infection* and for *gangrene,* one of the most serious complications of diabetes. It is generally believed that these complications appear most frequently in neglected diabetes of long standing. It seems possible that neglect of the feet, dermatophytosis and secondary infection in patients with compromised circulation are of greater importance. Loss of pulsations in the dorsalis pedis and posterior tibial arteries and cold feet should constitute a warning concerning the dangers of subsequent infection. Angina pectoris and *cardiac infarction* are extremely common in older diabetics. This is of importance in relation to the management of older patients with insulin.

Eyes. Retinitis may occur in diabetics with or without hypertensive vascular disease, and may appear as early as the second decade of life. This disorder is ten times as frequent in patients who have had their disease for fifteen years as it is in patients in whom diabetes has been known only one year. It is generally believed that the diabetic retinitis is most apt to develop in patients with poorly controlled diabetes or in those who have been given a diet high in fat and low in carbohydrate. The most characteristic lesion is aneurysmal dilatation of the finer blood vessels, often simulating punctate hemorrhages. Hemorrhages are also common and frequently occur in association with waxy and cotton-wool exudates. Later, proliferating retinopathy and advanced arteriosclerosis are found.

Cataracts may develop in young diabetics, but their incidence is extremely low. Senile cataract is common in older diabetic patients, but perhaps no more so than in nondiabetic persons of the same age group.

Nervous System. Rundles has reported 125 cases of diabetic neuropathy among 3000 diabetics. These include peripheral neuritis with motor and sensory changes most frequently involving the legs, as well as lesions of spinal nerve roots and autonomic disturbances involving the bladder and vasomotor apparatus. There are no clinical signs which, with any regularity, serve to distinguish diabetic neuritis from neuritis due to other causes. Associated with the diabetic neuropathies there is often an increase in spinal fluid protein, which may reach 200 mg. per 100 cc.

The basis for neurologic lesions is not definitely established. Vitamin B_1 deficiency has been implicated by some. Also a defect in vitamin B_{12} metabolism with an unusual degree of "tissue unsaturation" has been claimed only for diabetics who have associated retinopathy. Others are of the opinion that the diabetic neuropathies result from "ischemic" neuritis due to sclerosis of the vasa nervorum. In the opinion of Rundles the neuropathies are caused by other "metabolic disturbances" which appear in the course of poorly controlled diabetes. In support of this view is the fact that striking improvement frequently follows a period of adequate regulation of the disease. Probably multiple factors play a part in the genesis of the diabetic neuropathies. Mirsky has reported that diabetics, regardless of duration of their disease, intensity, or age at onset, exhibit a diminution in vibratory sense equivalent to that in nondiabetics two decades older. This suggests that neurologic lesions, like vascular lesions, may not be correlated with the disturbances in carbohydrate metabolism.

Diabetic neuropathies are encountered from the first decade on. In Rundles' series, however, about 17 per cent appeared in the sixth decade alone.

Skin. Furuncles and carbuncles are sufficiently frequent in patients with diabetes to make examination of the urine for glucose mandatory in any person suffering from these pyogenic infections. Pruritus of a generalized nature is an occasional complication of diabetes, but pruritus is much more commonly limited to the vulva. Whether the pyogenic infections of the skin and pruritus are to be correlated with elevated glucose content of the skin is not known. Pruritus vulvae is frequently associated with infection due to *Monilia albicans,* which appears to thrive on the sugar deposited locally from the urine.

Numerous observers have commented on the presence of xanthochromia in diabetes. Rabinowich, Ralli and others showed this to be the result of an increase in the circulating carotene which occurs because of an apparent decrease in the capacity of the liver of the diabetic to convert carotene into vitamin A. Xanthochromia is not to be confused with xanthoma diabeticorum, a relatively rare disorder characterized by nodules commonly on the elbows, ulnar surfaces of the forearms, and knees, and usually associated with hypercholesterolemia.

Tuberculosis. The incidence of pulmonary tuberculosis is about four times higher among diabetics than among nondiabetics. The two diseases occur together with sufficient frequency so that all diabetics should have roentgen ray study of the chest as part of their routine examination.

Course and Prognosis. At the present time diabetes mellitus must be looked upon as a chronic and incurable disease. There is a tendency for it to progress in intensity with time, but there are many exceptions to this generalization. The fluctuations in intensity of the disease in any patient have already been commented upon. Richardson found that in a group of 55 patients followed for more than five years, the insulin requirement increased in 21 and actually decreased in 10. In a group of 45 patients who did not require insulin for regulation, 21 were still able to remain sugar-free without insulin after five years of observation.

The average duration of life in diabetics in all age groups, according to Joslin, has increased from 4.9 years in pre-insulin days to about 13 years at the present time. The most striking increase in the anticipated span of life is in the young. For example, in an analysis of Joslin's material, it appears that the life expectancy of a child of 10 years with diabetes is 40 years, in contrast with the normal expectancy of 57 years. At 60 the anticipated duration of life is 10 years, in contrast to the normal of 16 years (Metropolitan Life Insurance Company).

The actual cure of diabetes mellitus is probably a rare occurrence. In the obese, as mentioned under Etiology, it is not unusual to find a reversion to normal carbohydrate metabolism with a return to a more normal weight. In these persons, diabetes should be considered "latent" rather than "cured," because a return of obesity is associated with a return of overt diabetes. In hyperthyroidism, likewise, relief of this disorder may cause mild diabetes to become "latent." With growths of the adrenal glands in which diabetes results from the elaboration of "anti-insulin," e.g., Cushing's syndrome, diabetes

may be relieved by removal of an adrenal cortical tumor.

Lukens and Dohan were able to cure diabetes induced in cats by means of anterior pituitary extract, provided the hyperglycemia was abolished before hyalinization of beta cells took place. This is not so in dogs. It is unfortunate but probable that man resembles the dog more closely than the cat in this respect and that his diabetes cannot be cured by the early alleviation of hyperglycemia.

Classification. Patients are usually classified as having mild, moderately severe or severe diabetes, and yet the basis for such classification is wholly arbitrary and quantitatively ill defined. There would be general agreement that a diabetic requiring only moderate restriction of his diet for adequate control of his disease could be termed as having mild diabetes. Furthermore, if, in the absence of insulin therapy, heavy glycosuria, loss of weight and acidosis tend to develop, all would agree that the disease is severe.

The dosage of insulin required for the regulation of diabetes also serves at times as a general guide for classification. However, it has been indicated elsewhere that certain endocrine and other factors determine insulin requirements, and hence exceptions to the use of insulin dosage as the grounds for classification have to be made. For example, a girl with Addison's disease and diabetes, who excreted 60 to 80 gm. of glucose daily without insulin, could scarcely be classified as having mild diabetes merely because, in these circumstances, her insulin requirement was only 4 to 6 units a day. Adding still further to the difficulty of definite classification of diabetes is the fact that the individual patient may fluctuate from one category to another. Thus mild diabetes may, in the course of an acute infection, become severe, only to revert to a milder form with subsidence of infection.

Diagnosis. The diagnosis of diabetes mellitus affords no difficulty when polyuria, polydipsia and polyphagia are associated with an elevation of the fasting blood sugar level and with glycosuria. Even in the absence of symptoms, glycosuria related to the ingestion of carbohydrate and a postabsorptive blood sugar concentration in excess of 120 mg. per 100 cc. constitute an adequate basis for the diagnosis. The presence of glycosuria is, however, not essential for the diagnosis, because the renal threshold may be significantly elevated in certain older diabetics. In this group the fasting blood sugar may be as high as 200 mg. per 100 cc., and glycosuria may appear only after meals if the blood sugar exceeds levels as high as 300 mg. per 100 cc.

Diabetes mellitus should be suspected in any person who exhibits glycosuria in relation to food intake on an unrestricted diet or whose venous blood sugar level rises above 170 to 180 mg. per 100 cc. at any time. In these patients the form of the blood sugar curve following either a carbohydrate-rich meal (containing potato, three slices of bread, a sugar-containing dessert and sugar in coffee) or a glucose tolerance test may prove helpful in establishing the diagnosis of latent diabetes. The *glucose tolerance* test is usually carried out by determining the blood sugar level before and after the oral administration of 1 to 1.75 gm. of glucose per kilogram of body weight in the fasting state. The blood sugar should be determined before, and 1 and 2 hours after the administration of glucose, and urine collected at these times should be tested for sugar. Normally, the blood sugar does not rise above about 150 to 170 mg. per 100 cc. in one-half to 1 hour after the ingestion of the glucose, and returns to a normal level in 2 hours, and the urine remains sugar-free. If higher levels are reached or *if the blood sugar does not return to normal in 2 hours, diabetes should be suspected.*

Beaser has pointed out that cognizance should be taken of the presence of "latent" diabetes characterized clinically only by a diabetic glucose tolerance curve and possibly transient glycosuria. When these occur, particularly in persons with a family history of diabetes, the avoidance of obesity and the restriction of dietary sugar may prevent the establishment of overt diabetes.

The *interpretation of the glucose tolerance test* is to a great extent dependent upon the conditions under which it is carried out. If this fact is not thoroughly appreciated, mistakes in diagnosis are bound to occur. The state of nutrition and the nature of the diet preceding the test are of prime importance. This is graphically demonstrated in Figure 84. Thus the curve characteristic of diabetes occurs in patients with undernutrition or in those who have maintained a diet low in carbohydrates, whereas in the same person after the liberal ingestion of carbohydrate for a few days prior to the test, normal responses are evoked. As has been mentioned before, this diabetic type of response following un-

dernutrition or the administration of insulin to the normal is characteristic of "starvation" diabetes. Likewise, as stated before, this temporary decrease in glucose tolerance may in part result from "rest" of islet tissue with a decrease in the elaboration of insulin, as shown by Best and Haist. It is well established also that the effectiveness of insulin in man and animals is in general reduced by starvation or by low carbohydrate diets, prob-

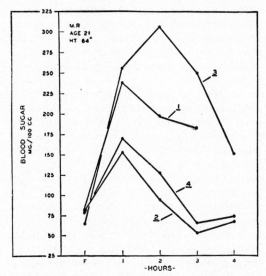

Fig. 84. Effect of diet upon the glucose tolerance curves (after Conn). *1,* Test done on admission in severe undernutrition. *2,* After two weeks, 3000 cals. 300 gm. CHO, 80 gm. P. *3,* After seven days, 1600 cals. 20 gm. CHO, 50 gm. P. *4,* After seven days, 3000 cals. 300 gm. CHO, 80 gm. P.

ably in relation to fatty liver, and on the other hand it is increased by the liberal ingestion of carbohydrate and by hyperglycemia. Whatever the ultimate explanation for these observations, it is important to bear in mind that *glucose tolerance curves typical of diabetes may signify undernutrition or carbohydrate starvation and not necessarily the presence of diabetes mellitus.*

Errors in the diagnosis of diabetes may occur from faulty appraisal of normal or low blood sugar values obtained after strenuous exercise. If a person, either normal or diabetic, exercises after the ingestion of carbohydrate, an appreciable reduction in blood sugar occurs in association with an increase in utilization of glucose.

Transient hyperglycemia and glycosuria occur in a good many circumstances and may not signify the presence of diabetes mellitus.

For example, as stated elsewhere, transient hyperglycemia and glycosuria occur frequently in hyperthyroidism. Hyperglycemia and glycosuria also occur after the injection of epinephrine and, on the same basis, during acute emotional strain or in the presence of certain tumors of the adrenal medulla. A few nondiabetic persons have a brief rise in blood sugar above their renal thresholds and excrete traces of glucose after the ingestion of large amounts of sugar—this is known as *alimentary glycosuria.* Hyperglycemia and glycosuria occur not infrequently in severe meningitis and in certain injuries to the brain. The history and other findings serve to differentiate these disorders from diabetes mellitus.

An unusual condition in which considerable quantities of glucose appear in the urine is *"renal glycosuria."* In at least certain cases this results from an inborn error of metabolism in which the normal reabsorption of glucose fails to take place in the renal tubules (Fanconi's syndrome). Patients with this disorder resemble animals poisoned with phlorizin in that they do not have hyperglycemia and the degree of glycosuria is essentially independent of the carbohydrate intake. Young people with alimentary glycosuria or renal glycosuria should be considered potential diabetics and should be reexamined at frequent intervals, particularly when a family history of diabetes has been elicited.

Lactosuria is not uncommon in pregnancy, but is not related to diabetes mellitus. Levulosuria, galactosuria, pentosuria and maltosuria are rare conditions not, as a rule, associated with elevation of the blood sugar. The nature of the sugar excreted should be determined in all cases of atypical glycosuria.

In children with marked hepatomegaly, glycosuria, ketosis and a blood sugar exhibiting swings from marked hyperglycemia to striking hypoglycemia, the diagnosis of von Gierke's disease (glycogen storage disease) should be seriously considered.

Treatment. During the past two decades the treatment of diabetes has become greatly simplified, and it should now be the responsibility of the family physician rather than the specialist to treat the numerous patients who seek his aid. Nevertheless it cannot be overemphasized that the successful treatment of diabetes continues to demand the closest attention to detail by both the physician and the patient.

The aim of therapy in diabetes mellitus should be directed towards maintaining health, happiness and normal nutrition on a regimen which keeps the patient approximately sugar-free. This can be achieved easily in the vast majority of patients with but little modification of the patient's way of life. In a few patients, the so-called "brittle" diabetics, satisfactory regulation is extraordinarily difficult even for the specialist to achieve and in these patients intermittent glycosuria is preferable to a life dedicated to the testing of urine.

The management of diabetes must be based upon two principles. The first is the establishment of a dietary regimen, with or without insulin, in accordance with the aims set forth for therapy. The second is the education of the patient so that he understands (1) the nature of the fundamental disorders in his disease, (2) the preparation and regulation of his diet, (3) the method of testing his urine for sugar and ketone bodies, (4) the technique of self-administration of insulin when this is required, and (5) the complications which may occur and how they should be met. The diabetic patient should be taught to assume the role of the physician and the latter should assume the role of the consultant in routine management of this disease. These principles are put into practice most simply and effectively and with the least loss of time if the patient is hospitalized for regulation and training at the time the diagnosis is established.

One of the first and most important questions which arise in the regulation of a diabetic is whether insulin will be required or whether dietary restriction alone will suffice to achieve the aims of therapy. Upon the decision reached will depend the amount and distribution of the carbohydrate in the diet, frequency of collection of urine specimens, the times of meals, the economic factor involved in the provision of insulin and, to a large extent, the education of the patient. Whether or not insulin will be required cannot be answered dogmatically, and the method of trial and error must frequently be invoked. This is particularly true in patients whose disease process, for one reason or an-

* The aim of maintaining the patient approximately sugar-free has been challenged by Tolstoi, who administers insulin and disregards the degree of glycosuria, provided that ketonuria and the loss of nitrogen do not develop. It remains for the future to determine whether or not this seeming laxity in management will add materially to the incidence of arterial disease, neuropathies and retinitis.

other, may at one time be severe and at another time mild. For example, in the presence of infection or hyperthyroidism, insulin therapy may be essential and yet, after subsidence of activity, dietary regulation alone may suffice. In spite of these apparent difficulties in arriving at an important decision, the following generalizations can be made and serve as useful guides: (1) the majority of older obese patients in whom the disease is essentially without symptoms do not require insulin; and (2) all diabetic children, young adults and most older patients who acquire the disease acutely with the characteristic symptoms of polydipsia, polyuria, rapid loss of weight and strength require insulin therapy. The percentage of patients with diabetes who can be regulated without insulin varies in different clinics according to the type of regimen established, the standards for "adequate" treatment, the intelligence of the patients as a group, and many other factors. According to Adlersberg and Dolger, 46 per cent of their series of 1131 patients more than 14 years of age did not require insulin and were treated with diet alone. These patients were undoubtedly in the older age group and were presumably overweight.

Dietary Treatment without Insulin. This form of treatment, as mentioned before, is applicable only to the management of the relatively mild diabetes encountered in obese patients, most of whom are more than 50 years of age. As stated under Etiology, the control of obesity in these patients usually suffices to render the urine sugar-free and to reestablish an essentially normal blood sugar level. It is rarely necessary, nor is it advisable, to attempt to reduce body weight all the way to the "ideal" value in these patients. Furthermore, reduction in weight should be gradual, since rapid reduction with extreme curtailment of carbohydrate may initiate ketosis and intensify the diabetic process. If regulation is not accomplished without the establishment of undernutrition, or if loss of weight is accompanied by significant loss of strength or marked ketosis, insulin therapy is indicated.

The most important rigid dietary restriction to be initiated is the *omission of free sugar from the diet.* This includes candy, cake, ice cream made with sugar, pastry, fruits preserved with sugar, jam, and so on. When sweetening is desired, saccharin should be used in the preparation of foods.

The diet should be limited as to its content of foods containing high concentrations of starch, e.g., bread, potato, macaroni, spaghetti, rice, cornstarch or tapioca. The patient should not be allowed more than three slices of bread daily and more than one small serving of any of these other foods mentioned. The reason for these limitations is the fact that the availability of glucose in foods having high concentrations of carbohydrates results in rates of absorption which may exceed the rate of utilization by the diabetic and therefore may give rise to hyperglycemia and glycosuria. The remaining carbohydrate of the diet should be in the form of vegetables and fruit with relatively low concentrations of carbohydrate, e.g., 12 per cent or less. It is desirable to have the daily carbohydrate ration divided approximately equally in the three meals.

Protein should be permitted as desired, but for most patients 1 to 1.5 gm. per kilogram of "ideal" weight is sufficient. Fats may be allowed in any form, but the total daily food intake should not exceed 1200 to 1500 calories. Care must be taken in the selection of foods in this limited regimen to provide for vitamin requirements.

When the desired reduction in body weight has taken place and the urine remains sugar-free, the caloric intake may be gradually increased to prevent further weight loss. If this increase in diet results in the reappearance of glycosuria or of a fasting or 2-hour postprandial blood sugar level in excess of perhaps 150 mg. per 100 cc., treatment with insulin becomes indicated.

Patients following this simple type of regimen should, during the period of desugarization, collect 24-hour specimens of urine to be tested for sugar and ketone bodies. After the urine becomes sugar-free, the patient should test an early morning specimen for glucose—this should then become a lifetime habit.

There is no need for frequent determinations of the blood sugar level in these patients. When the urine becomes sugar-free, it is well to determine the fasting level in order to establish whether or not an unusually high threshold is present. Thereafter it may be of interest to determine the fasting blood sugar level at intervals of about six months unless complications intervene.

Treatment with Insulin. When the decision to use insulin has been reached, time is saved if the patient is at once started on the *diet* which it is anticipated will meet his energy requirements and, as far as possible, his desires. The *amount of carbohydrate* which the diet should contain has long been a matter of controversy. In the opinion of the writer the satisfaction of the patient and his nutritional state are the important determining factors. Diets with 100 gm. of carbohydrate or less have no virtue and usually add to the difficulty of management rather than its simplification of two reasons: first, they tend to decrease carbohydrate utilization, and second, they decrease the cooperation of patients, the vast majority of whom desire a more liberal carbohydrate ration. Most patients are satisfied with diets containing 150 to 250 gm. of carbohydrate. Insulin-treated patients, as well as those being treated with diet alone, should not be permitted the use of free sugar.

The *distribution of carbohydrate* between the three repasts is a matter of detail, which, however, assumes great importance in successful regulation. The optimal distribution depends upon individual responses and still more upon the type of insulin used. There is, therefore, no hard and fast rule to be followed in the partition of the daily carbohydrate ration, but when the slow-acting protamine zinc insulin (PZI) is used, the majority of patients are best controlled when the carbohydrate ration is divided into $\frac{1}{5}$, $\frac{2}{5}$ and $\frac{2}{5}$ among breakfast, lunch and dinner or when part of the evening ration (e.g., a slice or two of bread and butter) is saved for a bedtime feeding. When globin or NPH insulin is employed, more frequently part of the noon ration is needed in mid-afternoon to avoid shock. If the carbohydrate of a patient receiving protamine zinc insulin is divided into thirds, it may be expected that the patient will experience hypoglycemia in the early morning hours and heavy glycosuria after breakfast. If a patient has been established on a regimen with regular insulin given twice daily (a regimen rarely indicated today), distribution of the carbohydrate ration into $\frac{2}{5}$, $\frac{1}{5}$ and $\frac{2}{5}$ usually proves the most satisfactory. When a mixture of regular insulin and protamine zinc insulin or NPH insulin is used or when globin insulin or the newer Danish zinc insulin mixtures are given, many patients are best controlled with carbohydrate divided equally among the three meals. However, individual variations are great and many patients require a part of the noon ration of carbohydrate in mid-afternoon

and others require part of the dinner ration at bedtime for satisfactory control as with PZI. The important point to be borne in mind is that *the distribution of the carbohydrate among the three meals, without any change in insulin dosage, often determines the success or failure of therapy*.

The amount of *protein* in the diet should be determined by the amount necessary to maintain nitrogen balance and normal nutrition and by the patient's desires. In most cases, amounts between 60 and 100 gm. daily prove adequate to meet these demands. Obviously the requirements are greatest during the period of growth, in the undernourished, and for hard physical work.

When the carbohydrate and protein rations have been decided upon, enough *fat* should be included to provide the calories necessary to fulfill energy requirements. If patients exhibit a distaste or intolerance for fat or if their desires for carbohydrate are not satisfied, the latter foodstuff should be increased and the fat correspondingly decreased. Most patients are best satisfied with diets containing between 80 and 125 gm. of fat daily. Rigid control of the fat intake is of considerably less importance for satisfactory regulation, as might be expected, than is control of the total carbohydrate intake and its distribution in the meals.

During the period of regulation in the hospital, it is most helpful to have the patient deviate as little as possible from his anticipated way of living, both with regard to physical activity and time of meals; otherwise many unnecessary adjustments of diet and insulin become essential when the patient returns to his home and normal existence.

In the education of the diabetic, regulated with insulin, it is essential that he be instructed promptly in the preparation of a standard diet (a sample of which is shown in the accompanying table) from which in the future he will be able to make indicated adjustments and add to the variety of his meals with the aid of tables of food values. (The *Diabetes Guide Book* of the American Diabetic Association will be found most helpful to physicians and patients in the preparation of menus.)

During the regulation of patients treated with insulin, the *urine* should be collected in four parts during each 24 hours; the first sample from before breakfast up to lunch time, the second from before lunch to before dinner, the third from before dinner to bedtime, and the fourth from bedtime to the next morning. Adjustments in insulin dosage, the type of insulin used and distribution of carbohydrate depend to a large extent upon a knowledge of the time of day at which heavy glycosuria tends to persist. Quantitative determinations of the sugar in the urine are not deemed essential for regulation of the patient.

The *type of insulin to be used in treatment* is to a great extent a matter of choice, but the majority of patients can be treated suc-

few days of regulation. For convenience, each voiding should be tested for sugar with Benedict's reagent. If a red or orange precipitate forms, 10 units may be given, and if a yellow or green color appears, 5 units should be administered. Further decisions concerning the type of insulin, its dosage and the distribution of carbohydrate depend on the response of the individual patient. During regulation, changes in insulin dosage should, when possible, be made not more frequently than every

Example of a Standard Diet

FOOD	TOTAL DAILY PORTIONS	GRAMS—EACH PORTION				GRAMS—TOTAL PORTIONS		
		Weight	C	P	F	C	P	F
Bread	5 slices	25	15	2	—	75	10	0
Oatmeal	¾ cup	20 dry	15	2	—	15	2	—
Potato	1 small	90	15	2	—	15	2	—
Fruit—10%	3	100	10	0	—	30	—	—
Vegetables—3%	5 servings	100	3	2	—	15	10	—
Milk	2 cups	240	12	8	10	24	16	20
Cream—20%	2 tbsp.	30	0	0	5	4	3	5
Butter	4 pats	5	—	—	5	—	—	20
Eggs	1	—	—	7	5	—	7	5
Meat	4 ounces	120	—	28	20	—	28	20

Approximate total grams... 180   70   70
Approximate total calories... 1650

cessfully and with the least inconvenience with a single dose of NPH, globin or protamine zinc insulin. Adlersberg and Dolger report satisfactory regulation of 79 per cent of 489 patients with the latter. Of these, 77 per cent required 40 units or less; about 10 per cent required 65 to 80 units. With the advent of long-acting insulin preparations and particularly with mixtures such as NPH, the former bugbear of two or three injections daily for routine management has been obviated in almost all cases. In patients requiring 40 units of insulin or less, a single injection of NPH is usually equivalent to the same dose of PZI and the fluctuations of blood sugar are less wide. Also, night hypoglycemic reactions are less frequent. These comments apply to the use of globin insulin and zinc insulin preparations also.

In apparently mild cases, treatment may be initiated with a dose of 10 to 20 units of long-acting insulin given subcutaneously, one half hour before breakfast; if the diabetes appears severe, it may be necessary to start with 40 units. When heavy glycosuria is present, time may be saved if supplementary doses of regular insulin are used in the first

other day, since time is obviously required for physiologic adjustment to each change. Except in the presence of heavy glycosuria, acidosis or recurrent hypoglycemia, changes in daily dosage in excess of 5 to 10 units should be avoided.

The intensity and persistence of glycosuria in patients with essentially normal renal thresholds are more important criteria for therapy than are blood sugar levels which may show wide diurnal fluctuations and may at any moment bear little relation to the over-all control of the disease. In elderly diabetics with unusually high thresholds, blood glucose determinations are obviously of importance. In these arteriosclerotic patients, some degree of hyperglycemia is preferable to hypoglycemia which often precipitates coronary insufficiency.

In rare instances patients acquire extraordinary *resistance to insulin* and may be given in excess of 2000 units in a day without significant effect on the blood sugar level or on glycosuria. Lowell found that one patient acquired a neutralizing antibody for insulin, which disappeared after the withdrawal of insulin and reappeared some time after insulin treatment was reinstituted. Local or generalized urticarial reactions constitute the most common allergic response to insulin. This reaction may vanish spontaneously or it may be controlled by antihistaminic drugs or by the use of zinc insulin preparations not containing protamine.

Hypoglycemic reactions are likely to occur from time to time in any patient treated with insulin. In most instances, reactions are mild, transient and easily controlled. Occasionally, particularly in patients receiving large doses of protamine zinc insulin, protracted or fatal reactions occur and are associated with punctate hemorrhages and other changes characteristic of cerebral anoxia. With intense and prolonged hypoglycemia there may be an increase in the number of cells in the spinal fluid, and changes in the electro-encephalogram may persist for days or weeks.

The *symptoms of hypoglycemia,* commonly known as *"insulin shock,"* do not make their appearance at any definite level of blood sugar, but the diagnosis should be considered doubtful if the blood sugar is over 70 mg. per 100 cc. In some patients the symptoms of insulin shock do not appear until the blood sugar falls to 40 mg. per 100 cc. or even lower. The symptomatology is extremely variable, but each person tends to follow a reproduceable pattern. The commonest complaints in mild shock are a "trembly feeling inside," an empty feeling in the epigastrium, profuse sweating, pallor, rapid pulse, weakness and transient loss of memory which develop in the course of 15 to 30 minutes. In some cases unfortunately there may be none of these prodromal symptoms; the attack may begin abruptly with disorientation, confusion, delusions, aphasia, ataxia, even loss of consciousness or generalized convulsions. A positive Babinski reaction and other local neurologic signs may be present. In patients using protamine zinc insulin, the onset with symptoms of headache, nausea and vomiting are common and tend to be insidious in their appearance and progression. It is important to bear in mind that *shock following protamine zinc insulin not infrequently appears as long as 24 to 48 hours after the last dose—particularly when large doses are given.*

The administration of sugar constitutes the *treatment of insulin shock.* Every insulin-treated patient should carry a lump of sugar to be taken if suggestive symptoms arise. This treatment or, better, a small glass of orange juice usually suffices to relieve mild symptoms in a few minutes. If the patient cannot be prevailed upon to swallow, 20 to 40 cc. of 50 per cent glucose may be given intravenously. When severe shock appears in patients taking large doses of insulin, shock is apt to recur and is often resistant to treatment, particularly if convulsions or loss of consciousness has persisted for some time. In these cases a 1000 cc. clysis of 5 per cent glucose may be needed to prevent the reappearance of hypoglycemia. As an emergency measure, 0.5 to 1 cc. of *epinephrine* may be given subcutaneously to raise the blood sugar temporarily.

Every diabetic treated with insulin should at all times be provided with an identification card stating that he has diabetes and takes insulin. This is absolutely essential, for patients have been killed when, on admission to a hospital in hypoglycemic coma, the presence of sugar in the urine has led to the administration of more insulin before the blood sugar has been determined. There should be no confusion between the recognition of hypoglycemic coma and coma due to acidosis, but a safe rule to be followed is to *administer glucose when in doubt* after a sample of blood has been taken for determination of sugar and carbon dioxide.

Treatment of Acidosis. When *severe* diabetic acidosis develops, immediate and intensive treatment is indicated, since recovery is the more likely, the shorter the duration of symptoms. The best treatment requires the coordinated effort of medical, nursing and laboratory groups in a hospital.

The treatment of diabetic acidosis must be directed primarily toward (1) the *restoration of salt and water* to the depleted circulating blood volume and interstitial spaces in order to arrest the progression of dehydration, circulatory collapse and renal failure which lead to death, and (2) *to correct simultaneously the glycosuria, ketosis and acidosis,* which, for reasons discussed elsewhere, give rise to the loss of inorganic base and water.

Upon admission, the precipitating cause for the development of acidosis should, if possible, be promptly determined from the history and physical examination. If an obvious infection, e.g., pneumonia, is present, its treatment may be initiated simultaneously with that of the acidosis. At the time of admission, blood should be obtained for the *immediate* determination of carbon dioxide or pH, sugar and urea and for grouping. Through the same needle, left in place, an infusion of 1500 cc. of physiologic sodium chloride solution should be started and completed in one hour, except in the presence of overt cardiac insufficiency, when it should be given more slowly and preferably with measurements of venous pressure. The patient should be given an initial dose of 100 units of regular or crystalline insulin subcutaneously. If the blood pressure is below 90 mm. of mercury, half of this dose should be given intravenously. If the blood glucose is in excess of about 700 mg. per 100 cc. an additional 100 units should be given at once. *Long-acting insulin should not be used in treating severe acidosis.* If gastric dilatation is present or acidosis is accompanied by recurrent vomiting, gastric lavage should be carried out with caution. Fluids orally should be withheld until nausea has disappeared. If the carbon dioxide is reported as less than 20 volumes per 100 cc. (9 millimols per liter), a single dose of 20 gm. of sodium bicarbonate in 1000 ml. of water may be given intravenously. Despite objection by some, this *limited use of bicarbonate* has distinct advantages. First, it replaces directly and promptly one salt lost from the body, i.e., sodium bicarbonate, second, it shortens the period of severe acidosis, which is particularly deleterious to all patients in shock, and third, the utilization of carbohydrate is decreased by acidosis. In addition to this therapy, a clysis of 1500 cc. of normal saline may also be given at the beginning of treatment. If the blood pressure does not rise, or if severe peripheral circulatory collapse and oliguria are present, the initial infusion should be followed at once by the administration of 500 cc. of whole blood.

After the initiation of therapy as outlined, insulin should be given hourly until ketosis has disappeared; in most cases 50 units an hour prove adequate. *Urine specimens* should be obtained hourly, by catheterization if necessary, for sugar and ketone tests. *Blood sugar and carbon dioxide determinations* should be made at least every 3 hours and, if possible, also a serum potassium determination. It is advantageous to give enough glucose intravenously to maintain the blood sugar at about 300 mg. per 100 cc. as long as ketosis persists, in order to increase the utilization of glucose and to avoid the possibility of superimposing hypoglycemic shock on coma due to ketosis and acidosis. Frequently, an infusion of 1000 cc. of 5 per cent glucose in

water, given about 3 hours after the initial infusion, is necessary to make adequate amounts of glucose available and to rehydrate the patient. This solution also decreases the possibility of developing metabolic acidosis due to excessive concentration of the chloride ion and further dehydration resulting from osmotic diuresis due to the excessive sodium ion given. Solutions of fructose have no practical advantage over those of glucose. A number of workers suggest the use of complex hypotonic solutions of sodium chloride, lactate and phosphate which may also include magnesium and potassium salts as well as some glucose. Whereas there may in some instances be theoretical reasons for their use, the mortality rates are not appreciably lowered by their employment. Probably all patients with severe diabetic acidosis have a fluid deficit in excess of 5 liters which should be replaced parenterally or orally in 24 hours.

Occasionally, significant *hypopotassemia* develops in the course of treatment of diabetic acidosis and results from continued loss of potassium in the urine and a shift of this ion to cells. Decrease in serum potassium may be accompanied by profound muscle weakness involving the extremities and at times the diaphragm, resulting in dyspnea. Restlessness, sweating and electrocardiographic changes may also be present. In rare instances patients die from cardiac arrest. This syndrome, which does not appear until after 3 or more hours of treatment with glucose and insulin, is alleviated or can be avoided by the administration of 2 gm. of potassium chloride given three or four times at hourly intervals by mouth. If oral medication is not feasible, 200 cc. of 1 per cent solution of potassium chloride may be given *slowly* intravenously. Preferable is an infusion of 1 liter of a solution containing 100 milliequivalents of sodium chloride and 40 milliequivalents of potassium chloride. *Potassium salts should not be administered in the presence of oliguria or earlier than 3 hours after the initiation of treatment of the acidosis* because of possible potassium poisoning. The fact that Joslin has successfully treated 90 consecutive patients suffering from severe acidosis without potassium salts indicates that the importance of hypokalemia is not great numerically. When nausea has disappeared and ketosis is greatly lessened, the patient may be given fluids by mouth on schedule. Water, broth, gruel, diluted milk or orange juice may be given in small amounts at a rate not exceeding 200 cc. an hour. Insulin at this time should be given in accordance with the degree of glycosuria, the urine being tested every 2 hours. If a red or orange precipitate appears, 20 units should be given, and if yellow or green, 5 to 10 units should be administered. A soft diet with a minimum of fat should be given for 24 to 48 hours after ketonuria disappears, and insulin should be administered in relation to the degree of glycosuria, as just stated. The patient may then be regulated on his usual diet.

The outline of therapy of *severe acidosis* proves satisfactory in the majority of patients, but many factors modify responses; consequently deviations from this regimen must often be made. For example, *wide variations in the amount of insulin required are encountered in different patients.* In the presence of persistent infection or hyperthyroidism several hundred units of insulin may be necessary, and the tendency for ketosis to recur is great. On the other hand, the writer had a patient 13 years of age who was admitted to the hospital in coma with a carbon dioxide of 15 volumes per 100 cc. who became completely free of ketone bodies and sugar-free with a total of only 85 units. In the majority of cases 300 to 400 units are required. In older persons cardiac failure and pulmonary edema are apt to develop with the liberal administration of fluid given intravenously. In these patients frequent examination of the chest for the appearance of basal rales and measurements of venous pressure serve as a useful guide. Digitalization may prove helpful in this group. If urinary suppression develops, it should be treated as indicated elsewhere in this volume.

In the presence of *mild or moderate acidosis,* as defined elsewhere, the patient should be put to bed, the fluid intake should be increased to about 3 liters a day, and sodium chloride, to about 10 gm. a day, should be taken in the form of broth and enteric-coated tablets. Carbohydrate in the form of fruit juices, toast, cereal, potato, rice and milk should be given up to 200 gm. a day, and fat should be reduced as much as possible in the diet. The urine should be examined every 2 hours, and regular insulin given at the rate of 20 units for a red or orange reaction and 10 for a yellow or green reaction. The basis for acidosis must obviously be sought and corrected if possible.

Treatment of Surgical Complications. Surgical procedures no longer constitute a great hazard to the patient with diabetes, provided that rigid supervision is exercised. It must be borne in mind, however, that surgical procedures and anesthesia are potentially capable of inducing ketosis. Immediately before operation an infusion of 1500 cc. of 5 per cent glucose in saline should be given, and the patient should receive 25 units of regular insulin subcutaneously. Another infusion and the same dose of insulin should be repeated after operation. The urine should be tested for sugar and ketones at 2-hour intervals. Regular insulin and not long-acting insulin should be given, as outlined in the treatment of mild acidosis. Unless there are specific contradictions, a light soft diet may be instituted on the second day, and, when the surgical condition permits, the patient should again be regulated on his normal diet. If an acute surgical condition, e.g., appendicitis, has been responsible for the development of severe acidosis, operation should be postponed and antibiotics administered until after peripheral circulatory collapse has been treated.

The treatment of *infections of the feet* has benefited greatly from the introduction of sulfonamide and penicillin therapy. Even in the presence of a seriously compromised circulation, there has been a striking decrease in the necessity for amputation.

Retinitis, Neuropathies and Arteriosclerosis. The most important measure in the management of these complications is that of possible prevention by adequate dietary control of the disease.

Pregnancy in Diabetes. Until recently pregnancy in diabetes has been associated with fetal mortality rates as high as 60 per cent in certain series and with definite risks for the mother, including predisposition to toxemia. With regimens including the rigid restriction of salt, the administration of diethylstilbestrol and progesterone and with cesarean section in selected cases, White reports maternal survival in 99.5 per cent of 181 cases and fetal survival in 84 per cent. There is not, however, general agreement concerning the value of hormonal therapy in pregnant diabetics.

Hygiene of the Diabetic. A great decrease in the death rate from diabetes can be brought about by early diagnosis of the disease, by frequent routine health examinations, and by prevention of complications through education of the patient and cooperation of the physician.

The patient should not be made unnecessarily introspective in the process of his education, but he should never forget that he is a diabetic, for laxness in attention to diet or to urine examination sooner or later results in serious consequences. Exercise in moderation is to be advocated, for it actually increases carbohydrate tolerance to a certain extent. Overfatigue, both physical or mental, worry, unhappiness and lack of "peace of mind" decrease carbohydrate tolerance. Any simple cold or other infection, when it develops, requires bed care, the liberal ingestion of fluid and the immediate attention of the physician. A patient should never for any reason lower his insulin dosage without first consulting this physician. Likewise, digestive "upsets" require the advice of a physician. Many cases of gangrene can be prevented in arteriosclerotic diabetics if they will care for their feet as well as they do their hands. Now that normal nutrition can be maintained by the use of insulin there would appear to be no obvious reason for a higher incidence of tuberculosis among diabetics than among other persons.

Prevention. Probably the most important factor in the prevention of diabetes mellitus is the prevention of obesity in the community in general. In people with a family history of diabetes, the avoidance of excessive weight is mandatory. Experience dictates that "casual" or "alimentary" and "emotional" glycosuria are often forerunners of overt diabetes and should be considered as such. Patients exhibiting these abnormalities should have 2-hour postprandial blood sugar determinations and should restrict the use of free sugar. "Screening" tests when widely applied will unearth many latent diabetics. How much this early detection will alter the course of the disease in general is not yet clearly established.

ROBERT F. LOEB

References

Adlersberg, D., and Dolger, H.: Insulin Mixtures in the Treatment of Diabetes. J.A.M.A., 128:414, 1945.
Best, C. H.: Aspects of the Action of Insulin. Ann. Int. Med., 39:433, 1953.
Conn, J. W.: Interpretation of the Glucose Tolerance Test. Am. J. M. Sc., 199:555, 1940.
Haist, R. E., Campbell, J., and Best, C.: The Prevention of Diabetes. New England J. Med., 223:607, 1940.
Houssay, B. A., and Biasotti, A.: Hypophysectomie et Diabete Pancreatique chez le Crapaud. Compt. rend. Soc. de biol., 104:407, 1930.
Joslin, E. P., Root, H. F., White, P., and Marble, A.: The Treatment of Diabetes Mellitus. 9th ed. Philadelphia, Lea and Febiger, 1952.
Long, C. N. H., and Lukens, F. D. W.: The Effects of Hypophysectomy and Adrenalectomy upon Pancreatic Diabetes. Tr. A. Am. Phys., 51:123, 1936.
Lukens, F. D. W., Dohan, F. C., and Wolcott, M. W.: Pituitary-Diabetes in the Cat: Recovery Following Phlorhizin Treatment. Endocrinology, 32:475, 1943.
Miller, M., Drucker, W. R., Owens, J. E., Craig, J., and Woodward, H., Jr.: Metabolism of Intravenous Fructose and Glucose in Normal and Diabetic Subjects. J. Clin. Investigation, 31:115, 1952.
Nabarro, J. D. N., Spencer, A. G., and Stowers, J. M.: Treatment of Diabetic Acidosis. Lancet, 1:983, 1952.
Peters, J. P.: Starvation Diabetes, the Reason for Use of Glucose in the Treatment of Diabetic Acidosis. Yale J. Biol. & Med., 17:705, 1945.
Stetten, D.: Metabolic Effects of Insulin. Bull. N. Y. Acad. Med., 29:466, 1953.
———, and Boxer, G. E.: Studies in Carbohydrate Metabolism. J. Biol. Chem., 155:231, 1944.
Wilkerson, H. L. C., and Krall, L. P.: Diabetes in a New England Town. J.A.M.A., 152:1322, 1953.
Young, F. G.: Permanent Experimental Diabetes Produced by Pituitary (Anterior Lobe) Injections. Lancet, 2:372, 1937.

SPONTANEOUS HYPOGLYCEMIA

Definition. The term "spontaneous hypoglycemia" denotes a depression of the blood sugar to abnormally low levels, usually in association with a characteristic group of symptoms, which occurs without the administration of exogenous insulin.

Etiology. Seale Harris was the first to call attention to the fact that spontaneous hypoglycemia might be recognized by symptoms resembling those which result from an excessive dose of insulin. In 1924 he wrote, "When I saw the insulin reaction in diabetic patients, I realized I had seen many patients (not taking insulin) who had complained of the same symptoms: i.e., hunger, weakness, and the anxiety neuroses." On the basis of symptomatology correlated with blood sugar determinations, Harris established the presence of spontaneous hypoglycemia in a number of patients. In 1927 Wilder first showed that this disorder could result from *hyperinsulinism.* He demonstrated the presence of a large amount of insulin in the liver metastases of a patient with carcinoma of the islands of Langerhans. Since that time numerous cases of spontaneous hypoglycemia have been reported. The following classification (modified after Conn) indicates the wide variety of disorders in which spontaneous hypoglycemia may be encountered:

I. Hypoglycemia associated with anatomic lesions —"organic"
  A. Hyperinsulinism
     1. Pancreatic islet-cell adenoma
     2. Pancreatic islet-cell carcinoma
     3. Diffuse hypertrophy or hyperplasia of pancreatic islet tissue
  B. Hepatic disease
     1. Toxic hepatitis
     2. "Fatty liver"
     3. Diffuse carcinomatosis
     4. von Gierke's disease (glycogen disease)
     5. Diffuse intrahepatic cholangitis
  C. Hypopituitarism (anterior lobe deficiency)—Simmonds' disease
     1. Destructive lesions, e.g., chromophobe adenoma and Rathke's pouch cyst
     2. Atrophy or infection
  D. Adrenal cortical insufficiency—Addison's disease
     1. Destructive granuloma—usually tuberculous
     2. Primary atrophy
     3. Destructive neoplasms
     4. Amyloid disease
  E. Hypothyroidism
  F. Lesions of the central nervous system, e.g., thalamic
II. Hypoglycemia without demonstrable anatomic lesions—"functional"
     1. Increased secretion of insulin by normal islet cells—autonomic imbalance?
     2. Decreased secretion of anterior pituitary or adrenal cortical hormones?
     3. Excessive oxidation or carbohydrate in severe muscular work
     4. Pregnancy and lactation
     5. Idiopathic hypoglycemia
     6. Malabsorption syndrome

The mechanisms producing spontaneous hypoglycemia in patients with pancreatic islet-cell tumors, with destruction of the anterior lobe of the pituitary gland or with loss of adrenal cortical or thyroid tissue, have a recognizable physiologic basis. Since hepatectomy is followed promptly by intense hypoglycemia, it might also be expected that patients with diffuse disease of the liver would have spontaneous hypoglycemia regularly. It is of interest, however, that, whereas disorders of the liver contribute significantly to the total number of cases of spontaneous hypoglycemia reported, its incidence in cirrhosis, infectious hepatitis and ascending cholangitis is surprisingly low. Fatty metamorphosis of the liver is perhaps a more frequent cause. Hypoglycemia occurs in all cases

of von Gierke's disease. In a few instances, hypoglycemia has been reported associated with lesions in the thalamus.

In the majority of patients with spontaneous hypoglycemia without demonstrable anatomic lesions, i.e., in cases of "functional" hypoglycemia, there continues to be speculation concerning etiology. It seems possible that an increase in secretion of insulin by the islet cells of the pancreas or a decrease in secretion of "anti-insulin" by the pituitary or adrenal glands or the pancreas may be of importance, but these changes, if they do exist, have not been demonstrated. It is conceivable, but not established, that primary disturbances in liver function alter the utilization of carbohydrate without the striking demonstrable changes which, for example, occur in von Gierke's disease. Hypoglycemia in pregnancy and lactation is possibly related to functional disturbances in the liver or in the endocrine glands which exert an effect on carbohydrate metabolism. Whatever may be the etiology of "functional" spontaneous hypoglycemia, its existence and importance cannot be doubted. The relative frequency of various causes for spontaneous hypoglycemia has been analyzed, and, according to Conn, 80 to 90 per cent of all cases result from one of three causes, namely, "functional" hypoglycemia, hyperinsulinism with a demonstrable pancreatic lesion, or organic disease of the liver.

Morbid Anatomy. It is clear from the classification of spontaneous hypoglycemia that a variety of pathologic lesions may be encountered. Whipple analyzed neoplasms of the islands of Langerhans present in a group of 149 cases of *hyperinsulinism*. In this group, 106 were benign adenomas, 15 were outspoken carcinomas, and the remaining 28 were questionably malignant. Islet tumors occur most frequently in the body or tail of the pancreas and are often multiple, but many escaping detection on surgical exploration are ultimately found to lie on the posterior surface of the head. As a rule the growths are small, averaging 1 to 2 cm. in diameter, but they may be much larger. Multiple adenomas of the beta cells associated with hypoglycemia and with functioning adenomas of the pituitary and parathyroid glands have been reported by Wermer. Few cases of hypertrophy of the islands of Langerhans have been well documented. The anatomic lesions of the liver, the anterior lobe of the pituitary gland, adrenal and thyroid glands responsible for the development of spontaneous hypoglycemia have already been mentioned.

Long-continued and intense hypoglycemia, regardless of the cause, gives rise to hemorrhages, cerebral edema and other lesions in the brain that are characteristic of severe cerebral anoxia.

Physiology. The concentration of glucose in the blood is the resultant of a number of physiologic and biochemical forces engaged simultaneously in the transfer of glucose to and from the blood stream. The body is normally protected against the development of hypoglycemia by various mechanisms discussed in the material on the physiology of diabetes mellitus. A number of physiologic factors are probably responsible for the wide range of clinical manifestations of hypoglycemia and also for their poor correlation with the actual level of blood glucose. These may include (1) the liberation of epinephrine; (2) cerebral anoxia, secondary to a decrease in blood glucose, which is the chief substrate for cerebral activity; (3) possible disturbances in the synthesis of acetylcholine; (4) hypokalemia in certain instances; (5) variations in threshold inherent in different persons; and (6) activity of the adrenal cortex, since Thorn and also Sprague have shown that cortisone alleviates the clinical manifestations of hypoglycemia even though the blood sugar level may remain below 40 to 50 mg. per 100 cc.

The basis for hypoglycemia in myxedema and cretinism is probably in part poor absorption of glucose from the gut. Other factors which may contribute to it remain unrecognized.

In severe liver disease, hypoglycemia may ensue from the depletion of glycogen stores. It may also result from the fact that the "anti-insulin" effects of anterior pituitary extract and adrenal cortical steroids and glucagon on carbohydrate metabolism are probably to a considerable extent dependent upon normal liver function. It is conceivable that there might be an increase in utilization of carbohydrate by the tissues in severe liver disease, as a result of a decrease in the degradation of fat which takes place chiefly in the liver. Finally, it is possible that degradation of insulin is diminished in severe liver disease.

In the course of severe physical exertion, glucose utilization is increased and may result in transient hypoglycemia. A decrease in blood sugar occurs in the diabetic as well as in the normal in exercise, and therefore may result from an increase in carbohydrate utilization by tissue cells independent of the elaboration of insulin by the pancreas.

Clinical Picture. The pattern of the clinical picture in hypoglycemia is extremely varied, but in a given person the same symptoms tend to recur, though they vary in severity at different times. The hypoglycemic syndrome is almost always episodic. The attacks usually occur before breakfast or several hours after any repast, and are frequently precipitated by physical exertion. The episodes vary greatly in duration and intensity. They may last but a few minutes and terminate either spontaneously or after the ingestion of food. On the other hand, they may be severe and last for hours or even days and prove resistant to treatment. Occasionally an attack ends fatally. The blood sugar level at which symptoms appear varies; some patients are devoid of symptoms until levels below 40 mg. per 100 cc. are reached, and others present classical symptoms with blood sugar concentrations of 50 to 60 mg. per 100 cc. The rate of fall of the blood sugar as well as the actual level reached may be a factor in determining the intensity of symptoms. The symptoms and signs of hypoglycemia are referable primarily to the vegetative and central nervous systems. Sympathetic disturbances include sensations of hunger, "trembling inside," pallor, sweating, tachycardia, nausea, chilliness and syncope. Signs and symptoms resulting from involvement of the central nervous system include muscle weakness, spasticity with hyperreflexia, Babinski sign and clonus, ocular palsies, generalized or focal convulsive seizures and episodes suggesting petit mal. Disturbances of the psyche such as apprehension, disorientation, confusion, delusions of grandeur, mania and coma are not rare. The electro-encephalogram often shows focal or widespread dysrhythmia, which is usually transient, but may persist for days or even weeks, with or without focal signs, after a prolonged and intense bout of hypoglycemia.

Diagnosis. To establish the diagnosis of spontaneous hypoglycemia it is essential to demonstrate a depression of the blood sugar level. It is of equal importance to ascertain its cause. In view of the fact that the periods of hypoglycemia are often transient, various means must at times be used for their detection. Four procedures may be recommended: (1) Of foremost importance is the determination of the blood sugar level before breakfast, although it may be normal in many cases. (2) A blood sugar determination should be made, if possible, at the onset of an attack. If the attack is convulsive in nature, the blood sugar toward the termination of the episode may be normal or even elevated. (3) The glucose tolerance test has limited value and is of use only in patients in whom the fasting blood sugar is normal or in whom it has been impossible to procure a sample at the beginning of an attack. The blood glucose curve may be normal, "flat" or diabetic in form during the first two or three hours, but if the blood sugar falls to levels of 50 mg. per 100 cc. or lower, 3, 4 or 5 hours after the "stimulating" dose of glucose, and particularly if the fall is associated with the development of characteristic symptoms, the diagnosis is established. (4) When hypoglycemia is not demonstrable by these means, a 24-hour fast should be instituted and blood sugar determinations should be made at 12, 18 and 24 hours. The prompt alleviation of symptoms and also modification of the electroencephalographic pattern in the direction of the normal with the administration of glucose affords strong evidence for the diagnosis.

The chief problem of diagnosis, from the standpoint of management of the patient, is to differentiate, if possible, *hyperinsulinism* due to organic disease of the islands of Langerhans, from *"functional"* hypoglycemia. Both these disorders often escape recognition for months or even years. As a general rule, the attacks in "functional" hypoglycemia tend to be less severe and of shorter duration than in hyperinsulinism due to organic disease of the pancreas. Furthermore, "functional" hypoglycemia is apt to occur in association with one of the neuroses.

Using criteria which demonstrate unequivocally the presence of severe hypoglycemia, Whipple found islet-cell tumors in 27 of 32 patients operated on at the Presbyterian Hospital. It is possible that adenomas may have been present in unoperated patients who presented less convincing evidence of hypoglycemia. At times it is essential to resort to surgical exploration to establish the diagnosis, but even this procedure is not wholly satisfactory, since small adenomas lying deep in pancreatic tissue easily escape detection. Hypoglycemia resulting from organic disease of the pituitary, thyroid or adrenal glands or of the liver usually occurs in association with other manifestations of disease of these structures and consequently presents little difficulty in diagnosis.

Treatment. The therapy of spontaneous hypoglycemia can be separated into (1) the treatment of the acute episode, and (2) the treatment of the underlying cause.

The management of the attack depends obviously upon its intensity and its response to therapy. Early and intensive treatment of hypoglycemia is of importance to prevent anoxic damage in the brain. Frequently, 10 gm. of sugar, orange juice, glucose as candy, or a glass of milk will relieve the symptoms and raise the blood sugar to a normal level. When hypoglycemia is more severe and the patient is unable to swallow, 0.5 to 1 mg. of epinephrine may be administered subcutaneously as an emergency measure, and 10 to 20 gm. of glucose should be given intravenously in 25 to 50 per cent solution. In cases of intractable or frequently recurring hypoglycemia, 1000 cc. of 5 per cent glucose can be given by hypodermoclysis. In these patients it is essential also to give, by gavage, hourly feedings containing both glucose and milk or a casein autolysate until symptoms have been relieved for some hours. When the patient is able to cooperate, oral feedings at 2-hour intervals should be instituted. Despite all therapeutic efforts, hypoglycemic attacks occasionally have a fatal outcome.

The management of the underlying causes is naturally dependent upon the nature of the lesion. If the diagnosis is believed to be *hyperinsulinism* due to an organic lesion of the islands of Langerhans, surgical intervention should not be delayed, since the frequent feedings necessary to ward off attacks often lead to the development of obesity, which adds greatly to the difficulties in ultimate surgical treatment. Also, the prolonged use of ACTH or cortisone, which may control symptoms, induces hyperadrenalism and does not resolve the underlying problem. Dilantin may be useful in controlling recurrent epileptiform seizures.

In patients with mild "functional" hypoglycemia, in whom the symptoms tend to recur just before meals, it is advisable to have the patient reduce his regular repasts and take supplementary feedings in the middle of the morning, afternoon and at bedtime. It is desirable to prescribe a diet high in protein for these patients and to reduce the intake of sugar. This regimen appears to be useful in some cases. When "functional" hypoglycemia is associated with a neurosis, it is possible that treatment of the latter will reduce the tendency to hypoglycemia if, as believed, it is the result of "autonomic imbalance."

Spontaneous hypoglycemia due to disease of the pituitary or adrenal glands is not benefited significantly by preparations of these glands now generally available, although adrenocorticotropic hormone administered in early hypopituitarism or cortisone in Addisonian patients with recurrent hypoglycemia may prove useful. Treatment is therefore limited to the direct restoration of the blood sugar as outlined previously. In cases resulting from disease of the liver or biliary tract, treatment should be directed toward correcting the underlying disorder.

ROBERT F. LOEB

References

Conn, J. W.: The Spontaneous Hypoglycemias. The Importance of Etiology in Determining Treatment. J.A.M.A., *115:*1669, 1940.

Gray, S. H., and Feemster, L. C.: Compensatory Hypertrophy and Hyperplasia of the Islands of Langerhans in the Pancreas of a Child Born of a Diabetic Mother. Arch. Path., *1:*348, 1926.

Harris, A.: Hyperinsulinism and Dysinsulinism. J.A.M.A., 83:729, 1924.

Howard, J. M., Moss, N. H., and Rhoads, J. E.: Collective Review: Hyperinsulinism and Islet Cell Tumors of the Pancreas. Internat. Obst. & Surg., 90:417, 1950.

Whipple, A. O.: Hyperinsulinism in Relation to Pancreatic Tumors. Surgery, 16:289, 1944.

Wilder, R. M., Allan, F. N., Powers, M. H., and Robertson, H. E.: Carcinoma of the Islands of the Pancreas. Hyperinsulinism and Hypoglycemia. J.A.M.A., 89:348, 1927.

DIABETES INSIPIDUS

Definition. Diabetes insipidus is a symptom complex resulting from a deficiency of antidiuretic hormone of the pars nervosa of the pituitary gland. The deficiency is manifested by the excretion of a large volume of dilute but otherwise normal urine and by an unrelenting thirst. The condition is chronic and is corrected by replacement therapy.

Incidence. Diabetes insipidus is a rare disease, with its onset more common in childhood than in adult life.

Physiology. The initial step in the formation of urine by the kidneys is the production in Bowman's capsule of a protein-free filtrate of plasma. As this filtrate progresses along the renal tubules, water and solutes are reabsorbed; the tubular reabsorption of water is, in part, facilitated by the antidiuretic hormone of the pituitary. In the absence of this gland less water is reabsorbed and a sustained diuresis results. In normal subjects the release of the antidiuretic hormone from the pars nervosa of the pituitary is regulated by its nerve supply, which originates, for the greater part, in the supraoptic nucleus of the hypothalamus and passes down the pituitary stalk to the neurohypophysis. The highly vascular supraoptic nucleus seems to be responsive to changes in the total osmotic pressure of the plasma, so that, in times of excessive water loss, as in copious sweating, a greater amount of hormone is released, with a resultant renal conservation of water and the excretion of a highly concentrated urine. On the other hand, the ingestion of large amounts of water reduces the total osmotic pressure of the plasma by dilution and thus suppresses the release of the hormone and causes diminished renal tubular reabsorption of water; the well known water diuresis results.

Morbid Anatomy. Any lesion which interferes with the innervation of the pars nervosa, the supraoptic-hypophysial system, leads to an anatomic degeneration and secretory paralysis of the gland. The lesion may be in the supraoptic nuclei, in the tuber cinereum, the pituitary stalk or in the pars nervosa itself. The reported causes of destruction of the supraoptic nuclei are tumors of the hypothalamus or optic chiasm, xanthomatosis of the hypothalamus, trauma and hemorrhage or infection, metastases or embolism; the pars nervosa is usually destroyed by trophic changes which result from the lesions described, but primary destruction may result from trauma, hemorrhage or more usually by neoplastic growth in or encroaching on the sella turcica.

Etiology. Diabetes insipidus may be either acquired or inherited. In the hereditary form there is a congenital absence of the supraoptico-hypophysial system, so that a polyuria exists throughout life, which may be of normal span. In the acquired form known causes include syphilis, tuberculosis, encephalitis, xanthomatosis, trauma or tumor; less frequently, mycotic infections, leukemia, Boeck's sarcoid, basilar meningitis and lymphogranulomatosis. In many cases the underlying cause of the polyuria is not demonstrated in life, and thorough postmortem examination has not revealed the basic lesion. It should always be kept in mind that polyuria is a symptom and merely applying a diagnosis of diabetes insipidus is not helpful; a thorough and repeated inquiry into the cause of the hypothalamico-hypophysial damage should be made.

Diagnosis. The onset may be acute or insidious, depending on the cause, and the daily turnover of water may be as great as 20 liters.

Diabetes insipidus must be differentiated from diabetes mellitus, nephritis, psychogenic water drinking and nephrogenic diabetes insipidus. The first two diseases can be distinguished by urinalysis; the third is less obviously different. Hickey and Hare devised a test of the functional integrity of the supra-optico-hypophysial system; after the onset of a water diuresis the patient is given by vein 0.25 cc. of a 2.5 per cent sodium chloride solution per kilogram of body weight per minute for 45 minutes to increase the total osmotic pressure of the plasma. In diabetes insipidus the polyuria is increased by the procedure; in psychogenic water drinkers the pituitrin released from the normal pituitary causes a sharp drop in the urine flow. All patients with a polyuria should be tested for a response to pituitrin (0.1 unit) to exclude those whose kidneys are refractory to the antidiuretic hormone.

Williams and Henry have described a syndrome, which they called nephrogenic diabetes insipidus and which is hereditary. It is transmitted by females, but appears only in males.

The urine in diabetes insipidus is pale, with a specific gravity of 1.001 to 1.008 and free of abnormal contents. The blood picture is usually normal, although findings related to the causative lesion may be found, as in leukemia. X-ray films of the skull may show erosion of the clinoid processes or the sella turcica with expanding lesions or cystic areas in osseous xanthomatoses, but more frequently there is no detectable abnormality.

Treatment. Replacement therapy is the logical treatment of diabetes insipidus. This is available in three forms—aqueous extract of posterior lobe, pitressin tannate in oil and dried posterior pituitary powder. The aqueous extract must be given at short intervals (4 to 12 hours) by subcutaneous injection or on

cotton pledgets inserted into the nose; side effects are disturbing. The less soluble pitressin tannate is suspended in oil for intramuscular injection, and a single dose is effective for one to seven days. The dried posterior pituitary powder is available in bulk or in capsules which fit into specially designed powder blowers for nasal insufflation. This form of administering the hormone has many advantages; it is cheaper, requires no sterile equipment and is painless. It is the method of choice and works satisfactorily in almost all cases except when upper respiratory infections diminish absorption from the nasal mucosa. During such episodes the hormone can be given in injections of the aqueous solution or the oily suspension.

KENDRICK HARE

References

Chambers, G. H., Melville, E. V., Hare, R. S., and Hare, K.: Regulation of the Release of Pituitrin by Changes in the Osmotic Pressure of the Plasma. Am. J. Physiol., *144*:311, 1945.
DeBodo, R. C., and Slater, I. H.: Diabetes Insipidus and Its Differential Diagnosis. In Soskin, Samuel, Ed.: Progress in Clinical Endocrinology. New York, Grune and Stratton, 1950, pp. 549–556.
Gilman, A., and Goodman, L.: The Secretory Response of the Posterior Pituitary to the Need for Water Conservation. J. Physiol., 90:113, 1937.
Hickey, R. C., and Hare, K.: The Renal Excretion of Chloride and Water in Diabetes Insipidus. J. Clin. Investigation, 23:768, 1944.
Kao, M. Y.-C., and Steiner, M. M.: Diabetes Insipidus in Infancy Resistant to Pitressin. Pediatrics, *12*:400, 1953.
Lewis, A. A. J., and Chalmers, T. M.: A Nicotine Test for the Investigation of Diabetes Insipidus. Clin. Sc., 10:137, 1951.
———, Ward, C. S., and Bishop, P. M. F.: Diagnostic Tests in Diabetes Insipidus. J. Endocrinol., 6:37, 1950.
Pender, C. B., and Fraser, F. C.: Dominant Inheritance of Diabetes Insipidus. Pediatrics, *11*:246, 1953.
Williams, R. H., and Henry, C.: Nephrogenic Diabetes Insipidus: Transmitted by Females and Appearing during Infancy in Males. Ann. Int. Med., 27:84, 1947.

HEMOCHROMATOSIS

Definition. Hemochromatosis (pigment cirrhosis, bronze diabetes) is a chronic disease characterized by the deposition of iron in body tissues with eventual fibrosis and functional insufficiency of organs severely involved. Etiologically, three types of hemochromatosis may be recognized: idiopathic hemochromatosis, transfusion hemochromatosis and dietary hemochromatosis.

Morbid Anatomy. At autopsy the unique finding in hemochromatosis is a bronze or ochre pigmentation of body tissues due to widespread deposition of hemosiderin. These iron deposits are heaviest in the liver, but are also prominent in the reticuloendothelial tissue, endocrine glands, striated muscle and skin. The liver is sclerotic and usually large (average weight, 2400 gm.). Fibrosis of the pancreas and of lymph nodes containing large amounts of iron is common. While there seems to be a general correlation between the amount of iron and the degree of fibrosis in an organ, exceptions in the case of the pancreas have been described.

Pathogenesis and Pathologic Physiology. Recently many of the unusual features of idiopathic hemochromatosis have been clarified. Fundamental studies in iron metabolism have demonstrated that the excretion of iron in man is negligible and that absorption rather than excretion controls the amount of body iron. In ordinary circumstances a "mucosal block" prevents excessive iron absorption. In idiopathic hemochromatosis this "mucosal block" is ineffective, and over many years surplus iron accumulates. The underlying cause for this uncontrolled absorption remains obscure. The gradual accumulation of iron accounts for the late appearance of symptoms, usually between the ages of 35 and 60 years. The predominance of hemochromatosis in the male (about 95 per cent) is understandable when one considers the difference in iron balance between the two sexes. While the male is unable to rid himself of iron once absorbed, the female does so continually through menstruation and pregnancy. Just as these iron losses greatly increase the incidence of iron deficiency among women, they also serve to decrease the frequency of hemochromatosis.

Tissue iron in idiopathic hemochromatosis represents iron absorbed and stored in a form available for hemoglobin formation rather than the product of abnormal tissue metabolism. The liver is the shock organ for such storage iron and may contain up to 50 gm. of iron as ferritin and hemosiderin. As the storage capacity of the liver is exceeded, iron spills over into other receptor tissues, particularly the endocrine glands of the body and the skin. The serum iron becomes elevated and saturates the iron-binding protein of the serum by which it is transported. Liver fibrosis is thought to be produced by the large amounts of iron which accumulate in the periportal areas of the liver lobule. The defect in absorption is not limited to iron, since other metals may be found in excess in the tissues. Indeed, an excess of copper was once considered to be the etiologic agent in idiopathic hemochromatosis, a hypothesis no longer tenable. In contrast to Laënnec's cirrhosis, alcoholism and diet do not appear to be important etiologic factors in the disease. Enough data are available to indicate a significant familial and hereditary tendency. Idiopathic hemochromatosis must be considered a rare disease, although undoubtedly more frequent than the reported autopsy incidence, which varies from 0.003 to 0.08 per cent.

Transfusion hemochromatosis appears to be pathologically indistinguishable from the idiopathic type. However, the excess iron in this instance gains entrance to the body through transfusion of blood. Probably in excess of 100 transfusions and an interval of several years are required to produce tissue damage comparable to that seen in the idiopathic form. Patients with what may be designated *dietary hemochromatosis* have been reported by Gillman and his co-workers. Extrinsic dietary factors are probably responsible for overcoming the "mucosal block" to iron absorption in these patients, as has been demonstrated experimentally. The iron distribution again is indistinguishable from that in idiopathic hemochromatosis. However, the liver damage is more likely produced by general malnutrition rather than by iron. The oral administration of medicinal iron to the anemic patient over many years may also lead to hemochromatosis.

Clinical Picture. The presenting complaints in idiopathic hemochromatosis may be related to skin pigmentation, diabetes, hepatomegaly, symptoms of severe liver disease, endocrine dysfunction and heart failure.

Pigmentation of the skin is of two types. In about half of the patients there is a bronzing due to increased melanin similar to that found in Addison's disease. In the remaining patients the skin acquires a blue-gray or leaden cast due to the deposition of iron. The pigment is distributed most prominently over the external genitalia, face, arms and in skin folds. Mucous membranes are involved in only about 15 per cent of the patients. The liver is usually palpable, and the spleen in about half the cases. The enlarged liver is frequently associated with upper abdominal pain, which may occasionally be excruciating and knifelike, simulating biliary colic or perforated peptic ulcer. There is frequently no indication of the severe liver disease other than general body wasting. Many patients, as a result of some acute illness or stress situation, suffer acute liver decompensation with coma and death rapidly supervening. Hemorrhage from a ruptured esophageal varix is less frequently encountered than in nonpigmentary cirrhosis, and evidence of increased collateral circulation is rare. Ascites may appear as a terminal event. Sexual impotence is a common complaint in the late phase of the disease, but may occur when the patient is otherwise asymptomatic. Testicular atrophy, loss of axillary and chest hair, and occasional gynecomastia may be regarded as related to liver dysfunction. The diabetes of hemochromatosis is mild at the onset, but becomes progressively more severe. A few patients are sensitive to insulin, but a greater number are relatively resistant, occasionally requiring several hundred units a day. Cardiac deposits of hemosiderin are frequently associated with arrhythmias and congestive heart failure which responds poorly to conventional therapy.

Diagnosis. There is little difficulty in recognizing the disease in the patient with the classic tetrad of skin pigmentation, liver disease, diabetes and cardiac failure. A high index of suspicion in the presence of any two of these four cardinal findings will frequently lead to the diagnosis. Laboratory studies center around the demonstration, *first,* of excessive iron stores, and, *second,* of evidence of hepatic, pancreatic or cardiac disease. Most conclusive is a needle biopsy of the liver, but the use of this diagnostic procedure must be limited because of the risk involved. (In this type of liver disease abdominal exploration and direct biopsy are even more hazardous.) An elevated serum iron and saturation of the iron-binding capacity of the serum are the most useful special laboratory findings in the demonstration of iron excess. Other tests employed, in order of their usefulness, are an examination of the sternal marrow for hemosiderin, skin biopsy, biopsy of gastric mucosa, examination of urinary sediment. Iron in the skin is of diagnostic significance when found in the epithelial cells of the sweat glands. Serum bilirubin is only slightly elevated (usually between 0.5 and 1.5 mg. per 100 cc.), and clinical jaundice is rare. In the early stages of the disease the blood hemoglobin concentration is somewhat above normal; later a mild macrocytic anemia is seen.

Prognosis and Treatment. The average duration of life after diagnosis has been lengthened from the eighteen months reported by Sheldon in 1935 to several years. With the advent of insulin, diabetes in the majority of cases is adequately controlled. Before the age of 40 most fatalities are ascribable to cardiac failure, between the ages of 40 and 60 to hepatic failure and infection, and over 60 to hepatoma.

Supportive therapy in idiopathic hemochromatosis is directed at management of the liver disease and diabetes when present. A high caloric diet (50 calories per kilogram) and supplementary B vitamins would appear beneficial. Insulin should be prescribed as required with this diet. It would appear wiser, in view of the liver disease, to allow some glycosuria than to risk hypoglycemia.

On the assumption that iron deposits are chiefly responsible for the tissue damage, specific therapy should be directed at the removal of iron through phlebotomy. In patients with idiopathic hemochromatosis, weekly phlebotomies of 500 cc. are well tolerated. Each phlebotomy represents the removal of 200 to 250 mg. of iron from the blood which is replaced by an equivalent amount of iron from tissue stores. In contrast to normal persons who rapidly become anemic on this regimen as their iron stores are depleted, patients with idiopathic hemochromatosis maintain their hematocrit between 35 and 45 per cent. Over a period of two to three years the bulk of iron deposits will be mobilized for hemoglobin production and removed by the bleedings. The reversibility of the process will depend on the amount of tissue damage present before the therapeutic procedure was undertaken and to what extent the iron *per se* is responsible for tissue damage. Experience with this form of treatment is sufficiently encouraging to indicate its routine usage, but as yet is too limited to permit evaluation of its long-term effect on the course of the disease.

CLEMENT A. FINCH

References

Davis, W. D., and Arrowsmith, W. R.: The Treatment of Hemochromatosis by Massive Venisection. Ann. Int. Med., 39:723, 1953.

Gillman, J., Mandelstam, J., and Gillman, T.: Comparison of Chemical and Histological Estimations of Iron and Copper Content of Livers of Africans in Relation to Pathogenesis of Cytosiderosis and Cirrhosis (Haemochromatosis). South African J. M. Sc., 10:109, 1945.

Granick, S.: Iron Metabolism and Hemochromatosis. Bull. New York Acad. Med., 35:403, 1949.

Rath, C. E., and Finch, C. A.: Serum Iron Transport. Measurement of Iron-Binding Capacity of Serum in Man. J. Clin. Investigation, 28:79, 1949.

Schwartz, S. O., and Blumenthal, S. A.: Exogenous Hemochromatosis from Blood Transfusions. Blood, 3:617, 1948.

Sheldon, J. H.: Haemochromatosis. London, Oxford University Press, 1935.

OBESITY

Definition. Obesity is that physical state in which the amount of fat stored in the body is excessive. It is a symptom which, because of its implications and consequences, commands the medical consideration accorded serious disease.

Incidence. Immoderate accumulation of adipose tissue may occur at any age, but is more common in middle life. Minor degrees of corpulence (10 or 15 per cent above optimal weight) are the rule rather than the exception after the age of 30 years. In the United States population of 160 million, it is estimated that 15 million are 10 per cent overweight and 5 million are 20 per cent overweight. Of these about 4 million are over 40 years old. Women are more frequently affected than men. Extreme obesity or localized distribution of the body fat is uncommon and suggests unusual etiologic factors.

Etiology. A plethora of calories is the only explanation of obesity. The law of the conservation of energy applies to the human body as surely as to any other machine which produces heat and performs work. When the intake of food, whether protein, fat or carbohydrate, exceeds in caloric value the expenditure as work and heat, the excess will be stored in the body tissues. Because of the relatively limited capacity of the body to store protein and carbohydrate, the greatest part of the excess is converted into and stored as fat. Thus too much of any type of food is fattening.

Pathologic Physiology. Numerous careful studies have conclusively demonstrated that changes in body weight can be accurately predicted when all metabolic influences are known and measured. The apparently paradoxical situation in which weight is maintained temporarily in spite of low caloric intake is explained by transient water retention. The immediate cause of obesity is always *a positive energy balance,* but there are many ways in which the balance may be tilted toward the positive side. Obesity is often divided into two types, exogenous and endogenous. This classification is not recommended, for all corpulence is exogenous (due to an oversupply of food) and likewise endogenous (the reason that the caloric intake is excessive lies within the patient's body).

Although one or more endogenous factors may be present, the intake of more food than is necessary is the cause of the excess fat deposit. Enforced inactivity from a broken leg does not cause weight gain, but the persistence of "normal" food habits (now excessive) is chiefly responsible. A psychoneurosis may among other symptoms be manifested by gluttony with resultant obesity, but a similar psychoneurosis may lead to anorexia and emaciation. The difference is in the food intake.

A positive caloric balance may result from an intake greater than normal or expenditure less than normal, or a combination of both these influences. Weight is maintained within normal limits in most persons without conscious attention to diet or exercise at least until the age of 30 or 35. Aberration from a desirable level of intake or from optimal expenditure of energy may result from either physiologic or psychologic disturbances or both.

Physiologic Factors. A number of the possible metabolic disturbances have been investigated and many attractive theories have been disproved. *Digestion* of food is not more complete, nor is *absorption* more efficient, in obese persons. *"Lipophilia"* of the tissues, consisting in an ability to take up fat more readily, or to retain it more tenaciously than normal, has not been demonstrated to account for the usual type of generalized adiposity. *Local factors* must, however, be invoked to explain the formation of lipomas, the occurrence of lipodystrophy (the commonest type consisting of a lean upper body and obese hips, thighs and legs) and the characteristic fat distribution of certain endocrine disorders.

A basal metabolic rate lower than normal, if coupled with an average normal food intake, causes fat storage, but *low metabolic rates* account for relatively few cases of obesity. The great majority of obese persons have rates within normal limits. Persons with severe hypothyroidism may be overweight if the appetite is good, but often the desire for food decreases in proportion to the metabolic rate. If the metabolism of food (*"the specific dynamic action"*) were accomplished with less than the usual expenditure of energy, obesity theoretically might result. Recent studies indicate no abnormality in this respect in those who become obese. The *total metabolism* of obese persons is higher, not lower than normal; so weight gain cannot be explained by conservation of energy in work or heat production.

Certain experimentally produced *destructive lesions of the hypothalamus* lead to the rapid development of obesity in animals. Two mechanisms within the hypothalamus appear to regulate food intake: if certain lateral centers are bilaterally destroyed, aphagia results; when the medial control centers are bilaterally destroyed, the lateral "feeding" areas are freed of their usual regulatory checking action, and hyperphagia and obesity result. The exact site of the hunger sensation accompanying hypoglycemia is not yet well understood. Persons with so-called "pituitary obesity" presumably suffer from a hypothalamic disturbance. Experimental pituitary destruction does not cause obesity unless the hypothalamus also is injured. Epidemic encephalitis may be followed by the development of obesity, and in such cases hypothalmic lesions have been found which resemble those known to cause experimental adiposity.

Certain *endocrine disorders* may predispose to obesity. Fröhlich's syndrome, characterized by hypogonadism and obesity, has been considered the result of *hypopituitarism,* but present evidence indicates that the glandular disturbance is not the cause of the obesity, but is an associated phenomenon. In *adiposogenital dystrophy* the excessive fat accumulation may result from hypothalamic disturbance, but its typical distribution is characteristic of hypogonadism, which may result from pituitary insufficiency. Clinically, destruction of the pituitary does not cause obesity, but pituitary cachexia (Simmonds' disease). In *Cushing's syndrome* there is a peculiar plethoric obesity confined to the head, neck and trunk. This syndrome, originally considered to result from pituitary basophilism, is apparently not caused primarily by pituitary disease, but by prolonged hypersecretion of the adrenal cortex. Similar obesity occurs in some cases of *hyperadrenocorticism* without evidence of pituitary disorder. Although a low basal metabolic rate cannot explain the usual type of obesity, *hypothyroidism* may be associated with gain in weight, partly due to water retention in the tissues, and partly to fat storage. The latter is particularly evident in deposits about the face, neck, supraclavicular regions, wrists and ankles. Functional or organic hypoglycemia (*hyperinsulinism*) is frequently associated with abnormal hunger leading to excessive food intake and obesity. In man as well as in animals, removal or destructive *disease of the gonads* predisposes to obesity. The disposition becomes more placid, there is less tendency to muscular exertion, and there is a moderate fall in the basal metabolic rate. Many women show such changes and gain weight after the menopause, and similar but less evident symptoms often occur in men as sexual activity wanes. The adiposity characteristic of hypogonadism involves chiefly the breasts, abdomen, hips and thighs. From these considerations it is apparent that it is inaccurate to speak of "endocrine obesity." The endocrine disorder does not cause the obesity, but may favor its development by increasing food intake or decreasing energy expenditure, or both. Localization of fat deposits is, however, specifically influenced by certain abnormalities of the internal secretions.

Limitation of energy output in the form of muscular exercise while eating habits remain unaltered causes weight gain and explains the obesity often developing after enforced inactivity following fractures, rest treatment of tuberculosis, poliomyelitis and other diseases.

Obesity occurs much more frequently among the members of certain families than among others. In animals the *hereditary influence* is clearer than among human beings, but even in the latter, evidence points to the inheritance of the tendency to obesity.

Psychologic Factors. Some persons enjoy food more than others because of habit or training, eat more than they require, and become fat. The food excess need not be great: 15 gm. too much of fat or its equivalent in other foods per day will lead to a gain of a pound a month, or 12 pounds a year. Family custom or imitation of elders often starts the habit. During periods of athletic activity or strenuous muscular work, habits of eating are often acquired which persist for years after the requirement for the high calorie intake ceases. (Normal rats can be trained to eat a whole day's food in one hour; such rats, like those with hypothalamic damage, convert carbohydrate to fat at excessively rapid rates.) The habit of overeating frequently is established after illness, when a concentrated, highly nutritious diet is encouraged. Preference for the richer, less bulky foods is often part of a behavior pattern dating from early life, sometimes started by the misguided anxious or overindulgent parent. Some enjoy exercise less and prefer sedentary occupations and will become obese even with an apparently normal diet. Such excessive food intake or low energy output, if only moderate in degree, can hardly be considered pathologic, for pleasure in eating and avoidance of exertion are universal human traits. The common moderate obesity of middle age probably results from the persistence of the dietary habits of youth coupled with an increasing disinclination to muscular effort, which in turn is due at least partly to diminution of gonadal secretion. The degree of overweight is seldom extreme, and reduction by formation of new habits is often easily accomplished.

When obesity is extreme, psychologic influences beyond such relatively normal limits are suggested. The majority of persons maintain approximately normal body weight without conscious regulation of food intake. Intake is by some mechanism balanced with the caloric requirements. Evidently the metabolic processes and nutritional status of the body normally regulate the psychologic drives which govern appetite, satiety and physical energy. These psychologic sensations may become deranged so that the usually automatic balance of the intake and outflow of energy is upset. Pleasure in eating may become a dominant personality trait. The sense of repletion after a meal may require an inordinate amount of food. The sensation of physical energy usually expressed in muscular activity may be depressed.

When social, business or sexual desires are unsatisfied, the enjoyment of food often becomes magnified in importance and serves as a substitute. Addiction to food, like alcoholism, is often a symptom of psychologic maladjustment. Placid daydreaming, in which desires are imaginatively fulfilled, may take the place of ambitious exertion, so that not only is the caloric intake increased, but energy expenditure is diminished. In addition, the resultant obesity makes the satisfaction of social and sexual desires less likely and physical exercise more difficult, more discouraging and more fatiguing. A vicious circle thus becomes established which favors further increase in the adiposity.

Obesity may not only be the result of defensive mental processes, but the obese state itself may appear desirable to the psychologically maladjusted person for use as a defensive or offensive weapon. It may serve as a defensive against undesired contacts or activities, for example, to avoid sexual advances of an unloved husband, or to escape work. In a positive direction, it may be useful to gain attention and is often used by children to demand solicitous care.

Combined Physiologic and Psychologic Factors. In the great majority of cases of obesity both physiologic and psychologic influences may be discovered. For example, adiposogenital dystrophy (secondary to hypothalamic disturbance and hypogonadism) leads to weight gain, and the psychic reaction to the sexual deficiency favors the substitution of eating for other satisfactions. Psychosomatic relationships are also clearly evident when the carbohydrate habit results in regularly recurring hypoglycemia due to functional hyperinsulinism with consequent hunger, more carbohydrate ingestion and obesity.

Morbid Anatomy. A certain amount of fatty tissue is a normal component of the body, furnishing important structural support and acting as a storehouse of energy. In extreme obesity the subcutaneous fat may be 10 cm. or more in thickness, and excessive fat deposits occur in the retroperitoneal tissues, omentum, mesentery, perirenal tissues, mediastinum and pericardium. Large deposits may occur in the fascial planes between the muscles, and fat infiltration may be found in the pancreas and heart. The liver may be enlarged, each liver cell containing a large fat vacuole.

Symptoms. Obesity causes dyspnea and fatigue, increasing in proportion with the degree of overweight. In extreme cases the bulk of the body may cause such mechanical limitation as to result in almost complete incapacity. Flat feet and arthritis of the knees and lower back are common and often serious. Maceration and infection of the skin beneath rolls of fat occurs. Corpulence increases the probability of cardiac failure in heart disease and exaggerates the symptoms resulting from an impaired circulation.

Diagnosis. Adiposity may be obvious from inspection alone, but determination of the *ideal weight* and the *degree of obesity* is desirable. This may be accomplished within approximate limits by reference to tables, or more exactly for each person by calculation

Prognosis. The prognosis can be treated from two viewpoints: (1) What is the likelihood of achieving an approximately normal weight? (2) What influence has obesity upon health and longevity?

1. Whether the obese person will accomplish satisfactory weight loss depends upon the effectiveness of treatment. The success of therapy depends upon discovery of the etiologic factors and their removal or control. The physician must find out why the positive

Ideal Weights for Men, Ages 25 and Over

HEIGHT (WITH SHOES)		WEIGHT IN POUNDS (AS ORDINARILY DRESSED)		
		Small Frame	Medium Frame	Large Frame
Feet	Inches			
5	2	116–125	124–133	131–142
5	3	119–128	127–136	133–144
5	4	122–132	130–140	137–149
5	5	126–136	134–144	141–153
5	6	129–139	137–147	145–157
5	7	133–143	141–151	149–162
5	8	136–147	145–156	153–166
5	9	140–151	149–160	157–170
5	10	144–155	153–164	161–175
5	11	148–159	157–168	165–180
6	0	152–164	161–173	169–185
6	1	157–169	166–178	174–190
6	2	163–175	171–184	179–196
6	3	168–180	176–189	184–202

Metropolitan Life Insurance Company, Statistical Bureau.

from skeletal measurements. Use of tables giving *average* weights at various ages and heights is misleading, for the optimal weight of an adult remains unchanged, but average weights increase in the middle decades. The use of the Wood-Baldwin tables for ideal weights of boys and girls is recommended (published by the American Child Health Association), and for ideal weights of men and women the tables published by the Metropolitan Life Insurance Company.

More important in diagnosis than detection of obesity and its severity is discovery of the etiologic factors. The various possible physiologic and psychologic disorders must be considered, and appropriate methods must be used to investigate the patient's history and habits, his physical characteristics and response to special tests. Psychiatric study often yields the solution and reveals the obesity as a symptom of a basic maladjustment.

energy balance developed and must know how to reverse the process. The patient must understand and cooperate. If both roles are not well performed, the outlook is poor; if they are well performed, establishing normal weight is not difficult.

2. Obesity, if persistent, impairs health and shortens life. Dublin and Lotka found that "the penalty of overweight is one-fourth to three-fourths excess in mortality." The hazard of obesity increases with its degree of severity and with the age of the subject, so that persons who are only 10 pounds overweight have an increase above the average death rate of 8 per cent; when 20 pounds overweight, of 18 per cent; 30 pounds overweight, of 28 per cent; 50 pounds overweight, of 56 per cent. Death from cardiovascular renal disease is 62 per cent more frequent in the obese than in persons of normal weight. Cirrhosis of the liver, ap-

pendicitis, biliary calculi, and liver and gall-bladder cancer occur about twice as often in the obese; cerebral accidents and puerperal complications about one and one-half times as often. Twelve per cent more of the obese die from accidents, possibly because of sub-normal agility. Gallbladder disease is especially frequent in those overweight. Obesity predisposes to diabetes, especially after age 40. The death rate from diabetes is about four times as great in the obese. The greater

ment which consists solely in giving the patient a low calorie diet outline is seldom successful. This is because the reasons for the positive energy balance are frequently multiple, and successful therapy requires removal of the causes, often both physiologic and psychologic.

Treatment may be divided into two phases: (1) elimination of etiologic factors, and (2) getting rid of the excess fat stores. For example, if hypogonadism is a causative influence,

Ideal Weights for Women, Ages 25 and Over

HEIGHT (WITH SHOES)		WEIGHT IN POUNDS (AS ORDINARILY DRESSED)		
		Small Frame	Medium Frame	Large Frame
Feet	Inches			
4	11	104–111	110–118	117–127
5	0	105–113	112–120	119–129
5	1	107–115	114–122	121–131
5	2	110–118	117–125	124–135
5	3	113–121	120–128	127–135
5	4	116–125	124–132	131–142
5	5	119–128	127–135	133–145
5	6	123–132	130–140	138–150
5	7	126–136	134–144	142–154
5	8	129–139	137–147	145–158
5	9	133–143	141–151	149–162
5	10	136–147	145–155	152–166
5	11	139–150	148–158	155–169

Metropolitan Life Insurance Company, Statistical Bureau.

the obesity, the poorer the prognosis following surgical operations. Resistance to infections such as pneumonia is decreased.

Treatment. Prevention or elimination of obesity depends upon instruction by the physician and dietitian, but the patient must carry out his own treatment. Therefore the *patient* must be impressed with the *seriousness* of the condition and provided with *specifice means* to combat it.

Prevention of excessive weight gain is preferable to and easier than treatment. Proper eating habits of those predisposed to obesity for any reason and of persons entering middle age should be established, and, unless contraindicated, moderate regular exercise should be encouraged.

Weight reduction may be accomplished by decreasing the food intake, by increasing the energy expenditure, or both. Although the immediate cause of obesity is always a caloric intake in excess of the requirements, treat-

use of gonadotropins or gonadal hormones is helpful; or if hypothyroidism is a factor, thyroid therapy is indicated; or if a psychologic difficulty is expressed in inordinate eating, its removal is necessary before the patient can reduce weight by dieting. Removal of stored fat may be accomplished by forcing its consumption for the production of body heat and energy. To achieve this, the caloric intake must be reduced or the metabolism accelerated, or both. Increase in energy expenditure may be induced by *exercise* when muscular exertion is not contraindicated by such complications as myocardial disease, orthopedic disorders, and so on. Definite amounts of moderate regular exercise such as walking, golf and swimming should be prescribed, since it not only increases caloric output, but improves muscle tone and general health. The value of exercise in weight reduction is, however, strictly limited, because activity stimulates appetite, and because mild exertion requires comparatively little energy expenditure. An average man walking 2½ miles, for example, uses only 120 calories, the content of one slice of bread. *Desiccated thyroid* will raise the metabolic rate and facilitate weight loss, but it should be given only when there is definite hypothyroidism, and then only in amounts sufficient to maintain a normal basal metabolic rate. Dinitrophenol will accelerate metabolism, but is toxic and should never be used.

Drugs to induce purging may reduce weight temporarily, chiefly through water loss, but the treatment of obesity is necessarily a prolonged process, and repeated catharsis is ineffective and harmful.

Diuresis with weight loss often occurs during therapy with low calorie, low salt diets. The use of diuretic drugs is usually not advisable unless indicated by the presence of edema.

Diet restriction is always necessary to induce weight loss (except in the mildest cases), no matter what caused the obesity. An allowance of 35 calories per kilogram of body weight is a maintenance diet for the average moderately active person. Limitation to 15 or 20 calories per kilogram of ideal weight provides a satisfactory reduction diet which will permit the patient to follow his usual occupation and to lose 1 or 2 pounds a week. For an ideal weight of 70 kilograms (154 pounds) this would amount to 1000 to 1400 calories daily. The protein allowance should be liberal (1 to 1.5 gm. per kilogram) because of the high satiety value of protein, its high specific dynamic action, and its importance in protecting tissues and building muscles. Carbohydrate should be taken chiefly in the low-carbohydrate bulky fruits and vegetables, and should total 0.75 to 1.5 gm. per gram of protein. The fat intake should be minimal, restricted primarily to the eggs and meat necessarily included in the liberal protein allowance, and amounting to about 0.5 gm. per kilogram of ideal weight. A widely applicable diet of this type providing approximately 85 gm. of protein, 35 gm. of fat and 105 gm. of carbohydrate (1075 calories) follows: 2 glasses of skimmed milk or buttermilk, 3 slices of whole wheat bread, 1 egg, 2 servings of lean meat, 1 potato, 4 servings of 1 to 8 per cent vegetables (raw cooked or in salads), 3 servings of raw or unsweetened canned fruit. The daily food allowance should be divided into three or four meals of approximately equal caloric value; omission of meals should

be discouraged. Such a diet should be adequate in calcium, iron and ascorbic acid, but, if followed for a long time, should be supplemented with concentrates of vitamins A and D and the B complex. Moderate restriction of water and sodium chloride is advisable for patients who tend to retain fluid.

Prescription of a diet does not ensure its observance. The patient must be instructed in the principles and details of the diet. The causes of excessive appetite must be eliminated if possible, and psychologic drives encouraging low caloric intake must be substituted: pride in appearance, desire for physical skills, wish to avoid physical disabilities and to prolong life.

Dietary instructions should be *written,* and must be explicit and detailed.

Most essential is *periodic consultation* with the physician to maintain morale, provide encouragement, record weight loss and improved body measurements, and to permit repeated instructions concerning diet and other details of treatment. Too often the obese patient is considered medically unimportant and uninteresting, is given inadequate instructions, and these only once, and then is cast adrift to fight his long and difficult battle alone. As in other conditions requiring prolonged therapy, dietary control and attention to psychiatric aspects, frequent advice from a sympathetic physician is vital. In obesity more than in any other common condition rather simple measures can result in great relief of symptoms and prolongation of life.

Formal *psychotherapy* is seldom required if prolonged cooperation with an understanding physician can be established. More deep-seated psychic disorders or habit patterns may require the attention of a trained psychiatrist.

Drug therapy in some cases helps to decrease appetite, especially amphetamine sulfate, 5 to 10 mg. one-half to one hour before meals, usually on arising, at 11 A.M. and 4 P.M. (not after 4 P.M., since it causes insomnia).

The physical and psychic effects of successful treatment are usually gratifying. Weight reduction often results in correction of menstrual disorders, diminution in hypertension, decrease in circulatory and cardiovascular strain with relief of dyspnea, fatigue and edema, decrease in joint pain, in the engorgement of venous varicosities, in the discomfort and disability from hernia, improvement in carbohydrate tolerance, and increase in physical and mental efficiency and in enjoyment of the normal pleasures of life.

CYRIL M. MACBRYDE

References

Armstrong, D. B., Dublin, L. I., Wheatley, G. M., and Marks, H. H.: Obesity and Its Relation to Health and Disease. J.A.M.A., *147*:1007, 1951.

Barr, D. P.: Health and Obesity. New England J. Med., 23:967, 1953.

Bruch, H.: Psychological Aspects of Reducing. Psychosom. Med., *14*:337, 1952.

Conn, J. W.: Obesity: Etiological Aspects. Physiol. Rev., 24:31, 1944.

Evans, F. A.: Obesity, in Duncan, G. G.: Diseases of Metabolism. 3rd ed. Philadelphia, W. B. Saunders Company, 1952, Chap. 9.

MacBryde, C. M.: Obesity, in Signs and Symptoms. Philadelphia, J. B. Lippincott Company, 1952, Chap. 27.

McLester, J. S., and Darby, W. J.: Nutrition and Diet in Health and Disease. 6th ed. Philadelphia, W. B. Saunders Company, 1952, Chap. 17.

Newburgh, L. H.: Obesity: Energy Metabolism. Physiol. Rev., 24:18, 1944.

Nutrition Symposium No. 6: Overeating, Overweight and Obesity. New York, National Vitamin Foundation, 1953.

Rynearson, E. H., and Gastineau, C. F.: Obesity. Springfield, Ill., Charles C Thomas, 1949.

THE LIPOMATOSES

Definition. The term "lipomatoses" is used here as a convenient if arbitrary classification of a group of probably unrelated disorders affecting the distribution or state of neutral fat deposits. The involved areas, although often multiple, are more or less discrete, as opposed to general metabolic or ·endocrine disturbances such as obesity and diffuse fatty infiltration.

Nodular, Circumscribed Lipomatosis. Single or multiple lipomas are of frequent occurrence, particularly in women. They are soft, slow-growing, ordinarily well encapsulated and discrete tumors arising usually from the subcutaneous fat, particularly of the shoulders, back, neck and proximal half of the extremities. They are usually asymptomatic, but if tender, large or unsightly they may be excised. Interstitial, visceral, thoracic, abdominal and nervous system lipomas also occur. A painful form of multiple, circumscribed, subcutaneous lipoma or neurolipoma was described by Dercum (Dercum's disease, adiposis dolorosa). Recently Smetana and Bernhard called attention to what they designated sclerosing lipogranuloma, the result of trauma, local ischemia and necrosis of fat deposits, with infiltration and fibrosis of the surrounding tissue; when amenable to surgery, such areas are best excised. Localized atrophy or spongy hypertrophy of fat at the site of insulin injections—"insulin lipodystrophy"— occasionally occurs in women and children; it can be avoided by varying the site of injection.

Diffuse, Symmetric Lipomatosis. Lipomatosis may be more extensive, symmetrically involving the neck ("fat neck," Madelung's neck) to form large, disfiguring masses which sometimes extend down over the shoulders and arms, or are occasionally segmentally distributed on the thorax. This disorder is more common in males. Extensive plastic revision may be required. In women a common form of symmetrical subcutaneous deposition of excessive fat in the buttocks and legs, with more or less dependent edema, has been designated lipedema of the legs by Allen and Hines.

Progressive Lipodystrophy (Barraquer-Simmons Disease). Progressive lipodystrophy is a disorder characterized by symmetrical and slowly progressive loss of subcutaneous fat from the face, in more severe cases also from the neck, arms, thorax and abdominal wall, with preservation or increase in the fat of the lower part of the body. Extensively affected patients present a bizarre appearance of emaciation of the upper portions of the body, particularly of the face, with contrasting pronounced obesity of the hips, buttocks and legs.

The cause of the disease is not known. Endocrine factors, particularly of the pituitary gland, and some intrinsic abnormality of fat tissue metabolism have been suspected. Because of the symmetric and sometimes segmental distribution, a neurotropic mechanism has been suggested. There appears to be no hereditary trait.

The onset commonly is between the ages of 4 and 8, young girls being chiefly affected, but the disorder may develop in adults. The rate of progressive involvement varies from one or two years to over a decade, but arrest may occur at any stage. The muscles, hair and sweat glands of affected areas are spared. Apart from weight loss and emotional disturbances attending disfigurement, there is usually no associated abnormality or incapacity. There is no known treatment.

Intestinal Lipodystrophy (Whipple's Disease). As described by G. H. Whipple in 1907, this disorder is "characterized by gradual loss of weight and strength, stools consisting chiefly of neutral fat and fatty acids, indefinite abdominal signs and a peculiar multiple arthritis." The underlying pathologic findings include a striking lipogranulomatosis of enlarged mesenteric lymph nodes and the presence of large, foamy macrophages, filled with an unidentified glycoprotein, in the tunica propria of the small intestine; cystic dilatation of the mesenteric lymphatics may also occur. These morphologic abnormalities induce or reflect a malabsorption syndrome resembling sprue.

The disease has a marked predilection for males, usually between the ages of 30 and 65. The onset is insidious, usually with diffuse abdominal discomfort and intermittent diarrhea, the stools later becoming bulky, frothy and foul-smelling, and containing large amounts of neutral fat and fatty acids. Sometimes the disease is ushered in with bouts of migratory polyarthritis which may, indeed, dominate the picture for several years. Intermittent fever, hypotension, hypochromic anemia, generalized lymphadenopathy, chronic cough, hypoalbuminemia and edema are common accompaniments. Ascites (sometimes chylous) and fibrous polyserositis may occur. Occasionally there is pronounced pigmentation of the skin, simulating Addison's disease, in the late stages; tests for adrenocortical function, however, give essentially normal results. X-rays show a typical "deficiency pattern" of the small bowel. The glucose tolerance curve is normal or flat, free acid in the gastric contents is diminished or absent, pancreatic secretion is preserved. Marked hypocholesterolemia and increased serum glycoproteins have been described.

The course is protracted and, with spontaneous remissions, characterized by progressive weakness and weight loss terminating in extreme debility and death, usually within five years of onset. The etiology is obscure. Some morphologic or metabolic defect in absorption from the small intestine, particularly of fat, is present but many features of the disease suggest a systemic rather than a localized disorder. Treatment is supportive and symptomatic. Corticotropin and corticosteroids have been found to induce amelioration of symptoms in some cases, and these agents should be given a protracted trial.

Relapsing Febrile Nodular Nonsuppurative Panniculitis (Weber-Christian Disease). This disorder in its most typical form is characterized by recurring febrile bouts associated with the appearance of crops of subcutaneous fatty nodules which are usually tender. The cause of the disease is not known. Necropsy findings indicate that the underlying abnormality may be not an entirely local disturbance confined to the panniculus, but a more generalized disorder of fat metabolism. Whether this is primary or secondary to small blood vessel disease is not clear. Kennedy and Murphy believe that the changes in adipose tissue are due to ischemia secondary to thrombosis or endarteritis of small vessels, with subsequent necrosis of fat cells and infiltration by macrophages and mononuclear cells. Weber found that administration of iodides could produce the manifestations in susceptible persons, but in most cases there is no history of exposure to iodides. Similar manifestations have been produced by trauma, repeated subcutaneous injections and local application of cold. Despite recent claims of a beneficial effect of penicillin, there is no convincing evidence of an infectious etiology.

The earliest morbid changes in the panniculus appear to be accumulations of lipophages, often associated with small vessel changes such as periarteritis and arteriolitis. Central areas of softening due to fat necrosis and edema then appear, along with increased numbers of fat-laden macrophages, lymphocytes, large mononuclear cells and sometimes many polymorphonuclear cells. Late lesions show a decrease in necrotic material and inflammatory cells with more or less fibrous tissue replacement. In cases coming to necropsy it is apparent that similar changes may involve fat deposits in addition to those in the subcutaneous layers—for example, pancreatic adipose tissue and omental, mesenteric, peripelvic, periadrenal and epicardial deposits. Moreover, extensive fatty infiltration and central necrosis of the liver, with hemorrhage, occur apparently quite regularly. Fatty and hydropic degeneration of the pancreas and adrenal cortex have been described, as have fat emboli in the lungs.

Although accounted a rarity, some 60 cases of Weber-Christian disease have been reported, most of them in recent years. The disorder has been described in patients ranging in age from 2 to 64 years. Females appear to be somewhat more frequently affected. Prodromal symptoms of malaise, fever, sore throat or arthralgia often precede the onset. Some 90 per cent of patients exhibit fever, which may precede the appearance of nodules and which usually persists until they regress, recurring with each new outcrop. Leukopenia is the rule and may be marked, although some cases have shown leukocytosis. Joint and muscle pains sometimes are generalized and severe, suggesting to some observers a possible relationship to dermatomyositis.

The subcutaneous nodules upon which clinical recognition largely depends appear most frequently on the thighs, also on other portions of the legs and on the arms and trunk; they are rare on the buttocks, breast, face, hands and feet. They are usually multiple, vary in diameter from about 1 to 10 cm., and are apt to be tender and sometimes spontaneously painful. The overlying skin may be inflamed. A nodule occasionally may rupture, exuding turbid, fatty material which yields no bacterial growth on culture. Involvement of internal fat deposits does not give these visible manifestations, of course, but may be responsible for obscure febrile episodes and abdominal pain.

The course is protracted and marked by remissions and exacerbations. There is no satisfactory treatment, although improvement of uncertain duration has been ascribed to sulfapyridine and penicillin. ACTH and cortisone have been tried but proved generally disappointing.

ALEXANDER B. GUTMAN

References

Beerman, H.: Weber-Christian Syndrome. Am. J. M. Sc., 225:446, 1953.

Harris, J. S., and Reiser, R.: Lipodystrophy. Am. J. Dis. Children, 59:143, 1940.

Hendrix, J. P., Black-Schaffer, B., Withers, R. W., and Handler, P.: Whipple's Intestinal Lipodystrophy. Arch. Int. Med., 85:91, 1950.

Jones, C. M., Benson, J. A., Jr., and Rocque, A. L.: Whipple's Disease. New England J. Med., 248:665, 1953.

Kennedy, R. J., and Murphy, L. R.: Weber-Christian Disease. Am. J. Med., 6:672, 1949.

Plummer, K., Russi, S., Harris, W. H., Jr., and Caravati, C. M.: Lipophagic Intestinal Granulomatosis (Whipple's Disease). Arch. Int. Med., 86:280, 1950.

Russo, F. R.: Whipple's Disease. Arch. Int. Med., 89:600, 1952.

Smetana, H. F., and Bernhard, W.: Sclerosing Lipogranuloma. Arch. Path., 50:296, 1950.

Wakeley, C., and Somerville, P.: Lipomas. Lancet, 2:997, 1952.

Whipple, G. H.: A Hitherto Undescribed Disease Characterized Anatomically by Deposits of Fat and Fatty Acids in the Intestinal and Mesenteric Lymphatic Tissues. Bull. Johns Hopkins Hosp., 18:382, 1907.

Wold, L. E., Hines, E. A., Jr., and Allen, E. V.: Lipedema of the Legs: A Syndrome Characterized by Fat Legs and Edema. Ann. Int. Med., 34:1243, 1951.

ATHEROSCLEROSIS

Definition. Atherosclerosis is a disease in which patches of lipid-containing material (atheromas) are deposited beneath the intimal surfaces of blood vessels. It is not to be confused with senile or involutionary arteriosclerosis in which loss of elasticity, ectasia and gradual infiltration by calcium, lipid and protein appear as inevitable consequences of the aging of arteries. Its development depends upon causes quite separate from those involved in Mönckeberg's medial calcification. Pathogenetically as well as anatomically it is distinct from the arteriolar sclerosis which characteristically accompanies prolonged hypertension. The distinction is significant because senile arteriosclerosis and medial calcification are not often demonstrably consequential in the production of symptoms, while the complications of arteriolar sclerosis although serious differ from those of atherosclerosis. In older persons, however, strict separation of the several forms of arterial disease offers difficulty since atheromatous deposits are seen in vessels which have already developed senile alterations, which exhibit variable degrees of medial calcification and which may show the characteristic arteriolarsclerosis of concomitant high blood pressure.

Incidence. Postmortem examinations indicate that in more than 50 per cent of North Americans who die before the age of 50 atheromatous plaques are demonstrable, and that among those who die after the age of 75 more than 90 per cent are moderately or seriously afflicted. That the disease does not spare American youth is indicated by recent studies of soldiers killed in combat in Korea. In 40 per cent of men averaging 22 years of age atherosclerotic plaques of some degree were found in the coronary arteries. The disease is so widely distributed as to suggest a defect inherent in mankind. Certain it is that clinical conditions otherwise regarded as normal permit extensive formation of atheromatous patches in blood vessels of a large part of the adult population of North America and northern Europe. The susceptibility of man is the more remarkable since other species of mammals have not been shown to develop spontaneous atherosclerosis.

Etiology and Pathogenesis. Although in man the tendency to atherosclerosis appears to be almost universal, the rapidity and extent of development of the lesions are modified by a variety of factors. *Race* appears to have an important influence on the degree of susceptibility. Of people living in the United States, Jews appear to be especially prone to the serious effects of the disease. Testimony of many observers indicates that Mongoloids, African natives and the Tamils of southern India are less affected than the Caucasians of the United States and northern Europe. Difficulty is encountered in interpreting the evidence concerning some of the supposed racial differences, since the influence of other factors such as longevity, eating habits, and the frequency and thoroughness of postmortem examinations cannot readily be evaluated. *Familial and hereditary influences* are potent factors in determining the rate at which atherosclerosis develops. Families afflicted with hypercholesterolemia, and especially those in which the cholesterol concentration is so high and persistent as to produce xanthomatosis, tend to develop extensive lesions and serious or fatal complications in early life. The degree of atherosclerosis increases with *age*. Plaques are seldom seen in the newborn although they may develop as yellow streaks in the aortas of unweaned infants within a few weeks following birth. Lesions tend to become more extensive with each succeeding decade, a circumstance which is in part the result of accretion of repeated deposits, but which may be attributable in some degree to changes in physical and chemical factors in the aging population. *Sex* appears to exert a significant influence on the rate of development. Women before the menopause seldom suffer from complications of the disease. When compared with men of like age they exhibit less atherosclerosis of the coronary arteries and possibly less deposit in the peripheral vessels. In older women this outstanding advantage appears to be lost, and in the later decades of life there is little difference between the sexes either in the extent and degree of the deposits or in the incidence of their serious consequences.

Some *physical factors* favoring the deposit of lipids in arterial walls have been well established. The lesions tend to occur earlier and to be more florid in areas of *intimal thickening*. They are exaggerated in locations where *syphilis* or other injury to the circulation within the arterial wall has previously occurred. That the deposit is to some extent dependent upon a minimum *blood pressure* is indicated by the fact that pulmonary arteries and veins do not become atherosclerotic unless their intraluminal pressure is materially increased by disease. In otherwise normal individuals the deposit is greatest at sites in the arterial system where the blood pressure is highest. Persistent *hypertension* exaggerates the tendency to atherosclerosis so significantly and constantly that in the past, high blood pressure has been regarded as a primary cause of the atheromatous changes.

Although physical factors are undoubtedly important in determining the location and extent of lesions, the fact remains that atheromas develop widely in arteries that reveal no evidence of preceding structural changes. Differences in blood pressure and the anatomy of arterial walls have failed to explain the variation and susceptibility between man and other mammalian species. Recently attention has been focused on the possibility that something in the *chemical composition* of the plasma of man makes him more vulnerable than other species. A number of factors have been emphasized. It has been suggested variously that the rate and extent of deposit might be dependent upon the cholesterol concentration in the plasma; that it might be more influenced by the cholesterol-phospholipid ratio; that it might depend upon the distribution of lipids between the several lipid-bearing proteins or lipoproteins of plasma; that it might depend upon the actual amount of the lipids combined with beta$_1$ globulins in the form of beta lipoproteins, or upon the concentration of specific forms of beta lipoproteins recognizable in the ultracentrifuge and designated as S_f 12-20 bodies. Investigations have shown that in several of these particulars the plasma of man differs from that of nonsusceptible mammals, and that the divergence is greatest in physiologic states and in diseases which appear to predispose to more rapid and more extensively atheromatous deposit. In general the recent observations lend strong support to the chemical hypothesis for the pathogenesis of atherosclerosis, although they do not establish any one chemical factor as solely responsible. It now seems not unlikely that atheromatous deposits are dependent upon chemical factors operative to some extent in all human adults but grossly exaggerated with familial predisposition and with a variety of diseases.

Pathogenetic significance has been attributed to other circumstances. There is some statistical evidence that *habitus* is important and that the disease appears earlier and more extensively in mesomorphic individuals. Heavy indulgence in alcohol over many years has seemed to afford some protection, while excessive use of *tobacco* has been urged as a contributing factor to the development or aggravation of complications. A low caloric vegetarian diet has been regarded as protective whereas consumption of animal fat has been thought to exaggerate the deposit. It has been stated and contradicted that the obese develop a greater degree of atherosclerosis than the spare. Abundant evidence supports the contention that overweight individuals suffer at an earlier age the serious consequences of the disease.

Pathology. Atherosclerosis is preeminently a disease of the aorta and its branches. It is minimal or absent in pulmonary arteries except in conditions such as mitral stenosis which cause pulmonary artery hypertension. It is not seen in the walls or veins except after injury from phlebitis or at sites of arterial venous aneurysms. It appears early on the posterior wall of the aorta at the openings of the intercostal arteries and also at the mouths of the coronaries. It is more abundant in the descending than in the ascending aorta, more evident in the abdominal than in the thoracic portion. Atherosclerosis is patchy in its distribution, and it is not an uncommon experience to discover extensive lesions in vessels of one organ with almost complete freedom from involvement in other parts of the vascular system.

The early atheromatous patch consists of cholesterol, cholesterol esters, phospholipids and neutral fat, together with a considerable amount of protein. When first deposited its composition mimics that of the blood. The earliest lesion appears as a yellow linear streak hardly raised above the surface, which may be seen even in unweaned infants. The deposit begins in the deepest part of the intima, and the lipid may be seen partly in the intercellular ground substance and partly in the intimal connective tissue cells, some of which are distended with fat to such a degree that they have been called foam cells, lipoid cells or lipophages. Gradually the fat extends to the surface of the intima. The connective tissue over the fatty area becomes thickened; necrosis may develop in the deeper part of the plaque; cholesterol crystals become more abundant because of the disintegration of cholesterol esters. The area becomes calcified and in some instances somewhat vascularized. The amorphous fatty tissue accumulates and at times to an extent which may cause rupture of the intima with ulceration and production of a site favorable to the formation of thrombi. In large vessels such as the aorta and its main branches intimal plaques have no appreciable effect on the lumen. In smaller vessels such as the coronaries or the arteries at the base of the brain, the plaques may accomplish almost complete occlusion and may lead to ischemia or infarction of tissue. More often, however, these accidents are dependent upon thrombosis or hemorrhage on the thickened or ulcerated surface of a narrowed vessel.

Clinical Manifestations. Extensive lesions may exist for long periods without producing clinically recognizable abnormalities. The disease need not be widespread, however, to produce serious symptoms. A single atheromatous plaque strategically placed may lead to a serious or fatal accident.

Clinical manifestations may be limited to fatigue and a diminished capacity to perform mental or physical tasks. Localizing signs may develop in any part of the body but are usually referable to disturbances in circulation of the heart, brain, extremities or gastrointestinal tract.

Manifestations Referable to Ischemia of the Heart Muscle. It is estimated that atherosclerosis of the coronary arteries is responsible for 25 to 40 per cent of all heart disease. The most distinctive clinical manifestations are angina pectoris and myocardial infarction. Pathologic experience indicates that 90 per cent of patients suffering from anginal pain exhibit at autopsy obstructive narrowing or occlusion of the main coronary arteries or their primary branches. Causes of myocardial infarction other than atherosclerosis of the coronary arteries are extremely infrequent. In the absence of angina pectoris or the signs of myocardial infarction, the presence of coronary atherosclerosis, even when it has produced extensive narrowing and multiple occlusions, may be clinically unrecognizable. Although bundle branch block and other disorders of the conduction system, ventricular tachycardia, diminished cardiac reserve and heart failure are common manifestations of the myocardial ischemia of coronary atherosclerosis, they occur also in hypertension and other conditions with sufficient frequency to rob them of diagnostic significance.

Manifestations Attributable to Atherosclerotic Disease of the Aorta. Even massive atherosclerosis of the aorta may be clinically unrecognizable except by roentgenographic visualization of intimal calcification. Rarely when combined with hypertension and dilatation of the aortic ring it may contribute to incompetence of the aortic valve. In syphilitic aortitis, atheromatous plaques tend to be excessive where the arterial wall and its internal circulation have been damaged by the spirochete. Saccular aneurysms are not attributable to atherosclerosis although their walls may contain many atheromatous plaques. Dissecting aneurysm, which was formerly attributed to channeling of blood beneath fractured calcified patches of atherosclerosis in the presence of hypertension, is now usually ascribed to cystic degeneration of the media.

Clinical Manifestations of Cerebral Atherosclerosis. Together, hemorrhage and thrombosis of cerebral vessels constitute 90 per cent of all cerebral vascular lesions. In both processes atherosclerosis is significantly implicated, for it is recognized as the most frequent cause of cerebral thrombosis, and traditionally hemorrhage has been thought to result from the rupture of an atherosclerotic vessel in the presence of hypertension. Furthermore, before actual blockage or hemorrhage occurs, progressive occlusion of vessels leads to ischemia with patchy degeneration of cortical cells and nerve tracts and disseminated areas of atrophy. Actual obstruction with or without thrombosis leads to small or large areas of softening. Numerous small lesions as well as larger ones may result in paralysis or in mental deterioration which clinically overshadows the loss in motor function. They cause diminution in intellectual capacity, impaired memory, especially for recent events and names, emotional instability, addiction to reminiscence with more or less confabulation. The victim becomes self-centered, hostile and sometimes paranoid with loosely constructed delusions. Actual dementia is not uncommon.

Manifestations of Atherosclerosis of Peripheral Arteries. Atheromatous disease is by far the commonest cause of arterial occlusion in the legs. Except in diabetes, symptoms referable to its presence are uncommon before the age of 55. In the arms serious impairment of circulation from atherosclerosis is not frequent, and the calcification which is so often demonstrable in the radial, ulnar and brachial arteries of older persons is usually attributable to medial rather than intimal disease. Obliterative lesions in the terminal branches of the posterior tibial and dorsalis pedis arteries produce symptoms which in their early stages consist of paresthesias, nocturnal cramps, weakness and chilliness of the legs and feet. Later faint discoloration of the ends of the toes may be followed by more serious circulatory disturbance or by dry or moist gangrene. In many patients the most troublesome symptom is intermittent claudication, which consists of cramping pain that appears with walking and subsides with rest. This may develop before the signs of complete arterial occlusion are apparent. Prominent physical signs are lack of pulsation in the peripheral arteries, blanching on elevation of the foot with slower than normal return of color with dependency. The veins remain collapsed for some time.

Manifestations of Atherosclerosis of the Mesentery Vessels. Digestive disturbances, including achlorhydria, intestinal atony and constipation which are frequent in the aged, have been attributed without convincing proof to the impaired circulation and ischemia of atherosclerosis. Thrombosis of the mesenteric arteries, like that of the coronary and cerebral vessels, may depend upon the formation of an intraluminal clot at the site of an atherosclerotic patch.

Diagnosis. As yet there is no adequate clinical or laboratory means of estimating the degree and extent of atherosclerosis, or even of recognizing its presence. Lesions may be suspected because of the visibility by roentgenographic examination of calcified lesions in the aorta and its main branches. Tests of tolerance to exercise and response to deprivation of oxygen, ballistocardiographic observations and electrocardiographic studies may permit the inference that the coronary circulation is insufficient. Careful measurement of the pulsations in the extremities may indicate defects which are most easily ascribable to atherosclerosis. Unfortunately, even with the use of all of these tests the existence of atheromatous plaques is usually not established until serious complications have already developed.

Treatment. In considering the treatment of atherosclerosis several objectives may be kept in mind: (1) It would be desirable to limit or prevent the deposit of lipids or to cause the disappearance of lesions already formed. (2) It would be an advantage to control hypertension, which is thought to accelerate the deposit and to favor rupture of atherosclerotic vessels. (3) Most desirable of all would be the prevention of intraluminal clotting which is responsible for most of the mortality and a large part of the morbidity of the disease.

The criteria for judging the degree to which any of these desirable objectives are achieved are unreliable. Since we do not have the means of recognizing the location and extent of atheromatous lesions, we cannot tell whether they are affected by therapy. Under the best circumstances judgment concerning efficacy of management would require statistical analysis of an immense experience.

A vast number of remedies have been suggested and tried. Of the more recent ones a word may be said. Neither the efficacy nor the rationale for administration of choline, methionine, lipocaic and inositol has been established. The use of heparin recently suggested with hope deserves further study. As yet its efficacy in accomplishing any of the objectives of treatment has not been proven. It has been shown that the administration of estrogen can modify the cholesterol concentration and abnormal lipid pattern of survivors of myocardial infarction to a degree which in many cases amounts to reestablishment of normal chemical conditions. It has not been demonstrated that the administration of a female sex hormone inhibits or prevents the development of atherosclerosis or exercises any influence on the incidence or severity of its complications. Side actions of estrogens, chiefly impotence and gynecomastia, are so undesirable as to preclude an extensive trial of these substances as therapeutic agents.

In patients who have suffered myocardial infarctions, carefully controlled anticoagulant therapy has aided in the prevention of still more serious complications. Success in this situation has suggested the more extensive use of anticoagulants in the prophylaxis of thrombosis in those who appear to be especially threatened by the degree and location of their atherosclerosis.

In recent years chief attention in the treatment of atherosclerosis has been focused upon the use of diets with chief emphasis on restriction of cholesterol, fat and caloric intake. Extensive trial of diets, low in cholesterol alone, has failed to show crucial changes in the cholesterol concentration of the plasma or in most of the essentially pathologic features of lipid composition in persons especially susceptible to the development of atherosclerosis. The restriction of fat and calories, on the other hand, appears to be somewhat more helpful. It has recently been reported by several observers that predictable reduction of serum lipids has followed the use of diets containing vegetable but no animal fat.

It is no new doctrine that gluttons have a relatively high morbidity and mortality from vascular disease, or that there is greater average longevity and relative freedom from vascular accidents among the spare and the frugal. More recent evidence has strengthened this traditional impression. It is stated with statistical support that the obese have a greater incidence of hypertension and that atherosclerotic plaques develop earlier and more abundantly in the overfed. Some evidence has been presented that life expectancy may be increased by correcting overweight. This circumstantial evidence seems to indicate that while waiting for more effective means of treatment, a low fat, low but adequate caloric diet may be advised with the expectation of partial protection against the rapid development of the complications of atherosclerosis. Since man is an atherosclerotic animal and since atheromas form to some degree in most individuals in middle and later life, this advice need not be limited to those already obese or to those who have disclosed the obvious presence or complications of atherosclerosis.

DAVID P. BARR

References

Adlersberg, D., Parets, A. D., and Boas, E. P.: Genetics of Atherosclerosis. J.A.M.A., *141:*246, 1949.

Ahrens, E. H., Jr., Blankenhorn, D. H., and Tsaltas, T. T.: Effect on Human Serum Lipids of Substituting Plant for Animal Fat in Diet. Proc. Soc. Exper. Biol. & Med., 86:872, 1954.

Barr, D. P.: The George E. Brown Memorial Lecture. Some Chemical Factors in the Pathogenesis of Atherosclerosis. Circulation, 8:641, 1953.

——: The Basis for Dietary Treatment in the Prevention and Control of Atherosclerosis. Am. J. Med., 13:663, 1952.

————, Russ, E. M., and Eder, H. A.: Influence of Estrogens on Lipoproteins in Atherosclerosis. Tr. A. Am. Phys., 65:102, 1952.

Enos, W. F., Holmes, R. H., and Beyer, J.: Coronary Disease Among United States Soldiers Killed in Korea. J.A.M.A., 152:1090, 1953.

Gertler, M. M., Garn, M. S., and Lerman, J.: The Interrelationships of Serum Cholesterol, Cholesterol Esters and Phospholipids in Health and in Coronary Artery Disease. Circulation, 2:205, 1950.

Gofman, J. W., and others: Blood Lipids and Human Atherosclerosis. Circulation, 2:161, 1950.

Kinsell, L. W., and others: Effect upon Serum Cholesterol and Phospholipids of Diets Containing Large Amounts of Vegetable Fat. J. Clin. Nutrition, 1:224, 1952–53.

Moschkowitz, E.: Arteriosclerosis. J.A.M.A., 143:861, 1950.

Wilens, S. L.: Bearing of General Nutritional State on Atherosclerosis. Arch. Int. Med., 79:129, 1947.

Wright, I. S., Marple, C. D., and Beck, D. F.: Myocardial Infarction. Its Clinical Manifestations and Treatment with Anticoagulants. New York, Grune and Stratton, 1954.

XANTHOMATOSIS

Definition. Xanthomatosis, as defined in this section, includes only those conditions in which deposits of lipid in tissues are dependent upon or accompanied by abnormally high concentrations of lipids in the blood. Not included are several clinical states which are sometimes given the name of xanthomatosis and are characterized by lipid-containing histiocytes or reticular endothelial cells but which develop without perceptible hyperlipemia. (See Niemann-Pick's Disease, Hand-Schüller-Christian Disease.)

In the discussion distinction is attempted because of differences in clinical manifestations between the xanthomatoses in which deposits appear to depend upon hypercholesterolemia and those which are associated with hyperlipemia. Chemically the separation of these two states cannot be sharply made, since many cases of hypercholesterolemia exhibit moderate increase in the plasma concentration of neutral fat and most cases of hyperlipemia have higher than normal plasma concentration of cholesterol.

Etiology and Pathogenesis. *Hypercholesterolemia.* The mean cholesterol concentration for young normal adults is about 200 mg. per 100 cc. with a rather wide range from 120 to 280 mg. per 100 cc. In older normal persons of both sexes the mean as well as the maximum concentrations are moderately increased. Although there are large differences between members of a group, the range of concentration in each individual is seldom more than ± 15 per cent under a considerable variety of life situations. Hypocholesterolemia, normocholesterolemia and hypercholesterolemia are relative terms and the dividing line between the normal and the pathologic is entirely arbitrary. In this discussion we have set 300 mg. per 100 cc. as the upper limit of normal but with the suspicion that values below this level may be consequential in the tendency to deposit of lipids in tissues.

Hypercholesterolemia has been observed under a variety of conditions, but may be classified rather simply as *familial* or idiopathic and *acquired,* either in the course of diabetes, nephrosis or myxedema, or as a consequence of hepatic and biliary tract disease.

By far the commonest cause both of excessive concentration of cholesterol in plasma and of xanthomatosis is *familial hypercholesterolemia.* That it is hereditary is attested by many observations of family groups in whom hypercholesterolemia, xanthomatosis, premature atherosclerosis and coronary heart disease are so frequently encountered as to be considered parts of the same genetic defect.

Hypercholesterolemia from secondary causes is seldom sufficiently severe or prolonged to cause deposit of lipids in the skin. When these do appear they take the form of eruptive xanthoma and usually consist of small papules, pinhead to pea size, subcutaneously located on the trunk and extremities and surrounded at their inception by hyperemic halos. In the arteries extensive deposit of lipids and the clinical complications of atherosclerosis may accompany both diabetes and nephrosis. In myxedema the pathologic evidence of more than usual atherosclerosis is less convincing, although relative frequency of angina pectoris in this condition has been noted.

The hypercholesterolemia and xanthomatosis which accompany hepatic and biliary disease is seen most often in cases of long-standing biliary cirrhosis. Higher than normal concentrations of plasma cholesterol are also frequently encountered in a variety of obstructive lesions of the biliary tract but seldom lead to xanthomatosis of the skin or tendon sheaths. In these conditions clinical complications of atherosclerosis are rare, although superficial deposits of lipids have been noted in the postmortem examination of the aorta and the endocardium.

Hyperlipemia. Like hypercholesterolemia the excessive accumulation of neutral fat in the blood may be due to primary or secondary causes. It may be simply classified as (1) essential familial hyperlipemia; and (2) acquired from nephrosis, diabetes, von Gierke's disease, chronic pancreatitis or a variety of miscellaneous conditions.

The family disease is regarded as a rarity. Only a few cases and one autopsy have been recorded. Since its presence does not interfere with the maintenance of apparently good health over long periods, there is reason to think that it is commoner than a review of the literature might indicate. Acquired hyperlipemia is seen more frequently. It is a part of the nephrotic syndrome where it is always associated with hypercholesterolemia. In a few diabetics hyperlipemia may be extreme, and when present is accompanied by greater than normal concentration of all other lipid components. Xanthomatosis accompanying hyperlipemia seldom involves the tendon sheaths but usually takes the form of the eruptive xanthoma that is seen in acquired forms of hypercholesterolemia. The lesions appear to represent a spillover from the hyperlipemic plasma into highly vascularized tissue. Similar forms have been occasionally noted in association with von Gierke's disease and in association with chronic pancreatitis.

Pathology. The lesions of xanthomatosis tend to be quite similar pathologically regardless of location. There is a deposit of lipid, and in the hypercholesterolemic families chiefly of cholesterol, in subcutaneous and cutaneous tissues, tendons and aponeuroses. Cholesterol crystals may be evident. Connective tissues containing fat and variously called xanthoma cells, foam cells or lipophages tend to accumulate. In some of the lesions there are giant cells (Touton cells) which contain several nuclei in an almost complete circle around an opaque cytoplasm. The lesions are most easily recognized in the skin and tendons, but those which develop in the structure of internal organs such as the heart and arteries do not differ materially from the superficial lesions. In the eruptive xanthomas much of the lipid is extracellular; foam cells are not numerous; giant cells are absent; little granulation tissue is seen.

Clinical Manifestations. In many cases both of hypercholesterolemia and hyperlipemia, clinical recognition must depend solely upon chemical tests unsupported by any obvious symptoms or physical signs. The condition of the patient during life may disclose no evidence of the underlying defect or its anatomic damage.

Xanthomatosis has been noted most often and in its most obtrusive clinical forms in association with familial hypercholesterolemia, although other forms of hypercholesterolemia and hyperlipemia may mimic the clinical picture of the familial disease. The lesions are various and have been given many names.

Xanthelasma is a term used to indicate collections of fat and cholesterol in the eyelids. Although these are frequent accompaniments of hypercholesterolemia and may be occasionally seen in association with hyperlipemia, it is important to remember that the lesions may be present in patients who exhibit no chemical defects. *Arcus senilis* in relatively young people, like xanthelasma, is a frequent accompaniment of hypercholesterolemia but may develop in people as in the Eskimos in whom no chemical defect in the plasma can be demonstrated. *Xanthoma planum* is the term reserved for flat or slightly raised lipid deposits seen in many parts of the body but with special frequency in the creases of the palms, in the folds of the elbows, in the creases below the breasts and in wrinkles or folds elsewhere. *Xanthoma tuberosum* is a name given to nodular lipid deposits in the skin. It appears in many places but may develop floridly on the buttocks, elbows, knees and hands. *Xanthoma tendinosum* is a term used to describe hard nodules of lipid deposits in the tendon sheaths of hands, forearms, ankles and many other sites.

It is to be noted that these different forms and localizations of deposits do not represent separate diseases. On the contrary, all of them may be evident in the same individual. The distinctions are not qualitative but are used entirely for descriptive purposes.

Vascular Involvement. Those who suffer from familial hypercholesterolemia and xanthomatosis may deposit cholesterol and develop collections of foam cells or lipophages beneath the intima of blood vessels and occasionally beneath the endocardium. These lesions cannot be strictly differentiated from the atheromatous patches which are found in persons who have normal concentrations of cholesterol in the plasma. They are notable chiefly because of their development in younger individuals and because of their greater degree and extent. The formation of xanthomas in the vascular system is usually localized to blood vessels and chiefly to the aorta and its branches, with frequent and early involvement of the coronary arteries. The deposits may be seen in pulmonary arteries and in a few cases have implicated the endocardium with or without involvement of the aortic, mitral and pulmonary valves. The evidence of ischemia, scarring and infarction of heart muscle is frequently encountered in these patients even in youth. Members of such hypercholesterolemic families often exhibit symptoms and signs of heart disease at an early age. Angina pectoris is frequent and was noted in one child at the age of 4. Several sudden deaths in children have been recorded.

In idiopathic familial hyperlipemia the deposit of lipids may not be limited to the formation of superficial xanthomas. Hepatomegaly, splenomegaly and enlargement of lymph nodes have been recorded. Foam cells have been found in biopsy specimens of the liver, spleen, lymph nodes and bone marrow. Abdominal pain variously ascribed to acute swelling of the liver and spleen and to pancreatitis has been frequent. Glycosuria of mild degree, not influenced by the administration of insulin, has also been reported. The relationship of familial hyperlipemia to atherosclerosis has not been established. The single autopsied case in an infant failed to show deposit in arteries. Recent reports of idiopathic familial hyperlipemia, however, have emphasized the coincidence of angina pectoris and myocardial infarction.

Treatment. In familial hypercholesterolemia the course of the disease and the development or persistence of superficial xanthomas are but slightly influenced by therapeutic measures. It cannot be shown that the cholesterol concentration of the blood is materially diminished by removing cholesterol form the diet. Even low fat, low caloric diets seem to have little effect on the chemical constitution of the blood. The administration of estrogens in most cases is followed by changes in the direction of normal plasma values. In no case of xanthomatosis, however, has estrogen accomplished complete restoration of a normal pattern.

In acquired hypercholesterolemia the chemical defects of the plasma as well as the xanthomatoses may be favorably influenced by specific measures. This has been particularly dramatic with the use of insulin in diabetic xanthomatosis, and with the administration of thyroid substance in the rare cases in which xanthomas develop in the course of myxedema.

The possibility of modifying conditions in essential familial hyperlipemia offers more encouragement. In this condition it appears that neutral fat accumulates in the blood partly because of a delay in the removal or metabolism of ingested fat. Spacing of fat ingestion with restriction for intervals of 24 hours or more has in some cases produced material reduction in the concentrations of neutral fat in the plasma. The administration of insulin is successful in controlling the hyperlipemia of diabetes but is ineffective in idiopathic familial hyperlipemia.

DAVID P. BARR

References

Movitt, E. R., Gerstl, B., Sherwood, F., and Epstein, C. C.: Essential Hyperlipemia. Arch. Int. Med., 87:79, 1951.

Schaefer, L. E., Drachman, S. R., Steinberg, A. G., and Adlersberg, D.: Genetic Studies on Hypercholesterolemia: Frequency in a Hospital Population and in Families of Hypercholesterolemia Index Patients. Am. Heart J., 46:99, 1953.

Thannhauser, S. J.: Lipidoses: Diseases of the Cellular Lipid. Metabolism. New York, Oxford University Press, 1950.

Wilkerson, C. F., Hand, E. A., and Fliegelman, M. T.: Essential Familial Hypercholesterolemia. Ann. Int. Med., 29:671, 1948.

ACIDOSIS

Definition. Acidosis is an abnormal condition caused by the accumulation in the body of excess acid or by the loss from the body of alkali. The more common cause is the accumulation of acid, that is, a state in which acids are formed or absorbed more rapidly than they can be destroyed or eliminated. This process may be considered to have produced a state of acidosis when it has caused either the bicarbonate of the blood to fall or the hydrogen ion concentration to rise above the normal limits.

Etiology. Acidosis is a symptom complex, not a disease in itself. Acidosis of clinical importance is observed chiefly in diabetes, renal disease, certain diarrheas and cyclic vomiting

leads to severe dehydrat
nephritis and diabetes, poly
excessive loss of water t
ventilation all contribute
The fluids of the body b
that blood volume may fa
at which the circulation ca

The larger part of the l
This comes almost entire
cellular fluids, which a
amounts of water, so that
of sodium in plasma and
may be reduced, normal, c
elevated. It is possible tha
of the normal small intra
of sodium leave the cells
contribute to the overall s

Considerable amounts
major intracellular base,
acidosis. The effect on pl
depend to a large exten
potassium, the severity o
the functional status of
in advanced renal disea
polyuria treated with pa
ing in potassium, the con
sium may be subnormal i
in cells. This is true als
tubular dysfunction, in
of potassium as well as s
be impaired. In most in
however, accompanied as
the discharge of potassiu
in elevated plasma potas
cially pronounced if exce
down and glycogen depl
lease of potassium from c
collapse is present. Du
large amounts of fluid ar
plasma potassium falls sl
continued urinary loss, d
of extracellular fluid v
into cells during resump
utilization. In infantile
acidosis, for example, s
quently falls below 2 mi
ing intensive treatment
cose, water and salts of
Muscular paralysis, card
even death have been
in plasma potassium. Ac
romuscular excitability.
dence that it impairs
hydrate. Chronic acidosi
decalcification of bones,
tures. It presumably affe
tions to varying degrees

in children. The etiology of diabetic acidosis is discussed in the chapter on Diabetes Mellitus.

Acidosis of varying degrees may complicate any diffuse renal disease when renal function deteriorates. It occurs commonly in advanced chronic glomerular nephritis, pyelonephritis and arteriolar nephrosclerosis, with nitrogen retention, less commonly in acute nephritis. Primary disorders of the renal tubules may produce acidosis without nitrogen retention, with variable disturbances of tubular function other than acidification.

Marked loss of alkaline intestinal fluids from biliary or pancreatic fistulas or in profuse diarrheas, especially Asiatic cholera and some childhood diarrheas, may produce acidosis. It also occurs in the peculiar cyclic vomiting of children. Severe acidosis may complicate implantation of the ureters into the sigmoid colon.

Acidosis may occur in pulmonary emphysema, bronchitis or extensive fibrosis, from impaired pulmonary exchange of gases. It does not play a considerable part in the symptomatology of these diseases.

Physiology and Chemistry. The body fluids are mildly alkaline and, even in the most extreme acidosis compatible with life, they remain on the alkaline side of neutrality; i.e., in acidosis the body becomes more weakly alkaline than normal. Reaction (degree of acidity or alkalinity) of fluids is customarily noted in terms of pH which is the negative logarithm of the H ion concentration. The H ion concentration of blood is something less than one ten-millionth normal. It may be described as having a hydrogen ion concentration of $10^{-7.4}$, or more conveniently as having a pH of 7.4. In adopting this logarithmic form of expression, however, it must be realized that a fall in pH from 7.4 to 7.2 represents a doubling of H ion concentration. The extremes of pH encountered in disease are something of the order of 7.0 and 7.7.

Normal body function depends on maintenance of the reaction of body fluids within relatively narrow limits, between pH 7.35 and 7.45. This regulation is dependent on the buffer properties of blood, regulation of carbon dioxide excretion by the lungs, and renal function.

Buffer Effect. Substances which, by their presence in solution, decrease the pH change caused by the addition of acid and alkali are called buffers. They are mixtures of a weak acid and its alkali salt or of a weak base and

its acid salt. The buffers of physiologic importance are mixtures of weak acids and their alkali salts. Those of significance are carbonic acid and $BHCO_3$*, B_2HPO_4 and BH_2PO_4, proteins (including hemoglobin and tissue protein) with base proteinate, and organic phosphates with their basic salts. Together, these comprise approximately one third of the alkali normally present in plasma, and probably a greater fraction of the alkali of the cells of the body.

Respiratory Regulation. In any mixture of a weak acid and its salt the pH of the solution is determined by (and in turn determines) the ratio of free acid to salt in the mixture. The reaction of blood, therefore, depends on the ratio of free carbonic acid to bicarbonate, $\dfrac{H_2CO_3}{BHCO_3}$, which at normal pH of 7.35 is about 1:20. The concentration of carbonic acid in this equation is directly related to the carbon dioxide tension in the blood. Since carbon dioxide, which is constantly formed in abundance in cellular oxidations, is excreted through the lungs, the carbon dioxide tension may be altered rapidly by change in respiration. Other factors being constant, the carbon dioxide tension of the blood decreases with deep respiration and increases with shallow respiration. The carbonic acid-bicarbonate buffer is thus much more effective *in vivo* than *in vitro*, since in the latter the addition of strong acid causes a comparable increase in carbonic acid, while in the former carbonic acid becomes decreased below its original level through increased pulmonary ventilation.

Renal Regulation. The metabolism of the ordinary diet yields phosphoric and sulfuric acid in excess of the available base of the diet. If this excess acid (equivalent to 400 to 800 cc. or more of tenth normal acid) were excreted as neutral sodium salts, the body would rapidly be depleted of base. There are two renal mechanisms for the excretion of acid without equivalent base. First, the renal tubules synthesize ammonia from plasma glutamine by the action of renal glutaminase and from amino acids by the action of renal amino acid oxidase. Second, the renal tubules convert the slightly alkaline glomerular filtrate into acid urine, which permits the excretion of weak acids, such as uric, citric and betahydroxybutyric in the free form. The cells of the distal tubules derive the hydrogen ions for

* B = base (sodium or potassium).

this purpose from (
can form rapidly fr
action of carbonic
urine which the k
pH of 4.8, at whi
amounts of strong
hydrochloric can e
base can be sparec
acids only by subst

Pathologic Phys
abnormally high
acidosis is almost
crease in the der
acid-bicarbonate r
carbonate is, howe
It is always cause
the body of an ex
bonic, or by the l
more commonly th

In the acidosis
bicarbonate is rec
tion of abnormal
sulfuric acids, be
number and effic
concentration of
vated for the sam
effect of poor fo
ketone production
ing upon bicarbc
sodium of plasn
mechanisms for
creting acids. Th
ney to acidify the
is much impaire
these mechanism
nephritis is a sm
these mechanism
parable degree. I
mal glomerular f
tubular function
ing acidosis. T
urine, together v
cretion of calciu
osteoporosis an
renal tubular f
of ammonia ar
phosphorus, pot
also be defective

Starvation ac
tance since it j
complicating fa
unavailability of
can be produce
of carbohydrate
tion. The redu
displacement b
acids. The incr

---

normal loss of alkaline intestinal secretions or with ureterosigmoid anastomoses depends on suspicion of the possibility. In renal disease, severe acidosis is manifest by hyperventilation, but moderate acidosis of long duration may be asymptomatic. Awareness of this possibility in patients with dwarfism or with unexplained decalcification of the bones may lead to the primary diagnosis of chronic renal disease, especially the type with renal tubular dysfunction, in which the urine may be free of albumin.

Prognosis. Death probably never results from acidosis *per se.* The prognosis depends first upon that of the underlying or complicating disease and, second, upon the state of the circulation. The outlook of the patient with the acidosis of advanced renal insufficiency is understandably poor. Recognition of asymptomatic acidosis in renal disease may improve prognosis in respect to decalcification of bones and may initiate therapy to accelerate growth if retarded. The outcome of acute diarrhea or cyclic vomiting is dependent less on the degree of acidosis than on the extent to which the circulation has been compromised by loss of water and salt and on the degree to which depletion of potassium has progressed. Sudden deaths during apparently successful therapy of infantile diarrhea have been ascribed to the development of subnormal levels of potassium in the plasma. Prognosis is improved by the prompt use of blood or plasma in combating circulatory collapse and by supplying potassium at the proper time. A rapidly fatal outcome in the acidosis complicating ureterosigmoidostomy is readily averted by simple measures.

Treatment. In acidosis due to excessive loss of alkaline intestinal secretions in diarrheal stools or from fistulas or surgical drainage, correction of the acidosis is usually less urgent than that of dehydration, circulatory collapse, starvation and potassium deficit. Physiologic saline solution is of prime importance to replace losses of water and electrolytes by parenteral routes. Approximately 80 cc. per kilogram of body weight is necessary to correct severe dehydration. Half of this should be given within the first hour or two if possible, and the remainder in the course of the next few hours. Sufficient glucose (or fructose or invert sugar) must be supplied to reduce protein breakdown and excessive ketone formation. For this purpose at least 2 gm. per kilogram of body weight should be

---

given daily, and it is probably advisable to give twice this much. This may be given as 5 or 10 per cent solution intravenously until oral feeding becomes possible. The glucose should be given in distilled water unless the plasma sodium is subnormal, in which case it may be given in physiologic saline solution.

Alkali may be used to speed relief of hyperpnea in the acidosis associated with diarrhea, especially in infants, in whom the renal regulatory mechanism is incompletely developed. Alkali may be given as bicarbonate (4 per cent intravenously) or lactate (one sixth molar subcutaneously or intravenously). Sodium lactate (molar or one sixth molar) and sodium bicarbonate (7.5 per cent) are available commercially in ampules. In the body the lactate is converted to glycogen, leaving the base available for neutralization of acid. Patients with acidosis severe enough to provoke recognizable hyperpnea may be given 7 cc. of 4 per cent bicarbonate (or 25 cc. of one sixth molar lactate) per kilogram of body weight with impunity. It is rarely necessary to give more to relieve the hyperpnea, and it matters little if plasma bicarbonate is not restored to normal levels immediately. Various preparations containing sodium, potassium, bicarbonate (or lactate), and chloride in proportion to those found in normal intestinal fluids are available commercially. These may be substituted freely, if desired, for physiologic saline in replacing current losses of intestinal fluids.

The intravenous drip has largely supplanted the subcutaneous route of administration. This is unfortunate, in the author's opinion. It has been demonstrated that the administration of fluids intravenously results, in the shocked subject, in a loss of plasma protein to the tissue, which may serve to deepen the shock. On the other hand, massive infusions of physiologic saline solution may be given subcutaneously with impunity. If the circulation is adequate, this is absorbed with extreme rapidity by the severely dehydrated patient, as much as 3 liters being commonly absorbed within 2 hours. Failure of the severely dehydrated patient to absorb subcutaneous fluid rapidly denotes circulatory collapse, and is an indication for prompt blood transfusion or administration of plasma. Glucose solutions should not be given subcutaneously, since they cause a temporary net loss of available salt to the tissue because salt diffuses into them more rapidly than glucose diffuses out. All these considerations, unimportant as they may seem in most cases, may be important in individual cases in tipping the balance into circulatory collapse, which is a prime threat to life. In the author's clinic, tranfusion of 500 cc. of blood is given as soon as possible if any evidence of shock is present.

The parenteral administration of potassium serves to minimize the risk of serious depression of plasma potassium during treatment with parenteral fluids and glucose and also speeds the restoration of normal cellular potassium. The potassium should not be given at the start of treatment, when plasma potassium is commonly normal or elevated, lest plasma potassium rise to the point at which fatal heart block ensues (approximately 10 mm. per liter). Ideally, it should be given only after a sharp depression of plasma potassium has been demonstrated by analysis. In the absence of facilities for such analyses, evidence of subnormal potassium levels may be detected by electrocardiographic changes. These are, in order of their appearance, prolonged Q-T interval, low T waves, sagging S-T segments, and depressed S-T take-off, the last occurring at levels of 1.5 mm. or less. In any event, potassium should not be given until sufficient saline and, if necessary, blood or plasma is given to insure adequate circulatory status and urine flow. If neither chemical determinations nor electrocardiograms are available, it is probably safe to give potassium 6 to 8 hours after the start of therapy, unless shock or anuria is present. For general use it is probably safest to use considerably less than the maximal amount of potassium tolerated. It is suggested that 0.1 to 0.15 gm. per kilogram of potassium chloride or 0.15 to 0.22 gm. per kilogram of buffered potassium phosphate (5.1 parts of dibasic potassium phosphate to 1 part of potassium dihydrogen phosphate) be given, and be repeated daily until feeding by mouth has been resumed. The salts may be kept in sterile packets to be added to solutions of glucose or physiologic saline and given intravenously over a period of not less than 4 hours. The buffered phosphate has the theoretical advantage of counteracting the deficit of phosphorus which accompanies that of potassium, although there is no evidence as yet that the deficit of phosphorus is of clinical significance. When feeding is resumed, there is no clear indication for supplementary potassium, since most foods contain it in abundance, although, in the opinion of some, complete recovery is speeded by the addition of potassium salts to the diet. If feeding can be resumed within 6 to 8 hours of the start of treatment, it is probably desirable to dispense with the parenteral administration of potassium, since both fruit juices and milk as well as most other foods contain considerable potassium, and supplementary potassium chloride can be given by mouth if desired. The risk, however slight, of producing fatal elevation of plasma potassium by parenteral administration is thus avoided.

Renal Acidosis. Acidotic hyperpnea should be allayed if possible by administration of alkali. This may be tolerated by mouth, but more often must be given intravenously (as 4 per cent bicarbonate or one sixth molar lactate). It is neither necessary nor desirable to restore the plasma bicarbonate to normal. Attempts to do so may precipitate tetany or edema. In the hyperpneic patient 7 cc. of 4 per cent bicarbonate or 25 cc. of one sixth molar lactate per kilogram of body weight may be given slowly. This must be repeated if hyperpnea persists or recurs. Smaller doses seldom give any relief. If tetany supervenes, administration of alkali must be slowed or stopped; if severe, especially with laryngospasm, 1 gm. of calcium chloride should be injected slowly intravenously (as 10 per cent solution), and repeated if necessary. Asymptomatic reduction of serum bicarbonate may be treated by daily doses of sodium bicarbonate or citrate sufficient to correct the deficit partially (2 to 6 gm. daily in divided doses). If heart failure makes the use of sodium salts undesirable, the potassium salts may be substituted, provided, of course, serum potassium is not considerably elevated.

The use of alkali is imperative in those cases of primary renal tubular disease in which prolonged, though often asymptomatic, acidosis contributes to the production of osteoporosis. These patients should also receive supplements of calcium lactate (2 to 4 gm. daily) and vitamin D (50,000 units daily). Some patients with renal tubular defect waste potassium sufficiently to cause muscular weakness and electrocardiographic abnormalities. Large supplements of potassium may prove necessary to compensate for this deficiency.

The acidosis of ureterosigmoidostomy is corrected by salt restriction, supplements of sodium bicarbonate or citrate, and care to evacuate the rectum frequently.

The treatment of diabetic acidosis is presented in the chapter on Diabetes Mellitus.

P. H. LAVIETES

References

Darrow, D. C., and Pratt, E. L.: Fluid Therapy. Relation to Tissue Composition and Expenditure of Water and Electrolyte. J.A.M.A., *143*:365, 432, 1950.

Gilman, A., and Brazeau, P.: The Role of the Kidney in the Regulation of Acid-base Equilibrium. Am. J. Med., *15*:765, 1953.

Mackler, B., Lichtenstein, H., and Guest, G. M.: Effects of Ammonium Chloride Acidosis on Glucose Tolerance in Dogs. Am. J. Physiol., *168*:126, 1952.

Pines, K. L., and Mudge, G. H.: Renal Tubular Acidosis with Osteomalacia. Am. J. Med., *11*:302, 1951.

Singer, R. B., and Hastings, A. B.: An Improved Clinical Method for the Estimation of Disturbances of the Acid-Base Balance of Human Blood. Medicine, 27:223, 1948.

Wilder, C. E., and Cotton, R. T.: Reabsorptive Hyperchloremic Acidosis Following Ureterosigmoidostomy. Report of a Severe Case Showing Disturbed Carbohydrate Metabolism. Am. J. Med., *15*:423, 1953.

ALKALOSIS

Definition. Alkalosis is an abnormal condition caused by the accumulation in the body of an excess of alkali or by the loss of acid, more commonly the latter. The bicarbonate of the blood is increased (with one exception which is described later) and its hydrogen ion concentration is usually diminished.

Etiology. Alkalosis may be produced by administration of alkali for gastric hyperacidity, especially if renal function is impaired either by primary renal disease or by dehydration. Loss of acid in excess of base in the vomiting of pyloric stenosis is the most common cause of alkalosis. Suction drainage of the stomach may likewise result in great loss of predominantly acid secretions. Severe alkalosis has been reported in infants who lose large amounts of acid in diarrheal stools. Alkalosis may result from loss of carbonic acid through hyperventilation in response to functional or organic disease of the central nervous system, or to anoxemia. In Cushing's syndrome, persistent mild alkalosis has been reported, associated with sub-normal plasma potassium. The administration of ACTH or cortisone may reproduce this. Depletion of potassium may also cause alkalosis. This may be clinically important in patients with large losses of intestinal secretions or in patients maintained for long periods by parenteral fluids lacking in potassium.

Pathologic Physiology and Chemistry. Alkalosis due to excessive loss of acid in intestinal secretions is always accompanied by severe dehydration. Base greatly in excess of acid is excreted in the urine as bicarbonate but subsequently acid urine may be excreted despite severe alkalosis. In alkali-excess alkalosis, change in pH is opposed by increase in carbon dioxide tension of the body fluids through diminished pulmonary ventilation. Conversely, the alkalosis of primary overventilation is tempered by decrease in the bicarbonate of the body fluids by selective retention of chloride. Renal tubular reabsorption of bicarbonate has been shown to be regulated by the carbon dioxide tension of the body fluids. This contributes to the paradoxical production of acid urine in gastric alkalosis, since the compensatory rise in carbon dioxide tension in turn increases tubular reabsorption of bicarbonate. Potassium deficiency and decreased glomerular filtration may also impair the ability to produce alkaline urine under these circumstances.

The most striking manifestations of alkalosis are those of neuromuscular hyperexcitability. These are indistinguishable from those of hypocalcemia, though there is no clear evidence that they exert their effect indirectly through calcium. That the influences of alkalosis and hypocalcemia are additive, however, is demonstrated by amelioration of hypocalcemic tetany by administration of acid or acidifying salts, and by the precipitation of tetany in hypercalcemic terminal nephritics by alkali administration.

In alkalosis the cells contain subnormal amounts of potassium and excessive amounts of sodium. This disturbance of composition is not necessarily associated with abnormal concentrations of sodium and potassium in the serum, and no symptoms can be directly attributed to it. The same factors which tend to depress plasma potassium during the treatment of acidosis also operate during the treatment of alkalosis. In addition, there is the substitution of sodium for potassium in the cells, requiring potassium for its correction.

Symptoms. The symptoms of alkalosis are those of the underlying disease plus those of tetany. Tetany is discussed in detail elsewhere in this volume. In alkali-excess alkalosis, respirations are shallow; in the alkalosis of primary hyperventilation they are abnormally deep.

Diagnosis. If the possibility of alkalosis is entertained in patients with vomiting and tetany, diagnosis presents no difficulty. The plasma bicarbonate is markedly elevated (to as high as 140 volumes per cent) and plasma chloride proportionately reduced. Serum calcium is within normal limits. In patients receiving alkali for gastric acidity, alkalosis should be suspected when vomiting increases or evidence of renal insufficiency develops, even in the absence of tetany, and confirmation should be sought by determination of plasma bicarbonate. Tetany in the presence of hyperventilation should suggest alkalosis. If this is of brief duration as in sighing or hysterical breathing, plasma bicarbonate and serum calcium are both within normal limits. In more prolonged hyperventilation, as in disease of the central nervous system, plasma calcium is again normal, but bicarbonate may be subnormal. Thus we have the paradoxical situation in which hyperventilation and reduction of plasma bicarbonate accompany alkalosis, and not acidosis. Determination of pH will, of course, make the differentiation, but this is usually not necessary if the possibility of alkalosis is entertained in such cases, and the usual causes of acidosis are excluded.

Prognosis. The prognosis is that of the disease which it complicates. Severe tetanic spasms of the larynx or skeletal musculature may contribute to a fatal outcome.

Treatment. The alkalosis which results from loss of acid secretions requires treatment no more urgently than does the accompanying dehydration and starvation. Carbohydrate must be supplied to reduce ketosis and protein wastage and precautions taken against circulatory collapse as described for acidosis. Approximately 80 cc. of fluid per kilogram of body weight is required to correct severe dehydration. In most instances physiologic saline suffices, chloride being selectively retained by the kidneys. If tetany is severe, it may be desirable to give some ammonium chloride initially. Two hundred to 500 cc. of 2 per cent solution may be given slowly intravenously, physiologic saline being given more rapidly at the same time. Instead of the ammonium chloride solution, one or two liters of a solution of potassium, sodium,

ammonium and chloride in concentrations devised to replace gastric losses may be used. After correction of the initial defect, such solutions may be used to replace continued losses of gastric secretions. Potassium is usually required in large amounts, not only to prevent the consequences of hypokalemia (as described under acidosis) but also to correct fully the large cellular deficit which is commonly present. Retention of more than 500 mEq. (38 gm. of potassium chloride) may be necessary before serum potassium rises into the normal range. When urine flow is good, there is no risk in giving large amounts of potassium parenterally or orally. It is of course desirable to control treatment by analysis of the serum for potassium and to follow electrocardiograms as described for the treatment of acidosis. Initial hypokalemia as well as marked cellular depletion of potassium is often marked in alkalosis complicating drainage of acid intestinal secretions, and the alkalosis can not be fully corrected until the potassium is restored.

In hyperventilation tetany, treatment of the underlying disease is the prime indication. Breathing mixtures of 5 per cent carbon dioxide in oxygen will afford relief of the tetany of primary hyperventilation, though this is hardly necessary in the hysterical group.

P. H. LAVIETES

References

Cooke, R. E., and Crowley, L. G.: Replacement of Gastric and Intestinal Fluid Losses in Surgery. A Preliminary Report. New England J. Med., 246: 637, 1952.

———, Seegar, W. E., Cheek, D. B., Coville, F. E., and Darrow, D. C.: The Extrarenal Correction of Alkalosis Associated with Potassium Deficiency. J. Clin. Investigation, 31:798, 1952.

Elkington, J. R., Squires, R. D., and Crosley, A. P., Jr.: Intracellular Cation Exchanges in Metabolic Alkalosis. J. Clin. Investigation, 30:369, 1951.

Kennedy, T. J., Jr., Winkley, J. H., and Dunning, M. F.: Gastric Alkalosis with Hypokalemia. Am. J. Med., 6:790, 1949.

DEHYDRATION AND FLUID BALANCE: PHYSIOLOGICAL PRINCIPLES

The term dehydration, as used in clinical medicine, refers to a condition in which the volume of body fluids, and particularly the volume of extracellular fluid, is diminished. Because of the multiplicity of derangements which may contribute to dehydration, and the varying severity and chemical nature of the disturbance, each patient constitutes an individual problem in evaluation and therapy. Therefore it is important that the *principles* involved in fluid and electrolyte balance be clearly understood.

The volume and the total concentration of dissolved substances in body fluid are the dimensions particularly pertinent to this consideration of fluid and electrolyte balance. The maintenance of composition with respect to specific electrolytes and the regulation of acid-base equilibrium, while of vital importance, and not infrequently disturbed in association with dehydration, is beyond the scope of the present discussion.

Normal Anatomy. Water constitutes some 55 to 60 per cent of the weight of an average normal individual, but varies in amount inversely with the body's fat content. The plasma and the interstitial fluid of tissues, which together constitute the extracellular fluid, comprise slightly more than one third of the body water; the remainder is within cells. The cell membranes may be regarded as freely permeable to water, but do not allow the *free* passage of strong electrolytes.

Water moves into and out of cells in response to changes in osmotic activity across the cell membranes. Water added to the extracellular compartment is rapidly distributed in the total body water. Conversely, if solute to which cell membranes are impermeable is added to the extracellular fluid, water is withdrawn from cells. In each case the total concentration is ultimately uniform throughout body water.

Extracellular fluid throughout the body is a phase of fairly uniform composition in which sodium ions and their complement of anions, chiefly chloride and bicarbonate, constitute all but a small fraction of the solute. Intracellular fluid varies somewhat from tissue to tissue, but, in general, contains little sodium and chloride. The major cation, potassium, is balanced probably largely by organic phosphates and the anionic groups of proteins. The disparity in electrolyte distribution across cell membranes is maintained by the metabolic activity of the cells.

Measurement of the Volume of Body Fluid and Its Compartments. Numerous procedures for the estimation of the volume of body water, extracellular fluid and plasma have been devised. For the most part these are clearly designed for investigative purposes and have little utility in the study and treatment of the individual patient. However, since certain generalizations concerning the behavior of body fluid compartments have been derived from studies using these techniques, it is well to be informed concerning their nature and limitations and hence the reservations necessary in their interpretation.

The estimation of *total body water* is usually based on the dilution principle. Satisfactory approximations can be made by determining the volume in which heavy water or antipyrine is distributed. Sufficient time must be allowed for complete distribution of the substance in body water and, in the case of antipyrine, to obtain an estimate of the rate of metabolic breakdown of the drug.

The volume of *extracellular fluid* has been estimated as the apparent volume of distribution of a number of substances, among them: thiocyanate, chloride, bromide, thiosulfate, sulfate (labeled with S^{35}), inulin, mannitol and sucrose. None of these substances can be considered to yield quantitatively reliable values for various reasons, including: failure to remain in an exclusively extracellular position, rapid excretion so that prolonged intravenous infusion under completely stable conditions is necessary during their equilibration in extracellular fluid, and failure to become evenly distributed in extracellular fluid within a time which can reasonably be devoted to the procedure. Since *intracellular fluid* is evaluated as the difference between total and extracellular volumes, the estimate is subject to summation and magnification of the errors of the two individual determinations.

The evaluation of *plasma volume* by dilution methods is subject to variable errors due to losses of dye (or tagged albumin) from the circulating blood, while estimates based on the use of tagged red cells require assumptions concerning the proportion of red cells to plasma in the body as a whole, a ratio not necessarily given by the hematocrit determined in peripheral blood.

Normal Fluid and Electrolyte Balance and Its Regulation. The body normally gains fluid and electrolytes from the exterior only through the gastrointestinal tract. Water is derived from the intake of liquids and from the food, both as preformed water and that obtained upon oxidation of the foodstuffs. Those electrolytes which are of major concern in fluid balance—sodium, potassium and chloride ions—are present as such in the food.

Fluid, electrolyte or both are lost to the environment through the lungs and skin, and in the feces and urine. Air is inhaled at the ambient temperature and humidity and exhaled saturated with water vapor at body temperature. Losses of water through the lungs are therefore increased by increased pulmonary ventilation and when the water content of the inspired air is low. No electrolyte is lost by this route.

Output of water through the skin, in the form of evaporation or as visible sweat, may vary in amount over a wide range. The salt content of sweat is appreciably lower than that of extracellular fluid and is subject to some physiologic regulation, being reduced when there is a stimulus for retention of salt in the body. In the absence of visible sweating, electrolyte loss through the skin is negligible.

Although up to 10 liters of isotonic fluid are secreted into the gastrointestinal tract each day, practically all of this water and electrolyte, in addition to that ingested, is normally reabsorbed into the body. The feces normally contain only a minimum of water, sodium, potassium and chloride.

Since losses through lung and skin are dependent on environment and the functions of respiration and temperature regulation respectively, and excretion in the stools is normally negligible, only the kidney can modify the output of salt and water in a manner directly subservient to the regulation of the volume and concentration of body fluids. In general, the concentration of body fluids is regulated by the retention or excretion of water, whereas volume is regulated by the retention or excretion of salt.

Regulation of body fluid concentration is initiated in the hypothalamus, where receptors responsive to changes in the effective osmotic pressure of body fluid regulate the release of antidiuretic hormone from the neurohypophysis. Secretion is increased when osmotic pressure is high, diminished when osmotic pressure is low. Antidiuretic hormone, in turn, causes the renal tubules to reabsorb water and excrete a concentrated urine. The water thus conserved dilutes the body fluid, reducing osmotic pressure. Since sodium salts contribute some 85 per cent of the total solute of extracellular fluid, the plasma sodium concentration is an excellent indicator of the effective osmotic pressure of the body fluids, except when a high concentration of some other solute to which cells are relatively impermeable (e.g., glucose) is present. Urea does not contribute to *effective* osmotic pressure since it permeates cells easily.

Regulation of the volume of extracellular fluid is accomplished by modification of the excretion of sodium and the anion which accompanies it. The chain of events in this homeostatic process is not clearly understood. Several contributory factors are recognized, including changes in the rate of glomerular filtration and variation in the secretion of adrenal steroids which regulate sodium reabsorption by the renal tubules. Other factors are probably also involved. Normally, losses or gains of sodium are not accompanied by appreciable changes in the sodium concentration of extracellular fluid, since operation of the hypothalamic regulators of water loss accurately maintains the total effective osmotic activity, and hence the plasma sodium concentration, at normal levels. Changes in sodium balance are, therefore, manifested largely as changes in extracellular fluid volume and, short of actual measurements of balance, are detected as changes in weight and by the clinical signs of changes in extracellular fluid volume.

Regulation of the volume of intracellular fluid is poorly understood. Most variations are probably associated with (1) changes in the organic components of cells and (2) dilution and concentration of cell solutes as a result of accession of water to or loss of water from the body.

Exchanges of Fluid and Electrolyte Between Intra- and Extracellular Spaces. In recent years, data have been presented which have been interpreted to indicate that, under the influence of certain stresses or the administration of adrenocortical hormones, there may be transfers of fluid and electrolyte from the intracellular space into the extracellular fluid which are not dependent upon exchanges with the exterior or changes in the osmotic pressure of body fluids. For the most part, these conclusions are based on the estimation of body fluid compartments and therefore subject to reservations on the basis of methodology. It is undoubtedly true that sodium can replace an appreciable fraction of the intracellular potassium when the body has been depleted of the latter, and that the sodium is extruded when potassium is again available. It is also probable that bone can serve as a source of cation in the presence of acidosis of the extracellular fluid (and, therefore, can presumably accept additional cation in alkalosis). Except for these considerations it is best to regard exchanges of fluid and electrolyte between compartments of the body water as determined by the organic constituents within cells, the movement of water in response to changes in total solute in one compartment or the other, and the capacity of cells to maintain, with the potassium available, the normal gradients of sodium and potassium across cell membranes.

Pathologic Physiology. The level of intake required to maintain fluid and electrolyte balance varies widely. The *minimum* intake of water under normal conditions is that required to replace losses through lung and skin and to put out, in a urine of maximum concentration, those solutes which must be excreted. In individuals with free access to water, the thirst mechanism is adequate to insure sufficient intake for maintenance of the normal concentration of body fluids. In the absence of abnormal output, small amounts of sodium and potassium are adequate to maintain balance and are obtained from any but the most restricted of dietary intakes. The presence of abnormal losses may, of course, greatly increase intake requirements.

Loss. Increases in output by any of the normal routes as well as from the development of abnormal routes may lead to deficits of fluid and electrolyte. While generally of minor importance relative to the other disturbances it accompanies, the loss of water by *evaporation* in hyperventilation is a factor which should not be neglected. The considerable losses of both water and salt which occur with profuse sweating are frequently of clinical consequence, while leakage of extracellular fluid through areas denuded of skin, as by burns, may lead to grave disturbances of fluid balance.

The *gastrointestinal tract* is a potential source of difficulty in the maintenance of fluid balance, since it is the route of normal replacement and since a large fraction of the body's extracellular fluid is secreted into and reabsorbed from it each day. Large losses of such fluid may occur with either diarrhea or vomiting, the latter being complicated in that it may cut off intake. The development

of fistulous connections between the gastrointestinal tract, liver or pancreas and the exterior commonly leads to very large deficits of fluid and electrolyte if adequate replacement is not undertaken.

Regulation is ultimately dependent upon *renal function* and since this function, with respect to fluid and electrolytes, represents the integration of a number of processes, each with its intrinsic mechanism and extrarenal regulator, it is subject to a number of disturbances, each of which may arise from either local or nonrenal causes. The initial process in urine formation, *glomerular filtration,* is dependent upon the anatomic and functional integrity of the glomeruli and upon the blood pressure. The energy is thus contributed by the heart. The restriction of glomerular filtration in the face of a falling cardiac output in dehydration and shock is often quite out of proportion to the fall in blood pressure, since compensatory vasoconstriction is often far more marked in the kidney than in the body as a whole. Although such reductions of glomerular filtration tend to minimize fluid output when fluid is badly needed, they seriously impair the capacity to maintain the composition of body fluids, and when renal vasoconstriction has been severe and prolonged, function may not be restored when shock has been alleviated.

Abnormalities of water excretion leading to dehydration with increased osmotic pressure or overhydration with decreased total solute concentration result from failure of the renal tubules to reabsorb water to form a hypertonic urine or to reject water in a dilute urine. The capacity to form a concentrated urine is vulnerable to many insults and is often the first function to be impaired in such disorders as nephritis and hypertensive disease, and one of the last to be restored following acute renal damage produced by shock or nephrotoxic agents. The defect is apparently in the intrinsic capacity of the tubules to transport water. Far less commonly, failure to form a concentrated urine is the result of a lesion in the hypothalamic-hypophysial system leading to diabetes insipidus. Whatever its cause, *incapacity of the kidney to form a concentrated urine* is a common source of fluid imbalance, since any interruption of intake, such as may be produced by vomiting, is likely to lead to rapidly developing dehydration with further impairment of renal function.

Although inability to form a concentrated

urine is usually due to organic renal disease, *failure to excrete a dilute urine* when body fluids are diluted is preponderantly attributable to functional, nonrenal disturbances. The intrinsic capacity to form a dilute urine is often maintained after organic renal disease has led to severe limitation of concentration. However, increased secretion of antidiuretic hormone which prevents the formation of a dilute urine may be produced by stimuli other than the normal one of a rise in the osmotic pressure of body fluids. Among such stimuli are a number of drugs (e.g., nicotine, morphine, barbiturates), emotional disturbances and operative trauma. Failure to excrete water normally is also observed in many patients with cardiac failure, or cirrhosis, and in adrenal insufficiency or severe salt depletion. Any of these disorders may be accompanied by dilution of the body fluids whether total volume is high, low or normal.

Impairment of the ability of the renal tubules to reabsorb sodium is occasionally a very striking feature of renal disease (so-called salt-losing nephritis) but it is best to consider some *limitation of the capacity to limit loss of sodium,* when intake is severely restricted, as an almost constant concomitant of advanced disease of the kidney. Less commonly, the tubules fail to reabsorb sodium because of failure of normal hormonal regulation (adrenal insufficiency). The loss of sodium leads to contraction of extracellular fluid volume and usually, but not necessarily, a fall in the sodium (total solute) concentration of extracellular fluid.

Abnormal losses of sodium with depletion of extracellular volume may also occur, even though the sodium transport mechanism and its regulation be fundamentally normal, when there is *massive excretion of solute* (e.g., glucose in uncontrolled diabetes) which, by osmotic effect, carries out increased amounts of electrolyte. This effect is greatly increased when the solute excreted is anion, for instance the keto acid of diabetic acidosis or the chloride from ingested ammonium chloride, since this must be balanced by the equivalent amount of cation. The tendency of such excretory loads to produce rapid sodium depletion is greatly magnified in the presence of renal damage with limited ability to reabsorb sodium and to form ammonia with which to replace it in the urine.

Clinical Manifestations. The clinical manifestations of loss of fluid and electrolyte are more or less independent of the nature of the defect which produces them, and, in general, are those of diminished extracellular fluid and circulating blood volume—weakness, anorexia, nausea and vomiting, circulatory insufficiency with failing renal function, and ultimately shock and coma. When loss of water predominates over that of solute and osmotic pressure rises, thirst is particularly prominent, although, to a lesser extent, a fall in volume alone may produce an increased desire for water.

Diagnosis. An exploration of the patient's *history* as to intake and output of fluid has much to contribute to the diagnosis of disorders of fluid balance and to the selection of appropriate therapy. Such an evaluation should include consideration of both the volume and the probable electrolyte content of fluids gained or lost by all of the normal and abnormal routes. Often, the presumptive diagnosis of dehydration can be made and proper therapeutic measures undertaken from such consideration alone.

On *physical examination,* the findings are largely those of diminished extracellular fluid volume: weakness and lassitude, thirst and dryness of the mouth (these particularly marked when body fluid concentration is increased), loss of skin elasticity, a sunken appearance of the eyeballs, weakness of the pulse and hypotension. In severe grades of volume loss, the signs of circulatory failure may advance to frank shock which may be accompanied by stupor or coma and severe oliguria or anuria.

Laboratory Findings. Changes in the effective concentration of body fluids are best evaluated by measurement of the plasma sodium concentration. Consideration must be given, however, to the concentration of other substances, particularly glucose, that may constitute an appreciable fraction of that solute which does not easily penetrate cells. When a flame photometer is not available for estimation of sodium, and there is no reason to suspect the presence of increased amounts of anions other than chloride and bicarbonate in the blood (as in ketosis or advanced renal insufficiency), determination of the plasma chloride and carbon dioxide content may give a useful approximation of the plasma sodium. The latter is about 10 mEq./1 higher than the sum of chloride and bicarbonate when both are expressed in mEq./1.

There are no wholly satisfactory laboratory methods for estimating the volume of extracellular fluid. Since changes in blood volume are frequently responsible for the severe clinical manifestations of loss of extracellular volume, a rough approximation of changes in plasma volume such as can be obtained from the hematocrit and from the plasma protein concentration may be useful. Only when changes from the normal are large (and usually only when the values are increased) can any weight be given to these determinations in evaluating the initial status of the patient. Thereafter, short-term changes in plasma volume can be followed, but it should be kept in mind that a rise in plasma protein means a decrease in the fluid of plasma only if the total circulating plasma protein has not increased. Similar consideration is necessary with respect to the hematocrit and circulating red cell mass.

The level of urea or nonprotein nitrogen in the blood is useful in following the effects of dehydration on renal function. Considerable elevation of these levels may result from dehydration even if the kidneys are intrinsically normal. However, the level of urea in the blood is dependent upon the rate of protein catabolism as well as on the function of the kidneys.

Treatment. Unfortunately, dehydration of clinical significance is not infrequently permitted to develop in individuals under medical care because attention is devoted to the underlying problem and fluid and electrolyte balance neglected, or because an adequate volume of fluid is administered, but the electrolyte content is inadequate. The prevention of such disorders of fluid balance may require only nursing attention to keep up fluid intake or the addition of salt to ingested fluid or food when loss of sodium is high. When losses are too large to be compensated by oral intake, or when gastrointestinal disorders render oral administration impracticable, parenteral fluid therapy may be required. The regulatory capacity of the kidneys makes it easier to maintain normal fluid balance than to correct it when depletion has progressed to impairment of renal function.

When dehydration is an established problem, the primary objective should be the prompt relief of circulatory insufficiency, if this is part of the clinical picture. Simultaneously, restitution of a normal volume and concentration of the body fluids, along with correction of other complicating disturbances, such as acidosis or alkalosis, should be pressed as rapidly as is compatible with safety. The

possibility of relieving the disorder responsible for precipitating the dehydration should not be overlooked, although delay, until the more serious aspects of the dehydration have been controlled, may be necessary. Milder dehydration without impairment of the circulation can often be treated by increasing the intake of fluid (to, perhaps, 3 liters per day) and sodium chloride (to, possibly, 10 gm. per day) by mouth.

The management of fluid balance by the parenteral administration of fluids should be guided by consideration of the volume and composition of the deficits in each of the divisions of the body fluid. In the presence of reasonably normal renal function some reliance can be placed upon the kidneys' capacity to retain selectively those components needed while discarding others—provided that *all* of the necessary materials are supplied in sufficient quantities, that the circulation is adequate for effective operation of the kidney, and provided that there is not present some powerful stimulus to retain some specific body fluid component. Excesses of water or sodium, for example, are often retained, presumably because of overactivity respectively of the hypothalamic hypophysial system and adrenal cortex, in severely ill patients or those who have recently undergone surgery, despite the fact that such retention may distort volume and concentration of body fluids.

The aspect of dehydration most threatening to the well being or even the survival of the patient is the diminution in blood volume. Restitution is most rapidly accomplished by the administration of whole blood and this is the treatment of choice in *severe dehydration* in which shock is present or threatening. While preparation for transfusion is in progress, treatment should be initiated with the administration of 1 to 2 liters of isotonic sodium chloride solution. If whole blood is not available, plasma or human serum albumin (diluted with isotonic saline to contain 5 to 7 per cent protein) may be used as a substitute, and they are especially indicated when there has been extensive exudation. However, the danger of hepatitis from pooled human plasma is to be weighed against the expected benefits.

Milder abnormalities of volume, concentration and acid-base balance can be controlled entirely by the administration of isotonic saline solution, leaving to selective renal activity the correction of minor deviations in these dimensions. When the deviations are more severe, more direct measures may be desirable. When *losses of water in excess of solute* have resulted in marked increases in concentration, 5 per cent glucose solution will serve as a source of water, since the glucose is rapidly metabolized. In some patients a marked *decrease of body fluid concentration* may be encountered, most often because losses of isotonic fluid have been inappropriately replaced with water or 5 per cent glucose. In such instances, there may be a place for hypertonic (2 per cent or 3 per cent) sodium chloride solutions, since the hypertonic fluids are considerably more efficient in restoring concentration than is isotonic saline. However, a low osmotic pressure (plasma sodium concentration) is often found in association with *increased* extracellular volume in cardiac failure, cirrhosis and advanced renal failure, and the use of hypertonic saline solutions in these conditions is more detrimental than helpful.

In dehydration with severe *acidosis,* restoration of acid-base balance may be hastened if isotonic (one-sixth molar) sodium lactate solution is used in place of sodium chloride, since oxidation of the lactate makes the sodium available as bicarbonate without interposition of renal activity. *Alkalosis* is sometimes treated by the intravenous administration of ammonium chloride, but the practice is to be discouraged as dangerous and rarely necessary. Ammonium ion absorbed from the gastrointestinal tract is fixed as urea in the liver, but, administered intravenously, it is distributed in the general circulation and may have marked toxic effects on the central nervous system. The possibility that potassium depletion may, in part, be responsible for alkalosis should be kept in mind.

The addition of potassium chloride to solutions for intravenous use has become common practice for the treatment of *potassium depletion.* This may, under selected circumstances, e.g., diabetic acidosis, metabolic alkalosis, be highly beneficial, but the dangers should be recognized and promiscuous use discouraged. The cardiotoxic effects of potassium are well known and should be avoided by keeping rates of administration low, by following the electrocardiogram for changes characteristic of potassium intoxication, and, if possible, by frequent determination of the plasma potassium concentration. Potassium should *not* be administered before an adequate level of renal function has been established.

Certain *precautions* to be taken in the intravenous administration of saline solutions are especially important in the treatment of patients who have or who are likely to develop cardiac insufficiency. The too rapid administration of fluids in such individuals may precipitate pulmonary edema. Keeping infusion rates low, periodic examination of the lung bases for rales, and frequent determination of the venous pressure may minimize the danger. In such individuals there may be occasion for subcutaneous administration of saline, but poor absorption may be anticipated in the presence of peripheral circulatory failure. Another occasion for caution is in the treatment of patients with renal insufficiency in which renal function cannot compensate for miscalculation of fluid requirements. This is particularly the case when renal shutdown is complete, even though this may have resulted from dehydration and shock. If, when blood pressure has been restored and the peripheral circulation is adequate, a flow of urine has not been established, the further administration of fluids will not "force open" the kidneys, and, indeed, attempts to do so may be fatal. Conservative, expectant treatment, with fluid and electrolyte intake carefully balanced to output, is required.

Specific consideration of the management of dehydration and disturbances in fluid balance is discussed under diseases in which these problems are of major importance, e.g., diabetes mellitus, adrenal insufficiency, uremia, etc. For normal values of blood constituents see tables at the end of this book.

ROBERT W. BERLINER

References

Black, D. A. K.: Sodium Metabolism in Health and Disease. Oxford, Blackwell Scientific Publications, 1952.

Moyer, C. A.: Fluid Balance. Chicago. Year Book Publishers, Inc., 1952.

Peters, J. P.: Body Water, The Exchange of Fluids in Man. Springfield, Illinois, Charles C Thomas, 1935.

AMYLOIDOSIS

Definition. Amyloidosis is a disorder characterized by the deposition in various tissues of amyloid, a protein-chondroitin sulfuric acid complex of obscure and probably variable composition. Four categories of amyloidosis are customarily distinguished: primary, secondary, amyloidosis associated with multiple myeloma, and localized amyloidosis.

Etiology. The cause of *primary systemic amyloidosis,* an uncommon disease of which some 75 cases have been recorded, is still completely obscure. It is not ordinarily associated with chronic infection, known disturbance in protein metabolism or other abnormalities.

Secondary amyloidosis classically is related to chronic suppuration, notably protracted tuberculous involvement of the lungs or bone, chronic osteomyelitis due to pyogenic organisms, lung abscess and bronchiectasis. It occurs also as a complication of many other conditions associated with extensive tissue destruction and infection, including malignant tumors, Hodgkin's disease, chronic ulcerative colitis and regional ileitis with fistulation, rheumatoid arthritis, chronic pyelonephritis, and paraplegia with suppurating decubitus ulcers and urinary tract infection; occasionally, also, in association with plasmacytosis and hyperglobulinemia in drug sensitivities. In recent years, owing to the advent of effective antibiotics, these latter associations with secondary amyloidosis have, indeed, superseded in frequency the classic occurrence with tuberculosis and pyogenic infections of lung and bone—such, at least, has been the experience of the author in a general hospital.

In view of the chondroprotein nature of amyloid and its not infrequent appearance in hyperimmunized animals with prolonged hyperglobulinemia, some investigators have related secondary amyloidosis to a disturbed protein metabolism associated with suppuration and tissue breakdown. The evidence for this relationship is not clear, however, and further investigation is needed.

The incidence of amyloidosis in *multiple myeloma* varies in different series, averaging about 15 per cent. Magnus-Levy stressed derivation of the amyloid from Bence Jones and related abnormal proteins in multiple myeloma, but most cases with extensive amyloidosis do not have conspicuous hyperglobulinemia. *Localized amyloid tumors* occur as isolated growths chiefly in the larynx, trachea and bronchi. A rare form limited to the skin has been described (lichen amyloidosis). There is no clue as to etiology.

Morbid Anatomy. The spleen, kidney, liver and the cortex of the adrenal glands are the most common sites of *secondary amyloid-*

osis, these organs characteristically being enlarged and firm, the involved areas homogeneously infiltrated and of waxy pallor. Lymph nodes, pancreas, gastrointestinal tract, prostate, thyroid and other organs may also show involvement. Microscopic examination indicates a predilection for the walls of capillaries and arterioles, earliest deposition occurring beneath the endothelial cells, in arterioles extending into the media. In the spleen, infiltration of amyloid begins in and around the malpighian bodies, giving rise to the typical sago spleen; in the liver, earliest involvement is subsinusoidal; in the kidney, amyloid first appears subendothelially in the glomerular capillaries, beneath the epithelium of Bowman's capsule and occasionally in the tubular epithelium beneath the basement membrane. In all organs, accumulation and expansion of these deposits in blood vessels and reticulum fibers lead to compression and atrophy of the tissue parenchyma until, in advanced cases, much of the substance may be composed of amyloid.

Iodine (Lugol's solution) imparts a deep brown color to secondary amyloid deposits; upon addition of sulfuric acid, a dark blue color forms, hence Virchow's designation of the substance as amyloid (starchlike). Congo red and eosin give an intensely pink color; with van Gieson's stain a yellow or brownish color is obtained. Amyloid stains metachromatically with methyl violet and crystal violet. These reactions are consistently obtained in secondary amyloidosis as encountered in man, and upon them rests the ultimate diagnosis.

In *primary systemic amyloidosis* the sites of predilection are cardiac, skeletal and smooth muscle, initially involving the interstitium and progressively compressing muscle fibers, with atrophy and replacement by amyloid. The myocardium characteristically is extensively involved, with cardiac enlargement. Macroglossia is common. The smooth muscle of many medium-sized and small blood vessels throughout the body is usually selectively involved. Skeletal musculature, including the diaphragm and the smooth muscle of the gastrointestinal tract, also the skin, may be diffusely affected. The spleen, kidney, adrenal gland and liver are more commonly involved than is generally stated. The skin may be diffusely infiltrated, particularly about the head and neck, hands and nails, often with local hemorrhages; or translucent papules and plaques of the skin and mucous membranes may appear. Staining reactions with iodine, Congo red and the metachromatic dyes are often erratic, apparently because of variations in chemical structure which have suggested the term "paramyloid."

In distribution and erratic staining characteristics, the amyloid deposits in *multiple myeloma* resemble primary more than secondary amyloidosis.

Symptoms and Signs. The onset and progression of amyloid disease are insidious. In *secondary amyloidosis* the clinical picture ordinarily is overshadowed by the inciting disease. Amyloid disease of the kidneys is most apt to become clinically apparent, with marked albuminuria, cylindruria, edema, hypoalbuminemia and more or less pronounced hypercholesterolemia—in severe cases the full-blown nephrotic syndrome. In exceptional instances obliteration of nephrons may become extensive enough to cause uremia. Diffuse involvement of the liver may be suggested by hepatomegaly with a firm, blunt, smooth, nontender liver edge. Ascites may occur, but jaundice and significant hepatic failure are rarely observed. In the author's experience there may be bromsulfalein retention and marked increase in serum alkaline phosphatase, apparently due to obstruction of intrahepatic excretory channels. Palpable enlargement of the spleen is uncommon despite the frequency of the typical sago spleen, which is usually only moderately enlarged; however, the diffuse type of splenic involvement occasionally results in marked splenomegaly. Manifestations of Addison's disease, if present, ordinarily are due to associated tuberculosis or to primary atrophy, only rarely to amyloidosis despite extensive replacement of the adrenal cortex bilaterally. Amyloidosis of the gastrointestinal tract may be associated with chronic diarrhea.

Whereas secondary amyloidosis may develop at any age, depending on the underlying disease, *primary systemic amyloidosis* occurs almost exclusively between the ages of 40 and 80. Males and females are about equally affected. The presenting symptoms are usually those of congestive heart failure with dyspnea, edema and fluid in serous cavities. Macroglossia may be striking, with dysarthria and dysphagia. Asthenia and weight loss are the rule in late stages. Deposits in the skin may simulate scleroderma, scleredema or myxedema. Hypertension, lymphadenopathy, pains in joints and extremities, and purpura occur.

Localized amyloid tumors of the larynx may cause hoarseness, and if large may result in obstructive dyspnea. They can be visualized by laryngoscopy or bronchoscopy and identified by histologic examination of biopsy specimens.

Diagnosis. Amyloidosis should be kept in mind as a possible complication of the suppurating diseases with which *secondary amyloidosis* is associated. Development of marked albuminuria or the nephrotic syndrome in the course of these diseases should raise the question of amyloid nephrosis. Needle biopsy of the liver or kidney may secure the diagnosis. Gingival biopsy is helpful, and biopsies of suspicious muscle or skin areas may be indicated.

The Congo red test, which depends upon rapid removal of the injected dye from the blood as a result of selective adsorption by amyloid deposits, is a useful but sometimes uncertain diagnostic method. Taran and Eckstein recommend standardization of the procedure by use of 1 cc. of a 1 per cent aqueous solution per 10 pounds of body weight. Adsorption of at least 90 per cent of the dye in one hour constitutes a positive test and good evidence for diffuse amyloidosis. A smaller percentage of dye is removed in nonamyloid cases or when the amyloid deposits are small or of a type that does not readily adsorb the dye. Untoward reactions to Congo red preparations recently available have been frequent.

Recognition of *primary systemic amyloidosis* is difficult, the cardiac manifestations closely simulating arteriosclerotic heart disease. Macroglossia may suggest the diagnosis, which depends upon biopsy, and even then may be uncertain because of erratic staining properties of the amyloid. The Congo red test frequently is negative or inconclusive for the same reason.

Prognosis and Treatment. The average period of survival from onset of symptoms in *primary systemic amyloidosis* is about three years. Death is usually due to intractable cardiac failure. Treatment is symptomatic.

In *secondary amyloidosis* therapy is aimed at the underlying suppurative disorder, and if this can be controlled by surgery or appropriate antibiotic therapy, as in localized tuberculosis or pyogenic infections, healing of early amyloid lesions may take place. It is claimed that this may be accelerated by use of crude liver preparations. Control of suppuration by treatment with antibiotics has a prophylactic effect on complicating amyloidosis, as indicated by a reduction in incidence in recent years.

ALEXANDER B. GUTMAN

References

Dahlin, D. C.: Secondary Amyloidosis. Ann. Int. Med., 31:105, 1949.

Editorial: Primary Systemic Amyloidosis. Ann. Int. Med., 38:620, 1953.

Goltz, R. W.: Systematized Amyloidosis. A Review of the Skin and Mucous Membrane Lesions. Medicine, 31:381, 1952.

Higgins, W. H., and Higgins, W. H., Jr.: Primary Amyloidosis; a Clinical and Pathological Study. Am. J. M. Sc., 220:610, 1950.

Pearlman, A. W.: Amyloidosis. A Clinical and Pathological Study of 135 Cases. Quart. Bull. Sea View Hosp., 6:295, 1941.

Schottenfeld, A., Arnold, L. M., Gruhn, J. G., and Etess, A. D.: Localized Amyloid Deposition in the Lower Respiratory Tract. Am. J. Med., 11:770, 1951.

Snapper, I., Turner, L. B., and Moscovitz, H. L.: Multiple Myeloma. New York, Grune and Stratton, 1953.

Stemmerman, M. G., and Auerbach, O.: Value and Limitations of the Congo Red Test for Amyloidosis. Am. J. M. Sc., 208:305, 1944.

Taran, A., and Eckstein, A.: Standardization of the Congo Red Test for Amyloidosis. Am. J. M. Sc., 203:246, 1942.

MELANOSIS AND MELANURIA

The brown or black pigments called melanins are high molecular polymers of oxidation products of ortho-dihydroxyphenol derivatives. They are formed for the most part from tyrosine, which is oxidized by tyrosinase to dihydroxyphenylalanine ("dopa"), then to a red quinone designated hallachrome, which is converted to indolequinones and finally polymerized to form melanins.

The melanins are elaborated by melanoblasts normally present in the skin and other organs. Abnormal deposition of melanins is called *melanosis*. Darkening of the urine due to excretion of these pigments is termed *melanuria*.

Increased pigmentation of the skin, mucous membranes or internal organs need not, of itself, have any deleterious connotation, as, for example, the tanning or freckling of the skin after exposure to ultraviolet rays, or the pigmentation particularly of the face (chloasma gravidarum) commonly accompanying pregnancy. Darkening of the skin also occurs after radiation therapy and after prolonged mechanical irritation (scratching due to vermin infestation or to other causes of pruritus) or prolonged administration of certain chemicals, notably arsenicals.

The chief importance of diffuse or localized melanosis lies in its frequent association with a variety of significant disorders. The melanosis of Addison's disease, for example, may provide an important clue to diagnosis even though the nature of the pigmentary disturbance remains obscure. The blue-black ears of ochronosis are characteristic of that disorder. Vitamin deficiencies in pellagra and sprue not infrequently are accompanied by increased pigmentation of the skin, particularly of the exposed areas. In neurofibromatosis (von Recklinghausen's disease) sharply defined areas of skin pigmentation characteristically are present even if subcutaneous nodules are inconspicuous or absent, and are an aid in diagnosis. Similar pigmented areas, usually more irregular in configuration, are apt to develop in involved neurodermal segments in fibrous dysplasia of bone. Familial polyposis of the small intestine, with early neoplastic degeneration, is sometimes identifiable by the presence of melanosis of the skin about the mouth and nose, with discrete areas of pigmentation of the buccal mucous membranes and on the hands.

Most important of all, however, is the occurrence of melanosis and melanuria in association with *malignant melanomas*. These tumors usually arise from a pigmented, flat, hairless mole or from the uveal tract and metastasize widely and rapidly. They are apt to elaborate melanin pigments in considerable quantity, many, however, as colorless precursor melanogens. In addition to pigmented metastases, there may be diffuse melanosis of the skin and other organs. In such instances the urine may contain a sufficient quantity of pigment to take on a brown or black color when voided; often, however, the urine turns dark only upon standing, due to the oxidation of melanogens. Addition of ferric chloride gives a dark brown or black precipitate; bromine water forms a yellow precipitate which darkens gradually. The dark color of the urine due to the presence of melanins should be readily distinguishable from that of hemoglobinuria, porphyrinuria and alkaptonuria by these and other appropriate tests.

Acanthosis nigricans is characterized by the appearance of soft, velvety, brownish-to-black verrucous plaques of cutaneous folds, characteristically present in the axillae but sometimes also involving the external genitalia, perianal area, nipples and umbilicus, and occasionally affecting the mucous membranes. There may be hyperkeratosis of the palms and soles, with papillomatous elevations elsewhere, often associated with local loss of hair. The juvenile form, usually present at birth, is benign. Onset after the age of 40 is associated in approximately one half of the cases with malignancy, preponderantly of the stomach but also arising from the uterus, liver, rectum, large bowel, ovary, breast and bronchi. These tumors are usually adenocarcinomas and highly malignant. The significance of this association is not known.

ALEXANDER B. GUTMAN

References

Curth, H. D.: Acanthosis Nigricans and its Association with Cancer. Arch. Dermat. & Syph., 57:158, 1948.

Lerner, A. B., and Fitzpatrick, T. B.: Biochemistry of Melanin Formation. Physiol. Rev. 30:91, 1950.

PORPHYRIA

Definition and Classification. Porphyria may be defined as a constitutional fault or "inborn error" in porphyrin metabolism. It is probably best to limit the term to cases in which uroporphyrin and/or porphobilinogen are excreted in great excess, since this characterizes the constitutional abnormality. Thus used, the term "porphyria" embraces two fundamentally distinct groups: (1) erythropoietic, (2) hepatic. The former is synonymous with what Günther described as porphyria congenita. The latter includes (*a*) the intermittent acute form, (*b*) the cutanea tarda type (Günther's "chronic" porphyria), (c) the combined or "mixed" type, (d) latent porphyria.

Incidence. The erythropoietic (congenital) form of the disease is distinctly rare. Many of the cases described in the literature as "congenital" porphyria are undoubtedly of the hepatic cutanea tarda type, differing fundamentally from the erythropoietic disease. The hepatic intermittent acute type is the most common form of porphyria. It has often been overlooked because of its close mimicry of various other pathologic states. During the past eighteen years, 74 cases of porphyria have been studied in Minneapolis. Of these,

but 2 were erythropoietic, thirty-six were of intermittent acute type, 15 were of the cutanea tarda type, 6 were combined and 15 were latent.

While it has been believed that striking differences in sex incidence exist between the congenital and acute types of porphyria, recent studies based on the above-mentioned fundamental classification fail to reveal any significant sex difference in the erythropoietic type, while the hepatic intermittent acute form is somewhat more common in females. The ratio in 97 cases was about 1.5:1.0. The cutanea tarda form is distinctly more frequent in males, a ratio of 19 to 4 being noted in 23 cases. The age at onset of manifestations is much earlier in the erythropoietic disease, usually in infancy or early childhood, the condition in some instances being evident at birth. In the hepatic forms, symptoms are rarely noted before puberty, the age at onset more often being in the third or later decades.

Etiology. Although porphyria is to be regarded as an "inborn" error of the metabolism, the erythropoietic or congenital type has been shown to be familial only in exceptional cases. By way of contrast, the hepatic forms, and especially the more common intermittent acute types, are commonly, perhaps uniformly, familial. The existence of a genetic trait in this form is clearly revealed if a careful search is made for latent or mild cases among other members of a family of any given patient.

Günther and others used the term "toxic" acute porphyria to imply that some cases were acquired, on the basis of chemical poisoning. There can be no doubt that acute attacks are often precipitated by chemicals in the hepatic intermittent acute form of the disease. Sulfonal, Trional, barbiturates and less frequently a variety of other chemicals, even including alcohol, have been implicated. Waldenström and others have clearly demonstrated that barbiturates may precipitate attacks in individuals having latent porphyria, previously free of symptoms. Such latent cases were identified because other members of the patient's families had manifest disease. The exact mechanism by which chemicals precipitate attacks is unknown. This variety of porphyria is to be distinguished sharply from the ordinary, symptomatic or *secondary coproporphyrinuria*. Coproporphyrin is normally present in urine and feces and is increased in a variety of pathologic states, in-

enough, the small amounts of uroporphyrin excreted in the intermittent acute cases are mainly zinc complex, while in the erythropoietic type it is present, chiefly at least, as the free porphyrin. The significance of the zinc complex is not clear. It has been observed, however, in cases of "mixed" type with photosensitivity, but during complete remission of abdominal or nervous symptoms; thus a causal relationship with the latter appears unlikely.

The urines from cases of the intermittent acute type need not be abnormally colored even during the acute attack, although in most cases the patient will have noticed a darkening of the urine at the outset. Porphobilinogen is usually present in large amounts at this time. If the fresh urine is normal in color, the diagnosis may be overlooked unless the chromogen is sought for. If the urine is allowed to stand in the light to bring about the characteristic darkening, the uroporphyrin (metal complex) spectrum is then readily detected. The porphobilinogen is demonstrable in fresh urine by means of the Ehrlich aldehyde test. The resulting red compound is chloroform insoluble, a fact which serves to distinguish it from urobilinogen aldehyde. Porphobilinogen, in addition to being a porphyrin precursor, gives rise to porphobilin, a dark brown, nonporphyrin pigment of unknown chemical structure. Probably because of its content of this pigment, the urine of the intermittent acute type of porphyria is darker, with more brown and less red color than that of the pure photosensitive types. Porphyria urine usually contains an excessive amount of coproporphyrin. The porphyrin and pigment content of the urine is much more complex in the intermittent acute than in the photosensitive type of the disease.

Differential Diagnosis. The possibility of porphyria should be borne in mind in the presence of any obscure nervous disturbance, especially unexplained peripheral neuritis, flaccid paralyses of extremities, bulbar palsy and hysteria. It should also be searched for in any instance of abdominal pain which is otherwise unexplained. Among other conditions, the disease has been confused in the past with gallstone colic, renal colic, appendicitis, bowel obstruction and lead poisoning. In the last, the urine regularly contains a marked increase of coproporphyrin, but rarely any marked excess of porphobilinogen or uroporphyrin, nor is the amount of copro-

porphyrin sufficient to color the urine red. In gallstone colic the urine Ehrlich reaction may be positive because of excessive urobilinogen. Confusion of porphyria with renal colic has usually been due to the belief, based on superficial examination, that the red urine was due to blood and the pain due to ureteral calculus. Careful examination of the urine will obviate this mistake. The lack of rebound tenderness and muscle spasm, together with the urinary findings, serves to distinguish porphyria from appendicitis. The leukocyte count is usually normal, but in exceptional cases may be considerably elevated. The roentgenographic findings aid in excluding bowel obstructions, the characteristic layering of the small bowel not being observed. Areas of marked alternating spasm and distention of the large bowel are rather common, especially of the transverse colon and splenic flexure.

Hypertension is noted in some cases, and it is of interest that lumen attenuation of retinal arteries of spastic type may be seen in such instances. During the acute attack the hypertension may be associated with oliguria, and these manifestations coupled with the dark urine may give rise to a superficial resemblance to acute glomerulonephritis. If the attack subsides and the disease becomes quiescent or latent, the blood pressure returns to normal and retinal vascular abnormalities may disappear entirely. Electrocardiographic changes are observed in some cases.

At times the persistent tachycardia and muscle weakness may be suggestive of hyperthyroidism, while at others weakness and pigmentation give rise to consideration of Addison's disease. The pigmentation is present in but a minority of cases. It is usually rather patchy in character, in some cases associated with intervening vitiligo. The nature of the pigment has not been determined. In one case seen by the writer the patient at an earlier age had had an appendectomy which failed to relieve the attacks of abdominal pain for which it was done; several years later she underwent a thyroidectomy because of tachycardia, weakness and nervousness; later still, in another hospital, she received salt and adrenal extract treatment for supposed Addison's disease, on the basis of weakness and mild pigmentation of the skin. Subsequently this patient had severe abdominal pain and paralyses of all four extremities, from which, however, she recovered completely. More than ten years later she had had no recurrence of symptoms, although the urine still contained small amounts of porphobilinogen and uroporphyrin.

Occasional cases are observed in which chronic constipation and longstanding abdominal pain are prominent and in which the urine contains a several-fold increase of coproporphyrin, but neither porphobilinogen nor uroporphyrin. A satisfactory classification of these cases is impossible at the present time, but it does not appear that they should be included in the category of true porphyria. As a matter of fact, they will not be recognized as involving any disturbance of porphyrin metabolism unless a quantitative study of coproporphyrin excretion is made.

Many cases of "hydroa aestivale seu vacciniforme" bear no relation to porphyria, although the skin lesions may be indistinguishable. In some of these it is evident that ordinary window glass prevents the photosensitivity, since it absorbs the exciting light (below 3000 Å). In the photosensitive types of porphyria the wave length of the light most important in inducing skin lesions is probably in the neighborhood of 4000 Å, with the result that window glass is not protective.

Prognosis. In the erythropoietic, photosensitive type the outlook for life is relatively good, the disease having a long chronic course and death being due to intercurrent affections of one kind or another. In some instances, however, severe anemia, hemolytic in character, is the most important governing factor in prognosis. In the intermittent acute type the mortality is relatively high, especially in cases with nervous system manifestations. In the past, a figure of 80 per cent within five years from the time of the first attack has generally been accepted, but our own experience indicates that the prognosis is distinctly better than this even in cases predominantly nervous in type. A further survey of this question is now in progress. In those cases in which only abdominal symptoms are present the outlook is distinctly better, although these cases, too, may develop nervous system involvement at any time.

Treatment. From the standpoint of photosensitivity this is purely preventive, consisting in protection from the light. As stated, ordinary window glass does not filter out the exciting light. There is some evidence that vitamin B_{12} is beneficial in reducing or eliminating photosensitivity in the hepatic cutanea tarda group. This deserves further trial.

Splenectomy is of value in at least some cases of the erythropoietic type with splenomegaly and hemolytic anemia. In one of our cases splenectomy has been followed by a complete symptomatic remission of the disease for a period of over four years. The anemia and photosensitivity have disappeared, and the porphyrin excretion, though still abnormal, has decreased remarkably.

Various methods of treatment have been advocated for the intermittent acute type, but none is of proved value except from the standpoint of temporary relief of pain in the abdomen and extremities. Calcium given intravenously has been reported to be beneficial. A number of investigators have stated that the administration of crude liver extract has resulted in improvement. The author's experience with both of these methods has been disappointing. Demerol, 50 to 100 mg. given hypodermically, has been of value in allaying pain, although its effect has seldom lasted more than 4 hours. In some instances it was clearly more effective than morphine, probably because of its antispasmodic as well as analgesic effect.

Tetraethylammonium chloride has been of definite value in reducing or eliminating pain. One injection of 200 to 250 mg. intravenously or 500 to 1000 mg. of the chloride intramuscularly has provided complete relief for as long as 12 hours in some cases. It is well to commence with a small dose as some cases are unduly sensitive and develop untoward hypotension. In some cases a beneficial effect is entirely lacking. Hexamethonium has been used in small amounts in two cases, but in both was followed by a profound drop in blood pressure again indicating that there may be an unusual sensivity in this disease.

In a number of instances, prompt remission has occurred following brief ACTH therapy. In others, no definite beneficial effect has been observed and in a few it has been thought that the effect was adverse, actually hastening the patient's demise. Present experience indicates that a brief trial of ACTH is warranted. If no definite benefit has been observed within a four-day period, it probably should not be continued.

Barbiturates should not be used, since there is definite evidence that they may precipitate or intensify the attacks. There is evidence also that other chemicals, including alcohol, are precipitating factors in some cases. Patients with latent porphyria should be given a written statement concerning the diagnosis and danger of barbiturates and other chemicals, to carry on their person at all times.

C. J. Watson

References

Brunsting, L. A., Mason, H. L., and Aldrich, R. A.: Adult Form of Chronic Porphyria with Cutaneous Manifestations. Report of Seventeen Additional Cases. J.A.M.A., 146:1207, 1951.

Cookson, G. H., and Rimington, C.: Porphobilinogen. Chemical Constitution. Nature, 171:875, 1953.

Denny-Brown, D., and Sciarra, D.: Changes in the Nervous System in Acute Porphyria. Brain, 68:1, 1945.

Dobriner, K., and Rhoads, C. P., The Porphyrins in Health and Disease. Physiol. Rev., 20:416, 1940.

Falk, J. E., Dresel, E. J. B., and Rimington, C.: Porphobilinogen as a Porphyrin Precursor, and Interconversion of Porphyrins, in a Tissue System. Nature, 172:292, 1953.

Schmidt, P. R.: Neurologische und psychische Störungen bei Porphyrinkrankheiten. Fortschr. d. Neurol. u. Psych., 20:422, 1952.

Waldenström, J.: Studien über Porophyrie. Acta med. Scandinav., Supp. 82, 1937.

————: Neurologic Symptoms Caused by So-called Acute Porphyria. Acta psychiat. et neurol., 14:375, 1939.

Watson, C. J.: Porphyria. Advances in Internal Medicine. Chicago, Yearbook Publishers, Inc., 1954, vol. 6.

————, and Larson, E. A.: The Porphyrins and Their Relation to Disease: Porphyria. Oxford Medicine, Vol. 4. New York, Oxford Unviersity Press, 1951, p. 228.

————, and Schwartz, S.: A Simple Test for Urinary Porphobilinogen. Proc. Soc. Exper. Biol. & Med., 67:393, 1941.

Diseases of the Ductless Glands

INTRODUCTION

The author will not write the conventional introduction. He will not give the Greek derivation for the word "hormone," coined by Starling; he will not discuss the experiments of Claude Bernard which led to the concept of an internal secretion; he will not delve into the earliest beginnings of endocrinology which had as their *raisons d'être* such ends as the procurement of a form of manpower safe for the harem, the salvaging of a male soprano voice for the choir, the increased palatability that a rooster attains when he turns into a capon, and so on. He will not trace experimental endocrinology from 1849, when Berthold studied the effect of the gonads on the secondary sex characteristics of fowl, for the next hundred years down to 1949, when attention was focused on cortisone and its pituitary stimulator, adrenocorticotrophic hormone (ACTH). But why mention such prosaic facts in 1955 when we are well into the schizo-atomic era and rapidly approaching, the author fears, the posthistoric era? It would be more in keeping to mention that a pellet of stilbestrol can now replace pregnancy as a promoter of lactation in cows. No, the author will not even list the names of describers of various endocrine syndromes—from Addison with Addison's disease in 1855, down past the almost simultaneous elucidation of hyperparathyroidism in 1926 both by Mandel and by Du Bois to—well—to whom? The author thinks of no recent unmasking of a new syndrome. Are we leaving an era behind?

Instead, he will discuss what endocrinology is, with special emphasis on what endocrinology is not, and then will comment on certain other aspects of the subject.

What Endocrinology Is. Endocrinology is an indivisible division of internal medicine and has to do with certain glands or tissues which secrete highly specific substances into the blood stream for use by other tissues. The only important thought in this definition is contained in the word "indivisible." It is impossible to separate endocrinology from internal medicine; by the same token it is impossible to be an endocrinologist without being an internist. The physician who calls himself an endocrinologist and confines his interest to such unfortunate members of society as might appear in the sideshow of a circus, never realizes that pneumonia, a broken leg and a bad burn involve important changes in adrenal cortical function (cf. "Alarm Reaction" of Selye), that the disturbance in homeostasis occasioned by chronic renal insufficiency is ameliorated by a secondary hyperparathyroidism, that the somatotrophic action of testosterone propionate may be made use of in many conditions other than male hypogonadism, and so on.

The author resents the tendency to limit the scope of endocrinology to those disorders of the internal secretions which are not clearly understood. Thus, once some division of endocrinology such as diabetes is put on a firm footing, it is removed from the section on endocrinology to the section on metabolic diseases.

What Endocrinology Is Not. Certain conditions often considered to be endocrinologic are probably not so at all.

First, in order of frequency, comes the fat boy who is slightly late in sexual development and whose genitalia are obscured by excess of fat. This patient, nine times out of ten, is labeled as having Fröhlich's syndrome, whereas in point of fact he is just a fat boy, whatever that is. If left alone, he will develop normally sexually and frequently will cease to be fat after puberty. True Fröhlich's syndrome is exceedingly rare and difficult to diagnose before the normal age of onset of puberty.

Then there comes the child who does not do well in school. There is a feeling among would-be progressive educators that such a situation demands a survey by an endocrinologist. In the author's experience there is only one endocrine abnormality which leads to mental retardation, namely, cretinism. The diagnosis of this condition is a problem for the obstetrician and the pediatrician, not for the endocrinologist. If it is not made in the first few weeks or, at the most, months of life, the damage is already done, and one might just as well not make the diagnosis. Parenthetically, it might be added that every physician should suspect cretinism in any child with an umbilical hernia at birth which persists after the first few weeks of life. Even juvenile myxedema is not associated with retarded mentality. To be sure, longstanding hypoparathyroidism leads to epileptic seizures and secondary mental retardation. The author has seen in consultation a number of children with poor school records and to date has been unable to make a diagnosis of endocrine disease in any of them. He is impressed by the fact that many of them have been "mirror readers."

Thirdly, the author has yet to see a homosexual patient in whom the trouble was based on faulty endocrine function or in whom the giving of a hormone influenced the direction of the libido. Of interest in this connection is an observation made by Dr. Anne P. Forbes and known in our clinic as "Forbes's law": A patient who complains of impotence or of lack of libido does not suffer from a hormonal lack; a patient with real endocrine insufficiency, e.g., eunuchoidism, has impotence and absent libido, but does not complain of them, but of something more trivial, such as being mistaken for a girl over the telephone.

A fourth type of case sent to the endocrinologist is the patient with some congenital disorder of the germ plasm, such as mongolian idiocy, Laurence-Moon-Biedl syndrome, and so on. Just why such conditions should be confused with endocrinopathies is not clear. It is probably connected with the belief that anything which is not fully understood belongs to endocrinology.

Finally, there are the patients with alopecia areata. The endocrines have something to do with certain types of hair; these patients have too little hair; therefore they are sent to the endocrinologist. However, the fact that this condition starts by being spotty is strong evidence against an endocrinologic etiology. It makes no difference that one spot may enlarge to the point where it covers the whole body; the disease is still a "spotty" one. Endocrinologic diseases are generalized, not localized; hormones do not stop in the midline or proceed down one limb and not the other. For example, Paget's disease of bone is not endocrinologic, since it is not generalized. Though it involve 95 per cent of the skeleton, there will still be a sharp demarcation between the uninvolved part and the Paget's disease. Postmenopausal osteoporosis, on the other hand, may be confined to the spine and pelvis and still be a generalized disease, since here there is a rhyme and a reason to the distribution. This discussion concerns the *primary* lesion produced by an endocrinopathy. Secondary complications can be spotty (e.g., gangrene of the toe in diabetes, bone cyst with hyperparathyroidism).

Failure of End Organs to Respond to Hormones. Since a hormone acts somewhere, it is obvious that one might get much the same clinical syndrome from failure of the end organ to respond to the hormones as one would get with absence of the hormone itself. For example, let us take "pseudohypoparathyroidism." Patients with this condition have the clinical and chemical findings that one associates with hypoparathyroidism, but they fail to respond to parathyroid hormone and their parathyroid glands not only are not absent, but may be hyperplastic. A second example is the failure of the American Indian to develop a beard. Recently a patient presented himself, his only complaint being failure to develop a beard. Elaborate studies were carried out with uniformly normal results. Finally someone had the wit to inquire about the patient's ancestry and found that he was part Indian.

Oophorectomy. The author feels that needless oophorectomy constitutes one of the greatest faults in medical practice. A normally functioning ovary, needless to say, is most essential for the future physical and mental well being of a young woman. Satisfactory as replacement therapy is, it will not produce ova or be a substitute for motherhood.

There are two chief reasons for unnecessary ovarian surgery. The general surgeon does not realize that the normally functioning ovary is a cystic organ; he performs an exploratory laparotomy for some sort of abdominal pain and finds nothing but cystic ovaries; out they come. For some reason the surgeon is never sued for malpractice because of this; the story would be different if, under somewhat analogous conditions, castration were resorted to in the male.

Metropathia hemorrhagica is the second big cause for unnecessary removal of the ovaries. This interesting condition can be treated medically in almost all instances.

Even after the menopause the author disapproves of oophorectomy. He feels that the ovary still functions to a certain extent after the periods have ceased and that one sees more severe osteoporosis after an artificial menopause than after a physiologic one.

Fat Distribution. Considerable space has been wasted in textbooks and writings on endocrinology about the distribution of fat. In the writer's opinion there are fat people and thin people, but with one exception the distribution of fat is of no diagnostic significance. The one exception is in Cushing's syndrome, in which there is a tendency for the face to be round ("moon-faced"); this roundness is probably due to a tendency to deposit fat in front of the ears. However, that a propensity to deposit fat around the hips or on the lower extremities or diffusely throughout the body or where you will has any diagnostic significance, is most unlikely; it almost certainly has nothing to do with pituitary disease.

Hirsutism without Virilism. Of the many thorns in the side of the endocrinologist the most aggravating is the patient whose life is made miserable by excessive hair growth on the face and elsewhere. In only one case in a hundred can the physician find an endocrine fault; and, what is worse, in only the small percentage of cases in which the hair is too much, not only where it should not be, but also where it should be, can the physician save his ego by asserting with any degree of confidence that the condition is not endocrinologic. The only treatment he can offer is symptomatic, which, in this instance, means the removal of the excess hair. The "Wonderstoen" helps in some, but most end up by turning to the painful, costly and not-too-successful method of electrolysis. For psychologic reasons the physician must never mention the words "beard" or "razor" or *anything* which suggests masculinity. It is probable that the best way to remove the hair is with a razor. What is needed more than any other one thing is a razor in disguise, e.g., an electric razor that has been camouflaged with some fancy embellishment and called an "electric depilator."

"Practical" versus "Theoretical" Knowledge. The subject matter of this paragraph is applicable to all internal medicine, but especially to endocrinology. The author is frequently asked in giving a talk to make it "practical" and not too "theoretical." By "practical" is usually meant "therapeutic"; by "theoretical" is usually meant "fundamental." The author has no patience with such a philosophy. One cannot possible practice good medicine and not understand the fundamentals underlying therapy. Few if any rules for therapy are more than 90 per cent correct. If one does not understand the fundamentals, one does more harm in the 10 per cent of instances to which the rules do not apply than one does good in the 90 per cent to which they do apply. The same policy carries over to medical education. There are those who advocate medical schools which will turn out practical physicians rather than "theorists." But they end by turning out a poorer grade of doctors. As with eggs, there is no such thing as a poor doctor, doctors are either good or bad.

FULLER ALBRIGHT

References

Albright, F.: Metropathia Hemorrhagica. J. Maine M.A., 29:235, 1938.
———, Burnett, C. H., Smith, P. H., and Parson, W.: Pseudo-Hypoparathyroidism—An Example of "Seabright-Bantam Syndrome." Endocrinology, 30:922, 1942.
———, Smith, P. H., and Richardson, A. M.: Postmenopausal Osteoporosis. Its Clinical Features, J.A.M.A., 116:2465, 1941.
Folley, S. J., and Malpress, F. H.: Artificial Induction of Lactation in Bovine by Subcutaneous Implantation of Synthetic Oestrogen Tablets. J. Endocrinol., 4:1, 1944.
Selye, H.: The General Adaptation Syndrome and the Diseases of Adaptation. J. Clin. Endocrinol., 6:117, 1946.

DISEASES OF THE THYROID GLAND

NORMAL PHYSIOLOGY OF THE THYROID

Among the principal functions of the thyroid gland are: the removal from the circulation of adequate amounts of iodine; the utilization of iodine in forming thyroid hormone; the storage of the hormone in combination with protein as colloid in the thyroid follicles; the breakdown of the hormone-protein combinations in the colloid; the delivery to the blood of the hormone in amounts sufficient for the needs of the tissues. Knowledge of the steps and mechanisms by which these functions are accomplished is still fragmentary, but is already helpful in the understanding of many clinical manifestations of thyroid disease.

Iodine and iodide are promptly absorbed from the gastrointestinal tract solely in the form of inorganic iodide. This is selectively concentrated or trapped by the thyroid cells, a function which is enhanced by the thyroid-stimulating hormone of the pituitary but inhibited or blocked by the action of thiocyanates. A second stage in the process is the oxidation of the trapped iodide into iodine and its combination with protein. This step can be inhibited or prevented by the action of thiourea compounds. Details of the actual formation of the hormone, thyroxin, are shrouded in mystery. The iodine alone or in organic form is incorporated with two molecules of tyrosine to form thyroxin, but whether this is accomplished directly through stages of monoiodotyrosine and diiodotyrosine or by direct addition of four atoms of elemental iodine to the thyroxin precursor, thyronin, is not as yet established.

Thyroxin combined with protein is stored as thyroglobulin which is broken down as is necessary to meet the hormonal needs of the tissues. Radioactive iodine studies indicate that normally the iodine leaving the gland in hormonal form approximately equals that which enters it in the form of inorganic iodine. The mechanism of breakdown of thyroglobulin to liberate active hormone is not known, although it is supposed that a proteolytic enzyme activated by thyrotropic hormone is involved. Following its liberation from the thyroid, thyroxin enters the circulation.

Until recently it was supposed that thyroxin was the only thyroid hormone and indeed the only iodinated compound in the circulation. Doubt was thrown on this concept when Gross and Leblond with chromatographic techniques observed a compound which could not be thyroxin and which Gross and Pitt-Rivers later identified as tri-iodothyronin. When this was assayed for its physiologic effects it was found to be three to five times more active than thyroxin. The relative roles of thyroxin and tri-iodothyronin in hormonal control of metabolic activities are as yet not clearly defined. Qualitatively their action appears to be identical, and the difference in effect seems to be confined almost entirely to potency and rapidity of action.

DAVID P. BARR

References

Gross, J., and Leblond, C. P.: Metabolites of Thyroxine. Proc. Soc. Exper. Biol. & Med., 76:686, 1951.

————, and Pitt-Rivers, R.: The Identification of 3:5:3 L-Triiodothyronine in Human Plasma. Lancet, 1:439, 1952.

————, and Pitt-Rivers, R.: Physiological Activity of 3:5:3 L-Triiodothyronine. Lancet, 1:593, 1952.

Harrington, C. R., and Barger, G.: Chemistry of Thyroxine. III. Constitution and Synthesis of Thyroxine. Biochem. J., 21:169, 1927.

Kendall, E. C.: The Isolation in Crystalline Form of the Compound Containing Iodin Which Occurs in the Thyroid: Its Chemical Nature and Physiological Activity. J. Biol. Chem., 20:501, 1915.

Rawson, R. W., and Rall, J. E.: Diseases of the Thyroid. In Duncan, G. G.: Diseases of Metabolism. 2nd ed. Philadelphia, W. B. Saunders Co., 1952.

SIMPLE GOITER

(Endemic Goiter, Colloid Goiter, Struma, Bronchocele)

Definition. Simple goiter is an enlargement of the thyroid, dependent upon a deficiency of iodine or upon the inability of the body to utilize iodine.

Etiology. For the most part the develop-

Page 730

ment of simple goiter is limited to localities in which the soil and drinking water are deficient in iodine. Among the districts of greatest incidence are the Alps, the Himalayas, the Pyrenees, the Carpathians, the Andean Plateau and the mountains of New Zealand. In the United States it is found chiefly in the Great Lakes Basin, in Minnesota, the Dakotas, the Pacific Northwest and in the valley of the Upper Mississippi. In a few areas almost the entire population is affected. In most, however, the distribution of goiter in the population reveals the influence of other factors. It is more common, and in some places seven times as common, in girls. The swelling most often makes its appearance at puberty and may tend to diminish or even to disappear at the age of 25 to 30. In temperate climates there is a seasonal variation with greatest incidence in late winter and spring.

From time to time so-called goiter epidemics have been observed in endemic areas. These have tended to occur in garrisons or institutions. Probably any conditions which increase the need for thyroxin and hence for iodine will augment the prevalence of goiter. Puberty, pregnancy, infectious disease are outstanding examples. Simple goiter can be exacerbated by diets which tend to produce rickets.

It has also been demonstrated that simple goiter may be produced by feeding cabbage and related vegetables. The fact that these foods contain considerable amounts of organic cyanide and that cyanides are powerful depressants of tissue oxidation led Marine to test the effect of various organic cyanides which were found also to produce simple goiter. It appears that through interference with the trapping of iodine by the thyroid gland, such factors may contribute both to variation in incidence of endemic goiter and to differences in the size and character of the thyroid glands in different persons.

Symptoms. There is a gradual enlargement of the thyroid, which may be subject to exacerbations and remissions with infections, with changes in seasons and in diet, with puberty and pregnancies and with other vicissitudes of life. In early cases the gland may be diffusely enlarged and smooth; later it tends to become nodular with irregular areas of hyperplasia and involution or from cyst formation, hemorrhage or calcification. In its growth the goiter may cause a distressing sense of fullness with difficulty in swallowing, or it may press on the trachea with resulting dyspnea on exertion. The trachea may be grossly displaced and at times narrowed. Paralysis of a recurrent laryngeal nerve may occur in uncomplicated simple goiter, but its appearance should be regarded as a possible evidence of malignancy. The health is usually not impaired and constitutional symptoms are lacking. The basal metabolic rate is almost always within normal limits, although late in the disease extensive changes may lead to thyroid insufficiency. Rarely Graves' disease may develop from simple goiter.

Prevention. Although the administration of iodine as a method of eradicating simple goiter was advocated as early as 1860, it was not until 1917 that the problem was attacked thoroughly and systematically. Prophylaxis depends simply upon the administration of iodine in sufficient amounts. Actually, very little is needed. It has been estimated that 25 to 50 mg. of inorganic iodine may be sufficient to supply an adult of average size for a year. For children between the ages of 5 and 15 years and for pregnant women, a larger dose of about 10 mg. per week is commonly advocated. This can be supplied approximately by giving 1 cc. of the syrup of hydriodic acid each week. Children may prefer chocolate-coated tablets made to contain 10 mg. of iodine. This represents a generous excess and is surely more than is needed by the general population, which probably could be well cared for with one-tenth to one-half as much. For the supply of entire communities various methods have been tried, and there is still discussion concerning the most effective scheme. Iodinization of table salt has been extensively tried. The amount of iodine added has varied in different countries, but in the United States has been about 200 mg. of potassium iodide per kilogram of salt. An average consumption of 10 gm. of salt would therefore provide 2 mg. of potassium iodide or 1.5 mg. of iodine per day. Iodinization of city water in concentrations of 1 part to 100,000,000 has been tried in some communities.

Treatment. If treatment with iodine can be instituted in the early or hyperplastic stages of development of simple goiter, curative effects, sometimes very dramatic, may be expected. Large doses are no more effective than small, and 10 to 15 mg. of inorganic iodine given every day for two or three weeks and repeated every three or four months for a year should be ample. For maximum reduction in size, at least a year of treatment is necessary. When the colloid stage of simple goiter has been reached, the benefit from administration of iodine is not often striking. All cases, however, should be given a thorough therapeutic trial.

Surgical removal of a simple goiter may be indicated either because of the size of the goiter or because the patient finds it unaesthetic or a psychologic handicap. The danger that cancer may develop in a nodular goiter must always be considered. Removal is especially indicated in goiters which surround the trachea or displace it far to one side and in those which are intrathoracic or press upon the great vessels of the neck. In preoperative management of simple goiter it is safer to administer iodine for a period of ten days or more, even though there may be no signs of thyrotoxicosis.

DAVID P. BARR

References

Kimball, O. P.: The Efficiency and Safety of the Prevention of Goiter. J.A.M.A., *91*:454, 1928.

Marine, D.: Etiology and Prevention of Simple Goiter. Medicine, 3:453, 1924.

————: Further Studies on Etiology of Goiter with Particular Reference to the Action of Cyanides. Proc. Soc. Exper. Biol. & Med., 29:772, 1932.

————, Baumann, E. J., Spence, A. W., and Cipria, A: Studies on Simple Goiter Produced by Cabbage and Other Vegetables. Proc. Soc. Exper. Biol. & Med., 26:822, 1929.

————, and Kimball, O. P.: Prevention of Simple Goiter in Man. Arch. Int. Med., 25:661, 1920.

HYPERTHYROIDISM

(Thyrotoxicosis, Toxic Goiter, Exophthalmic Goiter, Parry's Disease, Graves' Disease, Basedow's Disease)

Definition. Hyperthyroidism is the condition which results from an excessive secretion of the thyroid gland. Anatomically, it is associated with hypertrophy or hyperplasia of the glandular parenchyma. Clinically, it is characterized by an increased rate of oxidation in tissues, by disturbances in the vegetative nervous system, by abnormalities in creatine metabolism and frequently by exophthalmos and other ocular abnormalities.

Etiology. With the exception of exophthalmos, all the clinical manifestations of thyrotoxicosis can be produced by the administration of thyroid substance or of thyroxin. Furthermore, partial removal of the thyroid gland results in striking benefit or cure. It seems likely at present that hypersecretory activity of the thyroid gland is responsible for most of the clinical phenomena of the disease. The ultimate cause or reason for the continual overactivity of the gland is not manifest. It is known, however, that the function of the thyroid is controlled by an extremely labile and sensitive mechanism which is influenced by many circumstances. Hyperplasia of the gland may result from such widely different factors as environmental temperature, seasonal fluctuations, adolescence, pregnancy, infection, partial removal of the gland, lack of iodine, and emotional trauma. In general, anything which constitutes an increased demand or a lack of proper secretion may initiate hyperplastic changes. The disease may develop at any age, but has its greatest incidence in the third or fourth decade. It is much more common in women, the ratio in some nonendemic goiter areas being as high as 4 to 1. In those who have some predisposition, the state appears to be initiated or exacerbated by puberty or by successive pregnancies. The influence of the menstrual cycle is apparent in changes both in the size and activity of the thyroid gland. Many cases appear to develop immediately after acute infections, especially of the upper respiratory tract. History of repeated attacks of tonsillitis and the presence of large infected tonsils are frequently encountered in younger patients with hyperthyroidism. The high incidence of thyrotoxicosis in acromegaly has long been recognized, and it has been demonstrated that appropriate amounts of the thyrotrophic hormone of the pituitary gland can produce in normal animals practically all the changes of clinical thyrotoxicosis, even including exophthalmos, a symptom which has never been observed following the use of thyroxin. Prolonged anxiety, worry, grief and frustration, as well as acute emotional shocks, play an important role in the development and progress of the disease.

In individual cases difficulty is encountered in demonstrating the relative importance of the several factors. It would appear that functional variations in the state of the pituitary gland might be of the utmost importance in the etiology. Except in cases of frank acromegaly, however, its role is not often apparent. Estimation of its precise significance awaits quantitative determinations of thyrotrophic hormones in blood and urine. The multiplicity of factors influencing the activity of the thyroid gland indicates that hyperthyroidism in the sense of a variably increased activity of the gland is a part of the normal response to environment and to the vicissitudes of life and cannot in itself be considered in any sense a pathologic state. The distinguishing feature in Graves' disease is not alone the degree of hyperthyroidism, but much more its continuity over long periods of time and after supposed etiologic factors have been removed or controlled. It is a reasonable hypothesis that an interplay of several factors may initiate thyrotoxicosis, which then becomes a vicious circle in which circumstances ordinarily of minor significance assume a major role in the prolongation of abnormality.

Clinical Picture. The onset of thyrotoxicosis may be abrupt, following an infection, physical or psychic trauma, or without recognizable precipitating factors. More often it is insidious. The presenting symptoms may be any of the classic manifestations of the disease. Prominent among them are loss of weight and strength without impairment of appetite. Fatigue is an early and relatively constant symptom, but may be masked by a restless ambition which induces the patient to undertake many purposeless tasks. There is intolerance to heat and profuse sweating. Palpitation is a frequent presenting symptom. There may be a history of tremor, of increasing clumsiness and a tendency to drop things. Increased irritability with emotional outbursts and unexpected loss of temper is frequent. By no means constant are complaints relative to the appearance of the eyes or to the size and appearance of the neck. Retraction of lids and lid lag often precede by some time the actual protrusion of the eyes. If there is a goiter, there may be difficulty in swallowing and occasionally a tendency to hoarseness. Oligomenorrhea or even amenorrhea is not infrequent. In the more severe cases there may be attacks of vomiting and diarrhea with rapid and alarming loss of weight.

Occasionally the warning symptoms are minimal or are not heeded, and the patient presents himself only after a serious gastrointestinal crisis or cardiac failure has developed.

Physical examination usually reveals striking and characteristic signs. Emaciation is frequent. The skin is delicate, warm and moist. Hyperkinesis with purposeless movements at times almost choreiform in character may occur, especially during embarrassment or other emotion. The speech may occasionally be so uncoordinated as to make understanding difficult. The hands show a frequent, fine, intense tremor, greatly intensified by extending the fingers or by any display of emotion. Often there is an anxious expression.

In many cases the eyes are large and shining and exhibit a stare. Winking is infrequent (Stellwag's sign). The lids are retracted, and in the downward gaze the upper lid follows the eyeball jerkily or not at all (von Graefe's sign). There is a weakness in convergence (Moebius' sign), and in some of the more severe cases of exophthalmos there may be marked limitation of other movements of the eyeball. Less constant and of later appearance than the lid phenomena is protrusion of the eyeball. When this occurs, there may be also a puffiness of the lids and a fullness both above and below the globe due to increase in the contents of the orbit. In some cases and more often when other symptoms of thyrotoxicosis are minimal, the exophthalmos may be rapidly progressive and assume alarming proportions with injection and chemosis of the conjunctiva, edema of orbital tissues and varying degrees of ophthalmoplegia. This state is usually designated as malignant exophthalmos.

The thyroid gland at times may not be palpable, but is usually increased in size. In younger persons the enlargement tends to be diffuse, although it may not be entirely symmetrical. The surface is smooth, the consistency soft or elastic. A systolic thrill may be palpable and a corresponding bruit may be heard. This may have a variable significance and may depend either upon an increased vascularity of the gland or upon pressure of the goiter on one of the great vessels. In cases of long duration and in older people the gland is often nodular, usually because of irregular areas of hyperplasia or involution, but occasionally from the growth of adenomas.

In the early stages of the disease, circulatory changes may be limited to tachycardia, with or without the subjective sensation of palpitation, and to an increase in pulse pressure. There is an increase in cardiac output and an increased velocity of blood flow. In younger persons with otherwise normal hearts, cardiac decompensation is not frequent, but in older patients it may be the first recognized manifestation of the disease. Atrial fibrillation may be an early sign of failing circulation. Extrasystoles occur frequently, and atrial flutter is not uncommon. The pulse pressure is increased, usually because of an abnormally low diastolic rather than a raised systolic pressure.

Weakness of skeletal muscles is present to some degree in most patients and occasionally may be so severe as to suggest myasthenia gravis. Other forms of myopathy are occasionally associated with hyperthyroidism.

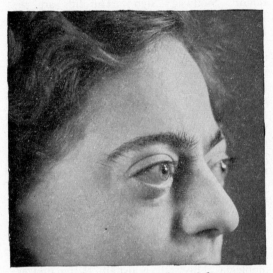

Fig. 85. Exophthalmos in Graves' disease.

The spleen can be palpated in a few cases, but the lymphoid hyperplasia observable in fatal cases is seldom sufficient to produce obvious physical signs.

Laboratory examinations are helpful in study of the disease. Elevation of the basal metabolic rate may be regarded as an almost constant sign of thyrotoxicosis. It must be remembered, however, that, according to the Du Bois standards, the normal range varies from minus 10 to plus 15. Increase in rate is therefore not always apparent. In a patient with a normal rate of minus 10, a strictly basal reading of plus 15 might indicate a significant degree of hyperthyroidism. In cases of great severity the recorded resting metabolic rate may be plus 100 or more. The usual range in cases of moderate severity is from plus 30 to plus 60.

Spontaneous glycosuria with variable degrees of hyperglycemia occurs in many cases. In most cases the ability to oxidize carbohydrate is not lost, and there is no evidence of a lowered renal threshold for the excretion of sugar.

There may be in hyperthyroidism some reduction in blood cholesterol, although the depression is not often sufficient to be of diagnostic value.

One of the more constant accompaniments of thyrotoxicosis is a spontaneous creatinuria on a creatine-free diet. When a test dose of creatine is given, the retention is less than occurs normally. These tests are not reliable in children and in some women who retain a tendency to lose creatine. They are invalidated by the administration of even small amounts of iodine.

The protein-bound iodine of the serum is elevated above the normal maximum level of 7.5 micrograms per 100 cc. Under ideal conditions this is a valuable diagnostic test, but its practical utility is impaired because values are distorted by previous ingestion of iodine and for long periods by the administration of Iodeikon, Lipiodol and other compounds containing protein-bound iodine.

In Graves' disease from 35 to 90 per cent of a test dose of radioactive iodine is taken up by the thyroid gland and only 5 to 40 per cent of the dose is excreted in the urine. This test is valid only when the patient has not recently received iodine.

Metabolic studies have demonstrated a tendency to a more or less constant loss of nitrogen which can be corrected only by an adequate caloric intake; also a negative calcium and phosphorus balance which, in long-continued hyperthyroidism, gradually leads to a demineralization of the skeleton.

Thyroid Crisis or Storm. Infections, anxiety or, most commonly, manipulation of the thyroid gland may initiate an acute exacerbation of thyrotoxicosis. This is characterized by increase in all the symptoms and signs of the disease with hyperpyrexia, extreme tachycardia and sometimes persistent vomiting. Such crises are the most dreaded features of thyrotoxicosis. They lead rapidly to profound exhaustion and carry a mortality of 60 per cent or more. By all the older observers of the disease they were seen not infrequently and particularly following operation. With appropriate preoperative use of iodine they have fortunately become rare.

Diagnosis. In the more typical cases, diagnosis should offer no difficulty. The combination of loss of strength and weight with preservation of appetite, with heat intolerance, tremor and hyperkinesis should be sufficiently suggestive. When this syndrome is accompanied by exophthalmos and goiter, there can be no doubt. The picture, however, is not always so obvious. Exophthalmos and other eye signs are not always present. The thyroid gland may not be enlarged, and in a few patients the signs of overactivity are not apparent. Diagnosis in such cases may be easily missed, and may still remain unrecognized even after the disease has caused serious heart failure.

Mistakes in diagnosis may also arise in confusing anxiety states and neurocirculatory asthenia with hyperthyroidism. These conditions are also characterized by palpitation, tachycardia, tremor and sweating. It is true that in the neuroses tachycardia may disappear during sleep or periods of apparent security, that the increases in pulse pressure are seldom impressive, that the tremor is coarse and less intense and that sweating palms are cold and fail to radiate the heat so characteristic of hyperthyroidism. It is also true that in psychoneuroses the basal metabolic rate is not elevated. Nevertheless differentiation of the two conditions may offer difficulties, and not infrequently neuroses have been wrongly diagnosed and treated as thyrotoxicosis.

In many cases, determination of the basal metabolic rate may solve the difficulty. In others, estimation of the degree of spontaneous creatinuria and of creatine retention, following a test dose of creatine, is indicated and may offer an important clue. Still another method of value in differentiation is a therapeutic test with iodine. To accomplish this the patient, who must not have had recent treatment with iodine, is carefully observed, under standard conditions, for a period of two weeks. Pulse rates, basal metabolic rates and creatine values are determined. Iodine is then administered for ten days, after which all observations are repeated. Patients with hyperthyroidism almost invariably show marked improvement, while those suffering from other conditions are not affected by the treatment. In many cases, masking of thyroid symptoms is attributable to the previous use or administration of iodine. Complete withdrawal of all contact with iodine will often result in exacerbation and permit establishment of the diagnosis.

Prognosis. Observations on the course of hyperthyroidism with no effective treatment have indicated that the disease is to a certain extent self-limited, that remissions are not infrequent and that the tendency is toward gradual arrest of symptoms in one to five years. Most of the so-called cured cases, however, continue to display residual symptoms of greater or lesser severity and are always subject to relapse. Complete spontaneous recovery must be extremely rare. Prognosis for spontaneous improvement is better in young patients and in those whose onset has followed remediable psychic or physical trauma.

Danger to the thyrotoxic patient consists chiefly in attacks of uncontrollable vomiting and diarrhea, in the occurrence of thyroid crises and in the strain which continuing overactivity throws upon the circulation. In patients more than 40 years of age, prognosis depends chiefly upon the state of the heart. In those with previous cardiac damage, early onset of atrial fibrillation and of other manifestations of decompensation is frequent. Without effective treatment heart failure tends to become progressive.

A few patients exhibit jaundice and other signs of hepatic disease. Both the incidence and mortality of acute infectious diseases is increased in thyrotoxicosis.

Treatment. Experience has shown that the course of thyrotoxicosis may be favorably modified by the use of small amounts of iodine, and can be interrupted temporarily or permanently by administration of thiourea and its derivatives or of salts containing radioactive iodine or by subtotal thyroidectomy. With improvement of other methods of treatment, irradiation of the thyroid gland by x-ray has been almost entirely abandoned in practical therapy. For optimal management the control of physical activity, diet, emotional factors and circulatory complications is of great importance.

The use of *iodine* alone seldom accomplishes permanent satisfactory control. In cases otherwise untreated it increases the iodine content of the thyroid gland and reduces the concentration of protein-bound iodine in the circulating blood. It effects involution and relieves congestion of thyroid tissue. It results in amelioration of the more acute manifestations of the disease. The amount of iodine required to cause remission is not great, and daily doses of 1 cc. (13 mg. of iodine) of syrup of hydriodic acid or 2 minims (18 mg. of iodine) of Lugol's solution are sufficient to produce optimal response. The rate of fall of the basal metabolic rate in a patient with Graves' disease given iodine is identical with that of a patient with treated myxedema from whom effective desiccated thyroid dosage is withdrawn. It would appear that in some unexplained manner the release of thyroid hormone is prevented by the administration of iodine. Ordinarily, maximal effect should be apparent in ten to fourteen days. Continuance of the same dosage tends to prevent critical episodes and in some mild cases may constitute sufficient protection over long periods.

Thiourea and its derivatives have in common the action of preventing production of thyroxin in the thyroid gland. They exert no effect on preformed thyroxin. In Graves' disease their use causes amelioration or complete correction of tremor, hyperkinesis and circulatory symptoms. They restore to normal the basal metabolic rate, elevate the cholesterol content of the blood and correct the creatine defect as well as the negative nitrogen and calcium balance. They lessen or control lid spasm, but do not diminish protrusion of the eyeballs. Complete control of the thyrotoxic state may be accomplished in some cases within three weeks but in others is long delayed. In patients with large nodular goiters a year or more of treatment may be required for complete control. It is doubted that any gland is truly insensitive to the action of the drugs. The interval depends to some extent upon the dosage and the method of administration, but chiefly upon the amount of thyroxin present in the body at the time the drug is started. Previous use of iodine tends to delay the effect. It has been found, however, that glands of patients treated solely by thiourea compounds tend to remain friable and vascular to an extent which interferes with surgical removal. The use of iodine for two weeks following attainment of a euthyroid state by a thiourea compound is helpful in increasing the firmness of the gland.

Many derivatives of thiourea have been tested, and great variations both in their potency and toxicity have been discovered. Fever, a variety of eruptions and depression of the bone marrow may accompany the use of any of the compounds. Thiouracil, the first of the derivatives to receive extensive trial, caused serious granulocytopenia or agranulocytosis in approximately 2.5 per cent of the cases in which it was exhibited. At present 6-n-propylthiouracil is the drug of choice, not only because of the relative lack of toxicity, but also because of the experience gained in

its use by many competent observers. Optimal dosage for establishment of antithyroid effect and for its maintenance must be established by careful observation of each individual patient. Usually daily administration of 150 to 300 mg. of 6-n-propylthiouracil is sufficient for detoxication. Because of rapid excretion of the drug, it must be given with great regularity at 8-hour intervals in doses of 50 to 100 mg. For maintenance of euthyroid state, 25 to 100 mg. a day may be necessary. The administration of an excess of the drug results in myxedema. Although not incapable of producing agranulocytosis, 6-n-propylthiouracil is a relatively safe compound and its long-continued use has been accompanied by few serious toxic reactions. Lasting remission of the disease is seldom induced by less than six months of therapy, but may be expected in approximately half of patients so treated.

Another relatively safe antithyroid drug concerning the use of which considerable experience has accumulated is 2-methyl-mercaptoimidazole, which appears to be effective in about one-tenth the dosage of propylthiouracil.

Radioactive iodine has been used in the treatment of Graves' disease since 1942. Although several isotopes of iodine have been tried, present practice is confined to the use of I^{131} which has a half life of eight days. In thyrotoxic patients who have received no iodine in the recent past, 50 to 90 per cent of the radioactive material is taken up by the thyroid gland, the remainder being rapidly excreted. Thus the effect of the preparation is exerted chiefly within the gland and, when sufficient amounts are given, results in inactivation or destruction of thyroid tissue. The dose must be carefully calculated. As an aid in determining the actual receptivity of the gland, a small tracer dose of radioactive iodine is given several days before the treatment is begun. Even with this information the calculation cannot be precise, since it must also depend upon a necessarily inexact estimation of the size of the gland. Radioactive iodine is administered as a single oral dose the full effect of which cannot be finally judged until at least two months have elapsed. In the reports now available a high percentage of improvement and cures have been recorded. Except for transient radiation sickness and a considerable incidence of long-sustained hypothyroidism, untoward effects have not been encountered.

Of all therapeutic expedients, *partial sur-*

gical removal has received the greatest attention and in the past has offered the most hope. With the best preparation and in the hands of the most expert surgeons the operative mortality has been reduced below 1 per cent with a relapse rate estimated variously between 5 and 20 per cent. Such a remarkable record represents an optimum which has been attained only when the best surgical skill and judgment has been combined with thorough understanding of the thyrotoxic patient and with meticulous attention to many details of preoperative and postoperative management.

With so many resources, the choice of treatment in the individual patient presents many problems. For large, unsightly goiters, particularly those in which pressure on surrounding structures is present or anticipated, surgical removal is indicated. Cancer of thyrotoxic glands is not common, but must be suspected in nodular glands, especially when single or multiple nodules are encountered in young people or when in any patient a portion of the gland is observed to increase in size. In such cases surgical removal becomes an urgent necessity. The indication is less apparent in older persons displaying multiple nodules, since these usually represent areas of localized hyperplasia, involution or cyst formation. The great majority of patients in whom neither the fear of cancer nor the size and appearance of the gland are important factors can be controlled either by radioactive iodine or antithyroid compounds as well as by surgical subtotal thyroidectomy. Other considerations, however, influence the final selection of therapy. The use of radioactive iodine is relatively new, its effects are irreversible, its late effects have not been evaluated, estimation of correct dosage is difficult, and facilities for determination of the receptivity of the gland for iodine are not everywhere available. In situations in which circulatory complications preclude subtotal thyroidectomy, the use of radioactive iodine usually is the therapeutic method of choice. In older patients whose goiters are neither unsightly or nodular it affords a satisfactory substitute for surgical treatment. Though 6-n-propylthiouracil is a relatively safe drug and will establish a euthyroid state in most patients, its administration requires careful and frequent supervision over a period of at least six months. In many cases this offers great difficulties, and unless cooperation and availability of the patient can

be assured, subtotal thyroidectomy must be regarded as preferable treatment.

When thyroidectomy is contemplated, a thyrotoxic patient should be under observation and preferably in a hospital for at least two weeks before the operation. Effective *rest* and *relaxation* are essential, and it should be the rule to spare the patient all unnecessary stress until the condition can be permanently remedied. The thoroughness with which rest must be enforced, however, will depend upon the age and general condition as well as upon the degree of hyperthyroidism. The young, previously healthy patient has large factors of safety which may resist without distress unmodified activity except in the severest grades of thyrotoxicosis. On the other hand, rigid protection is obligatory in older patients whose hearts have lost some of their initial reserve, in those whose illness is so severe as to threaten a thyrotoxic crisis, or in those suffering from infection or recent psychic or physical trauma. Even in the best circumstances appropriate relaxation is not always easy of accomplishment. Complete inactivity in seclusion may be impossible, and unwise attempts to enforce it too literally are among the causes of failure in management. For most patients, continuous recumbency is by no means necessary. Even in the very ill the avoidance of boredom is important as a means of controlling restlessness. Periods of complete rest should be frequent, but need not be continuous except in patients whose hearts are seriously incompetent. In the less severe cases, activity under strict observation is desirable, since its effect on pulse, blood pressure and respiration may offer a valuable indication of the ability of the patient to withstand the strain of operation.

Psychological factors are of great importance in the management of thyrotoxicosis, and attempts to control or remove anxieties constitute a main aim in treatment. Though formal attempts at psychotherapy may be inadvisable during the preoperative period, an understanding of the personal problems of the patient and a sympathetic and helpful attitude on the part of the physician confer significant therapeutic benefits. Thyrotoxic patients are often susceptible to suggestion and are influenced to an unusual degree by the mood of the physician. An attitude of gloom or uncertainty may be disastrous, while optimism and assurance often have dramatically beneficial effects.

Control of restlessness depends chiefly

upon reassurance, upon removal of causes of anxiety and the avoidance of boredom. In some cases, however, restlessness and insomnia persist in spite of the most enlightened management. For such, tepid sponge baths given morning and evening may be helpful. Phenobarbital in doses of 15 to 30 mg. four times each day is useful. For insomnia, the night dose may be increased to 60 or even 90 mg. Large doses of sedatives are seldom if ever indicated.

Undernutrition is usually evident. Even under complete resting conditions the thyrotoxic patient expends much more than a normal amount of energy. Moreover, all muscular work is performed inefficiently. In calculating a diet, it is usually safe to consider that at bed rest a patient with moderately mild thyrotoxicosis will require at least twice as much food as a normal person of the same size. A liberal supply of carbohydrate and protein is indicated. Excessive amounts of fat are undesirable, since they tend to cause diarrhea. All thyrotoxic patients tend to lose calcium and phosphorus and therefore need more than the normal intake of lime salts. Furthermore, it has been demonstrated that the requirement of thiamine is proportional to the caloric expenditure. It is likely also that in thyrotoxicosis an increased intake of pyridoxine and pantothenic acid is required to maintain normal nutrition.

All these factors must be taken into account in prescribing a diet. In addition to adequate calories, protein and carbohydrate, the diet should include each day 1 quart of milk, 10 to 20 mg. of thiamine hydrochloride and yeast or other vitamin supplements which will increase materially the usual intake of pyridoxine and pantothenic acid. Since the caloric needs of each patient cannot be calculated exactly, daily weight must be used as the best indication of the caloric sufficiency of any given diet.

Since Plummer's demonstration in 1923, iodine has been regarded as the prime essential in the preoperative treatment of Graves' disease. Now, by combining the use of 6-n-propylthiouracil with iodine, the benefits of both drugs may be obtained and preparation for operation can be more satisfactory than ever before. The drugs may be given simultaneously, but for promptest effect it is necessary to start the antithyroid drug several days before iodine is exhibited. In preparing a patient for operation, the combined treatment should be continued until a euthyroid state has been attained.

Statistical evidence indicates that the routine administration of large doses of digitalis is detrimental to patients with thyrotoxicosis and actually increases the mortality from surgical procedures. Tachycardia with regular rhythm and without cardiac decompensation is best controlled by rest and iodine. Congestive heart failure or cases of auricular fibrillation with very rapid pulse rate or continued or large pulse deficit require digitalis, which should be started early in the preoperative period in order that its benefits may be achieved and its possible toxic effects controlled before the time of operation. The preoperative use of quinidine for the control of auricular fibrillation is seldom if ever indicated.

With the combined use of protection, good psychologic management, adequate diet, iodine and 6-n-propylthiouracil, most patients can be satisfactorily prepared for the necessary surgical procedures. For the few who are too old or infirm or who have serious circulatory disease, a euthyroid state may usually be maintained by the continuance of adequate amounts of 6-n-propylthiouracil or by the administration of one or more doses of radioactive iodine.

DAVID P. BARR

References

Astwood, E. B.: Treatment of Hyperthyroidism with Thiourea and Thiouracil. J.A.M.A., 122:78, 1943.

von Basedow, C. A.: Exophthalmos durch Hypertrophie des Zellgewebes in der Augenhöhle. Wchnschr. f. d. ges. Heilkunde, 6:197, 1840.

Graves, R. J.: Clinical Lectures. London Med. & Surg. J., 7:516, 1835.

Hamilton, J. G., and Lawrence, J. H.: Recent Clinical Developments in the Therapeutic Application of Radio-Phosphorus and Radio-Iodine. J. Clin. Investigation, 21:624, 1942.

Hertz, S., and Roberts, A.: Application of Radioactive Iodine in Therapy of Graves' Disease. J. Clin. Investigation, 21:31, 1942.

McGavack, T. H., Chevalley, J., Shearman, A. M., Dreakter, I. J., and Stern, S.: Clinical Application of Certain Mercaptoimidazoles to Hyperthyroidism. J. Clin. Endocrinol., 10:813, 1950.

Magnus-Levy, A.: Ueber den respiratorischen Gaswechsel unter dem Einfluss der Thyroidea sowie unter verschiedenen pathologischen Zuständen. Berl. klin. Wchnschr., 32:650, 1895.

Means, J. H.: The Thyroid and Its Diseases. Philadelphia, J. B. Lippincott Co., 1948.

Parry, C.: Collected Works. London, 1825.

Plummer, H. S.: Results of Administering Iodine to Patients Having Exophthalmic Goiter. J.A.M.A., 80:1955, 1923.

Rawson, R. W., and others: Effect of Iodine on the Gland in Graves' Disease when Given in Conjunction with Thiouracil—a Two-Action Theory of Iodine. J. Clin. Investigation, 24:869, 1945.

Richardson, H. B., and Shorr, E.: The Creatin Metabolism in Atypical Graves' Disease. Tr. A. Am. Physicians, 50:156, 1935.

Solomon, D. H., Beck, J. C., VanderLaan, W. P., and Astwood, E. B.: Prognosis of Hyperthyroidism Treated by Antithyroid Drugs. J.A.M.A., 152: 201, 1953.

Williams, R. H., Clute, H. M., Anglem, T. J., and Kenney, F. R.: Thiouracil Treatment of Thyrotoxicosis. II. Toxic Reactions. J. Clin. Endocrinol., 6:23, 1946.

HYPOTHYROIDISM

Definition. Hypothyroidism is the functional state which results from a deficiency or complete lack of the thyroid hormone. When it is permanent and complete, as a result of destruction or removal of the thyroid gland, it may be correctly called *athyrosis*. It is not always complete and may develop as a temporary functional disturbance. It may start at any time, before birth, in infancy, childhood or adult life. Since the thyroid hormone is of great importance in growth and development, the effect of deficiency varies considerably at different ages of onset. For purposes of discussion, it has been customary to consider hypothyroidism under three separate headings of cretinism, juvenile myxedema and adult myxedema. A fourth category of hypometabolism or hypothyroidism without myxedema may be added.

Etiology. In regions of endemic goiter a lack of iodine in the mother's body may give rise to a lack of thyroid development during fetal life or shortly after birth. Some cases of hypothyroidism developing later in life are due to a primary atrophy of the thyroid gland, the cause of which is entirely unknown. Occasional cases have been reported following typhoid, influenza, pneumonia and syphilis. Destruction of the gland has occurred rarely from tuberculosis, actinomycosis and from gunshot wounds or other local injuries. The most common cause of hypothyroidism in adults is the surgical removal of too much thyroid tissue. Temporary hypothyroidism has followed the use of x-rays in the treatment of goiter or malignant disease of the neck. Approximately 80 per cent of the cases of spontaneous hypothyroidism occur in women, most often between the ages of 30 and 50. Diminished function of an anatomically normal thyroid gland may develop secondarily to the destruction or loss of function of the anterior lobe of the hypophysis (see Hypopituitarism, p. 756).

Symptoms and Signs. The manifestations of hypothyroidism vary both with the age of onset and the degree of deficiency.

Cretinism. When severe hypothyroidism develops during fetal life or early infancy, there is dwarfism and imbecility. Even in the earliest weeks of life some thickening of subcutaneous tissues, hoarseness of the cry and the characteristic facies of cretinism may be apparent to the experienced observer. By the second or third month the tongue may be large and the eyes appear far apart. The condition may escape detection during the early months of life and suspicion of the defect arise only when the child is late in sitting up, walking and talking. At this time the skin is rough and scaly and has a yellowish tint. The head is large, the face round and stupid-looking, with a wide flat nose, thick lips, open mouth and thick, partially protuberant tongue. Fat pads develop on the buttocks and back of the shoulders. Frequently there is a pot-belly with umbilical hernia. Legs and arms are short in proportion to the body. Dentition is delayed, and the osseous development remains at an infantile stage. Growth is slow. Mental deficiency varies from complete, helpless imbecility to moron levels. Hypothyroidism does not ordinarily interfere with sexual development.

Juvenile myxedema may be defined as hypothyroidism acquired by a previously normal child prior to the attainment of puberty and full growth. Symptoms vary with the age of onset. There may be dwarfing, retardation of osseous development and some degree of mental deficiency. Consequences are in general less disastrous than in the state of cretinism. Early recognition, however, is urgent if irremediable defects in physical or mental status are to be avoided.

Myxedema of Adults. Adult hypothyroidism often presents an appearance so characteristic that it may be recognized at a glance. Relatively constant among symptoms are weakness, lethargy, slow speech, nonpitting edema of the eyelids and of other tissues, dry, coarse, cold, pale skin, dry, brittle head hair which tends to fall, sparse eyelashes and eyebrows, a remarkable sensitivity to cold and decreased sweating. Speech may be thick because of enlarged tongue and swollen lips. The pitch of the voice is lowered, and there is a characteristic hoarseness. Constipation is a common and often troublesome symptom. The menses tend to be excessive and prolonged. Both menorrhagia and dysmenorrhea are frequent symptoms. The pulse rate is

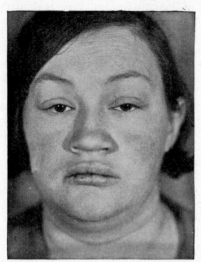

Fig. 86. Twenty-six year old woman with myxedema, before treatment. Basal metabolic rate, —36.

apt to be slow. The blood pressure is usually low, although in later stages of the untreated disease it may be permanently elevated. The circulation is indolent, and both the minute volume of blood flow and the stroke volume of the heart are greatly diminished. On the other hand, the apparent size of the heart as measured by percussion and the roentgenogram may be increased. Rarely the myxedema heart of Zondek with its great increase in transverse diameter is encountered. The electrocardiogram even in the earlier cases often shows flattening or inversion of the T waves with small P waves and QRS complexes of low potential. Dyspnea and dependent pitting edema may develop, but gross cardiac decompensation is rarely attributable to uncomplicated myxedema. Anemia is frequent. It may be hypochromic or may simulate pernicious anemia. Occasionally it is severe. Joints and muscles are often stiff and painful. Impaired hearing is characteristic of myxedema, and vertigo is not uncommon. Although placidity, sleepiness and indifference are usual, some patients may exhibit irritability and apprehension.

Hypothyroidism without Myxedema. The

edema which accounts for many of the usual clinical manifestations of hypothyroidism may not be evident in mild cases and may be minimal even in complete athyrosis. It is of special interest that myxedema is seldom a feature in the hypothyroidism which develops secondary to hypopituitarism. Boothby has suggested that the degree of accumulation of fluid depends upon the protein content of the diet, but this and other factors have not been quantitatively appraised.

Laboratory Aids. In all cases of hypothyroidism the oxidative rate is diminished. Complete athyrosis is usually accompanied by a metabolic rate of minus 35 to minus 45. In milder cases the decrease in oxidation is in proportion to the secretory defect. The serum cholesterol is significantly elevated and bears in general a reciprocal relation to the metabolic rate. The level of protein-bound iodine in the blood is greatly reduced, from a normal of 4.0 to 7.5 micrograms per 100 cc. to levels below 2.0 micrograms per 100 cc. Ingestion of any one of a large number of iodinated organic compounds may give spuriously high values of protein-bound iodine. Radioactive tracer techniques are of value in determining whether a thyroid gland

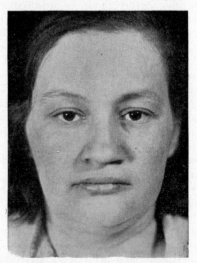

Fig. 87. Same patient as in Figure 86, two months later, after treatment with desiccated thyroid gland. Basal metabolic rate, —5.

is present and capable of utilizing iodine. Athyrotic patients concentrate practically no radioactive iodine in the neck region and excrete in the urine 70 to 95 per cent of the administered dose. The amount excreted in the urine may be diminished in patients with myxedema who have developed polyserositis. Endogenous protein metabolism is reduced, and there is a storage both of protein and water. The urine may contain albumin, but there is seldom any evidence of renal insufficiency. Gastric anacidity may be demonstrated in about half of the cases.

Diagnosis. Early recognition of hypothyroidism is always of the most practical importance, the urgency being greatest in infancy and childhood, when the lack of thyroid hormone leads to irremediable defects both in physical and mental development. In early infancy the clinical condition may not be immediately apparent even to experienced observers. Both intimate knowledge of normal development and close observation are necessary for its detection at a stage early enough to prevent dire consequences. Any physical or mental retardation should be regarded as possible evidence of hypothyroidism. Since basal metabolic rates cannot be reliably determined in infants, the level of cholesterol in the serum may be of the greatest diagnostic importance and may confirm clinical impressions that otherwise could be regarded only as suspicious.

Though myxedema in adults in its advanced form is one of the most evident of diagnoses, many cases, particularly of partial hypothyroidism, fail to show the typical signs. In cases of hypothyroidism without myxedema many of the usual manifestations are lacking. Such patients may be erroneously diagnosed and treated for suspected arthritis, obesity, nephritis or anemia for many months or years. In some, dryness and scaliness of the skin, sensitiveness to cold or inexplicable fatigue are helpful in early recognition. The basal metabolic rate is usually taken as the criterion of reference and has been responsible for the recognition of many cases of hypothyroidism which had defied clinical diagnosis. It must be remembered, however, that low oxidative rates may be encountered in conditions other than hypothyroidism. In such cases, determination of the level of serum cholesterol or the uptake of I^{131} may be helpful in the differential diagnosis.

Treatment. *Cretinism.* Prophylactic treatment of cretinism is important. In goiter districts iodine must be given to pregnant women. Early recognition of cretinism is essential, for, if the arrest in development has continued for a long time, it may be impossible to reestablish normal conditions. Thyroid, U.S.P., which is desiccated and standardized to contain 0.2 per cent of iodine in thyroid combination should be given in tablets by mouth. Estimation of correct dosage may offer difficulties, not only because of lack of objective criteria of improvement, but also because relatively few cretins are completely athyrotic. The dose of thyroid should be adjusted to the age of the patients. In infants of 2 to 4 months treatment may be started with daily doses as small as 6 mg. In a child of 2 to 4 years, 30 to 90 mg., and in a child of 6 to 12 years, 180 to 360 mg., may be necessary each day. It is to be remembered that in childhood the thyroid medication must not only correct the state of hypothyroidism, but must also promote growth. The effect of the medication may be detectable in three to five days. It displays itself by diuresis, loss of weight, sweating of a previously dry skin and increased physical activity. New growth of hair may be noted within a week. Previously subnormal temperature may be gradually elevated to normal levels. Further criteria are depression of the level of serum cholesterol and attainment of normal osseous development. After the initial loss of weight which accompanies diuresis there is a gain which may approximate that of normal growth. Toxicity from thyroid is difficult to recognize in infants, but is not infrequent even with moderate dosage.

Success in treatment depends upon the age at which it is started, upon the severity of the hypothyroidism and upon the adequacy of treatment. If the arrest in development has continued for a long time, therapy may be entirely unsatisfactory. If, on the other hand, thyroid can be begun in earliest infancy and continued without interruption, the chance of normal growth and development is good. In all cases, even in those who have passed the age of puberty, the effects of thyroid therapy should be tested. Some growth has been noted in cretins whose treatment was started when they were 20 years of age or over. Mental improvement is less striking; if the cretin is an imbecile, he is likely to remain one. In the older cretins even the most skillful treatment may result only in increased irritability and greater difficulty in general management. In cases in which athyrosis is not complete the use of iodine as the syrup of hydriodic acid in doses of 0.2 to 0.3 cc. may be followed by considerable improvement.

The treatment of *juvenile myxedema* does

not vary from that of cretinism. Although it is necessary that the dose be adequate, too rapid administration may be accompanied by acute nervousness and anxiety or even by alarming though temporary psychoses.

In *adult myxedema* the patient should be under strict surveillance during the beginning of treatment, since profound changes in general condition occur during the early stages of therapy; hospitalization is desirable whenever possible. Particular care must be exercised in those who have shown evidences of circulatory disease such as arteriosclerosis, hypertension, enlargement of the heart or angina pectoris. There is no agreement on the optimal thyroid dosage. In patients whose thyroid function is completely lost, even so small an amount as 15 mg. daily may cause perceptible changes in creatine metabolism and in clinical state. It is safest to start with relatively small daily doses of 15 to 30 mg., increasing gradually to 180 to 240 mg. if necessary to establish normal relations. Effects are not immediately apparent. They may be noted as early as three days, but are seldom easily detectable in less than five to seven days. The patient feels warmer and less sleepy. Speech and muscular movements are quicker. The basal pulse rate increases. Body temperature rises to normal levels. As in cretinism, there is an impressive diuresis with increased excretion of nitrogen. The level of cholesterol in the blood is diminished, and the basal metabolic rate gradually rises to normal. The facial appearance may be remarkably changed within ten days, and in a few weeks the patient may be almost completely restored to normal health. Adjustment of a maintenance dosage may take some time and require careful observation. The amount necessary to maintain an athyrotic patient in a normal state varies, but usually is between 120 and 180 mg. per day. Anemia is usually corrected by thyroid medication. When the anemia is markedly hypochromic, the administration of iron may be necessary as an adjuvant.

There is danger in suddenly increasing the metabolism of myxedematous patients whose myocardium has been damaged. Precordial distress or even sharp attacks of angina pectoris or of cardiac decompensation are not infrequent accompaniments of rapid elevation of the metabolic rate. Death has resulted from incautious therapy.

It has been shown that tri-iodothyronin administered intravenously exerts a prompter action than thyroxin. The maximum effect is achieved within 24 hours as compared with eight days for thyroxin. The offset is also much more rapid, with a maximum fall in sixteen days compared with a month for thyroxin. Although experimentally this preparation has been used in the treatment of myxedema, its utility for routine management has not been established.

DAVID P. BARR

References

Bomford, R.: Anaemia in Myxoedema, and the Role of the Thyroid Gland in Erythropoiesis. Quart. J. Med., 7:495, 1938.

Boothby, W. M., Sandiford, I., Sandiford, K., and Slosse, J.: The Effect of Thyroxin on the Respiratory and Nitrogenous Metabolism of Normal and Myxedematous Subjects. I. A Method of Studying the Reserve or Deposit Protein with a Preliminary Report of the Results Obtained. Tr. A. Am. Physicians, 40:195, 1925.

Burgess, A. M.: Myxedema—Controlled by Thyroid Extract for Fifty-two Years: Report of a Case. Ann. Int. Med., 25:146, 1946.

Committee of the Clinical Society of London: Report on Myxedema. London, Longmans Green and Co., 1888.

Davis, C. H.: Hypothyroidism as Problem in Women. Am. J. Obst. & Gyn., 46:85, 1943.

Fahr, G.: Myxedema Heart. Am. Heart J., 3:14, 1927.

Gordon, M. B.: Childhood Myxedema or So-called Sporadic Cretinism in North America. Endocrinology, 6:235, 1922.

Gull, W.: On a Cretinoid State Supervening in Adult Life in Women. Tr. Clin. Soc., 7:180, 1873.

Hurxthal, L. M.: Blood Cholesterol and Thyroid Disease. III. Myxedema and Hypercholesteremia. Arch. Int. Med., 53:762, 1934.

McGavack, T. H., Lange, K., and Schwimmer, D.: Management of the Myxedema Patient with Symptoms of Cardiovascular Disease. Am. Heart J., 29:421, 1945.

Means, J. H.: The Thyroid and Its Diseases. Philadelphia, J. B. Lippincott Co., 1948.

Murray, G. R.: The Life History of the First Case of Myxedema Treated by Thyroid Extract. Brit. M. J., 1:359, 1920.

Ord, W. M.: On Myxedema, a Term Proposed to Be Applied to an Essential Condition in the "Cretinoid" Affection Occasionally Observed in Middle Aged Women. Med. Chir. Tr., 61:57, 1878.

Rawson, R. W., and others: 1-Triiodothyronine versus 1-Thyroxine, A Comparison of Their Metabolic Effects in Human Myxedema. Am. J. M. Sc., 226:405, 1953.

Schwittay, A. M.: Occult Hypothyroidism in Wisconsin Women. Wis. M. J., 40:475, 1941.

Tagge, C. H.: On Sporadic Cretinism Occurring in England. Brit. M. J., 1:279, 1871.

Zondek, H.: Das Myxödemherz. Münch. med. Wchnschr., 65:1180, 1918.

THYROIDITIS

Infections of the thyroid are not common, and some of the pathologic states that have been included under the designation of thyroiditis may be neither infectious nor inflammatory.

Purulent thyroiditis with abscess formation is rare but has been seen as an unusual complication of a variety of regional and general infections. The condition offers serious threat because of the anatomic relation of the thyroid to fascial planes and the danger of extension of infection into the mediastinum. Opportunity for identification of invading organisms has been limited and the effectiveness of antibiotic and chemotherapeutic agents has not been satisfactorily evaluated. *Chronic specific infections* of the thyroid such as tuberculosis, syphilis and actinomycosis affect the gland so rarely that specialists of great experience may never encounter a case.

The clinical problem of thyroiditis is centered about the consideration of three forms of subacute or chronic disease, all of which are of completely unknown etiology.

The most common form of thyroiditis was first described in 1904 and again in 1936 by the Swiss surgeon, Guervain. It has been variously called **Guervain's thyroiditis** and subacute, pseudotuberculous and giant cell thyroiditis. It occurs at any age but has been seen six times more frequently in women than in men.

Pathologically, the gland is involved in a subacute inflammatory process which accomplishes extensive destruction. The acinar cells of the thyroid follicles disappear, and their former location is recognizable only by the persistence of colloid residue in which there are numerous, extremely large, multinuclear cells. During the acute phase there is considerable infiltration with round cells and polymorphonuclear leukocytes which occasionally form tiny abscesses. As the condition progresses, fibrous tissue reaction may be extensive. Although the lesions superficially resemble those of tuberculosis, no tubercle bacillus has ever been recovered.

The onset is sudden, with fever, rapid pulse, leukocytosis and increased sedimentation rate. The gland is exquisitely tender. Pain which may be severe is exaggerated by swallowing and is often referred to the ears and jaw. At first the tenderness may be confined to only one lobe but later it extends to other parts or to the entire gland. The thyroid enlarges but is seldom more than twice its normal size. Symptoms may suggest thyrotoxicosis but the basal metabolic rate is not elevated. The uptake of radioactive iodine by the thyroid is so greatly diminished as to resemble that of advanced myxedema. This has been found even in cases in which only one lobe of the thyroid appears to be involved.

Spontaneous recovery of normal function of the thyroid gland may be expected, although the condition may remain painful and troublesome for several weeks or months. The inevitably good prognosis and the irregular course of the disease have made judgment concerning the efficacy of therapeutic measures extremely difficult. Rapid improvement has been reported after a single exposure to 600 to 800 r of roentgen irradiation. The administration of 6-propylthiouracil has also been recommended. Recent reports indicate that the use of cortisone is regularly followed by prompt remission. Surgical intervention in this type of thyroiditis is not indicated.

A much rarer form of thyroiditis was described by Riedel in 1896 and is usually called **Riedel's struma.** It affects both men and women, usually after the age of 50. It develops insidiously without fever and at first may cause no symptoms. Ordinarily it affects only one lobe or part of a lobe, but even when sharply localized tends to extend outside of the gland to involve adjacent tissue. In its development it may invade adjacent structures, producing hoarseness and stridor or symptoms attributable to constriction of the trachea or esophagus. The involved portions are hard but not tender. It is less likely to be confused with other forms of thyroiditis than with cancer, from which in many cases it can be differentiated only by biopsy. Surgical treatment may be necessary for establishment of a diagnosis or for correction of pressure on surrounding structures.

The third form of thyroiditis was first described by Hashimoto in 1912. It is called also **Struma lymphomatosa.** It consists of a diffuse and extensive lymphoid infiltration of the entire gland. The condition is rare. The relatively few cases have occurred most often in women between the ages of 40 and 50. Its occurrence in men is extremely unusual. The onset is usually insidious, although fever with pain and tenderness over the gland has occasionally been noted in the early stages. In its chronic state it is almost completely asymptomatic except for the goiter which is firm, irregular in shape and often large enough to press without invasion on its surrounding structures. It is easily confused with simple multinodular goiter, while the hardness and bosselations of the gland may suggest the possibility of carcinoma. Strictly, differentiation from these two conditions can be made only by biopsy or operation. Spontaneous recovery cannot be expected and hypothyroidism secondary to the infiltration has been reported. Roentgen ray treatment is often beneficial. Surgery is not necessary except for diagnosis and occasionally because of the large size of the goiter.

DAVID P. BARR

References

Crile, G., Jr.: Practical Aspects of Thyroid Disease. Philadelphia, W. B. Saunders Co., 1949.

DeQuervain, F.: Die akute, nicht eitrige Thyreoiditis. Mitt. Grenzgeb. Med. Chir., Supplement 2, 1904.

———, and Giordanengo, G.: Die akute und subakute nicht-eitrige Thyreoiditis. Mitt. Grenzgeb. Med. Chir., 44:538, 1936.

Hashimoto, H.: Zur Kenntnis der lymphomatösen Veränderungen der Schilddrüse (Struma lymphomatosa). Arch. f. klin. Chir., 97:219, 1912.

Lasser, R. P.: Subacute Thyroiditis Treated with Cortisone. J.A.M.A., 152:1133, 1953.

Riedel: Die chronische zur Bildung eisenharter Tumoren führende Entzündung der Schilddrüse. Verhandl. d. deutsch. Gesell. Chir., 25:101, 1896.

Robbins, J., Rall, J. E., Trunnell, J. B., and Rawson, R. W.: The Effect of Thyroid-Stimulating Hormone in Acute Thyroiditis. J. Clin. Endocrin., 11: 1106, 1951.

MALIGNANT DISEASE OF THE THYROID

Cancer of the thyroid is not a common disease, and analysis of two large series of autopsies done in general hospitals indicates that it is a rare cause of death. Nevertheless the reports of surgical pathologists indicate the presence of recognizably malignant cells in 4 to 10 per cent of nodular goiters and 19 to 24 per cent of solitary nodules of the gland. These figures make imperative the consideration of possible cancer in any nodular goiter which is increasing in size or in any solitary nodule of the thyroid.

Many forms of epithelial tumors of the thyroid have been described and classification has offered great difficulty. Morphologically, tumors which present the histologic appearance of benign fetal adenoma may invade blood vessels with formation of distant metastases in the lung and skeleton, while others morphologically malignant in appearance may grow so slowly as never to cause clinical symptoms of cancerous invasion.

Of the malignant tumors of the thyroid, *papillary adenocarcinoma* is the most frequently encountered. It occurs characteristically but not exclusively in younger persons and is twice as frequent in women as in men. From a small and sometimes undetectable tumor in the gland, it may spread to adjacent lymph nodes, the tissue of which may be almost entirely replaced by the new growth. Such invaded lymph nodes have sometimes been mistakenly regarded as aberrant thyroid tissue in which primary malignancy has developed. Papillary adenocarcinoma may metastasize beyond the confines of the neck to the chest, where x-ray examination reveals miliary nodules fanning out of the hilum. Skeletal metastases are relatively infrequent. If detected early and adequately treated, the salvage rate in this type of cancer is high and the prognosis excellent. Even those who have pulmonary or skeletal metastases may live for many years.

Alveolar adenocarcinoma, another tumor of relatively frequent occurrence and of only moderate malignancy, is found more often in older people. It may metastasize both to regional lymph nodes and through the blood stream to the lungs and skeleton where its structure may at times simulate normal thyroid tissue. Hürthle cell carcinoma and solid adenocarcinoma are relatively rare tumors which have a moderate degree of malignancy. Small cell carcinoma (carcinoma simplex) and giant cell carcinoma which may spread with extraordinary rapidity constitute only a small percentage of the cancers of the thyroid. Epidermoid carcinoma and other highly malignant tumors such as fibrosarcoma and primary lymphoma have an extremely low incidence.

In general it may be said that highly malignant, undifferentiated neoplasms of the thyroid have slight if any endocrine function. The use of autoradiographic techniques has shown, however, that almost half of the specimens of thyroid cancer which have been studied pick up measurable amounts of radioactive iodine. Experience indicates that this ability is retained in those tumors which contain colloid-filled follicles and only rarely in those which do not contain colloid. In no instance has a malignant tumor concentrated as much as adjacent normal thyroid tissue.

Therapeutically an important advance has been the demonstration of an increased ability of several metastatic cancers of the thyroid to take up radioactive iodine following the removal or destruction of all normal thyroid tissue.

The clinical diagnosis of cancer of the thyroid offers great difficulties. The possibility of malignant growth must be considered in every nodular goiter. Nodules encountered in the glands of young persons and single nodules at any age should excite particular attention. Rapid growth of any part of the gland should be regarded usually as an indication for surgical treatment. Abnormal fixity of the thyroid, and involvement of the recurrent laryngeal nerves and nodules in the adjacent tissue, are signs suggestive of cancer, but too often indicate extensions which make complete surgical removal difficult or impossible.

Treatment consists in radical surgical resection of the cancerous tissue. This should usually be attempted even after extension of the growth to lymph nodes and other adjacent structures in the cervical region, and even when distant metastases are demonstrable. Roentgen irradiation is indicated in some in-operable cases and in selected cases as a postoperative measure. Treatment of the original growth and of metastases with radioactive iodine is still in the experimental stage. Treatment by radioactive iodine should be reserved for inoperable and metastatic thyroid cancer. It should not be used until a maximum pick-up of radioiodine has been demonstrated.

DAVID P. BARR

References

Cole, W. H., Slaughter, D. P., and Rossiter, L. J.: Potential Dangers of Nontoxic Nodular Goiter. J.A.M.A., *127*:883, 1945.

Fitzgerald, P. J., Foote, F. W., Jr.: Function of Various Types of Thyroid Carcinoma as Revealed by Radioautographic Demonstration of Radioactive Iodine (I[131]). J. Clin. Endocrinol., *9*:1153, 1949.

Rogers, W. F., Jr., Asper, S. P., Jr., and Williams R. H.: Clinical Significance of Malignant Neoplasms of the Thyroid Gland. New England J. Med., *237*:569, 1947.

Seidlin, S. M., Marinelli, L. D. and Oshry, E.: Radioactive Iodine Therapy. Effect on Functioning Metastases of Adenocarcinoma of the Thyroid. J.A.M.A., *132*:838, 1946.

VanderLaan, W. P.: The Occurrence of Carcinoma of the Thyroid Gland in Autopsy Material. New England J. Med., *237*:221, 1947.

DISEASES OF THE PITUITARY GLAND

INTRODUCTION

The organization of this brief account of diseases of the pituitary body follows conventional textbook lines. Those disorders long correctly attributed to this structure are of course included, together with a number of complex or imperfectly defined entities, such as anorexia nervosa, Fröhlich's syndrome and ateleiosis, to which pituitary defect contributes or is often supposed to contribute. Several questions of the responsibility of the pituitary body for diseases of the thyroid, adrenal cortex and gonads are dealt with in the sections on these dependent or semi-dependent glands. The clinical expressions of such disorders as Cushing's syndrome, Graves' disease and eunuchoidism are at least in substantial part due to variations in the secretion of these target glands. Some indications of the widely ramifying influences of the anterior lobe hormones are, however, included in this section.

A. T. KENYON

THE HORMONES OF THE ANTERIOR LOBE

Six separate agents have now been isolated in relatively pure form and have been found to repair the respective anterior lobe defects in hypophysectomized animals. In several instances administration to the normal animal produces specific exaggerations of structure and function. Each agent may be taken to constitute a fair representation of an anterior lobe hormone. It should be kept in mind, however, that in no instance is it certain that the actual secretion is at hand. The mere detection of such a hormone in the blood itself presents nearly insuperable difficulties as a rule, to say nothing of chemical identification and characterization.

In general, the properties of pituitary hormones in man must be inferred from the study of disease and from our knowledge of experimental research on lower forms. Desirable and, in the end, necessary information provided by the administration of pituitary principles to man himself has been difficult to come by. The recent accomplishments with adrenocorticotrophin (ACTH) constitute a dramatic exception and arouse hopes that the problems of the production of an abundance of sufficiently pure material for use in man can be solved for other hormones as well. Thus far, however, the results are often sadly disappointing, as witness the thirty-three years of labor between Evans and Long's growth-promoting extract, effective in rats, and today's unsuccessful use of better extracts in man. The reasons for failure are complex. Man is sensitive to the parenteral introduction of foreign protein and reacts often with inflammation, fever and malaise. Individualized states of allergy are relatively common. Large amounts of highly purified agents are accordingly required in man, placing prodigious demands upon the producer. It is possible, furthermore, that the protein hormones of the anterior lobe are more varied in chemical structure from species to species than is apparently true of insulin, for example. There are distinctive chemical differences in some instances between the most highly purified physiologic counterparts from differing species, as in the interstitial-cell-stimulating hormones from swine and sheep. Whether these differences are sufficient to foster antibody formation when the hormone is given to an alien species or not is unknown. In any event, anterior lobe hormones or closely associated proteins are commonly antigenic, and neutralizing antibodies (antihormones) arise to terminate physiologic effect after long-continued and repeated injection into another species. Such antihormones have been demonstrated in man, notably to several foreign gonadotrophins, but rarely or not at all to the native chorionic gonadotrophin. Antihormone formation may be expected against other pituitary hormones and may seriously limit long-term study and treatment. The extent to which these and other problems inherent in the use of injected protein hormones in man can be solved is tomorrow's story. As it stands, clinical research and treatment are still sorely handicapped.

The Growth or Somatotrophic Hormone. Its existence was inferred from knowledge of excesses and deficiencies of growth in man as exemplified by gigantism and dwarfism, and later from dwarfing following hypophysectomy (Aschner, 1910; Smith, 1926). Active extracts were first obtained by Evans and Long (1921), and a relatively homogeneous principle by electrophoretic, diffusion and solubility tests extracted by Li, Evans and Simpson (1944–45). It restores the defective growth of hypophysectomized animals (rats) and carries the growth of hypophysectomized or normal rats to gigantism. The growth in these circumstances is relatively harmonious. Skin, musculature, skeleton, viscera and the cardiovascular system grow together. There is little established influence on the brain and no or minimal effect on the adrenal cortex, thyroid or gonads, the proper targets of other anterior lobe hormones. In all probability this growth agent is the sole factor responsible for the distorted overgrowth of the soft tissues and certain bones induced in adult dogs by cruder extracts, changes constituting experimental acromegaly. The epiphyses of bones of dogs, unlike those of rats, close with maturity, providing a test animal similar to man.

As studied by metabolic techniques, the effects of the growth hormone are manifold. Nitrogen is quickly retained, expressing the deposition of new protein. This response should prove helpful in detecting the effects of growth hormone in man, but it has thus far not been obtained even with the best extracts used. Insulin is apparently a necessary cofactor for the nitrogen-retaining, i.e., growth, effect.

Many profound influences upon carbohydrate metabolism are produced by hypophysial extracts. Several of these influences are exerted by preparations comprised chiefly or entirely of the growth hormone. The physiologic mechanisms involved are complex and often a subject of disagreement. The reviews of Bennet and Evans in Pincus and Thimann, Soskin and Levine and Young will serve to introduce the reader to details. Roughly put, the animal lacking a hypophysis is exquisitely sensitive to insulin, cannot maintain its glycogen stores during fasting, and does not show the usual evolution of diabetes mellitus after pancreatectomy (Houssay phenomenon). Extracts restore the state prior to hypophysectomy and may furthermore induce an insulin-resistant diabetes in the normal animals of some species (dogs, for example), followed by islet cell degeneration and a permanent, insulin-sensitive diabetes enduring after cessation of treatment (Young's or metahypophysial diabetes). The growth hormone apparently serves to maintain one element of the fasting carbohydrate stores (muscle glycogen, glycostatic effect). It is, or else is closely associated with, the diabetogenic agent effective in the normal dog, in which it appears to act independent of the adrenal cortex. Thus it seems likely that the association of unusual growth and diabetes mellitus in acromegaly may well be due to excesses of a single agent, the capacity of the individual pancreas to secrete insulin determining whether diabetes will or will not occur.

The adrenal hormone secreted in response to ACTH is likewise diabetogenic in certain species (man and partially depancreatized or force-fed rat) and antagonizes the action of insulin. These are presumably the experimental analogues of the diabetes mellitus of Cushing's syndrome. The precise nature of the interrelationships between the activities of the growth hormone and those of the adrenal steroids on carbohydrate metabolism is obscure, and it is not clear whether the liability of patients with hypopituitarism to spontaneous hypoglycemia or their sensitivity to insulin is due chiefly to the lack of the one or of the other, or of both.

The amounts of the growth hormone circulating in the human system can be assessed now only by its effects. No workable biologic assay of the agent in body fluids is available, although its presence has been detected in the plasma of acromegalics. At the moment, therefore, estimates depend on a congeries of clinical and intrinsically nonspecific laboratory techniques. Though a good deal can be accomplished by sophisticated use of what we have, better methods are badly needed. The response of man to administered growth hormone, as stated before, has not yet been ascertained, even the best extracts being poorly tolerated or giving aberrant results.

The Lactogenic Hormone (Prolactin, Galactin). This is an agent necessary for lactation and apparently for the full growth of the mammae. Lyons' anatomic studies demonstrate a complex synergism among prolactin, ovarian and adrenal steroids and the growth hormone in the maturation of the lactating breast of the rat with a supplementary effect by the thyroid. Pure or highly pure protein agents obtained by Li, Simpson and Evans (1942) and by White, Bosnes and Long (1942) have the property of inducing survival and secretion by the transitory inactive corpus luteum of the normally cyclic rat. This is apparently an extraordinary example of the use by this organism of a single pituitary hormone for two distinct processes, one gonadotrophic, the other of somatic kind, but related to genital events. The term "luteotrophin" is often adopted for this agent to describe the gonadotrophic effect. It must be recalled, however, that such luteotrophic action is known only for the rat and has not been established as serving other species, such as man, whose corpora lutea normally exhibit a secretory life of some days. Clinical knowledge of prolactin is primitive. Assays of the hormone in body fluids are in the course of development. Administration of the hormone has neither been well controlled in the scientific sense nor productive of clear or useful results.

The Follicle-Stimulating Hormone (FSH). The best products from the chemical standpoint indicate a glycoprotein stimulating and necessary for the growth of the ovarian follicle, but requiring a cofactor provided by the luteinizing hormone (LH), at least for estrogen secretion and for ovulation. In the male, spermatogenesis is facilitated, although androgens alone, arising in response to LH, may suffice to support spermatogenesis in some species. In all probability there is some systematic scheme whereby FSH and androgens cooperate in the control of the seminiferous epithelium, with experimental conditions and species variations dramatizing first one aspect and then the other, but leaving the over-all pattern incoherent and inconsistent to us for the moment.

Deficiencies in FSH secretion contribute to the ovarian and testicular defects of hypopituitarism, yielding especially failures in development or maintenance of the follicular or seminiferous apparatus. In most instances peculiarities of LH secretion are involved as well, and independent and isolated disorder of FSH secretion is difficult to establish. The multiplicity of problems arising from the delicate interplay of these forces on the ovary during the menstrual cycle can be barely indicated here.

Normal human urine contains a gonadotrophin or gonadotrophins which may be increased to as much as tenfold or more by removal of the gonads or by the normal involution of the ovaries at the menopause. Unfortunately, this material has not been sufficiently purified to permit precise chemical definition. It has follicular growth-provok-

ing properties and excites estrogen secretion, and, if the analogy with anterior lobe extracts holds, may be dual in composition. Unlike chorionic gonadotrophin, abundantly secreted by the human placenta during pregnancy, it requires no pituitary cofactor for its influence on the ovaries, acting in hypophysectomized animals. Spermatogenesis and androgen production are facilitated by suitable doses in the male. The material may be assayed with fair efficiency either by its effects on the ovaries or by its indirect effects on the uteri of immature rats or mice. The results are of great value in determining whether the pituitary body or the gonads are primarily responsible for gonadal deficiency. High values bespeak primary gonadal defect, low values indicate pituitary defect if repeatedly obtained. Normal values are ambiguous. The administration of estrogens (or androgens in sufficient doses) inhibits the secretion of these materials by the anterior lobe.

The administration of foreign gonadotrophins to man for purposes of exciting the ovarian follicles to grow and to secrete estrogens has been disappointing. The difficulties may lie in the products, in antihormone formation, in imperfect knowledge of the character of the defect in the subject, and in failures to imitate nature's delicate synergism between FSH and LH. There is every reason to believe that all factors are involved.

The Luteinizing Hormone (LH) or Interstitial - Cell - Stimulating Hormone (ICSH). This is a glycoprotein, but purified (or pure) agents from swine (Chow et al., 1942) and sheep (Li et al., 1940–42) differ chemically. This hormone is a synergist and a companion hormone to FSH. It may cooperate with FSH in maturing the ovarian follicle and is essential to ovulation and formation of the corpus luteum. It is now usually held responsible in great part for estrogen secretion. In rats at least, continued secretory activity of the formed corpus luteum is attributed to luteotrophin (see Lactogenic Hormone) rather than to LH. The trophic influence of LH on the interstitial cells of the ovaries of rats, although used for assay, has not yet acquired real physiologic meaning. Luteinizing hormone is, however, a powerful stimulant of androgen production by the interstitial cells of the testes in all species studied. Deficiencies in hormone production by ovaries and testes in hypopituitarism are attributable to deficiencies in LH secretion. The gonadotrophic material in the urine of normal and castrate humans has some LH-like propensities despite the common practice of designating only the FSH-like properties. Assays are discussed under FSH. Luteinizing hormone of animal pituitary origin has not been successfully given to man, although the somewhat similar human chorionic gonadotrophin is quite potent.

The Thyrotrophic Hormone (TSH). This is probably a glycoprotein, although not yet obtained in pure form. It is effective in stimulating the release of stored thyroid hormone from the thyroid gland and probably in facilitating its manufacture as well. Its properties may not be solely thyrotrophic. Pituitary extracts rich in TSH evoke exophthalmos in several laboratory animals even in the absence of the thyroid. Thus the common association of hyperthyroidism and exophthalmos in Graves' disease may illustrate these two activities of a single agent. The matter is complex, however, since dissociation of these expressions of disease does occur and the two effects have not been proved due to a single chemical individual. Although thyrotrophic effects can be obtained from human blood and urine, sufficiently sensitive and simple methods of assay have not been perfected, so that thyrotrophic influences in routine study must be judged largely from secondary thyroid activity. Thyrotrophic hormone, which is active in man often for a limited period only, evokes increased uptake of radioactive iodine by the thyroid and elevated basal metabolic rate among other responses.

The Adrenocorticotrophic Hormone (ACTH). The activity resides in short peptide or polypeptide groupings. The protein structure identified by Sayers, White and Long (1943) and Li, Simpson and Evans (1943) no longer appears essential for activity but may be a carrier. The material stimulates the adrenal cortex of man to secrete an agent or agents with the properties of inducing sodium, chloride and water retention, potassium and uric acid diuresis, hyperglycemia and glycosuria that are resistant to correction by insulin, loss of nitrogen in the urine, modifications of circulating blood cells, elevation of urinary corticoids and 17-ketosteroids in man. In time these adrenal secretions give rise to the metabolic and clinical expressions of Cushing's syndrome. Great advances in our understanding of the nature of the adrenal steroids secreted under stimulation are now under way by virtue of microphysical and microchemical analyses of blood and of urinary products. While the effects of ACTH closely resemble those of cortisone or hydrocortisone, indications are growing that hydrocortisone (compound F of Kendall) is probably the steroid most involved in man. Others may well be involved. The rise in urinary 17-ketosteroids appears of a complex origin and is not to be taken as specifying solely the increased secretion of an adrenal androgen.

ACTH reproduces the extraordinary properties of cortisone in ameliorating both the local inflammation of rheumatoid arthritis and certain general reactions as fever, increased sedimentation rate, anorexia and malaise, discovered by Hench, Polley, Slocumb and Kendall (1949–50). This great work has been widely extended and its meaning closely examined although hardly fully explored. It appears that a multiplicity of host reactions in illness, including the articular and febrile elements of rheumatoid arthritis and of rheumatic fever, the cutaneous and systemic elements of lupus erythematosus, the bronchospasm and urticarias of allergic reactions, the colitis of ulcerative colitis and numerous other manifestations of obscure illness, may be ameliorated or abolished by ACTH as by cortisone. Temporary involution of lymphatic tissues in lymphomas may be induced. Signs and symptoms often recur at varying rates when treatment is stopped so that no cure occurs, and some balance must be struck between the manifestations of the original illness and hyperadrenocorticism in those requiring continued treatment with large doses. No elimination of a bacterial or viral agent of disease has been accomplished. The mechanisms of relief of symptoms are complex and probably vary from situation to situation. Reduction in the intensity of the inflammatory process with better preservation of vascular tone and reduction of exudate (Ebert and Wissler, 1951), modifications of the permeability of connective tissue ground substance, retardation of fibroblast proliferation, and reduction in the rates of release of antibodies are of significance. In lower forms the invasion of the host by bacteria and viruses is favored by these alterations in the mechanisms of protection. Under the conditions of work in man such potential dangers appear to materialize only occasionally. Defervescence, stimulation of appetite and enhancement of the sense of well being are often involved in the ameliorative process. It should be noted that no intrinsic defect in either the adrenal cortex or the pituitary-adrenal systems has been established in those systemic diseases ameliorated by cortisone or ACTH. Selye's concept of deranged adrenal function arising as a maladaptation to non-specific stress and resulting in widespread damage excited great interest and has been usefully provocative. It is now being subjected to searching inquiry and to qualification or challenge (Sayers, Bauer and Clark, Ingle and Baker). Details of the use of ACTH in the treatment of various diseases must be sought under those diseases influenced.

In ordinary circumstances the secretion of adrenocorticotropin is geared to a low level sufficient to maintain the necessary workaday activities of the adrenal cortex. With a number of diverse stresses, the common physiologic denominator of which is not now apparent, the pituitary-adrenal system is set in to high play. The resulting extraordinary increment in adrenal activity is of vital importance, and the vulnerability of man and animals with grave adrenal and pituitary deficiencies is in part due to its lack. Venning and Browne have provided numerous examples of enhanced corticoid excretion after operations, burns, fractures and the like, illustrating this process in man. Stress, however, is not indivisible. Damaging events are not alike insofar as the adrenal is concerned any more than they are in any other respect. More precise description of the circumstances requiring activation of the pituitary-adrenal axis in man are under way (Thorn et al., 1953). The usefulness of response to epinephrine in detecting the state of this mechanism is doubtful at this writing. The physiologic account of Baker and Ingle (1953) should be consulted.

Preparations of adrenocorticotropin are known as "corticotropin" to the Council on Pharmacy and Chemistry (see New and Nonofficial Remedies, 1953), and standardization is in terms of a powder which is accepted both as an international and as a U.S.P. standard. Assay is by depletion of the ascorbic acid content of the adrenals of hypophysectomized rats (Sayers). One milligram of the powder is 1 unit. Dosages at first amount to 10 to 50 I.U. daily intramuscularly, divided into four doses. Moderate guarded increase is feasible if necessary. Dosages of "purified corticotropin" are equivalent (clinical units) only when given intramuscularly

or subcutaneously. A single daily injection may be given with the longer acting preparations (in gelatin). Intravenous administration is possible but experience is limited and the hazards not completely assessed. Possible sensitivity should be tested for irrespective of the manner of administration. The hazards of treatment are largely those of hyperadrenocorticism. Alkalosis, potassium deficits, excessive salt and water retention may occur and can be minimized by salt restriction and the administration of potassium supplements. Glycosuria may occur. Psychoses occur from time to time. Other clinical phenomena of Cushing's syndrome appear with sustained use. Reduction in eosinophil counts by 50 per cent or more forms a useful guide to effectiveness if used with attention to normal variations. Discontinuance should always be gradual and carefully watched to allow the patient's own mechanism to take over if this is possible and to provide for orderly replacement when this mechanism is defective (as in hypopituitarism).

Chorionic Gonadotrophin. The placentas of several species constitute temporary but important organs of internal secretion with gonadotrophic properties so nearly like those of the anterior lobe that brief if incomplete notation must be given here. Chorionic gonadotrophin is apparently a glycoprotein, arising from the human placenta and excreted in the urine. It gives the classic Aschheim-Zondek test for pregnancy by its gonadotrophic properties in immature mice and the Friedman test by its capacity to evoke ovulation in the rabbit in heat. It is excreted in large amounts by men with testicular tumors (chorionepithelioma and others). It does not produce follicular growth in the ovary of the hypophysectomized rodent, differing thereby from pituitary and castrate urine factors. It is a powerful agent in protracting the life and function of the normal corpus luteum in women and in exciting androgen secretion in men with responsive testes. Its real usefulness in correcting disorders of the menstrual cycle is uncertain.

Pregnant Mare's Serum Gonadotrophin. This is a protein with both follicle-stimulating and luteinizing properties. It produces antihormones readily in man in contrast to human chorionic gonadotrophin. Its usefulness and effectiveness in man is a matter of disagreement.

A. T. KENYON

HYPERPITUITARISM

ACROMEGALY AND GIGANTISM

Definitions. Acromegaly is a chronic disease characterized essentially by the progressive and systematic overgrowth of many tissues in response to intense and long-sustained stimulation by the growth hormone of the pituitary body. The name designates the striking and presenting enlargement of the acral or terminal portions of the body, the hands, feet and certain elements of the face and head. Prior to normal ossification the youthful epiphysial cartilages are sensitive to increments in growth hormone, and *gigantism* may result, which is intensified if epiphysial closure is delayed. Some half or more of the recorded giants are acromegalic. It is the author's view that a serious reexamination of the etiology of gigantism is required in those instances (eunuchoid gigantism, and so on) in which excessive growth proceeds for some time without any vestiges of typical acromegalic transformations of the face and extremities. These rare entities will not be considered here.

History. Attention was focused on the disorder by Marie's description (1886) and fortunate choice of the name "acromegaly." The pituitary tumor was identified by Minkowski (1887) and Marie (1890). The concept of hyperpituitarism was advanced by Massalongo (1892) and Tamburini (1894). The American physician Woods Hutchinson (1895) early understood the anterior pituitary body as a prime regulator of growth. Several studies of the relationship of gigantism to acromegaly culminated in the work of Lannois and Roy (1903), who are credited with the modern view. Early discussions centered about the relative importance of hypopituitarism, hyperpituitarism, thymic hyperplasia (Fritsche and Klebs, 1884) and constitutional disorders of a generalized sort in explanation. The demonstration by Benda (1900) of eosinophile granules in the cells of pituitary adenomas, suggesting an active secretory process, and the growing appreciation that dwarfism on the one hand and acromegaly and gigantism on the other expressed opposite poles of pituitary activity, prepared minds for the modern experimental period. The earlier hypophysectomies by Aschner (1912) and Cushing and associates (1912) in dogs were followed by retardation of growth, and those of Smith, especially on rats (1926), provided a full demonstration of dwarfism and associated endocrine defects in a readily available animal that could be treated with small amounts of extracts. Much of the definitive experimental work since has been done on this species. Evans and Long (1921) first induced exceptional growth in normal rats with crude anterior pituitary extracts, and the repair of growth defects in hypophysectomized animals soon followed.

Li, Evans and Simpson (1944–45) finally isolated a protein that appeared homogeneous by numerous exacting physicochemical and biologic criteria. Appreciation of the influences of the hypophysis on carbohydrate metabolism was greatly advanced by the discovery of Houssay and Biosotti (1930) that hypophysectomy ameliorated pancreatic diabetes. (See discussion of the Growth Hormone, p. 746).

Etiology. Acromegaly and that form of gigantism properly associated with it (see Definitions) are due to hypersecretion from abundant neoplastic or hyperplastic eosinophile cells of the anterior lobe of the pituitary body. As the major and decisive effects are those of the growth hormone, this agent may accordingly be considered to come from these acidophile elements. Adenomas are most frequently described in autopsy or surgical material, although in large glands it may be difficult to say whether the origin was focal or diffuse. Microscopic eosinophile adenomas may be found in routine autopsies and may well represent sites from which larger tumors may arise. Rarely (Lewis, 1905), the gland may be of normal size, but contain an excess of active eosinophils. Since the normal mechanism controlling the growth and secretory activity of the eosinophils is poorly understood, and since disease has given no clear cue, it is difficult to guess the factors governing such an exceptional and abnormal transformation of cellular precursors into active eosinophils.

Acromegaly affects the two sexes equally. Gigantism affects the male chiefly. Over one half of the patients eventually considered acromegalic trace the onset to the third decade. The greatest incidence thus approximates the end of normal growth. The physiologic factors governing the termination of normal growth, however, are so poorly understood that it is impossible to assign them any clear influence on the processes leading to acromegalization. Gonadal deficiency arising in the course of pituitary disease may be expected to facilitate continued growth, especially of the long bones. Castration, however, does not commonly produce either gigantism or acromegaly, so that gonadal defect alone cannot be considered to bear primary responsibility. Though acromegaly may arise during pregnancy, the possible predisposing force of the physiologic hypertrophy of the anterior lobe at this time has not been ascertained.

It is a general rule that heredity must be given substantial weight in considerations of the cause of abnormal hyperplastic and neo-plastic processes. Concrete evidence here is surprisingly scant. Only 4 per cent of acro-megalics give a history of similarly affected individuals in the family, although in 20 per cent some note is made of large relatives (Davidoff, 1926). A hereditary predisposi-tion to diabetes mellitus as a complication seems clearer (Coggeshall and Root, 1940).

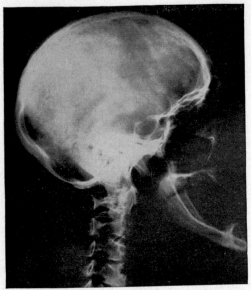

Fig. 88. Roentgenogram of skull of an acromegalic with verified eosinophile adenoma of the hypophysis. Note the ballooned sella turcica, thick skull, large frontal sinus and large mandible.

Pathology of the Pituitary Gland and Its Environs. The present section deals with the expanding gland itself and the mechan-ical consequences of such expansion. To avoid repetition, those aspects of morbid anatomy due to hormonal influences will be discussed later.

The *pituitary body* is usually large and the proliferative process considered adenomatous, although hyperplasia occurs on occasion. Al-though cellular aberrations are common with multinucleate cells and amitotic division, and the term "carcinoma" has been applied in some instances, metastases are rare. Spread is largely by direct extension of the main tumor mass. Eosinophils (acidophils, alpha cells) usually dominate the cellular popula-tion. Gonadal defects have been ascribed to the paucity of basophils. In some tumors eosinophile granules are sparse, indicating a transitional type between eosinophile and chromophobe adenomas, and the manifesta-tions of acromegaly are indistinct and ill defined. In others, degenerative changes and hemorrhage, leading to cyst formation, may come to predominate and the residual eosino-phils may be few. Thus even intense acro-megalization may come to a stage of arrest.

The growth of the tumor is typically slow and progressive. The sella turcica is visibly distended in the majority of instances and assumes a ballooned appearance from pres-sure within its confines (Fig. 88). The aver-age adult sella turcica measured by roent-genogram is 8 to 9 mm. in depth and 9 to 10 mm. in length. Upper normal limits are variously given as 10 to 12 and 12 to 16 mm. respectively.

These limits are usually but not necessarily substantially exceeded. The floor of the sella is commonly depressed, and the sphenoid cells may even be invaded. At first the dorsum sellae is displaced backwards. Together with the clinoid processes, it may eventually be eroded and destroyed. The diaphragma sellae is forced upwards and may be ruptured. Pressure is thus exerted upon the overlying optic chiasm and neighboring portions of the optic system. A number of other cerebral areas come to express damage in their own particular ways.

The tumor may appear stationary for years, accommodations to existing pressure takes place, and secretory activity declines into relative quiescence. Thus a stage of arrest which may last for almost any length of time supervenes. Irregularly phasic activity may recur from time to time.

Symptoms, Signs and Course. The out-ward appearance of the well advanced acro-megalic conforms, as a rule, to a single easily recognized type. There is thickening and coarsening of the features, notably of the lips and nose, with accentuation of the nor-mal eminences of the brow, nose and lower jaw. Mandibular prognathism is character-istic. The hands and feet are large, the thor-acic cage increased in size, the back stooped. These deformities are exaggerations of fam-iliar normal variations of man. The continued growth of connective tissue and bone tra-verses the path from the not remarkable through the merely peculiar to the obviously deformed so slowly and by such imperceptible gradations that the early phases escape identi-fication by the expert. Even the later phases may seem right and proper though unusual to the patient and his family. In gigantism accelerated longitudinal growth commonly appears in late boyhood and lasts longer than usual. The typical stigmata of acromegaly are superimposed in due time.

As this massive appearance emerges, a contrasting enfeeblement afflicts the victim. The disabilities are numerous. Muscular and ligamentous investments of the sella produces headaches, which may be referred to the temporal area or elsewhere and which may be intense and continuous enough to disturb sleep. On the other hand, the pain may be transient or even insignificant. As a

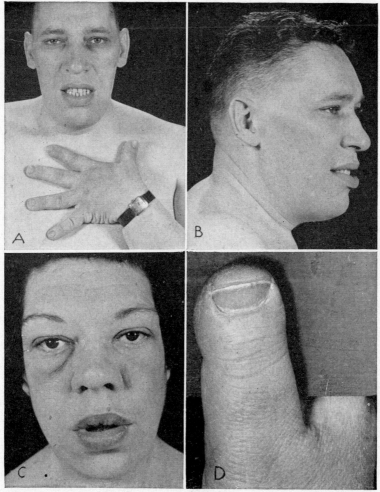

Fig. 89. Acromegaly. A and B, Note the large and elongated head, large hand, nose, ears and lips. There is also prognathism and slightly increased interdental spaces. C, Note the coarse features. D, Large, blunt-pointed thumb. (R. H. Williams: Textbook of Endocrinology.)

weakness is eventually the rule, although accounts of considerable early vigor are given. Amenorrhea or impotence commonly occurs. Excessive sweating is common. Diabetes mellitus supervenes in some 15 per cent or more. The hypertrophied and distended extremities may be painfully uncomfortable, the affected joints of the extremities and spine stiff and painful. Pain of neuritic character may occur. The expansion of the tumor against the bony result of pressure, *visual difficulties* progressing to blindness are common. Most typically the focus of pressure bears anteriorly impairing conduction in the decussating nasal nerve elements, yielding bitemporal hemianopsia with initial upper quadrant defects. Color vision is affected before form vision. Many varieties of visual defects occur, however, with blindness only in the affected eye and homonymous hemianopsia among them.

Choked disk is rare. As the growth extends, the brain suffers from direct encroachment of the tumor, from displacement and from obstruction to the ventricular systems. *Drowsiness, polydipsia* and *polyuria* may signify injury to the hypothalamus. Usually, after years of illness, death comes from the brain tumor, from cardiac failure, from diabetes, intercurrent disease or ultimate panhypopituitarism. The course is subject to great variations, and long or even permanent remissions can occur, leaving the structural changes to mark the hormonal influences of the past.

Hormonal Influences on Structure and Function. The greater part of the general somatic expressions of the disease are due to excessive secretion of the growth hormone of the pituitary body. Chondrogenesis is stimulated with manifold consequences. Increased proliferation of youthful epiphyseal cartilage elongates bones. Gonadal defect secondary to the pituitary disorder diminishes androgens and estrogens. Since these sex hormones tend to favor the ossification of the cartilages of the long bones, continued growth is favored by their lack. In the adult, residual cartilage responds to stimulation. The costal cartilages hypertrophy, thus contributing decisively to the *enlargement of the thorax;* a special form of arthritis follows proliferation of the deeper layers of joint cartilage; growth of nasal and ear cartilages contributes to the acromegalization of the face, and hypertrophy of the laryngeal cartilages makes for a *deep* and *husky voice.* Osteogenesis succeeds chondrogenesis in gigantic overgrowth. Osteogenesis from periosteum is greatly accelerated, but so accompanied by resorptive processes that systematic alteration in shape is accomplished, and the enlarged bones may come to be rarified rather than condensed. Although the skull may be thickened generally with expansion of the diploic portion, the frontal bone especially grows with protrusion of the supraciliary ridges and extraordinary excavation of the frontal sinuses beneath. The ramus of the mandible extends and the angle is blunted, thus advancing the lower jaw in the classic *mandibular prognathism.* Heaping of new alveolar bone separates the teeth. The bones of the hands and feet may be enlarged with *tufting of the terminal phalanges.* The vertebrae may come to be virtually enclosed by shells of new bone. Points of ligamentous and muscular insertions generally are accentuated by ossification within or about the attached structures, the ligamentous apparatus of the spine especially becoming affected.

Despite this extensive growth of bone, the actual enlargement of the body members is commonly due chiefly to proliferation of the soft parts, and in certain acromegalics it may be difficult to prove exceptional bone growth at all. The true skin thickens and considerable *hypertrichosis* is common. The sweat gland mass has been reported increased. Connective tissue in the skin and in the subcutaneous and submucosal regions grows in excess, giving the large broad hands and feet and the full lips and nose, increasing the flaccid cutaneous structures about the eyes, and producing the thickened corrugated "bull-dog" scalp. Hypertrophy of the soft parts about joints and fiber proliferation here and in the cartilage contribute to the arthritis. The *tongue* is often large with great hypertrophy of the papillae. Internal structures share the growth of these external and supporting tissues. The *liver* may be twice or more the normal size, and the lungs, spleen, pancreas and intestines enlarged. Grafflin's account, based on a model reconstruction, shows that renal growth depends on hypertrophy of individual nephrons. The *heart* may weigh as much as 1 kilogram, more than three times normal, with varying growth and fragmentation of individual muscle fibers. It is uncertain whether circulatory demand is sufficient to account for cardiac growth by work hypertrophy, and a primary influence of the growth hormone on the cardiac musculature may be involved. Curiously, although the giant rats responding to Li's growth hormone show substantial growth of skeletal musculature, there is no good evidence of sustained growth of this tissue in acromegalic man. The brain does not itself grow, although perineurium about peripheral nerves does proliferate, and certain ganglia have been reported enlarged.

Experimental research leaves little doubt that the associated growth of skeleton, connective tissue and viscera is due to the secretion of abnormal amounts of a single growth hormone. Similarly, thymic hypertrophy, known in acromegaly since Fritsche and Klebs (1884), and once considered as perhaps the primary factor, appears due to excesses of the growth hormone. The frequent diabetes may well be due to the growth hormone. This diabetes is variable in intensity, may or may not require large amounts of insulin for control, and may undergo spontaneous remissions. Pituitary extracts rich in the growth factor exert influences on carbohydrate metabolism opposed to those of insulin and create a strain upon the islet mechanism. The capacity of the patient's pancreas to secrete insulin would determine whether or not diabetes will transpire. Ultimate degeneration of the islets, analogous to that in dogs or cats (Young's or metahypophysial diabetes), may conceivably occur, but has not been established at autopsy.

Several other characteristics of the disease are less clearly due to excesses of the growth hormone or cannot be so accounted for at all. The *basal metabolism* is commonly increased to plus 15 or 25 or more. This contributes to the excessive sweating, but is probably not a sole and necessary cause. *Exophthalmos* is also common. These features, together with tachycardia and goiter, may combine strongly to suggest complicating Graves' disease, directing treatment toward the thyroid and suggesting excessive thyrotrophin as a factor in pathogenesis. Though Graves' disease certainly is present at times, the signs and symptoms suggesting it may often be misleading. Dissociation of these signs and symptoms is common, the goiters are often large and of a nodular colloid type, and thyroidectomy or the use of antithyroid drugs may prove disappointing. Obviously, workable assays for thyrotrophin would be most useful in analyzing this matter further. *Vascular hypertension* may occur in cases of long standing and may in part be due to sclerosis of small vessels, although the matter has not been carefully studied and other factors may enter in.

The participation of ACTH in the process of acromegaly is even more uncertain. Although moderate overgrowth of the adrenal cortex is common, studies of urinary 17-ketosteroids have not given high results, and the typical clinical expressions of Cushing's syndrome are rarely if ever intermixed with acromegalization. The hypertrichosis of acromegaly may be due to the growth hormone itself. Since adrenal hormones appear to be antagonists to the anabolic effects of the growth hormone on protein metabolism, a case could be made out for their reactive and compensatory hypersecretion, but the whole matter is uncertain, and satisfactory assays of urinary corticoids may give the answer. The *excessive lactation* in acromegalic women may or may not have to do with prolactin.

The *gonadal defects* in acromegaly and gigantism are presumably due to secondary damage to gonadotrophic elements of the pituitary itself, either by pressure from the tumor or by involution in some subtle consequence of eosinophil proliferation. No direct damaging effects of the growth hormone on the gonads are known with the better extracts. The occasional complicating myxedema may be interpreted along similar lines. Manifest general hypopituitarism may be an end result of exhaustion of the secretory elements and of their destruction by pressure and necrosis, but this time-honored concept could well stand modern documentation.

Diagnosis. A firm grasp of the clinical expressions of acromegaly is usually adequate preparation for recognition of the disorder. The appearance in the advanced stages is pathognomonic, but its early recognition may be difficult, and in some cases time alone may tell. A documented history of progressive and unusual increases in size is important; increasing shoe and glove size or the imperfect fit of old rings may be suggestive. Photographic records of changing features are most useful. On occasion the fullness of the lips and tongue, the huskiness of the voice and puffiness about the eyes suggest myxedema, but the pallor, loss of head and body hair, dryness of the skin and depressed heat production characteristic of hypothyroidism are usually absent in acromegaly. Paresthesias and pains about the joints and elsewhere may be considered "rheumatic" or arthritic, and the headaches may be wrongly assigned to that vast, obscure category of functional headaches including migraine. Roentgenograms of the skull usually, but by no means always, show typical excavation and enlargement of the sella turcica by the time the signs and symptoms cause concern. Later perimetric studies of the visual fields may show distortion from pressure, first in color fields, later in those for form.

Measurements of the secretory activity of the adenoma are indirect and imperfect. Albright has suggested that increases in serum inorganic phosphorus may serve to indicate excesses of the growth hormones. The method has experimental support and may well prove useful. The basal metabolic rate may be normal or elevated. Diabetic glucose tolerance curves or frank diabetes mellitus usually speak for hyperactivity, particularly if accompanied by any notable insulin resistance. serial evaluations of secretory activity, x-rays of the sella, visual studies and neurologic examinations are essential for years, once the disorder is established, for the appraisal of activity of the disease process.

Treatment. In embarking upon treatment it is necessary to judge the size of any existing pituitary adenoma and its rate of growth, to estimate the secretory activity at the time and to assess the extent of damage to the visual pathways and the brain.

Irradiation of the pituitary body by x-rays is preferred. Arrest of the process often occurs, as judged by improvement in the visual fields, headache and in signs of secretory activity. The imperfections of measurements and the exceedingly slow and variable course of the disease itself make evaluation difficult. Albright has recommended the use of large doses of diethylstilbestrol based on the capacity of estrogens in experimental animals to deplete the anterior lobe of eosinophils and to retard growth. A complete account of his results is not available as yet. Surgical removal of the adenoma is commonly reserved for those in which sight is threatened. All methods may fail, and lingering disability of varying degrees with uncertain or smoldering residual activity is common or perhaps the rule.

A. T. KENYON

CUSHING'S SYNDROME

See the discussion under Diseases of the Adrenal Glands (p. 777).

PRECOCIOUS PUBERTY

Certain tumors or inflammatory lesions of the hypothalamus evoke a true precocious puberty, presumably by evoking increased anterior lobe activity before its proper time. Somatic growth is accelerated and is accompanied by the attributes of advancing puberty appropriate to the sex. The ovarian follicles grow, ovulate and give rise to secreting corpora lutea in cyclic fashion. Similarly the seminiferous epithelium matures. The characteristic effects of estrogens or androgens on the secondary sex characters are seen. This harmonious association between the germinative and the secretory functions of the gonads differentiates this process as a rule from precocious development of gonadal or of adrenal cortical origin, since with these disorders early maturation of the germinal line rarely if ever occurs.

It would appear that all hypophysial elements necessary for well organized gonadal function come into play, i.e., FSH, LH and luteotrophin (see reservations under Lactogenic Hormone, p. 747). It is not clear that the growth hormone is secreted in excessive amounts. The unusual physical growth of the boys may be ascribed to the somatotrophic effect of androgens (Kenyon et al.), that of girls possibly to estrogens. Very small tumors have been found on occasion to be the primary lesion, permitting accurate localization of pressure. Characteristically, they lie against the hypothalamus just posterior to the attachment of the stalk. This strongly suggests that the brain is an important portion of the mechanism governing the onset of puberty. Unfortunately no experimental reproduction of this phenomenon has been achieved. It is probable, however, that the macrogenitosomia classically associated with pineal tumors is actually due to pressure on these hypothalamic centers. Wilkins (1950) may be consulted for further discussion.

A. T. KENYON

HYPOPITUITARISM

The greater part of our clinical information deals with gross destructive lesions of the pituitary body causing numerous defects. Isolated impairment of the capacity of the anterior lobe to make one hormone or a group of hormones, leaving the remainder of its functions intact, is poorly understood for the most part and imperfectly documented. Nevertheless there is ample reason for expecting such defects and for believing that they do exist. Smith and MacDowell demonstrated that dwarfism in a strain of mice was associated with a deficient development of the eosinophils and that the growth could be repaired by administered pituitary material. Gonadal peculiarities were less conspicuous. There is scant evidence for a corresponding deficiency in man, and yet the circumstances that dwarfism is often inherited and that the sexual development of such dwarfs may be satisfactory suggest such an explanation. In the absence of assays for the growth hormone and in the light of our incapacity to test accurately for response of tissues to this growth hormone, the matter rests unanswered. In a number of eunuchoids, however, without obvious general defects of pituitary origin, urinary assays for gonadotrophins are low and androgen secretion in response to chorionic gonadotrophin may be substantial. This provides excellent evidence for a relatively isolated pituitary deficiency, affecting the entire gonadotrophic complex. Genetic factors are probably responsible in part. The extension of such studies to other pituitary functions is badly needed and may be possible now as far as the adrenal cortex is concerned.

SIMMONDS' DISEASE

(Panhypopituitarism)

Definition. Primary chronic hypopituitarism involves defects in several pituitary functions, leading usually to more or less general disability. Usage of the term and the criteria for nomenclature are confused for historical reasons.

History. Simmonds (1914) described an autopsy on a woman with a history of puerperal sepsis and noted cachexia, with loss of weight and atrophy of the skin, loss of pubic hair, amenorrhea and splanchnomicria. He attributed the fibrosed pituitary body to septic embolism years before. He adopted the term "pituitary cachexia," emphasized cachexia as a cardinal feature, and subsequently pointed out that similar clinical states followed damage to the anterior lobe from other causes, including tumors. Subsequent authors continued this emphasis on cachexia, often meaning excessive weight loss, although brain surgeons, including Cushing, for years recognized a related state of geroderma, weakness, loss of pubic hair, and sexual defects in the victims of chromophobe adenomas of the pituitary body who might or might not have lost much weight. The emphasis on weight loss has led to the confusion of primary pituitary disease (called Simmonds' disease or pituitary cachexia) with anorexia nervosa in certain quarters. Sheehan (1937–49) has done much to straighten matters out. His major contributions have rested on his detailed description of fresh infarcts in the anterior lobes of women dying from collapse and hemorrhage at childbirth, relating these to the ultimate fibrosis described by Simmonds and others in those who survived such injuries, and in pointing out that cachexia in the sense of weight loss was a relatively infrequent expression of the disease. He suggested "postpartum necrosis" for the lesions arising at childbirth, but retained the name of Simmonds' disease for severe hypopituitarism of whatever origin. This work brought the general clinical consequences of postpartum necrosis close to experience with pituitary tumors. Albright's term "panhypopituitarism" has had considerable appeal and is appropriate when used to mean what it says. The writer will use the more noncommittal "Simmonds' disease" in Sheehan's sense, but the reader must expect a continuing change in terminology as knowledge grows and conventions shift.

Since the modern work on hypophysectomy, especially that of Smith (1926), appreciation of the dependence of the adrenals, thyroid and gonads on the anterior pituitary body has grown. Pathologic interpretations of the secondary atrophy of dependent endocrine structures have matured along corresponding lines. It is possible that this has led to neglect of the concept of Claude and Gougerot (1908) of multiple independent glandular sclerosis, which Simmonds (1914) explicitly distinguished from his disorder. Support, however, for the existence of pluriglandular sclerosis apart from primary hypopituitarism is not sufficient now for its presentation here.

Etiology and Pathology. Postpartum necrosis of the anterior lobe of the pituitary body is common in women dying from collapse or hemorrhage at childbirth. These infarcts, which may be tiny to nearly total, have been attributed by Sheehan (1937) to local thrombosis rather than to septic embolism (Simmonds, 1914). Strands of viable tissue often survive near the attachment of the stalk or along the capsule. Fibrosis supervenes, and years later contracted shreds of anterior lobe tissue may be found in those surviving such obstetric accidents. Direct damage to the pituitary body may occur following head injuries, hemorrhage into its substance being presumably decisive. Granulomas may occur and have been attributed to tuberculosis, rarely to syphilis. Fibrosis of a diffuse type distinguishable from the more sharply demarcated scars of infarction has been noted in both sexes since Claude and Gougerot (1908) and is of obscure origin, although thought syphilitic by some.

Tumors arising either within or outside the sella may compress and destroy the pituitary body. Of those arising within, chromophobe adenomas are the most common. Developing from stem cells of the secretory elements of the anterior lobe, they are nonfunctioning, save for rare and sparse eosinophile granulation which may be associated with some degree of acromegaly. Endocrine symptoms are therefore produced by impairment of the secretory elements. The sella is ballooned, the clinoid processes eroded, the visual system encroached upon, and the brain invaded much as in the eosinophile adenomas described under Acromegaly.

Craniopharyngiomas (a term not universally accepted), also known as Rathke pouch tumors, arise from fragments of the oral epithelium remaining from the primitive invagination. Although intrasellar on rare occasions, they are more likely to proliferate from the neighborhood of the upper suprasellar reaches of the stalk. They give symptoms often during childhood in contrast to chromophobe adenomas, which typically begin during adult life. Comprised chiefly of oral epithelium often with squamous cells or important dental elements (adamantinoma), these tumors show a strong disposition to necrosis and cyst formation, with points of calcification which may be recognized on roentgenograms. The sella is likely to be stretched anteroposteriorly with erosion of the clinoids, rather than first ballooned as with primarily intrasellar lesions, and the visual system is often affected early and irregularly. The brain is slowly distorted by progressive growth, and hypothalamic symptoms are common. Neurologic texts should be consulted for a discussion of other intracranial tumors which must be distinguished from craniopharyngiomas and which may produce similar damage directly or indirectly.

With gross injury to the hypophysis of whatever origin, the gonads, adrenal cortex and thyroid glands are likely to show atrophic changes and the liver and other viscera to be small (splanchnomicria) in contrast to the splanchnomegaly seen in acromegaly.

Symptoms, Signs and Course. At the time of postpartum necrosis, hypoglycemia may occur acutely, lead to coma and require urgent use of glucose for treatment. Otherwise the signs and symptoms of hypopituitarism evolve slowly, often over a period of years, by virtue of the gradual development of the responsible lesion. Gonadal functions seem most sensitive. After postpartum necrosis the menses often do not return. With chromophobe adenomas, amenorrhea is often the first stigma in women. If the effects of a craniopharyngioma or chromophobe adenoma appear at puberty, sexual development may be retarded, while growth continues for a while, giving a characteristic eunuchoid appearance to the victim. This, however, is rare. It is not usually possible to identify dissociation of gonadotrophic defects, follicle-stimulating and luteinizing hormones failing together. The atrophy of the gonads and dependent genitalia is profound in any severe grade of hypopituitarism.

Atrophy of the skin is common. There is infantile smoothness, dryness and a fine wrinkling which, when extreme, gives that appearance of precocious aging (geroderma) that so struck Simmonds. The subcutaneous fat is usually well preserved, although on occasion when weight loss is great it may largely disappear. Body hair is usually reduced, and loss of pubic hair, the beard and

axillary hair, given time and a severe lesion, is common and of diagnostic significance. These atrophic skin changes are partly due to reduction in androgen secretion, although the role of loss of the growth hormone is not clear. The skin is rarely puffy as in myxedema despite the commonly reduced basal heat production, which may reach levels as low as minus 40 for long periods. Rarely, however, typical myxedema appears (*pituitary myxedema*). Radio-iodine uptake by the thyroid gland and serum-precipitable iodine are decreased as in primary hypothyroidism. The skin is commonly pale with a faint yellowish cast, occasionally but by no means always due in part to a normocytic anemia, and tans poorly. Even with manifest suprarenal deficiency Addisonian pigmentation does not often occur. Thus the usual expressions of hypothyroidism and hypoadrenocorticism are qualified and blurred. This may be in part due to residual activity of these dependent glands forming minimal amounts of hormone apart from the influences of thyrotrophin and ACTH. It may also mean that the full expressions of thyroid and adrenal deficiencies as seen in primary disorders of these structures require anterior lobe influence on other systems of the organism. Such a requirement would be analogous to those for diabetes mellitus due to pancreatectomy and to diabetes insipidus due to destruction of the diencephalo-posterior lobe complex. The integrity of the anterior lobe appears essential for the evolution of both syndromes.

Weakness and loss of energy to the point of incompetence and mental apathy are common, although on occasion performance is amazingly good despite substantial endocrine deficits. Psychoses may occur. Hypotension is often present, with orthostatic exaggeration, and syncope may occur. Water diuresis is slow, little or no increase of urine volume occurring in 4 hours after the ingestion of a liter or more of water. Though adrenal cortical defects may contribute to these peculiarities and to the weakness as well, outstanding adrenal insufficiency is not regularly present. Abnormalities in the concentration of serum electrolytes typical of Addison's disease are not usually seen, but may often be brought out by salt restriction, as in the dangerous but revealing procedure of Cutler, Power and Wilder. Urinary sodium and chloride are then shown to be excreted in relatively high concentration despite reduction of blood levels, thus exhibiting the typical renal peculiarity of adrenal insufficiency (Loeb, 1933). On occasion adrenal insufficiency is manifest rather than latent, with all the cardinal signs of Addison's disease save pigmentation and leading to grave debility and death in crisis.

Eosinophilia of a relatively mild degree may exist in hypopituitarism. The level of circulating eosinophils is readily depressed by adrenal steroids bearing on oxygen on carbon-11. ACTH (25 units every six hours) may induce an eosinopenia through stimulation of the adrenal cortex in hypopituitarism and so testify to the reactivity of the dependent adrenal cortex. If adrenal atrophy is of long standing, however, the response to ACTH may be absent or imperfect until sustained treatment restores the tissue. Eosinopenia in response to epinephrine appears a less certain indicator of the integrity of the pituitary-adrenal axis than had originally been believed. Urinary corticoids are characteristically low in hypopituitarism. Urinary 17-ketosteroids may be low or virtually absent depending on the duration and extent of the adrenal and gonadal (testicular) defect. Hypoglycemia may be troublesome, emerging especially after prolonged fasting, and is often readily induced by small doses of insulin. This latter procedure is dangerous. As previously noted, both the growth hormone and the adrenal steroid or steroids governed by adrenocorticotrophin contribute to the control of carbohydrate metabolism and to opposition to insulin. It is not always clear how much loss of each contributes to the defects of hypopituitarism.

Anorexia to some degree is common, but the metabolic requirements are low, and conspicuous loss of weight may not occur. More rarely loss of weight is substantial and contributes an important element to an appearance of cachexia. Progressive obesity is rare in hypopituitarism alone and bespeaks hypothalamic injury when it does occur (see Fröhlich's Syndrome).

Save for the gonadal defects which are rarely absent in gross destructive pituitary disease, there is a great variation in the symptoms and signs of hypopituitarism, depending in part on the extent to which one or another pituitary secretory element is involved. Sheehan has estimated that the anterior lobe must be reduced to fragments for Simmonds' disease to be clear cut. Spontaneous recovery of one or another function after deficiency has been established, however, is not common,

since the capacity of the anterior lobe cells for regeneration is poor indeed, even if the responsible lesion provides the opportunity. With tumors, the endocrine aspects may be completely dominated by the mechanical effects of the neoplasm, and reduction in visual acuity to blindness, headache and the various other expressions of an expanding intracranial lesion come to preoccupy the patient and to demand concentrated attention.

Diagnosis. The milder forms of hypopituitarism are most likely to escape detection. The history of obstetric accident with collapse or hemorrhage points to the possibility of postpartum necrosis and should always be sought. Anorexia nervosa affects chiefly young females, and the considerable emaciation, the maintenance or increase of body hair, the restless behavior and the manifest emotional disorder form a general clinical picture usually quite distinct from that of Simmonds' disease. Genuinely retarded sexual development in either sex requires investigation of the possibility of gross pituitary disease. Amenorrhea in women of previously normal menstrual habit should lead to consideration of gross pituitary disease, and the presence of fine, hairless skin with reduction or loss of axillary or pubic hair is especially suggestive. Films of the sella usually show distinct ballooning and enlargement if a chromophobe adenoma is responsible. Calcification in the region of the sella suggests the possibility of a craniopharyngioma. Urinary gonadotrophin studies may be helpful, since the values are high in early natural menopause, low in primary pituitary disease.

The distinctions between primary hypothyroidism, primary adrenal insufficiency and Simmonds' disease are usually apparent, but may occasionally offer considerable difficulty. Typically, Simmonds' disease presents the depressed basal metabolism of hypothyroidism without the soft tissue swellings of myxedema and frequently with less elevation of serum cholesterol. Evidence of adrenal insufficiency of varying degree without pigmentation may occur in Simmonds' disease and is unusual in either primary thyroid or primary adrenal disease. Poor tolerance to thyroid in myxedema should lead to suspicion of anterior lobe deficiency and is caused, in all probability, by the associated adrenal defect. Definitive response to ACTH as determined by a fall in circulating eosinophils, a rise in urinary 17-ketosteroids, and so forth, precludes primary adrenal disease.

The several laboratory procedures useful in recognizing hypopituitarism have been referred to in foregoing sections. Wilkins or Williams may be referred to for further details.

Treatment. Chromophobe adenomas may be less sensitive to irradiation than chromophile tumors, but this therapy should be tried in the hope of arresting the process. Craniopharyngiomas are still less sensitive. Significant restoration of pituitary function is rare. Progressive loss of vision despite irradiation or other evidences of continued intracranial expansion may require attempts at surgical reduction of the tumor mass. By virtue of the location of the tumor, the approach is difficult, hazardous and often unsuccessful.

The endocrine defects are best managed by substitution therapy for the dependent glands. If the adrenal cortical defect is latent as is commonly the case, both the wisdom and the usefulness of vigorous treatment may be considered sub judice at this time. General well being is then the chief criterion of response and this is, of course, influenced by many factors including subjective ones. When the adrenal insufficiency is manifest under ordinary living conditions, the treatment corresponds to that for Addison's disease (see Addison's disease). Although sustained treatment with ACTH is feasible, injections must be given daily and cortisone, 12.5 to 50 mg. daily in divided doses orally, will usually be preferred. Desoxycorticosterone may still have a place. Salt supplements of 1 to 6 gm. daily may be used. Potassium deficits should be guarded against. It must be remembered that cortisone will depress residual adrenal function so that the gain from treatment must be clear and any discontinuance gradual and guarded. ACTH may be used to restore the depressed adrenal. In manifest crises of adrenal insufficiency treatment corresponds to those of primary Addison's disease. ACTH may be used to support and restore the adrenal cortex but it may not work quickly enough if the adrenals have long been atrophic and should not be counted on as a sole measure. Preparations of ACTH and their use are cited briefly under adrenocorticotrophin. In general the patient with hypopituitarism should be protected against those events known to put a strain on the pituitary-adrenal axis. ACTH may serve from time to time to aid in this protection when the strain such as a surgical operation is unavoidable.

Frequent findings of carbohydrate in day-to-day management and the use of intravenous glucose for emergencies may be essential for the control of hypoglycemia. Cortisone may be expected to protect against such hypoglycemic episodes and to contribute to their control. Thyroid may be helpful in sustained treatment but the reasonable integrity of the adrenal cortex should be assured or any deficiency provided for in advance. Dosage should be small at first (6 mg. to 15 mg. daily) and increased slowly to 30 or perhaps 60 mg. daily. On rare occasions unexpected collapse, apparently of adrenal origin, may follow vigorous treatment with thyroid. Androgens (testosterone propionate 25 mg. two or three times weekly by injection; methyl testosterone 20 to 50 mg. daily orally, perhaps somewhat less by linguets) may be used to enhance masculine secondary sex characteristics. Although anabolic effects of protein metabolism are demonstrable, opinion differs as to the general gain from such influences in adult Simmonds' disease. Interpretations of increased well being and strength are governed by subjective factors and are greatly affected by a complex metabolic situation. While chorionic gonadotrophin would appear more elegant than androgens, stimulating rather than replacing the testes, its advantages do not appear real enough at this time. Repair of sperm formation by this gonadotrophin has not been shown with any regularity. It should not be forgotten that some patients are best left untreated if the external demands can be adjusted to their capacities.

HYPOPITUITARISM DURING CHILDHOOD (INCLUDING ATELEIOSIS)

(Pituitary Dwarfism)

Gross pituitary defect arising during childhood is expressed by retardation of somatic growth in addition to the endocrine deficiencies previously cited. This impairment of growth is relatively uniform throughout the skeletal, visceral and cardiovascular systems yielding a small but relatively harmoniously developed person whose childish proportions and contours mark the time of growth arrest for years to come (Fig. 90). The cartilaginous epiphyses remain unossified for long periods. The secondary gonadal insufficiencies contribute in their own characteristic ways to the fixation of the sexual attributes of childhood. Later the atrophic skin may be wrinkled, superimposing an incongruous aspect of aging. The profound impairment of the development and function of the central nervous system seen in cretinism does not occur, nor does the myxedematous infiltration of the subcutaneous and submucous tissues so characteristic of juvenile myxedema appear to be frequent. The several metabolic consequences of adrenal defect are less conspicuous than in Addison's disease and must be sought. On occasion a pituitary tumor can be demonstrated; more often perhaps careful physiologic studies will create a strong presumption for pituitary responsibility.

Autopsy experience is limited. Craniopharyngiomas are the most common tumor (see Etiology of Hypopituitarism), and are rarely intrasellar (Erdheim). Cysts of a developmental sort are known, including those occurring between separated anterior and posterior lobe anlagen which remain in positions indicating arrest of embryologic procession (Priesel). Simmonds noted fibrosis of unknown origin. It is by no means clear that a full histologic account of the real varieties of pituitary defect has been given, and one misses descriptions of aplasia or hypoplasia of a pituitary cell line analogous to that in the hereditary dwarf mice of Smith and Mac-Dowell. Familial associations of growth defects are common in man.

The establishment of diagnosis based on etiology is especially difficult when growth alone is defective, sexual development normal and other endocrine disorders not conspicuous. Such dwarfs are often termed "primordial" and held to be small but otherwise normal persons analogous to the pygmy races of man. The term "constitutional" is often used to imply a peripheral tissue growth defect than a primary pituitary disorder. Though such interpretations are reasonable, it must be recalled that neither autopsy experience nor assays for growth hormone nor measurements of response to growth hormone suffice now to place them beyond question. Throughout the entire problem of dwarfism this interplay of tissue response and hormonal impetus is imperfectly understood. The term *ateleiosis* (Gilford), which is wisely nondescript, might well be reserved for the generality of dwarfs both with and without sexual defects until the extent of true hypopituitarism in explanation can be fully ascertained.

Wilkins' treatment of this problem should be consulted, together with his description of the differentiation between primary pituitary disease in girls and the much more common association between shortness of stature and ovarian agenesis, with consequent elevated urinary gonadotrophins. The associated, var-

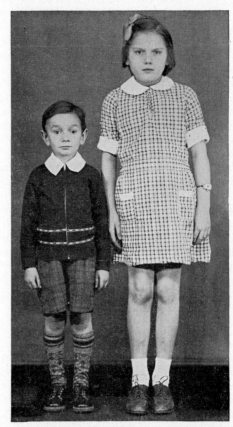

Fig. 90. Two children of the same age. The one on the right is normal. The one on the left had a craniopharyngioma at the age of 5. Note the complete cessation of growth.

iegated congenital defects are often those described by Turner, and there is now a tendency to call the entire group Turner's syndrome. In any event, this important syndrome well illustrates that the mere association of growth and sexual defects cannot prove anterior lobe responsibility for both.

The **treatment** of hypopituitarism in childhood is much the same as in adult life. Some increase in stature may be expected from the use of androgens, although full restoration of normal growth is not to be expected. Use of androgens in the female must be carefully guarded.

FRÖHLICH'S SYNDROME

(Adiposogenital Dystrophy)

Since Fröhlich's (1901) account of mild obesity and retardation of genital development in a boy with the visual field defects of a pituitary tumor, the association of obesity and hypogonadism has been termed Fröhlich's syndrome, although *adiposogenital dystrophy* is more precise. Erdheim's view that the progressive obesity is due to hypothalamic lesions rather than to hypopituitarism has received modern experimental support. Excessive eating is the most important factor in producing this obesity. Genital dystrophy has similarly been induced by circumscribed hypothalamic lesions, but in this instance secondary hypopituitarism presumably occurs. The term "Fröhlich's syndrome" may be properly applied to the pituitary or juxtapituitary lesions in which the association of obesity and hypogonadism is due to a common cause. Hypogonadism *per se* does not give rise to progressive obesity. Obesity in children before puberty should not be termed Fröhlich's syndrome, nor can hypopituitarism be often held responsible for their obesity. Obesity of hypothalamic origin will respond to dieting if appetite can be controlled.

ANOREXIA NERVOSA

Anorexia nervosa is a chronic disorder chiefly of young women and is characterized essentially by an obsessive aversion to food leading to emaciation. Amenorrhea is the rule. Gull described the disease and attributed it to a functional disorder of the nervous system, an interpretation which survives. The profound emotional and character disorder, the tendency to develop with the assumption of independent adult life, and the common history of grievous personal difficulties support this view, together with the recovery that may be made under fortunate medical and general environmental conditions. The few autopsies have shown no gross pituitary disease. The early onset of the amenorrhea in some instances before notable weight loss, but with the onset of emotional disturbance, suggests an interpretation analogous to that of the amenorrhea of psychoses. The deficiency in gonadotrophin secretion is thus considered secondary in part to starvation and in part to disturbed mental state. The basal metabolic rate is often markedly lowered.

The disorder may develop after dieting for obesity. The aversion to food is profound or, if hunger is experienced, satiety comes so quickly that eating provides little more than a nibbling of sweet, insufficient juices, perhaps enough to prevent ketosis, but far from enough to meet energy requirements. A variety of disagreeable abdominal sensations occurs, including nausea. Vomiting is common if food is forced, and is often self-induced. The loss of weight is extreme, often reducing the victim to the contours of her bony skeleton. Unlike in Simmonds' disease, however, sexual hair is retained, and even a fine general hypertrichosis may develop. Despite her pitiable plight the victim is often active or restless, with an even cheerful preoccupation with trivia. Sustained effort is difficult, and pressure, especially to eat, may lead to every variety of deceit to avoid compliance. Moderate anemia, hypoproteinemia and nutritional edema may develop. Death may occur from starvation after years of debility.

Treatment comprises reeducation of the patient with persuasion to eat, together with whatever gentle force the physician can command. Psychiatric care is desirable if judicious, but the results are variable. In a few hands they seem good indeed, but great patience is necessary and failure is common enough. Endocrine treatment has not been established as valuable.

A. T. KENYON

References

Bailey, P.: Intracranial Tumors. 2d ed. Springfield, Illinois, Charles C Thomas, 1948.

Bauer, W., and Clark, W. S.: The Relationship of the Adaptation Concept to the Connective Tissue Diseases. In Pincus, G., Editor: Recent Progress in Hormone Research. Vol. VIII. New York, Academic Press, 1953, p. 217.

Friedgood, H. B.: Endocrine Functions of the Hypophysis. New York, Oxford Medical Publications, 1946.

Ingle, D. J., and Baker, B. L.: Physiological and Therapeutic Effects of Corticotropin (ACTH) and Cortisone. Springfield, Illinois, Charles C Thomas, 1953.

Kenyon, A. T., Knowlton, K., and Sandiford, I.: Anabolic Effects of Androgens and Somatic Growth in Man. Ann. Int. Med., 20:632, 1944.

Nurnberger, J. S., and Korey, S. R.: Pituitary Chromophobe Adenomas. New York, Springer Publishing Co., 1953.

Pincus, G., and Thimann, K. V.: The Hormones. New York, Academic Press, 1949–50.

Rolleston, H. D.: The Endocrine Organs in Health

and Disease. London, Oxford University Press, 1936.

Sayers, G.: The Adrenal Cortex and Homeostasis. Physiol. Rev. 50:241, 1950.

Selye, H.: The General Adaptation Syndrome and Diseases of Adaptation. J. Clin. Endocrinol., 6: 117, 1946.

Sheehan, H. L., and Summers, V. K.: The Syndrome of Hypopituitarism. Quart. J. Med., 42:319, 1949.

Soskin, S., and Levine, R.: Carbohydrate Metabolism. Revised edition. Chicago, University of Chicago Press, 1952.

Sprague, R. G.: Effects of Cortisone and ACTH. In Harris, R. S., and Thimann, K. V., Eds.: Vitamins and Hormones. Vol. IX. New York, Academic Press, 1951, p. 265.

Thorn, G., and Forsham, P.: Metabolic Changes in Man Following Adrenal and Pituitary Hormone Administration. In Pincus, G., Editor: Recent Progress in Hormone Research, Vol. IV. New York, Academic Press, 1949, p. 229.

———, Jenkins, D., and Laidlaw, J. C.: The Adrenal Response to Stress in Man. In Pincus, G., Editor: Recent Progress in Hormone Research, Vol. VIII. New York, Academic Press, 1953, p. 171.

Wilkins, L.: Endocrine Disorders in Childhood and Adolescence. Springfield, Illinois, Charles C Thomas, 1950.

Williams, R. H.: Textbook of Endocrinology. Philadelphia, W. B. Saunders Company, 1950.

Young, F. G.: The Growth Hormone and Diabetes. In Pincus, G., Editor: Recent Progress in Hormone Research. Vol. VIII. New York, Academic Press, 1953, p. 471.

DISEASES OF THE ADRENAL GLANDS*

INTRODUCTION

The first known description of the adrenal glands is recorded in *Opuscula Anatomica Venetiis* (1563) by the great anatomist of the Renaissance, Bartholomaeus Eustachius Scantoseverinatus. It is of interest that Eustachius described these structures as glands, although their function was not at all understood. Thomas Bartholin and his father, Casper (1641), advanced the theory that a "dark excrementitious biliary humor" was purified or altered in some way within these glands to permit its passage through the kidneys. Meckel's studies in 1806 deserve particular consideration, because he introduced new methods of studying adrenal gland function by destroying the organ within living animals and by studying the organ in different types of animals. Meckel also advanced the idea that the adrenal glands were related to the gonads in a special manner, and he believed, with Autenreith, that the adrenal glands with the liver, spleen, thymus and thyroid were concerned with metabolic processes and that they served to regulate respiratory and tissue metabolism. It was not until 1855, however, in Thomas Addison's classic description of a clinical syndrome which resulted from destruction of the adrenal glands, that the vital function of these organs was really appreciated. Shortly thereafter Brown-Séquard demonstrated conclusively that complete removal of both adrenals was followed promptly by death of the experimental animal. The studies of Vulpian, Oliver, Schaeffer, Abel, Takamine and Aldrich ultimately resulted in isolation of epinephrine from the adrenal medulla, but since the relationship between medullary secretion and cortical secretion was not understood, it was with some disappointment that epinephrine was found to be ineffective in the treatment of patients with Addison's disease. This observation, however, stimulated further experimental work in which it was demonstrated that the complete removal of one adrenal,

accompanied by the destruction of the medulla of the remaining adrenal, did not give rise to the classic signs and symptoms of adrenal insufficiency. From these observations it appeared that the "life-maintaining" substance liberated by the adrenal was derived from the cells of the cortex.

In 1927 Hartman, MacArthur and Hartman, and Rogoff and Stewart independently reported the preparation of adrenal cortical extracts which were capable, on injection, of prolonging the survival period of adrenalectomized animals. In 1930 Swingle and Pfiffner, and Hartman and Brownell independently described methods of preparing adrenal cortical extracts of much greater potency. These extracts appeared to be capable of maintaining bilaterally adrenalectomized dogs and cats in good condition for prolonged periods. It was also noted that injections of these extracts in adequate quantities resulted in considerable improvement in patients with Addison's disease. However, difficulties encountered in the preparation of large quantities of potent extract and in the standardization of the hormone, in addition to the high cost of preparation, greatly limited adequate clinical trial. Furthermore, it was apparent at this time that, although improvement might be made in the methods of extracting hormone from the adrenal glands, it was doubtful whether the preparation of hormone from this natural source could ever provide an adequate quantity of potent material at a cost which most patients could afford.

The classic studies of Loeb and Harrop demonstrated the beneficial effect of sodium salts in the treatment of patients with Addison's disease. Not only was a diet of high sodium content beneficial, but the studies of Truszkowski and Zwemer and Wilder demonstrated the advantages of a low potassium intake in patients with adrenal insufficiency. From these observations it was evident that, in the clinical evaluation of adrenal cortical hormone therapy, the mineral content of the diet required great consideration.

In 1933 both Kendall and Grollman obtained crystalline material from adrenal cortical extracts. This material appeared to have cortical hormone-like activity. Somewhat later

* The author wishes to express his deep appreciation to Dr. John C. Laidlaw for his valuable assistance in the revision of this article.

Reichstein isolated a crystalline compound from the adrenal cortex which had cortical hormone-like activity and which he identified and named "corticosterone." Subsequently Kendall demonstrated that the active compound which he had described was identical with that of Reichstein's "corticosterone." In 1937 Steiger and Reichstein announced the synthesis from *stigmasterol* of a steroid compound, *desoxycorticosterone acetate*. This compound was found to have cortical hormone-like activity and was noted to be closely related, chemically, to progesterone. During the following year Reichstein and von Euw succeeded in isolating desoxycorticosterone from adrenal cortical extract. Finally, the development by Reichstein, Kendall and Sarret of procedures for placing an oxygen atom on the 11 and 17 carbon atoms of the steroid nucleus led to the preparation of cortisone and hydrocortisone for therapeutic use.

GEORGE W. THORN

DISEASES OF THE ADRENAL MEDULLA

The cells of the adrenal medulla are of ectodermal origin and arise, as do the cells of the sympathetic nervous system, from the primitive neural crest. The parent cell is the sympathogone. This cell may differentiate to form a sympathoblast or neuroblast, and finally a mature ganglion cell, or it may give rise to a chromaffin cell. The latter is so named because of the brown color which the granules of its cytoplasm assume when treated with chromic acid salts.

These cell types are found not only in the adrenal medulla but wherever sympathetic nervous tissue occurs, particularly in the ganglia and in the organs of Zuckerkandl at the bifurcation of the aorta. Tumors may develop from any of these cell types.

Hormones of the Adrenal Medulla. Epinephrine was the first hormone to be isolated (Abel, 1897) and chemically identified (Aldrich, 1901). However, it was not until 1949 that von Euler isolated norepinephrine from the adrenal medulla and from adrenergic nerve fibers, thereby establishing the existence of two medullary hormones. Structurally, these two hormones are catecholamines and differ only in the fact that norepinephrine lacks the N-methyl group possessed by epinephrine (Fig. 91). The

epinephrine and norepinephrine content of human adrenal medullary tissue has been estimated biologically by von Euler to be 2.4 to 4.0 mg. per gram, of which 10 to 30 per cent is norepinephrine. Weil-Malherbe and Bone with the aid of a sensitive fluorometric method have found the total plasma concentration of epinephrine and norepinephrine to be approximately 3 micrograms per liter; norepinephrine makes up approximately 80 per cent of this value. The urine normally con-

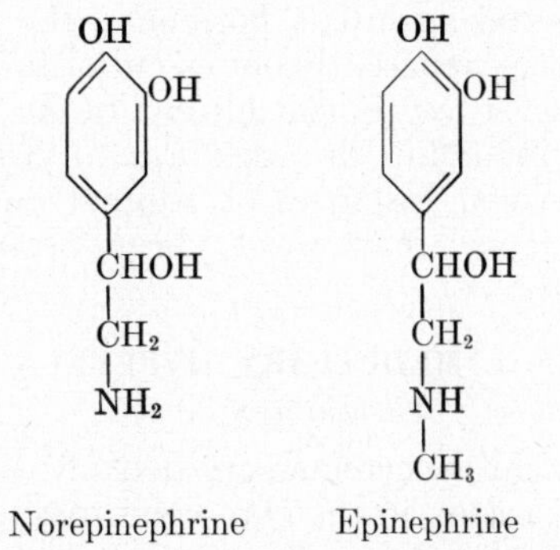

Fig. 91. Adrenal medullary hormones.

tains between 15 and 45 micrograms of catecholamines per day; 85 per cent of this is norepinephrine. The preponderance of norepinephrine in both plasma and urine in the face of a low norepinephrine-epinephrine ratio in the adrenal medulla is thought to reflect the liberation of additional quantities of this humoral agent from adrenergic nerve endings. In contrast to normal medullary tissue in which the predominant hormone is epinephrine, actively secreting adrenal medullary tumors, pheochromocytomas, often contain large amounts of norepinephrine.

Pharmacologic studies have shown highly important differences in the actions of epinephrine and norepinephrine. Both hormones raise the blood pressure but by different mechanisms. Epinephrine causes an increased cardiac output and, with the exception of the skin vessels, generalized vasodilatation. The cardiac rate increases, the systolic pressure rises, but the diastolic pressure shows little change. Norepinephrine, on the other hand, causes marked peripheral vasoconstriction with a rise in both systolic and diastolic blood pressure. The cardiac output is little altered and the heart rate may be slowed. Epinephrine has a prominent metabolic effect which is possessed to only a very limited extent by norepinephrine. It causes increased oxygen consumption with a rise in body temperature and basal metabolic rate. Furthermore, it accelerates hepatic glycogenolysis with a consequent rise in fasting blood sugar levels and often a diabetic type of glucose tolerance curve. Muscle glycogen is broken down more rapidly to lactic acid. Epinephrine will cause a significant fall in the level of circulating eosinophils but actual stimulation of the adrenal cortex has not been demonstrated to occur in man.

Despite the important physiologic effects of the adrenal medullary hormones, the adrenal medulla is apparently not essential for life. It is, however, a valuable adjunct to the adrenal cortex in aiding the organism to cope with acute stress. Instances of adrenal medullary insufficiency have not been recognized clinically.

ADRENAL MEDULLARY HYPERFUNCTION
(Pheochromocytoma)

Pheochromocytomas are actively secreting tumors arising in the chromaffin tissue of the adrenal medulla or the paraganglia of the sympathetic nervous system. The first description of the association of paroxysmal hypertension and pheochromocytoma was given by Labbé in 1922. In 1927, C. H. Mayo removed such a tumor and there followed complete relief of the associated hypertension.

Pheochromocytomas are comparatively rare. In 1950, Smithwick collected 270 cases from the literature (67 per cent demonstrated only at autopsy). A recent apparent increase in the incidence of these tumors may be accounted for by the use of new diagnostic agents, by careful search among hypertensive patients for curable forms of hypertension, and by the increased opportunity to detect chromaffin tumors when operations are being performed on the thoracolumbar sympathetic chain for the treatment of hypertension.

Pheochromocytomas occur in all age groups, but are more frequent in adults. There is no sex predilection.

Pathology. In 10 to 20 per cent of cases, the tumors are multiple. In a similar number of instances, the tumors have been found outside the adrenal, in chromaffin tissue in the paraganglia along the retropleural and retroperitoneal chains of the sympathetic nervous system, in the carotid bodies or the organs of Zuckerkandl. An associated neurofibromatosis has been observed in 5 per cent of cases. Approximately 10 per cent of the tumors are malignant and metastasize to regional and thoracic lymph nodes, liver and skeleton.

The tumors vary in size but are frequently quite small. They are usually lobulated, highly vascular and well encapsulated. The cut surface is yellowish brown in color and frequently shows evidence of hemorrhage and cystic degeneration. Microscopically, the tumor cells are large, irregular or polyhedral in shape and have a granular cytoplasm.

Clinical Picture. The manifestations of pheochromocytoma are the result of an increased secretion of norepinephrine and epinephrine. Two distinct syndromes occur: one associated with intermittent or paroxysmal hypertension and the other characterized by persistent hypertension.

In 35 to 50 per cent of cases, classic paroxysms, "adrenosympathetic crises," occur. These may be precipitated by such events as emotional upsets, physical exertion or changes in posture. Early, the attacks tend to occur at long intervals and last only a few minutes. Later, they may be more frequent and severe, lasting many hours. The attacks are characterized by severe anxiety, throbbing headache, forceful palpitation, tremulousness, visual blurring, nausea, sometimes vomiting, occasionally retrosternal chest pain, and a rise in blood pressure, which may attain a systolic level of 300 mm. of mercury or more. The diastolic blood pressure may rise to a level of 175 mm. of mercury. The extremities are cold and often pale, the neck veins distended, the pupils dilated, and the skin soaked with perspiration. Hyperglycemia and glycosuria during attacks are common. Prolonged episodes may terminate in a shock-like state with hyperpyrexia and hypotension. Death may occur from pulmonary edema, ventricular fibrillation or cerebral hemorrhage.

Unfortunately, in many cases of pheochromocytoma there is sustained hypertension. The course of the disease is not unlike that of essential hypertension with progressive cardiovascular, renal and retinal involvement. The basal metabolic rate is often elevated and frank diabetes may be encountered. Chemical analysis of tumors in these cases usually reveals a marked preponderance of norepinephrine.

Diagnosis. This may be established by the history of a typical attack or by deliberately precipitating an attack through change in position or direct pressure upon the tumor. In a small percentage of cases, a tumor or a displaced kidney may be palpated in the flank.

Pyelography may reveal depression of the renal shadow. Perirenal, and more recently presacral, insufflation of oxygen have been employed to outline a tumor mass.

Certain pharmacologic tests may be of considerable aid in the diagnosis of pheochromocytoma. Two types of test are used. In one, the provocative test, a paroxysm of hypertension is precipitated when the blood pressure has been normal. In the other, the blocking test, a fall in blood pressure is induced by the use of an adrenolytic compound when the pressure has been elevated. Of the provocative agents, histamine probably provides the most reliable response, but both false negative and false positive responses have been reported. *Histamine phosphate* when given intravenously in a dose of 0.01 to 0.025 mg. induces a flush, headache and a slight blood pressure fall in the normal subject. A rise in blood pressure significantly greater than the cold pressor response within two minutes of injection is considered a positive test. This occurs in many, but by no means all, cases of pheochromocytoma. Sometimes alarming rises in blood pressure occur which may be dangerous in patients with advanced arterial disease. In these instances Regitine, 5 mg., should be administered intravenously. *Methacholine hydrochloride* (Mecholyl), when given subcutaneously in doses of 12.5 to 25 mg. to a normal subject, produces salivation, sweating and a transient fall, followed by a mild rise, in blood pressure. A striking rise in blood pressure may occur when pheochromocytoma is present but, as with the histamine test, both false negative and false positive tests occur. Alarming reactions may be seen, and the subcutaneous administration of 1 mg. of atropine sulfate prior to the injection of the Mecholyl is recommended.

Of the blocking agents, Benzodioxane and Regitine are the most reliable. *Benzodioxane* (*piperoxanhydrochloride*) is structurally related to epinephrine. It exerts an antipressor effect while retaining certain sympathomimetic actions. When given intravenously over a two-minute period in a dose of 10 mg. per square meter of body surface, it causes agitation, tachycardia, flush, headache and dizziness. In the normal subject, there is a slight rise in blood pressure. When a pheochromocytoma is present, the pressure usually falls at least 35 mm. of mercury. False positive tests are extremely uncommon, although false negatives occur not infrequently. *Regitine* (*phentolamine*) has a similar antipressor action but does not yield unpleasant side effects. When given intravenously in a 5 mg. dose, a similar blood pressure fall occurs if a pheochromocytoma is present. Although insufficient time has elapsed for a definitive evaluation, preliminary experience indicates that Regitine is at least as effective as benzodioxane and possibly more reliable.

In the performance of the above tests, it is important to have the patient resting quietly to establish a good baseline blood pressure. When sedatives have been administered within 24 hours of the test, false reactions may occur. The responses in uremic patients are unreliable.

In 1950, Engel and von Euler observed a marked increase in the urinary excretion of catecholamines in the presence of pheochromocytoma. This finding has been confirmed by Goldenberg employing a fluorometric technique rather than a biologic assay. As further experience accumulates, it is probable that the determination of urinary catecholamines will become the most reliable single diagnostic procedure in pheochromocytoma.

Treatment. Surgical excision of the tumor may result in complete remission of symptoms, although in certain instances in which the hypertension has been persistent and of long duration little change in blood pressure may occur following operation. The transperitoneal approach allows satisfactory exploration of all possible tumor sites in the abdomen. Two serious events may occur during operation: (1) The blood pressure may rise to extreme heights or fatal cardiac arrhythmias may occur due to excessive discharge of medullary hormones; or (2) following resection of the tumor, the blood pressure may fall precipitously and profound shock ensue due to abrupt withdrawal of circulating hormones. Adequate preoperative sedation is important. Anesthetic agents likely to produce serious cardiac arrhythmias in the presence of high epinephrine levels—cyclopropane, ethyl chloride—should not be employed. Induction with Pentothal followed by intratracheal nitrous oxide—ether with high oxygen saturation provides satisfactory anesthesia. Ligation of the blood supply of the tumor before handling will reduce the likelihood of precipitating a hypertensive episode. The latter can be corrected by the use of intravenous Regitine which should be kept ready during the operation and administered when indicated. The precipitous fall in blood pressure which often occurs following ligation of the tumor vessels can be managed by the use of intravenous norepinephrine. During the postoperative period neosynephrine may be given subcutaneously to correct mild hypotensive episodes. Once the immediate postoperative period is over, patients usually do well and symptoms and hypertension disappear.

Because of the excellent results of surgical treatment, it is of the utmost importance to consider the possibility of pheochromocytoma in all hypertensive patients.

NONFUNCTIONING TUMORS ARISING FROM MEDULLARY TISSUE

These tumors may arise from any of the primitive or mature cells of the sympathetic nervous system and the adrenal medulla.

The *sympathogonioma* is a rare, highly malignant tumor which appears in early infancy or intrauterine life. It is a large, soft, cellular growth, which often shows evidence of hemorrhage and necrosis. It metastasizes early to retroperitoneal lymph nodes, liver and bone. The prognosis is poor.

The *ganglioneuroma,* on the other hand, is a small, well encapsulated, slow-growing tumor, which occurs in adults and is usually an incidental finding at post mortem. It contains many mature ganglion cells separated by a network of myelinated or nonmyelinated nerve fibers.

Neuroblastoma (Sympathoblastoma). This highly malignant tumor occurs almost exclusively in infancy and early childhood. Except for renal embryoma (Wilms' tumor), neuroblastoma is the commonest retroperitoneal, malignant tumor of children. In approximately 50 per cent of cases these tumors are extra-adrenal, arising retroperitoneally or retropleurally in the sympathetic chain, the celiac ganglia, the organs of Zuckerkandl, the cervicosympathetic ganglia or from the substance of the central nervous system. The tumor metastasizes early to regional lymph nodes, liver, bones and orbit. The older classification into Pepper and Hutchinson types is no longer tenable since the neuroblastoma arising from either adrenal may metastasize to the orbit or to the liver.

Pathologically, the tumors are large and cellular. The cut surface is firm, with many areas of hemorrhage and necrosis. The cells, which are oval with dark brown nuclei and thin rims of cytoplasm, are often arranged in rosette fashion and separated by fine fibrils.

The manifestations of a neuroblastoma may be those of a local tumor mass with abdominal enlargement, vomiting and pain; or they may be those of a generalized malignancy, with weakness, loss of weight, fever and anemia. In one quarter of the cases, there is generalized lymphadenopathy. In some instances, metastases may introduce the disease and the child may present swellings in the skull, proptosis and ecchymoses of the eyelids.

Radical surgery, followed by deep x-ray therapy, is the treatment of choice. Although the prognosis is poor, Farber reported 10 cures in 40 cases treated in the above manner and followed over a ten-year period. In some of these children, complete surgical removal of the tumor had not been possible.

GEORGE W. THORN

References

Cahill, G. F.: Surgery Involving the Adrenals. New York State J. Med., 53:308, 1953.
Engel, A., and von Euler, U. S.: Diagnostic Value of Increased Urinary Output of Nor-adrenaline and Adrenaline in Pheochromocytoma. Lancet, 2:387, 1950.
Gifford, R. W., Roth, G. M., and Kvale, W. F.: Evaluation of a New Adrenolytic Drug (Regitine ®) as a Test for Pheochromocytoma. J.A.M.A., 149:1628, 1952.
Goldenberg, M., Serlin, I., Edwards, T., and Rapport, M. M.: Chemical Screening Methods for the Diagnosis of Pheochromocytoma. I. Nor-epinephrine and Epinephrine in Human Urine. Am. J. Med., 16:310, 1954.
Howard, J. E., and Barker, W. H.: Paroxysmal Hypertension and Other Clincial Manifestations Associated with Benign Chromaffin Cell Tumors. Bull. Johns Hopkins Hosp., 61:371, 1937.
Marriott, H. J. L.: Editorial. Diagnosis of Pheochromocytoma. Ann. Int. Med., 39:1341, 1953.
Pack, G. T., Horning, E. D., and Ariel, I. M.: Neuroblastoma (Sympathicoblastoma). J. Neuropath. & Exper. Neurol., 11:235, 1952.
Smithwick, R. H., Greer, W. E., Robertson, C. W., and Wilkins, R. W.: Pheochromocytoma. New England J. Med., 242:252, 1950.
Thorn, G. W., Hindl, J. A., and Sandmeyer, J. A.: Pheochromocytoma of the Adrenal Associated with Persistent Hypertension. Case Report. Ann. Int. Med., 21:122, 1944.
Weil-Malherbe, H., and Bone, A. D.: The Adrenergic Amines of Human Blood. Lancet, 2:974, 1953.

DISEASES OF THE ADRENAL CORTEX

INTRODUCTION

During the past two decades, approximately thirty steroid compounds have been isolated from the adrenal cortex. Six of these, which are capable of maintaining life in adrenalectomized animals, have been identified: hydrocortisone (Compound F), cortisone (Compound E), corticosterone (Compound B), dehydrocorticosterone (Compound A), desoxycorticosterone (DOC) and the recently isolated aldosterone (electrocortin) (Fig. 92). These compounds, which possess an alpha-ketol side chain ($CO-CH_2OH$) at carbon-17, are termed "corticoids." Compounds A, B, E and F, which possess an oxygen atom at a carbon-11, are "11-oxygenated corticoids." Compounds E and F are "11, 17-oxygenated corticoids."

pound A) stand halfway between hydrocortisone and desoxycorticosterone in terms of the physiologic activities which they exhibit. Unlike hydrocortisone and cortisone, they do not induce an eosinopenia or lymphopenia. Although many steroids have been isolated from adrenal cortical tissue, it would appear from studies on adrenal venous blood that the human adrenal cortex secretes mainly hydrocortisone, corticosterone, aldosterone and an androgenic 17-ketosteroid, androstenedione; of these hydrocortisone is secreted in the greatest amount. Desoxycorticosterone does

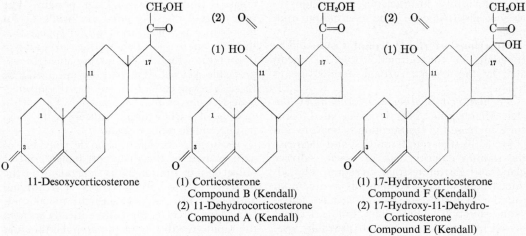

11-Desoxycorticosterone

(1) Corticosterone
Compound B (Kendall)
(2) 11-Dehydrocorticosterone
Compound A (Kendall)

(1) 17-Hydroxycorticosterone
Compound F (Kendall)
(2) 17-Hydroxy-11-Dehydro-
Corticosterone
Compound E (Kendall)

Fig. 92. Active adrenal cortical steroids.

Hydrocortisone (Compound F) and cortisone (Compound E) exhibit most of the known effects of the adrenal cortex when administered to adrenalectomized human subjects. While these compounds have a relatively weak electrolyte-regulating activity when given by mouth or by intramuscular injection, they are capable of producing a profound sodium retention when administered continuously by the intravenous route. Desoxycorticosterone, while strongly sodium retaining, has little effect on intermediary protein, fat and carbohydrate metabolism. Aldosterone (electrocortin), which is a derivative of corticosterone with an aldehyde group at carbon-18, has recently been crystallized from the amorphous fraction of adrenal cortical extract and from adrenal venous blood. This compound is twenty to thirty times as active in sodium retention as desoxycorticosterone and appears to be more effective than desoxycorticosterone in its influence on carbohydrate metabolism. Corticosterone (Compound B) and dehydrocorticosterone (Compound A) and dehydrocorticosterone (Com-

not appear to be a natural secretory product of the adrenal cortex.

The principal adrenal cortical hormone, hydrocortisone (Compound F), and its major metabolic products—tetrahydrocortisone, tetrahydrohydrocortisone, dihydrocortisone and cortisone—all possess a hydroxyl group at carbon-17 and are excreted in the urine both in the free form and as conjugates with glucuronic acid. These compounds are measured by methods which determine the "17-hydroxycorticoid" fraction. The urinary 17 ketosteroids of adrenal origin consist of two types of compound. One type is strongly androgenic, has no oxygen atom at the carbon-11 position and probably arises from androstenedione; the other is weakly androgenic, does have an 11-oxygen atom and is derived from hydrocortisone and cortisone. 17-Ketosteroids of the first type are also derived from the testicle.

The adrenal cortex is under the direct control of the anterior pituitary gland, the stimulus for its secretion being provided by adrenocorticotrophin or ACTH. ACTH appears to be secreted in response to a decreased level of circulating adrenal cortical steroids or to stimulation by a humoral substance produced in the hypothalamus. Administration of ACTH has been shown to produce an increased secretion of adrenal steroids and an intensification of those metabolic reactions known to be under their control. It is now well recognized that activation of the anterior pituitary-adrenal cortical system plays an essential role in the response of the organism to major stress. This is best illustrated by the marked vulnerability of patients with adrenal cortical insufficiency to a wide variety of disturbances in the external environment.

Functions of the Adrenal Cortex. The functions of the adrenal cortex as mediated by the adrenal cortical steroids are as follows:

Regulation of Sodium, Potassium and Chloride Metabolism. The 11-oxygenated corticoids increase the reabsorption of sodium and chloride by the renal tubules and decrease the sodium chloride loss in sweat, salivary gland and gastrointestinal secretion. The administration of these compounds results in an initial and inconstant rise of urinary potassium excretion. There may follow a brief period of potassium retention probably associated with the deposition of glycogen in the liver. Thereafter, one observes a continued loss of potassium. This is induced by the anti-anabolic action of these steroids which leads to liberation of nitrogen, potassium and phosphate from intracellular sources. Whereas all of the foregoing electrolyte changes may be observed following large doses of the 11-oxygenated corticoids, only part of the pattern is exhibited by desoxycorticosterone, which has no oxygen atom at carbon-11 and which lacks an anti-anabolic action and an effect on glycogen synthesis. Removal of the adrenals is followed by sodium chloride and water loss, potassium retention, dehydration and circulatory collapse.

Regulation of Water Balance. Water retention is observed following corticoid administration. This appears to be largely a reflection of sodium retention. Desoxycorticosterone favors initially an increase in extracellular sodium chloride and water, later an increase in intracellular water and sodium. The 11, 17-oxygenated corticoids, hydrocortisone and cortisone, appear to exert a regulatory effect on intracellular water, facilitating water loss from cells in the presence of excessive cellular hydration and increasing the water content of dehydrated cells. Although the mechanism of interaction is not known, it is generally accepted that the 11, 17-oxygenated corticoids antagonize the physiologic effects of the posterior pituitary antidiuretic hormone.

Regulation of the Metabolism of Carbohydrate, Protein and Fat. The 11-oxygenated corticoids, particularly hydrocortisone and cortisone, have an anti-insulin effect which decreases the peripheral utilization of glucose. An antianabolic effect leads to an increased gluconeogenesis from protein. The role of the 11-oxygenated corticoids in fat metabolism is not clear. It would appear that there is increased mobilization and utilization of fat which is not accompanied by appreciable ketosis. The net overall effect of these adrenal steroids is increased gluconeogenesis from protein and possibly fat with a sparing of carbohydrate utilization by those tissues which require insulin.

Androgenic Function. The development of axillary hair in the male and female and of pubic hair in the female is dependent on the presence of the adrenal cortex. The adrenal androgens also possess a protein anabolic effect. This effect is most dramatically seen in the rapid growth rate of the prepubertal child with the adrenogenital syndrome.

Regulation of Hematopoiesis and Tissue Reactivity. Only the 11,17-oxygenated corticoids, hydrocortisone and cortisone, exert significant hematologic effects. These consist of an eosinopenia in all probability due to increased peripheral destruction; a lymphopenia due to increased lysis of both fixed and circulating lymphocytes; a neutrophilia and a tendency to polycythemia. With large doses of hydrocortisone or cortisone, the reactivity of mesenchymal tissues to injury, irritants and foreign proteins (including microorganisms) may be greatly inhibited. As a result of this inhibitory effect on both fixed and mobile cellular defenses, inflammation is reduced but resistance to injury and infection may be seriously impaired.

Control of Pigmentation. Primary adrenal cortical insufficiency is accompanied by an increased deposition of melanin in the skin. Following bilateral adrenalectomy, this may be inhibited by the daily administration of hydrocortisone or cortisone. Desoxycorticosterone is ineffective in this regard. The absence of pigmentation in most cases of secondary adrenal insufficiency indicates that an intact anterior pituitary is necessary for this phenomenon to occur. There is evidence to suggest that, in the absence of the adrenal cortex, there is an increased secretion of a melanophore-stimulating substance from the anterior pituitary gland.

Effects on the Gastrointestinal Tract. Hydrocortisone and cortisone increase the secretion of hydrochloric acid and pepsin by the stomach and of the pancreatic enzymes as well. These steroids also appear to facilitate the secretion of bile and increase the absorption of fat from the intestinal tract.

ADRENOCORTICAL HORMONE AND CORTICOTROPIN PREPARATIONS AVAILABLE FOR CLINICAL USE

1. Hydrocortisone. This hormone is available as the free alcohol in ampules containing 100 mg., in 20 cc. of 50 per cent ethyl alcohol for addition to intravenous fluids. It can also be obtained as the acetate in crystalline suspension in saline (25 mg. per cubic centimeter) and in the form of scored tablets (10 and 20 mg.).

2. Cortisone. This hormone is available as the acetate: (*a*) as a crystalline suspension in saline which is suitable for intramuscular injection and of which 1 cc. contains 25 mg. of hormone, and (*b*) as scored tablets, 5 and 25 mg. for oral use.

3. Desoxycorticosterone. This hormone is available in four forms: (*a*) as the acetate dissolved in sesame oil for intramuscular injection, 5 mg. of the hormone in 1 cc.; (*b*) as the acetate in the form of tablets, known as linguets or buccalets, containing 2 or 5 mg. of the hormone in inert vehicles for direct sublingual absorption; (*c*) synthetic desoxycorticosterone trimethylacetate, a crystalline suspension of slowly hydrolyzed microcrystals acting for approximately four weeks after intramuscular injection, 25 mg. once a month being equivalent to 1 mg. daily of desoxycorticosterone acetate in oil; (*d*) sterile pellets of crystalline material weighing 75 mg. or 125 mg. and suitable for subcutaneous implantation; each pellet exerts the physiologic effect of daily injections of 0.06 cc. (0.3 mg.) and 0.1 cc. (0.5 mg.) of the solution in oil, respectively.

4. Extracts of Adrenal Cortex. Extracts of the adrenal glands of beef and hogs are available in aqueous solution (in 10 cc. and 50 cc. vials) for intramuscular or intravenous injection. They are assayed by biologic methods (1 cc. equals 0.1 mg. of hydrocortisone activity).

5. ACTH. ACTH is available as: (*a*) lyophilized powder, 10 to 40 U.S.P. units per vial, which can be administered in aqueous solution either intravenously or by intramuscular injection, by which route it has a duration of action of 6 to 8 hours; or (*b*) as a long-acting gel preparation (duration of action 18 to 24 hours), 20–100 "clinical" units per cubic centimeter; each "clinical" unit is equivalent to approximately one third of a U.S.P. or International Unit. Gel preparations must be kept refrigerated and warmed to 50° C. before being taken up in a syringe. Since ACTH is a polypeptide, sensitivity reactions may be encountered, particularly in patients with primary adrenal insufficiency who have not received cortisone.

HYPOFUNCTION OF THE ADRENAL CORTEX

The various types of adrenal insufficiency may be classified as follows:

1. Acute adrenal cortical insufficiency
   (*a*) Adrenal crisis (in patients with Addison's disease)
   (*b*) Adrenal hemorrhage
   (*c*) Surgical (following adrenalectomy or resection of hyperfunctioning adrenal tissue)
   (*d*) Iatrogenic—induced by ACTH, cortisone or hydrocortisone therapy
2. Chronic adrenal cortical insufficiency
   (*a*) Primary (Addison's disease)
   (*b*) Secondary (hypopituitarism)
   (*c*) Surgical (following adrenalectomy)
   (*d*) Insufficiency associated with androgenic adrenal hyperplasia

ACUTE ADRENAL CORTICAL INSUFFICIENCY

Adrenal Crisis. An adrenal crisis represents a severe acute exacerbation of Addison's disease. Although present-day substitution therapy has materially reduced the frequency of adrenal crisis, the advent of infection, trauma or gastrointestinal upsets in patients with Addison's disease, unless combated by an immediate increase in hormone dosage, may rapidly lead to the development of acute adrenal insufficiency. The classic manifestations of adrenal crisis are anorexia, nausea, vomiting, headache, diarrhea, abdominal pain, dehydration, hypotension, restlessness, marked weakness and lethargy. Hyperpyrexia, often extreme, usually occurs, but subnormal temperatures may be encountered even in the presence of infection. Ultimately, coma and vascular collapse ensue. It should be emphasized, however, that in well treated patients, especially those who have received desoxycorticosterone, hypotension and shock may only occur terminally. Laboratory study usually but not invariably reveals hyponatremia, hyperkalemia, hypoglycemia and azotemia.

The necessity for immediate and vigorous treatment of adrenal crisis is strongly emphasized. Therapy is directed at the provision of adequate adrenal cortical hormone, the control of infection and support of the cardiovascular system.

1. A continuous intravenous infusion of 5 per cent glucose in normal saline is started immediately. If available, 200 mg. of hydrocortisone (the free alcohol, not the acetate ester) is administered in 5 per cent glucose by a separate intravenous infusion. If an intravenous preparation of hydrocortisone is not available, cortisone acetate is given intramuscularly in an initial dose of 200 mg. (in four different sites) and 50 to 100 cc. of aqueous adrenal cortical extract is injected intravenously, followed by a continuous intravenous infusion of 100–200 cc. of extract in glucose and saline. Cortisone in a dose of 25 mg. is then administered intramuscularly every 6 hours until the patient is able to take medication by mouth. Thereafter, the hormone may be given orally, and the dosage gradually tapered to a maintenance level of 25 mg. per day.

2. Penicillin is given by intramuscular injection in a minimal dosage of 400,000 units every 6 hours.

3. If shock is profound or if hypotension persists, Neo-Synephrine may be injected subcutaneously in a dose of 0.3 to 0.5 mg. every 1 to 2 hours, or 5 to 10 mg. may be added to the intravenous infusion and the rate adjusted to maintain blood pressure at normal levels. Infusions of norepinephrine may also be employed to maintain the blood pressure. In the presence of extreme, persistent shock, it may be necessary to administer a transfusion of whole blood or concentrated serum albumin. Since the sodium-retaining effect of *intravenously* administered hydrocortisone is marked, it is usually not necessary to give desoxycorticosterone during the acute phase of adrenal crisis, unless the hypotension is refractory to other measures. In the latter situation, 10–20 mg. of the hormone may be injected intramuscularly initially and 2.5 to 5 mg. per day thereafter.

Adrenal Hemorrhage. The causes and manifestations of massive, bilateral adrenal hemorrhage vary with age. In the newborn infant, adrenal hemorrhage may occur during a prolonged and difficult labor, especially when asphyxia and traumatic resuscitation procedures are involved. In older children and adults, adrenal apoplexy is usually associated with overwhelming sepsis (Waterhouse-Friderichsen syndrome). Meningococcus has been the causative organism in approximately 75 per cent of cases; other organisms have been the staphylococcus, streptococcus and pneumococcus. In a few adult cases, adrenal hemorrhage has occurred as a result of anticoagulant overdosage.

Pathologically there is extensive bilateral adrenal hemorrhage which may occasionally rupture through the capsule of the adrenal into the peritoneal cavity. In those cases associated with a fulminating sepsis, a widespread capillary and arteriolar necrosis is frequently observed. Frank meningitis is rarely seen.

Acute adrenal insufficiency at birth produces the characteristic picture of acute shock; hemorrhagic manifestations are usually absent although in some cases a retroperitoneal mass may be palpated. Later in life, when the disease is associated with an overwhelming septicemia, there are extensive cutaneous petechiae and purpura. Early symptoms in these cases are increased irritability, nausea, vomiting, abdominal pain and headache. Shortly after the onset of the disease, a petechial rash appears which progresses to form a diffuse confluent purpuric eruption. Fever is present early and the temperature may rise to extreme levels. Intense cyanosis develops and finally circulatory collapse ensues. Death usually occurs within 24 to 48 hours after the onset of symptoms. As blood cultures are not always positive, specific therapy should not await the report of bacterial growth. In some cases the meningococcus can be seen on a Gram stain of fluid obtained from carefully punctured petechial spots.

The specific diagnosis of adrenal insufficiency under these circumstances is difficult to establish and must await the development of a rapid and practical method for blood corticoid determination. In the absence of such a method, blood eosinophil counts may be of help. While it is recognized that the occurrence of eosinopenia alone does not necessarily reflect increased adrenal cortical activity, a significant degree of eosinopenia ordinarily occurs during periods of severe stress in patients with intact adrenal cortices and is usually absent during equally severe stress in patients with adrenal insufficiency. Thus in the presence of fever, cyanosis, purpura and circulatory collapse, an eosinophil count of 100 cells per cubic millimeter is suggestive of adrenal cortical failure. In some cases of the Waterhouse-Friderichsen syndrome, a significant eosinopenia may occur during the first 6 to 12 hours after the onset of symptoms; later the eosinophil count returns towards normal levels.

Treatment is essentially similar to that outlined under Adrenal Crisis. Control of the infection is, of course, absolutely essential. Although formerly the Waterhouse-Friderichsen syndrome was uniformly fatal, in recent years several instances of recovery have been reported. It should be emphasized, however, that meningococcemia with purpuric rash may be associated with circulatory collapse in the absence of adrenal hemorrhage and without pathologic evidence of acute adrenal cortical insufficiency.

Acute Adrenal Insufficiency Associated with Surgery of the Adrenal Gland. This condition may occur following bilateral adrenalectomy or the removal of a unilateral adrenal cortical tumor which is associated with atrophy of the contralateral gland. Adrenal insufficiency should, of course, be anticipated under these conditions and adrenal cortical hormone replacement therapy instituted during and after operation as described in the section on the Treatment of Cushing's Syndrome (see table, p. 780).

Acute Adrenal Insufficiency Associated with ACTH or Cortisone Therapy. The commonest cause of acute adrenal cortical insufficiency is that which occurs in association with prolonged ACTH or cortisone administration. Here there is a diminished reactivity of the pituitary-adrenal cortical system due to pituitary inhibition in the case of ACTH administration and to both pituitary and adrenal cortical inhibition in the cases of cortisone treatment. When the stress of a severe medical illness or a surgical operation is imposed, the adrenal cortex may not respond adequately enough and a state of relative adrenal insufficiency may ensue. This may occur during the period of ACTH or cortisone administration or following the discontinuance of hormone therapy before the responsiveness of the pituitary-adrenal cortical axis has returned to normal. An adrenal crisis which may arise under these circumstances must be anticipated and supplementary hydrocortisone or cortisone administered until the period of stress has ended.

CHRONIC ADRENAL CORTICAL INSUFFICIENCY

PRIMARY FAILURE (ADDISON'S DISEASE)

"The leading and characteristic features of the morbid state to which I would direct attention are anemia, general languor and debility, remarkable feebleness of the heart's action, irritability of the stomach, and a peculiar change of the color of the skin occurring in connection with the diseased condition of the suprarenal capsule" (Thomas Addison, 1855).

Incidence and Etiology. True Addison's disease is a relatively rare condition, the incidence approximating one case per 100,000 population. There are two major causes of this condition: fibrocaseous tuberculosis of the adrenal gland and an idiopathic process of bilateral adrenal cortical atrophy. In earlier reports, the incidence of tuberculosis of the adrenal glands as a cause of Addison's disease was as high as 80 to 90 per cent. More recently, the incidence of tuberculosis has diminished in these patients and approximately 50 per cent of cases are nontuberculous in origin. In a small percentage of patients, other lesions may be encountered such as bilateral tumor metastases, leukemic infiltration, amyloidosis, hemochromatosis and histoplasmosis. Adrenal tuberculosis usually destroys both cortex and medulla, whereas in adrenal cortical atrophy the cortex is chiefly involved. In the latter condition, the gland is largely replaced by fibrous tissue and fat and only occasional strands of residual cortical cells may remain.

Clinical Picture. The onset of the disease is usually insidious. Occasionally, however, the first evidence of adrenal failure may be the development of crisis precipitated by an acute infection or a surgical operation. The predominant symptoms are asthenia, easy fatigability, weight loss, increased pigmentation of the skin and mucous membranes, gastrointestinal complaints including anorexia, nausea, vomiting, diarrhea and abdominal pain, and episodes suggestive of hypoglycemia. Increased irritability, nervousness, emotional instability, and periods of depression and negativism are not uncommon. Pigmentation usually appears early and is the most striking physical evidence of the disease. It usually presents itself as a diffuse tanning with increased pigmentation over pressure points such as the knees, elbows and knuckles. There may be bluish black pigmentation of the mucous membranes and multiple black freckles over the body. Not infrequently,

though 20 to 25 per cent of patients reveal adrenal calcification on roentgenographic examination, this finding is not pathognomonic of adrenal insufficiency. The basal metabolic rate is often between minus 10 and minus 20 per cent. The blood plasma volume is reduced. The electrocardiogram characteristically shows a low voltage and there is a decreased frequency of the waves on the electroencephalogram.

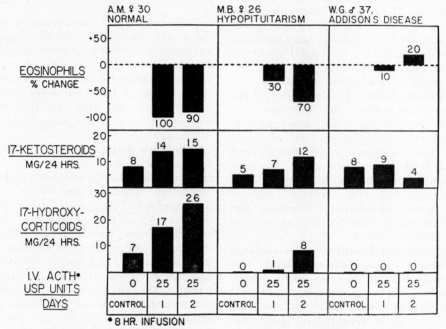

Fig. 93. Adrenal responses to intravenous ACTH.

vitiliginous areas or "leukoderma" may be noted. Most patients with Addison's disease will have hypotension and a small heart. Secondary sex characteristics are usually little affected except for the reduction of the growth of axillary and body hair. The menstrual cycle and gonadal function are ordinarily remarkably well maintained.

Laboratory Findings. There is a normochromic, normocytic anemia which becomes accentuated when rehydration is achieved. There is a tendency to lymphocytosis and moderate eosinophilia. In severe deficiency low serum sodium and chloride and a high serum potassium are observed. Hypoglycemia may occur during extended fasting or following high carbohydrate loads. Urinary 17-ketosteroid excretion is diminished in the male and may be virtually absent in the female. The level of urinary 17-hydroxycorticoids is generally below 2 mg. per day. Al-

Diagnosis. The most definitive diagnostic procedure is the demonstration of a lack of adrenal cortical response to the administration of pituitary corticotrophin (ACTH). In the 8-hour intravenous ACTH test, 25 U.S.P. units of the hormone are infused intravenously in 500 cc. of 5 per cent dextrose in saline over an 8-hour period on each of two successive days. Determinations of urinary 17-ketosteroids and 17-hydroxycorticoids are carried out on 24-hour collections on a control day and on each of the two days during ACTH administration. Blood is taken for an eosinophil count at the beginning and end of each infusion. Under these circumstances, a normal subject will exhibit an increase of 8 to 16 mg. per day in the excretion of 17-hydroxycorticoids and 4 to 8 mg. per day in the excretion of 17-ketosteroids, while patients with Addison's disease will show virtually no response. Normal subjects will respond with an eosinopenia of 80 to 90 per cent whereas Addisonian patients show little or no change. Patients with hypopituitarism and ACTH insufficiency exhibit varying responses depending upon the degree of adrenal cortical involution. When the intravenous ACTH test is repeated on three or more consecutive days, patients with Addison's disease continue to show no change, whereas those with secondary adrenal insufficiency reveal a gradual rise in 17-ketosteroid and 17-hydrooxycorticoid excretion and an increasing eosinopenia (Fig. 93).

An alternative method of testing adrenal cortical response consists in the intramuscular injection of 40 "clinical" units of ACTH gel twice daily over a two-day period. Urinary 17-ketosteroids and 17-hydroxycorticoids are determined on a control day and on each of the days of ACTH administration. Eosinophil counts are checked before each morning injection. Results are similar to those obtained with the intravenous ACTH test. Occasionally a false negative response is observed when extravascular inactivation of ACTH prevents the hormone from reaching the adrenal cortex. Thus with a negative response to the injection of ACTH gel, one should always resort to intravenous administration of the hormone.

The 4-hour ACTH test may be of value as a rapid screening procedure. In this test, the level of circulating eosinophils is determined before, and 4 hours after, the intramuscular injection of 25 U.S.P. units of ACTH in aqueous solution. A fall in circulating eosinophils exceeding 50 per cent of the initial value makes adrenal insufficiency highly unlikely. A fall of less than 50 per cent may be due to adrenal cortical insufficiency but can also be caused by inadequate adrenal stimulation due to extravascular destruction of ACTH. In the latter event, the more definitive ACTH tests described above must be employed.

Additional tests of adrenal cortical adequacy include the measurement of capacity for prompt water diuresis, which is lost in adrenal insufficiency but which is quite nonspecific (Robinson-Kepler-Power water test). The defect in salt-retaining capacity may be revealed by testing the ability of the patient to withstand sodium chloride deprivation (Cutler-Power-Wilder test). Gluconeogenesis may be assessed by testing the capacity of the patient to maintain a normal blood glucose concentration during a 24-hour fast. Since they may precipitate adrenal crisis, the salt withdrawal test and the 24-hour fast for hypoglycemic response should be carried out only in a hospital under competent supervision when other tests have failed to provide a definitive answer.

Treatment. As a result of the remarkable advances in recent years in the preparation of crystalline adrenal steroids, highly effective replacement therapy is now possible for patients with Addison's disease. The prognosis of such patients has been particularly improved since the advent of cortisone. The administration of this hormone leads to a restoration of appetite, muscular strength and body weight, and a general feeling of well being. The anemia is corrected, the tendency to hypoglycemia is reduced, the electrocardiogram and electroencephalogram return toward normal, the capacity to excrete an ingested water load improves, pigmentation is lightened and the capacity to withstand the stress of intercurrent infection and trauma is greatly enhanced. Adequate maintenance therapy is provided by an average daily dose of cortisone of 12.5 to 25 mg. by mouth. Alternatively, hydrocortisone may be administered in a dose of 10 to 20 mg. by mouth per day. Each of these hormones is best given in divided doses at 8 A.M. and 3 P.M. Similar doses of cortisone and hydrocortisone when given daily to patients with Addison's disease and active tuberculosis do not appear to promote the spread of the infectious process.

During periods of intercurrent illness, it is essential that the dose of cortisone be increased to a level of 75 to 100 mg. per day. If the administration of the hormone by the oral route is not possible, the aqueous suspension of cortisone acetate may be given intramuscularly in equivalent doses. Patients with Addison's disease who undergo surgery should be adequately prepared with supplementary hormone. It is recommended that for major surgery in Addisonian patients, a therapeutic program similar to that described for patients undergoing adrenal surgery for Cushing's syndrome should be instituted (see table, p. 780).

Unfortunately, the amounts of cortisone or hydrocortisone required to restore to normal the metabolism of carbohydrate, protein and fat are too small to assure normal electrolyte and water balance. Thus, adequate hydration and blood pressure stabilization require either the use of 10 to 15 gm. of supplementary sodium chloride per day or, in the vast majority of cases, the use of small amounts of desoxycorticosterone acetate (DCA) with a normal sodium and potassium intake. DCA may be employed in one of the following four ways. Treatment is ordinarily initiated by the daily intramuscular injection of the hormone in oil, 2.5 to 5 mg. per day. Basal weight, blood pressure and hematocrit are followed and the dose is adjusted to bring these measurements within normal limits. When the maintenance dose has been determined, the necessity for daily intramuscular injection may circumvented by the use of linguets, subcutaneous pellets or the long-acting injectable preparation desoxycorticosterone trimethylacetate. Linguets or buccalets of DCA may be used sublingually or in the buccal pouch. These require from 30 to 40 minutes to dissolve. They weigh 2 or 5 mg. and must be given two or three times daily. The dose required for proper maintenance is three to four times that of DCA in oil. Two types of pellets, weighing 75 and 125 mg., are available for subcutaneous implantation. The duration of effect is five and ten months, respectively. The smaller pellets may be implanted through a trocar; the larger require a surgical incision, with subcutaneous implantation. The effect of one 75 mg. pellet is equivalent to that obtained from the daily intramuscular injection of 0.3 mg. of DCA in oil; one 125 mg. pellet is equivalent to 0.5 mg. of DCA in oil. Three to five of the smaller and two to three of the larger pellets represent the average requirement.

At present, the preparation of desoxycorticosterone to be preferred in the treatment of most Addisonian patients is the long-acting trimethylacetate ester. The microcrystalline suspension of this compound contains 25 mg. per cubic centimeter. The administration of 25 mg. every three to four weeks corresponds approximately to the daily administration of 1 mg. of DCA in oil. This method of treatment can be instituted within a week after the establishment of the proper dosage of DCA in oil. It can often be started without prior treatment with DCA in oil by administering 2 cc. once a month and estimating the approximate dosage required by following the patient's weight, blood pressure and well being over consecutive months.

Manifestations of desoxycorticosterone acetate overdosage which must be carefully watched for in patients on prolonged therapy include edema, headache, hypertension and cardiac enlargement. Arthralgia and tendon contractures may also occur; these are rarely seen, however, when cortisone is given along with DCA. When DCA dosage has been particularly excessive, extreme weakness of the extremities, due to potassium depletion, may develop; an ascending paralysis, cardiac arrhythmias and even sudden cardiac arrest may occur. The treatment of DCA overdosage consists of the following: (1) discontinuance of DCA and doubling of the dose of cortisone if such is being given; (2) a low salt diet until sodium balance has been reestablished, as judged by clinical improvement; (3) oral administration of 3 to 5 gm. of enteric-coated potassium chloride per day; (4) administration of mercurial diuretics, cautiously and in divided doses, e.g., mercuhydrin 0.5 cc. every 12 hours for two to three doses.

Because of the relatively small doses of cortisone employed in maintenance therapy, undesirable effects such as are encountered in the treatment of collagen diseases are rarely seen. Gastric irritation occasionally occurs in patients taking cortisone acetate by mouth. This is overcome in most instances by giving the hormone during meals. Increased excitability and sleeplessness are only rarely encountered if the last dose of cortisone is given no later than 4 P.M. Psychotic reactions are quite uncommon, but occasionally occur even at low dosages. This demands reduction in dosage until the patient's psyche becomes stable. In view of this side effect, it is advisable to start therapy with a small dose (12.5 mg. per day) of the hormone.

Patients with Addison's disease and those who have undergone bilateral adrenalectomy should carry a card with them at all times bearing the doctor's name, telephone number and address, the patient's disease, his name and address, and that of the nearest of kin. In addition, the following sentence should be written: "In the event of illness, administer 25 mg. of cortisone acetate every 6 hours by mouth unless the patient is unconscious, when 200 mg. of the hormone should be given by intramuscular injection."

Prognosis. In the absence of active tuberculosis, the outlook is good with modern substitution therapy. On DCA alone, 5-year survival in a large group of patients was increased from 20 per cent in the salt treatment era to 50 per cent. Further improvement is to be anticipated now that cortisone and hydrocortisone are available. In the majority of instances it is no longer necessary to administer supplementary salt and dietary regulation is ordinarily not required. It should be emphasized, however, that the success of treatment largely depends, as it does in diabetes mellitus, upon careful education of the patient. It is absolutely essential that the potential threat of intercurrent stress and the necessity of administering increased quantities of cortisone during a period of stress be thoroughly appreciated by both the patient and his physician.

CHRONIC ADRENAL CORTICAL INSUFFICIENCY SECONDARY TO PITUITARY FAILURE

This condition is due to an anterior pituitary insufficiency of ACTH. It differs from primary adrenal insufficiency (Addison's disease) in that the electrolyte disturbance is usually less marked, the susceptibility to hypoglycemia is greater and pigmentation is minimal or absent. Associated deficiencies of gonadal and thyroid function are ordinarily present and in many patients dominate the clinical picture. The response to ACTH is typically delayed in proportion to the degree of secondary adrenal cortical atrophy (Fig. 93). Treatment involves the use of cortisone or hydrocortisone as described above for Addison's disease. Desoxycorticosterone is administered if there is a significant tendency towards salt loss. In addition, thyroid extract and testosterone are employed as indicated.

CHRONIC ADRENAL CORTICAL INSUFFICIENCY SECONDARY TO ADRENALECTOMY

Patients who have undergone total, and in many instances subtotal, adrenalectomy require adrenal cortical hormone replacement therapy similar to that described for Addison's disease. These patients, however, are particularly susceptible to the effects of cortisone deprivation. Moreover, they may tolerate larger quantities of cortisone than patients with Addison's disease and often only attain an optimal state of well being on doses of 37.5 to 50 mg. per day. In addition, their requirement for desoxycorticosterone is considerably more variable than is the case for patients with Addison's disease.

CHRONIC ADRENAL INSUFFICIENCY ASSOCIATED WITH CONGENITAL ADRENAL CORTICAL HYPERPLASIA

Congenital bilateral adrenal cortical hyperplasia causes pseudohermaphroditism in females and sexual precocity in males. Acute adrenal insufficiency may occur in these instances, especially in males. It is characterized by salt loss, dehydration and eventually circulatory collapse. More commonly the illness may pursue a subacute course, marked by periods of dehydration, rapid weight loss, vomiting, diarrhea and abdominal pain, usually in association with intercurrent infections. Hypoglycemia ordinarily does not occur. Treatment of acute adrenal insufficiency in these patients is the same as in other types of adrenal crisis. The use of cortisone in maintenance therapy is discussed below in the section on the adrenogenital syndrome. When cortisone alone does not control salt loss, desoxycorticosterone must be added to the therapeutic regimen.

HYPERFUNCTION OF THE ADRENAL CORTEX

The clinical picture of hyperadrenocorticism extends in a broad spectrum from Cushing's syndrome at the one end to the adrenogenital syndrome at the other. Cushing's syndrome is the expression of an excessive adrenocortical secretion of the 11, 17-oxygenated corticoids, hydrocortisone and cortisone, while the adrenogenital syndrome is the manifestation of an increased secretion of androgens from the adrenal cortex. Between these two extremes, there are many patients who present manifestations of each syndrome to a varying degree. Rarely, adrenal cortical hyperfunction may be associated with feminization in the male. Twelve such cases have been reported and all have been due to estrogen-producing, malignant adrenal cortical tumors.

CUSHING'S SYNDROME

This syndrome was first clearly recognized by Harvey Cushing in 1932. While admitting that certain of the cases were due to primary adrenal disease, adenoma or carcinoma, Cushing believed that in those patients with a pituitary basophil adenoma and bilateral adrenal cortical hyperplasia ("Cushing's disease"), the disturbance rested in the anterior pituitary.

Etiology. Cushing's syndrome represents the effects of a long continued, excessive secretion of 11, 17-oxygenated corticoids, hydrocortisone and cortisone, by the adrenal cortex. The adrenal lesion may be adenoma, carcinoma or bilateral hyperplasia; rarely unilateral hyperplasia may be found Much more normal or hyperplastic adrenals, there is a basophil adenoma in the anterior pituitary; in these cases, the primary lesion is believed to be in the pituitary from which there is increased secretion of ACTH.

Incidence. Cushing's syndrome is a rare disorder which occurs much more frequently

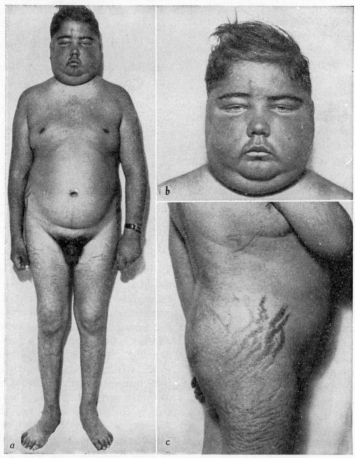

Fig. 94. Classical appearance of patient suffering from Cushing's syndrome due to bilateral adrenal hyperplasia. Note (*a, b*) the "moon facies," the truncal obesity and (*c*) the cutaneous striae over the lower abdomen and hips. (R. H. Williams: Textbook of Endocrinology.)

rarely, a tumor in aberrant adrenal cortical tissue (e.g., ovary) may be seen in association with bilateral atrophy of the adrenal glands. When congenital, Cushing's syndrome is almost always associated with bilateral adrenal hyperplasia. When the disease has its onset during the prepubertal period, the adrenal lesion is usually a malignant tumor. In 60 per cent of adult cases bilateral adrenal cortical hyperplasia is found, in 30 per cent an adenoma or a carcinoma, while in 10 per cent of cases the adrenal cortices appear normal. In many of the patients with in the female than in the male. Actively secreting adrenal cortical adenomas are practically confined to the female. The incidence of the disease is at its peak in the third and fourth decade. The syndrome appears to occur particularly frequently following pregnancy.

Pathology. Bilateral hyperplasia is characterized by symmetrical enlargement of the cortex with increased convolution of the surface. Not infrequently, a few hyperplastic nodules are present. Microscopically, the hyperplasia is particularly marked in the zona fasciculata. The single and, rarely, multiple adenomas are well demarcated and surrounded by a narrow rim of atrophied cortical tissue. Carcinoma of the adrenal cortex is often highly malignant, with spread of the tumor usually occurring by vein. The liver is a frequent site of metastases. When a unilateral adenoma or carcinoma is present, there is atrophy of the contralateral adrenal cortex due to suppression of the output of ACTH from the anterior pituitary. Hyalinization of the basophil cells (Crooke's changes) of the anterior pituitary is invariably present in Cushing's syndrome. Similar changes have been observed in patients who have received long-term cortisone therapy. In the presence of bilateral hyperplasia, basophil adenoma is frequently found. These tumors are small and enlargement of the sella turcica is exceedingly rare.

The most striking, generalized, pathologic change in Cushing's syndrome is protein depletion. There is osteoporosis and general muscle wasting. The blood vessels are fragile and frequently show changes secondary to hypertension. Widespread fatty degeneration is common. The kidneys reveal nephrosclerosis and calcinosis. The pancreas may show fatty necrosis and islet cell hyperplasia. Carcinoma of the pancreas and of the thymus has been found in a small number of cases.

Clinical Picture. The clinical picture of Cushing's syndrome is essentially the expression of an excessive secretion of hydrocortisone-like hormones (Fig. 94). The most striking feature is protein depletion which is evident in muscle, skin, blood vessels and bone. Marked weakness is associated with diminution of muscle mass. Fragility of the skin and blood vessels is evidence by depressed purple striae over the abdomen, thighs and upper arms, and increased susceptibility to bruises and ecchymoses. Osteoporosis leads to backache and dorsal kyphosis and compression fractures of the vertebrae are not uncommon.

Increased gluconeogenesis from protein, and possibly fat, leads to a diminished carbohydrate tolerance and, occasionally, diabetes.

There is a striking redistribution of fat with the obesity confined to the face, neck and trunk. The combination of supraclavicular fat pads combined with dorsal kyphosis give rise to the "buffalo hump" while the facial obesity is seen as the typical "moon face."

Facial plethora, hypertension and peripheral edema are common. Lability of mood is usually present and occasionally there may be an overt psychosis.

Female patients with Cushing's syndrome may show signs of masculinization, with hirsutism, acne, deepening of the voice, amenorrhea and enlargement of the clitoris. In these cases, there is probably an increased secretion of androgens as well as hydrocortisone-like hormones by the adrenal cortex.

The clinical course is characterized by progressive weakness, increased susceptibility to infection, the symptoms of which are often masked, and the appearance of fractures of the spine. Death occurs from vascular accidents, intercurrent infection or diabetic coma.

Diagnosis. The combination of marked protein depletion, the typical fat distribution and a diminished carbohydrate tolerance strongly favors the diagnosis of Cushing's syndrome. Sudden onset suggests an adrenal cortical adenoma or carcinoma; an insidious onset favors bilateral hyperplasia.

Definitive diagnosis of Cushing's syndrome requires the determination of urinary 17-ketosteroids and 17-hydroxycorticoids. The urinary excretion of 17-hydroxycorticoids is almost invariably increased. In general, the level of 17-ketosteroids is lower than normal in the presence of an adenoma, normal or slightly elevated with bilateral hyperplasia and above 30 mg. per day when the lesion is a carcinoma of the adrenal cortex. Differentiation of these lesions may be considerably helped by study of the patient's response to an 8-hour intravenous infusion of ACTH. Patients with bilateral hyperplasia tend to show a hyperactive response as measured by rises in urinary 17-ketosteroids and 17-hydroxycorticoids. When the lesion is a carcinoma, usually no response is observed. In the presence of an adenoma, the response may be normal or hyperactive. It is probable that the degree of autonomy of the tumor determines its response to ACTH stimulation.

In the presence of an elevated level of urinary 17-ketosteroids, further help in the differentiation of tumor and bilateral hyperplasia of the adrenal cortex may be obtained by following the urinary 17-ketosteroid excretion during the administration of cortisone acetate over a six-day period, 100 mg. per day by intramuscular injection. Under these conditions, patients with bilateral hyperplasia usually show a fall in 17-ketosteroid excretion, while those with an adrenal cortical tumor may show no change.

Diagnostically helpful laboratory findings are an eosinophil count below 50 per cubic millimeter, lymphopenia, neutrophilia and polycythemia. Glycosuria with diminished carbohydrate tolerance is of frequent occurrence; occasionally frank diabetes mellitus may be present. In a small number of cases there is a hypokalemic, hypochloremic alkalosis. Roentgenogram of the sella turcica is almost invariably normal. Films of the skull and spine show osteoporosis and compression fractures of the vertebrae may be

mencement of therapy. A fall in the titer of urinary 17-hydroxycorticoids and a rise in the level of circulating eosinophils are indications that therapy has been effective.

In more seriously ill patients (particularly those with marked mental changes or extensive protein depletion, e.g., severe osteoporosis with fractures), or in those early cases which have failed to respond to roentgen therapy, bilateral subtotal or total adrenalectomy is recommended. *Bilateral total adrenalectomy* is preferred for the following reasons: to prevent the recurrence of hyperadrenocorticism; to obviate the hazard of

---

Hormone Therapy for Complete Adrenalectomy—Cushing's Syndrome

Preoperative:
    Cortisone acetate: 100 mg., I.M.   12 hrs. and 2 hrs. preop.
Operation:
    (1) Hydrocortisone or cortisone 100–150 mg., I.V. During adrenalectomy and 6–12 hrs. postop.
    (2) Cortisone acetate: 50 mg., I.M. q.6h.
Postoperative:
    (1) Day 1
        Cortisone acetate: 50 mg., I.M. q.6h.
    (2) Days 2, 3
        Cortisone acetate: 50 mg., I.M. q.8h.
    (3) Days 4, 5, 6, 7
        Cortisone acetate: 50 mg., P.O. q.12h.
    (4) Days 8, 9, 10
        Cortisone acetate: 25 mg., P.O. q.8h.
    (5) Thereafter, taper cortisone acetate (P.O.) slowly to maintenance level.

---

found. An abdominal film may outline an adrenal mass while intravenous pyelograms may reveal depression of the renal shadow. Retroperitoneal pneumograms may be of value in the detection of an adrenal mass and the differentiation of adenoma or carcinoma from bilateral hyperplasia.

Treatment. Whatever the plan for specific therapy, it is well to administer potassium chloride, 6 gm. per day by mouth, in the presence of a hypokalemic, hypochloremic alkalosis, and to combat the protein depletion by the administration of testosterone propionate, 25 mg. daily by intramuscular injection.

Bilateral Adrenal Cortical Hyperplasia. When all efforts to detect the presence of an adrenal cortical tumor have failed and bilateral hyperplasia is suspected, *pituitary irradiation* may be instituted in those early cases which show minimal signs of protein depletion and only mild psychic involvement. A minimum dose of 3000 r should be delivered to the gland. Improvement occurs in approximately one quarter of these cases within three months following the com-

relying on a possibly insufficient remnant of adrenal cortex; because of the proven effectiveness of modern substitution therapy for adrenal insufficiency; and because aberrant adrenal cortical tissue may be present in an appreciable number of patients. Adrenal cortical hormone therapy is routinely instituted prior to operation and continued during and after surgery as outlined in the accompanying table. As intravenous solutions of hydrocortisone and cortisone have become available, the operative and immediate postoperative course has been greatly smoothed. In particular, the incidence of hypotensive reactions has been diminished. Occasionally, however, such reactions do occur and Neo-Synephrine or norepinephrine should be given intravenously at a rate sufficient to maintain the blood pressure at normal levels.

Patients who have undergone complete bilateral adrenalectomy must be treated in the same manner as are those with Addison's disease. Following operation, it is advisable to taper the dose of cortisone gradually over a period of four to six weeks to maintenance levels of 25 to 37.5 mg. by mouth per day.

Thereby, it may be possible to diminish the incidence and severity of the postadrenalectomy syndrome described by Kepler. This syndrome is characterized by nausea, vomiting, diarrhea, muscular tenderness and aching and arthralgia. Furthermore, the administration of desoxycorticosterone along with cortisone is not only unnecessary but contraindicated before the cortisone dosage has been tapered to 75 mg. per day. At this time, the need for the salt-retaining effect of desoxycorticosterone may be assessed by the daily determination of urinary sodium excretion.

Although the availability of hydrocortisone and cortisone has greatly facilitated adrenalectomy in patients with Cushing's syndrome, it must be emphasized strongly that these patients are extremely fragile and particularly prone to postoperative complications.

Unilateral Adrenal Cortical Adenoma or Carcinoma. When Cushing's syndrome is due to an adrenal cortical tumor, surgical removal is necessary. Because the uninvolved contralateral adrenal cortex is atrophied owing to suppression of ACTH secretion from the anterior pituitary, adrenal cortical hormone therapy must be instituted as described for patients undergoing bilateral total adrenalectomy for hyperplasia. Within two weeks after surgery, the status of the contralateral adrenal cortex is evaluated by the determination of urinary 17-hydroxycorticoids during ACTH administration and rapid tapering of cortisone dosage over a five-day period. The ACTH is given daily either in a lose of 20 U.S.P. units by intravenous infusion over an 8-hour period or in doses of 80 "clinical" units of the gel preparation in a single intramuscular injection. A gradual rise in the level of urinary 17-hydroxycorticoids during this period indicates that the remaining adrenal gland is functioning adequately. The ACTH dosage is then very gradually tapered to allow the inhibited anterior pituitary to return to normal. Occasionally, irreversible atrophy of the contralateral gland occurs and permanent substitution therapy, as for Addison's disease, is required.

ADRENOGENITAL SYNDROME AND ADRENAL VIRILISM

Apert, a French physician, introduced the term adrenal virilism in 1910 to designate a syndrome of masculinization in women which he related to alterations in adrenal cortical function. Its biologic counterpart, feminization in the male, has since been recognized as an extremely rare condition. Twelve such cases have been reported, and all have been due to malignant estrogen-producing tumors of the adrenal cortex.

Etiology. The manifestations of adrenal virilism are due to an increased secretion of androgens from the adrenal cortex. The adrenal lesion may be bilateral hyperplasia, adenoma or carcinoma. Adrenal virilism, which is evident at birth, is almost invariably due to bilateral hyperplasia. When the disease has its onset in later life, the lesion is usually a tumor, more frequently a carcinoma. It is not certain, at the present time, whether those cases with bilateral hyperplasia are due to a primary anterior pituitary disturbance with an increased secretion of ACTH.

Pathology. While it is difficult to correlate cytologic changes in the adrenal cortex with the type of endocrine disturbance produced, it is not uncommon to find in cases of virilization due to bilateral adrenal cortical hyperplasia that the overgrowth is primarily in the zona reticularis. The virilizing tumors are frequently highly malignant and metastasize chiefly to the liver and lungs.

Clinical Picture. As a result of their virilizing properties, an increased secretion of adrenal androgens may lead to female pseudohermaphroditism at birth, precocious puberty in the preadolescent male, and heterosexual development in the preadolescent and adolescent female. In addition to their androgenicity, these hormones possess a protein anabolic effect. Thus, while patients with Cushing's syndrome present evidence of protein depletion, those with the adrenogenital syndrome show signs of protein conservation, e.g., increased rate of growth in the prepubertal child and increased muscle mass in the adult. Heterosexual development in the young female is characterized by hirsutism, deepening of the voice, absence of breast development, enlargement of the clitoris and amenorrhea. It must be emphasized that when adrenal virilism is due to bilateral hyperplasia, particularly the congenital variety, the symptoms and signs of Addison's disease may be present. Such patients are particularly prone to develop evidence of salt deficiency.

At all ages, the psychologic and social problems associated with this disease must be given careful consideration.

Invariably in this condition, there is an

increased excretion of urinary 17-ketosteroids. High values (50 mg. per day or more) with an increased proportion of the beta fraction (largely dehydroisoandrosterone), in combination with high levels of urinary estrogens, are strongly suggestive of carcinoma of the adrenal cortex as opposed to hyperplasia or adenoma. In the presence of congenital adrenocortical hyperplasia, the blood ACTH level is high while urinary and blood levels of 17-hydroxycorticoids are low. The response of the latter to ACTH is subnormal or absent. The presence of a tumor may be detected by means of an abdominal film, intravenous pyelography or retroperitoneal pneumography.

Differential Diagnosis. Sexual precocity in the prepubertal male may be constitutional, owing to a pineal tumor, to lesions in the hypothalamus or to a Leydig cell tumor of the testes as well as to an adrenal cortical lesion. Heterosexual development in the prepubertal or adult female may be caused by a lesion in either the adrenal cortex or the ovary. The ovarian lesions include arrhenoblastoma, Leydig cell tumor, adrenal rests, luteoma and polycystic disease (Stein-Leventhal syndrome). Differentiation between ovarian and adrenal lesions as the cause of the virilizing syndrome may be helped by following the level of urinary 17-ketosteroids during the administration of cortisone. The hormone is administered intramuscularly in doses of 100 mg. per day over a period of one week. Should a dramatic fall in urinary 17-ketosteroid excretion occur, the causal lesion is presumed to be bilateral adrenal cortical hyperplasia. When a persistent depression of the urinary 17-ketosteroid level is not observed, it is presumed that the lesion is either an adrenal cortical tumor or ovarian disease. In this instance, the relatively simple operation of pelvic laparotomy is first performed. In the absence of a responsible ovarian lesion, the adrenals are then explored.

Treatment. Treatment of virilizing adrenal cortical tumor is surgical removal. In a few cases, atrophy of the uninvolved contralateral gland has been found and it is therefore wise in all instances to institute adrenal cortical hormone therapy as described previously for operation on patients with Cushing's syndrome due to tumor. When the lesion is a carcinoma with widespread metastases, postoperative x-ray therapy is advised, but it is usually of little value.

When adrenal virilism is associated with bilateral hyperplasia, a congenital condition which occasionally goes unnoticed until adulthood, the treatment of choice is cortisone suppression of adrenal androgen secretion. Therapy is usually initiated with intramuscularly administered hormone at a dosage level of 50 mg. per day for older children and 25 mg. per day for younger children and infants. Maximum suppression of urinary 17-ketosteroid excretion is usually seen within five to ten days. Thereafter, the dose of cortisone should be gradually tapered to that level which gives reasonable suppression of adrenal androgen secretion with minimal untoward side effects; of the latter, a diminution in the rate of growth is particularly to be watched for. For older children, maintenance doses of 50 mg. of cortisone every other day by intramuscular injection are usually optimal, whereas, in infants and younger children, smaller doses may be quite adequate. The amount of orally administered cortisone which is required for maintenance is approximately two to three times as great as that which is effective by the intramuscular route. In those cases of bilateral hyperplasia associated with adrenal insufficiency, cortisone alone may not control salt loss and desoxycorticosterone must be added to the therapeutic program. At the present time, it is too early to be certain whether the above treatment alone will prove adequate to control the disease. As further experience with this condition accumulates, bilateral adrenalectomy may prove to be a worth-while procedure in selected cases.

NONFUNCTIONING ADRENAL CORTICAL TUMORS

Benign, nonsecretory cortical adenomas are a frequent finding at autopsy. These tumors, which are rarely more than 2 to 3 cm. in diameter, are well circumscribed, yellow masses, similar in appearance to the normal adrenal cortex. They are seen more frequently in middle-aged or elderly subjects and in women more often than in men.

Nonfunctioning, primary adenocarcinomas are extremely rare. Unfortunately, the tumor is seldom recognized until it is large enough to be palpable or until metastases have occurred. It is often mistaken for a kidney and its true character may only be demonstrated by roentgenographic studies (pyelography, pneumography) or at operation. The tumor must be removed surgically. Pre- and postoperative replacement therapy such as is essential in patients with functioning adrenal cortical tumors is not necessary in these patients.

Carcinomas of the lung and breast frequently metastasize to the adrenal glands. Patients with these tumors may occasionally die of adrenal insufficiency induced by such metastases.

GEORGE W. THORN

References

Chemistry and Physiology

Loeb, R. F.: The Adrenal Cortex and Electrolyte Behavior. The Harvey Lectures, Series 37. Lancaster, Pa., Science Press Printing Co., 1942.

Mason, H. L.: Steroid Nomenclature. J. Clin. Endocrinol., 8:190, 1948.

Selye, H.: The General Adaptation Syndrome and the Diseases of Adaptation. J. Clin. Endocrinol., 6:117, 1946.

Thorn, G. W., and others: Medical Progress: Pharmacologic Aspects of Adrenocortical Steroids and ACTH in Man. New England J. Med., 248: 232, 284, 323, 369, 414, 588, 632, 1953.

Adrenal Insufficiency

Addison, T.: On the Constitutional and Local Effects of Disease of the Suprarenal Capsules. London, D. Highley, 1855.

Soffer, L. J.: Diseases of the Adrenals. Philadelphia, Lea and Febiger, 1952.

Thorn, G. W., Forsham, P. H., and Emerson, K., Jr.: The Diagnosis and Treatment of Adrenal Insufficiency. Springfield, Illinois, Charles C Thomas, 1950.

Thorn, G. W., and others: Advances in the Diagnosis and Treatment of Adrenal Insufficiency. Am. J. Med., 5:595, 1951.

Cushing's Syndrome

Albright, F.: Cushing's Syndrome. Harvey Lectures, Series 38, Lancaster, Pa., Science Press Printing Co., 1943.

Cushing, H.: The Basophil Adenomas of the Pituitary Body and Their Clinical Manifestations (Pituitary Basophilism). Bull. Johns Hopkins Hosp., 50:137, 1932.

Plotz, C. M., Knowlton, A. I., and Ragan, C.: The Natural History of Cushing's Syndrome. Am. J. Med., 13:597, 1952.

Sprague, R. G., and Kvale, W. F.: Management of Certain Hyperfunctioning Lesions of the Adrenal Cortex and Medulla. J.A.M.A., 151:629, 1953.

Steinbach, H. F., Lyon, R. P., Smith, D. R., and Miller, E. R.: Extraperitoneal Pneumography. Radiology, 59:167, 1952.

Adrenogenital Syndrome

Jailer, J. W., Louchart, J., and Cahill, G. F.: Adrenal Virilism. Diagnostic Considerations and Treatment. J.A.M.A., 150:880, 1951.

Wilkins, L.: The Diagnosis of the Adrenogenital Syndrome and Its Treatment with Cortisone. J. Pediat., 41:860, 1952.

Young, H.: Genital Abnormalities, Hermaphroditism and Related Adrenal Diseases. Baltimore, Williams and Wilkins Co., 1937.

DISEASES OF THE THYMUS GLAND

Many possible functions have been attributed to the thymus gland, but, thus far, none has been subject to proof. Classic extirpation experiments in a variety of animals have given no conclusive results. Extracts of many types have been tested, but the results have been variable. The planning of such experiments is exceedingly difficult because of the fact that, in our ignorance of the functions of the thymus, the conditions for making any effects recognizable have not been fulfilled. There are certain clinical relationships which suggest that the thymus has an endocrine function. Myasthenia gravis is associated in many instances with a tumor of the thymus. In many cases of hyperthyroidism, a disease associated with thymic enlargement, muscular weakness is a prominent feature; and the occasional development of myasthenia gravis in association with exophthalmic goiter is probably more than coincidental. Much discussion has taken place about the relationship of the thymus enlargement to sudden death in infants, particularly during anesthesia. Thus the function of this organ, and its relationships to clinical disease, are still for the most part shrouded in mystery.

Anatomy and Physiology. In the normal thymus of infants there is a well defined cortex consisting of closely packed masses of cells ("thymocytes"), resembling lymphocytes, and a medulla. During the process of differentiation into cortex and medulla, concentric masses of cells, the Hassall corpuscles, appear in the sheets of epithelial cells of the medulla. Opinion varies as to the nature of the thymocytes. Some observers contend that the thymocytes are in reality lymphocytes, and appear in the gland only after invasion from without. Others believe that the morphologic similarity does not establish their common identity. This group feel that the cell is formed *in situ* from thymic epithelium.

Near the age of puberty the gland becomes narrower and occupies a relatively smaller portion of the anterior mediastinum, although in actual size it may be larger than in the infant. As involution takes place, thymic tissue is replaced by adipose tissue which separates the lobules from each other. The

number of lymphocytes in the cortex and medulla decreases, but, in spite of these changes, thymic tissue can, with rare exceptions, be found in any person regardless of age, type of illness or cause of death. There may be an acceleration of involution brought on by illness, a so-called "accidental involution."

Animal experiments have demonstrated relationships of the thymus to certain of the endocrine glands. Castration and administration of thyroxin in rats cause comparable increases in the weights of the thymus, the lymph nodes and the spleen. Thyroidectomy and treatment with testosterone tend to decrease the weights of these structures. These procedures also prevent the increase in weight of the thymus which follows castration. There is a reciprocal relationship between the size of the adrenal cortex and the thymus. Deficient adrenal cortical secretion results in hypertrophy, and the injection of adrenocortical steroids or the adrenotrophic hormone of the pituitary results in a decrease in thymic weight. Rats exposed to low atmospheric pressures for more than two days exhibit an increase in adrenal weight and a significant decrease in the weight of the thymus and testes.

Evidence has been obtained by some investigators of a neuromuscular blocking effect in extracts of thymus and pancreas, while others have concluded that extracts of thymus from patients with myasthenia gravis are capable of inhibiting acetylcholine synthesis, in contrast to similar preparations from normal individuals.

Pathology. *Atrophy.* Nutritional atrophy is a common finding, since the thymus involutes rapidly during inanition and febrile illnesses which last for more than a few days. Nine days of starvation in the rabbit will reduce the thymus to 10 per cent of its original size.

Infections. Metastatic abscess formation in the thymus during bacteremia is rare. Tubercles are occasionally found in association with infection of the tracheobronchial nodes. Gummas of the thymus have been reported occasionally.

Neoplasms. No group of tumors has proved more difficult to interpret and classify than those of the thymus gland. The problems involved are those which have complicated the embryologic and histologic study of the gland. Because of this lack of specific knowledge of the true histogenesis of the constituents of normal thymus, the generic term "thymoma" has come into use, indicating only the primary source of a new growth from thymic parenchyma. A thymoma may originate from thymic lymphocytes, reticular cells, Hassall's bodies or the thymic stroma. Norris feels that the thymomas often associated with cases of myasthenia gravis should be regarded as adenomas produced by an extreme degree of local hyperplasia of the thymic epithelium.

Seybold and his colleagues have defined the thymoma as a slowly growing tumor which may arise from both the thymocytic and epithelial cells. The relative proportion of these cellular types varies greatly both in different tumors and in various regions of the same neoplasm. Features which they noted as commonly present were: dense fibrous capsule; distinct fibrous trabeculae; the palisading of epithelial cells about cystic spaces; foci of necrosis, cyst formation and calcification. Most of these tumors lie anterior to the aortic arch and base of the heart but may be located lower. They are usually round or oval, clearly differentiated from the remainder of the gland and may contain sufficient calcium to be seen radiologically. Tumors of the thymus are usually encapsulated but may be adherent to the surrounding organs, and invade the pericardium, pleura or lungs. Distant metastasis is rare.

Clinical Diagnosis of Thymus Enlargement. Neoplastic enlargement of the thymus of considerable size may occur without the production of any local signs and symptoms. If the enlargement is in the anteroposterior diameter, cough and hoarseness, pain in the chest and neck, dysphagia and compression of the large veins may develop. Pleural and pulmonary involvement with hydrothorax may occur, and extension through the chest wall has been described.

Other conditions which must be considered in differential diagnosis are tracheobronchial lymphadenitis, mediastinal pleurisy, paravertebral abscess, aneurysm of the aorta and other mediastinal neoplasms.

In the roentgenogram the shadow is more or less circular, sharply defined, and located just above the cardiac shadow. Lateral films will show that it occupies the anterior mediastinum. In advanced cases with extension to the pleura and lungs, a circumscribed shadow may not be visible. Other types of mediastinal tumor are likely to be found higher and may occupy the middle and posterior portions of the mediastinum. It is difficult at times to differentiate between a thymoma and an aortic aneurysm.

Because of the great variation in size of the organ in relation to age, physical condition and other factors, there is no satisfactory way of diagnosing diffuse enlargement of the thymus. Many of the tumors are so small that they are not recognized before operation or autopsy, and then only by careful search.

Diseases of the Thymus in Infants and Children. *Status Thymolymphaticus.* Most of the evidence at present indicates that the state of the thymus and lymphatic structures originally described as enlarged, and as associated with the syndrome known as "lymphatic constitution" or status thymolymphaticus, is in most instances within the limits seen in normally developed persons who have died of a variety of causes. In many of the cases described at autopsy there is adrenal atrophy which is known to be associated with enlargement of the thymus. If such a condition as status thymolymphaticus exists, and if it is related to certain instances of sudden death, there is no justification for the belief that radiotherapy or extirpation of the thymus would have prevented death. Coe described eight "thymic" deaths in 2500 operations in children less than 18 months of age. They were not due to anesthesia, or to obstruction of the respiratory tract. The outstanding characteristic was complete absence of respiratory effort, and ordinary methods of resuscitation were not beneficial. The heart continued to beat normally after respiration had ceased. He suggested that some curare-like substance might be released under these conditions, an interesting suggestion in view of the possible relationship of the thymus to myasthenia gravis.

The Thymus and Respiratory Obstruction. Chronic stridor, attacks of cyanosis and choking in infancy have often been attributed to the thymus. With modern diagnostic methods these symptoms are usually shown to be the result of other causes such as congenital hypotonia of the larynx, congenital obstructive anomalies of the respiratory tract, inflammatory lesions, tetany and other local or general conditions. At the age of 6 months both the body and the thymus have doubled in weight. The body has tripled in weight by the end of the first year; the thymus not until five years. Thus, after six months to one year the thymus becomes increasingly insignificant as a possible cause of respiratory obstruction. Enlargement of the thymus in the anteroposterior plane is most apt to cause respiratory obstruction, and careful roentgenograms in oblique as well as anteroposterior positions are necessary in evaluating it as a factor in any case. Bronchoscopy may show compression, and symptoms usually cease after radiation therapy. The diagnosis cannot be made with any certainty by physical examination.

Relationship of the Thymus Gland to Myasthenia Gravis. In over half of the reported autopsies of cases of myasthenia gravis some abnormality of the thymus has been described.

Of 60 patients at the Johns Hopkins Hospital who either had a thymectomy or came to autopsy, 53 per cent had a hyperplastic thymus with germinal center formation, 23 per cent a thymoma, which in one instance had metastasized to the pleura, 8 per cent a persistently enlarged thymus which was normal microscopically, and the remainder either a normal appearing thymus or no detectable thymic tissue. In spite of the greater number of female patients in this series (34 to 26), thymomas were more common in the males (8 to 6). In general, the patients who had a thymoma developed a more severe form of the disease with a higher mortality rate. Of these patients still alive and in whom the status of the thymus was known as a result of operation, 10 per cent had a thymoma, while of those patients who died, 38 per cent had a tumor. A large majority of the tumors were nonmalignant, encapsulated nodules of small size and of a soft hemorrhagic nature.

Myasthenia gravis is characterized by the occurrence of spontaneous remission in many of the cases, and by the repair of the defect in neuromuscular transmission immediately after an injection of neostigmine. This emphasizes the reversible character of the defect. These facts, coupled with the similarity between myasthenia gravis and partial curarization, suggest that some inhibitor substance released into the circulation in varying amounts might be responsible for the functional defect. No significant pathologic changes have been found in this disease other than those described in the thymus, which points to this organ as a possible source of such a substance.

In vitro studies have been made of acetylcholine synthesis in mixtures of frog brain and serum from normal persons and from patients with myasthenia gravis. The synthesis has been reported to be significantly less when the serum of patients with myasthenia gravis was used, particularly when the serum was from patients with a severe form of the disease. It has also been reported that when thymus tissue from a severe case of myasthenia gravis was added to the medium, there was a decrease in the amount of acetylcholine synthesized. These results suggest that there may be in the serum or thymus of patients with myasthenia gravis a substance capable of inhibiting the synthesis of acetylcholine. However, the results of other reported studies on the effects of body fluids and tissues on acetylcholine synthesis and on neuromuscular function have been so variable that no conclusions can be drawn at present as to the pathogenesis of myasthenia gravis and its possible relationship to the thymus gland. The usual *clinical picture* in myasthenia gravis is described in the section on Myasthenia Gravis.

Treatment. The indications for *roentgen ray therapy* have changed in recent years. "Prophylactic" irradiation to prevent "sudden death" is not warranted, and therapeutic irradiation for respiratory obstruction is indicated only after all other possible causes have been ruled out. Many tumors of the thymus are sensitive to irradiation, and remissions have been reported in myasthenia gravis following roentgen therapy. On the whole, however, this form of treatment has not been satisfactory.

The indication for *thymectomy* in *myasthenia gravis* cannot be clearly defined at the present time. Forty-three patients, 18 male and 25 female, have undergone thymectomy at the Johns Hopkins Hospital and have been observed from two to twelve years (average six years). The average duration of the disease at the time of surgery was three years, but one third of the patients were operated upon during the first year of their illness. In general, the course of the disease in these patients has been only slightly better than in those who had neither thymectomy nor irradiation of the thymus. Approximately the same proportion have died in each group and the number who had had striking remissions is similar. Perhaps a slightly greater number have improved and fewer patients have become worse since thymectomy, but the difference between this group and those not operated upon is disappointingly small. The course of female patients following thymectomy has been slightly better than that of the males, but this is also true of patients who were not operated upon. Younger patients have done better than older patients following the operation, but again so have younger patients not subjected to thymectomy. Patients with a thymoma have, in general, had a severe form of the disease which was not improved following thymectomy, but removal of the tumor should be carried out because of the occasional occurrence of metastases.

Viets and Schwab reported the results of operation in 78 patients. Most of the patients selected had had the disease for a considerable period, so that there would be a suitable basis for evaluation. Patients with a thymoma had no benefit from thymectomy. Of the patients who did not have a thymoma, the males did not appear to benefit from the operation, while the females did, 63 per cent improving, compared to 34 per cent in a control group. These authors conclude that thymectomy is indicated in female patients who do not have a thymoma.

Eaton and Clagett reviewed their observations involving over 300 patients seen since 1941. Of this series 62 patients had the thymus removed and were compared to a selected group of 56 patients not undergoing surgery. Their conclusions were that the chance of remission following surgery was 35.5 per cent, as contrasted to a 28.5 per cent chance that a similar remission would develop without operation. It is their belief that thymectomy probably does not exert a beneficial effect.

Recently, Keynes has reported the results in 155 patients with myasthenia gravis who were treated by surgical extirpation of the thymus. Of 120 patients who did not have thymic tumors and survived the operation, 79 (65 per cent) have shown a complete or almost complete remission of symptoms. He does not believe that these results could be accounted for as "spontaneous remissions." It is agreed that cases with a demonstrable

tumor in general do poorly if the primary treatment is operative. Keynes has recommended that surgical incision of a known tumor be preceded by irradiation.

It is still too early to make any final evaluation of these results. Thymectomy should certainly be considered in those cases in which the disease is severe and progressive without any tendency to remission. There is no method by which the results of the operation can be predicted.

A. McGehee Harvey

References

Bailiff, R. N.: Thymic Involution and Regeneration in Albino Rat Following Injection of Acid Colloidal Substances. Am. J. Anat., 84:547, 1949.

Boyd, J. D.: Development of the Thyroid and Parathyroid Glands and the Thymus. Ann. Roy. Coll. Surgeons England, 7:455, 1950.

Castleman, B., and Norris, E. H.: The Pathology of the Thymus in Myasthenia Gravis. A Study of 35 Cases. Medicine, 28:27, 1949.

Grob, D.: Course and Management of Myasthenia Gravis. J.A.M.A., 153:529, 1953.

———, and Harvey, A. M.: Abnormalities in Neuromuscular Transmission, with Special Reference to Myasthenia Gravis. Am. J. Med., 15:695, 1953.

Harvey, A. M., Lilienthal, J. L., Jr., and Talbot, S. A.: Observations on Nature of Myasthenia Gravis. The Effect of Thymectomy on Neuromuscular Transmission. J. Clin. Investigation, 21:579, 1942.

Hubble, D.: Cushing's Syndrome and Thymic Carcinoma. Quart. J. Med., 18:133, 1949.

Keynes, G.: The Results of Thymectomy in Myasthenia Gravis. Brit. M. J., 2:611, 1949.

Reinhardt, W. O., and Wainman, P.: Effect of Thyroidectomy, Castration and Replacement Therapy on Thymus, Lymph Nodes and Spleen in Male Rats. Proc. Soc. Exper. Biol. & Med., 49:257, 1942.

Schwab, R. S., and Leland, C. C.: Sex and Age in Myasthenia Gravis as Critical Factors in Incidence and Remission. J.A.M.A., 153:1270, 1953.

Seybold, W. D., McDonald, J. R., Clagett, O. T., and Good, C. A.: Tumors of the Thymus. J. Thoracic Surg., 20:195, 1950.

DISEASES OF THE PARATHYROID GLANDS

Introduction. Diseases of the parathyroid glands include primary hyperparathyroidism and hypoparathyroidism. For clinical purposes the latter includes "pseudohypoparathyroidism," although there is evidence that this is in reality an "end organ" disease rather than a true parathyroid disease. "Secondary" hyperparathyroidism is thought to play a part in the pathologic physiology of osteomalacia— a condition in which the parathyroid glands are found to be hyperplastic. This is further discussed in the chapter on Osteomalacia. In renal glomerular insufficiency, with elevation of the serum inorganic phosphate* and depression of the serum calcium, parathyroid hyperplasia is almost constantly seen. Some investigators attribute the osteitis fibrosa of this condition to "secondary hyperparathyroidism," others to the renal failure *per se.* (See the chapter on Osteitis Fibrosa Cystica Generalisata.) Space does not permit a discussion of the thoretic issues involved. However, there is general agreement as to the pertinent practical consideration: Removal of parathyroid tissue is *not* of benefit in renal osteitis, but rather the reverse.

This chapter is devoted to primary hyperparathyroidism, hypoparathyroidism and pseudohypoparathyroidism.

PRIMARY HYPERPARATHYROIDISM

Definition. Primary hyperparathyroidism is a condition in which chemical abnormalities of the serum and extracellular fluid result from overproduction of parathyroid hormone. Osteitis fibrosa cystica generalisata may or may not be present.

Etiology. The immediate causes of primary hyperparathyroidism are carcinoma, single or multiple adenomas of the parathyroid glands and "primary hypertrophy and hyperplasia" of all parathyroid tissue. As the name implies, the latter is an entity distinct from the "secondary" hyperplasia seen with osteomalacia and renal failure. If it involves a "trophic" stimulus, the source or nature of such stimulus is entirely obscure. Available evidence is strongly against the existence of pituitary parathyrotrophic hormones. The

cause of adenoma formation is also obscure. The relatively common association of pancreatic islet cell tumors and pituitary tumors with those of the parathyroid suggests a common etiologic factor, but throws no light on what it may be.

Incidence. Primary hyperparathyroidism is a relatively rare disease. After the chemical and clinical criteria for diagnosis had been established, and cases were being actively sought for at the Mayo Clinic and the Massachusetts General Hospital, it required twenty years for each clinic to accumulate 100 cases. Adenomas were found in approximately 90 per cent of these, and "primary hyperplasia and hypertrophy" in 10. Carcinoma is extremely rare. Adenomas appear about twice as frequently in women as in men.

Morbid Anatomy. Adenomas vary greatly in size, ranging from minute tumors, barely visible macroscopically, to large growths, displacing the esophagus, easily palpable *in vivo,* and resembling thyroid nodules. With primary hyperplasia and hypertrophy, the weight of the combined glands has ranged from 2 to 70 gm., with the upper glands quite consistently larger than the lower.

Microscopically, the functioning adenomas are composed of chief cells, water-clear (wasserhelle) cells, admixtures of the two, and, less commonly, of pale oxyphil cells. Among the chief cells, considerable variability in nuclear size, with "giant" nuclei, and multinucleated cells are not infrequent, and are not criteria of malignancy. With primary hyperplasia, all the parathyroid cells are very much larger than wasserhelle cells, and are also clear.

When the bones are affected they show osteitis fibrosa cystica generalisata, as discussed in the section on Diseases of Bones.

When the kidneys are affected they may develop nephrolithiasis or nephrocalcinosis, both frequently complicated by pyelonephritis.

Pathologic Physiology and Chemistry. As a result of overproduction of parathyroid hormone by the adenomatous or hypertrophied glands, there ensues (1) an increase in urinary phosphorus excretion and (2) a decrease in serum phosphorus. This results in a relative undersaturation of the extracellular fluids with respects to calcium phos-

---

* Hereafter, the serum inorganic phosphate will be here termed the "serum phosphorus" for the sake of brevity.

phate, with the result that (3) there is a rise in serum calcium. If the calcium intake is adequate, and the additional calcium available in the gastrointestinal tract, the bones are not affected. If it is inadequate, osteitis fibrosa generalisata develops. As a result of the rise of serum calcium, (4) the urine calcium rises. (An effect of the parathyroids directly on bone, independent of the renal effect, has been established. Such an effect alone will not explain the lowering of serum phosphorus, or the occurrence of severe hyperparathyroidism without bone disease.)

The cardinal biochemical signs of primary hyperparathyroidism are thus a lowered serum phosphorus, an elevated serum calcium and an elevated urine calcium. (A low calcium diet is generally employed for at least three days to evaluate urinary calcium excretion.) When the bones are affected, there is in addition an elevated serum alkaline phosphatase. (The urine phosphorus is not of diagnostic value after a "steady state" of disease has been reached.)

The signs of primary hyperparathyroidism become more difficult to interpret with the appearance of renal failure, a very common sequela if treatment is not instituted. Renal failure results in (1) a rise in serum phosphorus, (2) a relative supersaturation of the extracellular fluid with respect to calcium phosphate, (3) a fall of serum calcium and (4) a fall of urine calcium. It is apparent that a point will be reached when the diagnosis can no longer be made. At this point, however, removal of the tumor does little to improve the patient.

Symptoms. Symptoms in primary hyperparathyroidism may result from the hypercalcemia, the hypercalciuria and the bone disease when it is present. Hypercalcemia results in anorexia, weakness, fatigability, difficulty in swallowing, nausea, vomiting, constipation and hypotonicity of the muscles and ligaments, the last often resulting in striking "double-jointedness." These are presumably a reflection of the known effects of hypercalcemia in depressing the sensitivity to electrical stimuli of ganglia and peripheral nerves. The latter can be demonstrated directly by the use of Erb's test. Shortening of the Q-T interval in the electrocardiogram is found in some cases. Two lesions in the eyes result from hypercalcemia —"band keratopathy" in which bands of opaque material are found beneath Bowman's capsule in lines parallel to and within the limbus, especially in the palpebral fissure,

and conjunctival crystals located medially and laterally to the limbus, also in the palpebral fissure. Both lesions often require a slit lamp for recognition.

Hypercalciuria may result in nephrolithiasis, and the appearance of calcium oxalate or calcium phosphate stones is often the presenting symptom of the disorder. In other cases, nephrocalcinosis may result, with progressive renal damage. Infection of the urinary tract is common with both complications.

The bone disease, when it occurs, is osteitis fibrosa cystica generalisata. It is dealt with in the section on Diseases of Bones. Of special value in diagnosis are the loss of lamina dura about the teeth, the finding of subcortical bone resorption, and the presence of "cysts" and "brown tumors," especially the epulis of the jaw.

Differential Diagnosis. Hypercalcemia is found with vitamin D overdosage, with certain bone diseases—notably osteoporosis and Paget's disease—when the patient is immobilized, and, associated with renal damage, with prolonged excessive intake of calcium and alkali. In all of these the history is of paramount importance; in all of them the serum phosphorus is characteristically normal (although it may, rarely, be depressed with hypervitaminosis D). In osteoporosis the serum alkaline phosphatase is normal and in Paget's disease the x-ray picture is usually diagnostic. Hypercalcemia and hypercalciuria are also often found in multiple myeloma and in sarcoidosis. In these diseases, the serum phosphorus is characteristically normal, and the serum globulin frequently elevated. The serum alkaline phosphatase is almost always normal, in spite of bone disease, in the former, and is generally normal in the latter. Metastatic malignancy in bone may produce hypercalcemia and resemble hyperparathyroidism closely, as the serum phosphorus, although generally normal, may be depressed. In this as in all the above disorders, a *normal lamina dura about the teeth* helps to exclude hyperparathyroidism as the cause of the bone disease.

Hypercalciuria is characteristic of all hypercalcemic states except that due to prolonged excessive intake of calcium and alkali. Hypercalciuria without hypercalcemia occurs in "idiopathic hypercalciuria," a renal disease often accompanied by coccal infection, and in "renal tubular acidosis." In neither is the serum calcium elevated; in the latter, metabolic acidosis is present. When metabolic bone disease occurs in these conditions it is osteomalacia: the reader is referred to the chapter on the subject.

The differential diagnosis of osteitis fibrosa cystica is discussed in the appropriate place.

Prognosis. Primary hyperparathyroidism responds very satisfactorily to surgery. The frequency with which a second adenoma occurs in patients from whom one has been removed is greater than that with which primary hyperparathyroidism occurs in the population at large. When primary hyperplasia and hypertrophy has been present (and partial resection done), persistence of hypercalciuria, and recurrence of hypercalcemia, are common.

Treatment. The treatment of primary hyperparathyroidism is surgical. Search for adenomas often involves dissection of the mediastinum as well as the neck. Adenomas should be removed *in toto*. With primary hyperplasia and hypertrophy (the presence of which should be confirmed by frozen section), small (*ca.* 250 mg.) sections of two glands, with blood supply, should be left, and the rest removed. Postoperatively, severe tetany may be expected where there has been bone disease. It may require vigorous therapy with calcium by vein (e.g., 30 cc. of 10 per cent calcium lactate in 1000 cc. of normal saline) and by mouth (e.g., 6 teaspoons calcium lactate a day), and with vitamin D by mouth (e.g., 50,000 units a day) until the bone disease is healed. Therapy must then be promptly stopped before it results in hypercalcemia.

HYPOPARATHYROIDISM

Definition. Hypoparathyroidism is a condition in which chemical abnormalities of the serum and extracellular fluid result from underproduction of parathyroid hormone.

Etiology. The commonest cause of hypoparathyroidism is the inadvertent removal of or damage to parathyroid tissue during thyroid surgery. The resulting disease may be temporary, if enough tissue was left, or if edema and hemorrhage were precipitating factors. Rarely, hypoparathyroidism appears without apparent cause. Some cases are preceded by acute systemic infections, others are accompanied by mild infection of mouth, skin and nails with monilia. (It is not clear whether the monilia is a cause or a result of the disease.) In the latter group, familial incidence has been reported. The disease tends to develop in children under 15, or in adults over 40, and is rare between these ages, for reasons not apparent. The frequency of its co-

existence with Addison's disease is significantly above the probability of chance.

Incidence. "Idiopathic" hypoparathyroidism is a rare disease; only 34 cases had been reported by 1946. The incidence of postoperative hypoparathyroidism in various clinics naturally varies.

Morbid Anatomy. In "idiopathic" hypoparathyroidism the parathyroid glands have been reported to show complete or almost complete replacement of parenchymal tissue by fat. The finer blood vessels of the brain, especially those of the basal ganglia, may be surrounded by hyalin deposits which calcify. The bones may be abnormally dense.

Pathologic Physiology and Chemistry. As a result of a decrease in parathyroid hormone secretion, there ensues (1) a decrease in renal phosphorus excretion, (2) a rise in serum phosphorus. This results in a relative supersaturation of the extracellular fluid with respect to calcium phosphate, with the result that (3) there is a fall in serum calcium. As a result of the fall in serum calcium, (4) the urine calcium falls, reaching essentially zero at serum levels below 7 mg. per 100 cc.

The cardinal biochemical signs of hypoparathyroidism are thus an elevated serum phosphorus, a lowered serum calcium and a lowered urine calcium. (The urine calcium is occasionally normal or even elevated in hypoparathyroidism—a phenomenon often associated with coccal pyelonephritis or prolonged calcium chloride medication.) The lowered serum calcium results in increased excitability of peripheral nerves and ganglia, and hence in tetany and symptoms referable to hyperactivity of the autonomic system.

Symptoms. Most of the symptoms in hypoparathyroidism can be explained as results of the hypocalcemia; a few are unexplained. The most prominent manifestation of hypocalcemia is *tetany*. The first sign of this is often a sensation of numbness and tingling in the fingers and toes or about the lips. Laryngeal stridor, with prolonged "crowing" inspiration, dyspnea and cyanosis are not infrequently seen, occasionally leading to a mistaken diagnosis of vocal cord paralysis. As the tetany becomes more severe, cramps of individual muscles, and finally tonic contractions of muscle groups appear. In the hand and arm, this results in the characteristic "accoucheur's" position. Gastric pain, nausea and vomiting may accompany severe tetany. Generalized convulsions have frequently been described with severe hypoparathyroidism. In some cases there is an aura, tongue-biting, urinary and fecal incontinence, and post-seizure coma, and electroencephalograms support the impression that hypocalcemia is acting to "trigger" a preexisting grand mal. Others, in which both the seizure pattern and the electroencephalograms are "atypical," presumably represent a direct effect of hypocalcemia on the central nervous system. In all, great improvement occurs when the hypocalcemia is eliminated. The differential diagnosis of tetany is dealt with below.

Papilledema and increased intracranial pressure are relatively frequent accompaniments of hypoparathyroidism. They disappear with therapy. Calcifications about the smaller vessels of the brain, especially those of the basal ganglia, often visible in skull x-rays, are commonly seen in hypoparathyroidism. These do not regress with therapy. Neither of these lesions is found in hypocalcemia of other cause. Cortical cataracts are common in hypoparathyroidism, and in other disorders involving hypocalcemia. The underlying mechanism for all these lesions is obscure.

Defects in ectodermal structures that may be found in hypoparathyroidism involve the teeth, nails, skin or hair. When hypoparathyroidism develops before the permanent teeth are mature, they may show shortening and malformation of the enamel organ and shortening of the roots. The nails, which may be malformed and brittle, are sometimes infected with moniliasis, as mentioned above. The skin is sometimes coarse and dry, the head hair patchy and thin; the eyebrow, axillary or pubic hair may be scant or absent.

Diagnosis. A number of clinical tests may be employed to reveal the presence of "latent" tetany. Chvostek's sign is sought by tapping the finger over the facial nerve. A positive response consists of twitching of the muscles of the mouth, and, with severer cases, of the nose and eyelids. A positive Chvostek's sign is usually but not invariably present in tetany. A positive response occurs commonly in normal individuals. Trousseau's sign is sought by producing ischemia to peripheral nerves by inflating a pressure cuff on the arm above systolic pressure for 3 minutes. A positive response is frequently elicited in patients with latent tetany. Erb's sign is sought by applying a galvanic current to the skin over a peripheral motor nerve, and measuring the minimal current necessary to produce a muscle contraction upon cathode opening. With latent tetany, a response appears with 5 milliamperes or less.

The characteristic serum values have been discussed. The electrocardiogram may show a prolonged Q-T interval with hypocalcemia.

The combination of increased intracranial pressure, papilledema and a history of convulsions in hypoparathyroidism has often led to a mistaken diagnosis of brain tumor. The relationship of epilepsy to tetany has been discussed.

Prognosis. In the hypoparathyroidism which follows thyroid surgery recovery often occurs, even after weeks or months. Therapy should be carefully withdrawn at intervals in such cases until it is clear that no recovery will ensue. Idiopathic hypoparathyroidism requires continuous therapy, and if this is adequate, new cataracts should not develop. The prognosis of classic or atypical epilepsy in hypoparathyroidism is excellent if adequate therapy can be maintained.

Treatment. Acute hypocalcemic tetany requires prompt treatment with calcium intravenously (e.g., calcium lactate, 10 per cent solution, 10 to 30 cc. intravenously in 1000 cc. normal saline) given as often as necessary to control symptoms. Simultaneously, calcium (e.g., calcium lactate, 4 gm. 6 times daily) and vitamin D (e.g., 50,000 units daily) should be started by mouth. The dosages should be reduced when the serum and urine calcium are brought to normal, and maintained in quantities found adequate to keep them so. The Sulkowitch test for urine calcium, which the patient can perform, provides a useful index of the adequacy of therapy. AT 10 (Hytakerol) may be used (e.g., 0.5 to 1 cc. orally each day) in place of vitamin D for maintenance therapy. It has the advantage of more rapid action, the disadvantage of greater cost.

TETANY

The symptom complex of tetany and the diagnostic tests for latent tetany have been discussed under hypoparathyroidism. The present section is devoted to its etiology and differential diagnosis.

Tetany may be precipitated by hypocalcemia or alkalosis or both. Whereas low magnesium tetany has been described, its extreme rarity renders it negligible from the clinical point of view. In the accompanying table are summarized the causes of tetany, with the essential laboratory data.

The *causes of hypocalcemia* may be divided into those in which the calcium intake is inadequate, those in which gastrointestinal calcium loss is excessive, those in which urinary calcium loss is excessive, and those in which the serum phosphorus is elevated (and the serum calcium depressed presumably because the solubility product of calcium phosphate is exceeded).

Inadequate intake of calcium as a cause of hypocalcemia probably does not occur in the United States. Excessive calcium loss via the gastrointestinal tract occurs in hypovitaminosis D, in "resistance to vitamin D," in the sprue syndrome in which vitamin D and calcium soaps are lost because of steatorrhea, and in severe diarrhea in which calcium-containing secretions are lost. In all these

parathyroidism (see the section on Pseudo-hypoparathyroidism), and in virtually none in renal failure. In infants fed cow's milk, hyperphosphatemia with hypocalcemia and tetany has been reported in the absence of renal failure. Here the amount of phosphorus fed exceeds the amount filtered by the glomeruli at normal serum levels. In glomerular insufficiency, the tetany should respond to measures designed to lower the serum phosphorus, e.g., oral aluminum hydroxide; the therapy of hypoparathyroidism has been discussed.

Schema for the Classification and Differential Diagnosis of Tetany

CAUSE	SERUM				URINE	
	Ca	P	pH	CO_2	Ca	pH
Hypocalcemia						
Low Ca intake	low	low	normal	normal	low	indeterminate
High intestinal Ca loss						
1. Vitamin D lack	low	low	normal	normal	low	indeterminate
2. Sprue	low	low	normal	normal	low	indeterminate
3. Diarrhea	low	low	normal	normal	low	indeterminate
High urinary Ca loss						
1. Essential hypercalciuria	low	low	normal	normal	normal	indeterminate
2. Renal tubular acidosis	low	low	low	low	normal	indeterminate or high
Elevated serum P						
1. Hypoparathyroidism	low	high	normal	normal	low	indeterminate
2. Glomerular insufficiency	low	high	low or normal	low or normal	normal	indeterminate
3. Excessive ingestion	low	high	normal	normal	low	indeterminate
Alkalosis						
Respiratory	normal	normal	high	low or normal	normal	high
Metabolic						
1. Excessive alkali intake	normal	normal	high	high	normal	high
2. Persistent vomiting	normal	normal	high	high	normal	high

Ca   Calcium   P   Inorganic phosphate CO_2 Carbon dioxide content
    Note that in renal tubular acidosis and in renal insufficiency the serum acidosis tends to oppose the effect of hypocalcemia.

conditions the tetany should respond to measures designed to increase calcium absorption, e.g., vitamin D, calcium salts, control of diarrhea. Excessive calcium loss via the kidneys occurs in "essential hypercalciuria" and in "renal tubular acidosis," but tetany is rare in these conditions.

Elevated serum phosphorus and lowered serum calcium are found in hypoparathyroidism and in glomerular insufficiency; in the former, calcium is usually absent from the urine; in the latter, urinary calcium is often decreased but seldom absent. The two conditions are generally easily distinguished by the presence or absence of other signs of renal failure, e.g., nitrogen retention. The intravenous injection of 200 units of parathyroid extract should clarify the differential diagnosis if any doubt remains. This results in marked phosphaturia in hypo-

The *causes of alkalosis* may be divided into those in which respiratory loss of carbon dioxide is excessive, those in which alkali intake is excessive, and those in which loss of gastric acid is excessive. With potassium deficiency, as occurs, for example, in hyperadrenocortical states, alkalosis appears as hydrogen ions are transferred to the urine and into tissue cells. Tetany has not been reported with this form of alkalosis.

Hyperventilation is not infrequently a manifestation of psychoneurosis. With a sudden increase in respiratory rate, serum carbonic acid is lowered by loss of carbon dioxide in the lungs, the serum pH is elevated, and tetany may follow. The condition is readily remedied by having the patient breathe into a paper bag, or inducing him to decrease his respiratory rate. In this form of alkalosis alone serum bicarbonate is normal or low.

Excessive intake of alkali and excessive loss of gastric acid may produce alkalosis and tetany. The diagnosis, which should be clear if a history is obtainable, is supported by the finding of an elevated serum bicarbonate and an alkaline urine. The tetany should respond to measures designed to prevent vomiting and, of course, to cessation of alkali therapy.

PSEUDOHYPOPARATHYROIDISM

Definition. Pseudohypoparathyroidism is a condition in which the chemical abnormalities of hypoparathyroidism exist in the presence of normal or hyperplastic parathyroid glands and in the absence of renal glomerular insufficiency. It is generally part of a syndrome involving developmental changes of bone. An essential feature in its recognition is the demonstration of nonresponsiveness to parathyroid extract.

Etiology. Nothing is known of the etiology of pseudohypoparathyroidism. "Resistance" to parathyroid extract is found but circulating antibodies or precipitins have not been demonstrated. Certain elements of the disorder suggest a relationship to achondroplasia and myositis ossificans progressiva. Since the characteristic epiphysial changes and metaplastic bone growth are found in these conditions in the absence of serum chemical abnormalities, it appears that these features are related genetically but are not interdependent.

Incidence. Pseudohypoparathyroidism is a very rare disease, the incidence of which cannot be accurately evaluated. Since it was first described in 1942, a few new cases have been reported and a few cases formerly classified as idiopathic hypoparathyroidism have been reclassified under this heading.

Morbid Anatomy. The essential features of morbid anatomy are: the presence of normal or hyperplastic parathyroid glands, the short stature and round face found in most patients, the shortened metacarpals and metatarsals and ossifications in skin and tendon.

Pathologic Physiology and Chemistry. The sequence of chemical events in this condition is the same as that in idiopathic or postoperative hypoparathyroidism, and the cardinal biochemical signs are the same, with the significant difference that parathyroid extract given intravenously in a dose which produces marked hyperphosphaturia in the former conditions produces little or no change in urine phosphate in this one. As might be anticipated, it fails also to lower the serum phosphorus, or to raise the serum calcium.

Symptoms. The symptoms and signs of pseudohypoparathyroidism include all those of idiopathic hypoparathyroidism with the possible exceptions of papilledema and associated moniliasis. In addition, patients characteristically show short stature and roundness of the face.

In most cases certain of the metacarpal and metatarsal bones are abnormally shortened as a result of early epiphysial union. The corresponding shortness of fingers and toes is readily apparent. In many, there are found metaplastic islands of true bone in skin and connective tissues. As mentioned above, these features have suggested a relationship with achondroplasia and myositis ossificans progressiva. In Browne's case a mother and daughter both had stigmata of achondroplasia as well as multiple exostoses, and the daughter had, in addition, pseudohypoparathyroidism. Mental deficiency is present in most cases and does not depend upon a history of convulsions.

Diagnosis. This is established by finding the serum chemical abnormalities of hypoparathyroidism without those of glomerular insufficiency, and by demonstrating less than a twofold increase in urinary phosphorus excretion following administration of 200 units of active parathyroid extract intravenously. (The activity of the extract should be checked simultaneously in a normal subject.) The features discussed above may obviously be of considerable help in diagnosis. The demonstration of parathyroid tissue by biopsy establishes the diagnosis unequivocally.

Treatment. The treatment is that of hypoparathyroidism in general; larger doses of AT 10 may be required than are needed in idiopathic hypoparathyroidism.

F. C. BARTTER

References

Albright, F., and Reifenstein, E. C., Jr.: The Parathyroid Glands and Metabolic Bone Disease. Baltimore, Williams and Wilkins Co., 1948.

Bartter, F.: The Parathyroids. Ann. Rev. Physiol., 16:429, 1953.

Castleman, B.: Tumors of the Parathyroid Glands, Atlas of Tumor Pathology. Washington, D. C., Armed Forces Institute of Pathology, Section IV, Fasc. 15, 1952.

Elrick, H., Albright, F., Bartter, F. C., Forbes, A. P., and Reeves, J. D.: Further Studies on Pseudohypoparathyroidism: Report of Four New Cases. Acta endocrinol., 5:199, 1950.

Kramer, B., and Leibner, I. W.: Tetany—Biochemical and Clinical Considerations. M. Clin. North America, 36:875, 1952.

Snapper, I.: Medical Clinics on Bone Disease. 2nd Edition. New York, Interscience Publishers, 1949.

DISEASES OF THE SEX GLANDS

DISEASES OF THE MALE GONADS

ANATOMY AND PHYSIOLOGY

The testis consists essentially of two parts: (1) the seminiferous tubules, which produce spermatozoa, and (2) the interstitial cells, which produce androgen. There is some interrelation between the functions of these two structures. The production of androgen results in the development of secondary sex characteristics: namely, change in pitch of voice, growth of the penis, scrotum, prostate, seminal vesicles, epididymis, vas deferens, the musculature, body hair, beard and, to some extent, the skeleton, with a resulting modification in the contour of the body. There is a delicate balance between the anterior lobe of the pituitary and the gonads. The pituitary stimulates activity of the gonads, and production of sex hormones by the gonads inhibits the pituitary. The anterior lobe of the pituitary produces two gonadotrophic hormones. One causes development of the follicles in the ovary and influences the function of the seminiferous tubules in the testis ("follicle-stimulating hormone"); the other causes luteinization of the follicles in the ovary and stimulates the interstitial cells in the testis ("luteinizing hormone"). Menopausal and castrate urines contain primarily the follicle-stimulating material, whereas human pregnancy urine contains largely the luteinizing factor, which is available under a variety of trade names. Gonadotrophic material from the serum of the pregnant mare and commercial preparations from the pituitary itself contain both factors, with a preponderance of follicle-stimulating material. It is thus theoretically possible to stimulate the testis selectively, although in actual practice the gonadotrophic material from human pregnancy urine (chorionic gonadotrophin) is the only one with which adequate stimulation has been produced up to the present time. The material from the serum of the pregnant mare produces only slight stimulation. Pituitary preparations are not of much value at present, and the material from menopausal and castrate urines is not available in sufficiently large quantities.

The principal hormone of the testis is testosterone, which is secreted by the Leydig cells. Estrogen also appears to be produced by the testis. Most of the evidence indicates that its source is the Leydig cells, although some observers have reported data in favor of its secretion by the Sertoli cells. Estrogen is produced by the adrenal cortex in both sexes and in the female by the ovary as well. Some esters of testosterone are more potent than testosterone itself, and in clinical practice the propionic-acid ester (testosterone propionate) is most commonly used and is administered parenterally. Claims made in the last few years that methylandrostenediol and androstanolone will inhibit cancer of the breast without producing virilizing effects have not been substantiated by clinical observation. For therapeutic purposes, testosterone is made synthetically. A very large number of related compounds have been prepared by the degradation of sterols, but they are not used therapeutically. Testicular androgens are 19-carbon compounds, but estrogens are 18-carbon compounds. Adrenal steroids, including androgens produced by the adrenal cortex, and progesterone are 21-carbon compounds.

The simplest and most commonly used index of androgen production in clinical medicine is the determination of the amount of neutral 17-ketosteroids excreted in the urine over a period of 24 hours. In order to get a satisfactory figure for comparison, the average result obtained on two or three 24-hour specimens is used.

In both sexes, androgenic material is produced by the adrenal cortex, but there is no evidence that the human female produces testosterone. In young boys and girls from 6 to 10 years of age, very little androgen is found in the urine. At about the time of the onset of puberty or slightly before, a marked increase in the production of both androgen and estrogen occurs in both sexes. The excretion of 17-ketosteroids reaches a maximum of 15.0 mg. in 24 hours in the male and of 10.0 mg. in 24 hours in the female by the age of about 30 years or a little earlier. The excretion in the male then drops rapidly until it reaches a level of about 5.0 mg. in 24 hours by the age of 70 years. In the female the excretion decreases more gradually to a level of about 3.5 mg. at the age of 70 years, with a plateau of about 6.5 mg. in 24 hours between the ages of 35 and 55 years. Production of spermatozoa may diminish in later life, but the change is variable, and high spermatozoa counts are often found in men over 65 years of age. What role sex hormones play in sex differentiation has not been established, but they may be responsible in part for the early development of secondary sex characteristics.

WILLARD O. THOMPSON

ANOMALIES OF DEVELOPMENT

The undifferentiated sex gland develops about the fifth week from the medial surface of the mesonephros. Differentiation into testis or ovary occurs during the sixth or seventh week. Whether a male or female will develop seems to depend upon the type of spermatozoon with which the egg is fertilized, those with the so-called "X chromosome" giving rise to females. In some instances gonadal tissue of both sexes may appear in the same person. It may occur unilaterally or bilaterally and give rise to a true hermaphrodite, i.e., a person with the internal and external genitalia of both sexes. True hermaphroditism is rare and is not to be confused with the more common pseudohermaphroditism. A female pseudohermaphrodite is an individual in whom the sex organs are predominantly female but have some of the characteristics of the male sex. A male pseudohermaphrodite is one in whom the sex organs are predominantly male but have some of the characteristics of the female. Testicular tissue may appear in virilizing arrhenoblastomas of the ovary. The wolffian and müllerian structures both appear in each sex, possibly as relics of early vertebrate life when all organisms produced both sperm and eggs. If a testis develops, the wolffian body and duct give rise to a vas deferens, seminal vesicles, epididymis and ejaculatory duct. At the same time the müllerian structure atrophies, but vestiges remain (appendix testis and utriculus masculinus). From the urogenital sinus and genital tubercle there develop a prostate gland, Cowper's glands, a male type of urethra, a scrotum and a penis. If an ovary develops, the müllerian ducts

give rise to oviducts, uterus and upper vagina, while the wolffian structures atrophy. The urogenital sinus and genital tubercle develop into the lower vagina, female urethra, Bartholin's glands and external female genitalia. The differentiation of the external genitalia takes place a little later than that of the internal, and abnormal hormone stimulation may result in their assuming the characteristics of the opposite sex. Some investigators believe that in this way the development of pseudohermaphroditism may be explained. It follows that every person is, in a sense, bisexual throughout life. One sex usually predominates, but vestigial organs of the opposite sex remain, and their development may be stimulated by sex hormones. If this stimulation is applied sufficiently early in embryonic life, many interesting bisexual developments may result.

Wilkins has shown that in some cases of congenital adrenal hyperplasia with a high excretion of neutral 17-ketosteroids in the urine, the administration of cortisone will reduce adrenal cortical function through pituitary inhibition and permit secondary sex characteristics to develop in the female.

Many details of descent of the testis are still to be worked out. It lies just inside the internal inguinal ring; by the seventh month, at the lower end of the canal; and during the last month of intrauterine life it descends into the scrotum. The pouch of peritoneum which later becomes the tunica vaginalis precedes the testis into the scrotum. The gubernaculum is supposed to play an important role in directing the course of descent. It is early attached to the genital ridge as it develops downward and, in the beginning, has attachments to the abdominal muscles, the root of the penis, Scarpa's triangle, the base of the scrotum and the perineum.

WILLARD O. THOMPSON

PUBERTY AND ADOLESCENCE IN THE MALE

Following the disappearance of prenatal enlargement and engorgement, the genitalia remain relatively stationary in size until the eleventh to the thirteenth year, when the changes of puberty begin to appear in association with a marked increase in the excretion of androgenic material in the urine. What role, if any, the gonads play in somatic development from birth to puberty is unknown. During puberty the external genitalia gradually increase in size, the skeleton grows rapidly, and the emotional changes associated with the increase in sexual function appear. The prostate, which is usually not palpable in young boys, begins to develop, reaching its adult size about the same time as the external genitalia. Hair begins to appear on various parts of the body. The pubic hair at first is usually feminine in distribution, but after a period of several months fine short hairs begin to appear in the lower midline of the abdomen and then often all over the abdomen, chest, back, arms and legs. However, the amount of body hair is variable, many normal men having very little and exhibiting an almost feminine distribution of pubic hair. The beard appears as a fine fuzz and then gradually increases in length and stiffness. The pitch of the voice gradually becomes lower. Marked alterations in body contour may take place. The amount of fat in the abdomen and thighs may diminish and the shoulders become broader. The relation between the length of the trunk and the length of the extremities is affected, absence of testicular function during the age of normal puberty resulting in long extremities and a comparatively short trunk. Skeletal growth may at first be stimulated, but epiphysial union is nearly complete about the end of the puberal period. In men this usually occurs during the sixteenth or seventeenth year and in women between the fourteenth and sixteenth years. The epiphyses of the vertebrae, pelvis and clavicles do not unite until a little later. In man and lower animals, spermatogenesis occurs at a somewhat later time than the corresponding first menstruation or first estrus. Familial instances of puberty occurring prematurely at the age of 5 to 9 years are described, although the condition is rare. In a similar manner the onset of puberty may be greatly delayed, although this disturbance usually indicates a deficiency of pituitary function.

Puberty is a complex phenomenon involving the anterior lobe of the pituitary, the adrenals and the gonads. In the male the following hormones appear to be involved: (1) follicle-stimulating hormone (FSH), (2) luteinizing hormone (LH), (3) adrenocorticotrophic hormone (ACTH), (4) androgens from the adrenal cortex, (5) androgens from the testis.

The development of most of the secondary sex characteristics seems to depend upon the production of androgen by the testis. Androgen production by the adrenal cortex also appears to play some role. There is evidence that androgens from this source are involved in the development of pubic and axillary hair and in the maturation of bone in both sexes. It is still not clearly established just what role the adrenal androgens play in puberty, although there seems to be no doubt that they are involved. The old idea that puberty involved essentially stimulation of the gonads by the pituitary must be modified to include adrenal stimulation by the adrenocorticotrophic hormone.

It is not definitely established why puberty occurs when it does. According to Engle, the seminiferous tubules in the testis and the follicles in the ovary can respond to gonad activators only after the gonads have undergone a certain amount of ripening, which may be independent of the hypophysis. This conclusion does not appear to apply to the interstitial cells of the testis. They may be stimulated to increased activity at any age before puberty by gonadotrophic material from human pregnancy urine, and a condition produced which simulates premature puberty (see discussion of Precocious Sexual Development). The fact that these changes do not occur normally until the age of puberty suggests that the pituitary stimulus itself may be held in abeyance.

PRECOCIOUS SEXUAL DEVELOPMENT

In the course of treating young boys for undescended testes with chorionic gonadotrophin, rapid genital growth may be observed. The changes may be so great that a condition resembling premature puberty is produced. This phenomenon is illustrated in the accompanying photographs of a six and one-half year old boy who was treated for a right undescended testis and an inguinal hernia (Fig. 95). In the course of a few months his penis became as large as that of a normal adult male. There was an increase in the size of the scrotum and prostate, a growth of pubic hair, a marked increase in the frequency of erections, a change in the pitch of the voice and some growth of hair on the sides of the face, although a true beard did not develop. His height increased rapidly. The testes increased little if any in size during treatment, presumably because this material stimulates primarily the interstitial cells and not the seminiferous tubules. The right testis descended, but remained smaller than the left. The associated hernia did not disappear, but became strangulated and had to be corrected by operation. No change was noted in basal metabolism during treatment.

come shorter than he might otherwise have been, because of premature epiphysial union. If treatment with chorionic gonadotrophin is carried out for a sufficiently long period, young boys may sometimes be made tall for

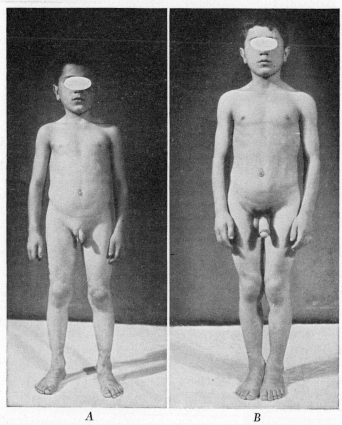

A   B

Fig. 95. Precocious sexual development and rapid skeletal growth during treatment with chorionic gonadotrophin.

A, Before treatment, age 6 years, 7 months. Weight, 19.5 kg. (43 pounds); height, 114.6 cm. (44¾ inches).

B, After eleven and one half months of treatment with chorionic gonadotrophin (total dose 56,570 rat units). Weight, 27.8 kg. (61¼ pounds); height, 128 cm. (50 inches). (Thompson and Heckel: J.A.M.A., Vol. 110.)

When treatment was discontinued, some regression in size occurred. The penis became slightly smaller and less engorged, but remained larger than before treatment was started. The prostate became flat and smaller in diameter, and the body weight and height, which had increased more rapidly than normal during treatment, increased only slowly for the next two and one-half years. The pubic hair decreased to about one third of its maximum amount. Precocious sexual development associated with interstitial cell tumors of the testis stimulates skeletal growth at first, but ultimately may cause the person to be-

their age, but the final height does not appear to be altered unless pituitary dwarfism is present.

The susceptibility to this growth stimulus varies markedly, but it appears probable that precocious genital growth may be produced with it in most normal young boys, if sufficiently large doses are used. Premature sexual development may also be produced in man by tumors of the adrenal cortex, occasionally by tumors of the testis, and also by lesions of the midbrain, which apparently result in pituitary stimulation. Its relation to tumors of the pineal gland is open to question. There are cases which can be explained only by a marked familial tendency to precocious development. The association of premature puberty with interstitial cell tumors of the testis is of interest in view of the fact that chorionic gonadotrophin is known to stimulate the interstitial cells. It is also of interest that, in patients showing precocious development of the genitalia associated with tumors of the adrenal cortex, the testis may show little or no increase in size and spermatogenesis may not occur. In such patients the development of secondary sex characteristics is caused by androgenic material produced by the adrenal cortical tumor.

In some instances a delay in the onset of puberty is seen in individuals who appear to be normal in other respects. Any delay in the onset of puberty beyond the fourteenth year makes it necessary to investigate very carefully the function of the anterior lobe of the pituitary. Like other biologic functions, puberty and adolescence may show a considerable amount of variation in the time of onset from individual to individual.

WILLARD O. THOMPSON

HYPERGONADISM AND HYPO-GONADISM

As with other glands of internal secretion, the testis may show various degrees of hyperfunction and hypofunction. States of hyperfunction associated with increased production of androgen undoubtedly occur, but are not clearly defined. It is difficult to differentiate the effects of overproduction of sex hormone from those of overactivity of the sympathetic nervous system. For the most part, disorders of function requiring treatment are those associated with hypofunction of the testis. In most instances both portions of the testis are affected.

PRIMARY AND SECONDARY HYPOGONADISM

The testis, like the ovary, may fail to function properly because of some defect inherent in the testis itself (primary hypogonadism) or because of lack of adequate stimulation, notably by the anterior lobe of the pituitary (secondary hypogonadism). As in the case of the thyroid, normal pituitary function is necessary for normal testicular function, and in its absence atrophy of the testes and geni-

talia occurs, with decrease in, or disappearance of, spermatogenesis and production of androgen. Secondary hypogonadism appears to be more common than the primary type, although there is some question at present just how some disorders should be classified. Cases of undescended testes in which descent is prevented by mechanical factors, and cases in which the testes are removed or destroyed by various agents, represent examples of the primary type; whereas all cases associated with hypopituitarism, and cases of undescended testes in which descent is prevented by some hormonal deficiency, appear to be of the secondary type.

The following types of primary hypogonadism may occur:

1. Deficient function of both the seminiferous tubules and the interstitial cells of Leydig (the most common type)
2. Deficient function of the seminiferous tubules and infertility with various stages of degeneration, as shown by testicular biopsy, and some production of androgen by the interstitial cells (rare)
3. Some production of spermatozoa by the seminiferous tubules with deficient production of androgenic material and eunuchoidism (rare, but observed occasionally).

The following types of secondary hypogonadism may occur:

1. Deficient production of both follicle-stimulating and luteinizing hormones (the most common type)
2. Deficient production of follicle-stimulating hormone with enough production of luteinizing hormone to stimulate development of secondary sex characteristics (not uncommon)
3. Deficient production of luteinizing hormone with enough production of follicle-stimulating hormone to stimulate spermatogenesis (rare, but does occur).

It is uncertain whether Klinefelter's syndrome belongs in the primary or secondary type of hypogonadism. The essential features of this syndrome are gynecomastia, azoospermia, without aleydigism, and increased secretion of follicle-stimulating hormone in the urine.

TYPES OF THERAPY IN HYPOGONADISM

Two types of therapy are now possible in hypofunction of the testis: (1) substitution therapy with androgens, and (2) stimulation therapy with gonadotrophic material. In substitution therapy the androgen is supplied artificially. With gonadotrophic material the testis is stimulated to increased activity so that the testis itself produces more androgen, and it is to be preferred in most instances in which the testis is capable of responding to stimulation.

Testosterone is the androgen most commonly used for substitution therapy. It may be administered in the following ways: (1) by the intramuscular injection of testosterone propionate in oil; (2) by the intramuscular injection of a suspension of free testosterone in water; (3) by the intramuscular injection of a suspension of testosterone phenyl acetate in water (not yet available commercially), which has a more prolonged effect than testosterone propionate; (4) by the oral administration of methyltestosterone; (5) by the buccal administration of tablets of testosterone propionate; and (6) by the implantation of pellets of testosterone propionate. The intramuscular injection of testosterone propionate in oil is the method usually used to produce maximal effects, although the comparative data available on the relative effectiveness of the various methods of administration are not entirely satisfactory. A summary of the effects of stimulation therapy with various types of gonadotrophin material is given in the section on Anatomy and Physiology.

SUBSTITUTION THERAPY WITH ANDROGENS

Androgen therapy has been reported of value in the following conditions: eunuchism; primary eunuchoidism; bilateral intra-abdominal cryptorchism, when there is no response to stimulation therapy; the adiposogenital syndrome associated with intra-abdominal cryptorchism, when there is no response to stimulation therapy; pituitary dwarfism; inoperable carcinoma of the breast; functional uterine bleeding; suppression of lactation; impotence from glandular causes; the male climacteric; fractures in old men; Cushing's syndrome; Addison's disease; hypopituitarism with secondary hypogonadism in old men; rheumatoid arthritis; and disseminated lupus erythematosus.

Androgen therapy must be thought of in terms of both its physiologic and pharmacodynamic effects. The doses required to produce physiologic effects, such as induction of sexual maturity, are much smaller than those required to produce pharmacodynamic effects, such as the temporary control of inoperable carcinoma of the breast. Androgens and estrogens are general metabolic stimulants which influence the function of all tissues in the body and are not merely materials which stimulate sex function.

EUNUCHISM

Definition. Eunuchism is caused by complete loss of testicular function from castration, inflammation or injury.

Pathologic Physiology. The basal metabolism often shows a moderate depression, but is usually not lower than minus 20 to minus 25 per cent. The excretion of neutral 17-ketosteroids in the urine is greatly decreased.

Symptoms. The symptoms depend to some extent upon whether the condition develops before or after puberty, the chief difference being the effect on body contour. The effect of loss of function on skeletal development does not show up until about the time of puberty, when the extremities become long in proportion to the comparatively short trunk, the voice remains high pitched, and other secondary sex characteristics fail to develop. The persons affected are often tall and have a narrow chest and shoulders. They are usually shy, effeminate and high strung. Pubic and axillary hair does not develop, and there is no growth of beard and no development of hair on the chest, abdomen, arms or legs. The genitalia remain infantile. The prostate is usually not palpable. The muscles are small and feminine in type. There may or may not be slight development of breast tissue, but it is much less marked than in persons of the adiposogenital type. Obesity may or may not be present. In fact, the patients may weigh less than normal in contrast to patients of the adiposogenital type, who may be excessively fat. When testicular function is lost after normal masculine development has taken place, the skeleton is not grossly affected and many of the secondary sex characteristics tend to persist. The penis and scrotum become smaller but may remain nearly as large as before loss of function, the prostate usually atrophies, the growth of hair on the face and in the pubic, axillary and other regions may decrease a great deal, but usually does not disappear completely. The pitch of the voice may become slightly higher, but usually retains much of its masculine quality. There is decrease in sexual desire, but ability to perform the sexual act may not be completely lost. There is a great decrease in bodily vigor, muscle strength and ambition, and the patient becomes somewhat placid and listless. There are sometimes nervous phenomena resembling those which occur during the menopause in women.

EUNUCHOIDISM

Definition. Eunuchoidism is the term applied to partial loss of testicular function.

ble attempts at function is often noted in the appearance of a few pubic and axillary hairs (Fig. 96). The interstitial cells are apparently less susceptible to damage from the environment of the abdominal cavity and may show a considerable amount of function, even though both testes remain in the abdomen. Between these two extremes all variations are possible. Eunuchoidism may also be present with both testes in the scrotum. The testes

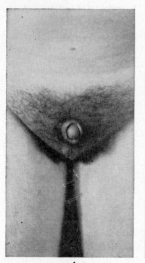 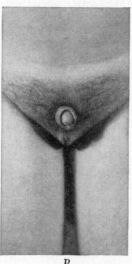 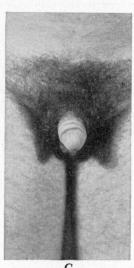

A   B   C

Fig. 96. Eunuchoidism (bilateral intra-abdominal cryptorchism) in a man aged 29, showing no effect from treatment with chorionic gonadotrophin, and a marked effect with testosterone propionate.

A, Before treatment. Patient had extremely small genitalia, and the prostate was not palpable. He was effeminate, smooth-skinned, had no beard, and no hair on his abdomen or extremities. There was a small amount of pubic hair. His voice was high pitched, and he had a marked inferiority complex.

B, After 1,024,00 rat units of chorionic gonadotrophin: practically no change in genitalia; prostate not palpable. He had gained 2.5 kg. Contrast this lack of effect with the marked effect of chorionic gonadotrophin in Figure 98.

C, After 8800 mg. of testosterone propionate: marked growth of genitalia; prostate 3 cm. in diameter; increased growth of hair on body and development of a more normal body contour in spite of a gain of 9 kg. The patient grew a beard, requiring him to shave every other day. His voice became masculine, and he became much more energetic and aggressive.

The decrease in function may vary from a slight deficiency to almost complete loss. The eunuchoid state may result from a primary defect in the testes themselves (primary eunuchoidism) or from inadequate stimulation of the testes by the anterior lobe of the pituitary (secondary eunuchoidism).

Pathologic Physiology. Moore has pointed out that the testes can develop normally only in the environment of the scrotum. When they remain in the inguinal canals or are deflected over the external oblique, they appear to function better than when they remain in the abdominal cavity. When both testes fail to descend from the abdominal cavity, virtually complete lack of testicular function often results. However, evidence of fee-

are usually small and show varying degrees of function.

Symptoms. When the secondary sex characteristics develop normally, the body contour is usually normal even though both testes remain within the abdomen; and when the secondary sex characteristics do not develop, the skeleton seems to assume the typical eunuchoid character. These facts indicate that androgen is necessary for normal skeletal growth.

TREATMENT OF EUNUCHISM AND EUNUCHOIDISM

Substitution therapy is required in all cases of eunuchism and most cases of eunuchoidism because of inability of the testes to respond to stimulation. Large doses of testosterone propionate are indicated (from 25 mg. three times per week to 25 mg. daily by intromuscular injection). The doses originally recommended (1 to 5 mg. daily) are inadequate. Oral administration of methyltestosterone produces a definite effect, but it is better in all eunuchs and eunuchoid individuals to give testosterone propionate parenterally until maximal changes have been produced. In order to simulate natural phenomena and to prevent the development of the skeletal characteristics of the eunuchoid state, it is desirable in all castrates and in all patients with bilateral intra-abdominal cryptorchism to begin treatment just before the onset of normal puberty, namely, at about the age of 12 years. When this is not done and the typical eunuch or eunuchoid changes have been allowed to develop, Thompson and Heckel have demonstrated the following effects with large doses of testosterone propionate:

1. The gradual appearance of the secondary sex characteristics of the adult male (Fig. 96). The infantile penis may become normal in size, the prostate develops, and hair grows in the pubic and axillary regions, on the face and on other parts of the body. The pitch of the voice rapidly assumes its characteristic masculine quality. Erections and seminal emissions become frequent. Priapism has been described.

2. A marked increase in appetite and body weight (as much as 40 pounds [18 kg.] in four months). The patients do not become obese, but show an increase in the size, firmness and strength of muscles.

3. An increase in basal metabolism of as much as 40 points.

4. An increase in vigor and sense of well being. The patients are capable of and have the initiative to do much more mental and physical work. They become more proficient in games involving muscle coordination and physical stamina.

5. Loss of their effeminate characteristics. Whereas before treatment they tend to run away from arguments and physical combat, after treatment they tend to welcome opportunities to demonstrate their physical prowess.

The response is determined not only by the substance given, but also by the susceptibility of the organ involved. There are thus variations in the amount of growth of the penis that may be produced with this material, and development usually stops before

the size becomes completely normal. The amount of development of secondary sex characteristics that can be induced is related to the age at which treatment is started. Maximal development can be induced only if treatment is started at the age at which puberty normally begins, namely, about the age of 12 years. The longer the treatment is delayed beyond this age, the less the response, although marked individual variations occur. A heavy beard may develop even when treatment is delayed until the age of 29. Observations appear to indicate that the rate at which development of secondary sex characteristics can be induced cannot be accelerated beyond a certain point. This is not surprising in view of the fact that the changes associated with normal puberty occur gradually over a period of several years. When there is complete lack of sex development, it is necessary to give intensive treatment for between two and three years, and then continue with maintenance therapy for the rest of the patient's life. In patients whose testicular function disappears after normal development has taken place, a shorter period of intensive therapy may be adequate. For maintenance therapy it is probably best to administer testosterone propionate intramuscularly in doses varying from 25 mg. once a week to 25 mg. three times a week. Patients may also be maintained with other forms of therapy previously described.

OTHER APPLICATIONS OF SUBSTITUTION THERAPY

The Male Climacteric. A condition characterized by various manifestations of hypogonadism and by vasomotor and emotional instability has been described in some older men. The condition is not common, and there is no definite epoch in the male like the menopause in the female. It has already been pointed out that the excretion of neutral 17-ketosteroids in the urine of men diminishes after the age of 30 years. More than 50 per cent of men over 70 years of age are reported to show spermatogenesis. Brown-Séquard and others have associated the fatigue and decreased vitality of advancing age with decrease in sexual vigor. However, the problem of aging is a complex one and probably involves all glands of internal secretion and the tissues which they stimulate. The diagnosis of the male climacteric should be made only after very careful study of the patient, because many disorders in older men may produce fatigue and decrease in sexual vigor and other manifestations of the climacteric. When a true climacteric is present in the male, there is a very definite and specific improvement during the administration of androgen.

Impotence. Impotence is a symptom and not a disease, and the most important consideration in its management is to determine its cause. Many cases are psychogenic in origin. When impotence is associated with a gradual decline in sexual function with advancing years, or when the onset is associated with injury to the testes or with atrophy secondary to hypopituitarism, then some improvement may be expected from glandular therapy. This may be of the substitution or stimulation variety, depending upon the capacity of the testes to respond.

Infertility. Infertility is a complex problem. The spermatozoa may be absent, greatly decreased in number or deficient in quality. Infertility may be produced by obstruction to the discharge of spermatozoa or by hypofunction of the seminiferous tubules. Testicular biopsy may yield valuable information concerning the condition of this portion of the testis. The treatment of infertility is not very satisfactory, but some improvement has recently been reported following the administration of chorionic gonadotrophin or large doses of testosterone propionate. In some men with very low spermatozoa counts, treatment with chorionic gonadotrophin may cause the count to increase sufficiently to make conception possible. The beneficial effect may be dependent upon the relation between the two functions of the testis, and optimal production of androgenic material by the testis appears to facilitate the production of spermatozoa. Equine and pituitary gonadotrophin, although theoretically desirable because of their content of follicle-stimulating hormone, are not very effective in stimulating spermatogenesis. The intramuscular administration of 25 to 50 mg. of testosterone propionate daily causes a marked depression in both functions of the testis. In men with normal and deficient spermatozoa counts, spermatogenesis disappears, and a biopsy of the testis shows a striking degeneration of the seminiferous tubules and a diminution in the number of interstitial cells. However, when treatment is discontinued, the testis gradually recovers over a period of about 18 to 24 months (so-called "rebound phenomenon"). The number of interstitial cells increases, the seminiferous tubules appear healthier, and the spermatozoa count may rise to a higher level than before treatment was started. As a result of such therapy, men with very low spermatozoa counts have gradually shown an increased count, and conception has become possible.

Benign Prostatic Hypertrophy. The experience of Heckel and Thompson with androgen therapy in benign prostatic hypertrophy has been disappointing. Since androgen causes development of the prostate, it is not easy to understand how its use in benign prostatic hypertrophy would be beneficial. It may also be emphasized that castration causes atrophy and that stimulation of the testes of young animals with gonadotrophic principles causes growth of the prostate.

Sex Hormones and Cancer. Interesting observations have been made on the effect of estrogens and androgens on carcinoma of the prostate and carcinoma of the breast. In 1941 Huggins reported that bilateral orchiectomy produced great improvement in patients with cancer of the prostate. The improvement consists in decrease in the size of the primary lesion in the prostate, disappearance of pain and great diminution in the x-ray evidence of metastases in the bones (notably those of the pelvis and spine). Definite improvement also follows functional castration with stilbestrol, although Huggins believes that bilateral orchiectomy produces better results. Five of 20 patients followed by Huggins for a period of five years after orchiectomy were reported to show no evidence of carcinoma. The acid phosphatase activity of the serum dropped to normal and remained there. The other 15 died of carcinoma of the prostate. Most of them had a remission which did not persist. Huggins has suggested that the differences in beneficial results may be explained by the hypothesis that some carcinomas of the prostate require androgenic material for their development, whereas others do not. Subjective improvement following surgical or functional castration with stilbestrol occurs in a much higher percentage of patients (about 80 per cent) than objective improvement (about 35 per cent). After initial improvement a relapse usually sets in, and death eventually occurs from carcinoma of the prostate. Up to the present time sufficient evidence has not been accumulated to indicate that cancer of the prostate has been cured in any patient by castration.

Huggins has recently reported that in patients with far-advanced cancer of the breast and prostate in whom other forms of therapy have ceased to be effective, a great deal of improvement may be produced by bilateral adrenalectomy. The status of this form of therapy is still to be determined.

Before Huggins' report on the effect of castration in patients with cancer of the prostate, Adair reported improvement in some patients with inoperable carcinoma of the breast during the administration of large doses of testosterone propionate (usually 300 mg. a week in divided doses). Among the beneficial effects noted were disappearance of pain, decrease in the x-ray evidence of metastases to bone, decrease in the size of the local lesion in the breast, increased appetite and gain in weight. Some masculinization occurred, with enlargement of the clitoris, lowering of the pitch of the voice and hirsutism. It is interesting that sexual desire was usually greatly increased. Subjective improvement occurred in a much higher percentage (about 75 per cent) than did objective improvement (about 25 per cent).

There is no evidence that carcinoma of the breast has ever been cured with androgen therapy. Patients eventually die in spite of initial improvement. In women several years beyond the menopause, in whom the metastases from carcinoma of the breast are found primarily in soft tissues, estrogen therapy appears to be more effective than androgen therapy. In women in this age group estrogen therapy also appears to have more effect on the local lesion in the breast. The explanation for this curious fact is not clear. It should be pointed out that glandular therapy should be used only in women with inoperable carcinoma of the breast. The treatment of an operable carcinoma is a radical mastectomy. Glandular therapy should be regarded as an adjunct to other forms of treatment, such as irradiation, and not as a substitute for them.

Miscellaneous Conditions. The administration of small doses of testosterone may be effective in the control of functional uterine bleeding. It is important to make an accurate diagnosis and avoid masculinizing changes. Estrogen therapy is more satisfactory for suppression of lactation than androgen therapy, because it will not cause any masculinizing effects. Androgens and estrogens cause retention of calcium, and their administration is sometimes of value in older men and women with fractures that do not heal well. Androgen therapy causes some retention of

nitrogen and may produce temporary improvement in patients with Cushing's syndrome. In patients with Addison's disease the administration of androgen, in addition to specific therapy, may produce more improvement than specific therapy alone. In Addison's disease the production of androgens by the adrenal cortex is greatly diminished or absent, and adrenal androgens play some role in the body economy. The administration of testosterone propionate in large doses may produce some improvement in patients with rheumatoid arthritis and disseminated lupus erythematosus, but cortisone and ACTH are much more effective therapeutic agents.

HARMFUL EFFECTS OF ANDROGEN THERAPY

It is uncertain whether permanent *injury to the testis* can be produced by the prolonged administration of large doses of testosterone propionate. After the administration of large doses for three months the testis not only gradually recovers, but eventually appears healthier than it was before treatment.

The administration of testosterone propionate commonly produces *acne* in both sexes, regardless of the age at which it is given. Acne can also be produced in young boys by the administration of chorionic gonadotrophin, which stimulates the production of androgen. Acne appears in both sexes without treatment at puberty when the production of androgenic material increases. There seems to be little doubt that there is some correlation between the concentration of androgenic material in the tissues and the development of acne vulgaris.

Masculinizing changes may be induced in women by the administration of androgens or by the development of masculinizing tumors of the adrenal cortex or of the ovary.

Pitting edema of the dependent portions of the body usually develops only when the dose of androgen is excessive. Testosterone propionate causes some retention of water, sodium and chloride. In this respect its effect is similar to that of estradiol, progesterone, desoxycorticosterone and cortisone, which have a similar molecular structure.

Hypermetabolism usually occurs only with large doses of testosterone propionate and methyltestosterone. The minimal amount necessary to induce sexual maturity may not affect the level of metabolism. The intramuscular injection of 50 mg. daily may cause the metabolism to rise to a level of plus 40 per cent. It has not been determined whether this increase in basal metabolism represents a direct effect on the metabolism of the tissues or a secondary effect by way of the pituitary or thyroid, or both.

STIMULATION THERAPY
UNDESCENDED TESTES
(*Cryptorchism*)

Definition. True cryptorchism is present when it is impossible, on repeated examination, to displace the testis into the scrotum in any position of the body. It is to be distinguished from pseudocryptorchism, in which the testes are migratory and move back and forth spontaneously from the scrotum to a higher level. The condition is bilateral in 25 to 40 per cent of the cases. The importance of failure of descent of the testis lies in the fact that the testis cannot function normally except in the environment of the scrotum.

Incidence. The highest recorded incidence for adults is 3.1 per 1000 reported by the U. S. War Department. The figures for children appear to be much higher, but it is not certain whether migratory testes are included in them. Drake reports 38 cases among 1050 boys from various schools, and Williams, 59 cases among 2104 boys in boarding schools. Both observers report descent in about two thirds of the cases during the school age.

Pathologic Anatomy. The testis may theoretically be stopped at any point along its so-called path of descent. In most instances undescended testes are found just inside the internal ring, in the inguinal canal, or deflected from the external ring in various abnormal positions, usually those in which fibers of the gubernaculum are found early in its development. The most common site of abnormal deflection is over the external oblique. Undescended testes are occasionally deflected toward the base of the penis and, in rare instances, in the perineum. In some instances "intra-abdominal" testes cannot be found at operation. Undescended testes may be associated with actual or potential hernias, and sometimes the patient first consults a physician because of strangulated hernia. The testis itself is often found to be defective at operation. Even after it has been brought into the scrotum with appropriate therapy, it remains smaller than the testis which has been there from the time of birth. The spermatogenic function of undescended testes is deficient.

Pathologic Physiology. The response to treatment in successful cases and the findings at operation in unsuccessful cases indicate that descent of the testis depends upon anatomic integrity of the parts involved and upon hormonal stimulation. There is some evidence that increased production of androgen from stimulation of the interstitial cell mass by chorionic gonadotrophin may play a role. Prenatal hypertrophy and postnatal involution of the interstitial cells of the testis have been demonstrated. There is an associated prenatal hypertrophy and engorgement of the genitalia and a postnatal decrease in size. The only mammals in which prenatal descent of the testis occurs are those in which chorionic gonadotrophin appears in the circulation during pregnancy, namely, in man and in the great apes. In other mammals descent occurs just before, or early in puberty, but in such animals precocious descent may be induced by administration of gonadotrophic material from human pregnancy urine. It follows that failure of descent of the testis may be caused by (1) an anatomic deficiency, or (2) a hormonal deficiency. With all the recent work on glandular therapy there has been too much tendency to neglect anatomic defects, which appear to play an important role in many cases of undescended testes.

Signs and Symptoms. The absence of one or both testes from the scrotum is usually first noted by the child's parents. Not infrequently a painful swelling representing an associated inguinal hernia first brings the patient to a physician. The effect of deficient testicular function does not become evident until about the time of puberty, although some patients with this disorder are rather effeminate before this age. The body contour of young boys with undescended testes is usually normal and only occasionally of the adiposogenital type. When the condition is bilateral and intra-abdominal and persists beyond the age of puberty, a eunuchoid condition commonly develops, although even the intra-abdominal testis may secrete enough androgen to preserve normal body contour. When the condition is unilateral and persists beyond the age of puberty, the testis in the scrotum usually produces enough androgen to cause normal development of secondary sex characteristics, although in some instances the testicular function is deficient and appears to be associated with hypo-pituitarism. The basal metabolism in patients with undescended testes is usually normal, but may be moderately depressed. In about one third of the cases the condition is associated with other abnormalities, among which may be mentioned hypospadias, slip-

be carefully manipulated on more than one occasion with the patient in the upright position. The location of an undescended testis cannot be determined accurately with the patient in the recumbent position, and a testis cannot be considered intra-abdominal unless it is impossible to palpate it by any method of

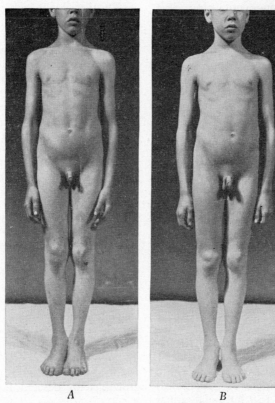

A   *B*

Fig. 97. Bilateral undescended testes. Growth of genitalia and descent of both testes during treatment with chorionic gonadotrophin.

A, Before treatment at the age of 10 years.

B, After 15,000 rat units of chorionic gonadotrophin, showing both testes in the scrotum. The left testis became migratory after treatment was discontinued.

ping of epiphyses, infantile sacrum, clubfoot, poorly developed abdominal muscles, pilonidal sinus and defective cerebral development.

Diagnosis. It is important to distinguish true cryptorchism from pseudocryptorchism. Migratory testes tend to remain in the scrotum after puberty and, therefore, require no treatment. It is common for the inexperienced observer to consider testes of this type as true undescended testes. In distinguishing between true cryptorchism and pseudocryptorchism it is important that the examiner have a thorough knowledge of the pathologic anatomy of undescended testes and that the testes

examination. A testis which appears to be in the abdominal cavity in the recumbent position is often found in the inguinal canal in the erect position or after straining. It may occasionally be impossible, because of retraction, to palpate testes that at other times can be felt. Testes which are deflected in abnormal positions, notably those over the external oblique, can usually be distinguished from those in the inguinal canal by the fact that they lie more superficially and can be moved readily under the skin. Those in the upper part of the canal can often be displaced into the abdominal cavity. It is important to define the position of the testis accurately because it has an important bearing on the response to glandular treatment.

Treatment. The best form of treatment at the present time appears to be the intelligent combination of glandular therapy and surgical procedures. The material most commonly employed in the glandular therapy of undescended testes is chorionic gonadotrophin. The preparations containing 500 and 1000 rat units per cubic centimeter are more practical than weaker concentrations. This material stimulates the interstitial cells of the testis to produce androgen. This in turn causes enlargement of all parts involved in descent and, if pushed too far, precocious sexual development resembling premature puberty (Fig. 95).

Hamilton has demonstrated that descent of the testis may be produced by androgen, but since this may injure the normal testis, at least temporarily, it is contraindicated unless both testes are within the abdominal cavity and incapable of responding to chorionic gonadotrophin. Gonadotrophic material from the pituitary and from the serum of the pregnant mare have also been reported to cause descent, but the data available are not very convincing. Since Schapiro's report twenty-four years ago a large number of observations have appeared on the use of chorionic gonadotrophin in undescended testes. Most of these reports appear to be overenthusiastic. A review by Thompson and Heckel about fifteen years ago of all available reports showed that descent was claimed in 61 per cent of the cases on the average, including successful results in 55 per cent of 150 intra-abdominal testes. In contrast to these high percentages of successful results, Thompson and Heckel were able to produce descent in only 20 per cent of all their cases and in only 27 per cent of those occurring in patients under 16 years of age. The difference in results may be attributed in part to their exclusion, except in the beginning of the study, of all testes of the migratory or retracted types.

In successful cases descent usually occurs within two months after starting treatment, although in occasional instances it may take as long as twenty-one months. It is easier to produce descent before, than after the age of puberty (27 per cent as compared with 6 per cent in the series of Thompson and Heckel). Descent has been produced, however, as late as the age of 32 years in a eunuchoid person.

The position of the testis has an important

bearing on the result of treatment. According to Thompson and Heckel, "Descent was produced in nine of twenty-one instances (43 per cent) in which the testis was in the inguinal canal, in only one of nine instances (11 per cent) in which it was deflected in an abnormal position outside the canal, and in none of twenty instances in which it was within the abdominal cavity." Descent was produced in one instance in which the testis was deflected in the fold of skin to the left of the scrotum. "Descent was not produced in any instance in which the testis was deflected over the external oblique muscle or toward the base of the penis. . . . Our failure to produce descent in our cases of intra-abdominal testes is in striking contrast to the results of some other observers. In five of our ten successful cases the testis could either be pulled into the upper end of the scrotum or to a level between the lower end of the canal and the upper end of the scrotum before treatment was started. In other words, the testes were of the type that commonly descends at puberty. In the other five cases there could be little doubt of the influence of the treatment in causing descent."

The influence of chorionic gonadotrophin on genital growth is more striking than its influence on descent of the testis. Marked development of the genitalia may occur without any change in the position of the testis, just as during normal puberty, illustrating the importance of anatomic factors in preventing descent. An example of genital growth with descent is recorded in Figure 97.

RELATION OF GLANDULAR THERAPY TO OPERATIVE PROCEDURES

Treatment with chorionic gonadotrophin may be of value before and after surgical procedures. Before operation it stimulates genital growth and makes it easier to bring the testis into the scrotum. This is important, because Thompson and Heckel have demonstrated that operative procedures are necessary in about three fourths of all cases of true cryptorchism. After operation the material may be of value in cases in which the testis is not brought to a sufficiently low level. When hernia is present, it is not corrected by glandular therapy, even if descent of the testis is produced.

When glandular therapy is not successful, orchiopexy will usually reveal anatomic factors which prevent descent. In 11 patients in the series of Thompson and Heckel these anatomic factors were found to be: "(1) fibrous bands (all patients); (2) shortness of the structures to which the cord and testis were attached, namely the peritoneal process, the transversalis fascia, the intercolumnar fascia, and the cremasteric muscle and fascia

Influences similar to those introduced artificially come into play during normal development and might be expected to result in descent of those testes not retained by mechanical factors. If no more is accomplished with glandular therapy than is accomplished by natural processes at a later age, it is perti-

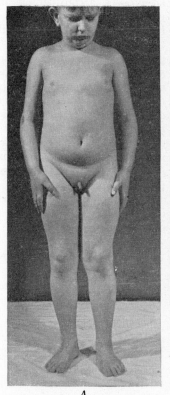 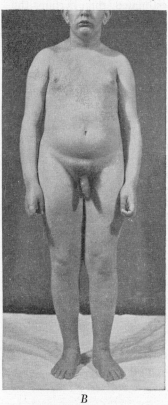

A   B

Fig. 98. Effect of chorionic gonadotrophin in a boy of the adiposogenital type.
A, Before treatment, at the age of 10 years; extremely small genitalia.
B, After 575,130 rat units of chorionic gonadotrophin.

(all patients); (3) abnormal direction of the peritoneal process (four patients), which in three patients was turned upward on the external oblique muscle, and in one lay over the rectus sheath; and (4) absence of the external ring (one patient)."

STATUS OF GLANDULAR THERAPY

The following facts suggest that chorionic gonadotrophin may cause descent only of those testes which would descend normally without treatment at the time of puberty: (1) the high percentage of failures with treatment. (2) In unsuccessful cases operation has shown anatomic factors which prevent descent. (3) The decrease in the incidence of undescended testes after the age of puberty in untreated cases.

nent to inquire whether the treatment is worth while. The crux of the problem is whether a testis made to descend at an early age with treatment is more likely to be normal than one which descends later without treatment. The consensus appears to be that the testis should be brought into the scrotum at an early age, although there is some difference of opinion on this question. The following points are in favor of glandular therapy:

1. It makes it possible to tell at an early age what patients will require surgical intervention by distinguishing between those in which descent is prevented by anatomic factors and those in which it is not.

2. It causes the testis to move into the scro-

tum at an early age without operation in one fourth of the cases.

3. It facilitates subsequent operative procedures by enlarging the parts involved, even when it does not produce descent.

If the importance of bringing the testis into the scrotum at the earliest possible age has not been overestimated, then perhaps the wisest course to follow in boys with undescended testes is to administer chorionic gonadotrophin cautiously and carry out operative procedures if descent fails to occur. The age at which treatment should be started is uncertain, but if it is to be given at all, it should probably be given early, perhaps at the age of 3 years. The effective dose and the duration of treatment vary from patient to patient. In successful cases, descent of the testis usually occurs within two months during the parenteral administration of from 100 to 500 international units three times a week. After the age of puberty larger doses (as much as 1000 international units three times per week) may be required. The patients must be observed carefully and treatment discontinued before genital growth becomes excessive. It has already been pointed out that, if treatment is pushed too far, a condition simulating premature puberty may result. However, a moderate amount of genital growth usually must be induced to accomplish the result desired. It must be emphasized that little is known about the effect of premature stimulation of the testis with this material on subsequent spermatogenesis and skeletal growth.

HYPOGONADISM SECONDARY TO HYPOPITUITARISM

The production of genital growth with chorionic gonadotrophin has an important application in the treatment of patients with the adiposogenital syndrome (hypopituitarism with secondary hypogonadism and obesity), commonly referred to in the past as the Fröhlich syndrome. Patients with this syndrome often have some degree of hypothyroidism with a low basal metabolism, and a few of them have hypoadrenalism of varying degree. There is a deposition of fat in the abdomen and thighs with a transverse ridge in the lower abdomen tending to produce an apron of fat, genu valgum, and, in males, the feminine type of breasts. The pituitary appears to be involved, and perhaps also the hypothalamic area. This condition is described in more detail in the section on the

Pituitary, but an example of what may be accomplished with chorionic gonadotrophin in a boy 10 years old is recorded here (Fig. 98), because of its bearing on the conditions already described. This material appears to be more effective before or during the age of normal puberty than after. Nevertheless, with large doses, a considerable amount of genital growth may be produced in older men with hypogonadism. It appears that the smaller the genitalia after the age of puberty, the greater the likelihood of influencing their size; and the more nearly they approach the normal in size, the less the likelihood of doing so. If treatment is given before the age of puberty, the fat in the abdomen and thighs may decrease markedly as genital growth occurs and the skeleton increases in length, so that normal body contour is produced. Adequate therapy usually results in increased physical and mental vigor. Lack of energy and ambition may be noted when treatment is discontinued, necessitating readministration of the material.

Willard O. Thompson

TUMORS OF THE TESTIS

Tumors of the testis are rare and occur mostly between the ages of 20 and 40 years. Their incidence is said to be higher in the cryptorchid testis than in the normal testis.

The tumors may be classified as follows:

Malignant:
1. Carcinoma
2. Embryonal teratoma or mixed tumor type, including chorionepithelioma
Benign:
1. Adult teratoma or dermoid
2. Adenoma of the seminal tubules
3. Interstitial cell tumor
4. Fibroma, lipoma, myxoma

The teratoma is the most common form of testicular tumor. Next is the carcinoma, which has its origin in the adult tubule cells. Malignant tumors of the testis are noted for early metastasis by way of the blood or lymph vessels.

The teratomas may form growths resembling rudimentary fetuses, including the chorion. These growths are counterparts of the chorionepitheliomas seen in the female and are just as malignant.

Feminizing Tumors of the Testis. Chorionepithelioma of the testis is especially interesting to the endocrinologist because, in about 10 per cent of the cases, there is evidence of a feminizing influence. This is expressed by enlargement of the breasts, sometimes painful and sometimes associated with the secretion of colostrum. Aschheim-Zondek tests often give positive results, and in some cases in which the pituitary has been examined, its cells have shown the condition typical of pregnancy. In some instances of feminizing tumors the histology is that of teratoma without the chorionic element.

Interstitial Cell Tumors. In any condition involving overgrowth of these cells, hypermasculinity would be expected, since they are the cells concerned with elaboration of androgen. It is only in children, however, that the masculinizing effect of these tumors can be noted. In adults the effects are not so spectacular, since the secondary sex characteristics are already present. In the infant or young boy the genitalia become as large as those of an adult, accompanied by the rapid skeletal growth, muscular development and voice changes that normally occur at puberty. Only rare instances have been noted in children, although several cases are recorded as developing after puberty.

Symptoms of Testicular Tumor. The enlargement is often painless, usually develops rapidly, and is firm and symmetric. There may be quiescent periods. There are apt to be enlarged inguinal lymph glands, and even the periaortic lymph glands in the abdomen are often involved early.

Diagnosis. Tumor must be differentiated from tuberculosis, which can usually be done by considering the personal and family history, and by the fact that in tuberculosis the epididymis and vas are usually hard and nodular. Syphilis, with a history of chancre, may cause some difficulty in differential diagnosis. If in doubt, the effect of antisyphilitic treatment should be evident within a short time. If there is difficulty in differentiating hydrocele from a tumor, transillumination should be used. Hydrocele and tumor may coexist.

Treatment. In the benign types, surgical removal is indicated. In the malignant types the only hope of cure is an early radical operation. This should be performed before metastases have formed. Irradiation should then be used. Teratomas are resistant to irradiation and should be treated by radical surgical removal unless metastases have developed. Malignant tumors of the testis are usually fatal, although life may be prolonged by treatment.

WILLARD O. THOMPSON

MISCELLANEOUS DISEASES OF THE TESTIS

ORCHITIS

A systemic infection, such as typhoid or pneumonia, may be followed by *acute orchitis* (inflammation of the testis), but the chief offender in this respect is mumps. Orchitis occurs in about 12 per cent of patients with this disease. There is marked swelling of one or both testes, which are sensitive to palpation. This lasts from three to five days, and is associated with a sudden rise in temperature. The importance of the condition lies in the fact that in about one third of the cases, atrophy of the testis occurs, with subsequent sterility. Damage to the testis is said to be prevented by the administration of stilbestrol.

Chronic orchitis, on the other hand, is not painful, although the testis slowly becomes swollen and hard. The most common cause is tertiary syphilis. It may also be caused by tuberculosis, glanders, leprosy and certain parasitic diseases.

Treatment is directed at the systemic disease of which the orchitis is a manifestation. In some instances it may be necessary to treat the condition surgically.

HYDROCELE

This is caused by excessive accumulation of fluid in the tunica vaginalis. It may be congenital. When acute, it is always secondary to inflammation of the epididymis or testis, for example, in syphilitic infection. The chronic type is usually seen in men of middle age. Hydrocele caused by such diseases as filariasis may reach an enormous size.

Treatment. If the condition is mild, no treatment is indicated. Immediate relief in acute cases can be produced by aspiration of the fluid. In severe cases, surgical procedures are often necessary.

CONDITIONS ARISING FROM INTERFERENCE WITH BLOOD SUPPLY

Extravasation of blood into the testes is usually caused by injury. Sometimes it occurs during breech deliveries. The blood supply may be cut off by torsion of the spermatic cord.

Infarction of the testis may occur. Often there is no apparent cause. It is accompanied by severe pain, nausea and vomiting and some fever, although the fever is not as high as that noted in mumps. The testicular swelling subsides within a week. Treatment is palliative.

ATROPHY

Atrophy may be caused by a variety of conditions, e.g., infections such as syphilis; derangement of function of some other gland of internal secretion, such as hypofunction of the pituitary; exposure to roentgen rays or radium; permanent interference with blood supply; or pressure such as that from large varicoceles. One of the most important causes is the orchitis associated with mumps.

Treatment. Either substitution or replacement therapy is indicated, the type depending on the capacity of the testes to respond. In most instances substitution therapy with androgen is necessary.

WILLARD O. THOMPSON

References

Adair, F. E.: Testosterone in the Treatment of Breast Carcinoma. M. Clin. North America, 32: 18, 1948.

Butenandt, A., and Hanisch, G.: Über Testosteron; Umwandlung des Dehydro-androsterons in Androstendiol und Testosteron; ein Weg zur Darstellung des Testosterons aus Cholesterin. H. S. Ztschr. f. physiol. Chem., 237:89, 1935.

Engle, E. T.: Male Reproductive System, in Cowdry's Problems of Aging. Baltimore, Williams & Wilkins Co., 1939.

Heller, C. G., and Nelson, W. O.: Classification of Male Hypogonadism and a Discussion of the Pathologic Physiology, Diagnosis and Treatment. J. Clin. Endocrinol., 8:345, 1948.

Howard, R. P., Sniffen, R. C., Simmons, F. A., and Albright, F.: Testicular Deficiency: A Clinical and Pathologic Study. J. Clin. Endocrinol., 10: 121, 1950.

Huggins, C., and Bergenstal, D. M.: Inhibition of Human Mammary and Prostatic Cancers by Adrenalectomy. Cancer Research, 12:134, 1952.

———, and Hodges, C. V.: Studies on Prostatic Cancer; Effect of Castration, of Estrogen and of Androgen Injection on Serum Phosphatases in Metastatic Carcinoma of the Prostate. Cancer Research, 1:293, 1941.

Laqueur, E., and others: Über männliches Hormon, Unterschied von Androsteron aus Harn and Testosteron aus Testis. Act. Brev. Neerland, 5:84, 1935.

Thompson, W. O.: Androgen Therapy. Ann. Int. Med., 30:55, 1949.

Thompson, W. O., and Heckel, N. J.: Precocious Sexual Development from an Anterior Pituitarylike Principle. J.A.M.A., 110:1813, 1938.

———: Undescended Testes; Present Status of Glandular Treatment. J.A.M.A., 112:397, 1939.

Wilkins, L., and others: Treatment of Congenital Adrenal Hyperplasia with Cortisone. J. Clin. Endocrinol., 11:1, 1951.

DISEASES OF THE FEMALE GONADS

INTRODUCTION

The ovary serves the function of procreation by providing the mature ovum and the hormonal secretions which prepare the uterus for its reception after fertilization. Under stimulus of the anterior lobe of the pituitary, it initiates and maintains the changes which begin with the onset of puberty and culminate in the full sexual development of the adult woman. These changes include the development of the genitalia and of the breasts and secondary sexual characteristics, and the attainment of adult psychosexual status. In the adult woman the ripening of the ovum is accompanied by the secretion from the follicular cells of estrogen, which causes growth of the endometrium and also prepares the vaginal wall for coitus. With the extrusion of the ovum the area of rupture closes, and the cells, previously follicular, take on the character of thecal cells to form the corpus luteum. These cells secrete progesterone, the function of which is to cause further growth of the endometrium and increased secretory activity in preparation for the nidation of the fertilized ovum. In the absence of conception the progestational endometrium breaks down, leaving only the basal layer. This is accompanied by the flow of nonclotting blood, i.e., menstruation.

The secretion of ovarian hormones is controlled by the gonadotrophic hormones. The present concept of this regulation, based largely on experiments in the hypophysectomized rat, may be briefly summarized as follows: The follicle-stimulating hormone, FSH, stimulates follicular growth, estrogen production by the follicle requiring the complementary action of small amounts of luteinizing hormone, LH. The increasing estrogen formation associated with follicular maturation reduces FSH formation and leads to a preponderance of LH. This alteration in the ratio of FSH and LH results in rupture of the follicle and its transformation to a corpus luteum whose persistence and secretion of progesterone are dependent upon the elaboration of pituitary luteotrophic factor, probably prolactin (Fevold).

Under the sequential influence of these ovarian hormones, the growth and development of the endometrium takes place according to a specific pattern. That associated with the first half of the menstrual cycle, up to the rupture of the ripened follicle, and resulting from the action of estrogens alone, is referred to as the interval, or better, the proliferative endometrium. It is characterized by the moderate amount of growth and vascularity and by straight, nonsecretory glands. Under the synergistic action of estrogens and progesterone during the latter half of the menstrual cycle, there is a further increase in height and vascularity, and in the growth of the glands which now assume a corkscrew appearance and acquire secretory activity. This is termed a glandular or secretory endometrium, or better still, a progestational endometrium because of its property of forming decidual tissue for the implantation of the ovum. The events in the ovarian cycle are reflected in the vaginal epithelium and can be observed by the examination of the vaginal fluid. A description of the cytology of the vaginal secretions during the menstrual cycle will be found in another portion of this section.

Menstruation may be broadly defined as spontaneous bleeding from the uterus which recurs in cycles as the result of desquamation of the endometrium. This desquamation can take place only if the endometrium has been built up previously by the action of estrogen, with or without progesterone. The latter is not essential, since menstruation can take place without ovulation and consequently without the production of progesterone. Menstruation is the result of two processes, the building up of the endometrium by the internal secretions of the ovaries, and the sudden drop in the level of these secretions.

The morphologic and the functional (Markee) characteristics of the vascular bed of the uterus have been well described, and their importance for menstruation pointed out. Two types of arteries furnish blood to the endometrium, both arising at right angles from the arteries in the subendometrial layer of the myometrium. The first type, or straight artery, supplies the basal portion of the endometrial glands and stroma and is independent of hormonal influences. The second type, the spiral artery, extends up through the endometrium to within a short distance of the surface epithelium and presents a typical corkscrew appearance, the number of whose coils varies with the stage of endometrial development. The growth, development and regression of the spiral arteries are conditioned by the action of the ovarian hormones. The study of the behavior of these vessels in ocular endometrial transplants in the monkey has disclosed a specific dynamic relation of the spiral artery to menstrual bleeding. The growth of the endometrial implant under the influence of endogenous or exogenous ovarian hormones is accompanied by a parallel but disproportionate growth of the spiral arteries which results in their progressive coiling. When the anabolic phase is interrupted by the cessation of ovarian secretary activity, or by hormonal withdrawal, characteristic changes take place in the behavior of the spiral arteries and in the endometrial implants. The initial change is a regression in the mass of the transplant through loss of interstitial fluid. This leads to the compression and progressive coiling of the spiral arteries and to vascular stasis, usually accompanied by general vasodilatation. About 4 to 24 hours before the first hemorrhage, intense vasoconstriction of the spiral arteries sets in, the site of vasoconstriction being located in the deepest portion of the implant. There is blanching of the area fed by the constricted vessel, indicative of local anoxia, which is in turn responsible for the endometrial necrosis and its eventual sloughing. In one after another of the constricted arteries, the blood flow is temporarily and briefly restored and bleeding occurs through the walls of the damaged vessels, with desquamation of the adjacent necrotic endometrium. Cessation of the bleeding takes place through final vasoconstriction of the arteriole and thrombus formation. Thereafter, rapid reepithelialization takes place from the residual basal portions of the uterine glands, which have been maintained intact by a continuous circulation through the straight arteries.

Particular stress is placed on the necessity of rapid regression of the endometrium as a preliminary to bleeding and desquamation. There are no fundamental differences between endometrial and vascular changes in ovulatory and anovulatory cycles, or after hormonal administrations, providing comparable endometrial growth has been achieved. It is still uncertain whether the profound changes just preceding and during menstrual bleeding are of general or local origin or both.

Menstruation runs parallel to ovarian activity, but is neither fundamental nor indispensable. It occurs only in primates and not in other mammals, whereas estrus and the rest of the ovarian cycle are common to all. That menstruation is not directly associated with ovulation can also be demonstrated in the human being. Anovulatory menstruation is now well known, and the reverse is shown by instances in which conception occurs without menstruation. Furthermore, a mass of evidence makes it clear that ovulation occurs, not simultaneously with menstruation, but approximately fourteen days from the onset of menstruation. This evidence is in general agreement, though obtained by various methods, such as examination of the vaginal secretions, determinations of the basal body temperature, endometrial biopsies, observations on ova in the tubes at operation, time of single coitus producing conception or by estimation of hormones in urine or blood. According to the evidence of the vaginal smears (Papanicolaou), ovulation takes place in most instances on the twelfth or thirteenth day, although wide variations occur in individual cases.

A. C. CARTER
E. SHORR

References

Fevold, H. L.: The Gonadotrophic Function of the Pituitary Gland. The Chemistry and Physiology of Hormones. Publication of the A.A.A.S., p. 152, 1944.

Markee, J. E.: Menstruation in Intraocular Endometrial Transplants in the Rhesus Monkey. Carnegie Inst. Wash. Pub. 518, Contrib. Embryol., 177:221, 1940.

Papanicolaou, G. N.: The Sexual Cycle in Human Female as Revealed by Vaginal Smears. Am. J. Anat. (supp.), 52:519, 1933.

METHODS OF STUDYING OVARIAN FUNCTION

The many methods currently available for the study of ovarian function will be discussed with respect to the value of the information they provide and their practicability, particularly for the general practitioner. They fall into two major categories: the first consists in measurements, chiefly in urine, of the several hormones concerned in the regulation of menstruation, the second in procedures for evaluating the effects of the ovarian hormones on various end organs.

Pituitary gonadotrophic activity is estimated by bioassay, usually in the mouse, of urinary gonadotrophins. The range of normal varies from 5 to 40 mouse units in 24 hours, and represents the combined effect of FSH and LH, since there is at present no satisfactory method for estimating them separately. Estrogens may be determined in blood or urine either by chemical methods or bioassay. The end product of progesterone metabolism, pregnanediol, can be isolated from urine as the glucuronide and measured with a fair degree of accuracy. The luteal phase of a normal cycle is associated with the excretion of 4 mg. of pregnanediol daily. The 17-ketosteroids, representing androgens chiefly of adrenal origin in women, are determined chemically, the normal range being 7 to 14 mg. per 24 hours. Of these hormonal analyses, that for gonadotrophin is of particular value for the assessment of the amenorrheas, both primary and secondary. Assays for 17-ketosteroids are of diagnostic value for certain syndromes to be described. The determination of the magnitude of estrogen excretion is without value unless a curve for the entire cycle is obtained, and, even under these circumstances, subject to such analytic inaccuracies and with such a wide range of normal values that it has fallen into disuse. For pregnanediol measurements to be of value, they should be obtained throughout the luteal phase.

In the second category, the end organ responses to the ovarian hormones, fall a variety of indices of more or less objective and quantitative character. An evaluation should be made of the extent of development of the secondary sex characteristics, such as breast development, the body contour, carrying angle of the arm, growth of axillary and pubic hair, the regression of the scalp hair line at the temples and the development of the external and internal genitalia. In skilled hands, useful information can be obtained from the histology of endometrial biopsies obtained at times in the menstrual cycle when proliferative and secretory patterns are normally present. Criteria for dating the secretory endometium have been provided by Noyes, Her-

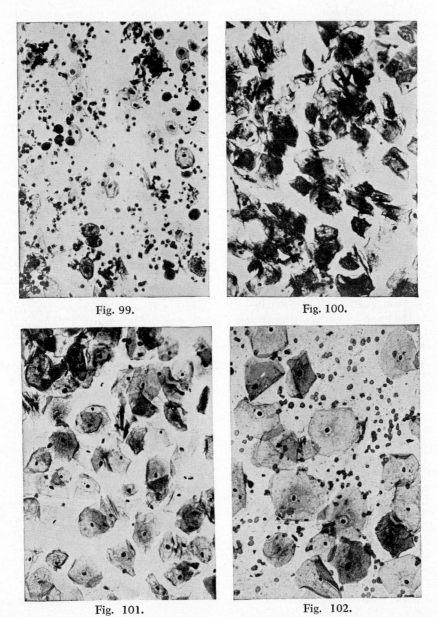

Fig. 99.   Fig. 100.

Fig. 101.   Fig. 102.

Figs. 99–102. Primary amenorrhea. The use of the vaginal smear as a guide to estrogenic therapy. (Papanicolaou and Shorr.) This serves to illustrate also the castrate and postmenopausal cases, in which the same initial smear and the same reaction to therapy are observed.

Fig. 99. Atrophic smear in primary amenorrhea.

Fig. 100. Change in smear following estrogenic therapy.

Fig. 101. Follicular smear, maximum effect induced by estrogenic therapy. This is referred to as a follicular reaction because it is the normal accompaniment of the full development of the ovarian follicle in a menstruating woman.

Fig. 102. Pseudomenstrual or withdrawal bleeding. This occurs regularly when treatment is stopped, at an interval which is usually five days after cessation of estrogenic therapy.

tig and Rock. The basal body temperature is widely used as an index of ovarian function, and particularly for estimating the time of ovulation. In our hands it has been more reliable when grossly abnormal cycles exist; the presence of entirely "normal" temperature curves are, however, frequently associated with demonstrably subnormal cycles.

Advantage can be profitably taken of the circumstance that the events of the ovarian cycle are reflected in the vaginal secretion and can be simply observed by examination of the vaginal secretions by the methods developed by Papanicolaou (1933) as modified by Shorr (Figs. 99-102). Smears can be obtained daily by the patient at home and without trauma. The staining techniques have been so simplified as to permit it to be an office procedure. The cytologic criteria for the evaluation of the vaginal smear picture have been quite securely established by a number of published studies (deAllende, Shorr and Hartman). Recognizing certain limitations, the vaginal smear furnishes an extremely satisfactory picture of ovarian function and serves as a sensitive guide for the most efficient use of therapeutic agents.

Special attention should be paid to two details of the technique. Cells which are allowed to dry even for an instant are tinted a yellow orange. Such slides are not diagnostic. To prevent drying, the pipet and the slide may be moistened in advance with physiologic saline solution. The other point is the use of the procedure recommended for the removal of red cells in the presence of uterine bleeding. These can be laked by the addition of enough concentrated hydrochloric acid to the alcohol-ether mixture to make a 0.25 per cent solution.

After the cessation of the menstrual flow, the epithelial cells stain blue-green and are relatively small with large nuclei. During the next five to eight days the epithelial cells become navicular in shape, then more square, and discrete in arrangement. The nuclei become shrunken and pyknotic, and the cells take on the brick red stain of cornification. They assume the typical appearance shown in Figure 101. Polynuclear leukocytes disappear, and the cells distribute themselves discretely in a thin layer of mucus. Occasionally red corpuscles are found. They may even be visible as overt bleeding and accompanied by pain, the well known "mittelschmerz."

The changes in the vaginal epithelium and secretions are the expression of follicular development in the ovary. They are the same as those which occur in other mammals under the designation of "heat" or estrus. The preovulatory phase lasts two to three days and the ovulatory peak one day, and is followed by a postovulatory reaction. This lasts usually one day, and is characterized by leukocytosis, by folding and clumping of the epithelial cells and usually by a reduction of the cornified cells. The luteal phase which follows lasts ten to fourteen days. The cytologic picture "may be divided into the early luteal phase lasting three to four days during which considerable cornification is likely to persist due to the shedding of the upper cornified layers previously built up under the influence of the estrogenic hormone, and the late luteal phase which is the expression of the growth and desquamation of the luteal epithelium resulting from the combined action of estrogen and progesterone" (Shorr). DeAllende, Shorr and Hartman have described and illustrated the various cell types of the menstrual cycle. The cornified cells of the luteal phase are usually clumped, crenated or folded, and present a variety of degenerative cytoplasmic changes. The noncornified elements are more varied, but show similar features, among which are wrinkling, curling of the edges, folding and granular deposits. At first, small pyknotic nuclei may predominate, but later the larger nuclei are in the majority, usually with degenerative features.

Other procedures which are used to study gonadal function in women are culdoscopy for direct inspection of the ovaries without laparotomy, hysterograms to outline the endometrial cavity and tubes, and tubal insufflation to ascertain their patency.

A. C. CARTER
E. SHORR

References

de Allende, I. L. C., Shorr, E., and Hartman, C. G.: Comparative Study of the Vaginal Smear Cycle of the Rhesus Monkey and the Human. Carnegie Institution of Washington, Publication 557, Contrib. to Embryol., *31:*1, 1943.

Noyes, R. W., Hertig, A. T., and Rock, J.: Dating the Endometrial Biopsy. Fertil. & Steril., *1:*3, 1950.

Shorr, E.: An Evaluation of the Clinical Applications of the Vaginal Smear Method. J. Mt. Sinai Hosp., *12:*667, 1945.

HORMONAL PREPARATIONS USEFUL IN THE MANAGEMENT OF OVARIAN DYSFUNCTION

Before discussing specific ovarian disturbances, consideration should be given to the basic principles which underlie the use of the hormonal agents currently available for their management. These basic principles are the same as with other diseases and their

is approximately 3000 rat units daily, with a range between 2000 and 4000 rat units; however, individual variations may be far greater and as much as tenfold (Fig. 103). Furthermore, with estrogens available for parenteral and oral use, the difference in the effectiveness of all estrogenic preparations by these two routes should be recognized and the marked loss of activity by the oral route borne in mind. This can be as great as 95

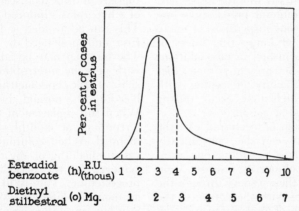

Fig. 103. Range of dosage required for estrus (development of a complete follicular reaction in the vaginal smear) in the human being. (Journal of the Mt. Sinai Hospital, Vol. 12.)

pharmacologic agents: to give enough of the preparation to produce the intended effect as demonstrated by objective criteria. The effects of estrogens, progesterone, androgens and gonadotrophic hormones can be assessed by the use of a variety of criteria which vary in specificity and ease with which they can be used. Qualitative information is provided by changes produced in breast development, bodily contour, sexual hair growth and withdrawal bleeding; more precise indices are furnished by endometrial biopsies and vaginal smears.

The Estrogens. Vaginal smears are particularly useful in regulating therapy with estrogens. Considerable confusion has been introduced in the use of this group of hormones through the failure to require that they be marketed in terms of biologic activity and because of marked individual differences in replacement requirements. These factors are less disadvantageous when the objective of treatment is symptomatic relief as in the menopausal syndrome; however, when replacement is the therapeutic goal they make it necessary to resort to an objective procedure such as the vaginal smear. The average estrous or full replacement dose in the human

per cent with some estrogens. The synthetic and natural estrogenic preparations currently available differ greatly in biologic activity on a weight basis, with an extreme variation of 240 fold. Examples of the relative biologic activity of a number of the more commonly used estrogens are given in the accompanying table.

Comparison of the Biologic Activity and Weight of Various Estrogens

(Based on Human Assay by Vaginal Smears)

	MG.	EQUIVALENT IN RAT UNITS
Intramuscular route		
Natural estrogens:		
α Estradiol benzoate	1.0	6000
Estrone	1.0	1250
Oral route		
Natural estrogens:		
α Estradiol	1.0	600
Conjugated estrone sulfate (Premarin, Konestrin)	1.25	800
Synthetic estrogens:		
Stilbestrol	1.0	1500
Monomethyl stilbestrol	1.0	500
Ethinyl estradiol	0.1	1000

With respect to the dosage schedule, vaginal smears have shown that the more frequently estrogens are given the more efficient they are. Convenience and efficiency are best achieved when the dose is given in the morning and at bedtime. Parenteral therapy is usually not necessary and is justified chiefly when a rigorous schedule of the treatment is desired. Most parenteral preparations come dissolved in sesame oil and the injection is best made intramuscularly into the upper part of the buttocks. Parenteral preparations are also available as aqueous suspensions of micro crystals. A number of long-acting esters of estrogens are also furnished in oily solutions for parenteral use. They present as their chief disadvantage the difficulty of coping with uterine bleeding which may occur during their sustained period of action.

The oral route is to be preferred. All the effects of estrogens can be conveniently achieved by this route providing one compensates for the loss of activity resulting from their inactivation in their passage through the liver. This loss varies with the nature of the estrogen. The choice of oral estrogen is dependent upon economic considerations. Synthetic estrogens, of which a large number are now available, are somewhat less costly, but they carry with them the disadvantage of producing unpleasant side reactions in many patients, particularly at full replacement dosage levels. These unpleasant symptoms include nausea, vomiting and drowsiness and, less commonly, vertigo and skin rashes. Permanent damage as a result of stilbestrol therapy has not been demonstrated. Derivatives of stilbestrol have been prepared with a view to diminishing its toxic effects. It is difficult to establish whether the reduced toxicity observed with some of these derivatives is actual or based on lower biologic activity per unit of weight. Ethinyl estradiol, a semi-synthetic estrogen, has the highest biologic activity per unit of weight. The toxic symptoms are the same as for stilbestrol but may occur less frequently.

All estrogenic preparations, particularly the synthetic estrogens, may produce hyperpigmentation of the nipples and areolae. This occurs commonly in the younger age group although it may be occasionally encountered in menopausal patients. The pigmentation will usually regress with continued therapy and always on discontinuing therapy.

The natural estrogens are devoid of toxicity whether given orally or parenterally. Most commonly used by the oral route are those consisting largely of the estrone sulfate. This latter preparation loses relatively little of its biologic activity by the oral route and is, hence, an economical form of natural estrogenic therapy.

Certain complications of prolonged estrogenic therapy should be recognized. If given continuously to a woman whose uterus is intact, bleeding may occur in the course of therapy or after its discontinuation as a result of a hyperplasia induced in the endometrium. This can be avoided or kept from being profuse and prolonged by several procedures. The estrogen may be administered cyclically with periodic interruptions to permit regression of the endometrium and withdrawal bleeding of a normal character and duration. When full replacement therapy is given, interruptions at monthly intervals are recommended. When continuous therapy is indicated, shedding of the endometrium can be achieved by the periodic administration of progesterone. This is likewise recommended at monthly intervals. When cyclic therapy is given, the following course should not be reinstituted until bleeding has ceased. This principle of giving treatment intermittently is more difficult to enforce with oral therapy; hence, only enough estrogen should be prescribed to give the intended course of treatment. More specific details of estrogenic regimens will be given in appropriate portions of this section.

The danger of the induction of cancer should not be overemphasized. The susceptibility of some animals to carcinogenesis by estrogens is not shared by monkeys in whom all attempts to produce cancer by estrogens have been unsuccessful. The reasons for these differences in susceptibility are not apparent. As regards the use of estrogens in women, it is perhaps relevant that the amounts employed are of the order of magnitude of those produced spontaneously throughout the reproductive period. It is a question therefore whether cancer in women is related to estrogenic activity or to some still unclarified derangement of steroidal hormone metabolism. Reports of carcinogenesis in the course of estrogenic treatment are so rare as to suggest that it occurs as a coincidence. The main concern in its use arises with respect to women with a family history of carcinoma.

Progesterone. There are two types of progesterone preparations, progesterone in oil for parenteral therapy and the orally active

therapy.
a day i
the orall
may be
therapeu
ally resu
course o
Funct
monly s
for consε
cedures
most cas
treatmen
the secti

Fluhmann
Diagnos
Saundeι
Shelton, E
Metabol
Mentall
Child. I
Shorr, E.:
Pediat.,
Shuttlewoι
Graphic
for Resε
Serial N
search C

I

If pub
considere
no organi
occasiona
ovary may
ual precο
genic effe
sexual deν
Rare case
nated ost
of peculiι
(Jaffe).
Theraμ
present.]
directed t
the patieι

Jaffe, H. L
Entity a

anhydrohydroxyprogesterone. No differences have been recognized in their action except for their relative effectiveness by weight. The orally active form is one tenth as active as progesterone in oil given parenterally. As with the orally active estrogens, anhydrohydroxyprogesterone is most efficiently given in two divided doses, on arising and at bedtime. Full replacement therapy with progesterone is usually achieved with doses of 10 mg. a day parenterally or its oral equivalent.

Androgens. When androgens are required they may be given intramuscularly as testosterone propionate in oil, as implanted pellets of free testosterone or orally in the form of methyltestosterone. Methyltestosterone is approximately one fourth as active by the oral route as is testosterone propionate given intramuscularly.

Gonadotrophic Hormone Preparations. The gonadotrophic preparations currently available have not proved therapeutically satisfactory. Chorionic gonadotrophic preparations have been used with some success in very large doses but with considerable doubt as to whether a normal stimulation of ovarian function was achieved. The highly purified pituitary gonadotrophic hormones such as crystalline FSH are of limited value as yet because of a rapid development of antihormones. This chapter in hormonal therapy has yet to be written.

A. C. CARTER
E. SHORR

PUBERTY IN THE FEMALE

Puberty is the change from childhood to maturity. The physiologic and psychosexual adjustments required during this process are difficult at best. The emotional disturbances occurring at this time are varied and often reawaken maladjustments which were present in early childhood. The problem is frequently complicated by the attitude of the parents, in particular the mother, who tends to reinforce the natural reluctance of the growing child to assume adult status.

To puberty in general is added the psychologic effect of the menarche itself, that is, of genital bleeding. To many girls this is alarming, particularly if unexpected. Often they think that the bleeding is the result of an injury.

Puberty is a gradual process which becomes complete only after the lapse of several years (Fluhmann). It is initiated by the pituitary gonadotrophic hormones. The first change is in the increase in the size of the follicles of the ovary, which leads to the secretions of estrogens at the age of 8 to 10, or three to five years before the menarche. At the age of 11 or 12 fat appears under the nipple and there is increased pigmentation of the nipples and areolae. Breast development continues, with estrogens stimulating duct and alveolar growth and progesterone lobular growth.

The changes in hair at puberty are marked: terminal hair replaces the vellus hair; pubic hair appears followed later by axillary hair; there is temporal regression of scalp hair. There is an increased bony growth with the appearance of a female carrying angle of the arms. The serum phosphorus and alkaline phosphatase fall at this time. The body musculature increases. Fat deposition increases about the abdomen, hips and mons veneris. The skin undergoes changes and with the appearance of the menarche acne is common, owing to increased follicular growth and increased secretions of the glands.

Further evidence of estrogenic activity is the menarche. Ovulations may or may not occur; anovulatory and irregular menstruation is common in the first few years after the menarche. Complete fertility and maturation may not be attained until the sixteenth to the nineteenth years. Thus the physiologic changes may require ten years. Psychosexual maturity comes last and may not be complete until the early twenties, even in well adjusted girls.

Anxiety of parents is usually aroused by absence of menstruation at the expected time, by failure to grow according to preconceived standards or by obesity. They usually attribute the last to endocrine disturbances. The probable age of onset of menstruation may be judged first from statistics and second from the age of menarche of the relatives. Statistically, a peak is observed at 13 years. The curve falls off rapidly in either direction. Five to 10 per cent of normal girls begin to menstruate between 11 and 12 years of age, but menarche before 10 or 11 years is outside the normal range. At the other end of the scale, more than 5 per cent of normal girls begin to menstruate at 15 to 16 years of age. Delay to 16, 17 or even 20 years is compatible with childbearing.

Anxiety concerning height is warranted if growth stops. Ordinarily this is not the case,

Ripley). The disease occurs most commonly in young single women, typically within half a dozen years after the onset of the menarche, and often preceded by evidence of ovarian insufficiency in the form of menstrual disturbances. Such persons lose appetite, or, more commonly, diet to reduce their weight for psychologic reasons. The dieting has a compulsive quality, as shown by the effect of attempts to increase the weight of the patient against her will. Such attempts are met by resentment, subterfuge or even attempted suicide. Compulsive behavior in other fields is also evident. Most of these patients have gastrointestinal symptoms, in the form of obstinate constipation leading to the inordinate use of cathartics, and often abdominal pain. On recovery of a normal degree of nutrition, menstruation is resumed, as a rule, but in many cases amenorrhea persists. Typical and extreme cases are unusual, but milder forms are fairly common.

At the other extreme, many women who are obese have ovarian insufficiency. It is all too customary to think of the glandular disturbance as primary and to ascribe it to the pituitary gland. More often, however, the obesity in itself has an adverse effect on ovarian function. Reduction in weight is difficult because the obesity often serves a psychologic purpose, but, when accomplished, the loss of fat is not infrequently accompanied by a resumption of menses. Conception following a long period of sterility is occasionally observed after weight reduction.

The amenorrheas are most readily classified according to the level of estrogen production and the presence or absence of cyclic changes. By means of the vaginal smears Shorr has distinguished four major types. The first of these is the *atrophic acyclic* type. This is characterized by the uniformly atrophic smear in which the predominance of deep cells indicates virtual absence of estrogenic hormone production. Most cases of primary amenorrhea exhibit this type of smear. They may excrete excessive amounts of pituitary gonadotrophins suggesting an associated developmental ovarian anomaly; in other cases the low level or virtual absence of urinary gonadotrophins indicates their pituitary origin. Other cases are associated with diseases such as diabetes mellitus or hypothyroidism which have arisen in childhood and have been inadequately treated. The atrophic acyclic smear also occurs in secondary amenorrhea and is generally indicative of a profound depression of pituitary gonadotrophic activity. It is usual with the syndrome of anorexia nervosa with amenorrhea. It is frequently present in amenorrhea secondary to arrhenoblastoma, virilizing tumors of the adrenal cortex and Cushing's syndrome, disturbances in which there is excessive elaboration of steroidal hormones capable of inhibiting pituitary gonadotrophic function. The prognosis for the initiation of normal spontaneous ovarian function in patients with this type of smear picture varies with the underlying condition. When congenital ovarian or pituitary defects are responsible, it is virtually hopeless. When due to poorly controlled juvenile diabetes mellitus or hypothyroidism, the amenorrhea will usually respond to the correction of these defects. In secondary amenorrhea this type of smear picture has a variable prognosis though, as a rule, the expectation of spontaneous resumption of menstruation is poor, except in the presence of arrhenoblastoma, adrenal tumor or hyperplasia, and worsens in proportion to the duration of amenorrhea. However, the prognosis, although not good, should be guarded.

The second type of amenorrhea, the *subfunctional acyclic* type, is characterized by a diminished level of estrogen secretion, with little day-to-day variations. This type of smear is characteristically seen in secondary amenorrhea. It indicates subnormal rather than absent ovarian function and presupposes some pituitary gonadotrophic activity, subnormal in amount and acyclic in character, provided no ovarian pathology exists. The prognosis for spontaneous resumption of menstruation is much better in secondary amenorrhea of this type than in those cases with atrophic acyclic smears.

In contrast with the preceding types, the third or *subfunctional cyclic* type presents a fluctuating type of vaginal smear picture with recurring episodes of cyclic ovarian activity resulting in varying degrees of cornification. These periods of cornification usually last from one to two weeks and are followed by rapid regression to smear types indicative of low estrogen production. These bursts of ovarian activity may occur at fairly regular intervals or may be widely spaced. In the regressive phase immediately following the peak of cornification, red blood cells are occasionally present in the vaginal secretions, a circumstance comparable to postovulatory bleeding. These episodes represent periods of anovulatory ovarian activity which are not prolonged or intense enough to produce endometrial changes sufficient to result in withdrawal bleeding. Cycles of this type are occasionally encountered in both the natural and surgical menopause, spontaneous symptomatic relief occurring during the phase of estrogenic activity. This type of amenorrhea is, with rare exceptions, related to the secondary group. It should, however, be suspected when there is significant development of secondary sexual characteristics in primary amenorrhea. The differentiation between primary amenorrhea due to ovarian or pituitary defects and that to delayed puberty can frequently be made by the recognition of subfunctional cyclic ovarian activity in the vaginal smear, since such activity often precedes the menarche by many months. The prognosis for spontaneous resumption of menstruation by patients exhibiting this type of smear picture is quite good, particularly if the cycles occur regularly.

The fourth or *hyperfunctional acyclic* type of amenorrhea is least common and related to the secondary amenorrheas. It is encountered almost exclusively in patients with a history of menorrhagia, and generally interrupts, for varying lengths of time, such bleeding episodes. The vaginal smear uniformly shows a significant degree of cornification with no luteal transitions throughout the period of amenorrhea. Eventually, this sustained estrogenic hormone production, presumably from a persistent functional follicle or series of follicles, is terminated by a bleeding episode from a hyperplastic endometrium. The significance of this type of amenorrhea lies in its inevitable production of endometrial hyperplasia and its consequences.

In addition to the hormonal assays and vaginal smears, much help can be gained in the evaluation of an amenorrhea by attention to the physical examination and notably the primary and secondary sexual characteristics. The development of the skeleton can be estimated by inspection of the carrying angle of the arms and the offset of the knees. The body contours, degree of breast development and distribution of body hair should be noted. The development of the external and internal genitalia should be observed and organic lesions sought for in the genital tract.

Amenorrhea associated with pronounced insufficiency of the thyroid gland with classic signs of myxedema requires no comment here. There is a group, however, in which the evidences of thyroid insufficiency are slight and atypical. They may have sparse hair, transparent appearance of the skin of the face and fullness of the tissues of the face and legs, muscular weakness and undue sensitivity to cold with or without depression of the basal metabolism.

Ovarian Insufficiency with Persistence of the Menstrual Cycle. This group comprises a great bulk of patients with ovarian insufficiency. They are characterized by disturbance of the menstrual function with alterations in the rhythm, duration or quantity of the menstrual flow. It is precisely in this group that it is most difficult to arrive at a diagnosis. The outward manifestations vary widely. The menses may become infrequent, scant, or of short duration, or the interval may be lengthened; the flow may also be excessive or prolonged. The diagnosis can often be established by serial vaginal smears, basal body temperatures or endometrial biopsies.

Treatment of Amenorrhea and Ovarian Insufficiency. Replacement therapy is only one aspect, although the most important initial step, in the treatment of ovarian insufficiency. It should be combined with treatment of disorders of nutrition, avitaminosis, constitutional disease and of disturbances of the other endocrine organs, especially the thyroid. Hygiene, psychotherapy, readjustment of habits, of living conditions and of emotional attitudes are of permanent value in the many cases in which there is a strong psychogenic component.

The pituitary and urinary gonadotrophic preparations now available are uncertain in their effects on ovarian function. For practical purposes treatment of amenorrhea is limited at present chiefly to replacement therapy with estrogens and progesterone.

The patient with primary amenorrhea is especially in need of treatment. Often she has a strong sense of inadequacy; naturally she fells incomplete as a woman. The status of a patient with inadequate physical and emotional equipment, in an adult world, is not enviable. *Replacement therapy with estrogens* should be given in full estrous doses, as judged by the vaginal smear, for fourteen to twenty-one days, so that withdrawal bleeding following the interruption of each treatment cycle will occur at approximately monthly intervals. When full replacement therapy is given, withdrawal bleeding will occur approximately five days after the last dose of estrogen. Progesterone may be added to the estrogenic regimen although there is little advantage to be gained save more regular withdrawal bleeding. Progesterone should be given during the last five days of estrogen therapy in amounts of 5 to 10 mg. or its orally active equivalent. The development of satisfactory secondary sexual characteristics as a result of this treatment can be expected to require several years, but once established, they persist. Thereafter, the continuation of this cyclic therapy is largely dependent on the attitude of the patient, who should also, in the course of the treatment, be gradually made aware of the purpose of the therapeutic regimen and its limitations with respect to spontaneous menstruation and childbearing. As a rule, spontaneous menstruation is not to be expected although, in rare instances, the ovaries may assume their own cyclic activity. Many patients will make excellent marital adjustments under these circumstances.

The treatment of amenorrhea occurring after puberty varies with the cause. In patients with anorexia nervosa, *psychotherapy* is effective in the milder cases, particularly those in which a situational factor is predominant. These patients benefit by the opportunity to talk out their personal problems. The more severe cases are the result of a prolonged and deep-seated neurosis, they are resistant to psychotherapy and improve, if at all, only after prolonged psychiatric care.

Women who stop menstruating when they become obese are best treated by reduction of weight. Amenorrhea in unsuspected thyroid insufficiency has also been referred to. The induction of bleeding is of value in many cases of secondary amenorrhea without obvious etiology and may be accomplished as described for primary amenorrhea. Not infrequently this is followed by spontaneous ovarian activity. In cases in which the vaginal smear shows some estrogenic activity, bleeding may frequently be induced by giving progesterone for a few days each month, just prior to the desired flow.

Secondary amenorrhea has also been treated by irradiation to the pituitary and ovaries or both (Israel). This method of therapy awaits further evaluation. A few cases of secondary amenorrhea with mild virilizing symptoms have been treated with cortisone. Further experience is needed in this group of patients.

Patients with mild ovarian insufficiency, as indicated by scant, irregular or infrequent menstruation, may be treated by replacement therapy when the symptoms warrant it. The demonstration of the insufficiency by the technique of the vaginal smears requires examinations over a long period. The treatment is complicated by the fact that, when the menstrual cycle is present, the use of the hormone, even in physiologic doses, may disturb it. Treatment with estrogens, progesterone, or both, in combination is best reserved for the postovulatory period and ending about two days before the expected onset of the next bleeding. In these cases of mild insufficiency, attention to psychogenic and dietary factors is particularly fruitful.

Amenorrhea due to secondary pituitary disease resulting from hormonal suppression such as the adrenogenital syndrome due to adrenal hyperplasia or tumor, Cushing's syndrome due to adrenal hyperplasia or tumor or arrhenoblastoma, may be treated in several ways. If a tumor is present and benign, surgical removal will lead to complete cure. When the adrenogenital syndrome is due to adrenal hyperplasia, the administration of cortisone, either intramuscularly or orally, is the treatment of choice (Wilkins et al.). The daily dosage of cortisone varies from 25 to 100 mg. orally or 25 to 100 mg. intramuscularly. Therapy can best be followed by the lowering of the 17-ketosteroid excretion and most conveniently by vaginal smears as well as by the clinical course of the patient.

A. C. Carter
E. Shorr

References

Israel, S. L.: The Empiric Usage of Low Dosage Irradiation in Amenorrhea. Am. J. Obst. & Gynec., 64:971, 1952.

Rahman, L., Richardson, H. B., and Ripley, H. S.: Anorexia Nervosa with Psychiatric Observations, Psychosom. Med., 1:335, 1939.

Richardson, H. B.: Simmonds' Disease and Anorexia Nervosa. Arch. Int. Med., 63:1, 1939.

Turner, H. H.: A Syndrome of Infantilism. Congenital Webbed Neck and Cubitus Valgus. Endocrinology, 23:566, 1938.

Wilkins, L.: Diagnosis and Treatment of Endocrine Disorders in Childhood and Adolescence. Springfield, Ill., Charles C Thomas, 1950.

————, and others: Treatment of Congenital Adrenal Hyperplasia with Cortisone. J. Clin. Endocrinol., 11:1, 1951.

THE STEIN-LEVINTHAL SYNDROME

This is a syndrome with a variable clinical picture including sterility, secondary amenorrhea or menstrual irregularities including menometrorrhagia, and is frequently associated with hirsutism, pain, acne and obesity. The ovaries characteristically are enlarged, have a thickened tunica albuginea and multiple cysts. The excretion of 17-ketosteroids and gonadotrophins is usually within normal limits. The diagnosis of bilaterally enlarged ovaries may be established by pelvic or rectal examination, culdoscopy, gynecography or pneumoroentgenography (Levinthal and Cohen).

Treatment. The treatment of choice is a plastic operation on the ovaries, either bilateral wedge resection or decapsulation of the ovaries (Stein et al. 1949).

A. C. CARTER
E. SHORR

References

Levinthal, M. L., and Cohen, M. R.: Bilateral Polycystic Ovaries, The Stein Syndrome. Am. J. Obst. & Gynec., 61:1034, 1951.

Stein, I. F., Cohen, M. R., and Elson, R.: Results of Bilateral Ovarian Wedge Resection in 47 Cases of Sterility. Am. J. Obst & Gynec., 58:267, 1949.

MENORRHAGIA

Functional uterine bleeding may be defined as that which occurs in excessive amounts or at unexpected times in the absence of organic disease. It is due to the dysfunction of one or more of the hormones, ovarian or pituitary, which are concerned in the ovarian cycle.

Much attention has been given to the histology of the endometrium in functional bleeding in order to determine whether the basis for the bleeding might reside in functional abnormalities in the endometrial pattern. Initial emphasis was placed on the association of such bleeding with hyperplasia of the endometrium resulting from the persistence of Graafian follicles which undergo atresia rather than corpus luteum transformation. In recent years this view has been superseded by the recognition that, although the majority of cases (23 to 68 per cent in reported studies) are associated with endometrial hyperplasia, functional bleeding may occur from all types of endometrial patterns (Hoffman). Of particular interest are the mixed endometrial pictures (33 per cent), designated by Traut and Kuder as irregular shedding or irregular ripening. In the former, the histologic picture of the glands and stroma indicates an abnormal type of regression; in the latter, an irregular development of the endometrium is evidenced by the presence of both secretory and proliferative types of endometrial glands.

By means of vaginal smears two major types of ovarian disturbance have been distinguished, both of which lead to functional bleeding (Shorr). The first is characterized by some degree of ovarian insufficiency, with recurrent menstrual bleeding. This type comprises most instances of bleeding in adolescents and during the menopause, but also occurs at any time between these phases. Such bleeding is thought to arise from an endometrium which fails to desquamate completely in successive cycles, and eventually becomes hyperplastic as a result of subnormal but long continued estrogenic stimulation.

The second type of menorrhagia, in contrast with the first, is characterized by excessive and sustained production of estrogen. Luteal activity is low or absent. This is the most common type of functional bleeding in the third or fourth decades. It may give rise to long periods of amenorrhea followed by excessive bleeding or else to periods of menorrhagia which are fairly regular. This type of bleeding suggests the persistence of one or more ovarian follicles or a succession of them, which failed to undergo luteal transformation.

Functional bleeding is common. At best it is a social and marital disability and at worst produces chronic anemia and, not infrequently, threatens life. The aims of treatment are to stop the acute bleeding episode, to restore a menstrual flow of normal quality and at normal intervals, and, if possible, to prevent operations on or irradiation of the pelvic organs and the distressing effects which often follow in their wake.

Treatment. The treatment recommended is based on the observations of Markee (1940) as to the sequence of endometrial events which occur during a normal menstrual cycle and lead to adequate desquamation of the endometrium previously built up by the ovarian hormones. His studies have shown that the denudation of the endometrium after a normal menstruation is dependent upon (1) an adequate mid-menstrual growth of the endometrium as a result of the action of estrogens and progesterone or estrogens alone, and (2) an abrupt regression of the endometrium resulting from a sharp decline in the production or supply of these ovarian hormones. In practice, the ovarian hormones are administered in such a way as to imitate the rhythm of the normal cycle with its rise in the hormonal level and the sudden drop which precedes menstruation. When the bleeding is of the first type mentioned which occurs with anovulatory cycles with low estrogen production, estrogens are given in amounts sufficient to build up the endometrium to the normal state of proliferation and then discontinued suddenly. Vaginal smears permit the ready estimation of the estrogenic dosage requirements. Somewhat more reliable effects with a close imitation of the normal cycle can be obtained if progesterone is given along with estrogen during the last five to seven days of the estrogenic regimen. Bleeding usually occurs about two days after the hormonal treatment is discontinued. The regimen should be resumed immediately after bleeding has stopped and interrupted two days before the next desired menstrual flow. In the second type characterized by high sustained estrogen production, only progesterone is required in its management. It is administered for a period of five to seven days, the last dose being given two days before the next desired menstrual flow. In both types of functional bleeding treatment may have to be continued for long periods of time and until a more normal type of spontaneous ovarian activity is resumed as shown by vaginal smears.

The dosage requirements for estrogens are those which achieve full replacement therapy as indicated by cornified vaginal smears. Progesterone may be given by injection or as its orally active form, anhydrohydroxyprogesterone. The usual progesterone dosage intramuscularly is 10 mg. daily for five to seven days at the times given above. When the orally active progesterone derivative is given, ten times the parenteral dose should be used.

An acute menorrhagic episode can usually be interrupted with somewhat higher doses of progesterone; 25 mg. intramuscularly daily is usually effective within four to five days. A flow of normal amount and duration will then generally occur two days after the last injection. Thereafter, the regimen as described above can be instituted for as long as required. Androgens have also been used to suppress severe functional bleeding; in sufficient doses they neutralize the peripheral effects of the ovarian hormones on the endometrium; and with prolonged administration they inhibit the gonadotrophic activity of pituitary. However, in the acute or chronic management of functional bleeding androgens are distinctly inferior to the procedures described above.

By definition the type of bleeding under discussion is that in which no gross lesions can be demonstrated. The presence of certain benign uterine lesions is not, however, a contraindication to hormonal therapy, since they may be unrelated to the functional bleeding. However, when an adequate trial of hormonal therapy fails it is usually because of the presence of an undetected organic cause for the menorrhagia. Since functional bleeding occurs in association with types of ovarian dysfunction that gives rise to menstrual irregularity or secondary amenorrhea, consideration should be given to the possible etiologic role of psychogenic factors, caloric undernutrition, avitaminosis and thyroid insufficiency. Such treatment has the advantage of being directed at the cause rather than the symptom.

A. C. CARTER
E. SHORR

References

Hoffman, J.: Female Endocrinology. Philadelphia, W. B. Saunders Company, 1944.
Traut, H. F., and Kuder, A.: Irregular Shedding and Irregular Ripening of the Endometrium. Surg., Gynec. & Obst., *61*:145, 1935.

PREMENSTRUAL TENSION

Premenstrual tension is the term applied to a variety of symptoms such as nervousness, irritability, depression, headache, nausea and tension which occur premenstrually and which usually subsides with or shortly after the onset of menstruation. There is no certain knowledge as to the manner in which these symptoms are related to the hormones involved in the ovarian cycle. Several theories have been advanced, such as exaggerated premenstrual increase in circulating estrogens and the effects of abnormal hormonal patterns on the retention of electrolytes and water, but none is substantiated by valid data. They have, however, served as the basis for a variety of therapeutic regimens. The authors' concept of premenstrual tension would place it in the same category as the menopausal syndrome, not only because of the similarity of symptomatology but because of its association with the waning phase of estrogen production during the menstrual cycle. We would accordingly consider the same predisposing factors as operative, namely, a psychologic and emotional maladjustment intensified by the temporary premenstrual reduction of estrogen in the organism.

Treatment. A wide variety of therapeutic regimens have been employed in the treatment of premenstrual tension with results difficult to evaluate. One type of therapy is aimed at the reduction of fluid retention by the restriction of sodium and water premenstrually, as well as by the addition of ammonium chloride and even of mercurial diuretics during this period. Progesterone and androgens have also been used during the second half of the cycle with claims of equal success. The type of therapy that has seemed most effective to the authors is the use of estrogens during the second half of the cycle, in amounts of approximately 2400 rat units daily. The estrogens are discontinued two days before the anticipated flow and resumed during the menstrual flow at a somewhat lower dosage level. This or any other temporary effective regimen should, however, not be used to the exclusion of the more fundamental psychotherapeutic approach.

A. C. CARTER
E. SHORR

DYSMENORRHEA

Primary, that is, functional or essential dysmenorrhea is the term applied to painful menstruation occurring in the absence of demonstrable organic pelvic disease. Although it is generally held that dysmenorrhea characteristically occurs in essentially normal ovulatory cycles (Novak and Reynolds; Wilson and Kurzrok), this is not invariably the case since it has been observed in women with proliferative, hyperplastic or atrophic endometrial patterns (Lackner et al.).

Because of its usual association with normal ovulatory cycles the possibility has been entertained that dysmenorrhea may result from abnormal uterine contractions which are dependent upon previous priming with both estrogen and progesterone. Studies of uterine motility in normal women have disclosed contraction patterns which are characteristic of the different phases of the menstrual cycle. The contraction waves during the follicular phase are frequent and of low amplitude; during the progestational phase there is a decrease in frequency but an increase in height and duration, a pattern that is also carried over into the early part of menstruation. Comparative studies of uterine motility during the menstrual phase of painless and dysmenorrheic cycles have yielded discrepant results which may stem from the techniques used. Woodbury and associates, using multiple small balloons and highly sensitive recording methods, found in dysmenorrheic women a variety of abnormal menstrual uterine contraction patterns, as well as intrauterine pressures often significantly elevated above normal and frequently above the arterial pressure, a circumstance which would interfere with uterine blood flow. These patients were also extremely sensitive to uterine distention at pressures which were tolerated without discomfort by patients with painless menstrual periods. Hence, the abnormal contractions in dysmenorrhea may be attributed to an increased uterine irritability due not only to the intrauterine pressure of menstrual debris but also to Pitressin-like and other hormonal factors involved in the menstrual cycle. However, no information is available as to the factors responsible for the increased uterine irritability in dysmenorrhea of which the abnormal uterine contractibility is the result. There is a growing tendency to regard dysmenorrhea as a psychosomatic problem and to emphasize the importance of psychotherapy in its management. This concept is not incompatible with the observed abnormalities in uterine contractions but would regard the heightened uterine irritability as secondary to psychic and emotional stress.

Treatment. A wide variety of therapeutic measures have been used in the treatment of dysmenorrhea. Analgesic drugs such as aspirin and codeine have been used with moderate success. Addiction to opiates should be avoided. The antispasmodic drugs have been used with little success. The more usual association of dysmenorrhea with ovulatory cycles has prompted the use of estrogens postmenstrually to prevent ovulation and to eliminate the effects of progesterone on uterine contractions during the subsequent menses. On the other hand, favorable results are also reported to follow the brief premenstrual administration of progesterone. Androgens have been used at all dosage levels and during all phases of the cycle, equally good results being claimed for all regimens. The success of such a wide variety of therapeutic measures, many with opposite physiologic actions, suggests that psychologic and emotional factors are prominent in the development and amelioration of this syndrome.

A. C. CARTER
E. SHORR

References

Lackner, J. E., Krohn, L., and Soskin, S.: The Etiology and Treatment of Primary Dysmenorrhea. Am. J. Obst. & Gynec., 34:248, 1937.

Novak, E., and Reynolds, S. R. M.: The Cause of Primary Dysmenorrhea with Special Reference to Hormonal Factors. J.A.M.A., 99:1466, 1932.

Sturgis, S. H., and Albright, F.: The Mechanism of Estrin Therapy in the Relief of Dysmenorrhea. Endocrinology, 26:68, 1940.

Wilson, L., and Kurzrok, R.: Studies on the Motility of the Human Uterus in Vivo. Endocrinology, 23:79, 1938.

Woodbury, R. A., Torpin, R., Child, G. P., Watson, H., and Jarboe, M.: Myometrial Physiology and its Relation to Pelvic Pain. J.A.M.A., 134:1081, 1947.

ENDOMETRIOSIS

Endometriosis is a condition in which tissue resembling endometrium occurs aberrantly, chiefly in the pelvic cavity. Although it may occur at any period during the menstrual life, it is most usual between the ages of 30 and 50. Although it may be asymptomatic in a large proportion of cases, endometriosis is frequently associated with menstrual disturbances, with infertility and with dysmenorrhea. The latter may be of all degrees of intensity and the pain is most commonly referred to the rectum and lower back. Dyspareunia and painful defecation are not uncommon. The pain is believed to be due to the increase in size of the implants of menstruation as well as to the pressure of retained menstrual blood in the cyst cavities. These may occasionally rupture with resultant peritoneal irritation. The masses are tender and painful to palpation. Diagnosis is occasionally difficult and may rest on history

and the presence of painful nodules, tenderness and thickening of the uterosacral ligaments.

Endometrial implants are most commonly found in the ovaries, uterine ligaments, cul-de-sac and the pelvic peritoneum covering the uterus, tubes, rectum, sigmoid and bladder. They not only resemble the uterine endometrium histologically but respond in like manner to ovarian hormone stimulation. Among the several current theories as to the genesis of these implants are tubal regurgitation of endometrial tissue, lymphatic dissemination of endometrial tissue and coelomic metaplasia. The last is favored although tubal regurgitation is regarded as an occasional mechanism.

Treatment. Treatment consists in the reduction of endometrial implants by hormonal measures, the surgical removal of the implants wherever possible, or more drastic surgical or roentgen castration for the purpose of removing the source of hormonal stimulation necessary for the survival of the implant. Hormonal regimens have been employed to produce atrophy of the ectopic endometrial tissue—androgens by the suppression of pituitary gonadotrophin secretory activity and by peripheral neutralization of the action of endogenous estrogens on the implant; and massive doses of estrogens for the purpose of producing exhaustion atrophy. The former regimen is more widely favored (Carter, Cohen and Shorr). Androgens are given in suppressive doses (25 mg. testosterone propionate intramuscularly or 100 mg. methyl-testosterone orally daily) for a period of four weeks starting mid-menstrually. This results in the early appearance of the next menstrual flow which is usually scant. The following period occurs approximately four weeks after androgen therapy is discontinued. Occasionally nonsuppressive doses of androgens over several months have been necessary to obtain a remission which may be permanent or last for several years. Should these measures fail then recourse can be made to surgery or irradiation as described above.

A. C. CARTER
E. SHORR

Reference

Carter, A. C., Cohen, E. J. and Shorr, E.: The Use of Androgens in Women. In Harris, R. S., and Thimann, K. V., Eds.: Vitamins and Hormones. Vol. 5. New York, Academic Press, 1947, p. 317.

THE MENOPAUSAL SYNDROME

The menopausal syndrome, whether due to the spontaneous aging of the ovary or induced by surgery or irradiation, is accompanied by at least two characteristic alterations in the hormonal environment, a profound reduction in estrogen production and a heightened excretion of urinary gonadotrophins. To this altered hormonal environment, a considerable percentage of women react by the development of a wide variety of symptoms which include vasomotor reactions, psychic and emotional instability and other functional disturbances; whereas the remainder make an uneventful or relatively asymptomatic adjustment to this episode (Shorr; Henry and Shorr). No measurable difference in the known hormonal changes of the menopause exists between the two groups. The opinion is widely held and would appear to be justified, that the psychologic and emotional status prior to the menopause is a major determinant in the subsequent adjustment to the new hormonal environment. The therapeutic effects of estrogens in ameliorating the menopausal syndrome is well established although some difference of opinion still exists as to the mechanism by which relief is achieved—whether by the restoration of a more adequate concentration of estrogens in the organism or the reduction to normal levels of the heightened gonadotrophin excretion. The weight of evidence favors the former concept. Symptomatic relief with estrogens may be experienced with little or no reduction in urinary gonadotropins (Heller et al.; Shorr, unpublished data). Furthermore, typical menopausal symptoms may occur with nonendocrine pituitary tumors in association with subnormal urinary gonadotrophin values as well as in young menopausal women in their twenties, in whom the amenorrhea is due to a depression of pituitary gonadotrophic function.

Symptoms. The most characteristic menopausal symptom is the hot flush. This consists in a sensation of warmth, starting somewhere in the trunk and spreading over the face, causing visible redness and often sweating. The latter is sometimes sufficient to require a change of clothing. The characteristic which differentiates the flushes from other vasomotor symptoms is the rapid onset and offset, usually within 5 minutes or less. These are repeated in severe cases many times a day. The flushes are often accompanied by dizziness, palpitation or exhaustion. Gastrointestinal symptoms and arthralgia are also observed. The next most common symptom is headache, which presents no unusual features. A frequent complaint is loss of well being often described by the patient as "not being herself." Nervous disturbances are extremely common, as illustrated by inability to cope with situations which formerly presented no special difficulty. Any preexisting emotional or psychic difficulty is accentuated, such as feeling of inadequacy, anxiety state or recurrent mild depressions. The women who have severe menopausal symptoms are for the most part those who have been maladjusted prior to the onset of the climacteric.

Treatment. The evaluation of therapeutic agents may be complicated by several circumstances. Occasional brief periods of spontaneous ovarian activity may occur which are associated with heightened excretion of estrogens, typical changes in the vaginal smear and spontaneous temporary symptomatic relief (Papanicolaou and Shorr). Of even greater significance is the frequency with which symptoms may be alleviated or aggravated by changes in the extent of stress to which the patient is exposed. It is thus important to consider such general measures as hygiene, psychotherapy, readjustments of habits, of living conditions and of emotional attitudes as being of permanent value in the many cases in which there is a strong psychogenic component. In a fair percentage of cases general measures plus mild sedation, phenobarbital 15 to 30 mg. three times a day, are sufficient to control the subjective symptoms.

The objective of hormonal treatment in the menopausal syndrome is to secure relief from the debilitating symptoms and to restore well being until such time as an adequate readjustment shall have taken place to the menopausal status. Androgens as well as estrogens are used for this purpose, the latter being preferable for reasons to be described. Estrogenic therapy should be given in amounts which achieve maximal well being, and subjective criteria are often adequate in themselves. However, symptoms due to ovarian insufficiency are often entangled with those of other origins, and the differentiation between the latter and those capable of relief by estrogens is often difficult. In these and other respects the vaginal smear can serve as a valuable adjunct to optimal management (Fig. 104). Once the full estrous smear has been obtained by adequate estrogen dosage, symptoms which still persist can be ascribed to causes other than ovarian insufficiency. Vaginal smears are also helpful in other ways; for example, they enable a physician to determine the degree of biologic replacement therapy requisite to produce symptomatic relief, information of some prognostic value with respect to the probable difficulty in the adjustment to be anticipated. They are also helpful in estimating how long uninterrupted treatment may be given without the induction of endometrial growth sufficient to lead to hyperplasia and bleeding. The higher the biologic effects, as evidenced by the vaginal smear, the shorter should be the period of uninterrupted therapy. Interruptions at three- to four-week intervals are recommended with the resumption of therapy not sooner than ten days afterwards, or until some symptoms recur. Advantage may be taken of this rest period to ascertain the rapidly and severity with which symptoms recur as a measure of the extent to which an adjustment is being made to the menopausal status. In severe

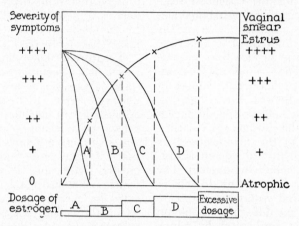

Fig. 104. A diagrammatic representation of the relation of the vaginal smear changes to the symptomatic effects of estrogens. A, B, C and D represent individual patients with different types of response. (Journal of the Mt. Sinai Hospital, Vol. 12.)

bleeding; the higher the degree of biologic replacement required for symptomatic relief, the shorter should be the duration of continuous treatment if bleeding is to be avoided. These evaluations cannot be made on the basis of dosage alone because of the wide individual differences in the biologic response to estrogens at any dosage level.

The general principles of treatment are as follows. Either parenteral or oral estrogen therapy may be employed; the latter is preferable. During the first course of treatment, enough hormone should be given to produce and sustain a follicular type of smear in order to obtain the maximal relief which estrogenic therapy can produce. This procedure also calls attention to those symptoms which cannot be modified or affected by hormonal therapy and for which other causes should be sought. Thereafter that dosage level should be selected which will produce the same optimal well being attained during the initial course. In those patients with an intact uterus, therapy should be given intermittently in order to avoid excessive endometrial

cases in which continuous therapy may be indicated, uterine bleeding must be anticipated as the price of comfort. In such cases, the bleeding can be kept within normal bounds by induced shedding of the endometrium through the administration of 50 to 100 mg. of anhydrohydroxyprogesterone orally or its parenteral equivalent for five consecutive days every four weeks. An indication for this regimen is the coexistence of menopausal osteoporosis for which continuous estrogenic therapy at high dosage levels is necessary to insure maximal lime salt storage. Even if the uterus has been removed, institution of occasional rest periods is recommended for the purposes cited above. The opinion is held by some that the adjustment to the menopausal status is hastened by the use of estrogens in amounts which ameliorate but do not abolish symptoms; this viewpoint is not supported by the authors' experience which has rather emphasized the advantages of well being as an aid to this readjustment.

Androgens may also be used for the management of the menopausal syndrome. They have the advantage of producing no endometrial proliferation and, hence, no bleeding. Androgens also have merit as a temporary measure after operations for endometriosis, and in young women with breast carcinoma and menopausal symptoms following castration. On the other hand, they have the disadvantage of inducing masculinizing phenomena when high doses are required for symptomatic relief as is often the case. Many women are also unable to tolerate the psychosexual effects of prolonged androgenic therapy. Although there are individual differences in this respect, these complications usually arise as a deterrent when 10 mg. or more of methyltestosterone is required daily for symptomatic relief. As with other uses of androgens, the orally active methyltestosterone is about one quarter as effective by weight as testosterone propionate in oil given intramuscularly.

Efforts have been made to develop a regimen based on the concurrent administration of both androgens and estrogens which would retain the merits of both hormonal agents without their disadvantages. These are based on the use of androgens and estrogens in a ratio which would neutralize the virilizing effects of androgens as well as the action of estrogens in inducing proliferation of the endometrium and subsequent bleeding. The results are only occasionally satisfactory when a fixed ratio of androgens to estrogens is used, since such fixed ratios fail to take into account the marked individual variations in the response to each of these hormonal agents. When combined therapy is attempted, it is necessary to adjust the dosage of each to the responsiveness of the individual patient.

A. C. CARTER
E. SHORR

References

Heller, C. G., Chandler, R. E., and Myers, G. B.: Effect of Small and Large Doses of Diethylstilbestrol upon Menopausal Symptoms, Vaginal Smear and Urinary Gonadotrophins in 23 Oophorectomized Women. J. Clin. Endocrinol., 4:109, 1944.

Henry, G. W., and Shorr, E.: Problems of Mental Adjustment at the Climacteric. Mental Health in Later Maturity. Pub. Health Rep., Suppl. No. 168, 125, 1941.

Papanicolaou, G. N., and Shorr, E.: The Action of Ovarian Follicular Hormone in the Menopause, as Indicated by Vaginal Smears. Am. J. Obst. & Gynec., 31:806, 1936.

Shorr, E.: The Menopause. Bull. New York Acad. Med,. 16:453, 1940.

Diseases of the Digestive System

DISEASES OF THE MOUTH, SALIVARY GLANDS AND PHARYNX

DISEASES OF THE MOUTH

Diseases of the oral cavity are not only numerous, but extremely varied. Many of them are pathologic entities arising primarily in the mouth, while others represent manifestations of some underlying systemic disorder. Because of the limitations of space it will be possible to discuss only the important features of the more common types of oral disease. Those rare lesions in the mouth which really are more of academic than of practical interest will be ignored.

In patients with oral conditions of uncertain diagnosis the importance of a general examination, including studies of blood and urine and a thoracic roentgenogram, cannot be overemphasized; frequently such an examination will reveal the nature of the pathologic changes in the mouth such as occur in cases of leukemia, anemia, tuberculosis, syphilis and other diseases. One cannot stress too strongly the value of securing a small specimen of tissue for microscopic study from any ulcer in the mouth which fails to heal in three or four weeks. Many of these ulcers are malignant neoplasms, and their early detection will greatly facilitate effective treatment.

DISEASES AFFECTING THE ENTIRE MOUTH

"Catarrhal" stomatitis refers to any generalized and simple form of inflammation affecting the oral mucosa. Although this inflammatory process usually is the result of poor oral hygiene or the excessive use of tobacco or alcohol, it may occur in debilitated persons and can be associated with measles, scarlet fever and other acute infectious diseases. The mucous membrane is red, and there is increased exudate from the mucous glands. Though the condition is not actually painful, it is uncomfortable and disagreeable to the patient. No particular form of treatment is necessary other than removal of the cause if possible; the condition subsides spontaneously. A mild alkaline mouthwash often is soothing. If the stomatitis is the result of poor oral hygiene, dental prophylaxis and education in proper care of the mouth are essential.

Aphthous stomatitis (canker sores, dyspeptic ulcers) is an oral condition characterized by the development of one or more vesicles, each of which ruptures and leaves a yellowish white, depressed, painful ulcer. These ulcers heal spontaneously within a few days unless they become secondarily infected. Aphthous ulcers occur singly or multiply. In many persons frequent periodic crops of these ulcers develop for months or years. There is no known cause for aphthous stomatitis, and there is no treatment which is of any value. The use of silver nitrate or any other caustic drug is to be condemned, for such agents cause necrosis in the bed of the ulcer, thereby producing an ulcer larger than that which was originally present. A mild alkaline mouthwash is soothing, and a solution of hydrogen peroxide diluted half with water is helpful in clearing up secondary infection. The patient should be told at the start that no treatment can effect a cure and that he must learn to live with the condition. He should not be given some form of mouthwash, diet or other form of therapy with the false hope that this will help to correct the disorder.

Ulceromembranous stomatitis (Vincent's angina, trench mouth) is an infectious and contagious disease affecting the oral and pharyngeal mucous membrane and particularly the gingival tissue. This disease produces characteristic ulcerations and is thought to be due to *Bacillus fusiformis* and *Borrelia vincentii*. These bacteria can be found in many normal mouths, particularly in pyorrhea pockets. Consequently a culture which is positive for these organisms does not necessarily indicate that the patient has ulceromembranous stomatitis. This diagnosis can be made only when there is clinical evidence of the disease.

The causative organisms can best be demonstrated by securing a small amount of the necrotic tissue in an ulcerated area and smearing this directly over a glass slide. *Bacillus fusiformis* and *Borrelia vincentii* stain easily and are not difficult to find.

The lesion produced by this disease usually is a very painful, superficial ulcer of irregular shape and covered with a whitish gray membrane that can easily be removed. These ulcerations are associated with much inflammatory induration of the surrounding tissues. On removal of the necrotic tissue the underlying bed will bleed easily. There is increased flow of saliva and a foul odor to the breath. Usually this condition is associated with a moderate amount of fever, which may rise very high in severe cases. Usually there is enlargement of the submaxillary lymph nodes. When the pharynx is involved, the patient may have difficulty in swallowing.

This condition must be differentiated from diphtheria. The diphtheritic membrane is more difficult to remove, and the constitutional symptoms are more severe than in ulceromembranous stomatitis. *Corynebacterium diphtheriae* is gram-positive, while the fusiform bacillus is gram-negative. This should be borne in mind when the smears are taken for microscopic examination of the etiologic organisms.

Ulceromembranous stomatitis can be easily confused with blood dyscrasias, particularly with acute and chronic lymphatic leukemia. As a matter of fact, the oral manifestations of these diseases often cannot be differentiated clinically. Consequently, even though Vincent's organisms are present, one should not make a diagnosis of trench mouth until a blood count has been made to rule out leukemia. The treatment of Vincent's infection formerly was a serious problem. However, penicillin now offers a rapid and effective means of curing the disease. Dental hygienic measures are essential to heal interproximal ulcerations (*pyorrhea pockets*) which, if allowed to persist, will cause occasional flare-ups of the disease.

Thrush (parasitic stomatitis) is a form of stomatitis due to the yeastlike fungus *Candida albicans,* which forms whitish, exudate-like patches on the mucous membrane of the mouth, tongue or pharynx. This condition occurs particularly in undernourished children and in persons who are debilitated from some chronic disease or some major surgical operation. On culture, the causative agent, *Candida albicans,* presents budding yeastlike growths and mycelial threads. This disease begins as small white spots which tend to coalesce and form large uneven patches on the surfaces of the oral mucous membrane. When the exudate-like membrane is wiped off with a cotton applicator, a bleeding excoriated surface is left. This condition usually is associated with a great deal of pain. The diagnosis is based on films made from the membrane and can be confirmed by culture.

In the treatment of thrush, one of the simplest forms of therapy is the use of a saturated solution of sodium bicarbonate as a mouth wash. Every hour the patient should take a mouthful of this solution and hold it for a few minutes before spitting it out. In young children the mouth should be swabbed out frequently with cotton applicators dipped in the alkaline solution. Unless the patient is in poor general condition, this form of treatment will cause prompt regression of the disease. For persistent areas of thrush which occur in debilitated subjects, it has been found that painting the patches with a 10 per cent solution of formalin often will cure the condition. The use of formalin in this manner is extremely painful and must be preceded by the application of a 10 per cent solution of cocaine hydrochloride to the oral mucous membrane.

Gangrenous stomatitis (noma, cancrum oris) is an uncommon disease which consists of a spreading form of gangrene which is usually due to a hemolytic streptococcus or to *Bacillus fusiformis* and *Borrelia vincentii.* This condition usually involves the cheeks, but may begin on the lips and invade the tissues of the palate and floor of the nose. It usually is associated with a high fever, rapid pulse and prostration; this is particularly true in children. However, in adults the disease may progress rapidly without causing any noticeable constitutional symptoms. Irradiation and penicillin or other antibiotics should be tried, but often seem to have little effect on this condition. One of the most effective forms of therapy consists in cleansing the involved area with a solution of one-half hydrogen peroxide and one-half Mercurochrome every 2 or 3 hours. Although this disease often is fatal in children, I have seen it brought under control in several adults merely by the use of hydrogen peroxide and Mercurochrome.

Infectious diseases produce oral manifestations too numerous to mention. The most common are Koplik's spots of measles, which are small whitish areas surrounded by a reddish areola, and the strawberry tongue (enlarged fungiform papillae) of scarlet fever. Small vesicles may occur in the mouth both in smallpox and in chickenpox.

Herpetic stomatitis is a form of herpes simplex similar to cold sores or fever blisters on the lips. In the mouth this form of stomatitis occurs usually on the palate and consists of a cluster of sharply defined vesicles which are located only on one side of the mouth and never cross the median line. Within a few hours they become ulcerated and painful. They heal spontaneously within a few days. There is no treatment of any value, although mild alkaline mouth washes may make the patient feel more comfortable.

Hypertrophic mucous glands of the palate frequently are noted under an upper denture which is not cleansed properly and more commonly in persons who use tobacco excessively. The glands appear as small inflamed elevations with a central pore (the duct). This condition does not require any treatment other than removal of the cause.

Erythema multiforme is a skin disease characterized by subacute papular or vesicular lesions symmetrically distributed and may be associated with lesions on the oral mucous membrane (Stevens-Johnson syndrome). In the mouth this condition is difficult to describe, but consists of bullous or vesicular lesions which change into superficial ulcerations; the lips become crusted. The constitutional symptoms are slight, and the disease is self-limited, lasting two to four weeks. It is likely to recur at about the same time each year. As far as the oral lesions are concerned, there is no treatment of specific value, but antibiotic therapy and simultaneous administration of an 11-oxysteroid may prove useful.

Pemphigus is a skin disease with oral manifestations consisting of bullous or bleb-like lesions which rupture and leave shallow painful ulcers. Such bullae occur spontaneously and at irregular intervals; usually they are about 5 mm. in diameter, but in many instances they can be easily overlooked. This disease usually is fatal, but there is at the present time some hopeful indication that certain antibiotics may prove beneficial. Cortisone and ACTH bring about dramatic improvement in pemphigus.

Fordyce's disease is a condition of the oral mucous membrane characterized by minute whitish or yellowish white granular areas, particularly on the buccal surfaces of the cheeks or on the lip. This condition is encountered in a great many mouths and is not pathologic. The granules merely are normal sebaceous glands. It is of no consequence and requires no treatment. Persons who are concerned over such areas in their mouths should be told that the condition is entirely normal.

Lichen planus is a skin disease with oral manifestations characterized by whitish areas on the tongue, lips or buccal surface of the cheek which must be distinguished from leukoplakia. Lichen planus never produces a uniform whitish patch as does leukoplakia, but consists of whitish threadlike lines, which tend to branch out or radiate away from a central point. At times, lichen planus of the oral mucous membrane undergoes superficial ulceration which is slightly painful. There is no treatment of any value for this condition. Local excision or destruction by electrocoagulation or the use of irradiation does not result in permanent cure. After such forms of therapy the lesions promptly recur. Lichen planus always should be distinguished from leukoplakia, and when the former condition is present, the patient should be reassured that it is of no consequence.

Leukoplakia is a thickening of the oral mucous membrane which occurs in some persons in response to any form of irritation, particularly tobacco. Leukoplakia is characterized by the appearance of whitish areas which cannot be dislodged from the mucous membrane. When superficial and thin, this condition requires no treatment; but when thickened and especially when papillary, malignant changes are likely to ensue. Consequently, thickened areas of leukoplakia should be removed, either by excision if practical or otherwise by electrocoagulation.

Traumatic ulcerations in the mouth are due to ill-fitting dentures or other prosthetic appliances, to the injudicious use of a tooth brush, to eating rough foods or to biting the cheek. These ulcers are simple inflammatory lesions which heal promptly with no treatment other than removal of the cause.

Syphilis in all its stages can affect the oral mucous membrane. Primary syphilitic lesions or chancres are not uncommon, and are characterized by painless ulcerations with an indurated base. These ulcerations develop within the course of a few days and are associated with enlarged cervical nodes, especially in the submaxillary regions. The sudden appearance of an ulcerated oral lesion associated with enlarged nodes in the neck should make one suspicious of syphilis, and scrapings from the lesion should be examined by the transillumination technique for *Treponema pallidum*. Secondary syphilis may cause whitish mucous patches on the oral mucous membrane and condylomas at the angles of the mouth. The tertiary stage of this disease may produce gummas, particularly of the tongue, and appear as punched-out looking ulcers that cannot be diagnosed with certainty until a biopsy is taken.

In syphilitic glossitis the mucous membrane becomes markedly atrophic; this process leads to the development of a thick form of leukoplakia, often with a crosshatched appearance. Leukoplakia developing on this basis is prone to become malignant, and the outlook in such cases is extremely poor. Syphilitic leukoplakia of the tongue should be removed by electrocoagulation early in the course of the disease.

Tuberculosis in the mouth may be primary or more commonly secondary to infected sputum from pulmonary tuberculosis. In either case the local lesions consist of sloughing superficial ulcerations, usually multiple, which are very painful. There is little evidence of inflammatory induration. The diagnosis may be suspected, but is not completely certain until a biopsy has been made. The use of streptomycin for primary tuberculosis of the mouth produces encouraging results and often is helpful in some secondary tuberculous ulcers in the mouth associated with pulmonary tuberculosis. However, in the latter circumstance the oral ulcers indicate a low degree of resistance to the disease, and consequently indicate a poor prognosis.

Actinomycosis is due to a yeast fungus producing a granulomatous lesion that can become secondarily infected with organisms which cause a purulent discharge. When the purulent material from an actinomycotic abscess is examined, the so-called sulfur bodies or *Actinomyces* are usually in evidence. The condition may occur as an acute phlegmon of the tongue, parotid region or neck and often follows a dental extraction. Actinomycosis may cause trismus, pain and swelling. The disease may be present as a hard inflammatory mass with multiple sinuses along the jaw or as a small nodule in the substance of the tongue. Purulent material from any abscess about the mouth or neck should be checked for *Actinomyces*. Actinomycosis can be successfully treated by large doses of penicillin, 1,500,000 units daily for three weeks, and after a rest period for two or three weeks the course can be repeated if necessary. In draining actinomycotic abscesses, drains should be left in place for several weeks. Potassium iodide, 10 drops three times a day and increased a drop every day, is extensively used, but its efficacy is questionable.

Blastomycosis is a chronic granulomatous disease due to a specific fungus which can affect the oral cavity. A typical lesion is a granular ulcerated growth which can be confused with a malignant process. Externally, such lesions contain small pustules. Tissue removed for microscopic examination will show a granuloma with marked epithelial hyperplasia; blastomycetes or budding fungi are usually in evidence or can be cultured. A solitary lesion in the mouth can be cured by electrocoagulation. However, the disease usually is systemic, often with pulmonary involvement. In these circumstances the prognosis generally is hopeless.

Histoplasmosis is a systemic infectious disease caused by the fungus *Histoplasma capsulatum*. In the mouth it produces a granulomatous ulcerated lesion which can be diagnosed with certainty only on microscopic examination. The oral lesion often is associated with cervical adenopathy and marked loss of weight. The disease is uniformly fatal.

DISEASES AFFECTING THE GUMS

Pyorrhea is an inflammatory condition of the gingival tissue and periodontal membrane. It results in resorption of bone of the alveolar process surrounding the roots of the teeth, and is associated with secondary infection. In many cases there is no apparent cause for the condition, while in some instances malocclusion and dental calculus are the causative factors.

Alveolar abscess is due to necrosis and infection of a dental pulp. The infectious process enters the pulp through an area of decay and results in an abscess, usually around the end of the root. As a result, there is external swelling and fluctuation of the overlying gingival tissue. In the lower jaw the abscess may present externally through the overlying skin. An alveolar abscess may be acute or chronic. It is surprising how frequently the possibility that a draining sinus in the maxillary area is due to a chronic dental abscess is forgotten.

Hypertrophic gingivitis or hypertrophied gingival tissue usually is the result of chronic irritation from mechanical causes such as ill-fitting dental appliances and of secondary infection. This condition is characterized by pedunculated or sessile enlargement of the gingival tissue. The enlargements are associated with much fibrous tissue and sclerosing periostitis, producing enlarged bony masses. The enlargements of the gum tissue are firm or hard; they are painless and bleed easily. This condition should be differentiated from chronic alveolar abscess with a draining sinus and from hypertrophy due to chronic lymphatic leukemia. In leukemia the gums usually are soft and bleed easily, and the histologic picture of blood smears is characteristic. Hypertrophic gingival tissue can be due to the long-continued use of Dilantin, which is employed as an anticonvulsant in epilepsy; meticulous mouth hygiene and massage of the gums tend to prevent some of this gingival thickening. Hypertrophic gingivitis is a dental problem, requiring the removal of the local irritant.

Bleeding gums are the result of engorgement and ulceration of the gingival tissue and are commonly due to pyorrhea. However, bleeding gums can accompany polycythemia, in which the oral mucous membrane may have an extremely red appearance. They can appear in Banti's and Gaucher's diseases, idiopathic aplastic anemia, purpura haemorrhagica and leukemia.

Scurvy is a dietary deficiency disease characterized orally by swollen and sore gingival tissue which bleeds easily. In advanced cases, hemorrhages beneath the oral mucous membrane are common.

Mercurial, bismuth and arsenical poisoning can produce oral manifestations, but are extremely uncommon today because of more effective methods of dealing with syphilis. Mercurial and arsenical poisoning can produce increased salivation, swollen gums which bleed easily, metallic taste in the mouth and in some cases ulceration of the gums. Bismuth can produce the so-called bismuth line, which is a bluish or black discoloration of the gingival margins of the gum tissue. The treatment of these conditions involves cessation of the use of such drugs. However, meticulous dental hygiene tends to prevent some of the severe stomatitis that can occur when such drugs are being used. BAL should be administered in severe cases.

DISEASES PECULIAR TO THE TONGUE

Geographic tongue is a condition peculiar to many normal tongues, and is character-ized by slightly elevated, irregular, gray rings surrounded by reddish areas on the dorsum, tip or sides of the tongue. This disorder comes and goes, and may make the tongue somewhat sensitive. It is of no consequence and does not require any treatment.

Scrotal tongue (beef tongue or fissured tongue) is not a pathologic but a normal condition in some persons. It is characterized by deep fissures and irregularities over the dorsum of the tongue, and should be no cause for concern.

Black tongue (lingua nigra) is a condition in which the papillae over the posterior portion of the dorsum of the tongue are greatly elongated and may appear black, brown or gray at times. The etiology is unknown. This condition should alarm neither the patient nor the physician. Although it cannot be eradicated, it does no harm.

Glossitis rhomboidea mediana is an inflammatory condition which covers a diamond-shaped area in front of the foramen caecum on the tongue. The etiology is unknown, and no treatment is required. It has been suggested in the literature that this disorder never becomes malignant. However, in this region of the tongue epitheliomas do occur which cannot be distinguished from glossitis rhomboidea. Consequently it is advisable in most cases to secure a small piece of tissue for microscopic examination.

Glossodynia or burning tongue is a functional disorder occurring in adults which produces a burning sensation that often is so severe as to keep the patient awake at night. A few such cases are due to pernicious anemia, in which there are atrophic changes in the mucous membrane of the tongue. Also the disorder occasionally can be due to arteriosclerosis in elderly persons. However, in the great majority of cases glossodynia is the result of a neurosis. In such cases the patient should not be given any form of medication, which not only is useless but also tends to keep him thinking about the condition. On the contrary, the neurotic basis for such a disorder should be discussed frankly with the patient; he should be taught to ignore the burning sensation, which often disappears after the patient no longer is concerned about it.

Moeller's glossitis consists of irregularly shaped red patches about the tip or margins of the tongue. These areas are sensitive and tend to produce a burning sensation. The etiology is unknown, and treatment is ineffectual. Moreover, this form of glossitis is of no consequence.

Macroglossia may refer to a congenital enlargement of the tongue, which in some instances protrudes from the mouth. Usually this condition is due to a lymphangioma that undergoes a gradual increase in size owing to repeated attacks of inflammation. The treatment of this condition is discussed in the section on Tumors of the Oral Cavity. Other causes of macroglossia are primary amyloidosis and acromegaly.

Pernicious anemia often produces pale atrophy of the mucous membrane over the tongue and is accompanied by a burning sensation as discussed under Glossodynia.

Sprue is a generalized disorder in which the tongue may be sore and red. The filiform papillae are enlarged, and in some cases small ulcerations are present.

Pellagra is a nutritional disorder often associated with redness and ulceration of the oral mucous membrane, while the tongue is somewhat swollen and bright red on the sides and tip.

TUMORS OF THE ORAL CAVITY

A wide variety of benign tumors occur in the oral cavity. Among the more common are submucous fibrous nodules which measure a few millimeters in diameter and which usually develop on the tongue or buccal surface of the cheeks. These nodules are due to trauma from biting the involved part. Simple excision is all that is necessary. Small papillary verrucous lesions are seen frequently on the tonsillar pillars. They consist of hyperplastic epithelium and can be removed by desiccation. Angiomas are not infrequently encountered in the mouth; in most instances they are better left alone. Epulis arising from the periodontal membrane is a common growth on the gingival tissue. There are four types: inflammatory, fibrous, angiomatous and the giant cell variety. An inflammatory epulis requires nothing more than removal of the growth. The other three types demand removal of the adjacent tooth in most instances if recurrences of the tumor are to be prevented.

Lymphangiomas of the tongue are rare, but produce marked deformity, the tongue being so large that it protrudes from the mouth. This type of tumor usually affects infants. Lymphangiomas should be scarred down by the insertion of radon seeds, and eventually can be partially excised to reduce the tongue to more normal proportions.

The *malignant tumors* which can affect the oral cavity are adenocarcinomas, melanoepitheliomas, hemangio-endotheliomas, plasmocytomas, rhabdomyomas and various sarcomas, such as small round cell sarcomas, fibrosarcomas, myxosarcomas, lymphosarcomas, chondrosarcomas and osteosarcomas. However, about 80 to 90 per cent of malignant neoplasms in the mouth are squamous cell epitheliomas. All these malignant tumors differ widely in their rate of growth and degree of activity. Usually they are graded on the basis of 1 to 4 according to Broders' classification, grade 1 being the least malignant and grade 4 the most malignant. Roughly, about 40 per cent of epitheliomas in the mouth are grade 1; 50 per cent are grade 2; 9 per cent are grade 3, and about 1 per cent are grade 4. Most epitheliomas of the mouth are rather inactive lesions which have a papillary or granular, ulcerated appearance. The less common high grade epitheliomas and sarcomas have a tendency to be much more vascular and friable than the low grade lesions and are subject to ulceration. In all these lesions, whether active or inactive, adjacent bone soon becomes invaded, as is evident on roentgenologic examination. Any solitary ulcerated lesion in the mouth which fails to heal in three or four weeks should be considered as possibly malignant until proved otherwise by microscopic examination. The low grade lesions, which are not particularly radiosensitive, are best treated surgically. Electrocoagulation in the form of surgical diathermy offers a simple method of treating the lesion and also the involved bone. Sequestra occurring as a result of this form of therapy can be removed with ease in two or three months. Highly active lesions in the mouth require irradiation therapy. In such cases, radon seeds or radium needles implanted throughout the growths are to be recommended in addition to external irradiation.

Grade 1 squamous cell epitheliomas in the mouth rarely if ever metastasize to the cervical nodes. Metastatic growths in the neck secondary to grade 4 lesions should be removed by block dissection of the nodes only when there is very limited involvement of the cervical nodes. Otherwise, for such grade 4 metastatic lesions, irradiation is usually preferable to surgical intervention. In general, cervical nodes involved by metastatic malignant growths from lesions that are grade 2 or 3 are best treated by block dissection of the cervical nodes. Many surgeons recommend a "prophylactic" dissection of the cervical nodes for most grade 2 or 3 epitheliomas in the mouth.

On the palate an adenocarcinoma should be distinguished from torus palatinus. The latter growth is not a tumor, but a congenital, osteoma-like overgrowth of bone in the median line. It requires removal only when it will interfere with the wearing of a full upper denture. Adenocarcinomas of the palate are not bony hard as is a torus. Usually, adenocarcinomas are well encapsulated, and in these circumstances they can be surgically enucleated without difficulty. When poorly encapsulated, they are better destroyed with surgical diathermy. In spite of any type of treatment, adenocarcinomas of cylindroma type are almost certain to recur, and then are best treated by the insertion of radon seeds.

JOHN B. ERICH

DISEASES OF THE SALIVARY GLANDS

Mumps (epidemic parotitis) is a communicable disease characterized by enlargement of the salivary glands in addition to other symptoms. This is probably the most common disease of the salivary glands. While the submaxillary and sublingual glands often are involved by the infectious process, the parotid glands are most frequently affected. Swelling of one gland followed by enlargement of another is usual. Sudden, painful, nonpurulent and unexplained enlargement of one or more salivary glands associated with leukopenia and increase in number of lymphocytes should be considered as mumps until proved otherwise. There is no treatment for involved salivary glands in mumps.

Acute inflammation of the salivary glands usually is due to a hemolytic streptococcal infection, which affects the parotid glands most frequently. The infectious process can reach the salivary glands through the ducts, through the blood stream or lymphatics, or by extension from adjacent structures. This condition is accompanied usually by a moderately high fever, rapid pulse, leukocytosis and more or less trismus. Pressure on the affected gland will usually induce a purulent discharge through the associated duct. Treatment consists in the use of antibiotics, usually penicillin. Therapeutic doses of irradiation sometimes are helpful if antibiotics fail. The duct of the involved gland never should be probed. If the infection is secondary to a calculus, the stone should not be removed until the acute process has subsided. External drainage is required only when an abscess forms and produces a subcutaneous area of fluctuation.

Chronic purulent inflammation of the salivary glands is likely to follow an acute infectious process and frequently is associated with calculi. The gland is enlarged, more or less tender and firm, and pus can be expressed from the duct. The chronic inflammatory process can become acute at irregular intervals. If it is due to a calculus, the stone should be removed. If the inflammatory process involves a sublingual or submaxillary gland, it generally is advisable to remove the gland surgically. When one of the parotid glands is involved, surgical extirpation of the gland is impracticable; instead, the use of therapeutic doses of roentgen rays or the preparation of a vaccine is to be recommended. An autogenous vaccine often will keep the condition under control, although "flare-ups" often arise when administration of the vaccine is discontinued. Antibiotics seem to be of no value in the treatment of chronic inflammatory conditions of the salivary glands.

Calculi in the salivary ducts are common. By obstructing the flow of saliva they tend to produce a somewhat painful swelling of the involved gland at mealtimes. A stone is extremely uncommon in the parotid duct, but is encountered not infrequently in the submaxillary duct. In the latter situation the stone usually can be palpated without difficulty. In any case the diagnosis is confirmed by evidence of the calculus on a roentgenogram of the affected area. It is well to mention that symptoms similar to those due to a calculus can be produced by inspissated mucus in the distal end of the duct. When calculi are present, the duct never should be probed. Stones in the submaxillary and parotid ducts should be removed through an incision in the mucous membrane parallel with the duct and over the stone. A calculus in the submaxillary gland or in the immediate proximal end of the duct seldom can be satisfactorily removed without considerable injury to the surrounding tissues. In these circumstances it is preferable to extirpate the entire submaxillary gland through an external incision rather than to attempt local removal of the calculus.

Tuberculosis is a rare condition of the salivary glands. It usually is secondary to tuberculous infection through the ducts or through the lymphatics from the tonsillar region. This condition cannot be diagnosed with any degree of certainty unless an abscess is present with a draining sinus from which infected material can be obtained for microscopic examination and culture. Often tuberculosis of the salivary glands is mistaken for a tumor or an inflammatory process of an overlying lymph node. The true nature of the condition is discovered on surgical exploration. In addition to drainage, the use of streptomycin has been effective in many cases.

Syphilis of the salivary glands is so rare that it need not be considered here. Its diagnosis can be suspected on the basis of positive blood serologic reactions and can be confirmed only on the basis of rapid response to antisyphilitic therapy. In most instances a definite diagnosis requires surgical exploration and biopsy of the mass.

Actinomycosis of the salivary glands is rather uncommon and is characterized by multiple abscesses and draining sinuses in the affected area. The diagnosis and treatment of this condition have been discussed under Diseases of the Mouth.

Mikulicz's disease is a rare condition involving the salivary and lacrimal glands. It is characterized by enlargement usually first of the lacrimal glands and subsequently of the submaxillary and parotid glands. Enlargement consists of a firm, painless swelling without systemic symptoms; the mass is not adherent to surrounding tissues. The etiology of this condition, which usually becomes progressively worse, is obscure. Tissue removed for microscopic examination may show a form of lymphoma. Mikulicz's disease must be differentiated from chronic lymphatic leukemia. Arsenic and potassium iodide are helpful in many cases of Mikulicz's disease, and roentgen therapy is an effective means of controlling the condition. Surgical excision of localized tumor-like enlargements, which do not encroach on the facial nerves, often will cure the disease. Doubtless some cases of *uveoparotid fever,* a form of sarcoidosis, have been designated Mikulicz's disease.

Ranula is a cystic enlargement of a portion of a sublingual salivary gland and appears as a soft, bluish, painless mass in the floor of the mouth. In general, a ranula is considered to be a retention cyst and can be removed most satisfactorily by destroying its lining with surgical diathermy. Many other surgical methods of treatment have been recommended for this condition, but they do not produce uniformly satisfactory results, and recurrences are common.

Ptyalism is characterized by excessive secretion of the salivary glands. It can be associated with any acute inflammatory condition of the mouth or may be entirely a neurosis, often accompanying hysteria. Treatment consists in removal of the cause if possible. When due to a neurosis, ptyalism cannot be effectively treated. Belladonna and atropine have been recommended for this condition, but these drugs should not be used indefinitely.

Xerostomia or dry mouth is a condition of obscure etiology characterized by decreased secretion of the salivary glands. No treatment which has been recommended is really effectual. This disorder sometimes is associated with dryness of the conjunctiva and other mucous surfaces (Sjögren's syndrome).

Benign and malignant tumors of the salivary glands are numerous, and the various types need not be considered here. Their diagnosis cannot be made with certainty except on microscopic examination after removal or biopsy. Most common and therefore perhaps the most important of the tumors which affect the salivary glands are the so-called mixed tumors. The majority of mixed tumors in the salivary glands are considered to be benign growths, although some pathologists consider them to be low grade adenocarcinomas. This is a controversial problem, through one finds that the majority of such tumors may recur locally but do not tend to metastasize to the cervical nodes. They begin as a small, movable, encapsulated nodule in the substance of the gland. Over a period of years they tend to grow and eventually become fixed. In the parotid area they can produce facial paralysis by encroachment on the facial nerve. Mixed tumors are most common in the parotid glands. If they are movable, they should be surgically enucleated, regardless of possible injury to the facial nerve. When they are fixed, surgical removal is not practicable, and the implantation of radon seeds throughout the mass is of great value in controlling the progress of the disease. It has been found that simple adenocarcinomas and those of mixed tumor type are not likely to recur if completely excised. However, adenocarcinomas of cylindroma type practically always recur in spite of radical surgical treatment. This is thought to be due to extensions of the tumor along the nerve sheaths far beyond the apparent limits of the growth. Recurring cylindromas should be treated by implantation of radon seeds rather than by attempts at surgical removal.

JOHN B. ERICH

DISEASES OF THE PHARYNX

The oropharynx, soft palate and fauces frequently are the site of traumatic injuries; this is true especially in children, who may fall on sharp objects held in their mouths. Lacerations so produced seldom require suturing, and the use of antibiotics will prevent subsequent infections in most cases.

Many diseases which involve the oral cavity also affect the pharynx. Particular reference here is made to thrush, Vincent's angina, blastomycosis, histoplasmosis, tuberculosis, syphilis, pemphigus, erythema multiforme, blood dyscrasias, leukoplakia and benign and malignant tumors. These conditions have been discussed under Diseases of the Mouth and need not be elaborated further here.

Acute pharyngitis also requires no detailed consideration here. It produces local and systemic symptoms much the same as those of acute tonsillitis. However, acute tonsillitis usually is the result of infection by hemolytic streptococci, pneumococci or other organisms sensitive to penicillin; in most instances the seriousness, duration and complications of acute tonsillitis are reduced to a minimum under penicillin therapy. On the other hand, acute pharyngitis frequently is due to influ-enzal or other penicillin-resistant bacteria; in these circumstances, sulfonamide drugs or Aureomycin will be found to be much more effective than penicillin. In all cases of acute pharyngitis it is well to give procaine penicillin empirically until a culture of the causative organism can be secured; if the inflammatory process then is found to be due to penicillin-resistant organisms, the antibiotic therapy can be changed accordingly.

Chronic pharyngitis usually occurs in adults and may be of three types: (1) hypertrophic with thickening and redness of the mucous membrane; (2) atrophic with thinning and atrophy of the pharyngeal mucosa; and (3) granular with hypertrophy of the lymph follicles. This disease produces sensations of fullness and soreness in the throat; often there is a feeling of dryness, or there may be an increase of thick mucus. Etiologically, the condition is due to excessive use of alcohol or tobacco, poor dental hygiene or postnasal drip from chronic inflammatory processes in the nose. The cure of chronic pharyngitis is difficult, but involves an attempt to remove the cause.

Neuroses of the pharynx are extremely common. The two most common functional complaints are burning and a sensation of fullness or of a lump in the throat (globus hystericus). After a thorough examination, if no lesion is present to explain such symptoms, one can be fairly certain that the disorder is psychogenic. Patients with such symptoms should not be given vitamins or other medication, which will in no way help the situation. On the contrary, the problem should be discussed frankly with them, and they should be taught to ignore such symptoms, which will soon disappear when the patient no longer is concerned or fearful of them.

JOHN B. ERICH

DISEASES OF THE ESOPHAGUS

The diagnosis of esophageal disease can ordinarily be made on the basis of excellent history alone. The demonstration of the exact nature and location of the esophageal disturbance must subsequently be determined by careful roentgenologic examination, with or without esophagoscopy and a study of biopsy material and cytologic preparations. Morbid conditions affecting the gullet are more apt to produce symptoms that are easily recognized and localized than those occurring in almost any other portion of the digestive tract. Clinical and experimental observations have shown that esophageal sensations are perceived at the level of stimulation or just above it. Furthermore, these sensations are usually felt under the sternum unless the stimulus is excessive, in which event they may extend laterally in a segmental distribution or go through directly to the back. At times esophageal pain may spread into one or both arms simulating angina, or it may radiate into the neck and postauricular area. In almost every instance, however, there is a recognized relationship between the development of symptoms and the ingestion of solid food or liquids. Symptoms of esophageal disease are fundamentally due to motor disturbances mediated by the autonomic nervous system. Undue stimulation caused by emotional disturbances may be quickly reflected by substernal distress arising solely from abnormal changes in smooth muscle tone or propulsive activity. Intraluminal overstimulation due to too rapid ingestion of food or to excessively hot or cold or bulky food may cause identical sensations. Experimentally they can be reproduced by cholinergic drugs, by balloon distention or by the local instillation of ice water or of inert solutions given at a rapid rate. The most sensitive or reactive portion of the gullet is that segment just above and including the cardiac sphincter, the latter being influenced in a striking degree by both sympathomimetic and parasympathomimetic impulses. It is supposed that propulsive movements and relaxation of the cardia are produced by normal vagal stimuli and that the latter is inhibited by sympathetic stimulation.

Sensory stimuli are normally carried seg-mentally over sympathetic fibers to the upper seven thoracic ganglia, and then through the dorsal roots to the spinal cord and higher centers. In all probability, other sensory pathways exist, inasmuch as cervicodorsal ganglionectomy does not abolish esophageal sensations, nor does cordotomy performed at the segment levels mentioned. The vagi almost certainly carry afferent sensory fibers.

Anatomically, the upper end of the esophagus is continuous with the pharynx. This fact is of clinical importance, inasmuch as normal pharyngeal activity (deglutition) depends upon the integrity of the glossopharyngeal nerves and therefore can be influenced by disease affecting these particular cranial pathways. A further important anatomic fact is that the lower portion of the gullet passes through the esophageal hiatus of the diaphragm and is in close relationship to the crura. Abnormal diaphragmatic activity may produce esophageal symptoms. Finally, it is to be remembered that adjacent mediastinal structures and thoracic organs, if diseased, can easily cause extraluminal irritation or compression, with resulting esophageal disturbances.

The nature of esophageal symptoms varies greatly. Difficulty in swallowing or a feeling of constriction at a certain point, beyond which ingested materials pass with difficulty, suggests actual obstruction. A sense of fullness or pressure experienced at or above a given level has a similar implication. Regurgitation of undigested food may occur, depending on the degree of constriction. In the presence of an esophageal pouch or diverticulum, food stasis may occur with eventual putrefaction, resulting in a foul odor to the breath or the regurgitation of putrid material. Intense substernal burning (heartburn) is essentially an esophageal symptom, usually secondary to spasm or very abnormal smooth muscle activity of the cardiac end of the organ. That it is largely independent of gastric secretory factors has been shown by several investigators and by the fact that it may occur in the presence of complete gastric achlorhydria. Actual pain of severe cramping quality may occur. It is nearly always due to intense local spasm with or without associated organic disease. As a rule, it is encountered along with focal ulceration or with some developmental abnormality that acts as a trigger point for the activation of increased motor activity. The pain and spasm may be transitory or may persist for hours. They are always initiated by the intake of food and may be sufficiently intense to require the use of morphine for relief.

Any striking degree of esophageal dilatation invariably implies long duration of the underlying obstructing condition. The greater the dilatation the less likelihood there is that pain will be present. Symptoms are usually limited to substernal sensations of fullness, an awareness of difficulty in getting ingesta past a certain point and regurgitation of undigested food. Because the gullet is the only pathway for ingested food, it follows that esophageal disease may be closely associated with nutritional problems of major importance.

Physical examination is chiefly of value in producing evidence of cervical or mediastinal pressure, tracheal displacement, metastatic nodes, neurologic abnormalities and general or specific nutritional deficiencies. It rarely provides direct evidence of esophageal disease. Specific diagnostic measures include radiographic studies of the thorax and the mediastinal structures, barium studies of the hypopharynx, esophagus and stomach, and esophagoscopy with tissue biopsy or smears for cytologic examination.

Esophageal disease may be conveniently classified as follows:

1. Disturbances of function (motor)
2. Developmental abnormalities
3. Neighborhood disease (extraluminal)
4. Inflammatory disease (intraluminal)
5. Degenerative (deficiency) disease
6. Neoplastic disease
7. Esophageal varices

Modern transthoracic surgery has made it possible to correct many previously intractable esophageal abnormalities or structural changes. A meticulous interpretation of symptoms is therefore a *sine qua non* of proper diagnosis and therapy.

DISTURBANCES OF MOTILITY

The most common manifestation of a motor disturbance is heartburn. It is frequently encountered in the early months of pregnancy and in hyperreactive individuals, particularly following too rapid ingestion of food or the taking of food when tense or fatigued. It is commonly associated with excessive smoking, owing conceivably to the sympathomimetic action of nicotine. It is relieved, in the absence of organic disease, by regulation of habits and by the use of antispasmodics or antacids. When it persists, consideration should be given to the existence of definite esophageal lesions or of disease of the stomach, duodenum or gallbladder.

Esophageal spasm may cause severe pain in the absence of organic disease. When encountered, it warrants careful study to rule out developmental abnormalities, which act as trigger points for abnormal motor disturbances, or the existence of an esophageal ulcer. In the absence of demonstrable organic lesions, treatment should be directed toward emotional control of the individual, dietary regulation, the avoidance of rapid eating, moderation in or prohibition of the use of tobacco and alcohol, the use of antispasmodics, including atropine, its derivatives and the slow-acting nitrites, before meals, and the administration of nitroglycerin and warm bicarbonate of soda solution immediately at the onset of pain.

Functional dysphagia and globus hystericus may occur in emotionally unstable patients of either sex. Fear of choking is often the most prominent symptom, with difficulty in swallowing either solid or liquid foods. Unless an esophagoscopic examination is carried out, these diagnoses are untenable and dangerous, inasmuch as serious organic lesions may be missed.

Difficulties in swallowing may be encountered as a result of focal neurologic disease, such as bulbar palsy due to any cause or tabes. Myasthenia gravis may also cause difficulty in swallowing as a result of fatigue of the pharyngeal muscles.

A quite different type of motor disturbance is that known as *achalasia of the cardia* (Hurst) or so-called *cardiospasm*. This disorder is usually encountered in young adults who are almost invariably overreactive neurotic individuals. In this condition there is the most striking dilatation of the esophagus due to the prolonged course of the disease. As the term implies, there is failure of relaxation of the lower segment of the esophagus just above the cardia, with resulting difficulty in the passage of food and secretions into the stomach. The fundamental cause is still not known. One theory is that there is degeneration or absence of the ganglion cells in Auerbach's plexus in the narrow segment; another hypothesis holds that vagal control of this segment is vestigial or inadequate. In any event, there appears to be a functional over-stimulation of the cardiac segment by sympathetic stimuli with resulting failure of normal relaxation. Dilatation above the cardia gradually appears, increasing with the months or years, and because of the stasis of food and secretions a local esophagitis develops, with initial swelling, congestion and subsequent fibrotic thickening and permanent constriction of the lumen. X-rays of the esophagus (Fig. 105) show varying degrees of dilatation and tortuosity, with a smooth, symmetrical, fusiform narrowing at the lower end. Esophagoscopy will characteristically show varying degrees of esophagitis in the lowest portion, occasionally with minute superficial erosions. *Early symptoms* are typically those of substernal fullness following hurried eating or the ingestion of bulky or very cold foods. Food seems to stick at a point about at the level of the xiphoid. Emotional tension aggravates the intensity and frequency of symptoms. Remissions are frequent. Subsequently dysphagia is more striking, and food is successfully ingested only by voluntary swallowing and straining. Regurgitation of food occurs if too much is taken, and eventually involuntary regurgitation at night may be experienced, with possible aspiration pneumonia. Because of difficulties of alimentation, severe malnutrition may result. Actual pain is usually not experienced. The diagnosis is usually evident, but the possibility of esophageal cancer must always be excluded. When actual persistent narrowing has taken place, esophagoscopy is indicated to rule out the presence of malignancy, and the taking of a biopsy from the stenotic area is frequently proper.

Treatment depends on the stage of the disease. In the early stages, dietary regulation is advisable, with avoidance of bulky, irritating or extremely cold foods and of alcohol. The proper handling of emotional difficulties is very important. At times the use of the nitrites before the intake of food is extremely helpful. In the later stages, careful bouginage by an experienced endoscopist is necessary to provide adequate dilatation of the fibrosed, constricted terminal esophagus. Successful dilatation may quite adequately control symptoms, although it may have to be performed at repeated intervals. Rarely attempts at mechanical dilatation are unsuccessful or

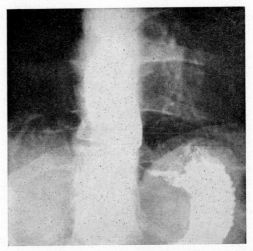

Fig. 105. Achalasia of the cardia.

dangerous, in which event esophagogastrostomy with resection of the stenosed area may have to be performed to permit adequate nutrition. Once dilated, the esophagus never returns to its original size.

CHESTER M. JONES

DEVELOPMENTAL ABNORMALITIES

Under this heading should be included congenital atresia of the esophagus with tracheoesophageal fistula, esophageal webs, diverticula, congenital short esophagus and paraesophageal hernia. The latter condition is included because many of the symptoms from such a hernia are essentially esophageal in origin. Previously hopeless, *atresia,* with or without a tracheobronchial fistula, can now be treated by skilled thoracic surgeons with some chance of success. Total regurgitation of food and an aspiration pneumonia in a newborn infant are the cardinal diagnostic points.

Esophageal webs represent redundant folds of mucous membrane capable of causing obstructive symptoms. Identification of the condition is made by esophagoscopy, and treatment consists in rupture of the web and subsequent bouginage.

Diverticula are of two types: pulsion diverticula and those due to external traction. The former are typically to be found at the pharyngo-esophageal junction (an area inadequately protected by the cricopharyngeal muscle layers) and at the point where the left bronchus crosses anterior to the esophagus and may cause pressure. Pouches also may occur as the result of local injury, as from a lye burn. Symptoms depend upon the size of the pouch, the amount of food stasis that occurs and, in the case of a large diverticulum, upon the fact that when full it may actually compress the adjacent segment of the gullet with consequent obstruction. Localization of symptoms is usually remarkably accurate. In the case of those diverticula at the pharyngo-esophageal junction, the full pouch may form a mass easily noted by the patient in the supraclavicular region. Small diverticula usually are symptomless, unless they act as trigger points in disturbing normal motility in overreactive individuals. Traction diverticula are lateral outpocketings as the result of an adjacent inflammatory cicatrizing process in the mediastinum. They are usually small in size and of little importance, except as noted above. Diagnosis of diverticula is easily made by roentgenography, and treatment, when necessary, can be successfully carried out by proper plastic surgery.

Congenital short esophagus is relatively uncommon. Symptoms are associated with the fact that the stomach is actually pulled up through the esophageal hiatus. Possibly as a result, there develops a gastritis in the herniated portion of the stomach and occasionally a peptic ulcer of the esophagus with more or less typical ulcer symptoms. This will be discussed later.

Paraesophageal hiatus hernia is a developmental defect due to a large esophageal hiatus. Symptoms when present are either epigastric distress, due to localized gastritis in the herniated portion of the stomach, or definite esophageal symptoms with substernal distress, dysphagia, regurgitation experienced in the horizontal position, and severe heartburn. Roentgen diagnosis is easy if the condition is suspected. Treatment includes intelligent psychotherapy, regulation of eating habits, antispasmodics and antacids. Intractable symptoms, including major bleeding, may occasionally require transthoracic surgical repair.

Chester M. Jones

NEIGHBORHOOD DISEASE

Neighborhood disease is obviously associated with mediastinal tumors, aneurysm of the aorta, metastatic disease causing enlargement of mediastinal glands, rarely extreme cardiac enlargement or pericardial effusion, and occasionally inflammatory disease of the diaphragmatic pleura which may cause esophageal compression or irritation. The cause of symptoms is usually apparent on radioscopic examination. Therapy should be directed toward the primary disease.

Chester M. Jones

INFLAMMATORY DISEASE

Inflammatory disease involving the esophagus usually is intraluminal. Perforation of the esophagus by instruments, ingested foreign bodies or caustics may result in an acute inflammatory process involving the interior and exterior of the tube. Such traumatic accidents, if not immediately fatal, may subsequently produce cicatricial strictures with varying degrees of obstruction. The acute reactions to trauma may include mediastinitis with fever, leukocytosis, and so forth. Treatment here consists in the careful feeding of bland foods, provided emergency surgery is not indicated, and the use of antibiotics. Residual strictures require the use of guided bougies and rarely resection of stenosed areas with anastomotic surgery.

Specific *granulomatous diseases,* such as syphilis and tuberculosis, rarely cause local ulceration, cicatrization and stenosis, with accompanying obstructive symptoms. *Scleroderma* may be the cause of multiple irregular constricting lesions in the esophagus. The diagnosis in each instance is made by recognition of other manifestations of the disease in question.

Peptic ulceration of the esophagus may occur. It is apt to appear in the congenital short esophagus, possibly because of the easy regurgitation of gastric juice that occurs in this condition. The ulcer is found near the cardia and produces symptoms of two types: one is characteristic of ulcer in general—pain after eating, relieved by food or antacid; the other is essentially esophageal and is due to the associated spasm, which may in itself cause severe, intractable pain and dysphagia. With recurrent attacks, stenosis of the esophagus typically develops, with frank obstruction. Diagnosis is made by radioscopic examination or by direct endoscopy. If routine measures employed in the treatment of peptic ulcer are not effective, the disease may progress until sufficient obstruction exists to warrant resection and esophagogastrostomy.

In general, it can be said that the condition is extraordinarily difficult to handle. Complications are those of peptic ulcer elsewhere.

Acute esophagitis not only may be associated with trauma from various causes but may accompany an acute infectious disease, such as diphtheria, smallpox, typhoid and thrush. It is, of course, a serious complication. *Chronic esophagitis* may be the commonest disease of the esophagus. In the majority of instances, it is directly related to other diseases of the digestive tract, especially to those in which vomiting or regurgitation of acid gastric secretions is of frequent occurrence. Thus many cases have been noted in association with hiatus hernia, esophageal ulcer, duodenal ulcer and, in recent years, with the operation of esophagogastroscopy. It eventually produces shortening and stricture at or near the esophagogastric junction, causing dysphagia and regurgitation, usually without nausea or real vomiting. Heartburn is common, and inability to belch is frequently noted. Diagnosis is by x-ray examination and esophagoscopy. Once the possibility of malignancy in the stricture is eliminated, successful therapy usually can be obtained by careful dilatation with a string-guided bougie. If dysphagia is unrelieved by this means, resection of the stricture and esophagogastrostomy are indicated.

CHESTER M. JONES

DEGENERATIVE DISEASE

Degenerative disease is associated with atrophic changes in the esophageal mucosa and is encountered in such deficiency states as *pellagra* and the so-called *Plummer-Vinson syndrome*. The substernal burning encountered in pellagra responds readily to niacin therapy; that of the latter may be helped by iron therapy.

CHESTER M. JONES

NEOPLASTIC DISEASE

Neoplastic disease of the esophagus is most frequently carcinoma. Other malignant or benign tumors occur, but are numerically of minor importance. The majority of esophageal cancers involve the lower and mid portions and are either squamous cell (esophageal) or adenocarcinomatous (gastric) in character. Symptoms are essentially those of an obstructing lesion. Early in the course of the disease substernal pain may be present, but, as a rule, difficulty in swallowing, loss of appetite and malnutrition are the characteristic symptoms, with later regurgitation, excessive thirst and constipation of marked degree. Bleeding, usually of a minor degree, may occur. An early diagnosis must depend

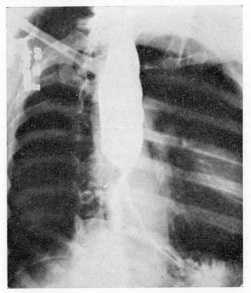

Fig. 106. Carcinoma of the esophagus.

upon an awareness of the significance of substernal distress in relation to the intake of food and anorexia. Roentgen ray studies, especially in older patients, are always warranted. It should be noted that in certain instances obstructive symptoms associated with an obvious esophageal constriction may have been present for a long time. Barium studies may show an irregular lesion or occasionally a symmetrical narrowing (Fig. 106). Esophagoscopy should be performed for the purpose of obtaining biopsy material from the stenosed area. The esophogoscopist should be prepared to dilate the constriction by means of a guided bougie in order to obtain an adequate biopsy from the center of the stricture.

Radical resection is dangerous, and cure is infrequent, especially in the later decades, but skilful surgery may produce palliation from the distressing dysphagia for two or more years in a reasonable number of patients. In inoperable cases, intensive radiation at times produces extraordinary temporary results, and complete relief of dysphagia can frequently be obtained by careful dilatation of the constricted area by guided bougies.

The other benign or malignant tumors of the esophagus are less common than carcinoma and involve the same diagnostic and therapeutic considerations.

CHESTER M. JONES

ESOPHAGEAL VARICES

Esophageal varices occur frequently, but are entirely asymptomatic until gross hemorrhage occurs. They result from any condition causing portal hypertension, either as the end result of chronic fibrosing diseases of the liver (cirrhosis) or of those conditions classified as congestive splenomegaly (so-called Banti's syndrome). In almost all such instances, careful x-ray studies reveal the varices. Aside from the immediate therapy of blood loss, treatment of the underlying condition includes a variety of procedures. Attempts to sclerose the dilated veins by intraesophageal injection are dangerous and at best palliative procedures. For intractable bleeding, transthoracic ligation of the varices may prove an immediate life-saving measure.

Elective shunt surgery (splenorenal anastomosis or portacaval shunt) may prove effective in lowering portal hypertension and thus in preventing future bleeding.

CHESTER M. JONES

References

Benedict, E. B., and Sweet, R. H.: Benign Stricture of the Esophagus. Gastroenterology, *11*:618, 1948.

Bockus, H. L.: Gastroenterology. Philadelphia, W. B. Saunders Company, 1944, Vol. 1, pp. 78–167.

Chamberlin, D. T.: Peptic Ulcer of the Esophagus. Am. J. Digest. Dis., *5*:725, 1939.

Harrington, S. W.: Pulsion Diverticulum of the Hypopharynx at the Pharyngo-Esophageal Junction. Surg., *18*:66, 1945.

Hurst, A. F., and Rake, G. W.: Achalasia of the Cardia (So-Called Cardiospasm). Quart. J. Med., *23*:491, 1930.

Jones, C. M.: Digestive Tract Pain. New York, Macmillan Company, 1938

Kampmeier, R. H., and Jones, E.: Esophageal Obstruction Due to Gummata of the Esophagus and Diaphragm. Am. J. M. Sc., *201*:539, 1941.

Linton, R. R.: The Surgical Treatment of Bleeding Esophageal Varices by Portal Systemic Venous Shunts. Ann. Int. Med., *31*:794, 1949.

Lockard, L. B.: Esophageal Tuberculosis. Laryngoscope, *23*:561, 1931.

Sweet, R. H.: Treatment of Carcinoma of the Esophagus. Surgery, *23*:952, 1948.

DISEASES OF THE STOMACH

Anatomic Variations. The shape and position of the stomach depend upon the constitutional type of the person, upon his adiposity, and upon the condition of his anterior abdominal musculature. In the relatively short, thick, sthenic person with tense abdominal wall, the stomach lies high in the left upper abdomen and is "steer horn" in shape, whereas in the long, lean, thin person, the greater curvature is likely to extend to the brim of the true pelvis in the shape of the letter "J." This condition is often called gastroptosis and a symptomatology erroneously ascribed to it. The important consideration is not *where* the stomach is, but *how* it functions. The vague digestive symptoms and disturbances often seen in these patients are not due to the location or position of the stomach.

CONGENITAL ANOMALIES

The three important congenital anomalies of the stomach are hypertrophic stenosis of the pylorus, diverticula and diaphragmatic herniation, including the so-called "thoracic stomach" with a short esophagus.

HYPERTROPHIC STENOSIS OF PYLORUS

Definition. Hypertrophic stenosis of the pylorus is an obstructive narrowing of the pylorus accompanied by, and apparently due to, hypertrophy of the pyloric muscle.

IN INFANTS

Hypertrophic stenosis is found most frequently in infants two or three weeks old, although it may occur at any time between the ages of ten days and three or four months. The condition is three or four times more common in males than in females. It is generally attributed to congenital hypertrophy with or without spasm. At operation or autopsy the pylorus is found to consist of an oval tumor of muscular tissue 2 to 3 cm. long and 1 to 2 cm. in width, hard, at times almost cartilaginous in consistency, and with no histologic evidence of inflammation. Patients are occasionally seen with the typical clinical syndrome, but operation reveals no

hypertrophy; the obstruction presumably is due, therefore, to spasm.

Symptoms and Diagnosis. The symptoms are projectile vomiting, constipation or obstipation, decreased urinary output and rapid loss of weight. Bile is rarely present in the gastric content. On physical examination the most characteristic feature is the demonstration of large peristaltic waves passing from left to right across a distended, globular stomach which fills the upper abdomen after eating. If the child is relaxed adequately, a tumor resembling a small peanut or marble may be palpated frequently, deep in the abdomen at the outer border of the right rectus muscle a few centimeters below or immediately under the costal border. The diagnosis of pyloric obstruction is confirmed by roentgenologic examination. When the factor of *spasm* predominates, a somewhat milder picture is seen. The vomiting tends to be explosive rather than projectile, the peristaltic waves are less marked, and a tumor is not palpated. The stools may be scanty, and soft rather than hard. These cases outnumber those of true hypertrophic stenosis of the pylorus by about 30:1 and usually respond well to medical treatment.

Treatment. In both types medical treatment should be tried first, provided the condition of the infant warrants it. Phenobarbital sodium, 0.125 grain, given immediately before each feeding, is effective, more so than atropine, but it may be combined with atropine, 0.001 grain. Atropine alone in large doses is undesirable because it may produce distention of the bowel, dryness of the nose and throat, and cerebral stimulation. The diet should consist preferably of breast milk or a prepared milk giving a fine curd. Thick cereal feedings may be used. The infant should be watched most carefully.

If a definite and favorable response is not secured within a few days, or if the symptoms grow worse, with dehydration and fever, operation should be performed at once. When a tumor is palpable, operation is, as a rule, required, and it may become necessary in cases in which a tumor is not palpable. The surgical procedure, known as the Rammstedt operation and consisting of a longitudinal incision through the pyloric muscle down to the mucosa, has a mortality rate in competent hands ranging from 2 to 6 per cent.

IN ADULTS

Hypertrophy of the pylorus is seen in adults with and without stenosis and with and without symptoms. The congenital origin of the hypertrophy has been questioned. It has been noted, however, that periodic attacks of nausea and vomiting are less frequent throughout childhood and later adult life in patients operated on in infancy for hypertrophic stenosis than in those treated medically. Cases of periodic nausea and vomiting have been described, beginning in childhood and continuing until old age, in which the pylorus is found to be markedly hypertrophied by the development of massive muscular bundles, apparently congenital in origin. On the other hand, in the adult, pyloric hypertrophy is often associated with some acquired gastric disease such as gastric ulcer or gastritis.

Symptoms and Diagnosis. The primary symptom is vomiting, with or without pain. The pain is usually due to an associated lesion such as gastric ulcer, for pyloric obstruction *per se* does not produce pain. The diagnosis of hypertrophic stenosis in the adult cannot or should not be made on clinical evidence alone. Roentgenologically, it may be evident from dilatation of the stomach, the abnormal width of the pylorus, and the crescentic indentation of the base of the bulb, although in some normal persons the pylorus is wide and a crescentic indentation may be made out in the base of the bulb. An important and difficult task is the differentiation of benign and malignant hypertrophy of the pylorus, the so-called *carcinoma fibrosum,* which usually begins in the pyloric end of the antrum. The history of such cases is usually of short duration, whereas in true hypertrophic stenosis it extends over many years. Roentgenologic evidence of neoplasm may be found in an infiltration of the antrum and an absence of the crescentic indentation of the bulb. In cases of pyloric hypertrophy associated with gastric ulcer, or of gastric ulcer associated with pyloric hypertrophy, the ulcer may produce little or no pain and be unsuspected until demonstrated roentgenologically or gastroscopically.

Treatment. Treatment depends upon the severity of the symptoms and upon the associated conditions present. If the stenosis is not marked, treatment may be unnecessary. If gastric ulcer is present, the usual ulcer management may be followed, unless the pyloric obstruction interferes. If there is any reasonable doubt as to the nature of the pyloric lesion, operation should be seriously considered. Exact differentiation is usually as difficult at the operating table as it is preoperatively, and hence as a rule in such questionable cases, if operation is undertaken, subtotal gastrectomy should be performed. In true hypertrophic stenosis, pyloroplasty or simple gastroenterostomy may be sufficient. Atropine is of no value in the differentiation of the various types of pyloric hypertrophy or in their therapy.

WALTER L. PALMER

References

Berk, E., and Dunlap, H. J.: Hypertrophic Pyloric Stenosis in Adults. Ann. Surg., *119*:124, 1944.
Vance, C. A.: Congenital Pyloric Stenosis. Ann. Surg., *119*:351, 1944.
Wakefield, H.: Hypertrophic Pyloric Stenosis in Adults. Gastroenterology, 2:250, 1944.

DIVERTICULA

Definition. A diverticulum is a pouch opening out from a tubular organ. True diverticula contain all the coats of the normal stomach and are either congenital or secondary to pulsion and traction; false diverticula lack the muscular coats and are attributed to weakening of the gastric wall from local disease, as in gastric ulcer.

Incidence and Location. True diverticula of the stomach are rather uncommon; false diverticula are rare. Both types are encountered, as a rule, accidentally in the course of a routine roentgenographic examination or at autopsy. They are seen most frequently roentgenologically in the region of the cardia, but any part of the stomach may be involved. Duodenal diverticula are more common than gastric. Congenital diverticula of the duodenum occur usually in the second and third portions, whereas acquired diverticula develop almost exclusively in the first portion. Practically all diverticula of the duodenal bulb are secondary to duodenal ulcer.

Symptoms. Gastric and duodenal diverticula rarely cause distress, although occasional cases have been described in which a marked inflammation was found about the duodenal diverticulum and relief of epigastric distress obtained by the removal or invagination of the diverticulum. The belching, discomfort or pain is usually to be attributed to the accompanying disease or to a functional disturbance independent of the diverticulum.

Treatment. Direct treatment of the diverticulum is rarely indicated. Concomitant diseases such as ulcer or carcinoma or concomitant functional disturbances should be treated appropriately. Relief from the distress is usually obtained without directing attention to the diverticulum. In rare cases, surgical treatment with excision or invagination of the diverticulum may be required.

DIAPHRAGMATIC HERNIA

Diaphragmatic hernia is discussed in the section on Diseases of the Diaphragm.

FOREIGN BODIES IN THE STOMACH

The foreign bodies most frequently swallowed are those taken accidentally by children, such as pennies and marbles, which in time pass through the stomach and intestine without harm. Sharp-pointed articles, such as needles, pins and especially open safety pins, are likely to penetrate the wall of the intestine and lead to peritonitis or abscess formation. In the insane the stomach may be found to contain a most varied assortment of nails, spoons, forks, knives and other objects which may remain for years without causing symptoms. Bezoars are conglomerations of swallowered foreign material such as hair and so forth. *Hair balls* are the most frequent and are found in women addicted to the habit of chewing the ends of their hair. *Gastroliths* have been reported from the long-continued use of calcium or magnesium powders. Spontaneous cholecystogastric fistula formation may lead to the extrusion of *gallstones* into the stomach.

Symptoms. Foreign bodies in the stomach rarely cause symptoms unless there is an associated ulcer or gastritis.

Treatment. Treatment is indicated only when definite distress is present or when the foreign body constitutes a real menace, as in the case of a needle or an open safety pin. The procedure indicated is usually surgical removal by means of laparotomy, for this is, on the whole, less dangerous, simpler and more effective than open-tube gastroscopy.

WALTER L. PALMER

Reference

Eusterman, G. B., and Balfour, D. C.: The Stomach and Duodenum. Philadelphia, W. B. Saunders Company, 1935, p. 259.

DISTURBANCES OF GASTRIC FUNCTION

SENSORY DISTURBANCES
HUNGER AND APPETITE

Hunger and appetite were interpreted by Beaumont and subsequent workers as sensations differing only in degree, but Cannon, and later Carlson, carefully differentiated the pleasant sensation of appetite, related to previous sensations of the smell and taste of food from the disagreeable and painful sensation of hunger, the essential factor of which, the epigastric hunger pang, was shown to be produced by contractions of the empty stomach. The average person in fasting does not distinguish sharply between hunger and appetite, for the accentuation of the appetite is interpreted merely as a portion of the total complex of hunger, which may be divided into the following components:

(A) Sensory:
1. Pleasant olfactory and gustatory sensations with their associated pleasant memories of the taste and smell of food, constituting appetite
2. Painful "hunger pangs" resulting from contractions of the empty stomach or intestines
3. An indefinite, unpleasant, generalized, steady and continuous sensation interpreted as hunger and vaguely referred to the abdomen
4. Accessory phenomena, such as lassitude, weakness, drowsiness, faintness, irritability, restlessness and headache

(B) Associative or Imaginative: The mind associates these various sensations with indefinite concepts of food or with definite images of specific foods.

The phenomenon of hunger is thus seen to be a complicated sensory and associative process, consisting in an accentuation of the pleasant sensation of appetite and the various unpleasant sensations of hunger, including the painful contractions of the empty stomach, and all associated with definite or indefinite concepts or imageries of food.

Excessive appetite and hunger occur in various conditions such as in convalescence from an acute infectious disease like typhoid fever. The digestive tract is then able to digest and absorb unusual amounts of food in order to restore rapidly the weight lost earlier. A similar condition may obtain in thyrotoxicosis, in which the requirement of food is maintained at a high level because of the excessive metabolism. In diabetes mellitus the glucose in the blood is not available to the tissues, and hunger and polyphagia result. In peptic ulcer the distress is often interpreted as hunger because the patient fails to differentiate it from a "hunger pang" or because it occurs when the stomach is thought to be empty and is relieved by foodtaking.

Bulimia, a term applied to an inordinate appetite and food intake, is a purely psychologic phenomenon. Continued excessive hunger and its resultant excessive ingestion of food lead eventually to obesity, except in diabetes mellitus or thyrotoxicosis.

Loss of appetite and of *hunger* is a variable but common symptom in disease of all kinds. When it appears suddenly in persons known to have been in good health, it is a highly important symptom that warrants a most thorough search for the cause. It is an early and prominent symptom in many cases of gastric or pancreatic neoplasm. Therapeutically, the primary indication is that of the underlying disease.

ANOREXIA NERVOSA

See section on Diseases of the Pituitary Gland.

SIMMONDS' DISEASE

See section on Diseases of the Pituitary Gland.

NERVOUS VOMITING

Nervous vomiting is, strictly speaking, neither a sensory nor a motor disturbance of the stomach, but it may be briefly considered here because it is a manifestation of a basic psychiatric problem similar to that of anorexia nervosa. It is in some respects more dramatic, but less subtle, than anorexia and more typically hysterical in nature, although the patent usually does not appear to be hysterical. The most characteristic feature is the continued, effortless vomiting of meals, usually immediately after eating, with no loss of weight. The patient complains bitterly, but looks well. Gastric and esophageal disease, particularly cardiospasm, should be excluded. The therapy is a psychiatric problem. Sedatives are valuable. Fluids should be administered parenterally for a few days until the acute phase has passed. The chronic forms of nervous vomiting may be very resistant to treatment.

WALTER L. PALMER

MOTOR DISTURBANCES

Gastric atony is not a clinical entity. The large sagging stomachs of gastroptosis may empty slowly, but they are not abnormal and do not give rise to symptoms. In pyloric obstruction the stomach is dilated but not atonic.

Hyperperistalsis and **hypertonicity** of the stomach are likewise not disease entities or the basis for symptoms. They are often found in tense, nervous persons, in patients with duodenal ulcer, gastric carcinoma, diabetes mellitus and other conditions, including complete achlorhydria.

Spasm of the entire stomach or of a segment of the stomach has been described in tabes dorsalis, in other lesions of the central nervous system, and also in the presence of extragastric abdominal conditions, such as cholelithiasis or pancreatic disease. The relationship of such spasm to abdominal pain is questionable, for the pain of tabetic gastric crises seems not to arise in the stomach itself, and segmented gastrospasm has been observed without pain. On the other hand, painful gastric spasm has been noted in the normal stomach. Localized muscular spasm is not infrequently seen with gastric lesions as in hour-glass contracture associated with benign ulcer, the contracture disappearing when the ulcer heals. Painless spasm of the pylorus, as evidenced by rather persistent closure, occurs frequently with intrapyloric peptic ulcer and also with gastric and duodenal lesions adjacent to the pylorus. Gastric ulcers several centimeters proximal to the pylorus on the lesser curvature are occasionally associated with a disturbance in the opening of the sphincter, presumably a reflex pylorospasm. Contractions of the pylorus and of the stomach are, on the whole, independent of the sensation of pain, but may be painful if sufficiently intense or if they occur in the region of an ulcer.

ACUTE DILATATION OF THE STOMACH

Definition. Acute dilatation of the stomach, or acute gastromesenteric ileus, is, as the name implies, a condition in which the stomach is extremely dilated, flabby, inactive, and contains 1500 to 4000 cc. of thin, slightly colored gastric and intestinal liquid content. The condition occurs chiefly as a postoperative or postpartum complication and is due to compression of the third portion of the duodenum between the spine and aorta posteriorly and the mesenteric root anteriorly. Gastric dilatation is in part secondary to the obstruction and in part induced by the depression in gastric tonus resulting from the general anesthesia. It is quite possible that the depression in gastric tonus precedes, rather than follows, the obstruction. Another important factor may be the maintenance of the dorsal position, for relief occasionally follows a change in position.

Symptoms. The symptoms are variable and apparently result from distention of the stomach, the loss of water and electrolytes, and toxemia of indefinite origin. The onset often is insidious, the symptoms not marked, and the severity of the condition not appreciated. Pain is often slight or absent. The more important symptoms are listlessness, apathy, lack of appetite, epigastric fullness, regurgitation, nausea and vomiting. The vomitus is usually dark brown, green or black, foul-smelling, and copious, consisting of large quantities of gastric biliary and pancreatic secretions. The abdomen is soft, distended, without visible peristaltic waves, and gives a succussion splash. The urine is scant. As the condition progresses, the signs of shock or collapse appear, a cold clammy skin, anxious facies, rapid pulse, low blood pressure, shallow, quick respirations, and delirium, followed by coma and death.

Treatment. Treatment consists in gastric lavage, the administration of large amounts of fluid parenterally, and frequent changes in position. In the modern hospital the routine postoperative use of the Wangensteen continuous suction apparatus has proved most effective. In some cases the suction must be continued for several days, but if the parenteral replacement of fluids is adequate, usually 2 to 4 liters per twenty-four hours, recovery occurs.

NORMAL AND ABNORMAL VARIATIONS IN GASTRIC SECRETION

Normal persons with essentially normal mucosa, gastroscopically, exhibit a wide variety of responses to histamine, ranging from complete achlorhydria with a pH of 8.7 to a highly acid juice with a hydrogen ion concentration of 0.1 (normal pH 1.0). These differing secretory rates are not to be correlated definitely with specific symptoms or diseases, except that chronic peptic ulcer does not occur in the continued absence of acid gastric juice, nor does pernicious anemia or combined column degeneration of the spinal cord occur in its presence.

There is a certain correlation between the number of parietal cells and the amount of acid secreted. Normal persons in the fasting state secrete an average of 660 mg. of hydrochloric acid per 12 hours, whereas patients with duodenal ulcer average 2240 mg.; patients with gastric ulcer average 450 mg.; and those with gastric cancer 245 mg. However, occasionally in normal persons and in patients with gastric ulcer or carcinoma the hypersecretion characteristic of duodenal ulcer is found.

ACHLORHYDRIA

Incidence. The complete absence of all gastric juice, *achylia gastrica,* is rarely seen, for some secretion containing ferments in small amounts is almost always present. The more exact terms achlorhydria and anacidity are preferable. Complete achlorhydria, as shown by the absence of acid in the gastric secretion even after the subcutaneous injection of histamine hydrochloride, so-called histamine-proved achlorhydria, occurs in approximately 10 per cent of all persons, in about 60 per cent of patients with gastric carcinoma, in nearly all cases of adenomatous polyps or gastric polyposis, and in all patients with pernicious anemia or combined cord degeneration.

Etiology. The anacidity is usually ascribed to atrophic gastritis, because such mucosal changes are found histologically in pernicious anemia. It has been observed, however, that in many cases of anacidity with gastric carcinoma the mucosa is not atrophic histologically, and no pathologic changes are evident to account for the achlorhydria. Similarly, in many cases of histamine-proved anacidity in apparently normal persons the mucosa as seen gastroscopically is essentially normal, or shows evidence of relatively slight or patchy inflammation. On the other hand, extensive atrophy of the gastric mucosa undoubtedly leads to a depression or suppression of gastric secretion, although surprising degrees of atrophy may be seen gastroscopically in stomachs found to secrete acid gastric juice.

Symptoms. Achlorhydria, *per se,* is not important clinically. It does not produce gastric symptoms. From the standpoint of digestion also it is not particularly important, for intestinal digestion almost completely compensates for the absence of gastric digestion. The stomach empties somewhat more rapidly in achlorhydria than it does when acid is present, but this process is not affected by the oral administration of acid. The term *gastrogenous diarrhea,* referring to diarrhea with achlorhydria, is not appropriate, for there is no satisfactory proof that the diarrhea is related to the achlorhydria. The functional diarrheas seen in patients with achlorhydria do not differ in their symptomatology or in their response to dietary management from those seen in persons with acid gastric secretion.

Treatment. The time-honored therapy is dilute hydrochloric acid given in doses of 1 to 4 cc. in a half to a whole glass of water before each meal. The results are often striking, but similar results may be obtained without the use of acid, suggesting that the real role of the acid is that of a psychotherapeutic agent. The amount of acid actually given is too small to alter materially the hydrogen ion concentration of the gastric or intestinal content.

Walter L. Palmer

References

Bloomfield, A. L., and Polland, W. S.: The Diagnostic Value of Studies of Gastric Secretion. J.A.M.A., 92:1508, 1929.

Cannon, W. B., and Washburn, A. L.: An Explanation of Hunger. Am. J. Physiol., 29:441, 1912.

Carlson, A. J.: The Control of Hunger in Health and Disease. Chicago, University of Chicago Press, 1919.

Kirsner, J. B., Nutter, P. B., and Palmer, W. L.: Studies of Anacidity: the Hydrogen-Ion Concentration of the Gastric Secretion, the Gastroscopic Appearance of the Gastric Mucosa, and the Presence of a Gastric Secretory Depressant in Patients with Anacidity. J. Clin. Investigation, 19:619, 1940.

Levin, E., Kirsner, J. B., and Palmer, W. L.: The Nocturnal Gastric Secretion in Patients with Gastric Carcinoma: A Comparison with Normal Individuals and Patients with Duodenal Ulcer and with Gastric Ulcer. Gastroenterology, 12:561, 1949.

Meyers, C. W.: A Study of Gastric Mucosa in Various Diseases Affecting the Upper Part of the Gastro-intestinal Tract. Gastroenterology, 10:923, 1948.

Wood, I. J., and others: The Relationship between the Secretions of the Gastric Mucosa and Its Morphology as Shown by Biopsy Specimens. Gastroenterology, 12:949, 1949.

NONSPECIFIC INFLAMMATION OF THE STOMACH

Definition. The term "gastritis" is usually applied only to acute or chronic nonspecific inflammations of the gastric mucous membrane, although, strictly speaking, specific lesions such as syphilis, tuberculosis and actinomycosis should be included.

Morbid Anatomy. Acute and chronic inflammation is the most frequent pathologic process of the stomach. Interstitial cellular infiltrations with collections of lymphocytes are almost invariably found in the wall of the stomach at autopsy. More marked alterations, such as hemorrhage in the superficial layers of the mucosa, erosion of the papillae, and infiltration of the submucosa, muscularis and serosa with lymphocytes, plasma cells and polymorphonuclear leukocytes, are frequently observed. Chronicity is evidenced by fibrous tissue proliferation in the gastric wall, atrophy of the mucosa, distortion or disappearance of the glandular structure, and transformation of the normal glandular epithelium, into the intestinal type with numerous goblet cells.

ACUTE GASTRITIS

Description. Acute gastritis was originally and beautifully described in 1833 by William Beaumont, who studied the mucosa of the stomach of his servant, Alexis St. Martin, through the fistula produced by a gunshot wound: "There are sometimes found, on the internal coat of the stomach, eruptions, or deep red pimples, not numerous, but distributed, here and there, upon the villous membrane, rising about the surface of the mucous coat. These are at first sharp pointed and red; but frequently become filled with white purulent matter. At other times, irregular, circumscribed, red patches, varying in size or extent, from half an inch to an inch and a half in circumference, are found on the internal coat. These appear to be the effect of congestion in the minute blood vessels of the stomach. There are, also, seen at times, small aphthous crusts, in connection with these red patches. Abrasions of the lining membrane, like the rolling up of the mucous coat into small shreds or strings, leaving the papillae bare, for an indefinite space, is not an uncommon appearance." These changes came often, lasted one day or more and disappeared.

Etiology. With regard to etiology, Beaumont states: "After excessive eating or drinking, chymification is retarded; and, although the appetite be not always impaired at first, the fluids become acrid and sharp, excoriating the edges of the aperture; and almost invariably produce aphthous patches, and the other indications of a diseased state of the internal membrane."

Symptoms. Beaumont's word again is authoritative: "These morbid changes and conditions are, however, seldom indicated by any ordinary symptoms, or particular sensations described or complained of, unless when in considerable excess, or when there have been corresponding symptoms of a general affection of the system. They could not, in fact, in most cases, have been anticipated from any external symptoms; and their existence was only ascertained by actual, ocular demonstration." These observations have been repeatedly confirmed.

Treatment. The treatment, as implied by Beaumont, is that of abstinence from dietary indiscretions, or perhaps indeed temporarily from all food. Healing of the lesions and a return to a normal mucosa invariably occur within a few days.

ALCOHOLIC GASTRITIS

So-called alcoholic gastritis is frequently diagnosed clinically on the basis of the clinical syndrome of nausea and vomiting after the ingestion of alcoholic beverages. After a drinking bout the vomiting may be so persistent that the patient is unable to retain food or drink of any kind for several days. The vomitus usually contains bile, considerable amounts of mucus, occasional flecks, streaks or even large amounts of blood. Hirsch, in a histologic study of the stomachs of 13 alcoholic addicts, 9 of whom had died of delirium tremens, found no evidence of an acute or chronic inflammation. Schindler and Gray, in a gastroscopic study of 100 such addicts, found the stomach to be normal in 55. The morning nausea is difficult to explain. It occurs as frequently when the stomach is normal as when it is diseased. The symptoms are more likely to appear if the first swallow taken is water than if it is alcohol. After two or three drinks of alcohol the nausea and vomiting usually disappear and do not recur until the following morning.

CHRONIC GASTRITIS

Pathologic features of chronic gastritis cannot be directly or precisely correlated with clinical syndromes. Indeed, the diagnosis of chronic gastritis should be made only on the basis of anatomic evidence obtained at autopsy or laparotomy, or by gastroscopy. The correlation between the pathologic and gastroscopic methods of study is fairly good. Gastroscopically, Schindler recognizes superficial, atrophic, and hypertrophic types of chronic gastritis.

SUPERFICIAL GASTRITIS

This condition is characterized gastroscopically by (1) reddening of the mucous membrane, (2) edema and (3) exudation. The mucosa is friable, small purpuric spots are common, and small erosions are not infrequent. The terms "hemorrhagic," "erosive," or "ulcerative" may be used to describe the various features present. The symptomatology, if any, of chronic superficial gastritis is still debatable, for no one has succeeded in establishing a definite gastric syndrome. The condition is not infrequently seen gastroscopically in patients without gastric symptoms. The etiology is unknown, and no treatment is indicated.

ATROPHIC GASTRITIS

Description. The characteristic gastroscopic features are (1) the gray or greenish-gray color, due to the thinning of the mucosa, in sharp contrast to the orange-red color of the normal stomach; and (2) the presence of branching blood vessels seen through the thin mucosa. The atrophy is usually rather localized and patchy in distribution but the entire mucosa may be involved.

Relation to Other Diseases. In pernicious anemia, during the phase of relapse, the entire mucosa is invariably atrophic, but marked improvement occurs after treatment with liver extract. The propriety of ascribing the atrophy of the gastric mucosa in this disease to "gastritis" is still debatable. In certain cases of iron-deficiency anemia the gastric mucosa is also atrophic and improves markedly in appearance after suitable therapy. Schindler considers that atrophic gastritis is usually the end result of a continued superficial gastritis. There is a great deal of evidence that atrophic gastritis may be the precursor of pernicious anemia, gastric polyposis and gastric carcinoma (see Fig. 107). An atrophic gastric mucosa is present in all cases of pernicious anemia, in a high percentage of those with gastric cancer and also in a rather high percentage of normal persons of comparable age groups. Konjetzny has presented histologic evidence of the transition from atrophic gastritis to benign and malignant epithelial neoplasia.

Symptoms. The symptoms, if any, are indefinite, although anorexia, heartburn and various "dyspepsias" have been described.

Treatment. There is no acceptable evidence that treatment is of value except in those cases associated with pernicious or iron-deficiency anemia. Hydrochloric acid may be given, but it is of psychotherapeutic value only. The possibility of carcinomatous metaplasia may be used as an argument for therapy in atrophic gastritis, but this is scarcely permissible until more is known with regard to the actual occurrence and incidence of such neoplasia and also the real value of any proposed therapeutic procedure.

HYPERTROPHIC GASTRITIS

Description. This condition is characterized gastroscopically by a velvety, slightly swollen, dull, loose, spongelike appearance of the mucosa, usually with the formation of granular nodules and larger nodes, as may be indicated by the commonly used adjectives "granular," "nodular," "verrucose" and "hemorrhagic." At times the polypoid nodes may be difficult to differentiate from true polyps and neoplastic infiltrations. Erosions and small ulcerations are frequent and usually multiple. The cause of hypertrophic gastritis is unknown.

Symptoms. There is evidence, both clinical and histologic, that the erosive and ulcerative forms of gastritis, particularly in the hypertrophic type, may cause symptoms consisting not only of epigastric distress identical with that seen in peptic ulcer, but also massive gastric hemorrhage.

Treatment. In such cases the distress disappears after the administration of a bland diet or the institution of a therapeutic program such as that used in peptic ulcer, a more or less conventional Sippy program, but the gastroscopic evidence of hypertrophic gastritis usually persists. Symptomatic relief, however, is all that is required, for it is not necessary to insist on disappearance of the lesion, as is the case in peptic ulcer. After intensive radiation therapy directed at the stomach, hypertrophic gastritis disappears and rarely recurs, but the condition is almost

never severe enough in itself to justify such treatment.

GASTRITIS OF THE POSTOPERATIVE STOMACH

This is not a separate type of gastritis, but it deserves special mention because of its severity and because it consists of a combination of the superficial and hypertrophic forms, with marked erosive and hemorrhagic features. In some cases the indefinite symptoms of epigastric distress and discomfort seem definitely attributable to the severe gastritis present. There is no specific therapy; hence the treatment must be symptomatic. When definite erosions and ulcers are present, the therapeutic problem is that of recurrent ulcer.

GASTRITIS SIMULATING CARCINOMA

Occasional cases of gastritis with giant enlargement of the rugal folds simulate neoplasm both roentgenologically and gastroscopically. In some, the polypoid or pseudopolypoid changes in the mucosa may be interpreted as precarcinomatous proliferations, as "gastritis not yet carcinomatous." The difficulty in excluding malignancy frequently leads to unnecessary resection.

WALTER L. PALMER

References

Beaumont, W.: Experiments and Observations on the Gastric Juice and the Physiology of Digestion. Plattsburgh, F. P. Allen, 1833.

Findley, J. W., Jr., Kirsner, J. B., Palmer, W. L., and Pullman, T. N.: Chronic Gastritis. Am. J. Med., 7:198, 1949.

Guiss, L. W., and Stewart, F. W.: Chronic Atrophic Gastritis and Cancer of the Stomach. Arch. Surg., 46:823, 1943.

Maimon, S. N., and Palmer, W. L.: Giant Hypertrophic Gastritis. Gastroenterology, 8:397, 1947.

Schindler, R.: Gastroscopy. The Endoscopic Study of Gastric Pathology. Chicago, University of Chicago Press, Revised 1949.

———, and Gray, S. J.: The Gastric Mucosa of Chronic Alcohol Addicts. J.A.M.A., 117:1005, 1941.

Warren, S., and Meissner, W. A.: Chronic Gastritis and Carcinoma of the Stomach. Gastroenterology, 3:251, 1944.

SPECIFIC INFLAMMATION OF THE STOMACH

CORROSIVE GASTRITIS

This type of inflammation follows the ingestion of corrosives, particularly acids, taken accidentally or with suicidal intent. Perforation of the stomach and death may ensue, or spontaneous recovery may occur. Pyloric stenosis may result either from the acute inflammation or from the connective tissue proliferation and require surgical relief.

PHLEGMONOUS GASTRITIS

This is an acute, infectious, usually pyogenic, inflammation of the stomach involving chiefly the submucosa. It occurs as a rare complication of septicemia or other infectious processes, as a rare surgical complication following operations on the stomach or other intra-abdominal organs, as a complication of peptic ulcer or, more frequently, of gastric carcinoma. Focal abscesses of the mucosa and submucosa are not infrequently seen in the gastritis associated with gastric carcinoma, but true phlegmonous gastritis is rare. The symptoms consist of the sudden appearance of acute epigastric pain and fever, often preceded by a chill, with vomiting, prostration, a rapid, weak pulse and rapid exitus. The diagnosis is rarely made ante mortem. The value of chemotherapy in this disease has not yet been established.

SCIRRHOUS OR SCLEROSING GASTRITIS

Leather-bottle stomach or *linitis plastica* is customarily considered to be of two types: benign and malignant. Gastric syphilis may produce a diffuse fibrosis of the stomach. The existence of any other benign type is debatable. The malignant type, due to scirrhous carcinoma, is rather common. The tumor cells may be extremely difficult to demonstrate histologically. The outstanding symptoms are moderate epigastric distress, inability to eat more than a small meal, regurgitation, belching and loss of weight (see Fig. 111). The course may be chronic.

GASTRIC SYPHILIS

Incidence. Syphilis of the stomach is relatively rare, but it occurs in all age groups and in both sexes, although it is more frequent in males.

Morbid Anatomy. As in all tertiary lues, the characteristic pathologic lesion is the gumma. Four different types are seen: (1) the solitary ulcerated gumma; (2) multiple ulcerated gummas forming a nodular serpiginous syphilid; (3) diffuse nodular nonulcerated infiltration; (4) chronic fibrosis. The first type simulates benign gastric ulcer in appearance, whereas the other three simulate carcinoma. Histologically, perivascular round cell infiltration, gummas, obliterating endar-

teritis and phlebitis, and, with the appropriate technique *Treponema pallidum,* may be demonstrated.

Symptoms. The symptoms are variable, but epigastric pain or discomfort is the outstanding feature. The distress may simulate peptic ulcer, but more often it suggests carcinoma in that it comes on immediately after eating and is accompanied by a marked loss of weight. A mass may rarely be palpable, but massive hemorrhage and acute perforation almost never occur. Achlorhydria is present in about 85 per cent of the cases; gastric retention is noted in about a fourth.

Diagnosis. The positive diagnosis of gastric syphilis is difficult. The Wassermann test is almost always positive in the blood or spinal fluid or both. Occult blood is not found in the stools. Roentgenologically, the lesion rarely consists of a penetrating niche, but usually suggests an infiltrative tumor. The most frequent location is prepyloric; the defect, concentric, symmetrical and relatively smooth. In some cases the middle of the stomach is involved in a dumbbell-shaped deformity, the central constriction being, as a rule, long and tubular, but occasionally forming a narrow hourglass. In a small percentage of the cases the stomach is diffusely involved. The gastroscopic picture is highly characteristic, although scarcely pathognomonic.

The problem of differential diagnosis arises almost exclusively in patients with a history or definite clinical evidence of lues, including a positive serology. Benign peptic ulcer and carcinoma are encountered in such patients much more frequently than is luetic involvement of the stomach.

Treatment. A syphilitic gastric lesion should respond rapidly to antiluetic therapy. If it does not, and if occult blood is present in the stool, carcinoma is almost invariably present. The diet is relatively unimportant. The pyloric stenosis may be sufficient to warrant gastro-enterostomy.

TUBERCULOSIS OF THE STOMACH

This process is usually demonstrated at autopsy as an accidental finding in patients dying from pulmonary tuberculosis. Clagett and Walters, however, found reports in the literature of 368 cases of clinically significant tuberculous gastric lesions of four pathologic types: (1) the ulcerating type; (2) the hypertrophic infiltrating type; (3) acute miliary dissemination; (4) extragastric lesions involving the stomach. In at least 80 per cent of the cases the ulcerating type is the one found. For some strange and unknown reason about 10 per cent of the tuberculous lesions are associated with gastric carcinoma. Clinically, it is not possible to differentiate tuberculosis of the stomach from benign ulcer, carcinoma or syphilis. As yet the gastroscopic differentiation of tuberculous ulcers has not been made, perhaps because of their rarity. A positive diagnosis is established only by the demonstration of tubercle bacilli in the lesions. Treatment is surgical, resection of the involved portion being the operation of choice.

LYMPHOGRANULOMATOSIS

Hodgkin's disease may begin in the lymphoid tissue of the stomach and simulate carcinoma clinically, roentgenologically and gastroscopically. The diagnosis is usually made by the histologic examination of the resected specimen or of an excised lymph node.

RARE INFECTIONS OF THE STOMACH

Actinomycosis and other fungus infections, *nonspecific granulomatous ulcers, diphtheritic lesions* and *agranulocytic ulcers* of the stomach are rare lesions seen at autopsy almost exclusively; hence they scarcely deserve clinical mention.

WALTER L. PALMER

References

Bearse, C., and Pollack, L. H.: Mycotic Infection of Stomach. Ann. Surg., 104:167, 1936.
Clagett, O. T., and Walters, W.: Tuberculosis of the Stomach. Arch. Surg., 37:505, 1938.
Eusterman, G. B., in Portis, S. A.: Diseases of the Digestive System. 3rd ed. Philadelphia, Lea & Febiger, 1953.
Konjetzny, G. E., in Henke-Lubarsch's Handbuch der speziellen pathologischen Anatomie. Berlin, Julius Springer, 1928, Vol. 4, p. 769.
Patterson, C. O., and Rouse, M. O.: Description of Gastroscopic Appearance of Luetic Gastric Lesions in Late Acquired Syphilis. Gastroenterology, 10:474, 1948.
Williams, C., and Kimmelstiel, P.: Syphilis of the Stomach. J.A.M.A., 115:478, 1940.

GASTRIC NEOPLASMS

MESENCHYMAL TUMORS

Definition. Pathologically, gastric neoplasms may be divided into those of mesenchymal and those of epithelial origin, but their clinical differentiation is difficult. The mesenchymal tumors consist of fibromas, myomas, fibromyomas, leiomyomas, myofibromas, hemangiomas, lipomas, angiomas, dermoid cysts and the malignant sarcomas, including the lymphoblastomas.

Symptoms. Symptoms appear only when the tumor ulcerates, bleeds, obstructs the outlet of the stomach or becomes so large as to be noticeable to the patient as an abdominal mass. The clinical picture is not characteristic. There may be no symptoms. Epigastric distress, if present, is usually not severe; it may be induced by the taking of food, relieved by food, or bear no relationship to food taking. The symptoms and signs of anemia are often present.

Diagnosis. Mesenchymal neoplasms occur in all age groups, but the finding of a gastric tumor in a patient in the first or second decade of life would be suggestive. The roentgenologic demonstration of a circumscribed, apparently intramural, nonulcerated mass would conform with the diagnosis of a relatively benign mesenchymal tumor such as a myoma or fibroma. Gastroscopically, such a diagnosis is indicated by the presence of intact mucosa overlying a smooth mass. When ulceration is present, the differentiation is more difficult, if not impossible. The roentgenologic and gastroscopic demonstration of marked mucosal infiltration with swollen distorted folds is suggestive of lymphoblastoma, but a similar picture may be produced by infiltrative carcinoma or hypertrophic gastritis. The gastric analysis is not significant, nor is the presence or absence of occult blood in the stool important except as it betokens the presence of a bleeding lesion.

Treatment. The treatment indicated in all cases is removal of the tumor. In the infiltrative sarcomas and blastomas, resection is often not feasible, but a biopsy either of the tumor itself or of a metastatic lymph node, perhaps a cervical node, is valuable. Lymphoblastomas and malignant mesenchymal tumors in general tend to be radiosensitive; hence surprising results may be obtained with radiation therapy.

EPITHELIAL TUMORS
BENIGN MUCOSAL NEOPLASMS

Definition. Benign epithelial or mucosal neoplasms include adenomas, papillomas and adenomatous polyps of various kinds. The distinction between benign and malignant new growths is of course a relative one, for most benign tumors are potentially malignant. The relationship of these lesions to atrophic gastritis, pernicious anemia and carcinoma will be discussed further in the article on Carcinoma (see descriptive legend of Fig. 108).

Symptoms. Pain is, as a rule, absent or slight, and present only if the polyp prolapses into or through the pylorus or is sufficiently large to be caught and pulled by gastric peristalsis. The usual symptoms are those of anemia, resulting from continued bleeding.

lengthening of the life span. Gastric cancer is almost unknown in the first decade of life, rare in the second, uncommon in the third decade and common indeed thereafter, from the age of 35 on. It occurs among all races of mankind in all parts of the world. It is unrelated to occupation, position in life, social status, contact with other patients or trauma. Heredity may be important, for families are not infrequently encountered in

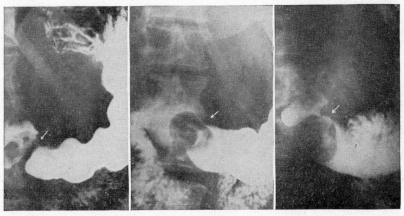

Fig. 107. Pedunculated gastric polyp in various phases of prolapse through the pylorus. The patient, a woman 44 years of age, had had indefinite abdominal distress intermittently for several years with occasional attacks of vomiting. There was no anemia.

Diagnosis. The syndrome of pernicious anemia may be simulated even to the extent of a high color index with definite macrocytosis. Achlorhydria is almost invariably present. The diagnosis is made by the roentgenologic or gastroscopic demonstration of a polyp (Fig. 107). Pernicious anemia and gastric polyposis may coexist. On the other hand, the chronic bleeding may rarely produce a blood picture simulating primary anemia, or the blood loss may modify the hematologic picture of pernicious anemia.

Treatment. Treatment consists in surgical removal. The polyp may be excised and the base cauterized, or a subtotal gastrectomy may be performed. The advantage of the latter procedure is that it protects the patient against carcinomatous change in the mucosa adjacent to the polyp. The prognosis is excellent.

CARCINOMA

Incidence. Cancer of the stomach kills more people than cancer of any other part of the body and, therefore, ranks high among the common causes of death. The incidence is increasing, apparently because of the rapid

which the incidence of carcinoma in the stomach or other organs is extremely high. On the other hand, gastric cancer is not infrequently observed in persons with no *known* history of cancer in the family.

Etiology. The cause of carcinoma is still unknown, but the gradually accumulating evidence seems to show that cancer is not congenital, that it does not develop from embryonal "rests," that it is not directly inherited, although a predisposition to it may be inherited, that it is an acquired disease, and that it is neither infectious nor contagious. Filterable viruses and various chemical carcinogenic agents are under active investigation as potential causes of carcinoma. Trauma is of etiologic importance only as far as it relates to the sequelae of corrosion of the mucosa, as in acid or alkali poisoning, or to the effect of the carcinogenic chemical agents. Gastric ulcer is generally considered to be a precursor of carcinoma, but the evidence is inconclusive. This problem is discussed in detail in the chapter on Peptic Ulcer.

Konjetzny and numerous other investigators contend that gastric carcinoma never develops in a normal mucosa and that it results from chronic atrophic gastritis with hyperplasia. The essential process is not the chronic inflammation, but the regenerative changes

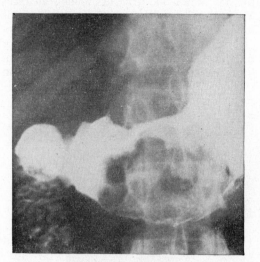

Fig. 108. Polypoid intraluminal gastric carcinoma. The patient, a man 58 years of age, had pernicious anemia in April, 1926, was operated on in November, 1926, because of a pedunculated polyp 6 by 4 by 3.5 cm. Sections of the polyp disclosed adenocarcinoma, but no tumor cells were found in the pedicle. In the spring of 1934 x-ray disclosed the polypoid intraluminal mass shown above. A subtotal gastrectomy was performed. Histologically, the tumor was found to be an alveolar colloid carcinoma. The need for persistent parenteral liver therapy continued, but in all other essential respects the patient remained in excellent health until May, 1943, when x-ray disclosed a recurrent polypoid growth in the fundus of the stomach. The patient continued his work as a general practitioner of medicine until moderate symptoms of esophageal obstruction appeared in January, 1946. Laparotomy disclosed a localized but inoperable carcinoma. Death occurred March 31, at the age of 78. Autopsy disclosed a recurrent adenocarcinoma of the stomach involving the adjacent tissues by direct extension, but with few metastases.

in the epithelium resulting from the chronic gastritis. In Konjetzny's extensive experience gastric carcinoma is always associated with such changes. The transitional stages from chronic atrophic gastritis with small areas of hyperplasia to papilloma and carcinoma have been clearly shown. There is abundant evidence to prove that carcinoma does not begin with a single cell, but that many cells throughout an area of variable size may undergo malignant neoplasia. Striking illustrations of these facts are seen in cases of multiple polyposis and frank multicentric carci-

noma. Chronic atrophic gastritis seems to bear a fundamental relationship to gastric polyposis and carcinoma and also to pernicious anemia. Rigler and his associates found the incidence of carcinoma in patients with pernicious anemia to be three times that of a control group. Varying views on the role of atrophic gastritis have been expressed by Warren and Meissner, Stout and others.

Special mention should be made of the experimental production of gastric adenocarcinoma in mice by the injection of methylcholanthrene by Stewart and Lorenz.

Morbid Anatomy. Carcinoma may develop in any part of the stomach, although fortunately for therapy the majority occur in or involve primarily the distal half or third. There are many types of gastric carcinoma, but for practical purposes the old classification of Borrmann and other pathologists is helpful. Four *macroscopic types* may be distinguished as follows:

1. The polypoid, mushroom, sharply circumscribed growth developing chiefly into the lumen of the stomach (see Fig. 108).

2. The ulcerated, circumscribed, dishlike tumor with clearly defined borders (see Fig. 109).

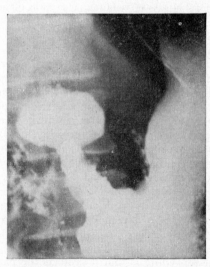

Fig. 109. Carcinoma of the antrum. The tumor was an ulcerated but sharply demarcated (type II Borrmann) alveolar carcinoma. At operation no metastases were found, and a subtotal gastrectomy was performed. Death occurred six and a half years after resection.

3. The ulcerated carcinoma with a definite wall or a sharp border on one side only, not sharply circumscribed, and infiltrating the gastric wall (see Fig. 110).

4. The diffuse infiltrating type, perhaps ulcerated superficially, without definitely palpable borders and often with thickening of the wall of the entire stomach (see Fig. 111).

Metastases tend to develop later in groups 1 and 2 than in groups 3 and 4, as expressed in the pathologic dictum: "Large primary growth, few metastases, small primary growth, many metastases."

The extent and the character of the ulceration may be affected by the gastric juice. When acid gastric juice is present, the base of the carcinomatous ulcer appears cleanly digested rather than necrotic, and its edge tends to be sharp rather than ragged and indefinite. The ulceration may rarely extend beyond the carcinoma into normal tissue and thus produce a lesion grossly indistinguishable from a benign ulcer.

The *microscopic types* of gastric carcinoma are variable and are not to be correlated with the macroscopic forms. All grades of differentiation are seen, from the highly differentiated cylindrical adenocarcinoma to the poorly differentiated or almost entirely undifferentiated cellular carcinomas resembling sarcomas. Broders classifies the malignancy on the basis of the degree of differentiation present histologically.

The tendency is for *metastatic lesions* to develop most rapidly in poorly differentiated tumors, least rapidly in the highly differentiated ones. The spread takes place by way of the lymphatics, the peritoneum or the blood. The adjacent lymph glands are usually first involved. Infiltration of the supraclavicular node, the so-called Virchow's node, is found in approximately 5 per cent at autopsy. Hepatic involvement, peritoneal and omental metastases, and direct extension into the esophagus are common.

The neoplasm rarely extends beyond the pylorus into the duodenum. Any adjacent organ may be involved by direct extension, particularly the pancreas, liver, colon, spleen or diaphragm. Peritoneal spread to the ovaries, the so-called *Krukenberg tumor,* invariably involving both ovaries, occurs in approximately 5 per cent of the cases. Similar implantation metastases occur in the male in the rectal pouch. Pulmonary metastases are less frequent than might be expected. Other rather rare but nevertheless definite sites of metastases are the navel, skin, brain and bone marrow.

Symptoms. The symptoms of cancer of the stomach are most indefinite; almost any *indigestion* in any person of cancer age is suspicious. Gastric carcinoma is a disease to be kept always in mind and to be excluded only with care and hesitation. The *onset* is indefinite; the symptoms are slight; the disease progresses so stealthily that it is neither suspected nor recognized until it is well advanced. The *duration* of symptoms is variable; usually it is a few months; occasionally it is two or three years; rarely it is several years, and then, of course, the question arises whether the early symptoms should not be attributed to some other cause. If so, the change in the distress picture may not be recognized by the patient. Remissions in the distress are rare, the course of the disease being almost invariably progressive.

Usually the patient is 40 or more years of age and previously has enjoyed excellent health. He first notices some *loss of appetite* and consequent *loss of weight and a very mild epigastric distress*. These symptoms are disregarded for a few weeks or months, but they progress, and in less than a year he seeks the advice of a physician. The weight loss then amounts to 10 or 20 pounds or more. The loss of appetite is definite, but the patient may not have noticed it. The *abdominal distress* consists of fullness or discomfort induced by eating, or of gnawing or aching epigastric pain which may appear at any time after eating, not infrequently is relieved by eating, and usually is relieved by induced or spontaneous vomiting. The pain may follow the identical pattern of peptic ulcer. In many cases, however, the distress of carcinoma is notably different from that of peptic ulcer in that it is present in the morning before breakfast, appears soon after eating, and is not completely relieved by food taking, alkali or even vomiting. *Nausea and vomiting* may occur regardless of the location of the lesion, but are much more frequent when the carcinoma obstructs the gastric outlet. More or less intractable vomiting of food and gastric juice may be the first symptom of small, early, intrapyloric tumors. The vomitus may or may not contain food, blood or bile, although the so-called "coffee-ground" emesis is particularly suggestive of carcinoma. *Hematemesis and melena* may be the first symptom of the disease or occur at any time during its course. *Anemia* is often, but not regularly, present, is almost invariably of the secondary type unless concomitant pernicious anemia exists, and is due to the continual loss of blood from the surface of the tumor. *Acute perforation,* although uncommon, does occur, and the surgeon may not suspect the carcinomatous nature of the lesion at the time of the repair. An elevation of temperature of 1 or 2 degrees F. is not infrequent. More marked *fever* does occur and is attributed to a coincident pyogenic gastritis, as is evidenced by the histologic demonstration of small abscesses, or rarely even by the presence of a phlegmonous gastritis.

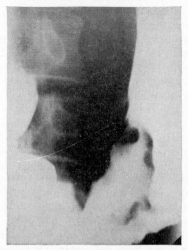

Fig. 110. Ulcerating carcinoma of the lesser curvature. The crater, lying beneath the line of the lesser curvature, is surrounded by the ragged nodular halo produced by the polypoid infiltrated wall.

Examination. *Physical Examination.* The physical examination is often negative, but it may reveal pallor, evidence of loss of weight, a palpable, movable, hard mass in the upper abdomen usually independent of the liver, a definite nodular enlargement of the liver, a hard enlarged Virchow's node, metastatic lesions in the ovaries or on the rectal shelf, or rarely in tumors of the fundus of the stomach, obliteration of Traube's semilunar space.

Laboratory Examination. The laboratory examination may disclose the presence of anemia. Free acid is present in the gastric content in about 40 per cent of the cases and after the injection of histamine hydrochloride subcutaneously may be found in rather high concentration, 75 to 100 clinical units (pH 1.3 to 1.0). Occult blood by the benzidine test is present in the gastric content and in the stool in 90 to 95 per cent of cases. Stool examination, therefore, gives valuable diagnostic evidence regarding the presence of carcinoma, but two possibilities must always be borne in mind: first, that occult blood, if present, may not be of gastric origin; and present, may not be of gastric origin; and

second, that carcinoma, particularly of the infiltrative and scirrhous types, may be present in spite of the continued absence of occult blood in the stool. Indeed, rarely after massive hemorrhage the occult blood in the stool may disappear completely for several weeks.

Roentgenologic Examination. The roentgenologic examination is probably more valuable in the diagnosis of gastric carcinoma than any other diagnostic method, sign or symptom. Although it is not infallible, it is constantly improving in accuracy as technique and equipment become better and the proficiency of the roentgenologist increases. The classic roentgenologic evidence of carcinoma is the filling defect, a rigid, constant, somewhat ragged alteration in the contour of a portion of the stomach. In the antrum, both curvatures are likely to be involved and the lumen raggedly narrowed by the infiltration of the wall (see Fig. 109). The polypoid tumor growing into the lumen appears as a nonopaque nodular mass when pressure is made on the barium-filled, or partially filled, stomach (see Fig. 108). Ulceration may be evident from collections of barium caught in the ulcer and typically presenting the appearance of the so-called meniscus sign of Carman (see Fig. 110). The normal mucosal pattern is almost invariably distorted or destroyed by the tumor, as may be seen from careful mucosal relief studies using small amounts of barium and graduated compression.

The roentgenologist not infrequently discovers a dilated stomach with hyperperistalsis, yet with obstruction so complete that he is unable to see any barium pass through the pyloric channel and hence is unable to ascertain the exact location or nature of the lesion. The problem in such a case is usually the differentiation of a pyloric carcinoma from a duodenal ulcer with high grade stenosis.

Gastroscopic Examination. Gastroscopy is of value in confirming the roentgenologic diagnosis of carcinoma, or not infrequently in providing definite evidence bearing on a questionable roentgenologic finding. Occasionally a tumor may be demonstrated with one method and not with the other. Gastroscopy may give important information with regard to the type of the tumor, its operability and the prognosis. Gastroscopically, tumors are seen in picturesque forms and in colorings much more brilliant than those seen at autopsy or in the resected specimen. The polypoid tumors are usually seen easily and are readily recognized, although occasionally it is difficult to differentiate them from benign tumors or hypertrophic gastritis. If ulceration is present, however, the carcinomatous nature of the lesion is apparent, for the irregular ulcer floor, covered with pieces of necrotic tissue, dirty gray, greenish gray, brown, red or violet in color, is surrounded by a thick wall usually dark red in color and sharply demarcated from the normal gastric tissue. When the margin of the ulcer is seen to fade gradually into infiltrated tissue which in turn blends imperceptibly with the normal gastric mucosa, the lesion is usually an infiltrating ulcerating tumor of type III or IV. Certain infiltrating carcinomas may be impossible to differentiate gastroscopically from lymphosarcoma, lymphogranuloma, leukemia, syphilis or hypertrophic gastritis.

Cytologic Examination. The positive diagnosis of cancer of the viscera by means of the microscopic identification of exfoliated cells has been revived in recent years by Papanicolaou and other workers. If appropriate methods are used with skill, tumor cells may be demonstrated in the gastric content of approximately 80 per cent of the patients found to have gastric cancer; incorrect positive diagnoses are rare. The procedure is very time-consuming and hence cannot be employed as a screening measure. In selected cases it often provides decisive and hence most valuable information.

Diagnosis. The importance of carefully examining all patients in middle life and beyond who have continued abdominal distress cannot be overemphasized. The symptoms of carcinoma, while usually suggestive, are not diagnostic. The physical and laboratory examinations may yield corroborative, although as a rule, not pathognomonic evidence. The roentgenologic and gastroscopic examinations give more exact and precise information. The diagnostic accuracy of the complete clinical study is great—so great indeed that "exploratory laparotomy" as a diagnostic procedure in gastric disease is rarely indicated. In fact, the evidence gained by palpation and inspection of the stomach at operation may be less reliable than that obtained preoperatively.

Course. The course of gastric carcinoma is invariably progressive; the symptoms are likewise progressive, although they may exhibit, in rare instances, remarkable fluctuations and remissions. The clinical course of the disease usually covers a period of twelve to thirty months, but it may be only a few weeks, almost "acute," or it may last several years, being in a sense "chronic." Death comes usually from inanition with prolonged anorexia, vomiting and weakness.

Prognosis. The prognosis depends upon the type and location of the tumor and upon the resistance of the patient. It is important to know that, in general, the polypoid, sharply circumscribed neoplasms growing into the lumen (type I of Borrmann, Moskowicz, Konjetzny, Schindler) (see Figs. 108, 109, 110) are much slower in their growth than are the infiltrative ones (types III and IV) (see Fig. 111), although exceptions do occur. Some papillomatous carcinomas metastasize early; conversely, the infiltrating carcinoma fibrosum, producing the so-called linitis plastica, may run a slow course, metastasizing late or not at all. The diffusely infiltrating carcinomas of Jarcho, on the other hand, produce very small local lesions and metastasize early, the metastatic tumors in the bone marrow or elsewhere giving rise to symptoms before the primary growth does so.

The histologic grading of malignancy (Broders) may be helpful in that, on the whole, the degree of differentiation and the grade of malignancy are inversely proportional to each other. Different sections from the same tumor, however, may disclose varying degrees of differentiation. Indeed, a highly differentiated colloid carcinoma may rarely be very malignant.

The location of the neoplasm is of prognostic importance in several respects. Carcinomas of the pylorus (intrapyloric tumors) produce obstruction and symptoms earlier than do those in the body of the stomach, and are easily resected. Tumors of the distal third of the stomach may be resected more easily than those of the middle third, and these in turn are much more easily resected than those of the upper third or cardia. Carcinomas of the greater curvature tend to be more easily resectable than those of the lesser curvature because the involvement of the deeper lymph glands occurs at a later stage in the disease, and also because the primary growth is, as a rule, most accessible.

The resistance of the patient to carcinoma is unpredictable, but there is evidence that the body does exhibit a certain ability to resist or even destroy cancer cells. Years after the resection of a gastric carcinoma cellular nests of carcinoma may be found "locked" in the scar tissue, no other metastases being demonstrable.

The prognosis is not influenced by sex and, on the whole, not greatly by age, although, in general, carcinoma is said to progress more rapidly in the young, more slowly in the aged. However, the longest cure in the Breslau clinic (twenty-one years) was

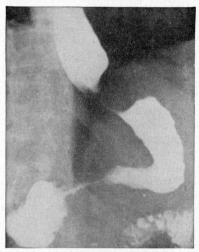

Fig. 111. "Leather-bottle stomach." Note the small, uniformly contracted stomach, giving the appearance of a stomach in miniature, the dilated esophagus, and the rather well-filled duodenum. Death occurred two months after the roentgenogram was taken.

observed in a young man 31 years of age. The duration of life after resection of a gastric carcinoma averages one to two years longer than in cases treated with palliative medical measures only or, indeed, with other forms of surgery. So-called three-year cures after resection are frequent; five-year cures are not infrequent; cures of longer duration do occur, as in cases shown in Figures 108 and 109. The most recent figures from the Mayo Clinic indicate a five-year cure rate of 14 per cent of 100 patients examined; in those surviving partial gastric resection the five-year cure rate rises to approximately 30 per cent.

Treatment. There is, at the present time, only one real treatment for gastric carcinoma, and that is surgical removal.

Contraindications to Operation. Definite contraindications are limited to the presence of proved metastatic lesions such as a carcinomatous peritonitis, neoplastic infiltration of the liver or metastases to the bone marrow. Great caution is necessary, for a nodular liver

may be a cirrhotic liver independent of the gastric tumor.

Resectability. The circumscribed polypoid type I carcinomas are usually resectable, whereas the infiltrative types III and IV are more likely to extend along the esophagus or to involve adjacent structures such as the liver or pancreas. The prognosis after resection is much better in types I and II than in III and IV, except for certain rare exceptions, such as the highly malignant papillomatous tumors on the one hand, and the slow-growing carcinoma fibrosum on the other. However, regardless of the gross or histologic appearance, all gastric carcinomas should, if possible, be resected, even a complete gastrectomy being justifiable. The presence of large lymph glands is not a contraindication to resection, because the enlargement may be inflammatory rather than neoplastic and because life is usually prolonged by resection even if lymphatic spread has taken place. Metastases in the liver or distant lymph nodes likewise do not necessarily constitute a contraindication to resection, for the operation may prolong life even in these circumstances and may lead eventually to a less agonizing death than that resulting from pyloric obstruction. In rare instances the patient may be definitely benefited by the removal of a gastric carcinoma, and simultaneous extirpation of metastatic lesions elsewhere such as ovarian (Krukenberg) implantations.

Mortality Rate. Statistics on operability and on surgical operative mortality are of little value because they are based upon three variables—the patient, the surgeon and the tumor. The mortality rate rises as the removal of the more extensive tumors in the more debilitated patients is attempted. Exploratory laparotomy *per se* has a definite hazard and little therapeutic value; gastroenterostomy has a certain palliative effect; *resection* alone offers the patient the chance of a cure. Consequently a high mortality rate with a high incidence of resection may be preferable to a low mortality rate with a low incidence of resection.

Radiation therapy has produced some striking morphologic changes in certain gastric carcinomas and has been found valuable in the treatment of lymphoblastoma and other malignant mesenchymal gastric tumors, but there is no satisfactory proof that it has ever cured a single case of gastric carcinoma. The nausea, vomiting and weakness resulting from the therapy usually accelerate the downward course of the patient. Radiation, therefore, cannot be recommended either as a therapeutic or palliative procedure.

Symptomatic treatment varies from day to day and from patient to patient. Rules cannot be laid down. The needs of the day must be met as they arise with the various diets, drugs and procedures available, but, above all, with kindness and sympathy, and with as much encouragement and cheerfulness as possible. The physician must endeavor to support the waning courage of the patient and thus help him carry on as bravely as possible.

The *diet* should be palatable and nutritious. Restrictions should not be imposed. In some cases, particularly those with acid gastric juice, the *antacid ulcer management program of Sippy* may afford partial or complete symptomatic relief for several weeks or months. Suggestion and other forms of psychotherapy are occasionally strikingly effective for a short time. Sedatives, analgesics, hypnotics and narcotics should be used unhesitatingly but judiciously. The parenteral administration of fluid, and rarely blood transfusions, may be indicated.

The Patient, the Physician and the Truth. The difficult question whether or not the patient should be told the true nature of his disease cannot be answered categorically. Patients and physicians have various opinions in this regard. The patient with carcinoma is not likely to accept the truth, if told it, as philosophically as he himself had planned. Certainly the patient should be told enough to ensure the proper treatment. Usually it is sufficient to state simply that an operation is necessary for obstruction or for tumor. A responsible member of the family should always be informed frankly and fully, not only of the presence and nature of the disease, but also of the prognosis and the therapeutic possibilities. The word "cancer" should not be used to the patient and usually not to the relatives if it can be avoided, for, to most people, it has only the most terrible connotations. The fear of cancer is so great that many patients, if told they have cancer, immediately abandon all hope and in utter panic refuse to make any attempt to deal with the disease intelligently. The public is not yet sufficiently aware that cancer may be curable. The patient told that he has a "growth" may well understand that he has a cancer, but he prefers not to press the point. The responsible relative is more likely to do so and of course

should be told. If, however, the patient refuses operation, and particularly if he does so when the physician considers that the tumor is likely to prove resectable, the facts should be presented fully and frankly. The patient may still refuse surgical treatment, and it is his privilege to do so, but usually he accepts the advice given. If he survives resection, it is better not to inform him of the likelihood of recurrence. If the tumor cannot be resected, it is not necessary to tell the patient that he is doomed. A certain vagueness leaves a ray of hope, whereas complete frankness may be terribly brutal. Honesty, as a moral law, does not justify brutality, and honesty, after all, is purely relative. The physician must remember also that mistakes are made, that his diagnosis may be wrong, and that strange things are seen in the practice of medicine. Usually the situation can be handled in such a manner as to avoid frank discussion of the nature of the disease, its course and prognosis. The patient may fear the worst, but usually finds courage to hope that the condition is not as bad as he fears. The physician with kindness, sympathy, courage and resourcefulness must travel the road with the patient, relieving his distress as much as possible and supporting his morale until finally the journey ends before the patient realizes that death is at hand.

Walter L. Palmer

References

Berkson, J., Walters, W., Gray, H. K., and Priestley, J. T.: Mortality and Survival in Cancer of the Stomach: A Statistical Summary of the Experience of the Mayo Clinic. Proc. Staff Meet. Mayo Clinic, 27:137, 1952.

Carey, J. B., and Hay, L.: Gastric Polyps. Gastroenterology, 10:102, 1948.

Konjetzny, G. E.: Der Magenkrebs. Stuttgart, Ferdinand and Enke, 1938.

Livingston, E. M., and Pack, G. T.: End Results in the Treatment of Gastric Cancer. New York, Paul B. Hoeber, Inc., 1939.

Proceedings of the Fifth National Gastrointestinal Cancer Conference. J. Nat. Cancer Inst., 13: 927, 1953.

Rigler, L. G., and Kaplan, H. S.: Pernicious Anemia and Tumors of the Stomach. J. Nat. Cancer Inst., 7:321, 1947.

Rubin, C. E., Massey, B. W., Kirsner, J. B., Palmer, W. L., and Stonecypher, D. D.: The Clinical Value of Gastrointestinal Cytologic Diagnosis. Gastroenterology, 25:119, 1953.

Schindler, R.: Gastroscopy: The Endoscopic Study of Gastric Pathology. Rev. ed. Chicago, University of Chicago Press, 1949.

Steiner, P. E., Maimon, S. N., Palmer, W. L., and Kirsner, J. B.: Gastric Cancer: Morphologic Factors in Five-Year Survival after Gastrectomy. Am. J. Path., 24:947, 1948.

Stewart, H. L., and Lorenz, E.: Adenocarcinoma of the Pyloric Stomach and Other Genetic Neoplasms in Mice Induced with Carcinogenic Hydrocarbons. J. Nat. Cancer Inst., 3:175, 1942.

Stout, A. P.: Gastric Mucosal Atrophy and Carcinoma of the Stomach. New York State J. Med., 45:973, 1945.

Templeton, F. E.: X-ray Examination of the Stomach, A Description of the Roentgenologic Anatomy, Physiology, and Pathology of the Esophagus, Stomach and Duodenum. Chicago, University of Chicago Press, 1944.

Walters, W., Gray, H. K., and Priestley, J. T.: Carcinoma and Other Malignant Lesions of the Stomach. Philadelphia, W. B. Saunders Company, 1942.

PEPTIC ULCER

(Digestive, Corroding, Eroding, Simple, Round, Perforating or Acid Ulcer)

Definition. Peptic ulcer is a sharply circumscribed loss of tissue resulting from the digestive action of acid gastric juice. The first clear description is usually attributed to Cruveilhier (1829), whose name it bore for many years as "the round ulcer of Cruveilhier," but Matthew Baillie pictured the lesion in a series of engravings published in 1799, and John Abercrombie wrote an excellent account of the symptoms in 1828.

Distribution. The geographic distribution of peptic ulcer is world-wide; it occurs in all races and in all occupations.

Incidence. The exact incidence in man is unknown, although it is estimated on the basis of autopsy statistics that approximately 10 per cent of all persons suffer at some time in their lives from a chronic gastric or duodenal ulcer. At autopsy the gastric lesion is more frequent than the duodenal, but duodenal ulcer is much more commonly encountered clinically. Males are afflicted about four times more frequently than females.

The lesion occurs at all *ages*. Acute ulcers are not uncommon in the newborn. Chronic ulcer is rarely diagnosed during the first decade of life, although its incidence is probably greater than is generally appreciated. Between the ages of 20 and 50 peptic ulcer is common; after 50 it is also frequent. Striking instances of a *hereditary* or *familial tendency* are encountered, but, perhaps, not more often than might be expected on the basis of coincidence. The typical ulcer patient is usually described as a lean person of a definite *constitutional type* contrasting with the short, stocky, obese, so-called "gallbladder type." As a matter of fact, peptic ulcer and cholelithiasis are seen in all constitutional types and not infrequently in the same person.

Morbid Anatomy. *Location.* Peptic ulcer occurs in the lower part of the esophagus, in the stomach, in the upper portion of the duodenum, in the small bowel, adjacent usually to a patent gastroenterostomy or a Meckel's diverticulum, and rarely elsewhere in the jejunum or ileum. The lesion occurs in constant association with normal or ectopic gastric mucosa. The vast majority of peptic ulcers occur along the lesser curvature of the stomach, the so-called "magenstrasse," or in the first 3 or 4 cm. of duodenum, the "duodenal bulb." The pylorus is not infrequently involved; prepyloric and postpyloric lesions are rather common.

Pathologic Description. Ulcers are usually single, but not infrequently are multiple, being present in both the stomach and duodenum or as multiple lesions in either organ, such as the so-called "kissing ulcers" of the anterior and posterior walls of the duodenum. Active and healed lesions may coexist. The average diameter of the gastric ulcer is 5 to 25 mm., although the lesions may be only 2 or 3 mm. in diameter or as large as 40 to 60 mm. In the duodenum and jejunum the diameter usually varies from 2 to 10 mm., sometimes reaches 15 mm., and rarely 20 or 30 mm. The depth is variable, often 10 to 20 mm. in the stomach, usually 2 to 6 mm. in the duodenum. The lesion differs from an erosion in that it involves not only the mucosa, but also the muscularis mucosae. Peptic ulcer is the result of a penetrating process beginning in the mucosa, invading the deeper layers of the gastric wall and, perhaps, perforating them completely. The border of the ulcer is sharp, and the surrounding mucosa may be normal or slightly inflamed, flat or slightly elevated, or even rounded, usually because of extensive edema of the submucosa or rarely of fibrous tissue. The floor of the ulcer is clean and consists of a thin layer of fibrinopurulent exudate overlying a narrow zone of fibrinoid necrois and a deeper zone of granulation and fibrous tissue. In chronic ulcer the muscular layer in the base is usually interrupted completely by fibrous tissue, and the blood vessels are thrombosed. The "life history" of an ulcer with its characteristic periods of remission and exacerbation is evidenced pathologically by phases of more or less extensive ulceration and more or less complete healing.

Carcinomatous Degeneration of Benign Ulcer. This subject has been a controversial one. It arises in connection with gastric ulcer only. Primary carcinoma of the first portion of the duodenum is rare, although carcinoma elsewhere in the duodenum is not so rare. Carcinoma of the jejunum adjacent to a gastroenterostomy stoma is also so rare that the question of malignant degeneration of a jejunal peptic ulcer has scarcely arisen. Although various explanations have been given for the alleged tendency of gastric ulcers to undergo malignant transformation, in contrast with duodenal ulcer, the evidence available suggests that benign peptic ulcer does not undergo malignant degeneration at all, but that gastric carcinoma, on the other hand, does at times undergo peptic digestion and may mimic the benign lesion in almost every respect. There is clear evidence that peptic digestion may almost completely destroy a gastric carcinoma and produce a lesion grossly identical with benign ulcer. It must be admitted, on the other hand, that the possibility of carcinomatous degeneration of a benign ulcer cannot be denied even though proof of its occurrence is lacking. From the practical point of view, however, the consideration is of little significance in comparison with the question whether a given lesion is benign or malignant.

Curling's Ulcer. Curling's ulcer is a special lesion, an acute gastroduodenal ulceration following extensive burns of the skin, described by Swan in 1823, later by Lang; Curling called attention to it in 1842. It occurs in both sexes at all ages, usually near the pylorus, may be single or multiple, usually causes pain, nausea and vomiting within a few days after the burn, and may be complicated by acute perforation or hemorrhage.

Association with Other Diseases. Peptic ulcer occurs in conjunction with practically all diseases, the notable exceptions being those characterized by a complete achlorhydria, particularly pernicious anemia and combined column degeneration of the spinal cord. Gastric carcinoma is rarely seen in the presence of an active or healed duodenal ulcer. Special reference should be made, perhaps, to the lesions occurring in patients with tumor of the brain, particularly after operation, although their exact frequency and significance are open to question. In pregnancy, ulcer rarely develops and the symptoms of ulcer, if present previously, usually subside. In diaphragmatic hernia, erosions or ulcers are likely to develop at the constricting ring. Renal calculi appear to be somewhat more frequent in patients receiving alkali therapy for peptic ulcer than they are in normal persons, although this point is not definitely established. Acute appendicitis is a common complication of antacid ulcer management, presumably because of the formation of enteroliths in the appendix followed by obstruction and resultant increase in the intraluminal pressure.

Etiology and Pathogenesis. Peptic ulcer is due to the digestive action of acid gastric juice, as illustrated by Claude Bernard's classic experiment on the frog's leg. The ability of the normal stomach to resist digestion is attributable, apparently, to the thin layer of mucus constantly secreted by the mucus-secreting cells.

The evidence that chronic peptic ulcer is in some way related to acid gastric juice seems conclusive. Clinically, chronic ulcer is found only in those portions of the digestive tract exposed to the action of acid gastric juice and only in persons whose gastric glands are able to secrete acid. It is highly significant that the 10 per cent of the population with histamine achlorhydria do not acquire ulcer. Experimentally, ulcer may be produced by various operations interfering with the normal neutralization of the acid by the duodenal content, by the administration of acid, or by the continuous stimulation of acid gastric secretion by means of the intramuscular injection of a mixture of histamine and beeswax. The pathologic, clinical and experimental evidence is in accord in indicating that peptic ulcer is a penetrative process beginning in the mucosa and dependent upon the destructive action of acid gastric juice. The explanation of the failure of the mucosa to withstand the acid attack in certain persons is not clear.

The factors responsible probably include lack of cellular resistance, an insufficient secretion of mucus, or excessive acid gastric juice, particularly during the night and during the fasting periods when the normal stomach secretes little acid (see p. 849). The central nervous system through the vagus may produce hypermotility and quantitative hypersecretion. Emotional factors may play a most important role, for Wolf and Wolff have demonstrated beautifully the response of the stomach to various psychologic states. It is premature, however, to conclude that peptic ulcer is a purely psychosomatic disorder.

Trauma. Direct epigastric trauma is occasionally followed by the prompt appearance of the symptoms of ulcer and indeed by its subsequent roentgenologic demonstration, but there is no other evidence that trauma plays any role in the pathogenesis in the vast majority of cases.

Symptoms. *Pain* is the outstanding symptom of ulcer, the four characteristic features being its chronicity, its periodicity, its quality and its relationship to food taking.

The *chronicity* of the disease is indicated by the fact that the average stated duration of the distress is six or seven years; in occasional cases the symptoms are of only a few days' or weeks' duration; in others they may have been present for forty or fifty years.

The *periodicity* of ulcer distress is striking. The usual statement is that the attacks come in the spring and the fall. As a matter of fact, the greatest incidence occurs in the months from October to March, inclusive, with an additional peak in June. The significant point is not the season of the year, but the periodicity of the distress. The symptoms may last for a few days, several weeks or several months, and the periods of remission be of similar duration. As time goes on, the tendency is for the periods of distress to become more frequent and of longer duration, whereas the remissions are less frequent and shorter. Precipitating causes of the exacerbations are usually listed as acute infections, worry and fatigue. These unavoidable accidents of living are so common and so universal that one doubts their causal relationship to the formation or reactivation of an ulcer.

The *quality* of ulcer distress, although rather variable, tends to conform to a definite pattern. It is, as a rule, a gnawing or aching sensation; sometimes it is described as burning, hurting, annoying or cramplike, or indeed as hunger. It differs from the intermittent pang of true hunger in that ulcer distress is almost invariably steady and continuous for periods of 15 minutes to an hour or more unless measures are taken to give relief. In severity the pain varies from a mild discomfort to acute pain. It is almost invariably epigastric, usually sharply localized to an area a few centimeters in diameter to which the patient points with the tips of the fingers. The pain may radiate around the costal border or through to the back or to the right lower quadrant or, rarely, to the navel or below. In duodenal ulcer the distress is likely to be located in the right epigastrium, in gastric ulcer in the left epigastrium, and in jejunal ulcer in the left mid-abdomen or even in the left lower quadrant. The presence of pain in the back suggests, but does not prove, the presence of chronic perforation.

The *rhythm of pain* in peptic ulcer is related to the digestive cycle and is the same for both gastric and duodenal ulcer. A detailed analysis of a "typical day" provides valuable information and should be incorporated in the history. Pain attributable to ulcer is almost invariably absent in the morning before breakfast, appears 1 to 4 hours after breakfast, and lasts 30 minutes or more, perhaps until relief is obtained at the noon meal. The distress recurs 1 to 4 hours later and is then usually more severe than in the forenoon. The afternoon pain may likewise disappear spontaneously, but more frequently definite measures are taken to bring relief, the patient having learned that the taking of food or alkali in adequate amounts, vomiting or rest usually affords relief. In the evening the pain may recur 1 to 4 hours after eating, but it is often less severe than in the afternoon. The same measures give relief. The patient may be awakened with pain, usually between 12 and 2 A.M. Rarely does nocturnal pain appear unless pain has been present in the evening, and rarely indeed does pain attributable to ulcer develop later in the night, unless it has been present earlier and relieved by food or alkali. The presence of nocturnal pain is often interpreted as evidence of pyloric obstruction or high grade stenosis, but it is also seen in nonobstructive acutely inflamed lesions with highly acid gastric secretion.

Mechanism of Pain in Peptic Ulcer. The normal gastric mucosa is insensitive to cutting, pinching, tearing or exposure to varying hydrogen ion concentrations. The inflamed mucosa, on the other hand, may be sensitive, apparently because of a lowering of the pain threshold. The pain of peptic ulcer depends primarily, therefore, upon the degree of inflammation present in or about the lesion. An acutely inflamed ulcer is highly sensitive to mechanical or chemical trauma in the form of peristalsis and spasm or changes in the hydrogen ion concentration. The role of acid gastric juice in the pathogenesis of peptic ulcer has already been presented, but it is important to point out that the acid juice evokes a chemical inflammation in the mucosal defect, lowers the pain threshold of the nerve endings and produces pain. When the moment, therefore, is dependent upon the presence of an inflamed lesion and acid gastric juice. Theoretically, the former could occur without the latter; practically it does not, probably for the reason that the inflammation

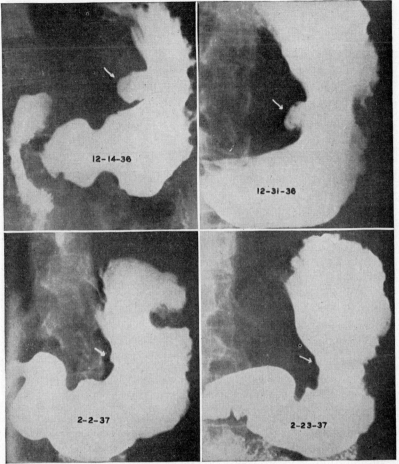

Fig. 112. Spectacular healing of gastric ulcer. The patient, a woman 63 years of age, gave a history of epigastric pain radiating through to the back between the shoulder blades, unrelated to food, relieved only by emesis, and accompanied by more or less persistent vomiting for sixteen days. Periodic postprandial epigastric distress had been present for eleven months, and several similar attacks had occurred in the preceding thirty-five years.

defect is protected from the action of the acid, the inflammation subsides, the sensitivity decreases and the pain disappears. The pain seems to arise directly at the site of the lesion, not in some distant part of the stomach or duodenum or through any vague reflex mechanism.

The concentration of acid at the time of the pain is not abnormal, nor is it greater than that present in the same stomach without pain when the ulcer is healed or in a healing phase. The presence of pain at any given

of peptic ulcer results from the continued action of acid gastric juice. The question is often raised why ulcers may be present, may bleed profusely and may perforate without antecedent pain. The only apparent answer is the rather vague and unsatisfactory one of a high pain threshold and low sensitivity.

Atypical Distress. The classic ulcer history as outlined is frequently not obtained. The usual reason is that the patient is a poor observer or that insufficient care has been taken in describing the symptoms. When a careful diary is kept or when the patient is hospitalized and the sequence of pain studied, it almost invariably conforms to the description given. Exceptions occur in acutely inflamed lesions, presumably with more or less *perigastritis* and *periduodenitis*. In such cases the pain may be only partially relieved by food taking or by alkali, or by the emptying of the

EMESIS may result from severe pain, although usually the vomiting is caused by obstruction—spastic, inflammatory or cicatricial. Painless vomiting may occur in high grade obstruction or more rarely in nonobstructive lesions, in which case it is presumably due to a reflex disturbance of the intrinsic neuromuscular coordination.

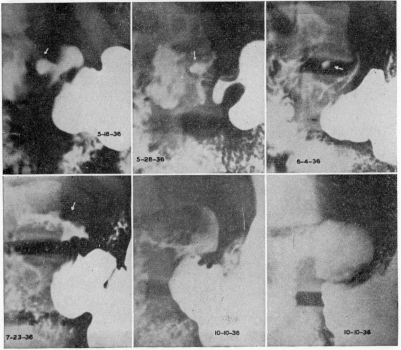

Fig. 113. Active duodenal ulcer showing an *en face* view of a large crater in an undeformed bulb. Under treatment the crater decreased rapidly in size from May until October and in healing left no residual evidence of deformity.

stomach; the incompleteness of the relief is due to a persistent soreness and tenderness which disappears in a few hours or days if neutralization of the acid is maintained.

The so-called *biliary* or *tabetic* types of ulcer distress in which there is a severe, steady, continuous pain accompanied by vomiting, and simulating both biliary colic and the gastric crisis of tabes dorsalis, constitute important variants of the usual picture. The attack may last for several days with continued pain, nausea and vomiting. The vomitus consists of clear or bile-colored, *highly acid* gastric juice, in marked contrast with the viscid emesis of continued biliary or tabetic vomiting.

Accessory Symptoms. NAUSEA is not a common symptom of ulcer, although it may occur and not be accompanied by pain.

WATER BRASH is a rather rare symptom consisting of a combination of excessive salivation and acid regurgitation, sometimes awakening the patient at night.

The APPETITE and WEIGHT are usually well preserved, but marked loss of weight, amounting to 30 to 40 pounds, may result from continued vomiting or the patient's fear of eating. On the other hand, the frequent ingestion of food in order to relieve the pain may result in a gain in weight.

CONSTIPATION is a common complaint, usually associated with a cathartic habit, the symptoms of which may completely obscure the distress of ulcer.

DIARRHEA is rare except in the presence of a gastrojejunocolic fistula which may develop gradually or suddenly after gastroenterostomy and without any pain whatsoever.

ANEMIA, if present, may develop gradually or acutely.

Examinations. *Physical Examination.* In peptic ulcer "the anamnesis is everything; the physical examination nothing" (Moynihan). Localized tenderness is not uncommon; occasionally the outline of a distended stomach may be made out and peristaltic waves observed; rarely a tender mass may be palpable.

Laboratory Examination. The demonstration of acid gastric juice is essential, because can be demonstrated in at least 90 per cent of the cases of active gastric ulcer, in from 50 to 70 per cent of those with active duodenal ulcer, and probably in the majority of cases of anastomotic ulcer. True craters may occur at any point along the lesser curvature of the stomach, in the bulb or even in the proximal part of the second portion of the duodenum. In profile the crater appears as a penetrating niche; *en face* it is a sharply outlined and circumscribed collection of barium,

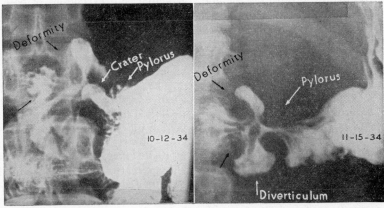

Fig. 114. Marked deformity of both curvatures of a large duodenal bulb although the lumen is still quite adequate. Between the pylorus and the deformity the duodenal bulb is rather ballooned out, producing a diverticulum-like appearance. The crater is usually found at, or just proximal to, the deformity. In this case the crater is immediately beyond the pylorus (left view). A month later no evidence of crater was found, although the deformity persisted.

chronic peptic ulcer does not occur in its continued absence.

Roentgenologic Examination. In peptic ulcer the roentgenogram is the most important diagnostic procedure. Mistakes are made, however, both of omission and commission. The roentgenologic evidence must be weighed and its value assessed by the clinician in conjunction with the other data available.

The roentgenologic signs of ulcer are usually divided into the direct or primary signs, and the indirect or secondary. The *primary signs* are relatively pathognomonic and consist of the demonstration of the crater of the ulcer or the deformity produced by it, or both; whereas the *secondary signs,* consisting of such nonspecific findings as gastric retention, altered peristalsis and localized tenderness, are relatively unimportant. In the stomach the crater is usually seen as a penetrating niche, in profile (Fig. 112), whereas in the bulb it is more frequently seen *en face* (Figs. 113, 114). The crater is the only definite roentgenologic evidence of active ulcer. It usually 2 to 10 mm. in diameter and surrounded by a clear halo. The gastric and duodenal folds typically radiate to it. As the ulcer heals, its site may be indicated by the radiating folds. In the stomach, healing rarely alters the contour of the organ, except in those cases in which an hour-glass contracture is seen, whereas in the duodenum the process typically causes some contraction and hence a deformity of one or both curvatures of the bulb (Fig. 114).

Gastroscopic Examination. This method often permits the demonstration of small lesions not visible roentgenologically. Its great disadvantage is that it permits no view beyond the pylorus or of certain "blind areas" in the stomach itself.

Diagnosis. The diagnosis of peptic ulcer is based upon the clinical syndrome described and upon the direct roentgenologic or gastroscopic demonstration of the lesion. The greater the skill of the roentgenologist, the less the frequency with which a positive diagnosis will be justified without confirmatory roentgenologic evidence. The differential diagnosis of a demonstrable gastric or duodenal lesion is usually not difficult, except for the differentiation of benign and malignant gastric ulcer.

Differentiation of Benign and Malignant Gastric Ulcer. The criteria available for the differentiation of these two lesions are of relative, not absolute, value. Certain signs are more or less diagnostic of gastric cancer, whereas none is pathognomonic of a benign process. Age is of some importance, although carcinoma may occur in the third decade and benign ulcer is not uncommon in the sixth and seventh. A long history of several years' duration suggests a benign lesion and a short one malignancy, but carcinoma may arise in a patient with chronic indigestion of whatever cause, and conversely benign ulcer often develops acutely and gives a short history. A qualitative or quantitative change in a chronic distress is sometimes considered evidence of malignancy, but this occurs in a benign lesion also. Periodicity is usual in ulcer, rare in carcinoma. The relationship of the distress to food taking, alkali or emesis, so classically typical or peptic ulcer, is likewise frequently seen in carcinoma. Loss of appetite is much more likely to occur in cancer, although marked loss of weight and strength may occur in both conditions. Hematemesis, coffee-ground vomitus and melena may be the initial symptoms in either. The continued presence of occult blood in the stool after two or three weeks of careful treatment is presumptive evidence of malignancy, whereas the continued absence of occult blood suggests that the lesion is benign, although exceptions of both kinds occur. The demonstration of histamine-achlorhydria speaks almost unequivocally against a benign ulcer. High acid values such as 100 or 110 after histamine (pH 1.0) are infrequently seen in carcinoma.

The *roentgenologic interpretation* of the nature of a gastric ulcer is valuable; it depends upon certain considerations such as location, size and depth, relationship to adjacent structures, and the character of the surrounding mucosal pattern. Ulcers of the greater curvature are more frequently malignant. Size is of relatively little value, for small lesions may be carcinomatous and large craters are often benign. The meniscus sign of Carman, consisting of an ulcer crater located beneath the level of the lesser curvature and demarcated by a zone of tumefaction appearing as a halo, almost invariably denotes carcinoma, for benign craters usually extend beyond the lesser curvature (compare Figs. 110 and 112). The halo, however, may be seen in both lesions, owing either to inflammatory swelling and edema or carcinomatous infiltration, or both. The rugae about a benign ulcer tend to converge or radiate in a starlike fashion, whereas in a carcinomatous ulcer they may be abruptly interrupted. Benign craters are usually smooth or slightly irregular, whereas malignant craters tend to be ragged and markedly irregular, but exceptions of both types occur. And last, but not least, under suitable therapy the crater of the benign ulcer diminishes rapidly in size and disappears completely, whereas carcinomatous craters decrease slightly and rarely disappear completely.

The *gastroscopic interpretation*, like the roentgenogram, is of great differential value in skilled hands, but it is not infallible. "The benign ulcer," according to Schindler, "is generally crater-like, rarely shallow; its floor is whitish-yellow, not often brownish in color, although after an acute hemorrhage it may be dark red; its edges are sharp, often partly undermined. The adjacent mucosa in early lesions is often normal; later there may be marked inflammation of the surrounding mucosa but rarely of the entire stomach. Converging folds occur. The carcinomatous ulcer, however, is characterized by less sharp edges so that the ulcer floor seems to blend with the mucosa. The floor is irregular and contains nodules, nodes, or ridges. It is occasionally whitish or yellowish in color, but more frequently brown, brown-red, violet, gray or a dirty color. The malignant ulcer is usually elevated and appears to lie on a hill, thus differing further from the benign ulcer. The adjacent mucosa may be nodular."

The various criteria outlined must be carefully evaluated in the consideration of any given case. The evidence may be sufficient to justify either a definite or a presumptive diagnosis of neoplasm and hence to indicate treatment as such, or it may be adequate to warrant a tentative diagnosis of a benign ulcer and provisional medical management; but conclusive clinical proof that the lesion is benign is obtained only by the roentgenologic and gastroscopic demonstration of complete healing. A sharply circumscribed penetrating lesion of the lesser curvature occurring in a stomach known to secrete acid gastric juice may be treated medically if its course is carefully studied. Relief from pain and gain in weight are to be expected, and in themselves are not very reassuring, but continued distress may be significant. The occult blood should disappear from the stool in two or three weeks if the lesion is benign, and should continue if it is malignant, but exceptions occur. If roentgenologic and gastroscopic studies made at weekly or biweekly intervals show that the crater is decreasing rapidly in size, and if it appears benign, medical treatment may be continued in the expectation that complete healing will be demonstrable within a few weeks. If, on the other hand, it changes very little, or appears to be malignant, a presumptive diagnosis of carcinoma should be made, and subtotal gastrectomy be carried out.

Prognosis. The prognosis in peptic ulcer is excellent for the immediate attack, but poor for the future, in that recurrence is the rule. The course of the disease is characterized by remissions and exacerbations. The "cures" for peptic ulcer are therefore infinite in number, for it is easy to be misled by the "therapeutic fallacy" and draw the erroneous *"post hoc ergo propter hoc"* conclusion.

Treatment. *General Considerations.* The therapy of peptic ulcer is essentially medical; surgery, if indicated, is usually undertaken for the complications of ulcer, less frequently for the lesion itself. The problem may be divided into two distinct phases: first, the healing of the ulcer, and second, the prevention of recurrence. On the whole, the former is accomplished very much more easily than the latter. In fact, healing frequently occurs spontaneously. Medical treatment cannot actually heal an ulcer; it can only endeavor to create the best possible conditions for the process of healing and thus facilitate it. Nature heals the ulcer. Complete healing is present only when the defect is closed and covered with a normal glandular mucosa. It is not possible for the clinician to know when this has occurred, but obviously it is at least many weeks after the disappearance of pain, of occult blood from the stool, and the vanishing of the roentgenologic crater. Treatment should therefore be continued for several months.

A further reason for prolonged treatment is the recognized tendency of ulcers to recur at the same site or a different site even after complete healing has taken place and regardless of the type of medical or surgical treatment given.

Rest is essential in the treatment of many diseases; in ulcer it is valuable, but often difficult to obtain. The rest should be, if possible, both physical and mental, the latter being even more important than the former. Occasionally a hunting or fishing trip proves more restful than a period of bed rest. Vacations often bring clearer perspectives and better attitudes. The use of tobacco and alcohol is to be discouraged.

Psychotherapy is essential. As a rule, the superficial psychotherapy and encouragement incident to the medical program to be outlined are adequate. Frequently, sedatives such as phenobarbital and sodium bromide are of value. In certain cases formal psychiatric care, perhaps including detailed and prolonged psychoanalysis, may prove helpful, but, unaccompanied by other medical treatment, it is not adequate therapy even though a remission of symptoms ensues.

Hospitalization with proper management is usually preferable to a vacation in the treatment of ulcer. Meticulous attention to the detailed program of therapy to be described not only creates the best conditions for the healing of the ulcer, but is of great psychotherapeutic value in establishing the patient's confidence in himself, in his treatment and in his doctor. In the hospital the patient learns that his condition is not unique, that the program of treatment can be carried out, and learns how to do it. Two weeks of hospitalization or of rest in bed at home is usually the minimum period permissible. In difficult cases a month or six weeks may be much more satisfactory, and occasionally a period of six months is desirable. Bathroom privileges may be allowed. The course of the lesion during this time should be determined at intervals by roentgenologic or gastroscopic studies. If possible, the patient should be kept away from work until the crater has disappeared. He must understand that he is confronted with a twofold problem, the healing of an ulcer and the prevention of its recurrence, and that certain restrictions and regulations of his life will be in order for an indefinite period, perhaps for life.

Acid Neutralization. RATIONALE. Sippy was the first to develop a program of therapy based on the premise that "the greatest known hindrance to the healing of peptic ulcer that is amenable to medical or surgical control . . . is the disintegrating and digestive action of the gastric juice." Once this is removed, "Nature . . . fills in the defect with granulation tissue and cicatrization of the ulcer may occur approximately as rapidly as it does elsewhere on other surfaces of the body." In all essential respects subsequent investigations have corroborated the original concept of Sippy. If it were possible, practical and feasible to bring about complete and permanent gastric anacidity, there would be no ulcer problem. Unfortunately there is no satisfactory method of attaining this goal. The "Sippy treatment" aims, however, at "maintaining an accurate neutralization of all free hydrochloric acid during the time that food and its accompanying secretion are present in the stomach." This goal also is somewhat difficult to attain, and the continued secretion of acid gastric juice during the night is even more difficult to control than Sippy appreciated. Nevertheless, the rationale of the program is valid, and it will be presented with the modifications indicated as the most practical and satisfactory type of management.

Neutralization of the acid gastric juice is maintained by means of the acid-combining power of food proteins and by the acid-neutralizing capacity of various types of alkali. It is important to point out two facts: first, that all foods and liquids when ingested stimulate the secretion of gastric juice, water being one of the most effective; and second, that the slight quantitative differences in secretion induced by various foods, as worked out by Pavlov, are not of much practical importance. Fats inhibit gastric emptying and secretion, but this factor is not as important in maintaining neutralization of the gastric content as is the acid-combining property of protein food.

DIET. The customary schedule consists in the administration of 90 cc. of equal parts of whole milk and 18 per cent cream hourly from 7 A.M. to 7 P.M. The caloric intake and the taste may be modified as desired by increasing the hourly milk and cream feeding, by adding malt or chocolate syrup, or by substituting whole milk or even skim milk for the milk and cream. Many patients state that they are unable to take milk or milk and cream, but few, indeed, are actually unable to do so.

Small additional feedings of soft foods may be given with or substituted for the milk and cream, beginning on the first day of treatment or a few days later. A good program is to begin with one feeding on the second or third day and add one every other day until six are being given. Orange juice and other fruit juices may be given as desired and often help to relieve the initial distaste for milk and antacid.

The gradual increase in the additional feedings has a definite psychologic value in that it enables the patient to see progress from day to day. In some instances, particularly in moderate obstruction, the six feedings may be too much and a three-feeding schedule may be maintained to advantage for several weeks, provided the caloric intake is adequate. Ordinarily the patient will be ready some time in the third week to resume a three-meal schedule. The hourly milk and cream should be continued between meals together with the antacid powders. The milk and cream may be omitted after the evening meal although the powders should be taken hourly until bedtime. Neutralizing food or medication is indicated during the night only if pain appears.

The diet consists of a fairly generous breakfast, with dinner at noon and a light supper not exceeding 400 or 500 cc. in total bulk. The average caloric and vitamin intake on the three-meal ulcer management program is adequate, but additional supplementary vitamins may be prescribed if desired. The patient is expected to follow the program outlined for a year or more, reporting to the office or clinic at monthly intervals for such changes as may be needed, for roentgenologic examinations, or for other subsequent studies as indicated.

ANTACIDS. Alkalis of various types, especially calcium carbonate, have been used in the treatment of indigestion from time immemorial. It may be used in hourly doses of 2 to 4 gm. Magnesium carbonate (2 gm.) powders may be substituted for the calcium as needed to regulate bowel function. Some patients do not require any magnesia powders; others require three, four or more. If too many are given, diarrhea and abdominal cramps ensue; if too few are taken, fecal impactions in the rectum or sigmoid may result. Aluminum hydroxide must be used in rather large amounts (30 cc. doses) if satisfactory neutralization is to be maintained.

The alkali should be given hourly during the day with/or between the feedings of milk and cream and should be continued until bedtime. The effectiveness of the antacid used in each case may be checked by determining the degree of neutralization in the gastric content obtained in samples aspirated at various times during the day.

ASPIRATION OF THE STOMACH. The routine gastric aspiration at bedtime decreases the period during which the ulcer is exposed to the action of the acid gastric content and affords valuable evidence regarding the rate of gastric emptying. As a rule, aspiration is not so important in gastric ulcer or in nonstenosing duodenal ulcer as it is in pyloric or duodenal lesions with marked narrowing of the channel, but occasionally nonobstructive lesions are associated with retention, due presumably to pylorospasm, hypertrophic stenosis of the pylorus, or to some disturbance in the reflex opening mechanism.

CONTROL OF THE NIGHT SECRETION. In patients with duodenal ulcer the stomach usually continues to secrete excessive quantities of highly acid gastric juice during the night; this secretion constitutes a hindrance to healing, occasionally prevents healing, and is difficult to control. In some patients the milk, cream and powder schedule may be continued through the night, or a continuous drip therapy be used.

CONTINUOUS DRIP THERAPY. The administration of food or antacid, or both, by means of a continuous drip through a nasal catheter has certain advantages as well as disadvantages. The feeding is in effect a fistula feeding, thus eliminating the important cephalic phase of gastric secretion. The Winkelstein formula consists of 1 liter of milk containing 5 gm. of sodium bicarbonate every 8 hours. Satisfactory neutralization can be maintained throughout the day and night. It is, as a rule, not feasible to continue this procedure for more than a week or two, after which a careful program should be followed. The disadvantage consists chiefly in the discomfort induced by the presence of the nasal catheter and the difficulty of adjusting the drip properly.

Complications of Antacid Therapy. ALKALOSIS. The term "alkalosis" is applied to an alteration of the electrolytes of the blood serum characterized by an elevation of the carbon dioxide content and the pH. The increase in the carbon dioxide is accompanied by a corresponding decrease in the chloride. Alkalosis may be produced by the administration of soluble alkali (sodium bicarbonate), in which case there is also an elevation of the fixed base (sodium) in the serum, or by depletion of chloride (low intake of salt, vomiting, aspiration of the stomach), in which case the fixed base of the serum is not elevated, but is, in fact, lowered. Since sodium bicarbonate is no longer prescribed as an antacid,

the first type of alkalosis is seen almost exclusively in persons who have acquired the "baking soda" habit. The second type is seen in patients with continued vomiting from obstruction at the outlet of the stomach, both benign and malignant, and in patients receiving frequent or continuous gastric aspiration.

In both types of alkalosis the kidney is not primarily involved even through there is a rise in the blood urea nitrogen and a decrease in renal function. The initial symptoms of alkalosis are loss of appetite with distaste for the milk and cream and powders. Nausea and vomiting may ensue. Weakness and lassitude may be marked, often accompanied by a dull headache and slight clouding of the sensorium. Tetany is rarely seen. Moderate alkalosis may be present without symptoms. Burnett and his associates have described an interesting syndrome with hypercalcemia without hypercalciuria but with renal insufficiency and calcinosis in patients with excessive intakes of milk and absorbable alkali over long periods of time.

Treatment consists in the discontinuance of alkali, if this is being given, and the administration orally or parenterally of large amounts of fluid and chloride. In mild cases, or as a prophylactic procedure, 5 to 10 gm. of sodium or ammonium chloride may be given daily in pills or capsules. Sodium chloride, 3 to 5 gm., may be added to the daily ration of milk and cream. More intensive therapy may be administered intravenously or subcutaneously. Sodium chloride in the form of a normal saline solution may be used in amounts of 1500 to 4000 cc. daily. Hypertonic saline should not be prescribed because sodium retention results in fluid retention. This may be sufficient to cause pitting edema; indeed, death may ensue from cerebral edema. Ammonium chloride is preferable and may be given safely intravenously as a 2 per cent solution in distilled water or in normal saline. The serum carbon dioxide is lowered at the approximate rate of one volume per cent for each gram of ammonium chloride. The results of treatment should be checked by daily determinations of the serum carbon dioxide, chloride and pH.

BOWEL DISTRESS. Abdominal distress during ulcer management is usually attributable to a functional disturbance resulting from improper regulation of the bowels. The powders and the diet should be manipulated in such a fashion as to produce daily formed stools.

FECAL IMPACTIONS. Special attention must be given to regulation of the bowels to prevent the formation of rectal or sigmoidal impactions of feces. This is best accomplished by alternating the calcium and magnesium powders until a mild diarrhea is produced and then determining just how many magnesium powders are required to maintain normal bowel function. When impactions form, they must be broken up digitally at once and removed manually or with large enemas. At times the rectum is filled with soft putty-like material which the patient is unable to expel. The enemas and rectal examinations should be continued until the rectum is proved to be empty. In rare instances a large calcium stool may lodge in the sigmoid, and the clinical picture of paralytic ileus develops. Watchful waiting with the application of hot stupes or an electric pad to the abdomen and, if necessary, the use of a Wagensteen or Miller-Abbott tube for the relief of the nausea, vomiting and distention, is rewarded in a day or two by the passage of the stool into the rectum, at which time it can be removed manually. Warm oil retention enemas may be helpful, but repeated large water or soapsuds enemas are likely to produce further distention of the abdomen without bringing the fecal mass down into the rectum.

RENAL AND UNRETERAL CALCULI. There is no satisfactory statistical proof that this complication is seen in greater than the normal frequency in patients receiving antacid therapy. Theoretically and practically there seems to be no contraindication to the use of the nonabsorbable salts of calcium, magnesium and aluminum.

ACUTE APPENDICITIS. This complication of antacid therapy is seen so frequently that the possibility must always be considered, although there is no statistical evidence that it occurs in greater than the anticipated frequency.

Inhibitory Drugs. BELLADONNA AND ATROPINE have long been used in the treatment of ulcer, and do inhibit, to a certain extent, gastric peristalsis thereby making possible neutralization of gastric acidity with smaller amounts of alkali. The development of more potent "cholinergic blocking agents" capable of inhibiting gastric secretion for prolonged periods after oral administration without disturbing side effects would be of great value. Belladonna and atropine in ordinary amounts have little or no influence upon gastric secretion in man. In recent years more potent drugs have been developed. The clinical usefulness of tetraethylammonium chloride or bromide and of the hexamethonium salts is limited by the side reactions. Banthine, a widely used drug, does reduce gastric secretion when administred intramuscularly but it is far less effective when taken by mouth; side effects are frequent and often uncomfortable. Many new preparations are undergoing clinical trial. Prantal, though well tolerated and inhibiting gastrointestinal motility, does not appear to influence significantly gastric secretion in patients with duodenal ulcer. The more recent compounds— Pamine, Pro-banthine, Monadral and Antrenyl—suppress gastric secretion after oral administration more effectively than earlier anticholinergic drugs. Thus far it has not been possible to dissociate completely the inhibitory effects on gastric motility and secretion and the systemic parasympathetic disagreeable or even severe side reactions such as blurring of vision, dryness of the mouth and difficulty in micturition. Although the ideal gastric antisecretory drug remains to be developed, some progress seems to have been made toward this ultimate objective. The currently available preparations are helpful adjuncts to the total therapeutic program.

X-ray Therapy. Radiation therapy is helpful as a means of inhibiting gastric secretion and thus facilitating healing. The radiation should be directed at the fundus and body of the stomach. The effect is variable and, as a rule, not permanent. If a phase of complete achlorhydria is produced, partial or complete healing invariably occurs, the degree depending apparently on the reparative ability of the tissue and the duration of the achlorhydria. Treatment is given daily for ten days through alternating anterior and posterior portals 13 by 13 cm., using 200 KvP, 20 ma., 1 mm. Cu plus 1 mm. Al filtration, HVL 1.5 mm. Cu, FSD 50 cm. The amount given is calculated to achieve a daily depth dose of 165 r in the gastric fundus; the total depth dose desired is 1650 r.

Surgery. Although uncomplicated peptic ulcer rarely requires surgical treatment, there are definite indications for certain surgical procedures. In some benign gastric ulcers the evidence suggesting malignancy is sufficiently great to warrant subtotal gastrectomy as the treatment of choice. In others the continued recurrence of the lesion under medical management justifies resection. The incidence of recurrent ulcer after subtotal gastrectomy for gastric ulcer is almost nil. Uncomplicated duodenal ulcer should not be treated by gastric resection because the incidence of recurrence is at least 10 to 12 per cent, probably higher; likewise gastroenterostomy is not indicated because of the great frequency of recurrent jejunal ulcer.

Dragstedt must be credited with a new surgical approach to the treatment of peptic ulcer —i.e., transthoracic or transabdominal *supraphrenic* section of both vagi. This procedure completely eliminates the cephalic phase of gastric secretion, markedly reduces the "night" or fasting secretion, and reduces the rate of gastric emptying. If there is stenosis of any significant grade, as is usually the case in patients with duodenal ulcer referred to surgery, the impairment of gastric emptying is increased by the procedure; hence it is advisable to perform a gastroenterostomy along with the vagotomy. If this is not done, abnormal gastric retention may result in the belching of foul-smelling gas or in diarrhea. In some patients—the exact number is as yet unknown, but perhaps between 10 and 35 per cent—the vagotomy is not complete as judged by the insulin test. In such persons the fasting secretion is not reduced; hence the desired result is not achieved.

Complications. *Perforations.* ACUTE PERFORATION. Acute perforation is the most dangerous complication of peptic ulcer and accounts for 65 to 85 per cent of the deaths from this disease.

DESCRIPTION. Moynihan's description of the clinical picture is superb:

The picture is so characteristic that error is hardly possible. . . . For the agony suffered by the patient is almost beyond belief, and is written on every line of a face that speaks of torture. The face is pale, haggard, anxious and appealing, the eyes wide and watchful, the brow and temples bathed in sweat, the hair soaked. The patient struggles for breath in short, panting respirations which are wholly costal, for the diaphragm, being an abdominal muscle, is fixed. Words spoken are jerked out in expiration only; every syllable is part of a deep moan. What strikes every onlooker is that the patient's body is rigid and motionless, no slightest movement dare be attempted. If an endeavor is made to touch the abdomen, the patient's hands are at once lifted in protest and in protection, but the chest and abdomen stay motionless. When examination is made, it is realized at once that the patient is cold; and the temperature will rarely be found more than 95° or 96° F. The abdomen is immobile, and the muscles are taut and rigid: "hard as a board" it is said, but if there is anything harder, it is the abdomen in this

time of catastrophe. A further examination of the abdomen will almost always show an area of greater tenderness and if possible, of added rigidity over the area involved in stomach or duodenum.

When the pulse is examined a great surprise is felt, for it is not increased in frequency nor diminished in volume, blood pressure is not diminished, and in a few cases that we have examined the blood volume is unchanged. There is, therefore, no "shock." . . . Shock is never a symptom of perforation. It is a symptom of peritonitis, which follows quickly upon leakage from the stomach or duodenum. In the patient's interest, no less than in the service of truth, we must discharge the word "shock" from its use in this connection.

The period of initial profound prostration varies in different patients and may be ascribed to variations in the size of the perforation, the character of escaping contents—especially in respect to acidity —the general condition of the patient and so forth. Within an hour or two it is followed by a period of reaction, characterized by an improvement in the appearance of the patient, pallor being replaced by flushing, lines of anxiety being smoothed away, and the body growing warmer. But the pulse steadily rises, the rigid abdomen becomes fuller and since the diaphragm is being pushed higher, respirations become shallower. . . . Fluids leaking from the stomach tend to trickle down to the right iliac fossa and to overflow into the pelvis. So there may be acute pain or tenderness in the right iliac fossa, and a careless diagnosis of appendicitis may be made. It is in this stage that the "absence of liver dullness" upon which so high a value has long been placed will be recognized. It is almost valueless. I very rarely percuss the abdomen, and I have been amused to see the liver percussed when it could be felt!

In untreated patients, generalized peritonitis usually ensues; the abdomen loses its "boardlike" character, but not its rigidity or tenderness; it becomes distended; the pulse becomes gradually rapid, weak, feeble; the respirations become more rapid and shallow; Hippocratic facies appears, and the patient dies the typical peritonitic death in the course of two to five days.

DIFFERENTIAL DIAGNOSIS. The differential diagnosis of acute perforation is rarely difficult. An "ulcer history" is present in 60 to 75 per cent of the cases. Biliary, renal and intestinal colic lack the boardlike rigidity. Perforation of the gallbladder, however, is usually indistinguishable from that of the stomach or duodenum except for the fact that it typically occurs during or after the apparent subsidence of an attack of acute cholecystitis. In coronary thrombosis not only is the rigidity absent, but usually there is some radiation of the pain to the precordium, sternum, neck or arms. In lobar pneumonia the temperature is elevated and the respiratory rate is increased. In the gastric crisis of tabes dorsalis the abdominal rigidity is absent; Argyll Robertson pupils are usually present. The onset of acute appendicitis is less sudden, the rigidity is less intense, the tenderness is most marked over McBurney's point. In mesenteric occlusion and intestinal obstruction the pain is rhythmical and intermittent, and the rigidity less intense. In ruptured ectopic pregnancy the pain and tenderness are in the lower abdomen, and the rigidity is only moderate.

The most difficult differentiation is that of acute pancreatitis. If the patient is a woman, the diagnosis of acute pancreatitis is much more probable, because 98 per cent of acute perforations in peptic ulcer occur in the male. Disease of the biliary tract is usually present in acute pancreatitis, but there may be no history of biliary colic. Marked shock is almost always present. The abdominal rigidity is not so intense or widespread, nor the tenderness so complete. Jaundice of slight degree is present in about one-half the cases, and often, at an early stage, the patient has a characteristic slate-blue tinge of color seen most distinctly in the lips, in the lobes of the ears, in the face and in the fingernails. The serum amylase during an attack is almost invariably elevated markedly, well above 500 Somogyi units.

TREATMENT. The urgent indication in acute perforation is immediate operation. Spontaneous closure does occur, but operation should never be deferred in the hope that it may take place. The earlier the operation, the better the prognosis, for few patients die if the operation is carried out within 10 or 12 hours. Rarely, when the patient is first seen several hours after the onset of symptoms and, from the rapid subsidence of the pain, the sharp localization of the tenderness and rigidity, and the excellent condition of the patient, it is apparent that spontaneous closure has already occurred, surgery may be deferred and the patient treated by starvation for two or three days before instituting ulcer management. In the vast majority of cases, however, operation should be performed at once.

In *subacute perforation* the clinical picture is similar but less intense. Spontaneous closure of the defect may occur as a result of fibrinous adhesions to omentum, liver, pancreas or other structure, and recovery ensue without surgical intervention. These so-called "formes frustes" perforations are more frequent than is generally recognized.

In *chronic perforation* the base of the ulcer is usually formed by the capsule of the pancreas or liver; rarely is the parenchyma of these organs attacked. Chronic perforation is of little clinical significance except when a gastrojejunocolic fistula is produced.

In *peptic ulcer of the esophagus,* perforation of an acute, subacute or chronic type may take place into the mediastinum, pleura or pericardium.

Massive Hemorrhage. DEFINITION. Massive hemorrhage may be defined as the vomiting of gross blood or the passage of tarry stools. The bleeding may be of all grades of severity, from the 60 cc. required to give a tarry stool without symptoms, to several hundred cubic centimeters resulting in severe collapse and even rapid death.

MORBID ANATOMY. Fatal hemorrhage is almost invariably arterial in origin, the pancreaticoduodenal, the gastric coronary or one of their main branches being eroded.

INCIDENCE. Probably 20 to 25 per cent of all patients with peptic ulcer experience massive bleeding at some time or other.

The MORTALITY RATE varies from 1.5 to 20 per cent or higher. It rises with age, being at least four times higher in patients over 50 than it is in patients under 50. It does not rise materially with recurring hemorrhages.

SYMPTOMS AND DIAGNOSIS. Since peptic ulcer is the most frequent source of hemorrhage in the digestive tract, it should be suspected in every case regardless of the presence or absence of pain. In gastric ulcer, hematemesis is usually present as well as melena; in duodenal ulcer it occurs in about one fourth of the cases. The patients usually give a history of epigastric distress of the ulcer type, but there may be no distress whatsoever at the time of hemorrhage or, indeed, previously.

The symptoms are faintness, weakness, dizziness, headache, perspiration, thirst, dyspnea, syncope and collapse, the severity depending largely upon the suddenness and severity of hemorrhage and the resultant rapid drop in blood pressure. Usually the vasomotor system regains its tone rapidly and the blood pressure rises, but in severe hemorrhage it remains low, the pulse more or less gradually increases in rate, and the patient continues in shock. The more marked and persistent the drop in the blood pressure and the more rapid and weak the pulse, the greater is the danger. In the first few hours the blood counts may be normal except for the moderate leukocytosis of hemorrhage. The drop in the red cell count and in the hemoglobin appears later as the total blood volume is restored by dilution. A moderate azotemia occurs owing to the absorption of protein from the blood in the intestine, the dehydration, and to decreased renal function as a consequence of the drop in the blood pressure.

PROGNOSIS. Recovery is the rule, but death may occur at any time, usually two to five days after the onset of symptoms, and results either from exsanguination or from intercurrent complications, such as pneumonia or perforation.

TREATMENT. The time-honored therapy in massive hemorrhage is bed rest, elevation of the foot of the bed, application of an ice-bag to the epigastrium, morphine in doses adequate to quiet the restlessness, and complete starvation for several days. Immediate feeding has been found to be superior to starvation. Blood transfusions allay the restlessness; hence morphine is rarely necessary. The blood pressure and the pulse rate should be watched carefully, readings being taken at hourly or half-hourly intervals. The blood count does not usually drop until several hours after the initial hemorrhage and hence is not as good an index of the severity of the bleeding as are the blood pressure and the pulse rate.

Blood transfusion is indicated when the pulse rate exceeds 120 per minute and the blood pressure drops below 90 or even 100 mm. of mercury. When the bleeding takes place slowly and continuously, the pulse rate and blood pressure may not reach these levels, and yet transfusion may be indicated because of the anemia. If the erythrocyte count is below 3,000,000 cells per cubic millimeter, transfusion is desirable; if it is below 2,000,000 cells, transfusion is imperative. Many patients recover spontaneously from such levels, but their margin of safety is narrow, and a relatively small hemorrhage may prove fatal. The blood should be matched most meticulously. Each transfusion should consist of 500 or 600 cc. of whole blood, and as many should be given as are necessary. The greater the number of transfusions required, the graver the prognosis, not because the transfusions are harmful, but because the great need for them constitutes evidence that a large vessel is bleeding.

Starvation is indicated only if the patient is vomiting, in which case it should be continued until this has subsided and the patient desires food. Dryness of the mouth may be relieved by cracked ice and by the daily subcutaneous (*not* intravenous) administration of small amounts (1000 to 1500 cc.) of normal saline with or without glucose. Occasionally, if the lesion, from previous roentgenologic examinations, is known to be duodenal and accompanied by considerable stenosis, starvation may be combined with continuous aspiration of the stomach through a Wangensteen tube. A surprising amount of highly acid gastric juice may be obtained. If the bleeding ceases promptly, the procedure may be continued.

Feeding and antacid ulcer management are, in the absence of vomiting, preferable to starvation. Milk and cream in equal parts, or whole milk, may be given in amounts varying from 30 to 120 cc., usually 90 cc., hourly from 7 A.M. to 10 P.M., and at 2-hour intervals through the night. Calcium carbonate, 2 gm., should be given hourly from 7:30 A.M. to 9:30 P.M. or on the hour with the milk, and during the night with the milk in 4 gm. doses, waking the patient if necessary. A sufficient number of powders of magnesium carbonate in doses of 2 gm., usually totaling 2 to 10 gm. daily, must be substituted for the calcium carbonate to prevent rectal impactions.

This progam is continued until the stools have been negative for occult blood by the benzidine test for at least two or three days and until the patient's general condition is good, at which time roentgenologic and gastroscopic examinations are in order to determine the location, nature and extent of the lesion, and the complications present. Aspiration of the stomach may then be carried out safely. If the occult blood in the stool does not disappear in the course of two or three weeks and if the patient is in good condition, the roentgenologic examination should not be further deferred. The risk of the procedure, if carefully carried out, is small, and it may be found that the bleeding lesion is not a benign ulcer, but a frank neoplasm, or varices of the esophagus.

Surgical treatment may be indicated in certain cases. Usually by the time the need for ligation of the artery has become apparent, the patient has become a poor operative risk and hence surgical intervention is further deferred. It may be difficult to find the bleeding vessel at operation and to deal with it adequately if found. There is evidence that immediate surgical treatment undertaken routinely in all cases of hematemesis and melena would increase rather than lower the mortality rate. On the other hand, it is possible to select the patients with rapid continued bleeding and to benefit them by surgical treatment. Gastroenterostomy alone is not effective. The bleeding vessel must be ligated. Subtotal gastrectomy may be advisable. In patients with recurring massive hemorrhage subtotal gastrectomy may be indicated after recovery as prophylaxis against further bleeding, although ulcer and massive hemorrhage do recur after this type of therapy as well as after other forms of medical and surgical treatment.

Acute Perforation and Massive Hemorrhage. These are, as a rule, independent complications of peptic ulcer. About 10 per cent of the acute perforations occur in patients who have experienced massive hemorrhage. Occasionally the two complications occur within a few days of each other.

Obstruction. DEFINITION. The term "obstruction," referring to obstruction to the passage of food from the stomach to the intestine, is loosely used. It is often applied to persistent vomiting, or the vomiting of food eaten the previous day, or the failure of the stomach to empty properly as evidenced by abnormal gastric retention of food or barium. The terms "obstruction" and "retention" are thus confused; they are not synonymous. Retention may be present in the absence of gastric disease. Obstruction *per se* may be due to spasm of the pylorus, to edema and inflammatory swelling about a pyloric or duodenal ulcer, to cicatricial stenosis or to a combination of these factors.

DIAGNOSIS. The mere retention of food or barium in the stomach for abnormal periods is not direct evidence of obstruction unless the retention is extreme. If food is retained in the stomach for 24 hours, as may be demonstrated by the vomiting of food taken the day previously, obstruction is almost always present.

The roentgenogram affords, on the whole, the most valuable evidence of obstruction, for it permits determination of the site of the lesion and usually of its nature, and also discloses the site of the obstruction, its nature, and the degree of stenosis. Pylorospasm, although it may occur with an ulcer at any point in the stomach or duodenum, is usually not important unless the lesion is intrapyloric. If the pyloric obstruction is due to a hypertrophic stenosis of the pylorus, surgical relief will frequently be required. Usually, however, the lesion is duodenal in location, and the question to be answered is the degree of cicatricial stenosis present. Often this cannot be settled until the initial spasm, edema and inflammatory swelling have subsided after a few days or even a few weeks of treatment. The lumen of the normal duodenal bulb has a diameter of 2 to 3 cm. If this is decreased to 5 or 10 mm., the stenosis is moderate; if to 2 to 4 mm., the stenosis is marked; and if the lumen is decreased to a hair line or to a diameter of 1 mm., the stenosis is high grade, usually accompanied by gastric dilatation, ballooning of the antrum, and hyperperistalsis. The maximum width of the channel should be determined fluoroscopically, not from the film, for the film may be exposed at the moment the muscle is in contraction, thus suggesting a much more marked stenosis than is actually present.

TREATMENT. Obstruction is the most frequent *indication for surgical treatment* in peptic ulcer. The term is relative, as has been pointed out previously; hence the indication is relative. In general, it is wise to try the effect of medical management for ten or fourteen days before arriving at a decision, for Sippy's original estimate that in 85 per cent of the cases the obstruction is due to spasm or inflammation is approximately correct.

The *location* and *nature of the obstruction* are important considerations. In duodenal ulcer, operation is definitely not indicated for obstruction if the maximum lumen through the deformity, as seen roentgenologically, is over 1 cm. in diameter; usually not if the lumen is over 4 or 5 mm. in diameter; and on the other hand, usually is indicated if the maximum lumen is less than 3 mm. in diameter. The width of the channel usually persists relatively unchanged as the ulcer heals; occasionally it increases; rarely does it decrease. In intrapyloric or prepyloric ulcer the obstruction and retention may decrease rapidly under management, or it may persist. The retention occasionally seen with ulcers of the lesser curvature of the stomach and due presumably to pylorospasm, disturbance of the neuromuscular reflex or associated hypertrophic stenosis of the pylorus, may be persistent and warrant surgical intervention.

Depending upon the surgeon and the conditions present, the *operation of choice* for obstruction is posterior gastroenterostomy, although some surgeons prefer a primary subtotal gastrectomy. The initial ulcers almost invariably heal after operation; the difficulty is to be found in the development of new ulcers later at the new stoma or in the stomach. Statistics on the *incidence of recurrent ulceration* vary, roughly, from 2 to 40 per cent. Subtotal gastrectomy results in a lower incidence of recurrence, although the initial mortality rate is higher. At the present time the procedure of choice appears to be posterior gastroenterostomy combined with supraphrenic vagotomy carried out through the abdominal incision by pulling the esophagus and the vagi down through the diaphragm sufficiently to permit section of the nerves. Regardless of the type of surgical procedure to be used, constant vigilance must be exercised to control dehydration, alkalosis with tetany and inanition.

Hour-glass contracture of the stomach usually results from longstanding chronic gastric ulcer, although a type of hour-glass deformity is seen in certain cases of carcinoma, lues and diaphragmatic herniation. It is a strange fact that hour-glass contracture is eight or nine times more frequent in females than it is in males. The incisura is sharp and narrow, involving the greater curvature almost exclusively and drawing it toward a point on the lesser curvature at which there may or may not be seen a penetrating ulcer of variable size, usually rather small.

The history is, as a rule, of many years' duration. Medical treatment usually suffices.

JEJUNAL ULCER

With the exception of the uncommon ulcer of Meckel's diverticulum and the rare primary ulcer of the jejunum associated with ectopic gastric mucosa, peptic jejunal ulcer is a complication of gastroenterostomy.

Incidence. Statistics vary greatly as to the incidence of the lesion, some authors reporting it to be as low as 1 or 2 per cent, while others find it as high as 40 per cent. The latter figure is more correct. Ulcer develops in a certain number of cases irrespective of the type of gastroenterostomy performed, irrespective of the type of anastomosis made, and irrespective of the suture material used. Jejunal ulcer is definitely less frequent after subtotal gastrectomy than it is after gastroenterostomy alone, and it is less frequent when the procedure is carried out for gastric ulcer than it is when carried out for duodenal ulcer. Jejunal ulcer practically never follows gastroenterostomy for gastric carcinoma.

Symptoms. The symptoms of recurrent jejunal ulcer resemble those of primary gastric or duodenal ulcer, although the relationship of the distress to food taking is likely to be less definite and the pain usually is referred to the left midabdomen or even to the left lower quadrant. Massive hemorrhage occurs frequently. Acute perforation is rare. Chronic perforation is common, particularly into the colon, producing even without pain a gastrojejunocolic fistula and severe diarrhea.

Diagnosis. Recurrent abdominal distress in a patient with a gastroenterostomy always suggests the presence of jejunal ulcer. Usually the lesion can be demonstrated roentgenologically; infrequently it can be seen gastroscopically also.

Treatment. Medical treatment is difficult. If it is undertaken, the course of the lesion should be followed closely by roentgenogram and gastroscopy. Surgical treatment is usually to be preferred, and in the case of gastrojejunocolic fistula is imperative. The gastroenterostomy may be simply undone, provided the channel through the bulb is adequate. A new duodenal ulcer may then develop. If a second gastroenterostomy is made at the time the first one is undone, a new jejunal ulcer is likely to develop. If subtotal gastrectomy is performed, the mortality rate is somewhat higher than it is for primary resection and there is a fair likelihood of recurrence after resection, for these are among the so-called "intractable" ulcers. The treatment of jejunal ulcers developing after resection is most difficult. It is in this group of patients that the most dramatic results of vagotomy have been seen.

POSTGASTRECTOMY SYNDROME
(Dumping Syndrome)

After partial or complete gastrectomy some patients develop the so-called "dumping syndrome" attributed, as Machella has shown, to the rapid emptying of the gastric stump and the resulting presence in the jejunum of irritating hypertonic solutions. The symptoms consist of faintness, weakness, warmth, sweating, nausea, palpitation, vertigo and collapse. They are not emotional in origin, but are due apparently to poorly understood reflex mechanisms. The pulse and blood pressure are usually moderately elevated. The symptoms vary greatly in severity, being scarcely recognizable in some individuals and in others completely incapacitating. The supine position usually affords partial or complete relief except in the severe cases in which vomiting is present. The syndrome may occur after gastroenterostomy alone, without resection, or it may be produced in the normal individual by the injection into the jejunum of sufficient amounts of hypertonic solution. Loss of weight occurs in the great majority of the patients often producing a difficult nutritional problem. The feces may be abnormally soft, even watery, containing excessive amounts of fat, protein and starch indicative of hypermotility.

In the milder forms treatment may be effective, but in the more severe instances nothing seems to avail. A simple gastroenterostomy may be undone; after partial gastrectomy a Bilroth I anastomosis may be feasible and may afford relief. Medical management consists of postprandial rest, a diet relatively high in proteins taken in frequent small feedings of dry foods, fluids between meals, sedatives and antispasmodics. Cortisone has not been found to be of value.

POSTVAGOTOMY SYNDROME

The introduction of vagotomy without the so-called drainage operations, gastroenterostomy with or without partial gastrectomy, was followed by the development in certain patients of symptoms attributable to continued gastric stasis: belching of foul-smelling gas, abdominal distention, occasionally nausea and vomiting, and more frequently diarrhea. These symptoms may be present in spite of marked gain in weight. Treatment with Urecholine may be satisfactory. The stomach tends to gradually regain its tone, motility and a satisfactory ability to empty, even though roentgen studies may show prolonged gastric retention after an indefinite number of months or years. If a stenosing duodenal lesion is present, gastroenterostomy is indicated; if not, time and patience will usually result in a spontaneous symptomatic recovery.

The addition of a gastroenterostomy or a partial gastrectomy to the vagotomy procedure may result in a combined dumping syndrome and postvagotomy state. The features of the dumping syndrome usually dominate the picture and require the appropriate treatment.

WALTER L. PALMER

References

Bonney, G. L. W., and Pickering, G. W.: Observations on the Mechanism of Pain in Ulcer of the Stomach and Duodenum. I. The Nature of the Stimulus. II. The Location of the Pain Nerve Endings. Clinical Science, 6:65, 91, 1946.

Dragstedt, L. R., and Woodward, E. R.: Appraisal of Vagotomy for Peptic Ulcer After Seven Years. J.A.M.A., 145:795–802, 1951.

Hurst, A. F., and Stewart, J.: Gastric and Duodenal Ulcer. London, Oxford University Press, 1929.

Ivy, A. C., Grossman, M. I., and Bachrach, W. H.: Peptic Ulcer. Philadelphia, The Blakiston Company, 1950.

Konjetzny, G. E.: Die entzündliche Grundlage der typischen Geschwürsbildung im Magen und Duodenum. Berlin, Julius Springer, 1930.

Machella, T. E.: Mechanism of the Post-Gastrectomy Dumping Syndrome. Gastroenterology, 14:237, 1950.

Portis, S. A.: Diseases of the Digestive System. 3rd Ed. Philadelphia, Lea & Febiger, 1953.

Report of the Committee on Surgical Procedures of the National Committee on Peptic Ulcer of the Amercian Gastroenterological Association. Gastroenterology, 22:297, 1952; 24:275, 1953.

Ricketts, W. E., Palmer, W. L., Kirsner, J. B., and Hamann, A.: Radiation Therapy in Peptic Ulcer. Gastroenterology, 11:789, 1948.

Sandweiss, D. J., Editor: Peptic Ulcer. Philadelphia, W. B. Saunders Company, 1951.

Sippy, B. W.: Oxford Medicine. New York, Oxford University Press, 1923, Vol. 3, p. 132.

Smith, L. A., and Rivers, A. B.: Peptic Ulcer. New York, Appleton-Century-Crofts, Inc., 1953.

Templeton, F. E.: X-ray Examination of the Stomach. Chicago, University of Chicago Press, 1944.

Wolf, S., and Wolff, H. G.: Human Gastric Function, An Experimental Study of a Man and His Stomach. New York, Oxford University Press, 1943.

DISEASES OF THE INTESTINES

DISEASES OF THE DUODENUM

Peptic ulcer is the most frequent affection of the duodenum. It usually appears in the first portion, the so-called duodenal bulb; it occurs rather often at the junction of the first and second portions; occasionally it develops in the upper part of the second portion of the duodenum and rarely as far down as the ampulla of Vater. Lesions occurring beyond this point are not simple peptic ulcers (see Peptic Ulcer).

Duodenitis is a term applied to a nonspecific inflammation usually seen anatomically as a part of the erosive gastritis of Konjetzny, a gastroduodenitis. Clinically, the diagnosis of duodenitis is made at times in patients who give a history of epigastric distress of the ulcer type and in whom the roentgenologist finds a duodenal cap which fills and empties rapidly, seems "irritable" and rather fuzzy in outline, but without definite deformity or crater formation. Not infrequently in such persons an ulcer crater or deformity is found months or years later. It is probable that the process represents an early phase of the acid attack on the mucosa and that the basic problem, therefore, is that of peptic ulcer (see Peptic Ulcer).

Diverticula of the duodenum may be divided into those occurring in the bulb and those in the remainder of the duodenum. The former are invariably secondary to peptic ulcer and do not cause symptoms. Diverticula of the second, third and fourth portions are usually considered as congenital, but the mechanism of their formation is not known; they are often found accidentally by roentgenogram and bear no relationship to the symptomatology present unless, as occurs rarely, they become the site of infection and inflammation.

Carcinoma of the first portion of the duodenum is a great rarity, scarcely more than a dozen cases having been reported in the medical literature of the world. In the other portions of the duodenum, however, the lesion is not uncommon (see Intestinal Neoplasms).

Stricture of the duodenum may occur at any level, most frequently in the first portion as a result of peptic ulcer. Congenital strictures usually involve the second portion, are often complete, and cause the death of the infant within a short time unless recognized and treated surgically. Extremely rare cases have been reported of incomplete congenital stricture discovered in adult life and producing intermittent attacks of nausea and vomiting. Duodenal obstruction may be produced also by external adhesions such as those resulting from an adhesive tuberculous peritonitis, severe cholecystitis, or neoplasm of the biliary tract.

Duodenal stasis is a term applied to instances in which considerable to-and-fro churning or "puddling" of barium with reverse peristalsis is seen roentgenologically in the second portion of the duodenum. It is a normal variant found most typically in lean, lanky persons with long abdomens.

Mesenteric duodenal ileus is a rare condition in which the third portion of the duodenum, caught between the spine posteriorly and the mesenteric vessels anteriorly, becomes partially or completely obstructed. The duodenum is enormously dilated. The symptoms are those of high intestinal obstruction with continued upper abdominal distress, nausea and vomiting, and loss of weight.

WALTER L. PALMER

References

Bockus, H. L.: Gastro-enterology. Philadelphia, W. B. Saunders Company, 1943–1946.

Kellogg, E. L.: The Duodenum. New York, Paul B. Hoeber, Inc., 1933.

VISCEROPTOSIS

(Splanchnoptosis, Glénard's Disease)

This is a term applied to prolapse or "falling" of the various viscera. It is not a disease entity, but rather a manifestation of a lean, lank body build with more or less relaxation of the abdominal wall. The stomach and transverse colon may extend down to the brim of the pelvis. Only two organs are ever affected seriously by ptosis: (1) the kidney with resulting attacks of Dietl's crisis, and

(2) rarely, indeed, the spleen, which has been known to become strangulated in the pelvis.

WALTER L. PALMER

DIARRHEA

Definition. Diarrhea consists in the evacuation of watery or unformed stools. It may be acute or chronic. It is a symptom present in many disorders and diseases; hence all cases should be studied carefully.

Etiology. The numerous causes of diarrhea may be partially classified and listed as follows:

Enteric infections such as bacillary dysentery, cholera, typhoid and paratyphoid fevers, food poisonings (usually staphylococcal), viral enteritis, and parasites, particularly E. *histolytica*

Food sensitizations, particularly shell fish, strawberries and eggs

Poisons such as arsenic, mercury, silver salts

Avitaminoses, particularly pellagra and sprue

Toxic, septic and metabolic states such as sepsis, measles, thyrotoxicosis, Addison's disease

Circulatory disturbances secondary to cardiac decompensation or cirrhosis of the liver

Emotional disturbances such as fear and grief

Incomplete intestinal obstruction

Nonspecific infections or inflammatory processes in the bowel such as regional enteritis and chronic ulcerative colitis

Neoplasms of the stomach, pancreas or intestines.

Symptoms. The clinical pictures seen in these different states vary a great deal, particularly in severity and duration, but nausea and vomiting, abdominal cramps, tenesmus and frequent watery stools more or less characterize them all. In the usual, so-called simple acute diarrhea the etiology is often not known and not discovered. The attack lasts one to three days, the stools vary from three or four to fifteen or twenty per day, usually watery, light brown, gray, or green in color, flaked with mucus, and often with a foul odor. Blood is rarely present. The intermittent cramps subside after the first day, as does the vomiting. The temperature is usually not elevated, although it may rise 1 or 2 degrees F., rarely higher. The leukocyte count is normal or slightly elevated. In severe cases the prostration and collapse may be profound.

Diagnosis. In simple acute diarrhea the diagnosis is made by the brief duration of the attack and by the failure to find a specific cause.

Treatment. In simple acute diarrhea, as in all diarrheas, rest is of great importance. It is well to keep the patient in bed and to allow no food for the first 24 hours. Normal saline with 5 per cent glucose may be given, if convenient, subcutaneously or intravenously in amounts of 1000 to 1500 cc. once or twice or even three times in 24 hours, depending on the degree of dehydration. Hot water, weak tea, broth or barley gruel may be permitted in small amounts after the nausea and vomiting have subsided and if the patient has a real desire for food. Boiled milk, toast, soft cooked eggs and custard may be given later. Hot stupes may be applied to the abdomen, although usually a hot water bottle or an electric heating pad is sufficient. Belladonna or atropine may be used but relatively little effect should be expected. When the pain is severe, codeine sulfate, 0.03 to 0.06 gm., or morphine sulfate, 0.008 to 0.015 gm., should also be given as needed. Paregoric and bismuth are commonly used; the effect is due entirely to the opium in the paregoric; few physicians know the amount of opium in paregoric; hence, one should prescribe opium directly or learn the opium content of paregoric! Calomel, a time-honored remedy, is best avoided, as is castor oil. The irritating substance is usually removed by the diarrhea in a short time. However, castor oil causes such a complete evacuation of the colon that it is frequently followed by a cessation of bowel movements for one or two days. Enemas or irrigations are not indicated. The patient should be advised to rest and to adhere to a bland diet until the bowel function has been normal for several days.

WALTER L. PALMER

References

Dack, G. M.: Food Poisoning. Chicago, University of Chicago Press, 1949.

Reimann, H. A., Hodges, J. H., and Price, A. H.: Epidemic Diarrhea, Nausea and Vomiting of Unknown Cause. J.A.M.A., 127:1, 1945.

CONSTIPATION

Definition. Constipation is defined as the passage of unduly hard and dry fecal material. The consistency of the stool is more important than the frequency of defecation or the quantity expelled. The average, normal person passes one well formed stool of good caliber daily, although people in the best of health may defecate only one, two or three times a week. Patients have various notions about normal bowel function and constipation; some expect a large watery stool after each meal; the majority consider themselves constipated if more than 24 hours elapse without a bowel movement. Those who complain of constipation usually are not constipated in the sense of passing hard dry stools, but rather in the sense of not passing the quantity of feces with the frequency they desire. True constipation without abdominal distress is, as a rule, atonic, whereas if abdominal pain or discomfort is present, the constipation is usually spastic or hypertonic.

Normal Intestinal Motility. The motility of the normal digestive tract varies considerably. The stomach empties in about 2 to 7 hours. Digestion in the small bowel takes place rapidly, the time required for completion after food leaves the stomach not exceeding 2 to 4 hours. The undigested residue enters the cecum in a liquid state. The chief change occurring in the colon is the absorption of water. Normally, as the food residue traverses the colon, its consistency increases so that a solid column is emptied into the pelvic colon from the descending colon. The defecatory reflex is initiated by the presence of a fecal mass in the lower sigmoid and rectum.

The rate of transit through the colon varies enormously, usually requiring from one to three days, but not infrequently requiring four or five days or longer. If the progress is so rapid that the residue is evacuated before the proper amount of water has been absorbed, the stool is unformed, mushy or watery; whereas if motility is slow, too much water is absorbed, and the stool is hard and dry. Diarrhea is thus defined as the passage of unformed, mushy or watery stools; constipation as the passage of stools that are hard and dry. The frequency of defecation is not of great significance; perhaps the average person expels one formed stool daily; many normal persons have two or three formed stools daily, and on the other hand, occasional persons habitually pass perfectly normal stools at intervals of two to seven days. The moderate amounts of gas evolved in the colon are usually absorbed by the blood; the quantity passed per rectum as flatus depends on the diet, on the amount of air swallowed, and on the rate at which the colon propels the gas along.

Atonic Constipation. This condition may be said to be present when, without abdominal distress, the fecal matter reaching the rectum is hard and dry. Symptoms arise from difficulty in expelling the large hard stools. Satisfactory bowel function can usually be obtained by including in the diet adequate amounts of the more laxative foods, such as oatmeal for breakfast, spinach and prunes daily, two other vegetables and two fruits either cooked or raw, fruit juices, whole wheat bread, honey and syrup.

The treatment of refractory cases is highly individual: some are helped by 1 or 2 ounces of brewers' yeast daily; some by mineral oil, agar or one of the various proprietary mechanical laxatives; some become regular cathartic habitués, using phenolphthalein (0.2 gm.) daily or aromatic fluid extract of cascara (4 cc.) with satisfactory results; some prefer oil retention enemas (3 oz.) at night followed by a small (1 pint) water enema the next morning if necessary. Glycerin rectal suppositories are frequently of value in overcoming rectal dyschezia and reestablishing the defecatory reflex.

WALTER L. PALMER

Reference

Bockus, H. L.: Gastro-enterology. Philadelphia, W. B. Saunders Company, 1943–1946.

IRRITABLE COLON

Definition. The most frequent cause of abdominal distress is disturbed intestinal motility, primarily in the colon, with more or less hyperirritability and hypersensitivity. In various sections of the world different names are applied to the syndrome, varying concepts are in vogue, and multitudinous types of treatment are prescribed.

None of the terms used to describe the functional bowel distress syndrome is entirely satisfactory. Perhaps "irritable colon" is the best, for the bowel is "irritable," as evidenced by the distress and by the abnormality of the stool. Similarly descriptive are the terms "unhappy" and "unstable" colon. The designation "spastic" or "hypertonic constipation" is usually only partially correct, for the "constipation" thought by the patient to be present is frequently absent. "Chronic functional colitis" implies a contradiction of terms.

"Cathartic colitis" is applicable in cases with a cathartic habit. "Spastic colitis" emphasizes the element of spasm rather than that of disordered function. "Mucous colitis" is applied to those cases in which large amounts of mucus are expelled, particularly the so-called mucus casts of the bowels. The presence of such casts of dried mucus and cellular debris stained with fecal content does not basically differentiate this condition from the other types, however, because the secretion of mucus is a normal response of the bowel to irritation. Less definite terms frequently used, such as dyspepsia, nervous indigestion, gastric neurosis, intestinal neurosis, and so on, do not have identical connotations, but fundamentally and practically the problems presented are the same and hence they may all be grouped together. The condition is characterized by an abnormal irritability of the bowel with resultant abdominal distress. The altered function consists of increased tone and motility with irregular and intermittent spasm.

Etiology. In the absence of disease, abnormal irritability may be related either to excessive irritants, such as laxative foods, cathartics and enemas, or to emotional disturbances, or to a combination of the two. The ability of castor oil and of fear to produce diarrhea is well established. The chronic effects of laxative foods and of the emotional reactions to the difficulties of life are, in certain persons, equally definite. Symptomatically, one sees all gradations from the chronic distress and diarrhea induced by the continued use of cathartics to the chronic complaints of the psychoneurotic. Usually it is difficult to differentiate sharply the physiologic and the psychologic or emotional factors, and indeed, as a rule, it is unnecessary to do so.

Most important and never to be forgotten is the fact that distress of bowel origin, and therefore, technically bowel distress, may accompany a variety of organic diseases. Thus the cramps of bacillary dysentery or of intestinal obstruction are "bowel," but obviously not "functional." Physiologic, "toxic," or reflex disturbances of the colon are seen in such diseases as pernicious anemia, thyrotoxicosis, pulmonary tuberculosis and pellagra.

Symptoms. The symptoms of functional bowel distress vary in severity from fullness and discomfort induced by the ingestion of food or drink to severe, cramplike abdominal pain. This tends to be generalized over the abdomen, may shift from point to point, and usually is more noticeable in the lower than in the upper abdomen. As a rule, defecation or the expulsion of flatus affords temporary relief; occasionally, however, the passage of a bowel movement inaugurates more vigorous cramps and tenesmus. Nausea is a frequent symptom. Many patients complain that they are unable to eat a full meal without experiencing an unpleasant sensation of fullness and distention, perhaps sufficient to force them to discontinue the meal. Belching, rumbling and gurgling in the abdomen, and excessive flatus are frequently noted.

Constipation is usually said to be present, the patient meaning that it is necessary to take laxatives or enemas in order to obtain a bowel movement. When one inquires as to how long the patient goes without a defecation, the typical response is: "I never let my bowels go more than a day without moving." Thus patients say they are constipated, whereas in fact they maintain a state of chronic diarrhea. Many patients are obsessed with notions concerning the desirable frequency of defecation, such as one after each meal, or with ideas as to the optimal quantity, assuring the physician dolefully that their bowels do not move "enough." Such patients are satisfied as a rule only by copious watery evacuations. Inquiry into the type of stool passed usually discloses the fact that some abnormality is present such as loose watery stools, unformed stools, narrow, ribbon-like or lead pencil-sized stools, or hard dry balls. The hard, dry, constipated stools, when accompanied by abdominal distress, are usually due to spasm—hypertonicity rather than atonicity.

Headaches, fatigue and countless other "nervous" manifestations frequently present in such cases are not to be interpreted as due to alleged "constipation" or "intestinal toxemia." These symptoms, as well as the bowel distress, are usually on a functional, "nervous" or emotional basis. It is surprising to note how frequently the therapeutic program outlined benefits them as well as the function of the digestive tract.

Physical examination usually reveals a well nourished person, but occasionally extreme grades of chronic malnutrition are noted. The colon is often palpable and tender, particularly the sigmoid portion. Proctoscopy discloses a normal rectum and sigmoid. The laboratory and roentgenologic findings are entirely normal. Frequently the colon, when examined with the barium enema, exhibits evidence of hyperirritability; waves of mass peristalsis may be noted, and the patient may complain of severe pain. However, these changes are not sufficiently constant, definite or regular in their appearance to justify reliance upon the roentgenologic diagnosis of an irritable colon.

Diagnosis. The diagnosis is based upon a history of catharsis or enema habit, dietary indiscretion or emotional strain, generalized or lower abdominal distress of the type described, abnormality of the bowel movement, and tenderness along the course of the colon.

Differential diagnosis involves, first, the search for organic disease of the digestive tract. *Carcinoma of the colon,* particularly of the rectosigmoid, should be excluded by digital examination, examination of the stool for occult blood, by roentgenogram and by proctoscopy. *Diverticulitis* may be detected by roentgenogram, although the mere demonstration of diverticulosis is not particularly significant. *Ulcerative colitis* may be detected proctoscopically. *Regional enteritis* may be suspected if the distress tends to be periumbilical or if there is roentgenologic evidence of a lesion of the small bowel. *Carcinoma of the stomach* occasionally produces diarrhea and lower abdominal distress, as does *carcinoma of the pancreas.* The pain of *peptic ulcer* may be masked by bowel distress which may persist after the ulcer heals. *Cirrhosis of the liver,* passive congestion of the liver, tuberculous and carcinomatous *peritonitis,* and other nondigestive diseases may be accompanied by these rather vague abdominal symptoms.

Gallbladder disease presents one of the most interesting diagnostic problems. Acute bowel distress may simulate biliary colic. On the other hand, patients with cholelithiasis not infrequently have two types of distress: (1) biliary colic and (2) so-called biliary dyspepsia, consisting of belching, upper abdominal fullness and distention and aversion for fried or fatty foods. The biliary colic is cured by cholecystectomy; the dyspepsia frequently is not and may be relieved even without cholecystectomy by the program used in the management of bowel distress. The latter statement applies also to the alleged dyspepsia of so-called noncalculous cholecystitis. In fact, it is doubtful whether gallbladder disease really produces dyspepsia at all. The problem is similar to that which arises in connection with the appendix. Acute and sub-

acute and so-called "interval" appendicitis produce the classic symptomatology of acute appendicitis. Chronic appendicitis, on the other hand, may be found pathologically in a high percentage of persons with bowel distress just as it may be found in a high percentage of normal persons. Removal of the appendix, or of a normal gallbladder or a diseased gallbladder, is followed by "good results" in some cases and by "bad results" in others, irrespective of the condition of the organ removed. The major psychotherapeutic effect of an operation must always be borne in mind and care exercised in the drawing of *"post hoc ergo propter hoc"* conclusions. The distress of these allegedly specific dyspepsias can usually be relieved by nonspecific measures.

A similar problem is presented by the gastritides found by the gastroscopists in approximately 40 per cent of all patients gastroscoped because of abdominal distress. Except for certain erosive forms the relationship between the disease and the distress seems highly questionable. Many of these patients present other manifestations of the irritable colon syndrome and respond well to management.

Some physicians regard all patients included in the "bowel distress" group as psychoneurotics. The great majority of them, however, pass for normal. Some are frank psychoneurotics; others are hysterical; a few are hopeless hypochondriacs; some are more or less profoundly depressed; some are psychotic.

Treatment. Actually, the first step in treatment is the relief of the patient's anxiety concerning organic disease. Definite reassurance that there is no cancer or ulcer or other serious condition cannot be given convincingly unless the examination has been detailed and careful. Some patients, however, react with disappointment, their thought being that they are ill, that they have pain, and yet nothing has been found to be wrong. It is then necessary to explain in detail the nature of the disorder, the cause of the pain, and to outline the procedures for obtaining relief. Superficial psychotherapy such as this is usually sufficient, but frequently a deeper analysis of the patient and his problems is required. In almost all cases in which the therapeutic program to be outlined is found ineffective, the cause will be discovered either as an unrecognized organic disease or a difficult, often insoluble psychiatric disorder.

tinence. There may be no pain at all and no abdominal tenderness, in marked contrast to the spastic bowel. In other cases cramps or tenesmus or both may be present and may be intense. Fever occurs in the more severe cases; leukocytosis is uncommon. Loss of appetite is frequent; nausea and vomiting occur occasionally. In the severe fulminating cases the onset is usually acute, and the course rapid and severe with continued diarrhea, inability to eat, fever, weakness, anemia and profound debility. Death may result from exhaustion or from perforation of the colon and generalized peritonitis. The course of the disease is exceedingly variable. In the less severe forms complete recovery may occur although relapse is frequent; occasionally a stage of complete invalidism is reached; intermediate grades of illness are common. In the phase of symptomatic remission, partial or complete healing may be evident proctoscopically. Radiologic evidence of improvement occurs much more slowly. The anatomic reversability of the inflammatory and ulcerative process is greater than is generally appreciated; spectacular changes are seen occasionally.

The more frequent complications are severe anemia, perianal abscess, perforation of the colon with local abscess formation or generalized peritonitis, stricture formation, polyposis of the bowel, and in about 3.2 per cent carcinomatous degeneration of the polyps. A certain number of patients have arthralgias, rheumatoid arthritis, various forms of erythema and occasionally uveitis.

Theories of Causation. In general the theories concerning etiology may be divided into those relating to (1) infection and (2) emotion. Pathologically and clinically, the disease is indistinguishable from chronic bacillary dysentery except by positive bacteriologic evidence. The well recognized difficulty encountered at times in isolating organisms of the dysentery group from cases of bacillary dysentery led early workers to look upon ulcerative colitis as chronic bacillary dysentery. Apparently in the tropics there are numerous cases of chronic dysentery in which no pathogenic organisms are demonstrable. An attractive hypothesis suggests that the disease process is initiated by a specific dysentery and maintained by ordinarily nonpathogenic organisms. Felsen presented evidence that ulcerative colitis developed in a small percentage of people afflicted with bacillary dysentery. Occasional cases of amebic colitis are seen in which the colitis persists after the eradication of the amebae. Numerous workers have found (a) that pathogenic organisms and parasites are present in only a small percentage of the cases of presumed nonspecific ulcerative colitis, and (b) that the serum of such patients does not contain in significant titer the antibodies of the known pathogens. Endless search has been made for other possible etiologic organisms. Hemolytic and nonhemolytic streptococci and staphylococci are occasionally found; diplococci and E. coli are invariably present; Bacterium necrophorum can usually be cultured if one uses the proper technique; but none of these organisms has as yet been accepted as the causative agent or proved capable of producing the disease with any regularity in the experimental animal. The lysozyme content of the stools is regularly increased but this is not of etiologic significance.

The concept of a *psychogenic cause* is based on certain clinical and experimental evidence. There is the well recognized capacity of fear to produce diarrhea. Many patients afflicted with ulcerative colitis have definite personality disorders. Occasionally the relation between an emotional disturbance and an exacerbation of the disease seems too direct to be merely coincidence. On the other hand, the so-called functional disorders of the colon almost never develop into ulcerative colitis, and, conversely, the latter usually develops in persons without previous digestive symptoms. Experimentally, Lium has produced ulceration of the intestinal mucosa as a result of spasm, but the significance of this observation remains to be determined.

Diagnosis. The diagnosis is established by a history of the symptoms described, by the demonstration proctoscopically of a diffusely granular, friable, superficially ulcerated and bleeding mucosa, and by the failure to find a specific cause for the inflammation. The stool and also rectal swabs should be cultured for pathogenic organisms and a careful search made for E. histolytica. Usually, if amebic colitis involves the rectum, the ulcers are easily identified by their sharply punched-out appearance, the peripheral red halo, and the areas of perfectly normal mucosa intervening between the ulcers, but occasionally the picture is confusing. The roentgenologic appearance of the bowel in the various types of ulcerative colitis is not pathognomonic. Classically, in the nonspecific type, the colon loses its haustral markings, decreases in caliber and length, and becomes somewhat fuzzy in outline. If the cecum and ascending colon are the portions of the bowel most extensively involved, the possibility of tuberculous enteritis or amebiasis should be seriously entertained. If the disease is limited to the rectum, sigmoid and lower descending colon, the roentgenologic appearance may be normal. Conversely, erroneous positive diagnoses may be made because the normal descending colon and sigmoid devoid of haustrations frequently present the straight tubelike appearance considered typical of ulcerative colitis.

teral administration of vitamins. When bleeding is present, a low prothrombin time is occasionally found, indicating a need for vitamin K, best given hypodermically to insure absorption. Belladonna may be used in large doses (40 to 120 drops a day) as tolerated. Phenobarbital, 0.03 gm. four times daily, is valuable for its general sedative effect and for its effect upon the bowel. Bismuth and chalk powders (bismuth subcarbonate, calcium carbonate, and calcium phosphate, each 1.5 gm.) are usually not of much value, but

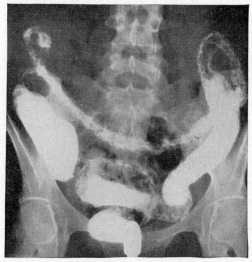 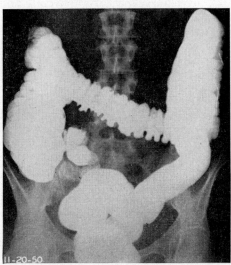

Fig. 116. Chronic ulcerative colitis. The roentgenogram on the left shows the shortened colon, devoid of haustrations, with an abnormal mucosal pattern throughout the transverse portion; the picture on the right, taken sixteen years later, discloses a longer colon of normal caliber with a return of haustra in the transverse section.

Lymphopathia venereum may produce a proctitis and sigmoiditis proctoscopically identical with the nonspecific form, but usually stricture formation is present. A history of buboes suggests, and a strongly positive Frei test almost proves, the diagnosis of lymphopathia venereum.

Treatment. There is no specific therapy. In the acute and subacute phases, rest in bed is important. The application of heat to the abdomen in the form of an electric pad or a hot water bottle is helpful. The diet should be as nonirritating yet as nutritious as possible. Meat and other proteins are well tolerated and most desirable. The patient's weight and caloric intake should be watched constantly.

Accessory food factors should be given as indicated to compensate for the low intake and the possibility of poor absorption. Deficiency states occur and require the paren-

may be tried. Opium may temporarily diminish the diarrhea, but it is not recommended because it increases the tonicity of the bowel. Occasionally, however, codeine in doses of 0.03 to 0.06 gm. when given with atropine or belladonna may be helpful.

Anemia is likely to appear early and to become profound, owing to the continued loss of blood. Iron is irritant to the bowel and should not be used. Transfusions of whole blood, 500 to 600 cc., should be given as frequently as necessary to maintain a normal blood picture. In some patients the bleeding is profuse and persistent.

Various soluble and insoluble sulfonamides have been tried extensively. As is usually the case in any chronic relapsing disease, "good results" have been reported. It is clear, however, that few if any miracles have been wrought, although some patients do seem benefited. The bacterial flora of the feces is altered markedly, the normal coliform organisms being replaced by cocci and the total bacterial count greatly reduced. These changes are transient and do not regularly affect the course of the disease. Other chemotherapeutic agents have been used with similar results. Streptomycin, given orally or parenterally, has only a transitory influence on the fecal flora. Penicillin may be of value, particularly in the few patients in whom hemolytic gram-positive organisms are found on fecal cultures. Chlortetracycline (Aureomycin), oxytetracycline (Terramycin) and neomycin are extremely irritating to many digestive tracts and apparently may even induce ulcerative colitis; hence, they should not be used in spite of the occasional report of a "good result." Fulminating staphylococcal gastroenterocolitis may follow the use of the broad spectrum antibiotics, the organisms being sensitive only to erythromycin. All in all, the various chemotherapeutic drugs should be used with great discretion in ulcerative colitis and with no expectation of the miracles seen in the treatment of lobar pneumonia and other specific infections.

It is too early to present a final appraisal of the value of corticotropin, cortisone and hydrocortisone. In many patients the effect is spectacular with a fall in temperature, decrease in the diarrhea, increased intake of food, improved sense of well being and subsidence of complications such as rheumatoid arthritis and uveitis. ACTH is more effective than cortisone. In acutely ill patients the slow intravenous administration of 20 to 40 units of corticotropin each 24 hours usually results in dramatic improvement. After a few days the intramuscular injection of 30 units every 6 hours may be substituted. Reduction in dosage should be carried out very cautiously and slowly. The various hazards of corticotropin therapy must be borne constantly in mind. Discontinuance of the hormone may or may not be followed by a recurrence of symptoms and exacerbation of the disease. In occasional instances the manifestations of perforation of the bowel with subsequent peritonitis seem to have been masked. Long-term therapy with ACTH gel or with cortisone in doses well tolerated clinically seems to have been of great value in certain patients. Emphasis should be placed, however, upon the fact that hormone therapy in itself is not the final answer to the problem of ulcerative colitis. The bowel must be given time to heal and every measure must be used that will facilitate the process in any way. Thus hormone therapy may be considered as a valuable but in some respects hazardous adjunct to the total treatment of the disease and the patient.

Surgery may be indicated for a variety of reasons: complete intractability, stricture formation, polyposis or neoplasm, perianal abscesses and fistulas, uncontrollable bleeding, persistent or recurring rheumatoid arthritis or iridocyclitis. The bowel does not heal after ileostomy; hence, the operation should include or be followed by colectomy in one or two stages. In fulminating cases in which surgical interference is undertaken as a life-saving measure, the risk of ileostomy combined with partial colectomy seems to be less than that of ileostomy alone because the diseased bowel is responsible for such great toxicity.

Finally, it should be emphasized that in few diseases is there required more patience and perseverance. The treatment, as in pulmonary tuberculosis, must be continued for months and years, most carefully and yet most tactfully. In few conditions is there more need for the art of medicine. Psychotherapy in certain patients appears to play an important role in the control of the disease.

WALTER L. PALMER

References

Bargen, J. A.: The Modern Management of Colitis. Springfield, Illinois, Charles C Thomas, 1951.
Bockus, H. L.: Gastro-enterology. Philadelphia, W. B. Saunders Company, 1943–1946.
Cave, H. W.: Late Results in the Treatment of Ulcerative Colitis. Ann Surg., 124:716, 1946.
Crile, G., Jr.: Treatment of Chronic Ulcerative Colitis. Gastroenterology, 23:533, 1953.
Daniels, G. E.: Psychiatric Factors in Ulcerative Colitis. Gastroenterology, 10:59, 1948.
Elitzak, J., and Widerman, A. H.: Non-Specific Ulcerative Colitis in Childhood. Am. J. Dis. Child., 62:115, 1941.
Felsen, J.: Bacillary Dysentery, Colitis and Enteritis. Philadelphia, W. B. Saunders Company, 1945.
Ginsberg, R. S., and Ivy, A. C.: The Etiology of Ulcerative Colitis, An Analytical Review of the Literature. Gastroenterology, 7:67, 1946.
Jones, F. A.: Modern Trends in Gastroenterology. New York, Paul B. Hoeber, 1952.
Kirsner, J. B., and Palmer, W. L.: Ulcerative Colitis. J.A.M.A., 155:341, 1954. Ulcerative Colitis: Therapeutic Effects of Corticotropin (ACTH) and Cortisone in 120 Patients. Ann. Int. Med., 41:232, 1954.
———, Palmer, W. L., and Klotz, A. P.: Reversibility in Ulcerative Colitis: Clinical and Roentgenologic Observations. Radiology, 57:1, 1951.

Klotz, A. P., Palmer, W. L., and Kirsner, J. B.: Aureomycin Proctitis and Colitis. Gastroenterology, 25:44, 1953.

Machella, T. E.: Chronic (Non-specific) Ulcerative Colitis: A Review of Medical Therapy. Am. J. Med. Sc., 222:579, 1953.

Terplan, K., Paine, J. R., Sheffer, J., Egan, R., and Lansky, H.: Fulminating Gastroenterocolitis Caused by Staphylococci. Gastroenterology, 24: 476, 1953.

REGIONAL ILEITIS

(Regional Enteritis, Regional Enterocolitis, Cicatrizing Enteritis, Crohn's Disease)

Definition. Regional ileitis is a granuloma of undetermined etiology involving sharply demarcated, single or multiple areas of the intestine. Pathologically, it is manifested by lymphatic hyperplasia and lymphedema, by ulceration and secondary infection of the intestinal wall, by cicatrization and localized perforation, abscess and fistula formation. The clinical course is one of a progressive nature or of relapses and remissions, with signs of chronic debilitating infection and increasing disturbance of intestinal function.

Etiology. Ileitis is a disease of youth, beginning usually before the age of 40. It is slightly more common in males. Infrequently, multiple cases have occurred in the same family. There is no known exemption of any race or culture and it is found in all geographic locations. The idea that physical trauma or emotionally charged life situations may precipitate the disease rests largely upon clinical and circumstantial evidence.

Its primary location in a mucous membrane, together with its microscopic pathology, certainly suggests a reaction to an invasive micro-organism; yet no specific agent has been successfully indicted. Despite the strong histologic resemblance, no relationship to tuberculosis or to Boeck's sarcoid has been established. The various bacteria which have been isolated from the lesions are apparently secondary invaders. Similar lesions have been produced experimentally by several agents which cause mesenteric lymphatic blockage. It is thus possible that regional ileitis is a nonspecific pathologic response to a variety of inciting agents.

Morbid Anatomy and Pathogenesis. The typical gross lesion occurs in a sharply demarcated segment of the terminal ileum, which is soggy and stiff, with a thickened wall and narrowed lumen. The mucosa is ulcerated, the serosa hyperemic and encroached upon by mesenteric fat. The mesentery and its lymph nodes are swollen and edematous. Dense adhesions, proximal dilatation of the intestine, and fistulas to the skin, to other loops of bowel and to other hollow viscera complete the picture. The process may extend proximally in the small intestine for a variable distance; or several sharply demarcated lesions ("skip areas"), separated by lengths of normal bowel, may be present. Extension to the proximal colon is less common, and isolated lesions of the distal colon, the duodenum or the stomach rarely occur.

The earliest microscopic lesion is swelling and proliferation of lymphatic endothelium in the lamina propria of the intestine, leading to lymphatic obstruction and lymphedema. This area is then infiltrated with eosinophils and lymphocytes, and a granuloma develops with giant cells but without caseation necrosis. Similar changes occur in the lymphatic channels of the submucosa, subserosa, mesentery, mesenteric nodes, and occasionally the liver. The mucosal lesions later become necrotic, ulcerated and secondarily infected. In later stages there is some repair by fibrosis.

Symptoms. The onset of symptoms of ileitis is most often insidious, rarely abrupt. Ordinarily, the illness increases in severity steadily or intermittently for several years before the diagnosis is made. The patient usually presents some combination of the following symptoms; any one of them may be the chief complaint.

Cramping or colicky *pain* occurs in the periumbilical region, the right lower quadrant or the suprapubic area. It usually follows meals, is accompanied by borborygmi and is relieved by a bowel movement or by vomiting. Afternoon *fever* of variable degree is present in the more active stages of illness, as well as slight or moderate leukocytosis and elevated sedimentation rate. Most cases have a *diarrhea* of two to six large stools daily, which are watery, mushy or semisolid, usually without visible blood or pus. A few patients remain constipated throughout. Though melena is rarely the presenting problem, the stools are often positive for occult blood. The earliest manifestations may be due to *fistulas*—perirectal abscess or fistula-in-ano, abscess of the abdominal wall, or dysuria and passage of gas by the urethra. In many instances the outstanding features are those of *general debility*: weakness, fatigue, moderate to severe weight loss, and in adolescents delayed somatic, skeletal or sexual maturation. The clinical picture is sometimes dominated by *emotional disturbances*—anxiety, tension, irritability, psychasthenia or frank psychotic episodes.

Physical signs of the disease are not numerous. In less than half of the cases, a tender fixed *mass* is found in the lower abdomen, most often in the right lower quadrant; it may be palpable on bimanual rectal or pelvic examination. It represents the involved loops of bowel, together with adherent organs. Many patients bear an *appendectomy scar*, the relic of earlier diagnostic confusion. The orifices of *fistulas* may be found in operative scars or other indurated portions of the abdominal wall, or in the perianal region. The abdomen may be distended, with exaggerated audible and visible peristalsis. The spleen is sometimes enlarged. The patient may be pale and emaciated, may have clubbed fingers, may have generalized edema or even ascites, and may present stigmata of vitamin deficiencies in the skin and mucous membranes.

Anemia, often present, may be either microcytic or macrocytic; hypoproteinemia may be severe. More rarely, defects in absorption may be revealed by a flat oral glucose tolerance curve, a flat vitamin A absorption curve or excessive fat in the stools.

Diagnosis. The clinical diagnosis of regional ileitis can be confirmed only by x-ray or by laparotomy. Either of these methods may fail, even in the presence of advanced disease. The typical roentgenologic appearance of an involved segment of bowel includes a narrowed lumen ("string sign"), ragged ulcerated mucosal surface and irregular polypoid filling defects representing the areas of surviving edematous mucosa. Minute hairlike outward projections often mark the internal orifices of fistulas, or an entire fistula may be traced. The common lesion of the terminal ileum can readily be shown by a barium enema producing an "ileal leak," and this procedure should be done first. The upper limit of the disease should then be established by the barium meal with serial studies of the small bowel. This study may show "skip lesions," and above these the delayed passage of barium through dilated loops, thus indicating the degree of obstruction present.

Differential Diagnosis. The problems of differential diagnosis are related to the various clinical forms of the disease. In *acute ileitis* the abrupt onset of severe right lower quadrant pain, with fever, tenderness and abdominal rigidity, at once suggests acute appendicitis, mesenteric adenitis or perforated diverticulum of the right colon. In ileitis nausea and vomiting are less likely, diarrhea more so; yet the diagnosis cannot be made safely without laparotomy. *Chronic terminal ileitis*, with its right lower quadrant mass and symptoms and signs of chronic inflammation and partial intestinal obstruction, must be differentiated from hyperplastic ileocecal tuberculosis. This disease, rare in the presence of a negative chest x-ray, involves the cecum more obviously than does ileitis. Occasionally, it is helpful to culture the stools for tubercle bacilli, provided the sputum is negative. Extensive tumors of the ileum, such as carcinoid or lymphosarcoma, may be distinguishable at times from ileitis only by histologic study of a resected specimen. Infrequently, regional ileitis extends to the proximal portions of the colon for a variable distance (*ileocolitis*). This process differs from ordinary ulcerative colitis in that the left colon is usually spared, and from "regional" or "right-sided" ulcerative colitis in that roentgenographic studies of the latter disease indicate only mucosal involvement of the terminal ileum, rather than the "string sign" of mural thickening and luminal constriction. Severe amebic colitis only rarely gives signs of ileal involvement, but appropriate stool examinations are indicated. Actinomycosis and tuberculosis should be carefully excluded. In *ileojejunitis* there may be multiple "skip lesions" or diffuse involvement of the small intestine extending as high as the second portion of the duodenum, and often sparing the terminal ileum. The roentgenographic appearances and the steatorrhea and signs of nutritional loss may closely correspond to those of idiopathic sprue, intestinal lipodystrophy or diffuse intestinal lymphosarcoma. In ileojejunitis, however, abdominal pain, fever and leukocytosis are more striking, defects in absorption are less marked, and careful roentgen study is likely to show one or more areas of luminal narrowing with proximal (often excentric) dilatation.

Prognosis. In all forms of regional ileitis the clinical course is variable, some patients having steadily progressing disability, others repeated relapses and remissions, and a few spontaneous resolution of disease. Spontaneous remission of symptoms is many times more common than disappearance of the roentgen signs or of the lesions themselves. In acute ileitis the majority enter promptly upon a prolonged remission of symptoms, and in many there is complete resolution of disease. In ileojejunitis as well, nearly one-half undergo marked spontaneous improvement or clinical remission. In chronic ileitis and ileocolitis lasting freedom from symptoms is rare, and anatomic reversal is almost unknown. Multiple clinical relapses occur in most cases, usually at intervals of less than four years, but occasionally after ten or fifteen years of well-being. Progression of disease in such cases usually eventuates in intestinal obstruction, formation of abdominal abscess or fistula, or general inanition. The gravity of the prognosis can usually be estimated from the previous record of extension to additional areas of bowel, the lack of response to ordinary medical and hygienic measures, and the present evidences of inflammation and penetration of the bowel wall.

Treatment. In the early stages of ileitis, or whenever signs of active inflammation predominate, conservative medical management is recommended. Relief of fatigue and lessening of emotional tension (e.g., by leaves of absence from college or business, or by the solution of marital problems) are important. Bed rest is required only during periods of fever or marked weakness. The diet should be high in calories and especially in protein (2 gm. a day per kilogram of *ideal* weight), and low in seasoning and cold fluids. In proportion to the degree of intestinal inflammation or cicatricial stenosis, dietary roughage should be reduced (in patients with poor teeth, a food mill or a Waring Blendor may be useful). Mixtures of the known vitamins should be given orally in amounts two to four times the normal daily requirements. In phases of severe depletion, transfusions and infusions of electrolytes or of human albumin may be desirable to restore normal blood levels. In diffuse ileojejunitis, anemia and deficiencies of minerals and vitamins should be corrected in the manner prescribed for sprue. Although the role of secondary bacterial infection is uncertain, many authorities recommend antimicrobial therapy in brief, repeated courses (e.g., phthalylsulfathiazole 1 to 2 gm. every 6 hours for three weeks, or chloramphenicol 0.5 to 0.75 gm. every 6 hours for ten days). Striking but temporary improvement is often achieved by corticotropin or by cortisone (the latter in divided doses totalling 300 mg. on first day, then 100 mg. daily for three weeks or longer, then gradual withdrawal); such a measure should, however, be reserved for those cases in which more conservative medical measures have failed and surgery is not indicated.

By such means, time is gained for the spontaneous resolution, partial or complete, of the inflammatory process. Surgical relief is best delayed until the full extent of the disease in the bowel has become apparent, and some degree of cicatrization has occurred. Earlier intervention is often dictated by a downhill course under medical management or by evidence of perforation or fistula formation.

Operation should include transection of the small bowel proximal to the highest recognizable area of disease, and anastomosis of the proximal end to the highest possible segment of colon. The usual procedure is thus an end-to-side ileotransverse colostomy. The need for resection of the intervening diseased bowel continues to be debated.

Postoperatively, most patients have a moderate diarrhea, but dramatic subsidence of other symptoms and a gratifying gain in weight. In 15 per cent or more, the disease may reappear, usually within six years, and in the few inches of ileum just proximal to the anastomosis. Treatment of recurrences involves the same medical and surgical principles as are outlined for the original lesion.

THOMAS P. ALMY

References

Chess, S., Chess, P., Olander, G., Benner, W., and Cole, W. H.: Production of Chronic Enteritis and Other Systemic Lesions by the Ingestion of Finely Divided Foreign Materials. Surgery, 27:221, 1950.
Crohn, B. B.: Regional Ileitis. New York, Grune & Stratton, Inc., 1949.
———, Ginzberg, L., and Oppenheimer, G. D.: Regional Ileitis—A Pathologic and Clinical Entity. J.A.M.A., 99:1323, 1932.
Garlock, J. H., Crohn, B. B., Klein, S. H., and Yarnis, H.: An Appraisal of the Long-Term Results of Surgical Treatment of Regional Ileitis. Gastroenterology, 19:414, 1951.
Kantor, J. L.: Regional (Terminal) Ileitis: Its Roentgen Diagnosis. J.A.M.A., 103:2016, 1934.
Sauer, W. G., Brown, P. W., and Dearing, W. H.: Experiences with the Use of Corticotropin in Regional Ileitis. Gastroenterology, 22:550, 1952.
Warren, S., and Sommers, S. C.: Cicatrizing Enteritis (Regional Ileitis) as a Pathologic Entity. Am. J. Path., 24:475, 1948.

APPENDICITIS*

Definition. Appendicitis, the most common major surgical disease, is an inflammatory lesion of the vermiform appendix. It may occur as an acute attack, acute appendicitis, which progresses to perforation or subsides spontaneously; as mild recurrent attacks, recurring appendicitis, or a so-called "chronic appendicitis."

History. Laurence Heister, in 1711, found an abscess of the appendix at autopsy which he described in his "Chirurgische Warnehmungen." From the time that Mestivier, in 1759, demonstrated at autopsy an appendiceal abscess originating from a pin in the appendix, the abscess having been surgically drained, 141 cases of disease of this viscus were recorded in the literature before the paper of Reginald Fitz in 1886. Fitz defined appendicitis and analyzed 257 cases of perforating ulcer of the appendix. Kelly states that "to Thomas G. Morton, of Philadelphia, belongs the credit for the first successful removal of the appendix, deliberately undertaken." That was on April 27, 1887. After this time the names of Ochsner, Murphy, McBurney and Deaver stand out as proponents of the surgical removal of the appendix, and they did much to increase the knowledge of appendicitis and its treatment.

Anatomy. Developing from a prolongation of the conical cecum in fetal life, the base of the appendix normally lies on the medial side of the cecum about 2 cm. below the entrance of the ileum. The taeniae of the colon converge at its base and continue on it.

The appendiceal artery is a terminal vessel without anastomosis. It passes posterior to the ileum in the appendiceal mesentery which arises from the posterior layer of the mesentery of the ileum.

The cecum and therefore the base of the appendix normally lie in the right iliac fossa. The appendix itself may lie in any direction from its base. Most frequently it lies inferior to the ileocecal junction. The retrocecal position follows in frequency. In children the appendix is commonly directed into the pelvis.

Etiology. Since the appendix is a blind tube the contents of which are discharged by peristalsis into the cecum, mechanical factors may play a part in predisposing to infection.

* The author wishes to express his deep appreciation to Dr. Brooke Roberts for his valuable assistance in the revision of this article.

The contents are, of course, heavily laden with bacteria, particularly those of the colon group. When the cecal outlet is blocked by fecal material, stricture or a concretion, a train of events is started which was described in the classic paper by Van Zwalenburg in 1905: "The efferent vessels which are within the resisting wall of the appendix will be more or less occluded by the greater pressure in the cavity. . . . Every atom of fluid which remains within the wall of the cavity adds its pressure to that already present and causes greater obstruction to the efferent current . . . now if this occurred in perfectly sterile surroundings this balance might be maintained for some time without material harm; enough fluid would filter through to maintain life in the cell. But our cavity is far from sterile. . . . With the circulation impeded, the tissue cells, deprived of their supply of food and oxygen, offer little resistance to the attack of germs." Wangensteen and his associates many years later confirmed and extended these observations on the obstructive mechanism in acute appendicitis. To this etiologic factor must be added the streptococcal infections which are frequent and which rise in frequency when acute respiratory infections are prevalent. These two factors may act simultaneously.

Symptoms and Physical Findings. The classic picture of appendicitis is that of pain, tenderness and spasm in the right lower abdomen. The localizing signs vary according to the location of the appendix, the extent of the disease and the individual reaction of the patient. Nausea and vomiting are usual but not constant symptoms. The temperature is usually elevated, but may remain normal for some hours after the onset of pain.

Pain. In acute appendicitis pain is almost without exception the first symptom. It frequently comes on suddenly and may be paroxysmal at first. The first pain commonly develops around the umbilicus or in the epigastrium and later localizes in the region of the appendix, typically in the right iliac fossa. The first pain occasionally arises in the area of the appendix itself. When there is distention and active peristalsis within the appendix, the pain may be crampy. Such pain is often associated with a fecalith. The later, more constant pain arises from irritation of surrounding peritoneum, and it is this irritation that produces the localizing signs. If the peritonitis extends, the signs spread with the process. If an abscess develops, tenderness becomes localized. Occasionally with an appendix which lies in the pelvis, tenderness may be elicited only on rectal or pelvic examination.

Rarely is acute appendicitis present with little or no pain. A history of nausea and tenderness upon pressure is, however, usually obtained. When intense pain suddenly disappears, perforation or gangrene of the appendix must be suspected. Sometimes a constant dull pain develops, gradually increasing in intensity. This is rare in children, but not uncommon in older patients.

When the disease is limited to the appendix, tenderness may be slight, but may be increased if pressure on the abdominal wall is suddenly released. This sign, rebound tenderness, is a valuable aid in diagnosis when signs of the disease are not well defined.

Nausea and vomiting are frequently present, but may be entirely absent. In children vomiting may be the first evidence of appendicitis.

Muscle Spasm. This reflex protection of the peritoneum, which must be distinguished from voluntary spasm, varies according to the degree of pain and the extent of peritoneal involvement. When present, it is one of the most reliable signs of acute appendiceal disease, although the degree of spasm may vary widely in patients with a similar involvement of the appendix. If the appendix lies low in the pelvis or if it is retrocecal, the spasm may be slight or may be posterior. If the diseased appendix lies in contact with the peritoneum of the anterior abdominal wall, the spasm may be marked from the beginning. With the spread of the infection to the peritoneum, the muscle spasm may be widely extended.

Delicate palpation will elicit this sign much more accurately than deep pressure.

Fever. There is nearly constantly some elevation of the temperature in acute appendicitis, but this may be slight. It is not uncommon to find the fever only 99° or 99.4° F., but it may be as high as 103° F. or higher. This is true in the acutely obstructed appendices with infection, and after perforation. The fever is more apt to be low than high. Chills are rare in uncomplicated appendicitis, but are relatively frequent when the vascular supply to the appendix becomes involved.

Leukocytosis. Leukocytosis of some degree is commonly found. This varies greatly, but as a rule a count of over 20,000 cells per cubic millimeter raises a question as to the diagnosis or strongly suggests perforation. Ten thousand or over should be considered suggestive in the presence of other symptoms and signs of appendicitis. In children the leukocyte count is frequently higher than in the adult. Polymorphonuclear leukocytosis may be present with a practically normal total white cell count. A normal white cell count does not preclude the diagnosis of acute appendicitis.

Differential Diagnosis. The differential diagnosis is influenced by age and sex.

In the child, fever and abdominal pain may be due to a *gastrointestinal disturbance* in which colic is present, but localized spasm and tenderness are usually absent.

Pneumonia with referred pain from diaphragmatic irritation may simulate appendicitis and presents one of the most difficult problems in differential diagnosis. Rapid respiration and absence of rebound tenderness aid in the diagnosis, but the most valuable sign is absence of tenderness or a mass on rectal examination. *Lymphadenitis* of the mesenteric glands presents a real problem in diagnosis, especially in the first attack. A more gradual onset, a low leukocyte count and more general tenderness lead one to suspect this condition, but accurate differential diagnosis is often difficult and at times impossible.

After puberty in the female a *ruptured graafian follicle* may be impossible to differentiate from appendicitis. If the hemorrhage is extensive, there may be faintness. A normal temperature, a high leukocyte count and the occurrence of the pain at the midperiod of the menstrual cycle are suggestive. However, this diagnosis is usually made after the abdomen is opened. *Torsion of an ovarian cyst* is also a diagnosis that is difficult to make before operation unless the cyst is large enough to be felt on rectal or vaginal examination.

A *ruptured tubal pregnancy* may, as a rule, be diagnosed from the history of missed menstruation, by the signs of intra-abdominal hemorrhage, by localized tenderness on vaginal examination and a history of some vaginal bleeding. Since this is also a surgical lesion, the diagnosis is of importance mainly because of the selection of the type of incision to be used.

Acute salpingitis with right-sided pain may be differentiated by the history of burning on voiding and a vaginal examination which will show a cervical discharge and localized tenderness in the pelvis. The sedimentation rate is greatly increased. The signs will usually be more pronounced than the general illness of the patient. In infection of a pelvic appendix giving as many signs and symptoms the patient is usually acutely ill.

Acute cholecystitis may offer a problem, for a high lying appendix and a low lying gallbladder may give tenderness in nearly the same region. In acute cholecystitis, however, the tenderness will be located along the lower border of the liver, and often the gallbladder can be felt. The reference of pain in gallbladder disease is usually to the back and right shoulder.

Diverticulitis of the colon usually occurs on the left side, and the onset of symptoms is more gradual. However, a *ruptured diverticulum* of the ascending, or even descending, colon and a ruptured appendix may have identical symptoms.

Ureteral stone and *infection of the right kidney* may give symptoms referred to the right lower quadrant, but the tenderness in kidney infection will be felt when the kidney is palpated, and the urine will, as a rule, contain blood or pus. The initial pain begins, as a rule, in the back and radiates to the suprapubic area.

An acutely inflamed appendix lying over the ureter may give rise to all these signs, however, and it is therefore better to operate in cases of doubt, for rarely does the patient in whom the diagnosis is incorrect die from the operation. If one waits until peritonitis more accurately leads to the diagnosis, the mortality must remain high.

Treatment. The treatment of acute appendicitis is surgical removal of the appendix as early in the disease as possible. If the patient is not seen before there are signs of abscess formation, the surgeon must make the decision as to the optimal time for operation and whether the appendix should be removed at the time the abscess is drained. There is no medical treatment for acute inflammation of this viscus. It is, of course, of first importance that, if appendicitis is suspected, nothing be given by mouth. Laxatives should never be given if there is any possibility of appendiceal involvement because of the danger of perforation.

Postoperative care, in the absence of peritonitis or other complications, is directed to maintenance of nutritional balance and the restoration of physiologic function. Patients may be fed as soon as they are able to digest liquids and solid food. It is not usually necessary to withhold oral fluids for more than 24 hours and food more than 48 hours. Most patients can be out of bed by the next day or even earlier if they so desire. Early feeding and early ambulation in the uncomplicated case not only reduce morbidity and mortality, but add to the patient's sense of well-being.

The reduction of mortality in appendicitis with peritonitis has been due more to careful postoperative treatment than to improvements in operative technique. In the presence of peritonitis one must attempt to maintain fluid and electrolyte balance, to prevent or limit the spread of the infection and the development of pulmonary complications. The patient is kept in the semi-Fowler position to aid respiratory exchange and possibly to aid localization of the infection in the lower abdomen. Sedation, deep breathing, frequent turning, "nothing by mouth," constant suction drainage of the stomach, intravenous solutions of glucose and electrolytes, antibiotics, and often blood are required in the treatment of peritonitis. It must be emphasized that chemotherapeutic and antibiotic agents do not take the place of sound surgical principles in the care of these patients.

Prognosis. The prognosis depends upon the extent of the infection at the time of operation, and it is for this reason that prompt diagnosis is of such importance. When the infection is limited to the appendix, there should be practically no mortality from this operation. The mortality is proportional to the extent of the spreading infection, and it must be remembered that perforation is not necessary for the presence of peritonitis. The rapid spread of peritoneal infection usually indicates perforation.

Chronic Appendicitis. True chronic appendicitis, that is, a continuous low grade infection, is a rarity, but may occasionally be seen as a part of the process of tuberculosis, amebiasis or similar chronic diseases.

Recurrent Appendicitis. Recurrent attacks of infection with residual scarring and adhesions are not rarities. Vague constant or burning pain in the right iliac fossa will seldom, if ever, be relieved by appendectomy, but if a patient has a history of repeated attacks of pain in the right lower quadrant with fever and nausea during the attacks, the diagnosis of recurrent appendicitis must be considered. If other causes for the pain can be eliminated, the appendix should be removed. In these cases the appendix may be found firmly bound down by adhesions or attached to other viscera.

Appendicitis in Children and in the Elderly. The cardinal symptoms of appendicitis are similar in the child and adult but are more difficult to elicit in the child because of lack of intelligent cooperation. The signs may be obscure in a crying infant. Frequently in a child the first sign noticed is vomiting or refusal of food, and all too often parents have given a cathartic before consulting a physician. A careful examination will usually elicit muscle spasm and tenderness. Rectal examination may be very helpful. Under the age of 2 appendicitis is not common, but of those children who have it, a relatively large proportion will have perforated appendices before they are seen by a physician. In the young child the omentum has not fully developed and cannot "wall off" a perforation as well as can a fully developed adult omentum.

In children acute mesenteric lymphadenitis is very frequent and may be difficult to differentiate from acute appendicitis. It is better to operate on a case of lymphadenitis than to fail to operate on a case of acute appendicitis.

Older patients may tolerate intraperitoneal inflammation with surprisingly little external manifestation and for this reason the early diagnosis of acute appendicitis is often missed in these patients. Anorexia and a vague persistent pain must not be overlooked in the older age group, and minor degrees of muscle spasm are far more significant than in young adults. Fever and leukocytosis, too, may be minimal in these patients. It is in the extremes of life that we find the highest percentage of perforations and the highest mortality from this disease.

I. S. RAVDIN

References

Bockus, H. L.: Gastro-enterology. Philadelphia, W. B. Saunders Company, 1944, Vol. 2.

Boyce, F. F.: Acute Appendicitis: Conservative Therapy Versus First Principles. Ann. Surg., *133*: 428, 1951.

Carp, L., and Arminio, J. A.: Acute Appendicitis in Chronically Ill Geriatric Patients. Am. J. Surg., 83:773, 1952.

DaCosta, J. C.: Modern Surgery—General and Operative. Philadelphia, W. B. Saunders Company, 1931.

Fitz, R. H.: Perforating Inflammation of the Vermiform Appendix. Am. J. M. Sc., 92:321, 1886.

Heister, L.: Medical, Chirurgical and Anatomical Cases and Observations, 1711.

Kelly, H. A., and Hurdon, E.: The Vermiform Appendix and Its Diseases. Philadelphia, W. B. Saunders Company, 1905, p. 44.

McLanahan, S.: Further Reduction in the Mortality in Acute Appendicitis in Children. Ann. Surg., *131*:853, 1950.

Mestivier: Observations on a Tumor Situated near the Umbilical Region on the Right Side, Produced by a Large Pin Found in the Vermiform Appendix of the Caecum. Jour. de med., Chir. et Pharm., *10*:441, 1759.

Reynolds, J. T.: Appendicitis: Basic Consideration in Choice of Therapy. S. Clin. North America, *24*:128, 1944.

Van Zwalenburg, C.: The Relation of Mechanical Distention to the Etiology of Appendicitis. Ann. Surg., *41*:437, 1905.

Wangensteen, O. H., and Bowers, W. F.: Significance of Obstructive Factor in Genesis of Acute Appendicitis: Experimental Study. Arch. Surg., *34*:496, 1937.

INTESTINAL OBSTRUCTION

Definition. Intestinal obstruction or ileus may be defined as a diminution, absence or reversal of the normal flow of the intestinal contents owing to partial or complete occlusion or to inadequate propulsion. Whereas in common usage the term usually signifies an actual mechanical hindrance to progression of intestinal contents, it should be realized that this is a restricted conception and that the condition may also be produced by disturbances of intestinal motility resulting from nervous or vascular influences.

Etiology. Undoubtedly the largest number of cases of intestinal obstruction are caused by mechanical agents which actually interfere with forward motion of the intestinal contents. This may be produced by various factors which can act by actually plugging the lumen, constricting the tube or compressing it from the outside. Accordingly, the various factors which may produce mechanical obstruction can be classified into three types: (1) intraluminal, (2) mural and (3) extramural. Examples of the first type, which has been referred to as obturation, are foreign bodies, gallstones, bezoars, enteroliths and worms. The mural type is typified by hernia, volvulus and compressive tumors. Ileus may also be produced by certain functional nervous disturbances resulting in peristaltic failure. Ileus may be classified into two types: (1) adynamic (inhibitive or paralytic) ileus and (2) dynamic (spastic) ileus. Failure of peristalsis may also be produced by vascular insufficiency in which the musculature of the bowel loses its capacity for contractile response. This is exemplified by mesenteric thrombosis and embolism.

It should be realized that, although intestinal obstruction may be produced independently by any one of these three principal mechanisms, i.e., mechanical, functional or vascular, it is possible and not infrequent that one becomes superimposed upon the other and that they even act concurrently. Moreover, the initial operation of one factor may not be sufficient to produce complete obstruction, but the additional effect of one or both of the other factors is enough to eventuate occlusion. Thus the original cause of obstruction may be an adynamic ileus following operation. If adequately treated early, this may be of no consequence, but if the distention is allowed to progress, a segment of bowel may become twisted and produce actual mechanical occlusion of the lumen, or the distention may be sufficiently extensive to produce circulatory embarrassment in the wall of the involved lumen. Similarly, in hernia, the lumen of the involved segment may be only partially occluded, but sufficiently to hinder the propulsion of the intestinal contents. The resultant stasis and dilatation cause interference with venous return, thus increasing the edema of the bowel wall; this further augments the constriction, resulting in complete occlusion and even strangulation. Hence, partial mechanical occlusion becomes converted into complete obstruction by the addition of the vascular factor.

Special Types of Obstruction. *Obturation Ileus.* Obturation ileus may be defined as that form of ileus in which a mechanical obstruction is caused by intraluminal agents. These may be of different types, such as gallstones, intestinal parasites, fecaliths, enteroliths, concretions, bezoars, food boli, miscellaneous foreign bodies, meconium and epithelial casts. This type is rare, comprising about 2 per cent or less of all types of ileus.

In the case of gallstone ileus, the stone is usually large and gains entrance into the gastrointestinal tract by passing directly from the fundus of the gallbladder into the duodenum by erosion and the production of a cholecystoduodenal fistula. In most instances of obturation ileus the obstruction occurs in the distal ileum because this is the narrowest part of the small bowel.

Congenital Atresia. By congenital atresia is meant an absence of the lumen due to some failure or arrest in the normal embryologic development of the intestinal tract. The condition appears about once in every 20,000 births.

Imperforate Anus. Imperforate anus and atresia of the lower portion of the rectum occur about once in 5000 births with equal sex incidence. Two types of imperforation are observed: (1) simple imperforation and (2) those imperfections associated with fistulous communications which are usually recto-perineal or, in the male, rectovesical and recto-urethral and, in the female, rectovaginal. The character of the obstruction varies from stenosis to atresia, with the rectum terminating as a blind sac for variable distances above the perineum.

Strictures. Intestinal obstruction may be produced by strictures which narrow or occlude the lumen. These strictures may be congenital or acquired, benign or malignant. The acquired cicatricial forms may follow mechanical or operative trauma, vascular injury, such as infarction, bacterial or inflammatory reactions. As a cause of intestinal obstruction they are relatively rare.

Any form of bowel ulceration with subsequent cicatricial healing may result in sufficient narrowing of the lumen to produce obstruction. Of these, regional enteritis, which is frequently multiple, is one of the most common. Other forms of ulcerative processes are those associated with tuberculosis, bacillary dysentery, ulcerative colitis and typhoid fever. Diverticulitis, especially of the sigmoid and occurring usually in older patients, may produce sufficient inflammatory reaction to cause obstruction. Benign rectal strictures are most commonly produced by lymphogranuloma inguinale.

Trauma incident to intra-abdominal operative procedures and faulty anastomoses may cause stricture formation. Accidental trauma also may give rise to the condition by vascular injury of the mesenteric vessels and production of hematoma or infarction. Traumatic stricture may also follow reduction of strangulated hernia, especially the femoral type. Irradiation therapy for pelvic malignancies has been known to produce obstruction by stricture formation.

The pathologic features are those of mechanical obstruction and the type of lesion producing the occlusion. Regional enteritis strictures are frequently multiple and most commonly involve the lower ileum and cecum. In ulcerative colitis and amebic lesions the strictures involve varying lengths of the colon. In practically all forms the degree of obstruction may vary from simple narrowing to almost complete occlusion. The obstruction is almost invariably of the simple type, and strangulation rarely complicates the condition.

Adhesions Ileus. Adhesions are responsible for approximately a third of all cases of intestinal obstruction, and the majority of these follow intra-abdominal operative procedures or infections. Of the operations, appendectomy is the most frequent and gynecologic procedures are next. Drainage of the peritoneum is believed to increase this liability. In addition to postoperative adhesions, ileus may be produced by congenital bands and adhesions such as the avascular fold between the terminal ileum and cecum, adhesions which follow endometrial transplants, tuberculous peritonitis and other nonoperative peritoneal infections.

Intussusception. Intussusception may be defined as the invagination of one portion of the intestine (the intussusceptum) into usually an adjacent, more distal, segment (the intussuscipiens). This is the descending type; the ascending or retrograde type is rarely observed. Intussusception comprises about 5 per cent of all cases of intestinal obstruction and is the most common cause in children. Approximately 75 per cent of the cases occur in children less than two years of age and 50 per cent in those less than one year. The ratio of males to females is about two to one. Other etiologic factors, particularly in adults, include the presence of Meckel's diverticulum, pedunculated tumors, carcinoma, inflammatory lesions and foreign bodies. Whereas usually there is no actual occlusion of the lumen in intussusception, the obstruction is due to the active contraction of the sheath, particularly at the neck. In addition to this, because of the tension of the mesentery of the intussusceptum and its compression, vascular disturbances are liable to occur early. Accordingly, the greatest pathologic changes are found in the intussusceptum, which soon becomes edematous, indurated and engorged with blood. There is excessive mucus secretion, extravasation of blood into the lumen, and eventually, especially in the irreducible form, ulceration, gangrene and perforation.

Neoplasms. Exclusive of hernias as a cause of intestinal obstruction, neoplasms comprise about one sixth of the cases and are among the most frequent causes in patients past middle life. These include benign and malignant tumors, the former arising most frequently in the small bowel and the latter in the colon. Lipoma, fibroma, adenoma and angioma comprise the benign tumors. The malignant tumors include primary and metastatic carcinoma and sarcoma. Primary carcinoma is by far the most frequent type of lesion and most commonly involves the colon. *Carcinoid tumors,* frequently referred to as argentaffinomas, usually occur in the appendix and lower ileum and give rise to obstruction. Whereas carcinoma situated in any part of the large bowel may produce obstruction, it is more liable to occur in the left half, and approximately half of the cases are in the sigmoid.

Occasionally, in both benign and malignant tumors the obstruction is precipitated by the development of intussusception, especially in the presence of polypoid growths. Volvulus may also occur. Inflammatory swelling and edema are particularly important factors in precipitating acute obstruction in carcinoma of the large bowel.

The pathologic features are those of mechanical obstruction and of the type of neoplasm concerned. In cases in which chronic obstruction has preceded the acute attack there may be hypertrophy and edema of the bowel wall above the site of obstruction. Because of the mechanism of the ileocecal valve in preventing regurgitation, colonic obstructions are converted into closed loops with consequent circulatory embarrassment or strangulation. Accordingly, gangrene and perforation are more liable to occur in these forms. Perforation may also be due to the malignant process.

Hernia. External hernias are by far the most frequent cause of intestinal obstruction, comprising almost 50 per cent of the cases. Inguinal hernias are the most frequent cause of intestinal obstruction, and of the hernial obstructions the next most frequent are femoral, umbilical and incisional. Hernias are of importance in the production of ileus, not only because of the mechanical obstruction offered by the presence of an intestinal loop in the hernia and compression at the neck, but also because of the liability of early vascular interference consequent to compression of the vessels in the mesentery. In addition to compression of the intestinal loop at the hernial orifice, an increased accumulation of gas and fluid in the imprisoned loop tends to produce an intramural strangulation.

Volvulus. By volvulus is meant torsion or twisting of a segment of bowel on its mesenteric axis, usually in a clockwise direction. Volvulus comprises about 10 per cent of all cases of intestinal obstruction. It is usually due to increased length or defective fixation of the mesentery, permitting abnormal mobility of the attached loop of bowel. The ileocecal area and sigmoid are the most frequent sites of involvement, the former being more common in children and the latter in adults. As a result of the torsion and consequent compression of the mesenteric vessels, especially the veins, circulatory disturbances occur early. Venous engorgement develops first, and hemorrhagic infarction finally occurs. The involved segment of bowel becomes edematous, discolored and eventually gangrenous and perforated. The distended loop, because of extravasation, usually contains more fluid than gas. There may be evidence of localized peritonitis and free peritoneal fluid.

Functional Obstruction. Functional obstruction may be defined as failure of normal propulsive peristalsis resulting from a disturbance in the nervous mechanism or contractile response. This type of intestinal obstruction may be classified into two forms: (1) adynamic (inhibition, paralytic) ileus, and (2) dynamic (spastic) ileus.

A mild form of ADYNAMIC ILEUS occurs after almost all intra-abdominal operations and is probably due to splanchnic irritation. This moderate degree of intestinal paresis is manifested by slight distention and inability to expel gas, and the subsequent gas pains indicate the return of peristaltic activity. Whereas adynamic ileus is observed most frequently following peritonitis and other intra-abdominal lesions such as strangulation of the omentum, renal and biliary colic, torsion of an ovarian cyst, retroperitoneal hematoma and infections, it may also occur after extra-abdominal lesions and systemic infections. It has been observed following fractured ribs or other bones, spine injuries and blunt trauma to the abdomen. Pneumonia, typhoid fever, meningitis and other infectious diseases may be associated with severe adynamic ileus. Embolism and thrombosis of the mesenteric vessels also produce this type of obstruction, and it may be superimposed upon or follow mechanical ileus. In these conditions there is the additional factor of circulatory embarrassment, which, by interference with the blood supply of the intestinal musculature, further reduces its capacity for contractile response. The common conception that in this condition the intestinal wall is paralyzed is erroneous, for it has been repeatedly demonstrated experimentally and clinically that after interruption of sympathetic impulses by splanchnic block or spinal analgesia, the ability of the intestinal musculature to contract is normal. Most observers believe that the condition is due to hyperactive sympathetic influence. Accordingly, the term "reflex inhibition ileus" is more accurately descriptive than paralytic ileus. Clinically, the condition is characterized by pronounced meteorism, due mostly to swallowed air, and, in contradistinction to mechanical obstruction, colicky pain is absent. Moderate tenderness may be present, and auscultation reveals a relatively silent abdomen. In contradistinction to the mechanical forms of ileus, these patients characteristically appear euphoric and exhibit less anxiety.

DYNAMIC or SPASTIC ILEUS is rare and, in contrast to adynamic ileus, is characterized by actual spastic contraction of a segment of the bowel, usually the colon. Various causative factors have been observed, including lead poisoning; injuries; irritating intraluminal contents or mural lesions such as foreign bodies, intestinal worms, ulcers; tuberculous peritonitis; neurasthenia and hysteria; renal colic; and infectious fevers.

Vascular Obstruction. Vascular obstruction usually results from interference with the blood supply to a segment of bowel. This is most commonly caused by occlusion of the mesenteric vessels. Arterial occlusion due to thrombosis and embolism is slightly more frequent than venous and affects the superior mesenteric artery more frequently than the inferior. Venous thrombosis is usually due to infection, especially of the portal radicals. The usual clinical manifestations are sudden acute abdominal pain, shock, vomiting, diarrhea and melena.

Pathologicophysiologic Changes in Ileus. In acute intestinal obstruction, especially if the obstructing lesion is located high in the intestine, there occur certain characteristic biochemical changes, consisting essentially of dehydration, hypochloremia, alkalosis, hemoconcentration, increased nonprotein nitrogen and urea, and possibly hypopotassemia. Most of these, at least the dehydration, dechlorination, alkalosis, hypopotassemia and hemoconcentration, can be explained on the basis of loss of fluid and electrolytes from the upper intestinal tract. It has been estimated that about 7000 cc. of fluids consisting of gastric secretions, succus entericus, bile and pancreatic juice are poured into the gastric and upper intestinal tract daily, and under normal conditions most of this is absorbed in the lower portions of the intestine. If there is interference with the normal transportation of these large quantities of fluid, stagnation and dilatation occur in the stomach and upper intestinal tract with consequent nausea and vomiting and loss of these fluids. The loss of fluids and electrolytes (the sodium and chloride ions) is largely responsible for dehydration. The alkalosis may be explained on the basis of the loss of chloride. In high intestinal obstruction there is a greater loss of chloride ion (because the vomitus contains a greater amount of gastric juice [and hydrochloric acid]) than sodium ion, and the relative excess of the basic ions, principally sodium, is compensated by an increase in bicarbonate ion with resultant alkalosis. The loss of potassium can greatly aggravate and even precipitate ileus, because muscle contractility is decreased in potassium deficiency. In this way the contractility and propulsive power of bowel musculature is further diminished. The hemoconcentration which is observed, particularly in high intestinal obstruction, may be due in part to the dehydration following the loss of fluids, but also in part to the loss of plasma into the lumen and the wall of the involved intestine.

In addition to the biochemical changes, practically all cases of ileus show a gradual accumulation of gas and fluid, proximal to the obstruction, which produces distention of the bowel. The gas in the dilated loops of bowel is to a large extent (about 70 per cent) due to swallowed air.

The *symptoms* and *prognosis* in acute ileus are largely dependent upon the viability of the bowel wall. In those cases in which there is interference with the blood supply to the intestine the patient is much sicker, appears much more toxic, and is more liable to die early than is the patient without strangulation. Also, everything else being equal, the higher the obstruction, the worse the prognosis and the more rapidly progressive the course. In the instances in which there is interference with the blood supply, whether it be mesenteric or intramural, there is transudation of fluid into the lumen and through the wall with transperitoneal absorption of

bacteria and other lethal agents. Obviously, as the intra-enteric pressure increases, interference with the venous return from the bowel wall increases, thus augmenting the capillary hydrostatic pressure and resultant filtration pressure. The associated anoxia produces increased capillary permeability, and all these factors result in considerable loss of plasma and aggravation of the ileus. If distention is permitted to continue long enough and there is sufficient intramural compression, actual necrosis of the gut may occur, particularly on the antimesenteric surface, where perforation is most liable to be found.

Symptoms. The symptoms of intestinal obstruction vary, and depend upon the degree and site of occlusion. In general, sudden acute mechanical occlusions located high in the intestinal tract produce more intense and earlier symptoms than other forms. Similarly, in strangulation the manifestations are more severe than in simple obstruction. Whereas such variations exist with the type and extent of obstruction, the cardinal manifestations, irrespective of the cause, are essentially pain, vomiting, distention and constipation.

Pain is usually the first symptom, especially in acute mechanical obstruction. It is characteristically intermittent and colicky, occurring in severe paroxysms with crescendo rises, and, after being sustained at a maximum intensity for several minutes, it ceases abruptly. Early, the pain may be located at the site of obstruction, but is frequently referred to the midabdomen. Between the paroxysms there is little discomfort except in the presence of strangulation. These paroxysms are usually more intense and frequent in small than in large bowel obstruction. As distention progresses and the contractile response decreases, the intensity and paroxysmal character of the pain recede. Whereas paroxysms of colicky pain are characteristic of mechanical obstruction, there is little or no pain in functional ileus.

Vomiting also varies in intensity and character, depending upon the type and site of obstruction. In general, the higher the obstruction, the earlier and more severe is the vomiting. After the stomach has been emptied of a previous meal by reflex vomiting, retching may be unproductive, or the vomitus may consist only of bile-stained gastric juice. This is soon followed by the regurgitation of a grayish, glairy material characteristic of intestinal contents, especially in high obstruction. If the obstruction is low, however, the appearance of this material may be delayed for hours. Although at first this material has a faint odor of moldy food, later it develops a fecal odor which is not necessarily an indication of colonic contents, for the fecal odor may be due to protein putrefaction occurring in the small bowel. Colonic obstruction, even when pronounced, is frequently associated with little or no vomiting except the initial reflex vomiting. This may be explained on the basis of the ileocecal checkvalve mechanism, which is usually competent and permits fluids and gas to enter the colon, but prevents their regurgitation.

Constipation is an eventual occurrence in all cases of ileus, but may not be significant early. Immediately after the onset of an acute obstruction, there may be one or two spontaneous bowel movements due to emptying of the intestinal tract distal to the obstruction. The presence of blood in the stools indicates strangulation; blood and mucus, intussusception.

Chronic intestinal obstruction may be due to many of the conditions which produce the acute type. It is most commonly caused by slow-growing benign or malignant neoplasms of the bowel which progressively encroach on the lumen, inflammatory and granulomatous lesions of the bowel, and intrinsic defects in neuromuscular mechanism such as Hirschsprung's disease. Characteristically, the onset is insidious, and the principal manifestation is constipation, which becomes progressively worse. Resort to laxatives and purgatives which produce temporary relief is frequent, but becomes increasingly necessary and progressively less effective. Recurrent attacks of abdominal discomfort, colicky pain and distention are common. In aged persons fecal impaction is not infrequent. The presence of hemorrhoids and blood-streaked stools may also be observed.

Physical Findings. Although the signs of acute intestinal obstruction are typical, there is some variation with the stage and site of obstruction. At onset the general appearance of the patient reveals no significant changes. As the disease progresses toward a more advanced stage and dehydration and other physiologic disturbances have occurred, the characteristic anxious expression with pinched facies, fast, thready pulse and cold, clammy extremities becomes evident. In strangulation, and in the late stages of other forms of obstruction in which there is vascular insuf-

ficiency of the involved bowel, shock may develop as the result of fluid and blood loss.

Abdominal distention due to dilatation of the bowel proximal to the obstruction is also an eventual occurrence in all cases of ileus. It is more likely to be pronounced in lower ileal and colonic obstructions, but in early, particularly in high obstructions, is characteristically absent. Although distention eventually becomes generalized, with barrel-like abdomen, it may be localized at first. Thus, in high obstruction, the distention may be limited to the upper abdomen, while in low colonic obstruction a prominent fullness appears on each side of the abdomen and extends across the abdomen along the course of the large bowel.

Visible peristalsis, which usually indicates hypertrophy of the bowel, is more characteristic of chronic obstruction, but may be present in acute ileus especially in patients with a thin abdominal wall. Furthermore, abdominal tenderness and rigidity are not prominent features of simple acute obstruction. Although there may be some tightening of the abdominal muscles during paroxysmal attacks of pain, the abdomen is relaxed between these attacks. Tenderness and rigidity indicate peritoneal irritation, and their presence suggests strangulation and peritonitis consequent to leakage or perforation.

Because of its early and constant character, auscultatory evidence of hyperperistalsis is particularly significant. The loud, whirring, gurgling sounds can frequently be heard readily without a stethoscope. However, auscultation with a stethoscope over various parts of the abdomen may be helpful, not only in diagnosing an acute ileus, but also in locating the obstruction. Characteristically, in intestinal obstruction these sounds (borborygmi) are heard with greatest intensity at the height of the paroxysmal attacks of pain. With progress of the ileus, the whirring sounds change to tinkling notes. In the late stages of obstruction and in adynamic ileus the abdomen is silent.

Roentgenographic examination is undoubtedly one of the most valuable diagnostic procedures in acute intestinal obstruction. A "scout" film taken with the patient in the prone position will aid in localizing the site of obstruction by revealing gas in the small intestine only in obstructions of the small bowel, and in the colon with relatively little in the small intestine in obstructions of the large bowel. Because the fluid in the various dilated loops of bowel will assume a level with the gas above, a skiagram taken with the patient in the upright position will reveal numerous fluid levels. Contrast substances should not be given by mouth in cases of suspected intestinal obstruction, but in obstructions of the colon a barium enema may be helpful in determining the site of occlusion.

Prognosis. The prognosis in intestinal obstruction depends upon a number of factors, among the most important of which are the type and extent of obstruction, integrity of the blood supply, and the time elapsing between the onset and the institution of therapy. Thus the mortality in obstructions due to external hernia is comparatively low, in spite of frequently associated strangulation, because the diagnosis can be made relatively early and rational therapy, i.e., operation, is usually not delayed. On the other hand, the mortality in obstructions due to mesenteric thrombosis and embolism is relatively high because the diagnosis is less obvious and necrosis, perforation, peritonitis and shock are likely to develop earlier.

Treatment. Whereas the treatment of acute intestinal obstruction may vary according to the type and degree of obstruction, in general the two principal therapeutic objectives consist essentially, first, in the correction of local and systemic disturbances produced by the obstruction and, second, removal of the obstructive agent and restoration of normal bowel function.

The systemic disturbances which may be pronounced, especially in high obstruction, consist essentially of dehydration, hypochloremia, hypopotassemia and hemoconcentration. These can be combated by the administration of *saline solution* and *other fluids* as soon as the diagnosis is established. Since potassium deficiency almost invariably exists in the presence of hypochloremia and alkalosis, parenteral fluids containing potassium are necessary. However, care must be exercised not to administer too much potassium because of the danger of increased muscle irritability, especially in the heart muscle. Elman et al. have showed that smaller amounts are required in patients who are in negative nitrogen balance because, as the result of excessive protein catabolism, large amounts of potassium are released from the cells. Although the loss of electrolytes is a more important factor in high obstruction,

dehydration plays a significant role in all obstructions. The required amount of fluids and saline must therefore be determined in the individual case and will depend upon the site, degree and period of obstruction. Elman et al. recommended the use of a solution containing 6.62 gm. of sodium chloride and 2.23 gm. of potassium chloride per liter of water. Periodic plasma chloride determinations will aid in gauging the salt requirements. Determinations of specific gravity of the plasma and the hematocrit will also indicate the degree of hemoconcentration or dehydration. Fluids can be administered in the form of 5 per cent dextrose solution. After the initial dehydration and hypochloremia have been combated, adequate hydration can be maintained by the simple method of determining urinary excretion. In the presence of normal kidney function sufficient fluids should be administered to permit daily urinary excretion of about 1200 cc. As shown by Coller and his co-workers, there is some danger of giving too much salt. Careful observation of the patient is necessary, particularly of one with poor urinary function, because of the likelihood of salt retention.

Because the patient often cannot take food by mouth for a number of days, *maintenance of caloric* and *nitrogen equilibrium* becomes important. Accordingly, intravenous feedings are necessary. The use of 10 per cent or even 20 per cent solution of dextrose administered slowly as an intravenous drip over long periods will aid greatly in meeting the caloric requirements. Nitrogen equilibrium may also be sustained by the intravenous administration of amino acids and plasma transfusions. Whole blood and especially plasma transfusions are particularly important in cases of vascular obstruction such as mesenteric thrombosis or embolism, and in acute mechanical obstructions such as volvulus, intussusception and hernias accompanied by strangulation. In such cases sufficient blood and plasma loss in the involved segment of bowel may produce serious blood volume reductions eventuating in "shocklike" manifestations. Obviously, this may be readily combated by the restoration of normal circulating blood volume with whole blood and plasma transfusions. The increasing significance of vitamin requirements has been recently demonstrated. In these cases the most important vitamins are B and C, which may also be administered intravenously.

The significance of distention has been emphasized and is undoubtedly one of the most important of the local factors requiring therapy. This may be realized by the fact that in spite of combating all the systemic factors mentioned and the maintenance of fluid and salt balance, life cannot be sustained long if acute distention of the small intestine remains unrelieved. The significance of *decompression,* therefore, becomes increasingly evident. Decompression may be achieved by means of intubation or enterostomy. Decompression by intestinal intubation is best accomplished by the use of a double tube or double lumen tube (Miller-Abbott) with an inflatable rubber balloon a few inches proximal to a perforated metal tip. Whereas this method of decompression is of inestimable value in cases of simple acute mechanical obstruction, it should not be attempted in strangulating obstructions or those limited to the colon by a competent ileocecal valve. Such cases require early operative intervention.

Of great value in the treatment of ileus is the administration of *morphine* or other opium alkaloids. Contrary to general conceptions, morphine exerts a powerful tonic effect on gut musculature and is helpful in combating intestinal distention and its consequent intramural strangulation both in mechanical and adynamic ileus. Extensive investigations have demonstrated that other drugs are of little or no value in ileus.

The second therapeutic objective, i.e., *removal of the obstructing agent* and *restoration of normal bowel function,* must be achieved for complete recovery. In the majority of cases surgical intervention is necessary; although in some cases of simple mechanical obstruction due to adhesions, hernia, volvulus or intussusception, and also in certain cases of inhibitive ileus the conservative management with decompression and other supportive measures referred to is sufficient to restore intestinal continuity. Conservative decompression should not be prolonged unduly, however, and if there is no appreciable improvement in 24 to 36 hours, operation should not be delayed. Immediate surgical intervention is necessary in strangulating obstructions and acute colonic occlusions with pronounced distention. However, even in such instances operation should not be attempted in the presence of considerable dehydration, shock or other complications of obstruction which would jeopardize the chance of recovery. For this reason it is de-sirable in all cases to improve the patient's general condition, before operation, by upper gastrointestinal decompression, hydration, transfusion and other supportive measures.

Once the decision of surgical intervention has been made, the type of procedure indicated will depend upon the condition found at operation. This, in turn, is greatly influenced by the viability of the bowel.

ALTON OCHSNER
MICHAEL E. DEBAKEY

References

Brady, L.: Mesenteric Vascular Occlusion. Arch. Surg., 6:151, 1923.

Cole, W. H.: Congenital Malformations of the Intestinal Tract and Bile Ducts in Infancy and Childhood. Arch. Surg., 23:820, 1931.

Coller, F. A., and others: Postoperative Salt Intolerance. Ann. Surg., 119:533, 1944.

DeBakey, M., and Ochsner, A.: Bezoars and Concretions. Surgery, 4:934, 1938; 5:132, 1939.

Dott, N. M.: Volvulus Neonatorum. Brit. J. Surg., 11:251, 1923; also Brit. M. J., 1:230, 1927.

Dragstedt, C. A., Lang, V. A., and Millet, R. F.: The Relative Effects of Distention on Different Portions of the Intestine. Arch. Surg., 18:2257, 1929.

Elman, R., Shatz, B. A., Keating, R. E., and Weichselbaum, T. E.: Intracellular and Extracellular Potassium Deficits in Surgical Patients. Ann. Surg., 136:111, 1952.

Ladd, W. E., and Gross, R. E.: Congenital Malformations of the Anus and Rectum. Am. J. Surg., 23:167, 1934.

———: Intussusception in Infancy and Childhood. A Report of 372 Cases. Arch. Surg., 29:365, 1934.

Ochsner, A., Gage, I. M., and Cutting, R. A.: The Value of Drugs in the Relief of Ileus, An Experimental Study. Arch. Surg., 21:924, 1930.

———: Effect of Morphine on Obstructed Intestines. Arch. Surg., 28:406, 1934.

———, and Granger, A.: The Roentgen Diagnosis of Ileus. Ann. Surg., 92:947, 1930.

Raiford, T. S.: Tumors of the Small Intestine. Arch. Surg., 25:122, 231, 1932.

Trotter, L. B. C.: Embolism and Thrombosis of the Mesenteric Vessels. Cambridge University Press, 1913.

Wangensteen, O. H.: Intestinal Obstruction. Springfield, Ill., Charles C Thomas, 1942.

Webb, C. H., and Wangensteen, O. H.: Congenital Intestinal Atresia. Am. J. Dis. Child., 41:262, 1931.

INTESTINAL NEOPLASMS

Incidence. The intestine is one of the most frequent sites of primary neoplasms; about 15 per cent of all cancers arise in the intestines. Slightly more than one half of all gastrointestinal tract tumors occur in the stomach, about two fifths in the colon and rectum and less than one tenth in the small intestine. Of all tumors in the gastrointestinal tract, about four fifths are malignant and one fifth benign. However, this ratio varies in different parts of the alimentary canal. Thus, although in the stomach about nine tenths of the tumors are malignant, in the colon and rectum about three fourths are malignant, and in the small intestine only slightly more than two fifths are malignant. About 45 per cent of all benign tumors and 37 per cent of all malignant tumors in the gastrointestinal tract are located in the large bowel, whereas only about one fourth of all benign tumors and less than 5 per cent of all malignant tumors are located in the small intestine. Of all intestinal (small and large bowel) neoplasms, slightly more than four fifths are located in the large bowel, and of the malignant tumors almost nine tenths are in the large bowel.

SMALL INTESTINE

BENIGN TUMORS

In the small intestine benign tumors are relatively more common than malignant neoplasms and tend to occur at younger ages than the latter. There is no significant sex incidence. Included among the benign tumors are adenoma, lipoma, fibroma, myoma, hemangioma, chylangioma, accessory pancreatic tissue, enterogenous cysts and gas cysts. Of these, *adenoma* is by far the most common and occurs most frequently in the ileum and next in the duodenum. Usually single, they may be multiple and polypoid. They vary in size from a few millimeters to several centimeters in diameter. Grossly they resemble other polyps, and histologically they are characterized by benign hypertrophy and hyperplasia of glandular epithelium of the mucous membrane. The potential danger of malignant change in benign adenomatous intestinal polyps should be remembered. *Lipomas* are believed to arise from the areolar tissue in the submucosa or subserosa, are usually single, tend to be pedunculated and are rarely more than a few centimeters in diameter. Pure *fibromas* are relatively rare. They may be sessile, pedunculated and project into the lumen or externally. The tumor appears as a discrete, freely movable, rather firm mass which microscopically shows connective tissue. *Myomas* grossly resemble other benign tumors, but histologically are characterized

by strands of smooth muscle fibers. Hyaline degeneration and hemorrhagic necrosis are common. *Hemangioma* and *chylangioma* are extremely rare in the small bowel. Chylangiomas are softer, more cystic, and gray or yellow in color. Accessory *pancreatic tissue* or aberrant pancreatic rests are believed to originate as misplaced pancreatic tissue and accordingly are found most frequently in the duodenum and upper jejunum. They appear as small, irregular, rather flattened submucous nodules closely resembling normal pancreatic tissue. *Enterogenous cysts* are extremely rare, and are believed to arise as a result of some anomaly of embryonic development.

Clinical Manifestations. The clinical manifestations are variable and depend upon location, type and character of the tumor. Many never produce symptoms and are recognized accidentally at laparotomy or autopsy. Symptoms are usually due to erosion or ulceration and consequent hemorrhage, or to intestinal obstruction produced by intussusception, or by gradual encroachment on the lumen. Tumors in the duodenum usually produce manifestations of progressive obstruction. Epigastric pain, nausea, vomiting and distention are prominent symptoms. Hematemesis and melena are not infrequent. As the obstruction increases, vomiting and distention become more pronounced. Abdominal tenderness is usually present, but rigidity is seldom elicited.

Diagnosis. This is based upon clinical manifestations and the roentgenologic demonstration of duodenal obstruction or a filling defect representing the tumor. In the jejunum and ileum the clinical manifestations are also usually those of obstruction caused by intussusception or gradual occlusion. Approximately a fourth of the cases of benign tumors in this segment of the bowel cause obstruction by intussusception, and in adults intussusception is most frequently caused by tumors in the ileum. In the other forms obstruction is produced by gradual encroachment on the lumen, and the symptoms are more insidious. The *physical findings* vary with the stage of the process; at first there are few signs except possibly some tenderness and, if the tumor is of sufficient size, a palpable mass. Roentgenologic examination, especially with the aid of a double lumen tube passed down to the site of obstruction, is of distinct value in the diagnosis.

Progress. In uncomplicated benign tumors of the small intestine this is relatively good. Complications such as hemorrhage, perforation, intussusception and complete intestinal obstruction increase the gravity of the condition.

Treatment consists in early and complete surgical extirpation. In some cases this necessitates intestinal resection.

MALIGNANT TUMORS

Malignant tumors of the small intestine include carcinomas, sarcomas and carcinoids or argentaffin tumors. Of these, carcinoma is probably the most common, with sarcoma next in frequency.

CARCINOMA

Carcinoma of the small intestine occurs more frequently in the male sex with the highest incidence in the fourth, fifth and sixth decades. The duodenum, especially the second or periampullary portion, is the region of greatest involvement. Several forms of carcinoma of the small intestine are recognized, depending upon their gross pathologic or histogenic characteristics. Histologically, these carcinomas are classified into four types: adenocarcinoma, medullary, scirrhous and colloid.

Clinical Manifestations. These are variable and depend upon the location, size and character of the tumor and the degree of malignancy. They are predominantly those of intestinal obstruction. A history of abdominal distress and pain is frequent. Pain is usually colicky and accompanied by nausea and vomiting. As the degree of obstruction progresses, these attacks increase in frequency and severity. Loss of weight and strength and even cachexia are characteristic of malignant growths. Tumors of the duodenum may produce hematemesis and melena or symptoms of duodenal ulcer. Those located in the periampullary region may produce biliary obstruction, and the consequent painless jaundice develops early. Malignant tumors of the jejunum and ileum produce symptoms usually of greater intensity, but similar to those described for benign tumors in this area with obstruction as the predominant feature. When the tumor becomes sufficiently large, a movable, palpable mass may be present. Roentgenography is of diagnostic value, especially with the aid of a double lumen tube which can be passed to the site of obstruction.

Prognosis. In primary carcinoma of the small intestine this is not good. Metastasis occurs early and extends first to the regional lymph nodes and peritoneum and then to the liver, lungs and other organs.

Treatment consists in radical resection when the tumor is removable. In the nonresectable tumors because of extensive metastasis palliative operations for relief of obstruction may be necessary.

SARCOMA

Sarcoma of the small intestine is about twice as frequent as sarcoma of the large bowel and occurs most commonly in males and in middle-aged persons. Depending upon their histogenesis, the various forms of sarcomas of the small intestine include lymphosarcoma, leiomyosarcoma, fibrosarcoma and neurofibrosarcoma. Lymphosarcomas comprise two thirds of the cases and leiomyosarcomas about one fourth. These tumors, especially lymphosarcoma, occur most frequently in the ileum and next in the jejunum. Lymphosarcoma is believed to originate in a simple lymphoid follicle or in lymphoid tissue located in the submucosa and in the early stage is localized in this region as a soft friable mass. It grows by spreading along the tissue spaces and soon infiltrates the muscularis and other tissue layers of the bowel wall. This tendency to invasion and destruction of surrounding structures is shown by the cylindrical or rigid tubelike character of the tumor growth. Ulceration is late, and when it occurs it is characteristically excavated. Obstruction may occur as a result of stenosis, intraluminal protrusion or external compression of the tumor, intussusception or kinking or by adherence of coils of intestine. Metastasis occurs to the regional lymph nodes in the mesentery and especially to the liver. Because lymphosarcomas infrequently encroach upon the intestinal lumen, extensive metastases are found before any symptoms are manifest. In fact an abdominal mass produced by the lymph node metastases may be the first manifestation. Melanosarcoma or malignant melanoma of the small intestine is rare and usually occurs in the rectum. It is usually multiple and appears as a polypoid or bosselated tumor with a bluish to black color.

Sarcomas of the small intestine produce **clinical manifestations** which vary from those of acute intestinal obstruction to symptoms of vague abdominal disorders. More commonly there is colicky abdominal pain accompanied by nausea and vomiting, some fever, gradual loss in weight, and secondary anemia. Occasionally the onset is sudden with manifestations of acute obstruction, perforation and severe hemorrhage. **Diagnosis** is difficult and is based upon the history of colicky abdominal pain, loss of weight and strength, the presence of secondary anemia and an inconstantly palpable tumor. Roentgenologic examination of the small bowel is of value especially with the aid of a double lumen tube which may be passed to the point of obstruction.

Prognosis is poor, since metastasis is frequent.

Treatment consists in radical extirpation when this is possible. Radiation therapy, especially for the lymphoid type, is of some value.

CARCINOID TUMORS

Carcinoid tumors, also known as argentaffin tumors because of their affinity for silver dyes, are believed to arise from what are known as the chromo-argentaffin cells of the normal intestinal mucosa, most numerously located in the appendix and terminal ileum and believed in some way related to the chromaffin system. These tumors occur most commonly in the ileocecal region, with the appendix and especially its tip as the most frequent site. Grossly, they appear as small, rather freely movable nodules varying in size from 0.5 to 1 cm. in diameter with a firm, somewhat rubbery consistency and a characteristically bright yellow color. Lying beneath the mucous membrane, they tend to obliterate the lumen of the appendix or bowel. Histologically, they are characterized by nests or columns of cells surrounded by a stroma of connective tissue and smooth muscle. The cells, which are fairly regular, contain distinctive nuclei and a granular cytoplasm with an affinity for silver. They are usually single and commonly regarded as benign, but should be considered potentially malignant because about a fifth of the cases show malignant characteristics with considerable enlargement of the original tumor and metastasis to the liver and regional nodes.

These tumors appear in either sex and at any age, but most commonly in young adults. Their **clinical features** depend to a great extent upon their location. In the appendix the manifestations simulate chronic appendicitis. In the small intestine they are symptomless unless they become of sufficient size to obliterate the lumen, and then the manifestations are those of intestinal obstruction. In the stomach, colon and rectum they produce symptoms resembling malignancy. The **prognosis** is relatively good especially if recognized before metastasis has become widespread. Recurrence is rare. A characteristic of carcinoids even in the presence of metastases is their relatively benign behavior. Not infrequently patients live many years with extensive liver metastases.

Treatment consists essentially in surgical excision.

COLON AND RECTUM

BENIGN TUMORS

Benign tumors of the colon include epithelial papilloma or adenoma, lipoma, fibroma, myoma, myxoma, adenomyoma and enterogenous and gas cysts. Of these, adenoma and lipoma are probably the most common.

Adenomas are polypoid tumors which may be sessile or pedunculated, single or multiple and limited to one segment of the bowel, or diffuse, producing generalized polyposis of the colon. The condition appears more commonly in males and in middle or late adult life, although the diffuse type, which is rarer, is encountered more frequently in younger persons. Enquist and State found adenomatous polyps in 18 per cent of all patients examined between the ages of 45 and 64. In a series of 900 polyps found in the entire large bowel, 868 (90 per cent) were in the distal 25 cm. of the bowel. Chronic inflammatory lesions of the bowel are believed to be of etiologic significance in the development of these neoplasms. According to Erdman and Morris, two types of adenomas of the colon may be recognized: those known as the adolescent or congenital type, which are disseminated, and those referred to as the adult or acquired type. The former appear as sessile or pedunculated, soft, round masses of variable size projecting into the lumen and uniformly distributed in the colon or rectum. The latter type is similar in gross appearance, but more frequently limited to one segment of the bowel, especially the rectosigmoid. Histologically, they consist of hypertrophic glands on a stalk of connective tissue with a rich vascular supply. Whereas both types may undergo malignant change, the adult type is more liable to be affected in this manner. The potentially malignant character of these adenomatous polyps should be emphasized, and many observers believe that all carcinomas of the large bowel arise from polyps.

Other benign tumors such as *fibromas, lipomas, myomas* and *angiomas* may also be polypoid in character. They may be sessile or pedunculated, single or multiple, and are usually symptomless, unless they encroach on the lumen or cause intussusception and obstructive symptoms. Hemorrhage may be caused by cavernous hemangioma. Adenomyoma is due to the implantation of endometrial tissue on the serosal surface of the bowel or the appendices epiploicae. As a result of deeper extension into the bowel wall, constriction of the intestine may occur.

The **clinical manifestations** of benign tumors of the colon vary with the type of growth, and the presence or absence of such complications as hemorrhage, intussusception or other obstructive features. Solitary pedunculated tumors may produce intermittent attacks of localized colicky pain. They are a frequent cause of intussusception, especially in the adult. Adenomatous polyps, especially the multiple forms, produce more characteristic symptoms. There is usually a history of repeated attacks of gastrointestinal upsets, with cramplike pain, diarrhea, hemorrhage from the bowel and the passage of mucus. In the diffuse forms the attacks are frequently associated with profuse hemorrhage and secondary anemia. However, even in the adult type moderate hemorrhage is common. Alternating attacks of diarrhea and constipation are not uncommon. Progressive loss of weight and anemia are indications of malignant change. In cases in which the tumor causes obstruction, the symptoms will depend upon the nature and degree of constriction.

The **diagnosis** of benign tumors of the large bowel is made on the basis of the clinical manifestations and the roentgenologic and proctoscopic findings. Solitary tumors that project into the lumen may be demonstrated by "double contrast" roentgenographic studies after the introduction of a radiopaque material and air. Multiple polyposis can usually be demonstrated either by this means or by proctoscopic visualization.

The **treatment** is essentially surgical and consists in excision. In case of obstruction, preliminary enterostomy may be necessary. Because of their potentially malignant nature, polyps should be treated by radical resection of the involved bowel (colectomy). The solitary type with a long pedicle may be excised at the base. Polyps limited to the rectum may be treated by fulguration through the proctoscope.

MALIGNANT TUMORS

Malignant tumors of the large bowel are among the most frequent tumors of the body. It is stated (Rankin and Graham) that carcinomas of the colon comprise 15 per cent of all carcinomas. In addition to carcinomas, other malignant tumors are sarcomas, of which lymphosarcoma is by far the most frequent. Sarcomas, however, occur most infrequently.

In the consideration of tumors of the large bowel, it is desirable to differentiate between the proximal and distal halves of the colon because they have different origins, different functions and different types of lesions. Carcinoma involving the right half, particularly the cecum, is likely to be fungating, so-called colloid carcinoma, with considerable mucus production, whereas those in the distal half are more often of the scirrhous type.

The involvement of different portions of the colon varies considerably according to reported statistics. Grinnell in a series of 2,152 cases of cancer of the large bowel found 17.2 per cent in the right colon (5.1 per cent cecum, 6.3 per cent ascending colon, 2 per cent hepatic flexure and 3.9 per cent proximal transverse colon); 39.5 per cent in the left colon (4.9 per cent distal transverse colon, 2.9 per cent splenic flexure, 4.9 per cent descending colon, and 26.7 per cent sigmoid flexure); and 43.3 per cent in the rectosigmoid and rectum. In a series treated at the Ochsner Clinic (Ochsner and Hines) the cecum was involved in 8.8 per cent, the ascending colon and hepatic flexure in 7.9 per cent, the transverse colon in 4.4 per cent, the splenic flexure and descending colon in 10.6 per cent, the sigmoid flexure in 24.3 per cent, the rectosigmoid in 16.7 per cent and the rectum and anus in 26.5 per cent.

The lesions of the large bowel more frequently affect males than females in a ratio of about two to one.

Carcinomas of the large bowel vary considerably in their gross appearance. They may be divided generally into three main types: (1) a large ulcerating, fungating tumor, with little evidence of obstruction (medullary); (2) a smaller tumor, which is characterized by overproduction of fibrous tissue, resulting in cicatricial contraction and early stenosis (scirrhous); and (3) a large tumor in which there is overproduction of mucinous material with little evidence of cellular activity (colloid).

Symptomatology. The symptoms vary considerably according to the location of the lesion. There is a fundamental difference in the symptomatology of neoplasia of the right and left sides of the bowel. On the right side the symptoms are those of disturbed function, and there is little or no evidence of obstruction, largely because the tumor is more likely to be fungating and soft and at the same time the contents of the bowel are fluid, whereas on the left side the tumor is of a cicatrizing type, i.e., scirrhous carcinoma. This, together with the fact that the contents of the bowel on the left side are solid, results in early obstruction. Patients with large, fungating, ulcerating tumors on the right side may suffer from a severe anemia and have alternating attacks of constipation and diarrhea. They vomit frequently, are conscious of a mass in the right lower quadrant, and occasionally have fever. The cause of the anemia, which can be very severe, is not known, but it is thought that it is commensurable with the size of the growth. The anemia may be so profound that it may simulate a primary anemia. In fact, in every unexplained severe anemia one should consider the possibility of a malignant disease of the right half of the colon, particularly the cecum. The symptoms of right-sided lesions so frequently simulate those of appendicitis that in approximately 18 per cent of cases the patient is operated upon for appendicitis. In lesions on the left side there is usually increased obstipation, a history of recurrent colicky pain, and also attacks of alternating constipation and diarrhea. Whereas in the majority of cases the symptoms are those of progressive intestinal obstruction, occasionally the first manifestation is that of acute obstruction. Distention and borborygmi are frequently associated with left-sided lesions. Blood and mucus may be present in the stool. Tumors of the transverse colon are readily recognized because of their superficial location and ease of palpation.

Careful examination of the abdomen and digital examination of the rectum as well as proctoscopic and sigmoidoscopic examinations should be done routinely in all patients suspected of having a malignant lesion of the bowel. As mentioned, approximately 75 per cent of rectal carcinomas can be palpated on digital examination. A lesion involving the rectum and rectosigmoid can be visualized by a sigmoidoscopic examination. Sigmoidoscopic examination is of value, not only in visualizing the tumor, but also in permitting biopsy.

In addition to proctoscopic examination, roentgenography is of inestimable value in the diagnosis of colonic malignant tumors, especially in those in and above the sigmoid. The barium should be introduced under fluoroscopic observation. In small tumors, particularly polyps, the use of the double contrast visualization, i.e., barium and air, is of utmost importance.

Prognosis. The prognosis of carcinoma of the colon is dependent upon several factors, which may be classified as (1) those which are uncontrollable and (2) those which are controllable. Under the first are the age of the patient, the lesion itself, and associated disease. The controllable factors are the duration, preoperative and postoperative management, anesthesia, operative management and complications. In 718 collected cases of carcinoma of the colon, the mortality rate following resection of the right-sided lesions was 19.6 per cent, whereas that following the resection of the left colon was 24.4 per cent.

Treatment. The treatment of malignant lesions of the large bowel is extirpation, and there are few places where surgical extirpation offers such good results as in the large bowel. In a series of 4561 collected cases of carcinoma of the large bowel, 58.5 per cent were operable. According to Jacobson, 75 per cent of the right-sided lesions, 80 per cent of transverse colon lesions, 63 per cent of splenic flexure and descending colon lesions, and only 30 per cent of sigmoid lesions were operable. The fact that carcinomas of the colon remain localized for long periods of time is demonstrated by the statistics of Larson, who found that of 210 cases of carcinoma of the colon coming to autopsy, 113 had either no metastases at all or only a few regional lymph nodes which were resectable. Of 3911 reported resections for carcinoma of the colon, 30.7 per cent had five-year cures.

ALTON OCHSNER
MICHAEL E. DEBAKEY

References

Cameron, A. L.: Primary Malignancy of the Jejunum and Ileum. Ann. Surg., *108*:443, 1938.

Enquist, I. F., and State, D.: Rectal and Colonic Polyps. Surgery, 32:696, 1952.

Erdman, F. J., and Morris, J. H.: Polyposis of the Colon. Surg., Gynec. & Obst., 40:460, 1925.

Grinnell, R. S.: Results in the Treatment of Carcinoma of the Colon and Rectum. Surg., Gynec. & Obst., 96:31, 1953.

Mayo, C. W.: Malignancy of the Small Intestine. West. J. Surg., 48:403, 1940.

Ochsner, A., and DeBakey, M.: Operability, Morbidity, and Mortality Factors in Carcinoma of the Colon. Am. J. Surg., 46:103, 1939.

————, and Mahorner, H.: in Pack, G. T., and Livingston, E. M.: Treatment of Cancer and Allied Diseases. New York, Paul B. Hoeber, Inc., 1940.

————, and Hines, M. O.: Carcinoma of the Colon. South. Surgeon, 12:269, 1946.

Rankin, F. W., and Graham, A. S.: Cancer of the Colon and Rectum. Its Diagnosis and Treatment. Springfield, Charles C Thomas, 1939.

————, and Mayo, C., Jr.: Carcinoma of the Small Bowel. Surg., Gynec. & Obst., 50:939, 1930.

AFFECTIONS OF THE MESENTERY

STRUCTURAL ABNORMALITIES OF THE MESENTERY

Variable structural abnormalities of the mesentery may occur and for the most part are due to failure or interruption of development at different embryologic stages. These consist essentially in abnormal lengthening or shortening of the mesentery, lack of fusion, or attachment to the posterior abdominal wall, clefts and fenestrations, and elongated folds and bands. Various pathologic states may occur as a consequence of these anomalies. Abnormal lengths of the mesentery permit the development of kinks and volvulus resulting in chronic recurrent partial obstruction or acute ileus and strangulation. Various degrees of intestinal obstruction and strangulation may also be produced by the herniation of small loops into abnormal clefts, fossae and elongated folds or bands. The clinical manifestations depend upon the type and extent of the anomaly, but in general are those of acute or chronic intestinal obstruction and usually appear in early life.

MESENTERITIS

The mesentery may become involved in the presence of general peritonitis just as the omental, visceral and parietal coats are involved in the inflammatory process. Rarely the inflammation is limited to the mesentery, and the condition is known as mesenteritis. The **etiology** is variable and may be due to tuberculous or pyogenic lymphadenitis, or to extension of infection from the adjacent intestine; the disease may follow accidental or operative trauma, or it may be hematogenous from distant foci. The **pathologic process** varies from a phlegmon or actual abscess formation to fibrous cicatricial thickening. The latter, referred to as chronic mesenteritis or mesenteritis retrahens, appears as a hard, thickened, shrunken, fibrous mass with radiating cicatricial bands which tend to distort the regional segment of intestine and thus affect intestinal motility. The **clinical manifestations,** which are not characteristic, are those of the primary disease, or they may simulate various acute and chronic abdominal diseases. **Treatment** is directed toward drainage of the abscess or release of intestinal obstruction.

MESENTERIC HEMORRHAGE

Spontaneous rupture of intra-abdominal blood vessels with mesenteric or subperitoneal hemorrhage is extremely rare. Arteriosclerosis and aneurysm are predisposing causes, and hypertension is frequently present. The vessels most commonly involved are branches of the celiac axis and superior mesenteric artery. The lesion consists of a hematoma which sometimes ruptures into the peritoneal cavity. The condition, frequently referred to as *abdominal apoplexy,* is more common in males and in advanced age. The **clinical manifestations** are sudden, dull, progressively increasing pain, nausea and vomiting, and, if the hematoma ruptures, sudden exacerbation of pain, shock and collapse. Abdominal tenderness and rigidity are variable in degree. **Treatment** is conservative or surgical, depending upon the extent and rate of hemorrhage.

MESENTERIC VASCULAR OCCLUSION

Mesenteric vascular occlusion is relatively uncommon, but probably occurs more frequently than is generally realized. It may develop in either sex or at any age, but the incidence is much higher in males and in advanced age groups. The **etiologic factors** are essentially embolism and thrombosis, inflammatory or degenerative processes obliterating the lumen, external pressure or constriction, and trauma. Of these, thrombosis of either arteries or veins and embolism of the arteries are the most common causes. Vascular diseases, such as endocarditis, degenerative heart disease, aortic atheromas, aneurysms, thromboangiitis obliterans, periarteritis nodosa, arteriosclerosis, especially of the mesenteric vessels, are frequent predisposing causes. Mesenteric venous occlusion is almost invariably due to thrombosis, and peripheral sepsis and portal obstruction are the most common predisposing causes. Septic processes which may contribute to mesenteric venous thrombosis include acute appendicitis, puerperal infections, phlebitis, pelvic inflammatory disease, diverticulitis and other inflammatory and suppurative processes in the peritoneal cavity. Portal obstruction may result from various conditions, including particularly cirrhosis of the liver, hepatitis and hepatic abscess, pylephlebitis and malignant diseases. Rarely certain blood diseases such as polycythemia and leukemia may be the responsible factors. Occasionally the condition appears as a postoperative complication, especially following appendectomy, hemorrhoidectomy or certain intestinal and pelvic surgical procedures. Mesenteric arterial and venous thrombosis also may be produced by external pressure or constriction from abdominal tumors, strangulated hernia, intussusception or volvulus.

Occlusion is more frequently arterial than venous and involves the superior mesenteric vessels much more commonly than the inferior. The pathologic changes depend upon the extent and character of the occlusion. Slow, incomplete occlusions limited to a few small branches may produce little or no pathologic change in the bowel wall because of the collateral blood supply. On the other hand, sudden complete obstruction of the main vessels is more liable to produce extensive changes. In either case the development of secondary thrombosis in the venous or arterial arcades is apparently the deciding factor and in the majority of cases leads to hemorrhagic infarction. The affected bowel becomes swollen, soggy and infiltrated with blood, and assumes a cyanosed, mottled, dark red or plum-colored appearance. The lumen, which is somewhat dilated, contains altered blood. The affected mesentery shows similar changes and appears thickened, cyanosed and rigid. The peritoneal fluid is usually increased and blood-tinged. Necrosis and perforation of the bowel are unusual, but peritonitis resulting from transperitoneal migration of bacteria through the devitalized bowel wall is common.

Symptoms. Clinically, the condition is characterized by an acute onset of violent abdominal pain, vomiting, disturbed bowel function, ileus and shocklike manifestations. Pain is the most constant and predominant symptom, occasionally develops gradually, but usually is sudden, agonizing and persistent, although frequently associated with severe colicky attacks. Vomiting occurs early and is pronounced for the first few hours. Constipation is common, although diarrhea associated with tenesmus or alternating constipation and diarrhea may be present. Melena is a fairly common occurrence. In the acute fulminating cases "shocklike" manifestations suggestive of internal hemorrhage are observed, and the patient appears pale, anxious and restless with a low blood pressure and a fast, thready pulse. Later the features of neglected intestinal obstruction appear. The physical findings usually do not conform with the severity of the symptoms. Early, the temperature may be normal or subnormal, and later, when peritonitis develops, becomes elevated. There is some abdominal tenderness and rigidity, but distention occurs late. A tumor is occasionally palpable, and free fluid in the abdomen may be demonstrable. The leukocytic count is always high.

Diagnosis is difficult, for early in its course the condition is easily confused with acute intestinal obstruction and may resemble numerous other acute abdominal catastrophes, such as intussusception, volvulus, acute pancreatitis, and perforation of an abdominal viscus. However, the condition should be suspected in a patient with the predisposing factors who suddenly exhibits acute violent abdominal pain associated with vomiting, shock, low temperature, high leukocytosis and melena. Aspiration of peritoneal fluid has been suggested as a diagnostic procedure, since the presence of a blood-tinged fluid is almost pathognomonic.

Treatment is surgical and consists essentially in resection of the infarcted segment of bowel and its mesentery with immediate or subsequent anastomosis, depending upon the condition of the patient. Blood and plasma transfusions are of inestimable value as preoperative and postoperative therapy. The **prognosis,** which depends upon the extent and period of involvement, is usually bad, the mortality ranging from 60 to 90 per cent.

MESENTERIC LYMPHADENITIS

Mesenteric lymphadenitis or lymphadenopathy has been classified into two types: the specific and nonspecific. The former occurs in association with certain specific infectious agents such as typhoid, tuberculosis or syphilis, and neoplastic diseases such as carcinoma, lymphosarcoma or Hodgkin's disease. In contradistinction to these forms, in which the causal agent of the lymphadenopathy is known, there is the type which has become recognized as a clinical entity and referred to as nonspecific mesenteric lymphadenitis because the etiology has not been definitely established.

Nonspecific mesenteric lymphadenitis occurs more commonly than is generally realized. The sex incidence is greater in females, and the age incidence is highest between 5 and 15 years. The **etiology** is controversial, and among the factors suggested are allergy, intestinal parasites, enteritis, absorption of bacterial toxins and stagnant material, upper respiratory infection, appendicitis, filterable viruses and specific bacterial infection. The two principal routes which permit involvement of the mesenteric lymph nodes are gastrointestinal and hematogenous. Whereas many believe that the appendix is the portal of entry, others consider the terminal ileum as the most important site of local absorption and the oropharynx as the origin of the swallowed causative agent. In the Tulane Surgical Laboratory, Plank investigated 65 cases of mesenteric lymphadenitis both histologically and bacteriologically. Enterococci were obtained in pure culture in 67 per cent and a gram-positive diplococcus in association with colon bacilli in 27 per cent. However, because the agglutination reactions and vaccine tests were negative, the assumption that these organisms were the definite causative agents was considered unjustified.

The **clinical manifestations** of nonspecific mesenteric lymphadenitis are fairly characteristic and closely resemble those of acute appendicitis. Pain is the most constant symptom, usually of a dull, aching character localized to the right, lower abdominal quadrant, but may be colicky and referred to the region of the umbilicus or right hypochondrium. The onset is frequently acute and usually of moderate severity, but recurrent attacks are common. Nausea and vomiting are fairly constant manifestations, but diarrhea and constipation are infrequently observed. Of the physical signs, abdominal tenderness is the most characteristic and is usually located in the right lower quadrant. Frequently the tenderness extends from McBurney's or Lanz's point upward and to the left along the course of the root of the mesentery.

It is usually of moderate severity, as is also muscular rigidity. Fever is characteristically of a low grade type with temperature ranging between 99° and 100° F. There is slight or moderate leukocytosis, and the differential count is usually within normal limits.

Treatment is symptomatic.

MESENTERIC SOLID TUMORS

Mesenteric tumors may be classified into *cystic* and *solid* forms. The former are about twice as frequent as the latter. The primary mesenteric solid tumors arise from the connective tissue, nerves and vessels between the mesenteric leaves and retroperitoneal space. In the latter instance the tumor assumes its mesenteric position by pushing its way forward between the mesenteric leaves. These tumors may be benign or malignant. Of the benign types the most common are lipoma, fibrolipoma, fibroma and fibromyoma. The malignant tumors include fibrosarcoma, liposarcoma, neurosarcoma, myosarcoma and lymphosarcoma. Lipomas are the most common of all solid tumors of the mesentery. The **clinical manifestations** are variable and depend upon the type, size and location of the tumors. In the benign forms there is frequently only a progressive, painless abdominal swelling. In some there is abdominal discomfort, nausea, vomiting and constipation. Tumors located near the bowel may produce intestinal obstruction. The malignant forms are frequently associated with progressive loss of weight and anemia. The mobility of these tumors is characteristic. **Treatment** is surgical and consists in enucleation or removal with resection of the adjacent intestine.

MESENTERIC CYSTS

Mesenteric cysts occur about once in every hundred thousand hospital admissions. They are found at all ages, but are most common in the fourth decade, and the ratio of females to males is about two to one. Various theories and classications have been presented to explain their pathogenesis. In general, it may be stated that they are of congenital or infectious origin. The *infectious types* are less common and may be due to echinococci or tubercle bacilli. The *congenital forms* may be simple embryonic cysts arising from serous or chylous structures or sequestration of embryonic diverticula during the development of the intestinal tract such as Meckel's diverticulum; or they may be neoplastic, arising from misplaced ovarian tissue (dermoids and teratomas) or from other urogenital tissue such as the wolffian duct and body and the müllerian body in the retroperitoneal area, or from the entoderm (enterocystoma). They vary in size considerably and may be unrecognizably small, or huge tumors which fill the abdominal cavity. Their location also varies, but they are found most frequently near the lower jejunum and ileum. Pathologically, the cysts are usually unilocular, although occasionally multilocular, and have a fibrous wall which may contain bundles of smooth muscle, giant cells and lymph follicles. Occasionally the cysts connect with the intestinal lumen by a duct. The contents of the cysts vary from a clear mucinous material to a yellowish, milky brown or sanguineous fluid. Rarely do the cysts undergo malignant degeneration.

The **clinical manifestations** are variable and there are no pathognomonic features. The **symptomatology** depends upon the complications produced by the cysts, the most frequent of these being intestinal obstruction. This may be of acute onset, but usually there is a history of repeated attacks of nausea, vomiting and colicky pain associated with chronic constipation and loss of weight and strength. Other complications are rupture with consequent peritonitis, and hemorrhage into and torsion of the cyst.

Diagnosis is rarely made preoperatively, but the condition should be suspected in the presence of a freely movable and cystic abdominal tumor associated with colicky pain and other manifestations of intestinal obstruction. Occasionally, roentgenographic studies are of value in delineating the cyst.

Treatment is essentially surgical, with enucleation as the procedure of choice. In some cases, because this is not feasible, or because of strangulation or malignant degeneration, intestinal resection with removal of the cyst-bearing area of the mesentery is necessary.

ALTON OCHSNER
MICHAEL E. DEBAKEY

References

Bockus, H. L.: Gastro-enterology. Philadelphia, W. B. Saunders Company, 1943–1946.

Cushman, G. F., and Kilgore, A. R.: The Syndrome of Mesenteric or Subperitoneal Hemorrhage (Abdominal Apoplexy). Ann. Surg., *114*:672, 1941.

Frazer, J. E., and Robbins, R. H.: One of the Factors Concerned in Causing Rotation of the Intestine in Man. J. Anat. & Physiol., *50*:75, 1915.

Harkins, H. N.: Mesenteric Vascular Occlusion of Arterial and of Venous Origin, Report of 9 Cases. Arch. Path., 22:637, 1936.

Meade, C. H.: Mesenteric Lymphadenitis Simulating Acute Appendicitis: A Quantitative Study of Size of Normal Lymph Nodes. Arch. Surg., 30:492, 1935.

Moore, T.: Mesenteric Vascular Occlusion. Brit. J. Surg., 28:347, 1940–41.

Morton, C. B.: Intra-abdominal Apoplexy. Arch. Surg., 36:723, 1938.

Ochsner, A., DeBakey, M., and Murray, S.: Pyogenic Abscess of the Liver. II. Analysis of 47 Cases with Review of the Literature. Am. J. Surg., 40:292, 1938.

Plank, J. R.: Non-tuberculous Mesenteric Lymphadenitis. Thesis, Tulane University, 1935.

Trotter, L. B. C.: Embolism and Thrombosis of Mesenteric Vessels. London, Cambridge University Press, 1913.

Wilensky, A. O.: General Lymphadenopathy with General Reference to Nonspecific Mesenteric Adenitis. Arch. Surg., 42:71, 1941.

DISEASES OF THE LIVER

INTRODUCTION

The liver is an integrated anatomic complex consisting chiefly of (1) parenchymal cells (polygonal cells), (2) reticuloendothelial elements (stroma and Kupffer cells) with intervening sinusoids and (3) biliary ducts. In the study of various hepatic disorders, each of these systems should be considered more or less as a functioning unit and the disease evaluated in terms of the extent of derangement of each. For example: Cases of cirrhosis of the liver with scarring due to chronic inflammation of the biliary radicles (biliary cirrhosis) differ in many essential features from cases of cirrhosis with primary injury to the parenchymal cells. In biliary cirrhosis, findings such as chronic jaundice, incomplete biliary obstruction, elevation of serum phosphatase and abnormal elevation of total serum cholesterol are common and characterize dysfunction of the biliary tree. The parenchymal cells may show but little involvement. On the other hand, cases of cirrhosis occur in which polygonal cell disintegration is a primary and active factor and in which there is little evidence of biliary disease. In these cases a positive cephalin flocculation or positive thymol turbidity is usually present and serves as an index of the activity of the process. The extent of the parenchymal damage may be determined by noting decrease in cholesterol esters in the blood or impairment of other metabolic functions of the liver, such as galactose tolerance or hippuric acid synthesis. Diseases of the reticuloendothelial elements may also lead to cirrhosis. They are less easily recognized and may give rise to a variety of clinical pictures, such as splenomegaly, hypochromic anemia, portal hypertension, hyperglobulinemia or acholuric jaundice. Many cases of cirrhosis and other disorders of the liver, especially when extensive or far advanced, show involvement of all the hepatic elements. In some instances, the scarring in cirrhosis may be static and represent merely an episode of the past, in which case the liver may show no functional derangement.

A careful history is usually essential for proper understanding of liver problems, since hepatic damage may develop from a great variety of injuries which augment one another. Factors such as hepatic circulation and oxygenation, adequacy of diet, exposure to toxins, the action of infectious agents, metabolic dyscrasias, neoplasms throughout the body and familial tendencies to liver disease should be especially evaluated.

Many lesions progress unrecognized unless jaundice or hepatic enlargement is present. Other clinical features that may indicate the presence of liver disease are irregularities of hepatic contour, firmness or tenderness of the liver, ascites, prominent collateral veins, hematemesis, splenomegaly, spider angiomas, unexplained anemia, digestive disturbances and lethargy or coma. Pain is rare in liver diseases except in those which cause a rapid stretching of the capsule, or in those involving the serous surfaces.

From a practical standpoint, in addition to the diagnosis, two problems are of paramount importance: (1) the severity of liver damage and (2) the trend of the disease process. A careful check-up at stated intervals of the physical abnormalities, and repetition of a selected group of laboratory tests, are often necessary before an adequate clinical appraisal can be made or the effect of various therapeutic measures determined.

FRANKLIN M. HANGER

JAUNDICE

Definition. Jaundice (icterus) is the yellowish or greenish staining of the skin, mucous membranes and certain body fluids with bile pigments. A persistent bilirubinemia of 1.5 mg. per cent or higher must be present before noticeable discoloration of tissues takes place. Bilirubinuria often precedes a noticeable yellow tint and may be the only indication of mild jaundice. Jaundice is usually a manifestation of some disorder of the liver or biliary tree, but also may result from excessive breakdown of hemoglobin within the body. Unless there is concomitant liver injury, however, the hemolytic type of icterus is characterized by an absence of bile in the urine, an indirect or delayed van den Bergh reaction in the serum, and increased urobilinogen in the urine and stools. (See also Congenital Hemolytic Icterus, p. 1146.)

Jaundice is best detected by examination of the sclerae by natural light. The yellow subconjunctival fat may sometimes cause confusion.

Mechanism of Jaundice. A precise explanation of all types of jaundice is impossible, since the processes involved in the formation and excretion of bile are not known. Bilirubin is derived chiefly from the iron-free porphyrin fraction of hemoglobin which is broken down in the bone marrow and other organs rich in reticuloendothelial tissue. It is liberated into the blood stream as a bilirubin-protein complex characterized by an "indirect" van den Bergh reaction with diazo reagent. The physiologic processes involved in the removal of bilirubin from the blood, the dissociation of the pigment-protein complex and the excretion of bilirubin as the sodium salt in the bile probably depend upon enzymatic activities of the parenchymal cells. Breakdown of red cells and the conversion of hemoglobin to bilirubin take place in the Kupffer system, but there is no evidence that Kupffer cells function in the transport of bile pigments from the blood to the biliary tract. The excretion of bromsulfalein and other colloidal dyes is probably similar to that of bilirubin in that all these are specific threshold substances to the hepatic cells. There is evidence that not all the constituents of the bile are excreted by identical mechanisms. For example, it is common experience to note disproportionate retention of bilirubin, alkaline phosphatase and cholesterol in certain hepatic disorders. Some observers also believe that specific absorption as well as excretion takes place in the liver and small biliary radicles during the elaboration of bile. The inspissated bile plugs of obstructive jaundice, the dilute bile common in hepatitis, and even certain forms of jaundice may in part represent imbalances in secretory or adsorptive activities of hepatic cells. Careful correlations between the histologic changes and various functional derangements have added somewhat to our knowledge of liver physiology, but cellular changes do not necessarily parallel enzymatic imbalances.

In the differential diagnosis of nonhemolytic jaundice it is of first importance to determine if icterus is due primarily (1) to mechanical impediment to the outflow of bile, i.e., obstructive jaundice; or (2) to functional or degenerative changes in the hepatic units, i.e., hepatogenous jaundice (hepatocellular jaundice). Differentiation on the basis of clinical features is sometimes helpful, but laboratory studies are often required. If properly selected, these tests may contribute useful information regarding the degree of active liver parenchymal damage and the status of metabolic and excretory functions of the liver. The following grouping of tests is arbitrary and represents oversimplification, but furnishes a practical approach to the study of jaundice and of disorders of the liver in general:

I. Tests for the detection of alterations in the serum proteins as a manifestation of active parenchymal liver damage:
   1. Determination of serum albumin and globulins
   2. Cephalin-cholesterol flocculation test
   3. Thymol turbidity test

Inflammatory processes within the liver are often manifested by changes in the serum proteins. In longstanding hepatitis the serum albumin tends to decrease below 4 gm. per 100 cc., while the serum globulins tend to rise above 2.8 per 100 cc. The cephalin flocculation test and the thymol test do not depend necessarily on quantitative changes in the serum proteins, but are means of detecting subtle alterations in the albumin and globulin fractions, which develop promptly with certain types of irritation and during active destruction of liver parenchyma. On the other hand, fatty and hyaline changes in the liver or degeneration from chronic anoxia or pressure often cannot be detected by these procedures. Diseases accompanied by chronic irritation of the reticuloendothelial system, such as infectious mononucleosis, acute leukemia, systemic infections, and so forth, may give positive tests in the absence of demonstrable liver disease because of the appearance of abnormal globulin constitutents in the serum.

II. Tests for the detection of impairment of specific metabolic functions of the liver parenchyma:
   1. Hippuric acid test
   2. Urobilinogen excretion in the urine

3. Galactose tolerance test
4. Cholesterol esters in the serum
5. Prothrombin content of the blood

In general the procedures in this category do not give results deviating significantly from the normal until extensive liver damage has occurred. When highly sensitive function tests are used, slight or irrelevant factors often cause deviations which prove quite misleading. Certain metabolic activities of the liver may be specifically affected by toxic agents.

The synthesis of prothrombin, for example, may be depressed by Dicumarol whereas all other hepatic functions are unimpaired.

III. Tests for determining the degree of imment of hepatic excretory function:
   1. Serum bilirubin with partition into the immediate direct and the delayed or indirect reacting fractions
   2. Bromsulfalein excretion
   3. Alkaline phosphatase in the serum
   4. Total serum cholesterol
   5. Bilirubinuria

Serum bilirubin measurements are of greater value in determining the degree of jaundice and following the course of the disease than in attempting to appraise the discoloration of the patient. The quantitation of bilirubin is preferable to using the time-honored icterus index scale (normal 8 units or less) in which nonbiliary pigments in the serum may give misleading readings. The bromsulfalein test is of little value in the presence of jaundice, but is extremely useful in recognizing hepatitis without icterus, cirrhosis of the liver and other diffuse hepatic lesions. Serum alkaline phosphatase levels usually parallel the obstructive factor of jaundice, whether the process is intrahepatic or extrahepatic. Elevation of phosphatase may occur without jaundice, with intrahepatic abscess or neoplasm, or with partial biliary tract obstruction. Serum phosphatase values are higher in children than in adults. In the presence of proliferative bone lesions which cause high blood phosphatase levels, the test is of little value in hepatic studies. Serum cholesterol levels are often conspicuously high when there are lesions involving the smaller bile ducts.

In special clinics all these tests, and many others, are often made. In ordinary practice, when laboratory facilities are limited, it is usually sufficient to rely on a few familiar, well tried techniques in each category, rather than attempt the entire assortment.

The data derived from liver function tests are of little value unless the method used is specified, variations in the normal range considered, and the factors that affect the accuracy of the test recognized and controlled. If the anatomic and functional derangements are complex and labile, with destruction and repair proceeding simultaneously, discrepancies between tests are common, and at times the results may be misleading.

It is essential to repeat the tests from time to time for proper diagnosis and to obtain better insight into the course of the disease.

OBSTRUCTIVE JAUNDICE

Etiology. Obstructive jaundice is caused by an impediment to the flow of bile anywhere along its course from hepatic lobule to duodenum. A rise in pressure in the biliary system causes a back flow of bile into the perilobular lymphatics and by this route into the blood stream (regurgitative jaundice). In chronic cases plugs of inspissated bile are common in distended bile capillaries, especially in a zone near the center of the lobule. These are probably a result of stasis and are not the cause of the obstructive process. In all types of uncomplicated obstructive jaundice the van den Bergh reaction is direct and immediate, indicating that the bilirubin present in the serum has been transformed from the indirect-reacting pigment into a metal-containing derivative with greater aqueous solubility and faster mobility during chromatographic separation. The validity of the van den Bergh reaction as a means of distinguishing and quantitating two forms of bilirubin in the blood has been rightly challenged by a number of observers. Artifacts are no doubt inherent in the procedure, but the presence of the prompt direct-reacting fraction is of unquestioned clinical significance. The rise of serum bilirubin is often slow and gradual, since the kidneys are capable of eliminating large amounts of the direct-reacting bile pigment when the renal threshold level of about 2 mg. per 100 cc. is exceeded in the blood. The bile salts formed in liver cells also increase in the blood and urine and are said to be the chief cause of the pruritus and bradycardia that often characterize obstructive jaundice. Alkaline phosphatase levels in the serum usually exceed 10 Bodansky units. A rise in the total serum cholesterol, especially in the free cholesterol fraction, is common in longstanding cases. The cephalin flocculation and thymol turbidity tests are usually negative, and serum proteins are but little affected except prothrombin, which is diminished unless vitamin K is supplied parenterally or orally with bile salts. When bilirubin fails to reach the intestines, or while certain antibiotics are being administered, urobilinogen practically disappears from the urine and stools.

Extrahepatic obstructive jaundice is usually due to occlusion of the common bile duct by gallstones, carcinoma of the head of the pancreas or of the ampulla of Vater and less commonly by chronic pancreatitis. It may also be caused by acute and chronic inflammation of the duct, stricture, spasm of smooth muscle (especially at the sphincter of Oddi), intestinal parasites within the lumen, pressure on the duct from without, or inflammatory and neoplastic processes in the duodenum.

Congenital malformations of the bile ducts. Obstructive jaundice with acholic stools may be observed in the newborn and in early infancy, due to a variety of intrahepatic disorders including viral and toxic hepatitis and functional excretory derangements associated with erythroblastosis and other hemolytic conditions. Only about one third prove to be caused by congenital malformations or absence of the biliary system.

The clinical features of congenital atresia are those of continued obstructive jaundice, which is most difficult to distinguish at first from less grave hepatic derangements. There is gradual enlargement and fibrosis of the liver and usually of the spleen. During the early stages the general nutrition may be good despite intense icterus, but gradually a cachectic state develops with gastrointestinal bleeding, intercurrent infections and manifestations of hepatic insufficiency. Congenital atresia usually terminates fatally within one or two years unless the cause of obstruction can be corrected surgically. Since exploration in the jaundiced infant entails considerable risk, it is best to delay operation for at least five months in the hope the icterus may be due to a functional derangement which will improve spontaneously. In cases of congenital atresia there is seldom sufficient duct tissue for any form of effective plastic procedure.

Intrahepatic obstructive jaundice, due to obstruction of finer intrahepatic biliary radicles, may result from a number of causes:

1. Acute or chronic cholangitis and cholangiolitis may be secondary to ascending infection along the biliary tract. Biliary cirrhosis may be an advanced stage of this process. Early recognition is important. Mechanical obstructions and gallbladder disease should be relieved surgically. Bacterial infection, if present, should be treated with sulfonamides or appropriate antibiotics.

2. Cholangiolitis may be due to drugs and toxins. This type of intrahepatic obstructive jaundice occurs most frequently during the first weeks of a course of an organic arsenical in patients who acquire an idiosyncrasy to the drug. Violent systemic reactions and increasing jaundice occur promptly after each subsequent injection. The lesion consists of a nonsuppurative cellular infiltration of the periportal areas and swelling of the walls of the finer bile radicles. Similar reactions occur rarely after intravenous gold therapy and after the administration of dinitrophenol, toluylene diamine, cinchophen and chlorpromazine. Jaundice may be protracted, but recovery usually takes place without special therapy. The offending drug should be discontinued indefinitely.

3. Primary cholangiolitis ("cholangie" of Naunyn, "primary intra-hepatic cholangitis" of Sigmund) may occur without exposure to known toxic agents, and is possibly a rare manifestation of infectious jaundice. High elevation of total serum cholesterol after a few weeks of symptomless obstructive jaundice may assist in the diagnosis of the condition, but recognition is difficult, and many protracted cases of this group are explored surgically. Spontaneous recovery usually occurs after many weeks of jaundice; some cases become chronic and terminate after many years with biliary cirrhosis. Relapses are not uncommon. Treatment is symptomatic.

4. Growing neoplasms within the liver, xanthomatosis and also various infectious processes which impinge upon the smaller bile ducts cause biliary obstruction. Increased intrahepatic pressure due to edema or congestion may also impede the excretion of bile.

Clinical Features. The symptoms of obstructive jaundice are variable and depend largely upon the cause and the degree of obstruction. Stones in the common duct are usually associated with pain, fever, and the like, but a significant number (about 5 per cent) cause no symptoms. Carcinoma of the head of the pancreas may be painless, but in about half the cases there is discomfort in the deep epigastrium or back. Itching may be severe and protracted and may precede the jaundice. Bradycardia is common. Loss of weight, anorexia, flatulence, diarrhea and progressive cachexia are often noted and may

many months. Jaundice may actually regress in intensity during longstanding cases of complete obstruction due possibly to secondary changes in the liver.

Treatment. The bleeding tendency in obstructive jaundice is promptly corrected by the daily oral administration of 2 to 4 mg. of menadione (vitamin K) with 0.2 gm. of a

Clinical Features of Possible Value in Distinguishing Hepatogenous from Obstructive Jaundice

	HEPATOGENOUS JAUNDICE (MEDICAL)	OBSTRUCTIVE JAUNDICE (SURGICAL)	
	Catarrhal Jaundice, Infectious Hepatitis, Acute Yellow Atrophy, Toxic (Chemical) Hepatitis	Complete, as in Carcinoma of Pancreas, Gallbladder, Bile Ducts and Liver (Primary)	Incomplete, as in Calculus in Common Bile Duct, Cholangitis, etc.
Age.........	80% under 40 years	80% over 40 years	80% over 40 years
Sex..........	Catarrhal jaundice, 67% males	Ca. of pancreas, 72% males	71% females
	Acute yellow atrophy, 76% females	Ca. gallbladder, usually female	
Initial symptom.......		Pain, 48%	Preceding indigestion
	Anorexia, nausea, vomiting or malaise, 60%	Insidious jaundice, 27%	
Jaundice.....	Rapid development	Progressive and gradual development	Jaundice intermittent or recurrent
Upper abdominal pain...	Present in 56%	Present in 65%	Present in 97%
Upper abdominal tenderness.......	Present in 55%	Usually absent	Present in 29%
Itching of skin	Often absent, usually mild	Usually present except with primary carcinoma of liver	Often absent
Loss of weight	Not striking	Average 20 pounds	Usually
Prodromal infection.....	Present in 25%	None	None
Epidemiology.	May be history of exposure to toxic agents, or of serum injection, or contact with cases	None	None
Fever........	Often present in prodromal period	Often present, except with carcinoma of pancreas	Often present
Spleen.......	Often palpable or enlarged by x-ray	Not palpable	Not palpable
Diabetes mellitus.......	Absent	With carcinoma of pancreas develops in 23%	Absent
Stools.......	Initially light, increasingly bile-stained	Permanently light	Intermittently bile-stained

be caused by the lack of bile salts in the intestines, which are important in the emulsification and absorption of fats and fat-soluble substances. The liver may be somewhat enlarged and tender in obstructive jaundice, and the gallbladder tense and distended, especially when the common bile duct is occluded by noninflammatory processes (Courvoisier's rule). The stools are "clay colored" and rich in fat when obstruction is complete. Malignancy of the head of the pancreas is often differentiated by absence of pancreatic ferments in the duodenal contents. Intermittent obstruction usually indicates a stone or inflammatory process. Longstanding biliary obstruction eventually leads to deterioration of liver parenchyma, but, in the absence of infection, normal liver functions may be maintained for

bile salt preparation, or by 2 mg. of the vitamin alone by subcutaneous injection. When liver injury is present, the response to vitamin K is much less dramatic.

Itching is often difficult to control. Refraining from scratching, soda baths, cooling sprays and lotions are of limited value. Injections of ergotamine tartrate, 0.5 mg., or dihydroxy-ergotamine may afford striking temporary relief. Methyltestosterone and cortisone have been effective in some cases. Hydrocholeretics, such as dehydrocholic acid, 0.25 gm. three times daily, are contraindicated in complete obstruction, but may be tried in cases of cholangitis with incomplete obstruction. The differentiation of extrahepatic obstructive jaundice from intrahepatic obstruction is important, since the

Laboratory Tests Commonly Used for the Differentiation of Hepatogenous from Obstructive Jaundice

TEST	METHOD	RANGE OF NORMAL VALUES	TREND IN HEPATOG-ENOUS JAUNDICE	TREND IN OBSTRUCTIVE JAUNDICE*
Serum albumin...............	Howe	4–5.6%	Decreased	Normal
Serum globulin...............	Howe	1.5–2.6%	Elevated	Normal
Cephalin flocculation...........	Hanger	Neg.–+	Positive	Negative
Thymol turbidity..............	Maclagan	0–4 units	Positive	Negative
Hippuric acid.................	Quick, 1.77 gm. i.v.	0.7 gm. excreted in 1 hr.	Diminished	Normal or slightly diminished
Urinary urobilinogen excretion...	Watson et al.	1 Ehrlich unit or less, in 2 hrs.	Increased	Absent in complete obstruction
Galactose tolerance............	Bassett and Althausen	Serum galactose less than 20 mg. % after 75 minutes	Increased in blood	Normal
Serum cholesterol esters........	Schoenheimer and Sperry	65–75% of total	Diminished	Normal
Plasma prothrombin time.......	Quick	12–18 sec.	Increased, little relief from vitamin K	Relieved by vitamin K
Serum bilirubin—prompt, direct.	Ducci and Watson, 1 minute	0–0.19 mg.	Rapid rise	Gradual rise
Serum bilirubin—total..........	Sepulveda and Osterberg	0.5–1 mg. %	Increased	Increased
Bromsulfalein retention.........	Mateer et al. 5 mg. per kilo, i.v.	0–10% after 30 minutes	Impaired excretion	Impaired excretion
Serum alkaline phosphatase.....	Bodansky	2–4 units	Less than 10 units	Above 10 units
Serum total cholesterol.........	Schoenheimer and Sperry	160–240 mg. %	Decreased	Increased

* Obstructive jaundice of long standing may develop changes similar to those of hepatogenous jaundice.

latter is seldom amenable to surgery. The differential diagnosis depends chiefly upon the history and clinical findings, since the laboratory features are identical. Abdominal exploration is indicated in all obscure cases of persistent or recurring obstructive jaundice.

HEPATOGENOUS JAUNDICE

Hepatogenous jaundice is the result of injury to the cells of the liver parenchyma. It is assumed that intact cords of polygonal cells form the walls of the bile capillaries; hence all pathologic processes disrupting these cells may lead to jaundice by permitting bilirubin in the biliary system to pass directly into the perilobular lymphatic spaces, and thence to the blood stream. It is probable that in some types of liver injury the cells are not actually destroyed, but may be altered functionally so that abnormal absorption and transportation of bile from the lumen of the liver cord to the lymphatic system takes place.

Causes of Hepatogenous Jaundice. Hepatic cells may be injured by diverse processes confined to the liver or in systemic derangements. Jaundice is not uncommon in the following diseases:

1. Infections due to certain viruses, protozoa, bacteria and helminths
    (a) *Viral:* Infectious hepatitis, yellow fever, infectious mononucleosis and primary atypical pneumonia
    (b) *Protozoal:* Weil's disease, malaria, amebiasis, relapsing fever and leishmaniasis
    (c) *Bacterial:* Pneumonia, typhoid fever and sepsis of all kinds; also infections of the liver, such as tuberculosis, mycotic disease, Boeck's sarcoid and suppurative processes
    (d) *Metazoal:* Schistosomiasis and infestations by other liver flukes
2. Chemicals and drugs

In this large list should be included chloroform, carbon tetrachloride and numerous other chlorinated hydrocarbons used in industry, or as insecticides; alcohol, cinchophen, yellow phosphorus, the sulfonamides, tannic acid, picric acid and many other coal tar derivatives, certain snake venoms and toxic mushrooms; also, certain heavy metals such as bismuth, arsenic, antimony, gold, lead and thorium; and, rarely, some of the biologically active steroids, such as methyltestosterone and synthetic estrogens.

3. Miscellaneous systemic reactions, such as severe toxemia of pregnancy, prolonged thyrotoxicosis, untoward immune reactions, anoxia, nutritional deficiencies, severe burns and hemolytic crises.
4. Injuries of unknown etiology, such as in progressive Laënnec's cirrhosis, periarteritis nodosa, and so on. Relatively minor injuries may precipitate jaundice when hepatic damage is already present.

ACUTE INFECTIVE HEPATITIS

(Acute Infectious Jaundice, Acute Catarrhal Jaundice, and Viral Hepatitis)

Catarrhal jaundice is a common clinical condition widespread in many regions, but more prevalent in localities where sanitary standards are low. The disease occurs usually sporadically or in small epidemics, but in times of war and mass migrations may involve thousands of subjects (camp jaundice).

Etiology. Infectious hepatitis is caused by a filterable virus present in the blood of patients for many days before the appearance of clinical manifestations, and for an indeterminate period after the onset of jaundice. Experimental transmission of the disease to human volunteers has led to the identification of at least two variations of viral hepatitis, i.e., infectious hepatitis, caused by virus A (I.H. virus), and serum hepatitis, caused by virus B (S.H. virus). These two forms of infection are not readily differentiated by clinical features, but are characterized by differences in incubation periods, by the routes of natural dissemination and by the specific immunity conferred by each virus. The two infective agents are similar in many respects. Both pass a Seitz E.K. filter, neither causes disease in laboratory animals, and both resist drying, freezing and heating at 56° C. for 30 minutes. Comparative resistance of the two viruses to other physical and chemical treatments has not been completely established, but fragmentary studies suggest survival after chlorination, 1 part per million, and exposure to tricresol 0.2%, ether 10%, merthiolate 1:2,000, and nitrogen mustard 500 mg. per liter. Virus B is inactivated in plasma containing sulfa mustard (0.005 M

final concentration). Both are transmissible to man through transfusions or through the administration of plasma, packed red cells, fibrinogen, thrombin or fraction IV. The agents are destroyed in the processing of Fibrin Foam, gamma globulin and albumin after heating at 60° C. for 10 hours. Plasma subjected to ultraviolet radiation or to storage at room temperature for long periods shows some decrease in infectivity, but no trustworthy method of sterilizing whole blood or plasma and many of its derivatives has yet been devised.

1. *Infectious Hepatitis.* The incubation period is relatively short, twenty to forty days. Infection is naturally disseminated by the fecal-oral route through the ingestion of contaminated food and water, and close personal contacts with carriers. The disease is also transmitted by exposure to infected blood. Virus A is demonstrable in the duodenal contents, stools and blood during the pre-icteric period and during the acute phases of the illness, but is probably absent in the nasal secretions, saliva and urine. The duration of infectivity is difficult to determine but probably terminates in most cases with the subsidance of acute symptoms. Carriers of virus A, however, have been identified, especially among children, as long as sixteen months after the initial infection.

2. *Serum Hepatitis.* The incubation period is relatively long, 60 to 160 days or more. The virus is found only in the blood, which may be infectious in minute amounts. Transmission occurs most frequently after transfusions or injections of materials containing human plasma, but has been observed after exposure to inadequately sterilized syringes, needles and surgical and dental equipment. The possibility of natural dissemination through insect vectors, sexual contact or placental transmission cannot be excluded. The majority of those individuals harboring virus B give no history of hepatitis and have no detectable evidence of hepatic disease, making the routine selection of safe blood donors an impossible task. The carrier state may persist indefinitely; an instance exceeding five years has been documented.

Infectious hepatitis has been recognized for centuries in this country and abroad, and recent studies on viruses A and B by no means exclude the existence of other related and unrelated icterogenic agents. The great increase in the incidence and severity of the disease in the past decade is generally ascribed to the growing use of parenteral injections and to the dissemination during World War II of strains of virus to which there was little acquired immunity. Sporadic catarrhal jaundice encountered before that time probably represented forms of mild endemic infection involving most of the population during early life, and only recognized in the occasional jaundiced patient. The immunity conferred by these infections was apparently lifelong and specific, but has offered little protection against the newly introduced prevalent strains. Sporadic cases of catarrhal jaundice are still common and the nature and source of infection may be difficult to determine.

Infectious mononucleosis may simulate viral hepatitis very closely. Many cases of hepatitis represent inflammatory and degenerative changes in the liver after exposure to various toxic agents. Some follow sore throats and other acute infections as an immune reaction similar to that occurring in the kidneys in acute nephritis. There is some evidence that previous exposure to noxious agents such as arsphenamine increases the severity of symptoms of viral hepatitis. In like manner, a recent prior attack of infectious hepatitis or a debilitating illness often augments the severity of a subsequent attack of serum hepatitis.

Pathology. The term "catarrhal jaundice" is a misnomer based on the assumption of Virchow that the primary lesion is an ascending catarrhal inflammation in the biliary tree. Such types of cholangitis and cholangiolitis do occur, but needle biopsies of the liver at various stages of the disease indicate the prime lesion to be injury and necrosis of parenchymal cells. The extent of cellular damage ranges from an occasional swollen or shrunken, pink-staining cell with disintegrating nucleus to massive central necrosis of practically every lobule of the liver. The Kupffer cells are often swollen and appear in masses along the walls of the sinusoids. Edema and cellular infiltration of the portal and periportal areas are also common. In rare instances the parenchymal damage is slight and periportal involvement marked.

The clinical picture and laboratory tests depend somewhat upon the hepatic structures involved. A positive cephalin flocculation reaction usually reflects parenchymal necrosis, whereas elevation of the serum alkaline phosphatase indicates a biliary obstructive factor. There is little correlation, however, between the histologic findings and the intensity of jaundice or disturbances in the metabolic function of the liver. In fatal cases parenchymal damage is usually extensive. When the disease process is confined to the portal and periportal structures— "cholangiolitic hepatitis"—the cephalin flocculation reaction is often negative and the elevated serum alkaline phosphatase, elevated serum cholesterol, itching of the skin and enlarged firm liver simulate the picture of extrahepatic obstructive jaundice. The larger bile ducts are usually not involved in infectious hepatitis; there is, however, evidence of gastritis and duodenitis by roentgenologic and gastroscopic examination in certain cases.

Clinical Aspects. In typical infective hepatitis there is usually a symptomless incubation period of twenty to 120 days, depending upon the type of infection and virulence of the agent. The *prodromal* or *preicteric stage* may be abrupt or gradual at onset. Fever and prostration are said to be more notable in infectious hepatitis than in serum hepatitis, but the two conditions cannot be distinguished on this basis. Transient skin rash, arthralgia and lymph node enlargement may appear during this stage and are thought by many to represent a sensitization of the host to the infecting agent. Other symptoms arranged roughly in order of frequency may be present: anorexia, which is a most important feature in differential diagnosis; malaise, distaste for tobacco, fatigability, headache, chilly sensations, nausea, vomiting, upper abdominal distress, pruritus, dark urine, light stools, constipation and diarrhea. Physical examination reveals little at this stage to distinguish hepatitis from many other acute febrile disorders, such as influenza, primary atypical pneumonia, malaria, infectious mononucleosis, encephalitis or gastrointestinal upsets. The liver may be somewhat enlarged and tender, especially to a jarring blow over the lower ribs. The spleen may be palpable, or found to be enlarged by roentgenogram, in about one fifth of the cases.

Laboratory values may be entirely normal at the pre-icteric stage, but elevation of serum alkaline phosphatase, bromsulfalein retention, a positive cephalin-cholesterol flocculation reaction and elevated urine urobilinogen may indicate involvement of the liver before the appearance of jaundice. Bilirubinuria, especially in morning specimens, may appear several days before jaundice, or even before hyperbilirubinemia occurs. Leukopenia with occasional large immature mononuclear cells is a finding often useful in distinguishing viral hepatitis from many other diseases causing jaundice. The pre-icteric stage averages about six days, but may vary from a few hours to three weeks. Jaundice is usually manifest early in severe cases, but fulminating infections may terminate fatally before icterus has appeared.

Icteric Stage. With the onset of jaundice the symptoms of the disease may abate promptly, but usually there are a few days of exacerbation in which lassitude, anorexia and nausea are striking. Right upper abdominal pain may be of such severity that a mistaken diagnosis of cholecystitis or other surgical conditions is made. The jaundice deepens rapidly, reaching a maximum within a week, and then fades gradually. The icteric stage lasts but a few days in mild cases, but may persist for six weeks or longer in patients with severe liver damage, or in those with a marked factor of biliary obstruction. Sudden reappearance of appetite and a return of the sense of well-being usually appear while jaundice is deepest and signalize the beginning of the recovery period. Spider angiomas are notably rare in acute hepatitis, and their appearance may signalize chronic inflammatory disease in the liver.

Laboratory Tests. During the icteric stage of hepatitis the cephalin flocculation and thymol turbidity tests are usually positive. A rise in serum alkaline phosphatase level to 15 Bodansky units or higher is not uncommon in viral hepatitis, especially at the onset. In contrast to extrahepatic obstructive jaundice, however, the alkaline phosphatase level decreases gradually in uncomplicated cases of hepatitis even while the serum bilirubin continues to rise. Most routine liver function tests (especially cholesterol ester determinations) indicate impairment of liver parenchymal activity. Urine urobilinogen, which is usually increased in the preicteric and convalescent stages of hepatitis, may be decreased as jaundice deepens because of the diminished amounts of bilirubin reaching the intestines at that time. The urine is dark, and the foam on shaking is discolored. Harrison's test or some other sensitive test should always be employed to identify suspected traces of bilirubin which might escape detection by gross examination.

Convalescence. The stage of convalescence and liver regeneration is often vague and difficult of clinical appraisal. Many patients are weak and depressed long after jaundice has disappeared. Some complain of flatulence and fat intolerance. The liver may remain enlarged and tender for many weeks, and at biopsy show persisting inflammatory lesions. In other cases, laboratory tests may indicate active parenchymal irritation and impairment of one or more liver functions long after clinical manifestations have subsided. Tolerance to exercise is often low in the convalescent, and undue exertion may cause exacerbation of symptoms and the return of abnormal laboratory findings. With proper care, eventual recovery usually takes place, but relapses and occasional cases of chronic hepatitis leading to coarse nodular cirrhosis have followed acute attacks.

Rarely, patients convalescing from hepatitis develop the picture of obstructive jaundice with itching, clay colored stools and elevated serum alkaline phosphatase, and negative cephalin flocculation. These attacks usually subside spontaneously and are attributed to accumulations of inspissated bile in the biliary tree.

The case fatality rate from hepatitis is less than 0.5 per cent. Severe acute cases can be recognized by rapidly deepening jaundice, a pungent amine odor to the breath, the appearance of neurologic symptoms such as coarse tremors, delirium, drowsiness and coma, and the development of a hemorrhagic tendency, unrelieved by vitamin K administration. Chronic cases also may succumb after a long lingering illness to hepatic insufficiency, intercurrent infection and inanition. Many patients with hepatitis, especially young children, are encountered in whom no jaundice develops. In different epidemics the incidence of nonicteric cases has varied from 28 to 80 per cent of the total number of infections. The symptoms are similar but somewhat milder than in the jaundiced group. The liver is usually enlarged and tender, or becomes so after exercise. Bromsulfalein retention is often present, and the cephalin flocculation is positive in about 85 per cent. Mild and unrecognized cases of hepatitis give rise to perplexing epidemiologic problems.

Prophylaxis. The dissemination of infective hepatitis is difficult to control because of the prevalence of unrecognized cases and because the disorder is probably most readily transmitted by subjects in the pre-icteric stage. The incidence of hepatitis among those receiving transfusions exceeds 3 per cent in certain clinics despite careful questioning and laboratory screening of all donors. The disturbing increase of healthy carriers emphasizes the curtailment of unwarranted transfusions and the use of human albumin and blood substitutes whenever practicable. Outbreaks of infectious hepatitis in dormitories and institutions have been found difficult to control by hygienic disciplines alone. Gamma globulin 0.01 cc. per pound (2 to 4 cc. for adults) has been shown by Stokes to be an effective measure in suppressing epidemics and preventing infection in those who have been recently closely exposed to fresh cases. Prophylaxis lasts for six weeks or longer and may be considered advisable for those traveling to countries where the disease is prevalent. Gamma globulin is of no value in the prophylaxis of serum hepatitis.

Management. Bed rest during the prodromal stage and during the period of increasing jaundice is most important, irrespective of etiology, since there is evidence that overexertion lengthens the clinical course and aggravates the severity of symptoms. The blood and stools should be regarded as infectious in the early stages of viral hepatitis. All needles and syringes should be thoroughly sterilized before further use, and aseptic precautions in handling excreta, bedding, and so forth, should be maintained at least until the fever subsides and jaundice begins to fade. The need for such precautions in the sporadic case of catarrhal jaundice has not yet been established, but seems advisable.

Dietary regulation is not an important factor in the treatment of acute hepatitis. Patients should be encouraged to eat bland food and suck hard candies. No particular value has been demonstrated in forcing high caloric or high protein diets. Fats, if well tolerated, may be added as the appetite returns. Small frequent feedings consisting of gruel, lean meats, milk, milk powder, cottage cheese and simple desserts are often better tolerated than large bulky meals. Liquids or semisolids are often more tempting than foods requiring chewing. Supplements of vitamins, lipotropic agents and intravenous amino acids are not indicated in acute cases and rarely in chronic cases except when the maintenance of nutrition becomes a serious problem.

For the vomiting patient or for one who is comatose or refuses food, slow infusions of 10 per cent glucose, 3000 to 4000 cc. daily, should be given. Human plasma or preferably blood transfusions are indicated for toxic cases with marked prostration or with hemorrhagic tendencies. Cortisone and ACTH are not to be recommended for the routine treatment of acute hepatitis. Symptoms may be temporarily abated, but relapses are notably high in the treated group. Brief trials of one of these drugs are indicated in cases failing to show improvement after an illness of six weeks or more, as convalescence may sometimes be hastened by 100 mg. a day of cortisone given for a period of five days. The indication for cortisone in fulminating and desperately ill cases of acute hepatitis has not been established. Recoveries have been reported in a few instances, but in the majority no benefit has been observed.

Gamma globulin fractions, useful in prophylaxis, have little therapeutic value. Alcohol and hepatotoxic agents should be avoided during the entire course of the disease. Barker and his associates have emphasized the importance of adequate rest during convalescence. The reappearance of an enlarged or tender liver, an exacerbation of jaundice, or unfavorable trends in the cephalin flocculation or various liver function tests are indications for further restriction of activity. Persisting positive flocculation tests months after subsidence of symptoms often indicate residual inflammatory foci in the portal triads, which, however, seldom lead to cirrhosis or to progressive and fatal hepatic tissue destruction. Constant bed rest is not indicated in these cases, but fatigue and strenuous work should be curtailed until complete recovery is established. The few patients who eventually have the chronic hepatitis syndrome may be recognized by increasing impairment of various hepatic function tests and the development of a firm, irregular liver. The factors leading to chronicity are not well recognized, but probably cannot be attributed to mismanagement so much as to the constitutional characteristics of the person. It is noteworthy that most cases of chronic hepatitis and nodular cirrhosis follow mild and atypical illnesses rather than a characteristic attack of hepatitis. No therapy has yet been found effective in modifying the unfavorable progression of well-established chronic hepatitis.

NONINFECTIOUS HEPATOGENOUS JAUNDICE (TOXIC HEPATITIS)

(Liver Injury Due to Chemical Agents)

The symptomatic and physiologic disturbances of "toxic hepatitis" vary considerably, depending upon the extent and cause of the liver injury, the amount of hemoglobin breakdown, and the involvement of other organs by the noxious agent. Shock and hepatic anoxia often augment the damage caused by toxic agents. Toxic necrosis may be difficult to distinguish from viral hepatitis since fever, deepening jaundice and enlarged tender liver are common to both. Leukocytosis points against a viral infection. The two conditions may also be difficult to identify by histologic examination, but cellular damage is more prone to show a zonal distribution, fatty infiltration is more prominent and secondary inflammatory reactions in the mesenchymal structures of the liver are less striking with toxic hepatitis. Lesions in the kidneys and skin, when present, are generally indicative of toxic processes.

Toxic hepatitis may develop acutely and jaundice and hepatic insufficiency may appear a few hours after exposure to the noxious agent such as phosphorus, arsenic and the chlorinated hydrocarbons. Smaller doses of the same toxic agents with repeated exposures may lead to more gradual liver injury with an insidious clinical course. In some cases fatty or hyaline degeneration develops; in others, cirrhosis; and in others, sudden massive cellular degeneration with jaundice appears weeks or months after exposure to the agent. Symptoms of chronic liver damage may consist of fatigability, nervousness and vague gastrointestinal complaints, or may be entirely lacking until jaundice or manifestations of extensive hepatic insufficiency develop. The liver may be somewhat enlarged and tender, but chronic liver injury due to chemicals may be difficult to recognize in the absence of jaundice. The cephalin flocculation test is often negative in these cases; it is not a reliable index of hyaline or fatty degeneration of liver cells. Cotter has noted that gradual decrease of cholesterol esters below 65 per cent of the total blood cholesterol may be the first indication of liver damage in those exposed to chemical hazards.

There is a marked individual variation in susceptibility to hepatotoxic agents. Persons with fatty livers are especially subject to injury by these substances, also patients with notable dietary deficiencies in carbohydrates, proteins and the vitamin B complex. Intercurrent infections, gastrointestinal upsets, gallbladder diseases and exposure to multiple toxins (including use of alcohol) often aggravate the severity and chronicity of symptoms.

Diagnosis. Hepatotoxic agents may be inhaled, ingested, absorbed through the skin or received by injection, and often careful and ingenious questioning is necessary to identify the offending substance and the mode of entry. A history of past arsphenamine administration, pills for arthritis (cinchophen), use of cleaning solutions, exposure to insecticides, and employment in chemical and electrical equipment plants, even months or years previously, may be significant in the appraisal of certain cases of hepatitis. It is often difficult to exclude the possibility of a superimposed virus infection.

Treatment. Therapy consists in stopping exposure to all liver poisons, including alcohol and drugs. The diet should be high in carbohydrate, moderately rich in proteins and low in fats with supplements of vitamin B complex. Methionine or choline, 2 to 4 gm. daily, may be tried, but these substances are much less effective therapeutically than when used prophylactically as lipotropic agents. Some authorities recommend frequent injections of crude liver extract. Rest in bed should be enforced until improvement is obvious. Fatiguing exertion should be avoided for many months. In severe cases continuous slow infusions of 5 per cent glucose in saline are indicated. Transfusions of whole blood or plasma are sometimes beneficial.

ACUTE YELLOW ATROPHY OF THE LIVER

Acute yellow atrophy of the liver is the designation usually applied to any severe form of hepatitis, either infective or toxic, characterized by rapid shrinkage in size of the liver, extensive necrosis of the polygonal cells, and the symptomatology of hepatic insufficiency.

Incidence. The disease is said to have become more common since chlorinated hydrocarbons and other hepatotoxic compounds have been widely used in industry and therapeutics. These toxic agents in sufficient amounts may cause liver necrosis directly, but in many instances are thought to condition the resistance of liver cells to further intercurrent injury. Various chronic infections and parasitic infestations, malaria, malnutrition, colitis, chronic fatigue, alcoholism and other disorders prompting fatty liver also predispose to extensive damage. Activation of autolytic processes within the damaged liver cells is probably an important contributing factor to the fulminating destructive process. The disease is most common in middle-aged women for reasons that are not obvious.

Clinical Features. At onset the clinical features are in no way different from those of infectious jaundice or toxic hepatitis. After a few days, however, jaundice continues to deepen, hemorrhagic tendencies appear, and the patient becomes lethargic, confused or comatose and exhibits neurologic signs such as tremors, rigidity, abnormal reflexes and convulsions which may be confused with meningitis or cerebral hemorrhage. The liver, which is normal in size or enlarged at onset, becomes soft, shrunken and tender, so that a blow over the lower right thorax causes the patient to cry out. The hemorrhagic tendency increases, with ecchymoses and bleeding from the mucous membranes. Breathing becomes deep and stertorous. The breath has a characteristic fishy odor (fetor hepaticus). The temperature is variable, but is often subnormal. The pulse becomes increasingly weak and rapid. Coma deepens and the patient dies in hepatic insufficiency, but the chemical factors precipitating death are not well understood.

The *laboratory findings* in acute yellow atrophy are those of hepatitis combined with evidence of marked breakdown of normal liver function. The cephalin flocculation test is positive, and there is at times sufficient reduction in serum albumin to promote ascites and generalized anasarca. The serum globulins are often elevated. The hippuric acid excretion, urobilinogen in the urine, galactose tolerance test, cholesterol ester determination and other liver function tests show extensive impairment. Lactic acid accumulates in the blood and deaminization is depressed, causing decrease of urea in the blood and urine and a rise in ammonia and amino acids. Deficiency of prothrombin and other factors in the clotting mechanism may give rise to spontaneous hemorrhage. Fibrinogen is decreased only as a terminal event. Hypoglycemia, which is observed in the totally hepatectomized animal, is infrequent. Serum bilirubin levels may rise rapidly to 20 mg. per 100 cc. or higher, with immediate direct van den Bergh reaction. The blood volume may increase 20 per cent or more. The urine is deeply bile stained and may contain red blood cells, albumin and casts. The stools may be acholic, but are often colored by bile-stained intestinal secretions and by bleeding into the gut.

Treatment. Acute yellow atrophy is usually fatal despite all therapy. Infusions of glucose, 5 to 10 per cent, totaling 3 to 4 liters daily by slow drip, should be given. Protein feedings should be curtailed, and amino acid supplements and ammonium salts are contraindicated, since they augment blood ammonia levels and intensify the neurologic disturbances. Whole blood transfusion and salt-free human albumin are indicated to maintain normal blood pressure levels. Sterilization of the gastrointestinal tract by the oral use of chlortetracycline (Aureomycin) or oxytetracycline (Terramycin) 1 gm. per day is sometimes of temporary benefit and at least curbs secondary infections. Cortisone has been employed in doses of 100 mg. to 1000 mg. daily, but its efficacy is dubious.

SUBACUTE YELLOW ATROPHY

Progressive hepatic insufficiency is frequently observed in subacute and chronic hepatitis. In these cases the course is less fulminating, rapid shrinkage of the liver is less common, but the symptomatology is in general the same as in acute yellow atrophy. Periods of temporary improvement may interrupt the downward trend. Ultimate recovery may sometimes take place after many discouraging weeks of severe "cholemia." Psychoses, mental depressions, transient ascites and marked weakness often feature the illness and early convalescence. The regenerated liver is often permanently scarred and coarsely nodular, but, if the disease process becomes quiescent, normal function is ultimately regained. Except for the possible development of portal vein hypertension, or superimposed hepatoma, patients with "inactive" cirrhosis have an excellent life expectancy despite diminished hepatic reserve.

Therapy consists of good nursing and maintaining adequate nutrition by frequent small tasty feedings and sparing the patient all fatiguing activities.

ACHOLURIC JAUNDICE

Jaundice with absence of bile in the urine and with a delayed or indirect van den Bergh reaction in the serum may result from (1) derangements of the liver or Kupffer cells leading to diminished or retarded removal of the bilirubin-protein complex from the blood, where it occurs as a natural product of hemoglobin metabolism (retention jaundice); or (2) from excessive breakdown of red blood cells within the body, leading to the formation of a bilirubin complex in quantities exceeding the excretion capacity of the liver (hemolytic jaundice). The intensity of jaundice is usually slight, and is often manifested only by a greenish discoloration of the sclerae. Massive or protracted hemolysis, however, may lead to hepatic injury with bilirubinuria and abnormal function tests. Serum bilirubin levels rarely exceed 9 mg. per cent, even in the severest cases. Itching and bradycardia are lacking, and symptoms, if present, are usually referable to the primary condition.

RETENTION JAUNDICE

All factors, physiologic or in disease, which cause sufficient rise of the bilirubin excretory threshold of the liver may induce acholuric jaundice. Icterus neonatorum, present in most infants during the first week of life, is probably the commonest example of this disorder.

Physiologic Hyperbilirubinemia (*Constitutional Hepatic Dysfunction with Indirect van den Bergh Reaction*). This condition occurs chiefly in a subclinical form and is detected during routine serum bilirubin determinations in normal healthy persons. In overt cases, jaundice is usually first noted in early youth and tends to become less striking with advancing years. Dameshek has described a familial type. Patients are usually symptomless, but may be thin, introspective and subject to fatigability, caused in part by the undue concern of physicians unfamiliar with the disorder. Icterus is seldom intense; it often becomes deeper after fatigue, exertion or intercurrent illnesses. The liver is normal in size and shows no impairment of function except a possible delay in the elimination from the serum of injected bilirubin. There are no abnormalities of the blood. The condition may be differentiated from familial hemolytic jaundice by the absence of anemia, splenomegaly, spherocytosis, reticulocytosis and normal fragility of red cells to hypotonic saline. It is also important not to confuse physiologic icterus with chronic hepatitis. The absence of prompt direct-reacting serum bilirubin and of bilirubinuria, and a normal cephalin flocculation test, tend to rule out parenchymal damage, but observations for many months and even biopsy may be required for the definite exclusion of a progressive degenerative process within the liver.

Increase of delayed indirect-reacting bilirubin in the serum may also be found in a variety of liver disorders such as hepatitis, prolonged obstructive jaundice, severe anemia, anoxia, toxic states, systemic infections and various hemolytic processes, in which impairment of hepatic excretory function is probably due to organic disturbances. Often both "regurgitative" and "retention" factors contribute to the development of hyperbilirubinemia in these conditions. Bilirubin due to the former is measured as the fraction giving a prompt direct van den Bergh reaction. The bilirubin resulting from "retention" factors is calculated as the difference between the total serum bilirubin and the prompt-reacting fraction. (Total bilirubin minus one minute reacting component.) The relative amounts of the two types found in the serum reveal little as to the nature of the hepatic disorder, since prompt direct-reacting bilirubin is subject to excretion by the kidneys in indefinite amounts, while the delayed indirect fraction is retained by the renal barrier.

CAROTENEMIA

Jaundice is not to be confused with carotenemia, which is a general term to denote excess xanthosis of the skin and increased lipochromes in the blood, secondary to the ingestion of carrots, squash, spinach, oranges, egg yolk and other sources of dietary pigment. Normal values of pigment are 0.07 to 0.19 mg. per 100 cc. of serum. The condition is usually harmless, but since pigmentation tends to parallel total serum lipids, its presence may denote hypothyroidism, diabetes and, rarely, nephrosis. The pigment in the blood causes an elevated icterus index but fails to give a positive van den Bergh reaction. Yellowish discoloration is deepest in the horny layers of the skin of the palms, soles, forehead, nasolabial folds, axillas and groin, but, in contrast to jaundice, does not appear in the conjunctivas or buccal mucous membranes. The pigment is secreted in the sweat and sebum and the staining of the skin is probably chiefly from this source.

HEMOLYTIC JAUNDICE

See the chapter on Hemolytic Anemia.

FRANKLIN M. HANGER

References

Jaundice

Barker, M. H., Capps, R. B., and Allen, F. W.: Hepatitis in the Mediterranean Theatre. J.A. M.A., *128*:997; *129*:653, 1945.

Eppinger, H.: Die Leberkrankheiten. Allgemeine und spezielle Pathologie und Therapie der Leber. Vienna, Julius Springer, 1937.

Gray, C. H.: The Bile Pigments. New York, John Wiley & Sons, 1953.

Hanger, F. M., and Gutman, A. B.: Post-arsphen-amine Jaundice Apparently Due to Obstruction of Intrahepatic Bilary Tract. J.A.M.A., *115:* 263, 1940.

Havens, W. P., Jr.: Infectious Hepatitis. Medicine, 27:279, 1948.

Havens, W. P., Jr.: Etiology and Epidemiology of Viral Hepatitis. Presented before the American Association for Study of Liver Diseases. Chicago, Oct. 29, 1953.

Mallory, T. B.: The Pathology of Epidemic Hepatitis. J.A.M.A., *134:*655, 1947.

Neefe, J. R.: Viral Hepatitis: Problems and Progress. Ann. Int. Med., 31:857, 1949.

Popper, H., and Franklin, Murray: Viral versus Toxic Hepatic Necrosis. Arch. Path., 46:338, 1948.

Stokes, J., Jr., and Neefe, J. R.: The Prevention and Attenuation of Infectious Hepatitis by Gamma Globulin. J.A.M.A., *127:*144, 1945.

Acholuric Jaundice

Dameshek, W., and Singer, K.: Familial Non-hemolytic Jaundice. Arch. Int. Med., 67:259, 1941.

Bibliography for Table on page 919

Bassett, A. M., Althausen, T. L., and Coltrin, G. C.: A New Galactose Test for Differentiation of Obstructive from Parenchymatous Jaundice. Am. J. Digest Dis., 8:432, 1941.

Bodansky, A.: Phosphatase Studies. II. Determination of Serum Phosphatase: Factors Influencing Accuracy of Determination. J. Biol. Chem., *101:*93, 1933.

Ducci, H., and Watson, C. J.: The Quantitative Determination of the Serum Bilirubin with Special Reference to the Prompt Reacting and the Chloroform-soluble Types. J. Lab. & Clin. Med., 30:293, 1945.

Hanger, F. M.: Serological Differentiation of Obstructive from Hepatogenous Jaundice by Flocculation of Cephalin-Cholesterol Emulsions. J. Clin. Investigation, 18:3, 261, 1939.

Hawkinson, V., Watson, C. J., and Turner, R. H.: Modification of Harrison's Test for Bilirubin in the Urine. J.A.M.A., 129:514, 1945.

Maclagan, N. F.: The Thymol Turbidity Test as an Indicator of Liver Dysfunction. Brit. J. Exper. Path., 25:234, 1944.

Malloy, H. T., and Evelyn, K. A.: The Determination of Bilirubin with Photoelectric Colorimeter. J. Biol. Chem., *119:*481, 1937.

Mateer, J. G., Baltz, J. I., Marion, D. F., and Mac-Millan, J. M.: Liver Function Tests. J.A.M.A., *121:*723, 1943.

Quick, A. J.: The Clinical Application of the Hippuric Acid and the Prothrombin Tests. Am. J. Clin. Path., 10:222, 1940.

Schoenheimer, R., and Sperry, W. M.: A Micro Method for the Determination of Free and Combined Cholesterol. J. Biol. Chem., *106:* 745, 1934.

Watson, C. J., Schwartz, S., Sborov, S., and Bertie, E.: Studies of Urobilinogen. V. A Simple Method for the Quantitative Recording of the Ehr-lich Reaction as Carried out with Urine and Feces. Am. J. Clin. Path., *14:*605, 1944.

CIRCULATORY DISTURBANCES OF THE LIVER

The liver is a highly vascular organ with a dual blood supply, the hepatic arterial system and the portal venous system. There are said to be shunts between the two systems as well a free mixing within the sinusoids. Both circuits are drained by a common venous system. Blood flow in the liver is said to fluctuate widely according to the organ's functional activity. It has been estimated that the blood flow through the liver of normal man at rest averages about 1500 cc. per minute, accounting for approximately 25 per cent of the basal cardiac output. During exercise this flow is sharply reduced. From 70 to 90 per cent of its circulation is mediated through the portal channels under normal conditions. Indeed, recent studies indicate that the normal dog can survive ligation of the hepatic artery.

Disturbances in circulation bring about functional changes in the liver. In both clinical and experimental *shock* there is evidence that the liver is damaged. In experimental hemorrhagic shock there is a sharp decrease in portal blood flow resulting in anoxia of the liver and widespread changes in metabolism. Likewise in *chronic passive congestion,* stasis and anoxemia may bring about functional and anatomic changes.

In addition, there are local vascular changes which affect the liver. In certain forms of *acute hepatitis* the sinusoids are constricted by swollen liver cells. It has been suggested that this interference with intrahepatic circulation may lead to massive necrosis. In advanced *cirrhosis* the main portal trunks are stenosed, the finer portal channels are obliterated and the blood flow is thereby greatly reduced. The cirrhotic liver depends chiefly on the hepatic arterial system for its effective blood supply. Local vascular diseases of the liver are rare. Of these, *thrombosis of the portal vein* is the most common.

PASSIVE CONGESTION OF THE LIVER

Etiology. Failure of the heart is the chief cause for passive congestion of the liver.

Pathogenesis. In the early stage the liver appears enlarged and its capsule tense. On section there is red and gray mottling, giving a "nutmeg" appearance. Microscopically, the central veins and capillaries are seen to be congested, and the liver cells in these areas are atrophied. Necrosis and hemorrhage take place in the central areas as congestion becomes more severe. The walls of the hepatic veins are thickened, and there generally is some increase of connective tissue about the central and periportal areas. Ultimately the liver becomes shrunken because of atrophy of parenchymal cells and condensation of tissue. In certain cases broad strands of connective tissue extend from one central vein area to another, giving the picture of false lobulation. This stage is termed congestive (cardiac) cirrhosis.

Symptoms and Signs. The primary disease (heart failure) dominates the clinical picture. Frequently there are no symptoms attributable to the liver itself, or merely a sense of heaviness in the right hypochondrium. The patient rarely has sharp pains that simulate gallbladder colic.

The liver surface feels firm, smooth and elastic. Tenderness over the liver, an inconstant feature, is said to be more frequent with rapid enlargement following acute cardiac decompensation. The venous pressure in the antecubital vein is elevated and the circulation time is prolonged. Ascites occurs in about one half of the cases. It is apt to be more prominent with severe or protracted congestive failure. Clinical jaundice is much less frequent and apparently bears no relation to the degree of passive congestion. The cause of jaundice in heart failure is not clear. It tends to be more intense in the presence of necrosis of liver cells. Splenomegaly is present in about one third of the cases. Although the esophageal veins may be widened, they do not form varicosities and they seldom if ever rupture.

Laboratory tests show evidence of functional impairment of the liver. As a rule there is slight elevation of serum bilirubin. In at least 75 per cent of the cases there is increased bromsulfalein dye retention and increased urobilinogen excretion in the urine, the degree of change bearing a correlation with the degree of congestive failure. In about one third of the cases there is a moderate decrease of serum albumin and increase of serum globulin. The serum alkaline phosphatase may be slightly increased. The function of the liver, as determined by the various tests, is restored to normal as cardiac compensation is achieved.

Treatment should be directed at the underlying disease.

CONGESTIVE (CARDIAC) CIRRHOSIS

Congestive cirrhosis is characterized by connective tissue proliferation chiefly about the central hepatic veins, in association with longstanding passive congestion of the liver. The histologic criteria for diagnosis have been the subject of controversy. Indeed, certain authorities do not accept congestive cirrhosis as a pathologic entity.

Occurrence. If the term "congestive cirrhosis" is restricted to those cases with extensive fibrosis about the central veins and distortion of the lobular pattern, the condition is seen in 5 to 10 per cent of patients dying of heart disease.

For the most part it occurs in patients who have had persistent or recurrent congestive failure for a year or more. It is associated most frequently with marked valvular deformity of rheumatic heart disease, somewhat less frequently with hypertensive heart disease, and only occasionally with other types of heart failure. Chronic constrictive pericarditis frequently is complicated by a severe grade of congestive cirrhosis.

Pathogenesis. Zimmerman and Hillsman have produced congestive cirrhosis in dogs by partial occlusion of the inferior vena cava in its thoracic portion. The prevailing opinion is that the combination of stasis and anoxemia leads to necrosis and connective tissue proliferation in the liver. There is little evidence to support a former concept that infection or "toxemia" plays a role in the pathogenesis.

Morbid Anatomy. The liver is of normal or somewhat reduced size, and its capsule is thickened. On cross section the liver appears finely nodular and mottled. Fibrosis is most marked in the central zones, but may also be present in the portal regions.

Physical Signs. Elevated venous pressure, cyanosis, palpable liver, ascites and dependent edema generally are present. The spleen is enlarged in about one half of the cases, and jaundice is present in about one third. Laboratory tests indicate functional impairment of the liver.

Diagnosis. The clinical picture may be indistinguishable from that of passive congestion. The liver tends to be smaller, and the spleen larger, in congestive cirrhosis than in passive congestion alone. Diagnosis here is based more upon inference than upon physical signs. A presumptive diagnosis of congestive cirrhosis may be made in a patient with congestive heart failure for a year or more who has either a small nonpalpable liver or a very firm liver, a palpable spleen and ascites, and who has no other apparent cause for liver damage. An occasional patient with Laënnec's cirrhosis has congestive heart failure. In these circumstances the differential diagnosis is difficult. Hematemesis and severe functional derangement are more characteristic of Laënnec's cirrhosis than of congestive cirrhosis.

As in chonic passive congestion, **treatment** should be directed at the underlying disease.

ARTHUR J. PATEK, JR.

References

Circulation of the Liver—General Considerations

Bradley, S. E.: Variations in Hepatic Blood Flow in Man during Health and Disease. New England J. Med., 240:456, 1949.

Ellenberg, M., and Osserman, K. E.: The Role of Shock in the Production of Central Liver Necrosis. Am. J. Med., 11:170, 1951.

Frank, H. A.: Present-Day Concepts of Shock. New England J. Med., 249:445, 1953.

Grindlay, J. H., Herrick, J. F., and Mann, F. C.: Measurement of the Blood Flow of the Liver. Am. J. Physiol., 132:489, 1941.

Himsworth, H. P.: The Liver and Its Diseases. Cambridge, Harvard University Press, 1947, pp. 19–48.

McIndoe, A. H.: Vascular Lesions of Portal Cirrhosis. Arch. Path. & Lab. Med., 5:23, 1928.

Wakim, K. G.: The Blood Supply of the Normal Liver. Proc. Staff. Meet., Mayo Clin. 28:218, 1953.

Passive Congestion and Congestive Cirrhosis of the Liver

Boland, E. W., and Willius, F. A.: Changes in the Liver Produced by Chronic Passive Congestion, with Special Reference to the Problem of Cardiac Cirrhosis. Arch. Int. Med., 62:723, 1938.

Chávez, I., Sepulveda, B., and Ortega, A. L.: The Functional Value of the Liver in Heart Disease. J.A.M.A., 121:1275, 1943.

Felder, L., Mund, A., and Parker, J. G.: Liver Function Tests in Chronic Congestive Heart Failure. Circulation, 2:286, 1950.

Garvin, C. F.: Cardiac Cirrhosis. Am. J. M. Sc., 205:515, 1943.

Katzin, H. M., Waller, J. V., and Blumgart, H. L.: "Cardiac Cirrhosis" of the Liver. A Clinical and Pathologic Study. Arch. Int. Med., 64:457, 1939.

Koletzky, S., and Barnabee, J. H.: "Cardiac" or Congestive Cirrhosis. Pathologic and Clinical Aspects. Am. J. M. Sc., 207:421, 1944.

Sherlock, S.: The Liver in Heart Failure. Relation of Anatomical, Functional and Circulatory Changes. Brit. Heart J. 13:273, 1951.

Zimmerman, H. M., and Hillsman, J. A.: Chronic Passive Congestion of the Liver. An Experimental Study. Arch. Path., 9:1154, 1930.

PORTAL HYPERTENSION

(Banti's Syndrome)

The syndrome of portal hypertension is characterized by splenomegaly, anemia, leukopenia, thrombocytopenia and attacks of gastrointestinal bleeding. Banti believed that the pathologic process, originating in the spleen, later involved the liver and produced cirrhosis. Subsequent studies, especially by Whipple and his associates, indicated that the syndrome embraced two separate groups of cases: (1) *Intrahepatic,* or cases in which the block is within the liver, due chiefly to cirrhosis; (2) *extrahepatic,* or cases in which the liver is normal and the obstruction resides in the portal vein or one of its radicles outside the liver. This type is due usually to thrombosis, trauma or pancreatic cyst.

As a result of the obstruction, esophagogastric varices form submucosally at the site of anastomosis between the coronary system, the azygos and diaphragmatic system of veins. They are seen in the lower esophagus and cardiac end of the stomach. The identification of varices by x-ray is a most important diagnostic procedure.

Catheterization of the hepatic vein has provided another diagnostic tool. By this means a direct measurement of portal venous pressure can be made. It can be used to differentiate between intrahepatic and extrahepatic block and also to determine the effectiveness of surgery to relieve the block.

The **treatment** of portal hypertension is a surgical problem. Methods have been devised to by-pass the venous obstruction by anastomosis of the portal vein and inferior vena cava or anastomosis of the splenic and left renal veins. The choice of operative procedure depends upon the nature of the obstructive factor, its location and the efficiency of the collateral circulation.

In a group of 43 cases with extrahepatic block, Blakemore reported an operative mortality of 6.9 per cent. In the presence of cirrhosis the surgical risk is formidable, especially when there are signs of hepatic failure such as jaundice or ascites. In a group of 117 cases with intrahepatic block (cirrhosis), Blakemore reported an over-all mortality of 21.9 per cent. The degree of hepatic failure preceding operation was the chief determinant of surgical mortality. With careful selection and preparation of patients the hazards of surgery are considerably less than the hazards of repeated gastrointestinal bleeding.

Arthur J. Patek, Jr.

References

Blakemore, A. H.: Portacaval Shunting for Portal Hypertension. Surg., Gynec. & Obst., *94:*443, 1952.

Child, Charles G., III: Hepatic Circulation and Portal Hypertension. Philadelphia, W. B. Saunders Co., 1954.

———, and Payne, M. A.: Portal Hypertension. Monographs in Medicine Series, *1:*132, 1952.

Linton, R. R.: Emergency Treatment of Bleeding Esophageal Varices and the Results of Portacaval Shunts in 90 Patients. New York State J. Med., *53:*2192, 1953.

Moschowitz, E.: The Pathogenesis of Splenomegaly in Hypertension of the Portal Circulation; "Congestive Splenomegaly." Medicine, 27:187, 1948.

Paton, A., Reynolds, T. B., and Sherlock, S.: Assessment of Portal Venous Hypertension by Catheterization of Hepatic Vein. Lancet, *1:*918, 1953.

Rousselot, L. M.: Combined (One Stage) Splenectomy and Portacaval Shunts in Portal Hypertension. J.A.M.A., *140:*282, 1949.

Thompson, W. P.: The Pathogenesis of Banti's Disease. Ann. Int. Med., *14:*255, 1940.

Whipple, A. O.: The Problem of Portal Hypertension in Relation to Hepatosplenopathies. Ann. Surg., *122:*449, 1945.

THROMBOSIS OF THE PORTAL VEIN

Etiology. Thrombosis of the portal vein may be caused by compression or stricture of the portal vein, by endophlebitis, by thrombocytosis or by combinations of these mechanisms.

Occurrence. The condition is uncommon. Lissauer reported 68 cases in 28,687 autopsies. In another series, Webster reported 21 cases in 6050 autopsies. *Cirrhosis of the liver* accounts for about one third to one half of the reported cases. Nevertheless, it is not a common complication of cirrhosis. In three large series comprising 1320 cases of cirrhosis (cited by Rolleston and McNee) the incidence of portal thrombosis was less than 2 per cent. In cirrhosis of the liver, stricture of the venous channels and portal venous stasis presumably lead to thrombosis. In *malignancy,* the next most common cause, thrombosis is produced by compression of the vein by tumor masses or by direct invasion of the vein. *Endophlebitis* generally is secondary to inflammation in adjacent structures, such as cholangitis, pancreatitis, duodenitis and splenic abscess. Occasionally it is a sequel to appendicitis. Portal vein thrombosis also is seen in conditions complicated by *thrombocytosis,* such as polycythemia vera and postsplenectomy.

Morbid Anatomy. The vein is distended by a clot, which may involve one or more branches. The character of the clot varies with the age of the lesion. The vein wall usually is thickened. In longstanding cases the portal vein may be transformed into a fibrous cord. At times the main stem and its branches are replaced by spongy cavernomatous tissue in which many small vessels partially take over the load (*cavernomatous transformation*). The liver is of normal size or small (atrophic), whereas splenomegaly is the rule. Collateral circulation is conspicuous in the esophageal and hemorrhoidal veins, and also at times in the veins of the anterior abdominal wall.

Symptoms. The classic signs of portal vein thrombosis—abdominal pain, hematemesis, splenomegaly and ascites—may develop rapidly or slowly. A moderate degree of fever may be present. The clinical course depends upon the extent of the lesion and the nature of the underlying disease. With extension of the thrombus to the mesenteric veins, there are signs of intestinal infarction, namely ileus, melena, diarrhea and terminal collapse. In *acute thrombosis* these changes may lead to death in a few days. In *chronic, partial thrombosis,* a more frequent form, recurrent abdominal pain and gastric hemorrhages may recur for months or years before failure takes place. Certain of the latter cases present the symptom complex known as *Banti's syndrome,* characterized by splenomegaly, anemia, leukopenia and thrombopenia.

Diagnosis is difficult. The demonstration of esophageal varices by x-ray is essential. The problem then involves differentiation between intrahepatic and extrahepatic obstruction of the portal circulation. In general, patients with extrahepatic venous obstruction present themselves at a younger age. The liver is not enlarged. Jaundice and other signs of hepatic failure are minimal. Ascites, however, may appear after hemorrhage. Upon catheterization of the hepatic vein the pressure is found to be normal, in contrast to the elevated pressure found with intrahepatic venous obstruction.

Intrahepatic obstruction is almost always associated with cirrhosis of the liver, and is far more common. In these patients it is impossible to determine whether signs of portal hypertension result from uncomplicated cirrhosis or from superimposed thrombosis. When signs of portal venous obstruction develop swiftly, thrombosis of the vein should be suspected.

Care should be taken to exclude other causes of splenomegaly such as leukemia, Gaucher's disease and lymphoma.

Treatment is outlined in the preceding section on Portal Hypertension.

ARTHUR J. PATEK, JR.

References

Kelsey, M. P., Robertson, H. E., and Giffin, H. Z.: The Rôle of Chronic Thrombosis of the Portal Vein and Its Tributaries in the Syndrome of Splenic Anemia. Surg., Gynec. & Obst., 85:289, 1947.

Klemperer, P.: Cavernous Transformation of the Portal Vein, in Relation to Banti's Disease. Arch. Path., 6:353, 1928.

Lissauer, L.: Beitrag zur Frage der Entstehung der Pfortaderthrombose. Virch. Arch. f. path. Anat. u. Phys., 192:278, 1908.

Rolleston, H., and McNee, J. W.: Diseases of the Liver, Gallbladder and Bile Ducts. 3rd ed. London, Macmillan and Co., 1929, pp. 91–107.

Ratnoff, O. D., Conley, C. L., and Berthrong, M.: The Differentiation Between Extrahepatic and Intrahepatic Obstruction of the Portal Circulation. A Clinical Study of the "Banti Syndrome." Bull. Johns Hopkins Hosp., 87:305, 1950.

Simonds, J. P.: Chronic Occlusion of the Portal Vein. Arch. Surg., 33:397, 1936.

Webster, L. T.: Portal Thrombosis. Bull. Johns Hopkins Hosp., 32:16, 1921.

THROMBOSIS OF THE HEPATIC VEINS

(Budd-Chiari Syndrome)

Etiology. Thrombosis of the hepatic veins may result from primary endophlebitis or may be secondary to inflammatory, cirrhotic or neoplastic changes in the liver. It also occurs in certain diseases characterized by multiple thrombosis, such as polycythemia vera and thrombophlebitis migrans.

Occurrence. It is a rare disease. In 86 cases cited by Thompson the average age was 34 years. There is no sex predominance.

Morbid Anatomy. The main sites for obstruction are at the junction of the hepatic veins with the inferior vena cava or in the smaller hepatic vein branches. Thrombosis of the hepatic veins often is associated with inflammation and thrombosis of the inferior vena cava. The obliquity of the hepatic veins entering the vena cava is believed to favor the localization near the ostia. Obstruction may be partial or complete. The pathologic changes in the liver vary with the extent and age of the process. In acute, complete occlusion there is marked engorgement of the liver with central hemorrhages, pressure atrophy, and necrosis. In recurring or partial thrombosis, areas of nodular regeneration are seen. In such cases collateral circulation is prominent.

Pathologic Physiology. Constriction of the thoracic inferior vena cava in the dog causes extreme congestion of the liver, enlarged hepatic lymphatics and ascites. It is felt that the dilated hilar lymphatics may contribute importantly to the formation of ascites in these animals. A similar mechanism may be operative in the human disease.

Symptoms. In the *acute form* the classic signs are sudden onset of epigastric pain, rapidly enlarging liver, ascites and collateral venous engorgement. Nausea and vomiting occur in about one fourth of the patients. Jaundice is mild or latent. Splenomegaly is not a feature. Hematemesis is rare. The abdominal pain may radiate towards the shoulder or back. The liver edge at first is smooth and tender, but later tends to become smaller, firm and nodular. Ascites usually recurs rapidly after paracenteses. The collateral veins are most prominent over the upper abdomen and lower thorax, and especially near the xiphoid process, where anastomoses take place. The flow in these veins tends to be *downward*. Moderate edema of the legs is seen in about one half of the patients. If this is extensive, other causes for edema should be considered, in particular thrombosis of the inferior vena cava. Hemoconcentration, as indicated by high hematocrit, may be striking. Shock, coma and death generally take place within a few days or weeks.

A *chronic form* is seen in patients with partial occlusion of the main veins or recurring thrombosis of the smaller branches. The symptoms are then gradual in onset, milder and intermittent. Such patients have been known to survive months or years before an acute and fatal episode supervenes.

In the **differential diagnosis,** portal vein thrombosis, carcinomatous and tuberculous peritonitis and adhesive pericarditis should be considered.

ARTHUR J. PATEK, JR.

References

Armstrong, C. D., and Carnes, W. H.: Obstruction of the Hepatic Veins (Chiari's Disease). Am. J. M. Sc., 208:470, 1944.

Hess, A. F.: Fatal Obliterating Endophlebitis of the Hepatic Veins. Am. J. M. Sc., *130*:986, 1905.

Kelsey, M. P., and Comfort, M. W.: Occlusion of the Hepatic Veins. Arch. Int. Med., *75*:175, 1945.

Thompson, R. B.: Thrombosis of the Hepatic Veins. The Budd-Chiari Syndrome. Arch. Int. Med., *80:* 602, 1947.

Volwiler, W., Grindlay, J. H., and Bollman, J. L.: The Relation of Portal Vein Pressure to the Formation of Ascites—an Experimental Study. Gastroenterology, *14*:40, 1950.

ASCITES

Ascites can be produced experimentally in the dog by constricting the inferior vena cava above the liver. This procedure not only causes a sharp increase of hepatic and portal venous pressure, but also results in retention of sodium, presumably due, at least in part, to hormonal imbalance. Constriction of the vena cava or the portal vein below the liver does not result in the formation of ascites unless the procedure is combined with plasmapheresis. Thus it appears that increased pressure in the hepatic and portal veins, retention of sodium and depletion of plasma proteins are factors in the experimental production of ascites.

Studies on human cirrhosis of the liver also have indicated that hormonal factors are responsible for the retention of sodium and water. It is not certain whether this retention is related to adrenal or pituitary activity, whether it is due to increased production or to decreased inactivation of the hormone. The relation of renal functions to the formation of ascites is as yet an unsettled problem. However, there is little doubt of abnormal retention of sodium. When sodium is administered to a patient with cirrhosis and ascites, almost none is excreted in the urine. Other studies have shown that there is a steady interchange of water, protein and electrolytes between the blood plasma and the ascitic fluid, that a state of dynamic equilibrium is maintained between the osmotic pressure of the plasma and that of the ascitic fluid. These studies suggest that the localization of fluid within the abdominal cavity is related to increased portal capillary pressure and to decreased osmotic pressure. It is evident that multiple factors are at play in the formation of ascites.

The control of ascites in patients with cirrhosis is aided greatly by restricting the intake of sodium. This measure acts presumably by inhibiting the antidiuretic hormone. With sodium restriction there is less frequent need of abdominal paracentesis, and there is conservation of the depleted protein stores. It is estimated that 1 liter of ascites contains the protein equivalent of about 200 cc. of plasma. To be effective in controlling persistent ascites the intake of sodium should be restricted to about 1 gm. of sodium chloride daily, and this should be combined with a diet rich in protein. Abdominal taps should be done before distention interferes with the appetite. Diuretics (ammonium chloride, 4 to 6 gm. daily; Mercuhydrin, 2 cc. twice weekly) are helpful adjuvants. With rigid restriction of sodium certain patients develop profound weakness and loss of appetite. Collapse after abdominal paracentesis has been attributed to the sudden depletion of sodium. Obviously in such patients a more liberal intake of sodium is needed. The place for cation exchange resins or for surgical measures to alleviate ascites has not been firmly established.

Arthur J. Patek, Jr.

References

Eisenmenger, W. J.: Role of Sodium in the Formation and Control of Ascites in Patients with Cirrhosis. Ann. Int. Med., 37:261, 1952.

James, A. H.: The Mechanism of Pleural and Ascitic Effusions with a Suggested Method for the Indirect Estimation of Portal Venous Pressure. Clin. Sc., 8:292, 1949.

Mankin, H., and Lowell, A.: Osmotic Factors Influencing the Formation of Ascites in Patients with Cirrhosis of the Liver. J. Clin. Investigation, 27: 145, 1948.

Post, J., and Patek, A. J., Jr.: Serum Proteins in Cirrhosis of the Liver. I. Relation to Prognosis and to Formation of Ascites. Arch. Int. Med., 69:67, 1942.

Ralli, E. P., Robson, J. S., Clarke, D., and Hoagland, C. L.: Factors Influencing Ascites in Patients with Cirrhosis of the Liver. J. Clin. Investigation, 24: 316, 1945.

Schilling, J. A., McCoord, A. B., Clausen, S. W., Troup, S. B., and McKee, F. W.: Experimental Ascites. Studies of Electrolyte Balance in Dogs with Partial and Complete Occlusion of the Portal Vein and of the Vena Cava Above and Below the Liver. J. Clin. Investigation, 31:702, 1952.

Volwiler, W., Grindlay, J. H., and Bollman, J. L.: The Relation of Portal Vein Pressure to the Formation of Ascites—an Experimental Study. Gastroenterology, 14:40, 1950.

White, A. G., Rubin, G., and Leiter, L.: Studies in Edema. III. The Effect of Pitressin on the Renal Excretion of Water and Electrolytes in Patients With and Without Liver Disease. J. Clin. Investigation, 30:1287, 1951.

CIRRHOSIS OF THE LIVER

There are several types of cirrhosis which are distinct in etiology, pathology and certain clinical features. The text of this chapter is based upon the following classification:

1. *Portal cirrhoses*
   Laënnec's cirrhosis
   Kwashiorkor
   Atypical
2. *Pigmentary cirrhosis*
3. *Hepatolenticular degeneration*
4. *Biliary cirrhoses*
   Obstructive (cholangitic)
   Primary (cholangiolitic)
5. *Postnecrotic cirrhosis*
6. *Congestive (cardiac) cirrhosis*
7. *Syphilitic cirrhosis*
8. *Zooparasitic cirrhoses*
   Distomiasis
   Schistosomiasis

LAENNEC'S CIRRHOSIS

(Atrophic or Hypertrophic Cirrhosis, Alcoholic Cirrhosis, Hobnail Cirrhosis)

Incidence. This is by far the most common form of cirrhosis. In the United States it is discovered in 2 to 3 per cent of all postmortem examinations, and in the Orient, Near East and South Africa the incidence post mortem is even higher (2 to 10 per cent). It is likely that environmental rather than constitutional factors determine the differences in racial incidence, as, for example, the predilection of cirrhosis for persons of Irish and Italian stock. Laënnec's cirrhosis occurs most often between the ages of 45 and 65 years. It occurs in men two to three times as frequently as in women.

Etiology. Several different agents apparently can produce the pathologic picture of Laënnec's cirrhosis, e.g., chronic poisoning by carbon tetrachloride and phosphorus. In certain instances it is associated with chronic ulcerative colitis and with hyperthyroidism. However, in the large majority of instances there is no known hepatotoxin. More than half of the cases in this country are associated with alcoholism. Malaria and enteric diseases are the chief predisposing factors in the Orient. The occurrence of syphilis in about 20 per cent of the cases is probably incidental. The role of infectious hepatitis has not been precisely defined. In most reported series a history of previous hepatitis is elicited in less than 10 per cent of the cases. However, in several series the incidence has been higher.

The possibility that nutritional deficiency might play an etiologic role was proposed on the basis of the frequent association of cirrhosis with alcoholism and nutritional deficiency and of the favorable therapeutic response of patients with cirrhosis to a highly nutritious diet. This hypothesis has been greatly strengthened by a number of experimental studies which have firmly established the importance of dietary factors in the pathogenesis of the disease. It has been shown that (1) cirrhosis can be produced in the laboratory animal by certain protein-deficient diets; (2) feeding of choline or methionine (its biologic equivalent) protects against cirrhosis; (3) feeding of diets rich in protein favors repair and regeneration of the damaged liver.

Pathology. The liver at autopsy is of variable size. In about half the cases the organ weighs less than 1500 gm. It is diffusely nodular and firm. The chief histologic features are dense perilobular connective tissue, degenerative changes of liver cells, dissociation of liver cords, areas of regeneration, fatty and cellular infiltration. It is generally believed that necrosis of liver cells precedes the overgrowth of connective tissue. The spleen, as a rule, is enlarged and firm, and the pancreas occasionally shows chronic interstitial fibrosis. Abnormalities other than those present in the liver are related chiefly to obstruction of the portal venous system and include ascites, varicosities of the esophageal veins, engorgement of the mesenteric veins, congestion and edema of the intestinal wall. In addition, changes resulting from malnutrition, hemorrhage and infection are frequent. Likewise endocrine changes, such as testicular atrophy and gynecomastia, are common associated findings.

Symptoms and Signs. Cirrhosis may provoke few symptoms. In about one third of the cases seen at autopsy the disease has been latent or unsuspected during life. Usually the patient gives a story of chronic alcoholism and malnutrition. His meals have been haphazard and his diet poor in meat and dairy foods. There may be considerable weight loss. Gradually there develops anorexia, nausea and vomiting. After a few months he observes abdominal fullness, due at first to flatulence and later to ascites. At this stage he is apt to seek medical aid.

Signs of failure of the liver are readily apparent. The patient is weak and mentally dull or confused. He complains of thirst and abdominal discomfort or pain. There is often a low grade fever. The sclerae are subicteric (jaundice is seldom conspicuous). The skin is dry and inelastic, and the body hair may be scanty. There are prominent venules over the face and telltale vascular spiders scattered over the head and upper body. The pulse is rapid, and breathing is shallow because of an elevated diaphragm. Occasionally there are signs of hydrothorax. Dilated collateral veins are seen over the bulging flanks of the abdomen and lower thorax. The liver, if palpable, feels firm and its surface rough or serrated. It may be moderately tender. The spleen is firm and easily palpable. Edema of the legs and occasionally of the scrotum may be present. Sometimes there is clubbing of the fingers. In an appreciable number of instances the first sign of cirrhosis noted by the patient is the appearance of icterus or the sudden onset of hematemesis. The incidence of symptoms and signs, as reported in two series of cases, is shown in the accompanying table.

Symptoms and Signs of Advanced Laënnec's Cirrhosis (Per Cent Incidence)

	PATEK ET AL.* 124 CASES	FLEMING AND SNELL† 200 CASES
SYMPTOMS		
Weight loss	89	58
Nausea and vomiting	51	30
Abdominal pain	50	46
Epistaxis	40	—
Hematemesis	34	13
SIGNS		
Ascites	93	100
Palpable liver	79	55
Edema	69	58
Jaundice	67	45
Vascular spiders	62	—
Dilated veins	61	34
Palpable spleen	55	32
Fever	49	—
Abdominal hernia	33	—
Clubbed fingers	18	—
Hydrothorax	17	—

* Series included 15 cases of postnecrotic cirrhosis.
† Series included only cases with ascites.

Certain of these signs are noteworthy. *Low grade fever* unaccompanied by leukocytosis and lasting for weeks or months has been observed in about one half of the patients. *Mental changes* unrelated to recent alcoholism have been seen in about one third of the pa-

tients. In most instances they were characterized by confusion and euphoria. The vascular *spider,* a tiny pulsating arteriole, is seen in about two thirds of the cases. Such vascular spiders are most frequently observed in the skin over the face and neck. The mechanism of their production is not entirely clear, but it may be related to the failure of the liver to metabolize estrogens. *Bleeding* phenomena, especially epistaxis, are seen in many instances. The bleeding tendency could be related to one or more factors that commonly are altered in the presence of liver disease. These include prothrombin, fibrinogen and accelerator globulin activity. A more important type of bleeding, however, results from rupture of veins in the lower esophagus due to portal hypertension. A profuse hematemesis of a liter or more is not unusual. In some patients there may be considerable hemorrhage from esophageal varices without emesis. The clinical picture presented by a patient who has experienced such an accident is identical with that observed in patients suffering from gastric or duodenal hemorrhage. With bleeding into the gastrointestinal tract there may be a sharp rise in the blood urea nitrogen.

The *bromsulfalein test* almost always shows increased retention of dye. The intravenous galactose test also shows increased retention in the large majority of patients. The serum cholesterol esters are generally reduced, whereas the total serum cholesterol may show little change. The serum alkaline phosphatase in general shows a moderate increase. Serum bilirubin and the icterus index show periodic elevations of moderate degree. Urinary urobilinogen is generally increased. The cephalin flocculation and thymol turbidity tests are usually positive. Serum proteins may be altered early in the disease. Characteristically, there is decreased serum albumin and increased serum globulin. Whereas the serum globulin is variable, the serum albumin values correlate fairly well with the clinical course. Thus a steady decrease in the concentration of serum albumin is of serious import. Blood counts frequently show macrocytic anemia and low grade reticulocytosis. The white blood count is normal or slightly increased. A sharp leukocytosis usually indicates the presence of some complication. Ascitic fluid has the characteristics of a transudate.

Diagnosis is obvious when the disease is advanced, but is difficult during the early stages, because symptoms may be vague or lacking. If a patient has gastrointestinal symptoms with a palpable liver or spleen, unexplained icterus, hematemesis or vascular spiders, an investigation of hepatic function should be conducted (see earlier in this section and Jaundice, p. 915). If the diagnosis of cirrhosis seems probable, the lower end of the esophagus should be visualized by fluoroscopy and roentgenography after the administration of barium in an effort to detect the presence of varices. Differentiation from other types of cirrhosis, particularly postnecrotic and pigmentary cirrhosis, may be difficult. *Postnecrotic cirrhosis* shows no sex predominance and occurs in a younger age group than the Laënnec type. A story of previous infectious hepatitis is characteristic, whereas alcoholism and malnutrition are not usual. The clinical features may be indistinguishable from those of Laënnec's cirrhosis. *Pigmentary cirrhosis* (hemochromatosis) occurs almost exclusively in males between 40 and 60 years of age. Signs of cirrhosis in a patient with bronzed skin and diabetes should suggest the diagnosis. The latter signs occur in about 75 per cent of the cases. A diagnostic test is the elevated serum iron. Biopsy of the skin and liver reveals the iron-containing pigment in most cases. *Carcinoma* of the liver, *schistosomiasis, polyserositis, amyloidosis* and *thrombosis* of the portal or hepatic veins also should be considered in the differential diagnosis. The expert use of puncture biopsy is of great help in puzzling cases.

Complications. *Intercurrent infections,* such as peritonitis, pneumonia and phlebitis, are encountered frequently. In the past these infections have accounted for about 25 per cent of the deaths from cirrhosis, but with the advent of penicillin and other new drugs, this danger has been lessened. Whereas active *tuberculosis* was formerly a common complication, it has been reported in only 2 or 3 per cent of the cases in recent series. *Abdominal hernias* occur in about one third of the patients who have ascites, presumably as a result of the increased intra-abdominal pressure. Five to 10 per cent of patients with cirrhosis have peptic ulcer. In certain instances hematemesis has been due to peptic ulcer rather than to the suspected rupture of a varix. *Portal vein thrombosis* occurs in about 3 per cent of the cases. It seems to be more frequent in patients who have undergone abdominal surgery. It also may be found in those with cirrhosis (4 per cent) who acquire *primary carcinoma.*

Prognosis. Cirrhosis of the liver does not necessarily imply a poor prognosis. In a considerable number of cases the disease remains latent throughout life. The prognosis is also not unsatisfactory for those patients with minimal or moderate involvement in whom the cirrhosis is recognized early and properly treated. However, when clinical signs of failure appear (such as ascites and jaundice), the outlook is grave. In an analysis of 386 cases it was found that 39 per cent of the patients survived one year after the onset of ascites, 21 per cent survived two years, and 7 per cent five years. Jaundice had a similar prognostic significance. In the case of hematemesis, about one third died from the initial episode and an additional third died by the end of the first year. The chief causes of death were cholemia, hematemesis and intercurrent infections.

The prognosis of this disease has become less grave since the introduction of dietary therapy. Beneficial results have been reported by the writer and his associates in a series of 124 patients fed on a highly nutritious diet supplemented by concentrates of vitamin B complex. After the onset of ascites 65 per cent survived one year, 50 per cent survived two years, and 30 per cent five years. Fleming and Snell and others have reported similer findings. In general it requires several months of treatment before significant changes occur. The first intimations of improvement are gain in appetite and a sense of well-being. More objective changes take place later, namely, subsidence of fever and disappearance of jaundice, ascites, edema and vascular spiders. There is a close correlation between the level of serum albumin and the clinical status, a sustained rise being a favorable sign. It is evident that early diagnosis and treatment of the disease will result in a better prognosis.

Treatment. When signs of liver failure appear, such as ascites or jaundice, the patient should be kept in bed most of the time. Alcohol should be prohibited. He should be urged to eat a diet rich in meat, fish, eggs, milk, fruit and green vegetables. A satisfactory regimen includes eggs for breakfast, meat at luncheon and supper, milk at each of three meals. At times it is necessary to feed a semiliquid diet consisting of such dishes as eggnog, puréed vegetables and meat for the patient who refuses solid foods. The diet should contain carbohydrate, 350 to 400 gm.; protein, 115 to 135 gm.; fat, 100 to 170 gm. There is no apparent intolerance to fat. A milk drink containing powdered brewers' yeast (15 to 25 gm.) may be given twice daily between meals. If powdered yeast is not tolerated, vitamin B complex may be substituted in the form of liquid concentrates. Thiamine chloride (10 mg. daily) and unconcentrated liver extract (5 cc. intramuscularly once weekly) are advised. Dietetic and nursing care during the period of decompensation should be meticulous and vigilant. It usually requires months to attain satisfactory results.

Beneficial results have been reported by some with the feeding of lipotropic substances, choline and methionine. It has been impossible to determine whether improvement was due to these factors or to the nutritious diets which they supplemented. Others have advocated the intravenous administration of liver extract, of concentrated human serum albumin solution and of amino acid hydrolysates. Broader experience is needed before these can be finally appraised. At present they may be considered as possible supportive aids when dietary measures have failed.

Only moderate restriction of salt and water is necessary in most patients with ascites. However, if ascites recurs persistently the intake of sodium should be curtailed further (see section on Ascites).

Hemorrhage from esophageal and gastric varices is a dread complication and the most common cause of death. Transfusions should be given without delay, and should be continued as long as there is evidence of bleeding. The patient should be given only light sedation since he has a tendency to lapse into cholemia. Esophageal tamponade by means of a rubber balloon has been life-saving in many instances. Direct ligation of esophageal veins also has been advocated as an emergency measure. For recurrent bleeding from esophageal varices the portacaval shunt is the procedure of choice. (See Portal Hypertension.)

The treatment of *hepatic coma* is unsatisfactory. Cholemia may be the terminal stage of progressive liver failure; it may appear abruptly during infection; it may follow hemorrhage. The outcome depends largely on the precipitating conditions. Tube feedings are indicated in these patients. In addition they may be given 1 or 2 liters intravenously of 10 per cent dextrose daily with added thiamine chloride (100 mg.), niacin (400 mg.) and riboflavin (100 mg.).

Arthur J. Patek, Jr.

References

Clinical

Armas-Cruz, R., and others: Portal Cirrhosis: An Analysis of 208 Cases, with Correlation of Clinical, Laboratory, and Autopsy Findings, Gastroenterology, 17:327, 1951.

Blakemore, A. H.: Indications for Portacaval Anastomosis—Analysis of Cases. Surg., Gynec. & Obst., 84:645, 1947.

Chalmers, T. C., and Davidson, C. S.: A Survey of Recent Therapeutic Measures in Cirrhosis of the Liver. New England J. Med., 240:449, 1949.

DeJosselin deJong, R.: Leberzirrhose. Compt. Rend. prem. conf. Intern. de Path. geog. Geneva. Kundig, 1931, pp. 38–120.

Fagin, I. D., and Thompson, F. M.: Cirrhosis of the Liver, an Analysis of 71 Cases. Ann. Int. Med., 21:285, 1944.

Fleming, R. G., and Snell, A. M.: Portal Cirrhosis with Ascites: An Analysis of 200 Cases with Special Reference to Prognosis and Treatment. Am. J. Digest. Dis., 9:115, 1942.

Henrikson, E. C.: Cirrhosis of the Liver. Arch. Surg., 32:413, 1936.

Karsner, H. T.: Morphology and Pathogenesis of Hepatic Cirrhosis. Am. J. Clin. Path., 13:569, 1943.

Patek, A. J., Jr., and others: Dietary Treatment of Cirrhosis of the Liver. Results in One Hundred and Twenty-four Patients Observed During a Ten Year Period. J.A.M.A., 138:543, 1948.

Ratnoff, O. D., and Patek, A. J., Jr.: The Natural History of Laënnec's Cirrhosis of the Liver. Medicine, 21:207, 1942

Experimental

Best, C. H., and Lucas, C. C.: Choline—Chemistry and Significance as a Dietary Factor. Vitamins and Hormones, 1:1, 1943.

Blumberg, H., and Grady, H. G.: Production of Cirrhosis of the Liver in Rats by Feeding Low Protein, High Fat Diets. Arch. Path., 34:1035, 1942.

Chaikoff, I. L., Eichorn, K. B., Connor, C. L., and Entenman, C.: The Production of Cirrhosis in the Liver of the Normal Dog by Prolonged Feeding of a High-Fat Diet. Am. J. Path., 19: 9, 1943.

Daft, F. S., Sebrell, W. H., and Lillie, R. D.: Production and Apparent Prevention of a Dietary Liver Cirrhosis in Rats. Proc. Soc. Exper. Biol. & Med., 48:228, 1941; 50:1, 1942.

György, P.: Experimental Hepatic Injury. Am. J. Clin. Path., 14:67, 1944.

———, and Goldblatt, H.: Treatment of Experimental Dietary Cirrhosis of the Liver in Rats. J. Exper. Med., 90:73, 1949.

Plough, I. C., Patek, A. J., Jr., and Bevans, M.: The Relative Effects of Protein, Choline, and Methionine in the Treatment of Experimental Dietary Cirrhosis in the Rat. J. Exper. Med., 96:221, 1952.

KWASHIORKOR

See under Deficiency Diseases, p. 627.

PIGMENTARY CIRRHOSIS OF THE LIVER

See Hemochromatosis, p. 686.

HEPATOLENTICULAR DEGENERATION

See under Diseases of Metabolism, p. 638.

BILIARY CIRRHOSES

OBSTRUCTIVE BILIARY CIRRHOSIS

Definition. This term is applied to patients with chronic jaundice and signs of liver failure caused by chronic obstruction and inflammation of the large bile ducts. It is a rare form. In 550 cases of cirrhosis of all types reported by Mallory, obstructive biliary cirrhosis accounted for 24 or 4.4 per cent.

Etiology. The chief predisposing conditions are stone in the common duct, carcinoma at the head of the pancreas, adhesions around the common duct, pressure from peribiliary lymph nodes, congenital atresia of the bile ducts, and parasitic infestation of the ducts. Rarely it is a sequel to primary chronic cholangitis (cholangitis lenta). In a series of 244 cases of obstructive jaundice, Gibson and Robertson reported 21 cases (8.6 per cent) of biliary cirrhosis. In 16 of these the primary lesion was benign and in 5, carcinomatous.

Pathogenesis. Some authors believe that bile stasis alone can produce the disease in man, whereas others stress the role of accompanying infection. There are experimental data to support either contention. However, in clinical experience the large majority of cases with simple obstruction do not develop biliary cirrhosis. The development of cirrhosis seems to be favored by longstanding partial or intermittent obstruction complicated by cholangitis.

Morbid Anatomy. Characteristically, the liver is dark green, firm, and its surface granular. There is increased connective tissue in the portal areas, with intralobular extension, and dilatation and proliferation of bile ducts, many of which contain plugs. The liver cells show degenerative changes and also areas of nodular regeneration. The spleen may or may not be enlarged.

Clinical Picture. This form of biliary cirrhosis is seen more often in women than in men. The average age at onset is about 50 years. In most instances there is a history of partial or intermittent obstruction for several years, associated with febrile episodes and occasionally chills. Anorexia and abdominal distention are frequent symptoms. The patient becomes increasingly weak, emaciated and listless. As the disease progresses, tests of liver function show severe derangement. (See Jaundice, p. 915.) Without surgical intervention the outcome is invariably fatal. Terminally, there may be hemorrhagic phenomena or ascites.

Treatment depends upon alleviation of the obstruction. Effective surgery can be curative in these patients even when there are signs of severe liver damage.

ARTHUR J. PATEK, JR.

References

Gibson, W. R., and Robertson, H. E.: So-called Biliary Cirrhosis. Arch. Path., 28:37, 1939.

Judd, E. S., and Counseller, V. S.: The Effects of Obstructive Lesions of the Common Duct of the Liver. J.A.M.A., 89:1751, 1927.

Mallory, F. B.: Cirrhosis of the Liver. New England J. Med., 206:1231, 1932.

Weir, J. F., and Snell, A. M.: Chronic Hepatitis with Jaundice (Biliary Cirrhosis). Am. J. Digest. Dis., 3:629, 1936.

PRIMARY BILIARY CIRRHOSIS

(*Primary Hypertrophic; Cholangiolitic; Hanot's Cirrhosis*)

Definition. A rare disease characterized by jaundice, pruritus, enlargement of the liver and spleen. It occurs predominantly in adult females.

Etiology. The etiology is unknown. Some writers have indicated that it may result from infectious viral hepatitis. However, the primary localization of the lesion in the small bile radicles rather than in the parenchymal liver cells throws doubt upon this hypothesis.

Pathology. The liver is greatly enlarged, firm and smooth. Whereas the larger bile ducts appear to be normal, the small radicles show the changes of cholangitis or pericholangitis. Additional features are an increase of connective tissue in a diffuse monolobular distribution, splenomegaly, and lymph node enlargement, particularly of the portal and mesenteric nodes. The liver cells are uninvolved until a late stage of the disease.

Symptoms and Signs. The onset generally is gradual with malaise which may exist for several months before attention is directed to the liver by the appearance of jaundice, pruritus, dark urine and pale stools. The patients seldom feel acutely ill. They have little or no fever. Except for the discomfort caused by the large liver, abdominal distress is not usual. The appetite and nutrition are fair. However, there is a tendency toward frequent stools and progressive weight loss probably related to malabsorption.

On examination the skin is usually pigmented. The melanosis apparently bears no relation to the degree of jaundice. Characteristically the liver is massive, firm, smooth, and in about two thirds of the cases there is splenomegaly as well. As the disease progresses, xanthelasma and xanthomatosis may appear as a result of extreme and protracted elevation of serum lipids. Occasionally there is clubbing of the fingers.

Laboratory findings suggest partial biliary obstruction. The blood serum values for bilirubin, alkaline phosphatase activity, cholesterol and total lipids are elevated. The urine bile and urobilinogen are increased, whereas the fecal urobilinogen is decreased. Elevation of the serum alkaline phosphatase and cholesterol may be extreme and may precede the development of clinical jaundice in some cases by months. Tests related to protein metabolism, such as measurement of the serum proteins, prothrombin time and cephalin flocculation reaction, are generally normal until late in the disease.

In the *differential diagnosis* extrahepatic biliary obstruction is chiefly considered. The onset of viral hepatitis at times may suggest biliary obstruction. This "cholangiolitic" phase, however, seldom exceeds a few weeks. Primary cholangitis, hemolytic jaundice and hemochromatosis also should be considered.

In most instances there is a slowly progressive, fatal course which may extend over a period of two to ten or more years. Terminally the symptoms and signs are entirely similar to those of advanced Laënnec's cirrhosis.

An occasional remission has been attributed to treatment with penicillin. It is difficult to determine whether the reported cases represent bacterial cholangitis or primary biliary cirrhosis. For intractable itching methyltestosterone (25 mg. daily) appears to be effective.

ARTHUR J. PATEK, JR.

References

Ahrens, E. H., Jr., Payne, M. A., Kunkel, H. G., Eisenmenger, W. J., and Blondheim, S. H.: Primary Biliary Cirrhosis. Medicine, 29:299, 1950.

Dauphinee, J. A., and Sinclair, J. C.: Primary Biliary Cirrhosis. Canad. M. A. J., 61:1, 1949.

MacMahon, H. E., and Thannhauser, S. J.: Xanthomatous Biliary Cirrhosis (A Clinical Syndrome). Ann. Int. Med., 30:121, 1949.

Ricketts, W. E., and Wissler, R. W.: Cholangiolitic Biliary Cirrhosis (Primary Biliary Cirrhosis). Ann. Int. Med., 36:1241, 1952.

Watson, C. J., and Hoffbauer, F. W.: The Problem of Prolonged Hepatitis with Particular Reference to the Cholangiolitic Type and to the Development of Cholangiolitic Cirrhosis of the Liver. Ann. Int. Med., 25:195, 1946.

POSTNECROTIC CIRRHOSIS

(Toxic Cirrhosis, Healed Yellow Atrophy, Coarsely Nodular Cirrhosis)

Etiology and Pathogenesis. Postnecrotic cirrhosis comprises about 5 to 10 per cent of the cirrhoses reported in the United States. The disease is a late result of extensive necrosis of the liver from various causes. Occasionally it is due to poisoning, as from cinchophen, carbon tetrachloride or phosphorus. More often it is a sequel to infectious viral hepatitis. Since complete recovery occurs in the vast majority of cases of infectious hepatitis, it seems plausible that an additional factor is involved in the pathogenesis of postnecrotic cirrhosis. The severity of the initial hepatitis seems to bear no relation to the subsequent development of cirrhosis. Indeed, in a significant number the initial hepatitis has occurred without jaundice and has been unrecognized.

Massive necrosis of the liver has been produced in the rat by feeding diets low in protein and specifically deficient in tocopherol or cystine. The lesions are prevented by appropriate supplements of tocopherol, cystine or methionine as a source of cystine. It has not been demonstrated that there is a human counterpart to this experimental disease.

Morbid Anatomy. The liver appears small and discolored. Its surface shows depressed areas and large nodules of varying size. On microscopic section there is evidence of preceding liver necrosis and regeneration. The depressed areas, which are composed of connective tissue and scattered bile ducts, probably represent collapsed stroma. The nodules consist of proliferating liver cells which lack the orderly arrangement of normal liver cells.

Fatty changes are seldom seen. The broad septums of connective tissue do not invade the lobules as in Laënnec's cirrhosis.

Symptoms. The disease occurs at all ages, with about equal frequency in either sex. The clinical picture at the outset may be that of acute hepatitis. However, instead of prompt recovery there may be persistence of symptoms for months. In other instances there appear to be recurrent attacks of acute hepatitis for months or even years before liver failure supervenes. Jaundice is a fairly constant sign. Abdominal pain and a bleeding tendency are frequently present, whereas ascites is not conspicuous until late in the disease. Laboratory changes are similar to those of Laënnec's cirrhosis but with some differences in degree. The serum bilirubin, serum globulin and serum alkaline phosphatase tend to be higher in postnecrotic cirrhosis. Failure in these patients may resemble acute yellow atrophy with its fulminating swiftness, or it may resemble the gradual progressive decline seen in other types of severe cirrhosis.

In the **diagnosis** the chief difficulty is in the differentiation from Laënnec's cirrhosis. The history of infectious hepatitis in a young adult should suggest the diagnosis whenever alcoholism and malnutrition are not features. In postnecrotic cirrhosis the liver tends to be smaller, and jaundice and purpura are more frequent than in Laënnec's cirrhosis. Ascites and esophageal varices are uncommon until a late stage in the disease. Once signs of failure appear, there is little or no response to dietary treatment.

Arthur J. Patek, Jr.

References

Baggenstoss, A. H., and Stauffer, M. H.: Posthepatitic and Alcoholic Cirrhosis: Clinicopathologic Study of 43 Cases of Each. Gastroenterology, 22: 157, 1952.

Bergstrand, H.: Ueber die akute und chronische gelbe Leberatrophie. Mit besonderer Berücksichtigung ihres epidemischen Auftretens in Schweden in Jahre 1927. Leipzig, George Thieme, 1930.

Bjørneboe, M., and Raaschou, F.: Pathology of Subchronic Atrophy of the Liver. Comparison with Laënnec's Cirrhosis. Arch. Int. Med., 84:933, 1949.

Himsworth, H. P.: The Liver and Its Diseases. Cambridge, Harvard University Press, 1947.

Kelsall, A. R., Stewart, A., and Witts, L. G.: Subacute and Chronic Hepatitis. Lancet, 2:195, 1947.

Krarup, N. B., and Roholm, K.: The Development of Cirrhosis of the Liver after Acute Hepatitis, Elucidated by Aspiration Biopsy. Acta. med. Scandinav., 108:306, 1941.

Mallory, F. B.: Cirrhosis of the Liver. New England J. Med., 206:1231, 1932.

Wilson, J. D., and Goodpasture, E. W.: Yellow Atrophy of the Liver. Acute, Subacute, and Healed. Arch. Int. Med., 40:377, 1927.

CONGESTIVE (CARDIAC) CIRRHOSIS

See Congestive (Cardiac) Cirrhosis, page 928.

SYPHILITIC CIRRHOSIS

(Hepar Lobatum)

In tertiary syphilis the liver may be the seat of single or multiple gummas, the healing of which results in deep broad scars and course lobulation. This lesion often is referred to as *hepar lobatum*. Hepar lobatum is an uncommon form of cirrhosis. Mallory cited only 28 cases (5 per cent) in 550 cases of cirrhosis. It also is an uncommon form of syphilis. In a series reported by Hahn there were 57 cases (4.9 per cent) of hepar lobatum or gumma in 1165 autopsies on adult syphilitics.

The clinical picture depends upon the extent and location of the lesions. Contrary to popular belief, hepatic syphilis rarely produces great enlargement of the liver or spleen. Because of its focal nature there are usually no signs of liver failure. The course of the disease is generally benign even in those who are untreated. On the other hand, if the process is extensive, the clinical picture may resemble that of Laënnec's cirrhosis.

The disease should be suspected especially in patients with gummas elsewhere in the body. Serologic tests for syphilis are almost invariably positive. The **diagnosis** can be established either by biopsy or therapeutic test. The latter is considered positive only if striking changes take place over a long period of time. In the **differential diagnosis** other forms of cirrhosis, carcinoma, abscess and cystic disease should be considered.

The **treatment** of hepar lobatum is essentially the same as the treatment of syphilitic gummas elsewhere (see p. 356), with the exception that arsenical compounds should not be used.

Arthur J. Patek, Jr.

References

Hahn, R. D.: Syphilis of the Liver. Am. J. Syphil., Gonor., & Ven. Dis., 27:529, 1943.

Karsner, H. T.: Morphology and Pathogenesis of Hepatic Cirrhosis. Am. J. Clin. Path., 13:569, 1943.

O'Leary, P. A., Greene, C. H., and Rowntree, L. G.:

Disease of the Liver. VIII. Various Types of Syphilis of the Liver with Reference to Tests for Hepatic Function. Arch. Int. Med., 44:155, 1929.

Symmers, D.: Anatomic Lesions in Late Acquired Syphilis. A Study of 314 Cases Based on the Analysis of 4880 Necropsies at Bellevue Hospital. J.A.M.A., 66:1457, 1916.

Tucker, H. A., and Dexter, D. D.: Treatment of Gummatous Hepatic Syphilis with Penicillin. Report of Two Cases. Arch. Int. Med., 78:313, 1946.

ZOOPARASITIC CIRRHOSIS

In regions where these diseases are endemic, cirrhosis may result from infestation by the liver fluke (hepatic distomiasis) or by the blood fluke (schistosomiasis). The former lodges in the bile ducts and thus provokes a cholangitic, biliary type of cirrhosis. Ova from the latter lodge in the portal venules and periportal tissues, giving rise to a clinical picture which simulates Laënnec's cirrhosis, with ascites, splenomegaly and anemia.

These diseases are discussed in detail in Metazoan Infections, pages 422 and 425.

Arthur J. Patek, Jr.

ABSCESS OF THE LIVER

AMEBIC ABSCESS OF THE LIVER

(Tropical Abscess)

About 5 per cent of patients with clinical signs of intestinal amebiasis exhibit hepatic complications, which may take the form of either focal hepatitis or liver abscess. In fatal cases of amebiasis roughly one third have shown liver abscess. Although the disease is prevalent in the tropics, it is not limited to these regions. Amebic abscess is discussed in detail in the section on Amebiasis (p. 394).

PYOGENIC ABSCESS OF THE LIVER

This is a suppurative process which originates from a bacterial focus, usually outside the liver. Pyogenic abscesses are generally multiple. The bacteria most frequently found are *E. coli* and gram-positive cocci.

Infection may reach the liver by way of the portal vein, bile ducts, hepatic artery, or by extension from an adjacent infected area. Infection via the portal vein may be due to septic emboli or to *pylephlebitis*. As a rule the primary focus is found in the gastrointestinal tract or pelvis, the most common source being appendicitis. Infection by way of the bile ducts commonly results from *suppurative cholangitis* associated with cholelithiasis and cholecystitis. Infection via the hepatic artery occurs in septicemia, but this is an infrequent cause of liver abscess. Rarely liver abscess results from trauma or a penetrating wound near the liver. When an amebic abscess becomes secondarily infected, the clinical picture resembles that of pyogenic abscess.

Symptoms. Extreme weakness, wasting, spiking fever with chills, sweats, nausea and vomiting, and abdominal distention are usual. The liver is almost always enlarged, painful and tender. A mild degree of jaundice is seen in about one half of the cases; it may be conspicuous when there is associated cholangitis. Ascites is seen occasionally in association with pylephlebitis. Leukocytosis is usually pronounced.

The **diagnosis** should be suspected in a patient who shows signs of sepsis together with enlargement and tenderness of the liver subsequent to a recent infection, such as appendicitis or cholangitis. The severe prostration, high fever, tendency toward chills and jaundice are more prominent in this disease than in amebic abscess.

The **prognosis** is grave. In a series of 432 cases collected from the literature by Ochsner, DeBakey and Murray, the case fatality rate was 79.6 per cent.

Treatment of pyogenic abscess was ineffective until the advent of sulfonamides and penicillin. The energetic administration of these drugs, together with appropriate surgery, will doubtless brighten the outlook in this disease.

Arthur J. Patek, Jr.

References

Flynn, J. E.: Pyogenic Liver Abscess. New England J. Med., 234:403, 1946.

Gamm, K. E.: Penicillin Therapy in Pylephlebitis. J.A.M.A., 128:1159, 1945.

Keefer, C. S.: Liver Abscess: A Review of 85 Cases. New England J. Med., 211:21, 1934.

Ochsner, A., DeBakey, M., and Murray, S.: Pyogenic Abscess of the Liver. II. An Analysis of Forty-Seven Cases with Review of the Literature. Am. J. Surg., 40:292, 1938.

NEOPLASMS OF THE LIVER

PRIMARY CARCINOMA OF THE LIVER

Primary carcinoma of the liver accounts for 5 to 20 per cent of malignant tumors in certain Asiatic countries, namely, Japan,

DISEASE

CYST

Simple hepati
developmental
hepatic bile cha
gle, small, subca
consequence. *Cy*
rare condition,
origin. It usually
cystic disease of
stances of large
ported, the cysts
rise to no sympto

Echinococcus
discussed in the
sites (p. 431).

FA

Definition. In
excessive depositio
Etiology. The
about 5 per cent fa
its fat content is i
corresponding incr
pathologic accumu
junction with alc
ciencies, severe a
betes mellitus;
such as chlorofor
certain infections
enteric diseases; an
toses.

Pathologic Phys
lieved that degene
transformed into f
which fat can accu
been demonstrated
(1) increased fat i
thesis of fatty acids
mine; (3) decrease
pids from the liver,
and other lipotrop
creased migration o
liver, as induced
pituitary substance.
notably pellagra, fa
to the lack of thiami
However, in most hi
pears to be increase
the depots to the live
There is evidence
tion of fat renders tl
jury from hepatotox

South China, the Malay States and the Philippine Islands. It is also prevalent among the Bantu natives in South Africa. In Europe and in the Americas it is uncommon, with an incidence of less than 0.5 per cent of all cancers. It is most frequent between 50 and 60 years, and it is seen predominantly in men.

Etiology. Irritation of the liver cells is believed to be the chief predisposing condition. Congenital rests, chemical irritants, parasitic infestations, cholangitis, cirrhosis and dietary deficiency have been suggested as specific contributory factors. Clinical and experimental evidence indicates that cirrhosis usually precedes the carcinoma.

Investigation in this field has been stimulated by the discovery of Yoshida, in 1932, that the feeding of certain azo dyes induces primary cancer of the liver in the rat. Subsequent studies by others have shown that dietary factors contained in yeast can modify or inhibit the development of the lesions.

Morbid Anatomy. Primary carcinoma of the liver usually is widespread, with nodules varying from a few millimeters to several centimeters in diameter. Occasionally it appears as a single mass occupying the greater portion of a lobe. The chief histologic forms encountered are the *liver cell carcinoma* (malignant hepatoma) and the *duct cell carcinoma* (malignant cholangioma). The *liver cell carcinoma,* believed to arise from the parenchymal cell, accounts for about 90 per cent of the cases and is seen predominantly in the male. *Duct cell carcinoma,* which presumably stems from the intrahepatic bile ducts, occurs more often in women.

There is no difference in the clinical picture presented by the two forms of carcinoma. In both types the tumor commonly spreads throughout the liver substance. *Venous thrombosis* in the portal or hepatic veins frequently results from invasion by tumor cells. In about one third of the cases metastases are found in the regional lymph nodes or lungs, less frequently in the ribs and vertebrae. Other metastases are rare.

Symptoms and Signs. Symptoms of primary carcinoma may be indistinguishable from symptoms of the cirrhosis which usually is also present. Weakness, loss of weight, gastrointestinal disturbances, ascites, jaundice, abdominal pain, fever and peripheral edema are characteristic of both diseases, but are not invariably present. In about one half of

the reported cases palpable liver, jaundice or ascites is described, and splenomegaly is present in about one third of the cases. Ascitic fluid may be hemorrhagic and, rarely, may contain tumor cells. Persistent dull pain in the region of the liver, radiating toward the back, is said to be more typical of carcinoma than of cirrhosis.

Laboratory findings usually indicate impaired liver function, but there are no tests specific for carcinoma. In certain cases the alkaline phosphatase is elevated out of proportion to the clinical jaundice.

Diagnosis. Carcinoma of the liver should be suspected in a patient with the symptoms described if there is an enlarging tumor mass; if there are hard, tender nodules on the liver surface; if the liver seems fixed to the adjacent organs; and if there is intra-abdominal bleeding. It should be emphasized that primary carcinoma is far less common than secondary carcinoma of the liver. The diagnosis may be established by biopsy.

Prognosis and Treatment. The clinical course seldom lasts more than a few months after the appearance of an abdominal mass or the signs of liver failure. Surgical excision of the tumor has been successful in a few instances. Medical treatment is limited to palliative measures and simple nutritious foods.

ARTHUR J. PATEK, JR.

References

Charache, H.: Primary Carcinoma of the Liver. Am. J. Surg., 43:96, 1939.
Ewing, J.: Neoplastic Diseases. 4th ed. Philadelphia, W. B. Saunders Company, 1940, p. 738.
Greene, J. M.: Primary Carcinoma of Liver; 10 Year Collective Review. Internat. Abstr. Surg., 59:231, 1939.
Kinosita, R.: Studies on Carcinogenic Azo and Related Compounds. Yale J. Biol. & Med., 12:287, 1940.
Orr, J. W.: The Histology of the Rat's Liver during the Course of Carcinogenesis by Butter Yellow (p-Dimethyl Aminoazobene). J. Path. & Bact., 50:393, 1940.
Warvi, W. N.: Primary Neoplasms of the Liver. Arch. Path., 37:367, 1944.
Wilbur, D. L., Wood, D. A., and Willett, F. M.: Primary Carcinoma of the Liver. Ann. Int. Med., 20:453, 1944.

SECONDARY CARCINOMA OF THE LIVER

Carcinomatous metastases to the liver are found at autopsy in about 30 per cent of all

patients
noma c
affects
and occ
In most
an orga
such as
gus, inte
invade t
noma of
ally retr
the lym
noma.
Morbi
greatly e
which pi
press and
In micros
dules res
mor mass
bilicated
rupture v
rhage. Ca
hepatic ve
Sympto
is gradual
primary gr
in bowel h
carcinoma
anemia ma
liver dama
nosis is fa
to be antic
few, if any
the presen
metastases
As the d
plains of ga
discomfort
drium or in
occurs in o
the first syn
volvement o
tive in type.
of the patien
and may co
per cent of
occur togethe
of these sign:
plastic invasi
both vein ar
usually large,
tenderness m
by areas of
enlarged. Fev
sionally is acc

Graham, R. L.: Sudden Death in Young Adults in Association with Fatty Liver. Bull. Johns Hopkins Hosp., 74:16, 1944.

Keefer, C. S., and Fries, E. D.: The Fatty Liver—Its Diagnosis and Clinical Course. Tr. A. Am. Physicians, 57:283, 1942.

Perlman, I., and Chaikoff, I. L.: Radioactive Phosphorus as an Indicator of Phospholipid Metabolism. V. On the Mechanism of the Action of Choline upon the Liver of the Fat-Fed Rat. J. Biol. Chem., 127:211, 1939.

Stetten, DeW., Jr., and Salcedo, J., Jr.: The Source of Extra Liver Fat in Various Types of Fatty Liver. J. Biol. Chem., 156:27, 1944.

AMYLOIDOSIS OF THE LIVER

See the chapter on Amyloidosis (p. 717).

DISEASES OF THE GALLBLADDER AND BILE DUCTS

INTRODUCTION

The central point of interest in this group of diseases is cholelithiasis. Gallstones are the most frequent source of symptoms referable to the biliary tract. They are commonly related to the development of a variety of abnormalities such as cholangitis, liver abscesses, jaundice and biliary cirrhosis. Furthermore, they are of undoubted significance in the etiology of primary cancer of the gallbladder and ducts. The early recognition of gallstones is therefore a matter of considerable importance. Modern methods, including cholecystography and microscopic examination of bile obtained by duodenal drainage, have aided greatly in the diagnosis. The history and physical examination, however, remain indispensable and often are sufficient in themselves to suggest strongly the presence of cholelithiasis.

Jaundice is often the outstanding sign of disease of the biliary tract. The jaundice associated with abnormalities of the bile ducts is of the regurgitation type. This is characterized by a prompt van den Bergh reaction and the presence of bilirubin in the urine, in contrast with retention jaundice, in which bilirubin alone accumulates in the blood because of faulty excretion by the liver cells. In the latter group, which includes hemolytic jaundice and certain milder forms of liver damage, the van den Bergh reaction is delayed or indirect, and bilirubinuria is absent. Regurgitation jaundice is often accompanied by varying degrees of pruritus, while retention jaundice is not. It may be emphasized that the two forms often occur simultaneously. As an example, cases of hemolytic jaundice complicated by common duct calculi may be cited. The regurgitation jaundice resulting from stone, cancer or stricture of the common bile duct is due to increased intrabiliary pressure. So far as can be determined, this results in injury of many of the smallest bile ducts within the liver. Bloom and others have shown that the bile escapes primarily into the adjacent lymphatic spaces, thence to the thoracic duct and circulating blood. Much experimental work indicates that regurgitation of bile may also occur as a result of increased permeability of the small bile ducts, particularly the ampullary portions of the bile capillaries. This change in permeability may occur without definite histologic change, and is caused by a variety of poisons and toxins. The jaundice which results may be spoken of as parenchymal in contradistinction to mechanical or obstructive jaundice.

Most cases of regurgitation jaundice are either parenchymal, calculous or due to biliary tract cancer. There are in addition certain forms of jaundice which are not readily classified with these three main groups, such as common duct stricture, pressure of benign tumors or cysts, Hodgkin's disease or leukemia, and parasitic disease. All of the latter, as well as the various types of parenchymal jaundice, are classified from a fundamental standpoint as members of the regurgitation jaundice group, but from the standpoint of prognosis and treatment, particularly the question of surgery, it is essential that parenchymal jaundice be distinguished from that due to common duct stone, cancer of the bile ducts and other extrahepatic biliary tract disease. This distinction is at times exceedingly difficult. It may be emphasized that in parenchymal jaundice, the van den Bergh reaction is commonly of the prompt direct type and bilirubin is present in the urine. In other words, these findings are often indistinguishable from those observed in extrahepatic biliary obstruction. In addition to a careful history and physical examination, the differential diagnosis may depend upon correlation of data gained in a number of different ways, including a composite liver function study, microscopic study of bile obtained by duodenal drainage, and the study of urinary and fecal urobilinogen excretion. Cholecystography as devised by Graham and Cole, or cholangiography, is often of decisive importance in cases without jaundice, while in patients with considerable jaundice the procedure is of relatively little value and is usually not carried out.

C. J. Watson

References

Bockus, H. L.: Gastro-enterology. Philadelphia, W. B. Saunders Company, 1946, vol. III, chaps. 78, 80, 81, 84, 98.

Graham, E. A., Cole, W. H., Copher, G. H., and Moore, S.: Diseases of the Gall Bladder and Bile Ducts. Philadelphia, Lea & Febiger, 1928.

Watson, C. J.: An Approach to the Distinction of Medical and Surgical Jaundice. Minn. Med. 32: 973, 1949.

CHOLELITHIASIS

(Gallstones, Biliary Calculus)

Etiology and Occurrence. The majority of human gallstones are composed chiefly of cholesterol. The concentration of cholesterol in the bile, as well as its stability of solution, is therefore of much significance. Several important factors may be mentioned.

Concentration of Bile. The bile is concentrated from five to ten times in the gallbladder, and the degree of concentration is increased when the rate of emptying is relatively slow. During pregnancy, for example, gallbladder function is distinctly sluggish (Boyden), with the result that stasis and further bile concentration are favored. As noted in the following, a concentrated bile may be sufficiently irritating to produce inflammation.

Cholesterol Content of the Bile. Hypercholesterolemia has been shown to be associated with an increased quantity of cholesterol in the bile. During the latter months of pregnancy, and for a time after delivery, hypercholesterolemia is marked. This, together with biliary stasis, as mentioned before, is probably important to the definite correlation that exists between pregnancy and gallstone formation. Hypercholesterolemia alone cannot be said to produce gallstones, since a number of diseases, such as myxedema and nephrosis, exhibit hypercholesterolemia, but in these cholelithiasis is no more common than in the normal population. Cholesterol is maintained in solution in the bile, at least in part, because of the presence of bile salts and fatty acids. It is probable that significant reduction in concentration of these substances tends toward precipitation of cholesterol. The concentration of bile salts, fatty acids and cholesterol in the bile depends in part on the normal function of the liver cells. In conditions associated with hepatocellular damage, the concentration tends to diminish. In spite of this fact gallstone formation has not been correlated definitely with parenchymal liver disease such as that due to various poisons and infections. Nevertheless, since gallstones may be present for long periods without manifestations, it is impossible to be certain that some previous toxic effect on the liver was not responsible for the onset of stone formation due to a temporary lowering of bile salt or fatty acid concentration in the bile. There undoubtedly are instances of liver damage in which the concentration of these substances is relatively much lower than that of cholesterol.

Inflammation. Naunyn believed that bacterial infection preceded all gallstones. He believed that stasis is usually preliminary to infection. More recent studies have emphasized that inflammation, chemical as well as bacterial, may relate in an important way to the genesis of gallstones. Thus, it has been shown that a chemical type of inflammatory reaction of a severe degree may occur in the gallbladder following a too great concentration of the bile (Womack) or if pancreatic juice enters the gallbladder (Andrews). The importance of inflammation to gallstone formation is as follows: (1) Small masses of exudate (leukocytes, fibrin, epithelial cells) serve as nuclei around which precipitation of cholesterol and other substances takes place. Precipitated protein favors the precipitation of calcium bilirubinate, either in crystalline or amorphous state. Inflammation may be the chief factor in the formation of multiple gallstones, in contradistinction to the solitary, large cholesterol stones which are usually regarded as metabolic and nonflammatory in origin. According to Aschoff, the latter commence with the precipitation of cholesterol on some one occasion, and any subsequent precipitation results simply in an increase around the solitary nucleus. After infection, however, there are multiple nuclei about which subsequent precipitation may take place. The equal growth around multiple nuclei accounts for the fact that the gallstones in any one gallbladder are commonly of the same general size. (2) Inflammation alters the bile salt and fatty acid cholesterol ratio in the bile. So far as can be determined at present, this is due to two factors. Inflammation probably accelerates reabsorption of these substances from the mucosa of the gallbladder. Inflammation tends to decrease their concentration because of suppression of liver cell activity. Whether it has any influence on cholesterol concentration is unknown. Chauffard believed that the frequency of gallstones after typhoid fever was related to hypercholesterolemia. It appears, however that biliary stasis, toxic suppression of bile salt and fatty acid formation, and multiple exudative nuclei are equally, or even more, important factors. Gallstones from patients who have

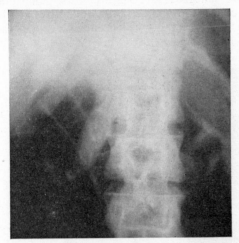

Fig. 117. Common duct visualized on flat film of gallbladder-common duct area, owing to presence of calcium carbonate precipitated in the bile. A calculus is seen at the ampulla. (This film was obtained through the courtesy of Dr. James Waring, University of Colorado School of Medicine, Denver, Colorado.)

had typhoid fever have been shown at times to contain viable typhoid bacilli.

Bilirubin Concentration. In conditions associated with a marked and prolonged increase in the amount of bilirubin excreted in the bile, such as hemolytic jaundice or anemia, there is a distinct tendency for bilirubin to precipitate as the calcium compound.

Calcium Carbonate. Phemister has emphasized the fact that obstruction of the cystic duct by one of the common variety of stones, or by carcinoma, may be followed by precipitation of calcium carbonate, in the form of a stone, a cast of the gallbladder or a soft milky suspension. On occasion the obstructed gallbladder is readily visualized owing to its content of precipitated calcium carbonate. Less frequently, the bile duct system is well outlined in this manner (see Fig. 117).

Predisposing Factors. *Age.* Clinical manifestations of gallstones are observed much more commonly after the age of 40, although they are frequently encountered in younger women who have had one or more

pregnancies. While it is probable that gallstones usually produce symptoms within a few months after their formation, many instances are encountered at autopsy in which no symptoms had been noted during life. This fact makes it difficult to establish the time of formation of gallstones, and impossible, therefore, to correlate them with age in any exact way.

Sex. From 5 to 10 per cent of adults of both sexes are found to have gallstones at autopsy. Chiefly because of pregnancy, perhaps also because of dietary factors, obesity and sedentary habits, the percentage is much higher among women than men, and is probably in the neighborhood of 20 to 30 per cent of women past 40 who have borne children.

Diet. No definite relationship is known, although it is true that gallstones are somewhat more common in obese persons. It may be true that overeating, particularly of fats, is important to the genesis of gallstones because of hypercholesterolemia. The relatively

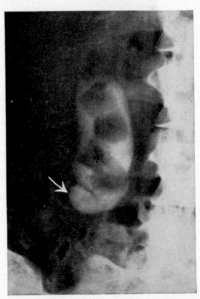

Fig. 118. Cholesterol stones in gallbladder partially filled with dye. Arrow indicates so-called phrygian cap. (Courtesy of Dr. Leo G. Rigler.)

rare occurrence of gallstones among Oriental people suggests that differences in diet may be of considerable importance.

Variety and Character of Biliary Calculi. Numerous classifications of gallstones have been suggested, of which the simplest and most useful, especially from a clinical standpoint, appears to be that which depends on whether the stone is relatively pure in composition, or a distinct mixture of two or more substances. On this basis, gallstones may be subdivided as follows: (1) pure stones, either cholesterol, calcium bilirubinate or calcium carbonate; (2) mixed stones including a preponderance of cholesterol, together with one or more of the other materials just referred to, as well as albuminate, cellular debris, and occasionally foreign

gallbladder probably produce symptoms by virtue of pressure or irritation of the wall of the viscus. Colicky pain such as characterizes stones in the ducts is not produced. Vague sensations of fullness, dull distress in the epigastrium or right upper quadrant, especially after eating, also pyrosis, sour eructations and flatulence are suggestive of gallbladder stones. Distress is often more noticeable after certain foods are eaten, notably pork, cabbage or fried foods. Other persons, however,

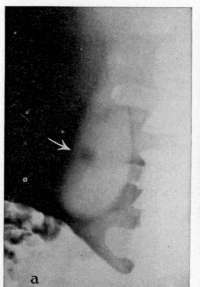 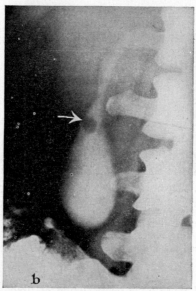

Fig. 119. *a,* Solitary cholesterol stone in dye-filled gallbladder. *b,* Displacement of stone into neck of gallbladder after contraction due to fatty meal. (Courtesy of Dr. Leo G. Rigler.)

bodies such as fragments of worms. Bacteria, especially viable typhoid bacilli, may be included (such persons are not necessarily infective carriers). In the mixed stones the proportion of the different chemical components is variable in different cases, cholesterol nearly always predominating to a marked degree. Calcium may be deposited as a shell about a stone composed of cholesterol and calcium bilirubinate. This is especially true in cases of cystic duct obstruction due to another stone. Such stones are distinctly radiopaque. Stones containing calcium bilirubinate are more difficult to visualize by roentgenography, while pure cholesterol is not distinguished except under optimal conditions by contrast with the dye used in cholecystography (see Fig. 119).

Symptoms and Signs. The symptoms of gallstones are dependent in considerable measure upon their location. Stones in the

with proved gallstones may not observe any qualitative food distress. The amount of food may or may not be of significance in various instances, although it is commonly noted that attacks follow a heavy meal. During pregnancy the symptoms are apt to be exaggerated, presumably because of increased biliary stasis.

The physical signs of gallbladder stones are few or none. There may or may not be tenderness over the region of the gallbladder. Rarely it is possible to palpate a stone or stones, especially if they compose a large mass adherent in the fundus of the thickened gallbladder.

Stones occluding the cystic duct commonly produce biliary colic. The gallbladder is often distended, at times enormously so, with a thin watery mucus. This distention is in contrast to the small or "atrophied" gallbladders usually noted in patients having common duct stone (Courvoisier). Chronic cystic duct obstruction may result in "hydrops" of the gallbladder of such extent that even several liters of fluid are found in the viscus at operation or autopsy, and in these cases it may extend well down into the pelvis. Of greater danger, however, is the accumulation of purulent exudate in the obstructed gallbladder. This condition of empyema may result in gangrene and perforation, with generalized peritonitis. The gallbladder in these circumstances may dilate considerably, even though the wall is markedly thickened. This is simply because of the considerable increase in intraluminal pressure, plus inflammatory softening of the gallbladder wall. A further discussion of this condition is found under the heading of Cholecystitis.

Stone in the Common Duct. More often than not, common duct calculi are multiple. Pain is produced when the stone or stones first enter the duct, after which there is stretching and smooth muscle spasm in an attempt to expel the stone. As the duct dilates, colic may disappear until such time as a stone enters the ampulla of Vater, when smooth muscle contraction again produces pain, which is often intermittent as the stone moves up and down in the lower end of the duct. A ball-valve action of this type usually results in jaundice of fluctuating intensity, and is often productive of suppurative cholangitis with chills and fever. The latter has been spoken of as "hepatic" intermittent fever (Charcot, Osler). The fever abates when bile drainage is reestablished, and recurs as the stone reenters the ampulla. Disappearance of fever and jaundice is usually not due to expulsion of the stone through the ampulla. More often it is simply due to a shift in position of the stone within the duct. Expulsion occurs at times, however, and in these cases the stone may be recovered from the stool. Except when the diagnosis of cholelithiasis is in doubt, examination of the stools for gallstones has relatively little value, since the finding of a stone gives no clue as to how many remain in the common duct or gallbladder. In doubtful cases the stools should be strained for stones after repeated duodenal instillation of magnesium sulfate.

Stones Impacted in the Ampulla of Vater. This condition is characterized by chronic jaundice and, as a rule, marked pruritus. Pain is often absent, but there is usually a history of colicky pain prior to the appearance of persistent jaundice. Chills and high fever may not be observed in these cases, although a low grade temperature elevation is not uncommon.

Physical examination reveals an enlarged liver, firm and often finely roughened, particularly if the jaundice is of long duration. At operation this is found to represent a mild degree of cirrhosis of biliary or obstructive type. The spleen is palpable with consider-

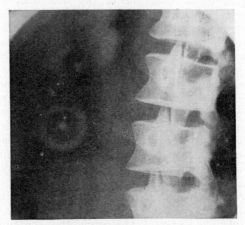

Fig. 120. Multiple gallstones of laminated type showing central calcification, intermediate cholesterol, and peripheral radiopaque area containing calcium.

able frequency, but not markedly enlarged. Ascites occurs rarely. Esophageal varices and hematemesis have been noted occasionally, but in such instances the question arises whether the cirrhosis was not coincidental and primary, rather than secondary to calculous biliary obstruction. Biliary or obstructive cirrhosis is undoubtedly related, not only to chronic biliary obstruction, but perhaps more closely to biliary tract infection associated with calculi. Graham has noted the association of cirrhosis with gallstones and biliary infection in persons who had not been jaundiced.

Gallstone Colic (Biliary Colic, Hepatic Colic). Attacks are usually abrupt in onset, often commencing several hours after a heavy meal and, as a consequence, most often occurring in the evening or during the night. The colic is due to smooth muscle spasm or stretching of either the gallbladder or ducts. The stone may be in the cystic or common duct, and the onset of colic follows shortly upon migration of the stone to a new location, either from the gallbladder to the cystic or common bile duct, or from the dilated common duct into the ampulla. The intensity of the colicky pain is variable in different attacks and depends in some degree upon the patient's sensitivity to pain. In general the attacks are severe, causing the patient to writhe, roll or double up, to walk about in anguish, to press his fists into his abdomen, or to shout or cry because of acute distress. In many cases these symptoms are accompanied by profound sweating. The pain is located in the right upper quadrant of the abdomen, at times somewhat near the midline. From the site of onset it radiates through to the back, usually beneath the right scapula, and sometimes to the right shoulder. The duration of the attack is variable, rarely more than several hours, often less. Vomiting is usual, and in many instances brings some degree of relief. In some cases the attacks recur frequently, in others after an intermission of months or even years. Fever and leukocytosis may or may not occur, depending upon the presence and degree of infection in the gallbladder, if there is a stone in the cystic duct, or in the bile ducts themselves if the stone is in the common duct. Slight or moderate icterus may be noted. The urine often contains bilirubin and/or urobilinogen within a few hours after the attack. This is a regular occurrence with common duct calculus, and is the basis for the important history of temporarily dark urine. The stools are often light in color from one to several days.

Complications. Internal biliary fistulas may open into the colon, duodenum or, rarely, the pylorus, also into the peritoneal or pleural cavities and the skin. Cholecystoduodenal fistulas permit passage of large stones into the small bowel, where they may produce intestinal obstruction. This is characterized by an irregular recurrence of vomiting and abdominal distention as the stone moves slowly along the small bowel, stopping at intervals until propelled further by increased peristalsis.

There are other complications in which both gallstones and associated infection play a common role, i.e., pancreatitis, both acute and chronic; peritonitis due to perforation of the gallbladder; cholangitis and liver abscesses; pylephlebitis; rarely thrombosis of the hepatic vein, or endocarditis.

Diagnosis. The dyspeptic symptoms due to stones in the gallbladder must be distinguished from those of *peptic ulcer*. Relief from food, milk or soda is rarely noted to any distinct degree in cases of gallstones, but is fairly characteristic of ulcer. The distress of ulcer is usu-

ally located in midepigastrium, while that due to gallstones is, as a rule, in the right upper quadrant of the abdomen. Dull pain caused by an irritable, *spastic colon* may be noted at times in the area of the gallbladder; this is usually distinguished on the basis of the history of marked constipation or diarrhea, relief of distress following bowel movement, and the occurrence of pain at other times in the region of the cecum, splenic flexure or sigmoid colon. Spastic colon and gallstones may be present in the same person, and there is little doubt that gallstones aggravate irritability of the colon.

Gallbladder stones are rarely palpable, and even in such instances, diagnosis must be confirmed by roentgenogram. Palpable stones usually contain enough calcium to permit visualization by means of a simple flat plate of the gallbladder region. Cholecystography is often necessary for the diagnosis of gallstones, particularly those composed chiefly of cholesterol, with little or no calcium. This method depends simply upon excretion of tetraiodophenolphthalein by the liver into the bile, with subsequent concentration in the gallbladder. The dye may be given by mouth satisfactorily. It is absorbed into the portal circulation, and about 96 per cent of it is excreted in the bile (Graham and Cole). If given in the evening, roentgenography the following morning will reveal the shadow due to concentrated dye within the gallbladder. A fatty meal or an egg yolk meal (Boyden) results in prompt contraction of the size of this shadow if the gallbladder function is normal. If the cystic duct is occluded or if the gallbladder has entirely lost its concentrating function, there may not be a sufficient concentration of dye to permit contrast with cholesterol stones; in this event the condition can be classified only as a nonfunctioning gallbladder in which stones may or may not be present. An upright film is occasionally of value in demonstrating cholesterol stones not otherwise evident. In the upright position the stones may be concentrated in a layer near the fundus of the gallbladder. Cholecystography is probably about 90 per cent efficient in the demonstration of gallstones. Duodenal drainage (Lyon) is often confirmatory in doubtful cases; it rarely yields positive information when the roentgenogram is negative, although the converse is often noted (Doran).

An important recent advance is the use of Biligrafin or Cholografin (the di-sodium salt of N, N'-adipyl-bis-(3-amino-2, 4, 6-triiodo)-benzoic acid), for intravenous cholangiography. This permits visualization of the bile ducts and detection of calculi, in the absence of jaundice.

Biliary colic is usually recognized without difficulty. *Renal* and *intestinal colic* rarely cause confusion. The pain of renal colic commences in the loin or flank and radiates downward, especially to the inner surface of the thigh, or to the genitalia; dysuria and hematuria are often present. The pain of intestinal colic (including lead colic and acute porphyria) is usually a more generalized crampy pain, often somewhat more marked below the level of the umbilicus. If due to intestinal obstruction, there is increasing emesis, distention of the abdomen, and the auscultatory finding of high-pitched or musical borborygmi in association with the colicky pain. If due to *lead colic,* the occupational history, the presence of a lead line on the

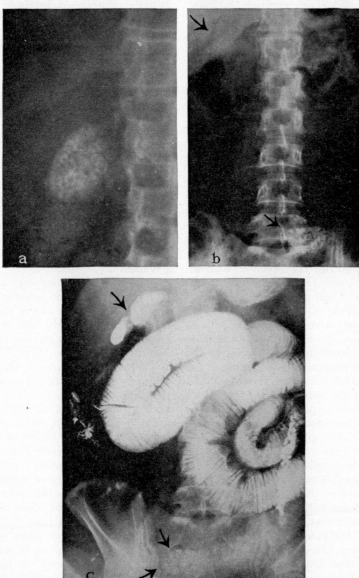

Fig. 121. *a*, Mass of calcified gallstones in the gallbladder as noted on 7/22/31. *b*, 8/18/32. Patient now has symptoms of bowel obstruction. Upper arrow indicates gas in the biliary ducts (due to cholecystoduodenal fistula). Lower arrow indicates the mass of calcified gallstones now in the small bowel. *c*, After barium meal; upper arrow indicates cholecystoduodenal fistula. Lower arrows indicate gallstones in the small bowel. Note distended loops above. (Borman and Rigler, Surgery, Vol. I.)

gums and the finding of basophilic stippling in the red blood cells are all of aid in diagnosis. The colic of *acute porphyria* may closely simulate gallstone colic; the presence of red urine, due to porphyrin (or of urine that becomes red on exposure to light), is of decisive importance.

The pain of acute *coronary thrombosis* may be confused with that due to gallstones. In some cases coronary thrombosis is productive of abdominal distress only, and this may be limited to the right upper quadrant or epigastrium. The electrocardiogram is of much aid in such instances. The presence of a pericardial friction rub is distinctive. Slight jaundice may follow an attack of coronary thrombosis, but is less common than with biliary calculus, and does not appear as a rule until several days after the attack, when it is often, but not always, associated with pulmonary infarct. Jaundice and dark urine (bilirubinuria) usually appear within 24 hours after a gallstone colic, if at all. Urobilinogenuria is usually noted shortly after a gallstone attack, but is delayed for 36 to 72 hours after a coronary thrombosis. *Biliary dyskinesia* (or dyssynergia) without gallstones is undoubtedly productive of biliary colic in rare instances. This term indicates a simultaneous spastic contraction of the gallbladder and sphincter choledochus, with resultant colicky pain. The cause of the condition is not clear. There can be little doubt that persistent distress after cholecystectomy, especially when stones were not found, is at times due to recurrent spasm of the sphincter of Oddi. Biliary dyskinesia is recognized by the fact that cholecystokinin, or substances such as egg yolk which stimulate its production, cause spasm of the sphincter of Oddi. With the duodenal tube in position, no bile can be obtained, but after instillation of magnesium sulfate, dark bile appears and the pain promptly abates (Ivy). Dyskinesia is not to be considered unless gallstones have been excluded by all possible means.

Marked jaundice due to *impacted stone* is at times confused with jaundice due to cancer of the biliary tract, including carcinoma of the head of the pancreas. A previous history of gallstone colic and jaundice is suggestive of calculous jaundice, but it must be borne in mind that cancer of the bile ducts is relatively common in persons with gallstones. Loss of weight is usually more profound in the presence of cancer of the biliary tract than in jaundice due to stone. The following features are of particular aid in distinguishing these conditions: (1) The palpation of a smooth, nontender, distended gallbladder. This is frequently possible in cases of cancer of the biliary tract, but very rare in jaundice due to stone in the common duct. Courvoisier found at autopsy that the gallbladder was atrophied in 70 of 87 cases of calculous jaundice, as contrasted with 17 in which it was dilated. This dilatation was marked in but two cases. Conversely 90 per cent of cases of obstructive jaundice of other cause, mainly cancer, exhibited distended gallbladders. The clinical value of palpating a distended gallbladder is probably even greater than Courvoisier's figures indicate. In the writer's experience, a distended gallbladder of the type mentioned has rarely been palpated in cases of jaundice due to calculus in the common duct. When found in association with complete biliary obstruction, the diagnosis of cancer of the biliary tract is relatively certain. (2) The presence of complete biliary obstruction as denoted by the finding of less than 5 mg. of fecal urobilinogen per day, over a four-day period, with less than 0.3 mg. of urobilinogen in the 24 hour urine. This finding is noted in over 90 per cent of cases of cancer of the biliary tract, and in less than 10 per cent of the cases of calculous jaundice (Watson).

Common duct stone may cause fever and pain, with little or no jaundice. In such cases significant elevation of the prompt direct-reacting serum bilirubin, and often marked increases of the serum alkaline phosphatase, are helpful in diagnosis.

Parenchymal jaundice may be confused with calculous jaundice. The term "parenchymal" applies to diffuse cellular liver damage, such as occurs with cirrhosis, acute or subacute atrophy and in many cases of so-called "catarrhal" jaundice (infectious hepatitis). In distinguishing jaundice due to hepatitis or cirrhosis, the following features are of importance: the history of exposure to persons having epidemic jaundice, or of the occurrence of jaundice in other members of the family in the recent past; the history of having received blood or blood products, especially pooled plasma, or of parenteral injection of any substance or needle puncture within the past six months, especially two to four months prior to the onset of jaundice; the history of chronic alcoholism; of ingestion of drugs, such as cinchophen, methyltestosterone, chlorpromazine or arsenic; of arsenical therapy for syphilis; or exposure to carbon tetrachloride. Further helpful features that may be mentioned are the presence of a small liver with or without ascites; the development of collateral circulation over the abdomen; enlargement of the spleen; hematemesis, and demonstration of esophageal varices by roentgenogram; the presence of *"spider nevi,"* which are much more often encountered on the face, back of the neck, shoulders, arms, hands or upper chest. In acute or subacute atrophy or diffuse necrosis of the liver the outstanding differential features are progressive increase of painless jaundice; demonstrable decrease in the size of the liver; early appearance of somnolence and coma; the "fetor hepaticus," or "amine" odor, a peculiar, musty-sweetish and pervading aromatic odor, quite characteristic of diffuse necrosis of the liver (Eppinger). This odor is noted at times in cases of advanced cirrhosis of the liver, and is observed in lesser degree in some cases of hepatitis.

Prognosis. Cholelithiasis of itself is rarely fatal, but death may be caused by complications, such as perforation of the gallbladder, cholangitis, liver abscesses or acute pancreatitis.

Treatment. The choice of medical or surgical treatment of gallstones depends chiefly on the patient's general condition. Cholecystectomy is the procedure of choice in cases in which the presence of gallstones is proved. Operation should not be undertaken simply because of pain suggestive of gallstones or gallbladder disease. Operation may be deemed inadvisable in proved cases because of advanced age, cardiac failure, renal insufficiency or other serious disease. In the usual case, however, cholecystectomy is indicated because of the many serious complications which gallstones may produce. Cases of cholelithiasis, when not treated surgically, are apt to have recurrent attacks in spite of medical management; operation has often been postponed until some dangerous complication has appeared, and the patient may now have reached an age which in itself materially increases the risk. Furthermore, the important relation of cholelithiasis to the occurrence of primary cancer of the biliary tract must be taken into account.

In cases of cystic-duct-stone colic when the presence of gallstones has been noted previously, or when it is readily established by a simple flat x-ray plate of the gallbladder region, early operation (cholecystectomy) is probably advisable, even as an emergency procedure, if the patient's general condition is suitable. In this way the development of empyema of the gallbladder may be avoided.

Medical. Control of the diet is of prime importance. Foods high in cholesterol, such as fat and eggs, should be eliminated or greatly reduced. Greasy or fried foods, pork products, rich dressings and cheese, spicy foods and alcoholic beverages are most likely to cause exacerbation of symptoms. Immediately after an acute attack it is desirable that the diet be limited to liquids, such as skim milk, milk soups and strained orange juice in small amounts. After a short time, cereals may be added, then rice and tapioca, later vegetables. Baked or mashed potato, spinach, carrots, string beans, asparagus, lettuce, celery, squash are tolerated best. Onions, sauerkraut, cabbage, turnips, radishes or cucumbers may cause recurrence of distress. Lean meat, including roast or boiled chicken, beef or lamb, may be eaten in moderation. Baked or boiled fish is usually tolerated. Butter and cream should be taken but sparingly; vegetable fat, particularly olive oil, probably has a beneficial effect in stimulating bile flow, without being productive of distress.

Bile salts at times appear to be beneficial. They should be used in fairly pure form, not simply as dehydrated bile, which may induce nausea and distress. Given in an amount of 0.2 to 0.4 gm. three times daily, bile salts often appear to prevent recurrences of symptoms for long periods of time.

Morphine is the time-honored remedy for biliary colic. Its use is still necessary in many instances, although there is little doubt that it increases spasm of the sphincter choledochus, thus increasing intrabiliary pressure (Walters; Bergh and Layne). Depending upon age and size of the patient, the dose of morphine to be given, hypodermically, usually varies from 0.01 to 0.02 gm. In severe attacks as much as 0.032 gm. may be required, within one hour, to bring relief. A very effective and rapid method is to inject 0.01 to 0.016 gm. of morphine intravenously. Nitroglycerin relaxes the sphincter choledochus and at times dramatically relieves biliary colic, but unfortunately is not trustworthy. To avoid the undesirable increase in intrabiliary pressure which morphine probably produces, nitroglycerin may be given simultaneously with morphine, the former by dissolving under the tongue, the latter hypodermically or intravenously

(Best). The nitroglycerin used should be the readily soluble hypodermic tablet, $\frac{1}{100}$ grain (0.65 mg.). Demerol, an analgesic and spasmolytic synthetic drug, given in an amount of 0.1 gm. hypodermically, will at times completely control the pain of biliary colic.

Milder attacks of colic are at times allayed simply by rest, the application of hot compresses to the abdomen, and the evacuation of gas by means of a tap water enema.

The treatment of pruritus associated with jaundice is not particularly gratifying. Calamine lotion or carbolic lotion, 1:60, is of aid in some cases. If it is known that the patient is not sensitive to procaine, benefit is at times noted following intravenous administration of 100 mg. of procaine hydrochloride. This should be given slowly in not less than 100 cc. of solution. Dihydroergotamine, given hypodermically in an amount of 1 mg., at times gives gratifying results, the duration of effect being from 4 to 12 hours, occasionally even longer. Thus far at least, the adverse vascular side effects of ergotamine have been rarely encountered with the dihydro derivative.

Surgical. Adequate preoperative preparation is of utmost importance. This is particularly true in jaundiced patients. The prothrombin time (Quick) should be determined, and, if significantly prolonged, synthetic 2-methyl-1, 4-naphthoquinone may be given either by mouth or intravenously. There are several water-soluble preparations of the synthetic naphthoquinone on the market which are entirely satisfactory. Given by mouth, an amount of 5 mg. daily is adequate. If given intravenously, 1 mg. of the active material per day suffices. The response of the prothrombin time to intravenous injection is of some diagnostic and prognostic value. In general it may be said that with relatively good liver function the prothrombin time will return to the control level within 6 hours after intravenous administration of 1 mg.; with poor liver function, especially with primary diffuse liver damage, the prothrombin time is unlikely to return to the normal range.

Operations on the biliary tract should be preceded by a diet plentiful in protein and carbohydrate, and low in fat. In general this diet should consist of approximately 300 gm. of carbohydrate, 100 to 150 gm. of protein, and a smaller amount of fat (50 to 80 gm.). If the patient is unable to eat a regular diet, it may nevertheless be possible to give frequent liquid feedings consisting of milk fortified with a powdered food of high protein and carbohydrate content. Foods of this type are available which contain 35 to 60 per cent protein and 40 to 65 per cent carbohydrate, and are at the same time rich in minerals and added vitamins. When mixed with milk, a food value of 1000 calories per liter or more can be attained. The studies of Ravdin, and of Whipple and his associates, reveal clearly that an adequate intake of protein is essential to the protection of the liver. While there is no doubt that glucose is of value, it is insufficient, in many instances, to prepare patients for operation simply by giving them intravenous glucose, as is often customary. This is especially true if the patient is malnourished, febrile, toxic or markedly obese. Such patients are apt to have fatty livers, a factor of great importance in operative mortality. The amount of glucose given intravenously is often not enough to supply the patient's caloric needs, much less to convert the fatty liver into one filled with glycogen. Further than this, the preoperative preparation should include, if at all possible, a plentiful supply of vitamins, especially B complex. Choline and riboflavin deficiency in particular have been implicated with respect to fatty infiltration of the liver. It is probably best to give these patients relatively crude sources of B complex, such as crude liver extract fortified with the known components such as thiamine, niacin and riboflavin.

Cholecystectomy in cases of proved gallstones effects a cure in most instances. The operative mortality rate is low in the hands of experienced surgeons, well below 1.0 per cent. The fatality figure is slightly higher for operations on the common duct.

Secondary operations are necessary at times because of postoperative stricture, unrecognized common duct stone, re-forming of stones in the hepatic or common bile ducts, adhesions or hernia. Common duct calculi are apt to be overlooked unless the common duct is opened and explored. This should be done if the patient is or has been jaundiced, assuming that operation has been decided upon. If possible, it is wise to have a cholangiogram made at the time of operation, before the abdomen is closed. After stones have been removed from the duct, T tube drainage should be carried out for a period of weeks or even months. Before the T tube is removed from the duct, a *cho-*

langiogram should again be made. This consists in injecting a radiopaque material, usually 50 per cent Diodrast, into the T tube, then taking an x-ray film of the area of the common duct and ampulla. Cholangiograms at times reveal unsuspected stones which were overlooked at operation in spite of opening the common duct. Best has described procedures intended to expel these stones into the duodenum. These include the in-

Gaebel, E., and Teschendorf, W.: Darstellung der Gallenwege mit Biligrafin (Schering). Röntgenblätter, 6:162, 1953.

Osler, W.: The Ball-Valve Gall Stone in the Common Duct. Lancet, p. 1319, 1897.

Ravdin, I. S., Royster, H. P., and Sanders, G. B.: Reflexes Originating in Common Duct Giving Rise to Pain Simulating Angina Pectoris. Ann. Surg., 115:1055, 1942.

Wakefield, Howard: Relationship of Gallbladder and Heart Disease. Medicine, 15:45, 1947.

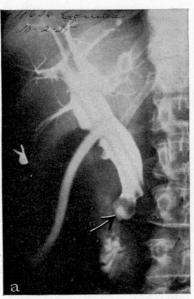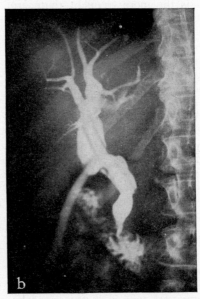

Fig. 122. *a*, Cholangiogram taken with T tube in common bile duct. Arrow indicates residual stone in lower end of duct. *b*, After removal of stone at a secondary operation. (Courtesy of Dr. Leo G. Rigler.)

jection of magnesum sulfate solution and of olive oil into the T tube; also the use of nitroglycerin.

Failure of cholecystectomy to relieve symptoms is much more common in cases in which gallstones were not demonstrated, either before or during operation. Some of these cases, at least, belong in the *biliary dyskinesia* group.

C. J. WATSON

References

Aschoff, L.: Lectures on Pathology. New York, Paul B. Hoeber, Inc., 1924, p. 206.

Bell, A. L. L., and others: Intravenous Cholangiography. Am. J. Surg., 88:248, 1954.

Bockus, H. L.: Gastro-enterology. Philadelphia, W. B. Saunders Company, 1946, vol. III, Chaps. 98, 102, 105.

Carter, R. F., and Gillette, Lee: Immediate Cholangiography. J.A.M.A., 143:951, 1950.

Comfort, M. W., Gray, H. K., and Wilson, J. M.: Silent Gallstone: Ten to Twenty Year Follow-Up Study of 112 Cases. Ann. Surg., 128:931, 1948.

CHOLECYSTITIS

Etiology. The age and sex incidence parallels that of cholelithiasis, except in typhoid epidemics, in which acute cholecystitis may occur in children of both sexes. Whether acute cholecystitis is more often chemical than infectious in origin is still controversial. There is strong evidence that undue concentration of bile (Womack) or regurgitation of pancreatic juice (Andrews) into the gallbladder may induce cholecystitis without the presence of bacteria. The majority of cases of acute cholecystitis are associated with cholelithiasis, and it is probable that gallstones are of much importance, both from the standpoint of obstruction and stasis, and trauma to the mucosa.

Acute cholecystitis may occur without gallstones. This is noted particularly as a complication in about 1 per cent of cases of typhoid fever, but may also be encountered in the wake of other acute infections.

Members of the colon-typhoid group are found most commonly when the contents of the acutely inflamed gallbladder are cultured. Staphylococci, pneumococci or streptococci are present much less frequently. It is probable that these organisms gain access to the gallbladder either by way of the blood stream or by ascent from the duodenum. Statistics as to which is the more frequent route are not available.

Chronic cholecystitis is to be regarded as the quiescent stage of the disease, after subsidence of acute manifestations. Subsequent acute attacks are apt to occur. There is usually, but not always, an associated cholelithiasis.

Morbid Anatomy. Acute cholecystitis varies in degree from a mild catarrhal type to an extremely dangerous, phlegmonous or gangrenous form. In the mild form the gallbladder is often moderately distended, the serosa exhibits injection of the blood vessels, the wall is somewhat tense and swollen, and the mucosa is congested, at times revealing small amounts of fibrinopurulent exudate on its surface. Microscopically, congestion and a moderate exudation of polymorphonuclear leukocytes in the submucosa and outer coats are observed.

The *phlegmonous* type is characterized by marked thickening of the gallbladder wall, at times attaining more than 1 cm. As a rule, the cystic duct is obstructed by stone, and the resulting pressure within the gallbladder is sufficient to cause distention, which may be considerable in some cases. The increase in pressure plus softening of the wall or outspoken gangrene constitute the chief dangers of this disease, i.e., perforation and peritonitis. This occurs with relatively greater frequency in patients more than 60 years of age. Perforation of the gallbladder with localized inflammation or pericholecystic abscess is much more common than was hitherto believed. In many cases, of course, the inflammation subsides without perforation. If the cystic duct remains closed, the distention of the gallbladder may persist, either as a low grade or subsiding empyema, or a hydrops.

In phlegmonous or acute suppurative cholecystitis, microscopic examination shows a diffuse exudate throughout the entire wall, composed of polymorphonuclear leukocytes and fibrin. Necrosis may be noted and is prominent in the gangrenous type. In chronic cholecystitis, perivascular foci of lymphocytes are seen in the serosa; there is often moderate thickening of the gallbladder wall, with some increase of connective tissue and extensive adhesions to adjacent organs.

In *cholesterosis,* or "strawberry" gallbladder, cholesterol esters are deposited just beneath the mucosa, and are seen grossly as numerous yellowish granules or streaks. The exact nature of cholesterosis is as yet unknown.

Symptoms and Signs. The symptoms of chronic cholecystitis cannot be distinguished from those of stones in the gallbladder. The manifestations of acute cholecystitis are in proportion to its severity. In the mild catarrhal form there may be nothing more than indigestion, moderate pain and tenderness in the right upper quadrant of the abdomen, slight fever and malaise. With more severe degrees of infection there is more marked pain and tenderness, and muscle spasm is elicited. Rebound tenderness in the right upper abdomen is noted in the more severe cases of suppurative cholecystitis. The spread of pain, tenderness and rebound tenderness over the abdomen generally indicates either that perforation has occurred or that there is an associated pancreatitis with areas of fat necrosis in the omentum and mesentery. The gallbladder is at times palpable in acute cholecystitis. As a rule it is rather vague and difficult to outline, principally because of tenderness and muscle spasm. At times, however, the gallbladder is felt more distinctly as a tender sausage-like mass, extending down below the right rib margin, slightly lateral to the midclavicular line. This type is more often palpated in patients suffering their first attack of cholecystitis, in which there has not been previous thickening of the gallbladder wall; for example, with typhoid fever.

Marked prostration often results from acute suppurative cholecystitis. The mouth temperature is commonly elevated to 102° to 104° F. Nausea and vomiting are frequently observed. Abdominal distention (ileus) is not uncommon. Jaundice may be present and, if at all prominent, indicates calculous obstruction of the common duct or the hepatic ducts. Slight jaundice is due in some cases to associated liver damage which results from the infection spreading via the lymphatics into the liver. The urine commonly contains increased amounts of urobilinogen, which usually disappear within 24 to 48 hours after the infection subsides. As a rule the attack of cholecystitis is relatively short, from a few hours to a few days. In some instance, however, empyema of the gallbladder may produce persistent pain and tenderness for weeks. A somewhat vague tender mass representing the subacutely inflamed gallbladder may be felt for an equal period of time, eventually becoming smaller and less tender, until finally it is no longer palpable. During the stage of acute inflammation, the leukocyte count is elevated to from 12,000 to 40,000, usually about 15,000, per cubic millimeter. This is a neutrophilic leukocytosis. It is of some value in determining the severity of the infection, particularly with reference to the question of operation, to follow the percentage of band forms, or the filament-nonfilament ratio.

Diagnosis. The location and character of the pain, and the history of previous attacks of gallstone colic or jaundice, are helpful in distinguishing cholecystitis from *ulcer*. After perforation has occurred, the symptoms and findings may be identical. The presence, however, of free gas in the peritoneal cavity, as determined by roentgenogram, is more likely to indicate perforation of the gastrointestinal tract than of the gallbladder. *Acute appendicitis,* particularly in persons with a high-lying cecum, may offer difficulty. The history of onset of diffuse abdominal pain with subsequent localization in the right lower quadrant, rarely higher, usually serves to distinguish appendicitis. Right *pyelonephritis* at times simulates cholecystitis with respect to pain. The maximal tenderness, however, is usually in the loin, and this fact, plus the urinary symptoms and findings, makes differentiation possible.

Prognosis. Except for complications, such as perforation and peritonitis, pancreatitis or liver abscess, the chances for immediate recovery are excellent. Subsequent attacks, however, are likely to occur.

Treatment. As already noted, cholecystectomy is recommended in definite instances of cystic duct stone colic before the appearance of the signs of cholecystitis, such as fever, marked tenderness and leukocytosis. There can be little doubt that operation at this time carries a relatively small risk and permits avoidance of complications. Admittedly, the signs of acute cholecystitis at times appear soon after the onset of pain. There is no general agreement as to early operation once these signs have appeared, although in recent years the trend has been in this direction. Glenn reported early operation in 350 cases of acute cholecystitis with but 6 deaths (1.7 per cent). He believed that 4 of the fatal cases might have been saved by still earlier operation, since the gallbladder in each of these was already gangrenous. Zierold, in experience to be published, has had but one death in 716 consecutive cholecystectomies, many of which were carried out in the presence of acute cholecystitis. It should be emphasized that in this study a relatively small operation was the rule with minimal incision and anesthesia (partly local) and no exploration. If conservative treatment is elected, it is usually desirable to wait several weeks after subsidence of acute symptoms before surgery is undertaken. If conservative measures fail to bring some degree of improvement within two to three days, and the severity appears to be such that perforation is feared, the procedure of choice is cholecystostomy. Extirpation of distended, empyematous gallbladders is not advisable. In older patients, in whom circulatory complications are often present, it may be possible simply to drain the gallbladder under local anesthesia. Later, depending upon the patient's general condition, cholecystectomy may be indicated.

Conservative measures during the acute stage include hot moist compresses to the abdomen; sedation by means of phenobarbital sodium subcutaneously, 0.13 gm. at intervals of 4 to 6 hours; and morphine, 0.01 to 0.016 gm., if necessary to relieve severe distress. Nitroglycerin, 0.65 mg., dissolved under the tongue, or Demerol, 0.1 gm. subcutaneously, will often aid in controlling pain and may be of value in relaxing the smooth muscle of the cystic duct. Nasal-suction siphonage may be necessary for abdominal distention and vomiting. In the severer cases, nothing other than ice chips should be given by mouth. Infusions of 5 per cent glucose in saline may be administered subcutaneously and intravenously. As the attack subsides, liquids by mouth may be started, and the diet as already described under the treatment of Cholelithiasis may be instituted. If the attack does not subside promptly, tetracycline and/or penicillin therapy may prove beneficial.

The treatment of chronic cholecystitis depends on several factors, the most important of which is the presence of gallstones. If these are demonstrated, cholecystectomy is usually the procedure of choice. This will depend again upon the patient's age and general condition; the operation should not be carried out in the presence of any serious constitutional disease such as myocardial or renal insufficiency. If there have been repeated, distinct attacks of acute cholecystitis, even though stones cannot be demonstrated, cholecystectomy is usually indicated during a quiescent period. Conservative treatment is to be preferred, however, in patients who complain only of dyspeptic symptoms, and in whom the cholecystogram has revealed nothing more than a reduced gallbladder function. There can be no doubt of the rare occurrence of mild chronic cholecystitis with apparently normal gallbladder function as determined by cholecystography. The symptoms in these cases are probably often on a dyskinetic basis, although there is some evidence that biliary dyskinesia also exists without any demonstrable pathologic change in the gallbladder or ducts. The results of operation in this group of cases are usually disappointing. Distress frequently recurs. Conservative treatment consisting of the diet already suggested for the management of cholelithiasis, together with bile salts, often enables the patient to avoid distress. The use of magnesium sulfate is at times beneficial, probably because of its relaxing effect on the sphincter of Oddi.

C. J. Watson

References

Bergh, G.: Critical Review of the Treatment of Acute Cholecystitis. Internat. Abstr. Surg., 66:29, 1938.

Bockus, H. L.: Gastro-enterology. Philadelphia, W. B. Saunders Company, 1946, vol. III, Chaps. 100, 101.

Glenn, F.: Conditions of the Biliary Tract Requiring Urgent Surgery. Am. J. Surg., 58:160, 1942.

Segal, H. L., Friedman, H. A., and Watson, J. S., Jr.: Problems in Diagnosis and Treatment of Non-Calculous Gallbladder. Am. J. Digest. Dis., 15: 321, 1949.

Senger, W.: The Unrelieved Cholecystectomized Patient. Rocky Mountain M. J., 39:106, 1942.

SUPPURATIVE CHOLANGITIS

Etiology and Occurrence. Suppurative cholangitis usually results from biliary stasis, due to stone or neoplasm, in persons who have had previous infection of the biliary tract. The condition is observed most often with common duct calculus, but is also seen at times with carcinoma of the gallbladder or bile ducts. In the latter cases of cholangitis there is nearly always an associated cholelithiasis. In contrast with these are the cases of carcinoma of the pancreas with biliary obstruction, in which cholangitis is relatively rare and in which there is usually not an associated cholelithiasis or previous biliary tract infection. Various pyogenic organisms are responsible for suppurative cholangitis. The colon bacillus and streptococcus are most common. Often these are present in the biliary tract prior to the onset of biliary stasis. In other cases the infection of the obstructed bile ducts is probably hematogenous, although this is a matter of some doubt. The occurrence of suppurative cholangitis in the absence of biliary obstruction is extremely rare.

Morbid Anatomy. The bile ducts, both intrahepatic and extrahepatic, are dilated above the area of obstruction, which is usually in the common bile duct. The ducts are also thickened because of inflammatory changes. In the liver there is periportal inflammation, often actually small abscesses. The periportal involvement is frequently of chronic suppurative type in cases of cholangitis due to calculous obstruction. Microscopically, the small bile ducts are seen at times to contain polymorphonuclear leukocytes, though more often the inflammation appears to be pericholangitic, the exudate being largely around the small bile ducts in the portal spaces. This consists of neutrophils in variable number, together with plasma cells and lymphocytes.

The term "cholangitis lenta" signifies a rare hematogenous form of suppurative cholangitis in the absence of biliary obstruction. Secondary endocarditis may occur (Pepper).

Symptoms and Signs. Jaundice, with or without colicky pain, chills and irregular but marked fever, usually of "spiking" type, are the outstanding features of suppurative cholangitis. The liver is usually enlarged and moderately tender. The spleen is occasionally palpable. There is marked neutrophilic leukocytosis. The urine contains bilirubin and, as a rule, much urobilinogen. The blood culture may be positive.

Complications. Metastatic abscesses may occur. Hemorrhage from the mucous membranes is likely to result from prothrombin deficit, if this cannot be corrected by administration of vitamin K. Hepatic coma is apt to precede death, which is due to severe liver damage and insufficiency, together with generalized toxemia.

Diagnosis. Suppurative cholangitis is likely to be present in any patient having jaundice, chills, fever, sweating, an enlarged tender liver and leukocytosis, especially if that patient has had previous jaundice or gallstone colics. Liver abscesses due to other causes, and suppurative pylephlebitis may give rise to confusion. The latter is suggested if there is free fluid in the abdomen. The stools should be examined carefully for amebas in order to exclude amebic abscess of the liver. Duodenal drainage may establish the presence of suppuration in the bile ducts, although the patient may be too ill to warrant the procedure.

Prognosis. The prognosis is much better than in former years, owing to antibiotic therapy. The establishment of adequate drainage or the beneficial effect of the newer antibiotics, especially tetracycline, may bring about prompt recovery.

Treatment. Temporary spontaneous improvement not infrequently occurs, particularly in the calculous cases in which obstruction is often partially relieved by the shifting position of a common duct stone. It is therefore best to support the patient for several days with fluids and glucose parenterally. The general condition may be improved by giving vitamins, especially B complex and K (2-methyl-1, 4-naphthoquinone), parenterally, together with protein either in liquid form, by mouth, or as plasma transfusions. Transfusion of blood is desirable if there is anemia or profound toxemia. Of the antibiotics now available, tetracycline is probably most likely to be beneficial. Streptomycin or pencillin may also be given. The sulfonamides are less valuable and somewhat more dangerous because of the possibility of additional liver injury. Operation should probably not be delayed for more than one week unless the infection is definitely subsiding. At the end of this time, T tube drainage of the common duct is usually advisable.

This subject is also discussed in the section on Diseases of the Liver (p. 917).

C. J. WATSON

Reference

Bockus, H. L.: Gastro-enterology. Philadelphia, W. B. Saunders Company, 1946, vol. III, Chap. 106.

CARCINOMA OF THE GALLBLADDER AND BILE DUCTS

Etiology and Occurrence. Carcinoma of the gallbladder is usually associated with gallstones, and is consequently observed more frequently in women. Carcinoma of the bile ducts is slightly more common in men; nevertheless, gallstones are not infrequently associated with this condition. In general, there can be little doubt that chronic irritation due to gallstones and associated infection is an important factor in the initiation of cancer of the gallbladder, and to a lesser degree of the bile ducts.

Morbid Anatomy. Carcinoma of the gallbladder may originate in any part of the viscus. If primary in the fundus, direct extension into the liver is common; tumors primary in the corpus or collum often invade the bile ducts. These differences in origin are of importance with respect to the presence or absence of icterus, also to the type of mass palpable in the gallbladder area during life. Tumors primary in the collum may cause simple distention of the gallbladder, while tumors of the fundus are often responsible for a hard nodular mass. Of interest is the fact that the gallbladder may be found to be markedly distended if the cystic duct is obstructed by a tumor. This is comparable to what has already been discussed in connection with calculous obstruction of the cystic duct, although the inflammatory changes with cancer are usually much milder; in these cases the lumen of the gallbladder is filled with thin, white mucus. In some instances carcinoma obstructing the cystic duct may bleed into the lumen of the gallbladder, thus causing marked distention. Microscopically, the tumor may be carcinoma simplex, adenocarcinoma or squamous cell carcinoma (metaplasia).

Carcinoma of the bile ducts is often of the scirrhous type and may be so small as to be confused with a benign fibrous stricture. Microscopic examination in such instances reveals nests of cancer cells interspersed with fibrous tissue. Suppurative cholangitis is seen at times above a primary carcinoma of the common duct or of the cystic duct at its junction with the common hepatic duct. Primary carcinomas are relatively frequent at this point. They may also occur in the lower end of the common duct. In rare instances, soft polypoid carcinomas occur within the common duct, and may exhibit ball-valve activity, much like a stone in the common duct.

Symptoms and Signs. Most of the patients have had previous symptoms of gallstones or cholecystitis. Carcinoma of the fundus of the gallbladder produces dull, constant pain and often tenderness, weakness and loss of weight, and a hard, nodular mass in the region of the gallbladder. Jaundice is usually present, but may appear relatively late. Once established, it deepens progressively, and complete biliary obstruction (less than 5 mg. of fecal urobilinogen per day) usually occurs. Jaundice appears relatively early with carcinoma of the corpus or collum of the gallbladder, and is usually the first symptom of primary carcinoma of the ducts. In some instances the latter may be masked by the presence of colic, chills and fever due to obstruction and cholangitis. Blood stream invasion by gram-negative bacteria, with the resultant clinical picture of bacterial shock, may follow a cholangitis of any cause. The jaundice occasionally disappears because of establishment of an internal biliary fistula.

The liver may be enlarged and nodular with any of these primary carcinomas. Enlargement due to metastases is somewhat more commonly encountered in cases of cancer of the gallbladder. Ascites is noted at times, owing to peritoneal involvement. As these conditions progress, there is deepening jaundice, cachexia and often a hemorrhagic tendency. Somnolence and coma, the "cholemic" state, usually precede death. The hemorrhagic tendency is due at least in part to prothrombin deficit. The jaundice may be of a deep olive type; this is said to be due to formation of biliverdin within the bile ducts, for which oxidative ferments liberated from the tumor cells are held to be responsible. Biliverdin icterus is strongly suggestive of carcinomatous biliary obstruction, although at times it is seen in cases of jaundice not due to cancer.

Diagnosis. In addition to these features, the evidence of complete biliary obstruction, as previously discussed, and the presence of a palpable gallbladder are of considerable importance. If the composite liver function study points more strongly toward obstructive rather than parenchymal jaundice, laparotomy is generally indicated. Experience has shown that needle biopsy of the liver is more dangerous in the presence of high grade biliary obstruction, owing to leakage of bile and bile peritonitis. In doubtful cases cholangiography through a small incision under local anesthesia has often proved very helpful. Peritoneoscopic cholangiography (Royer) is of much value in the hands of an experienced person.

Postoperative *stricture of the common duct* must be distinguished from cancer of the ducts. The history of onset of jaundice shortly after cholecystectomy usually serves to indicate the presence of the former condition. In many cases the general condition remains relatively good in spite of long-continued jaundice, in contrast with the progressively downhill course of cancer of the bile ducts. Traumatic stricture may or may not be associated with complete biliary obstruction, or with suppurative cholangitis. Nontraumatic benign stricture of the common bile duct of inflammatory origin is extremely rare (Walters).

Prognosis. Death usually occurs within a few months from the time of onset of symptoms.

Treatment. If the disease is obviously not too far advanced, operation should be carried out. In occasional cases it is possible to resect a small primary carcinoma of the common bile duct. A small number of cases have now been operated upon with longer survival and reasonable hope of cure. In patients in whom the tumor is inoperable, anastomosis of the gallbladder to the stomach or small intestine may prolong life or at least bring relief from otherwise intractable pruritus.

The preoperative preparation of these patients, especially the use of vitamin K, is the same as already described for stone in the common duct.

C. J. Watson

Reference

Stewart, H. L., Lieber, M. M., and Morgan, D. R.: Carcinoma of the Extrahepatic Bile Ducts. Arch. Surg., 41:662, 1940.

CONGENITAL ABNORMALITIES OF THE BILE DUCTS

Congenital Obliteration. This condition is probably due to developmental aplasia. The process is confined to the lower portion of the common bile duct in about 16 per cent of cases (Holmes), while in the remainder the ducts within the liver are also obliterated. The disease is characterized by deep jaundice coming on shortly after birth and gradually increasing. The stools are acholic, and contain not more than traces of urobilinogen. The urine contains much bilirubin and no urobilinogen. These features permit distinction from icterus neonatorum or erythroblastosis fetalis with jaundice. The liver is enlarged and usually exhibits obstructive or biliary cirrhosis. Surgical exploration should be carried out in the hope that the obliterative process is limited to the lower part of the common duct. Even when operation has been successful, however, the result has been but temporary. Infection of the biliary tract follows sooner or later upon anastomosis of the gallbladder to the stomach or small bowel.

Congenital Cystic Dilatation of the Common Bile Duct. This is a rare condition which is probably related to localized obliteration or stricture of congenital origin. Approximately 130 cases had been recorded in the literature up to 1942 (Glenn). In some cases no obstruction has been found. The cystic dilatation usually involves the middle and upper parts of the duct. The cyst at times attains the size of a full-term fetus. Clinical features suggesting this condition are recurrent attacks of jaundice, and often of paroxysmal pain, associated with a palpable cystic tumor, and appearing in childhood (McWhorter). The treatment is surgical.

C. J. Watson

References

Bockus, H. L.: Gastro-enterology. Philadelphia, W. B. Saunders Company, 1946, vol. III, Chap. 97.

Glenn, F.: Conditions of the Biliary Tract Requiring Urgent Surgery. Am. J. Surg., 58:160, 1942.

Lockwood, Bruce C.: Congenital Anomalies of the Gallbladder. J.A.M.A., 136:678, 1948.

McWhorter, G. L.: Congenital Cystic Dilation of the Common Bile Duct. Arch. Surg., 8:604, 1924.

DISEASES OF THE PANCREAS*

INTRODUCTION

Although affections of many major abdominal organs were well known to the ancients, those of the pancreas escaped detection until the nineteenth century. During this period, cysts, benign and malignant tumors and acute and chronic pancreatitis were accurately described. In addition, the enormous importance of the pancreas as an organ both of internal and external secretion was recognized. It was not, however, until this century that functioning tumors of the pancreas were identified. Furthermore, only during the past fifteen years or so has surgical extirpation of the pancreas and its tumors become practical.

PHYSIOLOGY OF THE PANCREAS

The external secretions of the pancreas are the most active and versatile of the digestive juices and contain enzymes for the digestion of all the principal foodstuffs. In the absence of specific stimuli, the pancreas secretes a continuous flow of pancreatic juice of low enzymatic content, the volume of which amounts to some 800 to 1000 ml. in 24 hours. Under the influence of hormonal or nervous stimulation, the amount of juice secreted as well as its concentration of enzymes may be greatly augmented.

Two major types of stimuli to the formation of pancreatic juice are recognized, nervous and humoral. Neurogenic stimuli, provoked by eating, are mediated through fibers of the vagus nerve. The juice secreted under this circumstance is high in enzyme concentration. When hydrochloric acid from the stomach enters the duodenum, secretin is liberated. This hormone, derived from upper intestinal mucosa, enters the blood stream directly and stimulates the pancreas to produce copious amounts of thin watery juice high in bicarbonate and low in enzymes. An intestinal phase of pancreatic secretion is also recognized. This is initiated by the entrance of gastric chyme into the intestinal tract. The

* The author wishes to express his deep appreciation to Dr. Harry Miller for his valuable assistance in the preparation of this article.

pancreatic secretions so evoked are characterized by a high enzymic content. A humoral agent, pancreozymin, has been extracted from intestinal mucosa, and is believed to be responsible for the intestinal phase of pancreatic secretion.

Pancreatic juice contains three proteolytic enzymes, the most important of which are trypsin and chymotrypsin. The former is secreted in an inactive form as trypsinogen which depends for its activation upon intestinal enterokinase. Chymotrypsin is secreted in inactive form and is activated only by active trypsin. In addition to these two common enzymes, carboxypeptidase is also present in pancreatic juice. Fats are hydrolyzed into glycerin and fatty acids by the pancreatic enzyme lipase. Raw starch is converted to maltose by means of pancreatic amylase. Additional pancreatic enzymes which are effective in carbohydrate digestion are maltase, lactase and sucrase. In addition to its enzymatic content, pancreatic juice is characterized by a high bicarbonate concentration which aids in the neutralization of the acid gastric juice. Insulin, the internal secretion of the pancreas, is elaborated by the beta cells of the islands of Langerhans and functions importantly in carbohydrate metabolism.

TESTS OF PANCREATIC FUNCTION

A number of tests have been developed which yield evidences of malfunction of the pancreas. The simplest of these involves little more than the gross and microscopic examination of the stool. In the absence of external pancreatic secretion, the stools are voluminous, poorly formed and of a foul and fetid odor. Excessive neutral fats, fatty acids and soaps are present (steatorrhea). The presence of large numbers of muscle fibers with well preserved cross striations indicates deficient protein digestion (creatorrhea).

Determinations of serum amylase concentrations are of diagnostic importance, especially in acute affections of the pancreas in which high values are obtained. High values are also present in mumps. Lesser elevations are inconstantly encountered in patients with tumors of the pancreas, with peptic ulceration penetrating into the pancreas, in the exacerbations of chronic pancreatitis, and also at times in cardiac infarction. Blood lipase levels can also be determined and are similarly elevated. The levels of these two enzymes in the urine can be ascertained and in many instances are diagnostically important because they frequently remain elevated longer than do those in the serum.

The secretin test of external pancreatic function provides useful and oftentimes diagnostic aid in chronic pancreatic disorders. After the administration of secretin, both the volume of pancreatic juice aspirated from the duodenum and its characteristics are determined. By demonstrating diminished amounts of enzymes in the secretions, important degrees of pancreatic damage are detected.

Charles G. Child, III

CONGENITAL ABNORMALITIES

Pancreatic Heterotopia. In about 1 per cent of individuals coming to autopsy, small nodules of typical pancreas are found in the wall of the stomach, duodenum, gallbladder or jejunum. These usually lie submucosally but on occasion are found within the muscularis or just beneath the serosa. A variety of disorders such as inflammation, cystic formation, ulceration and both benign and malignant tumors have been found in aberrant pancreatic tissue. Only a small percentage of individuals with this congenital defect develop symptoms related directly to the ectopic tissue. Ectopic islands of pancreas may become ulcerated, may bleed, may obstruct the pylorus or may cause intussusception.

Annular Pancreas. Pancreatic tissue partially or completely encircling the duodenum is referred to as annular pancreas. Symptoms appear in about 30 per cent of individuals with this anomaly. These are usually due to obstruction of the duodenum but may also be due to an associated peptic ulceration, pancreatitis or biliary tract obstruction. In some patients clinical manifestations of annular pancreas are present at birth; in others these do not appear until the fifth or sixth decades of life. The most common symptoms are nausea, vomiting and epigastric pain. The characteristic roentgenographic picture of this defect is narrowing and notching of the lateral duodenal wall. An asymptomatic annular pancreas does not require treatment.

Fibrocystic Disease of the Pancreas. Fibrocystic disease of the pancreas is an uncommon malady of childhood, the etiology of which is unknown. It is characterized by functional disturbances in the external secretory mechanisms of the pancreas and in the mucous glands of the gastrointestinal and respiratory tracts, and also of the sweat and salivary glands. The descriptive term "mucoviscidosis" has been applied to this disease. The diagnosis is generally made upon the basis of malnutrition, steatorrhea, chronic respiratory infections, and upon the demonstration of pancreatic insufficiency. A deficiency of trypsin in the pancreatic secretions is particularly important in this disease. In infancy, intestinal obstruction occurs due to the presence of thick viscid meconium. In later life, children with this ailment generally succumb to malnutrition or severe respiratory sepsis. They are also victims of salt loss through the skin in hot weather because of inability to regulate the sodium secretion by their sweat glands. The use of antibiotics and correction of sodium depletion has improved the prognosis.

Charles G. Child, III

DIETARY DEFICIENCY AND PANCREATIC DISEASE

In a number of areas of the world, particularly certain sections of Africa, a nutritional disease of children designated kwashiorkor has come to be recognized. This is asociated with mental retardation, pancreatic atrophy and fibrosis, fatty infiltration of the liver, edema of the extremities and a low serum albumin. The secretion of the pancreatic enzymes amylase, lipase and trypsin is reduced. Depigmentation of the skin and hair imparts a typical red color to these structures. Unless the disease is far advanced, its progress may be reversed by the addition of milk protein to the diets of afflicted children. Upon a diet so fortified, the normal secretions of the pancreas reappear and the other features of the disease regress. Because the caloric intake of these children is generally adequate, it is believed that this disease is primarily related to a deficiency in specific proteins. (See also Kwashiorkor under Deficiency Diseases, p. 627.)

PANCREATITIS

ACUTE PANCREATITIS

Acute pancreatitis is a serious and distinctive inflammatory reaction which presumably originates within the pancreas. It is characterized by an attack of excruciating upper abdominal pain which typically makes its appearance after a heavy meal and after the ingestion of alcohol. Its milder forms, often designated as acute pancreatic edema or acute interstitial pancreatitis, run a self-limited course and usually subside without evidence of permanent damage to the pancreas. Acute pancreatic necrosis, a severe form of the disease, is seen less often, pursues a fulminating course and is associated with profound prostration and extensive destruction of the pancreas.

Etiology. While it is generally accepted that the pathologic changes observed in acute pancreatitis are due to the effect of "activated" pancreatic enzymes upon the gland itself, the precise mechanisms responsible for the acute attacks remain controversial. A widely accepted explanation is "the common channel theory." This postulates that the junction of the pancreatic and common bile ducts provides a communication between the two systems that permits bile to enter the pancreatic ducts. This theory presupposes that bile within the pancreatic gland initiates the acute process. Spasm, edema and impacted biliary calculi have all been implicated as causes of ampullary obstruction capable of initiating reflux of bile.

The pathologic alterations in the pancreas occurring secondary to certain protein deficiencies as well as the experimental production of acute pancreatitis by d,l-ethionine, an antagonist to the essential amino acid methionine, suggest that dietary deficiencies may play an etiologic role in pancreatitis. Although alcohol is not a direct cause, alcoholism is considered a contributing factor in the etiology.

Morbid Anatomy. In milder cases of acute pancreatitis the gland is edematous and indurated but its lobular and microscopic structures are preserved. Fat necrosis, if present, is localized to the pancreas and immediately adjacent tissues. In more severe pancreatic inflammations, varying degrees of necrosis and hemorrhage into and about the gland are present. Severe pancreatitis is associated with the production of copious amounts of bloody peritoneal fluid and extensive areas of fat necrosis within the abdomen.

Symptoms and Diagnosis. The clinical picture of acute pancreatitis varies with the intensity of the pathologic process within the gland. In cases of acute pancreatic edema the symptoms are often mild and ill defined. Pain is the most important symptom and though this is usually localized to the left epigastrium, it may extend across the entire upper abdomen. Quite generally the pain is persistent, severe and unrelieved by the usual doses of narcotics. Vomiting occurs shortly after the onset of pain and often continues as long as the pain lasts.

The physical findings in patients with acute pancreatitis vary with the severity of the attack. Local epigastric tenderness over the pancreas may be the only sign that can be elicited during mild episodes, but during severe attacks the pain is intense and the muscles of the epigastrium are rigid. One of the characteristic features of severe pancreatitis is the accompanying shock. Such patients are frequently cyanotic and prostrate and show signs of peripheral vascular collapse, in part due to rapid depletion of plasma volume with the development of ascites. Their pulse rate is rapid and their blood pressure low. Fever is regularly associated with acute pancreatitis. Usually this varies from 100° to 103° F. and persists steadily throughout the attack without important variations. A common roentgenographic sign which is suggestive but not diagnostic of acute pancreatitis is segmental ileus involving the stomach, small intestine or colon.

Laboratory tests are important in establishing a diagnosis of pancreatitis. The most significant of these is the determination of serum amylase. This may show striking elevations within an hour or two after the onset of symptoms or may take 8 to 12 hours to reach diagnostic levels. In the course of an attack the concentration of this enzyme ordinarily returns to normal levels within 24 to 72 hours. Later, normal or subnormal values may be obtained even though the disease is actually increasing in clinical severity. The urinary amylase is also of diagnostic value. It usually becomes elevated 12 to 24 hours later than the serum amylase and high levels may persist for 24 to 72 hours longer than the serum elevations. The serum lipase is also elevated in patients with acute pancreatitis. A transient elevation in serum bilirubin is present in some cases of acute pancreatitis. In many patients with this disease elevations in the blood sugar and glycosuria are observed. A low serum calcium which results from the combination of large amounts of calcium with fatty acids in the areas of fat necrosis is sometimes an important laboratory finding in acute pancreatitis. A leukocytosis of 20,000 or greater is usually present during an acute attack of pancreatitis.

Complications and Prognosis. Following an attack of acute pancreatic necrosis, localized accumulations of necrotic debris and hemorrhagic exudate may become encapsulated and form a persistent pancreatic pseudocyst. Frank suppuration, however, does not commonly follow necrosis of the pancreas. Tetany due to a low serum calcium may, of course, make its appearance in patients with extensive fat necrosis. The prognosis for a patient with acute pancreatitis bears a direct relationship to the severity of the pathologic changes which occur. In patients whose disease does not progress beyond pancreatic edema, the mortality is negligible. When, however, appreciable degrees of necrosis appear, the mortality rate has been reported to be 30 per cent and higher.

Treatment. For many years, acute pancreatitis was generally regarded as an acute surgical emergency and an operative mortality as high as 50 per cent was reported. About twenty-five years ago, however, physicians and surgeons began to appreciate that the then current morbidity and mortality of acute pancreatitis was lower in patients not operated upon. This realization, together with the development of laboratory techniques whereby the diagnosis could be established early, led to the general adoption of a therapeutic program, the aims of which are diminution of pancreatic secretion, relief of pain and prevention of ileus. Food and fluids by mouth are withheld, ephedrine, atropine or methantheline bromide (Banthine) is administered parenterally, and continuous gastric suction is maintained. Spasm of the sphincter of Oddi may be relaxed by nitrites. Demerol is preferred to morphine for the relief of pain because the latter drug may, by producing spasm of the duodenum and sphincter of Oddi, intensify the disease process. Paravertebral, splanchnic and epidural nerve blocks are also effective in alleviating pain. If shock accompanies the acute attack, this must be appropriately treated. Deficits in serum electrolytes and body water must be corrected. Hypocalcemia should be treated with calcium gluconate or calcium chloride; hyperglycemia and glycosuria may require insulin for control. Broad spectrum antibiotics such as chlortetracycline (Aureomycin) or oxytetracycline (Terramycin), although not specific for pancreatitis, are important adjuncts to therapy which serve to minimize secondary infection. Only when the acute attack becomes complicated by obstruction of the biliary tract, by formation of an abscess or by extensive pancreatic necrosis, is surgical intervention necessary.

CHRONIC PANCREATITIS

(Chronic Relapsing Pancreatitis; Chronic Recurrent Pancreatitis)

Definition. For many years the term chronic pancreatitis has been applied to recurring or persistent inflammatory reactions within the pancreas. The milder forms, associated or not with affections of the biliary tract, are not so rare as are commonly supposed and are often unsuspected until identified either at operation or at autopsy. The more serious forms of pancreatitis are readily recognized and have been designated by Comfort and his associates as chronic relapsing pancreatitis. This disease, of unknown etiology, is characterized by recurrent attacks of severe upper abdominal pain and is associated with progressive destruction of the pancreas. Transient disturbances in the function of acinar and islet cells usually accompany the early stages of chronic pancreatitis. Eventually advanced malnutrition, greasy and bulky stools, and diabetes may become established features of the disease. Probably related to the demoralizing character of the pain, the disease may be accompanied by psychic disturbances; addiction to alcohol or narcotics is often an outstanding feature.

Morbid Anatomy. In the early stages of chronic pancreatitis, the gland is enlarged, indurated and irregularly nodular; later the pancreas becomes atrophic and ultimately presents as little more than a fibrous cord. Cystic degeneration and extensive calcification may also be features of advanced stages of the disease. Complications of the disease are stenosis of the common bile duct, the pancreatic ducts and the duodenum. In rare instances, occlusion of the portal vein occurs, and portal hypertension due to chronic fibrosing pancreatitis has been recognized.

Symptoms. Early in chronic pancreatitis, the episodes of severe pain are relatively brief. As the disease becomes established, however, the attacks of pain recur more frequently and tend to be more severe and protracted. Finally, intervals free of distress virtually disappear. The distribution of pain in chronic pancreatitis varies not only from patient to patient but from attack to attack in the same individual. In many it commences in the epigastrium and radiates through to the back or along one or both costal margins. Relief from pain is sought through sitting up, hunching forward and slowly rocking from side to side. So demoralizing is the pain that surcease is sought through morphine or alcohol. During an acute exacerbation, many of the physical, roentgenographic and laboratory features of acute pancreatitis are present. In the intervals between attacks patients with early relapsing pancreatitis often fail to manifest any clinical evidence of their disease. Eventually, however, such patients become malnourished, lose large amounts of weight and are unable to work. Abdominal examination is generally unrevealing unless cystic degeneration has produced a palpable mass in the epigastrium.

Diagnosis. In the patient with fully developed chronic pancreatitis a tentative diagnosis may be had with relative ease. Particularly is this true when malnutrition is obvious, when there is a long history of recurring acute attacks and when bulky and greasy stools foul in odor are passed. Should the patient also be diabetic and should pancreatic calcification be demonstrated on roentgenographic examination of the upper abdomen, a diagnosis of chronic pancreatitis is assured. In early or obscure cases of this disease, a diagnosis of chronic relapsing pancreatitis may be established only by observing the patient during one of his acute episodes.

In a certain number of individuals, chronic pancreatitis undoubtedly pursues a benign course in which symptoms and disabilities are negligible. On the other hand, few nonmalignant diseases can progress more relentlessly. Recurring attacks may become the rule, each one leaving its increment of pancreatic damage. Addiction to alcohol and narcotics is often a feature of the late phases of pancreatitis. If the progress of the disease is unstayed, patients become cachectic and ready prey to an overwhelming infection.

Treatment. As far as can be determined, medical therapy has little in a definitive way to offer the patient with advanced pancreatitis. Diabetes is readily controlled by insulin and troublesome steatorrhea minimized through the liberal use of pancreatic extracts. The severity and frequency of the attacks can be lessened if alcohol is relinquished and a diet adhered to which is high in carbohydrate and protein but low in fat. The acute exacerbations may be alleviated by constant gastric suction, administration of atropine and Demerol and institution of thoracolumbar nerve block.

That the surgical therapy in chronic pancreatitis is not universally successful is witnessed by the diverse number of operations which have been employed. Currently Mulholland believes that a large percentage of these patients will cease to have further attacks after division of the sphincter of Oddi. Bowers, on the other hand, advocates a Roux in Y choledochojejunostomy to divert bile away from the pancreatic duct. Partial gastrectomy, by diminishing the amount of hydrochloric acid and by diverting this from the duodenum, has also been reported to be effective in controlling the progress of this disease. It has long been held that one of the prerequisites to the cure of relapsing pancreatitis is the surgical correction of biliary tract abnormalities. All too frequently, however, such operations have had little effect on the course of pancreatitis except in the case of a patient with a common duct stone impacted in the ampulla of Vater.

In chronic pancreatitis with severe pain, sympathetic denervation of the upper abdomen affords relief. Subtotal and even total pancreatectomy have been performed as measures for relief from the dire effects of chronic relapsing pancreatitis. Although some striking successes have been reported, the surgical mortality after such radical procedures is high and too few cases are available for study to permit any final evaluation at this time. When viewed critically, chronic relapsing pancreatitis in all its protean manifestations must currently be considered a disease without decisive and effective treatment. Reasonable palliation and even cure, however, can sometimes be obtained by one or a combination of several judiciously selected operative procedures.

CHARLES G. CHILD, III

PANCREATIC CALCIFICATION

(Pancreatolithiasis)

Calcareous deposits within the pancreas have long been recognized and for years were considered to represent a specific disease. Recent evidence, however, indicates that in the majority of instances, pancreatic calcification is closely related to acute or chronic pancreatitis. Presumably inflammation within the pancreas produces stasis and an accumulation of protein debris in the ducts. These factors are considered responsible for the precipitation of calcium carbonate either as discrete calculi lying free in the ducts and acini or conglomerate masses of calcareous material forming casts of the pancreatic drainage system. The diagnosis of pancreatolithiasis can be established roentgenographically.

Although a few patients with this disorder are without associated symptoms, the majority have had, at one time or another, attacks of pain either suggestive or diagnostic of chronic relapsing pancreatitis. Furthermore, many patients with calcification of the pancreas are diabetic and give evidence of a deficiency in external pancreatic secretion. The problems of therapy in patients with this disease are primarily those of individuals with chronic relapsing pancreatitis. If symptoms are mild, only supportive therapy is required; if severe, pancreatectomy may become necessary. Only rarely has permanent relief been afforded by removal of one or more isolated calculi from the major pancreatic ducts.

CHARLES G. CHILD, III

PANCREATIC CYSTS

The term pancreatic cyst embraces a variety of tumefactions, each constituting a distinct clinical entity and each differing in nature and in derivation. Rarest of these cysts are those of developmental origin. Most commonly encountered are the so-called *pseudocysts* which develop as a complication of acute or chronic pancreatitis. The distinguishing features of pseudocysts are their lack of an epithelial lining and their thick fibrotic walls which are often densely adherent to adjacent structures. Pseudocysts commonly occupy the lesser peritoneal sac and present anteriorly through the gastrohepatic or gastrocolic ligaments. *Retention cysts* of the pancreas are due to obstruction of its ducts and are characterized by an epithelial lining as well as the accumulation of retained pancreatic secretions. Some, particularly those of the head of the organ, are considered inflammatory in origin, while others have been found secondary to cancer of the pancreas. Retention cysts are rare and, because they produce little reaction, insidiously enlarge to great size without seriously discomforting the patient. *Cystadenomas* of the pancreas are true proliferative neoplasms arising from pancreatic parenchyma. They are uncommon, constituting only 2 per cent of all pancreatic cysts. They are generally multiloculated and may reach large size before they are discovered. The majority arise in the body and tail of the pancreas and occasionally undergo malignant degeneration.

Symptoms and Diagnosis. The symptomatology of pancreatic cysts derives principally from their size, location and rate of growth. In an appreciable number of patients with slowly growing cysts the only complaint relates to the incidental discovery of a large upper abdominal mass. Epigastric pain which is occasionally referred to the back and left flank is the most common presenting symptom. Other symptoms, due chiefly to displacement or obstruction of adjacent organs, are nausea, vomiting, anorexia, postprandial discomfort, gaseous eructation and constipation. Jaundice due to pressure upon the common bile duct is sometimes encountered, and such unusual manifestations as hematuria, gastrointestinal hemorrhage and portal hypertension have all been described. Diabetes is encountered in about one tenth of the patients with pancreatic cysts. Upon roentgenographic examination of neighboring structures various types and degrees of pressure defects may be detected. A smooth compression defect of the stomach, duodenum or colon is the usual observation.

Treatment. The surgical treatment of pancreatic cysts may be relatively simple or may tax the surgeon's ingenuity and resourcefulness. In general, complete excision of the cyst in question must be considered the treatment of choice provided this does not subject the patient to excessive operative risks. Short of resection, tube drainage, external marsupialization with the abdominal wall, and internal drainage by means of an anastomosis between the cyst and stomach or small intestine, have all been employed with varying degrees of success. Resection of the cyst together with a portion of the pancreas is a surgical procedure generally reserved for cystadenomas and for cysts with complicated fistulas. More radical procedures are indicated for extensive cystadenomas which have undergone malignant degeneration.

TUMORS OF THE PANCREAS

ISLET CELL TUMORS

Benign and malignant neoplasms originating in the islands of Langerhans are rare, are encountered in all decades of life and occur with almost equal frequency in men and women. Most, but not all, of these tumors are associated with hyperinsulinism and hypoglycemia. The majority of islet cell tumors are benign adenomas which vary in size from 0.1 to 6.0 cm. Malignant tumors of this variety contrast sharply with their benign counterparts in that they are often large bulky tumors which metastasize and recur locally after unsuccessful attempts have been made to remove them.

Pathologic Physiology. Patients with functioning islet cell tumors manifest episodes of hypoglycemia induced by the large amounts of insulin which these tumors release into the blood stream. During the attack of hypoglycemia, oxidative processes within the brain are believed to be decreased to a degree at which cerebral function is impaired. The effects of hypoglycemia upon the central nervous system resemble those seen in hypoxia in that higher nervous centers are depressed. Normal cerebral function returns promptly after oral or intravenous administration of glucose. Through its capacity to increase blood sugar by mobilizing glycogen, the exhibition of epinephrine also terminates an attack promptly.

Diagnosis. Recurrent hypoglycemic seizures constitute the most important clinical manifestation of a functioning islet cell tumor. These are characterized by an initial period of hunger, soon followed by apprehension, agitation, weakness and excessive perspiration. Mental confusion, visual disorders, loss of consciousness or other neurologic disturbances such as transient hemiplegia may then make their appearance. Many patients discover that the attack can be prevented or terminated by the prompt ingestion of food, particularly of sugar. During an attack the blood sugar level usually falls below 50 mg. per 100 cc., and levels of 20 mg. per 100 cc. have been reported. Whipple believes that the following criteria should be met before a diagnosis of islet cell tumor is made: (1) that the attacks come on while the patient is fasting, (2) that the blood sugar be 50 mg. per cent or less during an attack, and (3) that the attack terminate with the administration of glucose. An important clinical aid in establishing a diagnosis of functioning islet cell tumor is the precipitation of an attack by a period of fasting. Exercise may hasten the onset of the typical seizure. Other causes of hypoglycemia must be eliminated before a diagnosis of functioning islet cell tumor is seriously entertained. Certain diseases of the pituitary, of the adrenals and of the liver, as well as functional hypoglycemia, must all be distinguished from islet cell tumors.

Treatment. The treatment of islet cell tumors is excision. When this is possible, the rate of cure is approximately 85 per cent. If a discrete tumor cannot be found, subtotal pancreatectomy may be advisable. In patients whose symptoms persist after removal of one tumor, reexploration in search of another is warranted. Not infrequently the adenoma may be small and lies in the posterior aspect of the pancreas and therefore easily escapes detection. Total pancreatectomy may become necessary when lesser surgical procedures have failed. Malignant islet cell tumors of the pancreas are treated by as radical excision as possible.

CANCER OF THE PANCREAS

Cancer of the pancreas is not rare since it accounts for 2 per cent of all deaths due to malignant disease. It seldom develops prior to the age of 30 years, and is seen principally in the fifth and sixth decades of life. It affects men more commonly than women. Diabetes mellitus appears to be a predisposing factor.

Morbid Anatomy. The majority of primary pancreatic cancers arise in the epithelium lining the ducts of the gland, while the remainder find origin in adjacent acinar tissue. Only rarely have squamous cell tumors or sarcomas of the pancreas been reported. Eighty per cent of malignant pancreatic tumors (excluding islet cell carcinomas) arise in the head of this organ while 20 per cent first appear in its body or tail. Pancreatic carcinomas characteristically infiltrate the gland and may early occlude one or more of its major ducts. For this reason a distinctive feature of pancreatic cancer is marked swelling and induration of the portions of the gland which are distal to the point of duct obstruction. As a group, pancreatic cancers are notorious for local extension, and for metastasizing early to regional lymph nodes as well as to more distant structures such as the liver and lungs.

Symptoms and Diagnosis. The cardinal symptom of pancreatic cancer is pain, despite the fact that painless jaundice has long been regarded as the distinguishing feature of the disease. Usually the pain originates in the upper abdomen, is often present in the back and occasionally is exaggerated at night. Dyspepsia, anorexia, weakness and mental depression are frequent concomitants. Progressively deepening jaundice, which usually appears some time in the course of the development of pancreatic cancer, is, of course, more frequent in tumors arising in the head of the gland than in those primary in the body or tail. Loss of weight constitutes a universal finding in pancreatic cancer, and a history of startling losses of as much as 50 pounds is not infrequent.

A palpable gallbladder, long regarded as an important feature of this disease, is found in about one quarter of patients with pancreatic cancer. Courvoisier's law, therefore, though it is valid enough in itself, is not as helpful clinically as is so commonly believed. Only in far advanced cases is a palpable tumor present. Recurrent migratory phlebitis has been described but is so rare as to have little diagnostic value. Roentgenologic examination of the duodenum occasionally reveals flattening of the mucosal folds, an "inverted 3 sign," enlargement of the duodenal sweep or evidence of invasion by tumor. Although roentgenography may be important in suggesting the diagnosis of pancreatic cancer, it usually does so only late in the course of the disease.

One of the tragedies of cancer of the pancreas relates to the fact that early in its course neither physical nor roentgenographic examination nor laboratory studies can be relied upon to indicate the true cause of the patient's persisting complaints. All too frequently cancer of the pancreas is considered only after jaundice appears. Late in the course of the disease, an enlarged liver, a palpable gallbladder, jaundice and a hard epigastric mass constitute a clinical picture the significance of which can hardly fail to be appreciated. Disturbances in carbohydrate metabolism, elevations in serum amylase and lipase, diminished secretion of pancreatic enzymes as determined by the secretin test, the presence of undigested meat fibers and excessive fat in the stools all have been invoked for their help in establishing a diagnosis early. When detected, abnormalities in pancreatic function provide strong presumptive evidence for a diagnosis of pancreatic cancer. Aspiration of malignant cells from the duodenum permits a positive diagnosis. Negative cytologic examination, however, is of little consequence. Despite the great amount of attention accorded pancreatic cancer in recent years, little important progress has been made in bringing patients with this disease under

treatment early in the course of their affliction.

Treatment. Twenty years ago Whipple and his associates demonstrated that removal of the head of the pancreas and contiguous structures was a practical procedure. The hope was then expressed that an operation was at last available which offered a chance of cure to patients with cancer involving the head of the pancreas. These original hopes, however, have failed to materialize, for the best that can be said for this operation today is that it prolongs life five to eight months and affords relief from pain and jaundice. Five-year survivors are few; perhaps no more than 4 or 5 have been recorded in the world literature. So poor in fact have been the results of pancreaticoduodenectomy that many believe the operation should be abandoned in the treatment of cancer of the pancreas. To the author, this seems to be an attitude of unwarranted defeatism. If pancreaticoduodenectomy is discarded, a few patients will be denied the possibility of cure and reasonable palliation will be withheld from an additional number. Decompression of the biliary tract alone is, of course, an important operation for the relief of jaundice and is widely applied in the presence of metastases.

When carcinomas of the body and tail of the pancreas are detected, they are generally so far advanced that resection is either impossible or obviously palliative. Recently total pancreatectomy and pancreatectomy together with resection of the portal vein have been employed as efforts to extend the surgical treatment of pancreatic cancer. Experience with these procedures is too limited to permit evaluation at this time.

CHARLES G. CHILD, III

References

Berk, J. E.: Diagnosis of Carcinoma of the Pancreas. Arch. Int. Med., 68:525, 1941.

Brunschwig, A.: The Surgery of Pancreatic Tumors. St. Louis, C. V. Mosby Co., 1942.

Cattell, R. B., and Warren, K. W.: Surgery of the Pancreas. Philadelphia, W. B. Saunders Company, 1953.

Child, C. G., Holswade, G. R., McClure, R. D., Jr., Gore, A. L., and O'Neill, E. A.: Pancreaticoduodenectomy with Resection of the Portal Vein in the Macaca mulatta Monkey and in Man. Surg., Gynec. & Obst., 94:31, 1952.

Comfort, M. W., Gambill, E. E., and Baggenstoss, A. H.: Chronic Relapsing Pancreatitis. A Study of 29 Cases without Associated Disease of the Biliary or Gastro-intestinal Tract. Gastroenterology, *6:* 239, 376, 1946.

Doubilet, H., and Mulholland, J. H.: Recurrent Acute Pancreatitis: Observations on Etiology and Surgical Treatment. Ann. Surg., *128:*609, 1948.

Elman, R.: Surgical Aspects of Acute Pancreatitis. With Special Reference to Its Frequency as Revealed by the Serum Amylase Test. J.A.M.A., *118:* 1265, 1942.

Mulholland, J. H.: Personal communication.

Opie, E. L.: The Relation of Cholelithiasis to Disease of the Pancreas and Fat Necrosis. Am. J. M. Sc., *121:*27, 1901.

Pratt, J. H.: Pancreatic Disease. J.A.M.A., *120:*175, 1942.

Whipple, A. O., Parsons, W. B., and Mullins, C. R.: Treatment of Carcinoma of the Ampulla of Vater. Ann. Surg., *102:*763, 1935.

Whipple, A. O.: Hyperinsulinism in Relation to Pancreatic Tumors. Surgery, *16:*289, 1944.

DISEASES OF THE PERITONEUM

INTRODUCTION

The peritoneum is a smooth, thin, normally glistening membrane lining the abdominal cavity and composed of cells of mesodermal origin. In covering all the abdominal viscera, it is thrown into numerous folds which give it a total area as great as that of the surface of the body. The peritoneal cavity is a peritoneal space, completely closed in the male, but in the female connected with the exterior through the fallopian tubes, uterus and vagina. Various portions of this cavity are roughly separable by certain anatomic structures into what are usually referred to as spaces, which assume some clinical importance in the localization of pathologic processes. The most cephalad is the subphrenic space above the transverse colon and roughly bisected by the round ligament of the liver. Somewhat more caudad, the subhepatic space lies between the liver and gallbladder above and the stomach, duodenum and hepatic flexure below. The lesser peritoneal sac posterior to the stomach communicates with the remainder of the abdominal cavity through the foramen of Winslow, and beneath the transverse colon lie the lumbar gutters on either side, each merging below with the corresponding iliac fossae. The pelvis constitutes the most dependent portion of the peritoneal cavity.

The retroperitoneal tissues are richly supplied with blood vessels forming part of the splanchnic bed and emptying either into the vena cava or portal veins, while the lymphatics, which are also numerous throughout, drain into the retroperitoneal nodes and thence into the cisterna chyli and thoracic duct. The spread of carcinoma from almost any viscera within the abdomen may be very great since it may travel through all of these channels.

Particulate matter and bacteria, when injected into the peritoneal cavity, can be recovered in the thoracic duct or blood stream within a half hour. Extravasated or injected blood clots slowly and is absorbed in its entirety, leaving the peritoneum unaffected unless infection, trauma or inflammation is also present.

The transudative and exudative properties of the peritoneum parallel the absorptive, and large amounts of fluid may accumulate in a relatively short period of time as the peritoneum, like other mesothelial membranes, responds to irritation or infection by the pouring out of fluid, at first of low specific gravity and containing few leukocytes, but becoming gradually more cloudy until it is frankly purulent, containing also fibrin, cell debris and finally numerous bacteria. By this route many of the constituents of the blood may be excreted, and Fine, Seligman and Frank have shown that by irrigation of the peritoneum, nitrogenous products equivalent to 20 to 25 gm. of urea may be removed from the blood stream in 24 hours, an amount approaching the total formation of this substance each day in the normal person and probably exceeding that synthesized by the acutely ill.

The powers of resistance and repair of the peritoneum are truly enormous. If the general condition of the patient is otherwise good and the injury not too prolonged or repeated too often, reexploration late after operations which have demonstrated the presence of blood, of gastric or small or large bowel content, has shown the peritoneum restored almost to its virgin state (Brunschwig).

Regeneration of Peritoneum. Brunschwig has observed clinically and in the experimental animal that when large peritoneal defects are created, reperitonealization takes place. He points out that the gross and microscopic appearance of this "new peritoneum" is identical with the normal peritoneum. He reasons that the reperitonealization occurs by "metaplasia" of connective tissue underlying the peritoneum and that the connective elements in the abdominal parietes are also capable of forming peritoneum under the proper stimulus. The fact that areas as large as the entire pelvis may be denuded of their peritoneum in radical operations in unusual instances of carcinoma, and that these same surfaces are to be found completely reperitonealized many months later, is indicative of the strong tendency of the peritoneum to regenerate. He visualizes the following steps: (1) In the area denuded of peritoneum granulation tissue appears; (2) the reperitonealization takes place by the growth of superficial areas of flat cells resting upon a fibrous tissue layer in which the capillaries, venules and arteries are irregularly dispersed.

The Diagnostic Value of Pneumoperitoneum. A 500 to 800 cc. pneumoperitoneum may safely be employed to diagnose and differentiate masses that may lie at or above the costal margin and in or below the diaphragm.

Maisel has reported that fluoroscopic study and roentgenographic examination performed with the patient standing will, by means of the pneumoperitoneum, outline the profile of the diaphragm disclosing defects, tumors and hernias of this structure. Thoracic and abdominal tumors that present at or in the diaphragm are differentiated and the peritoneum, therefore, aids in selecting the appropriate investigative incision. The mucosal pattern of the lower esophagus and the cardiac segment of the stomach may be studied in profile after a pneumoperitoneum by meals of a thick barium swallow. Tumors of the pancreas, liver, stomach, kidney and adrenal may be more carefully investigated when pneumoperitoneum is added to the plan of x-ray and contrast media studies.

FRANK GLENN

CONGENITAL ANOMALIES OF THE PERITONEUM

In the embryonic development of the intestinal tract, various folds or bands of peritoneum may be misplaced, or reflections from the abdominal wall may produce fossae which are abnormally deep, as, for example, near the ligament of Treitz or the cecum. Whether for this reason or because of mechanical or inflammatory causes, bands, membranes and so forth are present in about 15 per cent of newborn infants—most commonly about the colon, duodenum and gallbladder—and, although usually unimportant, may be responsible for obstructive symptoms in later life. Two of the better known of such bands are Lane's kink, a band between the terminal ileum and pelvic peritoneum which may cause acute angulation of the bowel beneath which loops of bowel may be caught, and Jackson's veil, a broad fold extending from the parietal peritoneum to the cecum or over the ascending colon and adherent to the

omentum. Less importance is attached to such congenital malformations now than formerly, and only when definite obstruction can be demonstrated by examination or roentgenogram is surgical attack warranted.

FRANK GLENN

GENERALIZED PERITONITIS

Peritonitis is an inflammation of the peritoneal cavity. It may be acute or chronic. The inflammation may be due to a number of causes. Peritonitis is almost always secondary to disease either of the abdominal organs or extending from elsewhere in the body by way of the blood stream. In a small number of cases it may appear to be primary, as, for example, in some cases of pneumococcal or streptococcal peritonitis in children, probably because the portal of entry is not recognizable.

So-called aseptic peritonitis is seen when urine, bile, pancreatic secretion or the contents of certain cysts are extravasated, but, except in the last instance, bacterial invasion or contamination occurs so promptly that the distinction from infectious peritonitis is rather artificial. More attention is being centered on the role of enzymes and of secondary anaerobic invasion in such cases in causing the rapid and enormous accumulation of fluid which may amount to as much as one third of the total plasma volume, and which is responsible for the rapid development of a shocklike picture and the relatively high mortality in these cases.

Etiology. The most common source of peritonitis is, of course, the intestinal tract, for, though normally impermeable to bacteria, any injury to the wall or impairment of viability through inflammation or interference with circulation may render it possible for bacteria to pass through the normal barrier and reach the peritoneal cavity. Perforations, as in appendicitis, peptic ulcer, diverticulitis or carcinoma, at once contaminate the peritoneal cavity, bringing about a localized or generalized peritonitis, depending upon the speed with which perforation actually occurs and the invasiveness of the infecting organism. The female pelvic organs may be the site of origin of peritonitis secondary to gonorrhea or sepsis associated with abortions or the puerperal state as well as of the tuberculous and pneumococcal forms.

Peritonitis complicating disease of the biliary tract is most often localized because of the anatomic features of this region, except that in elderly patients acute cholecystitis may be associated with gangrene of the fundus of the gallbladder which then perforates freely into the peritoneal cavity, giving rise to a generalized and rapidly fatal form of peritonitis. The name "primary peritonitis" is often applied to a form usually due to streptococci or pneumococci and occurring particularly in children, but even in this case the process is in reality secondary to a more generalized infection in which the bacteria reach the peritoneum from abscess or infected emboli in its immediate vicinity.

Clinical Findings. Certain visceral changes accompany peritonitis, the most frequent being actual invasion by the inflammatory reaction, causing disturbance of the motility of the intestinal tract, which is normally controlled partially by impulses transmitted by the vagus and sympathetic nerves and partially through the action of the intrinsic nerve plexuses. The reflex paralysis of the bowel occurs early in the course and has been thought of in the past as serving the useful purpose of aiding in the localization of the infection through promoting the formation of adhesions. Later, infiltration of the wall of the bowel may cause complete atony owing to the toxic effects of the infection, with marked distention of the bowel by fluid and gas, the latter produced in part by bacterial action in the stagnant intestinal contents and augmented by air swallowed by the patient. Paralytic ileus is looked upon at present as a serious complication of peritonitis and is believed to contribute materially to the mortality. Less commonly, diarrhea may accompany peritonitis, especially in children, and usually occurs when the condition is localized, often with abscess formation, and produces an irritation rather than paralysis of the bowel.

Symptoms and Signs. Since peritonitis is most often a sequel or complication of intraabdominal disease, its symptoms merge with or follow those of the antecedent condition, which also may determine their location and extent. It is of great importance, therefore, to recognize the onset of symptoms of peritonitis as distinct from those of appendicitis, cholecystitis, peptic ulcer or other lesions which may serve as its source.

PAIN of varying degree and extent is a most important symptom. At first poorly localized when only visceral peritoneum is involved, it becomes sharply defined as the inflammation reaches the parietal peritoneum. When such a catastrophe as perforation of a peptic ulcer results in the inundation of a large portion of the peritoneum with irritating gastric and duodenal content, the pain may be excruciating. Any movement accentuates the pain, and the patient usually resorts largely to thoracic respiration and lies with legs drawn up, although as ileus supervenes, the severe pain may subside and the patient may complain only of soreness or discomfort. In general, the pain is most severe near the source of the infection, but may also be referred to a distant site—as, for example, to the region of the trapezius when the diaphragmatic peritoneum is involved.

TENDERNESS. The commonest, indeed the most universal, feature of peritonitis is tenderness over the involved area, and such localization is an important diagnostic sign in determining the source of the infection. It can be elicited directly over the site of origin of the inflammation on abdominal examination and is present on rectal or pelvic examination in pelvic peritonitis. An extremely valuable and significant finding is so-called "rebound tenderness." This is provoked by making firm, deep pressure on some part of the abdominal wall at a distance from the suspected area and then suddenly withdrawing the palpating hand, thereby bringing about a sudden tensing of all the abdominal musculature. The resulting pressure exerted on the peritoneum as a whole will cause pain at the involved site, one of the earliest and most uniform indications of peritonitis or peritoneal irritation.

MUSCULAR RIGIDITY. Whenever the parietal peritoneum is irritated or inflamed, muscular rigidity is also present, most marked again over the site of origin of the peritonitis. This sign, however, is subject to confusing variation and often requires experience and skill in recognizing it, since, as the process progresses or in patients already debilitated, rigidity may be less marked or even absent. This feature must often be distinguished from rigidity arising from referred pain, as, for example, that seen in the upper abdomen in pneumonia or injury to the lower ribs with irritation of the intercostal nerves. Rigidity associated with referred pain is not as persistent and tends to disappear as continued firm pressure is exerted by the palpating hand. Careful examination will often reveal superficial hyperesthesia as well in such a case.

If the peritonitis is associated with perforation or rupture of a hollow viscus or when gas-forming organisms are responsible, free air may be demonstrable beneath the diaphragm in a film of the abdomen taken with the patient in an upright position. Absence of the normal liver dullness on percussion points to the same condition, but the sign is equivocal when marked distention of the bowel is also present.

NAUSEA and VOMITING are common and early signs of peritonitis even when not accompaniments of antecedent disease. Vomiting may arise as a reflex from the peritoneal irritation, and in such circumstances is forceful, the vomitus consisting of stomach contents. Later, as paralytic ileus ensues, small quantities may be vomited at frequent intervals as the intestinal content backs up into the stomach and is regurgitated without marked nausea or retching, large quantities of fluid and electrolytes being lost in this way.

FEVER. No particular temperature curve can be said to be characteristic of peritonitis. Sudden flooding of the peritoneal cavity yields a picture of shock or collapse with abnormal temperature, while accumulation of exudate often gives a gradual or "stair-step" rise. Chills and high fever are uncommon except in children. Low temperatures in the presence of widespread peritonitis are sometimes encountered in the aged or debilitated and are of grave prognosis.

PULSE. The pulse is almost always elevated in peritonitis, usually out of proportion to the temperature, and as toxemia increases and dehydration or diminished blood volume is produced, becomes still more rapid and of poor quality. An exception to this is seen in some cases associated with septicemia involving organisms of the colon-typhoid group, when little elevation of pulse rate may be seen or the patient may even show a bradycardia.

LEUKOCYTOSIS, often of 25,000 or more, with marked increase in polymorphonuclears, is the rule in generalized peritonitis, except in the aged or in the presence of overwhelming infection, when, as in the case of the temperature, a low level indicates a poor prognosis.

Diagnosis. The haggard, apprehensive, drawn expression known as *facies hippocratica* which was formerly considered characteristic of the disease has been largely eliminated by early diagnosis and the prompt institution of therapeutic measures. The former is made possible by understanding the basic features of conditions which may give rise to peritonitis and taking appropriate steps to detect its presence.

The *differential diagnosis* involves distinction from intrathoracic disease with involvement of the diaphragmatic or lower costal pleura which may give referred pain in the upper abdomen, retroperitoneal hemorrhage which also may cause distention and, less commonly, some rigidity. Mechanical intestinal obstruction has some features in common with peritonitis, notably distention, pain and vomiting, but the presence of audible borborygmi and absence of signs of inflammation aid in its distinction. Intraperitoneal hemorrhage as from a ruptured ectopic pregnancy may be confusing, though abdominal rigidity and tenderness are usually less marked and signs of acute anemia often supervene rapidly. Uremia, mesenteric lymphadenopathy and enterocolitis may be confusing, but each has characteristic and distinguishing features. Diabetes with acidosis and impending coma often causes abdominal pain, vomiting, tenderness, spasm and leukocytosis and must not only be distinguished from peritonitis, but also recognized as a complication when present as such.

Prognosis. A frequent, dreaded and highly fatal condition before the advent of modern antimicrobial therapy and before the derangements of fluid and electrolyte balance which accompany it were recognized, peritonitis, while still a serious condition, is far better understood and less likely to prove fatal than was formerly the case. The high mortality of certain surgical procedures such as combined abdominoperineal resection of the rectum for carcinoma, which was due largely to complicating peritonitis, has decreased almost to the vanishing point through appropriate postoperative control of intestinal flora by such agents as sulfasuxidine, streptomycin, Aureomycin and Terramycin, and the maintenance of therapeutic blood levels of the latter after operation. These same measures, together with adequate administration of whole blood, water and electrolytes, go far also to control peritoneal infection once it has occurred.

Treatment. If space permitted, it would be of interest to trace the evolution of the therapy of peritonitis, its transition from the most dreaded complication of intra-abdominal lesions or surgical procedures, save only septicemia, to its present status—a troublesome condition and one certainly to be avoided, but largely preventable in abdominal surgery and, when occurring, usually controllable if recognized in its early stages.

As suggested by this statement, whenever a condition such as diverticulitis, appendicitis or perforating ulcer is encountered, the prophylactic use of antibiotics, Aureomycin, Terramycin or penicillin and dihydrostreptomycin, will usually go far toward preventing the development of peritonitis. In turn, when major resections of the intestinal tract are contemplated, the administration of sulfasuxidine, with or without the addition of streptomycin, or the use of Aureomycin alone may so reduce the intestinal flora as to render gross infection of the peritoneum unlikely, provided careful surgical technique is maintained. The therapy of peritonitis, once it is established, involves at least two phases, the first directed at the contamination of the peritoneum itself and the other at correction of the derangements of the normal physiologic mechanisms which the peritonitis may have induced.

It has been known for many years that the peritoneum had enormous powers of resistance to infection and could overcome the grossest sort of contamination, provided the insults were not constantly repeated and the source of infection were eliminated. Thus, in peritonitis associated with perforated peptic ulcer, with ruptured diverticula of the large bowel, with perforated appendix, or arising whenever the irritative or actually infective content of any viscus is extravasated into the peritoneal cavity, definitive treatment must involve among other measures at least closure of the perforation or diversion of the contaminating material away from the peritoneal cavity. More and more the operative treatment of peritonitis is being restricted to the indications mentioned above. Drainage, except in cases of localized collections of purulent material or as a possible vent for the escape of material in the event of insecure or impossible closure of a contaminating source, has long since been abandoned.

Because peritonitis of intestinal origin is considered a mixed infection the virulence of which is due to the combined action of the various bacteria, the gram-positive species have been regarded as the pathogens. If possible, cultures of the infecting organisms should be tested for sensitivity to the various drugs to permit choice of the most effective ones, but even in the absence of this laboratory aid, there is today sufficient accumulated experience to justify embarking upon a therapeutic regimen with considerable assurance of a satisfactory outcome. Penicillin and dihydrostreptomycin were formerly considered highly satisfactory. At present, chlortetracycline (Aureomycin), by virtue of its potent and wide therapeutic spectrum, is superior. It has the additional advantage that it can be administered orally, usually 500 mg. every 4 hours until the temperature reaches normal and then the dosage is reduced to 250 mg. and continued for a week thereafter. If parenteral administration is desirable, it may be given intravenously in 5 per cent glucose in distilled water or in isotonic sodium chloride solution. Dosage is 500 mg. in 500 cc. of fluid given every 6 hours until the temperature reaches normal, and then it may be administered twice daily until the patient can take it orally.

When actual cultures of peritoneal exudate are available, the sensitivity of the organism present may be known and an appropriate antimicrobial agent selected. Without going into the details of the specific drug therapy, it is well to point out that oxytetracycline (Terramycin) is highly effective in the same diseases and by the same routes as Aureomycin. Likewise, streptomycin may be indicated and may be used in dosages of 1 gm. until the temperature reaches normal, and then 0.5 gm. twice daily for a week. Chloramphenicol, which has an equally wide therapeutic spectrum compared with Aureomycin and Terramycin, may be of great value when indicated. It may be administered orally beginning with 4 gm. as the initial dose followed by 1 gm. every 6 hours thereafter until the patient is afebrile. It is then reduced to 0.5 gram every 6 hours for one week. Penicillin and streptomycin, because they were used so extensively previously, are still preferred by some. The depot type penicillin can be given intramuscularly every 12 hours in dosages of 600,000 to 800,000 units. It should be continued for at least a week after the temperature becomes normal, reducing the dosage 50 per cent for a week thereafter.

The sulfonamides are being used less as more effectual antibiotics are developed. Sulfadiazine, sulfisoxazole and triple sulfonamides may be employed. Generally speaking, the beginning dose is 4 gm. followed by 1.5 gm. every 4 hours. Sodium sulfadiazine can be given intravenously in glucose and distilled water and is frequently employed in combination with other chemotherapeutic agents in desperate cases.

Attempts to sterilize the intestinal tract *prior to surgery* in order that postoperative infection be prevented have been highly successful. The effectiveness of these drugs depends upon their coming in contact with pathogens and remaining in contact with them for a sufficient period of time to prevent their growth. Mechanical factors, therefore, are significant in determining whether the pathogens and the drugs may be brought together under optimum circumstances. Thus, constipation and diarrhea may equally interfere with preoperative bowel preparation. Because of the multiplicity of the pathogens of the intestinal tract, those agents with the highest spectrum of effectiveness are desirable. The sulfonamides and later the antibiotics were used to reduce bacterial growth in the gastrointestinal tract. A combination of Aureomycin, streptomycin, penicillin and a sulfonamide has been widely used. It is likely, however, that Aureomycin alone in dosages of 750 mg. administered orally every 6 hours is the method of choice at present.

While active measures are being taken to overcome the infection, the secondary effects, such as ileus, accumulation of gas and fluid in the intestine, and loss of water, protein and electrolytes in the exudate, must be recognized and corrected. Ileus is best prevented or corrected by intubation of the stomach or bowel with the application of gentle suction, but care must be taken when this measure is used to keep accurate account of the quantity aspirated and to replace what is lost. Large amounts of chloride, sodium and postassium may be eliminated when continuous gastric suction is used, and these must be replaced, a difficult matter when oral administration is contraindicated. Chloride may be administered as sodium chloride if sodium retention has not occurred, in which case ammonium chloride in moderate and carefully controlled amounts may be given. Potassium is more difficult to administer parenterally, but may be given as modified Darrow's solution.

SPECIAL TYPES OF PERITONITIS

Streptococcal peritonitis due to beta hemolytic streptococcus may occur in so-called primary or secondary form. As indicated above, even when apparently primary, it is presumably always due to spread from some other focus by way of the blood stream from a portal of entry in the upper respiratory tract or in scarlet fever, measles, erysipelas or empyema. It may also occur as a complication of an operative procedure or a puerperal infection. The course is apt to be stormy, but the sensitivity of most of the strains of this organism to the modern antimicrobial agents has robbed this type of peritonitis of much of the gravity which used to attend it.

Pneumococcal Peritonitis. Another form of so-called primary peritonitis encountered most often in children and particularly in girls is due to the pneumococcus, and the portal of entry is frequently thought to be the pelvic organs. It may be seen more rarely as a complication of pneumonia. The onset is sudden, and the initial symptoms include vomiting, chills, high fever and diarrhea. The diagnosis is to be considered in peritonitis in female children without history of an antecedent intra-abdominal condition. Smears taken from the cervix of the uterus may be positive.

The prognosis was formerly extremely grave, some writers giving a hopeless outlook, but again, the modern antimicrobial agents are so effective that the condition yields to treatment in a high proportion of cases.

Gonococcal Peritonitis. This is a form complicating salpingitis and confined largely to the pelvis and lower abdomen, and may begin with fever, vomiting and intense pain a few days after the onset of a menstrual period, but the symptoms tend to subside fairly quickly and the signs become those of a localized pelvic infection. The diagnosis rests on the findings of positive cervical smears, and signs of inflammation on pelvic examination, together with a history of previous attacks and often of such symptoms as vaginal discharge or burning and frequency of urination as may be present with an active gonorrheal infection, and is to be distinguished from appendicitis. The extreme prostration and rapid pulse seen with other forms of acute generalized peritonitis are less commonly encountered. The treatment consists in the use of appropriate antibiotics and general supportive measures.

Tuberculous peritonitis is now a relatively rare manifestation of this disease and is most often seen in young women, in whom it may arise as part of a miliary dissemination or be secondary to involvement of some intra-abdominal organ. Characteristically, it may be encountered in a so-called "wet form," in which there is considerable fluid in the peritoneal cavity while the peritoneum itself is studded with countless small, grayish nodules beneath the real mesothelial layer. In another form the disease may be more localized with little fluid, the bowel being matted together with pockets of thick or even semi-inspissated pus between the folds of the mesentery.

Fever, malaise and signs of low grade intestinal obstruction may be present, and some loss of weight is the rule. In the "wet form," fluid is demonstrable on percussion or through the presence of a fluid wave. In the "plastic form" tenderness, a "doughy" abdomen and the presence of a mass are the characteristic findings.

The present treatment includes supportive measures and chemotherapy, and these usually produce marked benefit save when miliary dissemination is present or when the peritonitis appears as a terminal event. Complication of tuberculous peritonitis with a mixed flora from the intestinal tract through rupture of the bowel is an event of grave prognosis as a rule.

Localized peritonitis occurs about many foci of acute inflammation in the abdomen, as, for example, acute appendicitis, acute cholecystitis or perforating peptic ulcer, and may be thought of as an intermediary stage between infection limited to the involved organ and a generalized peritonitis. The course of the peritonitis follows that of the initial condition and usually subsides promptly after removal of the peritoneal source unless rupture or other gross contamination of the peritoneum has taken place, or the condition may become walled off as a localized intraperitoneal abscess.

Benign Paroxysmal Peritonitis. Reimann and others have recently (1945, 1948) reported a group of cases under the name of "benign paroxysmal peritonitis." Patients suffering from this condition appear very ill. During the attack, they have definite abdominal pain and tenderness with involuntary spasm of the abdominal muscles as well as rebound tenderness. Nausea, vomiting, malaise and leukocytosis may be present, and the temperature may range from 100 to 105° F. Attacks usually begin early in life and continue at irregular intervals for years. Most of the patients have been Jewish or Armenian. At operation a moderate amount of sterile, cloudy fluid is found, together with fibrinopurulent exudate, usually most marked

over the liver but found over other portions of the abdominal viscera. Lymph glands are not enlarged.

The cause of the disease is not known. The rapid onset and the rapid disappearance of symptoms with complete well being in the interval between attacks must be considered unusual for a bacteriologic process. Negative bacteriologic studies of the exudate, blood and bone marrow during the attack, coupled with its apparent unresponsiveness to chemotherapeutic agents, militate against its being of infectious etiology. Until more specific information concerning this entity is available, it may best be described as a paroxysmal peritonitis of unknown cause.

Pseudomyxoma peritonaei is a condition in which mucinous material, together with some cells, is scattered over the peritoneum from a focus in the appendix or ovary. In a typical case the source is a pseudomucinous ovarian cyst from which the content escapes and, being implanted over the peritoneum, continues to secrete. The mucus and cells causes a mild irritation with some exudation and the formation of adhesions, which in turn may cause symptoms of pain and low grade intestinal obstruction.

The differentiation from colloid carcinoma with peritoneal implants rests on the character of the cells present, which in true pseudomyxoma peritonaei do not have the characteristics of malignancy.

The treatment is extirpation of the original focus, after which the implants regress or disappear. The prognosis in such cases is usually good.

Whenever, following peritonitis, the temperature fails to subside to normal or, having subsided, then assumes a "stair-step" upward trend, **abscess** formation should be suspected. Rectal or pelvic examinations should be repeated daily, and the progress of the process followed. At first only local tenderness may be encountered, but as time goes on more and more induration develops and the tenderness increases, until finally the mass may be palpated abdominally as well either in the midline or in either lower quadrant as it extends upward toward the cecum or lateral to the sigmoid. Some spontaneous pain is usually present, and symptoms due to irritation of the rectum and bladder are frequent. In neglected cases involvement of the ureters with ascending infection and hydronephrosis can occur.

Pelvic abscess can be drained through the

vagina in the female, and in either sex drainage through a preexisting McBurney incision is the method of choice. Primary incision may be carried out through a muscle-splitting approach on either or both sides. Suprapubic drainage is to be avoided. Appropriate antimicrobial therapy should be continued or reinstituted when abscess formation is anticipated or known to exist, and carried on until cure is assured.

Subphrenic Abscess. Abscess formation in the subphrenic space, the anatomic boundaries of which are outlined at the beginning of this section, may occur through localization of a generalized peritonitis, by direct extension from the liver or kidney or possibly by lymphatic or hematogenous spread. Except for the rare instances associated with infected infarct of the spleen, perforation of a gastric ulcer into the lesser sac or extension from a left perinephric infection, all subphrenic abscesses are seen on the right. The majority are secondary to perforations of the stomach, duodenum or gallbladder and to appendicitis, and if to these sources is added liver abscess, the ultimate etiology of most subdiaphragmatic abscesses is accounted for.

The diagnosis of such abscesses is difficult so far as their location is concerned, though fever, leukocytosis, sweating and other signs of progressing sepsis should make one suspicious, particularly after one of the conditions mentioned above. Most of the old medical aphorisms have been discredited or at least modified over the years, but "pus somewhere, pus nowhere, pus under the diaphragm" remains useful today. The most important single finding, on fluoroscopic examination, is that of elevation and immobility of the right leaf of the diaphragm, sometimes with a small amount of fluid in the right costophrenic sulcus. The presence of gas-forming organisms in the abscess may permit the demonstration of a negative shadow beneath the diaphragm. Tenderness on pressure inward over the lower ribs or on heavy percussion is also significant.

Exploration is required for final diagnosis and drainage, and may be carried out anteriorly, posteriorly or transpleurally in stages according to the location of the abscess.

Other less common sites of secondary abscess formation include the lumbar gutters beside the spine, about the cecum, lateral to the sigmoid and between loops of bowel. In all, the general symptoms and signs of abscess formation are encountered, and those of obstruction of the bowel are not infrequent. A tender mass is usually palpable, though sometimes ill defined.

FRANK GLENN

MALIGNANT DISEASE OF THE PERITONEUM

Whereas primary tumors of the peritoneum are exceedingly rare, secondary carcinoma is often seen by the surgeon at the operating table. These secondary tumors are the result of transcoelomic dissemination from a primary tumor within the abdominal cavity. Those observed most commonly are tumors that are primary in the stomach, bowel or ovary.

The presence of secondary tumors in the peritoneum indicates an advanced process and more often than not it is associated with those debilitating changes that characterize advanced carcinoma. Secondary tumors of the peritoneum are to be found on both visceral and parietal surfaces and may or may not be more numerous in the vicinity of the primary tumor.

Ascites associated with secondary tumors explains in part the depletion of the protein stores in the body. Transudates and exudates may be present, depending on the trauma that these tumors are subjected to in the ordinary activity of the individual. With the exception of the clear cell tumors arising from the ovary, no treatment is effectual. X-ray therapy, chemotherapy and surgical drainage are seldom, if ever, employed successfully.

FRANK GLENN

ASCITES

The term ascites refers to the collection in the peritoneal cavity of fluid of low specific gravity, usually from 1.010 to 1.015, and containing few cellular elements. It may result from a variety of mechanisms which can best be considered as (1) general factors causing diffuse fluid retention in the body and (2) mechanical factors localizing fluid to the peritoneal cavity. In the former group hypoalbuminuria, renal retention of sodium, circulating antidiuretic substances and other hormonal products are contributing causes of generalized body retention of water. Portal hypertension, obstruction to hepatic lymphatic drainage and direct irritation of the peritoneum operate to localize the fluid to the peritoneal cavity. Clinically various combinations of these mechanisms are usually involved.

It is most often encountered in conditions associated with hypertension in the portal system due to cirrhosis of the liver, cardiac decompensation, right heart failure, or, more rarely, thrombosis of the portal or hepatic veins. Pressure on the vena cava above the entrance of the hepatic veins may also be responsible. The term is sometimes applied also to the fluid accumulation in the abdomen in cases of chronic or tuberculous peritonitis or malignant disease.

It is generally conceded that portal hypertension is an important factor in the production of ascites. However, chronic portal hypertension of major degree may exist in patients for many years without ascites formation. Conversely, ascites not infrequently is found in patients with normal portal pressure. These conditions can be demonstrated in the experimental animal by a variety of preparations. Therefore, it is apparent that portal hypertension usually acts in conjunction with other conditions to produce ascites.

Obstruction to hepatic lymphatics has been suggested as an important factor in ascites formation because of the marked increase in lymphatic drainage when the hepatic outflow tract is obstructed. The high protein content of hepatic lymph likewise corresponds to that of ascitic fluid under such conditions. This problem requires further clarification.

The symptoms of ascites itself are few save for the abdominal distention and feeling of weight and fullness of which the patients complaint. The abdomen is moderately or sometimes enormously distended, the skin appearing tense or shiny and often exhibiting lineae albicantes; the umbilicus sometimes is bulging, at other times stretched and flattened.

Dullness is present in the flanks as the bowel floats on the surrounding fluid, and a fluid wave can usually be demonstrated. The fluid itself is usually clear and light yellow save in instances in which the cisterna chyli or lower thoracic duct is invaded or ruptured, when the fluid may be milky or opalescent. Cells may be found in the centrifuged sedi-

ment, but care is needed in their identification, since elements desquamated from hypertrophic liver nodules may closely resemble those seen in certain neoplasms.

The treatment of ascites may be symptomatic, consisting of repeated paracenteses, or repeated injections of the mercurial diuretics, or may be directed toward elimination of the fundamental cause. When associated with neoplasms, the growth has almost always progressed beyond the point of cure. In ascites due to portal hypertension, one of the modern operative procedures aimed at diverting at least a portion of the portal stream into the vena cava may be indicated, such as splenorenal or portacaval shunt.

In many instances, when ascites is encountered with either hepatic or cardiac disease, hypoproteinemia is also present, and the correction of this defect by careful transfusion of blood, plasma or serum albumin as indicated may be an important feature of the therapy.

Localized irritation of the peritoneum by metastatic lesions or inflammation leads also to an accumulation of peritoneal fluid. The use of colloidal gold injected into the peritoneal cavity has been effective in control of such problems.

FRANK GLENN

References

Brick, I. B., and Cajigas, M.: Benign Paroxysmal Peritonitis: Surgical and Histologic Findings. New England J. Med., 244:786, 1951.

Brunschwig, A.: Regeneration of Peritoneum with Special Reference to Experimental and to Clinical Experience in Radical Resection of Intra Abdominal Cancer. J. Internat. Surg. Soc., 1953. In Press.

Daniel, O.: The Differential Diagnosis of Malignant Disease of the Peritoneum. Brit. J. Surg., 39:147, 1951–52.

Fine, J., Seligman, A., and Frank, H.: Peritoneal Dialysis for Acute Renal Failure. New York Med., 5:16, 1949.

Hughes, J. D.: Antibiotic and Chemotherapeutic Agents in Diseases of the Gastrointestinal Tract. J.A.M.A., 150:1456, 1952.

Maisel, B.: Personal communication, 1953.

Meleney, F. L.: Clinical Aspects and Treatment of Surgical Infections. Philadelphia, W. B. Saunders Co., 1949.

Payne, M. A.: Personal communication, 1953.

Pulaski, E. J., Seeley, S. F., and Matthews, C. S.: Streptomycin in Surgical Infections. Peritonitis. Surgery, 22:889, 1947.

Reimann, H. A.: Periodic Disease: Probable Syn-

drome Including Periodic Fever, Benign Paroxysmal Peritonitis, Cyclic Neutropenia and Intermittent Arthralgia. J.A.M.A., *136*:239, 1948.

Robbins, G., and Brunschwig, A.: Deperitonealiza-
tion: Clinical and Experimental Observations.
Ann. Surg., *130*:466, 1949.

Rutenberg, A. M., Jacob, S. W., Schweinburg, F. B.,

and Fine, J.: Aureomycin in the Treatment of Diffuse Peritonitis. New England J. Med., *246*:52,
1952.

Siegal, S.: Benign Paroxysmal Peritonitis. Gastroenterology, *12*:234, 1949.

Wegner, G.: Chirurgische Bemerkungen uber die
Peritonealhohle. Arch. f. klin. Chir., *20*:51, 1876.

Diseases of the Respiratory System

DISEASES OF THE NOSE

Under normal conditions air is warmed, moistened and cleansed during its passage through the nose. The mucous membrane of the nose is continuous with that lining the accessory nasal sinuses and is everywhere rich in mucous glands. If the nasal passages are obstructed by deflection of the septum, by hypertrophy of the mucous membrane of the turbinates, or by enlarged adenoids, the mucous glands may be stimulated to increased activity and chronically produce a catarrhal discharge. This catarrhal process may, by spreading to the mucous membrane of the eustachian tube, lead to changes in the middle ear that result in impairment of hearing. Obstruction of the nose favors pyogenic infection of the accessory nasal sinuses with such resulting symptoms as headache, chronic discharge of purulent material, much of which is swallowed, and the general disorders associated with focal infection.

Epistaxis is usually due to superficial ulceration of the anterior part of the septum. Hypertension, however, may cause rupture of the vessels in the posterior part of the nose and profuse hemorrhage. Hereditary multiple telangiectasis permits repeated hemorrhage that may lead to profound anemia. The telangiectatic areas in the nose and nasopharynx bleed more easily than those on the mucous membranes of the mouth or tongue. A blood-stained nasal discharge in a child always suggests enlargement and infection of the adenoids, nasal diphtheria, the presence of foreign body, or congenital syphilis; in adults it is frequently evidence of a new growth, blood dyscrasia, uremia or hypoprothrombinemia.

Adenoids and the tonsils constitute the most important parts of the ring of lymphoid tissue which encircles the pharynx and also includes the lingual tonsils, the lateral pharyngeal bands, the tissue in the fossae of Rosenmüller and scattered nodules beneath the mucous membranes of the posterior pharyngeal wall. The function of this tissue is presumably protective. Local as well as systemic disturbances may result from excessive enlargement or chronic infection of these structures. Hypertrophy of the adenoid tissue is the most common cause of chronic nasal obstruction in childhood. Structural changes and regional infections commonly follow, as well as constitutional disturbances such as listlessness and decreased appetite. Enlarged and infected adenoids are the most frequent cause of recurring otitis media and sinusitis in childhood, and insidious conduction deafness is a common complication. The frequency of recurrence of lymphoid tissue in the nasopharynx after adenoidectomy must be stressed, as well as its continued danger to the middle ear. The local use of small, carefully controlled doses of radium around the tubal orifices has proved to be the treatment of choice in these problems.

CLYDE A. HEATLY

INFECTIONS OF THE ACCESSORY NASAL SINUSES

Etiology. The most common cause of infection of the accessory nasal sinuses is *acute rhinitis. Abscesses* at the roots of the upper bicuspid and molar teeth may rupture into the maxillary sinus and produce infection which may give rise to no symptoms other than a chronic unilateral nasal discharge. Sinusitis may result from swimming or diving. Trauma, allergy and dietary deficiencies are important predisposing factors. Acute sinusitis may be induced by sudden changes in barometric pressure occurring during travel by air (aerosinusitis).

Symptoms. The nasal communications of the accessory nasal sinuses are narrow and easily obstructed by the edema and discharge of thick mucus that accompany acute inflammation. This obstruction gives rise to headache, which is the most characteristic symptom of acute sinusitis. The mucous membrane of the nasal passages and accessory nasal sinuses is innervated by the trigeminus nerve, and the pain of sinus infection is most commonly referred to the area of distribution of this nerve. Infection of the sphenoidal sinuses, however, may give rise to suboccipital discomfort.

The headache of acute sinusitis may be constant but it is characteristically more severe in the forenoon and disappears toward evening. It is commonly accompanied by tenderness on pressure over the affected sinus. Pain in the upper molar teeth is a frequent complaint in acute maxillary sinusitis and may be erroneously attributed to dental causes. In chronic sinus infections headache and pain are surprisingly infrequent except during acute exacerbations, and many so-called sinus headaches are actually on some other basis.

Diagnosis. Severe acute coryza or more general infection, such as influenza or pneumonia, is usually responsible for infection of an accessory nasal sinus. From 15 to 20 per cent of all infections of the maxillary sinus are of dental origin. X-ray shadows alone cannot differentiate between a sinus infection that is active and one that is clinically cured. The history, the presence of a discharge in the nose, the roentgenogram and, when possible, irrigation of the suspected sinus may all be necessary to establish diagnosis. The possible presence of an underlying allergy must always be considered. Chronic nasal allergy is commonly complicated by chronic bacterial infection caused by the profound changes produced in the nasal mucosa in the form of decreased ciliary activity, chronic edema and the formation of multiple polyps, all of which interfere with proper sinus ventilation and drainage. Repeated studies of the cytology of the nasal and sinus secretions are of great diagnostic value.

Treatment. The fundamental aim in the treatment of all forms of sinusitis is the establishment of free and adequate drainage. In acute sinusitis this may be accomplished in many instances by the local use of vasoconstricting solutions and external heat. Special measures such as the Proetz displacement treatment or irrigation of individual sinuses may be necessary. It is important to emphasize that the prolonged use of vasoconstricting solutions results in local irritation as well as vasomotor paralysis. Chronic infections usually require special surgical treatment which favors better drainage.

The widespread use of the sulfonamide drugs and the antibiotics has achieved great progress in the treatment of sinusitis and its complications. The organisms responsible for acute sinusitis are usually sensitive to these drugs, the use of which in conjunction with appropriate local measures to insure proper drainage has served to shorten the course and lessen the severity of these infections. The results in chronic sinusitis, however, have proved in the main disappointing, and their chief value in such cases has become recognized as an indispensable adjunct to surgical measures. The effects of the local application of these agents in the nose and sinuses are distinctly limited.

Infections of the Accessory Nasal Sinuses in Children. With the exception of the frontal sinuses, the accessory nasal sinuses are well developed at an early age. Sinusitis not infrequently complicates the exanthemas. Children who are subject to recurring respiratory infections often have foci in one or more nasal sinuses. Local treatment consisting of astringent and antiseptic nasal drops as well as gentle suction or irrigation will clear up many of the milder infections. The removal of infected tonsils and adenoids is regularly indicated. More rarely, improved drainage by conservative surgery will be necessary. It is of the utmost importance that any associated dietary deficiency or allergy be discovered and properly treated.

Complications of Sinus Infection. Extension of the nasal infection to neighboring structures such as the eyes, ears, throat or tracheobronchial tree is commonly observed. Alarming and often fatal intracranial invasion may also occur in the form of *meningitis, cavernous sinus thrombosis, epidural* or *frontal lobe abscess.* The prompt and intensive use of the sulfonamides as well as penicillin has greatly improved the prognosis in these serious complications, and numerous reports of cures have accumulated.

Osteomyelitis, a most important complication, may be precipitated by trauma or sinus surgery. The fulminating variety is frequently followed by involvement of the meninges or brain by way of a widespread thrombophlebitis. Edema of the soft tissues with characteristic doughy swelling is the outstanding clinical manifestation. Since the infecting organism is usually a staphylococcus or an anaerobic streptococcus, penicillin has proved especially effective and, given properly in the early stages of the disease, may greatly limit the area of bone necrosis. In advanced cases, however, radical surgery is necessary.

An *orbital cellulitis* or *abscess* may complicate an infection of the frontal or ethmoid sinuses, especially in childhood. Edema usually improves with conservative treatment, but external drainage is indicated by the presence of exophthalmos with limitation of motion. Needless infection of the orbital contents by premature incision must be carefully guarded against. Granulomatous lesions and arteritis may involve the sinuses as a part of Wegener's syndrome.

Retrobulbar neuritis in the past was frequently attributed to a posterior sinusitis because of rapid improvement following sinus surgery. Accumulated evidence, however, has raised grave doubts concerning the frequency of this causal relationship. Multiple sclerosis is the accepted cause of the majority of these disturbances, and hasty surgical intervention is to be avoided.

The frequent association of sinusitis with chronic diseases of the tracheobronchial tree —especially bronchiectasis as well as certain cases of asthma—has become well established. Proper treatment of the nasal infection is imperative in these cases.

CLYDE A. HEATLY

TUMORS OF THE NOSE AND NASO-PHARYNX

A wide variety of benign as well as malignant tumors arise in the nose, sinuses and nasopharynx. The maxillary sinus may be involved by cysts and tumors of dental origin. Osteomas are occasionally seen in roentgenograms of the frontal sinuses. Malignant tumors include most varieties of carcinoma and sarcoma. Benign tumors produce symptoms of obstruction. Malignant tumors are also characterized by pain, recurring epistaxis and, in their advanced stages, by progressive deformity of the nose, palate, cheek or orbit.

The finding of an easily bleeding polyp or mass in any of these areas requires a prompt biopsy taken deeply enough to secure representative tissue. The roentgenogram may assist by demonstrating bone destruction.

Enlargement of the cervical glands may be the first sign of a nasopharyngeal growth, although obstruction to breathing, a blood-stained nasal discharge, or ringing in the ear may be the initial symptom. Of 79 patients reported from the Mayo Clinic, only 38 had nasal symptoms. Invasion of the pterygoid fossa with fixation of the jaw, pain or anesthesia in the area of distribution of the second or third division of the trigeminus, invasion of the orbit with paralysis of certain of the extraocular muscles, and severe and constant headache from meningeal irritation are all common manifestations of malignant growth in the nasopharynx.

Pyogenic infection of the accessory nasal sinuses is usually associated with all new growths arising in the nose. Similarly, infection of the ear commonly accompanies new growths arising in the nasopharynx.

Treatment. Because of the anatomic relations, complete surgical removal of a malignant growth is seldom possible, and irradiation is the most desirable therapeutic measure.

CLYDE A. HEATLY

References

Boies, L. R.: Fundamentals of Otolaryngology. 2nd ed. Philadelphia, W. B. Saunders Company, 1954.

Morrison, W. W.: Diseases of the Ear, Nose and Throat. New York, Appleton-Century-Crofts, Inc., 1948.

Van Alyea, O. E.: Nasal Sinuses, An Anatomic and Clinical Consideration. Baltimore, Williams and Wilkins Company, 1946.

Ward, G. E., and Hendrick, J. W.: Diagnosis and Treatment of Tumors of the Head and Neck. Baltimore, Williams and Wilkins Company, 1950.

DISEASES OF THE LARYNX

INTRODUCTION

Stridor as a symptom may afford valuable clinical evidence as to the location of the lesion. *Inspiratory stridor* is particularly common in children and suggests laryngeal diphtheria, a foreign body, papilloma of the larynx, spasm, or incoordination of the muscles of the glottis—as in laryngismus stridulus. Almost any laryngeal irritation in a child may cause a glottic spasm, the most frequent manifestation being the crowing inspiratory stridor of catarrhal laryngitis (croup). *Expiratory stridor* suggests an obstructive lesion in the trachea or bronchial tree. This may be due to an inflammatory condition, as tracheal diphtheria, to asthma or pneumonia, or to pressure from mediastinal tumors. Aneurysm is a common cause of expiratory stridor in adults, while pressure due to tuberculous glands is frequently provocative of this symptom in children. It is important to emphasize that no patient with a marked stridor should be submitted to general anesthesia. A patient with stridor is forced to use all his accessory respiratory muscles, and a general anesthetic is liable to make the respirations cease abruptly.

Early and frequent examinations of the larynx are important in the three following conditions: (1) Pulmonary tuberculosis predisposes to catarrhal changes in the larynx; tuberculous laryngitis is an important complication and, if recognized in its early stage, may be cured by well directed measures. (2) The recurrent laryngeal nerves are in close approximation to the posterior capsule of the thyroid gland and may be injured by pressure exerted by an enlarged thyroid as well as by operative procedures on this gland. For this reason every patient with goiter should have a laryngeal examination both *before* and *after* operation. The prognosis of an operative lesion of the recurrent laryngeal nerve is favorable, provided the onset of the hoarseness is gradual and not immediate. (3) Hoarseness, when persisting in a patient over 40 for more than three weeks, is often due to cancer. If the condition is recognized early, the prognosis after operative removal and irradiation is good. If, however, examination is post-

poned until the appearance of evident clinical symptoms of malignancy, the chances of a permanent cure are greatly lessened.

CLYDE A. HEATLY

COMMON LARYNGEAL DISORDERS IN CHILDREN

ACUTE LARYNGITIS

The larynx in infancy and childhood is characterized by its relative smallness, its unusual irritability, and its tendency to dangerous edema as the result of acute infections or instrumentation. Direct laryngoscopy is essential to accurate diagnosis and is a most important advance over the inferential methods of former years. The clinical manifestations of nondiphtheritic and diphtheritic infections are so strikingly similar that a final diagnosis frequently depends on the results of this direct examination as well as on the cultures thereby made possible from the larynx itself. The spasmodic form of acute laryngitis (*croup*) differs from the more common acute catarrhal inflammations in its characteristic nocturnal episodes of harsh, metallic cough and often alarming inspiratory stridor and dyspnea, which are relieved by steam inhalations and emetics and leave few residual symptoms the following day. Acute infections of the larynx are so frequently complicated by varying degrees of obstruction that special consideration should be given to this difficult problem. The picture of *obstructive laryngeal dyspnea* should be completely familiar to every physician, for while the increase of dyspnea may be gradual, the transition to terminal asphyxia and collapse in childhood may be alarmingly sudden. The child is restless and anxious. Respirations are rapid, labored and accompanied by a harsh inspiratory stridor. Pallor is more common than cyanosis. The progress of the obstruction can best be followed by observing the degree of retraction about the thoracic cage, for, with progressing dyspnea, increasing retraction is noted in the suprasternal notch, the supraclavicular fossae, the intercostal spaces and the epigastrium. Cyanosis and apathy usually denote terminal exhaustion. Atropine, which thickens secretions, and opiates, which depress the respiratory center, must never be administered to these dyspneic patients.

Tracheotomy, through the second or third tracheal rings, should be carried out under local anesthesia in the presence of progressive and well established evidence of laryngeal obstruction. This procedure not only insures a proper airway and puts the inflamed larynx at rest, but also permits suction drainage of the profuse tracheal secretions which frequently complicate many of these cases and thereby constitute a continued source of danger from low obstruction (acute laryngotracheobronchitis).

CONGENITAL LARYNGEAL STRIDOR

This is characterized by the onset of stridor shortly after birth. The stridor is chiefly inspiratory, is aggravated by crying and tends to diminish or disappear during nursing or sleep. The voice sounds are unchanged, and cyanosis is seldom observed. This disturbance is caused by the vibrations of an elongated epiglottis as well as by the flabby structures of the upper rim of the larynx, and gradually disappears with the normal growth of the larynx, usually during the second year of life.

LARYNGISMUS STRIDULUS

(Laryngospasm)

Laryngismus stridulus in children may be defined as a laryngeal stridor of sudden onset, without fever. It is rare during the first three months of life, and most common in children from six months to two years of age. Boys are more frequently affected than girls. It is uncommon in breast-fed infants and is nearly always associated with rickets. The laryngeal spasm is a manifestation of the extreme irritability of the nervous system in tetany.

Symptoms. An attack is characterized by the sudden onset of inspiratory dyspnea without premonitory symptoms. Obstruction may be so marked as to cause temporary complete apnea with deepening cyanosis; unconsciousness, convulsions or death may follow in severe cases. Usually, however, after 15 or 20 seconds a characteristic deep inspiration shows that the glottic spasm has relaxed. There may be numerous subsequent attacks. The child may be normal between attacks or may show other evidences of tetany.

Diagnosis. The age of the patient, the absence of fever, the periods of apnea followed by a characteristic crowing inspiration, and the associated clinical signs of tetany (carpopedal spasm, Chvostek's and Trousseau's signs, and so forth) are pathognomonic. Since a foreign body lodged in the larynx may, however, produce almost identical symptoms, the larynx should be directly examined through a laryngoscope.

Treatment. During the attack artificial respiration and cold applications to the face and chest are most effective. Intubation and tracheotomy are rarely necessary. Later the fundamental metabolic disturbances must be treated.

FOREIGN BODIES IN THE LARYNX

The sudden onset of paroxysms of coughing and dyspnea in a healthy child suggests the presence of a foreign body in the larynx, trachea or bronchi. Immediate tracheotomy may be necessary. Metallic bodies such as coins may be localized with the fluoroscope. Since less opaque bodies, such as fish bones, may not be demonstrable by the x-ray, direct examination of the larynx and trachea is necessary. All examinations should be conducted without anesthesia.

PAPILLOMA OF THE LARYNX

Papilloma of the larynx in children, although benign, has a mortality almost equal to that of carcinoma of the larynx in adults. Fortunately, it is relatively rare. It may appear at any age and is much more common in boys.

The exact **etiology** is uncertain, although experimental studies suggest that an invisible, filterable virus is the direct cause. Both in structure and behavior the lesion resembles that of verruca vulgaris of the skin. Even very slight trauma may cause implantation of new growths on the surrounding mucous membrane.

Symptoms. The symptoms depend on the size and location of the tumor. Slowly developing but progressive hoarseness, a paroxysmal cough, and, at a later period, dyspnea, should excite suspicion of laryngeal growth.

Diagnosis. Direct inspection (without anesthesia) is necessary for positive diagnosis.

Treatment. Surgical removal by direct laryngoscopy is the treatment of choice, though recurrences may be expected over a considerable period. Tracheotomy may be necessary. Irradiation is to be used with caution because of its danger to the laryngeal cartilages. Recently the local application of estrogenic substances has been advocated.

CLYDE A. HEATLY

COMMON LARYNGEAL DISORDERS OF ADULTS

CATARRHAL LARYNGITIS

Acute catarrhal laryngitis is usually secondary to infection of the upper respiratory tract, but may be brought on also by irritation from improper use of the voice, as well as by excessive use of alcohol or tobacco, or by chemical fumes. The lesions in the larynx vary from slight subglottic hyperemia and edema to diffuse reddening of all the mucous membranes of the glottis, and shallow ulceration. Hoarseness is the most constant symptom, but in the more acute condition there may be aphonia and a dry burning sensation in the throat. Catarrhal laryngitis is differentiated from tuberculous laryngitis by the absence of pulmonary symptoms; *true tuberculous laryngitis is always secondary to a pulmonary lesion*. The **treatment** of simple catarrhal laryngitis consists in abstinence from speaking, with cold applications, benzoin inhalations, regulation of the surroundings so that the air is moist and of even temperature, and rest.

Chronic catarrhal laryngitis is due to long-continued irritation from any of the causes of the acute condition. The pathologic change which is usually most prominent in the posterior half of the larynx consists in thickening of the epithelium. This condition was originally described by Virchow as *pachydermia* and is not to be confused with carcinoma. The other lesions involve the vocal cords and the intrinsic muscles. In the larynx, as in the nose and nasopharynx, chronic irritation causes excessive secretion of thick glairy mucus which produces many of the symptoms of chronic laryngitis. The cause of such chronic discharge from the upper air passages, especially in pyorrhea, chronic tonsillitis, or sinusitis, demands proper treatment. Any excessive growth of epithelium between the posterior ends of the cords should be removed.

Tuberculous laryngitis is discussed in the chapter on Tuberculosis (p. 306).

Syphilitic laryngitis is discussed in the chapter on Syphilis (p. 351).

BENIGN AND MALIGNANT TUMORS OF THE LARYNX

BENIGN TUMORS

The most common of the benign tumors in the larynx are the polyp and the papilloma. The papilloma of the larynx in adults differs from that in children in that it is usually solitary and shows far less tendency to recur after removal; furthermore, it is frequently of tuberculous or syphilitic origin. The symptoms of a laryngeal growth depend upon its location. The long, pedunculated polyps that grow on the vocal cords cause attacks of paroxysmal coughing and hoarseness due to interference with accurate approximation of the vocal cords. Benign growths seldom cause bleeding, pain or dysphagia. They are best treated by local excision through the mouth, although larger tumors may require removal by an external approach.

MALIGNANT TUMORS

Cancer of the larynx is predominantly a disease affecting men over the age of 40. Epidermoid or squamous carcinoma is the most frequent morphologic variety. It may be divided anatomically into *intrinsic* and *extrinsic* forms. The majority of intrinsic growths originate on a vocal cord and cause increasing, persistent hoarseness as an early and significant symptom. The extrinsic tumors develop around the upper rim of the larynx, arising most frequently from the epiglottis and its appendages. Their early symptoms consist of ill defined soreness or mild dysphagia and are commonly mistaken for other causes. The appearance of an enlarged metastatic node in the upper cervical chain may be the earliest sign of these extrinsic neoplasms. Hoarseness, if present, occurs only in the late stages when extension to the glottis has developed. Intrinsic carcinomas are for the most part slow growing, well differentiated tumors which spread late because of the sparsity of the lymphatics of the vocal cords. Extrinsic cancers on the contrary are anaplastic, rapidly growing, ulcerating tumors which extend relatively early to the cervical lymph nodes.

Diagnosis. It is of the utmost importance to recognize carcinoma of the larynx early because only then can a cure be effected without radical, mutilating surgery. The physician must be urged to regard persisting hoarseness in an adult as strongly suspicious of cancer and to arrange for prompt examination of the larynx by an experienced observer. Vague discomfort or lump sensation in the region of the hypopharynx requires similar study. While the clinical diagnosis of malignancy can frequently be made by simple mirror examination, microscopic confirmation by biopsy is essential. A negative report should not be accepted as final in clinically suspicious cases and repeated biopsies may occasionally be necessary to establish the diagnosis. Tuberculous ulcers, gumma and leukokeratotic areas may closely simulate laryngeal cancer.

Treatment. Early removal of an *intrinsic carcinoma* and the affected cord results in a high percentage of cures. In more advanced cases total laryngectomy is necessary. *Extrinsic growths* are best managed by the improved methods of irradiation.

LARYNGEAL NEUROPATHIES

The muscles* that move the vocal cord are innervated by the recurrent laryngeal nerve, a branch of the vagus. This is frequently involved in pathologic processes, and hoarseness results. The common cause of a *recurrent nerve palsy* is an aneurysm of the arch of the aorta. Other causes are a mediastinal growth, tuberculosis of the apex of the right lung implicating the pleura, dilatation of the left auricle, as in mitral stenosis, carcinoma of the esophagus and thyroid, and metastasis and inflammation of the glands in the neck that involve the vagus. Postdiphtheritic and syphilitic neuritis may also cause

* The cricothyroid, a tensor muscle, is supplied by the superior laryngeal nerve.

laryngeal palsies. There are, too, so-called *"functional laryngeal palsies,"* which may be distinguished from the organic type by the sudden onset of complete aphonia without loss of ability to cough and laugh, and by the movements of the vocal cords revealed by the laryngeal mirror.

The recurrent nerve lies close to the posterior capsule of the thyroid gland, and the onset of hoarseness following thyroidectomy indicates that it has been injured. If the nerve is divided, hoarseness ensues immediately and may never entirely disappear. If the hoarseness comes on gradually, however, it may be due to stretching or edema of the nerve, and the voice will ultimately return to normal. If, during operation, both nerves are injured, but not divided, inspiratory stridor develops suddenly because of inability of the cords to open during inspiration. Temporary tracheotomy may be necessary.

The **prognosis** for complete restoration of function following postdiphtheritic paralysis is good. The laryngeal crises of tabes are really glottic spasms depending on syphilitic neuritis of the recurrent nerves. For this condition, also, tracheotomy may become necessary, since antiluetic therapy is not always effective.

CLYDE A. HEATLY

References

Jackson, C., and Jackson, C. L.: Diseases of the Nose, Throat and Ear, Including Bronchoscopy and Esophagoscopy. Philadelphia, W. B. Saunders Company, 1945.

Lederer, F. L.: Diseases of the Ear, Nose and Throat. Philadelphia, F. A. Davis Company, 1952.

DISEASES OF THE BRONCHI

BRONCHITIS

ACUTE BRONCHITIS

Definition. Acute bronchitis is an acute inflammation of the tracheobronchial tree, caused by infectious, physical or chemical agents, usually self-limited and resulting in complete healing and return to normal structure and function.

Etiology. In the common infectious form of the disease, acute bronchitis involves chiefly the larger and medium bronchi, up to the third or fourth division, and is part of a general acute upper respiratory infection. The onset is often the *common cold,* a virus disease, with malaise and coryza as the initial manifestations. Or one of the *influenza viruses* may start the infection, producing higher fever and more severe prostration at onset. Not infrequently the disease begins directly with a pyogenic infection of the nasopharynx, throat or bronchi, or one or more of the common pyogenic organisms may later dominate the picture: the *Streptococcus, Pneumococcus, Micrococcus catarrhalis, Hemophilus influenzae* or *Staphylococcus.* Upper respiratory infections of these types are highly contagious.

Acute bronchitis involving the larger and medium bronchi is usually a mild disease, but there is always the danger of extension of the infection into the lung parenchyma, causing pneumonia. This is more likely to occur in infants, in debilitated or elderly patients, or those with preexisting pulmonary disease or chronic cardiac disease. Contributory factors are exposure, chilling, fatigue, malnutrition, rickets. Like other respiratory infections, it is much more common during the winter months.

Frequently recurring attacks of acute bronchitis in an otherwise healthy person may be secondary to chronic sinusitis, or to hypertrophied tonsils and adenoids in children.

Bronchitis is an important factor in many of the specific infectious diseases. Whooping cough is itself an acute inflammatory disease of the tracheobronchial tree, due to *Hemophilus pertussis.* Bronchitis is a constant feature of the invasive stage of measles. It is a frequent early symptom in typhoid fever, is seen in typhus and occasionally in severe attacks of malaria. In diphtheria the diphtheritic membrane may extend down from the larynx into the trachea and bronchi. Primary atypical or virus pneumonia begins in some instances as a diffuse bronchiolitis; autopsied cases usually show a severe bronchitis and bronchiolitis. Acute stenosing laryngotracheobronchitis, a rapidly developing inflammatory process leading to laryngeal obstruction, should be mentioned, since the bronchi are also involved.

Spasmodic croup in children is a laryngeal condition, the trachea and bronchi being essentially unaffected.

Among the *mycotic* and *parasitic diseases,* an acute upper respiratory inflammation with bronchitis is a frequent type of onset in coccidioidomycosis of the lung. *Monilia* and other fungous infections can involve the bronchi. Trichinosis may be associated with bronchitis and bronchopneumonia if the trichinae invade the lungs.

Allergic factors are often significant in bronchial affections. Some persons are peculiarly susceptible to attacks of bronchitis, as if they were sensitized to bacterial protein. In bronchial asthma the patient is often so affected, and the acute bronchial and bronchiolar inflammation often aggravates the asthmatic state or precipitates an attack.

Physical and *chemical irritants* cause bronchial irritation and inflammation following inhalation. The irritant dusts, such as those of silica, or other mineral, metallic or vegetable dusts, often cause local irritation, with mucus formation and cough. This phenomenon is distinct from the chronic lymphatic and pulmonary changes of pneumonoconiosis. Tobacco smoke is a mild bronchial irritant for some persons. A patient who has suffered a severe burn will often have a complicating bronchitis of varying severity, due to inhalation of hot or toxic gases. Of the war gases, the direct irritants, such as mustard and chlorine, cause tracheitis and bronchitis, as contrasted with the slower-acting phosgene, which produces a delayed pulmonary edema. Among the many toxic and irritating inhalants encountered in industry may be mentioned the fumes of strong acids, ammonia, some of the volatile organic solvents, chlorine, hydrogen sulfide, sulfur dioxide, bromine and certain alkaloid dusts such as ipecac. A frequent form of reaction to these agents is initial cough, progressing to an acute obstructive asthmatic state, and eventually to frank pulmonary edema unless relieved.

"Smog," the chemical-laden atmosphere produced by factories, refineries and the like, can cause severe respiratory symptoms: cough, choking, asthmatic attacks, predisposing to bronchitis and bronchopneumonia, especially in elderly persons with chronic pulmonary diseases.

Morbid Anatomy. In the usual case of acute infectious bronchitis there is diffuse bilateral involvement, though it may be more marked on one side. The earliest change, in the larger and medium bronchi, is hyperemia of the mucous membrane. This is followed by desquamation of many of the superficial ciliated cells, edema and leukocytic infiltration of the submucosa, and swelling of the mucous glands. The bronchial lumen contains sticky mucoid or mucopurulent exudate, in which cellular debris and bacteria may be found. In the more severe cases, especially those associated with influenza, there may be extension of the inflammation into adjacent peribronchial tissues.

The bronchial damage produced by the war gases may be of any degree of severity, from a mild inflammation to the most violent and fulminating inflammatory edema and necrosis.

Pathologic Physiology and Chemistry. The normal tracheobronchial tree has a remarkable power of "self-cleansing," eliminating the innumerable bacteria and other small particulate matter that must come in with inhaled air. This is carried out in part by the pulmonary lymphatics, in part by phagocytic cells, and in part by the ciliated bronchial epithelium, which sweeps the normal mucus upward to the throat. There is also normally a bronchial and bronchiolar peristalsis, occurring in waves lasting 20 to 25 seconds. This helps to move particles headward. By reason of these functions, all the normal pulmonary tissues below the larynx are practically bacteria-free. Once this self-cleansing is interfered with, however, as in acute tracheobronchitis, the bronchi are readily invaded by bacteria.

Cough, the chief symptom of bronchitis, may be distressing, but it serves also an important physiologic function in eliminating

purulent secretions. Conversely, when there are regions in the lungs that are congested or poorly drained, as in bronchiectasis, pulmonary fibrosis and emphysema, or congestive heart failure, the likelihood of a persisting infection or of the development of bronchopneumonia is much increased.

In asthmatic subjects, bronchitis presents a special hazard. The intrabronchial exudate and submucosal swelling often occlude further the already narrowed air passages and precipitate asthmatic attacks.

There is little alteration in body chemistry in acute bronchitis. Pulmonary function, gas exchange, the oxygen and carbon dioxide values of the blood, remain normal unless there is an associated chronic pulmonary or cardiac disease or unless the bronchial airways become obstructed.

Symptoms. The symptoms of onset in acute infectious bronchitis are usually those of the acute upper respiratory infection, of which the bronchitis is a part: chilliness, malaise, pains in the back and muscles, headache, coryza, a dry scratchy throat, hoarseness or huskiness of the voice. There may be a mild or moderate fever, up to 101° or 102° F., with a corresponding rise in pulse rate and respiration. There may or may not be a moderate leukocytosis, up to 12,000 or 13,000 cells per cubic millimeter. Roentgenograms of the lung are negative.

The onset of cough commonly indicates the beginning of the acute bronchitis. This may be on the first day or may be delayed for several days. The cough is at first dry, irritative and nonproductive, and is associated with a substernal soreness or tightness. After a day or two there is some scanty viscid sputum, which later becomes looser, more abundant, and mucoid or mucopurulent in character. The fever and malaise subside in four or five days or sooner, though the cough and sputum may continue for two or three weeks.

The *capillary bronchitis* of infants is actually a form of bronchopneumonia, usually severe, sometimes fatal. The onset is usually acute, with fever, incessant cough, prostration and cyanosis. The diffuse bronchiolar obstruction produces a severe labored dyspnea, with marked retraction of the soft parts of the chest during inspiration.

Physical Signs. In the early stages of acute infectious bronchitis there may be no abnormal physical signs in the lungs. Frequently, however, scattered squeaking or sonorous rales can be heard, transitory in character. The disease may subside with no further development of physical signs. If the smaller bronchi are involved, however, either crackling or moist rales can often be heard at both lung bases posteriorly, and there may be some harshness of the breath sounds.

Diagnosis. The main problem in diagnosis is to rule out other more serious or more insidious conditions. Chief among these are pulmonary tuberculosis, acute pneumonia, left heart failure, acute pericarditis, acute or chronic sinusitis, bronchiectasis, bronchial asthma, foreign body in the lung, carcinoma of the lung; and, in children, measles, whooping cough, acute tonsillitis and acute otitis media. The other diseases mentioned under Etiology, in which bronchitis occurs, should also be kept in mind.

The development of pneumonia is the most common complication, and is to be suspected when there is higher fever, pulse and respiration, increased leukocytosis, and physical and roentgenographic signs.

If cough and symptoms persist, tuberculosis or other chronic pulmonary disease should be searched for. It should be noted that an apparently mild acute bronchitis may result in opening up an old caseous tubercular lesion, and so reactivate this disease.

Treatment. At the onset of an upper respiratory infection, with malaise and fever, the patient should be put to bed and should stay there until the fever has subsided. This is the most important feature of the treatment. It shortens the course of the disease, and usually prevents complications or sequelae. A single dose of procaine penicillin, 300,000 units, combined with 100,000 units of crystalline penicillin for quick initial effect, will often terminate the fever and prevent further bacterial invasion. Fluids should be forced to 3000 or 4000 cc. daily, with a simple bland diet. Aspirin, 0.3 or 0.6 gm., or aspirin, 0.3 gm., with acetphenetidin, 0.3 gm., given every 4 to 8 hours, relieves malaise and keeps the fever at a lower level. Codeine may be added if there is pain or severe malaise.

If there is a continued soreness in the anterior chest, a mustard plaster or flaxseed poultice will give relief. When the cough develops, steam inhalations with tincture of benzoin, oil of pine or other volatile counter-irritant are helpful. For a constant irritative cough, a steam kettle should be kept in the room continuously to humidify the air.

A cough mixture with codeine, or codeine itself, in doses of 0.015 to 0.06 gm., is often needed to control coughing spasms. A good mixture is elixir of terpin hydrate with codeine, 0.015 gm. per teaspoonful; or codeine, 0.015 gm., dilute phosphoric acid, 0.2 gm., syrup of wild cherry, to 4 cc. In the later stages an expectorant, such as terpin hydrate or ammonium chloride, may be sufficient, or the use of proprietary cough drops.

If the fever is high and does not come down within a day or two, especially if the sputum or throat culture shows a predominance of hemolytic streptococci, pneumococci or *Staphylococcus aureus,* continuous chemotherapy may be given, such as crystalline penicillin, 300,000 units every 12 to 24 hours; or procaine penicillin, 300,000 units every 24 hours; sulfadiazine, 1 gm. three or four times a day; Aureomycin, Terramycin or tetracycline, 250 mg. three or four times a day.

After a severe attack the patient should take a week or so of convalescence before returning to work. A roentgenogram of the chest should be taken if there is any question of pneumonia or other complication.

In asthmatic subjects bronchodilator drugs may be needed. Frequently one of the inhalation sprays (epinephrine, Vaponefrin) will be adequate; sometimes epinephrine hypodermically or aminophylline intravenously is necessary.

Prevention of the spread of acute respiratory infections is difficult, whether in office, institution, school or home. Those who are ill should, however, be isolated immediately in so far as possible, and put to bed in separate rooms, with separate toilet facilities. Children particularly should be kept away from all cases of acute cold, should avoid crowds in the winter season, and avoid both overheating and chilling or exposure.

The use of preventive cold vaccines has, generally speaking, proved disappointing. Influenza vaccine has been useful in stopping the spread of this disease in certain local epidemics.

CHRONIC BRONCHITIS

Definition. Chronic bronchitis is a longstanding disease of the tracheobronchial tree, with chronic inflammatory, fibrotic and atrophic changes in mucous membranes and deeper bronchial structures, frequently associated with pulmonary fibrosis, emphysema or other chronic pulmonary disease.

Etiology. Chronic bronchitis as an accompaniment or complication of other chronic pulmonary disease is fairly well understood. Low grade chronic infection, inadequate pulmonary drainage, mechanical distortions, inadequate circulation and tissue nutrition, leading to both atrophy and connective tissue replacement, are probably essential elements.

Thus one may find chronic bronchitis localized or diffuse, in most of the pulmonary fibroses, in chronic obstructive emphysema, chronic asthma, in pulmonary tuberculosis, bronchiectasis, chronic sinusitis and congestive heart failure. Wherever there is localized pulmonary disease, or inadequate bronchial drainage from any cause, there is apt to be a local region of chronic bronchitis, as in kyphoscoliosis, localized bronchiectasis, fibrocaseous tuberculosis, or bronchial narrowing or compression as from aneurysm or tumor.

Chronic bronchitis may also be an important initiating factor in the development of many cases of chronic asthma, emphysema or pulmonary fibrosis; and the bronchitis itself seems to be a result of oft-repeated attacks of bacterial infection, particularly those due to pneumococcus or *Hemophilus influenzae*.

Morbid Anatomy. The surface of the bronchial lumen is dark red, sometimes apparently trabeculated, and may be dry or covered with viscous mucus or pus. The bronchi are thickened and inelastic. Microscopically, the epithelium is deformed, with desquamation of surface cells. There may be epithelial hyperplasia in some places, denudation and atrophy in others. The same juxtaposition of hypertrophied and atrophied elements may be seen in the mucous glands and muscular layers. The submucosa usually shows fibrous hyperplasia. Varying degrees of peribronchial inflammation may be found.

In far advanced cases, autopsy may show fusiform dilatation of bronchial walls, with necrosis and small abscess formation in the bronchial and peribronchial tissues.

Though chronic bronchitis is typically a disease of elderly people, young persons with other chronic pulmonary disease are subject to it, and it is seen in children with debilitating disease such as rickets, or chronic respiratory conditions such as severe sinusitis, or bronchiectasis. Chronic bronchitis is one aspect of the severe progressive pulmonary manifestations seen in cystic disease of the pancreas in children.

Pathologic Physiology and Chemistry. The important dysfunctions caused by chronic bronchitis and its associated defects are those due to (1) inflammation and chronic infection of mucous membranes, with exudate and poor bronchial drainage; (2) tracheobronchial rigidity, or loss of elasticity; (3) obstruction of the air passages.

1. The chronic infective and degenerative changes in the bronchial walls both lead to mucus and pus formation and, in injuring the ciliary apparatus, destroy one important means of their elimination. Bronchial peristalsis is inhibited. Thus further stagnation and infection are promoted. Bronchial drainage becomes also more and more dependent on the physiologic function of coughing. In the presence of chronic congestion, as in longstanding congestive heart failure, these disturbances are further aggravated.

2. Fibrosis in the tracheobronchial walls destroys their normal elasticity. As Macklin has well shown, the normal tracheobronchial apparatus is extremely elastic and expansile, as indeed it would have to be, being an integral part of the expansile lung. The relative rigidity of the fibrotic bronchial tree thus diminishes the ventilatory capacity of the lung. If, as is frequently the case, there is in addition a diffuse intrapulmonary fibrosis, the breathing capacity becomes further diminished. This type of fibrosis, termed *restrictive* pulmonary fibrosis, is common; it is seen, for example, in many cases of fibrotic tuberculosis, and in silicosis, as well as in many "nonspecific" fibroses. Patients with this condition have little disability at rest or in mild exercise, but become dyspneic on more strenuous exertion, when their ventilatory capacities are strained to their limits.

3. Even more common are the disturbances produced by chronic *obstruction* of the air passages. Boggy, swollen mucous membranes, tenacious exudate, and frequently spasm of bronchial muscles may all be factors, and the effects are naturally most evident in the smallest air passages, those of the terminal bronchioles, with lumen half a millimeter or less in diameter. The condition thus becomes a part of a chronic asthma or chronic obstructive emphysema, with all the manifestations of these diseases.

Symptoms. A mild chronic bronchitis may exist for years with no symptoms at all, or at most a dry, irritative morning cough. In the more severe form, cough and sputum are prominent. These may occur only in the winter, or after an upper respiratory infection. As the condition progresses, year by year, cough and purulent sputum become more troublesome. Often, after a severe respiratory infection, such as an attack of bronchopneumonia, the chronic bronchitis will be abruptly much worse. The sputum may be scanty, or abundant, mucoid or purulent. Bloody sputum, foul sputum, or hemoptyses usually indicate some other disease, such as bronchiectasis, lung abscess or tuberculosis. Cough may be mild, or severe with paroxysms of several minutes' duration, persisting until sputum is raised and the air passages cleared.

When bronchial or bronchiolar obstruction develops, there is wheezing expiration, exertional dyspnea, often actual attacks of asthma. In the early stages, however, bronchiolar obstruction may cause only an increased and more frequent irritative cough.

Laënnec and other writers of the last century described a form of chronic bronchorrhea, with excessive amounts of thin or mucoid sputum, up to a liter and a half a day. This entity is practically unknown at the present time.

Chronic bronchitis as such is usually afebrile, and there is little or no change in the red or white blood cell count or erythrocyte sedimentation rate.

Additional symptoms are those of associated diseases, as indicated in preceding sections.

Physical Signs. Chronic bronchitis itself, except for cough and sputum, often gives no abnormal physical signs. Chest expansion and vital capacity may be somewhat diminished. Frequently, scattered rales are heard, which may be sonorous, wheezing, squeaking or moist in character, sometimes clearing after a vigorous cough. If bronchial exudate is abundant, or during or after a fresh respiratory infection, there may be numerous moist rales, chiefly at the bases posteriorly.

Persistence of localized physical signs suggests the presence of other disease, such as bronchiectasis, tuberculosis, bronchial carcinoma or chronic pneumonitis, the last often having a peribronchial distribution.

Clubbing of the fingers may occur in advanced chronic bronchitis with heavy infection and purulent sputum; but this sign usually indicates some intrapulmonary suppuration, bronchiectasis or else a marked anoxic state.

If there is restrictive pulmonary fibrosis without air passage obstruction, there will be exertional dyspnea, sometimes even dyspnea at rest. Breath sounds in this form are usually increased and harsh. An interesting physical sign, indicating inelasticity of lungs and bronchial tree, is the jerking downward of the trachea with each inspiration.

When chronic bronchitis is associated with chronic obstructive emphysema, as is frequently the case, the physical signs are predominantly those of the latter disease.

In the presence of congestive heart failure the signs of this condition dominate the picture. The congestive state usually both aggravates and prolongs the manifestations of chronic bronchitis.

A common clinical entity in elderly patients is a combination of chronic bronchitis, emphysema and arteriosclerotic heart disease with early cardiac insufficiency; and it may be difficult to evaluate each of these elements.

Diagnosis. As already indicated, many other diseases may simulate a simple chronic bronchitis, or may exist with it. Pulmonary tuberculosis should be searched for, in older as well as younger age groups, by sputum examination and roentgenogram. Carcinoma of the bronchus is another insidious and relatively common disease, which may exist for long periods with no symptom but cough. Other conditions are chronic sinusitis, bronchiectasis, lung abscess, chronic empyema, silicosis, mitral stenosis, aortic aneurysm, foreign body in the bronchus, Boeck's sarcoid, the various pulmonary fibroses, and the rarer mycotic and fungous infections.

Prognosis. Chronic bronchitis is usually a slowly progressing disease. It may continue essentially unchanged for many years, or may become progressively worse, especially if there are numerous exacerbations of acute respiratory infection. If serious physical disability develops, or progressive disease with fatal termination, it is almost always the result of pulmonary or cardiac complications.

Treatment. For the chronic cough, palliative remedies can be used as tolerated, such as cough drops, Stokes expectorant, or syrups containing ammonium chloride, potassium iodide, or other agents; and for severe or spasmodic coughing attacks, codeine or a codeine cough mixture may be used, as described under Acute Bronchitis. If the sputum is unpleasant in taste or odor, or actually foul, a deodorant may be tried, such as creosote, usually as an addition to the cough mixture. Postural drainage may assist in raising sputum and clearing air passages.

In children, special care should be given to the general nutrition. In particular, the patient should receive ample amounts of vitamins A and D, in cod liver oil or other suitable form.

Chronic bronchitis with bronchiolar obstruction calls for additional therapy. If there are asthmatic symptoms, or even in some cases with only increased irritative cough and slight dyspnea, bronchodilator agents may be tried, such as the bronchodilator sprays (epinephrine 1:100, Neo-Synephrin 1:100, Vaponefrin or Isuprel two or three times daily, and at bed time); ephedrine by mouth in doses of 25 or 50 mg., combined with a barbiturate if there is nervousness or restlessness. One of the antihistaminic drugs, by oral administration, may be tried. In more severe asthmatic states, epinephrine hypodermically may be needed, or aminophylline, 0.24 gm. by vein, or, for more sustained effect, 0.5 gm. by rectum. Courses of antibiotic therapy by aerosol inhalation may be useful in chronic or recurring infections.

Specific allergic sensitivities may be demonstrated in these conditions, and desensitization therapy is sometimes helpful.

In the way of general measures, the patient's activity should be regulated according to his tolerance, especially so as to avoid exposure and fatigue. Tobacco is often an irritant; if so, smoking should be stopped.

For prevention, the most important feature is avoidance of repeated acute infections. It is best if the patient can live in a mild equable climate, especially during the winter months. Some patients can tolerate small regular doses of an antibiotic or sulfa drug throughout the respiratory season, with apparently fewer infections.

FIBRINOUS BRONCHITIS

(*Plastic Bronchitis*)

Definition. This is a rare disease characterized by the formation of fibrinous or mucinous casts in parts of the lower bronchial tree, and expulsion of these casts in the sputum.

Etiology. The disease, though rare, has been recognized since the time of Galen, and more than one hundred cases had been reported in the literature before 1900. Walshe, in the last century, claimed to have had five cases under his own observation. It is said to occur more frequently in males, and between the ages of 10 and 30 years.

Cases of primary origin have been described; other cases apparently develop after some acute respiratory condition, such as measles or scarlet fever, or in association with chronic pulmonary disease. No specific bacteriologic agent has been recognized.

Morbid Anatomy. There are no specific pathologic lesions at the onset, the changes being those of acute bronchitis. Later the mucous membrane in affected regions may show both desquamation and ulceration. The characteristic development is the formation within the bronchial and bronchiolar lumen of casts of fibrinous or mucinous material enclosing varying amounts of cellular debris. When expelled from the bronchi, they can be floated in water. The larger casts are often laminated and hollow, the smaller solid, ending in spirals. A typical cast is an arborization 5 or 6 cm. in total spread. They may be, however, several inches in length. They are gray, white or pinkish, often blood-streaked, fairly firm.

Usually the lower lobes only are involved; not infrequently the condition remains unilateral.

Pathologic Physiology. The manifestations produced are those due to the mechanical effects of the cast: areas of atelectasis before dislodgment; coughing attacks as the material is brought up, often in violent paroxysms; occasionally suffocative if a large mass lodges in the larynx or larger air passages.

Symptoms and Physical Findings. In the acute form the symptoms at onset are those of acute bronchitis, with malaise, fever and cough, sometimes a chill, pleuritic pain or dyspnea. There is usually a moderate leukocytosis, in some instances eosinophilia. After several days the cough becomes severe and paroxysmal, the paroxysm subsiding with the expulsion of the cast. The coughing attack may be associated with dyspnea. There is often blood-streaking with the cast, and small hemoptyses are common. The casts may be brought up alone or surrounded by sputum; there may be Curschmann spirals or Charcot-Leyden crystals with them.

Physical signs in the lungs are usually minimal, as in acute bronchitis. Breath sounds may be suppressed in the region of cast formation, before dislodgment.

Roentgenograms show no characteristic features. Bronchograms are usually normal.

The attacks may continue for several days or several weeks, ending in complete recovery. Rarely, the lodgment of a large cast in the larynx has led to suffocation and death.

In the chronic form the early stages are usually similar to the acute, but the attacks recur at intervals of months or longer, and the condition may persist over many years. The chronically recurring attacks may lead to diffuse emphysema.

Diagnosis. The condition may be suspected in cases of bronchitis with severe paroxysms of cough ending in the raising of a heavy or solid mass of sputum, particularly if such attacks are of repeated occurrence. The diagnosis rests on the finding of the typical casts, by careful examination of the sputum, preferably by floating it on water.

Treatment. Therapy is largely symptomatic, to aid in expulsion of casts during attacks. Expectorants are usually recommended, such as potassium iodide (0.6 to 1 gm. three times a day). Steam inhalations may be helpful. If suffocation impends, bronchoscopy or even tracheotomy may be needed.

BRONCHIOLITIS FIBROSA OBLITERANS

Definition. This is a severe, usually fatal disease, characterized by widespread destructive lesions in the smaller bronchioles, followed by a rapidly progressing fibrosis, with narrowing and eventually occlusion of the bronchiolar lumen.

Etiology. The disease may be produced by inhalation of chemical irritants, such as strong acid fumes, sulfur dioxide or volatile solvents; it may follow acute infectious diseases, or occur in the course of a chronic bronchitis or asthma.

Morbid Anatomy. At autopsy the lungs are usually distended. Scattered throughout the parenchyma are grayish-white, firm, angular miliary nodules, 1 to 3 mm. in diameter. Within the center of each is a terminal bronchiole, its lumen narrowed and distorted or actually obliterated.

Microscopically, all stages of the disease process can usually be discerned. Beginning as a mild inflammation of the epithelium, there follows sloughing of the epithelial layer, edema of deeper layers with leukocytic infiltration. A dense fibrinous exudate forms, extending into the lumen, and this is progressively replaced by granulation tissue and then firm connective tissue. Other bronchioles may show repair, the lumen becoming relined with epithelium. The aveoli behind occluded bronchioles become atelectatic, hyalinized and filled with connective tissue. If the air passage is only partly occluded, the alveoli become emphysematous.

Pathologic Physiology. Cyanosis and dyspnea, the chief symptoms of the disease, can be readily understood from the pathology, with many bronchioles occluded, and others partly obstructed, rendering pulmonary ventilation both mechanically difficult and partly ineffectual.

Symptoms and Physical Findings. There is cyanosis, dyspnea with hyperventilation, and cough during the early days of the disease, when the bronchiolar epithelium is in the stage of inflammation and desquamation. Low grade fever occurs at this time, and rales are heard throughout both lungs. Then follows a temporary improvement, which may last one to three weeks. With the obliteration of the bronchioles, dyspnea and cyanosis recur, and coarse or crepitant rales are heard; in severe cases the patient becomes progressively weaker with shallow, labored respiration, and eventually succumbs. Roentgenograms show disseminated, more or less uniform nodular infiltration, usually indistinguishable from the changes of miliary tuberculosis. Some patients have survived, even after a stormy course.

Diagnosis. Only a few cases have been diagnosed during life. The disease should be suspected if, after exposure to some toxic and destructive inhalant, the patient exhibits intense cyanosis and dyspnea with x-ray shadows suggesting miliary tuberculosis.

Treatment. This is symptomatic. Oxygen in high concentration should be given continuously. If there is obstructed breathing, the bronchodilators (epinephrine, 1 cc. subcutaneously, or by inhalation spray; or aminophylline, 0.24 gm. intravenously or 0.5 gm. by rectum) may give relief. Sedation with codeine or morphia will probably be necessary, but should be given with caution, so as not to inhibit the cough reflex completely, or bring on respiratory failure.

BRONCHOPULMONARY SPIROCHETOSIS

(*Spirochetal Bronchitis, Castellani's Spirochetosis*)

Definition. This is an infection of the bronchial tree with a spirochetal organism, the disease being manifested by abundant mucopurulent sputum in which the spirochetes are found in large numbers.

Etiology. The spirochetal origin of this disease was established by Castellani in 1906. Several forms of spirochete have been described, of which the most characteristic is the *Spiroschaudinnia bronchialis*. This is a thin, delicate spirochete with numerous small uniform coils, one of the extremities blunt, the other pointed.

This condition has been reported chiefly in the Far East and in Europe; recently a number of case reports have appeared in the Central and South American literature.

Manson-Bahr has questioned whether the spirochetes in this condition are true etiologic agents or secondary invaders.

Symptoms and Physical Findings. There are acute and chronic forms. In the acute there is weakness, some fever and cough. The sputum may be scanty or abundant; mucoid, mucopurulent or hemorrhagic. The condition lasts about a month.

In the chronic forms there is usually chronic cough, with abundant mucopurulent sputum. The latter is at times blood-streaked or bloody, occasionally fetid. Small hemoptyses are common. There may be irregular fever, anemia and emaciation. The condition may persist for years. Roentgenograms may show widened hilar shadows, with some nodular shadows if there is associated bronchopneumonia. In uncomplicated cases, bronchograms are said to be normal; on bronchoscopy, mucopurulent secretion is found, but essentially normal mucous membrane.

Diagnosis. The sputum contains the spirochetes in large numbers, and these can be readily found by examination of fresh specimens in the dark field or with special stains (such as the Fontana-Tribondeau silver stain). The disease is usually diagnosed tuberculosis.

Treatment. Arsenic is said to be specific, resulting in cure or at least arrest of the process. It is usually given in the form of neoarsphenamine.

DICKINSON W. RICHARDS

References

Barach, A. L.: Physiologic Therapy in Respiratory Diseases. Philadelphia, J. B. Lippincott Co., 1948.

Boyd, W.: Textbook of Pathology. 6th ed. Philadelphia, Lea and Febiger, 1953.

Carlisle, J. M.: Pulmonary Edema after Exposure to Toxic Gases. J.A.M.A., 123:947, 1943.

La Due, J. S.: Bronchiolitis Fibrosa Obliterans. Arch. Int. Med., 68:663, 1941.

Logan, W. P. D.: Mortality in the London Fog Incident, 1952. Lancet, 1:336, 1953.

McVay, L. V., Jr., and Sprunt, D. H.: Antibiotic Prophylaxis in Chronic Respiratory Diseases. Arch. Int. Med., 92:833, 1953.

Neffson, A. H.: Acute Laryngo-Tracheobronchitis, a 25-Year Review. Am. J. M. Sc., 208:524, 1944.

Prentiss, A. M.: Chemicals in War. New York, Mc-Graw-Hill, 1937.

Reid, L. M.: Pathology of Chronic Bronchitis. Lancet, 1:275, 1954.

Seiler, S.: Bronchitis Plastica: Case with Recovery after Collapse Therapy. Schweiz. med. Wchnschr., 72:86, 1942.

Strong, R. P.: Stitt's Diagnosis, Prevention, and Treatment of Tropical Diseases. 7th ed. Philadelphia, Blakiston Co., 1944.

Stuart-Harris, C. H., Pownall, M., Scothorne, C. M., and Franks, Z.: The Factor of Infection in Chronic Bronchitis. Quart. J. Med., 22:121, 1953.

Walker, I. C.: Two Cases of Fibrinous Bronchitis, with a Review of the Literature. Am. J. M. Sc., 159:825, 1920.

Walshe, W. H.: Diseases of the Lungs. London, Smith Elder Co., 1871.

BRONCHIECTASIS

Definition. Bronchiectasis is a pathologic state of the lungs characterized by dilatation of the bronchi. The dilatation is associated with structural changes in the bronchial walls which are predominantly inflammatory, destructive or reparative, depending on the developmental stage of the process. The neighboring lung substance is usually involved in similar processes to a greater or lesser extent. The ectasia proper may be cylindrical, saccular or cystic in form. The principal changes affect the peripheral bronchi, the major divisions being but rarely involved. The disorder is of considerable prevalence. The incidence, based on recent area surveys in England, has been estimated to be between 1 and 3 per thousand of population. The involvement is bilateral in over half the cases.

Etiology. Bronchiectasis may develop as an obvious sequel of various pulmonary diseases such as bronchopneumonia, lung abscess, pulmonary tumors and tuberculosis; or it may be found without definite antecedent or predisposing pulmonary disease. The majority of cases are probably acquired, but it is agreed that congenital factors may occasionally be involved.

Pathogenesis. Destructive changes in the bronchial walls appear to be the most important factor in the pathogenesis of acquired bronchiectasis. These generally result from infection, although the inhalation of acid fumes or other chemical agents may cause similar effects. Mustard gas is a recognized cause. Bacteriologic studies, possibly because of the high prevalence of secondary invaders, have failed to establish any single organism or group of organisms as the usual cause. Combined pathologic and bacteriologic studies in early cases have indicated that the gram-positive cocci are usually present in abundance. Pneumococcal lobar pneumonia, however, is but rarely associated with the kind of destructive inflammation of the bronchial walls which leads to bronchiectasis. This is found more frequently in association with the bronchopneumonias and, especially, with frankly suppurative pneumonias such as result from bronchial obstruction by tumors or aspirated foreign bodies. The frequent development of localized bronchiectasis as a sequel of putrid or nonputrid abscess of the lung attests the importance of pulmonary suppuration in the pathogenesis of bronchiectasis. The etiologic importance of anaerobic organisms, including the fusospirochetal group, which are commonly present in bronchiectasis as well as in lung abscess, is uncertain. It is believed, however, that some of these contribute importantly to the necrotizing process.

The question whether, in addition to a destructive inflammation of the bronchial walls, mechanical factors are necessary to produce dilatation of the bronchi has occasioned much speculation. Laënnec, who first described the condition, suggested that the dilatation is caused by mechanical distention from the progressive accumulation of bronchial secretions in chronic bronchitis. Various other theories have been advanced, stressing particularly the differential intrabronchial pressure relations associated with cough and with bronchial obstruction and atelectasis. Traction on the bronchi resulting from pulmonary and pleural fibrosis has also been suggested as a possible actively distending force. Lisa and Rosenblatt critically reviewed these various theories in the light of recent experimental and pathologic data. These authors concluded that mechanical factors alone do not produce bronchiectasis and are seldom of importance even as contributory causes. According to this modern view, a necrotizing inflammatory process involving the walls of the bronchi is sufficient in itself to produce ectasia without the operation of mechanical forces other than those to which the bronchi are normally subject. Lindskog and Liebow reject this theory of destruction

and favor the traction theory, which maintains that bronchiectasis results from scarring in the parenchyma with consequent dilatation of the bronchi. In either view, however, necrotizing infection is the primary cause, and bronchial obstruction and atelectasis are important only insofar as they impair drainage and provide conditions which promote infection.

A primary causal relationship of upper respiratory infection, especially paranasal sinusitis, to bronchiectasis has been widely assumed, but such a connection is doubtful despite the frequent association of chronic sinusitis with bronchiectasis. There is, in fact, much evidence that the reverse relationship may exist and that chronic sinusitis can be considered a frequent complication of bronchiectasis. Both may develop simultaneously as sequelae of a severe pulmonary infection.

In children the first symptoms of bronchiectasis are frequently observed to follow measles, whooping cough or scarlet fever. In such instances its development may usually be attributed to the bronchopneumonic manifestations or complications of these contagious diseases. Similarly, the development of bronchiectasis following influenza is related to a secondary influenzal pneumonia, such as was prominently associated with the influenza pandemic of 1918.

Bronchiectasis may be found in association with chronic bronchitis, asthma and generalized emphysema. The causal relationships to these conditions are not clear, nor is the association as common as is often assumed because of the similarity of symptoms. In so far as they predispose to bacterial pulmonary infections, they may indirectly cause bronchiectasis, but they can exist for many years without any ectasia of the bronchi developing.

The frequency of bronchiectasis in early childhood suggests a congenital origin in many cases, but pathologic evidence to support the supposition is rare. A congenital origin has been attributed especially to the cystic form. Such cases are sometimes designated "congenital cystic disease of the lung," a term also frequently but erroneously applied to cases of bullous emphysema. There is no doubt that true congenital bronchial cysts occur in the lung and that they may be multiple. They have been found in infants that have died soon after birth, in the absence of infection. It is less certain, however, that all cases of the cystic form of bronchiectasis develop on a congenital basis or that congenital factors may be concerned in the development of this form only. Bronchiectasis is found in association with certain congenital anomalies and diseases. The triad of bronchiectasis, sinusitis and situs inversus (Kartagener) and that of cystic fibrosis of the pancreas, vitamin A deficiency and bronchiectasis (Andersen), though but recently described, are not rare. The exact nature of the relationship of bronchiectasis to these conditions has not been satisfactorily explained.

Morbid Anatomy. Although the characteristic change in bronchiectasis is ectasia of the peripheral bronchi, the bronchial tree is not necessarily the sole or even the primary site of the morbid process. The bronchiectasis is but one manifestation of a destructive and reparative process which involves the lung parenchyma as well as the bronchial walls in practically all instances. The associated parenchymal changes may be either concomitant or secondary, and not infrequently overshadow the bronchial pathology in degree. They consist of pneumonia, interstitial infiltration and fibrosis, pleuritis and pleural fibrosis, atelectasis, pulmonary carnification and emphysema. All the changes may be localized or diffuse. Frequently an entire lobe may be shrunken by fibrosis so that it presents an atelectatic appearance, even though its bronchi are patent. A thickening and distortion of the bronchial walls resulting from fibrosis is often conspicuous, together with the dilatation. The dilated bronchi may be but a few millimeters wider than their normal caliber, or they may be several centimeters across. Cylindrical, saccular and cystic dilatations may be present in the same lung or even in a single lobe. Characteristically, the disease is segmental, involving groups of adjacent bronchi. When multiple segments are involved, these are not necessarily adjoining, but may be scattered in several lobes, in one or both lungs. The dependent segments of the lungs are most commonly involved, including the right middle lobe and the lingular segment of the left upper lobe. When the apices of the upper lobes alone are involved, the bronchiectasis is generally regarded as post-tuberculous.

Miscroscopically, the muscularis of the bronchi is found to be the main site of both the early necrotizing bronchial inflammation and the later fibrous tissue replacement. In the most severe processes the bronchial wall is entirely destroyed, together with the neighboring alveoli, with resultant formation of a true cavity in the substance of the lung. Saccular or cystic bronchiectases generally arise from such extensive destructive processes, while the cylindrical dilatations result from those which are less severe. Both during the stage of active destruction and in the chronic cases of long duration, the bronchial lumina may be filled with purulent exudate. Bacteria are often present in this exudate and in the bronchial walls. It is rarely possible, even in early cases, to determine whether these are primary or secondary invaders.

Pathologic Physiology. The principal physiologic disturbance in bronchiectasis is impairment of the expulsive movements of the bronchi. The cough reflex, which acts in the major bronchi, is not primarily affected, but may be diminished in advanced cases in which sputum is copious. The cough mechanism may be further interfered with by associated parenchymal changes such as fibrosis and emphysema. The expulsive mechanisms of the peripheral bronchi are importantly and primarily affected. These mechanisms consist principally of the ciliary action of the epithelium and the peristaltic waves of the bronchial musculature. The anatomic changes in both the epithelial and muscular layers of the peripheral bronchi therefore interfere with the normal protective functions of these mechanisms and permit the accumulation of secretions as a nidus for bacterial growth. Emptying of the stagnant secretions from bronchiectatic sacs in dependent segments is consequently possible only by the aid of gravity and can be promoted by the maneuvers of postural drainage which are used therapeutically. The respiratory efficiency of the involved segments or lobes is impaired by the parenchymal fibrosis and emphysema. Vascular changes and disturbances of circulation also occur. Liebow and his co-workers have demonstrated extensive anastomoses between the bronchial and the pulmonary arteries which serve to shunt desaturated blood away from the involved parenchyma. This collateral circulation may impose a burden on the left side of the heart in consequence of the left-right shunt.

Symptoms and Signs. *Chronic productive cough* is usually the presenting symptom of established bronchiectasis. The quantity of sputum is variable. Frequently it is copious; production of several hundred cubic centimeters a day is common. A fetid odor is often conspicuous in extensive cases of long standing. It may so affect the patient's breath as to make his presence offensive even at some distance. A constant foul taste in the mouth may be complained of and may impair the appetite. The sputum is yellowish or of light greenish hue, and may, on standing, separate into three layers which are composed respectively of mucus at the top, a relatively clear intermediate fluid layer, and a thick bottom layer of pus and cellular debris. The quantity of sputum as well as the frequency of cough is often affected by posture and especially by change of posture. This accounts for the paroxysms of cough which commonly occur on arising in the morning and on reclining at night. There is frequently a history of repeated attacks of bronchopneumonia and of lesser febrile episodes which may have passed for attacks of simple bronchitis. It is rarely possible to date the onset from the history, since even the first remembered attack of pneumonia may be secondary rather than the originating one.

Hemoptysis is a common symptom, and profuse pulmonary hemorrhage may occur. There is a so-called "dry hemoptoic" type in which the first symptom is hemoptysis without any noticeable antecedent chronic cough. In some instances hemoptysis may recur at rare intervals for many years without other conspicuous symptoms. As a rule such "dry" types, if untreated, eventually develop chronic cough and expectoration as the result of infection.

Chest pain occurs usually only as the result of pleurisy or empyema complicating a pneumonic episode. Occasionally pain may be recurrently present, even in the absence of febrile exacerbations, and does not necessarily have the characteristic relation to respiration which is typical of acute pleurisy.

In rare instances there may be no respiratory symptoms and the disease is discovered in the course of a routine physical or x-ray examination. In such cases the disease is usually of limited extent, involving the small right middle lobe or a comparable segment of one of the other lobes.

The *general symptoms* are those of chronic infection and depend in degree on the extent and duration of the disorder. Good nutrition and normal vigor may be maintained for many years in those cases in which there is small production of sputum and in which episodes of pneumonia are infrequent. More often there are fatigability and gradual weight loss that progress to extreme weakness and emaciation in severe cases. Fever is usually absent in the intervals between bronchopneumonic exacerbations, but it may be continuous or recurrent over long periods and associated with chills or with night sweats. Dyspnea and cyanosis are late manifestations and depend less on the bronchiectasis itself than on the associated pulmonary fibrosis and emphysema. Rarely these may lead to cor pulmonale and right ventricular heart failure.

Progression of the disease occurs principally, if not indeed entirely, during the pneumonias which punctuate its course. These are usually of suppurative character and may lead to abscess formation. Death occurs usually from such pneumonias, which tend to increase in severity with successive attacks. Fatal hemorrhage may occur, but such a termination is unusual. The most important extrapulmonary complications are empyema and brain abscess. Either of these may be the immediate cause of death. Generalized amyloidosis may occur, but is rare.

Physical Signs. The physical signs are variable, but, except in cases of very limited extent, some abnormal signs usually can be elicited. In the absence of pneumonitis or other conspicuous associated parenchymal changes, these may consist solely of rales over the involved lung segments. The rales are usually subcrepitant in character and may be accompanied by rhonchi. The other signs which may be found depend on the nature and extent of the associated parenchymal changes, such as pneumonia, fibrosis, atelectasis and emphysema. Dullness to percussion, bronchial breath sounds and bronchophony may be present over consolidated or carnified segments. Sometimes, especially over saccular and cystic bronchiectases, the breath sounds are amphoric and the rales of consonating character, as over tuberculous cavities. Areas of hyperresonance may be found over segments which are emphysematous. Signs of displacement of the trachea and mediastinal structures may be present, depending on the amount and distribution of parenchymal and pleural fibrosis, and on the presence of shrunken or atelectatic lobes or segments of lobes. The variability of physical signs applies not only as between different patients, but may be noted in the same patient over a period of time. Such changes depend on the development of secondary inflammations in the lungs and also on the amount of accumulated secretions and the degree of bronchial obstruction which these produce. In those cases in which bronchiectasis develops secondarily to an organic bronchial obstruction, such as a tumor or aspirated foreign body, or secondarily to a lung abscess or diffuse aspiration pneumonia, the signs of bronchiectasis may be entirely obscured by those of the primary condition.

In addition to the signs in the chest the physical examination may reveal other important abnormalities. Prominent among these, and almost always present when the disease is extensive, are evidences of chronic infection in the upper respiratory tract. The maxillary sinuses are most often involved. There is chronic nasopharyngitis, usually of the hypertrophic type. With this the gag reflex is usually depressed or absent. Clubbing of the fingers and toes is frequently present to some degree, and severe grades of pulmonary osteo-arthropathy may occur.

Diagnosis. This rests principally on roentgen ray bronchography with the aid of iodized oil, a method introduced in 1922 by Sicard and Forestier. A preliminary simple roentgen examination, with standard postero-anterior and lateral or stereoscopic views should always be made. This may show no abnormal shadows in cases without pneumonitis or conspicuous fibrosis and emphysema. Usually there is some indication in the form of fibrotic strands, often following the course of the vascular trunks to the base, or small patches of infiltration. Neither such inconspicuous abnormalities nor more pronounced ones such as large areas of pneumonitis, annular shadows, marked fibrosis and contracted lobes are diagnostic. It is important to make the standard roentgenogram prior to bronchography, for subsequent to it some of the iodized oil may be retained and interfere with an accurate interpretation of pulmonary shadows. A preliminary bronchoscopy should be done if there is any indication of a tumor or other obstructive lesion in one of the larger bronchi, or for aspiration of secretions if these are not found to be draining freely with simple postural drainage. Since retention of secretions in the bronchi interferes with the entrance of the iodized oil, postural drainage should always be carried out immediately before bronchography is attempted. There are various satisfactory techniques for instillation of the oil both with and without the passage of a catheter into the trachea and bronchi. The most important consideration is the proper posturing of the patient so that adequate filling of the various pulmonary segments may be obtained. When lobectomy is under consideration, the entire bronchial tree should be outlined in this manner, in one or more sittings if necessary, and lateral or oblique views made as well as postero-anterior ones. The iodized oil must be especially prepared for the purpose. Recently water-soluble bronchography compounds have been introduced. The experience with these, however, has been in most respects less satisfactory than with the iodized oil and their use appears to be more hazardous.

There are certain *contraindications to the introduction of iodized oil in bronchography:* The procedure should not be performed during an attack of acute pneumonitis or within two or three weeks after such an attack, or any febrile episode presumably caused by the pulmonary lesions. A similar interval should be observed after hemoptysis. Bronchography should not be undertaken in the presence of congestive heart failure, severe generalized pulmonary emphysema or severe respiratory insufficiency from any cause. Active pulmonary tuberculosis with positive sputum usually contraindicates bronchography, especially if the disease is of the exudative type. Finally, if there is known hypersensitivity to iodine, or if there are other contraindications to absorption of iodine, the introduction of iodized oil is inadvisable, because a portion of the oil may be swallowed and iodine liberated by intestinal digestion.

As bronchiectasis may accompany other pulmonary diseases such as tuberculosis, pulmonary mycoses, emphysema, asthma, bronchitis and suppuration of the lung from various causes, it is always important that microscopic examinations and cultures of the sputum be made for completion of the diagnosis. Such examinations, especially those for tubercle bacilli, should be made before the Lipiodol studies are undertaken.

Differential Diagnosis. The differential diagnosis between simple bronchiectasis and other chronic pulmonary diseases is usually not difficult. The distribution of the signs over the dependent segments of the lungs generally serves to distinguish it from *pulmonary tuberculosis,* although tuberculosis limited to the lower lobes is not extremely

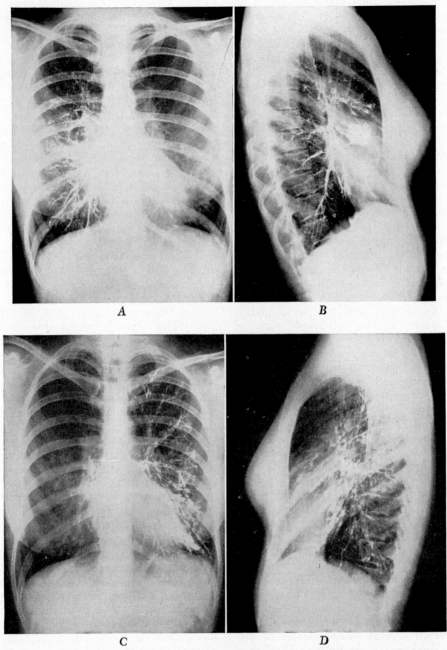

A   B

C   D

Fig. 123. Bronchiectasis. A, Postero-anterior projection of right bronchogram shows almost normal pattern because of shrinkage and medial retraction of involved segments.

B, The lateral projection of right bronchogram shows clearly the bronchiectasis in the right middle lobe. In addition to the pronounced change in the middle lobe, there is slight involvement of adjacent segments of the upper and lower lobes.

C, Postero-anterior projection, showing bronchiectasis on this side also, with conspicuous ectasia in some of the peripheral branches in dependent segments of the lung.

D, Lateral projection of left bronchogram, showing involvement to be principally of the lingular segment of the left upper lobe, but with the lower lobe also affected in its anterior basal branches.

rare and may occasionally be mistaken for bronchiectasis if careful sputum examinations are not made. The *obstructive suppurative pneumonias* associated with tumors and other stenotic processes of the bronchi may be distinguished by the signs of bronchial obstruction and by bronchoscopy. *Chronic bronchitis* with generalized fibrosis and emphysema, and asthma with severe bronchitis, may sometimes be associated with expectoration of sputum which in quantity and character resembles that of advanced bronchiectasis. The preponderance of signs attributable to secretions in the larger bronchi and to bronchospasm, together with absence of physical or roentgenologic signs of parenchymal infiltration, usually serves to differentiate these conditions. Bronchography to rule out the presence of some degree of associated bronchiectasis is inadvisable if there is much generalized emphysema. *Bullous emphysema* is usually distinguishable roentgenologically by its characteristic pattern, but may occasionally resemble cystic bronchiectasis. Differentiation in doubtful cases may readily be made by bronchography, since the bronchial communications of the bullous sacs are too narrow to admit the iodized oil. *Delayed resolution* of simple pneumonias may usually be differentiated by the history of a recent attack with typical symptomatology and the absence of history of several prior attacks and of chronic interim cough. When resolution is long delayed or when rales persist long after the clearing of the roentgenologic shadows, differentiation may be possible only by means of bronchography.

Prognosis. The prognosis of bronchiectasis depends on the extent of the original involvement and the degree of associated pulmonary infection. Until recently the average duration of life from the time of the onset of symptoms was generally estimated to be only ten or fifteen years. These estimates, however, were based on follow-up observations of hospitalized patients with extensive involvement, and relate to the prechemotherapy era. More recent evidence indicates the prognosis is by no means usually so poor, and that the common assumption that the condition is always progressive is not justified. Patients in whom the disease is of limited extent, and in whom it has been discovered before secondary infection is well established, are frequently observed for ten or more years without appreciable progression of the condition. The success with which

secondary suppurative pneumonias can be prevented by medical management importantly influences the prognosis, even when cure by excisional surgery is out of the question.

The *reversibility* of bronchiectasis in its early stages has been claimed to be demonstrable. The difficulty of interpreting slight degrees of cylindrical ectasia in bronchograms makes it uncertain whether such transient changes represent "true" or "false" bronchiectasis. There can be no doubt, however, that pneumonic or atelectatic conditions associated with bronchial distention or distortion may progress, if inadequately treated, to permanent bronchiectasis.

Treatment. Cure of bronchiectasis can be effected only by *resection* of the involved lobes or segments of the lung. The great advances of the last fifteen to twenty years in the surgical techniques of lung resection have made total and subtotal lobectomy a procedure of wide indications in the hands of experienced thoracic surgeons. Even the removal of a lobe on one side and one or more on the other has been accomplished successfully. There has been a progressive decline in operative mortality for unilateral resections, and in most leading clinics it is under 1 per cent. Every case of bronchiectasis, therefore, merits consideration of surgery, and resection is indicated in most children and young adults in whom the disease is unilobar. It is often indicated also when more than one lobe is involved, especially if the right middle lobe or the lingular segment of the left upper lobe is affected together with the lower lobe on the same side. In older persons, or in those with more extensive involvement, the indications for surgery are less clearly defined, but it may be undertaken in selected cases.

The *medical management* of bronchiectasis, though not curative, may accomplish much both in preparation for operation and in prolonging life and preserving the general health of those patients who are unsuitable for operation. Postural drainage is the principal measure for the accomplishment of these ends. In most cases the posture best suited for obtaining effective drainage is hanging head downward from the hips over the side of a bed or high chair. The trunk should incline perpendicularly to the floor and the position be maintained for 20 to 30 minutes. Dislodgment of secretions should be stimulated by deep breathing and by coughing. The postural drainage should be performed frequently during febrile exacerbations—at least four times a day and every 2 hours in severe cases. At night the foot of the bed may be elevated so that the patient sleeps on an incline of 15 to 30 degrees. In some instances the optimal posture for drainage may be best determined by trial. If the principal involvement is in anterior segments of the lung, maximal expectoration is sometimes obtained by lying on the back. Usually some declination of the head and shoulders below the horizontal is necessary.

In severe or neglected cases the accumulation of pus in the bronchi and associated edema of the mucous membranes may block drainage to such an extent that postural drainage does not suffice and bronchoscopic aspiration may be necessary. This usually does not need to be repeated if postural drainage is continued after the obstruction has been relieved. Postural drainage is important not only during exacerbations and febrile episodes, but even after the quantity of sputum has been reduced to a minimal output of only a few cubic centimeters daily. *Every patient with bronchiectasis who has any cough or expectoration whatever or who has ever had a secondary pneumonitis should practice postural drainage at least twice daily, on arising in the morning and before retiring at night.* Even if little or no sputum is obtained at the time, the secretions are usually loosened sufficiently to be coughed up and expectorated more easily afterward. In selected cases, recently developed cough machines have proved of great use in the removal of bronchial secretions.

The drug treatment of bronchiectasis consists principally of *antimicrobial* therapy. For this penicillin is usually the most effective agent, supplemented when appropriate by streptomycin, one of the broader spectrum antibiotics or, in special circumstances, the sulfonamides.

The dosage, routes of administration and combination of agents must depend on the clinical status of the individual case and the immediate purpose to be achieved, as well as on the bacteriologic findings. The immediate objectives of antimicrobial therapy are (1) treatment of acute febrile exacerbations and attacks of secondary pneumonia; (2) control of chronic symptoms and prevention of acute manifestations. An important element of both is the preparation of suitable cases for surgical resection.

In the *treatment of acute manifestations* with fever, penicillin is best given intramuscularly. In early or in mild infections 300,-000 to 600,000 units in a single daily dose of the slowly absorbed procaine penicillin may be sufficient. In the more severe cases, with extensive suppuration, it is best to administer potassium penicillin in aqueous solution every 3 or 4 hours in the total daily dosage of at least one million units (200,000 to 300,000 units, six to eight times daily). Supplementation by dihydrostreptomycin, 1.0 gm. intramuscularly once or twice daily, is indicated when cultures reveal the presence of *Hemophilus influenzae* or *Klebsiella pneumoniae,* or when penicillin-resistant gram-positive organisms are present in abundance. Results with penicillin and dihydrostreptomycin together are usually superior to those with any of the "broad spectrum" antibiotics (chlortetracycline, oxytetracycline, chloramphenicol, erythromycin), unless organisms predominate which are highly resistant to both of the former but highly susceptible to one of the latter. This situation pertains rarely.

Aerosol therapy may be used to supplement antimicrobial therapy by the usual routes. Penicillin and streptomycin are the antibiotics most often administered by inhalation. Ten thousand to 50,000 units of penicillin dissolved in 1.0 cc. of water can be nebulized and inhaled in approximately 10 minutes, and this may be repeated five or six times a day. Streptomycin (or dihydrostreptomycin) in dosage of 25 to 50 mg. per cubic centimeter may be administered in a similar manner. Alevaire, an aqueous solution of Triton WR 1339, may be administered as a detergent aerosol to liquefy thick viscid sputum. It may be used alone for this purpose, or may be employed as a vehicle for penicillin or streptomycin.

In the *control of chronic symptoms,* and in routine preparation for surgery, less intensive antibacterial therapy usually suffices. A reduction of cough and expectoration may be expected from a single daily injection of 300,000 units of procaine penicillin, or by the oral administration of relatively small doses (1.0 gm. per day in divided doses) of chlortetracycline (Aureomycin) or oxytetracycline (Terramycin). It may require a week or longer of such therapy to produce noticeable benefit. The improvement is usually not long sustained after daily treatment is discontinued, and such therapy is not a substitute for postural drainage which should always be continued concurrently. The use of antimicrobial therapy for extended periods is impractical and usuaally not well tolerated. Prevention of exacerbations is better accomplished by short courses, repeated frequently, than by uninterrupted long-term therapy. An exception is in the management of the cases in children of bronchiectasis and bronchopulmonary suppuration associated with cystic fibrosis of the pancreas. Many of these patients require sustained, almost year-around, antimicrobial therapy. In these patients chlortetracycline and oxytetracycline are well tolerated and they are effective, not only in controlling the respiratory tract infection but in improving the general condition and nutritional status. They are administered orally in doses of 7 to 30 mg. per kilo of body weight per day.

Cough mixtures have little place in the treatment of bronchiectasis. Except when cough is exhausting or causes pain, it is undesirable to suppress it. During acute exacerbations codeine in doses of 15 to 30 mg. may be given. Expectorants are usually ineffective. Creosote compounds and guaiacol were formerly much used, but have deservedly fallen into discard. Terpin hydrate in the form of the elixir is useful chiefly as a vehicle for codeine. Ammonium chloride, 0.3 gm., or the iodides of sodium or potassium, 0.3 gm., may be of temporary benefit when the secretions are tenacious.

The treatment of hemoptysis consists principally of complete rest in bed and reassurance. Sedation should be mild. Morphine, if used at all, should be given in a small dose of not more than 8 or 10 mg. and usually not repeated. Larger or repeated doses of morphine suppress respiration and cough and so tend to promote aspiration pneumonia and atelectasis from retained blood and clots. Rarely, hemorrhage may be so severe as to necessitate the induction of artificial pneumothorax, but this is to be avoided unless the hemorrhage is judged to be immediately threatening to life and otherwise uncontrollable.

The treatment of chronic paranasal sinusitis, which is almost always associated, should be conservative in most instances. Radical sinus surgery is no longer considered a necessary preliminary to lobectomy and is often disappointing in its results unless the bronchiectasis has first been eliminated or im-proved. Often there is striking improvement in the sinusitis after lobectomy, and surgical treatment of the sinusitis may then no longer be necessary.

In all cases of bronchiectasis the general health of the patient must be safeguarded with proper attention to diet, adequate rest and avoidance of unnecessary exposure to conditions which promote respiratory infections. When feasible, change of residence to a warm, dry climate may be advantageous. Should this be impossible, prophylactic chemotherapy may be considered, but usually careful regulation of living habits and special attention to continued periodic postural drainage as a matter of personal daily hygiene are sufficient to avoid the secondary infections that may lead to serious exacerbations and complications.

CARL MUSCHENHEIM

References

Adams, R., and Davenport, L. F.: The Technic of Bronchography and a System of Bronchial Nomenclature. J.A.M.A., *118*:111, 1942.

Alexander, J.: Roles of Medicine and Surgery in the Management of Bronchiectasis. Ann. Int. Med., *21*:565, 1944.

Finke, W.: Reversibility of Early Bronchiectasis: Its Implications for Therapy and Prevention. New York State J. Med., *51*:1163, 1951.

Liebow, A. A., Hales, M. R., and Lindskog, G. E.: Enlargement of the Bronchial Arteries and Their Anastomoses with the Pulmonary Arteries in Bronchiectasis. Am. J. Path., *25*:211, 1949.

Lindskog, G. E., and Liebow, A. A.: Thoracic Surgery and Related Pathology. New York, Appleton-Century-Crofts, 1953. Bronchiectasis, pp. 161–189.

Lisa, J. R., and Rosenblatt, M. B.: Bronchiectasis. New York, Oxford University Press, 1943.

McKim, Anson: Bronchiectasis as Seen in an Ambulant Clinic Service. A Follow-up Study of Forty-nine Cases over a Minimum Period of Nine Years. Am. Rev. Tuberc., *66*:457, 1952.

Miller, J. B., and Boyer, E. H.: A Nontoxic Detergent for Aerosol Use in Dissolving Viscid Bronchopulmonary Secretions. J. Pediatrics, *40*:767, 1952.

Peck, M. E., Neerken, A. J., and Salzman, E.: Clinical Experience with Water-Soluble Bronchography Compounds. J. Thoracic Surg., *25*:234, 1953.

Schwachman, H., Silverman, B. K., Patterson, P. R., and Zhentlin, L. J.: Antibiotics in Treatment of Pancreatic Fibrosis, with Emphasis on Terramycin. J.A.M.A., *149*:1101, 1952.

Wynn-Williams, N.: Bronchiectasis: A Study Centered in Bedford and Its Environs. Brit. M. J., *1*:1194, 1953.

FOREIGN BODIES IN THE BRONCHI

The aspiration of foreign bodies into the trachea and bronchi gives rise to a sequence of immediate and late manifestations, some of which are not easily recognized. Without a thorough understanding of these manifestations this important accident cannot be effectively treated and may even be wholly overlooked or confused with pulmonary diseases of entirely different nature. The pioneer work of Chevalier Jackson in the first quarter of this century stands as a monumental achievement, not only for his development of outstanding technical skill in the bronchoscopic manipulations for removal of foreign bodies from the lower air passages, but for his descriptions, worked out in collaboration with Thomas McCrae and others, of the diverse clinical effects of the aspiration of foreign bodies.

Definition. For practical purposes, any object or any solid or semisolid material which gains access to the bronchial system may be defined as a foreign body. It may be endogenous, as a broncholith which has ulcerated into a bronchus from a neighboring lymph node or an aspirated tooth, or it may be exogenous, as a particle of food or a metallic object. Dusts and liquids are not classed as foreign bodies, although their aspiration may also be followed by important and sometimes similar pathologic sequelae.

Etiology. Carelessness is generally the most important cause of foreign body aspiration. In adults the habit of holding in the mouth objects, such as nails, tacks and pins, that may be aspirated if the person is startled or makes a sudden movement is often responsible. In young children the tendency to put any object in the mouth may be irrepressible, but is often influenced by imitation of adults. A frequent cause in young children is nuts or candy containing nuts, which they cannot chew. Hurried eating is a common cause of aspiration of food particles. Aspiration of instruments or dental fillings in the course of dental operations, or during anesthesia, may occur unless special care is taken to avoid such accidents. The variety of objects which may be inhaled is almost unlimited. Pins, nails, screws and coins are the most frequent of the metallic objects. Among the foods small bones, nuts, beans and seeds are the most common. Some of the foods of vegetable origin are of special importance because of the severity of the inflammatory reaction which

they may set up. Of these, the most important is the peanut kernel. Jackson has designated the intense bronchitis which occurs in this group *"vegetal bronchitis,"* and that associated specifically with the aspiration of peanut kernels *"arachidic bronchitis."*

Exogenous foreign bodies are more common than endogenous and, as might be expected, are aspirated more frequently by children than by adults. Foreign bodies are more likely to enter the right main bronchus than the left, the proportion being variously estimated from two to one to five to one.

Morbid Anatomy and Pathologic Physiology. The pathologic changes resulting from foreign body aspiration depend not only on the chemical and physical characters of the body aspirated, but also on the site of lodgment and the length of time that elapses before it is removed or dislodged. Rarely a foreign body may be so large as completely to obstruct the trachea at or above its bifurcation and cause immediate suffocation without the development of any significant local pathology. A nonirritating smooth body which becomes lodged in such manner as to cause no trauma and little obstruction may remain for years without causing appreciable pathologic changes. Usually, however, the consequences of bronchial obstruction ensue: either immediate, if the object itself occludes a passage; or delayed, in which case the obstruction usually is secondary to traumatization, inflammation and infection of the mucous membrane. If obstruction is immediate and complete, the air in the lobes or segments distal to the occlusion is rapidly absorbed. The occluded lobe may collapse, with resulting simple atelectasis, or the alveoli may become filled by noninflammatory edema fluid, a condition sometimes designated "water-logged" or "drowned lung." Most often there is a combination of collapse and accumulation of fluid exudate in varying proportion. A check-valvelike mechanism may permit air to pass into but not out of the obstructed segment, and there then results obstructive emphysema, which, like atelectasis, may affect a lobe or an entire lung if the obstruction is in one of the major bronchi. If obstruction is partial or occurs gradually as a result of swelling of the mucous membrane or the growth of granulations, or if it persists for more than a short time, secondary effects of infection usually appear in the obstructed portion of the lung. There may be early development of massive suppuration and abscess formation, or the inflammation may be less acute and result in chronic fibroid changes and bronchiectasis. Shifting of a foreign body from one location to another is not uncommon, so that pathologic changes are not necessarily restricted to the region where the object finally rests.

Symptoms and Signs. Symptoms at the time of aspiration of a foreign body are variable, depending on the site and character of

"audible slap" synchronous with respiration or with cough, and a "palpatory thud" which is appreciated by placing the examining finger over the cricoid cartilage or the trachea. These signs result from movement of the foreign body with respiration and cough. Except for harshness of the breath sounds and coarse rales, there may be no other abnormal physical signs while the foreign body remains in the trachea.

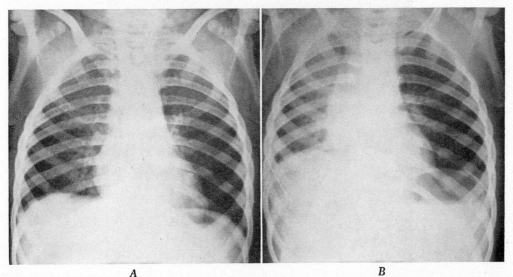

Fig. 124. *A,* Obstructive emphysema of left lung caused by foreign body (mashed potato) in left main bronchus. The hyperaeration is barely appreciable in the inspiratory phase. *B,* Expiratory phase, showing displacement of the mediastinum to opposite side and the more conspicuous hyperaeration of the left lung. These effects are due to trapping of air by the check-valve action of the bronchial obstruction.

the object and on the part of the tracheo-bronchial system which it reaches. A large foreign body which completely obstructs the trachea may cause immediate death from asphyxia. A small one which passes directly into a bronchus may cause little distress, and symptoms may be so slight as scarcely to attract attention. Usually there is choking, gagging, severe cough, dyspnea and cyanosis. These symptoms lessen if the object passes from the trachea into a bronchus. The distress is particularly severe if the body is movable. The cough associated with a foreign body in the trachea may, particularly in children, have a croupy character, which results from subglottic edema, or it may be paroxysmal and resemble that of pertussis. A loud wheeze, designated by Jackson as the "asthmatoid wheeze," is usually present. This may often be better heard by placing the stethoscope bell at the mouth than by auscultation over the chest. In addition, there may be an

After the passage of an object from the trachea into a bronchus there may be an entire subsidence of symptoms, and a quiescent period ensues lasting for days or weeks, to be followed by fever, return or exacerbation of cough, and appearance of expectoration. If the initial symptoms have been overlooked or if the possibility of a quiescent period is not appreciated, this phase may be mistaken for the onset of a simple pneumonia. The physical signs are variable, but the characteristic signs of pneumonic consolidation, such as bronchial breath sounds and bronchophony, are not found. If a major bronchus has been entirely occluded, there are the usual signs of an obstructed lobe or lung. These consist of decreased expansion, flatness to percussion, diminished fremitus, and absence of breath sounds. There are few or no rales. Usually some displacement of the mediastinum to the affected side occurs, the degree depending on whether simple atelectasis predominates or whether there has been considerable accumulation of secretions in the blocked segments of the lung parenchyma. If obstruction is partial, there is usually a constant sonorous rhonchus, more conspicuous during expiration, and sometimes best elicited by having the patient lie on the affected side. With incomplete obstruction, dullness, diminished breath sounds and coarse rales may be present, or there may be the signs of obstructive emphysema, with hyperresonance and markedly diminished breath sounds. When these signs of obstructive emphysema are present, a confirmatory shifting of the mediastinum with respiration may be elicited, especially on forced expiration. When there is little obstruction, the only abnormal physical signs may be rales over a small area. Such a patch then usually corresponds to the position of the foreign body. There may, however, be rales distant from the site of the foreign body. Such distant signs, which may even be on the opposite side, arise from shifting of the foreign body or from spread of infected secretions from the obstructed to other parts of the lungs.

A distinctive feature of the clinical picture resulting from aspiration of foreign bodies of vegetable nature, especially nuts, peas or beans, is the acuteness of onset of the general symptoms and the severity of toxemia. High fever rapidly develops with severe dyspnea and extreme cyanosis. There is marked secretion, and the severity of the symptoms appears to be due to the intensity of the tracheobronchitis from chemical irritation rather than to the mechanical effects of obstruction.

The late sequelae of foreign body aspiration are most commonly the formation of a bronchial stricture and the development of lung abscess and bronchiectasis. Less common complications are empyema and spontaneous pneumothorax.

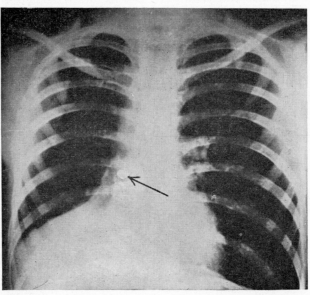

Fig. 125. Foreign body (aspirated tooth) in bronchus with resulting atelectasis of middle lobe. Note elevation of right hemidiaphragm, the contour of which merges medially with the dense triangular shadow of the shrunken lobe.

Diagnosis. Most important in the diagnosis is a careful history. Recognition of the possibility of a symptomless interval between the initial gagging and choking and the later symptoms resulting from obstruction and infection is important. The fact that there is sometimes little or no distress initially, and the possibility that an aspirated object may be believed to have been swallowed, must always be considered when the physical signs suggest the presence of bronchial obstruction. In children, diphtheria and pneumonia are the conditions most easily confused, but the differentiation is not difficult and depends on careful physical examination. In adults other causes of bronchial obstruction, such as bronchial tumors, may give identical physical signs, but here the more gradual onset and the more reliable history usually make differentiation easy. The roentgenogram is of great assistance, not only in the recognition of metallic and other opaque foreign bodies, but also in the diagnosis of nonopaque foreign bodies. In connection with the latter the various roentgenographic changes associated with bronchial obstruction, such as atelectasis, obstructive emphysema and obstructive edema or pneumonitis, are often so characteristic as to make confusion with simple pneumonias unlikely. Careful correlation of the roentgenographic appearance with the physical signs will make the differentiation between obstructive and nonobstructive processes certain in most instances. In the absence of a clear history of foreign body aspiration the cause of obstruction may be determined only by bronchoscopy.

Prognosis and Treatment. The prognosis is poor in most cases unless the foreign body is removed. Bronchoscopic removal is therefore indicated, whenever possible. Spontaneous expulsion by coughing is so rare that it should never be expected. The urgency of the indication for bronchoscopy is greatest when the clinical features indicate the presence of a movable foreign body in the trachea, for there is danger that it may become impacted in the larynx after cough. Digital removal or attempts to eliminate a foreign body by inversion of the patient should never be undertaken because of the same danger. The substances of vegetable origin also should be removed bronchoscopically as soon as possible. Because of the acuteness and severity of the toxemic and infectious complications in these cases the immediate prognosis is grave, and the shorter the stay of the foreign body the better the outlook. In other cases it is well to take time for thorough study, but usually no special preparation is necessary before bronchoscopy may be done. In infants and small children, especially, the occurrence of subglottic edema is common, and tracheotomy may be necessary. In cases of long standing with much suppuration, definite abscess formation or bronchiectasis, postural drainage is indicated after the foreign body has been removed. Whenever the presence of severe infection is manifested by high fever and leukocytosis, antimicrobial therapy is indicated as ancillary treatment. Penicillin in dosage of a million or more units daily, in divided doses administered intramuscularly every 3 or 4 hours, is usually the drug of choice. As in other suppurative mixed infections of the lung, aqueous solutions of potassium penicillin given frequently and in high dosage are more reliable than the slowly absorbed preparations of procaine penicillin which are generally used in simple pneumonias.

The surgical treatment of chronic lung abscess resulting from a foreign body that has not been promptly removed is similar to the treatment of chronic lung abscess from other causes, and usually consists of pulmonary resection.

CARL MUSCHENHEIM

References

Graham, E. A., Singer, J. J., and Ballon, H. C.: Surgical Diseases of the Chest. Foreign Bodies in the Respiratory Tract. Philadelphia, Lea and Febiger, 1935, pp. 525–531.
Jackson, C.: The Mechanism of Physical Signs of Foreign Bodies in the Bronchi. Am. J. M. Sc., 165: 313, 1923.
———, and McCrae, T.: Overlooked Cases of Foreign Body in the Air and Food Passages. Brit. M. J., 2:686, 693, 1925.
McCrae, T.: Lumleian Lectures on the Clinical Features of Foreign Bodies in the Bronchi. Lancet, 1: 735, 787, 838, 1924.

DISEASES OF THE LUNGS

PULMONARY FUNCTION IN HEALTH AND DISEASE

Introduction. The lungs, heart and circulation have together the primary bodily function of transporting the essential respiratory gases, oxygen and carbon dioxide, between the tissues and the outside atmospheric air. In this activity the lungs perform three basic services: (1) *ventilatory,* the displacement of air into and out of pulmonary tissues; (2) *alveolar,* the distribution of inhaled air to perfused alveolar spaces, and the conveyance (diffusion) of oxygen and carbon dioxide between alveolar air and pulmonary capillary blood; (3) *vascular,* the passage of the entire blood circulation through the pulmonary vascular bed. In addition, there is the subsidiary but important "self-cleansing" function of lungs and air passages, by which these structures are rendered and maintained free from foreign particles and bacterial invasion.

The pulmonary structures themselves are supplied by the bronchial circulation: the bronchial arteries branching from the aorta, and the bronchial venous flow emptying in part into the azygos system, in part by way of the smallest branches of the pulmonary veins directly into the main pulmonary vascular stream. This flow is estimated as about 2 per cent of total blood flow in normal subjects.

The pulmonary capillaries perform a secondary function at times in filtering out particles such as bacteria, small blood clots, fat emboli or air bubbles, that may have entered the venous blood. Whether there is any form of internal secretion from the lungs is not known.

Ventilation. Effective pulmonary ventilation depends upon patent airways; elastic and expansile lungs and tracheobronchial tree, to provide amplitude of respiration; terminal alveolar structures that can be evenly aerated, with alveolar walls that provide a large surface of well perfused capillaries; and an adequate musculoskeletal apparatus of chest wall and related structures, so as to move large volumes of air in and out of the lungs rapidly, under conditions of maximum stress.

The anatomic structures providing pulmonary ventilation may be divided into an upper and a lower half. The upper, consisting of the first five ribs, their spinal articulations and associated muscles, the upper sternum, and accessory neck and shoulder muscles, expands the upper lobes of the lungs (upper and middle on the right), largely through upward and forward movement of the anterior chest. This is the so-called upper-costal respiration, as described by Keith. The lower half, consisting of the sixth to tenth ribs and related structures, the diaphragm and abdominal musculature, expanding the two lower lobes, has a threefold type of movement: a lateral widening, a forward and upward movement anteriorly and the forward and downward piston-like movement of the dome of the diaphragm with each inspiration, accompanied by relaxation of the abdominal wall. These complex movements are called costodiaphragmatic respiration.

Lung Volumes. This is a general term, denoting the volumes of air contained in the lungs in different chest positions; also volumes of air that can be inhaled or exhaled from specific inspiratory or expiratory positions. The components of lung volume, according to a recently revised nomenclature, are shown in Figure 126, and may be defined as follows: *Residual volume* is the volume of air remaining in the lungs at the end of a maximal expiration. Its normal value is about 1500 cc. *Expiratory reserve volume* is the maximal volume of air that can be exhaled at the end of a normal quiet expiration. The normal value is about 1000 cc. *Tidal volume* is the actual volume of a single breath. Its normal value at rest is about 500 cc. *Inspiratory reserve volume* is the maximal volume of air that can be inspired, starting from a normal inspiratory position. Its normal value is about 3000 cc. *Vital capacity* is the maximal volume of air that can be exhaled after a maximal inspiration. Its normal average value is about 4000 to 5000 cc. *Total lung capacity* is the total volume of air in the lungs at maximal inspiration. Its normal average value is about 5500 to 6000 cc.

Vital capacity and other lung volumes, except residual volume, are readily measured by a spirometer. Normal values for vital capacity can be measured by West's simple formula: for males, V.C. (liters) $= 2.5 \times$ body surface in square meters; for females, V.C. $= 2.0 \times$ body surface. Baldwin's equation is more accurate (see Table 1).

per minute; for females, 100 liters per minute. The formula of Baldwin et al. is given in Table 1.

In determining the extent to which the ventilation in a given degree of exercise or physical stress encroaches upon the maximum breathing capacity, a useful concept is the *breathing reserve*. This function is the

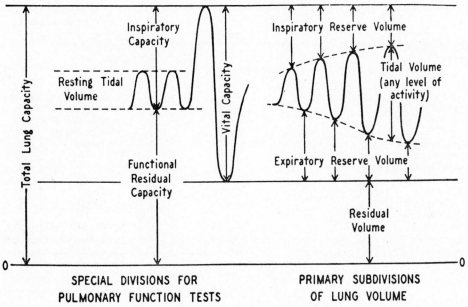

SPECIAL DIVISIONS FOR
PULMONARY FUNCTION TESTS

PRIMARY SUBDIVISIONS
OF LUNG VOLUME

Fig. 126. Subdivisions of the lung volume.

Residual volume can be measured by dilution, rebreathing a foreign gas in a closed circuit; or by "washing out" the nitrogen in the lung by a period of pure oxygen breathing, and measuring this nitrogen volume. The ratio of residual to total lung volume is a useful function, a significant increase indicating emphysema (see Table 1).

Maximum Breathing Capacity, and Graphic Registration of Breathing. The maximum breathing capacity, or maximum minute ventilation, is the maximum volume of air that can be breathed, by voluntary effort, per minute. Since it registers speed as well as amplitude of ventilation, it is a better index of ventilatory capacity than is the vital capacity. It can be measured either by collecting the expired air, or by having the subject rebreathe, through a system of low-resistance tubing, in and out of a small spirometer of about 10 liters' capacity and recording graphically the motion of the spirometer bell on a moving drum. The average normal value for males is 125 to 150 liters

maximum breathing capacity minus the individual's actual ventilation under the given conditions. In normal subjects, as well as in many forms of chronic pulmonary disease, the phenomenon of dyspnea is fairly well correlated with the breathing reserve. Dyspnea is first noticed when the breathing reserve is reduced to about 65 or 70 per cent of the maximum breathing capacity.

A simple index of speed, or conversely of retardation, of breathing is the timed vital capacity of Gaensler; normally 90 per cent of a vital capacity can be exhaled in 2 seconds, 100 per cent in 3 seconds (see Table 1). A similar measure is the air velocity index, % of predicted M.B.C./% of predicted Vit. Cap. If the actual M.B.C. is reduced more than the Vit. Cap., the patient's ventilatory defect is chiefly obstructive; if less, chiefly restrictive.

Ventilatory equivalent (Table 1) is the amount of ventilation needed for each 100 cc. of oxygen consumption; it is reduced in hyperpneic states.

Spirogram. The graphic registration of breathing on a moving drum is frequently valuable in recording exactly the pattern of a patient's respiration under various conditions. It registers accurately such changes as reduction in lung volumes in pulmonary fibrosis, the retardation of expiration in asthma and emphysema, the changes following surgery or the responses to medical therapy. It is thus both a qualitative and quantitative record of performance.

the lung's elastic recoil (elastance); (b) frictional and other resistance of moving tissues; (c) resistance of air flow in the air passages. Lung compliance is the reciprocal of elastance, and a normal average figure is 0.22; that is, 0.22 liters of ventilation for each 1.0 cm. H_2O change in intrapleural pres-

Table 1. Normal Values for Ventilatory Function Tests

TEST	MALE	FEMALE	UNIT OF MEASUREMENT
Maximum Breathing Capacity*†	100–150	70–120	l./min. at 37° C.
Vital Capacity*‡	3–5	2.5–3.5	liters
Total Lung Capacity	$\dfrac{\text{Vital Capacity}}{80} \times 100$		liters
Residual Volume**	20–35		% of Total Lung Capacity
Minute Ventilation, basal*	2.5–5.0		l./min./sq.m.B.S.***
Oxygen Uptake, basal*	110–150		cc./min./sq.m.B.S.
Ventilatory Equivalent, basal*	2.2–2.6		l./100 cc. oxygen
Alveolar nitrogen after 7 min. of oxygen breathing	less than 2.5		% nitrogen
Bronchospirometry, right lung			
Oxygen Uptake	52–58		% of total
Ventilation	52–58		% of total
Vital Capacity	52–58		% of total
Timed Vital Capacity*			
First second	at least 75		% of total Vital Capacity
First two seconds	at least 90		% of total Vital Capacity
First three seconds	100		% of total Vital Capacity
Air Velocity Index*	0.8–1.2		% of predicted MBC
			% of predicted VC

* Decreasing with age
** Increasing with age
*** Liters per minute per square meter body surface area
                            Regression Formulas:[2]

†	Males:	$[86.5 - (0.522 \times \text{age in yr.})] \times \text{sq.m. B.S.}$
	Females:	$[71.3 - (0.474 \times \text{age in yr.})] \times \text{sq.m. B.S.}$
‡	Males:	$[27.63 - (0.112 \times \text{age in yr.})] \times \text{height in cm.}$
	Females:	$[21.78 - (0.101 \times \text{age in yr.})] \times \text{height in cm.}$

Work of Breathing. An important recent development is the analysis of the work or effort involved in pulmonary ventilation; this has been shown to be in many instances well correlated with clinical dyspnea.

The simplest index of ventilatory effort is the intrapleural pressure. A normal resting ventilation of 5 to 8 liters per minute is accomplished by small change in intrapleural pressure, from about −3 cm. H_2O in expiration to −6 cm. H_2O in inspiration. Further analysis has been achieved by recording intra-esophageal pressures, which provide a measure of intrathoracic pressure change. The work of breathing has to overcome: (a)

sure. Marked changes in these relations take place in disease.

Alveolar Function. *Distribution of Inhaled Tidal Air; Intrapulmonary Mixing.* Of the 500 cc. of tidal air inhaled at each breath, about 150 cc. reaches only the pulmonary "dead space," i.e., the oronasal passages and tracheobronchial tree, and is thus exhaled again, without change. The 350 cc. of "effective tidal air" is, however, well distributed, in normal persons, throughout the pulmonary alveolar air spaces. Furthermore, at least some of the capillaries lining the walls of almost all ventilated alveoli are also perfused by the blood stream passing through the lungs. This statement has certain exceptions: In some normal persons at rest there are alveoli that are ventilated but not perfused.

In chronic pulmonary disease, particularly emphysema with its greatly distorted and dilated alveoli, this balanced relationship between ventilation and perfusion of alveoli breaks down, and there are both overventilated and poorly perfused alveoli, and other large stagnant alveolar spaces that are perfused with blood, but are inadequately ventilated. A simple test for the measurement of this important function is the "index of mixing," or "pulmonary emptying rate." The subject breathes pure oxygen for a period of 7 minutes; and the adequacy of mixing of air within the lungs is tested by the completeness with which the inert gas, nitrogen, has been washed out of an "alveolar" (i.e., deep expiratory) sample of air taken at the end of this 7-minute period. In normal persons, the nitrogen concentration remaining in the alveolar air after breathing pure oxygen for 7 minutes is less than 2.5 per cent. In moderate emphysema this residual nitrogen will be from 4 to 8 per cent; in some advanced cases from 10 to 15 per cent.

There are several other methods of measuring the distribution of inhaled air.

In pulmonary disease, uneven distribution of inhaled air with many alveoli inadequately aerated is obviously a potent cause of arterial anoxia.

Diffusion. In normal persons at rest the blood leaving the capillaries of the pulmonary alveoli is in equilibrium with the alveolar air, so far as partial pressures of carbon dioxide are concerned, such alveolar and arterial partial pressures being of the order of 37 to 42 mm. of mercury. There is an almost exact equilibrium also between alveolar oxygen tension and the partial pressure of oxygen in the blood leaving perfused pulmonary capillaries, alveolar oxygen pressures being not more than 1 or 2 mm. higher than that in the capillaries. In the arterial blood, however, the oxygen pressure is about 9 mm. of mercury lower than that of the alveolar air. This is due to a small amount of "venous admixture," some venous blood coming in by way of the bronchial circulation, as previously mentioned, and some from unaerated or poorly aerated pulmonary capillary blood.

The "oxygen diffusing capacity" is defined as the volume of oxygen absorbed per minute, per unit difference of mean partial pressures of oxygen between alveolus and pulmonary capillary; average normal value 15.

An average set of measurements of partial pressures of respiratory gases in air and

blood, in a normal man at rest, is given in Table 2. The "alveolar-arterial" (AA) oxygen gradient here is 103.5—94.2 =9.3 mm. Hg.

Respiratory Gas Exchange between Alveolar Air and Capillary Blood in the Lungs. The physicochemical processes whereby carbon dioxide is eliminated and oxygen taken up by the blood in the pulmonary capillaries may be outlined schematically as a series of steps. Actually, of course, all these processes take place not stepwise, but simultaneously.

1. When carbon dioxide, at a pressure of, e.g., 43 mm. of mercury in the venous blood, comes in contact with alveolar air having a carbon dioxide pressure of, e.g., 38 mm. of

Table 2. Partial Pressures of Respiratory Gases in Air and Blood (in mm. Hg)

(From Riley and Cournand, 1949)

GAS	INSPIRED (ATMOSPHERIC) AIR	ALVEOLAR AIR	ARTERIAL BLOOD	VENOUS BLOOD
Oxygen............	158.0	103.5	94.2	38.0
Carbon dioxide.....	0.03	37.8	37.8	42.5
Nitrogen..........	597.0	571.7	571.7	571.7
Water............	5.0	47.0	47.0	47.0
Total barometric pressure..........	760.0	760.0	750.7	699.2

mercury, there is a flow of carbon dioxide across the membrane which continues until equilibrium is established. This involves a redistribution of all carbon dioxide in the blood, both free and combined, the process taking place according to the well-known Henderson-Hasselbalch equation: $pH = 6.1 + \log \frac{BHCO_3}{H_2CO_3}$. Since the ratio of bicarbonate ($BHCO_3$) to dissolved carbon dioxide remains relatively constant, an approximate value of 20 to 1, this means that for every 1 cc. of carbon dioxide given up as carbonic acid, there will be 20 cc. eliminated from combination as bicarbonate.

2. Oxygen, at a pressure of 103 mm. of mercury in the alveolar air, passes into the blood, oxygenating the hemoglobin to 98 per cent of capacity. In other words, at this oxygen pressure 98 per cent of the blood hemoglobin is in loose combination with oxygen in the form of the specific chemical oxyhemoglobin, and 2 per cent exists as re-

duced hemoglobin. It requires about 140–150 mm. of mercury of oxygen pressure to "saturate" the blood hemoglobin, converting it 100 per cent into the form of oxyhemoglobin. ("Venous admixture" reduces arterial oxygen saturation to 96 per cent.)

3. Oxyhemoglobin, being more acid than reduced hemoglobin, holds more cell potassium, thus converting bicarbonate to H_2CO_3 for diffusion out as CO_2 gas.

4. The rate of the chemical reaction releasing CO_2 is much too slow for the short time (about 0.6 second) available for gas exchange in the capillaries. An enzyme, carbonic anhydrase, present in the red cell greatly accelerates this reaction, and CO_2 exchange thus proceeds in great part directly between red cell and alveolar air.

5. To maintain the Gibbs-Donnan ratio across the semipermeable membrane of the red cells, i.e.,

$$\frac{HCO_3\text{–plasma}}{HCO_3\text{– cells}} = \frac{Cl\text{–plasma}}{k_1 Cl\text{– cells}} = \frac{k_2 H^+ cells}{H^+ plasma},$$

bicarbonate ions enter the red cell (only partially restoring $HCO_3–$ concentration), and chloride ions leave the red cell. A small amount of water (about 2 per cent of cell water) leaves the red cell, as there has been a greater decrease in the total number of osmotically active particles within the red cell as compared with the plasma.

6. An additional quantity of carbon dioxide is given up directly by the hemoglobin, from combination as carbhemoglobin. This form of carbon dioxide, while only about 8 to 10 per cent of the total reservoir of carbon dioxide in the blood, is a labile form and provides about 25 per cent of the carbon dioxide exchange occurring normally under conditions of rest, in the pulmonary and tissue capillaries. This also is a rapid chemical reaction.

The decreased blood acidity from loss of carbon dioxide, when combined with the increased acidity from oxyhemoglobin formation, results in a small net change in pH (an alkaline shift to the extent of 0.02 increase in pH) as the blood changes from venous to arterial.

Respiratory Stimulus. The respiratory center is located in the reticular substance in the lower part of the medulla, anterior or ventral to the nuclear masses forming the floor of the fourth ventricle. While there is evidence for a further localization into a ventral inspiratory and a dorsal expiratory center, it now appears more probable that the essential rhythmicity of respiratory activity is inherent in all of this reticular substance.

When respiration becomes more active, with hyperpnea, excitatory impulses in the inspiratory center increase, both by increase in activity of previously functioning neurons, and by "recruitment" of previously quiescent neurons. In addition, expiration becomes a positive and active function.

As each inspiration proceeds, inhibitory impulses from all moving respiratory structures stream into the respiratory center by way of the vagus nerves, increasing with increasing chest and lung expansion, eventually stopping inspiration and initiating the expiratory phase of the cycle. The reverse occurs as expiration ends and the excitatory impulses of inspiration take over. This alternating inhibitory and excitatory activity is essentially that long known as the Hering-Breuer reflex.

The actual form of respiration is determined by many influences, voluntary and reflex, physiologic and pathologic.

Of the chemical regulators of respiration, the carbon dioxide tension of the arterial blood provides the dominant respiratory stimulus. Two other independent stimuli are recognized, blood acidity, and anoxia, the latter acting chiefly through the carotid sinus mechanism. These three can be shown to act additively upon the respiratory center. There are other stimuli to respiration, not yet identified, as for example in muscular exercise, where the levels of pCO_2, pH and arterial pO_2 all together do not nearly account for the actual ventilation observed.

An aspect of the CO_2 stimulus that is important in disease is that upon sustained exposure to low CO_2 tensions, the respiratory center becomes more sensitive to CO_2 as a stimulus; while upon sustained exposure to high CO_2 tensions the center becomes less sensitive.

Pulmonary Blood Flow. The entire cardiac output from the right heart, averaging 3.1 liters per minute per square meter of body surface, or about 5.4 liters per minute for a normal person at rest, is ejected into the pulmonary artery, and a slightly larger flow (augmented by a part of the bronchial circulation) empties into the pulmonary veins and left auricle.

The pulmonary arterial pressure is low, 18

to 28 mm. of mercury in systole, and 5 to 8 mm. in diastole. Pressure in the larger pulmonary veins and left auricle is about -2 mm. of mercury during inspiration and 8 mm. during expiration.

Thus the entire pulmonary circulation is a low-tension affair, indicating large channels of flow with low resistance.

Pulmonary Function in Muscular Exercise. In strenuous muscular exercise the oxygen consumption of the body per minute may increase from 250 or 300 cc. at rest up to 4000 cc. or higher. Pulmonary ventilation can also readily increase ten- or fifteen-fold, so that adequate aeration of the alveoli is rarely if ever a limiting factor in muscular exercise in normal subjects. Blood flow, however, probably does not increase much beyond 30 liters per minute, a sixfold rise. The additional transport of oxygen, between tissues and lungs, is achieved by a larger arteriovenous difference; in other words, more oxygen is withdrawn by the tissues from each unit of blood flowing, and the venous blood is thus more unsaturated as it arrives in the pulmonary circulation.

There is a marked widening of pulmonary vascular channels to accommodate this large increase in flow, so that pulmonary arterial pressure rises only slightly in moderate exercise, and always less than the increase in flow. It is astonishing that the lungs can ventilate 80 to 90 liters per minute while being perfused by blood at a rate of a pint a second.

An essential feature of this pulmonary vascular dilatation in exercise is the increased number and area of perfused capillaries, so that the "total diffusing capacity" of the lungs increases, reaching a maximum at an exercise of about 1500 cc. oxygen consumption per minute. A high pressure gradient of oxygen, moreover, between alveolus and pulmonary capillary is required in the exercise state, the "alveolar-arterial" oxygen gradient rising to 16 mm. Hg (normal resting 7 to 11) in mild exercise, and to 30 mm. Hg in moderately severe exercise.

A further consideration of importance in pulmonary disease is the large reserve of functioning tissue present in normal lungs. Recent studies have demonstrated that, after total operative removal of one lung, a person can perform maximal exercise with no loss of breathing capacity, and apparently with normal circulatory response, so long as there is no emphysema or other abnormality in the remaining lung. In special instances of pulmonary disease as much as two thirds or three quarters of total lung tissue may be completely functionless, yet with the patient suffering no physical disability on moderate activity, so long as the remaining lung tissue is normal.

Maintenance of Normal Pulmonary Structures: Self-Cleansing Function of Lungs. This function is of special importance to structures, such as the tracheobronchial tree and lungs, constantly exposed to unfavorable agents, physical, chemical and bacteriologic, that may enter with the inspired air.

The action of the ciliated cells in the respiratory mucous membrane, and such reflexes as sneezing, coughing and glottic spasm, are among the normal mechanisms for eliminating foreign materials from the tracheobronchial air passages.

Disorders of Pulmonary Function in Disease. Some of the more important diseases producing pulmonary symptoms or symptom complexes will be reviewed briefly.

Pulmonary Insufficiency: Methods of Measurement. As indicated earlier in this chapter, the methods most useful in the clinical analysis of pulmonary function are (1) lung volumes, especially vital capacity and residual air; (2) maximum breathing capacity and graphic registration of breathing; (3) "index of mixing"; (4) pulmonary ventilation and oxygen consumption, at rest and during and after a standard exercise period; (5) arterial blood, for carbon dioxide content, pH and oxygen saturation and capacity, an arterial sample being drawn at rest and another just after the standard exercise. Special techniques may provide additional important data: (6) bronchospirometry to measure the performance of each lung separately; (7) cardiac catheterization, for cardiac output, and pulmonary arterial and right heart pressures; (8) intra-esophageal pressures and ventilatory flow rates, to define effort of breathing.

Pulmonary Insufficiency: Classification. In accordance with the description of pulmonary functions, as given earlier, the forms of clinical pulmonary insufficiency may be broadly classified as in Table 3, together with the chief type of symptomatology produced by each.

This brief classification is oversimplified: certain categories are left out, such as the vascular or cardiac manifestations of pulmonary hypertension, and the symptoms, general and local, of pulmonary infection. Also, functionally a disease usually consists of more than one form of dysfunction. A physiologic analysis requires evaluation of all forms of insufficiency involved in a given case, and the relative importance of each.

Restrictive Ventilatory Insufficiency. This is perhaps the commonest clinical form of pulmonary insufficiency; it is certainly the form which is found more frequently by itself, as the sole cause of symptoms or disability.

Table 3. Forms of Pulmonary Insufficiency

DYSFUNCTION	TYPE	SYMPTOMS
Ventilatory Restrictive Obstructive Congestive	Mechanical	Dyspnea
Alveolorespiratory Distributive Diffusional	Mechanical, physico- chemical	Hyperpnea, anoxia

The intrapulmonary diseases causing restrictive ventilatory insufficiency are those associated with diffuse fibrosis of the lungs. A large proportion of cases of silicosis are in this group (excluding silicosis complicated by emphysema); nonemphysematous fibroid tuberculosis; pulmonary fibrosis secondary to bronchiectasis or other chronic infection, when not complicated by emphysema; some cases of sarcoidosis of Boeck; postradiation fibrosis.

The physiologic characteristics of this group are as follows: Lung volumes are more or less symmetrically reduced, in most cases. Maximum breathing capacity is reduced in almost all cases. The form of the spirogram is normal. There is a tendency to tachypnea and hyperventilation in the more advanced cases, more marked in exercise, probably owing to hyperactive Hering-Breuer reflexes. Correspondingly, blood carbon dioxide values are somewhat low, and arterial pH_S somewhat high.

Dyspnea on exertion, which is the chief symptom and occurs in the more severe of these cases, is associated with decreased breathing reserve, a combination of increased actual ventilation and decreased breathing capacity. Effort of breathing is increased, lung "compliance" much diminished.

The only other symptoms commonly found in this group are those due to bronchial irritation and chronic bronchitis in many cases, with cough and sometimes sputum.

Numerous extrapulmonary conditions may cause restrictive ventilatory insufficiency by diminishing breathing capacity, such as hydrothorax, pneumothorax, pleural fibrosis, kyphoscoliosis, arthritis of the spine, thoracoplasty.

Obstructive Ventilatory Insufficiency. Bronchial asthma and obstructive emphysema are the most important diseases in this group. The pathologic physiology in both is basically similar. Since the entire tracheobronchial tree dilates with inspiration, bronchiolar narrowing is relieved in the inspiratory state, and the patient tends to maintain this position and increase it during exertion. With the progressive loss of tissue elasticity and dissolution of alveolar walls that take place in emphysema, the hyperinflation becomes fixed. While the hyperinflated state relieves bronchiolar obstruction, it embarrasses the mechanics of breathing. The chronically contracted flattened diaphragm in particular reduces the costodiaphragmatic phase of respiration.

Residual volume is much increased (over 36 per cent of total lung volume), vital capacity reduced, maximum breathing capacity much diminished, to 30 per cent or 20 per cent of normal. The spirogram shows greatly retarded expiration, "trapping" of air on successive deep breaths and extreme hyperinflation on maximum ventilation. Distribution of inhaled air to the lungs is very uneven, as are the ventilation-perfusion relations generally; some regions overventilated and poorly perfused with blood (increased "dead space" ventilation), others perfused but non-ventilated (increased "venous admixture"). There is hyperpnea at rest and exercise in mild to moderate forms, and yet progressive arterial anoxia as the condition becomes more marked, aggravated in exercise; arterial oxygen saturation 90 to 80 per cent at rest, 70 to 60 per cent after exercise.

In advanced emphysema, elimination of carbon dioxide may be compromised and blood CO_2 increased. This engenders a vicious cycle: high arterial pCO_2 diminishes the sensitivity of the respiratory center, and CO_2 retention is thus further increased.

Loss of pulmonary compliance greatly increases effort of breathing, as does the increased resistance due to air-passage obstruction. Dyspnea, both exertional and at rest, is accounted for by the diminished ventilatory capacity, hyperventilation and increased ventilatory effort. The muscular act of breathing becomes asynergic and uncoordinated. Owing in part to marked diminution in the number of pulmonary capillaries, also sometimes to secondary pulmonary arteriosclerosis, the pulmonary arterial pressure is elevated in advanced cases of emphysema, and this may progress eventually to right heart failure with systemic congestion and edema.

Pulmonary arterial pressures of 60/30 or 70/40 are not infrequent.

From this will be seen that in emphysema, while obstructive ventilatory insufficiency is the primary and dominant form of dysfunction, practically all other forms are also involved. Thus the maldistribution of air, an alveolar respiratory dysfunction, leads to arterial anoxia, and in emphysema particularly, pulmonary vascular function is disturbed. In addition, the maintenance of pulmonary structures in these diseases is inadequate, and the cough and sputum of chronic bronchitis greatly aggravate the dyspnea and other symptoms.

In uncomplicated bronchial asthma, obstruction of air passages is the dominant factor, leading to increased ventilatory effort, poor air distribution and hyperpnea.

Congestive Ventilatory Insufficiency. This is suggested as a third category in the ventilatory group, to describe the phenomena in early or moderate left-sided heart failure, such as mitral valvular disease or left ventricular failure. These patients are dyspneic on exertion, yet have normal lung volumes and breathing capacity and are only slightly hyperpneic. It is found that the effort of breathing is increased in these patients during exercise, probably associated with increased pulmonary congestion in the exercise state.

In advanced left-sided congestive failure, vital capacity and maximum breathing capacity are also reduced. Pulmonary arterial pressures may increase to 100/50 or higher.

Alveolorespiratory Insufficiency. Abnormality in distribution of inhaled air has been sufficiently illustrated in the discussion of asthma and emphysema. However, the general phenomenon of inadequate aeration of alveolar capillaries that are being perfused with blood (venous admixture) is a cause of anoxia in many other diseases, such as acute and chronic pneumonia, carcinoma of the lung, bronchial obstruction or occlusion, or massive collapse of the lung. Arterial anoxia is common in pulmonary embolism with infarction.

Disturbance of diffusion of gases across the alveolocapillary membrane, when the alveoli themselves are well aerated, is found in pulmonary edema and in some forms of bronchopneumonia. When arterial anoxia occurs in congestive heart failure, it is often on this basis.

In addition there is a special group of fibrotic pulmonary diseases with particular thickening of the alveolocapillary surfaces, in which diffusional disturbance is paramount, the syndrome of diffusion insufficiency, or alveolar capillary block. This is a clinical entity, characterized by extreme hyperventilation, decreased vital capacity, but relatively normal maximum breathing capacity, and arterial anoxia, usually slight at rest, but markedly increased after exercise. Diseases producing this physiologic state include beryllium and other granulomatosis of the lung, scleroderma of the lung, some cases of sarcoidosis and certain rare forms of nonspecific pulmonary fibrosis.

Therapy. The principles of treatment follow the categories of pulmonary dysfunction as already described. For ventilatory insufficiency of the restrictive type, correction of anatomic faults can sometimes be achieved, such as removal of intrapleural air or fluid, surgery for spinal or chest deformities, an abdominal belt for a hypertonic flattened diaphragm. Restriction of physical activity may be necessary. For obstructive ventilatory insufficiency, bronchodilator agents are of primary importance. Expectorants are sometimes helpful to clear the air passages. Breathing exercises, if practiced persistently, may aid some patients. Positive pressure breathing is often valuable in severe asthma. In all dyspneic states not otherwise relieved, and for symptoms of anoxia, including cyanosis (i.e., in alveolar-respiratory insufficiency), oxygen therapy should be considered. With mild symptoms this may be more trouble than it is worth, but in the more severe forms it almost always gives relief, administered either intermittently or continuously.

In advanced pulmonary emphysema with both arterial anoxia and carbon dioxide retention, the effect of carbon dioxide as a respiratory stimulant is depressed, and such patients depend in part on their anoxic stimulus for this function. In such cases oxygen therapy may decrease ventilation further, and blood CO_2 may rise to toxic levels (90 to 100 volumes per 100 cc.), the so-called "CO_2 narcosis."

For such cases, and in fact for many patients in severe ventilatory insufficiency, artificial respirators, especially those providing inspiratory positive pressure ventilation, usually with oxygen or high oxygen mixtures, may give great relief clinically, even when used only at intervals during the day and for short periods.

DICKINSON W. RICHARDS

References

Austrian, R., and others: Clinical and Physiologic Features of Some Types of Pulmonary Diseases with Impairment of Alveolar-Capillary Diffusion. The Syndrome of "Alveolar-Capillary Block." Am. J. Med., 11:667, 1951.

Baldwin, E. deF., Cournand, A., and Richards, D. W., Jr.: Pulmonary Insufficiency. I. Physiologic Classification, Clinical Methods of Analysis, Standard Values in Normal Subjects. Medicine, 27:253, 1948. II. A Study of 39 Cases of Pulmonary Fibrosis. Medicine, 28:1, 1949. III. A Study of 122 Cases of Chronic Pulmonary Emphysema. Medicine, 28:201, 1949.

Comroe, J. H., Jr.: Methods in Medical Research. Vol. 2. Chicago, Year Book Publishers, 1950.

Cournand, A., Richards, D. W., Jr., and Darling, R. C.: Graphic Tracings of Respiration in Study of Pulmonary Disease. Am. Rev. Tuberc., 40:487, 1939.

Cournand, A.: Some Aspects of the Pulmonary Circulation in Normal Man and in Chronic Cardio-pulmonary Disease. Circulation, 2:641, 1950.

Fenn, W. O.: Mechanics of Respiration. Am. J. Med., 10:77, 1951.

Fry, D. L., Ebert, R. V., Stead, W. W., and Brown, C. C.: The Mechanics of Pulmonary Ventilation in Normal Subjects and in Patients with Emphysema. Am. J. Med., 16:80, 1954.

Fulton, J. F.: Textbook of Physiology. 17th ed. Philadelphia, W. B. Saunders Co., 1955.

Gaensler, E. A.: Analysis and Critique of Pulmonary Function Studies. Bull. New England M. Center, 13:49, 1951.

Gray, J. S.: Pulmonary Ventilation and Its Physiological Regulation. Springfield, Ill., Charles C Thomas, 1950.

Keith, A.: Mechanism of Respiration in Man, in Further Advances in Physiology. New York, Longmans, Green & Co., 1909.

Marshall, R., McIlroy, M. B., and Christie, R. V.: The Work of Breathing in Mitral Stenosis. Clin. Sc., 13:137, 1954.

Pappenheimer, J. R., and others: Standardization of Definitions and Symbols in Respiratory Physiology. Fed. Proc., 9:602, 1950.

Richards, D. W.: The Nature of Cardiac and of Pulmonary Dyspnea. Circulation, 7:15, 1953.

Riley, R. L., and Cournand, A.: "Ideal" Alveolar Air and the Analysis of Ventilation-Perfusion Relationships in the Lungs. J. Appl. Physiol., 1:825, 1949.

Riley, R. L., Shepard, R. H., Cohn, J. E., Carroll, D. G., and Armstrong, B. W.: Maximal Diffusing Capacity of Lungs. J. Appl. Physiol., 6:573, 1954.

CIRCULATORY DISTURBANCES IN THE LUNGS

PULMONARY EDEMA

Definition. An excess of serous fluid in the lungs, manifested chiefly by increased intra-alveolar fluid. It may be an acute condition, or subacute or chronic.

Pathology. Pulmonary edema, from one or another cause, is found in about 10 per cent of autopsies. The edematous lung is large and heavy; the cut surface exudes clear or pinkish fluid from alveoli and bronchi. In chronic edema the fluid is often gelatinous and confined to the lower lobes. Microscopically, the essential finding is the filling of alveolar spaces with edema fluid—homogeneous eosinophilic material, sometimes clear, sometimes mixed with erythrocytes, leukocytes or "heart failure cells." In the forms due to vascular congestion, capillary vessels are engorged, and there is often interstitial and pericapillary edema as well.

Physiology. Pulmonary edema develops from a variety of causes: hemodynamic, pulmonary, chemical, nervous and infectious. Normally, the main stream of blood flows through the pulmonary capillaries at mean pressures about 5 to 8 mm. Hg. above that of surrounding intrathoracic tissues, and only slightly above left atrial pressures. Plasma proteins, maintaining an oncotic pressure of about 25 mm.Hg, hold nearly all the blood water within the blood stream in its passage through the lungs, but small amounts are diverted to pulmonary lymph flow; it is not known how much of this is derived from pulmonary arterial and how much from bronchial arterial blood. The tracheobronchial tree is moistened with a thin layer of fluid that is gradually moved cephalad by the bronchial ciliated cells.

The commonest cause of pulmonary edema is hypertension in the pulmonary capillary bed secondary to left heart failure; left ventricular failure and mitral stenosis are typical examples. The degree of pulmonary edema is not strictly proportional to pulmonary capillary pressure, and there are thus other factors, but in general pulmonary capillary pressures in excess of 35 mm.Hg, or pulmonary arterial diastolic pressures in excess of 40 mm. or 50 mm.Hg, when due to left heart failure, are apt to be associated with more or less pulmonary edema. Pulmonary congestion and edema are important factors in advanced cardiac dyspnea.

Increased intra-alveolar and intrabronchial fluid induces cough and dyspnea, and hinders oxygen uptake. Arterial anoxia also probably increases movement of water out of the blood into lymphatic channels.

The second common cause of pulmonary edema is damage to the alveolar-capillary membrane, with increased permeability, encountered especially in infection (pneumonia) and chemical injury.

A third and highly important cause is inadequate tracheobronchial drainage. This is almost always a factor in any severe pulmonary edema, and may be produced by inadequate cough reflex, inadequate mechanics of cough, general weakness and prostration, aspiration, overdose of sedative and various neurologic conditions, especially those with stupor or coma.

Clinical Forms. 1. *Cardiocirculatory:* heart disease; renal disease; shock. Pulmonary congestion secondary to left ventricular failure, or to mitral valvular disease, may be mild and transient, or progressive and chronic, or recurrent. Mild attacks may be brought on in such cardiac patients by sudden undue exertion, and will consist of cough, dyspnea, sometimes pinkish frothy sputum, basal or diffuse pulmonary rales. Such attacks usually subside promptly with rest, in an hour or so, sometimes in a few minutes. More severe and persisting pulmonary edema occurs with more severely damaged hearts, or after some sudden episode, as paroxysmal fibrillation or a myocardial infarction. Paroxysmal nocturnal dyspnea is often on this basis. Symptoms may start with cough, oppression in the chest or dyspnea. At the height, the patient's respiration is labored and gasping and audibly moist, cough is frequent with frothy sputum, cyanosis marked, chest full of coarse bubbling rales, heart sounds labored or faint, pulse rapid and uneven. The patient may succumb in such an attack, in a matter of hours or even minutes.

Cardiac asthma is in large part a manifestation of acute pulmonary congestion, although clinical signs of acute bronchiolar obstruction may predominate.

The body water balance is an important factor in the production of pulmonary edema, an excess rendering patients much more susceptible. Patients with chronic cardiorenal disease, especially if uremic, often develop a subacute, more or less symptomless pulmonary edema. Hypoproteinemia may be a contributing factor in these cases. The most frequent immediate cause of death in "lower nephron nephrosis" with anuria is pulmonary edema. It occurs not infrequently, even with relatively normal hearts, in elderly patients given too much intravenous fluid, as for example, following a surgical operation.

Chronic pulmonary congestion and edema, on the basis of intractable heart failure, is often associated with other chronic pulmonary changes: alveolar thickening, interstitial fibrosis and pulmonary arteriosclerosis.

Traumatic or hemorrhagic oligemic shock is ordinarily not associated with pulmonary edema. When the latter occurs, one may suspect some thoracic or cardiac complication.

2. *Pulmonary:* infection, infarct, chronic pulmonary disease. In lobar pneumonia, pulmonary edema is ordinarily not seen early in the disease; it occurs rather as a late serious or terminal event. In acute bronchopneumonia, especially the influenzal forms, the lungs may be edematous almost from the onset, sometimes with a hemorrhagic edema. This is presumably due to direct injury of the alveolar membranes.

Pulmonary embolism with infarction of the lung may produce an acute pulmonary edema. The condition occurs occasionally, following rapid removal of pleural or abdominal fluid. The exact mechanisms involved in these forms of pulmonary edema are not known.

In chronic pulmonary diseases, such as emphysema, asthma, the fibroses, or bronchiectasis, pulmonary edema occurs chiefly when cough is ineffectual, secretions cannot be raised and an asphyxial state supervenes.

3. *Pulmonary drainage:* asphyxial, aspirational, neurologic. The importance of maintenance of the patency of pulmonary airways has already been stressed. When they become clogged with exudate, owing to inadequate cough reflex, pulmonary aeration fails and the alveoli soon fill with edema. Overdosage with morphine in asthmatic or emphysematous subjects causes pulmonary edema by this means. Terminal pulmonary edema is in part on this basis, as is much of the so-called "cerebral" pulmonary edema.

There are, of course, other factors in these forms, of which left ventricular failure is probably the most important.

Aspiration of vomitus can lead to pulmonary edema in comatose or prostrated patients. This is one of the frequent causes of sudden exitus in severe traumatic shock.

4. *Chemical:* industrial; war gases; blast injury. The chief industrial pulmonary irritants are: gases—ammonia, chlorine, bromine, phosgene, sulfur dioxide, arsine, the nitric oxides; the fuming mineral and volatile organic acids; dusts and vapors of corrosive agents, such as the oxides, sulfides and chlorides of phosphorus. Workers exposed to irritants often develop a persistent cough and are found to have rales at the lung bases ("wet lungs"). Removal from exposure brings prompt relief. Occasionally acute symptoms develop, including severe cough, asthmatic dyspnea, frothy sputum and frank pulmonary edema. This also responds to adequate therapy.

War gases in general are of two types, the immediate irritants and corrosives such as chlorine, producing a violent tracheobronchitis, and the slower acting, such as phosgene ($COCl_2$) or nitric oxide, causing in 3 to 8 hours a severe hemorrhagic pulmonary edema.

Blast injury to the lung consists of multiple small pulmonary hemorrhages. The symptoms are hyperinflation, cyanosis, intense dyspnea, chest pain and hemoptysis. Fatal cases terminate in shock and intractable pulmonary edema.

Lung burn from inhalation of hot gases is a common cause of traumatic pulmonary injury. Pulmonary edema may develop promptly, or after a delay of 12 to 24 hours.

Treatment. Mild attacks of pulmonary edema pass off by themselves, but in the severe and progressive forms, vigorous treatment is essential and often life-saving. Rational therapy depends on accurate evaluation of the type of pulmonary edema present:

1. *Cardiocirculatory:* (*a*) Sedation—morphine, 15 mg.; sometimes demerol, 50 to 200 mg., or other sedative will suffice. (*b*) Oxygen inhalation, with mask, concentration 75 to 100 per cent. Adequate volume inflow must be assured. Expiration against positive pressure of 2 to 5 cm. H_2O is of definite aid in clearing pulmonary rales. (*c*) Circulating blood volume should be decreased, by venous tourniquets on limbs, or phlebotomy of 250 to 500 cc., which may bring dramatic

improvement; later by mercurial diuretics. (*d*) Rapid digitalization is indicated in frank heart failure, as by intravenous Digoxin. (*e*) Inhalation of alcohol vapor can be tried.

2. *Pulmonary:* (*a*) Sedation for pulmonary edema in pneumonia, but the cough reflex must be protected. In asthma or emphysema, morphine must be used very cautiously, if at all. (*b*) Oxygen inhalation is indicated for cyanosis or dyspnea. Positive pressure is more effective in asthma and emphysema than in the pulmonary edema of pneumonia. (*c*) Bronchodilators should be used if bronchospasm exists. (*d*) Vigorous antibiotic therapy is given as required.

3. *Pulmonary drainage:* (*a*) Maintain airways. (*b*) Maintain cough reflex. (*c*) Active suction of the tracheobronchial tree may be lifesaving in patients choked with exudate, or bronchoscopic suction may be used if needed. (*d*) Avoid morphine or other repiratory depressant in these cases.

4. *Chemical:* (*a*) Sedatives, morphine or demerol. (*b*) Oxygen, with positive pressure as needed. (*c*) Bronchodilators according to indication.

References

Barach, A. L.: Physiologic Therapy in Respiratory Diseases. Philadelphia, J. B. Lippincott Co., 1948.

Friedberg, C. K.: Diseases of the Heart. Philadelphia, W. B. Saunders Co., 1951.

Goodman, L., and Gilman, A.: The Pharmacologic Basis of Therapeutics. New York, The Macmillan Co., 1941.

Gorlin, R., and others: Studies of the Circulatory Dynamics in Mitral Stenosis. II. Am. Heart J., *41:* 30, 1951.

Luisada, A. A., Goldman, M. A., and Weyl, R.: Alcohol Vapor by Inhalation in Treatment of Acute Pulmonary Edema. Circulation, 5:363, 1952.

Paine, R., Smith, J. R., Butcher, H. R., and Howard, F. R.: Heart Failure and Pulmonary Edema Produced by Certain Neurological Stimuli. Circulation, 5:759, 1952.

Underhill, F. P.: The Lethal War Gases. New Haven, Yale University Press, 1920.

Weiss, S.: Pulmonary Congestion and Edema. Bull. N. Y. Acad. Med., *18:*93, 1942.

PULMONARY HEMORRHAGE

Bleeding from the lungs occurs from a great variety of causes, some of serious prognostic consequence, others benign. The term hemoptysis, "spitting of blood," is literally not quite synonymous; but hemoptysis is usually considered to mean a hemorrhage from some pulmonary structure.

The problem in pulmonary hemorrhage is

chiefly one of etiologic diagnosis, less often of direct therapy.

Nonpulmonary Causes of Blood in Sputum. (*a*) *Upper respiratory.* The commonest cause of mild streaking or small amounts of blood in the sputum is some nasopharyngeal or oral inflammation or ulceration, the blood collecting locally, or dropping down into larynx or trachea: epistaxis, upper respiratory infection, other nasopharyngeal lesion, bleeding gums. Occult bleeding from the larynx is infrequent, but may occur from local inflammation, tuberculosis, carcinoma or other tumor. (*b*) *Gastrointestinal.* Hematemesis, bleeding from esophagus, stomach or duodenum, can usually be identified by the patient as vomiting, but may be difficult to differentiate from pulmonary bleeding, especially in very ill patients who have both vomited and aspirated blood.

Pulmonary Diseases. In spite of reduced incidence and severity of the disease, tuberculosis is still a major cause of pulmonary hemorrhage, extending in severity from the smallest amounts to death from rapid exsanguination. Slight hemoptyses may be due to local inflammation, small ulcers or the irritant effect of coughing; but the more severe are caused by actual erosion of a pulmonary blood vessel. Blood lost in a typical attack of moderate severity will range between 30 cc. and 300 cc. Hemoptysis in tuberculosis often comes on without warning; its occurrence indicates a caseous process of rather long standing, though sometimes its origin cannot be found by physical signs or x-ray.

Other common causes of pulmonary hemorrhage, mild or profuse, are: bronchiectasis, which may bleed in the "dry," asymptomatic phase as well as in the symptomatic; abscess of the lung or other pulmonary suppuration; chronic bronchitis and emphysema (infrequent); bronchogenic carcinoma; traumatic injury to chest or lung; familial telangiectasia.

In Abbott's study of 497 cases of pulmonary hemorrhage due to pulmonary diseases, bleeding occurred in 54 per cent of cancers, 49 per cent of abscesses, 45 per cent of bronchiectases, 44 per cent of pulmonary infarcts and 36 per cent of cases of pulmonary tuberculosis.

The pneumonias vary considerably in their tendency to bleed. As an initial or very early symptom, blood-streaked or frankly bloody sputum is common in most forms. The characteristic rusty sputum may come early, but often only after the first or second day. Persisting hemorrhagic sputum is seen in streptococcal and influenzal pneumonias. Frank hemorrhage occurs not infrequently in Friedländer bacillus pneumonia.

Among the less common pulmonary causes of severe hemoptyses one may list: foreign body in the lung or bronchus, benign bronchial adenoma and hemangioma of the lung. Blood-tinged sputum or mild hemoptyses are seen in acute bronchitis, whooping cough, membranous diphtheria and various pulmonary fungus diseases.

Cardiocirculatory Diseases. Mitral stenosis and pulmonary infarct are the most frequent circulatory conditions associated with pulmonary hemorrhage. In mitral stenosis the characteristic lesion is a rupture of dilated bronchial veins at the surface of the bronchial lumen. It indicates a considerable degree of mitral narrowing and pulmonary congestion. The hemorrhage may be mild or profuse, occasionally even fatal. Blood loss of 200 to 500 cc. is not unusual. It may recur at frequent or only long intervals. It is more likely to take place in the early or middle stages of decompensation, while the right ventricle is still competent, than in the stage of advanced right-sided and left-sided insufficiency.

Of the typical symptoms of pulmonary embolism and infarction, i.e., sudden pain in the chest, fever, cough and hemoptysis, the latter occurs in about half of all cases, as already noted. The amount is usually not great, but may continue, as blood-streaked or bloody sputum, over several days.

In aneurysm of the aorta, bleeding into the lung is of two types: streaking or small hemoptyses due either to pressure on a bronchus, or oozing of the aneurysm; and gross rupture of the aneurysmal wall. The latter provides a sudden and quite characteristic picture: the patient sits up abruptly, staring and terrified; there is a tremendous gush of blood from his mouth, and he falls over dead.

Congestive heart failure with pulmonary congestion and pulmonary edema will produce brownish or pinkish sputum, but usually not gross hemoptysis unless there is an associated pulmonary infarct. In systemic arterial hypertension, the pulmonary vascular pressures are normal, in the absence of heart failure, and pulmonary hemorrhage is not usually encountered.

General Diseases. Systemic diseases with bleeding tendencies may be the cause of pulmonary bleeding, for example, purpura, hemophilia, leukemia, granulocytopenia, nephritis.

Of the drugs commonly used in therapy, the most important are the anticoagulants, overdosage with which not infrequently induces hemoptyses.

Occasionally pulmonary hemorrhage may occur, even repeatedly, with no adequate cause found, either general or local. It has been described during menstruation in women without pulmonary disease, a form of so-called "vicarious" menstruation.

Symptoms and Signs. A small or moderate hemoptysis is initiated by a sensation of congestion or fluid in the air passages and is brought up with a slight cough. This is repeated at frequent or infrequent intervals depending upon the severity of the hemorrhage. The patient is usually anxious and apprehensive; he can sometimes tell from which side the bleeding is coming, though there is usually no actual pain. Physical examination may show rales or other signs on the affected side, but often does not.

The blood may be bright red, liquid and frothy, or in clots. Blood from the lung is sometimes swallowed, and later vomited, as dark or coffee-ground material.

Massive hemorrhage may lead to death by exsanguination, or suffocation from blood clots in the bronchi; there may be massive collapse of a lung or lobe, or aspiration pneumonia.

Diagnosis. History, physical examination, roentgenography and bronchoscopy are the chief diagnostic aids, each disease obviously having its own indications and manifestations. Bronchoscopy should not be done during profuse hemorrhage, but when diagnostic localization is important, the procedure is sometimes best carried out while the bleeding is still in progress.

A pulmonary hemorrhage of any severity is usually associated with some aspiration of blood, either unilateral or bilateral. This may give a diffuse shadow by roentgenogram. In tuberculous cases it often leads to a diffuse nodular bronchogenic spread of the disease.

Treatment. The principles of treatment of any considerable hemoptysis are: (*a*) Absolute rest in bed. (*b*) Enough sedation to allay anxiety and prevent severe coughing spasms, but not to suppress the cough reflex completely. Morphine, 0.01 gm. or 0.015

gm., is often needed at first, with Demerol or codeine as continuation. (*c*) The patient should lie preferably on the affected side, to prevent aspiration to the other side. (*d*) An antibiotic such as penicillin, 600,000 units twice a day, should be given to prevent pneumonia. (*e*) With aspiration of blood, oxygen therapy may be needed, or suction of air passages. (*f*) Various forms of collapse therapy have been used, in intractable hemorrhage, or even surgical removal of the lesion. These are special surgical problems for each case. (*g*) In tuberculous cases, active antibiotic therapy should be instituted at once.

References

Abbott, O. A.: Clinical Significance of Pulmonary Hemorrhage: Study of 1316 Patients with Chest Disease. Dis. of Chest, *14*:824, 1948.

Ferguson, F. C., Kobilak, R. E., and Deitrick, J. E.: Varices of Bronchial Veins as Sources of Hemorrhage in Mitral Stenosis. Am. Heart J., *28*:445, 1944.

PULMONARY EMBOLISM, PULMONARY INFARCTION AND THROMBOSIS

Definition. Pulmonary embolism is the lodgment of a clot or other foreign matter in a pulmonary arterial vessel. Pulmonary infarction is the hemorrhagic necrosis of a part of the lung parenchyma, due to interruption of its blood supply, usually as a result of embolism. Pulmonary thrombosis is the formation of a thrombus *in situ* in any pulmonary blood vessel.

Morbid Anatomy. Pulmonary embolism is found in about 10 per cent of all autopsies, and causes 2 to 3 per cent of deaths. Forty per cent of pulmonary emboli occur postoperatively, 30 per cent in medical cardiac cases, 30 per cent in medical noncardiac cases. Pulmonary embolization leads to infarction in 60 per cent of noncardiac cases, and in 90 per cent of cardiac. Eighty per cent of emboli in noncardiac cases come from phlebothrombosis in the extremities and about 10 per cent from thrombophlebitis. In cardiacs, about 25 per cent come from intramural cardiac thrombi, chiefly right atrial.

An embolus may be of any size, from microscopic to a huge long "saddle embolus" that lands astride the pulmonary artery bifurcation. Emboli may be single or multiple, occurring simultaneously or sequentially, involving small regions of the lung, or disseminated throughout. When infarction occurs, it may be of transitory nature ("incomplete") because of incomplete loss of blood supply, or, more commonly, complete with hemorrhage and necrosis. The most massive emboli may cause acute edema rather than hemorrhage, death occuring without a well formed infarct.

Pulmonary infarcts, ill defined anatomically in the first 24 hours, later become identified by x-ray, in typical cases, as wedge-shaped shadows. The lesion is always in contact with a pleural surface, peripheral or interlobar. It is dark red and airless; the chief microscopic manifestation is hemorrhage, both intra-alveolar and interstitial. "Incomplete" infarcts may disappear in two or three days, with reestablishment of the circulation; "complete" usually last two or three weeks, healing by fibrosis, ending as an irregular linear scar. Very large infarcts may persist for weeks or even months. Fibrinous pleurisy, or pleural effusion, serous or serosanguineous, are associated conditions in 30 to 40 per cent of cases.

Pulmonary thrombosis occurs most often as extension of previously existing lesions: emboli, invading tumor, narrowed vascular lumen or arteriosclerotic plaques. There may be extensive spread, both distal and proximal, of the thrombotic process from the original lesions. Systemic arterial embolization originates rarely from pulmonary venous thromboses, chiefly in cases of advanced tuberculosis.

Other pulmonary arterial emboli include: fat emboli following fracture of a long bone, especially the femur; air emboli, from neck operations, technically faulty infusions or attempted thoracentesis; the "chokes," multiple air embolization from air or nitrogen bubbles released into the tissues and blood following too rapid decompression from high to low atmospheric pressures; septic emboli from an infected venous focus, often with abscess formation; tumor emboli from a tumor, such as a hypernephroma or hepatoma, invading a systemic vein; or foreign body emboli, such as the multiple cotton or lint emboli in narcotic addicts using the intravenous route.

Physiology. Cyanosis and arterial anoxia, frequent symptoms in pulmonary embolism with infarction, are not wholly understood. It is known that an anastomatic circulation with the bronchial arteries develops readily; there may be pulmonary arterial-pulmonary venous shunts. Dyspnea, of the tachypneic, hyperpneic type, is probably associated with the anoxia; there may be "reflex" and other factors. Shock, when it occurs, is due in part to failure of venous return to the left heart, and in part to general disturbances in vasomotor tone. With multiple pulmonary emboli, the syndrome of acute right-sided heart failure may develop.

Symptoms and Signs. Phlebothrombosis and thrombophlebitis, especially of the deep veins of the leg, are the chief sources of pulmonary embolism. There are numerous predisposing conditions: prolonged bed rest—more of a risk in the obese; the postpartum state; postoperative states; many cardiac conditions, such as congestive heart failure, auricular fibrillation, myocardial infarction or subacute bacterial endocarditis.

The common symptoms of pulmonary embolism with infarction are: sudden chest pain, sometimes pleuritic, sometimes continuous and simulating cardiac or upper abdominal pain; moderate rise of temperature and pulse rate; cough, bloody sputum, mild leukocytosis and later increased sedimentation rate. There may be a local patch of crepitant rales, or a friction rub, but as often no chest signs. Systemic symptoms may predominate: weakness, nausea, sweating. A pleural effusion, small or moderate in size, often develops in the first few days, either serous or serosanguineous, and persists for several days, sometimes for a matter of weeks. The roentgenogram shows typically a wedge-shaped shadow, but it may be rounded, or a hazy density, especially if there is pleural fluid. Not infrequently the roentgenogram shows nothing.

With larger infarcts, fever, prostration, hemoptysis, cyanosis and dyspnea are likely to be more pronounced, and local signs of pneumonitis are usually found. A moderate jaundice may develop, especially in cases in congestive heart failure. With massive infarction there is profound shock, acute right-sided heart failure, or not infrequently sudden exitus. Apprehension is a characteristic symptom in pulmonary embolization.

While the venous thrombosis that is the source of the embolus can often be identified, frequently it cannot be, even by careful clinical search. There is also a clinical entity in which single or multiple pulmonary embolization occurs in apparently healthy young individuals. If such cases come to autopsy, thrombophlebitis may be found in pelvic or prostatic veins. Another quite rare condition is progressive diffuse pulmonary embolization, continuing for months or years, and ending in cor pulmonale with extreme right-sided failure, accompanied by severe dyspnea and cyanosis.

The electrocardiogram will show but little in smaller infarcts, but in the larger will usually show, at an early stage, wide large S_1, Q_3 present, T_3 and sometimes T_2 inverted. These changes are often transitory, disappearing in a few hours, or a day or two.

Clinical Course. The average pulmonary embolus with infarction runs a moderate febrile course for a few days, followed by clearing of roentgenographic and physical signs in one to three weeks, and absorption of pleural fluid, if this has been present. Some of the numerous clinical variations have been described above.

Diagnosis. Many clinical conditions can be confused with pulmonary embolization with infarction. The type of pain particularly will simulate a number of other conditions. Thus, in the differential diagnosis should be included: bronchopneumonia, pleurisy, pericarditis, spontaneous pneumothorax, myocardial infarction and acute upper abdominal conditions. Pulmonary embolism and infarction should be suspected in chest pain without known cause, atypical pleural effusion or bronchopneumonia, and should be watched for most closely in any lingering low grade unexplained fever during a postoperative course.

Treatment. Prophylactic measures include those directed toward prevention of thrombophlebitis and phlebrothrombosis, and toward diagnosis and treatment of these conditions when present. Movement of the lower extremities by exercises in bedridden patients, avoidance of "jack-knife" postures with venous pooling of blood, and early ambulation, are in the former category; and anticoagulant therapy, occasionally paravertebral block, or surgical venous ligation in the latter.

With an established pulmonary embolus and infarct, symptoms of the existing lesion should be treated and a second embolus prevented if possible. Bed rest in the sitting position, an analgesic or narcotic if the pain is severe, antitussive for cough, occasionally chest strapping for pleurisy, and prophylactic antibiotic (e.g., penicillin 600,000 units once or twice daily) will take care of the immediate symptoms of the average embolus with infarction. All sudden effort should be avoided, especially straining at stool. So far as possible colonic lavage should be substituted for the bedpan and enema during the first and second weeks following the embolization.

Anticoagulant therapy should be given, such as: heparin, 50 mg. intramuscularly or intravenously, every 4 hours for the first two days; Dicumarol, 200 to 300 mg. initially on the first day, followed by 50 to 100 mg. a day, or whatever dose will keep the prothrombin time (normal 10 to 15 seconds) around 25 to 30 seconds. This must be tested daily for the first week, two to three times a week subsequently. This therapy should be continued for three to six weeks, longer if there continues to be evidence of peripheral venous thrombosis, or if repeated pulmonary embolization occurs. The chief contraindication is, of course, excessively low prothrombin time with the development of a bleeding tendency. Vitamin K_1 oxide, 100 mg. intravenously, will stop such bleeding in 4 to 12 hours. Anticoagulant therapy has significantly reduced incidence and mortality of pulmonary embolism and infarction. A more complete description of the therapeutic use of anticoagulants is given in another chapter.

In more severe and extensive pulmonary infarction, cyanosis and dyspnea may require continuous oxygen therapy, by mask or tent, with positive pressure if there is pulmonary edema. Atropine is often recommended, in doses of 0.6 mg., or papaverine, 30 mg., repeated every few hours, to reduce bronchial spasm and bronchial secretions. The effectiveness of these medications is difficult to assess. Pleural effusion is rarely massive, but may need tapping, either for diagnostic or therapeutic reasons. With acute right heart failure, digitalization is indicated, but usually does not help very much. In the shock associated with massive infarction, the prognosis is usually rather poor, but not hopeless. Norepinephrine, 8 to 10 mg. in a 500 cc. or 1000 cc. slow intravenous infusion, may sustain the arterial blood pressure through the critical period. Venous pressure is usually already high and transfusion thus not indicated.

References

Hampton, A. O., and Castleman, B.: Correlation of Postmortem Chest Teleroentgenograms with Autopsy Findings. Am. J. Roentgenol., 43:305, 1940.

———, Prandoni, A. G., and King, J. T.: Pulmonary

Embolism from Obscure Sources. Bull. Johns Hopkins Hosp., 76:245, 1945.

Heckscher, H.: Mobilizing Treatment of Thrombophlebitis. Acta med. Scandinav., 138:293, 1950.

Roe, B. B., and Goldthwait, J. C.: Pulmonary Embolism: a Study of Postmortem Material at the Massachusetts General Hospital. New England J. Med., 241:679, 1949.

Zimmerman, L. M., Miller, D., and Marshall, A. N.: Pulmonary Embolism. Surg., Gynec. & Obst., 88: 373, 1949.

PULMONARY ARTERIOSCLEROSIS AND PULMONARY ARTERIAL HYPERTENSION

The forces that produce either hypertension or arteriosclerosis in the pulmonary circulation appear to be entirely distinct from those that produce the corresponding conditions in the systemic circuit. Thus, with uncomplicated essential hypertension, or with systemic arteriosclerosis, the pulmonary circulation is ordinarily normal; and pulmonary vascular disease is similarly not usually associated with any lesions in the systemic circuit. The two can, of course, coexist.

Pulmonary arterial pressures normally range from about 18/7 mm.Hg to 30/10 mm. Hg at rest, rising somewhat during moderate or severe exertion. Conditions causing a rise in pulmonary arterial pressure, by increased vascular resistance or congestion, include: (a) left ventricular failure, or mitral valvular disease, with inadequate left atrial emptying and rise in pulmonary venous pressure; (b) marked decrease in total pulmonary capillary bed, as in emphysema, and some of the pulmonary fibroses; (c) extensive loss of actively perfused total lung substance, as in widespread tuberculosis or other fibrotic or destructive disease; in severe kyphoscoliosis; or in certain already damaged lungs, following radical pulmonary surgery; (d) obliteration of vascular channels as in multiple pulmonary embolism; (e) diffuse pulmonary arteriosclerosis. In addition, (f) the large increase in bronchial artery blood flow that is found in certain cases of advanced bronchiectasis may contribute to an elevated pulmonary arterial pressure. Increase in blood flow may also contribute to pulmonary hypertension, as in the "high output failure" of cor pulmonale, or the greatly increased pulmonary blood flow seen with patent ductus arteriosus, interatrial septal defect or large interventricular septal defect.

The anatomic changes of pulmonary arteriosclerosis involve both larger and smaller vessels. The typical lesion is a concentric fibrotic thickening of the intima in a small artery or arteriole, greatly narrowing or obliterating the lumen. These usually develop slowly but progressively along with or following the rise in pulmonary arterial pressure, though there is much individual variation. Sometimes the intrinsic pulmonary disease favors pulmonary arterial change, as in radiation pleuropneumonitis. The factor of persistently increased pulmonary blood flow also tends to increase this anatomic vascular change, as in the congenital heart lesions already mentioned. It is not known just why this vicious cycle develops, in response to these underlying hemodynamic phenomena.

Mild pulmonary emphysema or fibrosis usually does not increase pulmonary arterial pressures. With the more severe forms pressures rise to the range of 40/20 to 60/30. At these pressures or higher, the evidences of cor pulmonale begin to be apparent: enlargement of the pulmonary artery at its base, later the right and left branches; right ventricular hypertrophy; electrocardiographic changes of right axis deviation. Accentuated second pulmonic sound is a useful but not always reliable sign of pulmonary hypertension. Pulmonary congestion from left heart failure, as in mitral stenosis, results also in progressive increase in pulmonary arterial pressures; in advanced failure as high as 115/70, occasionally to 150/100. The strength and relative competence of the right ventricle is obviously a dominant factor in extreme pulmonary artery hypertension.

In the most advanced stage there is marked enlargement and failure of the right ventricle, with liver enlargement and edema, sometimes associated, in the pulmonary cases, with polycythemia and hypervolemia. Patients with congenital heart lesions at this stage may develop a sudden right-to-left shunting of blood, if right heart pressures exceed those of the left. The symptoms are sudden intense cyanosis and loss of consciousness ("cyanose tardive"); the condition may also become continuous, but the prognosis is always poor.

Primary Pulmonary Hypertension. This is a rare disease, though a number of cases have been described recently, consisting of a progressing diffuse pulmonary arteriosclerosis and pulmonary hypertension, without other disease, either pulmonary or cardiac. It may occur at any age. Symptoms are dyspnea, weakness, dizzy attacks, syncope on exertion, chest pain, orthopnea and hemoptysis. Pulmonary arterial pressures are high, and the patient may succumb in right-sided heart failure. Autopsy shows narrowed sclerotic pulmonary arterioles.

References

Brill, I. C., and Krygier, J. J.: Primary Pulmonary Vascular Sclerosis. Arch. Int. Med., 68:560, 1941.

Cournand, A.: Some Aspects of the Pulmonary Circulation in Normal Man and in Chronic Cardiopulmonary Diseases. Circulation, 2:641, 1950.

Dresdale, D. T., Schultz, M., and Michtom, R. J.: Primary Pulmonary Hypertension. I. Clinical and Hemodynamic Study. Am. J. Med., 11:686, 1951.

Harvey, R. M., Ferrer, M. I., Richards, D. W., Jr., and Cournand, A.: Influence of Chronic Pulmonary Disease on the Heart and Circulation. Am. J. Med., 10:719, 1951.

Liebow, A. A., Hales, M. R., and Lindskog, G. E.: Enlargement of the Bronchial Arteries and Their Anastamoses with the Pulmonary Arteries in Bronchiectasis. Am. J. Path., 25:211, 1949.

PULMONARY ARTERIOVENOUS FISTULA

(Hemangioma of the Lung)

This is a relatively rare condition consisting of a cavernous hemangioma, with direct communication between a pulmonary artery and pulmonary vein, this part of the pulmonary circulation thus by-passing the alveoli. The pathologic entity may be solitary but is frequently a part of a generalized hereditary hemorrhagic telangiectasia. Multiple pulmonary lesions are found in about 50 per cent of cases.

Clinical manifestations depend upon the size of the communication, and the amount of blood shunted. Symptoms include cyanosis, dyspnea, hemoptysis, dizziness, chest pain, palpitation, headaches and paresthesias. Cyanosis is usually marked with advanced clubbing of fingers and toes. There is often, but not always, a murmur heard over the chest near the tumor; it may be systolic or continuous. There is polycythemia and increased blood volume commensurate with the arterial anoxia. Arterial oxygen saturation is apt to range around 75 per cent, but may be lower. X-ray or fluoroscopy shows a rounded or lobulated lesion in the lung field, which is often pulsatile. The hilar blood vessels on the same side are also enlarged and pulsating. Most fatalities that have been reported have been from massive pulmonary hemorrhage.

Polycythemia vera and congenital heart disease are the conditions most likely to be confused with pulmonary arteriovenous fistula.

Treatment is surgical. Most lesions can be successfully removed by segmental resection or lobectomy. After removal of the lesion, all clinical manifestations usually regress to normal.

DICKINSON W. RICHARDS

References

Burchell, H. B., and Clagett, O. T.: The Clinical Syndrome Associated with Pulmonary Arteriovenous Fistulas, Including a Case Report of a Surgical Cure. Am. Heart J., 34:151, 1947.

Wintrobe, M. M.: Clinical Hematology. Philadelphia, Lea and Febiger, 1952.

PULMONARY ATELECTASIS

Definition. There is some confusion, as well as difference of opinion, as to the meaning of the term atelectasis. The word by derivation (ἀτελής, ἔκτασις) signifies "incomplete extension or expansion." Referred to the lung parenchyma, this would imply only a shrinkage of alveolar spaces. The term as ordinarily employed today, however, implies also an airless or nearly airless lung, which is thus functionless. "Partial" and "complete" atelectasis are sometimes used to refer to incomplete and complete airlessness, in a retracted and shrunken lung or part of the lung. It may be difficult to draw a dividing line between a simple contracted region of the lung and a "partial" atelectasis.

In the normal lung, practically all alveoli are patent, even during rest, and are ventilated by a quiet tidal breath.

Acute Atelectasis. Conditions leading to acute atelectasis are those involving (1) bronchial obstruction, (2) exudative or inflammatory intrapulmonary processes or (3) poor chest wall expansion.

1. All the causes of bronchial obstruction need not be enumerated. Once a bronchus is even partially obstructed, aeration of the lung is diminished, and poor drainage of bronchial secretions aggravates the airless, atelectatic state in the lung distal to the obstruction. With complete obstruction, the circulating blood rapidly removes the contained air and complete atelectasis occurs. The lung or lobe shrinks to small size, producing a strong negative intrathoracic pressure on all sides.

2. While atelectasis sometimes takes place with a completely dry lung, as in a total therapeutic collapse by pneumothorax, there

is usually a considerable amount of excess pulmonary interstitial and intra-alveolar fluid. This is aggravated in the presence of any infection.

Atelectasis occurs in varying degree in the acute pneumonias; when shrinkage of the lung and "silent" physical signs are marked, an independent element of bronchial obstruction is to be suspected.

3. Inadequate chest wall expansion is a potent cause of pulmonary atelectasis, seen most significantly in acute paralyses, such as poliomyelitis. Prolonged hypostasis from lying supine in bed, and injuries or operative deformities of the chest, are further causes.

Symptoms of acute atelectasis vary from none, if the region involved is small, to severe dyspnea, cyanosis and cough if a large part of a lung is affected. The signs are chiefly suppression of breath and voice sounds, and displacement of diaphragm, chest wall and mediastinal structures toward the lesion. There is dullness to flatness on percussion if the process is extensive. Roentgenography shows a homogeneous airless density, and will often define exactly the part of the lung involved. With re-aeration of the lung, rales and breath sounds are heard again, and the lung re-expands.

Massive Collapse of the Lung. This is an acute lesion, developing usually after an operation, especially an upper abdominal operation. Pathologically, the lobe or lung is greatly shrunken, the alveoli are airless, contain some increase in serous fluid, and usually not much evidence of infection. There are often bronchial exudate and plugs, but it is not clear whether these are primary or secondary factors. The pathogenesis is not wholly understood, but poor aeration of the lung postoperatively, and bronchial obstruction, are important elements.

Clinical manifestations begin 24 to 48 hours after operation. There is dyspnea, tachypnea, cyanosis, prostration and often some lower chest pain. The patient is usually apprehensive and prefers sitting up in bed. Temperature may be from 100° to 104° and pulse 110 to 130; there may be a leukocytosis. The physical signs show heart, mediastinum, diaphragm and chest wall moved toward the shrunken lung, with little or no respiratory movement. There is relative hyperinflation of the opposite side. Breath and voice sounds are absent or faintly bronchial, and there is dullness to flatness on percussion over the atelectatic lung.

Most patients survive, but the lesion is occasionally fatal. With re-aeration of the lung, all symptoms subside in a few days.

The best *treatment* is prevention: careful anesthesia, with assurance that the lung is left filled with air (*not* oxygen) after anesthesia; change of the patient's position, assistance in eliminating sputum or mucus, and breathing exercises postoperatively. After the lesion has developed, oxygen, antibiotics, change of position, lying especially with the affected side up, encouragement to cough, and if necessary bronchoscopic suction or mechanically induced cough, are the chief therapeutic procedures.

Chronic Atelectasis. Many chronic pulmonary conditions lead to partial or complete atelectasis. Of the lesions causing bronchial obstruction, bronchogenic carcinoma, external pressure from a gland or tumor, or kinking in a greatly distorted lung or chest, are among the more common. The fibrotic lesions of tuberculosis or advanced silicosis, and the constricting action of a chronic pleurisy may lead also to shrunken and airless or nearly airless regions of the lung. There are often adjacent areas of emphysema. Kyphoscoliosis of advanced degree almost always produces atelectasis in parts of one or both lungs. There is a "middle lobe syndrome," consisting of a shrunken completely atelectatic right middle lobe, caused sometimes by pressure of a gland upon the middle lobe bronchus, but more often by an apparently nonspecific chronic inflammatory process with fibrosis and occlusion of the bronchus. This condition can be cured by lobectomy.

References

Christopher, F., and Shaffer, J. M.: Postoperative Atelectasis. Am. J. Surg., 32:195, 1936.
Dripps, R. D., and Deming, M. V.: Postoperative Atelectasis and Pneumonia. Ann. Surg., 124:94, 1946.
Xalabarder, C.: What Is Atelectasis? Tubercle, 30:266, 1949.

PULMONARY FIBROSIS

Definition. While the term pulmonary fibrosis is usually applied, in pathology and medicine, to cases of widespread or diffuse fibrosis in the pulmonary tissues, it is obvious that any laying down of scar tissue in the lung can properly be considered an example of the process.

The present chapter is in two parts. In the first, brief reference is made to the more important forms of clinical pulmonary fibrosis, both localized and diffuse. These are, of course, covered more fully under their own specific chapter headings.

As the second half, a description is given of a group of diseases recently identified, physiologically as well as pathologically, and variously termed "acute diffuse fibrosis of the lungs," "diffusion insufficiency" or "the syndrome of alveolar-capillary block."

Morbid Anatomy and Physiology. *Localized Fibrosis.* The infiltration of fibrous tissue into a region of the lung, from whatever cause, is almost always associated with marked reduction in its function. If there is also bronchial obstruction, there is obviously no aeration; pulmonary arterial flow usually ceases as well. If air passages remain open, some ventilation of the region may continue, providing that the scar tissue has not destroyed pulmonary expansibility; but here also pulmonary blood flow becomes greatly diminished or absent. Any ventilation of such a lung is therefore essentially functionless or "dead space" ventilation. This can often be measured in a single lung by the technique of bronchospirometry.

Diffuse Fibrosis. The consequences of diffuse fibrosis through the lungs depend upon its distribution in pulmonary tissue. With peribronchial, septal, or other "interstitial" fibrosis, the effect is a restriction of lung volumes and ventilatory capacity; if there is obstruction of air passages, either from bronchiolar narrowing or partial obstruction from pressure or angulation, the various dysfunctions of obstructive ventilatory insufficiency develop; thickening of alveolar capillary membranes produces the manifestations of diffusion insufficiency. This general subject is discussed in the chapter on Pulmonary Function in Health and Disease.

LOCALIZED PULMONARY FIBROSIS

Pulmonary Infarct. With embolization of a pulmonary artery, the affected part of the lung becomes hemorrhagic and airless. It is ordinarily triangular or polyangular in form, and so appears in the roentgenogram. The bronchial arteries dilate as the pulmonary circulation is cut off, and bronchial artery–pulmonary artery anastomoses are formed. A pulmonary infarct heals by progressive shrinkage to a narrow irregular cicatrix, clinically invisible and often difficult to find even at autopsy.

Pulmonary Atelectasis. Pulmonary fibrosis with atelectasis, a shrunken, airless segment of lung or entire lobe, occurs by way of infection and connective tissue infiltration, or by way of primary air passage obstruction. As examples of this type of lesion may be mentioned: localized tuberculosis; other localized chronic infection; bronchial stenosis or obstruction from a tumor, gland, foreign body, aneurysm or other solid structure; kyphoscoliosis with distortion and compression of local regions.

Sacculated Bronchiectasis and Chronic Lung Abscess. These are special cases of pulmonary atelectasis, in which localized suppurative disease of the lung is associated with much surrounding fibrosis.

Chronic Pleurisy, Pleural Fibrosis, Chronic Hemothorax, Chronic Empyema. These conditions frequently lead to a progressing unilateral pulmonary fibrosis. The plastic type of pleurisy that behaves in this manner is most often of tubercular origin. The tendency of chronic hemothorax to progress to fibrosis is a strong argument for surgical removal of the blood clot before organization has taken place. The characteristic lesion in this group is a constricting pleural fibrosis, with extension of fibrous tissue inward along the septums of the lung, ending in a fibrothorax, often a functionless lung, and marked shrinkage of the thorax and displacement of its contents toward the affected side. There may be moderate or considerable exertional dyspnea.

Pneumonectomy. After total removal of a lung, the large unilateral dead space is filled partly by displacement of the chest wall, mediastinal structures and contralateral lung, and partly by serum and loose areolar connective tissue. If the opposite lung is normal, it can assume both the larger space and larger function remarkably well. If there is a tendency to emphysema, this is exaggerated and symptoms may develop. Secondary thoracoplasty is sometimes carried out to reduce the intrathoracic dead space.

Organizing Pneumonia. Infrequently, and for reasons not well known, the intra-alveolar exudate in lobar pneumonia does not resolve and absorb, but becomes infiltrated with fibroblasts and ends in a fibrotic chronic pneumonitis. There is moderate but not extreme shrinkage of the lobe. Signs are those of chronic consolidation: dullness, loud or bronchial breath sounds, often coarse or medium rales.

Hemoptysis. Profuse hemoptysis with aspiration is rapidly absorbed, unless a secondary infection develops, as may occur typically in tuberculosis, with bronchogenic spread following the hemorrhage.

DIFFUSE PULMONARY FIBROSIS

The Aging Lung. Beginning in the third decade of life, pulmonary function steadily deteriorates, even in normal healthy subjects. Such functions as vital capacity, breathing capacity and maximum diffusion capacity decrease, and residual air increases, slightly at first, then more significantly. Even arterial oxygen saturation in the aged may be 93 per cent or 92 per cent, compared with the younger normal of 96 per cent. These changes are in most instances due to the usual atrophic phenomena of age, but subclinical fibrotic lesions doubtless frequently play a part.

Chronic Bronchitis. This is probably the commonest single cause of progressively developing diffuse pulmonary fibrosis, whether of the restrictive interstitial or the obstructive emphysematous form. The lesions responsible are in part the peribronchial fibrotic changes, extending further into pulmonary septums, and in part the thickened mucous membranes, with bronchiolar narrowing and poor bronchial drainage. An especially severe form is that associated with cystic disease of the pancreas in children.

Pneumoconioses. Post-Irradiation Fibrosis. These are lesions due to physical irritants, with at first slight, then more dense diffuse fibrosis in interstitial, perivascular and septal pulmonary tissues. The fibrosis is typically nodular in the pneumoconioses, linear in radiation fibrosis. Physiologically there is restriction of lung volumes and breathing capacity. Dyspnea is the outstanding symptom in severe cases, but considerable roentgenographic change may exist, especially in the pneumoconioses, with essentially no symptoms.

Sarcoidosis. This disease, whose primary pathology is a diffuse granulomatosis, has several pulmonary forms: (*a*) glandular, with enlarged mediastinal lymph nodes; (*b*) interstitial fibrosis of the usual restrictive type; (*c*) emphysematous; (*d*) alveolar thickening, with diffusion insufficiency; (*e*) combinations of these lesions.

Emphysema and Fibrosis. Chronic pulmonary emphysema, either diffuse, bullous or localized, is very frequently, but by no means always, associated with one or another form of pulmonary fibrosis. Chronic bronchitis and tuberculosis are diseases perhaps most frequently associated with the emphysematous change.

Chronic Congestive Heart Failure. Longstanding left-sided heart failure, with chronic pulmonary congestion, is often associated with chronic pulmonary changes: deposition of hemosiderin, fine diffuse fibrosis and pulmonary arteriosclerosis. This is seen characteristically in mitral stenosis with chronic heart failure.

Lymphoma, Diffuse Metastatic Carcinoma, Metastatic Sarcoma, Leukemia, Lupus Erythematosus, Scleroderma of the Lung. All these widespread conditions in the lung are frequently associated with more or less diffuse fibrosis.

LOCALIZED AND DIFFUSE PULMONARY FIBROSIS

Tuberculosis. The acute exudative forms can absorb without scarring. The essential chronic lesion, however, is the tubercle, and if this undergoes any significant degree of caseation necrosis, it heals by fibrous tissue infiltration. Tuberculosis may give almost any form of pulmonary fibrosis: the small healed primary lesion, the localized infiltrate or scarred functionless segment of lung at an apex, the dense fibrosis with necrosis and cavity formation, the diffuse interstitial fibrosis, the chronic shrunken wholly functionless fibroid lung, the acute hematogenous disease with "diffusion insufficiency" pattern on physiologic study, the acute bronchogenic spread. With the fibrosis in the more chronic lesions there is often calcification.

Fungus and Parasitic Diseases. In most pulmonary diseases due to fungus and allied agents, there is more or less pulmonary fibrosis associated with the chronic or healed lesion. Among these may be mentioned histoplasmosis, coccidioidomycosis, moniliasis, and the rarer conditions such as actinomycosis, streptothrix infection, blastomycosis, sporotrichosis, aspergillosis, hydatid cyst.

CHRONIC FIBROTIC PULMONARY DISEASE WITH IMPAIRMENT OF ALVEOLAR-CAPILLARY DIFFUSION; DIFFUSION INSUFFICIENCY; SYNDROME OF ALVEOLAR-CAPILLARY BLOCK

These terms describe a group of diseases, recently defined clinically, which have different pathologies and pathogenesis, but common symptoms and physiologic characteristics, and a similar clinical course.

Morbid Anatomy. Schjerning, and later Brauer and Knipping in Germany, about thirty years ago, noted alveolar thickening associated with clinical cyanosis in certain pneumonias in the influenza epidemic, and called this condition "pneumonosis." They postulated a defect in oxygen diffusion. In 1944 Hamman and Rich described three cases characterized by progressive dyspnea, cough and cyanosis, diffuse roentgenographic changes, and ultimately right heart failure, showing at autopsy a marked diffuse fibrosis involving all interstitial pulmonary tissues, and especially a fibrous thickening of alveolar membranes. This lesion they termed "acute diffuse interstitial fibrosis of the lungs." No physiologic studies were carried out.

In the last five years a considerable number of subacute or chronic pulmonary conditions have been found to fall in this general pattern. One of the more common is a diffuse form of fibrosis, often apparently starting from a "nonspecific" or "virus" type of pneumonia, and continuing, subacutely or recurrently, eventually forming a dense fibrotic thickening of alveolar walls, not unlike the disease described by Hamman and Rich. Another not infrequent type is a diffuse granulomatosis of the lung, as in beryllium poisoning, or sarcoidosis, or certain granulomatous conditions of unknown etiology. Here the basic lesion is a small granuloma consisting of epithelioid and giant cells, with much surrounding fibrosis, the process infiltrating alveolar septums and interstitial tissues generally. Still other conditions lead to this syndrome: scleroderma of the lung, reactions to certain chemical irritants like the sulfur oxides and the rare diffuse alveolar cell carcinoma of the lung. Physiologically, acute diffuse miliary tuberculosis may behave similarly.

Physiology. The diffuse fibrosis limits ventilatory amplitude, and lung volumes are diminished. There is no air passage obstruction, however, and maximum breathing capacity is nearly normal and alveolar spaces well aerated. The essential defects in pulmonary function are of two types: (1) increased alveolar-arterial oxygen gradient and decreased oxygen diffusing capacity due to impaired diffusion across thickened but partly functioning alveolar walls; (2) disturbed ventilation-perfusion relationships, such that many alveoli are ventilated with no perfusion (dead space ventilation), and others are perfused but all air interchange blocked off by excessive fibrous tissue infiltration (increased venous admixture). The measurable changes in cardiopulmonary function, other than lung volumes and breathing capacity, are: marked hyperventilation and tachypnea, normal arterial O_2 saturation and slightly low CO_2 at rest, arterial O_2 unsaturation in exercise, moderate pulmonary arterial hypertension.

Symptoms and Signs. Symptoms may begin insidiously, or following a pulmonary infection, with frequent cough, early associated with progressively increasing dyspnea on exertion. Cyanosis may be noted during exercise; at rest cyanosis is a late symptom. Dyspnea, of the rapid tachypneic type, becomes more urgent, and eventually requires bed rest or hospitalization. There may be recurring febrile episodes. Disability may develop in a month or gradually over many months.

On examination there is tachypnea, hyperpnea, poor excursions of the chest, usually loud hilar breath sounds and hilar or basal medium rales. The second pulmonic sound is frequently accentuated. Clubbing of the fingers is seen in most cases. There is no polycythemia, and leukocytosis only with secondary infection. Serum globulin may be increased in the sarcoidosis group. Roentgenogram may show linear shadows with hilar exaggerations, or diffuse nodular infiltration, or a fine nodular and reticular pattern.

Course. This varies with the etiology. The scleroderma and "nonspecific" fibrosis cases pursue a more or less relentless course, which may, however, run on for years, with exacerbations during pulmonary infections. Eventually the dyspnea and cyanosis require bed rest and then oxygen therapy. The need for oxygen may become continuous. Death occurs from (a) progressive anoxia and respiratory failure, (b) intercurrent bronchopneumonia, (c) cor pulmonale and right-sided heart failure.

The granulomatoses are more variable in their clinical course. With berylliosis, as well as sarcoidosis, about a third tend to recover spontaneously, a third become chronically incapacitated and a third grow progressively worse and die.

Diagnosis. In the early stages, the important question is that of diagnosis. The symptoms, type of tachypneic dyspnea, x-ray findings and arterial anoxia in exercise (post-exercise O_2 saturation usually between 80 per cent and 60 per cent) with low or normal CO_2, are the key manifestations.

Treatment. Limitation of activity is all that is needed at first, plus perhaps some prophylactic antibiotic. Later, oxygen will be needed, at first intermittently, later continuously (nasal catheter provides 30 to 35 per cent inhaled O_2 concentration, tent 40 to 45 per cent, masks up to 70 or 80 per cent). Some antitussive may help the cough, with sedation as indicated. In the later cyanotic stage, the patient may lose appetite and weight.

For the granulomatous cases, cortisone or corticotropin may provide great relief, even a considerable clinical reversal of the disease. It should be given in vigorous doses at the start, 300 mg. of cortisone the first day, 200 mg. the second, then reducing gradually to a daily maintenance dose between 100 mg. and 50 mg., or even 25 mg., as low as possible for moderate physical activity. Cortisone may have to be continued for many months. Some cases of granulomatosis, especially long-standing cases, will not respond to this therapy, but it is worth trying in all cases, so long as tuberculosis can be ruled out.

If there is right-sided heart failure, this should be treated by: low sodium regimen, mercurial diuretics, phlebotomy if there is frank congestive failure with edema and increased blood volume, digitalization, oxygen therapy, prophylactic antibiotics.

DICKINSON W. RICHARDS

References

Austrian, R., and others: Clinical and Physiologic Features of Some Types of Pulmonary Diseases with Impairment of Alveolar-Capillary Diffusion. The Syndrome of "Alveolar-Capillary Block." Am. J. Med., 11:667, 1951.

Baldwin, E. deF., Cournand, A., and Richards, D. W., Jr.: Pulmonary Insufficiency. II. A Study of 39 Cases of Pulmonary Fibrosis. Medicine, 28:1, 1949.

Hamman, L., and Rich, A. R.: Acute Diffuse Interstitial Fibrosis of the Lungs. Bull. Johns Hopkins Hosp., 74:177, 1944.

RADIATION PLEUROPNEUMONITIS

(Radiation Fibrosis)

Although the lung as a tissue is only moderately sensitive to the effects of x-ray, radiotherapy in heavy dosage may cause severe damage. Long continued or intensive courses of treatment for primary, metastatic or suspected metastatic cancer of breast, lung, esophagus or other thoracic structure are the common cause of pulmonary radiation fibrosis. Total dosages may range from 1000 r to 15,000 r.

Early pathologic changes consist in a hyalinization around the alveolar walls, later a more fixed and diffuse fibrosis. The smaller blood vessels may be involved. The pleura sometimes becomes densely fibrotic. Grossly, there is a progressing shrinkage, with atelectasis. Symptoms, when the condition is widespread, are increasing dyspnea, dry cough and cyanosis. There may be terminal cor pulmonale and right-sided heart failure. Physiologically, the dominant picture is shrinkage of lung volumes and ventilatory insufficiency. Treatment is symptomatic.

More acute reactions, simulating acute pneumonitis, with fever, prostration and extreme dyspnea, may develop progressively in two or three weeks following heavy x-ray dosage, especially with high voltage therapy. The acute reaction may regress, at least in part; it sometimes responds favorably to cortisone or corticotropin.

DICKINSON W. RICHARDS

Reference

Warren, S., and Spencer, J.: Radiation Reaction in Lung. Am. J. Roentgenol., 43:682, 1940.

LIPOID PNEUMONITIS

(Lipid Pneumonia, Paraffinoma of the Lung)

This is a chronic pneumonitis, due to the presence of nonabsorbable oil in the lungs. It is produced by long-continued use of oily nose drops, or by direct intralaryngeal application, or by regurgitation and aspiration of ingested mineral oil, cod liver oil, or the like. The condition is found most often in debilitated elderly persons, or malnourished infants. It has become less common in recent years. Pathologically there may be only mild edema, with macrophages, around the oil particles, or fibrosis, or a more cellular granulomatous reaction. Roentgenographic changes vary from exaggerated linear markings to massive conglomerate shadows. Symp-

sue, dissolution of alveolar walls and interstitial fibrosis result in a fixation of the state of hyperinflation. The position of hyperinflation has unfavorable effects on chest mechanics. This is seen chiefly in costodiaphragmatic respiration, due to the chronically hypertonic flattened diaphragm. With inspiration further contraction of the diaphragm produces little or no downward movement, but only contracts inward, thus actually pulling in the sides and front of the lower chest on inspiration. In extreme cases the lower lobes lose almost all expansion. The upper chest is held in upward and forward position, but upper costal breathing still functions.

An additional dysfunction that develops is a true hypertonicity and loss of synergy of the respiratory muscles. Breathing is often jerky and spasmodic. Hypertonic neck muscles help to bend the neck forward and exaggerate the characteristic upper dorsal kyphosis.

The effects on lung volumes are marked. Residual air (the volume in the lungs on deep expiration) is much increased, often twice normal. Vital capacity is decreased, often to 1500 cc. or less. Bronchioles become further narrowed during expiration, with retardation and prolongation of the expiratory act. The slowing of respiration causes maximum breathing capacity to be even more decreased than vital capacity, sometimes to 20 or 15 liters per minute. Efforts at deep breathing result in trapping of air in dilated air spaces, and additional hyperinflation. Coughing may produce the same effect.

Loss of elasticity of lung tissue, and bronchiolar obstruction, greatly increase the work of breathing. Intrapleural pressures show wide swings, from -5 cm. of water in inspiration to as much as $+10$ or $+14$ cm. of water during expiration.

Within the lung, alveolar function is deranged. Some alveoli are overaerated with inadequate blood perfusion (increased "dead space" ventilation); other stagnant spaces are perfused but not aerated, causing arterial anoxia, which is made worse during exercise. With further progression of the disease, carbon dioxide elimination by the lungs is compromised. There occurs, first, an increase in carbon dioxide tension in alveolar air and blood. This results, in turn, in bicarbonate retention by the kidneys, so that blood CO_2 rises still further, and a state of chronic hypercapnea ensues.

In the early and moderate stages of emphysma, patients characteristically hyperventilate, with prolonged expiration. Hyperventilation, increased ventilatory effort and greatly decreased breathing capacity readily explain the dyspnea which is the major symptom. In the most severe emphysema, with profound anoxia, hypercapnea and respiratory acidosis, the respiratory stimulus is depressed (owing to chronically elevated blood CO_2 tension), and a tendency to hypoventilation provides a vicious circle in the pathophysiologic complex.

The effects of emphysema on the pulmonary circulation are variable. Some mild to moderate cases have normal pulmonary arterial pressures. In most moderate and severe cases there is pulmonary arterial hypertension, pressures increasing from the normal 25/8 mm. of mercury, to 40/15, 60/30 mm. or even higher. Pulmonary arteriosclerosis is a frequent but not constant complication. Other factors are the greatly decreased pulmonary capillary bed, and possibly also the hypertensive effect of anoxia on the pulmonary circulation.

One of the severe stages of emphysema is that associated with cor pulmonale and right heart failure. This may occur acutely, most frequently as a complication of an intercurrent pneumonia. Or chronic cor pulmonale may develop, a clinical picture consisting in marked arterial anoxia and hypercapnea, polycythemia, increased blood volume, hypertrophy and dilatation of the right ventricle, increased venous pressure, and eventually the full picture of right-sided congestive failure. Cardiac output is usually decreased in acute cor pulmonale. In chronic cor pulmonale, when the patient is in congestive failure, cardiac output is frequently (but not always) increased above normal, returning to normal with clinical improvement, i.e., with improved arterial oxygenation, decreased blood CO_2, decreased blood volume and decrease in polycythemia.

Symptoms and Signs. The common symptoms of chronic obstructive emphysema are dyspnea on exertion, cough, asthmatic attacks and cyanosis. The onset of symptoms is usually gradual and insidious. A chronic cough from an associated infection, such as sinusitis or bronchitis, or recurring asthmatic episodes are often the initial manifestations.

As the emphysematous state progresses, the patient will exhibit exertional dyspnea, often ascribed at first to poor physical condition, smoking or advancing years. Sometimes dyspnea is first noted abruptly during or after an acute bronchopneumonia. In general, the condition is aggravated by respiratory infections and is worse during the winter months.

Physical signs at this time will show well developed anatomic changes. In the asthenic type of person, there is upper dorsal kyphosis, the upper chest is raised anteriorly, the lower chest narrow, the diaphragm position low, with poor expansion, and the abdominal wall protuberant with poor muscular tone. In the sthenic person, the spine is more often straight, and the chest wide and voluminous (barrel chest), the abdominal wall retaining a good muscular tone.

Chest movement is chiefly upper costal in form. Deep breathing reveals prolonged wheezing expiration. The percussion note is hyperresonant, and fremitus often decreased. The breath sounds may be exaggerated at the hili, but characteristically diminished elsewhere, with prolonged expiration. Rales are variable: there may be none, or scattered asthmatic squeaks and wheezes, or dry fine rales at the bases, or, if there is associated bronchitis or bronchiectasis, moist rales localized or at both bases. The heart borders may be difficult to define and heart sounds faint because of overlying lung, often best heard below the xiphoid.

A roentgenogram of the chest shows overaerated lung fields, sometimes individual bullae, diaphragms flattened and low in position (best seen in lateral view), heart shadow "vertical."

As the disease advances, dyspnea becomes more marked, expiratory and asthmatic in type, at times paroxysmal. Coughing attacks are frequent, especially during the night and in the early morning, until sputum is raised and the air passages cleared. The cough is deep, hard and spasmodic, and may set off asthmatic seizures. Cyanosis usually becomes apparent at about this time, worse after exertion or coughing spasms. Physical examination shows more pronounced respiratory difficulty, with hypertonic accessory muscles of respiration, and jerky, poorly coordinated respiratory movements.

In its final stage, chronic emphysema may terminate either by way of extreme pulmonary insufficiency, or may develop cor pulmonale with secondary right heart failure. In the former the patient becomes completely incapacitated. He is both dyspneic and orthopneic, sits leaning forward, with shoulders raised, his respirations consisting of an inspiratory gasp, and prolonged wheezing expiration, interrupted by cough. Sputum is often purulent, and difficult to raise. Cyanosis is present, often marked. There may be intractable asthmatic attacks lasting for days. Bronchopneumonia is a frequent terminal event. In the intervals between attacks of acute respiratory failure, symptoms of chronic anoxia may be dominant: weakness, fatigue, loss of appetite, indigestion, insomnia, loss of memory, mental depression. Clubbing of fingers and toes may be present if there is associated bronchiectasis.

The cases that go on to chronic cor pulmonale are characterized by the development of marked arterial oxygen unsaturation and cyanosis, and progressive enlargement of the right ventricle. The second pulmonic heart sound is usually accentuated. With progression of the syndrome there occurs increasing polycythemia and greatly increased blood volume. This clinical picture is often referred to as the Ayerza syndrome. Eventually the right heart goes into frank congestive failure, with liver enlargement, increased venous pressure and peripheral edema. Right ventricular hypertrophy and dilatation may cause marked cardiac enlargement, both to right and left. The heart rate is rapid, sometimes with a gallop rhythm. Auricular fibrillation is rare. Clubbing of the fingers and toes is common with this syndrome. Death usually occurs with the patient in right-sided congestive failure; death is sometimes, however, unexpectedly sudden, the patient being found dead in bed, after having been up and around a few hours before.

In elderly patients with emphysema there is not infrequently an independent arteriosclerotic heart disease, and it may be difficult to evaluate the factors of left ventricular and of right ventricular failure when both are present together.

Course and Complications. The clinical course in chronic diffuse emphysema, while always protracted, is also extremely variable. Mild forms continue for years, causing only slight symptoms during or after respiratory infections, and with little or no progression of the disease process. Other cases, particularly those associated with severe chronic bronchial asthma, show a relentless progression, with fatal termination after perhaps three or four years of incapacitating pulmonary insufficiency. There are all variations between these extremes.

Complications include nasal sinusitis, chronic bronchitis, bronchiectasis, bullous emphysema, cor pulmonale and spontaneous pneumothorax. Many forms of pulmonary fibrosis, secondary to nonspecific infection, to tuberculosis or to silicosis, may be associated with obstructive emphysema, with clinical manifestations a combination of the restrictive ventilatory insufficiency of fibrosis and the obstructive ventilatory insufficiency of emphysema.

Treatment. Much can be done for the symptomatic relief of the patient with obstructive emphysema. The principles of therapy are to improve pulmonary ventilatory function, and to treat promptly or, better, to prevent recurring respiratory infections.

Bronchodilator agents are the mainstays of therapy for most patients with obstructive emphysema. In early stages, ephedrine by mouth (25 to 50 mg. two to four times a day) may be adequate. Antihistaminic drugs are often useful as adjunct therapy. Epinephrine by subcutaneous injection (0.3 to 1 cc. of 1:1000 solution) usually relieves asthmatic attacks. Probably the most useful single agents are the bronchodilator sprays, consisting of epinephrine solution, 1:100, or its equivalent. From four to twelve deep inhalations of the orally administered spray will usually be followed by marked relief of obstructive breathing and dyspnea. This can be used up to five or six times daily. More frequent dosage is often followed by tolerance to the drug, or by local drying and irritation of mucous membranes. A convenient schedule is an inhalation regularly morning and night. Bronchodilator spray may be combined or alternated with antibiotic aerosol spray if chronic infection is a factor.

If the patient has definite asthma and known allergic sensitivities, courses of desensitization may be tried.

For those with persistent cough and tenacious sputum, it is most important to raise the sputum effectively, and clear the air passages. Bronchodilator sprays are often helpful, expectorants are worth trying. Antitussive agents, such as codeine, should be used so far as possible in the irritative, nonproductive stages of coughing.

Breathing exercises are occasionally of value for patients whose mechanics of respiration are uncoordinated. Diaphragmatic function should be encouraged. A simple exercise is to have the patient lie on the bed with hands on his abdomen and practice breathing with the diaphragm only, continuing for 15 to 30 minutes. In longstanding cases, an extended course of exercises reeducating the patient to diaphragmatic breathing may be effective, but more often the patient becomes discouraged and stops.

For asthenic subjects with poor abdominal tone a well fitting lower abdominal belt may provide improvement in ventilatory function, by forcing a flattened diaphragm up into the thorax. The pressure should be applied below the umbilicus. The effect can be observed under the fluoroscope. Vital capacity is sometimes increased by as much as 1 liter by a properly fitted belt.

Acute respiratory infections must be treated promptly with adequate bed rest and antibiotic therapy, and with attention to chronic sinusitis, bronchitis or bronchiectasis if these are complicating factors.

Many patients with chronic emphysema are greatly benefited if they can spend the winter in a mild climate, removed from respiratory epidemics.

The use of respirators, chiefly those providing intermittent positive pressure for inspiration, has been effective in many instances, either the type with automatic inspiratory cycling (starting when expiratory pressure in the airways reaches zero), or the type requiring the patient's own inspiratory effort. Breathing with the respirator for periods of one-half to one hour three times daily often improves the patient from a bedchair to mild ambulatory activity. Oxygen or an air-oxygen mixture may be used, depending on the degree of anoxia.

Cortisone or corticotropin may help considerably some patients with moderately advanced emphysema, especially those with asthmatic attacks. After a few days on larger doses, a maintenance of 50 mg. of cortisone daily (less if possible) is usually well tolerated. The side effects of hyperadrenalism must be watched for.

Advanced obstructive emphysema, when in the stage of severe pulmonary insufficiency, demands well planned and vigorous treatment. The patient is usually most comfortable with a high Gatch bed, or leaning forward on a bed table.

Clearing of air passages is most important. Aminophylline, 0.25 gm. administered slowly, intravenously, is an effective bronchodilator. Epinephrine, 1:1000, 0.5 to 1 cc. subcutaneously, will usually bring some relief unless the patient has established a tolerance. The inhalational sprays, with epinephrine, Vapo-nephrine or similar agents, are best administered by vaporizing 0.3 to 1 cc. continuously with a stream of air or oxygen from a tank, and having the subject inhale the vapor by mouth. An effective procedure is to have the patient sit up, take an inhalation, then an expectorant, then cough vigorously and raise sputum; this is repeated several times a day.

The elimination of bronchial secretions is also important. If the patient becomes exhausted, and the cough reflex ineffectual, actual asphyxia may occur. In extreme cases tracheobronchial suction, bronchoscopic suction, or even tracheotomy, may be required.

Anoxia is a major element in these cases, and oxygen therapy will usually be indicated. Oxygen in adequate concentrations, from 40 to 50 per cent, can be given by nasal catheter, mask or tent, and either continuously or intermittently, depending on the need.

For severely obstructed cases, particularly those in status asthmaticus, oxygen may have to be administered by mask under positive pressure, either expiratory positive pressure or continuous positive pressure. Sometimes high concentrations, up to 60 or 70 per cent, are necessary. This will usually provide adequate aeration and relieve cyanosis and anoxia.

In advanced emphysema with anoxia and CO_2 retention, much of the total respiratory stimulus may be that of anoxia. On oxygen breathing, respiration will then be reduced, and CO_2 accumulate further in the blood. If arterial blood CO_2 content exceeds 85 or 90 volumes per 100 cc. (40 mEq.), or about 100 volumes per 100 cc. in venous plasma, then CO_2 in the tissues exerts a narcotic effect, and the patient becomes stuporous or comatose. This "CO_2 narcosis," while not common, does occur from time to time in oxygen-treated emphysema cases of severe degree—always those with already high blood CO_2 levels.

The aim of treatment is better pulmonary ventilation, to eliminate CO_2. The respirators, above-mentioned, are often very useful. Occasionally a patient will have to be placed in a Drinker respirator for several days.

Patients with severe pulmonary insufficiency are restless and uncomfortable and usually need sedation. Barbiturates can be given with relative safety. Morphine, however, must be used with great caution: at most a single dose in 12 hours. Repeated doses will inhibit respiration and the cough reflex, producing accumulated bronchial secretions and asphyxia which may be rapidly fatal. Chronic asthma is also the largest single cause, among nonfatal organic diseases, of narcotic addiction.

The most frequent terminal complications in advanced emphysema are (1) bronchopneumonia, and (2) cor pulmonale with acute or chronic right-sided congestive heart failure.

Treatment of cor pulmonale includes all the measures to relieve pulmonary insufficiency, as well as therapy for congestive heart failure. Digitalization, low salt diet and diuretics should be given as indicated. Diamox, 250 mg. twice a day, may be of adjuvant value as a diuretic. If there is frank congestive failure with a coexisting polycythemia, a phlebotomy of 500 cc., repeated every few days, to a total removal of 1500 to 2000 cc., is often of great value. Next to actual blood volume measurement, the hematocrit is the best index of adequate blood removal.

NONOBSTRUCTIVE (SENILE, POSTURAL) EMPHYSEMA

While the nonobstructive or atrophic aspects are a part of diffuse emphysema generally, the senile lung may be a distinct entity. In its milder form senile emphysema is no more than the normal aging process, pulmonary tissues sharing loss of elasticity and resilience commensurate with similar changes in other tissues. Thus statistics of normal subjects show slowly progressive loss of vital capacity and maximum breathing capacity and relative increase in residual air, with advancing age.

As a pathologic condition, senile emphysema consists in marked loss of elastic tissue, degeneration of alveolar walls and diffuse coalescence of alveolar spaces, producing in extreme cases a typical "honeycomb" lung. This may cause symptoms of advanced pulmonary insufficiency.

Special forms of degenerative, nonobstructive emphysema have been described: emphysema of the lower lobes from widening of the lower thorax secondary to abdominal from depressed diaphragms secondary to obesity (Tendeloo); postural emphysema hypotonic abdominal wall (Kerr); emphysema from a stiffened spine and elevated ribs, with enlarged thorax (Alexander).

BULLOUS EMPHYSEMA; AIR CYSTS OF LUNG

Large emphysematous bullae may be single or multiple. In general this condition conforms to one of three types: (a) bullae with free bronchial communication, the remainder of the lungs being normal. These give few or no symptoms unless they become very large. In the latter case surgical removal may be considered. (b) A bulla (solitary air cyst) or bullae, with narrowed bronchial communication, allowing air passage only inward, during inspiration, the remainder of the lungs being normal. These form tension cysts of increasing size, gradually displacing lung and mediastinum. Treatment is surgical, usually requiring lobectomy or pneumonectomy. (c) Bullae of various sizes, with the remainder of the lungs emphysematous, sometimes called "vanishing lung," an atrophic process perhaps akin to the "senile" emphysematous lung. Surgical removal of bullae, if they are expansile, causing compression, may occasionally bring improvement, but more often does not.

LOCALIZED ("COMPENSATORY") EMPHYSEMA

Several types of localized emphysema are of clinical interest.

Small, thin-walled emphysematous vesicles occur not infrequently at the pleural surface of otherwise normal lungs. Rupture of one of these is the commonest cause of spontaneous pneumothorax in apparently healthy persons (Kjaergaard).

Localized emphysema occurs adjacent to regions of atelectasis or fibrosis, or in lungs subjected to anatomic distortion, as in kyphoscoliosis.

The situation following lobectomy or pneumonectomy is interesting. If the remaining lung is normal, it expands into the additional space without development of fixed emphysema and without disturbance of pulmonary function. But if there is a tendency to diffuse emphysema or if it develops later, pneumonectomy will aggravate the condition, and loss of function results. Such a condition has been called "compensatory" emphysema, obviously a misnomer.

DICKINSON W. RICHARDS

References

Baldwin, E. deF., Cournand, A., and Richards, D. W., Jr.: Pulmonary Insufficiency. I. Physiological Classification, Clinical Methods of Analysis, Standard Values in Normal Subjects. Medicine, 27:243, 1948.
———: Pulmonary Insufficiency. III. A Study of 122 Cases of Chronic Pulmonary Emphysema. Medicine, 28:201, 1949.
———: Pulmonary Insufficiency. IV. A Study of 16 Cases of Large Pulmonary Air Cysts or Bullae. Medicine, 29:169, 1950.
Barach, A. L.: Physiologic Therapy in Respiratory Diseases. Philadelphia, J. B. Lippincott Co., 1948.
Comroe, J. H., Jr.: Methods in Medical Research. Vol. 2. Chicago, Year Book Publishers, Inc., 1950.
Cournand, A., Himmelstein, A., Riley, R. L., and Lester, C. W.: A Follow-up Study of the Cardiopulmonary Function in Four Young Individuals after Pneumonectomy. J. Thoracic Surg., 16:30, 1947.
Ferrer, M. I., and others: Some Effects of Digoxin upon the Heart and Circulation in Man. Digoxin in Chronic Cor Pulmonale. Circulation, 1:161, 1950.
Kjaergaard, H.: Spontaneous Pneumothorax in the Apparently Healthy. Copenhagen, Levin and Munksgaard, 1932.
Loeschcke, H.: Das Lungenemphysem, in Henke, F., and Lubarsch, O.: Handbuch d. spez. Path., Anat., u. Histol., 1928, Vol. 3, page 612.
Segal, M. S., and Dulfano, M. J.: Chronic Pulmonary Emphysema: Physiopathology and Treatment. New York, Grune and Stratton, 1953.
———, Salomon, A., and Herschfus, J. A.: Treatment of Chronic Pulmonary Emphysema. Am. Rev. Tuberc., 69:915, 1954.
Smart, R. H., Davenport, C. K., and Pearson, G. W.: Intermittent Positive Pressure Breathing in Emphysema of Chronic Lung Diseases. J.A.M.A., 150:1385, 1952.

ABSCESS OF THE LUNG

A pulmonary abscess is a suppurative focus within the lung associated with necrosis. Although many inflammatory processes such as pneumonitis and bronchiectasis may show microscopic evidence of abscess formation, only those lesions in which the abscess is a predominant gross pathologic finding are classified clinically as pulmonary abscesses. When necrosis of tissue is the outstanding feature of the lesion, the term gangrene of the lung has been used. Because such marked necrosis of lung tissue is usually associated with serious bacterial invasion, especially with anaerobes, pulmonary gangrene has become rare since the advent of antibiotic therapy. Most cases of gangrene of the lung can be considered to be pulmonary abscesses in which vascular thrombosis is a prominent feature. Only rarely does gangrene of the lung occur without significant infection, because either the bronchial or the pulmonary vascular system alone can maintain the viability of the lung.

Etiology. Pulmonary abscesses are caused by a variety of pyogenic bacteria. Those organisms which tend to cause tissue breakdown are most likely to result in abscess formation. The staphylococcus, streptococcus, Friedländer bacillus, pneumococcus (rarely), actinomyces and various anaerobes including the fusiform bacilli and spirochetes are among the pathogenic bacteria found. The cultures from a pulmonary abscess often yield several types of bacteria, and therefore it may be difficult to ascertain the etiologic role of each. Symbiosis may be a factor. Following chemotherapy the bacterial flora may change because the reduction or elimination of the predominant organisms favors the emergence of secondary invaders. Thus fungi have become of greater etiologic importance since antibiotic therapy. The lesions caused by *Mycobacterium tuberculosis* are clinically not considered as pulmonary abscesses, although purulent foci may develop with caseation necrosis. A pyogenic pulmonary abscess can develop, however, as a complication of tuberculous bronchostenosis.

The bacteria responsible for a pulmonary abscess may reach the lung through aspiration down the tracheobronchial tree, via the blood stream, or by penetrating trauma or extension of an adjacent suppurative focus. Infected material aspirated from the upper air passages may lodge in a small branch bronchus and produce an acute inflammatory process. Partial obstruction of a bronchus favors a retention of secretion and suppuration in the corresponding bronchopulmonary segment. Tumors of the bronchus, foreign bodies and various stenotic bronchial lesions frequently are responsible for abscess formation. Infected pulmonary emboli or secondary infection of an infarct may produce a lung abscess. Suppuration may also result from secondary infection of a pulmonary hematoma or from penetrating trauma. Pulmonary abscess may result from the extension of a suppurative focus from beneath the diaphragm into the adherent basal portion of the lung. Amebic abscesses may reach the lung by this route. Likewise a mediastinal abscess or perforating lesion of the esophagus may cause an abscess of the lung by direct extension.

Pulmonary abscess rarely occurs as a complication of pneumococcal lobar pneumonia unless secondary invasion by other organisms occurs. Friedländer pneumonia by contrast is frequently associated with abscesses which may be large and chronic.

Incidence. The incidence of primary abscess of the lung has been greatly reduced since the introduction of effective chemotherapeutic and antibiotic agents for the treatment of pneumonia, or as a prophylactic measure in any case of bronchial infection. By contrast, secondary pulmonary abscesses resulting from bronchial obstruction are becoming more frequent because of the increasing incidence of bronchogenic carcinoma. Since most primary pulmonary abscesses begin as an area of acute inflammation which only later results in tissue necrosis, effective antibacterial therapy may prevent an area of suppurative pneumonia from progressing to abscess formation. The incidence of pulmonary abscess secondary to foreign body has been reduced by earlier endoscopic removal of aspirated objects.

Pulmonary abscesses are more frequent in individuals with oral sepsis and in persons subject to spells of unconsciousness. Epileptics and severe alcoholics are particularly prone to pulmonary suppuration. Aspiration into the lungs may also occur during general anesthesia, but such an occurrence is becoming less frequent owing to improvements in anesthesiology.

Pathology. The location of pulmonary abscesses varies depending on the etiologic factors. Abscesses produced by aspiration are most common in those portions of the lung which are dependent in the recumbent position. The apical portions of the lower lobes and the posterior segments of the upper lobes are the most frequent sites of such abscesses. Moreover, the angles of the main bronchi in relation to the trachea favor aspiration into the right side. Pulmonary abscesses secondary to infarction are more common in the basal portions of the lower lobe. Abscess of the lung secondary to bronchial obstruction by tumor may occur in any portion of the lungs, and therefore a pulmonary abscess located anteriorly or at the pulmonary apex is likely to be secondary to bronchial obstruction, because aspiration and embolic abscesses are less common in those sites.

An area of pneumonitis which progresses to significant tissue necrosis results in a lung abscess. The nature of the predominant bacteria and the degree of localized vascular thrombosis determine the extent of the abscess formation. The pathologic findings vary from lesions with a large area of pneumonia surrounding one or more pulmonary abscesses of varying size, to cases in which necrosis of a large segment of lung tissue has resulted from a pyogenic process with much vascular thrombosis. Foul pus usually indicates the presence of anaerobic infection. In an acute abscess a piece of necrotic pulmonary tissue may be found free or partly sequestrated within the abscess cavity. The degree of bronchial communication will determine the ease with which purulent material may drain from a pulmonary abscess and air may enter the cavity. With good bronchial drainage in the acute phase, the abscess may progressively diminish in size and heal with only a residual fibrous scar. Edema and granulation tissue in the bronchus often interfere with bronchial drainage. Spontaneous resorption may occur occasionally. If a pulmonary abscess becomes chronic, an increasing amount of fibrosis develops in the adjacent lung tissue and bronchiectasis of varying extent is usually found. The bronchial epithelium tends to grow into a chronic cavity if the infection is not too active. When lined by epithelium, spontaneous obliteration of the cavity can no longer be expected.

A cavity resulting entirely from destruction of lung tissue must be differentiated from a small suppurative defect which is markedly enlarged owing to localized obstructive emphysema. If a ball-valve mechanism develops in a bronchus proximal to any pulmonary defect caused by dissolution of lung tissue, air tends to be trapped distal to the site of bronchial narrowing, and the defect in the lung may become inflated by a positive pressure within the cavity resulting from straining or cough. Although such an occurrence is more frequent in tuberculosis than in suppurative disease of the lung, it may occur with pyogenic infections, especially staphylococcal pneumonia. A single roentgenologic observation may not permit differentiation between a large pulmonary abscess resulting from extensive necrosis and a cavity produced largely by the hyperinflation of a small pulmonary defect. The latter type of cavity might readily collapse or be absorbed when the draining bronchus either opens more widely or becomes occluded.

A pulmonary abscess may rupture into the pleural space and produce a pyopneumothorax, or the infection may extend to the pleura without gross rupture and result in empyema. Rupture into the pleura is relatively uncommon in spite of the peripheral location of most aspiration pulmonary abscesses, because the localized pleuritis which usually forms seals the suppurative area from the free pleural cavity. Occasionally a lung abscess ruptures into the esophagus or some other adjacent organ. Brain abscess, either single or multiple, may be a hematogenous complication of pulmonary abscess.

Symptoms. The symptoms at the onset of the illness are usually considered to be due to an acute bronchitis or pneumonia with cough, malaise and fever. Chest pain is frequently present owing to the development of pleuritis over the area of pulmonary involvement. Chills and night sweats may occur. The nature of the sputum may warn the clinician that the process is not a simple pneumonia. Purulent expectoration is often present after the first few days, but when an abscess has developed distal to a bronchial obstruction, purulent sputum may be late in appearing or not be manifest because of interference with bronchial drainage. Foul sputum is quite typical but is less common if antibiotic therapy has been employed in the early stages of the pneumonitis, and its occurrence will depend upon the nature of the primary organism and secondary invaders. The degree of malaise and fever is influenced by the causative bacteria, by antibiotic therapy, and by whether the abscess is secondary to bronchial obstruction. A pulmonary abscess distal to a bronchogenic carcinoma sometimes causes little malaise because a less virulent infection is present. Hemoptyses of varying amount may occur with a pulmonary abscess, and occasionally there are massive hemorrhages when much gangrene is present. A chocolate-colored sputum due to a mixture of blood and pus may be noted; an underlying neoplasm or an amebic abscess should be ruled out in such cases. The untreated pulmonary abscess often leads to progressive loss of weight and strength with anemia. Clubbing of the fingers may be noted after two or more weeks of illness.

The course of a pulmonary abscess developing after aspiration is considerably influenced by the adequacy of bronchial drainage. If the purulent material drains into the larger bronchi and can be expectorated, spontaneous healing may occur. Such drainage of purulent material into the bronchial tree does at times result in bronchogenic spread of infection into other portions of the lung. The occurrence of such spill-over abscesses is relatively uncommon under antibiotic treatment.

The patient with an acute lung abscess usually appears acutely ill and is febrile. Dyspnea is usually not prominent except with massive involvement. In the absence of pleural complications the physical signs may be meager. Slight dullness and rales may be noted. Early in the course of the disease a localized pleural friction rub may be present. Localization of the site of the abscess, if pleural pain and chest wall tenderness are absent, is often difficult by physical examination alone. Auscultatory signs of cavitation are often absent. Clubbing of the fingers is common in the subacute and chronic abscess. Leukocytosis is common, depending to some extent on the infecting organism, and anemia often develops with persisting infection.

Diagnosis. The possibility of an abscess of the lung should be considered when a patient who is acutely ill begins to expectorate pus. It is of the greatest importance to differentiate a primary pulmonary abscess from suppuration distal to a bronchial neoplasm. If the history does not suggest the possibility of aspiration of infectious material into the lungs or an embolic origin, and the area of involvement corresponds to a bronchial segment, the possibility of a primary neoplasm is very real. Purulent expectoration of long duration is often due to bronchiectasis but a chronic lung abscess must also be considered.

Roentgenologic studies are an important aid in the diagnosis of pulmonary abscess but the radiologic findings may not be diagnostic. When the films demonstrate an intrapulmonary cavity, particularly with a fluid level, and the patient is expectorating foul sputum, the diagnosis of abscess is quite certain. If the sputum is not foul, bacteriologic examination may differentiate between a pyogenic abscess and tuberculosis. If poor bronchial drainage from a lung abscess exists, the roentgenogram may fail to demonstrate the presence of a pulmonary cavity because of the failure of air to enter the abscess. In such cases the abscess appears as an area of homogeneous density on the film, and radiologic differentiation from a pneumonic area is difficult. In chronic cases bronchograms may differentiate bronchiectasis from a chronic pulmonary abscess.

Bronchoscopic examination is indicated for both diagnostic and therapeutic purposes. By bronchoscopy a foreign body, neoplasm or bronchial stenosis may be visualized if the lesion is not too peripheral in location. Bronchoscopy may faciliate bronchial drainage, and the cultures of the secretion obtained at bronchoscopy will give more reliable bacteriologic data than the examination of sputum which is contaminated with mouth organisms.

Exploratory needle puncture through the chest wall is contraindicated because of the danger of spread of the infection, especially into the pleural space. Bronchograms are usually inadvisable in the acute phase but are often important later to determine whether any residual cavitation or bronchiectasis remains.

Posteroanterior and lateral roentgenograms of the chest should be taken weekly during the acute phase of the illness. Bucky films may aid in the visualization of cavitation. If the suppurative process does not respond to antibiotic therapy as anticipated, the possibility of bronchial obstruction must be reconsidered.

Bronchiectasis in an advanced stage is often associated with abscess formation. Such patients usually have a history of chronic cough often dating to childhood or a history of previous pneumonias. In some instances, however, it may be difficult to determine whether the bronchiectasis is secondary to a chronic abscess or vice versa. Great care should be taken in obtaining a history about any possible aspiration, especially in children. Details of the onset of the illness can be most helpful in clinical evaluation.

In pulmonary tuberculosis the onset is usually less acute except when an acute tuberculous pneumonia is present. In uncomplicated tuberculosis the sputum is not foul and is usually not profuse unless the disease is widespread. The radiologic findings usually aid in differentiation. Sputum examinations for tubercle bacilli are indicated. The differentiation of a primary pulmonary abscess from an infected bronchogenic cyst may be difficult but the history and roentgen findings may distinguish the two lesions. Thoracotomy is indicated in such cases for diagnosis as well as therapy.

Treatment. The initial treatment of pulmonary abscess hinges on whether the lesion is secondary to a bronchial obstruction. Therefore early bronchoscopic examination is indicated. Antibiotic treatment with broad spectrum agents should be started at once in all cases. When the abscess is secondary to a neoplasm, pulmonary resection is indicated after a brief period of preoperative antibiotic preparation. Foreign bodies can usually be removed endoscopically. Suppuration distal to a bronchial stenosis is treated by surgical excision of the involved portion of the lung.

Antibiotic and chemotherapeutic agents are the chief measures employed for an acute primary pulmonary abscess. Aerosol therapy may be employed to supplement the systemic administration of antibiotics. Bacteriologic examination of the sputum or bronchial secretions obtained at the time of bronchoscopy may aid in the selection of the best agents for the individual patient. The sensitivity of the organisms to various chemotherapeutic agents should be determined. Because of the possibility of development of drug resistance and changing bacterial flora, it may be advisable to culture the secretions again in a few weeks and repeat the sensitivity tests. Such examinations may indicate that a different antibiotic should then be employed. Prolonged treatment for several weeks or even a few months may be indicated in order to avoid relapse. Clinical improvement is usually noted within a few days of the institution of drug therapy, and surgical drainage of an acute pulmonary abscess is rarely necessary. Postural drainage may be helpful.

The degree of response of a pulmonary abscess to antibiotic therapy and the amount of pulmonary damage will determine whether surgical treatment is indicated. If the pulmonary cavity disappears and no significant pneumonitis or bronchiectasis remains, only medical measures are necessary. If cavitation or other irreversible changes in the lung persist, surgical excision of the diseased part, usually by lobectomy or segmental resection, is indicated. The risk is low and the results good. If a pulmonary abscess does not heal

within a month or two, fibrosis of the pericavitary tissue and partial epithelization of the cavity wall may interfere with subsequent closure. Such chronic cavities should usually be resected surgically.

Localized obstructive emphysema as seen especially with staphylococcal pneumonia of infancy and childhood must not be confused with lung abscess, since these hyperinflated lesions are reversible and do not require surgical excision.

HERBERT C. MAIER

References

Drake, E. H., and Sones, F. M.: The Management of Lung Abscess with Special Reference to the Place of Antibiotics in Therapy. Ann. Int. Med., 35:1218, 1951.

Potts, W. J., and Riker, W. L.: Differentiation of Congenital Cyst of Lung and Those Following Staphylococcic Pneumonia. Arch. Surg., 61:684, 1950.

Shaw, R. R., and Paulson, D. L.: Pulmonary Resection for Chronic Abscess of the Lung. J. Thoracic Surg., 17:514, 1948.

Waterman, D. H., and Domm, S. E.: Changing Trends in the Treatment of Lung Abscess. Dis. of Chest, 25:40, 1954.

CYSTIC DISEASE OF THE LUNGS

The term "cystic disease of the lungs" has been applied to a rather wide variety of pulmonary lesions characterized by the presence of air- or fluid-containing spaces within the lung. Since the etiology, pathologic findings and clinical course may vary widely depending on specific features of the "cystic" lesion, it is important to differentiate various types.

Congenital cystic disease of the lung is relatively rare. It is due to embryologic maldevelopment of the lungs. Congenital cysts may be single or multiple, fluid- or air-containing. Such cysts are sometimes associated with anomalies of the lobar development of the lung together with anomalies of the pulmonary or bronchial vessels. If such cysts become distended, dyspnea and cyanosis may be present. Frequently the first symptoms are those of secondary infection to which such lesions are prone. The lesion may simulate an encapsulated empyema. Surgical excision is usually indicated (Fig. 127).

Most lesions designated as cysts of the lung are not congenital but are acquired secondary to infection, partial bronchial obstruction and obstructive emphysema. It is undesirable to designate a pulmonary lesion as a cyst or "cystic condition" merely because a rounded cavity containing air or fluid is seen on a roentgenogram. Saccular bronchiectasis which gives a roentgen appearance of multiple "cyst-like" spaces should be considered as a type of bronchiectasis and treated as such. An epithelialized chronic abscess cavity in the lung is not a pulmonary

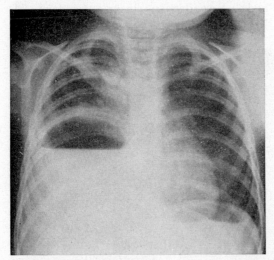

Fig. 127. Large congenital cyst at the base of a right lung in a 34 month old child. History and findings simulate an encapsulated empyema. Cured by lobectomy.

cyst although the radiologic features are sometimes similar. Bullous emphysema and subpleural blebs are locally advanced lesions of pulmonary emphysema. The localized obstructive emphysema which is not uncommon during the course of staphylococcal pneumonia in childhood may be confused with congenital cysts of the lung. Adequate differentiation can usually be made because serial roentgenograms often show rapid changes in the size of the air spaces associated with staphylococcal pneumonia as contrasted with the more stationary appearance of congenital cysts. Such air spaces developing in the course of staphylococcal pneumonia require no surgical therapy unless there is severe dyspnea. Cysts of the lung also occur in echinococcosis.

Some air cysts may enlarge to tremendous size owing to the development of a check-valve mechanism in the draining bronchus. Such tension cysts must be differentiated from tension pneumothorax and may produce severe dyspnea and cyanosis which re-

quires emergency thoracotomy with drainage or excision of the involved portion of the lung. Sometimes the entire lung is compressed and collapsed by a cystic lesion which occupies only a segment of one lobe.

HERBERT C. MAIER

References

Caffey, J.: Natural Regression of Pulmonary Cyst during Early Infancy. Pediatrics, *11*:48, 1953.
Cassels, D. E., Fitz, J. M., and Adams, W. E.: Congenital Cystic Disease of the Lungs. J. Pediat., 35:585, 1949.
Cooke, F. N., and Blades, B.: Cystic Disease of the Lungs. J. Thoracic Surg., 23:546, 1952.

NEW GROWTHS IN THE LUNGS

BENIGN TUMORS

Benign tumors of the lung are relatively uncommon and some neoplasms which were previously regarded as benign are now known to have malignant potentialities. Most important of these is the *bronchial adenoma,* which is most common in young women but may occur in both sexes at any age. This neoplasm usually arises in one of the larger bronchi but frequently extends outside the bronchial wall. The growth often manifests itself by wheezing or recurrent pneumonia in the portion of the lung distal to the bronchial obstruction. Severe hemoptyses may occur. The tumor itself is often not detectable on routine roentgenograms because of its location in the region of the root shadows at the hilum of the lung. The roentgenogram may demonstrate only the secondary pneumonitis, when present, unless bronchography or tomography is employed to delineate the endobronchial portion of the tumor (Fig. 128). A bronchial adenoma can usually be visualized through the bronchoscope, but biopsy must be done with caution as severe bleeding may occur. The treatment of choice is removal by bronchotomy or lobectomy, although pneumonectomy is occasionally required because of secondary suppuration and the location of the growth. The prognosis after surgical removal is excellent.

A benign pulmonary tumor which must be differentiated from bronchogenic carcinoma is the *chondromatous hamartoma.* This neoplasm usually consists largely of cartilage but microscopically also contains other tissues indicating an embryonal aberration, as implied by its name. A hamartoma is usually located close to the pleural surface of the lung and rarely compresses a segmental bronchus. Thus symptoms are mild or absent. The tumor is often an incidental finding on roentgen examination but a positive diagnosis is not possible from the roentgen shadow. Local surgical excision is indicated.

Other benign pulmonary tumors are very rare. These may arise within a bronchus or in the interstitial tissue of the lung. They

CARCINOMA OF THE LUNG

Carcinoma is by far the most common primary tumor found in the lung. Sarcoma arising from the bronchi or the interstitial pulmonary tissue is very rare and simulates the clinical features of carcinoma. Primary lymphosarcoma of the lung is a rare lesion which has a better prognosis than bronchogenic carcinoma. Hodgkin's disease may involve the lungs as well as the hilar lymph nodes. Secondary carcinoma or sarcoma of the lung is a frequent sequela of neoplasms

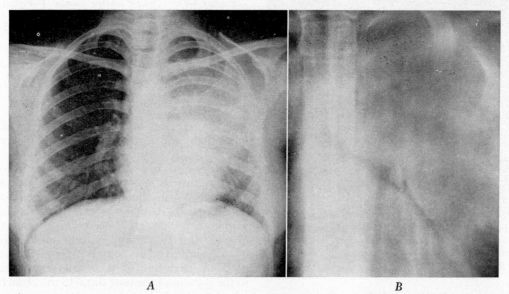

A   *B*

Fig. 128. A bronchial adenoma obstructing left upper lobe bronchus. *A*, Routine roentgenogram demonstrates an airless consolidated left upper lobe but does not indicate the cause of consolidation. *B*, Tomographic x-ray photograph of same patient shows endobronchial tumor projecting from orifice of left upper lobe.

include the neurofibroma, lipoma, leiomyoma, fibroma and endobronchial chondroma. If the growth projects into a bronchus, the symptoms of wheezing, cough and suppuration secondary to the bronchial obstruction may be present. The radiographic findings of bronchial stenosis and bronchoscopic examination with biopsy establish the diagnosis in the endobronchial lesions. When the tumor does not arise in or press upon the wall of a large or intermediate sized bronchus, the lesion may be an incidental finding on a roentgenogram. Symptoms may be minimal or absent unless the tumor attains large size and causes dyspnea. The endobronchial tumors can be removed bronchoscopically or by surgical bronchotomy. Resection of the involved portion of the lung is otherwise indicated.

in other organs and the differentiation from primary tumor is considered in the section on Diagnosis.

Etiology. The essential cause of neoplasms of the lung is unknown but contributory factors include various types of chronic irritation. Exposure to radioactive substances and certain chemicals such as chromate compounds accounts for the high incidence of cancer of the lung in special occupations. A frequent history of heavy cigarette smoking among males with squamous carcinoma of the lung is noteworthy. An analysis of etiologic factors must take into consideration the possibility that different types of primary pulmonary neoplasms may well have varied and multiple causes.

Incidence. Bronchogenic carcinoma has shown a startling increase in incidence during the past few decades. It has become the most common cause of death from cancer among males in some American cities and is also common in rural areas. A comparative study of various types of primary neoplasms of the lung reveals that the greatest increase has occurred in squamous and undifferentiated carcinoma among males. Carcinoma of the lung occurs among males and females in a ratio of at least 6 to 1. Adenocarcinoma of the bronchus, which accounts for only a small percentage of the cancers among men, is the most frequent primary pulmonary neoplasm in females. Most persons with bronchogenic carcinoma are over 45 years of age, but some cases, especially of adenocarcinoma and undifferentiated carcinoma, occur in a younger age group.

Morbid Anatomy. The vast majority of primary cancers of the lung arise from the bronchial epithelium and are therefore called bronchogenic carcinoma. A few originate from the bronchial mucous glands. In males most bronchogenic cancers are squamous or epidermoid, or undifferentiated because of their anaplastic nature. Adenocarcinoma is relatively uncommon as a primary pulmonary tumor in males whereas it is more common than the squamous or epidermoid cancers in females. In both sexes an alveolar cell tumor may occasionally occur.

Bronchogenic carcinoma arising in a bronchus of large or intermediate size often produces sufficient bronchial narrowing to cause a secondary pneumonitis, bronchiectasis or abscess in the corresponding portion of the bronchial tree. The neoplasm also extends into the pulmonary tissue or may involve other adjacent structures. The pleural cavity, mediastinum, chest wall, base of the neck and diaphragm may be invaded by direct extension depending upon the primary location of the tumor. Metastases in the mediastinal lymph nodes are frequent, and infiltration of the wall of the esophagus, pericardium and heart may occur. Metastases in the opposite lung occur much more frequently with adenocarcinoma and undifferentiated carcinoma than with the squamous cancer. Extrathoracic metastases to the cervical lymph nodes, liver and brain are of particular clinical importance. Anaplastic growths may show widespread metastases.

Symptoms. The symptomatology of bronchogenic carcinoma is influenced considerably by the location of the growth in reference to the bronchial tree (Figure 129). Relatively small tumors in a main bronchus may cause a cough which may be nonproductive at first. In contrast, a carcinoma which involves only a bronchus of small size in the peripheral portion of a lung may be asymptomatic until it attains considerable size. There-

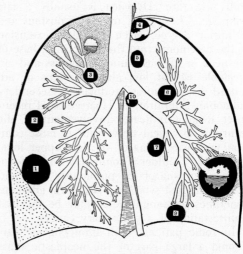

Fig. 129. The pathogenesis of symptoms and signs in primary carcinoma of the lung. *1*, Tumor near the pleura may produce pleurisy and serous or bloody pleural effusion. *2*, In this area a tumor may be "silent" for months. *3*, If a bronchus is occluded, atelectasis and dilatation of the distal bronchi may occur with bronchiectasis, pneumonitis or abscess formation. *4*, A tumor in the apex may cause erosion of a rib, paralysis of the sympathetic trunk causing a Horner's syndrome, pain in the arm and partial paralysis of the ulnar and median nerves by invading the first dorsal root of the brachial plexus, and invasion of adjacent structures. *5*, Pressure here may cause paralysis of the recurrent laryngeal and phrenic nerves. *6*, Incomplete obstruction of a large bronchus often causes unilateral wheezing and may cause obstructive emphysema. *7*, Ulceration of the bronchial mucous membrane gives rise to blood-streaked sputum or recurrent hemorrhages. *8*, Tumors may undergo central necrosis with abscess cavitation, and bronchial fistula. *9*, Irritation of the diaphragmatic pleura may cause pain of typical phrenic nerve distribution. *10*, Invasion of the esophagus with obstruction or ulceration may occur. (E. D. Churchill, in Christopher's Textbook of Surgery.)

fore the complete absence of symptoms is entirely consistent with a diagnosis of cancer of the lung.

Cough is the most common symptom of cancer of the lung, but, since most persons with primary pulmonary carcinoma are heavy smokers who have a chronic cough antedating the disease, the significance of this symptom may not be appreciated. Mucoid or mucopurulent sputum, sometimes with blood streaking, may appear. A hemoptysis may be the initial symptom. Localized wheezing may indicate partial bronchial obstruction. Fever may be present owing to secondary pneumonitis, but a septic appearance and chills are rare. Dyspnea is usually a late symptom. Chest pain, unless inconstant and of minor degree, often indicates extension of the carcinoma into the chest wall, base of the neck or mediastinum. Weakness and appreciable weight loss also are signs of advanced disease unless produced by secondary pulmonary suppuration. Hoarseness of recent onset usually indicates involvement of the recurrent laryngeal nerve and is most common with carcinoma of the left upper lobe. Pain in the shoulder is common with bronchogenic carcinoma of the pulmonary apex and may be the first symptom. A pleural effusion, sometimes serosanguineous, may be the first manifestation of a pulmonary cancer.

In some patients with bronchogenic carcinoma a large part of the neoplastic mass may extend outside the lung and invade adjacent structures. When the upper portion of the mediastinum is thus involved, the presenting symptoms may be swelling of the neck and face with venous engorgement caused by neoplastic compression or invasion of the superior vena cava—the "superior mediastinal syndrome." Dyspnea from tracheal compression and dysphagia from esophageal involvement may be present. Occasionally the earliest recognized symptoms may be from a brain metastasis. A small percentage of persons with bronchogenic carcinoma have joint symptoms simulating those of rheumatoid arthritis. The associated clubbing of the fingers which this group of patients with pulmonary osteoarthropathy manifest should lead to a careful radiographic search for an intrathoracic neoplasm. As such persons may have a small peripheral bronchogenic carcinoma, pulmonary symptoms may be slight or absent for a considerable time. The periarticular swelling and tenderness disappear dramatically following excision of the pulmonary tumor.

There are often no *physical signs* of pulmonary cancer in the earlier stages. Localized wheezing may indicate the presence of a lesion causing partial bronchial obstruction. Such wheezing may disappear as the obstruction becomes more complete. Dullness may

result from the pulmonary consolidation distal to the bronchostenosis or from a large peripheral tumor. Rales of an associated pneumonitis and various alterations in breath sounds are sometimes noted. Signs of pleural effusion usually indicate neoplastic involvement of the pleura or rarely an associated empyema.

The life expectancy in untreated primary pulmonary cancer varies considerably. Although many patients die within a year of the onset of notable symptoms, others may survive for a somewhat longer period. In rare instances the growth may be radiographically demonstrable for a few years before symptoms develop.

Diagnosis. Roentgenographic examination of the chest is the most important diagnostic step in the detection of tumors in the lung. Since pulmonary cancer is often in an advanced stage before significant symptoms are recognized, routine roentgen studies at half-yearly intervals are necessary if it is hoped to discover such neoplasms early. Although the film may thus alert the physician to the presence of a pulmonary lesion, the roentgen appearance alone may not permit a positive diagnosis in the earlier phases of the disease in many instances. Moreover, in some cases of bronchogenic carcinoma the lesion may escape detection because of its small size or its location close to the hilum of the lung, or obscuration by the cardiac shadow or dome of the diaphragm. Special radiographic techniques such as tomography are sometimes helpful. The data obtained by roentgenography should be interpreted in conjunction with the information gained from the history, physical examination and special laboratory studies. Bronchoscopic examination is indicated in all except the very peripheral lesions and permits the visualization and biopsy of tumors in the larger bronchi. The cytologic study of the bronchial secretions obtained at bronchoscopy and of sputum may demonstrate tumor cells even though the neoplasm is not visible through the bronchoscope. Negative bronchoscopic and cytologic findings do not rule out a neoplasm (Fig. 130).

Among the non-neoplastic pulmonary lesions which can simulate cancer of the lung are solitary tuberculous lesions, chronic lung abscess, bronchial erosion by lymph nodes, lipoid and interstitial pneumonia and pulmonary infarction. The scattered infiltration usually seen in the tuberculous lesions permits radiographic differentiation from a tumor in most instances. If only a solitary rounded tuberculous focus is seen on the roentgenogram, the appearance may be similar to that of a benign tumor or peripheral carcinoma. Since noncavitary tuberculous lesions do not necessarily produce a sputum with tubercle bacilli, only pathologic examination of the surgically excised nodule will establish the diagnosis. Chronic lung abscess may be confused clinically and radiographically with either a central excavated carcinoma or abscess distal to a bronchogenic cancer, but prompt surgical excision is indicated in either condition. Erosion of the wall of a bronchus by a diseased or calcified lymph node may cause severe hemoptyses and the signs of an endobronchial lesion. Bronchoscopy, bronchography and tomography aid in differentiation but doubt may remain prior to surgical exploration. Lipoid pneumonia may be suspected from a history of use of oily nose drops or inhalation of mineral oil owing to impaired gag reflex. Pulmonary infarction must be carefully differentiated from neoplasm since surgical exploration is contraindicated and is more hazardous in thromboembolic conditions.

Since the lungs are one of the most frequent sites of metastases from various primary neoplasms in other organs, the differentiation of primary pulmonary cancer from metastases is most important. Metastases are less likely to cause bronchial symptoms or hemoptysis. If the neoplasm is solitary and involves a bronchus, a primary bronchogenic carcinoma is most probable. When multiple nodules are present in the lungs, the pulmonary lesions are usually metastatic. Alveolar carcinoma of the lung, however, may be multicentric. A solitary nodule in the lung field might be either a primary or metastatic lesion. If the history and the physical and radiologic investigation of other portions of the body fail to demonstrate a primary neoplasm elsewhere, the pulmonary mass should be treated as a primary lung tumor. Since multiple primary tumors are not uncommon, a solitary mass in the lung of a person with a past history of cancer should not lead to the assumption that the lung lesion is necessarily a metastasis.

Treatment. Surgical excision of the lobe or the lung containing the pulmonary cancer together with the regional lymphatics is the preferred treatment if distant metastases or other evidence of inoperability cannot be definitely demonstrated. Because the majority

of patients with bronchogenic carcinoma are in the older age group, many have pulmonary emphysema of varying degree antedating the cancer. Since the physiologic adjustment to pneumonectomy is markedly influenced by the presence of severe emphysema in the remaining lung, less extensive surgical procedures such as lobectomy may be preferable in emphysematous patients if the location of

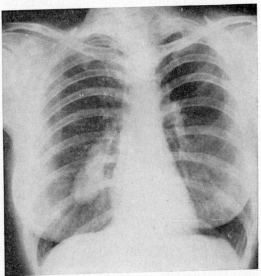

Fig. 130. Carcinoma of the lung which was not visible bronchoscopically. A sharp margin to the density on the roentgenogram does not indicate that the tumor is benign.

the carcinoma permits. If primary carcinoma of the lung is to be removed surgically before metastases have occurred, exploratory thoracotomy for removal of a roentgenologically demonstrated pulmonary lesion must often be undertaken without a positive preoperative diagnosis. When conclusive evidence of distant metastases is present, surgical therapy is no longer indicated. Evidence of mediastinal involvement by direct extension as seen with vena caval obstruction may likewise contraindicate operation unless the diagnosis of bronchogenic carcinoma is not established. Many patients with bronchogenic carcinoma already have an extension of the neoplastic process into the mediastinal structures at the time of exploratory thoracotomy. The prognosis in this group is poor even though a radical operation might still be technically feasible.

Radiation therapy, preferably with high voltage technique, is frequently employed as a palliative measure. Occasionally intensive radiation treatment for possible cure is indicated. Nitrogen mustard may cause temporary regression of some pulmonary cancers. Antibiotics ameliorate the effects of the secondary suppuration in many inoperable cases.

When a patient with a successfully treated primary carcinoma or sarcoma in some other portion of the body later develops an apparently solitary nodule in the lung, tomographic roentgenograms should be made to determine whether only a single nodule is present. Surgical excision of a pulmonary metastasis is occasionally warranted.

TUMORS OF THE TRACHEA

Tumors of the trachea are rare. The various types of neoplasms which are encountered in bronchi may also rise in the trachea. Because wheezing is a frequent sign of tracheal narrowing by tumor, most such patients are erroneously diagnosed as having bronchial asthma. The history of recent onset of fairly constant wheezing, perhaps with a dry or slightly productive cough, is an indication for bronchoscopy to establish the diagnosis. Roentgenograms of the chest are usually negative unless an extratracheal extension of the tumor has occurred or tomographic films demonstrate the lesion. The treatment is either by endoscopic removal, radiation therapy or surgical excision, depending on the nature and extent of the neoplasm. The prognosis depends largely on the time of correct diagnosis and the malignancy of the growth.

HERBERT C. MAIER

References

Ariel, I. M., Avery, E. E., Kanter, L., Head, J. R., and Langston, H. T.: Primary Carcinoma of the Lung. Cancer, 3:229, 1950.

Blades, B. B.: Surgical Management of Tumors of the Lung Discovered in X-ray Surveys. J.A.M.A., 154:196, 1954.

Churchill, E. D.: Primary Carcinoma of the Lung. J.A.M.A., 137:455, 1948.

De Bakey, M. E., Ochsner, A., and De Camp, P. T.: Primary Carcinoma of the Lung. Surgery, 32:877, 1952.

Moersch, H. J., and McDonald, J. R.: Bronchial Adenoma. J.A.M.A., 142:299, 1950.

Overholt, R. H., and Schmidt, I. C.: Silent Phase of Cancer of the Lung. J.A.M.A., 141:817, 1949.

Rubin, M., and Berkman, J.: Chondromatous Hamartoma of the Lung. J. Thoracic Surg., 23:393, 1952.

PNEUMONOCONIOSIS
(Pneumoconiosis)

Definition. Pneumonoconiosis is a generic term comprising all the chronic fibrous reactions arising in the lung as a result of the prolonged inhalation of excessive quantities of injurious mineral dusts, such as those of sand, granite, flint, asbestos. The term is used at times to describe pulmonary fibroses resulting from inhalation of dusts which are mixtures of substances in which the relative pathogenicity of each constituent is undetermined. Many of the pneumonoconioses are scarcely to be considered as diseases, since they may be present without producing symptoms or impairing physical efficiency, as in the case of anthracosis, chalicosis, siderosis, and so forth. On the other hand, dusts containing high concentrations of finely divided silica produce serious forms of pulmonary fibrosis of great medical and economic importance (silicosis). Admixture of alumina, carbon, gypsum and hematite with silica in dust results in a modification of the reaction to silica, retarding or inhibiting its noxious effects.

The silicates vary greatly in pathogenicity —some are apparently inert, others mildly pathogenic, while still others may even exert a retarding effect upon the action of free silica. Of the fibroses caused by silicates, that due to asbestos (abestosis) is probably the only one of importance, though certain investigators believe that some of the sericites are pathogenic.

As a rule the effects of inhalation of organic dusts are not included in the scope of the pneumoconioses. Such dusts may excite allergic reactions, they may introduce infection, or result in local irritant or toxic actions.

SILICOSIS

Definition. Silicosis is a chronic condition of the lungs caused by inhalation of air containing finely divided particles of silica (silicon dioxide) in sufficient quantity and over a sufficient period of time to produce fibrous nodules in the walls of the alveoli, which are readily recognizable in roentgenographs of the chest and in pathologic specimens. Clinically, the process is recognizable as a disease only in its advanced stages, either by increased dyspnea on exertion or by the symptoms of tuberculosis, to which it predisposes.

Etiology. Silica is widely distributed in nature, since it makes up a large part of the rocks and minerals which form the earth's crust. It occurs free as silicon dioxide and combined in the forms of silicates. Quartz, which is one of the most common forms of free silica, occurs abundantly in granite and other rocks. In consequence of this one might expect a high incidence of silicosis among workers in mines and tunnels and in stone cutters. There are, however, a great number of other industrial processes in which workers may be exposed to dust containing considerable amounts of free silica. Among these are listed the manufacture and use of abrasives, sandblasting, chipping, buffing of metals, metallurgic processes, ceramic manufacturing, glass making, enameling and the molding of metals. In 1930 it was estimated that more than a million industrial workers were potentially exposed to a silicosis hazard, and that half of this number were exposed to truly dangerous quantities of airborne silica.

Knowledge concerning the pathogenic effects of free silica in dust has come from several sources. Methods have been devised for counting dust, listing the number of particles, the distribution of their sizes and their composition. These data are correlated with the health records of the workers, including their death rate from tuberculosis, and with the incidence of pneumonoconiosis as revealed by x-ray survey.

Another important source of knowledge concerning the injurious effects of dust uses a technique in which animals are kept in dusts of known concentration for long periods of time so that the pathologic changes produced in their lungs may be observed. From studies of this kind it appears that the relative dangerousness of dusts is roughly proportional to the concentration of free silica in the different varieties. Other constituents of the dust either are inert or exert a modifying effect upon the reaction of the lungs to the free silica.

The size of the particles is important. It is doubtful whether particles larger than 10 microns enter the finer air passages. The greatest danger, therefore, lies in particles less than 10 microns, and it is probable that the most dangerous size is that less than 3 microns. There are several reasons for this: The larger particles settle out of the atmosphere more quickly than do finely divided particles. Also, the injurious effect of silica is believed to be exerted after partial solution; in other words its injurious effect is chemical rather than mechanical.

Information from field studies in various parts of the world indicates that a normal man might work in pure crystalline silica dust for many years without impairing his health, provided the concentration did not exceed 5,000,000 particles per cubic foot of air as determined by the lightfield counting method. Cummings has called this the "primary threshold." The duration of exposure is, of course, a most important factor. The rate at which silicosis develops under the same conditions varies with different persons. In general it may be said that in persons working in dust containing 5,000,000 particles of pure silica per cubic foot it would require from five to twenty years for the development of demonstrable silicosis. The rate of development, however, does not appear to vary directly with the concentration of silica, but increases slowly with elevations of the dust concentration up to a certain level, at which a marked acceleration is noted. Concentrations of dust in which there are more than 100,000,000 particles per cubic foot of air are extremely hazardous, and Cummings has called this the "secondary threshold," a value above which silicosis might be expected to develop with great rapidity. Under such conditions nodular fibrosis might occur in as short a time as two years. As a general rule, from fifteen to twenty years' working exposure to 15,-000,000 or 20,000,000 particles of pure crystalline silica is required to produce demonstrable silicosis.

Predisposing Causes. Reports from many parts of the world indicate that all races are susceptible. Sex is not a factor—women acquire the disease when exposed to the same conditions as men. The age factor is difficult to evaluate. Among predisposing causes, past and present respiratory infections are of great importance, particularly those of the nasal sinuses. Emphysema, old pleurisies, pneumonia and bronchitis are important in so far as they impair the dust-removal mechanism of the lung. The efficiency of the filtering mechanism of the nose appears to play an important role. Some observers believe that mouth-breathers are more susceptible than those with normal nasal passages. The fact remains, however, that individual variations in susceptibility are poorly understood.

Silicosis and Tuberculosis. In England the tuberculosis rate is higher among workers in dusty trades, being three to ten times as high as the rate for both employed and retired males. Gardner has made the statement that "At least 75 per cent of the human beings who develop silicosis die of tuberculosis, which may make its appearance at any stage of the disease." Such a statement, however, requires some qualification. In anthracosilicosis and siderosilicosis of coal and iron miners the action of silica is somewhat modified, the disease requires a longer time to produce disability, and the incidence of active tuberculosis is less than in the case of unmodified silicosis.

Modifying Factors. Apart from the modifying effect of coal dust and iron ore on the reaction to silica, there is increasing evidence that other dust constituents are not entirely inert. In a study of the gypsum industry Gardner found evidence of a protective action of gypsum dust when it is mixed with silica. Surveys of the cement industry have revealed a low incidence of silicosis among the workers. Some have taken this to mean that there is a protective substance, but it seems more likely that the low incidence of silicosis is due to the small amount of free silica in cement dust. Rapidly developing silicosis in the abrasive soap industry has been attributed to the accelerating effect of alkali. This conclusion should be accepted with reservations, since it is also possible that the rapid development is due to an extraordinary proportion of particles of silica less than 0.5 micron in size, the enumeration of which is not possible by the lightfield method.

Morbid Anatomy. For purposes of description it is important to distinguish between the lesions of simple silicosis and silicosis with infection. In *simple silicosis* the essential lesion is the silicotic nodule. Typical nodules are 2 to 5 mm. in diameter and are scattered more or less uniformly throughout the parenchyma of the lung, under the pleura and in the nodes at the hilum. They are avascular, laminated fibrous whorls and, when disseminated, are usually situated at the entrance to a lobule. They punctuate the perivascular lymphatic pathways between the alveoli and the hilum and between the alveoli and the pleura at the periphery of the lung. There is frequently associated a perilymphatic fibrosis. The alveoli may be thick-walled and dilated. The lymph nodes at the root of the

lung are usually fibrosed and in their periphery may show typical laminated whorls. As the process advances, these minute miliary nodules may become agglomerated and ultimately may form dense, fibrous rubbery masses of tissue replacing considerable numbers of lobules. As fibrosis and atelectasis progress in the more fibrous portion of the lung, the remaining portions may undergo considerable emphysematous change, often with the formation of large blebs. The pleura usually shows thickening and is frequently adherent.

In the advanced forms with dense fibrosis and emphysema, hypertrophy of the right ventricle is often observed, associated with some tendency to dilatation of the pulmonary conus.

Silicosis with Infection. All the usual manifestations of tuberculosis may occur, and the tuberculous infection may be extensive enough at times to obscure the underlying silicosis. The combination frequently presents the picture of an organizing pneumonic area about the silica nodule, which thus appears larger and less sharply circumscribed than in simple silicosis. The coalescence of such nodules leads to larger, dense fibrotic masses.

Symptoms. Simple silicosis may progress to advanced stages with no symptoms other than a tendency to shortness of breath. This is noted at first on moderate exertion, but as the disease progresses it may occur on less and less severe exertion. It is not accompanied by orthopnea, unless asthmatic paroxysms intervene. The occurrence of orthopnea suggests an associated cardiac condition. Riddell has pointed out that if severe dyspnea is produced by effort in two patients, one with silicosis and one with heart disease, the silicotic will be able to lie flat immediately after and the cardiac patient will not.

Cough, with uncomplicated silicosis, is not a prominent symptom. When it occurs, it is noted chiefly in the morning and is either dry or slightly productive of mucoid sputum. Cough may occur while actually working in dust, owing to irritation of the nose and throat without reference to the existence of silicosis. Men who have worked for a day in dust usually expel dust-discolored sputum on the following morning.

When cough is a prominent symptom, it is almost sure to denote complicating infection; in such cases it is usually more or less productive. Even when tuberculosis is present, tubercle bacilli are difficult to find in the sputum unless cavitation has occurred, and this is usually a late phenomenon. The fibroid tuberculosis most frequently accompanying silicosis may not be characterized by much fever or night-sweats, tachycardia or weight loss. This is not an invariable rule, but its frequent occurrence gives the impression that the silicotic fibrosis retards the symptoms of tuberculous activity.

The physical diagnosis of simple uncomplicated silicosis is practically impossible. The physical signs in simple silicosis are those of emphysema: hyperresonance on percussion, diminished intensity of breath sounds with prolongation of low-pitched expiration. Occasional rhonchi and fine and scattered medium coarse rales are heard in the interscapular regions and bases. When signs other than these are elicited, they are indications of a complicating infection rather than of the underlying silicosis. One is repeatedly surprised by the great discrepancy between physical signs and the extensive pulmonary disease revealed by roentgenographs.

Pathologic Physiology. Measurements of the total air capacity of the lungs (vital capacity plus residual air) show considerable variation. In general, the total capacity and vital capacity (VC) tend to be reduced and the residual air (RA) increased above predicted values. These values, taken singly or together, have proved to be less useful in evaluating the degree of impairment of functional capacity than the measurement of the maximal breathing capacity (MBC), which is affected by all the accessory mechanisms of breathing as well as by those within the lungs. Patients with emphysema and fibrosis have been found to hyperventilate relative to normal persons performing the same amount of external work. The more they hyperventilate, the more the respiratory reserve is diminished, especially when the total ventilatory capacity (MBC) is less than normal.

The voluntary maximal breathing capacity has been found to show the best single correlation with the degree of emphysema. If maximal breathing capacity is less than 40 liters per minute (or decreased more than 60 per cent of the predicted value), emphysema is found to be a significant factor in impairment of pulmonary function.

Roentgenograms of the chest do not afford a reliable means of evaluating functional impairment in silicosis. Extensive silicosis may be revealed when working capacity is only moderately impaired, while on the other hand minimal silicotic shadows may be seen in a person who is highly disabled. The variable factor is the degree of emphysema, which is frequently difficult to evaluate by roentgenograms alone.

As fibrosis and emphysema advance in the progress of silicosis, the oxygen saturation of the arterial blood may decrease, resulting in cyanosis; the carbon dioxide tension of the arterial blood may become elevated and compensated by an increase in the alkaline reserve. Recent studies reveal that anoxia excites vasopressor activity of the pulmonary arterioles, increasing the peripheral resistance to the right ventricle. The elevation of carbon dioxide tension has been shown to be an important factor in maintaining venopressor activity. Thus both factors probably contribute to the elevation of blood pressure in the right side of the heart and pulmonary artery, with the right ventricular hypertrophy and pulmonary arteriosclerosis which lead ultimately to failure of the cor pulmonale.

Diagnosis. The two essentials to a diagnosis of silicosis are an accurate occupational history and characteristic roentgenographic findings. The occupational history should cover all occupations in which the patient has been engaged and the duration of employment in each. In connection with those occupations which are dusty, as much information as possible should be obtained as to the amount and character of the dust and the extent to which protective devices were used.

The roentgenographic findings have certain characteristics which, when taken with a reliable occupational history and the clinical findings, warrant making a probable diagnosis of silicosis. The roentgenogram alone cannot decide the diagnosis, since a number of conditions may give similar appearances.

In roentgenograms of the lungs in simple silicosis there are seen discrete, round shadows not exceeding 5 to 6 mm. in diameter, having clear-cut borders. They are fairly uniformly distributed in each lung. The visualization of the process is greatly enhanced by stereoscopic viewing of the roentgenograms. In addition to these appearances, enlargement of the shadows of the tracheobronchial nodes is noted.

In infective silicosis, in addition to the picture of simple silicosis the following changes may be seen: localized discrete densities; mottling, in which the shadows vary in size and have ill defined borders; soft nodulation, in which the nodules have fuzzy borders with irregularity in distribution.

In advanced cases massive dense shadows appear with surrounding portions of increased radiotranslucency, caused by dense fibrosis and adjacent emphysema. Frequently seen also are evidences of pleural thickening and adhesion and "tenting" of the diaphragm.

tumors, the mycoses and tularemia must be excluded. The roentgenographic appearances in cases of beryllium granulomatosis, sarcoidosis and histoplasmosis will rarely be confusing to the diagnostician.

The finding of silica particles in the sputum is of little value in diagnosis unless the patient has been excluded from all contact with silicous dusts for some time.

Prophylaxis of silicosis is one of the major concerns of the industrial physician in charge

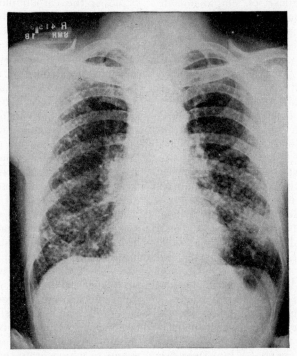

Fig. 131. Silicosis, showing beginning agglomeration in the left lobe, with resulting secondary emphysema (dark area just above left leaf of diaphragm).

The diagnosis of silicosis is impossible before the discovery of shadows of silicotic nodules. Before this stage is reached a positive or even probable diagnosis cannot be made. Developing silicosis may be suspected when serial roentgenograms show progressively increasing densities and serial measurements show decreasing maximal breathing capacity, when the occupation is known to involve a dust hazard, but the diagnosis should not be made until nodular shadows are seen.

Differential diagnosis involves the exclusion of other causes which may give similar roentgenographic appearances. Simple diffuse nodular silicosis must be differentiated from miliary tuberculosis by the absence of fever, tachycardia and wasting which characterize the latter. Similarly, metastatic

of workers in dusty trades. Systematic studies should be made of the air-suspended dusts at breathing levels of the workers. When excessive dust concentrations are found, and especially when the percentage of free silica is high, cooperation of managerial and engineering departments must be enlisted to improve ventilation and remove dust.

Many devices are now available for the protection of workers in rockdrilling, sandblasting, chipping and grinding, and foundry work. These protections are constantly being improved.

It is important not only to see that adequate devices are provided, but to insist upon their use, and frequent inspection in order to keep them in usable condition.

Periodic examination of workers exposed

to dangerous dusts is highly important. The exclusion of men with open tuberculosis is a great protection to other workers. Serial roentgenograms should be made at intervals.

In 1937 Denny, Robson and Irwin of Toronto claimed that inhalation of grease-free metallic aluminum powder, in particle sizes below 5 microns, prevented silicosis. In later work its action was attributed to the conversion of aluminum to hydrated alumina, which reduced the toxicity of quartz in tissues by flocculation, absorption of silica, but chiefly by coating the quartz particle with gelatinous hydrated alumina. Gardner, Dworski and Delehant verified the general conclusion of Denny, Robson and Irwin that aluminum in proper form constitutes an effective inhibitor of quartz in a living host, but suggest that an amorphous hydrate of aluminum may have certain advantages over the metallic powder. No harmful effects on normal animals have been observed, though excessive concentrations may unfavorably influence native susceptibility to tuberculosis in animals. Gardner cautions that the prophylactic use of alumina should never become a substitute for accepted methods of dust control.

Treatment. Gardner finds that inhalation of hydrated alumina in established cases of silicosis causes retrogression of immature silicotic lesions and prevents the further enlargement of fully developed fibrous nodules. Canadian observers report a high incidence of symptomatic relief of dyspnea, cough and chest pain, and in some instances improvement in respiratory functional tests. In view of the protracted nature of the disease, it is premature to attempt a full evaluation of the therapeutic effects of aluminum in this disease. Infective silicosis should be dealt with as tuberculosis. The **prognosis** in many cases of silicosis with tuberculosis is not as hopeless as many have assumed it to be. When tuberculosis occurs with a modified silicosis in an iron or coal miner or a foundry worker, suitable treatment may cause arrest of the disease. It is probable that the use of antibiotics such as streptomycin, and possibly chemotherapy, will improve the outlook in many cases.

Among copper and gold miners, sand-blasters and granite cutters, the outlook is serious if tuberculosis develops. It is important, however, for the patient to receive the same treatment as he would if silicosis were not present.

ASBESTOSIS

Asbestosis is a form of pneumonoconiosis produced by the inhalation of dust containing asbestos or rock wool fibers. The fibrosis of the lung differs from that of silicosis in that it is not nodular, but distributed in collar-like fashion around the atria and the respiratory bronchioles. The fibers find their way along the interlobular septa and into the pleura, outlining polygonal figures of blue-black color. Under darkfield illumination luminous asbestos fibers may be seen. Asbestosis bodies, which consist of such fibers on which iron-containing material is deposited, may be seen in sections as clubbed or beaded shapes. These are also seen in sputum from time to time.

Symptoms of disability, dyspnea and cough appear relatively much earlier in the course of the disease than is usual in uncomplicated silicosis.

Diagnosis depends upon the history of exposure; the appearance of an irregular reticular fibrosis in the lung roentgenograms, which has no specific features, and the finding of asbestos bodies in the sputum. Confirmation at autopsy depends upon the demonstration of the asbestos fibers and bodies in the tissues undergoing fibrosis.

WILLIAM S. McCANN

References

Drinker, P., and Hatch, T. F.: Industrial Dust. New York, McGraw-Hill Co., 1936.

Fourth Saranac Laboratory Symposium on Silicosis. Edited by B. E. Kuechle, Employers Mutual Liability Insurance Co., Wausau, Wisconsin.

Gardner, L. V., Dworski, M., and Delehant, A. B.: Aluminum Therapy in Silicosis. J. Indust. Hyg. & Toxicol., 26:211, 1944.

Lanza, A. J.: Silicosis and Asbestosis. New York, Oxford University Press, 1938.

Motley, H. L., Lang, L. P., and Gordon, B.: Pulmonary Emphysema and Ventilation Measurements in 100 Anthracite Coal Miners with Respiratory Complaints. Am. Rev. Tuberc., 59:270, 1949.

DISEASES OF THE PLEURA

PLEURISY

Introduction. The term "pleurisy" is used to denote any inflammation of the pleural serous membranes. The inflammation may be an early or late fibrinous pleurisy or an acute or chronic pleural effusion. The former is known as *"dry pleurisy"* or pleuritis, and the latter is known as *"wet pleurisy"* or pleural effusion. Acute fibrinous pleurisy is often the forerunner of pleural effusion. If dry pleurisy is not acute and is not the forerunner of pleural effusion, it has little clinical significance. As a painful complication of pneumonia, dry pleurisy is troublesome, but if it does not progress to effusion, its effects are usually transitory.

The pleural cavity is a closed sac, enclosing the lungs. Its normal communication with the environment is only through the blood and lymph system. It may become affected from disease agents brought to it by the blood or lymph, or by direct contiguity from neighboring structures such as the lungs, the lymph nodes and the ribs. As the pleura is a serous membrane in contact with both the systemic and the pulmonic circulations, it is often affected by physiologic changes in these systems. Interference with the pleural lymphatic circulation and drainage may be produced by malignant tumors or by pressure or injury to the vena cava or thoracic duct.

The only primary tumor of the pleura, mesothelioma, is extremely rare, and the tumors of the pleura, like infections of the pleura, are practically all metastatic or arise by direct extension from contiguous structures.

The pleura is a tolerant structure that tends to heal rapidly. It tends to wall off infections so long as the visceral and parietal surfaces are not separated artificially. Separation of the pleural surfaces by air or fluid permits widespread infection of the whole pleural cavity. Removal of the separating medium aids the pleura in localizing the infection, which then may be drained surgically. This localization also helps to stabilize the mediastinum, which may be dangerously shifted before pleural adhesions are present.

The normal pleura is a paper-thin, transparent, flexible and elastic membrane. It is smooth and well lubricated by a thin covering of lymph. Inflammation robs it of all these properties, and the deposition of fibrin from blood or the inflammatory products of effusion may thicken the pleura as much as 1 or 2 cm. It may become inelastic, unyielding and tough as leather. The contraction of the pleura by fibrosis during healing pulls the ribs together and may appreciably decrease the thoracic volume. If the exudate is completely absorbed, the two pleural leaves may become fused. The resulting reduction in respiratory capacity may be great.

Pain of Pleural Origin. As the visceral pleura is insensitive to pain, the lung may be penetrated through the visceral pleura without the production of pain. The only immediate indication of wounding the lung with a needle may be cough and the spitting of blood. The parietal pleura, on the other hand, is richly supplied with pain fibers. The nerve supply to the pleura of the thoracic wall is from the intercostals, and pain is sharply localized to the area of irritation. The phrenic nerve supplies the dome and central portion of the diaphragm as well as the pleura over the pericardium. Irritation over this area gives a typically referred pain into the neck and shoulder. The peripheral portion of the diaphragm is supplied by the lower intercostals in a roughly crescentic-shaped band which extends over about a third of the diaphragm posteriorly and is narrowed to 2 or 3 inches laterally. Painful sensations arising from this outer band of the diaphragmatic pleura pass along the intercostals to the posterior cord. There, irritation of the same and adjoining spinal segments may result in referred pain to the surface areas supplied by the lower intercostals. Peripheral diaphragmatic pleurisy, then, might be the cause of pain over the abdominal wall from the xiphoid to below the iliac crest. This fact has been responsible for the unfortunate and not uncommon mistake of diagnosing cholecystitis and appendicitis before the causal diaphragmatic pleurisy is discovered.

Significance of Pleural Pain. There are

many instances of chronic or intermittent pleural pain for which no cause is demonstrable. Some of these are presumably caused by hidden inflammatory lesions, the residual traces of which are demonstrable in the pleural adhesions frequently encountered on postmortem examination of adults. The scars may represent healed tuberculosis. The very chronicity of the symptom, in the absence of diagnostic findings, suggests its benign character.

Persistent pain may be the initial symptom of any of the thoracic maladies responsible for pleurisy. In primary tuberculosis, pleural effusion may be preceded by pain for several months before the cause is demonstrable by physical examination or roentgenogram. Such pleural pains have sometimes been prematurely dismissed with a diagnosis of "pleurodynia," a presumed entity. All pleural pain deserves thorough study until its cause is found or prolonged observation has rendered its significance less. A pulmonary infarct or a pneumonia may be ushered in by pain, and pain is the second most common symptom of carcinoma of the bronchus.

Pain is a prominent factor in the reduction of vital capacity and the production of dyspnea. The patient fears to take a deep breath. Restriction of respiratory motion by pain is also a factor in impairing the mechanism of cough and bronchial drainage. This sets the stage for bronchial blockage, atelectasis, "wet lung" pulmonary abscess and bronchiectasis. Diaphragmatic pain produces similar results whether the cause is intrathoracic or subdiaphragmatic, as in liver or perinephric abscess. Pain, therefore, may be indirectly responsible for postoperative atelectases and pneumonias.

Thus the relief of pain must be undertaken with these factors in mind. The reason for emptying the bronchi must be explained to the patient. The physician or nurse should assist the patient to raise blood or mucus by placing firm pressure over the painful area during efforts to cough. Strapping of the chest helps to relax the spasm produced by the pain, but interferes with physical examination and the interpretation of the roentgenogram. Codeine in 30 to 60 mg. doses every 3 to 4 hours does suppress the cough along with the pain. Opiates must be used with caution when there is material in the bronchi to be evacuated. Intercostal nerve block with an anesthetic agent such as pro-caine relieves pain and does not interfere with cough.

JOHN B. BARNWELL

PLEURAL EFFUSION
(Serofibrinous Pleurisy, "Wet Pleurisy," Hydrothorax)

Definition. The term "pleural effusion" is properly limited to inflammatory nonpurulent exudates appearing in the pleural cavity in the course of pleural infections. Thus an effusion is usually the sequel to acute fibrinous pleurisy. In a loose sense, the term is used to denote any collection of fluid in the pleural cavity, regardless of origin.

Dynamics of Pleural Effusion. The visceral pleura, over the outer surface of the lungs, and the parietal pleura, over the inner surface of the thoracic cage, are normally in constant contact. The surfaces are well lubricated and move freely over each other in respiration. The point of greatest cross movement is low in the anterolateral chest, where, on inspiration, the ribs flare out the parietal pleura while the descending diaphragm pulls the lower lung downward across the ribs. The point of least friction is anteriorly in the second interspace region. These facts are of importance when it is realized that a needle point thrust through a lower anterior interspace may be dragged a distance of 2 to 3 inches across the visceral pleura with each inspiration.

When the thorax is opened, the healthy lung collapses to its maximum contractility about the hilus. This constant pull of the lung away from the thoracic wall results in a *negative* or *subatmospheric pressure* in the pleural cavity. The pressure is in the order of -14 (inspiration) to -8 (expiration), measured in centimeters of water. Posture has an effect on the degree of negative pressure attained. The weight of the heart produces a higher negative pressure in the uppermost side when the patient lies on his side. Negative pressure is of some significance in the formation of transudates in the pleural cavity in conditions characterized by stasis of the pulmonary circulation or low osmotic pressure of the blood. The pressure is of greater significance in keeping the lungs inflated, the vena cava dilated, and in the rhythmic suction action of respiration upon the return flow of blood to the heart.

The appearance of fluid in the closed pleural sac *has two effects on pressure.* (1) The mere volume of the fluid partially collapses the lung and by that much relaxes the pull of the lung, thus reducing the negative pressure. Sufficient fluid may form to produce actual positive pressure, since the space is confined by the relatively unyielding bony cage. (2) The hydrostatic pressure exerted by the weight of the fluid has its effects upon adjacent structures. Pleural fluids lie in the bottom of the pleural cavity and the lungs float in the fluid. Change of posture results in a change of the position of the fluid. This change of fluid position requires a number of minutes, depending upon the viscosity of the fluid and the presence of pleural adhesions. When air is present above the fluid, the change is instantaneous, and the quick movement of the fluid under air can be heard, particularly if the patient is shaken ("succussion splash"). Fluid without air moves slowly, since the lobes have to float through the fluid to attain the uppermost part of the thoracic cage. The friction produced between pleura and fluid is an effective brake on expansion of the lobes. That is why a lung collapsed by inelastic and viscous fluid has less respiratory function than a lung collapsed to the same degree by elastic and relatively frictionless air (pneumothorax).

The factors of viscosity of fluid, friction retarding free pulmonary expansion and restriction of thoracic wall motion are in themselves enough to reduce respiratory function to the point of dyspnea on exertion. The added factors of loss of pulmonary volume, pressure on the vena cava and displacement of the heart and mediastinum, by their additive effects may result in the rapid appearance of extreme degrees of orthopnea and cyanosis. Fluid by its volume and weight may invert the diaphragm so that diaphragmatic contractions decrease the thoracic volume in inspiration. This can be observed fluoroscopically in pressure pneumothorax. The same pressure effects are present in hydrothorax, but are difficult to visualize fluoroscopically, since the fluid obscures the diaphragm. Death may result from these pressure effects alone if prompt aspiration is not done for relief.

Etiology. A sharp distinction should be made between those pleural effusions arising as a complication in the course of some disease, and those "primary" pleural effusions which appear to be the first manifestation of any disease process. Unfortunately, few statistical studies are able to make a sharp distinction, and exact information on the frequency of different etiologic agents is lacking. It is true that the disease which the pleurisy is complicating must often be named by hindsight. It is also true that a "primary" pleural effusion is nearly always due to some lesion in the lung or neighboring structures, which is primary in fact. The purest form of primary effusion is that found on routine physical or roentgenographic examination of apparently healthy persons. The next category most nearly deserving of the term "primary" effusion is represented by those patients whose presenting complaints are referable only to the presence of a pleural effusion. When the real cause of the effusion is not immediately apparent from the roentgenogram, the physical examination and the history, these two groups may be said to represent true primary pleural effusion.

The more common causes of *"primary" pleural effusion* depend mainly on the patient's age and the endemic diseases of his community. In most communities tuberculosis is the cause of primary pleural effusion in the great majority of persons less than 30 years of age. In persons of cancerous age, carcinoma of the bronchus and metastases from other malignant growths become more prominent as an etiologic factor. Pleural effusion due to tuberculosis is often an early sign of the disease, while that due to malignancy is always a late sign. Primary atypical or virus pneumonia may first show itself as pleural effusion and present a difficult problem. Pleural effusion occurs infrequently as the presenting manifestation of pulmonary abscess, pneumococcal or streptococcal pneumonia, rheumatic fever and fungous infections such as actinomycosis. It is also uncommon for pleural effusion to be the first recognized effect of subdiaphragmatic abscess and perinephric abscess.

The more obvious complicating or "secondary" pleural effusions are those arising in pneumonias, pulmonary infarcts, septicemias, pulmonary abscess, pulmonary tuberculosis and actinomycosis.

Noninflammatory transudates are most frequently encountered in the course of illnesses such as cardiac decompensation, renal disease, cirrhosis of the liver or nutritional deficiencies and anemias.

Clinical Investigation of Pleurisy with Effusion. The cause of many pleural effusions becomes obvious from the usual methods of examination. This is particularly true of those collections of fluid arising as a complication of an illness of known etiology. Whether the fluid be a transudate or exudate, the complication is to be anticipated in certain of the diseases already listed. In others, however, the underlying condition responsible for the effusion is difficult to determine. Therefore, certain points, some of them minor, need attention in the investigation of a pleural effusion.

History. It must be realized that asymptomatic pleural effusions are occasionally encountered on routine examination of apparently healthy groups. On careful questioning, the patient may admit some pain in the past few months, some discomfort, or slight dyspnea on exertion. In others, pain may have been present at some time previously. When instructed to take a deep breath, pain or discomfort may be provoked. In general, the appearance of fluid separates the pleura and lessens the pain. In some patients the pain is intense for some days or weeks before the effusion appears. The temperature is often slightly elevated to 99° or 99.5° F. For those with referred pain from diaphragmatic pleurisy, the problem of diagnosis is much greater. The symptomatic picture and the diagnosis in most of these cases is developed by hindsight.

In striking contrast are those who exhibit an acute fulminating clinical picture of pain, elevation of temperature to 104° or 105° F., dyspnea (due both to the pain and the presence of the fluid), night-sweats, anorexia and weight loss. Such an onset suggests a pyogenic infection rather than the more sluggish or chronic tuberculosis. The violence of the onset does not, as a matter of fact, differentiate the etiologic agent.

The history may throw some light on etiology when the patient is seen some time after the onset. Rapid and severe loss of weight is more often associated with carcinoma than with tuberculosis, which is more apt to give chronic underweight. A history of repeated aspirations of large amounts of fluid is less apt to mean tuberculosis than Hodgkin's disease or chylothorax, conditions in which fluid forms at a faster rate. The rapidity of change from clear fluid to pus may be helpful in diagnosis. In tuberculosis it occurs over weeks and months; in pneumonia, in a matter of days.

Physical Examination. A pleural rub may precede any other evidence of a pleural effusion and, as fluid forms, the rub disappears, the breath sounds become distant to absent, the percussion note dull to flat, and in large effusions the mediastinum is shifted and the diaphragm depressed. Tenderness in the interspaces may precede the rub and all other evidence of pleurisy.

ADDITIONAL FINDINGS. Besides locating the pleural fluid, complete physical examination may disclose other signs of a decompensated heart or the presence of renal disease. The finding of a sentinel node above the clavicle may suggest a carcinomatous metastasis. Examination of the larynx may disclose paralysis of the recurrent laryngeal nerve as additional evidence of carcinoma, or it may show the ulceration of tuberculosis. Clubbing of the fingers or toes suggests carcinoma or empyema. The appearance of shock, thready pulse and air hunger suggests hemothorax. The signs of air over fluid, such as the succussion splash, are evidences of bronchopleural fistula from any cause. Fistula in ano suggests tuberculosis as associated with the pleurisy. Tumefactions on the chest wall or sinus tracts may give opportunities for biopsy.

Roentgenologic Diagnosis. In the search for the cause of pleurisy it should be remembered that the roentgenogram may remain negative for some days or weeks before the fluid rises above the dome of the diaphragm and appears as a curve swinging from diaphragm to axilla. Before the characteristic picture appears, the diaphragm may become slightly elevated, and a slight blunting of the costophrenic angle is noted. On fluoroscopic examination, restricted motion is noted in inflammatory pleurisies, while complete paralysis may be found in the presence of a metastasizing carcinoma. Different postures of the patient may be used to demonstrate the shifting motion of the shadow cast by the fluid. With the patient recumbent, a moderate amount of fluid may spread itself over the posterior chest wall so as to form only a poorly defined haze. Posterolateral films may show the fluid, but make it difficult to localize, and lateral or oblique views may be needed. Preliminary fluoroscopy may be helpful in determining the best oblique view to obtain. When small amounts of fluid are present, it may be possible to see enough of the lung or mediastinal contour to visualize the lesion and thus gain some impression of its etiologic features. When the effusion is large, the lung and adjacent mediastinum may be completely hidden by the density of the fluid.

Serial roentgenograms taken over a period of time often disclose the primary lesion responsible for the effusion when this is not apparent on the admission films. Examination of roentgenograms made months or years before may disclose the presence of chronic tuberculosis in an area of lung which is hidden by the fluid. X-ray surveys in schools, industry and the Federal services, particularly Selective Service, have now covered a large part of the population of the United States and Canada. These sources of information should be sought. Serial roentgenograms, taken while the patient is under observation, may also disclose a lesion not apparent on the initial roentgenogram. A tuberculous lesion, too small to be visualized when the effusion first appears, may subsequently become readily demonstrable. The differential diagnosis between acute and chronic lesions may be made on the manner and rate of change in the roentgenographic shadows. In acute lesions, such as atypical pneumonias, roentgenograms taken every few days may serve to differentiate the lesion from tuberculosis.

Exploration. Aspiration of the fluid is a type of exploration which establishes the presence of fluid and provides material for diagnostic tests. When enough fluid is present to hide the lung and mediastinal contour from roentgenographic observation, removal of the fluid allows a better view. The best roentgenographic view of the pleura is obtained, however, when all the fluid is withdrawn and replaced with an amount of air (300 to 600 cc.) sufficient to keep all the pleural surfaces separated by an inch or more. Demonstrable lesions of the pleura may then be examined by thorascopic inspection or even biopsy, though the latter procedure is rarely indicated except in obscure cases. If the pleural cavity is kept dry by aspiration and the lung allowed to expand, the lung may also be more satisfactorily examined by roentgenogram. If fluid is allowed to reaccumulate, however, its presence causes shadows that may be confused with pulmonary lesions.

When roentgenograms have been taken shortly before the onset of the effusion, showing the lung, mediastinum and pleura free of abnormal shadow, the method is not needed to visualize these structures, and aspiration for diagnostic purposes need not be combined with air replacement. The appearance of pus, opalescent fluid or any fluid other than "clear" fluid in the aspirating syringe is definite contraindication to air replacement. Furthermore, when the amount of fluid is small or difficult to localize, exploration with a needle is likely to injure the lung, and the diagnostic aspiration might not yield results commensurate with the risk.

Character of the Fluid. The pleural transudates found in cardiac decompensation, nephritis, cirrhosis of the liver and nutritional deficiencies are low in protein (0.5 to 1.5 gm. per 100 cc.), have a specific gravity usually below 1.015, contain few cellular elements and do not clot. Inflammatory exudates usually contain 3 to 6 gm. of protein per 100 cc., a specific gravity above 1.015, white blood cell counts of 100 to 10,000 per cubic millimeter; and the fluid may clot readily. Most primary effusions are clean, translucent, straw-colored or amber, but they may be blood-tinged, serosanguineous or even bloody. Bright blood appearing only at the beginning or end of an aspiration may be due to blood escaping into the clear fluid from an injury to an intercostal vessel or lung. Both accidents are not uncommon, and the latter is particularly apt to occur when the amount of fluid in the chest is small and the lung is near the needle point. An evenly mixed bloody fluid is common in carcinoma and unusual in tuberculosis, but is not diagnostic of either condition. Pure blood is sometimes found in the pleural cavity. It usually results from the rupture of a vessel by tearing of an adhesion in spontaneous pneumothorax, or external trauma. If the accident is old, the blood appears dark and diluted, or it may be clotted and difficult to aspirate.

Inflammatory exudates due to tuberculosis are high in lymphocytes (up to 90 per cent) and low in polymorphonuclear cells (up to 10 per cent). In the fluids complicating acute pneumonias the polymorphonuclear cells predominate. The distinction between the pleural fluid of effusion and the pus of empyema is based loosely on its gross appearance to the naked eye. Pleural fluids are translucent; the pus of empyema is opaque. The time after onset when the fluid is seen is important, since in acute pneumonias it may change rapidly from clear fluid to pus. In tuberculosis repeated aspiration over days, weeks or months shows only a slow change in the character of the fluid. Actinomycosis produces a much more rapid transition to pus than does tuberculosis, and the sulfur bodies of actinomycosis may be apparent on inspection with the naked eye.

A milky fluid, with fat globules seen on the stained slide, is found in chylothorax. Occasionally, in old effusions, a brownish fluid suggesting cholesterol deposition may be observed.

Examination of the Fluid. The *specific gravity* of the fluid should be determined, the *color* noted, and a tube of the well mixed fluid allowed to stand to determine *clotting.* The *cell count* of the unsedimented fluid should be determined and the centrifuged sediment stained by Wright's stain for differential cell count, and by the Gram and Ziehl-Neelsen stains for bacteria. The sediment should also be fixed in paraffin blocks and sections prepared. The latter should be searched for malignant cells, particularly if the patient is in the cancerous age or the effusion is not otherwise explained. In some laboratories the Papanicolaou stain, without paraffin fixation, is used to identify malignant cells, but in either case the specimen should be prepared while it is still fresh, and before cellular detail is lost. Even the certain demonstration of malignant cells among the normal cells in pleural fluid does not identify the site of the primary tumor. Furthermore the differentiation between normal cells and those exfoliated by mesothelioma, the rare and only primary tumor of the pleura, is an uncertain diagnostic procedure. The heavier fluids and pus should be cultured for aerobic and anaerobic bacteria. In the translucent fluids of the primary effusion, tubercle bacilli are not usually demonstrable by staining, but must be sought by repeated culture on special culture media or by inoculation of a guinea pig. Positive cultures, however, are regarded as characteristic in most laboratories and need not be confirmed by animal inoculation, unless the appearance of the colonies is atypical or there are conflicting clinical or other laboratory data in the case.

The single culture of a small amount of sediment from a small amount (10 to 15 cc.) of fluid gave many negative results in the past. The more recent practice of repeatedly culturing large amounts of sediment from large amounts of fluid (100 to 500 cc.) has resulted in the detection of tubercle bacilli in approximately 70 per cent of primary pleural effusions in young persons. In tuberculous empyemas, cultures for anaerobes and aerobes should be repeated at intervals, since mixed infections may occur. These are usually the result of a bronchopleural fistula, the appearance of which changes both the treatment and the prognosis. The bacteriologic findings in the fluid may change with time. Fluid that is sterile for pyogens may have become so because of chemotherapy by sulfonamides or antibiotics. In these circumstances it becomes difficult to differentiate between an acute pyogenic pleurisy and a tuberculous pleurisy which would also be sterile for pyogens. Therefore, cultures should be made before the use of chemotherapy. In suspected or doubtful cases the fluid should be cultured on Sabouraud's media for fungi.

The blood count and the hemoglobin should be determined in bloody effusions. The fat content may be measured in chylothorax. Estimation of protein content serves to distinguish exudates from transudates. It is reported that the simultaneous determination of the blood sugar and pleural fluid sugar shows the latter far below the blood sugar in tuberculous pleurisy. This procedure might also be helpful in distinguishing any exudate from a transudate in borderline cases. Other than this, chemical study of pleural effusions is not of much value in clinical practice.

Other Laboratory Data. Sputum, if present, should be stained for pyogens and appropriate cultures made. It should also be stained for evidence of Loeffler's eosinophilia. Repeated concentration and cultures for tubercle bacilli may be needed for diagnosis. Cultures for fungi may be needed, but their pathogenicity should be demonstrated by animal inoculation before etiologic significance is assumed.

Culture or guinea pig inoculation with a series of fasting gastric washings, taken before the patient arises, may serve to demonstrate tubercle bacilli and establish the diagnosis. The finding of tubercle bacilli in the urine, other excretions or sinus tracts also points to the tuberculous nature of the pleurisy.

Leukocytosis is highly uncommon in tuberculosis, even in tuberculous empyema, while it is to be expected with pleurisies complicating acute pneumonias and in the presence of hemothorax.

The tuberculin test separates those persons

who might have some form of tuberculosis from those who, in all probability, are not infected with tuberculosis. When patients with obscure pleural lesions have resided in endemic areas, the skin tests for coccidioidomycosis, echinococcus, tularemia and histoplasmosis may serve a similar purpose.

Serologic studies are not of much use in the diagnosis of pleurisy, except that of tularemia.

Bronchoscopy. If, upon the completion of the clinical investigation, the effusion is still unexplained, bronchoscopy must be considered. This is particularly true if there are any indications of bronchogenic carcinoma such as evidence of partial or complete bronchial obstruction. Unexplained wheezing or localized rhonchi constitute strong indications for bronchoscopy. This procedure should be performed in all patients with sanguineous pleural effusions.

Unexplained Pleural Effusion. Cases remain that defy etiologic diagnosis. Tuberculosis develops in a certain number of these patients in the ensuing five years. If all patients with unexplained pleural effusions were thoroughly investigated for tuberculosis, the incidence of this disease as a late sequel of pleurisy would be considerably less than the 40 per cent which is generally quoted. Proper treatment includes strict bed rest until it has been demonstrated that all the cultures and guinea pig inoculations are negative. This requires a period of at least six weeks from the last obtainable fluid. If at that time at least three negative cultures have been obtained, the tuberculin test is still negative, and no abnormalities are demonstrable on x-ray examination of the lung, the patient may be followed on an ambulatory basis. Roentgenograms should be taken at three-month intervals for a year and at six- to twelve-month intervals for the next five years. If, however, the tuberculin test was positive on first investigation or has been positive during the period of observation, the patient should be treated as tuberculous, regardless of the negative cultural findings.

Treatment. All the conditions giving rise to pleural effusion demand bed rest. This is fundamental, and all the diagnostic investigation should be carried out with the patient at bed rest unless a tumor is established as the cause. This is true even of the occasional case discovered accidentally in routine roentgenograms. In such instances it is impossible to know how long the effusion has been present or how rapidly it may increase after its discovery. However, the primary consideration is that the treatment of the underlying, and as yet unknown, cause of the effusion probably requires bed rest.

Regardless of the cause, the treatment of the effusion itself demands some consideration. As soon as the cause is discovered, its treatment should modify these considerations. Since the effusion itself collapses the lung, partially splints the chest wall and diaphragm, and may place pressure upon and displace the mediastinal structures, the symptoms of dyspnea may demand its immediate removal. Such removal is for symptomatic or pressure relief and should be carried out gently and gradually to permit of physiologic readjustments. Depending upon the size of the effusion, in some instances removal of 500 to 1000 cc. may serve only to restore the mediastinal displacement, while in others it may result in a considerable reexpansion of a compressed and diseased lung. Sudden reexpansion of the lung may produce cough, distress and even pulmonary edema. The aspiration should be stopped short of this or the volume made up by replacement with air. The procedure may have to be repeated at intervals, depending upon the rapidity of fluid formation. Aspiration of a large inflammatory effusion will frequently reduce the temperature response and make the patient more comfortable.

The sequelae of an inflammatory or bloody effusion must be considered in relation to immediate treatment. Fluid keeps the lung collapsed, and deposits of fibrin form upon the pleural surfaces, thickening them and tending to make them inelastic and incapable of permitting later pulmonary expansion. Removal of the fluid promotes reexpansion of the lung and leaves less fibrin to be deposited upon the pleura. For unknown reasons most of this deposition is upon the parietal pleura, which, in itself, hinders further lymphatic absorption and splints the chest wall. Subsequent organization and contraction of this fibrin deposit result in pulling together of the ribs, deformity of the chest wall and moderate to severe scoliosis. This, however, is not always permanent, but may be reversible.

If clear fluid is not absorbed or aspirated, it may become purulent. Pus, if not aspirated, tends to find an outlet. This may be by rupture through the visceral pleura, producing bronchopleural fistula, or penetration through the parietal pleura, producing empyema necessitatis or pleurocutaneous sinus. Large undrained pleural fluids have been known to remain unchanged for a number of years before rupture has occurred through the bronchus or chest wall.

Studies of Tillett and Sherry suggest that the interpleural injection of the streptococcal enzymes streptokinase and streptodornase may cause lysis of fibrinous adhesions and cellular debris and promote healing in hemothorax and purulent pleurisy. The pancreatic enzyme, trypsin, in purified form has been used for the same purpose.

Most primary effusions, however, tend to absorb spontaneously on bed rest. This is particularly true of small effusions, and this consideration should be weighed against the meddlesome aspiration of small effusions that are likely to be absorbed spontaneously. There is also to be considered the possible danger of injury to the lung in aspiration of small effusions. These considerations of treatment, however, should not interfere with the employment of diagnostic aspirations.

In most instances of primary pleural effusion treated with or without aspiration there is little residual pleural scarring, and this is usually confined to the costophrenic angle. Nevertheless, in almost all cases there remains the necessity of treating the primary lesion in the lung or elsewhere. In effusion due to tuberculosis the successful management of the pleural fluid is only the beginning of the treatment, and the chemotherapeutic regimens presently in use for pulmonary tuberculosis are now generally started with the establishment of the etiologic diagnosis of the pleurisy.

JOHN B. BARNWELL

References

Berlines, K.: Hemorrhagic Pleural Effusions: An Analysis of 120 Cases. Ann. Int. Med., 14:2266, 1941.

Blackford, S. D., and Casey, C. J.: Pleuropulmonary Tularemia. Arch. Int. Med., 67:43, 1941.

Capps, J. A., and Coleman, G. H.: An Experimental and Clinical Study of Pain in the Pleura, Pericardium and Peritoneum. New York, Macmillan Company, 1932.

Claggett, O. T., McDonald, J. R., and Schmidt, H. W.: Localized Fibrous Mesothelioma of the Pleura. J. Thoracic Surg., 24:213, 1952.

Falk, A.: The Prognostic Significance of Idiopathic Pleural Effusion. Dis. of Chest, 18:542, 1950.

Graham, G. G., McDonald, J. R., Clagett, O. T., and Schmidt, H. W.: Examination of Pleural Fluid for Carcinoma Cells. J. Thoracic Surg., 25: 366, 1953.

Hartzell, H. C.: Spontaneous Hemopneumothorax: Report of Three Cases and Review of Literature. Ann. Int. Med., 17:496, 1942.

Jaksman, W. E.: Chylothorax: Brief Review of Literature; Report of Three Non-Traumatic Cases. Ann. Int. Med., 21:669, 1944.

Liebow, A. A.: Tumors of the Lower Respiratory Tract. Washington, D. C., Armed Forces Institute of Pathology, 1952.

Perlmutter, M.: Thecoma of the Ovary Associated with Pleural Effusion and Ascites; Meigs Syndrome. Ann. Int. Med., 20:132, 1944.

Phillips, S. K., and McDonald, J. R.: An Evaluation of Various Examinations Performed on Serous Fluids. Am. J. M. Sc., 216:121, 1948.

Reiser, H. G., Roettig, L. C., and Curtis, G. M.: The Tryptic Debridement of Fibrinopurulent Empyema. Surgical Forum, 1950 Clinical Congress of the American College of Surgeons. Philadelphia, W. B. Saunders Co., 1951, p. 17.

Roper, W. H., and Waring, J. J.: Primary Serofibrinous Pleural Effusion. Tr. Nat. Tuberc. A., 48:150, 1952.

Tillett, W. S., Sherry, S., and Read, C. T.: The Use of Streptokinase and Streptodornase in the Treatment of Chronic Empyema. J. Thoracic Surg., 21: 325, 1951.

Vincent Memorial Hospital: The Cytologic Diagnosis of Cancer, Philadelphia, W. B. Saunders Co., 1950.

PNEUMOTHORAX

Definition. Although by literal definition pneumothorax means air in the chest ($\pi\nu\epsilon\acute{\upsilon}\mu\alpha$ = air; $\theta\acute{\omega}\rho\alpha\xi$ = chest), for centuries the term has been used to designate the presence of air in the pleural cavity. The condition was, until recently, encountered most frequently as the induced *therapeutic* or "artificial" pneumothorax formerly used extensively in the treatment of pulmonary tuberculosis. *Induced* or "artificial pneumothorax" is also used as a *diagnostic* procedure: to visualize pleural lesions by roentgenogram or by thoracoscopy, to replace fluid for better visualization by x-ray, and occasionally as a preoperative procedure for pulmonary, mediastinal or pleural biopsies and resections.

Types. *Accidental* or *traumatic* pneumothorax is less frequently encountered in civilian practice than other types. There are three mechanisms in its occurrence which should be distinguished. Should the parietal pleura be opened without injury to the visceral pleura during an operation on the chest wall, the lung shrinks away from the thoracic wall and air enters the pleural cavity from the outside. With repair of the opening in the parietal pleura, the air will be absorbed from the pleural cavity or may even be aspirated. If an accidental opening is made into the parietal pleura in a bronchoscopy or esophagoscopy, air also will enter the pleural cavity from the outside. Although the site of the injury is usually not seen and is not subject to repair, the mechanism is the same, and air may be absorbed or may have to be aspirated until the wound heals. If the perforation is bilateral, the symptoms may be acute and the aspiration of the air must be carried out promptly. In a stab or bullet wound, air will also enter from without, but, in addition, will enter the pleural cavity from the lung which has been punctured. One of the commoner forms of accidental pneumothorax is that produced by needle injury of the lung during aspiration of air or fluid or during the administration of therapeutic pneumothorax. Traumatic fracture of a rib may produce injury to both the parietal and visceral pleura and may be considered along with other chest wall penetrations. The third factor involves the entrance of air into the pleural cavity from the lung.

Spontaneous Pneumothorax. This term has been used to designate a variety of conditions caused by a number of different factors. One universal factor is pneumothorax; the other is that the pneumothorax is not intentionally produced, is not "induced" or so-called "artificial," and is not a result of trauma. Pneumothorax of this sort should be separated sharply into two major groups. The first group comprises the pneumothoraces which appear in the *tuberculous* patient in the absence of operation or injury. This group is usually easily identified. The pneumothorax is produced by the ulceration of a tuberculous lesion through the visceral pleura before adhesions can be formed. The condition occurs in rapidly advancing cases that already have gone to cavity formation. In the vast majority of instances the patients present the classic symptoms of advancing tuberculosis. Moreover, a purulent empyema is produced as a result of the rupture of the cavity into a previously uninvolved intrapleural space. This group can be identified by (1) symptoms of tuberculosis before the "spontaneous pneumothorax"; (2) the temperature and other signs and symptoms of active tuberculosis when the pneumothorax

appears; (3) clinical evidence of empyema or at least pleural effusion; (4) the x-ray appearance of hydropneumothorax; and (5) x-ray evidence of tuberculosis in the partially collapsed lung or in the contralateral lung. The condition is a serious and often fatal complication of pulmonary tuberculosis. Before the days of modern therapy, about 3 per cent of the deaths from tuberculosis were brought about in this rather dramatic manner. The accumulation of these cases in autopsy statistics led to the old belief that tuberculosis was the cause of the great majority of spontaneous pneumothoraces. Few of the true spontaneous pneumothoraces ever reach the autopsy table.

PNEUMOTHORAX SIMPLEX, SPONTANEOUS PNEUMOTHORAX IN THE APPARENTLY HEALTHY AND SIMPLE SPONTANEOUS PNEUMOTHORAX. These are terms used to differentiate a second group from the described entity caused by tuberculosis. In a general hospital on a university campus the majority of this second group are healthy students, and many of them are athletes. There are no prodromal symptoms such as fever, cough and loss of weight. In a person enjoying good health there is sudden chest pain, tightness in the chest and dyspnea which may proceed to orthopnea and cyanosis. Sometimes there is a sensation of pleural rubbing without pain. The mechanism is the rupture of an emphysematous bleb in the visceral pleura. Occasionally the condition may be simulated by the distention of a bleb, without rupture, until it fills the hemithoracic cage. In either event the lung is partially or completely collapsed by atmospheric air. The predisposition to rupture results from either a congenital anomaly or a pulmonary infection which has resulted in a scar so situated that a one-way valve is present at the bronchiolar or alveolar entrance. Inspiration results in an enlargement of the bleb, while the valve prevents egress of air on expiration. The bleb finally bursts and permits alveolar air to enter the pleural cavity. The healed pulmonary infection resulting in the one-way bronchiolar valve may have been of a tuberculous origin. Other than this, tuberculosis is not usually involved in the production of this group of "pneumothorax simplex."

Clinically, these patients suffer only from the initial pain of the tear and from the pressure effects of the air in the pleural cavity. Rarely, the condition is complicated by hemothorax, but otherwise there is no evidence of toxemia. In further contrast to the pneumothorax caused by tuberculosis, the pleural cavity in simple pneumothorax is free of reaction and fluid does not usually develop, even though the opening in the pleura fails to heal and the condition becomes chronic or recurrent. Cough, if present, is due to the collapse of the lung and distortion of the bronchi by pressure. The cough is relieved completely by removing the air from the pleural cavity.

The accident has occurred at rest and under all manner of activities. It is usually associated with effort against a closed glottis such as hard coughing or straining at stool. However, the initiating act may be as simple as reaching across a table, or there even may be no inciting act.

Valvular Pneumothorax. Any pneumothorax with an opening in the visceral pleura and without an opening in the chest wall large enough to permit free egress of air may become a valvular pneumothorax. Synonyms are *"tension pneumothorax"* and *"pressure pneumothorax."* This condition may complicate any of the pneumothoraces, including accidental, traumatic, simple, and that due to tuberculosis. The lips of the opening in the visceral pleura form a valve which is opened by inspiration and closed by expiration. Air is thus sucked into the pleural cavity at each inspiration and is trapped there on expiration. The rapid respiration produced by the collapse may result in an extremely rapid accumulation of air under high positive pressure. In addition to the pulmonary collapse, the circulation is embarrassed by cardiac displacement and pressure on the vena cava. The diaphragm may be inverted downward and its contractions further reduce the thoracic volume. In extreme cases death may result in a matter of 10 minutes. The complication of hemothorax renders the condition doubly hazardous. Fortunately, after the development of a certain amount of pressure, many of the valves are forced shut, and the condition usually remains stationary or gradually subsides with absorption of air and healing of the tear in the pleura.

Hemopneumothorax. In any of the pneumothoraces described previously, some bleeding into the pleural cavity may occur, either from intercostal vessels or vessels in the lung. Bleeding from the intercostals occurs more frequently than from the lung. In an induced pneumothorax, bleeding is rare and is almost always due to an injured intercostal vessel. In spontaneous pneumothorax the bleeding is usually from a vascular adhesion which has been torn. Hemopneumothorax is more often found in traumatic cases than in any other. In addition to the signs and symptoms of the pneumothorax, there are the effects of hemorrhage. Pyogenic infection is an additional factor in some, particularly the traumatic cases. Some febrile response is to be expected, but the incidence of infection was surprisingly low in our battle casualties.

Diagnosis. The side of the pneumothorax is a little more prominent and moves less with respiration. In valvular pneumothorax these distinctions are more evident. The interspaces are filled and do not retract with inspiration. The percussion note is hyperresonant. The breath and voice sounds are absent, and the coin sign is present. Percussion, palpation and inspection will give evidence of displacement of the mediastinum and depression of the liver border. A peculiar accompaniment of the heart sound known as "pericardiac knock" is sometimes present with a left-sided pneumothorax unaccompanied by fluid.

The roentgenogram shows a fading-out of normal lung markings well within the periphery of the chest wall, and often the thin line of the visceral pleura separating lung from pneumothorax may be seen. In small pneumothoraces the routine roentgenogram taken in inspiration may not disclose the pneumothorax, but a roentgenogram in expiration may sufficiently exaggerate the air pocket so that the pneumothorax is demonstrable.

In a closed pneumothorax the percentage of oxygen is maintained at about 3 per cent. Any rise of the oxygen above 5 per cent would mean that outside air has recently been added. Such a finding is an indication that an opening in the visceral pleura is present unless air has recently been introduced through a needle. Gas analysis is particularly useful in determining an intermittent opening in the lung. The determination of intrapleural pressures before and after the introduction or withdrawal of air is also useful for diagnosis. Large amounts of air do not change the intrapleural pressures if the communication between lung and pleural cavity is patent.

Treatment. Tension pneumothorax requires immediate relief by removal of air until breathing returns to normal. If symptoms recur or the intrapleural pressure becomes positive, the simplest measure is to leave a blunt-ended needle or cannula protruding only slightly into the pleural cavity. The cannula should be connected by rubber tubing to a water trap with the end of the tube only 1 cm. below the water surface. Intrapleural pressure greater than 1 cm. will be bubbled through the water in each expiration. With healing of the tear in the lung the air is absorbed and the lung re-expands.

In simple pneumothorax without tension little treatment is needed. It is advisable to keep the patient on limited activity until the pneumothorax is absorbed and the lung is expanded. This usually occurs within three weeks. It is doubtful if strict rest is required. The avoidance of strain or overexercise may be sufficient. Persons with pneumothorax should be warned that ascent to a high altitude may result in an enlargement of the air pocket which was originally trapped at the greater atmospheric pressure of the lower altitude.

Some cases of simple pneumothorax remain chronic because the lung is not relaxed in a way that will permit healing of the fistula. In some, adhesions attached to the edge of the fistula prevent its closing. In these the adhesions may be cut. In others the pulmonary area containing the fistula may have to be excised and the wound closed surgically.

JOHN B. BARNWELL

References

Dolley, F. S., and Brewer, L. M.: Diagnosis and Treatment of Chronic Spontaneous Pneumothorax. West. J. Surg., 58:463, 1950.

Emerson, C. P.: Pneumothorax, An Historical, Clincial and Experimental Study. Johns Hopkins Hosp. Rep., 11:1, 1903.

Kjaergaard, H.: Spontaneous Pneumothorax in the Apparently Healthy. Arch. Med. Scandinav., Supplement 43, 1932.

Ornstein, G. G., and Lercher, L.: Spontaneous Pneumothorax in Apparently Healthy Individuals. Quart. Bull. Sea-View Hosp., 7:149, 1942.

Ross, J. B., and Fullerton, C. W.: Spontaneous Pneumothorax—Some Congenital Aspects. Tr. Am. Clin. & Climat. A., 55:239, 1939.

Waring, J. J.: Spontaneous Pneumothorax. Office of Medical Information, National Research Council, Washington, D. C., July 1944. (See references.)

UNCOMMON PLEURAL AFFECTIONS

Echinococcus cyst is not seen often in North America. It may be attacked surgically by complete exterpation. Various fungi attack the pleura, among them the *Actinomyces,* the *Aspergilli,* the *Coccidioides immitis* and *Histoplasma* bodies. There are antigens for diagnostic skin tests, and cultural methods are available for identification of most of these organisms. As a rule these infections are not checked by the usual anatomic barriers, but steadily progress through the tissues to produce tumefaction and sinus tracts, usually multiple, upon the chest wall. Pleural fluid may be clear initially, but becomes opaque and purulent in a matter of weeks. The sulfur granules grossly observable in actinomycotic fluid are usually diagnostic. Actinomycosis, particularly, produces a highly vascular reaction in contrast to the avascularity of tuberculosis. The amount of bleeding encountered in probing is therefore frequently significant in diagnosis. The infection is spread along aspirating needle tracks and is usually not amenable to local treatment. Therefore the treatment is that of the general treatment for these conditions.

JOHN B. BARNWELL

EMPYEMA

(Suppurative Pleurisy, Purulent Pleurisy, Purulent Pleural Effusion, Pleuritis Purulenta, Empyema Thoracis, Infected Pleural Effusion)

Definition. Empyema in its broadest sense refers to the presence of pus in any one of several cavities of the body in addition to the thorax, such as gallbladder, paranasal sinuses, pericardium and others. However, when used without anatomic identification, it regularly refers to the presence of thick, purulent exudation of inflammatory origin located in the pleural cavity.

There are both acute and chronic forms of empyema which not infrequently present different types of diagnostic and therapeutic problems.

Pathogenesis and Etiology. Developmentally, acute empyema occurs (1) by extension in association with spreading acute inflammations, such as from pneumonia due to pneumococcus, hemolytic streptococcus or *K. pneumoniae;* (2) by extension via mechanical transfer following rupture through the visceral pleura of miliary or solitary pulmonary abscesses located near the periphery of the lung, such as *putrid empyema* occurring in association with aspiration pneumonia and due to *anaerobic (micro-aerophilic)* streptococci, or a mixed flora consisting of fusiform and spirochetal organisms together with other gram-positive and gram-negative cocci of oral or dental origin; (3) from rupture of miliary or solitary abscesses due to hemolytic staphylococci (more commonly seen in pediatrics); (4) as part of septicemias of diverse bacterial etiologies with metastatic localization in the pleural area.

Chronic empyema is encountered (1) as the chronic stage of the acute forms; (2) in tuberculosis, following pneumothorax, or rupture of subpleural caseation, or in association with the appearance of bronchopleural fistula (see chapter on Tuberculosis); (3) in granulomatous diseases of fungal etiology, such as actinomycosis and others (see sections on fungous diseases); (4) postoperatively following thoracic surgery with intrapulmonary infections; (5) in subdiaphragmatic suppurative diseases with extension to the pleura through lymphatics or by perforation of the diaphragm.

Incidence and Significance in Internal Medicine. Formerly the most definite data concerning empyema were available from its incidence following pneumococcal pneumonia (approximately 5 to 6 per cent) and its high incidence in epidemics of acute hemolytic streptococcal infections of the respiratory tract. Although no figures are currently available, it is apparent that the occurrence of pneumococcal and hemolytic streptococcal empyema has been drastically reduced, that the other types listed also occur less frequently, and that the decline is directly referable to the widespread and effective use of first the sulfonamide compounds and later the antibiotics in the treatment of acute infections of the pulmonary tract. As a result, the role of the internist in minimizing the occurrence of empyema is of special importance through affording well planned medical treatment of the severe pneumonias which ordinarily precede empyema. In addition, the potentialities of the medical methods of the treatment of empyema, after it is established, by local intercostal aspira-

tions and injections have broadened the responsibility of internists in a field of therapy that was formerly exclusively surgical. Empyema is, therefore, a particularly striking illustration of a disease in the management and understanding of which modern procedures have added a new significance for internal medicine.

Symptoms and Physical Signs. *Acute empyema* usually makes its appearance before the disease on which it is superimposed has subsided. Consequently, the signs and symptoms of the latter, such as dyspnea, productive cough and purulent sputum, may continue to be present. The polymorphonuclear leukocytosis of the preceding infection (12,000 to 20,000 white blood cells per cubic millimeter) either continues or, if decreasing, may increase again. Unilateral thoracic discomfort and even pain, the appearance of fever of the intermittent type, and sweating are common findings. Anemia and loss of weight begin to be manifest.

The classic physical signs of pleural effusion are present, consisting of limited respiratory movement of the affected side, absence of tactile fremitus, flatness to percussion and absent breath sounds. However, in contrast to a massive effusion, the signs in empyema may be limited to a small area so that tactile fremitus and breath sounds are not completely absent and the percussion note is dull rather than flat. Egophony is frequently noted at the periphery of the collection of fluid, and, if consolidation of the underlying lung persists, distant bronchial breathing is detectable. A small loculated empyema, particularly when located in a pleural fissure, may produce no positive signs.

The physical findings in *chronic empyema* are similar to those described, with variations referable to the type of chronic infection present. Specific symptoms may be minimal except for those associated with a state of chronic invalidism.

Diagnosis. The procedures of greatest importance for the final diagnosis are x-ray or fluoroscopic examination followed by thoracentesis performed with due attention to appropriate technical details. In many instances the correct appraisal of a patient's status is unduly deferred as a result of procrastination from day to day in deciding to attempt aspiration, the success or failure of which gives the pathognomonic answer.

From the standpoint of technique emphasis should be placed on (1) the selection of the proper intercostal space and the posterior, lateral or anterior location of the pocket as determined by physical and x-ray examinations; (2) use of needle (15 to 17 gauge) that will permit removal of a sample of fluid even if grossly thick; (3) care that the needle is tightly fitted to the syringe so as to prevent introduction of air into the pleural area; (4) avoidance of puncture of the lung.

The characteristics of the fluid to be observed and evaluated are gross appearance, sediment, microscopic examination for cellular and bacterial content, and culture. The range is from moderately cloudy material with fibrinous webs forming on standing, to thick, grayish-green, coarsely sedimenting specimens. The former usually represents a sterile pleural reaction to a neighboring area of acute inflammation and subsides with the recrudescence of the collateral disease; the latter type of fluid indicates a suppurative process located in and on the pleura itself.

Great significance is attached to the bacteriologic examination, since the determination of the presence of viable bacteria and their species identification are of special importance both in evaluating the underlying pathology and in determining therapeutic management. In general, the thicker the exudate, the greater is the likelihood of viable bacteria being present. However, there are notable exceptions. For example, in the early stages of acute hemolytic streptococcal empyema the fluid is characteristically thin, but organisms, seen on direct smear, are abundantly present. Later the exudate becomes thicker.

Of special interest is the not infrequent observation made in recent years that specimens of thick purulent exudates are obtained from cases of empyema (nontuberculous) and are sterile on culture. It appears highly probable that, since empyema usually occurs in association with severe infections, the treatment with large doses of penicillin over extended periods of time has sterilized the area before the diagnosis of empyema is established. Sterile empyema is characterized by the presence of a well defined pleural shadow on x-ray examination, and the physical signs of a pleural effusion, but with considerable modification of the general reaction to suppuration as observed in the preantibiotic period. It is in a sense a new clinical entity created by modern antibacterial therapy.

Treatment. In empyema the immediate objectives are the eradication of the infection and the elimination of both the solid sediment adherent to the pleural surfaces and the free fluid. The ultimate objective is to promote expansion of the underlying lung, to obliterate the pleural space, and restore maximum pulmonary function.

In cases of empyema due to gram-positive cocci (pneumococcus, hemolytic streptococcus and hemolytic staphylococcus), penicillin introduced intrapleurally is highly efficacious in eradicating the infection. The instillation of 50,000 to 200,000 units of penicillin, depending on the size of the empyemal area, given on alternate days for three doses is a satisfactory procedure. Twenty-four hours after each treatment, aspiration is performed with special attention to cultures in order to determine the persistence or disappearance of organisms. Once sterility has been accomplished and aspirations have been continued until only minimal quantities of fluid are obtained, the subsequent clearing of the pleura with expansion of the underlying lung has been found to follow over the ensuing three to four weeks. Mobility of the patient is desirable during the convalescent period.

Infecting strains of hemolytic *Staphyloccus aureus* are particularly prone to develop fastness to penicillin. The increasing occurrence of strains of staphylococci refractory to the antibacterial effects of penicillin and other antibiotics in widespread use (Aureomycin and Terramycin) has recently been stressed by Finland and Haight. Consequently the antibiotic of choice as determined by sensitivity tests may be found among some of the newer agents, such as Magnamycin, erythromycin, and others.

The treatment of empyema may require surgical intervention in order to procure adequate drainage through open or closed thoracotomy. If loculations develop or other circumstances intervene that render sterilization and intercostal aspiration ineffective, surgical procedures should be undertaken.

In putrid empyema the possible need for surgical drainage is not infrequently required as an emergency. However, antibiotics, penicillin in cases due to anaerobic streptococcus, have proved effective in many cases and obviated the necessity of surgery. Not infrequently phlegmons and cellulitis of the extra-thoracic soft tissues have occurred along the track of the aspiration needle. The use of large doses of penicillin via the systemic route has reduced this complication.

An additional method in the medical management of empyema has recently been developed by the use of *streptokinase-streptodornase* (prepared by Lederle Laboratories under the trade name of Varidase), in causing rapid lysis of the solid sediments of purulent pleural exudations and thereby affording increased aspiration of the pleural cavity. The enzymatic liquefaction of the purulent exudation followed by aspiration of the thinned material makes possible a more rapid and greater evacuation of the pleural spaces which, freed of the exudate, are capable of permitting rapid reexpansion of the compressed lung. Ultimate recovery has been hastened both by medical enzymatic management, and also by the use of the enzymes in association with closed surgical thoracotomy as reported by Finnerty.

The following procedures are recommended.

1. *Intrapleural Dosage:* The content of one or two ampules of Varidase (each vial containing 100,000 units of streptokinase plus 25,000 units of streptodornase) is injected into a single site after removal of the amount of exudate that may be easily withdrawn. The dosage should bear a relation to the size of the empyemal cavity, varying from one-half the content of a single vial into areas containing less than 50 ml. to 2 vials into large areas containing several hundred ml. of exudate. If the empyema is massive, multiple simultaneous injections may be required at the first treatment. The quantity of enzymatic solution per dose averages 10 to 20 ml.

2. Aspirate by thoracentesis 12 to 24 hours after the injection. Subsequent aspirations are done as indicated. The guide to the effect of the treatment is decrease in amount of aspirated fluid associated with thinning. X-ray evidence of clearing also occurs. Repetitions of treatment may be required to effect maximal clearing. In cases of unusually longstanding chronic empyema the thick deposit on the pleural surfaces may be largely composed of material other than fibrin and desoxyribose nucleoprotein. Consequently, in such cases, even after many series of injections, a residual pleural peel is left that is not amenable to this type of lysis.

3. Quantitative determinations of the rate of decrease or disappearance of the local bacteria are valuable in estimating the effect of the therapy.

4. Supplementary appropriate antibiotics administered either systemically or locally may be given. The enzymatic débridement alone has effected sterilization in several instances.

WILLIAM S. TILLETT

References

Finland, M., and Haight, T. H.: Antibiotic Resistance of Pathogenic Staphylococci. A.M.A. Arch. Int. Med., 91:143, 1953.

Finnerty, J.: The Use of Streptokinase-Streptodornase in the Treatment of Thoracic Empyema. Surg., Gynec. & Obst., 97:220, 1953.

Graham, E. A., Singer, J. J., and Ballon, H. C.: Surgical Diseases of the Chest. Philadelphia, Lea and Febiger, 1935.

Hirshfeld, J. W., Buggs, C. W., Abbott, W. E., and Pilling, M. A.: Value of Penicillin in the Treatment of Empyema. J.A.M.A., 128:577, 1945.

Josey, A. I., Trenis, J. W., and Kammer, W. F.: Treatment of Postpneumonic Thoracic Empyema with Sulfonamides, Penicillin and Repeated Thoracenteses. Ann. Int. Med., 23:800, 1945.

Keefer, C. S., and others: Penicillin in the Treatment of Infections. J.A.M.A., 122:1217, 1943.

Maier, H. C., and Grace, E. J.: Putrid Empyema. Surg., Gynec. & Obst., 74:69, 1942.

Rudensky, H., Sprong, D. H., Jr., and Woods, C. C.: The Medical Treatment of Acute Empyema. J.A.M.A., 128:573, 1945.

Tillett, W. S., McCormack, J. E., and Cambier, M. J.: The Use of Penicillin in the Local Treatment of Pneumococcal Empyema. Bull. New York Acad. Med., 20:142, 1944; J. Clin. Investigation, 24: 595, 1945.

———: Sherry, S., and Read, C. T.: The Use of Streptokinase-Streptodornase in the Treatment of Postpneumonic Empyema. Journal of Thoracic Surgery, 21:275, 1951.

DISEASES OF THE MEDIASTINUM

INFECTIONS OF THE MEDIASTINUM

ACUTE MEDIASTINITIS

Acute infection of the mediastinum is most frequently the result of trauma. Infection may be introduced from without as in gunshot or stab wounds, or from within as in perforation of the trachea or esophagus by foreign bodies or instrumentation. When not directly or indirectly caused by trauma, it is almost always secondary to infections in neighboring structures, but may develop in the course of a general infection with septicemia. Infection may extend into the mediastinum from the neck as in Ludwig's angina or retropharyngeal abscess; it may extend from the esophagus (as in perforation of a carcinoma of the esophagus); it may arise from pneumonia or empyema; or osteomyelitis of various parts of the thoracic skeleton may be the source.

Acute nonsuppurative mediastinitis may accompany pericarditis, pleurisy, pneumonia or an infection in the neck. The symptoms are usually mild and consist in an abrupt increase of fever accompanied by pain beneath the sternum or between the shoulder blades, painful cough and discomfort on swallowing. Physical examination may reveal slight fullness in the suprasternal notch, tenderness over the sternum and crepitations along the sternal borders; or there may be no positive signs. The symptoms may subside spontaneously in a few days, and there are no sequelae.

In **acute suppurative mediastinitis** there is rapid spread throughout the mediastinal tissues from the point of origin of the infection, and the symptoms are severe, consisting of high fever, chills, severe prostration, painful shallow respiration and pain on swallowing. The pain is referred beneath the sternum or, in posterior mediastinitis, between the shoulder blades. On physical examination there may be, in addition to the signs noted in the nonsuppurative form, evidence of compression of the mediastinal organs. Signs of subcutaneous emphysema in the neck and upper chest, characterized by crepitation over these areas, may be present.

These result from escape of air from the trachea or esophagus into the adjacent tissues, which occurs most commonly in cases due to large perforations of the upper esophagus.

The *course* in acute suppurative mediastinitis is usually fulminating. Before the antibiotics became available, for use in conjunction with surgery, the case mortality was high. The complications of secondary perforation into the esophagus, the pleural cavity or a bronchus are still major hazards, particularly in neglected or inadequately treated cases.

Acute mediastinal abscess formation results from localization of an infection either in the anterior or the posterior mediastinum. The anterior abscesses are caused most commonly by extension of infections of the neck, posterior ones by perforation of the esophagus. Either may arise from suppuration of lymph nodes in pulmonary infections. The symptoms and signs of mediastinal compression commonly associated with abscesses vary according to the location. Pressure on the superior vena cava causes cyanosis, dilatation of the veins of the neck and thorax, exophthalmos, suffusion of the conjunctivas, and edema of the face and neck (*superior vena cava syndrome*). Pressure on the aorta and its branches causes inequalities in the pulsations of the carotid and radial arteries. Pressure on the heart, inferior vena cava or pulmonary artery causes cardiac dysfunction and congestive signs. Pressure on the trachea causes stridor, dyspnea and cough. Pressure on the esophagus causes dysphagia and pain on swallowing. Pressure on the thoracic duct may result in chylothorax or chylous ascites. Pressure on the vagus nerve may cause bradycardia; on the phrenic nerve, paralysis of the diaphragm; on the recurrent laryngeal nerve, paralysis of the vocal cord; on the stellate ganglion, or the roots of the cervical sympathetic, Horner's syndrome. Instead of these paralytic signs there may be irritative signs from nerve involvement, such as hiccups from irritation of the phrenic nerve, or pupillary dilatation instead of the miosis associated with Horner's syndrome. In addition to such signs of compression and nerve involvement, there may be localized redness and edema of the skin with tenderness in the suprasternal notch, in the supraclavicular spaces, about the sternum and xiphoid, or in the back, depending on the site of presentation of the abscess. In the larger abscesses there may be dullness to percussion anteriorly or posteriorly to either side of the midline. The roentgenogram may be helpful in revealing the presence and location of an abscess. In acute suppurative mediastinitis it may reveal nothing or may show diffuse widening of the mediastinal shadow.

Treatment. Acute nonsuppurative mediastinitis usually requires no treatment beyond that of the primary condition. Treatment of acute suppurative mediastinitis and of acute mediastinal abscess is surgical.

Preparatory to surgical drainage, and as concurrent treatment, antimicrobial therapy is always indicated. Penicillin is usually the drug of choice; it should be given in the water-soluble form in a dosage of 100,000 to 200,000 units intramuscularly every 3 or 4 hours. When penicillin-resistant organisms are present or suspected, supplemental therapy with other appropriate antimicrobial agents should be given. Dihydrostreptomycin, 1.0 gm. intramuscularly twice daily, should be given routinely in addition to penicillin whenever the source of the infection favors the presence of mixed pyogenic organisms, as in perforation of the esophagus.

CHRONIC MEDIASTINITIS

Chronic diffuse inflammation of the mediastinum is rare. It usually arises either as a sequel of acute suppurative mediastinitis or in association with chronic infections of neighboring structures. **Chronic fibrous mediastinitis** may thus occur following or in conjunction with pericarditis, aortic aneurysm, pleurisy, empyema, pulmonary infections of various kinds and infections of the thoracic skeleton. Thrombosis of the superior vena cava and of the innominate veins is sometimes associated with fibrous mediastinitis. This is reported particularly in cases thought to be of syphilitic origin.

Localized chronic mediastinitis or abscess is almost always tuberculous, actinomycotic, blastomycotic or syphilitic. Tuberculosis is the most frequent cause of chronic mediastinitis of this type, and the origin is usually a *tuberculous mediastinal and bronchopulmonary lymphadenitis,* which may occur alone or in association with other lympho-hematogenous forms of tuberculosis. The tracheal and tracheobronchial lymph nodes become enlarged, sometimes massively so, and may caseate, become matted together and break down. When liquefaction occurs, perforation into a bronchus is most common, but perforation into the mediastinal connective tissues may occur with formation of a cold abscess. As in all tuberculous abscesses, the tendency to burrowing and sinus formation is marked. A tuberculous mediastinal abscess may also arise from extension into the mediastinum of a tuberculous infection in the sternum, costal cartilages or spine.

The symptoms and signs of chronic mediastinitis, abscess and mediastinal lymphadenitis are variable, depending on the nature of the infection and the part of the mediastinum which is invaded. The cases of tuberculous mediastinal lymphadenitis may be symptomatically entirely latent, until the lymph nodes attain large size, or there may be mild constitutional symptoms. When the nodes become large, they may compress the bronchi or trachea sufficiently to cause cough and stridor. Signs of secondary pulmonary involvement from the bronchial obstruction may then appear. Symptoms and signs of superior vena cava compression are rare unless there has been invasion of the mediastinal connective tissues. These and other signs of mediastinal compression and nerve involvement may occur, however, in chronic mediastinitis and chronic abscess just as they do in association with acute abscesses and with mediastinal tumors.

Widening of the area of mediastinal dullness to percussion may be elicited when the mass is large and located in the anterior mediastinum. There may be dullness to either side of the vertebral column or of the sternum with alterations in the breath and spoken voice sounds.

The roentgenogram reveals the presence, size and location of any discrete lesions, or it may show diffuse widening of the mediastinal shadow. In the absence of fever or other constitutional symptoms of infection, differentiation between chronic infectious processes and tumors of the mediastinum is often difficult. In the tuberculous cases, evidence of tuberculosis elsewhere may clarify the diagnosis. The tuberculin test is helpful chiefly in children and young adults. Transient enlargement of mediastinal lymph nodes occurs in the course of various acute infectious diseases, particularly in children, and may be differentiated from tuberculous lymphadenitis by the slighter enlargement and early regression. The mediastinal lymph node enlargement of Hodgkin's disease and other lymphomas, as well as of sarcoidosis, may, in the absence of enlarged superficial lymph nodes suitable for biopsy, be undifferentiable from tuberculous lymphadenitis without exploratory operation. Diagnostic trial of x-ray therapy is rarely justified. The new technique, introduced by Daniels in 1949, of scalene lymph node biopsy may be tried, or, if this is unrevealing, an exploratory thoracotomy for removal of a lymph node from the mediastinum itself may be necessary. When chronic cutaneous fistulas are present, microscopic examination of the pus is necessary to differentiate between tuberculosis and the mycoses. Diagnosis of syphilis of the mediastinum is most difficult, because a positive serologic test is not by itself strong evidence that the mediastinal lesion is syphilitic. Even a response to antisyphilitic treatment is no longer a certain criterion, since the most effective treatment with penicillin is not specific for syphilis alone.

Treatment. The treatment of chronic mediastinitis depends on the nature of the infection. In the tuberculous cases long-term antimicrobial therapy with isoniazid or with streptomycin and para-aminosalicylic acid is essential. These drugs should be given in the same manner and for as long a period as for pulmonary tuberculosis. Dietary and rest treatment are also indicated, at least until any sinuses have healed and the enlarged lymph nodes have regressed to a maximal degree, which usually means to the extent that they are no longer visible roentgenographically. Surgical excision of sinuses or drainage of cold abscesses is rarely necessary in conjunction with such long-term drug therapy. The treatment of actinomycosis and blastomycosis of the mediastinum, formerly most unsatisfactory even with extensive surgery, has been improved in recent years. For actinomycosis penicillin, in high dosage and for extended periods, is the best single therapeutic agent. Sulfonamides and iodides may be given in addition. When surgery is necessary the medical treatment should, according to Smith, be continued for six months afterward to prevent relapse. Blastomycosis responds well to stilbamidine. This treatment should be administered only with full understanding of the toxic side effects. Most recently 2-hydroxystilbamidine, which appears to be less toxic, has been used successfully. Syphilis of the mediastinum, especially the gummatous form, responds readily to penicillin. Dramatic improvement may be expected with as little as 600,000 units daily. The optimal duration of therapy has not been determined. As in other forms of late syphilis, a total dose of 9,000,000 units (600,000 units daily for fifteen days) may be considered a minimal basic schedule. Treatment should be continued longer if symptoms or any signs of mediastinal compression or superior vena cava obstruction persist.

CARL MUSCHENHEIM

CYSTS AND TUMORS OF THE MEDIASTINUM

Mediastinal Cysts. Simple cysts derived from the thymus, the esophagus or the bronchi occur in the mediastinum. They are commonly lined with ciliated epithelium, contain fluid, and in most instances are bronchogenic. The simple thin-walled cysts, as well as the less common cystic lymphangiomas, are usually small, but may attain considerable size and extend into either pleural cavity. They usually cause no symptoms unless infection supervenes, when they may rupture into a bronchus and simulate lung abscess or empyema with bronchopleural fistula. Occasionally they may cause pressure symptoms and signs simulating those of solid tumors or aortic aneurysm. *Echinococcus cysts* are rare in the mediastinum. When present, they may be hour-glass extensions of echinococcus cysts of the spine. *Dermoid cysts* and cystic teratomas are the most important of the mediastinal cysts. These arise typically in the anterior mediastinum. Though present from birth, they grow slowly and usually do not cause pressure symptoms until adult life, if at all. They occasionally rupture into a bronchus, become infected, or undergo malignant degeneration.

Tumors of the Mediastinum. *Benign connective tissue tumors* of the mediastinum include fibromas, chondromas, xanthomas, lipomas, ganglioneuromas, neurinomas and neurofibromas. Of these, the fibromas and neurofibromas are the most common; they arise typically in the posterior mediastinum.

Benign solid tumors of the mediastinum, like the cysts, are discovered most frequently in the course of routine physical or x-ray examinations and do not cause thoracic symptoms until they have attained large size. A special group of so-called hourglass tumors which extend into the vertebral canal, or arise there and extend into the mediastinum, may produce symptoms and signs of spinal cord compression. These are most commonly neuro-

Symptoms and Signs. The symptoms and signs of mediastinal cysts and tumors depend mainly on their size and on the pressure which they may exert on vital structures situated in the mediastinum. Such manifestations of mediastinal compression differ in no way from those previously described in connection with mediastinitis and mediastinal abscesses. In the case of malignant tumors the effects of paralysis of various intrathoracic

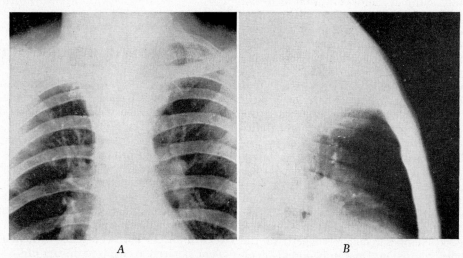

A   *B*

Fig. 132. Retrosternal goiter. *A,* Note displacement of trachea to the right in the postero-anterior projection. *B,* In the lateral projection, the anterior location of the tumor in the superior mediastinum.

fibromas, but they may be composed wholly of either neural or non-neural elements.

Malignant tumors and neoplastic diseases involving the mediastinum usually arise elsewhere, or are diffuse processes involving the lymphoid tissues throughout the body, such as lymphosarcoma, Hodgkin's disease or lymphatic leukemia. Mediastinal carcinoma is always secondary to carcinoma of the lung, thymus, esophagus or some more remote organ. Sarcomas of the mediastinum, as distinguished from lymphosarcomas, may arise as primary tumors from connective tissue elements in the various mediastinal and neighboring structures or by malignant degeneration of benign connective tissue tumors.

Intrathoracic (retrosternal) goiter and *tumors of the thymus,* though not usually classed as tumors of the mediastinum, are actually situated in the anterior mediastinum and may produce pressure effects similar to those from other tumors in this location. Tumors of the thymus are discussed in the section on Diseases of the Thymus Gland.

nerves (i.e., the vagus, phrenic, cervical sympathetic and recurrent laryngeal) may be the result of destructive invasion rather than pressure. In addition to the symptoms and signs resulting from disturbance of particular mediastinal structures there are those resulting from encroachment on the lungs and bronchi. The earliest symptoms may indeed be cough and dyspnea. Thymic tumors and substernal extensions of thyroid enlargements are particularly prone to cause tracheal compression in which severe dyspnea is associated with stridor. The cough associated with mediastinal cysts and tumors is usually nonproductive of sputum, unless bronchial obstruction is of sufficient degree to cause secondary suppurative disease in the lung. In case of rupture of a cyst into a bronchus, however, large amounts of sputum may be coughed up. When dermoid cysts have ruptured, the sputum may contain hair or other elements of the contents of such cysts. Pain occurs infrequently in association with benign tumors, but is commonly present with malignant tumors. The same may be said for hemoptysis. The physical signs attributable to the tumor mass itself depend on its size and location. There may be a bulging of the chest wall over the tumor, and transmitted pulsations from the heart or great vessels may be appreciable, simulating aneurysm. Tracheal tug is occasionally present, though more rarely than occurs with aneurysm. Signs of pleural effusion may accompany those of the tumor and may cause confusion as to the exact limits of the tumor mass itself.

Diagnosis. The x-ray and fluoroscopic examinations are of prime importance in determining the size, location and probable nature of mediastinal tumors. Lateral or oblique views are usually necessary in addition to the conventional postero-anterior projections. Bronchoscopy is helpful only when the symptoms and signs indicate the probability of intrabronchial involvement, either by primary bronchogenic carcinoma or by secondary invasion of a malignant growth from an adjacent lymph node. When mediastinal lymphadenopathy is present without enlargement of superficial lymph nodes suitable for biopsy, or without other manifestations of Hodgkin's disease or lymphosarcoma elsewhere in the body, differentiation from tuberculous lymphadenitis or Boeck's sarcoid may be impossible except by biopsy of scalene or mediastinal lymph nodes. The exact nature of benign tumors and cysts can often be determined only by surgical removal. Differentiation of mediastinal tumors from aortic aneurysms and from vascular structures in the lung roots is usually possible on the basis of history, physical signs and x-ray appearance. In doubtful cases angiocardiography will reveal whether or not the mass is vascular. This method is also helpful in determining whether a solid tumor at the lung root obstructs the pulmonary artery or its branches, and thus gives important information relative to its probable malignancy and operability.

Treatment. Benign tumors and cysts of the mediastinum should usually be removed, even if causing no symptoms, when they are discovered early in life. In skilled hands the surgical risk is small and the probability of growth with eventual development of pressure symptoms, or of malignant changes and other complications, is indeterminable without histologic diagnosis. Substernal or intrathoracic goiter also should be removed in most cases, especially if there are any symptoms or signs of tracheal or superior vena cava compression. Malignant mediastinal tumors are usually inoperable. Roentgen therapy is effective, especially in Hodgkin's disease and in lymphosarcoma, and may significantly prolong life in these conditions. In other malignant processes, such as metastatic carcinomas, it is of value mainly for palliation.

CARL MUSCHENHEIM

MEDIASTINAL HEMORRHAGE

Hemorrhage into the mediastinum occurs as the result of trauma, or from spontaneous rupture of an aneurysm of the aorta or one of its branches. Crushing injuries of the chest, with or without fracture of the sternum and ribs, may cause rupture or laceration of large vessels. The resulting hemorrhage or hematoma may compress the heart, trachea or great vessels, either alone or in association with tension pneumothorax and mediastinal emphysema, both of which also may occur in such injuries. The occurrence of hemorrhage alone is rarely recognized during life.

CARL MUSCHENHEIM

MEDIASTINAL EMPHYSEMA

Definition. Mediastinal emphysema, or pneumomediastinum, is defined as the presence of air in the tissues of the mediastinum.

Pathogenesis. Air may gain access to the mediastinum in several ways: (1) directly from the trachea, main bronchi or esophagus if these are torn or perforated as the result of injury; (2) by penetration of air through the interstitial tissues of the lung (interstitial pulmonary emphysema) to the lung root following rupture of alveolar walls, with or without associated spontaneous pneumothorax; (3) by extension, downward, from the neck of subcutaneous emphysema resulting from a chest wound; and (4) by direct suction from open wounds in the neck. Mediastinal emphysema is particularly common in association with tension pneumothorax, either spontaneous or traumatic.

Symptoms and Signs. The symptoms of

mediastinal emphysema itself may be slight if, as frequently happens, the air readily escapes to the subcutaneous tissues of the neck and thence over the body or downward into the retroperitoneal tissues. The spontaneous or traumatic pneumothorax which is commonly associated may, however, produce severe distress, especially if it is a tension pneumothorax. There may then be pain, extreme dyspnea, tachycardia, suffocation and shock. Rarely, though perhaps oftener than recognized, mediastinal emphysema may itself cause pain and symptoms of mediastinal compression. The pain is typically precordial and may be of sufficient severity to simulate that of coronary occlusion. The cardinal sign is the presence of air in the subcutaneous tissues of the neck which may be readily appreciated by palpation. The mediastinal air collection itself may give rise to obliteration of the area of cardiac dullness, and to crepitations over the mediastinum synchronous with deglutition, with respiration or with the heart beat. Hamman has described loud crunching and clicking sounds synchronous with the heart beat, which may be audible at some distance from the patient, in cases of *spontaneous mediastinal emphysema* (Hamman's syndrome). Such sounds may, however, be due in part to left-sided spontaneous pneumothorax which is present in many of these cases. The roentgenogram is of limited value in confirming the presence of suspected mediastinal emphysema, especially when there is associated pneumothorax. It may, however, especially in lateral views, reveal the mediastinal air collection and always reveals clearly any associated subcutaneous emphysema in the neck or over the chest.

Treatment is usually not necessary or is that of the underlying cause. When tension pneumothorax is present, this should be relieved by removal of air from the pleural space. Aspiration of air from the anterior mediastinum itself may be necessary as an emergency procedure, especially in pneumomediastinum of the newborn.

CARL MUSCHENHEIM

MEDIASTINAL HERNIA

Herniation of the thin septum of pleural reflections in the superior anterior mediastinum occurs commonly in association with pneumothorax on either side, and occasionally with large air cysts or bullae in the parenchyma of the lung. The condition is actually one of gaseous displacement rather than a true hernia. It usually causes no symptoms, and its chief importance lies in its recognition by roentgenogram and its differentiation from pneumothorax or air cyst in the opposite side of the chest. Mediastinal hernia is usually associated with displacement of the entire mediastinum, but may occur even when other mediastinal structures are fixed in a central position by pleural fibrosis and adhesions.

CARL MUSCHENHEIM

References

Dotter, C. T., and Steinberg, I.: Clinical Angiocardiography. Ann. Int. Med. 30:1104, 1949.

Hamman, L.: Spontaneous Mediastinal Emphysema. Bull. Johns Hopkins Hosp., 64:1, 1939.

Heuer, G. J., and Andrus, W. D.: The Surgery of Mediastinal Tumors. Am. J. Surg., 50:143, 1940.

Keefer, C. S.: Acute and Chronic Mediastinitis. Arch. Int. Med., 62:109, 1938.

Leather, H. M.: Syphilitic Mediastinitis. Lancet, 2: 116, 1953 (July 18).

Lindskog, G. E., and Liebow, A. A.: Thoracic Surgery and Related Pathology. New York, Appleton-Century-Crofts, 1953.

Schoenbach, E. B., Miller, J. M., and Long, P. H.: The Treatment of Systemic Blastomycosis with Stilbamidine. Ann. Int. Med. 37:31, 1952.

Shefts, L. M., Terril, A. A., and Swindell, H.: Scalene Node Biopsy. Am. Rev. Tuberc. 68:505, 1953.

Smith, D. T.: The Diagnosis and Therapy of Mycotic Infections. Bull. N. Y. Acad. Med., 29:778, 1953.

Snapper, I., and McVey, L. V., Jr.: The Treatment of North American Blastomycosis with 2-Hydroxystilbamidine. Am. J. Med., 15:603, 1953.

Touroff, A. S. W., and Seley, G. P.: Modern Surgical Management of Mediastinal Tumors and Infections. J.A.M.A., 154:230, 1954.

Veal, J. R., and Cotsonas, N. J., Jr.: Diseases of the Superior Vena Caval System with Special Consideration of Pathology and Diagnosis. Surgery, 31:1, 1952.

DISEASES OF THE DIAPHRAGM

Disturbances of the diaphragm result most commonly from (1) disease in adjacent viscera or serous cavities; (2) interference with its nerve supply; (3) developmental defects; and (4) trauma. Their importance derives from its dual function as a muscle of pulmonary ventilation and as the septum which separates the thoracic and peritoneal cavities and their contents. The muscle fibers of the diaphragm, which converge from their circumferential origins to insert into the trilobed central tendon, are anatomically considered to form a single muscle, but their motor nerve supply is derived from the paired phrenic nerves. Each half of the diaphragm functions, therefore, as a separate muscle and may become immobilized, or otherwise disturbed, without importantly affecting the function of the other half. The sensory nerve supply is derived partly from the lower thoracic nerves and partly from the phrenic nerves. Diaphragmatic pain is consequently referred both to the lower chest and upper abdominal wall by the former and to the neck and shoulder by the latter. The derivation of the phrenic nerves from the third, fourth and fifth cervical nerves is embryologically explained by the principal origin of the diaphragm from the fourth cervical myotome. Congenital hernias and other developmental defects which are encountered clinically are results of more complex embryologic factors. Failure of fusion of the cervically derived septum transversum of the embryo, which later forms the major anterolateral portion of the diaphragm, with other embryonic elements; failures of maturation of the various parts of the diaphragm; excessive degeneration of muscular elements in the formation of the central tendon; and delay in descent of the stomach are the most important causes of such developmental defects.

INFLAMMATION OF THE DIAPHRAGM

Inflammatory involvement of the diaphragm arises most commonly on its pleural surface as part of a generalized or localized pleurisy or empyema. Localized diaphragmatic pleurisy is not rare, especially in the early phase of development of acute tuberculous pleurisy with effusion. Symptoms and signs of diaphragmatic pleurisy may also appear as the initial manifestations of pneumonia, pulmonary infarction and other pulmonary inflammations. Less often, infection may extend to the diaphragm from other neighboring organs, or a generalized infection may become localized in this structure. Infiltration of the muscle of the diaphragm occurs in trichinosis, and the trichinae are often particularly numerous in this location.

Symptoms and Signs. Pain is the principal symptom of diaphragmatic irritation. It is characteristically related to inspiration. When it arises in the central portion of the diaphragm, it is referred, because of the phrenic innervation, to the neck and shoulder along the trapezius ridge. When the source of irritation is not centrally localized, the pain is referred also to the lower part of the chest and, not infrequently, to the epigastrium and hypogastrium. Dyspnea is usually not marked in unilateral inflammation, but breathing may be restricted because of the pain. Restriction of motion in acute processes results mainly from reflex splinting, in chronic processes from adhesions and pleural thickening. Elevation of the hemidiaphragm and diminished excursion may be recognized by percussion, and the breath sounds over the lower part of the lung are diminished. A pleural friction sound and tenderness over the lower rib interspaces are not uncommon findings when the inflammation is pleuritic. Roentgenograms and fluoroscopy are useful to confirm the presence of elevation and restriction of motion, and to reveal any associated pleural effusion or pulmonary pathology.

Treatment consists principally of measures to control pain. Adhesive strapping over the lower hemithorax often affords a considerable measure of relief. Codeine in doses of 0.03 gm. may be given every 3 or 4 hours if the pain is severe. Appropriate treatment of the underlying cause, including specific chemotherapy, is also indicated.

SUBDIAPHRAGMATIC ABSCESS

(Subphrenic Abscess)

Subdiaphragmatic abscess is one situated beneath either or both halves of the diaphragm. Usually it is unilateral, and the right side is affected more often than the left. On either side the abscess may be suprahepatic or infrahepatic, most often suprahepatic. It usually occupies but one of the spaces formed by the hepatic ligaments, but it may be multilocular within such space or multiple, occupying two or more of the anatomic subphrenic spaces. On the right side a subphrenic abscess is sometimes retroperitoneal, situated behind the coronary ligament of the liver or between its layers.

Etiology and Morbid Anatomy. Appendicitis was formerly considered the most common cause of right-sided abscesses. In more recent experience, both right and left abscesses arise most frequently by spread from neighboring intra-abdominal infections. Whether from a neighboring or distant focus, the abscess is usually secondary to suppuration or perforation of an abdominal viscus. It may be a localized and encapsulated residue of a general peritonitis, and, in its most common intraperitoneal form, it is essentially a localized peritonitis. In approximately 10 per cent of cases it is "primary," and no antecedent causal lesion is found. In another 10 per cent there is an associated liver abscess, usually with suppurative pylephlebitis, but this is more often concomitant or secondary to the subphrenic abscess than is the primary disease.

Whether on the right or left side, a subphrenic abscess is in intimate relation to the under surface of the diaphragm, and the accumulation of pus tends to elevate and restrict the motion of this structure. These effects are usually more pronounced with right-sided abscess than with left, because of the greater confinement of space above the massive and relatively immobile right lobe of the liver. On either side perforation into the pleural cavity is frequent, with formation of an empyema. Further extension of the infection to the lung may then occur, or this may arise directly when the pleural space is obliterated by adhesions. Even without perforation there is frequently a secondary pleural effusion, which may be serous and sterile on culture. Involvement of the pericardial sac by extension of inflammation or

by perforation is relatively rare. Curiously, extension of infection in the reverse direction, from above the diaphragm to the subphrenic region, is extremely rare.

Symptoms and Signs. Since subphrenic abscess usually occurs as a sequel or complication of some abdominal infection, the onset of general symptoms is rarely abrupt, but occurs as an exacerbation or renewal of symptoms of sepsis such as fever and chills. The most important localizing symptom is pain, characteristically located in the chest over the lowermost ribs. Depending on the location of the abscess, the pain may be anterior, posterior or lateral, or it may be referred to the shoulder. The most typical physical signs occur in right-sided abscess in which the liver is pushed down and the hemidiaphragm is pushed up. The liver, though palpable, is not tender unless it is itself the site of an abscess. There may be some bulging of the lower part of the chest, and the respiratory movements are diminished. Local tenderness is commonly present. The elevation and limitation of motion of the hemidiaphragm are evident by percussion and auscultation and by fluoroscopy. Differentiation from pleural effusion may be difficult, especially since this may be present as a complication. In many instances the abscess contains gas, and the signs may then simulate those of localized pneumothorax or hydropneumothorax. All the signs are usually less pronounced with left-sided abscess. Confirmation of the diagnosis depends on aspiration of pus through a needle. Such aspiration should usually not be done except on the operating table with all preparations completed for immediate surgical drainage.

Prognosis and Treatment. The prognosis of subphrenic abscess is grave unless the diagnosis is established early. Treatment is surgical, supplemented by appropriate antibacterial chemotherapy.

Carl Muschenheim

PARALYSIS OF THE DIAPHRAGM

Paralysis of the diaphragm results from any process which interrupts its motor innervation. Anterior poliomyelitis involving the cervical cord at the level of origin (C3, 4, 5) of the phrenic nerves is the most frequent cause of bilateral paralysis, and this is always serious. Bilateral paralysis of the diaphragm is not necessarily fatal, however, if the intercostals and the accessory muscles of respiration are not also impaired. Unilateral or hemidiaphragmatic paralysis is most commonly caused by intrathoracic tumors, either by pressure on the phrenic nerve or its actual destruction by malignant growth. Less common causes of phrenic paralysis are mediastinitis, mediastinal abscess and inflammations of the mediastinal pleura.

Surgical interruption of the phrenic nerve, by avulsion of crushing, has in the past been much used in the treatment of pulmonary tuberculosis. This operation is no longer in great favor because of the considerable resulting impairment of pulmonary function, which is often permanent, even when only the nerve crushing procedure has been performed.

Symptoms and Signs. Bilateral paralysis causes severe dyspnea and the use in breathing of the accessory muscles of respiration. Paralysis of either hemidiaphragm may cause no dyspnea at rest or even with moderate exertion unless there are additional causes of respiratory insufficiency. On examination, reversal of the respiratory motion of the upper abdomen will be found with recession rather than bulging in inspiration. There is elevation of the lower border of pulmonary resonance because the diaphragm has ascended and the normal respiratory excursion is absent. The breath sounds over the entire lung are diminished. Fluoroscopy reveals not only the elevation and absence of normal excursion, but also the presence of paradoxical motion if the phrenic paralysis is complete.

Prognosis and Treatment. In bilateral paralysis the prognosis is usually grave, and the use of the Drinker or another form of respirator may be necessary. Unilateral phrenic paralysis usually requires no treatment. Its presence in cases of bronchogenic carcinoma of the lung is an unfavorable prognostic sign with respect to operability, since it indicates probable extension to lymph nodes and invasion of the mediastinum.

CARL MUSCHENHEIM

DIAPHRAGMATIC SPASM, TIC, AND FLUTTER

HICCUP
(Clonic Spasm)

This common symptom consists in an involuntary spasm of inspiratory movement of the diaphragm checked suddenly by closure of the glottis. There is usually a succession of such spasms, often caused by rapid eating, which usually subside spontaneously within a few minutes. Hiccup is of medical importance only when it is persistent.

Persistent hiccup occurs most often in a setting of serious illness, yet the causes are usually obscure. The center for the reflex is considered to be in the upper cervical segments of the spinal cord. Afferent stimuli are transmitted principally by the vagus and by sensory fibers of the phrenic nerve. The efferent path is primarily the phrenic, but the accessory muscles of respiration may also participate. It is thought that both central and peripheral causes can be responsible for persistent hiccup.

Gastric irritation, from gastritis or gastric dilatation, is a frequent and well established cause. Irritation of the intestine, the peritoneum, the pleura, the mediastinum, the pericardium or the diaphragm itself is another apparent peripheral cause. The most common central causes are uremia and diseases of the central nervous system, especially epidemic encephalitis. In rare cases no associated disease is found, and the condition is thought to be psychogenic. Persistent hiccup may follow surgical operations, but here also the exact cause is most often obscure. It is no more frequent after operations in the thorax than in the abdomen, and apparently no more frequent after operations in the abdomen than in the pelvis.

Treatment. In persistent hiccup the simple maneuvers which usually suffice to stop a mild attack, such as holding the breath or drinking cold water, are rarely effective. Firm traction on the tongue may be tried, or pressure on the phrenic nerve in the neck. Rebreathing into a paper bag should next be tried. If all these methods fail, a gastric aspiration and lavage is indicated. If the hiccup still persists, administration should be started of 5 to 10 per cent carbon dioxide in oxygen by mask for 5 to 10 minutes at a time, or until the patient becomes dizzy. If the hiccups recurs, the inhalation should be repeated. Too long administration of carbon dioxide will cause unconsciousness and convulsions. *It is imperative, therefore, that the administrator be a physician or experienced nurse and be in constant attendance during the administration.* Finally, if all other methods have failed, and the patient is seriously weakened by persistence of the hiccup, surgical exposure and injection of one of the phrenic nerves may be necessary. Usually the left nerve is selected. The procedure, though it may not stop the hiccup, will usually reduce the violence of the spasm.

Tonic spasm occurs in rabies, tetanus, strychnine poisoning, eclampsia, encephalitis and epilepsy; less commonly in asthenia and emphysema. The symptoms are pain and dyspnea. The spasm may usually be stopped by application of counterirritation over the lower chest and epigastrium.

TIC AND FLUTTER

Diaphragmatic *tic* is characterized by rapid rhythmic motion of the diaphragm with rates up to one hundred or more per minute. Both halves of the diaphragm are usually involved. Many of the reported cases have been in postencephalitic patients or in hysteria. In addition to the rapid respirations, the symptoms are pain in the lower chest and along the costal margins. Tetany rarely occurs despite the rapid respiratory rate, which is usually compensated by the small volume of tidal air.

Diaphragmatic *flutter* is a more rapid rhythmic motion, with rates about three hundred per minute. It usually involves only one half of the diaphragm. The cause is unknown. Severe pain, sometimes simulating that of coronary insufficiency, is the predominant symptom.

Treatment. Persistent tic or flutter can be relieved only by blocking the phrenic nerve. Injection, freezing or crushing are preferable to avulsion.

DIAPHRAGMATIC HERNIA

Definition. Diaphragmatic hernia is defined for practical purposes as any condition in which there is protrusion of abdominal contents into the thoracic cavity through an abnormal opening in the diaphragm. In this common use of the term no distinction is made between "true" hernias, which have a hernial sac, and "false" hernias without such a sac. The presence of a sac cannot, in fact, be determined except at operation.

Etiology and Morbid Anatomy. Diaphragmatic hernias are either traumatic or nontraumatic. The nontraumatic hernias are classified as congenital or acquired. Congen-

ital hernia is met with principally in infants, many of whom die within a few days after birth. Acquired nontraumatic hernia is, like the congenital, attributable to developmental defects, but the herniation does not occur until after birth and usually causes no symptoms until adult life.

Esophageal hiatus hernia, in which a portion of the stomach herniates through the esophageal hiatus of the diaphragm, is the most common type of acquired hernia. Harrington found it between three and four

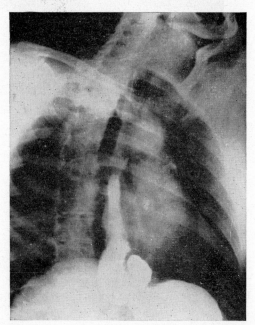

Fig. 133. Small esophageal hiatus diaphragmatic hernia of para-esophageal type.

times as common as the total of all other types of herniation that required surgical treatment. The *other common sites* of nontraumatic hernia are (1) the pleuroperitoneal hiatus (foramen of Bochdalek), (2) the gap left by partial absence of the diaphragm, usually situated in the posterior portion of the muscle, and (3) an anterior substernal opening (foramen of Morgagni).

In esophageal hiatus hernia the entire stomach may be contained within the hernial sac, but usually only a part is so contained, and other abdominal viscera are rarely involved. Congenital and traumatic hernias, on the other hand, not infrequently contain the entire stomach as well as other abdominal viscera—omentum, colon, small intestine, spleen, liver, pancreas and kidney.

Esophageal hiatus diaphragmatic hernias

are classified for surgical purposes into several distinct types, depending on the relative positions of the hernial sac and the lower end of the esophagus. The most important distinction to be made is between the various types of true hiatus hernias, which have a sac, and the false hernia associated with congenitally short esophagus. In this malformation the stomach does not reach its normal position below the diaphragm, but is held suspended partially within the thorax in the

carceration or strangulation of the hollow viscera. The symptoms in *congenital hernia* are often even more severe than in the cases of traumatic hernia, and the majority of infants with such defects die of respiratory and cardiac embarrassment soon after birth. Sometimes, however, extensive herniation may produce slight symptoms, and these patients may survive into childhood or adult life without disability unless intestinal or gastric obstruction develops.

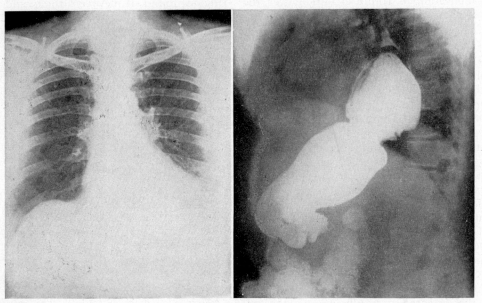

Fig. 134. Partial thoracic stomach with congenitally short esophagus. (Diaphragmatic "hernia," short esophagus type.)

posterior mediastinum. The condition is less common than true hiatus hernia, and the two conditions may be clinically and roentgenologically indistinguishable. However, they require different methods of operative repair.

Symptoms. The clinical symptoms of diaphragmatic hernia differ in the various types. They are in general more severe in the traumatic and congenital cases in which multiple abdominal viscera are more frequently involved in the hernia.

In cases of *traumatic hernia* the immediate symptoms are usually those of respiratory, gastric and circulatory embarrassment. They consist typically of pain, severe dyspnea, hiccup, vomiting and shock. If the patient survives the initial acute condition, there may later be gastrointestinal hemorrhage or symptoms of intestinal obstruction from in-

The symptoms of *esophageal hiatus hernia* may begin in childhood or at any later time. They are variable because of the progressive character of hernias of this type. Mild epigastric distress is usually the initial symptom. It occurs during or shortly after meals, may radiate through to the back, and is often accompanied by hiccup and gaseous eructations. As the condition progresses, the attacks become more severe, and there may be agonizing pain, radiating to the interscapular region or to the trapezius ridge, on the left, and down the arm. Gaseous eructations, which usually relieve the pain, may become difficult. The attacks of pain usually occur at intervals of weeks or months, but may become constant, with exacerbations whenever food is taken. Vomiting may then become severe, and there may be hematemesis or melena. Such hemorrhage is usually an indication of incarceration of a portion of the stomach in the hernial sac, with formation of a traumatic ulcer. Severe anemia may result from occult hemorrhage in some of these patients. In some instances the predominating symptoms are those of esophageal obstruction with dysphagia and regurgitation. Dyspnea, tachycardia and palpitations resulting from the presence of the herniated portion of the stomach within the thorax frequently accompany the other symptoms, especially after meals and in the recumbent posture.

Physical Signs. Abnormal signs are usually absent unless the hernia is large. When present, they consist in limitation of respiratory motion on the affected side of the chest, limitation of the diaphragmatic excursion, displacement of the heart, and abnormalities to percussion and auscultation of the chest which may be variable. Gas in the hollow viscera displaced into the chest causes a tympanitic note, and there may be borborygmi. The tympani may alternate with flatness to percussion when the gaseous contents are replaced by fluid.

Diagnosis. In most cases roentgenography is necessary to establish the diagnosis. This may be obvious with larger types, especially if there is incarceration. Small reducible hernias require special care and manipulation in observing the passage of the barium meal, or they may be overlooked. Hernia of the colon cannot be excluded without a barium enemia. *Symptomatically, "periesophageal," or hiatus hernia, may closely simulate such different diseases as peptic ulcer, cholecystitis and angina pectoris.* If the true condition is suspected, differentiation by roentgenography may be readily made. Roentgenographically, diaphragmatic hernia must be differentiated from eventration of the diaphragm, hourglass stomach, cardiospasm, and stricture or carcinoma of the esophagus. Esophagoscopy may be necessary to exclude the last. Moreover, stricture of the lower part of the esophagus may be associated with esophageal hiatus hernias; Harrington recommends that esophagoscopic examination be made in all cases of diaphragmatic hernia prior to surgical intervention.

Treatment. Traumatic and congenital hernias should be treated surgically whenever possible. The colon and small bowel are usually involved in such hernias and there is danger of intestinal obstruction. In hiatus hernia the advisability of surgical intervention depends on the severity of symptoms and the extent of herniation of the stomach. If a third or more of the stomach is involved, operation is usually indicated even in the absence of signs of incarceration or fixation. Many smaller hernias require no treatment, or the symptoms may be controlled by conservative measures. These consist in eating small meals, moderate exercise, avoidance of recumbency after meals and, sometimes, a bland diet similar to that given for peptic ulcer.

CARL MUSCHENHEIM

EVENTRATION OF THE DIAPHRAGM

This is a condition characterized by relaxation and atrophy of either half of the diaphragm. It differs from paralysis of the diaphragm in that it is apparently congenital and the atrophy is not dependent on any demonstrable involvement of the phrenic nerve. There is no defect in continuity, as there is in diaphragmatic hernia, but the affected leaf may be paper-thin because of complete degeneration of the muscle. As a result of the relaxation there is a marked elevation of the diaphragmatic septum, so that abdominal viscera may occupy the thorax on the affected side. In some instances it is associated with aplasia of the corresponding lung.

Symptoms and Signs. The symptoms are usually slight or absent. Some patients complain of vague gastric distress. Usually the condition is detected by routine physical or x-ray examination. The physical signs resemble those of acquired phrenic paralysis or, if the elevation is extreme, of diaphragmatic hernia. Differentiation from the former depends on the absence of any intrathoracic or cervical disease which might compromise the phrenic nerve. Differentiation from congenital diaphragmatic hernia depends on roentgenographic study with barium meal and enema.

Treatment. Treatment is usually not necessary, unless there is respiratory difficulty associated with another cause, such as emphysema. In such situations stabilization by plication of the atrophic diaphragm, or by its reinforcement with tantalum gauze mesh, may significantly improve the pulmonary function.

HEPATODIAPHRAGMATIC INTERPOSITION OF THE COLON

Interposition of a segment of the transverse colon between the right leaf of the diaphragm and the liver is a rare condition which may cause right lower thoracic or upper abdominal pain and obstipation. Usually the interposition is intermittent. Gas in the affected segment may cause obliteration of the area of liver dullness and on roentgenography may simulate free air beneath the diaphragm. Its chief importance lies in the differentiation from pneumoperitoneum secondary to perforation of an abdominal viscus, and in the differentiation from a gas-containing right subphrenic abscess.

CARL MUSCHENHEIM

References

Bailey, H.: Persistent Hiccup. Practitioner, *150:* 173, 1943.

Bisgard, J. D.: Congenital Eventration of the Diaphragm. J. Thoracic Surg., *16:*484, 1947.

Goodman, M. J.: Paroxysmal Flutter of Diaphragm Simulating Coronary Occlusion. J.A.M.A., *116:* 1635, 1941.

Handron, C. J.: Diaphragmatic Tic. Ann. Int. Med., *14:*1909, 1941.

Harley, H. R. S.: Subphrenic Abscess. Thorax, *4:*1, 1949.

Harrington, S. W.: Various Types of Diaphragmatic Hernia Treated Surgically. Report of 430 Cases. Surg., Gynec., & Obst., *86:*735, 1948.

Kizer, R. E., and Cook, J. C.: Lesions of Diaphragm with Special Reference to Eventration. Am. J. Roentgenol., *52:*611, 1944.

Diseases of the Kidneys

RENAL PHYSIOLOGY AND TESTS OF RENAL FUNCTION

The treatment of renal disease requires a background of physiologic knowledge. The kidney is the organ mainly responsible for the maintenance of the constancy of the volume and composition of body fluids. The constant chemical structure of body fluids, as revealed by analysis of blood or plasma, is normally protected from disastrous disorder by the selective functions of the kidney. The composition and the volume of materials taken in by the human organism may vary greatly from time to time. A nice adjustment by the kidney of the amount of each substance excreted is necessary to keep the balance between intake and output which is required if the internal fluid environment is to be constant.

The treatment of the patient with renal disease from the physiologic standpoint often involves the problem of adjusting the diet or intake in order to compensate for the inability of the diseased kidney to retain or excrete quantities of substances requisite for balance. Thus the behavior of the kidney in any patient must be interpreted with regard to the tasks it must perform as a result of changes in composition and the amount of the patient's intake, and also with regard for changes in the composition of the blood due to extrarenal disease. The total metabolic balance of the body, the concentration of materials in body fluids, and the functions of the kidney are mutually interdependent; deviations in one are reflected in the other.

In the performance of some of its functions the kidney is influenced by secretions of the endocrine glands, particularly of the adrenal and posterior pituitary. Renal function is also dependent on an adequate blood flow and intravascular pressure and is therefore modified by functional abnormalities of the heart and blood vessels. The administration of many drugs may cause marked and sometimes specific derangement of its functions.

In order to determine precisely enough for clinical purposes the degree and type of abnormality, it is necessary to apply various renal functional tests. An understanding of the physiological meaning of these procedures, of the limits of normal variation, and of the accuracy of the methods is necessary. The basic principles and interpretation of these methods will be discussed rather than the details of procedure.

Renal Physiology. The normal kidney is composed of millions of functional units, the nephrons. The process of urine formation may be divided into two phases, each associated with one of the two main divisions of the nephron. The first phase is filtration of the plasma, which takes place in the glomerulus. Through the glomerular capillaries there normally is filtered an essentially protein-free fluid containing the same concentrations of substances as is present in plasma. (Exception is made for materials which may be bound to the plasma protein and therefore not freely diffusible, and for small differences in concentrations of electrolytes due to adjustment of equilibrium between the plasma and the protein-free fluid, the so-called Donnan effect.) For the process of *filtration* an effective head of pressure must be maintained in the glomerular capillaries. This must exceed the opposing forces of the osmotic pressure of the plasma proteins and pressure of the surrounding tissue. Without filtration there can be virtually no urinary excretion, since, in the human kidney, urine formation results first from the process of filtration and secondly from modification of the filtered material by *tubular reabsorption*. A few normally occurring substances—ammonia, potassium, creatinine and certain foreign substances, notably the dyes and drugs used for renal function tests—are actively *secreted* by the renal tubular cells. The effective filtration pressure in the glomerular capillaries is transmitted to the afferent arteriole of the glomerulus via the renal artery and its intrarenal branches. The effective pressure in the glomerular capillaries is finally adjusted by a balance of the degree of construction of the vascular inlet, or the afferent arteriole, and the outlet, or efferent arteriole, of the glomerulus. Upon leaving the glomerulus, the blood courses through a network of peritubular vessels, where it takes up material reabsorbed through the tubular cells and finally empties into the renal vein. Obstruction to outflow of filtrate in the tubular lumen or back pressure in the urinary tract will oppose the process of filtration and the flow of blood through the glomerular capillaries.

In the average normal-sized man under basal conditions, the blood flow through the kidneys is 1200 cc. per minute, which is about one fourth to one third of the total output of the heart. The normal renal plasma flow is 650 cc. per minute. Of this 650 cc. of plasma, 130 cc. per minute, or 20 per cent, is filtered through the glomeruli. Thus the normal glomerular filtration rate (GFR) is 130 cc. per minute; the normal renal plasma flow (RPF) is 650 cc. per minute; and the filtration fraction (FF) is 0.20, or 20 per cent of the plasma flow.

A comparison of the enormous amount of plasma filtrate produced in 24 hours by the glomeruli with the amount of some of the substances in a normal 24-hour urine specimen reveals the importance of the second phase of urine formation. This phase of urine formation is the tubular reabsorption of part of the substances in the filtrate from the tubular lumen. For example, water is filtered through the glomeruli normally at 130 cc. per minute, or 187 liters per day; but a normal daily urine volume is only 1 to 2 liters. Therefore, only roughly 1 per cent of the filtered water escapes, and 99 per cent is reabsorbed. Other examples of substances which are in large part reabsorbed are sodium and chloride ions. A normal daily output of sodium chloride is roughly 10 gm. The renal tubules accomplish this rate of excretion by allowing only the amount of sodium and chloride in 1 cc. of glomerular filtrate to escape every minute. Since there are 130 cc. of fluid filtered per minute, there must be at least 99 per cent reabsorption of the filtered sodium chloride.

The process of urine formation which requires the filtration of roughly one hundred times the amount of water and salt that finally excreted seems a wasteful procedure. Therein, however, is one explanation of the capacity of diseased kidneys with markedly reduced function frequently to maintain adequate output of sodium chloride and water. A reduction in glomerular filtration rate to as little as 10 per cent of normal, or about 10 to 15 cc. per minute, still presents to the tubules ten times more water and salt than need be excreted to maintain equilibrium between intake and output. In these circumstances the renal tubular cells must reabsorb a smaller than normal proportion of the amount presented to them. Thus in any case the output of sodium chloride and water and other important plasma constituents is the net result of the two phases of renal function—filtration and reabsorption —and depends on a balance between glomerular and tubular function.

Any imbalance of these two phases of renal function may lead to abnormal retention or abnormal loss. Sodium is the main positive ion in the electrolyte structure of all extracellular fluids. The concentration of sodium in extracellular fluid is maintained within narrow limits of variation.

In most circumstances continuously varying proportions of sodium and water are both ingested and lost through other channels such as sweat. The task performed by the kidney is to adjust selectively the amount of sodium and water excreted. For example, if the intake of water is high and that of salt low, the kidney is required to conserve salt and excrete water. The renal tubular cells are stimulated in these circumstances to reabsorb nearly all the sodium and to reabsorb less of the water presented to them by the glomeruli. The result is a more dilute urine. The ability of the kidney to elaborate a dilute urine is therefore an important protective mechanism for the conservation of salt in the presence of excess water. Loss of this mechanism is found in varying degrees in some types of chronic nephritis. The result is loss of body salt with accompanying dehydration. Obviously, since this type of patient cannot conserve salt, "routine" treatment for kidney disease by restriction of salt intake might prove disastrous. Eventually, not only would dehydration occur from loss of body fluids, but the concentration of sodium would fall.

On the other hand, there are situations in which the kidney may be confronted with an intake of excess salt in proportion to water. Then the task is for the tubules to reabsorb more of the water and less of the sodium. The result is a more concentrated urine. The ability of the kidney to elaborate a concentrated urine is therefore a protective mechanism for the elimination of excess salt in the presence of relatively little water or, conversely, for the conservation of water in the presence of excess salt. Loss of this mechanism is also found in some cases of nephritis when there is damage to the renal tubules. A result of impairment of this function may be the retention of salt and water when the intake of salt is excessive. For a damaged kidney, an average salt intake may be excessive and lead to increased extracellular fluid with edema and sometimes to a rise in the concentration of sodium.

An excellent illustration of loss of the ability to adjust water and salt excretion is the common complaint by the nephritic patient of an increased volume of overnight urine. The symptom of nocturia represents inability of the damaged kidney to produce the concentrated urine excreted overnight, an adaptation which normally allows the excretion of solids with a minimum of water.

Renal Function Tests. The test designed to measure *concentration and dilution powers* is usually carried out by giving the patient food and no fluids for a 12-hour period, followed by a period of high water intake. Under the stimulus of restricted water the specific gravity of the urine should normally rise to the level of 1.025 to 1.030, and with excess water fall to 1.003. When the kidney can produce neither concentrated nor dilute urine, the specific gravity is said to be "fixed" and is characteristically fixed at 1.010 to 1.012. This is the specific gravity of plasma minus its protein, or of the glomerular filtrate. Fixation of specific gravity represents inability of the renal tubules to perform the work of altering the proportion of solids to water in the filtrate.

It is common to find that urine specimens obtained at random have a higher specific gravity than those obtained during test conditions. A single test is, therefore, not conclusive, nor is it necessary if random specimens have shown an adequate range of concentration and dilution. Normally, young people are capable of producing urine of specific gravity up to or above 1.025, whereas in elderly people it may not rise much above 1.018.

The specific gravity is governed normally, not only by the amount of salts, but also of other solids and particularly urea. To attain maximum specific gravity, the renal tubules must be under the stimulus to conserve water and to reject or excrete sodium chloride, and there must be sufficient urea. All three of these circumstances are not always

successfully combined during an applied concentration test, but may coincide when random specimens are obtained. In diabetes and nephrosis the specific gravity may be elevated by sugar or protein in the urine.

Other important factors beside the concentrating power of the tubules govern the renal *excretion of sodium and water* and affect the body fluid economy. Some of these factors are little understood. For example, the kidney in the nephrotic stage of nephritis fails to excrete sodium even though there may be several liters of edema fluid. The retention of salt by the kidney may be so marked that a reduction in the patient's intake to less than 1 gm. a day is necessary to prevent further accumulation. At any time the same patient may spontaneously have a diuresis.

It is not known what factors influence the glomerular-tubular balance and determine whether in nephritis the disease is the so-called "salt-losing" or "salt-retaining" type. Even in the presence of disease the amount of salt and water in the diet can frequently be adjusted to maintain body balance successfully. A few careful repeated clinical observations are usually sufficient to guide the dietary adjustments of salt and water. The daily urine volume and specific gravity, the daily body weight, and the salt and water content of the diet can be accurately estimated with minimal laboratory assistance. The general appearance of the patient with particular attention to the state of hydration and the arterial and venous blood pressures should be followed. Actual chemical determination of the total urinary output of salt and of the salt content of the diet are refinements rarely necessary, but may be helpful in difficult situation. Standard diets with foods of known salt content are readily available and sufficiently accurate for most purposes. Changes in the blood hematocrit are helpful in estimating changes in hydration. Defects in the composition of body fluids may be revealed by determination of the serum sodium and chloride concentrations. Interpretation of serum sodium and chloride concentrations is difficult, since abnormal salt retention may be accompanied by either low or high values. In some cases there may be so-called "dry salt retention" resulting from renal retention of salt without sufficient water. In contrast, there may be marked retention of sodium with massive accumulation of edema fluid containing an abnormally low concentration of sodium as is commonly found in the nephrotic stage of nephritis. Sometimes low sodium and chloride concentrations are caused by the prolonged use of low salt diets.

Other factors controlling the renal excretion of sodium chloride and water are better understood. The posterior portion of the pituitary gland secretes a potent antidiuretic hormone which acts upon the renal tubular cells, causing increased reabsorption of water and resulting in diminished water excretion. Failure of normal posterior pituitary function results in uncontrolled water excretion characteristic of diabetes insipidus. The daily urine volume may reach 10 to 15 liters, but can be kept within the normal limits of 1 to 2 liters by the administration of posterior pituitary extracts.

The secretion of the adrenal gland is necessary for normal tubular reabsorption of sodium and chloride. Destruction of the adrenal gland as is present in Addison's disease causes loss of sodium chloride in the urine and the sequelae—dehydration with low serum sodium and chloride plasma concentration. The loss may be replaced by increasing the intake of sodium chloride, or the effect of the adrenal cortex on the tubules may be replaced by the administration of desoxycorticosterone acetate (DOCA).

As part of its task of maintaining a constant composition of body fluids, the kidney must excrete any excess of acid or alkali which has been absorbed or produced by the body. The problem of maintaining a normal reaction or pH in body fluids is shared by both the kidney and the respiratory apparatus. Some adjustments in pH can be made by the liberation of carbonic acid through the lungs which will compensate for the accumulation of nonvolatile or "fixed" acids. Conversely, the accumulation of excess fixed cation can be partially neutralized by the retention of carbonic acid. Many acid substances—for example, lactic acid—when accumulated, are temporarily accommodated by the displacement of carbonic acid through the lungs, and finally are absorbed and utilized by the tissues, particularly the liver. However, the main burden of acid-base regulation is accomplished by the kidney.

There are three fundamental *mechanisms by which the kidney excretes acid,* and these mechanisms reside in the renal tubular cells. In most circumstances the problem is to dispose of excess acid, or to produce an acid urine, since most diets contain an excess of acid-producing substances. Normal blood is slightly alkaline, having a pH of 7.4. Usually the task is to excrete acid with minimal loss of cation, which for practical purposes means without undue loss of sodium, since sodium is the most abundant basic ion available to the kidney.

The first mechanism consists in the exchange of hydrogen ions by the renal tubular cells. An illustration of this mechanism may be written as follows:

$$\text{Na Ac} \quad + \quad \text{H}_2\text{CO}_3 \quad \rightarrow$$
in glomerular   produced
filtrate   by tubule

$$\text{H Ac} \quad + \quad \text{NaHCO}_3$$
excreted   reabsorbed
in urine   into blood

The sodium ion is conserved by reabsorption with bicarbonate, which is produced by the tubule, and the hydrogen ion is excreted with the fixed acid ion (Ac). This mechanism is capable of excreting most of the excess acid encountered in normal circumstances, and produces acid urine. A specific enzyme, carbonic anhydrase, in the renal tubular cells accomplishes the production of bicarbonate necessary for the reabsorption of sodium. Poisoning of this enzyme with resultant inability of the tubule to conserve fixed cation is caused by the administration of sulfanilamide and related compounds.

The second mechanism for eliminating fixed acid is the production and secretion of ammonia by the renal tubular cells. This mechanism is illustrated by the following formula:

$$\text{Na Ac} \quad + \quad \text{NH}_3 + \text{H}_2\text{CO}_3 \quad \rightarrow$$
in glomerular   produced
filtrate   by tubule

$$\text{NH}_4\text{Ac} \quad + \quad \text{NaHCO}_3$$
excreted   reabsorbed
in urine   into blood

The manufacture of ammonia allows the excretion of the fixed anion as the ammonium salt, the fixed cation being retained. In normal circumstances only a small amount of ammonia is produced, but under conditions of high acid intake the production of ammonia will rise rapidly, allowing the elimination of acid without loss of fixed cation. Acidification of body fluids is thus prevented.

In the diseased kidney both the ability to

secrete acids and to produce ammonia may be marked diminished. The patient is then unable to preserve the normal alkalinity of the blood, and the administration of acids is detrimental. To alleviate the burden of acid excretion on the kidney, it may be necessary to give a diet containing only neutral or alkaline-producing foods (alkaline ash diet).

The third mechanism for excreting fixed acids does not conserve base, and functions when and if the capacity of the kidney to eliminate acid by the other mechanisms is exceeded. The acid is excreted as the salt of the fixed base sodium. When the kidney is diseased or under conditions of abnormally high intake of acid, the loss of sodium may result in loss of body fluids with dehydration and acidosis. Failure to conserve fixed cation frequently causes loss not only of sodium but also potassium and calcium ions. Loss of potassium under some circumstances may be sufficient to cause serious low potassium toxicity; loss of calcium may lead to demineralization of bone and fractures.

The loss of sodium caused by administration of excess acid is the physiologic basis for the efficacy of the acid salts as diuretics. For example, large doses of ammonium chloride are sometimes used to remove edema fluid. After absorption by the intestinal tract, the ammonium ion is metabolized and the patient has an excess of the fixed acid chloride ion. The load of chloride exceeds the capacity of the kidney's first two mechanisms for excreting acid, so that large amounts of sodium are carried out by the chloride ion. Water excretion rises parallel with sodium excretion, and the edema fluid is removed.

The *mechanism of action of the mercurial diuretic* drugs is also to cause a loss of sodium chloride. The effect of the drug is to inhibit temporarily the reabsorptive function of the renal tubular cells so that large amounts of the glomerular filtrate are lost in the urine. The mercurial drug inhibits specifically the reabsorption of the chloride ion. Thus the administration of chloride in the form of ammonium chloride augments the mercurial diuresis by increased obligatory chloride excretion. Conversely it is thought that refractoriness to mercurial diuretics is sometimes due to low chloride concentrations in the body fluids.

Besides the concentration test, the determination of blood urea concentration, of phenolsulfonphthalein (PSP) excretion and of the urea clearance is useful in estimating renal function. Other renal function tests using mannitol, inulin, Diodrast or para-aminohippuric acid for clearance determinations have been devised in recent years. These clearance determinations have yielded much basic information concerning the circulatory pattern of the kidney in health and diseases, but as routine tests are too tedious and technically difficult. Mannitol or inulin clearance is used to measure glomerular filtration rate, and Diodrast or para-aminohippuric acid clearance to measure renal blood flow.

The *blood urea concentration* is primarily governed by the rate of excretion of urea by the kidney and is a valuable index of renal function. The normal blood urea concentration is from 8 to 20 mg. per cent. An elevation or a change in blood urea is not always due to changes in kidney function. A low protein diet or the storage of protein in tissues will lower, whereas a high protein diet or breakdown of tissues will elevate, the blood urea. The rate of excretion of urea is influenced by the urine volume. A high urine volume increases the rate of excretion of urea and lowers the blood concentration, whereas a low urine volume decreases urea excretion and increases blood concentration. The finding of a high blood urea concentration in the presence of a normal or low intake of protein and with a normal or high urine volume means abnormally low renal function. In the presence of cardiac failure or circulatory insufficiency, a moderate elevation of blood urea may occur which is not due to intrinsic renal damage, but to inadequate blood flow to the kidney.

The nonprotein nitrogen (NPN) concentration of the blood is frequently used instead of the blood urea nitrogen (BUN) concentration as a test of renal function. In renal insufficiency the elevation of nonprotein nitrogen is due principally to a retention of urea. The normal blood nonprotein nitrogen concentration is from 20 to 35 mg. per cent. Other nonprotein nitrogenous substances in blood, such as creatinine, uric acid and amino acids, may also be elevated in renal insufficiency, but they represent a relatively small part of the increase in nonprotein nitrogen.

The restriction of protein intake will reduce the blood urea concentration. Changes in the blood urea are good criteria by which to regulate protein intake. Sometimes the blood urea will rise sharply after an episode of fever or intercurrent infection in a patient with renal insufficiency due to breakdown of body proteins.

Determination of urea clearance is a common and useful test of renal function. An explanation of the significance and interpretation of the urea clearance is best approached by comparison with the inulin clearance, which measures specifically one phase of renal function, the glomerular filtration rate. Inulin is an inert injectable carbohydrate which is freely diffusible through the glomerular capillaries and is not reabsorbed or secreted by the renal tubules. These facts allow the use of inulin clearance to measure glomerular filtration rate. For example, suppose the plasma concentration of inulin were 1 mg. per cubic centimeter, and 100 mg. were excreted in each minute. The conclusion would be that 100 cc. of plasma per minute containing 1 mg. in each cubic centimeter had been filtered through the glomeruli in order to produce 100 mg. in the urine. This simplified calculation defines the concept of clearance. The clearance is the volume of plasma which contains the amount of the substance excreted per minute. In the specific case of inulin, the volume of plasma cleared is the volume which has been filtered through the glomeruli. The inulin clearance in the average normal man is 130 cc. of plasma per minute. Inulin clearance is constant under basal conditions and does not vary with urine volume, since the renal tubules can reabsorb more or less water independently of the amount of inulin excreted.

Urea is also a substance which is freely diffusible like inulin. But when the urea and inulin clearances are determined simultaneously, the urea clearance is always lower than the inulin clearance. Also, the urea clearance is not constant with varying urine flow. The urea clearance is lower than the filtration rate because part of the urea is reabsorbed through the renal tubules with water and does not escape in the urine.

Since the clearance of urea varies with water excretion, there must be correction for the effect of unequal urine flows if the test is to be comparable in different patients and in the same patient at different times. The relationship of urea clearance to urine flow is such that when the urine flow is above 2 cc. per minute, the clearance is *maximal* and nearly constant. As the urine flow falls below 2 cc. per minute, the clearance diminishes in proportion to the square root of the urine flow. By use of the square root relationship, the clearance may be made comparable in patients with urine flows below 2 cc. per minute. This is called the *"standard"* clearance.

It is wise to avoid the use of the *"standard"* urea clearance calculation if possible. The correction for urine flow by using the square root relationship is only an approximation and may not be accurate at low urine flows. The division between maximal and standard clearances by the value for urine flow of 2 cc. per minute is rather arbitrary. A more important objection to the use of "standard" clearances is that greater errors of urine collection are likely to be made when small volumes are voided. If possible, the patient should be given enough fluids to maintain the urine flows above 2 cc. per minute.

If the urea clearance calculations from two consecutive one-hour collection periods do not agree within 10 per cent, the error in the performance of the test is usually caused by incomplete emptying of the bladder. Collection of urine by catheterization will avoid such errors, but is not a justifiable routine procedure.

The normal maximal urea clearance for an average-sized adult is 75 cc. per minute; the standard clearance, 54 cc. per minute. The range of normal variation is large even when correction is made for variation in body size. A maximal clearance below 55 cc. per minute, or 75 per cent of normal, is considered abnormally low in a young person. In older people, particularly those above the age of 60 years, the maximal clearance may be reduced to 45 cc. per minute, or 60 per cent of the average normal.

Over long periods of time the urea clearance is the most important factor governing the blood urea concentration. When other factors such as protein intake and urine flow are adequate and fairly stable, the blood urea concentration increases as the urea clearance decreases. As a general rule, when the urea clearance falls to 50 per cent of normal the blood urea is always above the normal range, but is usually not higher than twice normal until the clearance is depressed to 30 per cent. Below 30 per cent renal function the blood urea rises more precipitously to levels of three to ten times the normal value.

The *test of renal function by determining the amount of phenolsulfonphthalein ex-*

creted after injection is frequently used. Phenolsulfonphthalein is a foreign dye which is excreted by renal tubular secretion. Less than 10 per cent of the phenolsulfonphthalein in urine is excreted by glomerular filtration, because most of the dye is loosely combined with serum albumin and therefore cannot pass the glomerular capillary membrane. It is easily measured in the urine by comparing the red color of diluted alkalinized urine with standard solutions.

The principal factor governing the amount of phenolsulfonphthalein excreted is the amount of functioning tubular tissue. Other factors may cause variation in excretion. Diminished blood flow to the kidney will lower excretion by reducing the rate of delivery of the dye to the tubules, as in congestive cardiac failure or states of peripheral circulatory insufficiency. If the dye is administered intramuscularly, delayed absorption may retard excretion. The dye is best given intravenously. In diseases producing low serum albumin concentration, unusually high excretion of phenolsulfonphthalein may occur, owing possibly to less dye being bound to albumin and therefore more available to the secreting renal cells. A significant fraction of the phenolsulfonphthalein injected is removed by the liver. In some cases of cirrhosis of the liver the phenolsulfonphthalein in excretion is unusually high, probably because of less uptake by the damaged liver.

After intravenous injection there is a period of time required for the first dye to appear in the urine. Since the circulation from the vein to the renal artery requires only a fraction of a minute, the 'appearance time' is almost entirely the time required for the dye to travel from the renal tubules through the calyces, renal pelvis and ureters to the bladder. The faster the urine flow, the more rapid the appearance. With normal kidney function, a normal urinary tract and a moderate urine flow, the appearance time is 3 to 4 minutes after injection. However, a slow urine flow or especially a dilatation of the urinary tract will delay the appearance time for as long as 10 to 15 minutes. Best results are obtained if the urine output is kept high by hydrating the patient before the test to minimize delay in appearance and also to increase the accuracy of the urine collection. When the urine volume is small, it is difficult to obtain complete and prompt voluntary emptying of the bladder.

In order to judge if the urine flow is adequate or if there is any error in collection, the volume of each specimen should be recorded as well as the dye content.

The urine is collected for 2 hours after injection of the dye, and the normal excretion is at least 70 per cent of the amount injected. As with the urea clearance test, there is a wide range of normal variation, and older people normally may not excrete more than 60 per cent in 2 hours.

The collection and analysis of fractional specimens during the 2 hours is of some aid in interpreting the test. Normally, the majority of the total 2-hour output is excreted in the first half hour, and each successive fractional period contains much less dye than the previous one. When renal function is diminished, as in Bright's disease, the amount of dye in each period is more nearly equal. In cases of severe functional damage the rate of excretion is nearly constant, and the total for 2 hours may not exceed 10 per cent of the amount injected. The finding in a later period of a larger quantity of dye than in an earlier period indicates either inaccuracy in collection of urine by failure to empty the bladder, or delay in passage of the dye from the kidney to the bladder. Such a delay is found in cases of hydronephrosis, or when there is a large residual urine volume in the bladder. Collection of the urine by inlying catheter is sometimes necessary in order to obtain accurate results.

The phenolsulfonphthalein test is valuable for determining the function of each kidney separately by collecting the urine from the upper urinary tracts with inlying ureteral catheters. That a diminution of total renal function may be due to unilateral disease must always be considered. Unilateral loss of *renal function may also be revealed by the use of intravenous pyelography.* The radiopaque substances injected for pyelography are secreted rapidly like phenolsulfonphthalein by the renal tubular cells. Normally, enough radiopaque material is secreted to outline the urinary tract in the x-ray film. Absence of dye concentration unilaterally in the roentgenogram in a patient with slightly or moderately reduced phenolsulfonphthalein excretion indicates a nonfunctioning kidney.

A patient with one completely nonfunctioning kidney may have only slight reduction in total function because of compensatory hypertrophy of the normal kidney. If there is bilateral renal damage, as in Bright's disease, the secretion of radiopaque substance is not likely to be sufficient to show by roentgenogram if the total two-hour phenolsulfonphthalein excretion is less than 30 per cent, and particularly if, in addition, the urine specific gravity fails to rise above 1.012 during a concentration test.

Because of the many factors which normally cause variation in the blood urea, and the wide range of variation of the normal urea clearance and phenolsulfonphthalein excretion, these tests of renal function are less useful for detecting mild degrees of renal damage than for following changes in the renal function in one patient by repeated observations. In Bright's disease there may be definite impairment of concentrating power and abnormalities of salt and water balance and composition of body fluid, although the urea clearance and phenolsulfonphthalein excretion are only slightly or doubtfully diminished. In some cases of the nephrotic type of nephritis with marked edema the urea clearance and phenolsulfonphthalein excretion may show supernormal values. In most instances the presence of albumin in the urine is the earliest sign of impaired renal function.

By repeated observations of the blood urea or nonprotein nitrogen concentration, as well as of the clearance tests and the phenolsulfonphthalein excretion, the progress of the disease may be followed and the effect of therapy evaluated. In cases of marked renal insufficiency other abnormalities are found in the composition of blood. The serum phosphate concentration rises and the calcium falls. The serum potassium may rise to levels which produce cardiac and peripheral muscular weakness. Acidosis will be revealed by a lowered carbon dioxide-combining power of the blood.

ELLIOT V. NEWMAN

References

Berliner, R. W., Kennedy, T. J., Jr., and Orloff, J.: Relationship Between Acidification of the Urine and Potassium Metabolism. Am. J. Med., *11*:274, 1951.

Bradley S. E.: Medical Progress; Modern Concepts of Renal Structure and Function in Chronic Bright's Disease. New England J. Med., *231*:421, 452, 1944.

Gamble, J. L.: Chemical Anatomy, Physiology and Pathology of Extracellular Fluid. Cambridge, Harvard University Press, 1947.

Peters, J. P.: Body Water; the Exchange of Fluids in Man. Springfield, Ill., Charles C Thomas, 1935.

Shannon, V. A.: The Excretion of Phenol Red by the Dog. Am. J. Physiol., *113*:602, 1935.

Smith, H. W.: The Kidney, Structure and Function in Health and Disease. New York, Oxford University Press, 1951.

Van Slyke, D. D.: Renal Mechanisms Controlling Composition of Body Fluids. Chem. Rev., *26*:105, 1940.

———: The Effect of Urine Volume on Urea Excretion, *26*:1159, 1947.

URINARY SUPPRESSION

Definition. Urinary suppression is the complete (anuria) or partial (oliguria) failure of the kidneys to excrete water and normal urinary solutes.

Physiologic Considerations. The normal person excretes in the urine any excess of ingested water above his losses of water through lungs, skin and gastrointestinal tract. If no excess of water is available, the kidneys excrete the minimal volume of urine in which can be concentrated the necessary excretory products. Butler and Gamble found that a healthy young man, fasting and without water intake, was obliged to excrete at least 500 cc. of water per day in the urine and a liter through skin and lungs. The feeding of glucose would theoretically further lower the volume by reducing the quantity of solutes to be excreted, but such a situation is not likely to be met with in practice. From a practical standpoint, a daily urine volume less than 1 liter is undesirable, while suppression of urine may be said to be present when less than 500 cc. is excreted in a day by an average adult.

Etiology. 1. Dehydration, loss of plasma or blood and circulatory collapse are followed by reduction or cessation of urine flow, by impairment of kidney function and, if allowed to persist in a severe form for some hours, by serious renal injury.

2. Shock associated with trauma, burns, infection and other causes of tissue necrosis is likely to be followed by acute renal tubular injury with oliguria. Anesthesia and surgical procedures may be precipitating factors in seriously ill patients. Obstetric complications (septic abortion, premature separation of the placenta, toxemias, postpartum hemorrhage) may be followed by acute renal tubular injury, and rarely by bilateral cortical necrosis of the kidneys.

3. Transfusion reaction and other causes

of rapid intravascular hemolysis are important causes of serious renal injury with urinary suppression.

4. Poisoning and allergic reactions due to drugs (especially the sulfonamides), metallic and industrial poisons, especially mercury and carbon tetrachloride, and other irritants make up another important group.

5. Acute glomerulonephritis is sometimes followed by a fall in urinary output and occasionally causes a serious and prolonged suppression of urine.

6. Other forms of acute renal injury may be followed by oliguria or anuria. Among these may be mentioned acute, ascending pyelonephritis, sometimes leading to necrotizing papillitis in patients with diabetes or urinary tract obstruction; acute, diffuse, arteriolar inflammation or necrosis (e.g., periarteritis nodosa); embolism or thrombosis of the renal arteries or veins; and the "hepatorenal syndrome" of patients with severe hepatic insufficiency.

7. Absence or loss of virtually all functional renal tissue is seen in congenital malformation, in the last stages of chronic renal disease, and rarely after removal of a diseased kidney without assurance of adequate remaining renal tissue.

8. Reflex anuria may follow trauma, stone or instrumentation of the urinary tract.

9. Obstruction of both ureters or renal pelves is occasionally encountered because of crystallization of sulfonamides from the urine. It may also be caused by malformations, multiple calculi, carcinomatous invasion or surgical injury.

10. A moderate, persistent oliguria is frequently noted during the rapid accumulation of edema in severe heart failure or in the nephrotic syndrome.

Pathologic Anatomy and Physiology of Acute Tubular Necrosis. Oliver's dissections of nephrons have demonstrated the presence of two types of anatomic lesion. Changes characteristic of the specific disease or toxic agent may be present. In many forms of acute renal failure of various etiology, ischemia is thought to be responsible for the bloodless glomeruli and the focal necrosis which may involve any segment of the tubule. Regeneration of tubular epithelium proceeds rapidly in the days following the injury, but the cells regain a normal appearance only after several weeks. Restoration of function may be impaired by obstruction of tubules by debris and proliferating epithelium.

During the oliguric phase, physiologic measurements suggest a marked reduction in renal blood flow and tubular function, with back-diffusion from the glomerular filtrate in the damaged tubules. The urine resembles an ultrafiltrate of plasma in electrolyte content and in the poor concentration of waste products. Specific gravity is fixed near 1.010, and variable amounts of protein, red blood cells and other abnormal formed elements may appear.

The consequences of suppression of urine depend (1) on water balance and (2) on the accumulation of metabolites in the body. Water intake in excess of losses leads to edema, hypertension, cardiac failure or signs of water intoxication. Injudicious administration of parenteral fluid is usually responsible. The quantity of solute excreted in the small volume of dilute urine is so small that azotemia develops at a rate proportional to tissue breakdown and protein metabolism.

One distinctive penalty of suppression of urine is the accumulation of potassium in the extracellular fluid. Potassium is present in most natural foodstuffs and is released from the cells during starvation. If this excess cannot be excreted in the urine, the potassium concentration of the extracellular fluid rises to abnormally high levels (8 to 12 mEq. per liter) with consequent muscular paralysis and cardiac failure. Bywaters pointed out that this picture is especially likely to develop in the crush syndrome, when large quantities of potassium are relased from injured and ischemic muscle. Specific measures are necessary to avoid or to control potassium intoxication.

At the end of one to two weeks, urine begins to appear in gradually increasing amounts. The first urine secreted reflects the impaired tubular function in its dilute, neutral character. Little effect on the azotemia is evident until the volume reaches 1 or 2 liters per day, when the concentrations of urea and all the other waste products in the blood fall rapidly. Even after a profuse urinary flow appears and good excretory function is established, the kidneys may still fail in their important functions of regulating hydration and total base concentration. After another week or two, these functions usually are regained. In the course of weeks or months, all measurable renal functions usually return to normal.

Clinical Picture. The patient may offer no complaints during the first days of acute renal failure. In patients who are seriously ill after injury, operation or infection, a record of urinary output should be kept in order to detect urinary suppression, which may be the only early sign of serious renal involvement. In the *crush syndrome,* for example, local injuries and vascular collapse command immediate attention, while an equally dangerous suppression of urine may not become apparent for some time. *Retention of urine* may be distinguished by palpation or by catheterization of the bladder. *Injury or rupture of the urinary passages* must be considered if urine does not appear after trauma.

In another group of patients, for example, in *sulfonamide nephrosis,* once the initial reaction or intoxication is past, the patient may feel quite well for a number of days. At first there are no disturbing symptoms, although the daily rise in the concentration of blood urea, creatinine, phosphate and all the other wastes goes on. The patient may complain of lumbar aching or of burning about the bladder. There may be some puffiness about the eyes, and the blood pressure may rise slightly above normal. Finally, full-blown signs of azotemia appear. Muscular twitching, confusion, stupor, convulsions and even pericarditis may be seen. The rapidity of development of this picture varies greatly.

Potassium intoxication may appear at any time after the first week of urinary suppression, or may be precipitated earlier by the administration of potassium salts or by the liberation of large amounts of potassium from injured muscle, hemolysis or other sources. When the serum potassium concentration exceeds 7 to 8 mEq. per liter, characteristic electrocardiographic changes begin to appear. As the serum potassium rises, the T wave becomes high and peaked, the QRS complex becomes broad and slurred, the P wave disappears, bradycardia and arrhythmia may appear, and, finally, at high potassium concentrations, the complexes resemble those of ventricular tachycardia or fibrillation. Cardiac failure with temporary dilatation and systolic murmurs has been described, or extreme bradycardia with circulatory collapse may be the terminal event. Flaccid muscular paralysis may occur when the serum potassium reaches 8 to 12 mEq. per liter.

The *early diuretic phase* usually begins during the second week after the renal injury. The volume of urine increases daily. Little clinical improvement can be expected until the urine volume has been maintained above 1 or 2 liters for several days. Abnormalities in hydration and in concentration of electrolytes in the serum may appear at this time, owing to deficiencies of renal tubular function. Disturbances of cardiac action, peripheral circulation, cerebral function or neuromuscular conduction appear if dehydration, sodium depletion or excess, or potassium depletion are allowed to become extreme.

Prognosis. The duration of suppression of urine is variable, lasting from a few hours to seven weeks. Diuresis occurs most commonly either immediately after rehydration and treatment of shock or after a delay of one to two weeks.

Between 60 and 85 per cent of patients with acute renal failure survive on conservative management. A fatal outcome may be the result of coexistent disease.

Infection and other factors favoring protein catabolism may greatly accelerate the onset of uremia, so that chemical abnormalities incompatible with life may occur within a few days of the onset.

It is probable that reasonable restraint in the administration of fluids will prevent the rapid development of cardiac failure which has frequently occurred in overhydrated patients.

Treatment. The first object of treatment is to minimize the extent of renal damage as far as possible. When dehydration or shock is a factor, *replacement of lost fluid and blood* is urgent. *British anti-lewisite* (BAL) may be helpful in mercury poisoning as late as 4 or 5 hours after ingestion, but is of limited value after anuria is established. *Alkalis* may be helpful in the early stages of transfusion reaction or sulfonamide precipitation, but serve only to produce alkalosis if renal insufficiency prevents their excretion.

In many cases, little or no urine is excreted despite restoration of the circulation to normal and despite the supply of an adequate quantity of fluid and electrolytes for proper hydration. It is then advisable to *limit total fluid intake to 1 liter per day,* plus any estimated excess due to profuse sweating, vomiting, diarrhea or other loss. Excessive quantities of fluid have been given frequently in the past without appreciable effect on urine volume. The seriously injured kidney fails to respond to overhydration or diuretics, which can do nothing but harm. Many deaths during the first week of anuria are attributable to heart failure following persistent overhydration.

In order to minimize protein catabolism, *glucose* is added in 20 to 40 per cent concentration to the liter of fluid. If this solution is administered very slowly into a large vein, venous thrombosis can usually be avoided. Water-soluble vitamins should be given parenterally.

If the patient desires to take the prescribed water by mouth, and if he is able to retain and absorb it, there is no objection. As long as the stomach will retain carbohydrate in the form of sweets, they may be given at will. Since potassium intake is presumably undesirable, most natural foodstuffs are eliminated unless specially prepared. Fruit juices contain considerable amounts of potassium.

Administration of *sodium chloride or lactate* should be used only if absolutely necessary: for example, to replace continuous loss of gastric or intestinal fluid. Moderate reduction of the serum sodium level or CO_2 content does not require treatment. Anemia and hypoproteinemia are usually less of a hazard than the possibility of pulmonary edema after transfusion.

Since infection is a serious complication in the azotemic patient, the prophylactic use of an antibiotic has been suggested. After the usual initial dosage, the frequency of administration should be reduced to avoid unnecessarily high blood levels in the absence of renal excretion.

Digitalis should be given at the first evidence of cardiac enlargement or pulmonary congestion.

Three methods to serve as emergency substitutes for functioning renal tissue are being studied:

1. In the "artificial kidney" heparinized blood runs from an artery through cellophane tubing, where it is dialyzed against a bath of approximately the electrolytic composition of normal extracellular fluid. Glucose is added to the bath to balance the osmotic pressure of the blood proteins, and calcium salts are replaced by separate injections, since they are not soluble in the usual dialyzing fluid. The blood is reinjected after dialysis and the elimination of clots and bubbles. Several types have proved to be effective dialyzers, eliminating moderate amounts of urea and other wastes from the body, with temporary symptomatic improvement. Disadvantages are the technical complexity requiring a trained team, and the necessity for heparinization with risk of bleeding, especially in postoperative cases.

2. In *"peritoneal lavage"* the peritoneum is perfused between two incisions with a solution similar to that used in the bath of the artificial kidney. Large volumes of sterile solution must be prepared, to which the sodium bicarbonate and antibiotics are added after sterilization. Dialysis is temporarily effective in removing waste products and in restoring a normal electrolytic balance. After continuous dialysis for a day or two, effectiveness decreases, peritonitis becomes more likely, and colic or meteorism may occur.

3. *Intestinal irrigation* is an attractive method because of apparently greater safety, but is technically difficult and generally less effective. The irrigation may be conducted between intestinal tubes (e.g., Miller-Abbott) or enterostomies. The upper intestine appears to be the most efficient site for exchange. In an effort to prevent excessive absorption, magnesium salts are usually added to the fluid. Effectiveness has been limited by technical difficulties in most reported cases. It seems possible to eliminate potassium by this route, even though the effects on azotemia are not impressive.

None of these methods have as yet been proved to affect the ultimate outcome of acute renal insufficiency. At the present writing it would seem best to treat patients conservatively unless some pressing indication exists.

Potassium intoxication may be prevented in most cases by the avoidance of exogenous potassium, by the daily administration of glucose in dosage sufficient to minimize endogenous release of potassium, and by the administration of a cation-exchange resin in the sodium and ammonium form (50 gm. of potassium-free resin daily in divided doses by mouth or in retention enemas given as soon as the serum potassium rises above 6 mEq. liter). The development of clinical evidences of potassium intoxication in spite of this regimen may be considered an indication for dialysis by one of the three methods described above. Medical countermeasures, such as the intravenous injection of solutions containing sodium chloride, calcium salts, or glucose and insulin, offer only temporary relief.

During the *early diuretic phase,* fluid administration should be increased to match the urine volume, with due regard for the state of hydration. Measurement of the concentration of sodium (or chloride) and potassium in the urine is valuable in estimating the quantity of electrolyte to be replaced and in avoiding marked deviations of the volume and composition of extracellular fluid. The replacement solution should contain some sodium lactate as well as sodium chloride, potassium chloride and glucose. Determinations of serum levels of sodium, potassium and bicarbonate serve as a measure of the adequacy of replacement. Although this program may seem elaborate, experience has indicated that many patients develop dangerous dehydration and hypochloremia unless accurate control is maintained, while other patients show hyperchloremia or potassium depletion.

When diuresis has been established for five to ten days, the patient is usually able to take increasing amounts of fluid and food by mouth, and intravenous therapy can be gradually eliminated. A high fluid intake and a high calorie, low protein diet should be given until renal function returns to a satisfactory level. Good general care and reasonable restriction of activity are advisable during this period. Although demonstrable impairment of renal function may persist for many months or years, a functional level compatible with normal life and activity is usually reached within a month after diuresis begins.

JOHN A. LUETSCHER, JR.

References

Bull, G. M., Joekes, A. M., and Lowe, K. G.: Renal Function Studies in Acute Tubular Necrosis. Clin. Sci., 9:379, 1950.

Bywaters, E. G. L.: Ischemic Muscle Necrosis: Crushing Injury, Traumatic Edema, the Crush Syndrome, Traumatic Anuria, Compression Syndrome: A Type of Injury Seen in Air Raid Casualties following Burial beneath Debris. J.A.M.A., 124:1103, 1944.

Finch, C. A., Sawyer, C. G., and Flynn, J. M.: Clinical Syndrome of Potassium Intoxication. Am. J. Med., 1:337, 1946.

Gamble, J. L.: Physiological Information Gained from Studies on the Life Raft Ration. The Harvey Lectures, 1946–47. Lancaster, Pa., The Science Press, 1947, p. 247.

Lowe, K. G.: The Late Prognosis in Acute Tubular Necrosis: an Interim Follow-up Report on 14 Patients. Lancet, 1:1086, 1952.

Merrill, J. P.: The Use of the Artificial Kidney in the Treatment of Uremia. Bull. New York Acad. Med., 28:523, 1952.

Oliver, J.: Correlations of Structure and Function and Mechanisms of Recovery in Acute Tubular Necrosis. Am. J. Med., 15:535, 1953.

Stock, R. J.: The Conservative Management of Acute Urinary Suppression. Bull. New York Acad. Med., 28:507, 1952.

NON-PARASITIC CHYLURIA

Definition. Chyluria denotes the passage of chyle in the urine. Chylous urine contains large amounts of albumin and fat, and may be translucent, milky or the consistency of thick cream.

Etiology. Chyluria results from obstruction in the lymphatics between the intestine and thoracic duct with retrograde dilatation of retroperitoneal and pelvic channels, insufficiency of the lymphatic valves and finally rupture into some part of the urinary tract. The most usual site of rupture is probably into the renal pelvis, at the fornix calyces, the site of "pyelolymphatic backflow" occasionally seen in retrograde pyelograms. Increased intrapyelocalyceal tension due to faulty urinary drainage may be a contributing factor. In a few cases a fistula has been demonstrated between dilated lymphatics and the bladder or posterior urethra. The commonest cause of lymphatic obstruction causing chyluria is, of course, the reaction produced by the filarial worm, W. bancrofti. It cannot be excluded in any patient who has ever been in an endemic area, for symptoms may not develop for some years after exposure, when no microfilariae can be demonstrated in the blood, and when even the adults have died. Other conditions which produce strangulation of important lymph channels are infiltrating growths and infections, especially tuberculosis, occasionally pregnancy and rarely trauma.

Symptoms. The only constant symptom is the passage of milky urine. The onset is usually sudden. The chyluria may be intermittent, or it may persist for years without materially compromising the health of the patient. The loss of chyle is rarely sufficient to interfere with nutrition of itself. Admixture with blood gives the urine a pink color. The amount of chyle in the urine is increased by exercise and by a high fat diet. Renal function is not impaired. Other symptoms present are due to the underlying disease. The urine often forms a semisolid gel on standing. Microscopically, chylous urine does not show fat droplets, and the fat cannot be removed by centrifugation, but is extracted by ether. Chyluria must be differentiated from severe pyuria and lipuria. In the former pus cells are seen under the microscope, in the latter fat droplets or crystals.

Treatment is largely unsatisfactory. A low fat diet will diminish the amount of chyle in the urine. Treatment should be directed primarily to the underlying condition.

J. M. HAYMAN, JR.

References

Kutzmann, A. A.: Non-parasitic Chyluria. Ann. Surg., 82:765, 1925.
Lazarus, J. A., and Marks, M. S.: Non-parasitic Chyluria with Special Reference to Traumatic Chyluria. J. Urol., 56:246, 1946.

PNEUMATURIA

Definition. Pneumaturia is the passage of urine containing air or gas.

Etiology. Pneumaturia may occur following injection of air into the bladder for diagnostic purposes, as a result of a vesico-vaginal or vesico-intestinal fistula, or from the presence of gas-forming bacteria in the bladder or urinary tract. The organisms most commonly involved are the colon bacillus, *B. lactis aerogenes, B. aerogenes capsulatus* and yeast. Infection of the bladder mucosa with gas-forming organisms may lead to the formation of small blebs, ranging in size from 1 to 3 mm. in diameter, giving the bladder a silvery appearance at cystoscopy, and releasing gas into the bladder on rupture. Half of the 36 reported cases of primary pneumaturia occurred in diabetics. The gas is alway carbon dioxide. Urinary retention has been considered an etiologic factor in almost all cases; it may be due to a cord bladder, diverticula, cystocele, prostatic enlargement or stricture. Pneumaturia has been reported about twice as frequently in women as in men, and is more common after the age of 50.

Symptoms. There are no symptoms due to pneumaturia itself. Those present are due to the underlying infection or other structural change. The gas is passed at the end of voiding, but the patient is not always aware of the passage of gas from the bladder. Its presence is often first detected by catheterization or by x-ray. A round or piriform gas shadow in the suprapubic region which does not resemble gas in a distended rectosigmoid should suggest pneumaturia. Gas in the bladder as a result of fistulas is usually accompanied by some fecal material, or the leakage of urine into the vagina or colon. The diagnosis is confirmed by cystoscopy or the injection of a dye into the bladder.

The treatment of pneumaturia is that of the underlying fistula, and of the obstruction and infection. The control of diabetes mellitus, if present, is essential.

J. M. HAYMAN, JR.

References

Arthur, L. M., and Johnson, H. W.: Pneumaturia: Case Report and Review of the Literature. J. Urol., 60:659, 1948.
Fineman, S., Ferber, W. L., and Roginsky, D. N.: Primary Pneumaturia, with a Report of Two Cases. Radiology, 59:63, 1952.

PORPHYRINURIA

Please refer to the chapter on Porphyria.

HEMOGLOBINURIA AND MYOHEMOGLOBINURIA

HEMOGLOBINURIA

Definition. Hemoglobinuria is the appearance of free hemoglobin in the urine and is a sign that red cells have been hemolyzed abnormally in one of three places, namely, in the urine, in the kidney or in the blood stream. Hemoglobinuria itself is not a disease but a sign of a variety of pathologic processes or disease entities which all result in the liberation of free hemoglobin that gains access to the urine. The color of hemoglobin attracts attention, may be confused with other pigments in the urine and is frequently associated with morbid processes of grave prognosis. From the single observation of hemoglobinuria, it may not be possible, without other information, to determine its cause. The mechanisms and diseases resulting in abnormal hemolysis and hemoglobinuria can be classified by the anatomic site of hemolysis and in some instances by the process causing hemolysis.

Hemoglobinuria from Hemolysis of Red Cells in the Urinary Outflow Tract. Rarely, hemoglobinuria occurs from the osmotic rupture of red cells that have been excreted into a urine that is hypotonic with a specific gravity of 1.006 or less. The combination of prolonged hematuria and chronic low specific gravity of the urine produces hemolysis of red cells and the liberation of hemoglobin in the urinary outflow tract, and may occur in such a condition as the lower nephron nephritis complicating therapy with certain of the sulfonamide drugs. In this syndrome, red cells may be detected in the urine if centrifuged promptly but they may also be absent because of hemolysis. Since the hemoglobin has been released in the urinary tract, there is no free hemoglobin in the plasma and no hemosiderinuria.

Hemoglobinuria in Infarction of the Kidney. Hemoglobinuria may occur in infarction of the kidney, and may be unilateral in origin if only one kidney is affected. In this condition it is presumed that hemolysis occurs in the infarcted area of the renal parenchyma so that hemoglobin gains access to the urine from the local lesion.

Hemoglobinuria from Intravascular Hemolysis of Red Cells. If hemoglobin is released into the blood stream by the hemolysis of red cells from any cause, or by the experimental infusion of a solution of hemoglobin, a series of events occur that are reproducible and may aid diagnosis. Hemoglobin in the plasma causes a color varying from faint pink to deep red depending on the concentration, which can be measured quantitatively by the benzidine reaction. There is some increase in the indirect-acting plasma bilirubin. Some of the hemoglobin is converted to methemalbumin which appears in the plasma but does not pass into the urine. Methemalbumin (not to be confused with methemoglobin) is a combination of the heme portion of the hemoglobin with the albumin of serum, is golden to brown in color, reacts with benzidine and is distinguishable spectroscopically from the several forms of hemoglobin and from other heme or pyrrol pigments. The occurrence of methemalbumin in plasma or serum, even in the absence of demonstrable hemoglobin, and many hours after a suspected hemolytic episode, is pathognomonic for intravascular hemolysis.

Hemoglobin is passed from the plasma into the nephron in spite of its large molecular weight of 68,000, appearing in the urine roughly as a threshold substance when the hemoglobinemia reaches approximately 50 to 130 mg. per 100 cc. or more of free hemoglobin in the plasma, depending on preexisting hemoglobinuria or albuminuria. The color

of the urine will vary from pink to deep red with oxyhemoglobin, from purple to black with reduced hemoglobin, from light tan to dark brown with methemoglobin. Hemoglobin may be excreted in the urine in varying amounts for years in certain chronic hemolytic anemias, in extreme amounts in instances of hemolytic reactions in disease or in hemolytic transfusion reactions. The passage of hemoglobin by the kidney is accompanied and followed by albuminuria, hemosiderinuria, by hemoglobin casts and by precipitates of hemoglobin. The tubular epithelium of the kidney converts hemoglobin to hemosiderin as a continuing process, and some of the hemosiderin is excreted into the urine. Renal shutdown and lower nephron nephrosis occur in some but not in all instances of acute intravascular hemolysis and hemoglobinuria. Chronic intermittent hemoglobinuria can be tolerated by the kidney for years, as in paroxysmal nocturnal hemoglobinuria.

EXAMPLES OF HEMOGLOBINURIA FROM INTRAVASCULAR HEMOLYSIS

Exercise-March Hemoglobinuria. Transient hemoglobinemia, sometimes accompanied by hemoglobinuria, occurs in normal men with considerable frequency after strenuous runs. This intravascular hemolysis is comparable in its benign nature to the albuminuria of exercise. In march hemoglobinuria, the occurrence of hemoglobin in the urine is always associated with hemoglobinemia and with moderate increase in plasma bilirubin (indirect-acting). In this syndrome, exercise such as walking or running in the lordotic position produces intravascular hemolysis and hemoglobinuria but exercise in the kyphotic position does not. There is no anemia and the condition is benign. The mechanism of the hemolysis in exercise is not known and is not associated with myohemoglobinuria.

Intravenous Distilled Water Hemoglobinemia Accompanying Transurethral Resection of the Prostate. It has been established that the intravenous injection of from 600 to 900 ml. of distilled water causes hemoglobinemia and hemoglobinuria, presumably from osmotic rupture of red cells intravascularly in plasma which has been rendered hypotonic. This mechanism probably explains the intravascular hemolysis and hemoglobinemia reported in transurethral resection of the prostate in which distilled water was used for irrigation of the bladder and was shown to gain access to the blood stream, presumably through veins injured in the operation.

Defects in Red Cells. Acute hemoglobinemia and hemoglobinuria occur following thermal burns in which the red cells, injured by heat, are rendered spheroidal and increased in susceptibility to osmotic and mechanical fragility. In paroxysmal nocturnal hemoglobinuria, methemalbumin is present chronically in the plasma, associated with intermittent hemoglobinemia that may be greater during sleep. Hemosiderinuria is perpetual and hemoglobinuria is intermittent, frequently nocturnal, reflecting the level of plasma hemoglobin. In this disease the essential abnormality is an acquired defect in the red cells which are hemolyzed more readily at an acid pH in fresh serum from the patient or from normal subjects. Although many features of this disease have been described, the abnormality of the red cells and the requirements of serum in the hemolytic mechanism are not understood.

Hemolytic Agents. Intravascular hemolysis with episodes of hemoglobinuria occurs in paroxysmal cold hemoglobinuria in which a true hemolysis in the plasma causes hemolysis of red cells after chilling and rewarming. Infrequently, a true hemolysin, more effective at an acid pH, occurs in acquired hemolytic anemia and may be responsible for episodes of marked hemoglobinemia and hemoglobinuria. In some transfusion reactions, isohemolysins as well as isoagglutinins are demonstrable in instances of intravascular hemolysis. Certain venoms of spiders and snakes produce intravascular hemolysis and hemoglobinuria.

Agglutinins and Antibodies on Red Cells. In severe hemolytic transfusion reactions, marked intravascular hemolysis occurs, in the absence of demonstrable isohemolysins, with isoagglutinins including anti A, anti B, anti Rh and other immune isoagglutinins. Minor degrees of hemoglobinemia, hemoglobinuria and hemosiderinuria are described in acquired hemolytic anemia associated with demonstrable globulin on the red cell (Coombs test) and with an agglutinin in the plasma in some instances.

Chemical Agents. Hemoglobinuria occurs from arsine poisoning which produces extreme increase in the osmotic fragility of red cells. With certain sulfonamides, quinine, paraminophenol, hydroquinone and certain oxidant compounds, severe intravascular hemolysis has occurred with increase in osmotic fragility of red cells and marked hemolytic anemia.

Infections. Blackwater fever, a syndrome of extreme hemoglobinemia and hemoglobinuria in malaria, occurs in some instances with large infestations of the red cells by the plasmodium. In Oroya fever (Carrión's disease) hemoglobinuria occurs with marked infection of the red cell by the rickettsia-like organism, *Bartonella bacilliformis*.

Favism. Acute hemolytic anemia with hemoglobinuria may occur from ingestion of the fava or horse bean (*Vicia faba*) in susceptible patients.

MYOHEMOGLOBINURIA

Definition. Myohemoglobin, also called myoglobin, is a protein occurring in the muscle sarcoplasm, serving as a respiratory pigment. It constitutes about one quarter of the total hemoglobin of the body and has properties similar to those of blood hemoglobin. Both are combinations of protoporphyrin with iron, forming heme which is combined with a specific globulin. Both are intracellular proteins and should not be found free in plasma or urine. Hemoglobin of blood has a molecular weight of 68,000 and has four iron atoms per molecule, whereas myohemoglobin weighs 17,500 and has only one iron atom per molecule. Myohemoglobin apparently is not metabolized, as is blood hemoglobin in the normal destruction of red cells. However, myohemoglobin may be released under unusual circumstances from the muscle and appear free in the plasma. Methemalbumin and bilirubin have not been found in such instances. In studies on animals, myohemoglobin is cleared from the plasma at a low concentration and approximately twenty-five times more rapidly than is blood hemoglobin, presumably because of the smaller size of the myohemoglobin molecule. In the urine, myohemoglobin is indistinguishable in appearance from hemoglobin, occurs in pigment casts, as brown crystals resembling red cells, and is associated in some instances with the development of renal shutdown and lower nephron nephrosis as observed in hemoglobinuria. A patient subject to ischemic muscle necrosis from any cause, such as trauma, may appear in good condition at first but may develop the hypotension of shock, oligemia with edema of the traumatized muscle and later oliguria and anuria. Myohemoglobinemia and myohemoglobinuria are not associated with anemia or changes in blood hemoglobin.

Ischemic Muscle Necrosis: Crush Syndrome. Myohemoglobinuria may occur following crushing injury to muscle or soft compression of muscle for periods of 2 hours, as observed in air raid casualties following burial beneath debris, or following traffic, industrial, mining accidents or mob stampedes. On release of the pressure of the burial, myohemoglobin is released into the plasma and passed into the urine, frequently with the development of anuria or impairment of renal function.

Ischemic Muscle Necrosis: Injury or Thrombosis of a Main-Limb Artery. Myohemoglobinuria may follow trauma to a main-limb artery including rupture, spasm or obstruction of the vessel as a result of accidents. It may also be associated with nontraumatic thrombosis of the femoral artery, the muscle showing pathologic and chemical changes similar to those of crush injury.

Spontaneous Myohemoglobinuria. Spontaneous myohemoglobinuria, with the passage of brown or dark red urine, is extremely rare and is associated with symptoms related to the muscles. A benign form is described in which attacks of transient myohemoglobinuria could be induced by strain on the quadriceps muscles associated with pain and a short period of weakness. Another form of unknown origin, acute paralytic myohemoglobinuria, may be fatal with renal failure, or recovery may occur in spite of recurrent attacks. In this condition, there are episodes of passing dark urine in association with attacks of pain, hard swellings and paralysis of muscles, followed by atrophy and contracture. Because of the dark urine and pain, the condition may be confused with acute porphyria, or the renal failure with "bloody" urine may be mistaken for nephritis with hematuria. In one family, a boy 10 years of age had repeated attacks over a period of six years of muscular pain and inability to walk, with myohemoglobinuria and creatinuria established during one episode. Progressive muscular dystrophy occurred in 8 male members of his family in three generations. The syndrome of acute paralytic myohemoglobinuria with renal fail-

ure occurs in horses that are subjected to strenuous exercise following a rest period.

Haff Disease: Myohemoglobinuria Associated With Poisoning. The ingestion of fish poisoned with resinous acids from the industrial wastes of cellulose factories has occurred in the bay area (Haff) of Königsberg, Germany, and has been associated with paroxysmal attacks of pain, stiffness and paralysis of muscles with myohemoglobinuria and with renal failure in some instances. Skeletal muscles showed blanching.

Symptoms and Signs. If hemoglobin arises in the urinary outflow tract, no symptoms occur from the passage of this pigment in the urine. Intravascular hemolysis, if chronic and moderate in degree, as in paroxysmal nocturnal hemoglobinuria, may cause no symptoms except those of anemia. When the intravascular hemolysis is large in amount or acute, or following the injection of stroma-free hemoglobin, there may be no reaction or there may be varying degrees of symptoms such as chill, nausea, vomiting or pain in the loins. These symptoms and signs are masked by anesthesia so that a hemolytic transfusion reaction may escape detection unless the plasma or urine is observed. The first urine samples after a hemolytic episode may be "dark," "bloody" in appearance from the content of hemoglobin and may be followed after a few hours, in some instances, by oliguria or anuria which may continue for days. Since hemoglobinuria and myohemoglobinuria are signs rather than diseases, the symptoms and signs of the underlying illness must be sought. The symptoms and signs of myohemoglobinuria have been described as related to muscle injury.

Diagnosis. Hemoglobinuria may be overlooked by the patient and the physician if it is small in amount, or may be mistaken for hematuria and lead to examination of the urinary tract by cytoscopy. Since the color may be brown with methemoglobin or reddish brown with mixtures of oxyhemoglobin and methemoglobin, the urine may be suspected to contain bile, urobilin or porphyrin. Relatively simple screening tests are available to identify certain of the pigments in the urine, or to distinguish them from hemoglobin or myohemoglobin. The first tests are the centrifugation of a fresh sample of urine to detect the presence of red cells and to observe the specific gravity to determine whether it is enough (above 1.006) to prevent osmotic hemolysis of free cells in the urinary tract. The plasma may be examined for the presence of free hemoglobin or methemalbumin. See p. 1097 for method.

Hemoglobin and Myohemoglobin. The heme portions of hemoglobin and myohemoglobin are both detected by the color reactions with benzidine and guaiac. The amount of hemoglobin can be measured quantitatively by benzidine dihydrochloride. However, benzidine and guaiac do not react with non-iron-containing pyrrol compounds such as the porphyrins, the several forms of bilirubin and their derivatives. Hemoglobin and myohemoglobin are separated and identified only by refined spectroscopic methods, by locating the alpha band of absorption. This is a marked limitation in methodology. Clinically, however, intravascular hemolysis as a cause of hemoglobinuria is usually associated with hemolytic anemia, is characterized by hemoglobinemia, by variable icterus and by the presence of methemalbumin in the plasma for a period of a day or longer. Methemalbumin can be detected by the color reaction with benzidine dihydrochloride. Myohemoglobinemia is cleared rapidly by the kidney and is not associated with the formation of methemalbumin in the plasma, with icterus or with anemia.

Hemosiderin. Hemosiderin may appear as a brownish or brownish green precipitate in urine and is readily detected, since it forms jet black ferric sulfide particles with ammonium sulfide solution and gives the Prussian blue reaction with potassium ferrocyanide. Hemosiderinuria is usually a sign of hemolytic anemia, occurs regularly in instances of hemoglobinemia, but also occurs in occasional patients with hemochromatosis without anemia. It has not been described in myohemoglobinuria.

Bile in the Urine. The passage of bilirubin into the urine gives a brown to almost black appearance which may be confused with other pigments. The Harrison spot test for bilirubin is simple and specific.

Urobilinogen and Urobilin. Urobilinogen and urobilin, like bilirubin, are chains of four pyrrol nuclei from the opened ring of the protoporphyrin of hemoglobin. These derivatives are not formed from hemoglobin in the urine, but may be increased in some instances of increased intravascular hemolysis in which conversion of hemoglobins to bilirubin is increased. Urobilinogen is a colorless precursor of urobilin and reacts with Ehrlich's aldehyde reagent. Urobilin and stercobilin are oxidized from the urobilinogen forms and contribute to the yellow, amber and brownish color of urine and may be increased in hemolytic anemia. The urobilins are remarkably nonreactive, give a green fluorescence with alcoholic zinc acetate and may be reduced to the urobilinogen form for measurement.

Porphyrins, Porphobilinogen and Porphobilin. Any abnormal reddish color in the urine may be suspected to be porphyrins but porphyrinuria is rare. The porphyrins are ring compounds containing four pyrrol nuclei, are pink to red in high concentrations, but rarely appear in the urine in enough concentration to give it color. The porphyrin ring of hemoglobin is not excreted as such but is converted to bilirubin. The porphyrins are identified by extraction and spectroscopic analysis. Porphobilinogen is *not* a porphyrin, does not occur with hemoglobinuria or myohemoglobinuria, but does appear in variable amounts in the acute episodes of certain of the porphyrias. Porphobilinogen is a colorless monopyrrol which reacts with Ehrlich's aldehyde reagent and is distinguished from urobilinogen aldehyde which is soluble in chloroform, whereas porphobilinogen aldehyde is not. Porphobilinogen condenses in the urine to chains of four or more pyrrol rings, forming the pigment porphobilin which is not a porphyrin but a compound resembling urobilin. Porphobilin may be formed in the urinary tract or on standing in acid urine and, depending on the concentration, may appear pink, red, brown or black. Porphobilin, which may be confused with the heme pigments, is remarkably nonreactive, does not react with benzidine or guaiac, and is precipitated by alcoholic zinc acetate whereas urobilin gives fluorescence with it. In the porphyrias, whether or not there is accompanying porphobilinogen or porphobilin, there is no hemoglobinemia, hemoglobinuria or hemosiderinuria. There may be hemolytic anemia in some instances of photosensitive or congenital porphyria, an extremely rare condition.

Other Colors and Pigments. Following the ingestion of a large meal of beets, the vegetable pigment from the beet is excreted in the urine and appears as a red color that has been confused with hemoglobin. The beet pigment does not react with the reagents previously mentioned. Red color in urine may be given by phenolphthalein in alkaline solution, and by Congo red, when these are used in diagnostic tests. Certain drugs such as antipyrine, pyridium or santonin may give a pink or red color to urine. Urorosein, a derivative of indol, is pink to red in acid urine and may occur in diseases of the liver and certain dietary deficiencies. In alkaptonuria, an inborn error of tyrosine metabolism, homogentisic acid is excreted in the urine, which turns black on standing. Melanin pigments or precursors in the urine may cause the urine to turn brown or black on standing and thus indicate the presence of melanosarcoma. None of these substances reacts with benzidine or guaiac as do the heme pigments.

Treatment. There is no specific treatment for hemoglobinemia and hemoglobinuria or for myohemoglobinuria. However, in crush injury and in instances in which hemoglobinuria may be anticipated or has just occurred, the administration of fluid and alkali may protect the kidney and prevent shut-down by providing diuresis of alkaline urine. A dosage of 4 gm. hourly of sodium bicarbonate by mouth up to 30 gm. in 24 hours and 3 liters of fluid should keep the urine alkaline. However, if oliguria or anuria is established, this diuretic treatment is of no avail and is contraindicated. The treatment of shock is essential if present in injuries such as crushing of muscles or thermal burns. The treatment of the underlying disease or process depends on the mechanism which has released the heme pigments into the urine. The complications of release of heme pigments include severe anemia in some instances of hemoglobinuria, renal failure and shut-down in some instances of hemoglobinuria and myohemoglobinuria. The renal problem is discussed elsewhere.

THOMAS HALE HAM

References

Bywaters, E. G. L.: Ischemic Muscle Necrosis. Crushing Injury, Traumatic Edema, the Crush Syndrome, Traumatic Anuria, Compression Syndrome: a Type of Injury Seen in Air Raid Casualties Following Burial Beneath Debris. J.A.M.A., *124:*1103, 1944.
Crosby, W. H., and Dameshek, W.: The Significance of Hemoglobinemia and Associated Hemosiderinuria, With Particular Reference to Various Types of Hemolytic Anemia. J. Lab. & Clin. Med., *38:*829, 1951.

Gilligan, D. R., Altschule, M. D., and Katersky, E. M.: Physiological Intravascular Hemolysis of Exercise. Hemoglobinemia and Hemoglobinuria Following Cross-Country Runs. J. Clin. Investigation, 22:859, 1943.
Ham, T. H.: A Syllabus of Laboratory Examinations in Clinical Diagnosis. Cambridge, Harvard University Press, 1950.
Kreutzer, F. L., Strait, L., and Kerr, W. J.: Spontaneous Myoglobinuria in Man. Description of Case with Recurrent Attacks. Arch. Int. Med., *81:* 249, 1948.
Ross, J. F.: Hemoglobinemia and the Hemoglobinurias. New England J. Med., 233:691, 732, 766, 1945.

HEMOLYTIC TRANSFUSION REACTIONS

Definitions. Red cells may be destroyed following transfusion by intravascular or extravascular hemolysis. *Intravascular* hemolytic transfusion reactions usually occur promptly during or immediately following the transfusion with the release of free hemoglobin into the plasma, frequently with hemoglobinuria. Such reactions are potentially dangerous because "lower nephron" nephrosis develops in some patients as manifested by oliguria or anuria and uremia. Transfusion reactions with *extravascular hemolysis* are usually gradual over days or weeks, occur without hemoglobinemia or hemoglobinuria, and without the danger of "lower nephron" nephrosis. The hemoglobin pigment is converted presumably by the reticuloendothelial system to bilirubin which is excreted as bilirubin derivatives in the feces.

Mechanisms. Intravascular hemolytic transfusion reactions result from the following known mechanisms. (1) Intravascular hemolysis of the donor's red cells occurs from transfusion of incompatible blood as a result of isoantibodies in the recipient's serum. These antibodies may be agglutinins, hemolysins, incomplete antibodies, or a combination of antibodies that may be inherent to the individual or may result from isoimmunization by previous transfusions, injections of blood or from pregnancy. The antibodies include those of the ABO system, the Rh system and other rarer blood groups. These hemolytic reactions are the most dangerous because of the extremely rapid and massive hemolysis that can occur from the large pool of patient's antibodies reacting with the donor's red cells. Such reactions from the administration of grossly incompatible blood result most frequently from such mistakes as giving of the wrong bottle of blood to a patient. Usually the proper blood grouping and compatibility tests will detect blood samples that would be hemolyzed when transfused. The amount of free hemoglobin in the plasma varies from a trace, giving only a pink color to the plasma, to an extreme amount, giving a dark red color and representing as much as 0.5 to 1.0 gm. or more of free hemoglobin per 100 cc. of plasma. Many patients tolerate hemoglobinuria without renal shutdown, but the occurrence of renal complications cannot be predicted in a given patient who is experiencing hemoglobinuria.

(2) Intravascular hemolysis of the recipient's own red cells may occur rarely in the ABO system from transfusing incompatible antibodies from the donor, including agglutinins or hemolysins or both. This has been described in instances when large amounts of group O blood, containing high titers of anti-A and anti-B isoantibodies, are transfused into patients of blood group A, B or AB. The rate and amount of hemolysis in this situation is usually much less marked than described in (1), and fewer renal complications occur. In paroxysmal nocturnal hemoglobinuria, transfusions are frequently associated with marked hemoglobinemia, and hemoglobinuria, with destruction of the patients' cells occurring by an unknown mechanism probably related to factors in the serum and the patient's red cells. (3) Intravascular hemolysis of the donor's red cells may occur from blood that has been stored for prolonged periods and is related to changes inherent in the cells and not to incompatibilities based on isoantibodies.

In extravascular hemolytic transfusion reactions the donor's red cells are removed in a period of days or weeks without hemoglobinemia or hemoglobinuria. Such hemolysis may be associated with incomplete isoantibodies of unknown origin in the recipient's serum. In some of these instances the Coombs test shows the presence of antibody globulin on the patient's red cells.

The events which occur following intravascular hemolysis with the consequent appearance of hemoglobin, increased bilirubin (indirect) and methemalbumin in the plasma, and the appearance of hemoglobin and hemosiderin in the urine have been described on page 1092. The clinical symptoms and signs appear similar for intravascular hemolysis of red cells and for experimental observations of the intravenous injection of stroma-free solutions of hemoglobin.

Diagnosis. The transfusion should be stopped at once in any patient showing a chill, pain in the back or signs of shock. If a patient is under anesthetic the only reactions that may be manifest when incompatible blood is injected may be increasing tachycardia and shock. These signs are consistent with the occurrence of an intravascular hemolytic transfusion reaction but are not pathognomonic and may be produced by reactions to pyrogens. Samples of blood should all be saved for immediate rechecking of blood groups and compatibility tests. The direct proof, however, for an intravascular hemolytic transfusion reaction requires the demonstration of hemoglobin or methemalbumin in plasma or hemoglobin in the urine. The test for hemoglobinuria has been outlined on page 1095. A blood sample can be taken immediately after transfusion or at intervals for the detection of free hemoglobin in the plasma. One procedure is as follows: Venous blood is collected with minimum trauma in a syringe and needle that have been rinsed in physiologic saline. Nine parts of blood are introduced gently down the side of a tube containing one part of an aqueous solution of sodium citrate, 3 gm. per 100 cc. The sample is mixed by gentle tilting of the tube, is centrifuged immediately, and the plasma removed. The plasma can be inspected for the presence of hemoglobin pigment by its pink to red color or it can be examined chemically for hemoglobin by the benzidine method. Plasma samples can also be observed for increase in bilirubin. Methemalbumin in the plasma will remain for many hours to several days, may be diagnostic and can be suspected by its gold to brown color and its reaction (heme) with benzidine and guaiac.

The diagnosis and treatment of "lower nephron" nephrosis are discussed elsewhere.

THOMAS HALE HAM

References

Mollison, P. L.: Blood Transfusion in Clinical Medicine. Oxford, Blackwell Scientific Publications, 1951.
Soutter, L., Allen, F. H., Jr., and Emerson, C. P., Jr.: Medical Progress, Blood Grouping, Blood Banking and Blood Transfusion. New England J. Med., 245:367, 410, 456, 1951.

NEPHRITIS

(Bright's Disease)

Introduction. In 1836 Richard Bright wrote: "It is, indeed, an humiliating confession, that, although much attention has been directed to this disease for nearly 10 years . . . yet little or nothing has been done toward devising a method of permanent relief, when the disease has been confirmed; and no fixed plan has been laid down, as affording a tolerable certainty of cure in the more recent cases."

More than a hundred years later we must amplify this apology of Bright with the equally humiliating confession that we, today, cannot cure the disease. Furthermore, the mechanism of its progression or of spontaneous healing remains obscure. Finally, the establishment of its diagnosis is at times impossible. Hence a textbook discussion of Bright's disease must in part be indefinite in its statements, unsatisfactory as to the statistical study of its incidence, course and outcome, and speculative concerning its nature and the therapeutic measures to be used. Despite this apparent state of confusion, and in all fairness to the innumerable studies devoted to the subject of nephritis, it should be recognized that the importance of the relationship of certain infections to the onset and course of the disease has in a measure been clarified. Also, the development and application of quantitative biochemical methods have contributed enormously to our understanding of the pathologic physiology of Bright's disease, upon which is based rational therapy.

Definition. The term "nephritis" embraces a number of disease states of unknown etiology, which may be acute or chronic and which are characterized by proteinuria and cylindruria and often by hematuria. In addition to these signs of local renal dysfunction which are dependent upon bilateral nonsuppurative inflammatory or degenerative kidney lesions, edema, hypertension and nitrogen retention are frequently present. Many of the manifestations, both local and systemic, are referable to disturbances in the vascular system.

Classification. The present status of the classification of nephritis has been best described by Addis, who says: "Every student of Bright's disease constructs his own classification to meet his own individual interests

and needs." In the absence of an etiologic basis for the classification of Bright's disease, most terminologies have been of a descriptive clinical or anatomic nature. With the present limitations of our knowledge, the chief aim in developing a classification is to find terms which may for the time being serve as labels characterizing for the pathologist and clinician the general aspects of Bright's disease in its various forms. The following classification in simplified form is in common use today. In the light of the foregoing discussion, it must be considered purely tentative.

A. Glomerulonephritis:
   1. Acute form
   2. Chronic form
      (a) Following known acute form
      (b) Without known preceding acute form
B. Arteriolar nephrosclerosis
C. Nephroses
D. Miscellaneous nephritides

Consideration of the various subdivisions of these larger classes will follow in their respective sections.

GLOMERULONEPHRITIS

Etiology. In a vast majority of instances acute glomerulonephritis follows *infection of the upper respiratory tract,* and in cases in which careful bacteriologic and immunologic observations have been made it has become apparent that the hemolytic streptococcus (Group A of Lancefield), above all other organisms, is of prime importance. For example, Longcope reported the presence of hemolytic streptococcal infection in 85 per cent of the patients with acute nephritis studied by him. In the series of Seegal, Lyttle, E. N. Loeb and Jost, the serums in 76 of 80 consecutive patients with acute nephritis contained a sufficiently high titer of antistreptolysin to be indicative of a recent hemolytic streptococcal infection. From these observations and many similar ones we find that disease of the upper respiratory tract, be it tonsillitis, pharyngitis, sinusitis, the common cold, "grippe," peritonsillar abscess, scarlet fever, rheumatic fever, and so forth, is usually associated with streptococcal invasion when it is followed by acute glomerulonephritis. The observations of Rammelkamp, Weaver and Dingle, as well as those of Wertheim, D. Seegal and others, indicate that infection with type 12 and perhaps type 4 hemolytic streptococcus is "especially likely to be followed by acute glomerulonephritis." Types 18 and 25 also appear to be nephritogenic but not to the same degree as type 12. It is probable that some strains of type 12 streptococcus as well as other types may not be nephritogenic. In contrast to acute glomerulonephritis, the experience of Rammelkamp indicates that there is no type specificity found in streptococcal infections preceding the onset of acute rheumatic fever. The mechanism of microscopic hematuria in 15 per cent of patients is probably merely another manifestation of the hemorrhagic diathesis in the rheumatic state. The 2 or 3 per cent developing associated acute glomerulonephritis may have both diseases initiated by a type 12 or some other nephritogenic strain.

That the streptococcus is not invariably the *infective agent* associated with the onset of acute nephritis seems apparent from the fact that most observers have a number of cases in their series which are thought to be associated with pneumococcal or gram-negative coccal infections, various pyogenic infections, enteric fevers or with no demonstrable infectious process at all. It must be kept in mind, however, that in many of these cases the presence of associated hemolytic streptococcal infection has not been eliminated by adequate bacteriologic or immunologic methods. Despite this criticism, it is certain that infectious agents other than the hemolytic streptococcus are occasionally associated with the onset of acute nephritis.

In addition to the factors already mentioned, certain *chemical poisons* such as carbon tetrachloride, pentachlornaphthalene and mercury salts cause renal irritation with proteinuria, hematuria and oliguria which may resemble the clinical picture of acute glomerulonephritis. Furthermore, when certain sulfonamides have been administered, hematuria, oliguria, nitrogen retention and edema may appear, and at times these drug effects are indistinguishable from nephritis which might be induced by the underlying infection. The confusion concerning the nature of the toxemias of pregnancy is so great that their consideration contributes little or nothing to a discussion of glomerulonephritis. Bacterial endocarditis and other septic states are not infrequently associated with embolic and local inflammatory lesions in the kidney, and occasionally typical glomerulonephritis is superimposed on these lesions. This is most frequently seen in cases of infection with *Streptococcus viridans.*

The foregoing discussion has dealt with the etiology of *acute* glomerulonephritis, in which the intimate association of this disease with hemolytic streptococcal infection has been stressed. Nevertheless, the severity and the course of the nephritis are entirely independent of the severity of the preceding infection. The role of acute infectious processes in the etiology of *chronic* glomerulonephritis is much less certain, although an exacerbation of the disease not infrequently accompanies or follows intercurrent streptococcal infection. In the studies of Seegal and his colleagues one or more exacerbations were seen in 13 of a series of 68 patients observed for one to eight years. In all, bacteriologic or immunologic evidence indicated that the exacerbations *may* be initiated by streptococcal infection; however, in 5 of 28 exacerbations no evidence of streptococcal infection was obtained. Ellis and others believe that two forms of chronic glomeronephritis occur. Type I represents the outcome of acute glomerulonephritis which has not healed. Type II is considered to be represented by patients exhibiting an insidious onset without recognized preceding infection, and those characterized by the nephrotic state and distinguished histologically by the predominance of intercapillary rather than intracapillary lesions. The validity of this concept of two independent types of chronic glomerulonephritis is not established. However, the strongest point in favor of the Ellis hypothesis is the great infrequency with which the nephrotic syndrome follows documented acute glomerulonephritis. Our ignorance concerning the etiology of chronic glomerulonephritis is well illustrated by the fact that the simple question of the frequency with which acute nephritis becomes chronic is answered by investigators in the field with the greatest divergence of opinion. For example; Addis, and also Longcope, state that more than 40 per cent of patients suffering from acute nephritis acquire the chronic form of the disease, whereas Richter and others find the acute disease progressing in less than 20 per cent. Still more puzzling is the experience of Snoke, who states that, among a large series of children with acute nephritis studied by him in California, the incidence of progression to the chronic form of the disease was 39 per cent. In studying a similar group of children in Rochester, New York, he found progression from the acute to the chronic form in only 10.6 per cent. This confusion arises in part from the fact that many patients with "acute" nephritis probably represent exacerbations of previously unrecognized latent chronic nephritis.

Mechanism of Glomerulonephritis. In the foregoing discussion the frequent association of infection with the onset of acute glomerulonephritis has been emphasized, but this knowledge has not fundamentally advanced our understanding of the mechanisms involved in the production of the disease. Thus many important and intriguing questions remain unanswered.

Bacteriologic studies of recent years have shown conclusively that actual invasion of the kidneys by the infectious agent does not occur in acute or chronic glomerulonephritis, except in the presence of bacterial endocarditis or sepsis. Furthermore, evidence points against the concept of immediate damage to the kidneys by the bacterial products, because of the fact that acute glomerulonephritis almost invariably follows rather than accompanies the acute infection. For example, the acute nephritis of scarlet fever develops classically ten to twenty days after the onset of the exanthem and a considerable time after the subsidence of the febrile reaction. Similar time relationships obtain in acute nephritis following tonsillitis and other infectious processes. In 1912 Escherich and Schick expressed the view that this time relationship suggested the possibility that glomerulonephritis was not induced by infection *per se,* but by the immune reactions resulting from the infection. Since that time, Friedemann, Longcope and others have come to a similar conclusion. This concept may offer a satisfactory explanation for some of the obscure phenomena observed in the disease and is at the present time receiving support from laboratory investigation.

Many attempts to produce in animals disease pictures analogous to acute and chronic glomerulonephritis in man have failed or have proved inconclusive. However, Doan has been able to establish in monkeys a clinical picture closely resembling human nephritis with intranasal reinoculation of a group C streptococcus. In 1928 Masugi demonstrated that an antikidney serum, produced by the injection of rat kidney emulsion into rabbits, when injected into rats gave rise to acute or chronic nephritis. These observations were confirmed by Arnott and others, and have been greatly extended by Smadel and Farr, who showed that the injection of one, two or three doses of rabbit anti-rat kidney serum into rats, in the course of a few days, induces acute nephritis. Some of the animals so treated recover in about three weeks, while others may develop a full-blown nephrotic syndrome and either recover or emerge from the nephrotic phase, progressing in the course of time with the appearance of hypertension and nitrogen retention. This suggests that a variety of disease patterns may be induced in different individuals by the same noxious agent. Thus it is conceivable that the so-called Types I and II chronic nephritis may be due to a difference in host response rather than in etiology.

Smadel and Farr have found that in one strain of rats the course of the disease initiated by nephrotoxin immune serum may be altered by the amount of protein in the diet. If this be restricted, the nephritis tends to heal; whereas if the amount of protein in the diet be increased, the nephritis becomes progressive. Thus the question of the possible deleterious effect of large amounts of protein, stressed by earlier workers, is again raised. B. Seegal and E. N. Loeb found that nephritis, indistinguishable from that produced by kidney antiserums, can also be induced by means of placental antiserums in the rat. Pressman has shown that the globulin fraction of antikidney serums tagged with I^{131} is localized primarily in the glomeruli, as determined by radio-autographs. Ferrebee has shown that isolated rat glomeruli adsorb the nephrotoxic agent, whereas tubule cells do not. Krakower and Greenspon have more recently shown that the basement membrane of glomerular tufts is twenty times more antigenic than are the combined visceral epithelial and endothelial cells of the glomeruli. Hill and Cruickshank employing fluorescin-marked immune globulin have confirmed and extended these findings.

If these observations concerning the nephrotoxic action of antikidney and antiplacental serums be applicable to man, we can hypothesize that an infectious agent, such as the hemolytic streptococcus, stimulates production of nephrotoxic immune bodies within susceptible persons. These may then give rise to acute or chronic glomerulonephritis. It is in relation to the latter form that we may find in these laboratory studies a possible explanation for those cases of progressive chronic glomerulonephritis in which most rigid clinical, bacteriologic and immunologic studies fail to produce evidence for the persistence or recurrence of streptococcal infection to account for the relentless progression of the disease. Unfortunately, none of the experimental studies throws light on the obscure fact that most cases of chronic glomerulonephritis begin insidiously and without apparent relation to a recognized preceding infectious process. These facts do not, however, exclude the possibility that the chronic glomerulonephritis may, nevertheless, find its origin in an unrecognized attack of acute nephritis. It is of interest that Lange has reported the presence of high titers of antibody to human kidney in both chronic and acute glomerulonephritis in man. The foregoing highly speculative discussion has no practical application, but shows the trend of present-day thought in relation to the mechanism of one of the commonest and most obscure of human maladies.

Predisposing Factors. The role of *sex* in the susceptibility to glomerulonephritis is of interest in that there is a striking consistency in the preponderance of the disease among males in a ratio of approximately 2 : 1. No satisfactory explanation is offered for this unequal distribution.

Age. Glomerulonephritis is essentially a disease of children and adults in the earlier decades of life, the acute form being more common in children than adults. The Seegals and Lyttle reported that 70 per cent of their cases occurred before the age of 21. The *incidence* of the disease in the acute form cannot be determined with any degree of accuracy, because those patients without extrarenal symptomatology frequently do not come to the attention of a physician; even when they do, there is difficulty in establishing the diagnosis in these mild forms. Among the cases diagnosed in general hospitals, the Seegals and Lyttle found that among 35,000 admissions to medical wards the incidence was 0.62 per cent in Northern hospitals, while in hospitals of Louisiana and Texas the incidence was approximately the same, being 0.47 per cent. Since the disease in its chronic form frequently begins insidiously, the proof of its relatively early onset in life is best established by the age at death. Of 57 autopsied adult cases at the Presbyterian Hospital, 35 died before the age of 40. In a similar group, but including children, Fishberg reports that 42 of 54 patients also died before the age of 40.

Climate. As mentioned before, the Seegals found the incidence of acute glomerulonephritis to be independent of latitude. These same investigators found that in the Southern states, as well as in the North, the disease reaches its greatest incidence at that season of the year when disease of the upper respiratory tract and streptococcal infection are at a peak. The role of nephritogenic types of hemolytic streptococci in the etiology of acute nephritis has now been reported widely through the world.

Exposure to Cold. Many years ago exposure to cold was thought to have great significance in relation to the onset of acute nephritis. These instances became progressively fewer, perhaps because the time interval between infection and the appearance of nephritis is better appreciated and because more careful bacteriologic and immunologic studies are made.

Familial Susceptibility. Nine of 57 patients at the Presbyterian Hospital who came to autopsy because of chronic glomerulonephritis gave a family history of Bright's disease. Ernstene reported a family in which 6 of 10 children had acute glomerulonephritis secondary to upper respiratory infection. It seems probable that multiple cases of acute glomerulonephritis occurring within a family are the result of infection with a nephritogenic strain of streptococcus, e.g., type 12.

Morbid Anatomy. At autopsy the kidneys in *acute glomerulonephritis* are normal in size or slightly enlarged. They are usually pale in color and may show punctate hemorrhages on their smooth surfaces. Microscopically, the earliest and most intense changes are found in the glomeruli. These include thickening of the basement membranes with proliferation of the endothelium and leukocytic infiltration to a degree which may render them wholly ischemic. These changes may be correlated with the observed decreased filtration rate present despite over-all hyperemia of the kidneys. The interstitium is infiltrated with leukocytes, and the tubule cells show varying degrees of swelling and lipoid deposits, and the lumina contain blood, leukocytes and cellular debris. If acute glomerulonephritis heals, there is no evidence of residual damage.

When glomerulonephritis becomes *chronic,* the kidneys may at first show increased pallor and enlargement. Ultimately, however, they contract as a result of scarring and may be reduced to one fourth the normal size. The glomerular tufts may develop adhesions and the capsule proliferate to form the so-called "crescents." Finally, glomeruli become hyalinized, and many disappear in the process of fibrosis. Some tubules become dilated and cystic, while others vanish. The interstitium shows progressive fibrosis and chronic inflammation. The arterioles may show marked thickening, and in the end stages it is frequently impossible to determine whether the underlying basis for the renal disease has been glomerulonephritis, chronic pyelonephritis or primary arteriolar disease.

ACUTE GLOMERULONEPHRITIS

Clinical Picture. The "classic" picture of acute glomerulonephritis is seen frequently in children and in young adults, following infection with a nephritogenic strain of hemolytic streptococcus. The patient usually complains of hematuria, puffiness of the face, headache and a decrease in urinary output. In the fulminating form of the disease, edema may become generalized, visual disturbances may occur, hypertension may become extreme, and dyspnea marked; delirium, convulsions, coma and death may ensue. This dramatic sequence of events may be accompanied by fever, anorexia, vomiting, anuria and varying degrees of nitrogen retention. The foregoing description comprises, perforce, a composite picture of the more striking features of acute glomerulonephritis. However, it should be emphasized that the "classic," i.e., the unmistakable, picture is rarely encountered in medicine. More frequently, one or more symptoms or signs dominate the disease. For example, in many patients with acute nephritis, edema may be the only complaint or objective physical finding. In others gross hematuria alone may attract attention to the disease. A few complain of weakness or backache. In still others it is important to recognize that there may be no symptoms and no abnormalities on physical examination, or they may be so mild and transient that they entirely escape detection. The diagnosis in these cases, which are numerous, is made possible only by examination of the urine.

In Richter's series of hospitalized patients *edema* was present in two thirds of the cases of acute nephritis. It usually begins about the eyes, and the face becomes puffy and pasty in appearance. This is frequently most apparent when the patient awakes in the

morning. In many cases the edema involves the dependent parts, and in some it becomes generalized, occasionally being accompanied by effusion into the serous cavities; it usually appears early in the disease, though it may appear at any time. The development of edema is due to at least four factors: (1) A decrease in urine formation due to decrease in glomerular filtration; (2) increase in reabsorption of sodium salts and water by the tubule cells; (3) congestive heart failure with elevation of hydrostatic pressure in many cases; and (4) possibly an increase in capillary porosity due to generalized capillary damage. It is of interest that the serum protein level in acute nephritis with edema is rarely reduced below 5.5 per cent, although the albumin fraction may be significantly lowered with some increase in globulin.

Variations in the elevation of *blood pressure* in acute nephritis are great. The pressure may never exceed normal limits in the entire course of the disease. On the other hand, in about 25 per cent of the cases there is a moderate transient elevation of either the systolic or diastolic pressure, or both. In about 10 per cent the systolic pressure reaches 180 to 200 mm. of mercury, and the diastolic pressure may be maintained well above 110 mm.

In acute nephritis the elevation of blood pressure, like the development of edema, usually begins early in the disease, but may appear some time after the onset. Progressive elevation of pressure usually precedes the appearance of cerebral and cardiac symptoms. The pressure may fluctuate widely from day to day, suggesting that arteriolar spasm is probably the chief underlying mechanism involved. In a few cases an extreme degree of hypertension is associated with an acute necrotizing arteriolitis.

Closely allied with changes in blood pressure in acute nephritis are the *cerebral manifestations* of the disease. When the pressure begins to rise rapidly, severe headache, nausea and vomiting, somnolence or mental confusion may develop. Finally, generalized clonic convulsions may occur. These episodes were present in 10 per cent of the series studied at the Peter Bent Brigham Hospital. Their mechanism is not understood, but they are not dependent upon nitrogen retention. They are probably due in part to cerebral ischemia associated with arteriolar spasm and hypertension and with more or less cerebral edema. Convulsions may occur once or may recur at frequent intervals, as in a status epilepticus. Death is not uncommon after recurrent convulsive seizures. *Visual disturbances* occur with these attacks of so-called "hypertensive encephalopathy." The commonest of these is blurring vision. Amaurosis is transient and occurs in about 2 per cent of hospital cases. The *eyegrounds* in acute nephritis are usually normal, but many changes may occur. Papilledema is not unusual and is most frequently seen with elevation of blood pressure, with or without hypertensive cerebral episodes. The retinal arteries appear pale and narrow when hypertension is marked. Hemorrhages into the retina are not unusual and are probably another manifestation of general capillary damage in acute nephritis. Exudate is rarely present. Occasionally the complete picture of edematous disks, vascular changes, hemorrhages and exudate is seen in the fundi of patients with acute nephritis. The author has seen one patient who had acute nephritis associated with massive edema, hypertension, nitrogen retention, a series of epileptiform convulsions, papilledema, retinal hemorrhages and "macular stars" of exudate. Fourteen years later that patient had no evidence of nephritis or hypertension, and his eyegrounds were normal but for slight pallor of one optic disk.

The *heart* frequently suffers to a greater or lesser degree in the majority of cases of acute nephritis. Whitehill, Longcope and Williams found that "myocardial failure varies in its severity in direct proportion to the severity of acute nephritis." Thus 53 of 59 patients with severe nephritis had some evidence of cardiac insufficiency. Among mild cases 12 of 35 had some circulatory disturbance. The abnormalities encountered range from mild electrocardiographic disturbances without symptoms to extreme congestive failure associated with dyspnea, orthopnea, tachycardia, gallop rhythm, pulmonary congestion and elevation of venous pressure. Cardiac insufficiency is the commonest cause of death in acute glomerulonephritis. Fatal insufficiency may be precipitated by the exertion associated with convulsive seizures.

With the progressive development of massive edema, fluid may collect in the pleural cavities, and the *lungs* may show the presence of rales at the bases. The patient may become dyspneic because of decreased lung elasticity. When cardiac insufficiency supervenes, frank pulmonary edema, as has been mentioned, may occur. Edematous patients not infre-

quently acquire secondary bronchopneumonia.

The presence of *anemia* early in the course of acute nephritis is distinctly unusual and, when present, should arouse suspicion of a chronic process with a superimposed acute exacerbation. When acute nephritis persists over a period of many weeks, particularly if renal bleeding or severe and persistent infection plays a prominent role, varying degrees of secondary anemia may develop. The white cells in acute nephritis are normal unless infection complicates the picture.

The *urine* volume in acute nephritis may be normal throughout the course of the disease. On the other hand, it may decrease in amount abruptly at the onset of the disease and may present either a smoky or definitely bloody appearance. Anuria occurs in about 5 per cent of hospitalized patients with acute nephritis and is a serious manifestation. The oliguria encountered may not be associated with outspoken edema for some time, although it represents retention of fluid in the interstial spaces. The reasons for the appearance of oliguria and anuria are those mentioned in the discussion of edema. There is usually little interference with the ability of the kidneys to concentrate early in the course of acute nephritis; consequently the *specific gravity* of the urine is, as a rule, maintained at normal levels. Protein is regularly present in the urine in acute nephritis, and the diagnosis of the disease is untenable in its absence. The amounts present are extremely variable. Proteinuria is frequently the last manifestation of the disease to disappear in the process of healing. According to Blackman, patients in whom a large amount of the urinary protein is globulin have a poor outlook for recovery.

Hematuria, either gross or microscopic, is present in acute glomerulonephritis with such regularity that the disease, in the classification of Addis, has been termed "acute hemorrhagic nephritis." In the absence of gross or microscopic hematuria, the diagnosis of acute glomerulonephritis must be held in doubt. The amount of blood in the urine is extremely variable. In about 40 per cent of the cases gross hematuria is recognized. This symptom is present, as a rule, for only a few days, but may recur from time to time in the course of the disease. Microscopic hematuria often persists for months and may continue long after routine examination fails to reveal proteinuria, although, as stated before, in other cases protein is the last to disappear. A moderate number of leukocytes are usually present in the sediment, but frank pus is not encountered. Casts of various kinds are always present in acute nephritis. Most characteristic and important diagnostically, if present among these formed elements, are red blood cell casts. Nevertheless, other cellular casts, granular, hyaline and waxy casts may be present in varying numbers.

Renal function as measured by tests other than routine urine examination is normal in about 50 per cent of patients with acute glomerulonephritis. In others, varying degrees of nitrogen retention are observed, but the blood urea nitrogen rises above 100 mg. per cent in less than 5 per cent of the cases. The higher values are usually associated with oliguria and hypertension, but it should be emphasized again that the convulsions of hypertensive encephalopathy occur independently of azotemia and may be fatal without any nitrogen retention. When nitrogen is retained in appreciable amounts, there may be a decrease in the rate of excretion of phenolsulfonphthalein, and the urea clearance test may show a striking decrease in kidney function. Accompanying these marked changes may be retention of creatinine and uric acid and the development of acidosis due primarily to phosphate and sulfate retention. Only 2 to 3 per cent of patients with acute nephritis die of true uremia. Whereas there is often a decrease in the total renal plasma flow in acute nephritis, this is not depressed to the same extent as is glomerular filtration; therefore, relative hyperemia is present. The marked depression of renal function occurring in a number of cases is not necessarily associated with progressive disease. On the contrary, it is usually a reversible disorder which may disappear in the course of a few days.

Diagnosis. In the "classic" case of acute glomerulonephritis diagnosis affords no difficulty. However, when protein, casts and red blood cells appear in the urine in unmistakable but small quantities, after or during an acute infection with the hemolytic streptococcus or other organisms and unaccompanied by edema, hypertension or nitrogen retention, the problem becomes more difficult. Certain authors escape this diagnostic difficulty by applying the term "focal nephritis" to these cases. In the writer's opinion this does not advance our knowledge or clarify the situation. If the urinary findings described persist over periods of one or two weeks, it seems likely that acute glomerulonephritis is present. If the microscopic hematuria, casts and protein disappear in a shorter time, it is best to admit that the diagnosis remains in doubt and that the findings may result from increased permeability of renal capillaries due to "irritation," passive congestion, embolic phenomena or to causes unknown. It should be emphasized that numerous blood pressure determinations, repeated urine examinations and a careful record of body weight aid tremendously in detecting transient abnormalities which may establish the diagnosis in mild cases. Fischel and Gajdusek have demonstrated that the level of complement in the blood serum is reduced in overt acute glomerulonephritis. This may be a useful aid in diagnosis.

The difficulty in establishing a diagnosis in borderline cases is emphasized by the studies of the urine in scarlet fever carried out by Lyttle. This investigator applied to 68 patients with scarlet fever Addis' quantitative method for the determination of protein, casts and cells in the urine. He found in all the cases that a moderate transient increase in all elements, above accepted normal levels, occurred between the eighth and the forty-fifth days after the onset of the disease. He found similar changes in the urine following other forms of streptococcal infections, but not with any regularity after infection due to other organisms. The type of streptococci were not identified in these studies. To state, on the basis of these findings, that all patients acquire nephritis after scarlet fever or other streptococcal infections seems to the author unanswerable, and whether the difference between this micronephritis or "renal irritation" and true outspoken acute glomerulonephritis is qualitative or quantitative cannot be settled at the present time. The difficulty in differentiating acute glomerulonephritis from the effects of certain sulfonamide drugs upon the kidney has already been emphasized.

In cases of acute glomerulonephritis in which gross hematuria persists, particularly when associated with dysuria and pain in one or both costovertebral angles, urologic aid may become necessary to establish the diagnosis. If the amount of protein in the urine is massive and red blood cell casts are present, and if edema or hypertension is found, the diagnosis is simplified. In the absence of these signs it may be necessary to resort to cystoscopic examination or intravenous pyelography to eliminate the presence of tumor, stone, tuberculosis, pyelonephritis, and so forth.

The differentiation between *orthostatic proteinuria* and acute glomerulonephritis arises only in those patients who have virtually no red cells in their urinary sediments. In the absence of other signs and symptoms of nephritis and in the presence of proteinuria which appears only in the erect position, a diagnosis of orthostatic proteinuria becomes justifiable with repeated observations, particularly when occurring in a thin child or in an adolescent.

The differential diagnosis between acute and chronic glomerulonephritis is of great importance because of the difference in prognosis. Nevertheless, this is at times impossible, particularly when an exacerbation of chronic nephritis follows an acute infection and resembles in all respects the disease in its acute form. In this situation a record of a urine examination just before the onset of the symptoms, or the presence of signs of advanced renal disease, will help to distinguish between the acute and chronic forms. Furthermore, the exacerbation usually appears within two or three days after the onset of infection in contrast to the long latent period characteristic of acute nephritis. In the absence of these aids the diagnosis becomes dependent upon the subsequent course.

In embolic acute nephritis, in which there are manifestations only of proteinuria, casts and hematuria, unless diffuse glomerulonephritis supervenes, the diagnosis is dependent upon the demonstration of blood stream infection by culture.

Prognosis. Less than 5 per cent of patients with acute glomerulonephritis die of this disease. In fatal cases, death results from one or more of the following causes: (1) hypertensive encephalopathy associated with convulsions; (2) cardiac decompensation frequently terminating in pulmonary edema; (3) uremia; and (4) bronchopneumonia, or sepsis.

Most patients who acquire acute glomerulonephritis recover completely, although authorities differ widely as to the actual percentage. In children it is generally conceded that the prognosis is particularly good. The course of the disease may last but a few days or may persist for more than a year and yet terminate in recovery. Perhaps the most frequent duration of acute nephritis among hospitalized patients is about two months. It is important to recognize that the duration of acute glomerulonephritis and the ultimate outcome in terms of healing or of the development of chronic nephritis are independent of the severity of the preceding infection and the apparent severity of the disease as measured by the degree of proteinuria, hematuria, hypertension or edema. In other words, the clinical course in one patient, while distinctly alarming, may terminate favorably within two or three weeks, whereas in another patient an apparently benign clinical course may progress to fatal chronic nephritis. Although it is apparent that the ultimate outcome in acute nephritis cannot be predicted, the impression has been gathered that healing is most frequent when the onset of the preceding infection is accompanied by severe constitutional reaction. The persistence of heavy proteinuria for more than three or four months suggests a worse prognosis than does persistent microscopic hematuria. At this point it should be emphasized that when a patient recovers completely from acute glomerulonephritis, i.e., when the urine becomes free from protein, red blood cells and casts, on repeated examinations, permanent immunity is almost invariably established, regardless of the frequency or severity of subsequent streptococcal infections, probably because of the persistence of circulating antibodies to the nephritogenic organism which initiated the disease.

Treatment. In the absence of specific therapy the treatment of nephritis must be largely symptomatic and, in so far as possible, based on recognized physiologic or biologic principles. *Bed rest* is the first and most important therapeutic indication. Ideally, perhaps, the patient should be kept in bed until all symptoms and signs of acute nephritis have disappeared. Practically, bed rest should be continued until all the general manifestations have disappeared. In spite of the fact that small amounts of protein and a few red blood cells may continue in evidence in the urine for six months or a year after the onset of the disease, it is usually impossible to keep the patient at rest for this length of time. If the urinary findings persist after two months and the extrarenal signs have vanished, and if the erythrocyte sedimentation rate has returned to normal, the patient may be allowed up. If this change is associated with an increase in proteinuria or hematuria, further bed rest is indicated. Exposure to chilling and exposure to persons with upper respiratory infection should be avoided. The *dietary restrictions* in acute glomerulonephritis depend to a large extent upon the presence or absence of oliguria, edema, hypertension and nitrogen retention. Even in the absence of these findings the *restriction of sodium chloride* or bicarbonate is indicated, since sodium salts constitute the chief "building block" of edema fluid. In the presence of anuria or severe oliguria, the daily fluid intake should be limited to less than 1000 ml. in excess of the combined volume of urine and vomitus. Foods and fluids containing potassium salts and protein should be avoided, and glucose in amounts of 100 gm. or more should be given daily orally or by drip through a nasogastric tube if gastric intolerance is marked. Only when necessary should 100 gm. of glucose be given slowly intravenously. This regimen tends to retard the development of azotemia and hyperkalemia. Caloric intake may be further augmented by the addition of emulsified fat, although the oral administration of fat is limited by its tendency to increase nausea. The application of the artificial kidney in these anuric patients probably rarely modifies the prognosis. In milder forms of the disease a salt-poor diet containing perhaps 50 to 60 gm. of protein a day seems to be the only dietary indication. There is, however, no sound clinical evidence to suggest that the amount of protein in the diet in any way influences the course or outcome of acute glomerulonephritis.

Medication. In the presence of hypertensive encephalopathy the daily administration of 15 to 30 gm. of magnesium sulfate by mouth and the slow intravenous administration of 25 cc. of 10 per cent solution of the same salt may have some effect in lowering the blood pressure and in preventing convulsive seizures. When these measures fail, the intravenous injection of hypertonic glucose solution, barbiturates, venesection and lumbar puncture are resorted to, but usually without striking benefit. Diuretics have no place in the treatment of acute nephritis and at times appear to add to the renal damage. Therapeutic hyperthermia is distinctly dangerous in that it not infrequently contributes to cardiac insufficiency, which should be treated with accepted methods. Cortisone and antihistamines serve no useful purpose in the treatment of acute nephritis.

The *surgical treatment* of acute nephritis consists in decapsulation of the kidneys, on the theory that the resulting decrease in tension permits greater blood flow. Most reports suggest that the results obtained by this method in the treatment of anuria are disappointing.

In view of the intimate relation between streptococcal *infection* and the etiology of acute nephritis, it is logical to eliminate all active and potential foci. When nephritis follows tonsillar infection, these structures should be removed when the general manifestations of nephritis have disappeared. In other cases, tonsillectomy may be postponed until later in convalescence. Acute exacerbations of nephritis frequently follow tonsillectomy and are usually characterized by an increase in hematuria. These "flare-ups" of the disease subside, as a rule, in a few days. This radical point of view toward tonsillectomy is justified only by the fact that many capable observers still stress the relationship between persistent infection and the progressive nature of the nephritic process in many cases. Further study may show, however, that this relationship is coincidental rather than causal, and the writer, from his experience, must confess that he has never been convinced that tonsillectomy has significantly altered the outcome of acute glomerulonephritis.

In view of the close association of streptococcal infection and acute glomerulonephritis, the role of *chemotherapy* deserves consideration. Evidence suggesting that penicillin or the sulfonamides influence the course of acute glomerulonephritis is not convincing. Nevertheless, penicillin should be administered to treat active infection if it persists when acute nephritis is first recognized. The use of penicillin or other antibiotics is preferred to that of the sulfonamides, since the latter are apt to cause further renal damage. *It now seems probable that treatment of hemolytic streptococcal infection initiated on the first or second day of the disease and continued until throat cultures are negative will prevent both acute glomerulonephritis and rheumatic fever.* Other antibiotics are less effective.

CHRONIC GLOMERULONEPHRITIS

Clinical Picture. The clinical picture of chronic glomerulonephritis is even more variegated than is that of the acute form of the disease. Only a small minority of cases is observed to develop from an attack of typical acute glomerulonephritis, after an acute infection with the hemolytic streptococcus. The majority of patients with chronic glomerulonephritis first seek medical aid because (1) they have noted the insidious onset of edema, primarily dependent in nature; (2) they complain of recurrent headaches which are usually associated with hypertension; (3) they have dyspnea which may be exertional or paroxysmal in nature and is also, as a rule, related to the presence of hypertension; or (4) they have been discovered, on routine examination, to have proteinuria. This last group comprises about 10 per cent of a series studied at the Presbyterian Hospital. Probably weakness, lassitude and loss of weight are the commonest of all symptoms, but they are characteristic of chronic disease in general and thus lose special diagnostic significance.

To cases in which proteinuria and cylindruria alone determine the presence of chronic glomerulonephritis, the term *latent nephritis* has been applied. Either with or without persistent or recurrent infection, the disease in a number of these patients becomes active, as determined by episodic increases in the number of red blood cells excreted in the urine. With this increase in activity there may appear any or all of the symptoms and signs characteristic of outspoken acute nephritis, and the patient may die with convulsions or in true uremia. Autopsy in these instances shows the presence of subacute nephritis. This active phase of chronic nephritis may, on the other hand, again become latent, only to recur repeatedly. In the following months or years, hypertension, anemia, nitrogen retention and, finally, the fullblown picture of uremia will terminate the disease, unless the course be intercepted earlier by fatal cerebral hemorrhage or cardiac failure. Few patients are observed to enter the *nephrotic state,* described fully in conjunction with the nephroses, and remain waterlogged for months or years. These patients either die of intercurrent infection, e.g., bronchopneumonia, or their edema subsides. When the edema decreases, the disease may again become latent with little or no demonstrable impairment of renal function. More frequently, however, the loss of edema presages further advance of the disease. As fluid vanishes, the blood pressure in time begins to rise, and the development of this *hypertensive phase* is often accompanied by severe headaches and varying degrees of *cardiac insufficiency.* Progressive failure in renal or cardiac function, or both, then terminates

the disease. Many patients pass directly into the hypertensive phase without ever having had more than minimal edema of the ankles or face. In a few instances the advance of chronic nephritis is so gradual and so devoid of symptoms that a patient comes first to the ophthalmologist, complaining of blurred vision, and then in the course of a few weeks dies in uremia.

The patient with chronic glomerulonephritis, on inspection, not infrequently presents the picture of health. In the nephrotic stage, striking pallor accompanies the edema and probably results, in part, from the wide separation of skin capillaries by edematous tissues. In the terminal stages of chronic nephritis the patient presents a classic appearance. He looks weary, and pallor, now due to anemia, is accompained by a characteristic sallow tint. His rest is frequently disturbed by muscle cramps. The skin becomes dry and atonic and, in advanced uremia in the colored race, more frequently than in the white, is often covered by the so-called "urea-frost." Widening of the palpebral fissures and the "china-blue" sclerae commonly appear with the advance of hypertension. The breath develops a typical odor, wrongly termed "urinous." Fibrinous pericarditis, occasionally accompanied by fibrinous pleurisy, appears in about 40 per cent of patients within two weeks of death. Muscular twitching, occasionally due to tetany, occurs with great regularity and when acidosis is marked, hyperpnea appears. Pruritus leads to uncontrolled scratching by the stuporous patient. Bleeding from the nose or gastrointestinal tract is a common terminal manifestation. In addition to dyspnea and Cheyne-Stokes breathing, probably the most distressing subjective symptoms are those of complete gastric intolerance coupled with thirst. Most patients die in coma, but 15 of 57 patients at the Presbyterian Hospital who died of this disease and were examined post mortem had had terminal generalized convulsions, and in 9, pulmonary edema was present.

The frequency with which *edema* appears in chronic glomerulonephritis is indicated by the fact that among 67 patients who died of the disease at the Presbyterian Hospital, this manifestation was recorded at some time in the records of 57. It was mentioned as being facial in 27 instances and dependent in 49. The edema, which appears during acute exacerbations, is probably caused by the factors mentioned in the discussion of Acute Nephritis. In the nephrotic phase the most important factor is a decrease in the albumin fraction of the serum proteins. The reader is referred to the chapter on Nephrosis for further information.

In all of 57 patients with chronic glomerulonephritis examined post mortem at the Presbyterian Hospital, some degree of *hypertension* had been present. On the other hand, in the so-called "latent phase" of the disease the blood pressure may remain normal for many years. For example, in a patient seen in the Presbyterian Hospital with edema, hypertension, nitrogen retention, proteinuria and hematuria, the blood pressure now, twenty-two years later, is normal, and only proteinuria and cylindruria persist. In another patient, refused a position because of proteinuria fifteen years ago, the blood pressure is normal despite the fact that edema and headache required hospitalization eleven years ago and that the patient has had many subsequent respiratory infections due to the hemolytic streptococcus. Thus it is apparent that hypertension, though it may occur early in the disease, at which time it fluctuates considerably, is a relatively constant finding only as chronic nephritis progresses to its termination. The height of the level attained is variable, but involves both the systolic and diastolic pressures. In 39 of a group of 57 patients studied post mortem, the systolic pressure was above 190 mm. of mercury, and in 16 of the group it reached levels higher than 230 mm.

Disorders of the *heart* appear late in the course of chronic nephritis and are usually associated with the presence of hypertension. In a patient in whom the disease progresses rapidly, hypertension and cardiac insufficiency may develop within a few months after the apparent onset of the disease. On the other hand, chronic glomerulonephritis may be present for many years before any elevation of blood pressure or impairment of cardiac function takes place. Cardiac hypertrophy and dilatation may develop slowly or rapidly after the appearance of hypertension, but neither the degree of cardiac embarrassment nor the size of the heart can be directly correlated with the height of the arterial pressure or with its duration. Hence it is fair to suspect that factors other than work contribute to cardiac hypertrophy in chronic nephritis.

In the series of patients studied post mortem at the Presbyterian Hospital, more than 90 per cent had complained of dyspnea. This was usually exertional in nature, but about 20 per cent of the patients also complained of paroxysmal dyspnea and had terminal pulmonary edema. In a number of patients, even in the absence of frank signs of left ventricular insufficiency, there may be elevation of the venous pressure which contributes to edema. In the uremic state, gallop rhythms are frequently heard, and, as has been stated before, about 40 per cent of the patients have a sterile fibrinous or serofibrinous pericarditis. There are no characteristic electrocardiographic changes associated with the cardiac insufficiency of chronic nephritis, but left ventricular preponderance naturally appears at times. The heart at post mortem weighed more than 400 gm. in 70 per cent of the Presbyterian Hospital cases, thus corresponding to the enlargement found on x-ray examination.

The *cerebral* manifestations in chronic nephritis should be considered primarily in conjunction with hypertension. Many patients without edema or hypertension complain of headache, which, in view of its frequency without renal disease, seems often falsely attributed to nephritis. About 30 per cent of patients with chronic glomerulonephritis are entirely free from headache, while, in the remainder, it may be mild and infrequent even though hypertension be present. On the other hand, almost daily headaches torture some patients for long periods of time; they may occur at any time of day and are accentuated by fatigue. Sometimes pain is present on awakening in the morning and disappears a few hours later. The mechanism of this distressing symptom is not understood, particularly as it comes and goes without necessarily being associated with any change in arterial tension. Classic hypertensive encephalopathy culminating in convulsions is rare but usually fatal in chronic nephritis. The epileptiform seizures seen in the terminal stages of the disease are probably related to renal failure with the retention of substances leading to increased irritability of the nervous system, but at times they are expressions of hypocalcemic tetany.

The majority of patients with chronic glomerulonephritis complain of some *visual disturbance* late in the disease. This is usually characterized by blurring of vision and less frequently by blindness. Ophthalmoscopic examination reveals arteriolar changes in most patients in whom hypertension has been established for some time. Edema of the optic disks or retinas appears in more than half the patients, and exudate and hemorrhage have approximately the same incidence. These changes in the fundi may occur singly for years and may vary in degree from time to time, but when all the changes enumerated are present, the duration of life is, as a rule, less than two years.

The *blood* in chronic glomerulonephritis may remain normal for many years, but anemia finally develops in most patients. Thus, in the Presbyterian Hospital series, the red blood count was less than 3,000,000 per cubic millimeter in about 60 per cent of the patients in advanced stages of the disease. Many factors contribute to this anemia. Among them are hemorrhage, aplasia of the bone marrow and arrested maturation as well as a hemolytic factor. The development of anemia is usually gradual, and yet the writer has seen the hemoglobin fall more than 30 per cent in twelve days, without hemorrhage, without increase in bilirubinemia, without increase in reticulocytes and in the face of repeated transfusions. The white blood cells show no particular change from normal except in advanced uremia, when brisk leukocytosis is common. The hemorrhagic diathesis seen in uremia results from an increase in capillary fragility. Bleeding from the nose or gastrointestinal tract or purpura develops terminally in about two thirds of the patients. The changes in the serum proteins and lipids in the nephrotic phase of glomerulonephritis are described elsewhere, inasmuch as they are qualitatively and quantitatively the same as in true nephrosis. In advanced glomerulonephritis the serum proteins may be normal or decreased in amount.

The *urine* in chronic nephritis varies in its characteristics, depending upon the degree of activity of the disease. In the latent phase, proteinuria may be minimal or marked, and cylindruria is variable, and, by arbitrary definition, red blood cells in the urinary sediment, if present at all, are few in number. When the nephritis is active, red blood cells are numerous and the urine has the characteristics of that seen in acute nephritis; it may be smoky in appearance or even grossly bloody. Microscopic hematuria may be recurrent and transient in nature or may persist over a period of years. In general, cases in which red blood cells persist in large numbers run a relatively rapid course. How-

ever, the writer has seen one patient who, under almost constant observation, showed persistent and marked microscopic, and at times macroscopic, hematuria for twelve years before she succumbed to her disease. In the nephrotic phase of chronic nephritis the urine contains large amounts of protein, whereas red cells though occasionally numerous, are at times present in only small numbers, thus making it difficult in the latter case to distinguish it from true nephrosis. As nephritis progresses, and usually when the kidneys have become reduced in size through extensive fibrosis, the specific gravity becomes fixed between 1.008 and 1.012. In this advanced stage, proteinuria, cylindruria and microscopic hematuria frequently decrease strikingly. The late changes in renal function receive their physiologic explanation through the fact that few glomerular units are capable of function and tubular degeneration prevents normal reabsorption and secretion.

As the ability of the kidneys to concentrate gradually diminishes, the patient compensates for this physiologic defect by increased thirst and increased ingestion of fluid. *Nocturia,* i.e., nocturnal polyuria, ensues and occasionally constitutes the presenting symptom in patients whose disease has progressed silently to an advanced degree.

Renal function may decrease rapidly and a patient may die in uremia in the course of a few months after the onset of the disease. On the other hand, in many cases of chronic glomerulonephritis there may be normal renal function for many years as measured by the usual tests. Thus the ability to concentrate is gradually impaired and the urea clearance decreases, as does the excretion of phenolsulfonphthalein or other dyes. These are reflections of severe impairment of glomerular filtration, renal blood flow and tubular function. As impairment of function advances, particularly if the fluid intake of the patient be restricted, accumulation of the end products of nitrogen metabolism gradually takes place over a period of many months. In other patients the specific gravity of the urine may remain fixed for months or years without associated nitrogen retention; and then, either with or without the development of cardiac insufficiency, or in the presence of infection, or after an operation, renal decompensation may occur rapidly and the patients die in uremia in the course of a few weeks. In exceptional cases severe renal decompensation, as indicated by nitrogen retention, may be present for years. For example, the author had a patient who, after six years of active glomerulonephritis, proved post mortem, reached a point where her excretion of phenolsulfonphthalein in two hours was nil, her blood urea was 90 mg.

in association with tubular defects, hypokalemia may be present.

Diagnosis. The diagnosis of chronic glomerulonephritis is usually simple and is based on the continued presence of proteinuria, cylindruria and varying degrees of microscopic hematuria, either with or without

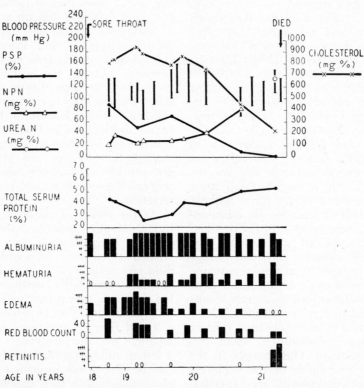

Fig. 135. Chronic glomerulonephritis with rapid progression. This patient's disease began with classic acute glomerulonephritis. The nephrotic state then developed, and, as it abated, rapidly progressive and fatal renal insufficiency ensued in less than two years.

per 100 cc. and her creatinine was 6 mg. per 100 cc. She worked most of the time during the next six years, and annual observations showed persistence of markedly impaired renal function with further accumulation of urea in the blood. Late in her disease she had also an acidosis, which is common terminally. These cases of prolonged renal insufficiency, when they occur early in childhood, produce *dwarfism* associated with osteomalacia and are described as *renal rickets*. The nature of the chemical disturbances occurring in advanced nephritis is discussed in the chapter on Uremia. Hyponatremia, hyperkalemia, hypocalcemia and hyperphosphatemia are common electrolyte disturbances, as is acidosis. Infrequently and

extrarenal manifestations of the disease. Not infrequently persistent proteinuria alone constitutes the only evidence of the disease for many years. In a number of circumstances, however, the diagnosis is difficult, and yet it is important from a practical standpoint, for prognosis and therapeutic indications may depend upon it. It has already been pointed out that the differential diagnosis between acute nephritis and an exacerbation of chronic nephritis is at times impossible. Nevertheless, marked enlargement of the heart, extreme degrees of hypertension, thickened and tortuous arteries, changes in the eyegrounds, severe anemia, marked lowering of the serum proteins and fixation of the specific gravity of the urine point definitely to a chronic process, although they do not, in rare instances, preclude the possibility of the acute form with a subsequent favorable outcome. The differentiation of the nephrotic phase of chronic glomerulonephritis and true nephrosis is also difficult. In both of these, depression of the basal metabolic rate, lipemia, hypoproteinemia characterized by hypalbuminemia and heavy proteinuria occur. Marked elevation of the blood pressure, enlargement of the heart, gross or marked microscopic hematuria and changes in the eyegrounds make chronic glomerulonephritis the more likely diagnosis. The age of the patient also lends some significance, since true nephrosis among adults is extremely rare. Even these criteria fail at times. Among the writer's patients was a boy of 15 who was proved at autopsy to have pure nephrosis, despite the elevation of blood urea to 100 mg. per 100 cc., and despite the fact that his blood pressure reached a level of 160/100 and that occasional red cells were present in the urinary sediment. The differentiation between orthostatic proteinuria and nephritis is discussed elsewhere.

In all patients presenting the picture of advanced renal insufficiency the possibility of renal disease other than nephritis must be borne in mind. Bilateral pyelonephritis with or without stones, periarteritis nodosa, bilateral renal tuberculosis, hydronephrosis due to ureteral or prostatic obstruction and advanced polycystic disease of the kidneys may all terminate in uremia. Hence, when confronted with advanced renal disease in which the etiology is not certain, it is often impossible to characterize the renal lesion without knowledge of the natural history of the disease and the application of the appropriate urologic techniques.

Prognosis. The prognosis in chronic glomerulonephritis is ultimately bad, but the speed with which the disease reaches its fatal termination is extremely variable. It is practically impossible to estimate the probable life span of a patient on the basis of a single set of clinical observations and tests of renal function, and it is not infrequently difficult to estimate it even with the aid of repeated observations over a period of months or years. For example, a patient may be seen in an acute exacerbation of the disease and then may enter the latent phase and lead a normal and useful existence for many years before his disease reaches the uremic state. On the other hand, another patient may have

nephritis of apparently identical severity and yet his disease may progress to its termination in a few weeks or months. The variations in the course of the disease and the attendant difficulties in predicting the rate of progression are depicted in Figures 135–137.

Despite these discouraging comments, there are features of the disease which distinctly facilitate prognosis. If the disease is accompanied by progressive elevation of the blood pressure, the outlook for more than a few years is poor. When progressive cardiac insufficiency develops, a return to a more benign course is distinctly unusual. The presence of choked disks, arterial changes, hemorrhages and exudate in the eyegrounds offers, as a rule, a prognosis of less than two years. The progressive development of anemia likewise indicates that an advanced stage of the disease has been reached. Pericarditis is an ominous sign, and its appearance is almost invariably terminal. Single tests of renal function, except relatively late in the course of chronic glomerulonephritis, offer little of prognostic value, but repeated observations made in the course of the disease may reveal a curve indicating the velocity of its progression. When the urea clearance is reduced to minimal values, when the excretion of phenolsulfonphthalein is virtually zero and nitrogen retention increases progressively, the prognosis can often be measured in months instead of years. It must be recognized, however, that there are many exceptions to the general statements, as shown by Figure 137, as well as another of the writer's patients who was able to continue work for six years after her excretion of phenolsulfonphthalein and the level of blood urea and creatinine suggested a prompt demise. Another patient, whose blood urea was 500 mg. per cent and who had profound anemia, left the hospital after treatment with transfusions and infusions and worked for eight months before death occurred.

Treatment. In the latent stage of chronic nephritis there are no therapeutic indications other than warning the patient against overfatigue and ridding him of obvious foci of infection, particularly in the upper respiratory tract. Certainly dietary restriction is not indicated when the only pathologic manifestations are proteinuria and cylindruria. Patients in this phase of the disease should be instructed to seek medical aid if symptoms or signs develop, and they should be seen by their physician routinely, at perhaps yearly intervals, in order to have the status of their disease appraised. This annual survey should include examination of the urine, a blood count, blood urea and serum protein determinations as well as a physical examination with emphasis laid on the heart, blood pres-

the basic principles involved. The custom of forcing the protein intake beyond the body requirements, in the writer's experience, has failed to attain its theoretical end, namely, that of raising the serum protein level. Addis believes that it is of vital importance to keep the protein of the diet at the lowest possible

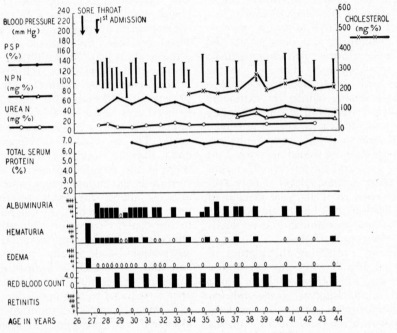

Fig. 136. Chronic glomerulonephritis with slow progression. This patient's disease began with typical acute glomerulonephritis. In contrast to the case illustrated by Figure 135, the nephrotic phase was absent and, except for some reduction in phenolsulfonphthalein (PSP) excretion, there was no evidence of progression over seventeen years of observation.

sure, eyegrounds and presence of edema. Abnormalities found in the course of these studies may necessitate the instigation of active therapeutic measures. If activity develops as determined by hematuria, particularly if associated with edema and hypertension, bed rest is indicated and the treatment is that of acute nephritis. The patient should be urged to remain in bed at least until the generalized signs have disappeared and, if possible, until microscopic hematuria becomes minimal.

In the nephrotic phase, also, bed rest is indicated, since this tends to inhibit the development of edema. It is in this phase of chronic glomerulonephritis that the most definite indication for dietary regulation is encountered. Rigid salt restriction and the incorporation of enough protein in the diet to maintain nitrogen equilibrium constitute

level compatible with nitrogen equilibrium. In the opinion of the writer, the evidence presented does not warrant this rigid restriction of protein. Details of this aspect of therapy are discussed in conjunction with the nephroses. Patients in the nephrotic state are especially susceptible to infection of the respiratory tract, which should be treated promptly with an antibiotic active against the invading organism.

The symptomatology associated with *hypertension* is particularly distressing to patients. The *headaches,* sleeplessness, nervousness and irritability are trying. Sedatives, particularly chloral hydrate in small doses, are useful in the treatment of these symptoms. Daily periods of rest and the avoidance of unnecessary physical exertion which may add further cardiac strain are also of great importance, as is the prevention of obesity through dietary restriction. The treatment of hypertensive encephalopathy has been discussed in the chapter on Acute Nephritis. The use of antihypertensive drugs in severe chronic nephritis with renal decompensation is of no value and may prove harmful.

venous pressure, especially when associated with pulmonary edema, phlebotomy may afford relief. This procedure naturally has no place when anemia is present. The use of diuretics, particularly the mercurials, is contraindicated in the presence of advanced

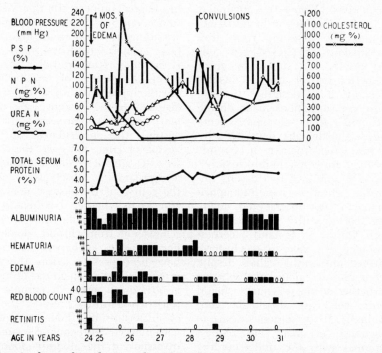

Fig. 137. Chronic glomerulonephritis with prolonged renal insufficiency. This patient's disease was first recognized with the appearance of the nephrotic phase. He had advanced renal insufficiency for five years. Despite marked nitrogen retention and convulsions five years before, he is still able to continue working full-time.*

Cardiac insufficiency, whether incipient or outspoken, demands bed rest, and the principles involved in its treatment are those which apply to cardiac decompensation in general. The problem of fluid regulation is difficult because some limitation is indicated in congestive heart failure, whereas with renal insufficiency, enhanced by the inability to concentrate, the liberal ingestion of fluid should be maintained to curb nitrogen retention. In such a situation the treatment of the cardiac insufficiency deserves first consideration, and moderate restriction of fluid, perhaps to 2500 cc. a day, may be tried. Salt restriction and a "cardiac diet" with an allowance of about 50 gm. of protein a day should be tried. Digitalis and sedatives are indicated as in other congestive disorders of the heart. In the presence of an elevated

renal insufficiency, since these substances not infrequently induce hematuria or anuria or may cause severe sodium depletion in advanced nephritics who already fail to reabsorb sodium salts adequately. Though cardiac insufficiency causes some depression of the excretion of phenolsulfonphthalein as well as of urea, its effect on renal function is not extreme. For example, if the "phthalein" excretion in 2 hours is less than 30 per cent and if the blood urea is higher than about 75 mg. per 100 cc., it is probable that nephritis is present in addition to congestive heart failure. In these cases of cardiac decompensation, in which the integrity of the kidney is in doubt, the use of diuretics should be undertaken with caution. Rigid salt restriction in the absence of edema and heart failure is unwise as it often increases nitrogen retention by decreasing glomerular filtration.

The treatment of the *anemia* of chronic

* Figures 135 to 137 were prepared by Dr. Richard Keating and Dr. William Watson.

nephritis is both important and difficult. Profound anemia contributes to weakness, cardiac insufficiency, edema and probably to the degree of renal failure. The effects of large doses of iron and of liver extract are notoriously disappointing, as might be anticipated from the fact that the anemia is essentially aplastic in type. When the anemia is hypochromic, perhaps because of hemorrhage, some benefit may be expected from iron therapy. Transfusions of packed red cells offer the best results, but should be given slowly. If hypertension or cardiac insufficiency be present, it is desirable to have venous pressure determinations made during transfusions in order that pulmonary edema may be avoided. Cobalt salts have been reported to relieve the anemia of chronic nephritis but they are often highly toxic.

Pregnancy, as a rule and for reasons unknown, intensifies chronic glomerulonephritis. If pregnancy is not interrupted, many patients either abort or suffer a toxemia after the fifth month. On the other hand, a certain number of women are able to reach term and are delivered of healthy babies despite the presence of chronic glomerulonephritis. In deciding whether or not pregnancy should be terminated, each case should be considered individually. If the patient's desire to continue pregnancy is great, her request should be granted with the understanding that premature labor may have to be induced promptly if the blood pressures rises, edema increases or other signs of toxemia begin to appear.

The problems concerned with the management of advanced nephritis are discussed in the chapter on Uremia.

ARTERIOLAR NEPHROSCLEROSIS

Hypertensive vascular disease terminates in cerebral hemorrhage, cardiac insufficiency or uremia. Here we are concerned with that 10 per cent of patients whose disease leads to renal insufficiency. The term "arteriolar nephrosclerosis" is applied to involvement of the renal area by hypertensive vascular disease, giving rise to disturbances in renal function associated with the development of a clinical picture identical with that of chronic glomerulonephritis.

Etiology and Mechanism. The etiology and mechanism of hypertensive vascular disease are discussed in the chapter on Vascular Hypertension.

Clinical Picture. The clinical picture of arteriolar nephrosclerosis is dominated by the various manifestations of hypertension. For months or years, depending upon the rate of evolution of the disease, the urine shows no abnormalities. Then, if cardiac or cerebral complications do not terminate the disease, proteinuria and cylindruria of varying degrees appear. In this stage, hypertension alone, with the symptoms and signs attending it, serves to distinguish the disease from glomerulonephritis in the latent phase. If the progress of arteriolar nephrosclerosis is rapid, the picture of rapidly advancing nephritis appears within a few months. If the disease is of the "benign" type, renal function may not be compromised for many years despite the persistence of albuminuria. Sooner or later, however, the clinical picture seen in advanced glomerulonephritis makes its appearance. Observations made early in the course of the disease may give the only clue as to whether a patient with advanced nephritis is suffering from arteriolar nephrosclerosis or from chronic glomerulonephritis. For example, if hypertension is known to have been present before the appearance of proteinuria, the diagnosis of nephrosclerosis is obvious, whereas in chronic glomerulonephritis proteinuria precedes the development of hypertension. The nephrotic syndrome with marked depression of serum proteins and inversion of the albumin-globulin ratio also serves as a distinguishing feature, since it does not occur in arteriolar nephrosclerosis; e.g., the serum protein concentration was found to be greater than 5 per cent in 16 of 17 patients dying of the disease at the Presbyterian Hospital. *Edema* occurs in about 70 per cent of patients with nephrosclerosis and is due either to associated cardiac insufficiency or to the fact that the remaining glomeruli are incapable of function adequate to maintain water balance.

It is often stated that the presence of *hematuria,* either gross or microscopic, is much more characteristic of glomerulonephritis than of nephrosclerosis, but of 46 patients dying of the latter condition 3 had gross hematuria, and red cells were found microscopically in the urine of 32. It can be shown statistically that the *degree of hypertension* tends to be greater in nephrosclerosis than in chronic glomeronephritis. In the Presbyterian Hospital series of patients with nephrosclerosis examined post mortem, 26 of 37 patients had a systolic pressure above 230 mm. of mercury. Thus the incidence of hypertension of this order of magnitude is greater in this group than in the corresponding group with chronic glomerulonephritis. However, in an individual patient the blood pressure level can have no differential diagnostic significance. The blood pressure shows wide fluctuations, depending upon the mental state and the amount of physical activity, but, as the disease progresses, the favorable effect of rest becomes less apparent. *Cardiac hypertrophy* occurs with great regularity in arteriolar nephrosclerosis. *Dyspnea* and *congestive heart failure,* with or without pulmonary edema, are equally common in both diseases. *Headache,* as might be anticipated, is one of the commonest complaints and had been present in 80 per cent of the series studied post mortem at the Presbyterian Hospital. It varies in intensity, as is true in glomerulonephritis. The *eyegrounds* showed definite arterial changes in over 90 per cent of the Presbyterian Hospital series. Exudate, hemorrhages and papilledema were each present at some time in about 70 per cent of the patients dying of arteriolar nephrosclerosis. Many statements in the literature suggest that the retinopathy of arteriolar nephrosclerosis may be differentiated with great regularity from the changes present in chronic glomerulonephritis with hypertension, but in the experience of the writer, this is not so. The *anemia* associated with advanced nephrosclerosis may be of the same severity and type as that present in glomerulonephritis, although it appears to occur a little less frequently. Disturbances in *renal function* are naturally dependent upon the extent of the arteriolar nephrosclerotic process, but when the disease progresses to an advanced stage, the loss of the ability to concentrate, the depression of urea clearance and excretion of phenolsulfonphthalein and the retention of the end products of nitrogen metabolism occur just as in late glomerulonephritis. There is greater relative depression of renal blood flow than of glomerular filtration rate in patients with early arteriolar nephrosclerosis. The opposite is found in glomerulonephritis, but has no practical significance.

Diagnosis. The diagnosis of arteriolar nephrosclerosis is suggested by the presence of hypertension antedating the appearance of proteinuria and cylindruria, terminating in uremia. The difficulties, both clinical and pathologic, encountered in differentiating this disease from chronic glomerulonephritis have been discussed. They are of only academic importance, since the prognosis and therapy of both disorders are essentially the same when that stage is reached in which identical physiologic disturbances are present.

Arteriolar nephrosclerosis may result from pyelonephritis; when this is suspected, urologic studies may clarify the diagnosis. Unfortunately, when the stage of arteriolar nephrosclerosis has been reached, the mechanism of its production alters neither therapy nor prognosis.

Prognosis. Patients suffering from arteriolar nephrosclerosis die eventually of uremia unless cardiac insufficiency or cerebral hemorrhage terminates the disease. The disease may be rapidly progressive, running its course in a few months, or it may progress gradually over a period of many years. In a number of cases it may change its nature abruptly, the slow progress of the so-called "benign" form becoming accelerated and the rapid downhill course of the so-called "malignant" type then leading to uremia in the course of some weeks.

As is also true of glomerulonephritis, no prognosis can be given on the basis of a single series of observations unless the picture of advanced nephritis is present. In the absence of demonstrable renal insufficiency, it is frequently impossible to prognosticate the course of arteriolar nephrosclerosis even with observations extending over some years. The height of the blood pressure is occasionally believed to have prognostic significance, but the rate of progression of renal insufficiency can in no way be correlated with the degree of hypertension. For example, the writer had a patient whose blood pressure at 33 years was 268/160. Her eyegrounds at this time showed arteriolar changes, and her urine contained a little albumin. This patient was seen regularly over a period of twelve years, after which time her blood pressure was still above 250 mm. of mercury. Her urine continued to show only a faint trace of albumin, her blood urea was normal, and at autopsy (death resulted from cerebral hemorrhage) only moderate nephrosclerosis was present.

Treatment. In the absence of any specific therapy, the medical treatment of nephrosclerosis resolves itself into the management of hypertension and of chronic nephritis, both of which are discussed elsewhere in this volume.

A considerable variety of surgical measures has been introduced in the treatment of hypertensive vascular disease. The most promising of these consists in the resection of the splanchnic nerves. In selected cases this approach to therapy appears to offer the patient more than does the alternative laissez faire attitude. The rice diet of Kempner may reduce the blood pressure and serum cholesterol level in patients with arteriolar nephrosclerosis. On the other hand, nephritic patients maintained on this regimen may suffer severe sodium depletion. Furthermore, nitrogen retention may actually be enhanced through a further decrease in glomerular filtration. The value of chemical agents in reducing blood pressure is discussed in the section on Vascular Hypertension.

MISCELLANEOUS NEPHRITIDES

ACUTE INTERSTITIAL NEPHRITIS

This constitutes an anatomic rather than a clinical entity and is characterized by a diffuse infiltration of the renal interstitium with red blood cells, polymorphonuclear cells and lymphocytes. Edema of the tissues may be present also. There are no characteristic glomerular or tubular lesions. This disorder of the kidneys is usually associated with severe sepsis or with diphtheria and constitutes a postmortem finding without known clinical significance.

TRANSFUSION NEPHRITIS

This type of nephropathy (not nephritis) usually follows transfusion from a donor whose blood is incompatible with that of the recipient, although occasionally no incompatibility can be demonstrated by the usual methods of blood grouping. There is usually a chill after transfusion. The patient then may have hemoglobinemia and hemoglobinuria, and jaundice may appear. In the next 24 to 48 hours, oliguria, complete anuria and edema make their appearance. The classic picture of uremia develops and may end fatally in ten to twenty days. A number of patients recover spontaneously even though almost complete anuria persists for ten to twelve days. Anatomic examination reveals that the kidneys are swollen. Histologically, the capsular spaces and, more particularly, the tubules are found to be filled with precipitated hemoglobin. The glomerular tufts are often ischemic, and the interstitium is edematous. The treatment of oliguria or anuria is discussed in the chapter on Urinary Suppression.

FOCAL NEPHRITIS

Probably most cases of so-called "focal nephritis" (characterized by albuminuria, cylindruria and microscopic hematuria without extrarenal signs and symptoms) are either true glomerulonephritis, as has been intimated elsewhere, or are embolic in nature, appearing in the course of infection. In other cases probably nephritis is not present at all, and the albuminuria, cylindruria and microscopic hematuria merely represent the result of increased capillary porosity occurring in febrile disease.

SYPHILITIC NEPHRITIS

Rich has described a characteristic histopathologic picture in the kidneys of a number of patients with tertiary syphilis. These changes consist in a diffuse infiltration of the interstitium with lymphocytes, macrophages and plasma cells. The process characteristically shows encroachment of these cell accumulations upon the tubules in which there may be deposits of cholesterol crystals. In later stages, scarring of the interstitium, atrophy of tubules and hyalinization of glomeruli take place. The clinical picture in these cases is indistinguishable from that of certain cases of chronic glomerulonephritis or of arteriolar nephrosclerosis. If the etiology of an existing nephritis could be established as syphilitic, active specific therapy might alter the course of the disease. In patients presenting the clinical picture of arteriolar nephrosclerosis combined with syphilis, an intensive course of penicillin may be indicated.

ARTERIOSCLEROTIC NEPHRITIS

Arteriosclerosis of the larger branches of the renal artery at times gives rise to areas of fibrosis in the renal parenchyma, characterized on gross examination by large depressed scars. It is extremely rare to find the functioning renal tissue reduced by this degenerative process *per se* to the point of serious renal insufficiency, even though the kidney reserve may be definitely compromised. Using inulin and Diodrast clearances, Shock has found that normal persons over 60 years of age reveal an average decrease in glomerular filtration of 40 per cent and a decrease in Diodrast clearance of about 55 per cent.

RADIATION NEPHRITIS

Following the exposure of the renal areas to radiation in dosages usually exceeding 2500 r, there may appear acute radiation nephritis after a latent period of about eight months. This may subside or give rise to a progressive chronic nephritis. Radiation nephritis is characterized by edema, hypertension, anemia, varying degrees of azotemia, proteinuria, cylindruria and some red cells in the urinary sediment. In some patients "malignant" hypertension supervenes.

CAPILLARY GLOMERULOSCLEROSIS

(*Kimmelstiel-Wilson Syndrome*)

See section on Diabetes Mellitus.

ORTHOSTATIC PROTEINURIA

(*Orthostatic Albuminuria, Postural Proteinuria*)

Orthostatic proteinuria is a physiologic disturbance in which protein appears in the urine in the erect lordotic position and at times in the supine lordotic position. The proteinuria disappears when the subject lies flat or assumes the kyphotic position. In Bull's classic studies postural proteinuria could be induced in the erect lordotic position in about 75 per cent of normal males 14 to 16 years of age, in about 30 per cent of men between 20 and 30 and in only 10 per cent of older men. It can be induced in females as well as males and contrary to general impression it is independent of body fluid. The concentration of protein may be in excess of 600 mg. per 100 cc., but in the majority it is less than 100 mg. per 100 cc. When postural proteinuria is induced, there is an accompanying increase in all the formed elements in the urine. The induction of orthostatic proteinuria in some patients is accompanied by temporary decreases in effective renal blood flow and filtration rate, and it is believed to result primarily from renal venous congestion. Follow-up studies of patients exhibiting the disorder give no evidence that they tend to develop nephritis or other renal diseases.

The differentiation of postural proteinuria and latent glomerulonephritis is of great importance. In the latter condition proteinuria does not disappear in the recumbent position whereas it does in the former. Indeed, Bradley has shown that it may actually increase in total amount. To establish the diagnosis of orthostatic proteinuria, the patient should retire at nine after emptying the bladder. Without assuming the upright position he should void at midnight and this specimen should be discarded. He should then void again in the morning before arising and this specimen should be tested for protein. If absent, orthostatic proteinuria is probable and nephritis unlikely. It should be recognized, however, that patients with nephritis may have superimposed postural proteinuria.

ROBERT F. LOEB

References

Addis, T., and Oliver, J.: The Renal Lesion in Bright's Disease. New York, Paul B. Hoeber, Inc., 1931.

Bradley, S. E., Bradley, G. P., Tyson, C. J., Curry, J. J., and Blake, W. D.: Renal Function in Renal Diseases. Am. J. Med., 9:766, 1950.

Bull, G. M.: Postural Proteinuria. Clin. Sc., 7:77, 1948.

Fishberg, A. M.: Hypertension and Nephritis. 4th Ed. Philadelphia, Lea and Febiger, 1939.

Hill, A. G. S., and Cruickshank, B.: A Study of Antigenic Components of Kidney Tissue. Brit. J. Exp. Path., 34:27, 1953.

Rammelkamp, C. H., Jr., and Weaver, R. S.: Acute Glomerulonephritis. The Significance of Variations in the Disease. J. Clin. Investigation, 32:345, 1953.

Wertheim, A., and others: The Association of Type-Specific Hemolytic Streptococci with Acute Glomerulonephritis at the Presbyterian and Babies Hospitals, New York, N. Y., 1936–1942. J. Clin. Investigation, 32:359, 1953.

THE NEPHROSES

Friedrich Mueller suggested the term "nephrosis" in 1905 to designate such degenerative lesions in the kidney as could not properly be called nephritic, i.e., inflammatory. Since he did not include vascular lesions, the term came to imply disease of the renal tubules. Based on this histologic connotation, numerous clinical conditions known to cause tubular damage have been classified as nephroses. However, a more clinical concept, the nephrotic syndrome, is now the common denominator in classifying the nephroses.

If the presence of the nephrotic syndrome be accepted as the essential criterion, the nephroses include (1) true or lipoid nephrosis; (2) the nephrotic stage of chronic glomerulonephritis; (3) amyloidosis of the kidney; (4) syphilitic nephrosis; (5) intercapillary glomerular sclerosis (Kimmelstiel-Wilson's syndrome); (6) renal vein thrombosis (rare); (7) Tridione toxicity; (8) disseminated lupus. The nephroses which do not manifest the nephrotic syndrome, such as acute tubular necrosis, are discussed in the chapter on Urinary Suppression. The nephrotic stage of chronic glomerulonephritis, amyloidosis of the kidney and intercapillary glomerular sclerosis are discussed in the chapters dealing with renal disease. Disseminated lupus is discussed in the section on Collagen Diseases. The nephrotic syndrome related to intercapillary glomerular sclerosis is always associated with diabetes mellitus, but the pathogenesis is obscure. Syphilitic nephrosis occurs during the secondary and tertiary stages and is usually reversible by antiluetic therapy. Tridione nephrosis appears to be relieved by withdrawal of the drug. Thus it is seen that this syndrome can be caused by a series of widely different underlying disease processes. Their only common component is some degree of affection of the kidney. However, renal function shows no constant alteration, either qualitative or quantitative.

The Nephrotic Syndrome. The nephrotic syndrome may be defined as a clinical state characterized by the presence of edema, albuminuria and decreased plasma albumin. There is usually, in addition, an elevation in the concentration of blood lipids and cholesterol and commonly a lowered basal metabolic rate. The original simple hypothesis that the edema is due to lowered plasma osmotic pressure because of hypoalbuminemia, which in turn is dependent on proteinuria, no longer adequately explains all the facts. However, its importance as a stimulus to the study of pathogenesis in this syndrome cannot be overestimated, and a great credit is due to Epstein, who propounded the theory in 1917. The components of the nephrotic syndrome will be discussed separately, but their considerable interdependence is obvious.

Edema. In spite of many contradictory factors, the Starling hypothesis as applied to the hypoalbuminemia deserves first mention as an explanation of the forces tending to increase extracellular fluid in nephrotic patients. Anasarca can be produced in animals by depletion of the plasma proteins, and there is a gross correlation between serum albumin levels and rate of edema formation. It is assumed that the final equilibrium point is determined by a balance between plasma oncotic pressure in the capillaries and increased tissue tension due to the edema fluid. That decreased plasma osmotic pressure is not the sole factor or, at times, even a significant one is proved by occasional instances in which diuresis and loss of edema occur with no measurable change in serum albumin levels.

The influence of sodium chloride ingestion on the accumulation of edema was recognized long before the Starling hypothesis was introduced into this field, but the mechanism of this influence remains unsolved. Frequent suggestions that the kidney in nephrosis has a specific defect as to sodium excretion (e.g., abnormal tubular reabsorption) have not been established. On the contrary, it has been shown that the nephrotic patient handles ingested sodium in a manner entirely analogous to that of the normal person, except for quantitative differences. This fact is most effectively demonstrated when the normal subject is given salt after he has been on a restricted sodium intake.

Since no extracellular fluid can exist without a certain concentration of electrolytes, largely sodium, it seems reasonable to assume that any tendency toward the accumulation of edema would require proportionate amounts of sodium and that, therefore, if this were unavailable, the process would be more or less inhibited. It has, in fact, been demonstrated by animal experiments that plasma osmotic pressure may be carried to a relatively low level without edema if sodium be eliminated from the diet, and that edema appears promptly when salt is added. This benefit from salt restriction is seen in practically all types of edema and is true of the nephrotic patient.

Although a few observations in capillary wall permeability would implicate it in the production of nephrotic edema, this evidence is not sufficiently conclusive for final acceptance.

Proteinuria. Large quantities of protein (averaging 5 to 10 gm., but reaching 30 gm. or more a day) are constantly found in the urine of patients suffering from the nephrotic syndrome. These proteins are qualitatively identical with those found in the plasma, but albumin predominates so that the electrophoretic pattern of the urine resembles that of normal plasma. It is probable that some defect in the glomerulus is responsible for the proteinuria.

Hypoproteinemia. The characteristic decrease in serum proteins is found essentially in the albumin fraction. The commonly advanced explanation of this lowering of the serum albumin (sometimes as low as 1 gm. per cent) is based on the heavy albuminuria. Although this loss probably plays an important role, it is generally conceded that some other mechanism, such as interference with protein synthesis, is required to cover all the facts. However, current knowledge of albumin synthesis and destruction is too limited to justify specific suggestions. It is of some therapeutic import that a protein intake in these patients which is adequate to produce a positive nitrogen balance, will not influence the serum albumin concentration.

Lowered Basal Metabolic Rate. Although the basal metabolism is usually low in the nephrotic syndrome, the thyroid gland itself apparently maintains relatively normal function. Radioactive iodine (I^{131}) uptake is not decreased and is sometimes elevated. Furthermore, the thyrotrophic hormone of the pituitary gland provokes a normal increase in serum protein-bound iodine. However, the concentrations of protein-bound iodine in the blood are consistently low, owing in part, probably, to its loss in the urine, for significant amounts may be recovered from this source in nephrotic persons.

Increase in Blood Lipids and Cholesterol. Although Richard Bright first described this curious disturbance of lipid metabolism, it has remained a mystery, and no hypotheses of sufficient validity to record have appeared. The plasma may be milky and the cholesterol may reach levels over 1000 mg. per cent. It is probable that lipid abnormalities have a causal relationship to the arteriosclerosis commonly found in nephrotic persons coming to autopsy after the disease has been present for a prolonged period of time.

Therapy. The nephrotic syndrome, whenever it occurs, has certain common therapeutic approaches. Of course, the underlying disease should have first consideration when possible; in syphilitic nephrosis, for example, treatment other than antispirochetal is rarely necessary. But in a majority of cases the basic disease is not amenable to such easy solution, and attention therefore must be concentrated mainly on the removal of edema, the principal source of discomfort. The need for sodium in the accumulation of extracellular fluid presents the same indication for a low sodium diet as in other forms of edema, and the sodium chloride intake should not exceed 1 gm. a day, with careful avoidance of all other sodium-containing substances.

Methods for the elimination of edema may be classified as (1) those influencing renal function, such as the mercurial diuretics; (2) those altering plasma osmotic pressure (plasma expanders), such as infusions of dextran or salt-free human albumin; and (3) nonspecific measures, such as artificial fever from intravenous typhoid vaccine or induced measles (in children mainly) and ACTH or cortisone. For further discussion see treatment of True Nephrosis.

TRUE OR LIPOID NEPHROSIS

Definition and Incidence. True nephrosis is a chronic disease of variable duration in which the nephrotic syndrome exists without evidence of specific underlying disease. Although some writers have denied that there is such a separate entity, asserting that careful histologic search will demonstrate glomerular damage, an increasing volume of opinion is sustaining the opposite point of view. The good prognosis, the peculiar susceptibility to pneumococcal infections prior to the use of antibiotics, the higher incidence in children and the clear-cut lack of renal histopathology early in the course are characteristics not found in other examples of the nephrotic syndrome. It is only fair to add, however, that satisfactory differential diagnosis may require many months of observation.

Nephrosis is a rare disease in adults. During thirteen years of an active special clinic for the study of renal disease, only three or four cases were discovered. On the other hand, the pediatrician finds that, though it is not a common disease in children, it is in no sense a rare one. There is no known sex predominance, nor have any facts as to racial or geographical distribution entered the literature.

Etiology and Pathogenesis. The relationship to infection seen in glomerulonephritis and amyloidosis does not appear to be present in true nephrosis; indeed, no convincing etiologic hypothesis has ever been propounded. Moreover, no unifying mechanism capable of explaining all the characteristic features is apparent in these cases. The high blood cholesterol and the presence of lipoid deposits in the kidneys have caused some writers to suggest that true nephrosis is the result of an obscure disturbance in lipoid metabolism. This has led them to designate it as "lipoid nephrosis." An hypothesis that would satisfactorily elucidate the mechanism of such pathogenesis has not been advanced.

Pathologic Anatomy. Abnormalities in the glomerular basement membranes have been rather consistently demonstrated in nephrosis by the use of trichrome stains. This is true in experimental nephrosis in animals as well as in the human disease. Late in the course, the convoluted tubules of the kidney are often dilated, their cells show advanced degenerative changes, and large quantities of lipoid substances may be deposited in them. There are no consistent changes outside the renal area and the cardiovascular system remains normal except for atherosclerosis.

Clinical Picture. The average case of true nephrosis (and there is little deviation from this average) is characterized chiefly by the insidious development of generalized edema, first gravitational, and later an anasarca with fluid in the serous cavities. There are no typical symptoms other than the mental and physical discomfort dependent on the monotonous and interminable existence of distended, water-logged tissues. The duration of the disease varies from a few weeks to a few years, but the patient eventually recovers and in most instances remains permanently well. There may be several remissions during the course of the disease, but the albuminuria rarely disappears until the cure is complete.

Physical examination in cases of true nephrosis is negative except for massive edema. Arterial blood pressure is rarely elevated, but occasional readings above 150 mm. (systolic) do not necessarily imply the presence of glomerulonephritis.

The *urine* always contains large quantities of albumin. There may be few or many white blood cells, but rarely red blood cells. Casts may or may not be found. Doubly refractile lipoid bodies are seen in the urinary sediment in many of these cases. They are not of special diagnostic significance, for they appear in the nephrotic stage of glomerulonephritis also.

Chemical examination of the *blood* uniformly reveals a low total serum protein content (usually below 4 per cent), and partition of these proteins shows that the serum albumin is greatly reduced with little accompanying change in the globulin fraction. Lipemia in persons with albuminuria has long been observed. Bright, in describing a "typical patient," said, "The serum is milky."

There is an increase in both fats and lipids, but for practical purposes an estimation of blood cholesterol is the most satisfactory clinical test. Most cases have more than 300 mg. per cent of cholesterol in the blood, while some may have above 1000 mg. Blood urea and total nonprotein nitrogen concentrations are normal in most cases, but a transient elevation of blood urea is not evidence against the diagnosis of true nephrosis. Serum chlorides are above normal, if altered at all, whereas sodium and bicarbonate concentrations are little changed. The erythrocyte sedimentation rate is greatly increased. This is probably dependent on the changes in the protein and lipoid contents of the plasma and cannot be interpreted as evidence of infection.

The lowered *basal metabolic rate* so commonly a part of the clinical picture of nephrosis occurs in the nephrotic stage of glomerulonephritis, and its significance has been discussed earlier. Patients with this finding can take large quantities of thyroid extract with little effect on their disease or in some cases on the basal metabolic rate itself.

Diuresis may occur spontaneously, or a remission may follow an unrelated intercurrent infection such as tonsillitis. It should be noted that these remissions may occur with little or no change in the serum protein levels, a fact which indicates that other forces than those dependent upon a lowered osmotic pressure must play a role. After the edema has gone, it is usually apparent that great loss of weight has taken place. At times the convalescent patient is genuinely emaciated. Part of this weight loss may be due to loss of appetite, a complication not infrequently seen in prolonged cases when the patients become greatly discouraged with the apparently endless edema.

Differential Diagnosis. True nephrosis may be confused with any other type of nephrosis exhibiting the nephrotic syndrome. The Wassermann test and other clinical manifestations of syphilis help in the diagnosis of syphilitic nephrosis, as does the fact that the beneficial response to antiluetic therapy is striking. In amyloidosis of the kidney there is usually some other manifestation of amyloid disease, or the focus of infection causing amyloid changes is so apparent that classification is relatively easy. If further diagnostic aid is required, an estimation of the rate of disappearance of Congo red from the blood stream is helpful. This substance, when injected intravenously in appropriate amounts, disappears rapidly in cases of amyloidosis. The rate is accelerated in true nephrosis also, but when 60 per cent or more has vanished in one hour, it is valuable evidence in favor of extensive amyloid infiltration.

The most difficult differential diagnosis, and one that at times is impossible, lies between true nephrosis and the nephrotic stage of glomerulonephritis. A satisfactory past history of acute glomerulonephritis, contemporary evidence of acute glomerulonephritis (hematuria or red blood cell casts) or signs of advanced chronic glomerulonephritis (hypertension, anemia, decreased renal function) would eliminate any indecision. But many of the patients with glomerulonephritis display every part of the pattern observed in true nephrosis with no evidence whatsoever of renal damage other than albuminuria. Then the final outcome of the disease gives the sole answer. Sooner or later, the patient who has uncomplicated nephrosis is likely to recover, but if terminal uremia develops, the underlying process is probably glomerulonephritis.

Prognosis. As has been stated, the prognosis of true nephrosis is relatively good. The writer has seen the duration of the disease vary from several weeks to several years. In spite of their susceptibility to secondary infection, over half of the patients recover and remain well. Although other infections do occur, a large majority is due to the pneumococcus, and peritonitis due to this organism is a common complication. The use of antibiotics in the treatment of pneumococcal infections has altered most favorably the mortality statistics of this disease.

Treatment. The general treatment suggested for the nephrotic syndrome is advisable in true nephrosis. Sodium chloride and sodium bicarbonate are in common use both in food and as home remedies; in either instance they should be carefully excluded. The so-called "salt substitutes" are usually sodium salts of organic acids and are, therefore, likewise to be avoided. As was pointed out when discussing the nephrotic syndrome, excessive protein feeding does not alter the serum protein levels. Protein restriction, however, is obviously contraindicated, for the protein needs of the nephrotic patient are somewhat increased by the excessive loss of protein in the urine.

The value of bed rest is a practical judgment to be made in the individual case according to the amount of edema and general well-being of the patient. Thyroid administration is a common custom when the basal metabolism is low. It is difficult to see any benefit from it.

When an extreme degree of edema produces symptoms, the various types of therapy mentioned under the Nephrotic Syndrome should be tried. Mercuhydrin, 1 or 2 cc. intramuscularly, is the simplest and generally the most effective, although the potential renal toxicity of organic mercurial compounds must be borne in mind. If good diuresis results, it may be repeated once or twice a week. Sometimes the effectiveness of a mercurial diuretic is enhanced by administering 3 to 4 gm. of ammonium chloride during the two or three preceding days. A new and promising diuretic agent is the carbonic anhydrase inhibitor acetazoleamide (Diamox). Its use and its limitations are not yet clearly defined.

The sudden loss of edema that follows acute infections led to the use of fever produced by intravenous typhoid vaccine and induced measles, and both have been successful at times. The use of substances that influence the osmotic pressure, the so-called plasma expanders, gives only temporary benefit. The safest and most economical material for this purpose is dextran. Salt-free human serum albumin is very expensive and no more effective. At the present time, ACTH or cortisone offer the most satisfactory palliative therapy for nephrotic edema. The current dosage is a minimum of 20 units of ACTH gel twice a day or 200 mg. of cortisone a day (50 mg. four times a day) for ten to fourteen days. The possible unpleasant side effects of this type of therapy are well discussed in the writings of Luetscher and others. No evidence that hormone treatment alters the life history of any type of the nephrotic syndrome is available as yet.

Dana W. Atchley

References

Bradley, S. E., and Tyson, C. J.: The Nephrotic Syndrome. New England J. Med., 238:223, 1948.
Epstein, A. A.: Concerning the Causation of Edema in Chronic Parenchymatous Nephritis: Method for its Alleviation. Am. J. M. Sc., 154:638, 1917.
Loeb, R. F., and others: On the Mechanism of Nephrotic Edema. J. Clin. Investigation, 11:621, 1932.
Luetscher, J. A. Jr., Deming, Q. B., Johnson, B. B.,

and Piel, C. F.: Advances in Management of the Nephrotic State. J.A.M.A., *153*:1236, 1953.

Starling, E. H.: On the Absorption of Fluids from the Connective Tissues Spaces. J. Physiol., *19*: 312, 1896.

UREMIA

Definition. Uremia may be defined as a clinical pattern associated with renal insufficiency and nitrogen retention. Although the uremic syndrome rarely occurs without evidence of maximal impairment of renal function, it has, nevertheless, been long recognized that extreme degrees of nitrogen retention may not be accompanied by uremic symptoms and that there is no constant correlation between the degree of nitrogen retention and the severity of the symptoms. The renal insufficiency can be derived from any of the various sources of kidney damage, such as nephritis, bilateral renal infection, mechanical obstruction of the ureters, polycystic kidneys and poison.

In addition to these organic conditions, there are many situations in which renal function is inhibited by physiologic disturbances originating outside the urinary tract. The terms *extrarenal* or *prerenal uremia* have been coined to designate this group. A contraction of the circulating blood volume with consequent decrease in renal circulation is the usual causative mechanism, dependent most commonly upon dehydration, sodium loss, hemorrhage or shock. Attention to the primary disease condition will solve the uremia unless it has been present so long that permanent renal damage has been established.

The first obligation of the physician in appraising a patient with uremia is to determine whether there is an underlying process which is amenable to treatment. In such circumstances renal insufficiency may be reversible and complete cure a possibility. The most scientific approach to the uremia itself would be a futile effort if bilateral obstruction to the ureters were neglected. A thorough urologic study is indicated whenever the diagnosis is in any way uncertain. Furthermore, the attitude of the clinician toward painful and drastic procedures in patients whose kidneys have been damaged acutely by a poison should be different from his point of view when treating the irreversible terminal stages of chronic glomerular nephritis. In the latter instance, comfort is the prime consideration; whereas in the former, life is at stake, and no effort can be spared.

The uremic state manifests itself in many ways, but, for purpose of exposition, one may indicate two major types of effect on the organism. In one group are found the relatively well understood physiologic complications of advanced renal insufficiency: acidosis, dehydration, potassium retention and disordered calcium metabolism. On the other hand, there are a large number of symptoms and signs that are apparently "toxic" in origin, although the nature of these poisons has defied analysis. In this latter group are found such phenomena as headache, vomiting, itching of the skin, pericarditis and anemia.

Manifestations Due to Renal Insufficiency. The *acidosis* which occurs when the kidneys are damaged is dependent upon the important role that the kidney plays in relation to the acid-base regulatory mechanism of the body. The normal kidney has the faculty of manufacturing ammonia to serve as base for the acids that must be eliminated via the renal route. In this way inorganic base is saved and the excretion of excess acid is furthered. Phosphate excretion also aids in this process by virtue of the ability of the kidney to form urine in which the ratio of the acid sodium phosphate to the alkaline phosphate is higher than that which occurs in the blood. When the kidney fails to synthesize adequate amounts of ammonia, and phosphate excretion is pathologically diminished, two of the important stabilizing forces of the acid-base equilibrium are impaired and acidosis occurs. The sulfate ion also is poorly handled by the damaged kidney, so that sulfate as well as phosphate retention is observed in uremia. Acidosis is occasionally so marked that low levels of blood bicarbonate are reached and characteristic hyperpnea may appear. Severe acidosis augments certain of the toxic symptoms such as anorexia and nausea. The electrolyte balance is altered in the same direction by loss of sodium. Such base loss is not uncommon and is due, in part at least, to the polyuria caused by loss of the power of urinary concentration. These profound changes in the extracellular electrolytes are undoubtedly reflected within the cell, producing abnormal conditions which may be responsible for many of the manifestations of uremia.

Sodium depletion and the loss of water which occurs with it as part of hyposthenuric polyuria lead to *dehydration,* one of the commonest and most distressing symptoms in uremia. Anorexia and vomiting markedly augment this tendency. Replacement of salt and water in such an event offers an unusually fruitful type of therapy in this distressing syndrome.

Retention of potassium during the uremic state may reach serious proportions and be a cause of death. Concentrations over 7 mEq. per liter may be dangerous and require active therapy. With modern methods of analysis, the levels of sodium and potassium in the blood are easily obtainable in an increasing number of laboratories. These levels should be carefully followed and serve as a continuous guide to therapy. If chemical quantitation is unavailable, the characteristic changes found in the electrocardiogram may be helpful in discovering potassium retention.

The serum calcium levels in uremia are often significantly below normal. This change is ascribed to the increased phosphate content of the blood and may also be due to a lessening of the percentage of plasma protein if such decrease be present. Obvious clinical *tetany* is an occasional complication to be found in the uremic state, and certain workers feel that much of the muscular irritability and convulsive tendency is due to a disturbed calcium metabolism. Tetany may be precipitated easily in severe uremia by relatively small doses of sodium bicarbonate, given to combat acidosis.

Profound disturbances in the osseous system may result from prolonged exposure of the body to these alterations in calcium and phosphate metabolism, and to chronic acidosis. Before puberty they result in *renal rickets* and in later life in a type of *osteitis fibrosa cystica* with more rarely *calcinosis universalis.* An accompanying hypertrophy of the parathyroid glands often occurs, and it is probable that the bone pathology is due in large part to secondary hyperparathyroidism. Serum calcium levels often return to normal under the influence of an increased production of parathormone.

Urea retention is the most classic physiologic result of renal insufficiency. It is, by definition, always present in uremia, and may play a minor role in the causation of such symptoms as headache and nausea. Ingestion experiments on human subjects do produce such effects, but the blood urea concentrations in uremia evince no consistently parallel relationship to these symptoms.

Creatinine, uric acid, amino acids and other end products of protein metabolism are retained in the blood in uremia. Their individual or collective relationship to the development of the syndrome is still in doubt.

"Toxic" Manifestations. It would be impossible to report the varied investigations devised to discover the poison that seems to play such an important role in uremia. Urea was the first chemical entity proposed, but it has long since been discarded as of no etiologic significance. Various extracts derived from the blood of patients suffering from this syndrome have been injected into animals, and certain toxic effects have been ascribed to them; however, no convincing solution has yet been presented.

The earliest and most *characteristic symptoms* of the uremic state are weakness and anorexia. The patient tires easily and finds active life an increasing effort. Anorexia is an important influence favoring weight loss; in fact, it may be the only cause of the emaciation seen terminally. Nausea and vomiting are constantly lurking in the background, and, when vomiting finally appears, it is difficult to control.

Headaches may appear early, but though they are not infrequent, their severity has been somewhat overemphasized. Most uremic patients, however, complain of "dull sensations," scarcely painful, in the cerebral area.

Disturbances in the mental state are varied and, when present, offer evidence of advanced disease. Restlessness and insomnia may be practically uncontrollable in one patient, whereas another will remain in deep coma. Muscular twitching or convulsions are further evidence of central nervous system involvement, although tetany may be responsible for a certain amount of muscular hyperirritability. It is possible that the itching of the skin should be classified with the symptoms related to the nervous system.

Stomatitis, diarrhea with ulcerative colitis, and membranous lesions of the larynx and trachea are occasional examples of the widespread damage that can appear in the uremic state.

Severe *anemia* appears at some time in most cases of uremia. It is not benefited by the substances which are specific for pernicious anemia. Iron administration is equally futile. Hemorrhagic tendencies are occasionally seen in severe cases. At the Presbyterian Hospital an elevated prothrombin time has been observed in a number of patients who exhibited these hemorrhagic tendencies but probably has no causal relationship to them. *Pericarditis* is a common late complication. No evidence of bacterial infection is available to explain the mechanism of the inflammatory changes. It would seem to be another example of "toxic" damage.

The clinical picture of uremia is hardly a characteristic one. There may be only one symptom or sign, or many. Indeed, nearly all the various manifestations that have been enumerated may be present together. In addition, cardiac insufficiency, coronary disease, cerebral accidents and visual damage may appear, owing to underlying glomerulonephritis or hypertensive vascular disease.

Pseudo-uremia. It is necessary to interrupt discussion of the uremic state in order to mention a syndrome of headache, hypertension, convulsions and other cerebral manifestations that occurs in two diseases more or less unrelated. This syndrome may be confused with true uremia, but careful differentiation is necessary for proper prognosis and therapy. In acute *glomerulonephritis* there may develop a rapid elevation of blood pressure accompanied by severe headache, papilledema, nitrogen retention, coma or convulsions. This condition is believed, by some, to be dependent upon edema of the brain. It usually yields promptly to such measures as intravenous hypertonic glucose solutions, phlebotomy or even lumbar puncture. The parenteral administration of magnesium sulfate represents another effective therapeutic approach. Pseudo-uremia is not a bad prognostic sign if the patient survives the immediate attack; in fact, such cases seem to evolve less often into chronic glomerulonephritis.

The other example of false uremia is seen in *hypertensive vascular disease*. It is less explosive in form here than when it is found in acute glomerulonephritis. Headaches, retinal pathology and convulsions may occur, but nitrogen retention is not a necessary or frequent accompanying sign. There may be other cerebral manifestations such as personality and memory changes or transient paralysis, and the suggestion that there are alterations in the cerebral circulation due to vascular spasm or actual damage seems reasonably supported by the evidence at hand. Fishberg uses the term "hypertensive encephalopathy" to cover the pseudo-uremia of both acute glomerulonephritis and hyper-

tensive vascular disease on the assumption that they have a common pathogenesis.

Prognosis. The prognosis of true uremia is dependent upon the underlying cause of renal insufficiency. When this cause is amenable to treatment, as in prostatic obstruction, the outcome is favorable. When, however, the basic problem is insoluble, as in chronic glomerulonephritis or nephrosclerosis, the onset of uremia is an indication that a fatal termination is not far distant. An increase in blood urea levels may precede such an outcome by many years and during the course of the disease correlate quantitatively in a most unsatisfactory manner with the seriousness of the condition. Retention of creatinine, on the other hand, is found more frequently in the terminal stages of uremia and hence is a bad prognostic sign. Other unfavorable manifestations are severe anemia, pericardial friction rub or convulsions. Prognosis as to duration of life should be guarded, for an occasional patient who apparently is in the terminal stage will have a long remission, remaining in a state of chronic uremia for several years.

Treatment. Therapy in uremia is wholly palliative. An understanding of the disturbed physiologic mechanisms suggests certain rational therapeutic approaches. If a patient is depleted of salt and water, replacement should be effected by intravenous or subcutaneous saline solution. A saline infusion of 1500 cc. will often prove of extraordinary benefit, but cardiac damage is so common a complication of the uremias that it is necessary to exercise great care not to overload the heart. The infusion should be given slowly and the patient constantly supervised for signs of heart failure. When possible, the function of the right heart should be measured by frequent venous pressure observations during the course of the injection. A rapid rise in venous pressure indicates the necessity for changing from the intravenous to the subcutaneous route. In the presence of manifest cardiac insufficiency, clysis is the preferable technique. The parenteral administration of salt solution should continue until urine volume is definitely increased or the appearance of edema proves that the fluid intake has exceeded the remaining functional capacity of the kidney to excrete water.

The chief indication for active treatment of acidosis is the presence of distressing hyperpnea. It may occasionally be combated by the ingestion of bicarbonate of soda by mouth, although great caution should be taken to avoid the production of vomiting or alkalosis. In the presence of nausea the intravenous route of administration is preferable, and 300 to 500 cc. of sixth-molar sodium lactate may be given. Further treatment should be controlled by the response of the blood bicarbonate levels, recognizing the fact that there may be a quick transition from acidosis to alkalosis in the patient with advanced renal failure. The oral administration of aluminum hydroxide is recommended by some clinicians as a measure to combat acidosis because it decreases the absorption of phosphate in the gastrointestinal tract. Tetany is an indication for intravenous calcium therapy (calcium chloride, 10 to 20 cc. of a 5 per cent solution), and some clinicians recommend the use of this therapy for twitching and convulsions, even when tetany cannot be proved. Loss of concentrating ability by the kidney necessitates a constantly high fluid intake in order to maintain an adequate urine volume. Fluid intake therefore should be carefully regulated.

Potassium retention may be combated by the use of glucose infusions accompanied by insulin. This stimulates potassium removal during glycogen storage. Carboxylic resins (hydrogen or sodium cycle) by both the rectal and oral routes are effective agents for the lowering of potassium blood levels.

The dietary problem in uremia consists chiefly in overcoming a more or less severe anorexia. Any food that will interest the patient without upsetting his gastric equilibrium is valid material for his menu. Protein restriction should be enforced as far as is practicable within the limits established by an interest in the total welfare of the patient. No degree of salt restriction is indicated in the absence of edema; it is not only of no value but may be harmful. A new drug, chlorpromazine (Thorazine), has proved of value in combating the nausea so frequently encountered in the uremic patient.

The only effective treatment for the anemia is transfusion. The use of this expensive procedure in a purely palliative role is a matter for practical decision in relation to individual problems. Usually, liver extract and iron do not help the uremic patient suffering from anemia. Cobalt salts may be tried.

One of the most perplexing situations that can arise in the treatment of uremia is found in the incorrigibly restless patient. Fortunately, this is an infrequent complication. Large doses of chloral hydrate, bromides, barbiturates (Nembutal is physiologically the safest in renal insufficiency), morphine and hyoscine may be of little or no avail. Even intravenous paraldehyde may be of only temporary aid.

When cardiac insufficiency complicates the uremic state, all other therapy must be considered secondary to the treatment of this defect. It is unwise, however, to bleed a uremic patient with anemia unless there is a grave emergency. Digitalis, morphine and oxygen are used here in a fashion identical with that recommended in the absence of renal insufficiency.

Purgation, colon irrigation and sweating are not only incorrect in theory, but in many instances are actually harmful to the very sick patients subjected to these drastic measures.

In recent years the use of peritoneal lavage or of some form of the so-called artificial kidney has been recommended in the treatment of uremia. These procedures have no place in the management of uremia resulting from progressive renal disease.

Dana W. Atchley

References

Albright, F., Drake, T. G., and Sulkowitch, H. W.: Renal Osteitis Fibrosa Cystica. Bull. Johns Hopkins Hosp., 60:377, 1937.

Fishberg, A. M.: Hypertension and Nephritis. Philadelphia, Lea & Febiger, 1939, Chapter 10.

Harrison, T. R., and Mason, M. F.: The Pathogenesis of the Uremic Syndrome. Medicine, 16:1, 1937.

TOXEMIA OF PREGNANCY

(Preeclampsia and Eclampsia)

Definition. Toxemia of pregnancy (preeclampsia and eclampsia) is a disorder characterized by an elevation of blood pressure or albuminuria accompanied by salt and water retention occurring only during the last half of pregnancy and often disappearing before and always shortly after delivery. If convulsions or coma do not occur, it is called preeclampsia; if they do occur, eclampsia.

Etiology. Despite an enormous amount of investigation, its cause and pathogenesis are not understood. Though distinct from acute glomerulonephritis, both have many resemblances. Indeed, the only method of clinical differentiation in pregnant women is by urinalysis. Microscopic hematuria is regularly present in acute glomerulonephritis and consistently absent in the toxemia of pregnancy. Casts are present in both.

Morbid Anatomy. Histologically, the most characteristic lesions are degenerative changes in the epithelium of the glomerular tufts and renal tubules and a thickening of the basement membrane of the glomerular tufts. Liver lesions are inconstant, but, when present, consist in changes in the periphery of the lobule. Placental lesions are characterized by infarction and premature syncytial degeneration.

Incidence and Predisposing Factors. The incidence of this disease appears to be about 5 to 8 per cent of all pregnancies. If hypertension is present before (and during) the first half of pregnancy, the incidence of a superimposed toxemia of pregnancy becomes about 50 per cent; i.e., preexisting hypertensive disease is a strong but not invariable predisposing factor to preeclampsia and eclampsia. Generalized edema is another important predisposing factor. It is the rule rather than the exception for generalized edema to appear in normal pregnancy. The cause of this fluid retention in pregnancy is presumably hormonal and is aggravated by at least two factors: (1) hypoalbuminemia, which is a manifestation of hemodilution and in many patients is exaggerated by an inadequate protein intake; and (2) sodium chloride, which is now restricted in the diet from the onset of pregnancy in all leading clinics. This generalized edema is rarely in itself of any seriousness. Its importance, however, lies in the fact that, should hypertension appear in the latter half of pregnancy, the severity of the hypertensive process closely parallels the degree of water and salt retention. Other predisposing factors are age, heredity, diabetes mellitus and twin pregnancies.

Clinical Course. The blood pressure of normal women in the first half of pregnancy is entirely within the normal range. Any elevation that occurs represents hypertension present before the onset of pregnancy. The same is true of albuminuria. The importance of establishing a blood pressure and albuminuria baseline in the first half of pregnancy is therefore obvious. As soon as the twentieth week of pregnancy appears, the mother is a potential candidate for toxemia of pregnancy, the first recognizable manifestation of which is either a rise in blood pressure or an increase in the amount of albumin in the urine above the levels previously observed.

At the onset there are frequently no symptoms, and it is only by measuring the blood pressure and testing the urine that the diagnosis can be made. Depending a good deal on the amount of water retention, the symptoms are frontal headaches, scotomas, dimness of vision, diplopia, nausea, vomiting, dyspnea, orthopnea and manifestations of pulmonary edema. Preceding the development of convulsions and coma (eclampsia), such neurologic abnormalities as dullness of intellect, tinnitus, deafness, abnormalities of taste and smell, delirium, excitement and mania, or somnolence and stupor may occur. During the hours, days or weeks when these symptoms have been developing, blood pressure has steadily risen, albuminuria has increased, and generalized edema with concomitant oliguria and eventually anuria has become more prominent. The patient may lapse into coma interspersed with recurrent convulsive seizures. Death usually occurs during a convulsion or as a result of circulatory collapse and shock.

At any time the process may reverse itself or become reversed by the institution of appropriate therapy. In other cases, despite the implementation of all known therapeutic procedures, the course is progressively downhill and can be reversed only by terminating pregnancy. After delivery, little if any change is observed for 12 to 24 hours, during which time convulsions may still occur, frequently for the first time. After 12 or 24 hours, diuresis occurs, and with the mobilization of fluid during the next 24 hours all symptoms may become exaggerated. Thereafter, symptomatic improvement is progressive. The diuresis may be rapid or require a week or more for completion. The behavior of the blood pressure is variable. It may return to the level that was present before pregnancy immediately, in a few weeks, or only after a period of months. The same is true of albuminuria. Postpartum sequelae depend more on the duration than the severity of the vascular disease during pregnancy. In those instances in which the hypertension or albuminuria, no matter how mild, persisted for more than about three weeks during pregnancy, the blood pressure and urine may never return to their former level. The patient then has permanent hypertensive or renal disease (post-toxemic hypertension or albuminuria), which, over the course of years, runs a course identical with that of hypertensive disease from other causes or similar to that of chronic nephritis.

During the acute phases of this disorder there are no important changes in blood chemistry except for hyperuricemia until oliguria becomes pronounced. Renal function during the acute stages is characterized by a normal renal blood flow and a decreased glomerular filtration. Hepatic function is normal except terminally.

Treatment. Treatment is prophylactic and therapeutic. Prophylaxis depends upon the control of generalized edema. To this end, a high protein diet (100 gm. daily) and restriction of sodium to not more than 2 gm. daily are prescribed throughout pregnancy. If hypertension or abuminuria appears in the second half of pregnancy, therapy again depends largely on the control of water retention, which is best accomplished by bed rest, strict salt restriction and, if tolerated, a high protein diet. Various diuretics have been used, but not with great success. If convulsions or coma supervenes, therapeutic principles consist in (1) heavy sedation for convulsions, (2) intravenous therapy to maintain electrolyte balance in the presence of oliguria and anuria—an exceedingly difficult problem, (3) digitalization for congestive heart failure and (4) the use of depressor drugs for the control of blood pressure. (5) All measures failing, evacuation of the uterus is invariably followed in 24 to 48 hours by a dramatic disappearance of the disease. The reader is referred to standard obstetrical textbooks for the details of management.

LEWIS DEXTER

References

Dexter, L., and Weiss, S.: Preeclamptic and Eclamptic Toxemia of Pregnancy. Boston, Little, Brown & Co., 1941.

Dieckmann, W. J.: The Toxemias of Pregnancy. St. Louis, C. V. Mosby Co., 1941.

Page, E. W.: The Hypertensive Disorders of Pregnancy. Springfield, Ill., Charles C Thomas, 1953.

ANOMALIES AND MALFORMATIONS OF THE KIDNEYS

Definition. Anomalies of the kidney include deviation from the normal in number, structure and position, the result of arrested or faulty embryonic development.

Etiology. The metanephros, or permanent kidney, develops from a bud on the posterior wall of the wolffian duct, and the metanephrogenic cap of mesoblast. The former grows cephalad and forms the ureter, kidney pelvis and, by dichotomous branching, the collecting ducts. From the last develop the convoluted tubules. Failure of union of these with the collecting ducts has been postulated as a cause for congenital cystic kidney, but this is probably erroneous. The kidney pelvis is opposite the second lumbar vertebra in a 9 to 10 mm. embryo, and nearly maintains this position in the adult. With the straightening of the back and development of the pelvic curvature, there is a tremendous lengthening of the ureter, often spoken of as the "ascent" of the kidney. The various anomalies of the kidney can be traced to interruption or aberration of development; they are more common in males, and tend to run in families.

Morbid Anatomy. *Bilateral absence* (agenesis) of the kidneys occurs in about 0.4 per cent of stillbirths, usually in males. *Congenital absence of one kidney* is found about once in 1000 autopsies, is more common in males and on the left side. The ureter is usually absent. The solitary kidney is hypertrophied and often diseased. The presence of both kidneys should always be established before nephrectomy, since more than one patient has died from the removal of a solitary kidney. *Hypoplasia* of one kidney is not uncommon. Only about 51 cases of *supernumerary* kidneys have been reported.

The important abnormalities of form are due to fusion of the kidneys, which may be at the upper or, more commonly, the lower poles (*horseshoe kidneys*); throughout (*cake kidney*); or the upper pole of one kidney may be fused with the lower pole of the other. Persistence of *fetal lobulations* is common and of no significance. *Polycystic kidney* should also be included among congenital malformations.

One (usually the left) or both kidneys may lie in the true pelvis or in the iliac fossa (*ectopic kidney*). When such an ectopic position is congenital, the ureter is short and is distinguished from movable kidney by this fact and the fact that it cannot be replaced in the normal position. Occasionally both kidneys lie on the same side of the spine. *Aberrant blood vessels* are extremely common, but only of surgical interest, except when they cause hydronephrosis by pressure on the ureter.

Anomalies of the ureter are not infrequent, and include bifurcation, at times with two pelves, complete double ureter, implantation in an abnormal position in the bladder or other part of the lower genitourinary tract.

Symptoms. The frequency of renal anomalies (8 per cent of routine autopsies) and the increased susceptibility to disease of anomalous kidneys indicate the clinical importance. Symptoms are usually due to infection, stone or obstruction, and are apt to become manifest in early adult life. In children, anomalies of the vesical neck may cause enuresis, which may be treated as a behavior problem while irreparable damage to the kidney is going on. Asymptomatic duplication of the ureter is of no clinical significance. A horseshoe kidney may occasionally give rise to abdominal symptoms owing to pressure of the isthmus on vessels and viscera. A pelvic kidney may interfere with parturition.

Diagnosis. A presumptive diagnosis of an ectopic or fused kidney can sometimes be made by palpation of a mass. Intravenous or retrograde pyelography, however, is essential for accurate identification.

Treatment. In horseshoe kidneys, division of the renal isthmus and nephropexy may give relief from abdominal pain. Plastic operations or removal of diseased anomalous kidneys in isolated instances has been beneficial. The advent of the modern urinary antiseptics has given better control of infections, but complete cure of the infection is difficult when drainage is poor.

J. M. HAYMAN, JR.

References

Benjamin, J. A., and Tobin, C. E.: Abnormalities of Kidneys, Ureters, and Perinephric Fascia: Anatomic and Clinical Study. J. Urol., 65:715, 1951.
Campbell, M.: Anomalies of the Kidney. New York State M. J., 51:493, 1951.
Carlson, H. E.: Supernumerary Kidney, Summary of 51 Reported Cases. J. Urol., 64:224, 1950.
Nation, E. F.: Horseshoe Kidney, a Study of Thirty-Two Autopsy and Nine Surgical Cases. J. Urol., 53:762, 1945.
Smith, E. C., and Orkin, L. A.: Clinical and Statistical Study of 471 Congenital Anomalies of Kidneys and Ureter. J. Urol., 53:11, 1945.
Smith, H. G.: Bilateral Renal Agenesis. Canad. M. A. J., 65:149, 1951.
Thompson, G. C. V., and Feddersen, A. S.: Congenital Anomalies of Clinical Interest. M. J. Australia, 1:360, 1950.

CIRCULATORY DISTURBANCES OF THE KIDNEY

Chronic passive congestion occurs most frequently in association with chronic myocardial disease, occasionally from obstruction of the inferior cava or from pressure upon the renal veins themselves. *Infarcts* may arise from thrombosis in the course of senile atherosclerosis, but are usually due to embolism. They appear as wedge-shaped lesions with the apex toward the medulla, either uniformly red or with a gray necrotic center and hemorrhagic border. Healed infarcts are represented by deep scars. Symptoms of small infarcts are often lacking or are overshadowed by those of acute infection or endocarditis. Larger ones give rise to sudden pain in the flank and hematuria. There is no special treatment, and the prognosis is good as far as the kidney is concerned except when one of the main renal arteries is blocked. Multiple large bilateral infarcts occasionally result in sufficient destruction of renal tissue to lead to uremia. *Bilateral cortical necrosis* of the kidney is a rare condition occurring usually in the toxemias of pregnancy, but occasionally during infectious diseases or after trauma. The cortex of both kidneys is yellowish, greasy and necrotic, sprinkled with hemorrhages and accompanied by thrombosis of the intralobular arteries. The symptoms are anuria or marked oliguria, albuminuria, hematuria and nitrogen retention. The etiology is unknown, but has been ascribed to vasomotor disturbances with vasoparalysis and secondary thrombosis.

Acute Tubular Necrosis. This subject is discussed fully in the section on Urinary Suppression.

J. M. HAYMAN, JR.

References

Darmady, E. M., and others: Traumatic Uraemia. Lancet, 2:809, 1944.

Duff, G. L., and More, R. H.: Bilateral Cortical Necrosis of the Kidneys. Am. J. M. Sc., *201:428*, 1941.

Dunn, J. S., and Montgomery, G. L.: Acute Necrotizing Glomerulonephritis. J. Path. & Bact., 52:1, 1941.

Hunter, R. B., and Muirhead, E. E.: Prolonged Renal Salt Wastage in Lower Nephon Nephrosis. Ann. Int. Med., 36:1297, 1952.

Lucké, B.: Lower Nephron Nephrosis. Mil. Surgeon, 99:371, 1946.

Oliver, J., MacDowell, M., and Tracy, A.: The Pathogenesis of Acute Renal Failure Associated with Traumatic and Toxic Injury. Renal Ischemia, Nephrotoxic Damage, and the Ischemuric Episode. J. Clin. Investigation, 30:1307, 1951.

Strauss, M. B.: Acute Renal Insufficiency Due to Lower Nephron Nephrosis. New England J. Med., 239:693, 1948.

Trueta, J., and others: Studies of the Renal Circulation. Springfield, Ill., Charles C Thomas, 1947.

NEPHROPTOSIS

(Movable Kidney)

Definition. The normal kidney is not fixed, but moves slightly with respiration and with changes of bodily position. These normal movements are slight. When the displacement is sufficient to allow the lower pole to be palpated on inspiration, the kidney is said to be *movable*. With greater degrees of mobility the kidney may descend so that the fingers meet above it, or it may fall as low as the iliac fossa. *Floating kidney* is one which has become intra-abdominal and has acquired a more or less complete peritoneal covering. Movable kidney is to be distinguished from ectopic kidney, which is congenital and cannot be replaced in the renal fossa.

Etiology. Constitutional factors are important. These include a shallow paravertebral fossa, often associated with a long flat chest, narrow subcostal angle, and ptosis of other viscera (Glénard's disease), defects in the perirenal fascia and lack of perirenal fat. Faulty posture, relaxed abdominal wall following pregnancy, and repeated trauma from coughing, straining, and so forth, are contributory causes. Nephroptosis occurs in about 20 per cent of women and 2 per cent of men, rarely during childhood, most frequently between 20 and 40 years of age. In women the right kidney is movable about five times as frequently as the left, while in men one side is as frequently affected as the other.

Morbid Anatomy. A movable kidney may be perfectly normal and symptomless. When pathologic changes occur, they are the result of interference with the blood supply or kinking of the ureter, and are due to congestion or hydronephrosis.

Symptoms. The great majority of movable kidneys give rise to no symptoms. Many patients, particularly women, who present vague gastrointestinal, dyspeptic or nervous symptoms have a movable kidney. But the relation of such complaints to the kidney is highly problematical, and frequently calling the patient's attention to the kidney only aggravates the symptoms. The degree of mobility has no relation to the type or severity of symptoms. These are due to disturbance of the blood supply, giving congestion and pain, or to obstruction of the ureter. The pain is a dull ache or dragging sensation, located posteriorly in the loin or in front over the kidney, and is relieved by lying down. It may not be present in the morning, but comes on during the day and is aggravated by exercise, menstruation and constipation. Less commonly the pain is acute, colicky, severe, and associated with nausea and vomiting or symptoms of shock, retention of urine and increase in the size of the kidney (*Dietl's crisis*). When the occlusion of the ureter is relieved, the pain ceases abruptly and is followed by the passage of large quantities of urine. Occasionally, colicky pain of similar severity may be due to twisting of the kidney pedicle with obstruction of the renal veins. Other symptoms accompanying movable kidney, as fever, pyuria and frequency, are due to complicating infection or to stone.

Diagnosis. The position and mobility of the kidney are determined bimanually with the patient both recumbent and standing. Intravenous pyelography, with films taken in two positions, is helpful. More important than the determination of mobility is the question whether it is the cause of symptoms. Urinalysis is of little help, for it is usually normal. When symptoms are of renal origin, they are relieved if the kidney is replaced, or can be reproduced by injecting fluid into the ureter. Dietl's crises must be differentiated from attacks of renal colic due to stone: the rarity of hematuria and frequency of polyuria at the end of an attack in the former, and the shadow of the stone on the x-ray film in the latter, usually suffice.

Treatment. In the majority of cases no treatment is necessary. When symptoms are

definitely related to the kidney, an effort
should be made to return it to its normal
position and keep it there. Postural exercises,
increased diet in an effort to add to the
perirenal fat, and an abdominal belt with or
without a special pad below the kidney are
conservative measures which are often successful. Pyelitis, if present, should be treated.
Surgical fixation (nephropexy), which fell
into disrepute because of many failures to
relieve symptoms, has a definite place in selected cases. Operation for a movable kidney
will not relieve psychoneurotic symptoms.
Surgery should be restricted to patients whose
symptoms are known to be of renal origin and
in whom medical treatment has failed. The
chief indication is obstruction to the ureter
and abnormality in the outline of the renal
pelvis on urography.

J. M. HAYMAN, JR.

References

Fish, G. W., and Hazzard, C. T.: Nephroptosis. J.
Urol., 41:336, 1939.
Hinman, F.: Principles and Practice of Urology.
Philadelphia, W. B. Saunders Company, 1936.
McCann, W. S.: Orthostatic Hypertension: Effect of
Nephroptosis on Renal Blood Flow. J.A.M.A.,
115:573, 1940.
Miller, C. O.: Nephroptosis, New Etiologic Concep-
tions. J. Internat. Coll. Surgeons, 15:219, 1951.

HYDRONEPHROSIS

Definition. Hydronephrosis is dilatation
of the pelvis and calyces of the kidney, with
pressure atrophy of its substance.

Etiology. Obstruction of the urinary tract
causes the greatest degree of hydronephrosis
when it is partial, gradual or intermittent.
The obstruction may be anywhere along the
urinary tract. When below the bladder, as in
prostatism or urethral stricture, the lesion is
bilateral, infection is predominant, and the
degree of hydronephrosis less marked. The
cause of the obstruction may be outside the
urinary tract, as neoplasms, adhesions, operative trauma, aberrant blood vessels or pressure from a pregnant uterus. The common
causes of acquired obstruction within the
urinary tract are stone, stricture, spasm,
foreign body and tumor. Many cases are due
to congenital abnormalities in the ureter or
urethra. Displacement of a movable kidney
may be responsible. Occasionally no obstruction can be found.

Morbid Anatomy. The degree of dilatation of the pelvis and distortion of the kidney
varies enormously. At times the sac may contain several liters of fluid. As the size of the
sac increases, the papillae first become flattened, then the renal cortex is thinned, until
finally it is represented only by a thin shell
of tissue. The fluid in the sac is more or
less like urine, but contains far less urea than
normal urine. Secondary infection and calculus formation are common occurrences.

Symptoms. There may be no symptoms
from a sight degree of hydronephrosis. When
the disease is more advanced, the outstanding
sign is palpable enlargement of the kidney.
Other symptoms are pain and tenderness.
When the obstruction is persistent, subjective symptoms are slight and may be limited to dull pain. The kidney seldom attains
a large size, and the urine is normal, for,
since the ureter is blocked, no urine is derived from the affected side. If the obstruction is intermittent, there may be attacks of
pain, accompanied by a definite increase in
the size of the kidney and by oliguria, with
polyuria when the pain is relieved. Accompanying this, there may be hematuria. When
such attacks are severe, they are usually due
to a movable kidney and are known as *Dietl's
crises.* When the degree of hydronephrosis is
more than minimal, the function of the affected kidney is diminished and in advanced
cases may even be abolished. Hypertrophy of
the other kidney may compensate for this defect, so that symptoms of renal insufficiency
do not develop. In bilateral hydronephrosis,
kidney function is much diminished and
uremia may develop. When the obstructed
kidney becomes infected (pyonephrosis),
fever, leukocytosis and pyuria are present in
addition.

Diagnosis. The intermittent type of hydronephrosis is recognized by the association
of pain and renal tumor with oliguria and
their simultaneous disappearance. When the
renal mass is large, it may be mistaken for a
kidney tumor, neoplasm of the retroperitoneal glands, encysted ascites or enlarged gallbladder. In women, ovarian cyst
may cause confusion, but is usually more
movable. Accurate diagnosis depends upon
pyelography, either intravenous or retrograde.

Prognosis. This depends much upon the
cause and degree of the hydronephrosis.
When unilateral and of moderate degree, the
condition may never produce serious trouble.
Spontaneous cure, however, does not occur.

When bilateral, there is always danger of uremia. Finally, there is always the specter of infection with the development of pyonephrosis.

Treatment. The cause of the obstruction should be removed, if possible. This may involve dilatation of a ureteral stricture, removal of a calculus or fixation of a movable kidney. The sac can frequently be drained by means of a ureteral catheter. If useful function has been destroyed, it is usually better to remove the kidney.

J. M. HAYMAN, JR.

BACTERIAL INFECTIONS OF THE KIDNEY AND URINARY PASSAGES

(Excluding Tuberculosis)

Definition. The term *bacterial infections* is used to describe diseases due to the actual presence of bacteria in the kidney and urinary passages.

Etiology. Bacteria may reach the kidney by way of the blood stream (*hematogenous infection*), by way of the ureter or periureteral lymphatics (*ascending infection*), or possibly directly from the intestines by way of lymphatics, especially those which run from the ascending colon and hepatic flexure to the right kidney. Hematogenous infections are by far the most frequent. While bacilluria may occur, as in typhoid fever, without detectable evidence of renal infection, the kidney does not filter bacteria, and their presence in the urine indicates some degree of renal damage. Infection of clinical importance occurs when bacteria come in overwhelming numbers, or continuously, or are particularly virulent, or because of lowered resistance of the urinary passages due especially to obstruction. The physiologic hydronephrosis of pregnancy frequently predisposes to pyelonephritis. Trauma, either from without or as a result of instrumentation of the urinary tract, is a predisposing factor. Infections of the kidney may be caused by almost any organism, but more than half of them are due to *Escherichia coli*. Next in frequency are staphylococci and streptococci, more rarely *Proteus vulgaris* and *Pseudomonas pyocyaneus*. In rare instances, infection of the kidney may result from invasion by *Actinomyces* and parasites such as Filaria, Bilharzia or Strongyloides. Infections of the cortex of the kidney are usually due to pyogenic cocci, while those of the portions of the kidney nearer the pelvis and of the pelvis itself are usually due to the colon bacillus.

Morbid Anatomy. The pathologic changes in the kidney and pelvis vary with the infecting organisms and the route of invasion. Hemolytic streptococcal sepsis usually produces a focal glomerulonephritis or an acute interstitial nephritis. In subacute bacterial endocarditis there are the characteristic focal embolic lesions in the glomeruli. Staphylococcal infection is usually manifest as small abscesses, most abundant in the cortex. The rare unilateral *renal carbuncle* is usually associated with furunculosis, whitlow or some suppurative lesion of bone or joint. Small abscesses may undergo resolution; otherwise they tend to increase in size, coalesce, and may rupture either into the perirenal tissue, leading to the formation of a *perirenal abscess,* or into the renal pelvis, when pyuria will appear.

Other infections involve the renal pelvis (*pyelitis*) and *medulla*. These are usually due to *Escherichia coli,* and may be either hematogenous or ascending. It was formerly believed that *pyelitis* and *pyelonephritis* were distinct entities, but it is probable that infection of the pelvis rarely if ever occurs without some involvement of the collecting portion of the kidney tissue. Clinically, the term "pyelitis" is used to describe those cases in which the infection is not severe enough to lower the function of the involved kidney.

Pyelonephritis may be acute or chronic, and unilateral or bilateral. In the acute stage, ureter and pelvis show various degrees of inflammation; the mucous membrane is red and thickened and at times shows small ulcers or a pseudomembrane. While the kidney may appear normal grossly, microscopic examination reveals scattered patches of cloudy swelling, necrosis, or suppuration in the papillae and pyramids of the medulla. When the disease is chronic, the kidney presents areas of cloudy swelling, suppuration or scar formation, the intervening parenchyma remaining comparatively normal in appearance. At times, the involved areas resemble chronic glomerulonephritis or arteriolar nephrosclerosis. Under such conditions the kidneys are small with narrowed cortex, and show distortion, flattening and reduction in size of the thickened pelvis. Dilatation of the ureter may or may not be present. When destruction of kidney substance is sufficiently extensive, death in uremia is inevitable.

Necrotizing renal papillitis is an unusual condition characterized by necrosis of the tips of the papillae or even the greater portion of a pyramid, which may at times slough into the lumen of the kidney pelvis. It occurs most commonly in patients with diabetes or urinary obstruction or both. There is some evidence that the primary cause is occlusion of multiple small blood vessels, precipitated by a toxic-infectious process. It should be suspected when pyuria and uremia become worse in spite of the control of diabetic acidosis, or in any patient developing fulminating renal failure, with oliguria, nitrogen retention and pyuria.

Symptoms. The symptoms of abcess of the kidney depend on their size and number. Small abscesses occurring in the course of septicemia may give no localizing symptoms. The sudden onset of chill, fever, pain in the loin, and tenderness on palpation of the kidney or in the costovertebral angle should arouse suspicion of renal suppuration in the presence of known infection elsewhere in the body. The urine may present no abnormalities save for the presence of the infecting organism on culture. Extension of the infection into the perirenal tissue (*perirenal abscess*) gives pain and later swelling in the costovertebral angle, pain on motion of the trunk, or spasm of the psoas muscle. The more chronic cases often present considerable diagnostic difficulty, being confused with biliary disease when the right kidney is involved, or with splenic lesions when the left.

The symptoms of *acute pyelonephritis* vary greatly. There may be no constitutional symptoms and no manifestation other than albuminuria and pyuria with some frequency or burning on urination. In the so-called typical attack the onset is sudden, or may follow a few days of malaise with chill, fever of 39° C. or more, headache, prostration, pain in the loin which may radiate along the course of the ureter, and leukocytosis as high as 20,000 per cubic millimeter or higher. In some cases leukocytosis is absent. The sudden onset of pain in the back, fever and leukocytosis may resemble that of lobar pneumonia; if the pain is along the course of the right ureter, it may be mistaken for acute appendicitis. Chills and remittent fever may last several days. The urine contains bacteria, albumin and varying amounts of pus. The largest amounts of pus are found when the renal pelvis and ureter are predominantly involved. The reaction of the urine is neutral or acid when *Escherichia coli* is present, alkaline with *Proteus vulgaris*. Red cells are frequent in the sediment, but gross hematuria is rare.

Chronic bilateral pyelonephritis is more common in women, and often begins as an acute pyelonephritis in childhood or during pregnancy. In men it is usually associated with retention of urine secondary to hypertrophy of the prostate gland. The clinical picture is variable, and frequently the symptoms are so mild that the disease escapes recognition until the terminal stage. A history of an acute attack followed by persistent albuminuria with intermittent pyuria should arouse suspicion. Recurrent bouts of fever with headache, lumbar pain and costovertebral tenderness are increasingly common as the disease progresses. The urine is dilute, increased in volume, and contains a variable amount of pus and albumin. As the disease progresses, renal function becomes impaired, and uremia ultimately terminates a picture which may be identical with that seen in other forms of chronic Bright's disease. The progress of the disease is slow, and patients may present elevation of blood nitrogen for years while remaining in relatively good health. Hypertension occurs in only one quarter of all cases, but in those cases with impairment of renal function it is present in 50 per cent. Usually the hypertension is not of the malignant type, the majority of cases showing a systolic pressure of less than 180. Edema is rare except that due to heart failure. *Chronic unilateral pyelonephritis* can usually be distinguished from bilateral involvement only by urologic study. Nephrectomy, however, has rarely been beneficial, for even where the disease has been unilateral at first, by the time it is discovered there is sufficient nephrosclerosis on the other side to make operation inadvisable.

Diagnosis. The diagnosis of renal infection is rarely difficult if its presence is suspected. Unexplained fever, chills or malaise, bladder symptoms, such as frequency, burning or dysuria, should lead to further study. Pus and bacteria in the urine, obtained by catheter in the female, are convincing evidence of renal infection. These urinary abnormalities serve in particular to differentiate infections of the kidney from acute disease of other abdominal organs, such as the gallbladder or appendix. In tuberculosis of the kidney the onset is insidious and gross hematuria more frequent, while dysuria and frequency are more prominent. Bacteria are not found by ordinary methods, but tubercle bacilli can be demonstrated in a smear of the urinary sediment, culture, or by guinea pig inoculation. All patients presenting evidence of urinary tract infection of uncertain cause should have the benefit of x-ray examination in order to rule out stone as a predisposing factor, and, if the infection persists, urologic study, including pyelograms to detect renal anomalies or partial obstruction with hydronephrosis. Culture of the urine is essential for an accurate diagnosis of the infecting organism. It is often impossible to diagnose a cortical abscess early in the disease, until it ruptures into the pelvis, discharging pus in the urine, or spreads into the perirenal tissues. The diagnosis of perirenal abscess may be extremely difficult. In the presence of pain in the costovertebral angle, with muscle spasm and scoliosis, the demonstration of a high fixed diaphragm, and obliteration of the psoas shadow or irregularity in the outline of the kidney by x-ray examination, are helpful. Treatment, of course, is surgical. Urinary tract infections, however, frequently occur with few or no symptoms. If the symptoms are unrecognized, serious hypertensive vascular disease may result. With some effort on the physician's part they may be recognized while still curable. Bacilluria, even in the absence of symptoms, is probably significant and requires investigation and treatment. Satisfactory care of urinary tract infection cannot be attained until any obstruction present is corrected.

Prognosis. The prognosis in acute pyelonephritis is excellent, the attack usually lasting one or two weeks. The severity of constitutional symptoms, however, bears no relation to the time necessary for the disappearance of bacilluria and pyuria. In pyelonephritis secondary to obstruction of the urinary tract or stone, the chronic form of the disease develops with great regularity unless the underlying cause is removed.

Treatment. Acute pyelonephritis with fever should be treated by bed rest, a soft diet and liberal amounts of fluid, 3000 to 4000 cc. daily. If the urine is highly acid, the intense urgency and dysuria can often be relieved by making the urine alkaline.

The introduction of the sulfonamides and the antibiotics has almost entirely displaced the older urinary antiseptics, such as methenamine, pyridium and mandelic acid. Methenamine (0.5 to 3 gm., three times a day) is occasionally useful for continued administration in the low grade infections of elderly debilitated patients. Streptomycin in doses of 1 or 2 gm. daily is useful in infections with gram-negative organisms, but is frequently ineffective because of the rapid development of bacterial resistance. Chlortetracycline (Aureomycin) and oxytetracycline (Terramycin), 2 gm. daily for seven days, are effective in a high proportion of infections due to both gram-positive and gram-negative organisms. Frequently a combination of antibiotics or an antibiotic and a sulfonamide is more effective than a single agent. The sensitivity of the organisms should be determined by *in vitro* tests.

In general, the sulfonamide compounds have proved highly satisfactory. The chief route of excretion is through the kidneys; the concentration of these drugs in the urine is ten to thirty times that in the blood. It is probably the blood concentration rather than that in the urine which is of greater importance, since the infection is in tissues and not in the lumen of the urinary passages. The sulfonamides are effective against both gram-positive and gram-negative organisms. There does not appear to be any qualitative difference among the sulfonamides with respect to specificity for certain organisms, nor is the reaction of the urine significant. These drugs should be administered with caution because of their toxicity. Sulfanilamide causes no renal complication, but the others may cause toxic damage to the renal tubules or obstruction of the renal pelvis or ureter from precipitation of the less soluble acetyl derivatives. Therefore fluids should not be restricted when these drugs are used. Urine volume should be at least 1000 cc. daily. Administration of 2 to 4 gm. daily of sulfadiazine or Gantrisin in divided doses is usually sufficient. The drug should be continued until two catheterized specimens of urine taken at four-day intervals are found to be sterile on culture. Absence of pyuria alone is not a criterion of cure. Usually a course of from one to two weeks suffices.

Like the sulfonamides, penicillin is many times more concentrated in urine than in blood. It is apparently much less effective than the sulfonamides in *E. coli* infections, but is of value in coccal infections, particularly those due to *Streptococcus faecalis*, strains of nonhemolytic streptococci, which are sulfonamide-resistant but penicillin-sensitive, and for *Proteus vulgaris.*

Satisfactory treatment of cases of *acute pyelonephritis* associated with stone or obstruction to the urinary passages may be impossible until these have been corrected by surgical means.

The treatment of *chronic pyelonephritis* consists primarily in prevention and in the removal of obstruction and stones. For the acute exacerbations of infection the sulfonamide derivatives appear to offer the best results and may at least delay the progress of the disease to the stage of serious renal failure. If urologic study shows that the pyelonephritis is unilateral and that function of the other kidney is good, surgical removal of the infected kidney should be considered.

The treatment of *perinephric abscess* and *renal carbuncle,* like other accumulations of pus, is surgical drainage.

Infections of the Bladder. The bladder mucosa is strikingly insusceptible to infection, so that in almost every instance *cystitis* is secondary to infection higher in the urinary tract, to obstruction to the outlet of the bladder with retention of urine, to genital infection, or to trauma from stone or contaminated instruments. When the primary cause is removed, the infection clears up spontaneously. The bacteria found are those mentioned under pyelonephritis. In rare instances the gonococcus invades the bladder, the lesions being almost entirely confined to the trigone. The pathologic changes are those of acute and chronic inflammation. The symptoms are frequency, pain and pyuria. Urination is more frequent during the day than at night. The pain is usually described as burning, is referred to the meatus, and only gradually subsides after micturition has been completed. In addition to variable amounts of pus, there is not infrequently some blood present, especially in the last urine voided. In chronic cystitis all symptoms are, as a rule, much milder. Accurate diagnosis depends upon cystoscopic examination. The most effective treatment consists in removal of the underlying cause. Palliative measures include abundant fluids, alkalinization of the urine, hot sitz baths, irrigation of the bladder and the instillation of the antiseptics, such as colloidal silver preparation or 1:10,000 silver nitrate. Gantrisin or one of the antibiotics may be helpful.

J. M. HAYMAN, JR.

References

Alexander, J. D., Eisenberg, G. M., and Flippin, H. F.: Combined Antibiotic Therapy in Refractory Urinary Tract Infections. J.A.M.A., 152:1302, 1953.

Knutsen, A., Jennings, E. R., Brines, A. O., and Axelrod, A.: Renal Papillary Necrosis. Am. J. Clin. Path., 22:327, 1952.

O'Conor, V. J.: Urinary Antiseptics: Past and Present: Fact and Fancy. Urol. Survey, 3:75, 1953.

Rhoads, P. S., Billings, C. E., and O'Conor, V. J.: Antibacterial Management of Urinary Tract Infections. J.A.M.A., 148:165, 1952.

Saphir, O., and Taylor, B.: Pyelonephritis Lenta. Ann. Int. Med., 36:1017, 1952.

Silberstein, J. S., and Paugh, J. T.: Necrotizing Renal Papillitis. Ann. Int. Med., 38:689, 1953.

Weiss, S., and Parker, F., Jr.: Pyelonephritis: Its Relation to Vascular Lesions and to Arterial Hypertension. Medicine, 18:221, 1939.

NEPHROLITHIASIS

(Renal Calculus)

Definition. This condition consists in the formation in the calyces or pelvis of the kidney of concretions of crystalline urinary constituents, which may be held together by a stroma of organic material.

Etiology. Nephrolithiasis is about three times as common in males as in females, and is most frequent between the ages of 30 and 50. It is said to be infrequent in the Negro. Heredity is unimportant except with cystine stones, which occur with a hereditary disturbance of metabolism. Calculi are commonly composed of *uric acid, urates, calcium oxalate, calcium phosphate* or mixtures of *calcium* and *ammonio-magnesium phosphate,* more rarely of *calcium carbonate, cystine* or *xanthine.*

Calculi are formed from urinary constituents which remain in solution under normal conditions; why they precipitate in some persons to form stones is obscure. The theory that the constituents of the urine are kept in solution by the protective action of nonprotein colloids and that stone formation results from a disturbance of this equilibrium has not been supported by experimental work. A number of contributory factors are recognized. These include climate, diet, hyperparathyroidism, disorders of metabolism, and local conditions in the urinary tract, especially stasis, infection and marked changes in the reaction of the urine. Stones are more common in hot, dry climates, where the urine volume is small, than in more humid regions.

The relation of *oxaluria* to the formation of calcium oxalate stones was well demonstrated during World War II. Many persons continue to show calcium oxalate crystals in their urine for years without symptoms. The calcium oxalate is generally precipitated after the urine has been passed and cooled, whether the reaction is acid or alkaline. In troops living in a hot dry climate, with inadequate water intake and a diet containing vegetables with a high oxalate content, oxalate crystals may be precipitated in the urinary tract. These crystals are irritants, and may produce gross hematuria, symptoms of renal colic or an epididymitis and cystitis. On cystoscopy there is an intense trigonitis, and oxalate crystals can be seen embedded in the mucosa. The fibrin formed as a result of bleeding provides a matrix for the formation of calcium oxalate stones. Unless obstructive calculi have been formed, the symptoms of oxaluria are relieved promptly by an increased fluid intake.

Excessive ingestion of nucleoproteins may favor the formation of uric acid stones. A high incidence of stone is reported in districts where the water contains a large amount of calcium carbonate. Experimentally, stones can be readily produced in rats by diets deficient in vitamin A. But it is not clear whether these are due primarily to the vitamin deficiency or to infection, changes in the epithelium of the pelvis, relative excess of vitamin D, or some other factor. The relation of vitamin A deficiency to nephrolithiasis in man is undecided. Probably inadequate or unbalanced diets are of more importance in the formation of stones in children than in adults. The work of Albright has established the high incidence of stone in hyperparathyroidism with its accompanying hypercalcemia. These patients may or may not show osteitis fibrosa cystica or osteoporosis. This suggests studies of blood calcium and phosphorus in all cases of renal stone. The influence of abnormal metabolism is also seen in the high incidence of stone in gout, and in the rare cystine stones. Feeding cystine to cystinuric patients, however, does not increase the excretion of cystine, but the administration of the sulfur-containing amino acids, methionine and cysteine, causes a marked increase in cystinuria. Urinary stasis, whether the result of obstruction in the lower urinary tract or of prolonged confinement to bed, favors the formation of stones. Infection not only provides a nidus of bacteria, but, be-cause of the frequent association of alkaline urine, favors the precipitation of phosphates. If urea-splitting organisms are present, recurrence of stone is likely in 75 per cent of cases. Randall believes that calculus formation is dependent upon a preexisting renal lesion and has demonstrated areas of calcifica-

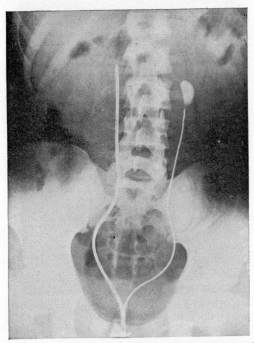

Fig. 138. Retrograde urogram, showing large oval calcium carbonate stone at the left ureteropelvic junction. (Courtesy of Dr. Harry Hauser.)

tion, without evidence of inflammation or infection in the renal papilla. He believes that it is upon a nidus of this type that calculi of various composition develop.

In *nephrocalcinosis* there is diffuse calcification in the renal parenchyma, chiefly in the pyramids, associated with hyperchloremia, lowered plasma bicarbonate, polyuria and a low fixed specific gravity. It is due to the deposit of calcium in damaged cells of the distal tubule. A number of cases have followed the use of sulfonamides.

Morbid Anatomy. The size of the concretions varies from small particles like sand (*urinary gravel*) to large oval or branching (*stag-horn*) calculi which fill the whole renal pelvis and branch into the calyces. Stones may continue to be formed and passed for years without serious kidney damage and with no more inconvenience than the attacks of renal colic. Much more frequently, however, movements of the stone lead to trauma to the pelvis or ureter with severe colic, hemorrhage and secondary infection. Persistent obstruction of the ureter leads to hydronephrosis or pyonephrosis with destruction of the kidney. Stones are bilateral in about 10 per cent of cases, and then almost always associated with

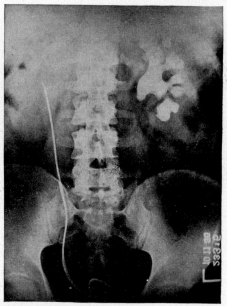

Fig. 139. A large calcium carbonate stag-horn stone in the pelvis of the left kidney. (Courtesy of Dr. E. Freedman.)

infection. A stone rarely persists in a normal bladder. If the nucleus comes from above, the potential vesical calculus is usually passed; retention and growth in the bladder result from obstruction, giving urinary stasis and residual urine. Trauma, inflammation of the bladder and infection follow.

Symptoms. These vary with the size, shape and position of the stone. Minute, smooth stones or gravel may be passed without symptoms. A smooth stone fixed in one of the calyces, and unaccompanied by infection, may remain for years without giving rise to either signs or symptoms. Even a large calculus filling the entire pelvis may be symptomless. The most common symptom is intermittent dull pain in the flank or back, intensified by motion or a sudden jolt. Abnormalities in the urine occur at one time or another in 80 per cent of cases; of these albuminuria, which may be minimal, is the most constant, while hematuria and pyuria each occur in about half the cases. The classic attack of *renal colic* occurs when a stone is small enough to enter the ureter and large

enough to obstruct it. The pain is of excruciating severity, begins in the back or flank, and radiates first across the abdomen and then down along the course of the ureter to the genitalia and inner aspect of the thigh. The pain is frequently sufficiently severe to induce nausea, vomiting, profuse sweating, faintness and shock. If there is infection, there will be fever and leukocytosis in addition. There is often frequency and urgency, but the quantity of urine passed is small. An attack may last only a few minutes, but usually persists for several hours. A patient may have but one attack of colic and pass the stone without further difficulty, or with multiple stones there may be repeated attacks over a period of years. After the attack is over the patient frequently complains of soreness along the course of the ureter, and tenderness on palpation. Albuminuria and microscopic hematuria are almost invariably present during the acute attack and may persist for several days.

Diagnosis. In patients suffering from typical attacks of renal colic, the diagnosis can be made with comparative ease from the clinical history and is supported by the presence of blood or numerous crystals in the freshly voided urine. A catheter specimen should be obtained in women. Nevertheless, the diagnosis can only be established by x-ray or pyelographic study, for the pain is frequently not referred in the usual manner and may simulate that of appendicitis, gallbladder disease, peptic ulcer, coronary thrombosis or even of disease of the vertebrae or spinal cord. Similar colicky attacks of pain also occur in Dietl's crisis, ureteral spasm and stricture, and in pyelonephritis and renal tumor if the ureter is obstructed by pus or clotted blood.

At times the shape and type of the shadows seen on an x-ray plate are characteristic. Cystine stones often coalesce to form large stones of a homogeneous, waxlike appearance. Calcium oxalate stones may have a snowflake form with spicules radiating from a central focus. Lamellar stones are usually phosphate in composition. Large stag-horn stones are calcium phosphate, calcium carbonate or cystine. Frequently the shadows are inconclusive. Suspicious shadows may represent concretions in a vein or in the gut rather than in the urinary tract. Uric acid, urate and cystine stones often fail to give a visible shadow, while denser calculi may be obscured by bone. Intravenous pyelography

curved indentatio
cysts.

Prognosis. In
rapidly fatal. In
for years, and
uremia or cerebr
Occasionally inte
gressive renal fa
years.

Treatment.
medical, identica
nephrosclerosis.
spond to rest. Pur
pressure on the
not proved succe
not be performed
reason, such as ir
rhage, and then
has been shown
to be only moder
process.

Other Forms
cysts are commor
of arteriolar ne
nephritis. They a
tubules by fibrosi
rare, occur usuall
from the surface
produce a dull,
panied by a palpa
ally yellow, res
lymph. It is not
either congenital
struction and isch
factors responsible
or the rapid incre
sists in complete re
age with destruct
brane. *Echinococc*
ney in 2 per cen
unilateral and gi\
slow-growing tun
If rupture is into
sage of the cyst
often provokes t
hematuria, and f
found in the uri
cyst ruptures into
leading to pyone\
tured cysts are pr
fore require nephi

Bell, E. T.: Cystic
Path., *11*:373, 19

---

may outline the stone, but frequently ureteral catheterization and retrograde pyelography are necessary.

Prognosis. The prognosis in patients with nephrolithiasis is extremely variable, depending upon the size, shape and position of the stone, and the presence of obstruction and of infection. Small stones retained by gravity in the lower calyx may do no harm, intermediate-sized ones should be watched at intervals by means of the roentgenogram, while stones more than 1 cm. in length are unlikely to pass spontaneously. Irregularly shaped stones are less likely to be passed. All stones tend to grow as long as urine is secreted by the kidney. It is the general opinion that any stone retained in the upper urinary tract ultimately leads to the destruction of the kidney. Renal calculus is one of the most common causes of infection and hydronephrosis, which may give rise to renal insufficiency, uremia, generalized sepsis, or, less frequently, ulceration and perforation of the renal pelvis or ureter. When anuria persists for more than a few hours, the outlook is grave in the absence of surgical intervention. When the conditions responsible for the formation of a stone persist after its removal, recurrences are likely.

Treatment. Although therapy depends upon the size and location of the stone and the presence of such complications as hydronephrosis, infection and renal insufficiency, general measures are of importance. Fluid ingestion should preferably exceed 3000 cc. daily in order to reduce the concentration of the urine. The diet of patients with oxalate or uric acid stones should contain minimum quantities of these substances. Such measures would be of more avail if stone formation were simply a matter of urinary concentration. Cystine stones may frequently be dissolved by making the urine alkaline.

For the pain of renal colic, morphine in large doses is usually required. A hot tub bath or local application of heat may help. Atropine or nitroglycerin may be tried. The intravenous injection of 15 cc. of 10 per cent calcium chloride has been recommended, but is not without danger.

Though expectant treatment may be adopted when there is a small stone and no infection in the hope that it will pass spontaneously, the vast majority of cases require special surgical and urologic procedures. At times a stone can be removed by dilatation of the ureter or other manipulation with the

---

ureteral catheter. Stones in the pelvis can often be removed by pyelotomy, but when there is marked renal destruction and large or multiple stones, nephrectomy is advisable. In spite of the best surgical technique and careful after-treatment, recurrences are seen in about 16 per cent of aseptic and 30 per cent of infected cases. The recurrence of phosphate stones may be suppressed by the ingestion of 40 to 120 cc. of aluminum hydroxide gels daily, the amount depending upon the dietary intake of phosphorus.

J. M. HAYMAN, JR.

References

Albright, F., Sulkowitch, H. W., and Chute, R.: Nonsurgical Aspects of the Kidney Stone Problem. J.A.M.A., *113*:2049, 1939.

Black, J. M.: Oxaluria in British Troops in India. Brit. M. J., *1*:590, 1945.

Brand, E., Cahill, G. F., and Harris, M. M.: Cystinuria. J. Biol. Chem., *109*:69, 1935.

Butt, A. J., Hauser, E. A., Seifter, J., and Perry, J. Q.: Renal Lithiasis: New Concept Concerning Etiology, Prevention, and Treatment. South. M. J., *45*:381, 1952.

Carroll, G., and Brennan, R. V.: The Role of Infection in Nephrolithiasis. J. Urol., *68*:88, 1952.

Engel, W. S.: Urinary Calculi Associated with Nephrocalcinosis. J. Urol., *68*:105, 1952.

Marshall, V. F., and Green, J. L.: Aluminum Gels with Constant Phosphorus Intake for Control of Renal Phosphate Calculi. J. Urol., *67*:611, 1952.

Randall, A.: Recent Advances in Knowledge Relating to the Formation, Recognition and Treatment of Kidney Calculi. Bull. New York Acad. Med., *20*:473, 1944.

Suby, H. I.: Dissolution of Urinary Calculi. J. Urol., *68*:96, 1952.

Wardlaw, H. S. H.: Observations on Incidence and Composition of Urinary Calculi. M. J. Australia, *1*:180, 1952.

AMYLOID DISEASE OF THE KIDNEY

(Amyloid Nephrosis)

This condition is discussed in the chapters on Amyloidosis and on the Nephroses.

CYSTS OF THE KIDNEY

By far the most common type of cyst of the kidney of clinical importance is *congenital polycystic disease*. In this condition the normal renal tissue is in large measure encroached on and replaced by multitudes of

cysts o
heredit
is prob
nant. S
fancy
years c
rare in

Fig. 1
cystic k
flattenin
due to th

althoug
than th

Etio
ease wa
voluted
tubules
the cys
parts o
fants th
while i
with ex

Mor
normal
pendin
scattere
three
much l
and kn
jecting
tissue s
giving
amount

Unfortunately, these are rarely present early, or they are so trivial that they are neglected by the patient and overlooked by the physician. Hematuria is the most constant and outstanding symptom of tumor of the kidney. In the renal cancers of adults it is usually the earliest symptom, but in Wilms' tumor in children, it is a relatively late manifestation. The bleeding generally comes on insidiously and is characteristically intermittent, lasting only a few hours or days. Pain, occurring in 60 per cent of cases, is frequently inconstant and vague, but may be colicky because of passage of blood clots, or dull and aching as a result of distention of the pelvis or capsule. Neuralgic pains, which may be severe, usually mean local spread of the tumor to adjacent nerve trunks. Pressure on neighboring viscera may also produce pain, gastrointestinal symptoms being not uncommon. Metastases to bones, especially the vertebrae, femur, humerus and skull, may give rise to pain in those regions. Metastases to lungs are usually silent. A palpable mass is present in less than 20 per cent of early cases, but, as the tumor grows progressively, can often be felt before death. The growth generally preserves the usual shape of the kidney, and may be uniformly smooth. Often it is irregular, lobulated or nodular. When the tumor is large, the flank is deformed, and the shape of the mass may be apparent on inspection. Small tumors are frequently movable, but the larger ones are generally fixed. Varicocele may result from direct pressure of the growth on the left spermatic vein or from complete blocking by infiltration. In rare instances marked circulatory disturbances with edema and ascites may occur from obstruction of the vena cava. Fever is said to be present in 20 per cent of cases, in those in which no signs of infection can be detected. Hypertension is found in 50 per cent of cases, but is presumably coincidental, since removal of the affected kidney produces no consistent alteration in blood pressure.

Prognosis and Treatment. The sole treatment of malignant renal tumor is nephrectomy, which, to be curative, depends on early and accurate diagnosis. Examination of smears of the urinary sediment by the Papanicolaou technique may be helpful in early diagnosis. Radiation, in the opinion of most observers, plays only an auxiliary role. The presence of metastases or marked functional impairment of the opposite kidney contraindicates surgery. X-ray of the lungs and long bones for metastases should be performed in every case before surgery is attempted. The *prognosis* of renal tumors is poor. Less than 20 per cent of patients recover from malignant renal disease. The immediate operative mortality is about 15 per cent; 20 per cent are found to be inoperable; and about 45 per cent die of metastases within a year or two.

J. M. HAYMAN, JR.

References

Davis, D. M.: Diagnosis of Renal Tumors in the Adult. Radiology, 54:639, 1950.
Foot, N. D., Humphreys, G. A., and Whitmore, W. F.: Renal Tumors: Pathology and Prognosis in 295 Cases. J. Urol., 66:190, 1951.
Harrison, J. H., Botsford, T. W., and Tucker, M. R.: Use of Smear of Urinary Sediment in Diagnosis and Management of Neoplasms of Kidneys and Bladder. Surg., Gynec. & Obst., 92:129, 1951.
Prather, G. C.: Differential Diagnosis between Renal Tumors and Renal Cysts. J. Urol., 64:193, 1950.
Riches, E. W., Griffiths, I. H., and Thackray, A. C.: New Growths of the Kidney and Ureter. Brit. J. Urol., 23:297, 1951.

Diseases of the Spleen and Reticulo-endothelial System

DISEASES OF THE SPLEEN

INTRODUCTION

The spleen, in the present state of medical knowledge, has come to assume a pathologic significance out of proportion to its known physiologic importance in human health and longevity. Under normal conditions the spleen is a relatively small organ, weighing in the adult from 75 to 150 gm., and reflecting from time to time a variable amount of reserve blood in its capacious sinuses and parenchymal spaces. Its reservoir function for red blood cells was experimentally studied and firmly established by Barcroft and his collaborators in the early 1920's. The extirpation of the spleen, however, in many animal species, and the accumulated experience of emergency splenectomy for traumatic rupture of the normal human spleen have fully confirmed the fact that this organ is *not* essential to the ordinary maintenance of health and life at any age in any species.

On the positive side, an increasingly critical analysis of hitherto obscure human disease syndromes has resulted in a rapidly growing clinical appreciation of the insidious threat to well-being and survival which is inherent in this organ. Its pathologic physiology may arise either on an inherited or an acquired basis, and is independent of the gross size of the organ. When such splenic dysfunction remains unrecognized in the patient, either chronic invalidism or acute fatal hemoclastic crises may result.

It is a biologic axiom that the structure of and cells comprising any given tissue or organ are directly related to and responsible for its physiologic functions; and the pathologic corollary to this axiom is that, given any known normal organic function, the clinical diagnostician may expect to find sooner or later a corresponding pathologic hypodysfunction or hyperdysfunction. John H. King in 1914 pointed out that "there is

. . . considerable evidence to show that the spleen may have a marked influence on hemolysis. To such a condition the term 'hypersplenism' may be applied. . . . If it can be shown that important clinical symptoms consistently point to a hyperfunction of the spleen, and that these symptoms disappear or are strikingly mitigated when the spleen is removed from the body, an important step will have been taken toward defining the changes in function of the spleen." In the interim since 1914 the inter-relationships between splenic structure, splenic function and splenic disease have become increasingly evident, largely through the type of human studies anticipated by King.

The spleen presents four rather obvious anatomic and histologic subdivisions, upon which its functioning is dependent and from which pathologic manifestations may be expected to arise: (1) the smooth muscle capsule and trabeculae which make this organ physiologically contractile and expansile; (2) the vascular system with fenestrated sinusoids and a vast network of dilated capillaries ideally placed and space for the temporary sequestration of cellular reserves from the circulating blood; (3) the lymphoid system, identical in every respect with lymphopoietic tissue elsewhere in the body; and (4) the reticuloendothelial system, comprising physiologic phagocytes, morphologically similar, but because of their location frequently dissimilar, to the reticuloendothelial cells distributed elsewhere in the body in quantitative pathologic phagocytosis.

The Spleen and Its Muscular Capsule. To the anatomic spongelike character of the splenic parenchyma may be attributed at least a part of the explanation of the specific relationship which this organ bears to a variety of human pathologic syndromes. Unlike lymph nodes and liver, the spleen has a smooth muscle–reinforced capsule and penetrating intraparenchymal trabeculae, which provide a mechanism for the rhythmic physiologic contraction and relaxation of this organ. Intrinsic epinephrine-induced contraction of the spleen occurs after voluntary muscular exercise, after hemorrhage and after psychic stimulation. The diagnostician may take advantage of this neuromuscular mechanism to obtain a nonsurgical "biopsy" of the potentially mobilizable splenic cell content at any moment by securing serial peripheral blood cell and blood volume studies before and after the injection of epinephrine.

both animal and human material. Our present concepts derive from these several basic studies. Using gelatin to induce erythrocyte rouleau formation, and saponin to produce less elastic spherocytes in rabbits, Björkman found that the pulp cords contained few, and the blood sinuses most, of the red cells, whereas in the untreated controls there was a more equitable distribution between pulp and sinuses. This was interpreted to mean that small changes in the size and shape of suspended particles or aggregations of particles are important to their vascular filtrability. By injecting intravenously starch granules measuring 1 to 5 microns in diameter and identifying their intravascular versus extravascular posi-

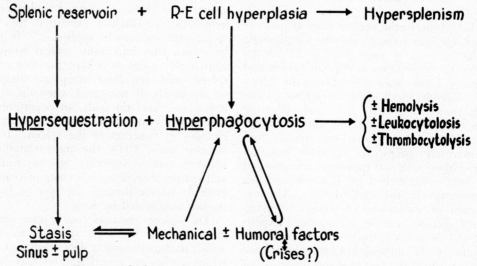

Fig. 141. The hypersplenic mechanism; theoretical considerations.

The Spleen and Its Vascular Sinuses. The ability of the spleen to change its volume has been known for a long time, and the direct relationship which has been repeatedly observed to be present between changes in splenic volume and circulating blood cell volume has inevitably focused attention sharply upon the nature and character of the intrinsic vascular pattern which must govern this reversible reservoir activity, and, as a direct corollary, the extent and effect of such temporary storage on the integrity of the involved blood cells. Increasingly ingenious methods have been developed for studying this most vascularized organ in the body.

Proceeding from the older fixed tissue techniques of Mall, and of Mollier, Knisely perfected (1936), and Whipple and associates at the Columbia Spleen Clinic (1941) applied, the procedures for direct observation by transillumination of the living intact spleen in a number of animal species. Björkman (1947) in Faraeus Clinic, Upsala, then followed with a series of penetrating observations, utilizing

tion, it was possible further to measure the approximate size of the suspected interendothelial stomas under various conditions. Under physiologic conditions 95 per cent of the starch granules 1 micron or less in diameter were found to have passed into pulp cords, whereas 80 per cent of those 5 microns and larger were still within the sinuses. However, after inducing an acute splenic tumor by experimental streptococcal infection, or by intoxication with a hemolytic agent, only 50 per cent of the larger starch granules remained within the sinuses. An *acquired* enlargement of the vascular stomas, in these pathologic circumstances, was hypothesized. An *inherited* increase in mean diameter of these same vascular stomas might well govern the ease with which normal-sized or microcytic blood cell elements become subjected to the extravascular influences of the splenic parenchyma.

Transferring his experimental observations to selected human autopsy material, Björkman found evidence to support the concept of an identical human splenic vascular mechanism, in which in acute splenic tumor there is sinus dilatation with an accelerated intercourse of both plasma and corpuscular elements between sinuses and pulp cords, via broadened and distended stomas. Conversely, in chronic cardiac decompensation and hepatic cirrhosis there is a pathologic modification with an increasing number of longitudinal anastomoses between the normally annular fibrils in the capillary sinus and venous walls, which tend toward a compensatory preservation of the tightness of the sinus filter in resistance to a mounting portal hypertension.

It has been found that there is marked variability in the extent and degree of sinus development in the spleen in different animal species (Snook, 1944). This may well explain the discrepant emphases which for the past hundred years have been given by different investigators in the study of an organ in which it now seems certain that both sinuses and pulp cords are important circulatory reciprocals. Man is classified among those species with a spleen rich in vascular sinusoidal structures. Thus the currently available evidence supports the concept (Fig. 141) that the human spleen has a semi-open circulation, controlled by a filter mesh mechanism in the sinus wall, which under many diverse pathologic conditions may be altered, in the direction of either greater or lesser selective or nonselective permeability to the cellular elements of the blood. This circulatory mechanism, unique as compared with all other organs and tissues, operates to separate the cells from the plasma and thus to concentrate in the spleen, both within and without the sinuses in varying degree and quantity, blood cells of various types and quality. The more disturbed the circulatory equilibrium, and the more profound and prolonged the stasis, the more the spleen seems to lack discrimination and to withhold and destroy morphologically normal as well as obviously fragile, senile and damaged elements. Both mechanical and chemical factors are accentuated in their respective influences on premature aging, including changes in the spherocytic fragility of the cells.

The Spleen and the Reticuloendothelial System of Cells. The reticuloendothelial system of phagocytic cells (Aschoff, 1913) extends throughout the organs and tissues of the entire body, but these functionally important, protective and conservational elements are more richly distributed within the parenchyma of the spleen than in any other organ in the human body. The so-called reticuloendothelial system is made up of "specific endothelia" and "reticulum cells," each endowed with general structural as well as special regenerative and phagocytic capacities. The fixed endothelial cells lining the vascular and lymphatic sinusoids, or anchored in midstream as in the liver, have a marked physiologic, protective and phagocytic capacity, both *in situ* and as free desquamated clasmatocytes or macrophages. The reticulum cells of the adult areolar connective tissues behave as do primitive mesenchymal elements with embryonic developmental potentialities. They give rise to the "primitive free cells" from which the blood monocytes of Schilling (1913) normally differentiate and mature.

In appropriate circumstances this focus of embryonic-like mesenchymal tissue in the adult spleen may revert to its earlier *in utero*, pancellular, hematopoietic function, and provide an essential, compensatory, extramedullary, ectopic center of blood cell formation (so-called agnogenic myeloid metaplasia). In other circumstances there may be a tremendous increase in the number, phagocytic activity and probably specific antibody productivity of the reticuloendothelial cells in a normal-sized or enlarged spleen, which, when combined with hypersequestration of entrapped and therefore hypersusceptible blood cell elements, may contribute to a circulating cell deficit despite an all-out hyperplastic bone marrow attempt at compensation (Fig. 141).

Wright and his associates (1953) have recently standardized a quantitative *in vitro* test for the determination of the relative erythrophagocytic index of splenic reticuloendothelial macrophages in a tissue culture medium. The extreme sensitivity of this index to increased human red cell susceptibility to phagocytosis reflects alterations in erythrocyte integrity under a great variety of human pathologic conditions and is further evidence of the potential importance of the role of the reticuloendothelial cells, and particularly of the splenic phagocytes, in the circulating cellular equilibrium of any patient.

The Spleen as a Lymphatic Organ. The lymphopoietic foci in the splenic parenchyma, made up of typical lymph sinuses, follicles and the germinal centers of Fleming, reflect and parallel the general lymphocytic responses elsewhere throughout the body, participating in the hyperplastic reactions in giant follicle lymphoma, chronic lymphatic leukemia, lymphosarcoma, infectious mononucleosis, serum sickness and other types and varieties of protein sensitizations, and in the hypoplastic inhibition of virus, chemical and irradiation intoxications.

The Spleen as a "Hormone"-Secreting, Antibody-Producing and Enzyme-Concentrating Organ. The basic mechanism or mechanisms which govern the reciprocal spleen-marrow relationships responsible for the constantly shifting cellular equilibria in the circulating blood are still in question. A hormonal influence arising within the spleen and carried via the blood stream to the bone marrow, and acting to inhibit the maturation and/or delivery of the definitive cellular elements normally developing there, has been

Primary hypersplenism (inherited hyperinstability)
  Spontaneous or precipitated by infections, trauma, pregnancy

  1. Congenital hemolytic icterus ⎫
       ↕   ⎪
  2. Thrombocytopenic purpura   ⎬ *a.* Chronic
       ↕   ⎪ *b.* Acute crisis
  3. Splenic neutropenia   ⎪
       ↓   ⎪
  4. Splenic panhematopenia   ⎭

Fig. 142. Primary hypersplenism.

hypothesized ("splenin," "thrombocytopen" and so on). The only cytologic source of such a "hormone" would appear to be the splenic representatives of the reticuloendothelial phagocytes, since there are no histologically distinct cellular elements comparable to those identified with a hormone-secreting function in other endocrine organs.

Specific globulin-antibody formation has been attributed to the reticuloendothelial cells, which, arising from and acting upon individual blood cell types, may explain the "sensitization-like" withholding phenomena via specific agglutinins and cytolysins on erythrocytes, granulocytes and thrombocytes, respectively, or collectively in the various hypersplenic syndromes.

The possible role of lytic enzymes has also been repeatedly explored. After Maegraith's isolation of a specific hemolytic enzyme, Ponder identified this agent as lysolecithin and the enzyme responsible as lysolecithinase. Originally discovered in normal blood serum by Bergenhem and Fahraeus and considered to be produced in the tissues generally, its lytic activity is dependent upon its concentration at any one time and place, which in turn is the resultant of the rate of production, the degree of circulatory stasis and the effectiveness of specific or nonspecific inhibitors. The spleen parenchyma is unique in meeting every condition for lytic enzyme con-

centration. Scheff and Awny (1949), using lecithin substrate plus fresh splenic tissue obtained surgically, report quantitatively higher titers of lysolecithinase activity uniformly in those patients with hypersplenic syndromes, as contrasted with similarly studied normal human splenic tissues. This is consistent with the observations of Hicks and Opie (1942), who demonstrated in the spleens of rabbits an increase in enzymatic proteolysis directly proportional to the evidence of heightened phagocytic activity.

Dyssplenism. From the foregoing functional analyses, it is now possible to hypothesize and to anticipate a variety of basic dysplenic disturbances, which explain a number of clinical syndromes not heretofore understood or successfully controlled.

To recapitulate, the mammalian spleen presents a unique anatomic structure, in which complex mechanical and chemical factors unite to influence blood cell formation, blood cell storage, and the physiologic phagocytosis of damaged and senile blood cells for the purpose of conservation of iron and other essential hematopoietic rebuilding blocks. This being true, it may be conceded that a congenitally inherited cellular or structural defect could precipitate an accentuation or diminution in any one of these functional objectives with the development of a corresponding specific pathologic syndrome. Also, when the spleen becomes involved secondarily in a general constitutional disease process, it may be anticipated that this delicately balanced splenic equilibrium will be upset at least occasionally.

Hyposplenism. Spontaneously occurring, progressive, atrophic, fibrosing autosplenectomy and surgically acquired asplenism fortunately are fraught with no known danger to, and no specific pathologic symptomatology in, the individual. An asymptomatic panpolycythemia, moderately participated in by all marrow elements, and with increased erythrocyte resistance, usually follows removal of the normal spleen. These phenomena, described independently by Frank and by Krumbhaar and therefore known as the Frank-Krumbhaar law, result from the removal of the local reservoir, from spherocytoid and other premature aging influences of the splenic sinusoidal-parenchymal filter on the circulating blood elements, and/or by the elimination of hypothetic splenic inhibitory hormones on marrow hematopoiesis. Progressive atrophic fibrosis

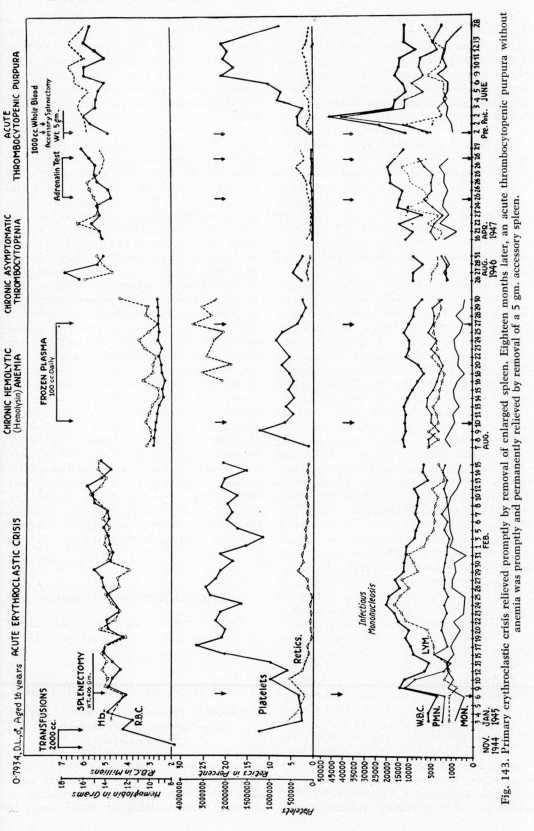

Fig. 143. Primary erythroclastic crisis relieved promptly by removal of enlarged spleen. Eighteen months later, an acute thrombocytopenic purpura without anemia was promptly and permanently relieved by removal of a 5 gm. accessory spleen.

of the spleen is not infrequently encountered in sickle cell anemia of long standing (as little as 10 gm. found at autopsy in one of our observed cases), more rarely in other conditions, without necessarily eliminating the hemolytic phenomena. Cooley's erythroblastic and target cell anemias show increased hypotonic erythrocyte resistance, and usually fail to reflect the improvement which follows regularly upon splenectomy in the true hypersplenic states.

The Hypersplenic Syndromes, as now recognized in terms of the pathologic exaggeration of one or more of the physiologic functions of this organ, may be considered under two main subdivisions: (1) primary hypersplenism, and (2) hypersplenism secondary to other diseases, when and as they involve the spleen.

Primary hypersplenism may be defined as a hyperfunctional instability of this organ, inherited either as a mendelian dominant chromosomal gene factor or as a recessive character of infrequent or sporadic expressivity. In such circumstances spontaneous hypersplenic episodes involving any one or more of the circulating blood cell elements may occur unrelated to any demonstrable environmental cause. Such physiologic stresses as extreme fatigue, emotional crises and normal pregnancy, or minor infections and traumas, will precipitate more or less severe exacerbations resulting in chronic invalidism or in acute hypersplenic crises in susceptible patients. Within this category should be considered (1) congenital hemolytic icterus, (2) thrombocytopenic purpura hemorrhagica, (3) splenic neutropenia and (4) splenic panhematopenia. Though these several clinical syndromes have been previously considered as characteristically distinct and separate etiologic entities, it is seldom that we encounter a "pure" hemolytic or an unadulterated thrombocytopenic or a strictly neutropenic episode. The predominant clinical picture may reflect anemia with or without jaundice or purpura, or Ludwig's angina and infection, but each one of these dominant symptom complexes more often than not will be found to have a subclinical, if not clinical, circulating cytopenia involving one or more of the other elements of marrow origin (Fig. 130). At different stages in the clinical course of the same patient (Fig. 131) differing degrees of panhematocytopenia may be observed, reflecting a variable idiosyncrasy of the pathologic spleen for withholding cells

which have entered the circulation from a hyperplastic bone marrow. Irrespective, however, of the degree and extent and variety of cytopenia, or of the clinical acuteness of the symptom complex, the response to splenectomy is equally prompt and sustained when "hypersplenism" is the basic etiologic mechanism.

Basic Diagnostic Criteria. The following repeatedly observed and consistently verifiable objective findings are common to all "hypersplenic" syndromes and constitute the *sine qua non* for the identification of this mechanism. (1) Specific compensatory cellular hyperplasia is always present in the marrow without maturation arrest or delivery "block" of the element or elements, nevertheless specifically reduced or absent in the peripheral blood. (2) Positive epinephrine contraction of the spleen reveals, by indirect peripheral blood studies preoperatively, and by direct comparative splenic artery and vein studies at the time of surgery, the extent, specificity and temporary reversibility of any cellular hypersequestration which is present. (3) Immediate supravital cellular studies of splenic tissue removed at the time of surgery demonstrate marked reticuloendothelial cell hyperplasia and specific hyperphagocytosis of the definitive elements abundant in the spleen, deficient in the circulation and hyperplastic in the marrow. (4) Prompt, permanent restoration of the normal hemolytopoietic equilibrium, both central and peripheral, usually follows surgical removal of all splenic tissue, including increased *in vivo* survival times for "marked" transfused normal erythrocytes.

CHARLES A. DOAN

THE HEMOLYTIC ANEMIAS

The hemolytic anemias reflect a variety of mechanisms and are discussed in detail on page 1179.

CONGENITAL HEMOLYTIC ICTERUS

(Acholuric Hemolytic Jaundice, Hereditary Spherocytosis, Hemolytic Splenomegaly)

Definition. Congenital hemolytic jaundice is an inherited gene-factor trait with mendelian dominance and high expressivity, the clinical manifestations of which may be latent, chronic or acute. When active disease is present, it is usually characterized by a varying degree of splenomegaly; by a spherocytic, microcytic, hemolytic type of anemia with an accompanying reticulocytosis greater than anticipated for the degree of anemia; by a striking increase in erythrocyte osmotic and mechanical fragilities; by acholuric jaundice; and by a varying degree of thrombocytopenia and neutropenia.

History. First observed by Murchison in 1885, established as a clinical entity by Hayem thirteen years later, and its familial occurrence reported by Minkowski at the turn of the century, hemolytic jaundice still remains, nevertheless, an all too frequently unrecognized hypersplenic state, despite signs and symptoms which should make the mechanism and diagnosis readily apparent. With Chauffard's report of the then unique observation of increased *in vitro* erythrocyte fragility to hypotonic saline solution, the congenital syndrome became known as the Chauffard-Minkowski type in contradistinction to the sporadic or acquired type. Many of the patients with clinical hemolytic jaundice "acquired" in the later decades of life, in which no history of past personal or previous familial incidence is obtainable initially, really prove on examination to have all the stigmata of the congenital type, and when blood relatives are available for supplemental blood studies, additional instances of mild clinical or subclinical hemolytic anemia are regularly revealed.

The current development of new laboratory tests for "blocking antibodies," utilizing serum albumin, the Coombs test and the trypsin sensitization test as modified by Wheeler, have been thought by some investigators to separate more clearly the "acquired" from the "congenital" forms of hemolytic anemia; but the observations of Wright and co-workers in this laboratory tend to assign quantitative rather than qualitative significance to these differences, and the underlying mechanisms, if they are distinct, require further clarification. For further details, see the discussion of Acquired Hemolytic Jaundice elsewhere in this volume.

With Widal's early emphasis on acute clinical exacerbations with "crises of deglobulization" came a universal warning from the surgeons to avoid splenectomy at such times. This was based upon the assumption that the hyperfragile spherocytes represented the inheritance of a defective bone marrow incapable of producing normally resistant biconcave erythrocytes (Haden, and others, 1934). More recently Owren (1948) has attributed acute erythroclastic crises in congenital hemolytic icterus to the sudden development of a panmarrow aplasia. In 1935

it was concluded, after several years of controlled studies in this laboratory and clinic, that the acute erythroclastic crises which characterize the clinical course of this disease are the result of an acute exacerbation of splenic erythrocyte hypersequestration and destruction, the marrow showing maximum compensatory erythropoietic hyperplasia at the normoblastic level without maturation arrest or toxic inhibition. That maximum red cell delivery is in fact occurring is attested by the reticulocytes, which represent at such times not infrequently more than 90 per cent of all circulating cells, and by direct contrastive splenic artery versus splenic vein studies. When such a mechanism is present, splenectomy is mandatory and may be life saving.

Etiology and Mechanism. Since obvious signs and symptoms of hemolytic jaundice may be present at birth (to be differentiated from icterus neonatorum and erythroblastosis) or may first appear in any subsequent year or decade, the identification of this disease in any particular patient must be based on objective laboratory data. Furthermore, the frequency and severity of the clinical disease vary so widely from family to family that it may be necessary to secure the appropriate laboratory studies in a representative sampling of blood relatives before affirmative proof of its hereditary characteristics can be firmly established. The incidence and distribution of hereditary stigmata in one representative family involved 9 of 14 persons in four generations. In so far as such evidence can affirm, a true inheritance of the tendency extended unbrokenly through each generation available for study, though only in the third and fourth of these generations was spontaneous disease sufficiently severe to produce invalidism and require splenectomy for the restoration of health.

Rather than inheritance as such, then, it is the specific modus operandi of the inherited mechanism responsible for this particular type of hemolytic anemia which has remained long in question. There being in both health and disease a reciprocal functional relationship between bone marrow and spleen, the relative role of each organ in any given syndrome in which qualitative and/or quantitative circulating cellular disequilibriums occur presents an immediate, important, but now resolvable problem. Presumably the red blood cell stigmata which characterize this disease could be the result either of a primary inherent defect in erythropoiesis or of secondary extramedullary influences on basically sound, circulating erythrocytes. It is difficult to demonstrate microcytic, spherocytic hyperfragility of the reticulocytes obtained directly from the marrow in these patients. Postsplenectomy circulating erythrocytes tend to return to normal contour, size and resistance. Observations of normal survival time for transfused erythrocytes from normal donors in patients during acute hemolytic crises, in contradistinction to a shorter survival time for the inferior product of their own marrow, have not been confirmed in our laboratory or in that of Dameshek. Rather, evidence directs attention to the potential dangers of increasing the hemosiderin and bile pigments from borrowed red cells destroyed prematurely during a crisis—especially if urinary alkalinization has not been accomplished to minimize hemosiderin crystallization in the loops of Henle—and of subsequent lower nephron nephrosis. Pigment gallstones are a frequent complication of long-continued hemolytic anemia. Complete and permanent hemolytopoietic remission follows complete removal of all splenic tissue in congenital hemolytic icterus, with a completely normal bone marrow response to every subsequent stress and strain to which the average human being may be subjected throughout a long life (Lord Dawson of Penn, The Hume Lectures, 1931).

Turning now to the evidence in support of a major role for the spleen in this disease, consider first its unique structure and vascular pattern, ideal for its physiologic cellular reservoir function. All cells coming from the bone marrow enter the spleen. Many remain for indefinite periods. Any disproportion between normal sinusoidal versus pulp storage of erythrocytes via enlarged vascular stomas facilitates prolonged stasis and direct contact between red cells and phagocytic clasmatocytes. Deplasmatization increases intercellular friction with changes in mechanical fragility; the loss of potassium by "stored" erythrocytes and other electrolyte disequilibriums lead to increased osmotic fragility; pathologic concentrations of lysolecithin and lycolethecin-like, normal products of the reticuloendothelial cells occur; polyhemagglutinin and hemolytic "blocking" antibodies, experimentally derivable from the reticuloendothelial phagocytes, may act to accentuate the vicious cycle of specific erythrocyte hypersequestration and hyperphagocytosis and so precipitate more or less severe crises. All these factors, each of which is capable of influencing the degree of cell withholding and the speed of cell destruction, have been shown to be present within the spleen in hemolytic icterus. The sudden and dramatic termination of a true erythroclastic crisis on the operating table at the moment of ligation of the splenic pedicle, after observing the splenic artery to be carrying many more erythrocytes to the greatly enlarged spleen than were being released via the splenic vein, is the final therapeutic test of the role of the spleen in this spleen-marrow mechanism (Fig. 144).

Symptoms and Signs. Signs may be present at birth or may first develop in infancy, adolescence, maturity or old age, and the symptoms vary markedly in severity. There may be no detectable clinical jaundice; when present, the icterus is never intense and characteristically is temporarily intensified by minor infections or traumas. Jaundice may be initially precipitated or exaggerated in women during normal pregnancy. A moderate anemia, reflecting in severity the hemolytic activity of the spleen, contributes to the sallow pallor and ease of fatigue. Upper left quadrant fullness or discomfort, or an acute painful episode, may lead to the discovery of enlargement of the spleen or its infarction, and upper right quadrant pain is typical of pigment cholelithiasis, a common complication of chronic, longstanding disease.

Laboratory Diagnosis. Much more specific are the laboratory signs. Qualitatively, there is a striking microcytosis of the red cells, usually, though not always, with more reticulocytes demonstrable than in any other comparable type or degree of anemia (98 per cent in one 4-year old child in acute hemoclastic crisis). The spherocytosis is attested by the increased osmotic and mechanical fragility of the erythrocytes. Moderate neutropenic leukopenia and thrombocytopenia are the rule rather than the exception, owing partly to the normoblastic myelophthisis in the marrow and partly to splenic hypersequestration. Cellular studies of the marrow confirm the peripheral blood interpretations of specific normoblastic hyperplasia at the expense of the other normally occurring elements, and without inhibitory, destructive maturation arrest or leukemic infiltrative phenomena. An epinephrine test usually reveals the degree and specificity of cellular sequestration in the spleen. The total circulating

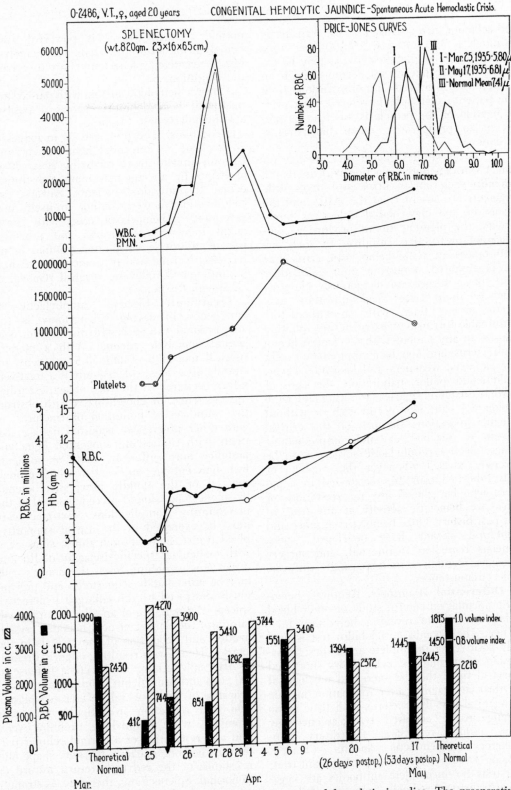

Fig. 144. Spontaneous acute erythroclastic crisis in congenital hemolytic jaundice. The preoperative epinephrine test with blood volume studies revealed the excessive critical retention of erythrocytes by the spleen. Splenectomy was followed immediately by cessation of both cell retention and cell destruction. Price-Jones curves show gradual return of erythrocytes toward normal size and shape postoperatively.

red cells not infrequently increase transitorily as much as 750,000 to 1,560,000 per cubic millimeter in prediction of what may be expected at the time of splenectomy. Such an epinephrine induced autotransfusion from the patient's own splenic reservoir just prior to ligation of the pedicle is much to be preferred to preoperative donor blood transfusions.

Chemical studies reveal an elevated indirect van den Bergh reaction with increased urobilin excretion in urine and stools. Bile pigments are absent from the urine, and the stools are not clay-colored unless, as rarely occurs, the pigment stones produce a complicating obstructive jaundice. In such circumstances an acute hemoclastic crisis may be precipitated, requiring both gallbladder and spleen surgery in dangerously close sequence. Such "crises deglobulization" may occur at any time, with or without determinable intrinsic or extrinsic precipitating causes, in any patient with congenital hemolytic icterus, and may be asymptomatic except for anorexia, weakness and lassitude. Fever, mild icteric pallor, palpitation, the signs of cardiac dilatation, nausea, vomiting and acute abdominal pain may occur with or without splenic infarction. Because of the critical threat to survival at such unpredictable times, elective prophylactic surgery is to be strongly advised whenever the stigmata of this inherited trait are recognized in a patient who has shown any manifestations of excessive hemolytic activity at any time in his past history. Once hemolytic jaundice and profound anemia have developed, spontaneous remission is unusual, and surgery becomes mandatory in increasingly unfavorable circumstances.

Differential Diagnosis. Acquired hemolytic anemia, on careful study of other blood relatives, fails to reveal a hereditary incidence. The Coombs antiglobulin test is usually positive for incomplete antibodies; transfusion of normal red cells shows shortened survival time; there is increased mechanical erythrocyte fragility after incubation in true congenital hemolytic icterus with little or no change in the "acquired" types; splenectomy may induce remission. Hereditary nonspherocytic hemolytic anemia (Haden, Major) occurs as a mendelian dominant trait; all tests for incomplete antibodies are negative; transfused red cells from normal donors have a normal survival time, but patients' erythrocytes are short-lived when given to a normal recipient; there is powerful autohemolysis *in vitro;* the Ham acid-hemolysis test is negative; splenectomy fails to correct the condition.

Chronic hemolytic anemia with paroxysmal nocturnal hemoglobinuria shows a positive acid-hemolysis test (Ham).

Prognosis. The prognosis as to longevity is excellent in congenital hemolytic icterus. Chronic invalidism or recurring acute crises of hemolytic anemia may mark the clinical course in individual patients. Always, any complication, however minor in itself, may precipitate a hemoclastic crisis with consequent increased seriousness and prolongation of otherwise self-limited traumas or infections. Normal and permanent health may be anticipated following surgical removal of all splenic tissue.

Treatment. Elective, prophylactic or emergency life-saving splenectomy is the only rational and successful therapy for congenital hemolytic anemia. With a modern surgical mortality of only 0.5 per cent, including all causes, splenectomy is a relatively safe procedure. In the face of acute cardiac incompetence, of cholelithiasis with obstructive jaundice, of nonunion of fractures, or with other progressive acquired disease, patients with underlying congenital hemolytic jaundice may suffer an acute or subacute hemolytic episode, an event in which prompt reversal of the rapidly progressive anemia by splenectomy should precede control of the precipitating complications. Extreme care must be exercised in the use of supportive blood transfusions at such times, since even with meticulous specific isoagglutin, Rh and direct cross-matching tests, the donor's cells may be immediately sequestered and precipitously destroyed by the enlarged hyperactive spleen. Maintenance of an alkaline urine will minimize the danger of acid hematin crystallization and deposition of the crystals in the loops of Henle with resulting oliguric uremia.

After splenectomy an effective increase in red cells and hemoglobin is immediate; disappearance of jaundice, fall in elevated plasma iron and reduction in reticulocytes occur promptly, with diminishing urobilin excretion and restoration of a normal cellular pattern in the bone marrow; the size, shape and resistance of the red cells return toward or to normal. Splenectomy, therefore, is strongly advised whenever this congenital trait has been definitely established in a patient at any age.

Recurrences—Accessory Spleens. Rarely, some months or years after successful splenectomy with complete clinical and hematologic remission, there may be a hypersplenic recurrence, either typical of the initial syndrome, with spherocytic anemia, reticulocytosis and normoblastic hyperplasia of marrow, or characterized—as in one instance (Fig. 143) in our own series of cases—by an entirely different clinical syndrome, a profound thrombocytopenic purpura without hemolytic anemia, the marrow showing a typical compensatory megakaryocytosis. When an accessory spleen, weighing 5 gm., was removed, complete hematologic and clinical recovery ensued. Because of the bizarre locations in which satellite spleens have been found on the basis of early embryonic migrations, viz., retroperitoneally, embedded within organs such as the pancreas or stomach, or in the scrotal sac, it is wiser in such circumstances to attempt to localize aberrant splenic tissue through Thorotrast visualization. The fact that such hypersplenic activity is always found in association with greatly increased numbers of highly phagocytic clasmatocytes, and that these same reticuloendothelial cells segregate and concentrate the Thorotrast, probably accounts for the ease and specificity of demonstration of such small islands of splenic tissue by the roentgenologist.

Even though the Kupffer cells of the liver and the reticuloendothelial cells elsewere in the body are identical in origin with and apparently similar in function to the reticuloendothelial cells in the spleen, removal of all splenic tissue fortunately brings complete erythrolytopoietic reequilibration in the patient. This strongly points to the unique reservoir function of the spleen for all blood elements, but more particularly for erythrocytes, as an essential factor in facilitating or precipitating hyperphagocytosis in both primary congenital and secondary acquired hemolytic jaundice.

CHARLES A. DOAN

SECONDARY "ACQUIRED" HEMOLYTIC ANEMIA

Hypersplenic Type. The finely balanced equilibriums between red cell storage and conservational reticuloendothelial cell phagocytosis of old, damaged or otherwise abnormal circulating erythrocytes, both primary functions of the normal spleen, provide the basis for an inherent erythrolytic functional instability of this organ which may be revealed in many pathologic circumstances of widely divergent etiology. Any circulatory or parenchymal involvement of the spleen potentially, if not actually, alters the structural relationship between the sinusoids and pulp spaces, resulting in varying degrees of retention, hypersequestration and premature destruction of the erythrocytes entering via the splenic artery.

With no past personal or family history of hemolytic anemia and without the usual stigmata of the congenital trait in the patient or his blood relatives, the physician on occasion will encounter an "acquired" or secondary hemolytic anemia with negative Coombs' test, high reticulocytes, hyperplastic normoblastosis in the marrow, and epinephrine test evidence of hypersplenic withholding of red cells. In such circumstances, whether the splenomegaly be on the basis of congestive failure, infection, Gaucher's disease, any of the chronic leukemias, Hodgkin's syndrome or other constitutional disease involving the spleen specifically, the induced hypersplenic anemia can be stopped only by prompt splenectomy.

The specific mechanism must be individually determined in each patient whenever any anemia occurs, and the attempt should then be made to correct the anemia as such as an important adjunct in the treatment of the primary disease.

Nonhypersplenic or "Combined" Type. In addition to the hemolytic syndromes just described, there occur more or less acute hemolytic episodes, associated with a positive Coombs' test titer, presenting as a critical complication in the course of a variety of constitutional diseases. The bone marrow shows a simple, uncomplicated, normoblastic hyperplasia with all of the other chemical functional test findings of a hemolytic anemia mechanism.

In such patients either adrenocorticotrophic hormone as Acthar Gel, 50 to 100 mg. parenterally, daily, or cortisone, 300 to 400 mg. orally for two days, with gradual reduction thereafter, should be tried until a maintenance level of 50 to 100 mg. per day is established. The response is usually first reflected by a beginning fall in the elevated circulating reticulocyte percentage followed by a steady rise in the peripheral red blood cell count to normal. The recovery may be maintained with or without continuing therapy. If after ten days a reversal of the hemolytic anemia trend has not begun, serious consideration should be given to splenectomy. In a certain proportion of these cases combined surgical and medical management is necessary to reestablish a normal hemolytopoietic equilibrium. Also, a relapse may occur following a more or less complete recovery, while cortisone therapy is still being administered, in which case splenectomy may offer the only recourse.

CHARLES A. DOAN

PRIMARY HYPERSPLENIC THROMBOCYTOPENIC PURPURA

(Werlhof's Disease, Essential Constitutional Thrombopenic Purpura, Thrombocytolytic Purpura, Idiopathic Purpura Haemorrhagica)

Definition. Spontaneous purpuric manifestations of skin and mucous membranes may reflect platelet, plasma and/or capillary defects. When the circulating blood platelets are discovered to be low or absent, and bone marrow studies reveal compensatory megakaryocytic hyperplasia without cell damage or decreased platelet potential, the accompanying purpura, whether acute or chronic, is most frequently due to a hypersplenic mechanism. When unassociated with or secondary to any other discoverable disease or coagulation defect, this purpuric syndrome is known as primary hypersplenic thrombocytopenic purpura hemorrhagica. It is usually characterized by a prolonged bleeding time, positive tourniquet test, an essentially normal coagulation time, but with delayed and incomplete prothrombin consumption time and noncontractile clot. The onset and course of the clinical disease are unpredictable, and may be marked by spontaneous showers of petechiae, ecchymoses, bleeding gums, epistaxes, menorrhagia and more or less severe hemorrhages of the genitourinary and gastrointestinal tracts, and of the central nervous system.

. **History.** This constitutional, purpuric syndrome falls into the classification "morbus maculosus hemorrhagicus," which was first differentiated and described by Werlhof (1735). Krauss (1883) and Denys (1887) noted independently the characteristic decrease in platelets, and Hayem (1895) observed the delayed retractility of the soft clot. Duke (1912) reported a prolongation of the bleeding time. The Rumpel-Leede capillary resistance test demonstrated the associated vascular phenomena.

Frank (1915) was the first to suspect the spleen of playing a role in this type of purpura. Kaznelson (1916), just a year later, hypothesized a direct thrombocytolytic mechanism within the spleen itself, and the first successful splenectomy for thrombocytopenic purpura was performed in that year on his advice. Since this demonstration of the potential benefits to be derived from splenectomy in selected cases of purpura, statistical studies (1916–1928) revealed more than 90 per cent recoveries in the clinically chronic thrombocytopenic purpuras, but more than 90 per cent fatalities in those patients with acute clinical syndromes and subjected to splenectomy *without* preoperative blood transfusions. With the increase in use and improvement in techniques for preoperative fresh whole blood transfusions, a better understanding of underlying mechanisms and a correspondingly greater accuracy in differential diagnosis within the wide range of purpuric syndromes, splenectomy has now become as safe and certain in the acute splenic thrombocytopenic crises as in those patients showing more chronic clinical manifestations.

Etiology and Pathologic Physiology. As the definition implies, this purpuric syndrome behaves and responds as though related primarily to a malfunctioning spleen rather than to an underfunctioning bone marrow, or to disturbances in other coagulation factors readily proved to be normal. Appropriate studies of the intact spleen (epinephrine test) reveal a reversible hypersequestration or direct "shunt" increase of circulating platelets. At the operating table it is possible to demonstrate far more platelets entering this organ via the splenic artery than can be shown leaving via the splenic vein—until a sharp splenic contraction is accomplished by intra-arterial epinephrine injection or by mechanical manipulation, when a reversal of the original afferent and efferent cellular disequilibrium is observed. Supravital studies of freshly removed splenic tissue reveal large foci of agglutinated platelets both within and without the highly phagocytic clasmatocytes far more often than can be demonstrated in fixed sections. Likewise, direct microscopic studies of living bone marrow preparations from the "typical" case of this type show increased numbers of megakaryocytes of all ages, many of the larger, more mature cells showing active cytoplasmic fragmentation with shedding of normal-appearing platelets. Within seconds or at most a few minutes after ligation of the splenic pedicle, the oozing blood in the operative field clots firmly for the first time, and peripheral blood studies at this time show a sharp, subsequently sustained increase in circulating platelets. Any subclinical neutropenia or mild hemolytic anemia which may have been associated is promptly corrected.

Symptoms and Signs. Recurrent capillary hemorrhages of skin and mucous membranes, with or without spontaneous bleeding of the gums, epistaxis and menorrhagia in the female, distinguish clinically the more chronic forms of hypersplenic thrombocytopenia from the purpuric syndromes resulting from other mechanisms. The purpuric signs will be found to fluctuate from time to time in direct relationship to the circulating platelets. The cutaneous manifestations may be extensive, but more frequently consist of a few scattered petechiae with an occasional large ecchymotic area. Slight trauma markedly increases these signs. Bleeding may occur into any tissue, and repeated occult blood loss as well as obvious hemorrhage may lead to clinical anemia. It is usual to obtain a history of easy bruising, with frequent but not severe bleeding and petechial "showers" over many years. Clinical exacerbations with more profound thrombocytopenia occur at the menstrual periods, during pregnancy or in the puerperium and associated with mild infections. Intracerebral or meningeal capillary hemorrhage may be accompanied by transitory sensory, motor, mental or meningismal disturbances, and the danger either of progressive scarring or of fatal hemorrhage into a vital area demands prompt prophylactic surgery as soon as the hypersplenic mechanism has been established. The spleen, in our experience, is never grossly enlarged in primary thrombocytopenic purpura.

In the *acute* thrombocytopenic crisis the hemorrhages may begin abruptly without previous warning, or they may reflect a sudden acute exacerbation of the more chronic syndrome. No enlargement of the spleen is present to direct attention to this organ. Acute generalized bleeding, both internal and external, when it develops, presents the most dramatic and urgent medical and surgical emergency with which any physician can be faced. An exact differential diagnosis is mandatory in the shortest possible time, since blood transfusions in the presence of a fulminant hypersplenic mechanism may fail to establish the platelets above a critical level, even temporarily. Signs of increased intracranial pressure may develop before the diagnostic procedures are completed, thus requiring emergency spinal tap and drainage.

Diagnosis. At the present time, when certain acute infections, some chemotherapeutic agents, as well as many industrial toxins, may precipitate a thrombocytopenic purpura secondary to bone-marrow damage, it is essential to know the number and quality of the megakaryocytes in every patient with such a purpuric crisis. A careful and thorough examination immediately of aspirated marrow from sternum and, if necessary, from other skeletal sites should be undertaken, preferably with living cell techniques, to evaluate megakaryocyte integrity, platelet potential and actual thrombocyte production. This is the most important single differential diagnostic test, and when a healthy compensatory megakaryocytosis is found, removal of the spleen will be followed by an increase in circulating platelets and clinical recovery. Such a study will reveal any toxic destruction or depression of the marrow leading to a hypoplastic subcellularity, or expose an acute leukemic myelophthisic displacement of megakaryocytes.

In the clinically subacute and chronic thrombocytopenic syndromes, an epinephrine-induced contraction of the spleen may be invoked to confirm further the direct bone marrow observations of compensatory megakaryocytosis with increased platelet production. Vitamin C, prothrombin and fibrinogen levels should be determined to assure their normality. Hemorrhages which result from telangiectatic foci can be readily differentiated. A mild hemophilic trait rarely may be confused with chronic, intermittent thrombocytopenic purpura, either when the platelets are found to be within the lower limits of normal, or when the coagulation time in a mild hemophiliac is temporarily within physiologic limits. Antigenic hypersensitization of the megakaryocytes may precipitate a transitory allergic thrombocytopenia with or without eosinophilia of blood and bone marrow; a study of the marrow cells will reveal the toxic nuclear and cytoplasmic vacuolization of the megakaryocytes and frequently of some of the other developing cells.

Prognosis and Treatment. Fatal internal hemorrhage is always a potential possibility; therefore the prognosis should be guarded in any purpuric syndrome. Carefully matched fresh blood transfusions must be given repeatedly. When a peripheral hypersplenic mechanism is established, the surgical removal of all splenic tissue may be life-saving, and is usually followed by immediate and sustained thrombocytosis and a dramatic clinical remission (Fig. 145). Rarely remissions do not follow, or relapses occur when accessory splenic tissue has been overlooked or is subsequently demonstrated embedded in other organs, such as the pancreas. Such ectopic foci are capable of precipitating a cytopenic develop with a corresponding persistence and chronicity of purpuric signs and symptoms. Thorotrast visualization of such reticuloendothelial cell concentrations or biopsy tissue studies will confirm the diagnosis. Surgical

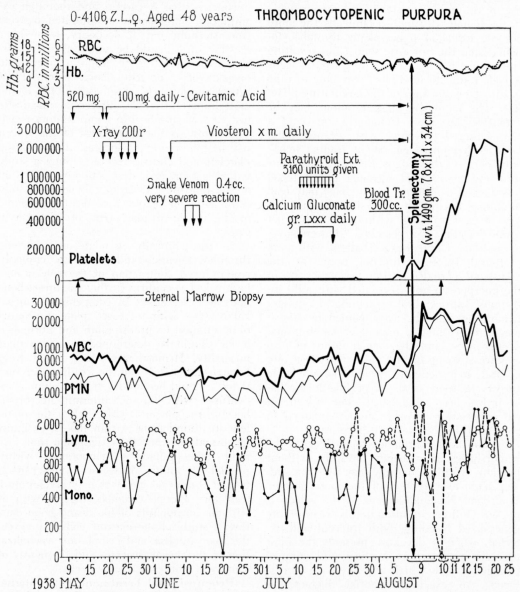

Fig. 145. Chronic primary splenic thrombocytopenic purpura with megakaryocytic hyperplasia of marrow. Failure of all medical treatment to effect hematologic or clinical remission was followed by complete and permanent restoration of the platelets to normal after splenectomy, with disappearance of all clinical symptoms.

episode similar to that provoked by the original spleen. Or a generalized reticuloendothelial cell hyperplasia and hyperphagocytosis, involving the Kupffer cells of the liver and the phagocytes in lymph nodes, bone marrow and diffuse connective tissues, may reexploration must be undertaken in those instances in which both x-ray and marrow findings point to a localized ectopic hypersplenic mechanism.

The role of ACTH and cortisone in the control of purpura haemorrhagica has been found in most clinics to be more variable than that of splenectomy. Harrington et al. (1951) have demonstrated the presence of a circulating thrombocytopenic plasma factor in 6 patients with the classic idiopathic or primary purpuric syndrome, in 2 of whom purpuric episodes recurred following splenectomy. Plasma from these patients in amounts of 100 to 300 cc., when given intravenously to normal human subjects, induced a significant thrombocytopenia lasting from four to six days, with clinical, hematologic and bone marrow findings similar to those existing in the donor patients. Cortisone and ACTH failed to prevent or alleviate the syndrome in 1 patient in this series. Stefanini and associates have confirmed these findings and have demonstrated a thrombocytopenic factor in normal human blood plasma and serum.

Studies in this laboratory have shown a positive Coombs' test for "blocking" erythrocyte antibodies in occasional patients with thrombocytopenic purpura, and it is in these patients that cortisone or ACTH seems to exert the best temporary effects. The development of anti-platelet substances following repeated transfusions has been cited as the acquired immunochemical mechanism which produces progressively shorter platelet survival times in some patients. It seems likely that there are at least two possible interacting mechanisms in this syndrome: One comprises the so-called "hypersplenic" platelet-sequestering and/or megakaryocytic-suppressive activities of a pathologic spleen, which are dramatically and permanently "cured" by successful splenectomy; the other is mediated by a circulating "thrombocytopenic plasma factor," which may be so high in titer in some patients as to continue its influence even after splenectomy, responding, on occasion, to ACTH and/or cortisone.

In our experience the former mechanism is much more commonly encountered than the latter, and the response to splenectomy may be the only way to make the differentiation.

Other methods of treatment such as x-ray, vitamins C and K, parathormone, calcium and rutin have proved ineffective. However, other potentially important defects in the coagulation mechanism must always be suspected and corrected when discovered, even when thrombocytopenia is obvious.

Charles A. Doan

PRIMARY SPLENIC NEUTROPENIA

History and Definition. When the modern studies of congenital hemolytic anemia and thrombocytopenic purpura began to point toward a splenic hypersequestration mechanism rather than to defective bone marrow production, the possibility of the granulocytes also becoming involved at times in this same general process had to be entertained. We had noted the frequency of an associated mild neutropenic leukopenia in our patients with hemolytic jaundice, more particularly during acute hemoclastic crises. It was during 1937 that the first clinical cases were recognized with primary neutropenic syndromes in this clinic, and since that time many similar cases have been recorded in the medical literature. This syndrome is defined by its name—a profound, clinically significant neutropenia due solely to hypersequestration and hyperdestruction of granulocytes by and within the spleen, despite compensatory marrow myelopoiesis and without demonstrable evidence of any other related organic pathologic process. As in the other hypersplenic dyscrasias, the granulocytopenic syndrome may manifest itself either by chronic recurrent clinical signs or as a fulminant septicemic crisis.

Diagnosis and Pathologic Physiology. There is usually an initially small spleen with progressive enlargement as the acute syndrome develops; in the more chronic cases the spleen may fill the entire abdomen. Oral ulcerations, conjunctivitis, refractory ulcers of the lower extremities, ulcerative enteritis and cystitis fail to respond to antibiotic therapy. There may be an associated thrombocytopenia and mild anemia of secondary hemolytic type. A profound granulocytopenic leukopenia is the rule with less than 1000 circulating leukocytes, of which only 1 to 10 per cent are granulocytes. A study of the marrow *always* reveals a nontoxic, nonleukemic, compensatory myeloid hyperplasia, together with normal though relatively reduced erythropoiesis and megakaryocytosis. An epinephrine-induced contraction of the enlarged spleen will be accompanied by a transitory increase in circulating neutrophils to normal or, at times, to a considerably higher than normal peak. All liver function tests are normal, and there are no arthritic manifestations of Felty's syndrome. Subleukemic leukemia, hypoplastic anemia, Schultz syndrome of malignant neutropenia are readily differentiated.

Prognosis and Treatment. Successful splenectomy is immediately and permanently curative. Irradiation, pentnucleotides, yellow bone marrow, spleen extracts and folic acid have all proved ineffective in influencing beneficially this syndrome.

CHARLES A. DOAN

PRIMARY CONGENITAL SPLENIC PANHEMATOPENIA

Definition, Pathologic Physiology and Treatment. Reference has already been made in this section to the occasional pancytopenic instability of the spleen in hemolytic anemia, thrombocytopenic purpura and splenic neutropenia. These mixed cell, peripheral hypersequestration phenomena, found always in direct association with a compensatory marrow hyperplasia, have only served to emphasize further the unique and unpredictable capacity of this vascular organ to precipitate a variety of cytopenic crises. It has seemed logical, therefore, to look for and to expect to find an occasional syndrome in which all three of these elements of bone marrow origin are equally susceptible of hypersequestration by a spleen in which there is histologic evidence of reticuloendothelial cell hyperplasia and nondiscriminatory cellular hyperphagocytosis.

In the fall of 1943 such a patient was first seen and studied in this Clinic. A girl, 14 years old, had been known to have a peripheral circulating pancytopenia since the first blood study made six months after birth. Infancy and childhood were spent as a semi-invalid with constant medical attention for skin infections, chronic anorexia, insomnia, diuresis, extreme weakness and pallor with emotional instability because of limitation of physical activities, without mental retardation. On admission 36 per cent of 1600 total white blood cells were mature neutrophils; total red blood cells were 1,030,000; hemoglobin, 3.5 gm., reticulocytes, 3 per cent; platelets, 200,000; normal corrected sedimentation index; normal erythrocyte fragility and van den Bergh reaction; normal prothrombin, blood urea nitrogen and blood sugar; phenolsulfonphthalein excretion 85 per cent; x-ray and electrocardiogram within physiological limits; serology normal. The bone marrow showed compensatory pancellular hyperplasia, and the epinephrine test was followed by an increase from 1450 to 10,250 white blood cells; 800,000 to 1,700,000 red blood cells; hemoglobin, 5.3 to 6.5 gm.; platelets, 313,000 to 911,000 per cubic millimeter. A 475 gm. spleen was removed without complications October 21, 1943, the white blood cell count increasing immediately postoperatively from 2100 (798 polymorphonuclear) to 17,000 (7140 polymorphonuclear); red blood cell count from 1,000,000 to 2,180,000 (without transfusion); hemoglobin from 4.3 to 7.8 gm.; platelets from 292,000 to 1,521,000. Only pancellular hypersequestration, reticuloendothelial cell hyperplasia and hyperphagocytosis without ectopic hematopoiesis were observed in both supravital and fixed tissue preparations from this spleen; sections from liver and lymph node biopsies revealed no pathologic process. The prompt hematologic reequilibration was accompanied by an equally prompt, dramatic and complete clinical recovery, which has been maintained uninterruptedly throughout the subsequent years to date.

Occasionally there may occur a pancytopenic crisis which requires emergency splenectomy—the criteria of differential diagnosis being the same as those already indicated for the more chronic syndrome.

To be differentiated are panhypoplasia and leukemic panmyelophthisis of the marrow, either of which may simulate primary splenic panhematopenia in terms of circulating blood elements. The prognosis in the latter is obviously excellent, in sharp contradistinction to the other two.

CHARLES A. DOAN

SECONDARY ACQUIRED HYPERSPLENISM

Clinical evidence has steadily accumulated through the past two decades that the spleen as well as the bone marrow is involved in a large number of patients who show a pathologic decrease in one or more of the essential circulating blood elements. While the marrow must always be appraised and its functional integrity accurately judged, a secondary acquired hypersplenic factor is being found frequently as an unexpected complication in an ever larger number of nonhereditary pathologic conditions. Referring to the discussion earlier in this section of the unique structure and function of the human spleen, we find in Björkman's crucial experimental studies the basic common denominator for a reasonably satisfactory explanation of the observed clinical facts.

Von Haam and Awny (1948) have divided secondary hypersplenism into six pathologic groups, in all of which hypersplenic syndromes indistinguishable from those already described on an inherited or congenital basis have developed.

1. Under *congestive splenomegaly* are included myocardial decompensation, Banti's

syndrome secondary to portal cirrhosis and hypertension, and acquired hemolytic icterus. More than 65 patients have been subjected to splenectomy in this group.

2. The *infiltrative splenomegalies* are represented by the xanthomatoses, with special reference to Gaucher's disease. Five of these patients have benefited from splenectomy with the correction of a profound panhematopenia and are living normal healthy lives at the present time, even though typical lipid-containing cells may be demonstrated in the bone marrow at any time. Two young women patients have married since splenectomy and have given birth to normal infants, without any evidence of progressive disease in the marrow or of transmission of the trait to the offspring.

3. During the course of chronic leukemia of any of the three main types there may develop suddenly an acute *hemoblastic splenomegaly* independent of any other evidence of leukemic exacerbation elsewhere in the body. The marrow will reflect this abnormal peripheral demand and destruction by a compensatory hyperplasia of the elements specifically depressed in the blood, without any evidence of myelophthisic displacement or replacement phenomena. In such circumstances —usually an acute hemolytic anemia—splenectomy is indicated and is usually successful in reestablishing the previous equilibrium, which is then maintained by whatever therapy has proved previously effective for the leukemia.

4. Splenomegaly secondary to *chronic infections,* such as tuberculosis, syphilis and moniliasis, has been identified on occasion with a characteristic hypersplenic cytopenia. Surgical removal of this focus of disease not only immediately releases the essential cellular products from the bone marrow more fully to the blood and tissues generally, but at the same time the primary disease may be more effectively treated by the specific agents indicated. Boeck's sarcoidosis and Hodgkin's syndrome, both granulomas of as yet undetermined and unproved etiology, are placed nevertheless in this same general category inasmuch as they have many features in common with the chronic tissue reactions already mentioned, and splenomegaly is a common finding. In 7 instances in which these conditions involved the spleen, an acute thrombocytopenia, granulocytopenia, or hemolytic anemia developed in which splenectomy was followed by an immediate and sustained re-

equilibration of the circulating elements. Bone marrow studies showed preoperatively the characteristic compensatory hyperplasia of the deficient circulating cells in every instance. The primary disease process progressed or regressed independently of the surgery, consistent with the effectiveness of the general therapeutic measures instituted.

5. *Neoplastic involvement* of the spleen is rare, but in one patient with retotheliosarcoma, one with multiple myeloma, four with follicular lymphoblastoma, and in two patients with large primary nodular hemangiomas of the spleen in our series, chronic hypersplenic cytopenia had made invalids of the patients, and splenectomy relieved all current symptoms with full clinical and hematologic remissions, which have persisted several years after the original surgery. Some 200 primary tumors of the spleen have been reported in the literature, and Krumbhaar found 40 secondary malignant tumors metastatic to the spleen in his series of postmortem analyses.

6. Finally, splenomegaly secondary to *progressive myelofibrosis* is usually the principal site of ectopic compensatory hematopoiesis. At times, however, the spleen participates in the fibrotic process, and hypersequestration and hyperphagocytosis of mature blood elements may supersede the hematopoietic potential. When such a hemolytopoietic imbalance occurs, splenectomy results in the reestablishment of an adequate cellular equilibrium. In two instances sustained benefit followed removal of all splenic tissue. In four other patients, studies revealed an almost absolute aplasia of the marrow with complete dependence upon spleen and liver for all current hematopoiesis. In such circumstances, even though recurrent hemoclastic crises do develop from time to time, secondary to the splenomegaly, removal of the spleen will only increase the need and frequency for blood transfusions and is definitely contraindicated. The spleen eventually fills the entire abdomen and makes for extreme discomfort. Even partial or complete intestinal obstruction may supervene. But when in a single organ both production and destruction are concentrated, the physician may be confronted with an insoluble dilemma.

Generalized Reticuloendotheliosis. In one other instance the physician is faced with an as yet insoluble problem. In 5 of some 375 patients with hypersplenic syndromes studied in this Clinic, removal of all discoverable splenic tissue has failed to relieve the evidences of excessive stress and bring the peripheral demands within the functional capacity of the bone marrow. In these instances the liver and mesenteric lymph nodes have been greatly enlarged, distended with blood, and purple in color; and biopsy studies have revealed greatly engorged sinuses with a generalized reticuloendothelial cell hyperplasia and hyperphagocytosis of platelets and erythrocytes, despite compensatory normoblastosis and megakaryocytosis in the marrow. A precarious balance with ebb and flow of signs and symptoms results clinically, with the cautious use of fresh whole blood transfusions in purpuric emergencies. Irradiation, radio-isotopes, Thorotrast or other phagocytizable inhibitors of reticuloendothelial cell hyperactivity have thus far failed to accomplish a satisfactory remission.

Relative Hypersplenism. In certain patients who have experienced permanent marrow damage from industrial or other toxins, but in whom progressive mesenchymal destruction has been halted by removal from the environment, the reservoir function of the normal spleen may be sufficient to continue the state of marrow decompensation. If, after a period of supportive therapy, the marrow still fails to produce sufficient cells, splenectomy may tip the balance and permit marrow recompensation.

Contraindications to Splenectomy. Emphasis has been placed on exact diagnosis in the hypersplenic states. Splenectomy may be life-saving. It also can be catastrophic if it is invoked when there is (1) any acute or chronic bone marrow damage, (2) myelofibrosis, (3) osteopetrosis, (4) panmyelophthisis or (5) ectopic splenic hematopoiesis plus secondary hypersplenism.

CHARLES A. DOAN

MISCELLANEOUS ABNORMALITIES OF THE SPLEEN

Movable Spleen. As part of a general visceroptosis, or secondary to an abdominal malformation, or as an adaptation to slow or rapid enlargement, the spleen occasionally presents a problem of identification. If the characteristic shape and notches can be palpated, diagnosis is easy. Usually any upper left quadrant mass, if it is the spleen, moves with respiration and displaces the resonant intestine downward and medially so that a flat percussion note is elicited, in contradistinction to the findings if it is a tumor arising retroperitoneally. An injection of epinephrine will usually elicit a sharp, transitory contraction of an enlarged spleen. The spleen may enlarge medially and still not be palpable below the left costal margin, where it usually presents when pathologic changes occur. Contrast x-ray films will help in such circumstances.

Torsion of the Pedicle is a complication of *lien mobile,* which may cause sudden, acute abdominal pain and distress, with rapid enlargement of the spleen and signs of shock. Immediate surgical exploration and relief is mandatory.

Rupture or tear of the normal spleen usually results from severe upper abdominal injury, such as frequently occurs in an automobile collision. Shock usually develops rapidly or after a brief latent period from internal hemorrhage, and a boardlike rigidity of the abdominal musculature is of diagnostic significance. A delayed reaction is sometimes encountered, when a subcapsular hemorrhage occurs at the time of the trauma only to rupture some hours or days later accompanied by agonizing pain and shock which resemble the symptoms of torsion with signs of internal hemorrhage.

Spontaneous rupture occurs only in diseased spleens, secondary to an infarct, abscess or acute infectious splenic tumor. Pain in the left scapular region and nonshifting paravertebral dullness are of diagnostic significance. A marked leukocytosis and rapidly developing anemia follow, and, if splenic sepsis is present, signs of general peritonitis will ensue promptly. Surgical intervention should be made as soon as the diagnosis is suspected and established.

Acute Splenic Tumor. Because of the vascular-parenchymal relationships peculiar to the spleen, and its high complement of reticuloendothelial cells with their protective function in infections and toxemias, active congestion with gross splenomegaly occurs most frequently in these circumstances. The passive congestion of chronic myocardial failure and progressive hepatic cirrhosis results in the "cyanotic induration" of the pathologist's description. Only occasionally are complaints referable to the spleen made in these circumstances. Unless a hypersplenic cytopenia is precipitated, the successful treatment of the underlying condition is sufficient to control such splenic tumors.

Abscesses occur rarely in the spleen, and are usually the result of a septic infarct. One patient with chronic ulcerative splenitis suggestive of acid-fast etiology and showing hypersplenic cellular manifestations was found at surgery to have a large adhesive subdiaphragmatic abscess involving the entire upper pole of the spleen and yielding a pure strain of monilia on culture. With antibiotic therapy and chemotherapy now being used early in all the infectious states formerly associated with abscess formation, the spleen, always relatively resistant, should become involved still less frequently in the future.

Infarction of the spleen occurs frequently, both as reflected by the symptomatic complaints of patients with known splenic disease and as revealed at the postmortem table. When caused by a sterile embolus, the infarct may produce a transitory perisplenitis, with or without mild symptoms, and terminate in a localized atrophic fibrosis. Septic infarctions from infected emboli are exceedingly rare. Thrombosis of the splenic artery or retrograde thrombosis in the vein may be the source of some splenic infarcts. Bed rest and symptomatic treatment with sedation are indicated.

Nonparasitic Cysts of the Spleen. A recent review records 169 cases of nonparasitic cyst of the spleen, 21 per cent with a true secreting membrane, 10 per cent of the epidermoid variety. Occurring predominantly in women in the child-bearing age, the symptomatology is that of an upper left quadrant tumor usually readily identified as spleen. Surgical removal is indicated with or without manifestations of a hypersplenic syndrome.

Chronic Splenomegaly. The spleen, with its elastic muscular capsule, capacious parenchymal spaces, rich vascular supply and lymphopoietic follicles, enlarges readily and becomes the secondary site of many constitutional diseases. The earlier stages of congestion with reticuloendothelial cell and lymphopoietic hyperplasia are readily reversible, but the later malpighian atrophy and fibrosis may render the splenomegaly irreversible, but the later malpighian atrophy and important to determine whether the enlargement is serving a protective reservoir function, as in the leukemic states, or whether it is the site of a primary or metastatic locus of disease from which further dissemination may be expected, as in primary Hodgkin's disease of the spleen. Finally, there is the possibility that the spleen has reassumed its important embryonic compensatory hematopoietic potentialities, as in myelosclerosis. In any case, under any and all of these several causes for general enlargement there is an accentuation of the inherent instability of the spleen, with its tendency to withdraw, to withhold and to destroy the circulating elements of the blood. When this reservoir function becomes pathologic in degree, splenectomy is necessitated, irrespective of the cause of the splenomegaly.

Cirrhotic Splenomegaly (Banti's Syndrome). Splenomegaly may be an early and prominent manifestation of hepatic cirrhosis. Whether or not the obstruction to the portal circulation is the sole cause, or only one contributing factor in the early vascular congestion of the spleen, hypertrophy quickly develops, with evidences of hypersplenic cellular hypersequestration. Perisplenitis with peritoneal adhesions, and greatly dilated vasa brevia, make surgery unusually hazardous in the late cases. Only when a profound leukopenia or hemolytic anemia develops should surgery be undertaken. Early recognition and intelligent medical management usually will prevent progressive hepatic scarring, functional decompensation and the secondary hypersplenic syndrome.

Thrombosis of Splenic Vein. Sometimes difficult to differentiate from Banti's syndrome is partial thrombosis or progressive phlebosclerosis of the splenic vein. Involvement of the mesenteric veins will result in hemorrhoidal varicosities; and if the portal vein is implicated, jaundice may develop with ascites and a *caput medusae,* and other signs of collateral circulation will appear. The spleen becomes greatly congested and enlarged, the vasa brevia (gastric veins) are dilated, and more or less severe recurrent gastric hemorrhages occur. Anemia and leukopenia may be severe in this chronic Banti-like syndrome.

In acute thrombosis sudden severe abdominal pain, pallor, weakness and signs of vascular collapse may precede or accompany fatal gastric hemorrhage.

Diagnosis is difficult. Recurrent splenic episodes are significant, and if and when a correct diagnosis has been made, emergency splenectomy should be performed.

Amyloid Splenomegaly. Amyloid disease, secondary to chronic disease elsewhere, occurs more frequently in the spleen than in any other organ in the body (Krumbhaar). The Congo red test, where positive, may be of diagnostic value. The elimination of chronic pulmonary infections, osteomyelitis and other chronic conditions by modern therapeutic measures should see the gradual disappearance of amyloidosis as a significant pathologic problem.

The Malaria Spleen. In some parts of the world where malaria is endemic, a large, hard, pigment-laden spleen is found in a majority of the native population. Its reservoir function for erythrocytes makes it also a reservoir for intracellular parasites, difficult of therapeutic sterilization. When the plasmodia are difficult to demonstrate in blood films, an epinephrine test will frequently visualize circulating parasite-containing erythrocytes at the height of the splenic contraction. Perisplenic adhesions in the more chronic cases render splenectomy difficult; but both on the grounds of chronic hypersplenism and as a means of accomplishing the elimination of a large focus of parasites, removal of the spleen is frequently indicated and is followed by decreased morbidity and mortality.

Kala-azar is one of the commonest causes of splenomegaly in the Orient. The splenic enlargement is due to an extensive hyperplasia of the reticuloendothelial cells, within which are found the *Leishmania donovani* parasites. Splenic puncture is diagnostic. When hypersplenic pancytopenia develops to complicate this condition, splenectomy promptly restores the circulating elements to normal.

CHARLES A. DOAN

References

Aschoff, L.: The Reticulo-Endothelial System. New York, Paul B. Hoeber, Inc., 1924.

Barcroft, J., and others: Contributions to Physiology of the Spleen. J. Physiol., 60:433, 1925; 74:299, 1932.

Björkman, S. F.: The Splenic Circulation. Acta med. Scandinav., 128:1947, Suppl. 191.

Dawson, Lord, of Penn: The Hume Lectures on Hemolytic Jaundice. Brit. M. J., 1:921, 963, 1931.

Doan, C. A.: The Spleen and Reticulo-Endothelial System, in Sodeman, W. A.: Pathologic Physiology. Philadelphia, W. B. Saunders Company, 1950.

————: The Etiology and Management of the Hemorrhagic Diatheses. Ann. Int. Med., 35:967, 1940.

————: Hypersplenism. Bull. N. Y. Acad. Med., 25:625, 1949.

————, and Wright, C. S.: Primary Congenital and Secondary Acquired Splenic Panhematopenia. Blood, 1:10, 1946.

Emerson, V. P., Jr., Shen, S. C., Ham, T. H., and Castle, W. B.: The Mechanism of Blood Destruction in Congenital Hemolytic Jaundice. J. Clin. Investigation, 26:1180, 1947.

Harrington, W. J., Minnich, V., Hollingsworth, J. W., and Moore, C. V.: Demonstration of a Thrombocytopenic Factor in the Blood of Patients with Thrombocytopenic Purpura. J. Lab. & Clin. Med., 38:1, 1951.

————, Sprague, C. C., Minnich, V., Moore, C. V., Aulvin, R. C., and Dubach, R.: Immunologic Mechanisms in Idiopathic and Neonatal Thrombocytopenic Purpura. Ann. Int. Med., 38:433, 1953.

King, J. H.: Studies in the Pathology of the Spleen. Arch. Int. Med., 14:145, 1914.

Knisely, M. H.: Spleen Studies. Anat. Rec., 65:23, 1946.

Krumbhaar, M. H.: Functions of the Spleen. Physiol. Rev., 6:160, 1926.

MacKenzie, D. W., Jr., Whipple, A. O., and Wintersteiner, M. P.: Studies on the Microscopic Anatomy and Physiology of Living Transilluminated Mammalian Spleens. Am. J. Anat., 68:397, 1941.

Owren, P. A.: Congenital Hemolytic Jaundice. Blood, 3:231, 1948.

Parnes, I. H.: Nonparasitic Cysts of the Spleen. J. Mt. Sinai Hosp., 16:245, 1949.

Scheff, G. J., and Awny, A. J.: Lecithinase Activity in Splenic Dyscrasias. Am. J. Clin. Path., 19:615, 1949.

Stefanini, M., and others: Studies in Thrombocytopenic Purpura: J. Clin. Investigation, 31:665, 1952; Proc. Soc. Exper. Biol. & Med., 79:663, and 81:230, 1952; Blood, 7:53, 1952.

Wright, C-S., Dodd, M. C., Brandt, N. J., Elliott, S. M., and Bass, J. A.: Erythrophagocytosis: Standardization of a Quantitative Tissue Culture Test and its Application to Hemolytic, Malignant and Infectious Diseases. J. Lab. & Clin. Med., 41:169, 1953.

————, Bundham Sundharagiati, Bass, J. A., and Bunner, A. E.: Review of the 1952 Hematology Literature. Arch. Int. Med., 92:357, 1953.

————, Mabry, S., Carr, R. D., and Perry, A. M.: Survey of the 1953 Hematology Literature. Arch. Int. Med., 94:648, 806, 995, 1954.

DISEASES OF THE RETICULOENDOTHELIAL SYSTEM

Diseases of the reticuloendothelial system include those which primarily affect the lymph nodes, eosinophilic granuloma, the Letterer-Siwe syndrome, and an apparently heterogeneous group of disorders characterized by accumulation of lipids in reticuloendothelial cells. The classification is not altogether consistent since it is no more logical to place lymphosarcoma under this heading than it would be to include the leukemias.

CONDITIONS PRIMARILY AFFECTING LYMPH NODES

The conditions primarily affecting lymph nodes are often collectively called malignant lymphomas, but objection to this term is raised by those workers who doubt that Hodgkin's disease is a malignant neoplasm. For that reason, the more general designation used here seems preferable. Further difficulty occurs when one attempts to divide these conditions into specific diseases. For instance, the term lymphosarcoma is often used generically to cover lymphocytic, lymphoblastic and reticulum cell types of sarcoma. Furthermore, many pathologists believe that reticulum cell sarcoma is indistinguishable from Hodgkin's sarcoma, and a few argue that the various lymphomas are so closely interrelated that transition from one type to another is a common occurrence. Precise classification at present, therefore, is impossible, and must wait until morphologic evidence can be supplemented by a better understanding of etiology and of cellular physiology. Division into lymphosarcoma, reticulum cell sarcoma, Hodgkin's disease and follicular lymphoma is a compromise, but it has the virtue of being simple and clinically serviceable.

LYMPHOSARCOMA AND RETICULUM CELL SARCOMA

The clinical manifestations, diagnosis and treatment of lymphosarcoma and reticulum cell sarcoma are so similar that it is profitable to consider them together in order to avoid unnecessary repetition.

Definition. Lymphosarcoma is a disease characterized by neoplastic proliferation of lymphocytes in lymph nodes, spleen and the lymphoid tissue of other organs. Almost any portion of the body may be involved either by direct extension or by dissemination through the blood stream or lymphatic channels. The same may be said for reticulum cell sarcoma except that it is the reticulum cell which undergoes neoplastic change. Symptoms are determined largely by the sites at which lymph node enlargement is greatest, and by the structures subjected to pressure, obstruction and infiltration by the sarcomatous tissue. Terminally, cachexia, fever, anemia, hemorrhagic manifestations and susceptibility to infections are common.

Incidence. Lymphosarcoma and reticulum cell sarcoma are not common, but neither are they rare diseases. Their distribution is world-wide, although their incidence seems to be somewhat less among nonwhite than among white races. Males are affected about twice as frequently as females. Both diseases occur at all ages, but their incidence rises sharply after the age of 40. In 1949 there were 2354 deaths reported in the United States from lymphosarcoma, or 15.8 deaths per million of the population. The corresponding figure for reticulum cell sarcoma is 383 total deaths, or 2.58 per million of the population. The actual difference in incidence is probably less than these figures indicate bcause many pathologists classify their cases of reticulum cell sarcoma as types of lymphosarcoma.

Etiology. Nothing is known about the etiology of these two diseases except that they seem to be malignant tumors. No predisposing factors have been recognized although a disease at least similar to lymphosarcoma has been produced experimentally by exposure of animals to estrogens and carcinogenic hydrocarbons. Lymphosarcoma in mice is transmissible.

Pathologic Anatomy. The involved lymph nodes enlarge, have a thickened capsule, are usually discrete, but may become matted together, particularly in the retroperitoneal area where large tumor masses may form. When sectioned, the grayish white, granular parenchyma bulges slightly above the cut surface. The normal histologic architecture is destroyed by what appears to be an almost solid sheet of the sarcomatous cells. Many pathologists differentiate between a large and a small cell, or a lymphoblastic and lymphocytic type of lymphosarcoma. This differentiation is of no clinical significance, however, because the course of the disease seems to be unrelated to the cell type. In reticulum cell sarcoma, the predominant reticulum cell is larger than a lymphocyte, has a large nucleus with a delicate chromatin network, a single prominent nucleolus, and moderately abundant pale-staining cytoplasm. Reticulin fibers may or may not be demonstrable with special staining techniques. In both types of lymphoma, mitotic figures are numerous, the marginal and medullary sinuses are invaded, and the cells may extend through the capsule to surrounding tissue or adjacent nodes. Similar changes may occur in any organs which normally contain lymphocytes or reticulum cells. In addition, the diseases may spread, apparently by metastasis, to any tissue. With serous membrane or meningeal involvement, the tumor may grow as thick sheets of cells rather than as nodular masses.

Clinical Manifestations. The most common and usually the earliest symptom is enlargement of lymph nodes in the cervical, axillary or inguinal regions. The nodes are firm, discrete, and are not painful unless growth has been rapid or an adjacent nerve is infiltrated. Enlargement may at first be unilateral and confined to one chain of nodes, or it may occur in several areas at about the same time. Mediastinal or retroperitoneal nodes may be the first to enlarge so that the presenting symptoms may be those of mediastinal obstruction, back pain or abdominal discomfort. It is not unusual for the primary site to be extranodal in tonsils, the nasopharynx, spleen, stomach, jejunum, ileum, rectum, and elsewhere. Primary lympho- or reticulum cell sarcoma of the stomach and rectum produces symptoms which may be clinically indistinguishable from those caused by carcinomas originating in these two organs.

After an initial period, very brief or prolonged for many months, during which the disease seems to be fairly localized, the sarcomatous involvement becomes more generalized. The patient complains of fatigue,

develops anorexia, loses weight and becomes debilitated. More specific symptoms are extremely variable, being determined by the tissues infiltrated, compressed or obstructed by the sarcomatous process. Enlarged mediastinal lymph nodes may produce cough, substernal pain, dysphagia, paralysis of the recurrent laryngeal nerve, and evidences of superior vena caval obstruction. Pulmonary involvement, nodular or of a diffuse miliary type, may cause atelectasis, cough, dyspnea and cyanosis. Pleural effusion is relatively common, may be unilateral or bilateral, may be chylous in type, particularly in lymphosarcoma, and is often incapacitating. Cardiac manifestations are rare, but there may occasionally be pericarditis with effusion or myocardial infiltration.

Lesions in the gastrointestinal tract may be secondary as well as primary. They may occur in the stomach, jejunum, ileum, cecum and rectum. The nodular masses may be large enough to feel; pain, hematemesis or melena, weight loss and evidences of chronic obstruction are the principal manifestations. Mesenteric nodes may become large enough to be palpated, and peritoneal infiltration may cause ascites. Rarely, the lacteals may be so extensively involved in lymphosarcoma that fat absorption is impaired and steatorrhea results. Jaundice may result from the intrahepatic obstruction of a segment of the liver by an enlarging nodule, or rarely from obstruction of the common bile duct by nodes at the hilum of the liver. The spleen is often not palpable during the early stages of the disease, but later it usually enlarges enough to extend below the costal margin and occasionally may become very large. Pain may occur in the left upper quadrant of the abdomen and the spleen may temporarily become very tender as the result of splenic infarction or perisplenitis. Retroperitoneal nodes may become so large that they can be palpated as a nodular matted mass just beneath the anterior abdominal wall. They may then produce a sense of fullness in the upper abdomen, interfere with eating, cause severe pain by pressure on spinal nerves, cause partial obstruction of the inferior vena cava, displace one or both kidneys and occasionally obstruct the ureters. There may be infiltration of the kidneys, bladder or prostate with resultant enlargement, pain, hematuria and retention of urine. Rarely, sarcomatous nodules may be found in the thyroid gland. The adrenal glands may become infiltrated so extensively that symptoms of adrenal cortical insufficiency are precipitated.

Osteolytic lesions develop not infrequently, particularly in lymphosarcoma. Bones most commonly involved are the vertebrae, pelvis, ribs and femurs but lesions may be found at any site including the skull. Pain, limited usually to the area affected, may be severe, and pathologic fractures may occur. Occasionally, enlargement of a bone may occur locally at the site of involvement.

Pruritus may be troublesome, but is less common than in Hodgkin's disease. Nodular infiltration in the skin or subcutaneous tissue is not unusual; there may be anywhere from one or two to hundreds of nodules scattered over a large portion of the body's surface. The nodules are usually dusky red or purplish in color; they may be small, discrete and nontender or they may enlarge to 5 cm. or more in diameter. In the latter case, they may extend several centimeters above the normal surface of the skin, may ulcerate and be painful.

All patients with lymphomas seem particularly susceptible to herpes zoster; those with lymphosarcoma and reticulum cell sarcoma are no exception. The lesions may involve the areas of distribution of any nerves in the body and tend to be severe. The pain may last for weeks or months during which time it may overshadow all other clinical manifestations.

The nervous system may be affected in other ways. Enlarged mediastinal nodes may cause Horner's syndrome by involving the cervical sympathetics, or vocal cord paralysis by pressure on the recurrent laryngeal nerve. Pressure on or infiltration of the brachial plexus and spinal nerves may lead to very distressing pain or paresthesias. Acute or subacute compression of the spinal cord, from collapse of an involved vertebra, or from pressure by subdural or epidural tumor masses, is not at all uncommon. The paraplegia, sensory loss and sphincter paralysis which follow may develop within a few days or may appear more slowly. Severe back pain often precedes the appearance of these symptoms. At times, the paraplegia comes on so quickly as to suggest interference with the blood supply to the cord. More rarely, there may be meningeal invasion, with or without cranial nerve paralysis, which causes headache, slight neck rigidity, evidences of increased intracranial pressure, mental

changes and even hemiparesis. A few instances have been reported of primary reticulum cell sarcoma of the brain; symptoms were those of a brain tumor and depended on localization.

Ultimately an anemia develops which contributes to the sense of weakness, and exaggerates any shortness of breath that may otherwise be present. Petechiae and bleeding from mucous membranes may also occur as the result of thrombocytopenia.

Diagnosis. The diagnosis of lymphosarcoma and reticulum cell sarcoma can be established only by biopsy. Clinical manifestations are not sufficiently distinctive to permit differentiation from other lymphomas, sarcoid, tuberculosis of lymph nodes, tumors in the mediastinum or abdomen, and other conditions. Laboratory procedures may be helpful in eliminating some but not all of the diseases which must be considered in the differential diagnosis, and there are no specific diagnostic tests other than biopsy. The lymph node to be removed for microscopic study should be selected with care, properly fixed and stained. Enlarged cervical, axillary and femoral nodes are satisfactory, but those in the inguinal regions are so frequently the site of chronic inflammatory changes that they should be avoided if others are accessible. Nodes in the posterior cervical chain should also be avoided if possible because of the danger of cutting the spinal accessory nerve during their removal. When this happens, there may be enough pain and weakness of the shoulder girdle to be partially disabling. Early in the course of lympho- and reticulum cell sarcoma, the histologic changes may not be distinctive enough to permit a diagnosis. Under these circumstances, if there are nodes in other areas, a second biopsy should be done. When enlargement seems limited to mediastinal nodes, biopsy of scalene lymph nodes may be attempted or a thoracic surgeon should be consulted about the possibility of obtaining tissue from the mediastinal lesion directly. If the only involved nodes are in the abdominal cavity, exploratory laparotomy should be done. Unless these precautions are taken to establish the diagnosis before treatment is begun, other diseases which can be treated more satisfactorily will mistakenly be regarded as lymphomas, therapy will be less intense because of the uncertainty, and the patient or his family is subjected to additional unnecessary anxiety.

Other diagnostic procedures are of value chiefly in recognizing sites of involvement. Roentgenographic studies of the chest, gastrointestinal tract and skeletal system are particularly helpful. Lateral or oblique views of the barium-filled stomach may reveal enlarged retroperitoneal nodes. Pyelograms may help to define a lower retroperitoneal mass or to identify lesions in the genitourinary tract. Cytologic examination of pleural or ascitic fluid may show great numbers of lymphocytes or reticulum cells. Spinal fluid studies may reveal a block when there is compression of the cord, or pleocytosis when the meninges are infiltrated.

Hematologic studies of the peripheral blood and bone marrow are usually of little diagnostic value except to rule out leukemia. In reticulum cell sarcoma, reticulum cells may be found in increased number in the marrow and a few young monocytes or reticulum cells may appear in the peripheral blood; the abnormalities, however, are usually not sufficiently definitive to be diagnostic. More frequently, in both lymphosarcoma and reticulum cell sarcoma the differential leukocyte count is normal except for an occasional myelocyte. The total white blood cell level is usually normal although a slight leukocytosis or a slight leukopenia may be present. Platelet levels tend to be within the normal range. Normocytic, normochromic anemia of moderate degree is common.

There are two important exceptions to the above statements which can best be classified as hematologic complications. Infrequently, late in the course of lymphosarcoma, peripheral blood and bone marrow changes similar to those of acute lymphocytic leukemia may appear (the leukosarcoma of Sternberg). The bone marrow becomes replaced by lymphosarcoma cells, the white blood cell count may rise to high levels, almost all of the leukocytes in the peripheral blood are abnormal lymphocytes, anemia becomes severe and thrombocytopenia may be profound. Of more practical therapeutic importance is the development of secondary hypersplenism or dysplenism. This complication may occur at any time in the course of any lymphoma to cause hemolytic anemia, often of severe degree, marked depression of the white cell count, thrombocytopenia or any combination of the three. The spleen is enlarged and the bone marrow precursors of the involved cellular elements are normal or even increased in number. With hemolytic anemia, the Coombs' test is frequently but not invariably positive.

Treatment. Deep roentgen ray therapy to lymph nodes and other areas of involvement is the treatment of choice. The exact method of administration and the dosage schedule must be decided by the radiotherapist, but the physician has three responsibilities: (*a*) to guide the radiologist in the selection of sites for therapy; (*b*) to make certain that treatment stops short of severe depression of the bone marrow; and (*c*) to decide when additional irradiation is necessary. If enlargement is limited to one group of nodes, little is to be gained by irradiating all lymph node areas; it is probably best to restrict the irradiation to the sites affected. When there is bone pain, nerve infiltration, or spinal cord involvement, considerable relief may follow local x-ray treatment. Irradiation to the pleura tends to be more effective if pleural fluid is first removed. An alternative and sometimes more effective way of treating pleural lesions is to instill, after first having removed as much fluid as possible, 100 millicuries of colloidal radioactive gold into the pleural cavity.

Roentgen irradiation frequently causes edema of the sarcomatous tissue during the first day or two. For that reason, one must proceed cautiously when signs of mediastinal obstruction are present or therapy is directed to spinal cord lesions. In general, treatment should be discontinued if the white cell count falls below 2000 per cubic millimeter or the platelet count decreases to less than 100,000 per cubic millimeter—to be resumed, if the radiotherapist so advises, after recovery from the marrow depression has occurred. Exceptions must be made at times, but the risk must be appreciated; with severe leukopenia antibiotics should be used prophylactically.

The clinical remissions produced by x-ray therapy vary greatly both in completeness and duration. At times, the patient may become asymptomatic for months or even years, while in other instances additional nodes enlarge before treatment at one site has been completed. When the remissions are good, the physician should observe the patient at intervals of two to six weeks in order that recurrences may be detected promptly.

Eventually, roentgen irradiation loses its therapeutic effectiveness. Nitrogen mustard or triethylene melamine may then be given (for method of administration, see under Hodgkin's disease) but results are usually disappointing. Cortisone in a dose of 100 mg. per day may afford temporary relief for short periods of time and may decrease bleeding by its effect on capillary permeability. Other chemotherapeutic agents (i.e., folic acid antagonists, 6-mercaptopurine) are even less satisfactory; they should be administered only when other measures have failed or when the changes of acute lymphocytic leukemia appear terminally in lymphosarcoma.

Anemia, thrombocytopenia or leukopenia may occasionally develop as a manifestation of abnormal splenic function (hypersplenism) even when the sarcomatous process otherwise seems to have responded satisfactorily to treatment. Under these circumstances, splenectomy may be followed by a return of the blood to normal, and may afford the patient additional months of comfortable, active life. Anemia may also appear late in the course of lympho- or reticulum cell sarcoma because of the general debility of the patient or because of extensive bone marrow invasion; transfusions should then be given as necessary for general supportive care.

Cases have been described in which very long remissions or apparent cures have followed surgical excision of a primary lesion. Many students of the disease argue that if patients are followed long enough, recurrence can always be observed. Until this dispute can be settled by further clinical study, it is difficult to justify subjecting patients to radical surgical procedures. On the other hand, if the primary involvement is localized in an area where it can easily be removed, the author believes it should be excised and the area then treated by irradiation. Many students of the disease, however, prefer to treat such localized lesions with a "tumor" dose of x-irradiation alone in the belief that there is just as much likelihood of eradicating the tumor in that manner.

Prognosis. Lymphosarcoma and reticulum cell sarcoma are fatal diseases at the present time. The average survival time from onset of symptoms is approximately two to two and a half years, with variations that range from only a few months to ten years or longer. If treatment is begun when lesions are localized to skin, the tonsils, the stomach, the intestinal tract or to one or two lymph nodes, the course of the disease tends to be longer than if dissemination has occurred before therapy is initiated. In general, the course in reticulum cell sarcoma tends to be somewhat more rapid than in lymphosarcoma.

HODGKIN'S DISEASE

Definition. Hodgkin's disease is a disease of the lymph nodes and non-nodal lymphatic tissue; reticulum cells are more specifically affected than are lymphocytes; most students regard it as a neoplastic disorder but there are vigorous proponents of an infectious etiology. Lymph node enlargement may initially be painless, insidious and localized to one group of nodes, but eventually the involvement becomes more generalized. Systemic reactions, particularly fever, are more prominent than with lympho- and reticulum cell sarcoma. Other symptoms are determined largely by secondary effects from pressure, obstruction or infiltration. The disease is regarded as being uniformly fatal, although a few isolated instances of apparent cure from early excision and treatment of a primary site have been reported.

History. Thomas Hodgkin in 1832 described 7 patients having in common lymph node and splenic enlargement, cachexia and a fatal termination. Twenty-three years later, Wilks concluded a detailed study of Hodgkin's cases, added 11 of his own, and named the condition "Hodgkin's disease." It is of interest that Fox later obtained the tissue from 3 of Hodgkin's original cases, and on the basis of microscopic examination accepted two as examples of Hodgkin's disease but regarded the third as lymphosarcoma. Some writers believe that the first recorded description should be attributed to Malpighi (1661), who observed "grape-like clusters of nodular splenic lesions" and enlarged lymph nodes in postmortem material. Scores of other names have been applied to the disease. Most of them, however, have carried the implication that the process is either a malignant neoplasm or an infectious granuloma. None has been generally accepted, and the term "Hodgkin's disease" now seems firmly established.

Incidence. Hodgkin's disease occurs among all races, but seems to be more frequent among the white races. Males are affected almost twice as commonly as are females. Although the disease occurs in children, it is unusual before the age of twenty. Its incidence increases gradually with advancing age to reach a peak value of about 60 deaths per million of the white male population at the sixth decade. In 1949, the number of reported deaths from Hodgkin's disease in the United States was 2476 or 16.6 per million of the total population.

Etiology. The etiology of Hodgkin's disease is unknown. All attempts to transmit it have been unsuccessful. The two principal opposing views are that it is (*a*) an infectious granuloma or (*b*) a true malignant neoplasm of lymphatic tissue.

Proponents of an infectious etiology point to the similarity between the granulomatous changes found in Hodgkin's disease and those characteristic of tuberculosis, brucellosis and other granulomas known to have an infectious origin. It is argued that the occasional patient in whom the disease lasts for twenty-five or more years does not behave as if he had a neoplastic disorder. Various workers have cultured from affected lymph nodes tubercle bacilli, particularly of the avian strain, Brucella organisms, diphtheroids, *Cryptococcus neoformans* and viruses. In each instance, however, subsequent work has indicated that the infectious agent was a contaminant, had secondarily invaded the involved tissue, or could not be established as the causative factor.

Greatest support for a neoplastic etiology comes from the infiltrative character of the lesions late in the course of the disease, and from the morphologic similarity they have to reticulum cell sarcoma. The tumor pathologist insists that Hodgkin's disease is a malignant neoplasm; if a virus or some other infectious agent should subsequently prove to be the etiologic factor, that would not necessarily invalidate the neoplastic hypothesis since some of the experimental, transmissible animal sarcomas have an established viral etiology.

Pathologic Anatomy. The lymph nodes in Hodgkin's disease are firm, may be as large as 4 to 6 cm. in diameter, and are usually discrete until late in the disease when invasion of the capsule causes them to become matted. Involvement of other tissues may occur either from direct invasion or by the development of lesions whenever accumulations of lymphocytes or reticulum cells are found. The histologic pattern is complex. The definitive landmark is the Reed-Sternberg cell, a cell apparently of reticulum origin, 10 to 40 microns in diameter, with a folded or multilobulated nucleus, coarse chromatin, prominent nucleoli and abundant cytoplasm which may show either acidophilic or basophilic staining reactions. Occasionally, the Reed-Sternberg cell may be multinucleated. In addition to these giant cells and lymphocytes, the nodes may also contain polymorphonuclear neutrophils, eosinophils, plasma cells and a hyperplasia of reticulum cells. The normal architecture of the node becomes destroyed and the capsule may be infiltrated. Necrosis and an increase in fibrous tissue are often present.

Early in the disease, the microscopic changes may be so indefinite that a diagnosis cannot be made with certainty. At times the histologic pattern so closely resembles lymphosarcoma, reticulum cell sarcoma or giant follicular lymphoblastoma that many pathologists believe these diseases may transform into Hodgkin's disease, or vice versa. The complexity of the microscopic pathology is further emphasized by Jackson and Parker's suggestion that three types of Hodgkin's disease can be recognized: paragranuloma, granuloma and sarcoma. They believe there may be transformation of the paragranuloma to granuloma, and then to sarcoma, but they are of the opinion that the reverse does not occur. It is claimed that there are important clinical correlations with these three types: i.e., paragranulomatous lesions are localized to lymph nodes and are compatible with a benign course until transformation takes place; Hodgkin's granuloma may involve any organ of the body, with the exception of the central nervous system, and is frequently widespread; Hodgkin's sarcoma is the most malignant, frequently has its origin in retroperitoneal lymph nodes, and may involve even the central nervous system. This division of Hodgkin's disease into three types, however, has been challenged by many pathologists who believe the variants may all be present at the same time and, with the exception of sarcomatous changes, are not associated with any important clinical correlations.

Clinical Manifestations. Painless enlargement of peripheral lymph nodes is usually the presenting complaint. The first nodes to be involved are most frequently those in the cervical region, with axillary and inguinal nodes following in that order. They are initially discrete, but matting may occur later. The nodes feel firm or rubbery. If enlargement has been rapid, they may be tender. Not infrequently, however, mediastinal or retroperitoneal lymph nodes may be enlarged before those in the peripheral areas; under these circumstances, the first symptoms may be those of mediastinal obstruction, substernal pain, abdominal pain, anorexia or awareness of an abdominal mass. In Hodgkin's disease, lesions do not originate in extranodal sites as often as in lympho- or reticulum cell sarcoma.

Tonsillar involvement is unusual. Lesions within the chest occur at some time during the course of Hodgkin's disease in more than half the patients. In addition to mediastinal lymph node enlargement, there may be infiltration of the pulmonary parenchyma, metastasis-like pulmonary nodules in which cavitation may occur, pleural invasion with effusion, and more rarely myocardial invasion. Prominent symptoms are cough, stridor, dyspnea, pain, cyanosis of the areas drained by the superior vena cava, and dysphagia. These symptoms may be incapacitating and so difficult to control that they overshadow all other manifestations of the disease.

The gastrointestinal tract is less frequently infiltrated in Hodgkin's disease than in lymphosarcoma and reticulum cell sarcoma, but lesions in the stomach are not rare. It is more common for a sense of fullness to result from pressure on the stomach by retroperitoneal nodes. The retroperitoneal mass may displace one or both kidneys, infiltrate spinal nerves or adjacent vertebrae, obstruct the ureters or the inferior vena cava, and grow so large that it is palpable in the epigastrium. Epigastric or back pain may be severe. A retroperitoneal mass, not otherwise palpable, can sometimes be felt by the examiner if the patient lies on his arms folded behind his back at the level of the upper lumbar vertebrae so that the vertebrae and retroperitoneal structures are forced anteriorly. The spleen becomes palpable in at least 50 per cent of cases. Partial or complete obstructive jaundice may be caused by nodules within the liver or occasionally by nodes at the hilum. Ascites may follow peritoneal invasion.

Lesions of Hodgkin's disease have been found in the uterus, ovaries, breast and prostate; symptoms are those of tumors occurring in these organs. Bone pain and tenderness may be very severe. Both osteoplastic and osteolytic changes can be demonstrated roentgenographically in about 15 per cent of patients; they are most frequently located in the pelvis, vertebrae, ribs and femur.

Changes in the nervous system and in the skin are similar to those described for lymphosarcoma and reticulum cell sarcoma. Pruritus, however, deserves special emphasis because it is more common and may be so severe as to be the patient's major complaint.

Generalized pigmentation, caused by melanin deposition, may also be pronounced enough to cause bronzing or even a Negroid appearance to the skin. Herpes zoster is fairly common.

Systemic manifestations are more prominent in Hodgkin's disease than in the other lymphomas. In the granulomatous and sarcomatous types of the disease, anorexia, lassitude, weight loss, night sweats, fever and chills may appear rather early. The fever may be mild or severe, and not infrequently is of the Pel-Ebstein type in which the temperature rises during a period of five or six days to about 40° C., remains for several days at this level, declines to normal during another period of five or six days, and then repeats the cycle. Fever tends to be particularly troublesome when there is pulmonary or retroperitoneal involvement, and is sometimes a prominent symptom when no enlarged nodes can be located by physical examination or the usual roentgenologic techniques. At times, patients with Hodgkin's disease may have fever of 38 or 39° C. and be totally unaware of the temperature elevation. Tachycardia is often present. Anemia develops except during the early stages of the disease. It exaggerates the weakness, lassitude, dyspnea, and causes pallor. Petechiae and bleeding from mucous membranes appear if the platelet count falls to low levels. Both anemia and thrombocytopenia may be manifestations of hypersplenism. Patients with Hodgkin's disease seem peculiarly susceptible to infection, probably because leukopenia may occur and because antibody production is impaired. It is said that tuberculosis follows Hodgkin's disease like a shadow. This susceptibility to infection may in part explain the large number of organisms (diphtheroids, *Cryptococcus neoformans,* etc.) which have been cultured from Hodgkin's tissue.

A strange symptom, apparently peculiar to Hodgkin's disease, is the occurrence of pain after the ingestion of alcohol at one of the sites of Hodgkin's involvement, such as peripheral lymph nodes, mediastinum or bone. In one series, it was observed in 9 of 62 patients. The pain is produced by relatively small amounts of alcohol, begins as soon as absorption occurs, and persists for 30 to 60 minutes, i.e., until the greater part of the alcohol has been oxidized. The symptom tends to disappear when remissions are induced by x-ray therapy.

Diagnosis. Although occasionally lymph

node enlargement, Pel-Ebstein fever and pruritus may strongly suggest that a patient has Hodgkin's disease, the diagnosis can be established only by biopsy. The same precautions about selecting lymph nodes for study which have been outlined for lympho- and reticulum cell sarcoma should be used. If

Roentgenographic studies of the chest, gastrointestinal tract, genitourinary system and bones are helpful in localizing involvement when symptoms point to these areas.

Hematologic changes are not definitive. The total white blood cell count may be normal, low or elevated, but leukocytosis of

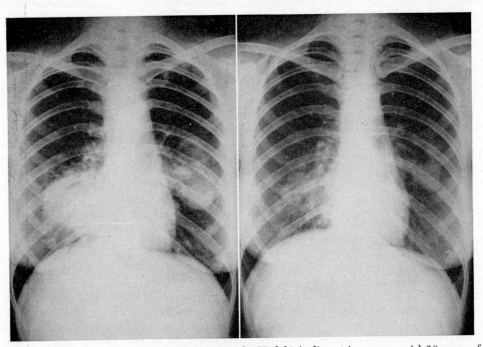

Fig. 146. Pulmonary and mediastinal involvement by Hodgkin's disease in a young girl 20 years of age. Pulmonary lesions had become refractory to x-ray therapy after having responded satisfactorily on several previous occasions. Roentgenogram at left was taken shortly after completion of last course of roentgen irradiation. There had been no decrease in the size of the infiltrations; cough, dyspnea and fever continued. Nitrogen mustard therapy was followed by prompt symptomatic relief and diminution in the size of pulmonary infiltrate. Roentgenogram on right was made three weeks after nitrogen mustard had been given.

several lymph nodes are enlarged in the area selected for biopsy, the surgeon should be urged to select not the most superficial, but one of the larger nodes which may have been involved for a longer period of time. This recommendation is made because the microscopic diagnosis of Hodgkin's disease may be difficult early in the course of the disease, particularly in nodes that have only recently increased in size. If the only detectable nodal involvement is in the mediastinum or retroperitoneal region, a decision must be reached about the advisability of an exploratory operation. Unless clear contraindications exist, it is usually wiser to proceed with the exploration and to establish the diagnosis with certainty because of the disadvantages of giving intensive irradiation therapy unless the diagnosis is certain.

moderate degree is most frequently found. The differential count usually shows an increase in granulocytes, lymphopenia, and an increase in monocytes. The band or nonsegmented granulocytes may or may not be elevated. Eosinophilia sometimes occurs, but its frequency has been exaggerated in the literature. When an anemia develops, it is usually normocytic normochromic with moderate to advanced degrees of aniso- and poikilocytosis. Recent studies have shown that it is often chiefly hemolytic in nature, the result of an extracorpuscular factor. Thrombocytopenia may occur late in the course of the disease, and along with hemolytic anemia may be a manifestation of abnormal splenic function. When the bone marrow is extensively involved, myelocytes and nucleated red blood cells may be found in the peripheral blood, and both anemia and thrombocytopenia may be severe. Studies of aspirated bone marrow usually contribute little except to confirm the presence of megakaryocytes and of erythroid hyperplasia in patients who develop hypersplenism, but occasionally Reed-Sternberg cells may be identified.

Other laboratory procedures are usually of little help. Plasma globulin may be elevated enough to give total plasma protein levels above the normal range. The basal metabolic rate not infrequently is in the range of plus 10 to 20. Pleural or ascitic fluid may have the characteristics of either a transudate or an exudate. With central nervous system involvement, spinal puncture may reveal a block, and/or the fluid may show both an elevation in protein plus pleocytosis.

Treatment. X-ray therapy remains the treatment of choice for Hodgkin's disease. The comments already made regarding x-ray therapy in lymphosarcoma and reticulum cell sarcoma apply equally well; a high degree of cooperation between the radiotherapist and the physician is essential to proper management. The remissions induced by irradiation vary greatly from a few weeks to months or rarely even years. Radioactive phosphorus is not a satisfactory substitute for x-ray therapy because so much of the isotope is taken up by bone marrow that a hypoplastic anemia almost invariably results when doses adequate to treat the involved lymph nodes are given.

Nitrogen mustard has proved a valuable adjunct to roentgen irradiation. Four-tenths of a milligram per kilo of body weight, given intravenously in two to four divided doses on successive days, constitutes a course of therapy. The total amount given in a course should not exceed 40 mg. It is most easily administered in the following manner. An intravenous infusion of physiologic saline or of 5 per cent glucose in water is begun. The nitrogen mustard from one or two 10 mg. ampules is then dissolved in approximately 10 cc. of saline; the calculated dose is injected without delay into the tubing through which the saline or glucose solution is running. Because patients so frequently suffer from nausea and vomiting for a variable period after the injection, one may minimize their discomfort by giving the nitrogen mustard at bedtime, approximately an hour after they have been given a sedative such as 1½ to 3 grains of a rapidly acting barbiturate. The therapeutic effects may be dramatic and prompt. Fever which has been persistent for days or weeks may disappear within a few days. Enlarged lymph nodes, spleen, or areas of infiltration in organs may seemingly melt away. Unfortunately, the remissions produced by nitrogen mustard usually last for only four to six weeks, and the drug is toxic to bone marrow. Leukopenia and thrombocy-

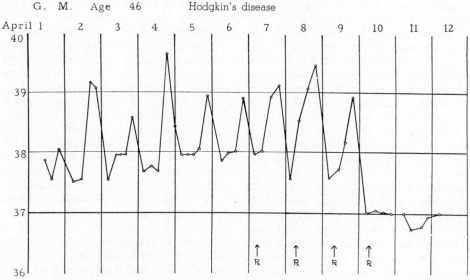

Fig. 147. Temperature response in a patient with Hodgkin's disease to administration of nitrogen mustard, 0.1 mg. per kilo body weight on each of four successive days (indicated by arrows). At times the temperature may not return to normal until several days after the course of therapy has been completed.

topenia almost invariably appear by the end of one week and persist for about ten to fourteen days. Usually, these complications are not severe enough to cause symptoms, but white blood cell counts below 1000 cells per cubic millimeter and platelet levels below 50,000 per cubic millimeter do occur. Petechiae and bleeding from mucous membranes may be troublesome. In spite of these disadvantages, however, nitrogen mustard is a most useful drug. Patients who no longer respond to x-ray therapy may be greatly improved after mustard. The dose may be repeated at intervals of six weeks or longer; eventually it, too, loses its effect. Patients treated in this manner for several months may again become sensitive to roentgen irradiation. In addition, nitrogen mustard may be used in patients who have marked constitutional symptoms but in whom one cannot identify a particular area to irradiate. When enlarged lymph nodes are so located that the edema which often follows x-ray therapy may produce further damage—i.e., with partial obstruction of respiratory passages or of the superior vena cava—nitrogen mustard is often particularly useful either in full dose, or at a level of only 0.2 mg. per kilo of body weight so that irradiation may be employed shortly after the nodes have decreased in size.

Triethylene melamine has a similar effect and may be administered as a substitute for nitrogen mustard. It is given orally in a dose of 5 mg. approximately one hour before breakfast, daily or every other day for a total of three or four doses. Larger amounts must be administered with great care because triethylene melamine temporarily damages bone marrow. Some hematologists have tried to work out a maintenance schedule, but the dose is so difficult to regulate that the drug is more safely given in short courses at intervals of four to six weeks. An occasional patient can tolerate as much as 5 mg. per day for several weeks and responds to that amount more satisfactorily than to smaller doses, but the risk of aplastic anemia is considerable.

None of the other chemotherapeutic agents is particularly useful in the management of Hodgkin's disease. Cortisone will occasionally control constitutional symptoms such as fever and anorexia for short periods, but is of little other value. When hypersplenism develops, splenectomy may restore the red cell or platelet levels to normal. General supportive care should include transfusions and antibiotics when needed. Salicylates must be used with caution. Occasionally, acetylsalicylic acid even in low dosage will cause a sudden drop in temperature in patients with Hodgkin's disease from 40° C. to levels as low as 35° C. and precipitate a state of shock.

Prognosis. The average survival time of patients with Hodgkin's disease is probably between twenty-four and thirty months after the onset of symptoms. Exact figures are difficult to obtain because the disease often begins so insidiously that the patient is unable to date its onset. The course may be as short as four to six months or so benign that it stretches to more than twenty years. In general, if the disease is localized to one chain of lymph nodes when treatment is first started, the duration tends to be longer than if there is early dissemination. Patients in whom pulmonary infiltration or extensive retroperitoneal involvement occurs usually have shorter survival times, but exceptions to this generalization are not infrequent.

It is difficult to demonstrate statistically that therapy prolongs life, although every physician with extensive experience in the treatment of Hodgkin's disease can recall instances in which life was almost certainly extended for significant periods of time. No doubt exists, however, about the fact that intelligent therapy makes patients much more comfortable, often symptom-free for long periods, so that the life they do have is more useful, more enjoyable.

The claim has been made that early surgical removal or intensive roentgen irradiation of a primary site of Hodgkin's involvement has resulted in apparent cures of the disease. In most of these reports, however, the periods of observation have not been greater than five to ten years, and the possibility of recurrence at a later date has not been eliminated. But whether cures have been obtained or not, the long remissions which occasionally occur after a localized, primary lesion has been treated in this manner make the procedure very worthwhile.

FOLLICULAR LYMPHOMA

(Giant Follicular Lymphoblastoma, Brill-Symmers Disease)

Follicular lymphoma is a primary disease of lymph nodes of unknown etiology characterized by hyperplasia of lymph follicles and a moderately benign course, but with a tendency to undergo transformation to a sarcomatous or leukemic process. It is distinctly less common than Hodgkin's disease or lymphosarcoma, occurs more frequently in males than in females by approximately a 2 to 1 ratio, and is more common above the age of 40 although cases in children have been recognized.

The enlarged lymph nodes may have a diameter of 5 or more centimeters, are usually discrete and not tender. Lymph follicles within the node are often so large that they appear prominent when a microscopic section is examined without magnification. The follicles are more numerous than normal, vary in size and shape, are distributed throughout the substance of the node rather than being limited primarily to the periphery, and are surrounded by a zone of closely set small lymphocytes. Trabeculae are obscured and lymph sinuses are usually obliterated.

Constitutional manifestations are infrequent. Skeletal and visceral involvement are unusual. Symmers has observed that the primary lesion may rarely be located in the lymphoid tissue of the appendix. Splenic enlargement is common and may be of great degree. Retroperitoneal lymph nodes are frequently affected.

Diagnosis can be established only by lymph node biopsy. The disease is best treated by x-ray therapy and often responds so well that remissions of long duration are produced. The two most common complications are: (1) hypersplenism resulting in hemolytic anemia, leukopenia or thrombocytopenia; and (2) transformation of the disease to produce follicular sarcoma or the hematologic changes of lymphocytic leukemia. Hypersplenism should be treated by splenectomy. It is still not clear whether all cases eventually undergo sarcomatous or leukemic change, or whether some are cured when irradiation therapy is instituted early. The latter probably is true.

MYCOSIS FUNGOIDES

Emphasis has already been given to the fact that cutaneous manifestations of various kinds occur in the diseases which primarily affect lymph nodes. Mycosis fungoides, however, deserves separate discussion because it is often regarded as a distinct dermatologic entity yet frequently terminates as a lymphoma. The disease is of unknown causation, is relatively rare, is more common in men than in women, usually affects adults after the age of 40 years, and tends to run a

chronic but progressive course. It may be divided into three stages: first, one characterized by generalized pruritus and an erythematous, eczematous or exfoliative dermatitis; second, a stage in which infiltrative plaques occur; and third, a stage of tumor formation. The disease may begin with any one of these manifestations, however, and may exist without the others. In the first stage there is hyperplasia of the epidermis with a dermal perivascular infiltrate of lymphocytes, reticulum cells and eosinophils. In the tumor stage, the infiltrate may still be pleomorphic or the histologic structure may resemble reticulum cell sarcoma or lymphosarcoma.

Lymph node enlargement may or may not be present. The involved skin feels thick or leathery and has a dusky red hue. When these changes are associated with a generalized erythema, patients may look like a boiled lobster. Pruritus may be so intense and persistent that it overshadows all other symptoms. When the changes resemble those of exfoliative dermatitis, skin infections and fever are not uncommon. Individual lesions may be circinate or arcate in shape. Lymphocytosis may cause moderate elevations of the white blood cell count. While many patients with mycosis fungoides, after a period of years, develop the histologic and clinical manifestations of lymphosarcoma, reticulum cell sarcoma, Hodgkin's disease or lymphocytic leukemia, others die before these changes have occurred and a few appear to recover. For this reason, one must be cautious at present about assuming that a clinical diagnosis of mycosis fungoides is necessarily synonymous with a proved diagnosis of a malignant lymphoma.

Remissions of varying duration are often produced by x-ray therapy. If satisfactory improvement is not obtained, nitrogen mustard or triethylene melamine, administered in the same manner as for Hodgkin's disease, should be tried.

CARL V. MOORE

References

Andrews, G. C.: Diseases of the Skin (Mycosis Fungoides). 4th Ed. Philadelphia, W. B. Saunders Co., 1954, pp. 719–725.

Bayrd, E. D., Paulson, G. S., and Hargraves, M. M.: Hodgkin's Specific Cells in Bone Marrow Aspirations. Blood, 9:46, 1954.

Berman, L., Klein, A. A., Linn, H. J., and Bates, G. S.: Hypersplenism Associated with Follicular Lymphoblastoma. Blood, 5:286, 1950.

Bichel, J., and Bastrup-Madsen, P.: Alcohol Pain in Hodgkin's Disease. Lancet, 1:764, 1953.

Elliott, G. V., and Wilson, H. M.: Mesenchymal Tumors of the Stomach. Arch Int. Med., 89:358, 1952.

Evans, T. E., and Doan, C. A.: Giant Follicular Hyperplasia: A Study of Its Incidence, Histopathologic Variability, and the Frequency of Sarcoma and Secondary Hypersplenic Complications. Ann. Int. Med., 40:851, 1954.

Gilliam, A. G.: Age, Sex and Race Selection at Death from Leukemia and the Lymphomas. Blood, 8: 693–702, 1953.

Henstell, H. H., Tober, J. N., and Newman, B. A.: The Influence of Nitrogen Mustard on Mycosis Fungoides. Blood, 2:564, 1947.

Hoster, H. A., Dratman, M. B., Craver, L. F., and Rolnick, H. A.: Hodgkin's Disease. Cancer Research, 8:1, 1948.

Jackson, H., Jr., and Parker, E., Jr.: Hodgkin's Disease and Allied Disorders. New York, Oxford University Press, 1947.

Sparling, H. J., Jr., Adams, R. D., and Parker, F., Jr.: Involvement of the Nervous System by Malignant Lymphoma. Medicine, 26:285–332, 1947.

Symmers, D.: Lymphoid Diseases. Arch. Path., 45: 73–131, 1948.

Wintrobe, M. M.: Clinical Hematology. 3rd Ed. Philadelphia, Lea & Febiger, 1951, p. 890.

———, and Huguley, C. M., Jr.: Nitrogen-Mustard Therapy for Hodgkin's Disease, Lymphosarcoma, the Leukemias and Other Disorders. Cancer, 1:357, 1948.

EOSINOPHILIC GRANULOMA, LETTERER-SIWE DISEASE, HAND-SCHÜLLER-CHRISTIAN DISEASE

These three syndromes, originally regarded as distinct entities, are probably interrelated manifestations of a single malady for which the common denominator is a histiocytic proliferation of unknown etiology. Lichtenstein has recently suggested that "histiocytosis X" be used as a generic name to cover all three. Until etiology is defined, it would be a mistake to accept the interrelationship as proved, but both the clinical and the morphologic manifestations seem to fade into each other. The clinical and pathologic manifestations of the three disorders appear to be determined largely by the location of the lesions and their acuteness or chronicity.

Eosinophilic granuloma is a comparatively benign disorder characterized by single or multiple skeletal lesions occurring in children and young adults. Histologically, the lesion consists primarily of a proliferation of histiocytes and eosinophils. It begins in the marrow but gradually erodes the cortex so that ultimately the bone expands at the area of involvement. The granulomas may retain their original character for years, but eventually at least in some of the foci, fibrosis occurs, the number of eosinophils diminishes, and the histiocytes tend to be converted into lipophages. Lesions occur in the skull, ribs, pelvis, vertebrae, humerus and femur; they are rare in the distal ends of extremities. Pain and swelling are common complaints, but the foci may be silent. Patients are usually free of any constitutional symptoms although they may have mild degrees of fever and eosinophilic leukocytosis. Pathologic fractures may occur. Roentgenograms show round or oval areas of destruction, often with a punched-out appearance. The lesions usually respond well to curettement or to x-ray therapy so that the prognosis tends to be good. During the past decade an increasing number of reports have described mucocutaneous, lymph node, pleural and pulmonary sites of extraskeletal involvement. Pulmonary infiltration may occur before any skeletal lesions can be identified, and is at first an interstitial infiltration by eosinophils and histiocytes. Later, the granulomatous areas become large enough to form nodules. The roentgenographic changes are those of a diffuse, bilateral, interstitial pulmonary infiltration. In at least one instance, diabetes insipidus has been reported as a complication of eosinophilic granuloma.

The *Hand-Schüller-Christian syndrome* is characterized by multiple round defects in the skull, unilateral or bilateral exophthalmos, and diabetes insipidus with or without other signs of pituitary failure. It is a relatively chronic disorder which affects children principally, but may be found in young adults and rarely in older people. The pathologic lesion is a histiocytic granuloma in which the histiocytes contain so much cholesterol that they become foam cells. Lichtenstein believes that the granulomas initially contain very little cholesterol, that eosinophils may at first be prominent, and that lipidization is a late, secondary change. He argues that there is no reason to postulate an abnormality of lipid metabolism in reticulum cells. Thannhauser, however, believes that the cholesterol esters in foam cells result from a faulty metabolism of cholesterol within the cells. It is of interest that the plasma cholesterol value is usually normal. Lesions are by no means limited to the skull; they may appear in other bones, the skin and the viscera. Cutaneous involvement, often as a papular eczema-like eruption or as xanthomas, occurs in about one third of all cases. Visceral changes may be found in the lung, liver, spleen, kidneys, perirenal fat, walls of the larger blood vessels and in the brain. Diffuse pleural and interstitial pulmonary infiltration, leading eventually to fibrosis, honeycombing of the lungs and episodes of spontaneous pneumothorax, is not uncommon in adults afflicted with the disease. If new skeletal lesions are biopsied early, the histologic picture may at times be indistinguishable from eosinophilic granuloma. The disease is best treated by x-ray therapy to the areas involved. While the response is often very satisfactory, new foci tend to appear elsewhere. At least one-third of the cases terminate fatally, but recovery, apparently complete, does occur. Secondary changes caused by the disease often lead to difficult therapeutic problems, i.e. diabetes insipidus. Pulmonary fibrosis may cause pulmonary insufficiency or right-sided heart failure. In an occasional patient with Hand-Schüller-Christian syndrome in whom the tempo of the pathologic process is accelerated terminally, the clinical manifestations come to resemble those of Letterer-Siwe disease.

The *Letterer-Siwe syndrome* is more acute, is largely limited to young children below the age of 3 years although occasional cases are observed in young adults, and is characterized by the development of multiple areas of proliferating histiocytes in the visceral organs. Secondary precipitation of cholesterol esters in the histiocytes to form foam cells usually does not occur. Clinical manifestations consist of a purpuric or ecchymotic cutaneous eruption which sometimes ulcerates superficially, a persistent, spiking, low grade fever, enlargement of liver, spleen and lymph nodes, hyperplasia of the gums, and a progressive anemia. Normoblasts may be found in the peripheral blood. Skeletal lesions cause localized areas of bone destruction, have a predilection for the calvarium, and roentgenographically resemble those of Hand-Schüller-Christian disease. The essential pulmonary change is one of diffuse histiocytic infiltration. In some instances, when the visceral lesions are quite characteristic, those in the bones may show the presence of some foam cells. Diagnosis can usually be made by biopsy of bone marrow or lymph nodes. Therapy consists of supportive care, antibiotics to control secondary infection and roentgen irradiation to the skin and other areas of involvement. The disease is usually fatal but patients rarely may recover or the process may become chronic so that it comes to resemble the Hand-Schüller-Christian syndrome.

CARL V. MOORE

References

Lichtenstein, L.: Histiocytosis X. Integration of Eosinophilic Granuloma of Bone, Letterer-Siwe Disease, and Hand-Schüller-Christian Disease as Related Manifestations of a Single Nosologic Entity. A.M.A. Arch. Path., 56:84, 1953.
May, I. A., Garfinkle, J. M., and Dugan, D. J.: Eosinophilic Granuloma of Lung. Ann. Int. Med., 40:549, 1954.
Snapper, I.: Medical Clinics on Bone Diseases. 2nd Ed. New York, Interscience Publishers, Inc., 1949, pp. 185–198.

GAUCHER'S DISEASE

Definition. Gaucher's disease is a rare, familial disorder of cerebroside metabolism characterized by abnormal storage or retention of cerebrosides in reticuloendothelial cells. In adults, clinical manifestations may appear so gradually that it is difficult for patients to date their onset; the course is usually protracted. Proliferation of the abnormal cells causes progressive splenomegaly, hepatomegaly and skeletal lesions. In addition, pigmentation and evidences of hypersplenism often occur. Patients most often die of intercurrent infections or other pathologic processes, but if they survive until the terminal stages of Gaucher's disease itself, cachexia may become extreme. In children, the course of the disease may be moderately acute.

History. Gaucher described the entity in 1882, observed the characteristic large, pale cells in the spleen, but regarded the disease as a malignant epithelioma. Marchand in 1907 concluded that the Gaucher cells were filled with a semisolid hyaline substance. Six years later, Mandelbaum and Downey identified the cells as reticulum cells and suggested that their abnormal appearance might be the result of a metabolic abnormality. Epstein and Lieb independently in 1924 showed that the hyaline substance was a lipid, kerasin, which contains nitrogen but not phosphorus.

Incidence. This comparatively rare disease affects both sexes equally, and may develop at any age even though it usually begins during childhood or early adult life. A large percentage of the cases occurs among Jewish people. A family history of the disease can often be obtained but involvement is usually limited to one generation. Groen has postulated that Gaucher's disease is a mutation transmitted as a simple dominant hereditary trait.

Pathologic Anatomy. The distinctive hallmark of Gaucher's disease is the Gaucher cell: a round or polyhedral, pale reticulum cell 20 to 80 microns in diameter with a small, eccentrically placed nucleus and a wrinkled cytoplasm which contains an irregular network of fibrils. A few cells may have two or more nuclei. The cytoplasm is largely filled with two cerebrosides: kerasin (galactosido-cerebroside) and glucoside-cerebroside. These substances are chemically inert and do not stain with any of the lipoid stains; with Mallory's aniline blue orange G stain, the cytoplasm becomes deeply blue. Thannhauser postulates that the reticulum cells are the site of the metabolic abnormality and synthesize the cerebrosides, whereas other workers believe that kerasin is formed as the result of a general disturbance of lipid metabolism and is stored only secondarily in reticulum cells.

Proliferation of the Gaucher's cells is responsible for enlargement of the spleen, liver and intrathoracic and intra-abdominal lymph nodes. The spleen may become tremendous in size. The architecture of these organs is altered by the infiltration, but there is little fibrous tissue reaction. Hemosiderin may be increased both in these sites and in the skin. Gaucher's cells are also scattered diffusely throughout the marrow, and in some areas, particularly the distal ends of the femurs, form tumor-like accumulations which may expand and erode the cortex. The brain is frequently involved in infants, with a proliferation of glial cells and degenerative changes in the pyramidal cells of the cortex; infiltration by Gaucher's cells has been observed in the region of the pituitary and hypothalamus. Infiltration of the lungs, kidneys, thymus, tonsils, adrenals and lymphoid tissue of the intestinal tract has also been described.

Clinical Manifestations. The course of Gaucher's disease is extremely variable. In children it may progress rapidly, but more often, particularly in adults, the patient has no symptoms for a long period of time except for awareness of a progressively enlarging mass in the left upper quadrant of the abdomen. The spleen may become very large and the liver is usually palpable. Pigmentation is more frequently limited to exposed surfaces of the skin, but may be generalized. A brownish wedge-shaped thickening of the subconjunctival fibrous tissue (a pinguecula) often appears. The bases of these wedges are located near the cornea with the apices pointed toward the inner or outer canthi. Pingueculae usually develop first on the nasal and later on the temporal side. Bone pain or aching and pathologic fractures may appear at sites of skeletal lesions. With marked destruction of the head and neck of the femur, walking may become progressively more difficult. Anemia may cause weakness, and when hemolytic, mild jaundice; thrombocytopenia may be responsible for hemorrhagic manifestations. While neurologic symptoms are unusual, they may constitute the dominant features in infants afflicted with the disease: strabismus, retraction of the head, laryngospasm, dysphagia, spasticity of the extremities, exaggerated deep tendon reflexes, and at times a complete loss of sensation.

Diagnosis. Gaucher's disease can most easily be diagnosed by finding the abnormal cells in bone marrow aspirates. Biopsy of liver or spleen can also be made, but marrow is more easily obtained. Hepatic function tests usually remain normal even when the liver is heavily infiltrated. Blood lipids are normal. Roentgenograms show cortical thinning and erosion at areas of involvement. Compression of vertebrae may be identified. The most common roentgenographic changes, however, occur in the femur: a bottle- or Erlenmeyer flask–shaped lesion in the distal end, and erosion with compression of the head and neck.

A high percentage of patients with Gaucher's disease develop hematologic changes of hypersplenism at some time during the course of their disease: a hemolytic anemia, leukopenia, thrombocytopenia, or any combination of the three. The peripheral cytopenia is accompanied by a normal or increased number of the progenitors of the involved formed element in the marrow. At times, a normocytic normochromic anemia may be myelophthisic, caused by extensive replacement of marrow by the Gaucher's cells.

Treatment. There is no satisfactory treatment for Gaucher's disease. X-ray therapy is frequently given to skeletal lesions, but does not seem to arrest the slow destructive process. When hypersplenism occurs, splenectomy should be done. It will correct the hemolytic anemia, the leukopenia or the thrombocytopenia caused by the abnormal splenic function, and is therefore of great value. There is no convincing evidence, however, to indicate that splenectomy otherwise influences the course of the disease.

Prognosis. In infants and small children, the disease may have a relatively acute course and cause death within a matter of months. Among older children and adults, the course tends to be protracted so that it extends over many years. Most older patients die of intercurrent diseases rather than as the result of the Gaucher disorder, *per se.*

NIEMANN-PICK'S DISEASE

Niemann-Pick's disease is a rare disease of infancy characterized by the widespread involvement of organs with abnormal reticulum cells which contain a phosphatid lipid, possibly sphingomyelin. It has a marked predilection for the Jewish race and is more common in females. Like Gaucher's disease, it is occasionally found in siblings. The abnormal cell is about 40 microns in diameter, contains one or two eccentrically placed small nuclei, and has a cytoplasm filled with hyaline droplets which give it the appearance of foam or a honeycomb. The cytoplasm stains with sudan III and other fat stains.

The liver, spleen and lymph nodes become enlarged. Digestive disorders and weight loss tend to be severe. The skin has a waxy, brown hue. Mental development ceases. Ophthalmoscopic examination frequently reveals a cherry red spot in the region of the macula lutea.

Anemia may be severe, and moderate thrombocytopenia is often found. The total white cell count may show either a leukopenia or a leukocytosis. There frequently is a moderate lymphocytosis or monocytosis. The blood cholesterol may be elevated. Diagnosis is made by identifying the abnormal cells in bone marrow obtained by aspiration. Treatment is unsatisfactory. Splenectomy produces only temporary improvement at best. Death usually occurs within a few months. Infections commonly complicate the last few weeks of life.

CARL V. MOORE

References

Chargaff, E.: A Study of the Spleen in a Case of Niemann-Pick Disease. J. Biol. Chem., *130*:503, 1939.

Medoff, A. S., and Bayrd, E. D.: Gaucher's Disease in 29 Cases: Hematologic Complications and Effect of Splenectomy. Ann. Int. Med., *40*:481, 1954.

Pick, L.: Niemann-Pick's Disease and Other Forms of So-called Xanthomatosis. Am. J. M. Sc., *185*: 601, 1933.

Reich, C., Seife, M., and Kessler, B. J.: Gaucher's Disease: A Review and Discussion of Twenty Cases. Medicine, 30:1, 1951.

Snapper, I.: Medical Clinics on Bone Diseases. 2nd Ed., pp. 201–207. New York, Interscience Publishers, Inc., 1949, pp. 201–207.

Diseases of the Blood

INTRODUCTION

The blood normally consists of a circulating liquid plasma in which, because of its turbulence, is maintained in suspension slightly less than an equal volume of corpuscles: red cells, white cells and platelets. A vital function of the circulating red blood cells is to hold in nondiffusible form the hemoglobin essential for the transport of oxygen. For the white blood cells the blood stream serves merely as a means of transportation to the locus where they are to act as phagocytes and assist in the defense against infection. The platelets are allied with the vascular endothelium in subtle ways necessary for the maintenance of its integrity. Enzyme systems in the plasma provide a second line of defense for the blood vessels, converting soluble fibrinogen to fibrin at the site of an injury.

Disorders of the blood and blood-forming organs result in abnormalities of the corpuscular composition (anemias, leukemias, agranulocytosis and erythrocytosis) or of the coagulating ability (prothrombin deficiency and hemophilia) of the blood, and in "spontaneous" lesions of the small blood vessels (purpuras), permitting hemorrhage. In addition are included conditions developing when the precursors of the adult leukocytes exhibit neoplastic growth, usually (leukemias) but not necessarily (Hodgkin's disease) affecting significantly the morphologic composition of the blood stream. In disease, histologic changes occur, especially in the bone marrow, lymph nodes or spleen, as well as in the circulating blood. Conditioned by the fundamental features of the underlying blood dyscrasias, there may develop the secondary manifestations of deficient oxygen transport, infection, hemorrhage, or invasion of vital organs by neoplastic processes.

As in any branch of medicine, correlation of laboratory findings with the results of history and physical examination is often essential for accurate diagnosis. At least an initial determination of the hemoglobin level and an inspection of a blood film should be routine procedures in every patient. The microscopic examination of the blood and, latterly, of biopsy specimens of the blood-forming tissues has rightly occupied the attention of those interested in the study of blood dyscrasias. Quantitative methods for describing the average volume, diameter and hemoglobin concentration of the erythrocyte have replaced earlier qualitative estimates. Supravital staining of reticulocytes, quantitative determinations of fecal urobilinogen and studies of red blood cell survival after transfusion into normal or abnormal subjects allow estimates of the rate of red blood cell production and destruction. Additional physiologic orientation has developed, exemplified by the effectiveness of liver or iron therapy in appropriate types of nutritional anemia. Also it is recognized that exposure, in occupation or through chemotherapy, to certain compounds containing the benzene ring may result in hemolytic or aplastic anemias, agranulocytosis, thrombocytopenic purpura or even leukemia. The recent renewed and intense interest in both normal and pathologic physiology of hemostasis and blood coagulation has led to a complex literature, but also to a better understanding of these subjects.

The treatment of blood dyscrasias presents as striking contrasts in effectiveness as are found in any field of medicine. Replacement of specific nutritional deficiencies by therapy with liver and stomach preparations (vitamin B_{12}), with folic acid or with iron is highly efficacious in appropriate nutritional macrocytic and hypochromic anemias, but is useless in other types of anemia. Splenectomy removes the chief hemolytic organ in congenital hemolytic jaundice and so is regularly effective. It may be useful in certain acquired types of hemolytic anemia, especially when the spleen is large and the fragility of the red blood cells is increased. Splenectomy is the measure most likely to be permanently successful in the treatment of thrombocytopenic purpura. It fails in certain acute types, and in any case the beneficial results may be only temporary. Splenectomy is also effective in certain patients with neutropenia and splenomegaly.

Irradiation is a purely palliative, though

often valuable, procedure. For reducing the local lesions of lymphosarcoma or of Hodgkin's disease, x-ray therapy must be intensive. In the chronic leukemias the use of small amounts of more general irradiation, given at regular intervals of a week or two, is a suitable and safer method. Radioactive phosphorus, another form of irradiation, has not yet been shown to have significant advantages over properly applied x-ray therapy in leukemia.

Chemotherapy may be dramatic in the treatment of hemolytic anemias such as those resulting from the use of quinine therapy in malaria, the use of sulfonamides in infections, or in the anemias resulting from the development of antibodies (e.g., Coombs'). A current revival of chemotherapy of leukemia, originally used in the form of benzol and potassium arsenite, has employed nitrogen mustards, urethane, folic acid and purine analogues and adrenocorticotrophic hormone and cortisone. The analogues and steroids have exhibited temporary benefit in acute leukemias, especially of children. Likewise in vascular and thrombocytopenic purpuras corticosteroid action may be symptomatically useful alone or as a means of preparation for splenectomy.

Transfusion is a helpful but purely passive form of therapy except when used in erythroblastosis fetalis as an "exchange transfusion" in order to remove abnormal plasma antibodies and to supply Rh-negative red blood cells. By transfusion the blood volume may be augmented in severe hemorrhage, and the hemoglobin may be increased in anemias with critically low values. In thrombocytopenic purpuras, platelets can be temporarily added to the blood stream, and in hemophilia the normal plasma globulins will reduce the clotting time of the blood for several hours. Transfusion does not raise the leukocyte count detectably. In addition, specific or general therapeutic measures of value in other types of disease have their indications and their propriety in the treatment of patients with blood dyscrasias. Important among these is the alleviation of fear, which unfortunately is sometimes of iatrogenic origin.

W. B. Castle

References

Castle, W. B.: Disorders of the Blood, in Sodeman, W. A.: Pathologic Physiology: Mechanisms of Disease. Philadelphia, W. B. Saunders Company, 1950.

Daland, G. A.: A Color Atlas of Morphologic Hematology: With a Guide to Clinical Interpretation. Edited by T. H. Ham, Cambridge, Harvard University Press, 1951.

Downey, H.: Handbook of Hematology. New York, Paul B. Hoeber, Inc., 1938.

Whitby, L. E. H., and Britton, C. J. C.: Disorders of the Blood. 6th ed. Philadelphia, Blakiston Company, 1950.

Wintrobe, M. M.: Clinical Hematology. 3rd ed. Philadelphia, Lea & Febiger, 1951.

THE ANEMIAS

Definition. Anemia may be said to be present when the concentration of hemoglobin in the peripheral blood falls below the normal range of 14 ± 2 gm. per cent for adult females and 16 ± 2 gm. per cent for adult males. In children average values are 2 or 3 gm. lower. When anemia is present, the red cells are usually but not always reduced below their normal ranges of 4.8 ± 0.6 and 5.4 ± 0.8 million per cubic millimeter for adult females and males, respectively. The normal mean corpuscular volume is 87 ± 5 cubic microns. The mean corpuscular hemoglobin concentration is 34 ± 2 per cent and is never exceeded except occasionally in congenital hemolytic anemia.

Pathologic Physiology. The accurate maintenance of the normal concentration of hemoglobin (and of red cells) in the peripheral blood stream implies a critical adjustment of production to the rate of blood loss. Anemia results when (a) red cell production, though increased, is less than the rate of increased red cell loss or destruction, or (b) red cell production is less than the normal rate of red cell loss or destruction.

If the hemoglobin becomes constant at an anemic level the rates of production and destruction of hemoglobin have again become equal. In anemias due to (a) this rate may be 6 to 8 times the normal. In anemias due to (b) this correspondence in rate may result either from some increase of blood production (anemic anoxia) or some decrease in blood destruction (reduced red cell mass). In anemias due to (b) in addition to decreased production the defective *quality* of red cells may condition some degree of increased red cell destruction, e.g., pernicious anemia.

The rate of red cell production appears to be intimately related to the oxygen content of the arterial blood. Beyond this the controlling mechanism is poorly understood and may be operative directly in the bone marrow or remotely through humoral mechanisms. Experimentally and clinically either a fall of hemoglobin concentration (hemorrhage) or oxygen unsaturation of the arterial blood (anoxia) causes increased red cell production. Conversely, a rise in hemoglobin concentration (transfusion) or a rise in oxygen tension (oxygen inhalation) of the arterial blood causes decreased red cell production. The red cells normally enter the blood stream after the loss of the nucleus characteristic of their precursors in the bone marrow, but while some still contain material demonstrable by staining with brilliant cresyl blue as "reticulocytes." Increased red cell delivery to the circulation can be detected by the rise of these cells after a hemorrhage or an acute hemolytic episode, or, for example, when nutritional arrest of red cell production is abolished by therapy with liver extract or iron.

Although in experimental animals dietary deficiency of many substances, including amino acids, vitamins and minerals, decreases red cell or hemoglobin production, in therapeutic practice only iron, folic, folinic and ascorbic acids, vitamin B_{12}, and rarely perhaps, in infants, copper result in increased erythropoiesis in anemias. Each of these substances is effective only when a specific deficiency is present although in pernicious anemia large doses of the nucleic acid precursors uracil and thymine have been found also to be active. By abolishing the deficiency, the bone marrow then becomes able to respond to the stimulus of the anemic anoxia. Anemia and nutritional deficiency contribute jointly to the hyperplasia and immaturity of the erythroid cells of the marrow.

After a lifetime of 100 to 120 days, the red cells become mechanically fragile and are then probably ruptured by the traumatic motion of the circulation. This releases daily about 7 gm. of the iron-porphyrin-globin compound called hemoglobin. Increased destruction of red cells as a cause of anemia may be the direct result of hemolytic systems demonstrable in the blood *in vitro*. It may result from osmotic or chemical lysis or perhaps from phagocytosis during sequestration of red cells in the spleen or other tissues, or from rupture of mechanically fragile red cells in the moving circulation. Abnormal red cells are rarely so osmotically fragile as to lyse in isotonic plasma, and are usually mechanically fragile. The reverse is not necessarily so. When hemolysis is especially rapid, as in a transfusion reaction, hemoglobinemia and hemoglobinuria may result. In most chronic processes only an increase in the indirect-acting serum bilirubin appears. This is derived from the splitting off of the iron and the opening of the porphyrin ring of the hemoglobin in the cells of the reticuloendothelial system. In either case excess bilirubin leads to increased excretion of urobilinogen in the feces and is not reused for the formation of hemoglobin. The iron is largely retained by the body and is reutilized in the formation of new hemoglobin. Histologically, excess iron deposition appears as hemosiderin, especially in the cells of the reticuloendothelial system of liver, spleen and marrow.

Symptoms and Signs. The decreased ability of anemic blood to transport oxygen leads to such general symptoms as headache, poor appetite, fatigue and tendency to fainting. Compensation is achieved partly by increasing the velocity and volume of blood flow and partly by removing more oxygen from the blood as it traverses the tissues. Because of the low hemoglobin level the latter causes no visible cyanosis. The former causes the heart to beat more rapidly; its diastolic size and stroke volume may be increased. Roaring in the ears, a wide arterial pulse pressure and capillary pulsation indicate diminished peripheral resistance. In patients with underlying disease of the coronary vessels, angina pectoris or congestive failure may develop. However, especially in young subjects, compensation for the anemia may be so effective that no discomfort at rest is experienced with one fifth, and locomotion is possible though difficult with only one tenth of the normal hemoglobin concentration. With moderate anemia, dyspnea, orthopnea or cough is noted only on exertion or with excitement. When present at rest, together with restlessness, circulatory decompensation is imminent. In chronic anemia, effective renal blood flow is reduced, presumably as a device for diverting blood to other tissues. Polyuria, hyposthenuria and moderate azotemia and proteinuria result. Edema is partly correlated with severe anemia. More often it appears as a feature of congestive failure or of hypoproteinemia. Purpura or ecchymoses are frequently due to thrombocytopenia; and lesions of the oral cavity, rectum or vagina may result from granulocytopenia. Such disturbances of platelet or white cell formation accompany the depressed or disturbed red cell formation causing the anemia. The relatively few symptoms and signs characteristic of special types of anemia will be discussed later. Of necessity, therefore, emphasis in the differential diagnosis of the anemias rests on laboratory studies.

ANEMIAS DUE TO INCREASED ERYTHROCYTE LOSS OR DESTRUCTION

ANEMIAS OF ACUTE ERYTHROCYTE LOSS

Red cell loss as classified in Table 1 occurs as a result of bleeding from either internal or external sources. When sudden and copious, it causes a corresponding reduction of the circulating blood volume. This, if sufficiently great, produces shock manifest by pallor, sweating, restlessness, tachycardia and low blood pressure. The entry of tissue fluids tends gradually to restore the volume of blood indispensable for an effective circulation. This dilutes the red cell and hemoglobin concentrations progressively in parallel fashion, sometimes for a day or two. Rarely, after the hemorrhage there is a transient rise of leukocytes. The platelets are usually not significantly altered. A few normoblasts may appear in the peripheral blood, but the reticulocytes do not increase until the second or third day, and then reach a peak value only on the fifth to seventh day after the hemorrhage. At this time there may be some macrocytosis of the red cells. At first the red cell and hemoglobin concentrations rise together, but after two or three weeks the rate of hemoglobin regeneration may lag behind that of the red cells, especially if the patient has a partial iron deficiency as a result of previous blood loss. When extensive bleeding occurs into a tissue or body cavity, as sometimes in scurvy or hemophilia, the early effects are similar to those of external blood loss except that slight jaundice may occur; the late effects differ only in that the iron is conserved and not lost from the body as with external hemorrhage. In both, the normoblasts of the bone marrow become increased in number.

The treatment of acute blood loss is really the treatment of shock. This involves control of the hemorrhage appropriate to the cause and prompt restoration of blood volume, in an emergency with saline or gelatin solution or plasma. Transfusion of whole blood is of course the ideal treatment. Iron therapy is not necessary in the early stages of the rapid erythropoiesis that follows even severe hemorrhage. Moreover, iron may be irritating to a bleeding lesion of the gastrointestinal tract and may obscure signs of further bleeding or cause falsely positive appearances and chemical tests for blood in the stools.

ANEMIAS OF INCREASED ERYTHROCYTE DESTRUCTION

Increased red cell destruction causes within a few days both morphologic and functional hyperplasia of the bone marrow. The pre-

Table 1. Classification of Anemias Due Mainly to Increased Erythrocyte Loss or Destruction (Bone Marrow Physiologically Hyperactive)

I. ACUTE ERYTHROCYTE LOSS
  (a) Hemorrhage, external
  (b) Hemorrhage into tissue

II. INCREASED ERYTHROCYTE DESTRUCTION
  (a) Extrinsic causes:
      Septicemias: streptococcus, Welch bacillus, malaria, bartonella
      Chemicals: lead, arsine, aniline derivatives, sulfonamides, venoms
      Heat: thermal burns
      Immunity, natural: transfusion of foreign red cells or plasma
      Immunity, acquired: Rh factor, favism, pollens, drugs
  (b) Intrinsic causes:
      Abnormal erythrocytes: congenital hemolytic (spherocytic and non-spherocytic) jaundice, sickle cell anemia, thalassemia, paroxysmal nocturnal hemoglobinuria
      Abnormal plasma: paroxysmal (cold) hemoglobinuria, cold, warm and acid-activated agglutinins, hemolysins
      Myelophthisic hemolytic anemia, liver cirrhosis

dominant erythroid cell is the normoblast, but younger forms are frequently seen in severe and chronic anemias of this type. Almost without exception the reticulocytes are elevated, and the granulocytes and platelets are either normal or increased in the peripheral blood. The survival time of transfused normal compatible (unagglutinable) or of the patient's own (Cr^{51}-labeled) red cells permits the best estimate of the rate of cell destruction. Increased bilirubin-globin in the serum and urobilinogen in the feces are consistent findings when hemolysis is active. The iron-containing pigment, hemosiderin, is usually found in increased amounts in the bone marrow. Manifest hemoglobinemia with resulting hemoglobinuria usually indicates a fulminating process.

The patient exhibits a combination of pallor and jaundice. Fever in the absence of demonstrable infection is a frequent finding when the hemoglobin level is low. The spleen and liver are frequently enlarged. The role of the spleen in increased red cell destruction is discussed on page 1146. This is rarely if ever the result of a *primary* splenic hyperfunction, but is rather due to the *secondary* effect of spherocytes, sickling, plasma-agglutinins or nonspecific increase in splenic size and filter capacity, such as by infiltration with Gaucher cells. Aside from general symptoms compatible with the degree of anemia, the clinical condition of the patient depends chiefly on the nature of the underlying cause of the anemia.

Extrinsic Causes of Increased Erythrocyte Destruction. Extrinsic causes of increased red cell destruction given in Table 1 may be distinguished by appropriate evidence. Thus, *septicemias* such as bacterial endocarditis, malaria or bartonella infections produce typical hemolytic anemias recognized by the demonstration of the specific organism in the blood stream. *Chemicals* such as arsine, naphthalene, quinine, acetanilid, phenylhydrazine or sulfonamides, particularly sulfanilamide, cause in some persons the formation of oxidant compounds that result in acute hemolytic anemia, sometimes with hemoglobinuria. Para-aminophenol, both in experimental animals and *in vitro,* causes increased osmotic and mechanical fragilities of the red cells. Such changes may be transiently observed in patients. Refractile (Heinz) bodies may be seen within the red cells in wet preparations. Methemoglobin is almost always present, and a marked leukocytosis with an outpouring of immature granulocytes and sometimes of myelocytes is not uncommon. In *burns,* local heating of the blood produces anemia at first characterized by dividing and spheroidal red cells with increased osmotic and mechanical fragilities. Ingestion of *fava beans* or even inhalation of pollen from the flowers of these plants causes acute hemolytic episodes, especially in children who have become sensitized. Little more is known concerning the hematologic findings in such patients. *Fuadin* therapy may develop plasma antibodies against red cells. Treatment is by removal of the offending agent and transfusions of whole blood or red cells until hemolysis abates.

Natural isoantibodies against red cells cause, in minutes or hours, lysis of donor's red cells resulting in hemoglobinemia and frequently hemoglobinuria. Lysis may follow transfusion of red cells containing A or B agglutinogens into a recipient whose serum contains a corresponding agglutinin. Depending partly upon the rapidity of blood destruction, symptoms and signs such as back pain, chill, fever, vomiting, circulatory collapse and anuria may appear somewhat in this order of increasing gravity. Similar clinical effects occur, even when the blood is entirely compatible as to major blood groups, if the plasma of an Rh-negative recipient contains acquired *anti-Rh antibodies* as a result of previous transfusion or pregnancy. The immunologic and therapeutic aspects of such hemolytic transfusion reactions are described on page 1096. Such mistakes with potentially tragic consequences can happen whenever more than one bottle of blood or more than one potential recipient is present in a hospital. When the donor's blood contains high titers of anti-A or B agglutinins, as in some samples of group O blood, the transfusion may result in the gradual destruction over days of the donor's red cells carrying the A or B agglutinogen. This difficulty can be avoided by adding A and B (Witebsky) substances to the donor's blood before use, but the doctor should always ask himself "Is this transfusion necessary?"

Erythroblastosis fetalis, the hemolytic anemia of the newborn, may occur when the father, though of the same major blood group as the mother, transmits the dominant Rh-positive gene to the fetus. As a result either of previous transfusion with Rh-positive blood or of previous Rh-positive pregnancies, a small proportion of Rh-negative mothers have anti-Rh antibodies in the plasma. In subsequent pregnancies these anti-Rh antibodies again increase and may enter the fetal circulation by traversing the placenta. If the father is heterozygous for the Rh factor, subsequent fetuses have a 50 per cent chance of being Rh-negative and therefore of being unaffected.* The severest affection appears as fetal hydrops with death before or shortly after birth. The hemolytic anemia is commonly manifest a few hours after birth by elevated bilirubin-globin and signs of rapid red cell regeneration, including many reticulocytes and nucleated red cells in the peripheral blood. In addition to marked bone marrow hyperplasia, pronounced extramedullary blood formation results in enlargement of the liver and spleen. The anemia becomes more severe, the reticulocytes and nucleated

---

* For more than this greatly over-simplified presentation, the reader is referred to the references.

red cells fewer after birth, probably because of the normal loss of the anoxic stimulus to increased erythropoiesis following the initiation of pulmonary respiration. In less marked instances the anemia may not develop significantly until several days or even weeks after delivery. In other infants the additional complication of kernicterus or bile staining of the basal ganglia of the brain may or may not be accompanied by marked jaundice. Treatment of the severely affected infant at birth includes "exchange transfusions" involving the removal of circulating anti-Rh antibodies by alternate venesection and infusion of Rh-negative blood in amounts of 10 cc. or more by means of an inlying catheter in the umbilical vein. In less severely affected patients transfusion of Rh-negative blood suffices. Despite expert and immediate attention at birth, unfortunately some of the anemic and fortunately nearly all the infants with extensive brain damage expire. No effective prophylactic measures have been developed other than in some instances the early delivery of the baby.

Intrinsic Causes of Increased Erythrocyte Destruction. Intrinsic causes of hemolytic anemias may be divided as in Table 1 into (a) abnormal red cells and (b) abnormal plasma.

Abnormal Erythrocytes. Abnormal red cells are responsible for the anemias of congenital hemolytic jaundice, sickle cell anemia, thalassemia major and chronic hemolytic anemia with paroxysmal nocturnal hemoglobinuria. In the first three, the hereditary abnormal morphology of the red cells seemingly constitutes the primary fault; in the last, the abnormally sensitive red cells are hemolyzed by a normal plasma factor, apparently a metal-requiring stromatolytic enzyme. In these anemias, transfused compatible normal red cells have been shown to survive normally. On the other hand, the patient's red cells are rapidly destroyed when transfused into normal subjects. In addition, rare instances of hereditary hemolytic anemias fulfilling these criteria have been reported, in which either numerous stippled or oval-shaped red cells are present.

CONGENITAL HEMOLYTIC JAUNDICE. The clinical features of congenital hemolytic jaundice, which is transmitted as a mendelian dominant by either parent, are described on page 1146. The pathologic basis of the anemia is the abnormal degree of red cell spheroidicity easily observed in wet or stained preparations.

Certainty of diagnosis depends on the demonstration of such cells with increased osmotic fragility in the blood of relatives with or without significant clinical anemia. Such a findng in the patient, though highly suggestive, sometimes occurs in acquired hemolytic jaundice. Increasesd osmotic fragility is invariably accompanied by increased mechanical fragility of the red cells. Both abnormalities are remarkably enhanced by sterile incubation of the blood for 24 hours. Studies of patients with congenital hemolytic jaundice into whom compatible normal red cells have been transfused a few days prior to splenectomy indicate that the normal red cells both in the peripheral blood and in the splenic pulp remain essentially unchanged. However, the proportion of and also the osmotic and mechanical fragilities of the patient's red cells in the splenic pulp greatly exceed those in the peripheral circulation. Thus, selective retention in the spleen, because of their abnormal spheroidicity, and separation there from the plasma presumably cause effects upon the patient's red cells similar to those of sterile incubation *in vitro*: markedly increased osmotic and mechanical fragilities of the red cells of the patient as compared to those of incubated normal red cells. Recent studies indicate that many of the so-called "hemolytic crises" are in reality sudden depressions of red cell formation by the bone marrow in association with grippe-like infections. Because of the brief life span of the red cells, this promptly results in an increase in the severity of the anemia in this as well as in other kinds of hemolytic anemia.

After splenectomy, the beneficial effects of which are described in the section on Diseases of the Spleen, the osmotic and mechanical fragilities of the circulating red cells decline toward, but do not usually reach, entirely normal values (see Fig. 148). Indeed, in some instances slightly increased reticulocyte and serum bilirubin values indicate persistence of a mild hemolytic process accompanied by an insignificant degree of anemia.

SICKLE CELL ANEMIA. Sickle cell anemia occurs in the United States in only about 2 per cent of Negroes exhibiting the characteristic red cell anomaly. Recent studies indicate that the anemic subjects are those in whom both parents, always asymptomatic, carry the trait. The probability is that half of the children of such parents will be homozygous and so have the disease. A few instances of sickle cell anemia in white persons have been reported. These are usually children of parents heterozygous for sickle cell trait and thalassemia, respectively. Affected subjects are frequently of asthenic habitus, with slender extremities and chronic leg ulcers. They experience symptoms felt. Indeed, it is likely to be reduced by infarction to a fibrous structure less than 50 gm. in weight. Multiple thromboses and infarcts of many organs, including the long bones, lungs and central nervous system, give rise to a variety of clinical manifestations which prove fatal to many patients before 10 years of age, and to nearly all before they

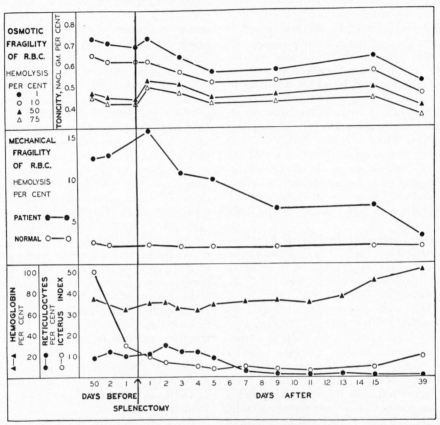

Fig. 148. Effect of splenectomy upon mechanical fragility of red cells of a patient with congenital hemolytic jaundice. The usual decline of the serum bilirubin and reticulocytes followed by a gradual elevation of the hemoglobin is shown, as well as the gradual reduction in the increased osmotic fragility of the red cells toward normal. Note especially the progressive and striking decline of the increased mechanical fragility of the red cells toward, but not entirely to, normal. (Reproduced from a figure kindly supplied by Dr. Shu Chu Shen.) (W. A. Sodeman: Pathologic Physiology: Mechanisms of Disease.)

corresponding to a moderate, fairly constant degree of anemia. The clinical course is punctuated by so-called "crises" during which fever and attacks of pain in the limbs or abdomen appear. Cardiomegaly with systolic or even apparently presystolic murmurs is common. Roentgenograms of the skull sometimes indicate gross extension of the marrow through the outer table of the skull and give the characteristic hair-on-end appearance. In children the spleen and liver are frequently palpable. In adults the spleen is almost never reach the age of 40. The anemia is normocytic and slightly hypochromic, with slight decrease in the maximal range of osmotic fragility of the red cells. Leukocytosis accompanies the crises, which sometimes appear to follow mild local or systemic infections. Red cell destruction is usually not significantly increased, but prothrombin decrease may precede and thrombin increase accompany crises. The usual stained blood smear in sickle cell disease shows a few "fixed" sickled or oatshaped red cells. In some patients, such cells are absent. This is always the case in sickle cell trait. However, when a drop of blood of either type is mixed with a drop of a 2 per cent solution of sodium metabisulfite (reducing solution) on a glass slide under a cover slip, sickling appears within 15 minutes.

The entire disease picture is the result of the characteristic behavior of the red cells that is associated with an abnormal type of hemoglobin. Parallel orientation and aggregation of the atypical S type hemoglobin molecules cause changes in red cell shape typified by the immediate development of sickle- or oat-shaped forms whenever the blood is exposed, as normally in the capillaries, to tensions of oxygen of 35 to 40 mm. of mercury or somewhat less. Electrophoretic studies show that S type hemoglobin comprises 75 per cent or more of the hemoglobin of homozygotes, but only from 25 to 45 per cent of the hemoglobin of those with the trait. In the S-thalassemia combination the predominance of S type hemoglobin is perhaps due to its more rapid formation. Molecular orientation of reduced S type hemoglobin is inhibited by normal hemoglobin and especially by fetal hemoglobin, but is enhanced by the abnormal hemoglobin of thalassemia and perhaps less so by types C and D hemoglobin. These rare abnormal hemoglobin types may be found in the blood of one of the parents of a child with sicklemia whose other parent carries the gene for S type hemoglobin. Measurements *in vitro* show that as sickling increases, the viscosity of the blood and the mechanical fragility of the red cells progressively increase. These phenomena lead to the multiple venous thromboses and infarcts and to the hemolytic anemia characteristic of the active disease. As oxygen tensions well below the physiologic range for capillary blood are required to cause sickling of the red cells of patients with the trait, such red cells survive normally when transfused into normal subjects or into patients with sickle cell disease.

Recognition of the existence of sicklemia helps to prevent mistakes in diagnosis such as an acute surgical emergency requiring laparotomy. Treatment of crises, which usually last only a few days, is generally symptomatic. Oxygen administration is rarely helpful, since it suppresses erythropoiesis in the bone marrow rather than sickling in the peripheral capillaries. Transfusion, however, provides red cells that will not sickle and consequently diminishes the abnormal physical characteristics of the capillary blood.

THALASSEMIA. *Cooley's anemia* and *familial microcytic anemia,* respectively, are the two forms, major and minor, of so-called thalassemia. This term, derived from the Greek word for sea, indicates the prevalence of this disorder among the populations of countries bordering the Mediterranean: Italian, Greek, Syrian or Armenian. When both parents carry the minor trait, the affected children exhibit a severe anemia which is usually fatal during childhood. In such parents the anemia is slight and resembles somewhat that of a mild iron deficiency.

The blood picture in the major disorder is one of a severe microcytic, hypochromic anemia with elevated reticulocytes, "target" and stippled cells. Individual red cells show great variation in size and especially in degree of hemoglobin concentration. The strikingly decreased osmotic fragility in the maximum range is due to the fact that the red cells are "flatter" than normal. Numerous normoblasts and sometimes erythroblasts and often a granulocytic leukocytosis, sometimes with myelocytes, are seen in the peripheral blood. The serum iron is elevated and the iron-binding capacity fully saturated. The bilirubin of the serum is slightly or moderately increased, as is the urobilinogen in the feces. Unlike the usual hemolytic anemias, however, there is little evidence of hemosiderin deposition in spleen, liver and kidneys. No hemolytic mechanism has been convincingly demonstrated. The mongoloid facies is due in part to the enlargement of the marrow cavities of the cranial bones. This also gives rise to the "hair-on-end" appearance of the calvarium and to thinning of the cortex of the long bones and trabeculation seen in x-ray pictures. The spleen is frequently enlarged, the liver moderately.

Thalassemia minor is ordinarily not a cause of symptoms, and is usually compatible with normal development and adult activities. However, in some individuals, the hemoglobin may be definitely reduced and splenomegaly and slight bone changes upon x-ray examination may be present. Indeed, clinically and hematologically a marked case of the heterozygous may resemble a mild case of the homozygous condition. In thalassemia minor, although cell survival may be short, the peripheral blood is lacking in the usual signs of increased red cell destruction. The hypochromia and microcytosis should not cause confusion with iron deficiency anemia if the high serum iron and the racial and familial aspects of the case are recognized. The occasionally somewhat elevated red count is accompanied by a moderately reduced hemoglobin level and thus should not lead to the erroneous diagnosis of polycythemia. Iron therapy is beneficial in neither form of the disease unless iron deficiency is a complication. Splenectomy is usually ineffectual in the major disorder but may justifiably be undertaken when the spleen is large and the maintained hemoglobin level is so low as to be incapacitating.

PAROXYSMAL NOCTURNAL HEMOGLO-BINURIA. This is a rare sporadic form of chronic hemolytic anemia with marked perpetual hemoglobinemia. During sleep the plasma hemoglobin level rises and causes hemoglobinuria to develop or to increase during some hours. A brown, less commonly reddish, color is consequently most noticeable in the morning urine. The immediate cause of the increased red cell destruction is the abnormality of the patient's red cells which renders them susceptible to lysis by a factor common to the plasma of the patient and of most normal persons as well. The appearance and the osmotic and mechanical fragilities of the red cells are normal.

Adults in the third decade are those most commonly affected, but incidence at any age except in young children has been reported. As a rule the anemia progresses and the condition is fatal after several years. Rarely partial or complete recovery does occur. The anemia is usually well marked and is normocytic or slightly macrocytic and normochromic with elevated reticulocytes but not always to the degree seen in congenital hemolytic jaundice. The plasma hemoglobin ranges from 25 to 150 mg. per 100 cc., partly in the form of methemalbumin which together with the moderately elevated bilirubin often gives the plasma a brownish color. The fecal urobilinogen output is not necessarily increased, and reticulocyte levels and radioactive iron turnover studies indicate less than the expected rate of hemoglobin and red cell production for a purely hemolytic anemia. The frequently observed moderate leukopenia and thrombocytopenia may suggest the erroneous diagnosis of refractory rather than hemolytic anemia. They offer a contrast to the findings in most hemolytic anemias and are thought to be due to the common suscepti-bility of the abnormal leukocytes and platelets to the action of the hemolytic plasma factor. Infections are frequent, but purpura is rare. As in any patient with chronic hemoglobinuria, the urinary sediment displays leukocytes or desquamated renal tubule cells containing brown hemosiderin granules which readily take the iron stain. Unless compensated by iron or by transfusion therapy, this chronic urinary loss of iron may result in depletion of iron deposits elsewhere than in the renal tubules. The liver and spleen are sometimes moderately enlarged.

The specific diagnostic test for the disease is hemolysis of the patient's red cells by slightly acidified patient's or normal serum (Ham test). The reaction is inhibited by oxalate or citrate. The red cells are apparently destroyed by a metal-requiring stromatolytic enzyme which is activated in vitro by a slight fall in pH. This presumably occurs in the relatively stagnant capillaries of some organs during sleep. The degree of hemoglobinemia and consequently of hemoglobinuria is enhanced by the administration of acid salts or inhibited, for example, by hyperventilation of the patient in a respirator. Inhibitors of this hemolytic system are said to exist in the plasma and to be destroyed by thrombin with consequent increase in hemolytic activity affecting platelets as well as red cells. Clinically, infection, trauma, anxiety, menstruation and whole blood transfusion appear to cause episodes of increased hemolysis. Dicumarol inhibits the thromboses of the systemic and portal veins characteristic of the disease, perhaps by diminishing the platelet-agglutinating tendency of the plasma. In some patients Dicumarol raises the platelet count and inhibits the hemolytic process as well. Heparin accelerates the latter as may normal plasma.

Thrombosis is the most serious complication of the disease. It may sometimes be combated by Dicumarol therapy which may also improve the hemoglobin level. Splenectomy is of no value against the anemia and increases the risk of thrombosis. Alkalinization is only temporarily effective, and its discontinuance results in increased hemolysis. Because normal red cells survive normally in these patients, packed red cell transfusions are useful in order to avoid low hemoglobin levels that incapacitate the patient. Saline washing of the cells to be transfused may be required to prevent increasing the destruction of the patient's red cells by the normal plasma introduced. ACTH, cortisone and Dicumarol do not obviate such plasma transfusion reactions.

Abnormal Plasma. Abnormal plasma is primarily responsible for several types of acute and chronic hemolytic anemias classified in Table 1.

PAROXYSMAL (COLD) HEMOGLOBINURIA. This is a rare but clinically dramatic consequence of transient and often occult hemoglobinemia, which causes manifest hemoglobinuria. Two entirely different mechanisms for the sudden increased red cell destruction may be involved in different patients and can be demonstrated under experimental clinical conditions.

The first mechanism depends upon a hemolysin present in the patient's serum which is activated by cooling and rewarming of the blood without agitation. This increasingly rare variety of hemoglobinuria is a late manifestation of syphilis, congenital or acquired, in patients with a positive Wassermann reaction. Characteristically, transient hemoglobinemia and consequent hemoglobinuria develop following exposure to a temperature of 18° C. or lower. Unless severe attacks occur repeatedly at short intervals, the acute hemolytic anemia is mild and soon disappears. Its immediate cause is the presence of a serum hemolysin capable, in the presence of complement, of sensitizing normal red cells at 16° C. or below and of hemolyzing them thereafter at body temperature. This, the so-called Donath-Landsteiner reaction, is diagnostic for the condition. The patient's serum upon chilling and incubation also causes clumping of leukocytes and phagocytosis of red cells of normal subjects of the same blood group.

Within several minutes or a few hours after exposure to cold or to cool damp conditions the patient experiences malaise, chilly sensations, headache, pain in the back and fever, which may sometimes even exceed 104° F. Sometimes urticaria, edema or vesicles appear on the cooled skin surfaces, probably due to a local dermolytic action of the hemolysin. The next specimen of urine passed may be dark red or brown and may contain hemoglobin, methemoglobin, sometimes a few red cells and granular and pigment-containing casts. The casts may not at first show a positive iron stain. In a day or two the urine becomes normal in color, and the patient may appear to be transiently jaundiced. In milder attacks or in those induced by immersion of an arm or leg in cold water, hemoglobinemia followed by bilirubinemia but not necessarily by hemoglobinuria may be observed. At the time of the onset of hemolysis, leukopenia with relative lymphocytosis develops accompanied by erythrophagocytosis in blood samples upon incubation. The treatment of the disorder is avoidance of exposure to cold until adequate therapy of the underlying syphilis has been achieved, preferably with penicillin. Clinical relief but not necessarily complete disappearance of the hemolysin is to be expected.

The second mechanism involves no hemolysin but instead a cold agglutinin which causes clumping of the red cells. These strongly agglutinated cells in chilled blood are abnormally susceptible *in vitro* to mechanical trauma which in the patient is presumably induced by the motion of the circulation. Clumps of red cells may be seen in cooled conjunctival and nail bed capillaries, and by obstructing the flow of blood probably give rise to Raynaud-like symptoms or even to gangrene of the digits. Sometimes local purpura and urticaria are observed. In some patients, in whom the cold agglutinin is active also to some extent at body temperature, there is a background of chronic hemolytic anemia which may exhibit moderate increase in severity during cool weather. On this may be superimposed episodes of acute hemolysis and hemoglobinuria following greater chilling of the patient. Usually the basis of the disorder is unknown. However, cold agglutinins not infrequently develop in atypical "virus" pneumonia which when in high titer have occasionally resulted in hemolytic anemia and even more seldom in cold hemoglobinuria. The best treatment is the avoidance of exposure to cold in anticipation of spontaneous decline of cold agglutinin titers.

ACQUIRED HEMOLYTIC JAUNDICE. The term *acquired hemolytic jaundice* is used here in a limited sense to designate a group of uncommon, acute or chronic hemolytic anemias exclusive of congenital hemolytic jaundice and of hemolytic anemias related to the various causes already discussed. Onset may be at any age and is without familial association. The clinical course, in contrast to that of congenital hemolytic jaundice, is rarely benign. These anemias are often without recognizable causation or red cell abnormality, other than a short survival time of patients' and of normal donors' cells as well. They are, however, sometimes associated with liver cirrhosis, Hodgkin's disease, leukemia, sarcoid, carcinomatosis, disseminated lupus erythematosus and ovarian cysts and teratomas. The spleen is often enlarged, sometimes to a considerable degree. Fever is a frequent finding.

Significant anemia is rare in acute hepatic cell injury, but a chronic hemolytic anemia without relevant plasma abnormality or positive Coombs' test is frequently present in patients with Laënnec's cirrhosis. However, the hemoglobin is rarely less than 50 per cent of normal unless nutritional deficiency is a causative factor or bleeding from varices has occurred. The mean corpuscular volume usually falls between 90 and 110 cubic microns. The reticulocytes are not impressively increased nor are the red cells "flattened" unless acute liver cell damage or obstructive jaundice exists. In such patients the shape of transfused normal red cells becomes so modified within a few days. The leukocytes and platelets may be somewhat decreased as in patients with hepatic or splenic enlargement due to other causes. The bone marrow is predominantly normoblastic rather than megaloblastic unless coincidental folic acid or vitamin B_{12} deficiency is present, as shown by a partial response to such specific nutrients. Cessation of alcohol ingestion often causes an early reticulocyte response but shortened cell survival is the major cause of the usual anemia. Ordinarily the anemia lessens spontaneously as the patient's liver function improves sufficiently to allow him activity enough to make more circulating hemoglobin useful to him. Consequently transfusions are indicated only when hemorrhage occurs.

The blood picture and bile pigment values are those of acute or chronic hemolytic anemias except when modified by the signs of an underlying blood dyscrasia such as leukemia. Frequently, the red cells exhibit increased mechanical fragility and sometimes also increased osmotic fragility. Characteristic of these patients as a group is the fact that their *washed* red cells are agglutinated by an antiserum developed against human serum or human globulin in rabbits (Coombs test). This indicates that some type of serum globulin has been adsorbed on the red cells, but not necessarily because of an immune mechanism. In a few observations it has been shown that normal red cells do not survive satisfactorily after transfusion into such patients and acquire within a few hours the property of being agglutinated in the Coombs test. Autoagglutination of the red cells is a common finding and may interfere with blood typing. This tendency is increased if the serum is acidified with carbon dioxide. In these circumstances the serum will also agglutinate normal red cells, which then become positive in the Coombs test. Rarely, it is possible to demonstrate a hemolysin active at a low pH. In many of these patients cold agglutinins are found in the serum, and when in high titer probably explain the occasional clinical observation of urticaria or Raynaud-like phenomena in the fingers on exposure to cold.

The paradox of hemolysis without demonstrable hemolysins is frequently involved in hemolytic transfusion reactions due to an incompatibility among blood groups and practically always when the incompatibility is due to Rh sensitization. It is also a challenging problem in erythroblastosis fetalis and in the majority of patients with acquired hemolytic jaundice. Common to all is some type of agglutination phenomenon. In the experimental animal increased osmotic fragility of the red cells regularly follows the injection of anti-red cell immune serum containing agglutinins as well as hemolysins. It also follows the injection of incompatible plasma of high agglutinin titer or even characterizes incompatible red cells when injected into human subjects. However, neither the immune serum nor the serum of the injected animal or patient can increase the osmotic fragility of red cells *in vitro*.

By dilution of the anti-red cell immune serum in the serum of the animal prior to its use it is possible to inject concentrations of the hemolytic serum that are *entirely sublytic in vitro*. Nevertheless, their agglutinating power for red cells both *in vitro* and *in vivo* is well retained; and they readily produce hemolytic anemia in the experimental animal. Perfusion of blood containing red cells agglutinated by such serums through the liver causes retention and subsequent increase in their osmotic and mechanical fragilities. Minced liver and other tissues cause similar changes when incubated with normal red cells. From this evidence it is conjectured that in clinical circumstances agglutination of red cells may lead to their sequestration in the liver, spleen and other tissues and to local ischemia and release of substances by the tissues that in turn cause damage to red cells in the adjacent tissue capillaries. This is consistent with the occasional clinical findings of central necrosis or fibrosis of the liver and the consistent congestion and infarction of the splenic pulp in patients with acquired hemolytic jaundice.

Splenectomy has been found to be a useful treatment in only about half the patients with acquired hemolytic jaundice. Rarely is the improvement as prompt as in congenital hemolytic jaundice; usually it is delayed over a matter of weeks and may even then not result in a complete restoration of normal blood values. The titer of the Coombs test may greatly diminish, disappear or not be significantly altered. Although the spleen has been shown to contain substances capable of endowing normal red cells with the ability to react positively in the Coombs test, such substances are doubtless produced elsewhere in the body by the cells of the reticuloendothelial or lymphoid systems. Depending on the underlying conditions, x-ray, nitrogen mustards, adrenocorticotrophic hormone or cortisone may be useful by suppressing their formation, or as a preliminary to splenectomy. In patients with chronic lymphatic leukemia or Hodgkin's disease who have severe hemolytic anemia, splenectomy is justified, for it may produce a striking decrease in red cell destruction. In some patients the removal of a cystic tumor or, regularly in alcoholic cirrhosis, abstinence has had a similar effect, sometimes associated with signs of increased red cell production as well. Transfusions can preserve life until other measures become effective or until spontaneous improvement occurs.

ANEMIAS DUE TO DECREASED ERYTHRO-CYTE PRODUCTION

In Table 2 these are classified according to various causes for failure of the bone marrow to produce sufficient red cells or hemoglobin to keep pace with the normal rate of red cell destruction. In general, although subject to exceptions, the diminished functional activity of the bone marrow is expressed in the peripheral blood by few reticulocytes, granulocytes and platelets. Sometimes only erythropoiesis appears to be significantly affected. In other instances abnormal leukocytes may indicate a primary disturbance of their progenitors in the marrow as the cause of the anemia. In order to determine the nature of its functional inadequacy, biopsy of the bone marrow by needle or trephine is often of particular value in these anemias.

Table 2. Classification of Anemias Due Mainly to Decreased Erythrocyte Production (Bone Marrow Physiologically Hypoactive)

I. NUTRITIONAL DEFICIENCY
  (a) Vitamin B_{12} (macrocytic anemia)
      Defective diet: nutritional macrocytic anemia, sprue
      Deficient gastric (intrinsic) factor: pernicious, tapeworm and pregnancy macrocytic anemias
      Intestinal impermeability: sprue, steatorrhea, stenosis and short circuits of gastrointestinal tract
  (b) Folic acid (macrocytic anemia)
      Defective diet: megaloblastic anemia of infants, tropics, pregnancy
      Intestinal impermeability: megaloblastic anemias of sprue, steatorrhea, blind loops and stenoses of gastrointestinal tract
  (c) Folic and ascorbic acids (macrocytic anemia)
      Defective diet: megaloblastic anemia of infants, adult scurvy
      Defective metabolism: liver disease (?)
  (d) Iron (hypochromic anemia)
      Requirement increased: growth
      Loss increased: menstruation or pregnancy, chronic hemorrhage, Banti's syndrome
      Intake decreased: defective diet, gastric anacidity, diarrhea, steatorrhea

II. ENDOCRINE DEFICIENCY
  Thyroid or pituitary hormones

III. TOXIC INHIBITION
  (a) External poisons: benzol, arsphenamine, insecticides, antileukemic drugs
  (b) Internal toxins: chronic infections, renal failure, cancer (local or metastatic)

IV. PHYSICAL INJURY
  X-rays, radium, radioactive phosphorus

V. MECHANICAL INTERFERENCE
  (a) Inadequate marrow capacity: anemia of newborn and of prematurity
  (b) Myelophthisis: leukemia, myelofibrosis, osteosclerosis, metastatic carcinomatosis, primary xanthomatoses

VI. IDIOPATHIC FAILURE
  Refractory (aplastic) anemias of children and adults

NUTRITIONAL DEFICIENCY OF ERYTHROPOIESIS

Nutritional deficiency is an important cause of deficient erythropoiesis. Well established clinical varieties are known to result from lack of metabolically available vitamin B_{12}, pteroylglutamic acid, ascorbic acid or iron, individually or in various combinations. In any given patient the dietary defect may be of more than one substance and in addition, specific and nonspecific gastrointestinal defects of absorption may play primary or secondary roles of greater or less importance in different patients. It is possible that liver cirrhosis disturbs the conversion of folic acid to its metabolically active form, the *citrovorum factor* or folinic acid.

Deficiency of the Anti-pernicious Anemia Vitamin B_{12} Principle. Deficiency of vitamin B_{12} (cyanocobalamin and its congeners) is common to pernicious and related macrocytic anemias. Experiments concerned with the growth requirements of certain Lactobacilli and of chicks and rats show that this red, cobalt-containing vitamin is present in many foods of animal origin such as milk, eggs, skeletal muscle and liver. Observations in patients with pernicious anemia have shown that the characteristic lack of gastric secretion deprives them of a thermolabile substance (intrinsic factor) apparently specifically required for the efficient absorption of vitamin B_{12} (extrinsic factor) when present in the relatively low concentrations found in most foods. Whether this is the result of an interaction between vitamin B_{12} and the gastric juice or whether the gastric juice specifically catalyzes some absorptive process in the intestinal wall remains unknown. However, if vitamin B_{12} is injected parenterally, without contact with gastric juice, it is invariably more active in promoting erythropoiesis than when orally administered with gastric juice. Liver is an example of a sufficiently concentrated source of vitamin B_{12} to allow some absorption without the mediation of intrinsic factor. Desiccated hog stomach is hematopoietically effective because it contains both vitamin B_{12} and intrinsic factor. The latter has recently been stated to be intimately associated with mucoprotein fractions of human gastric juice.

Diets low in animal protein may directly fail to provide sufficient vitamin B_{12}. Total gastrectomy or the gastritis that frequently precedes the development of cancer of the stomach (rather than the cancer itself) is probably responsible for the occasional development of pernicious anemia. During pregnancy gastric acidity and sometimes intrinsic factor secretion are progressively inhibited until after delivery. In Addisonian pernicious anemia, the gastric mucosal atrophy causing achylia is probably the result of a hereditary genetic defect. The presence of the broad tapeworm in the upper intestine in some way disturbs the action of an already limited secretion of intrinsic factor and so precipitates the macrocytic anemia found in a small percentage of the many persons, chiefly in Finland, bearing this parasite. Chronic intestinal disease, idiopathic steatorrhea or diarrhea such as occurs in sprue prevents the adequate absorption of vitamin B_{12} even when intrinsic factor is present in the gastric juice. Intestinal short circuits and stenoses and especially blind loops of bowel are presumably effective either by disturbing assimilation or by promoting competitive utilization of vitamin B_{12} by intestinal bacteria.

Both *in vivo* and *in vitro* the numerous megaloblasts in the extensive deep red bone marrow of pernicious anemia are rapidly matured by vitamin B_{12}. However, the circulating red cells of the untreated patient are defective, for they have a short survival time when transfused into normal persons. Moreover, there is accumulating evidence that normal red cells do not survive normally in the untreated patient. The anemia is thus due both to "maturation arrest" and to increased red cell destruction, which is, however, not so great as bile pigment excretion measurements suggest. Studies with isotopic nitrogen indicate that in pernicious anemia as much as half the excess urobilinogen in the feces results from a breakdown of heme molecules from sources other than circulating red cells.

Addisonian pernicious anemia is uncommon in persons under 35 years of age. It affects both sexes equally and occurs mainly in the northern part of the temperate zones of Europe and North America. In the United States the mixed racial population renders less characteristic the classic impression that the disease is prone to affect blue-eyed persons whose hair has turned gray prematurely and who have a wide jaw angle and are of "large and bulky frame." Negroes and Chinese are sometimes affected. Pernicious anemia is one of the few anemias with symptoms sufficiently characteristic in many instances to permit an almost certain diagnosis. Thus the condition should always be considered when a patient complains of persistent, symmetrical paresthesias of the toes or fingers. If, in addition, a sore tongue or mouth together with variable degrees of epigastric distress, "gas," constipation, or looseness of the bowels is described, pernicious anemia can be diagnosed with practical certainty. Such symptoms, though usual, are by no means invariably present. Even in patients with little or no anemia, they are promptly relieved by specific treatment.

The physical examination displays pallor, sometimes with some jaundice of the skin and sclerae, although this is not invariable. Characteristically, the tongue either shows atrophy of the papillae of the tip and sides

almost invariably somewhat reduced. In rare patients a combination of vitamin B_{12} and of iron deficiency expresses itself as a slightly macrocytic and mildly hypochromic anemia. Bone marrow puncture invariably indicates a cellular marrow characterized by numbers of megaloblasts when the anemia is severe. In patients in remission or without significant anemia, the bone marrow picture is not diagnostic.

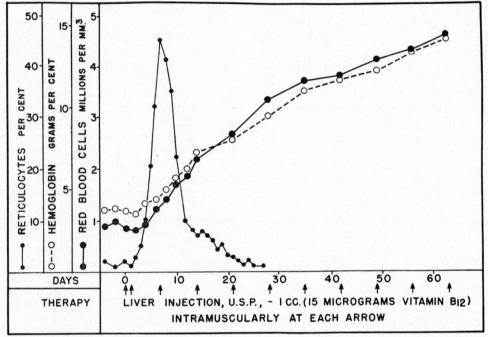

Fig. 149. The response of the blood to vitamin B_{12} in a case of pernicious anemia.

or an intensely red, inflamed surface with vesicles or shallow ulcerations. Today splenomegaly is an unusual finding. More often the liver is slightly enlarged. Combined system disease of the spinal cord in the fully developed disastrous form that may result unless specific treatment is promptly instituted is described on page 1553.

The anemia, when well established, is macrocytic and normochromic. Characteristic red cells are oval macrocytes; but small irregular forms are common as in many severe anemias. Reticulocytes are few. Nucleated red cells, including megaloblasts of Ehrlich, are seen in the peripheral blood of severely anemic patients. There is usually definite leukopenia with a diminution of the percentage of granulocytes, most of which are unusually large, adult forms with many subdivisions of the nucleus. The platelets are

Other macrocytic anemias sharing in common the response to vitamin B_{12} have been already referred to. Combined system disease of the spinal cord is virtually confined to patients with achylia gastrica. Lingual and gastrointestinal disturbances, however, are common to all, but of varied severity in different clinical syndromes. The overlapping in blood picture and bone marrow findings among these conditions is complete. In general, associated or secondary nutritional disturbances are common in patients with defective food intake or diarrhea. In pernicious anemia the diet is not ordinarily strikingly defective until the anemia is severe. Occasionally the disease may be precipitated by a change to a defective diet, whether resulting from loss of a husband or of a set of dentures.

Pernicious and related macrocytic anemias exhibit low levels of serum vitamin B_{12} (microbiologic test) and respond to the parenteral administration of vitamin B_{12} itself, or vitamin B_{12} in the form of highly refined liver extracts, as illustrated in Figure 149. In the severely anemic patient, 15 micrograms of vitamin B_{12} or its equivalent as Liver Injection U.S.P. may be given intramuscularly at once and repeated every 2 hours for three or four doses. Thereafter it is reasonable to continue the patient on a schedule of injections of 30 micrograms of vitamin B_{12} or its equivalent as Liver Injection U.S.P. at weekly intervals for two months. In usual circumstances normal red cell values are achieved after about six weeks, irrespective of the height of the initial red cell count. Thereafter the patient with Addisonian pernicious anemia and most cases of sprue should receive injections *indefinitely* at intervals of no longer than one month at the rate of at least 1 microgram of vitamin B_{12} a day.

Diagnosis is best established by the characteristic reticulocyte response within ten days following the administration of the specific nutrient. In practice, inspection of two or three reticulocyte preparations will often suffice for this demonstration. Lack of such evidence leaves the need for and type of future treatment uncertain. The granulocytes and platelets also increase early in the remission. The first detectable sign of improvement may appear within 48 hours. It frequently consists in a slight improvement in the patient's color, usually with no change or even a slight fall of the hemoglobin concentration. Shortly thereafter jaundice begins to diminish, the patient's appetite and strength are greatly improved, and within a week he may become ambulatory. At this time edema of the lower extremities is often transiently observed. Orally administered medication is not recommended unless it is impossible for the patient to receive injections.

If the patient has combined system disease the dosage of liver extract or of vitamin B_{12} should be doubled on a purely empirical basis, as also for such complications as acute or chronic infection or advanced arteriosclerosis. With a complicating iron deficiency, a condition rarely present initially in pernicious anemia but not infrequently in related macrocytic anemias, and in any of these during the latter stages of red cell recovery, the oral administration of ferrous sulfate, 0.3 gm. three times a day, is indicated. As an adjuvant in the treatment of sprue, described on page 627, folic acid, U.S.P., in oral doses of 5 to 10 mg. daily may be given to patients who must receive regular injections either of vitamin B_{12} or of liver extract at intervals of less than a week in order to control the diarrhea. Because combined system disease has frequently appeared to progress in patients with pernicious anemia treated exclusively with pteroylglutamic acid, this agent should not ordinarily be used in the treatment of pernicious anemia.

Deficiency of Folic Acid. Folic acid occurs naturally in a variety of foods, mostly in the form of "conjugates" of pteroylglutamic acid containing seven rather than only one molecule of glutamic acid. Hematologic studies of monkeys and later work on the growth requirements of chickens, rats and Lactobacilli eventually led to the synthesis of pteroylglutamic (folic) acid. This yellow substance was then unexpectedly found to be active in pernicious and related macrocytic anemias. Subsequently it was shown that in the group of patients now under discussion, failure to respond to purified liver extract or to vitamin B_{12} in usual doses is followed by prompt hematologic and clinical improvement with orally administered crude liver extract or pteroylglutamic acid. The practical therapeutic implications are obvious.

A distinction between these patients and those with pernicious and related macrocytic anemias first appeared when patients in India with macrocytic anemia failed to respond to a parenterally administered purified liver extract in dosage usually effective in pernicious anemia. As since noted in many other localities, these patients were usually but not exclusively women in the last trimester of pregnancy, whose diets had been grossly defective, often as a result of anorexia or vomiting. However, in these patients dietary defects have not always been noted, and steatorrhea, occult or otherwise, has been found in some patients. In some cases of tropical sprue, folic acid deficiency may be primary or secondary to disorder of the small intestine. Experimentally, infections have been shown to reduce the folic acid content of the liver and to produce megaloblastic marrows in monkeys upon limited folic acid intake. These findings may be especially significant in macrocytic anemias of infants.

Differentiation from macrocytic anemias responsive to vitamin B_{12} on ordinary clinical grounds is not necessarily possible. In general, however, glossitis is infrequent and neural manifestations lacking. Free hydrochloric acid is usually present in the gastric contents. The macrocytosis of the red cells is usually not so marked as in classic pernicious anemia, and hyperbilirubinemia is not usual. In some patients the red cells are slightly small and definitely hypochromic. Leukopenia and thrombocytopenia are usual findings. The bone marrow in the anemic patient is definitely megaloblastic and indistinguishable from that of pernicious anemia. Serum vitamin B_{12} levels are, however, in the normal range.

Deficiency of Folic and Ascorbic Acids. In some patients of the types just described, an additional dietary deficiency of ascorbic acid may condition the primary deficiency of folic acid because ascorbic acid is required for the conversion of pteroylglutamic acid to its metabolically active form, the citrovorum factor or folinic acid. In adult patients with nutritional macrocytic anemias, normal serum vitamin B_{12} levels, signs of clinical scurvy and no ascorbic acid in the leukocytes, administration of ascorbic acid potentiates the hematopoietic effects of small amounts of orally administered pteroylglutamic acid and augments the output of folinic acid in the urine. Failure of this process is presumably the basis of the megaloblastic anemias that have appeared sporadically in infants fed exclusively on unsupplemented formulas based on dried milk preparations deprived of ascorbic acid in the manufacturing process. The majority are between 5 and 11 months of age; about a quarter show clinical signs of scurvy. The hematopoietic response to either folic or folinic acid is often dramatic, as in adults with scurvy and macrocytic anemia. Rarely in some of the latter, when presumably the deficiency of ascorbic acid is the controlling deficiency, response occurs to ascorbic acid alone. In some patients with liver cirrhosis and macrocytic anemia the dietary deficiency has not been impressive, leading to the suspicion that metabolic conversion of folic acid may be defective because of the damaged liver.

Deficiency of Iron. Deficiency of iron is a frequent cause of microcytic hypochromic anemia, usually with little alteration in leukocyte or platelet levels in the peripheral blood. In some chronic cases moderate leukopenia is found. The bone marrow is somewhat more cellular than normally, with erythropoiesis predominantly at the normoblast level. If causes of hypochromia other than iron deficiency, such as chronic infection or thalassemia minor and sicklemia, can be excluded, a successful response to iron administration can be predicted with certainty. This is heralded by beginning clinical improvement and a prompt reticulocyte response, and is followed by restoration of normal blood values by the end of six to ten weeks. Whereas the laboratory diagnosis of hypochromic anemia is clear-cut, the clinical manifestations of the patient are relatively nondescript except for the occurrence of glossitis, dysphagia, "indigestion" and the brittle and flat fingernails characteristic of the chronic hypochromic anemia of adult women. Occasionally the spleen may be palpable.

Iron, once absorbed from the blood or derived from the catabolism of hemoglobin, is not excreted in significant amounts in the feces or urine unless hemoglobinuria is present. Thus, iron deficiency develops only from adventitious iron loss relative or absolute and resulting in a quantitative decrease in the amount of iron available for hemoglobin production. Clinically, this may occur in infants without external bleeding who have received a poor endowment of iron from the mother, usually because she was herself anemic. In older children the annual iron requirements of growth range from approximately 200 down to 80 mg. during the sixth year of life. Thereafter there is a gradual increase to about 350 mg. a year in the male and to nearly 500 mg. in the female at the end of the pubertal growth spurt. In the adult male there is no further iron requirement unless overt or occult bleeding, usually from the gastrointestinal tract, occurs as the result of such causes as varices, ulcers, parasites, cancer or hemorrhoids. In the female, however, during the entire reproductive period the annual loss of iron amounts to about 300 mg. due to menstruation. The child receives at birth from the mother a somatic inheritance of about 375 mg. Diets low in iron-containing foods, as well as lack of hydrochloric acid in the stomach resulting in failure of the food iron to be ionized and subsequently reduced by the weak acids of the food, are the usual causes of a limited assimilation of iron.

Assimilated iron is not a catalyst, but a quantitative component of the increased hemoglobin formed in hypochromic anemia following its administration. In practice the daily oral administration of about a gram of ferrous sulfate divided into three equal doses and given immediately after meals is highly effective. Liver extracts, vitamins, copper, molybdenum or arsenic have no adjuvant value. Cobalt, a nonspecific erythropoietic stimulant, is not indicated because replacement therapy with iron is sufficiently effective. In rare instances iron may not be well tolerated when given orally in sufficient doses to be effective. Iron combined with sucrose, in the form of a suitable preparation of saccharated iron, may be given in considerable amounts by intravenous injection without undue discomfort. This procedure, however, will rarely be needed and, if carried to excess, could lead to undesirable degrees of hemosiderosis.

ENDOCRINE DEFICIENCY OF ERYTHROPOIESIS

Anemia due to endocrine deficiency, unless complicated by other factors, is never severe; it is usually normocytic and normochromic in type with little alteration in leukocyte or platelet values. Most common in association with hypothyroidism, anemia also accompanies insufficiency of the anterior pituitary and of the adrenal cortex. What little information is available indicates that the bone marrow is somewhat hypoplastic.

In myxedema, perhaps because of the frequent association of achylia gastrica, the usual type of more severe anemia is hypochromic; but macrocytic anemia has also been observed. These varieties of anemia clearly represent deficiencies of iron and of vitamin B_{12}, respectively, superimposed on thyroid deficiency. Thyroid deficiency alone apparently limits chiefly the ceiling of hematopoiesis, because active initial responses to iron or to liver extract may be induced. Final restoration of normal red cell and hemoglobin levels, however, requires the additional administration of thyroid extract, often for several weeks. The anemia of thyroid deficiency is of obscure cause, but may be the result of erythropoiesis retarded in rate, as are the growth and function of other body cells in this disease. The treatment of the mild anemia of endocrine disorders is largely incidental to the management of the conditions themselves. Recently it has been claimed that sheep pituitaries contain an independently effective erythropoietic factor.

TOXIC INHIBITION OF ERYTHROPOIESIS

Certain anemias are considered to be due to toxic inhibition of the erythropoietic function of the bone marrow, by substances either absorbed from external sources or elaborated internally. Benzol, a volatile solvent useful in industry, still unfortunately sometimes affects groups of workers. However, many other cyclic compounds are suspect in individual instances: arsphenamine, volatile insecticides, hair dyes, photographic developers, atabrine, chloramphenicol and Tridione. Characteristically, affected patients exhibit normocytic, or even frequently somewhat macrocytic, normochromic anemia. Reticulocytes are few. The associated granulocytopenia may lead to local infections, especially of the oral cavity. Thrombocytopenia, when severe, results in bleeding into skin and mucous membranes. Modern studies indicate that such a peripheral blood picture is common to the bone marrow hypoplasia found in a few patients as well as to the more frequently found marrow hypercellularity with immaturity of the predominating cells. Moderate splenomegaly, usually without lymph node enlargement, is sometimes observed. A hemolytic process, best demonstrated by shortened red cell survival, may also be present. In some patients with chronic anemia the marrow eventually becomes frankly leukemic; and in others fibrosis and even osteosclerosis seem to be terminal pathologic sequences. These last can be demonstrated only by trephine biopsy.

The toxic nature of the anemia is suggested by a history of exposure to drugs and by the finding of an excess of coproporphyrin type III in the feces, indicating, as in lead poisoning, a perversion of hemoglobin synthesis. In acute poisonings spontaneous recovery sometimes occurs. Little can be done for these patients if profuse hemorrhage appears. Modern chemotherapy permits some control of infections secondary to granulocytopenia. Without these complications maintenance of a sufficiently elevated level of hemoglobin to permit light work is often possible for a considerable period of time by the systematic use of sufficiently frequent single transfusions. A thorough therapeutic trial with orally administered liver extract or with both folic acid by mouth and liver extract or vitamin B_{12} by parenteral injection should always be carried out. However, unless a fortunate mistake in diagnosis has been made, these measures are usually ineffectual. ACTH and cortisone may be useful in a few patients, and in these splenectomy may also either help to increase the period of red cell survival or possibly, by improving erythropoiesis, reduce the need for transfusions. Cobalt therapy is useless.

Chronic uremia is the best example of a cause of anemia due to toxins of internal origin. A severe normocytic normochromic anemia often develops when the nonprotein nitrogen of the blood has been over 100 mg. per 100 cc. for several weeks or more. In some patients, as in nephrectomized dogs, red cell survival is shortened. The nature of the toxic substances is unknown. The polymorphonuclears may show "toxic" granulation. Otherwise the leukocytes and platelets in the blood stream and the morphology of the bone marrow are little altered from the normal. Although most common with chronic nephritis, congenital cystic kidneys, pyelonephritis or chronic prostatic obstruction produces the same result. Unless urinary obstruction can be mechanically relieved, neither can the anemia. With severe anemia, transfusion may increase the comfort of the patient somewhat, but renal function is rarely improved and other aspects of uremia are usually limiting factors upon his activities.

Rheumatic fever, tuberculosis and other chronic granulomas are examples of clinical causes of the anemia associated with chronic infection. Usually normocytic and slightly hypochromic, the red cells may be normochromic and even slightly macrocytic. Unless another cause for anemia, such as chronic blood loss, is also present, the hemoglobin is rarely less than 60 per cent of normal. Leukocytosis with basophilic granules in the granulocytes is common because of the underlying infection. Rarely the platelets are reduced with resultant purpura. Although the plasma iron values are usually low because of deviation of iron to the tissues, this is not the cause of the anemia. Serum copper and erythrocyte protoporphyrin are increased. More significant, perhaps, is the recent experimental evidence indicating a disturbance of folic acid metabolism as a result of chronic infection in monkeys. Cancer, especially when massive in primary or secondary deposits, and Hodgkin's disease with extensive visceral involvement are associated with a similar type of anemia. A superimposed infection can sometimes clearly be shown to inhibit the action of liver extract or of iron in anemias that would otherwise respond rapidly to these agents. For obvious reasons, elimination of the infection is the treatment desired. Cobaltous chloride given orally in daily doses of 60 to 120 mg. will in many instances abolish the mild anemia of chronic infection or of cancer, will sometimes significantly relieve the anemia of chronic uremia, but will usually cause anorexia or nausea. As with the use of transfusions, the resulting improvement in the patient's color is more gratifying to observers than of value to the patient.

PHYSICAL INJURY OF ERYTHROPOIESIS

Except as a result of accidental exposure in industry or medical practice, physical injury of erythropoiesis by roentgen rays or radioactive material is fortunately rare today. When irradiation is used in a carefully controlled fashion in the treatment of neoplastic disease, the development of anemia is usually the result of the uncontrolled progress of the underlying disorder. The biologic effects of irradiation usually occur only where the energy is delivered. Thus, alpha and beta particles which can traverse only a few millimeters of tissue are harmful only when derived from internally absorbed radioactive substances, whereas the penetrating x and gamma rays or neutrons are a danger from external exposure. In common, their injurious effects, judging from the peripheral blood picture only, are greatest on lymphocytes and lymphoid structures, next upon granulocyte production and least upon red cell formation. Actually, the adult circulating cells of the blood are not affected, and the lymphocyte and erythrocyte precursors are about equally radiosensitive. Yet the hundredfold greater life span of the erythrocyte compared to the lymphocyte makes it appear otherwise. Shielding of the spleen has recently appeared to promote bone marrow recovery in otherwise totally irradiated experimental animals, and experimental reduction of tissue oxygen tension diminishes the damage from the ionizing effects of irradiation.

Every precaution must obviously be taken to prevent exposure, particularly repeated chronic exposure, to penetrating rays and particles. Especially disastrous is the absorption of sources of long-lived irradiation, for example, radium, which behaves somewhat like calcium and is deposited in the bones. Studies of one such extensive exposure occurring in workers applying radium-containing luminous paint to watch dials showed transient polycythemia, then a blood picture, when fully developed, closely resembling that of pernicious anemia. The bone marrow was at first hypercellular because of increase of young forms of all marrow cell types. Later it became fibrotic and hypocellular. Finally, osteogenic sarcomas developed in several persons. The incidence of leukemia in radiologists is said to be eight to ten times that in members of other medical specialties, and only after five years had elapsed following the atomic explosion at Hiroshima was an increased evidence of leukemia in the irradiation-exposed individuals noted. Transfusions for the anemia or hemorrhagic manifestations and chemotherapy for secondary infection are the only useful forms of treatment of the hematologic effects of both acute and chronic exposure to irradiation.

MECHANICAL INTERFERENCE WITH ERYTHROPOIESIS

It is convenient, though probably in many instances inaccurate, to consider certain anemias as due to mechanical interference with erythropoiesis. However, in the premature infant the entire bone marrow as well as the liver and spleen is hematopoietically active. Because at birth, with the establishment of pulmonary respiration, the bone marrow is deprived of the erythropoietic stimulus of the relatively anoxic placental blood, it is possible that this organ is no longer sufficiently active to maintain the high hemoglobin concentration found at birth. This may account for the progressive and completely refractory normocytic, normochromic anemia of moderate degree that develops in the first weeks of life of many premature infants, only to disappear spontaneously after the third or fourth month. It is of interest that a similar less marked fall in hemoglobin occurs in the normal infant; and especially that in infants who exhibit chronic anoxia of the arterial blood after birth, because of a congenital heart lesion, the usual decline in circulating hemoglobin concentration and marrow cellularity may not occur.

The peripheral blood picture of patients whose bone marrows have been more or less extensively invaded by leukemic or cancerous cells differs characteristically from that of patients whose erythropoietic functions are depressed by nutritional deficiency or toxic inhibition. Thus, in classic instances of myelophthisic anemia there are usually signs of disturbed erythropoiesis while the anemia is yet relatively slight: irregularities of red cell size and shape, showers of nucleated red cells and of reticulocytes. Moreover, granulocytopenia and thrombocytopenia may appear together or separately and either early or late in the disease process without the more consistent relation to depressed erythropoiesis usually seen in anemias resulting from toxic suppression of marrow function.

Examination of the bone marrow of patients with the rare syndrome of marble bone disease, or that described as osteosclerotic anemia, leaves little doubt as to the pathologic importance of a diffuse replacement of normal marrow activity by fibrous or osteoid tissue. In lymphatic leukemia, when anemia is established, a rather uniform invasion by lymphocytes is commonly observed. The invasion by myeloma cells is less uniform. The purely mechanical hypothesis seemingly does not suffice, however, to explain the effect of miliary tuberculosis, Hodgkin's disease and some instances of myelogenous leukemia. Early in the development of the last condition transient polycythemia has often been observed. Later, when anemia has developed, there is rather constantly evidence of increased myeloid and also erythroid activity in the bone marrow. Suggestive in this connection is the experimental evidence that the presence of necrotic tumors entirely outside the bone marrow and also injections of extracts of leukemic urine and of various normal organs as well as of nucleic acid will produce myeloid hyperplasia of the bone marrow. The anemia of metastatic cancer may be well marked without evidence of marrow involvement, blood loss or hemolysis. These observations suggest the possibility of a chemical influence conceivably producing maturation arrest of erythropoiesis to some extent. Also to be borne in mind is the evidence for a latent hemolytic process, especially in lymphatic leukemia, lymphosarcoma or Hodgkin's disease.

Usually the clinical characteristics of the underlying disease, be it metastatic cancer, leukemia or xanthomatosis, will suggest an explanation of the accompanying anemia. Otherwise, if the characteristic findings in the peripheral blood of myelophthisic anemia are kept in mind, a diagnosis will be established by bone marrow needle or trephine biopsy. Treatment obviously depends on the nature of the primary process. Usually irradiation, nitrogen mustard, folic acid analogues or other methods of suppressing the invading cells, together with transfusion, may produce temporary improvement or at least palliative prolongation of life. Splenectomy may be useful when hemolysis is important.

IDIOPATHIC FAILURE OF ERYTHROPOIESIS

Many mildly anemic patients present this problem. It is difficult of analysis because of the lack of striking morphologic changes in either blood or bone marrow and because of the difficulty of evaluating the effectiveness of therapeutic measures. Combinations of malnutrition and low grade infection are perhaps most commonly at fault. These patients should not be confused with the adult young to middle-aged female patient who complains of chronic fatigue and experiences vaguely defined symptoms referable to a variety of body symptoms and who exhibits a low normal hemoglobin level sometimes accompanied by a low blood pressure. Whether these individuals, like patients with neurocirculatory asthenia, have an organic or a functional basis for their complaints is unclear. What is certain, however, is that their hemoglobin level is itself not the cause of their symptoms nor is it improved nor are the patient's symptoms alleviated by the indiscriminate use of vitamins, liver extract or iron, individually or in combination.

The fulminating and fatal idiopathic aplastic anemia affecting especially young adults and manifested by fever, stomal ulcerations and bleeding from the mucous membranes as described by Ehrlich is not now commonly encountered. Possibly this is because such patients are now diagnosed as acute leukemia as indeed the clinical picture would suggest. However, acute transient suppression of erythropoiesis by viral infections is readily detectable in chronic hemolytic anemias with short red cell survival.

Seemingly idiopathic chronic aplastic anemia, frequently but not always accompanied by hypoplasia of the bone marrow, is probably sometimes the unrecognized result of exposure to cyclic organic compounds in industry, home, or even the hospital. In other patients, however, a history of such exposure cannot be elicited and the slowly progressive clinical course resembles that of patients with a history of such toxic exposure as described on page 1192. Study of the peripheral blood of these patients likewise discloses a normocytic or slightly macrocytic normochromic anemia with leukopenia and thrombocytopenia. The bone marrow picture varies from hypoplasia to hyperplasia with cellular immaturity. Sometimes reticulocytes are increased for some days and may be accompanied by normoblasts in the peripheral blood. Cases

have been reported by Fanconi in which pigmentation, gonadal hypoplasia and other developmental anomalies appear in siblings during childhood. The so-called "pure red cell anemia" of children does not exhibit decreased levels of circulating leukocytes or platelets and may disappear spontaneously at puberty. Association with thymic or other mediastinal tumors has been reported.

Ordinarily the mainstay of treatment in chronic aplastic or refractory anemia is a systematic transfusion schedule ideally employing only packed red cells from fresh bank blood. A few such patients have recently been reported to respond to cortisone and in one infant the cellular marrow so induced thereafter responded to vitamin B_{12}. In severely anemic patients splenectomy may be justified on the theoretical grounds of removing either an inhibitory influence on the marrow or an effective filter for circulating blood elements. Preliminary benefit from cortisone appears to intimate that splenectomy is likely to be useful, but this is the exception rather than the rule in this group of patients. Repeated transfusions carry the risk of producing hemosiderosis.

W. B. CASTLE

References

Pathologic Physiology

Blumgart, H. L., and Altschule, M. D.: Clinical Significance of Cardiac and Respiratory Adjustments in Chronic Anemia. Blood, 3:329, 1948.

Castle, W. B., Ham, T. H., and Shen, S. C.: Observations on the Mechanism of Hemolytic Transfusion Reactions Occurring without Demonstrable Hemolysin. Tr. A. Am. Phys., 63:161, 1950.

Crosby, W. H.: The Limit of Hemoglobin Synthesis in Hereditary Hemolytic Anemia: Its Relation to the Excretion of Bile Pigment. Am. J. Med., 13: 273, 1952.

Dacie, J. V. and White, J. C.: Erythropoiesis with Particular Reference to Its Study by Biopsy of Human Bone Marrow: A review. J. Clin. Pathol., 2:1, 1949.

Finch, C. A., and others: Iron Metabolism: The Pathophysiology of Iron Storage. Blood, 5:983, 1950.

Grant, W. C., and Root, W. S.: Fundamental Stimulus for Erythropoiesis. Physiol. Rev., 32:449, 1952.

Rimington, C.: Haems and Porphyrins in Health and Disease. I. Acta med. Scandinav., 143:161, 1952.

Watson, C. J.: Some Newer Concepts of the Natural Derivatives of Hemoglobin. Blood, 1:99, 1946.

Increased Erythrocyte Loss or Destruction

Bauer, J.: Sickle Cell Disease: Pathogenic, Clinical and Therapeutic Considerations. Arch. Surg., 41: 1344, 1940.

Becker, R. M.: Paroxysmal Cold Hemoglobinurias. Arch. Int. Med., 81:630, 1949.

Cappell, D. F.: The Blood Group Rh. Brit. M. J., 2: 601, 1946.

Chini, V., and Valeri, C. M.: Mediterranean Hemopathic Syndromes. Blood, 4:989, 1949.

Crosby, W. H.: Paroxysmal Nocturnal Hemoglobinuria: Relation of the Clinical Manifestations to Underlying Pathogenic Mechanisms. Blood, 8: 769, 1953.

Dacie, J. V., and de Gruchy, G. C.: Auto-antibodies in Acquired Anemia. J. Clin. Pathol., 4:253, 1951.

Dameshek, W., and Schwartz, S. O.: Acute Hemolytic Anemia. Medicine, 19:231, 1940.

Kaplan, E., Zuelzer, W. W., and Neel, J. V.: Further Studies on Hemoglobin C. II. The Hematologic Effects of Hemoglobin C Alone and in Combination with Sickle Cell Hemoglobin. Blood, 8: 735, 1953.

Mackell, J. V., Rieders, F., Brieger, H., and Bauer, E. L.: Acute Hemolytic Anemia Due to Ingestion of Naphthalene Moth Balls. Pediatrics, 7:722, 1951.

Singer, K.: Problems of Erythrocyte Disintegration with Particular Reference to the Life Span of the Red Cell. J. Lab. & Clin. Med., 30:784, 1945.

Wagley, P. F., Shen, S. C., Gardner, F. H., and Castle, W. B.: Studies on the Destruction of Red Blood Cells, VI. The Spleen as a Source of a Substance Causing Agglutination of the Red Blood Cells of Certain Patients with Acquired Hemolytic Jaundice by an Antihuman Serum Rabbit Serum (Coombs' Serum). J. Lab. & Clin. Med., 33:1197, 1948.

Whipple, A. O.: The Problem of Portal Hypertension in Relation to the Hepatosplenopathies. Ann. Surg., 122:449, 1945.

Young, L. E., Christian, R. M., and Izzo, M. J.: Some Newer Concepts of "Congenital" and "Acquired" Hemolytic Anemias. M. Clin. North America, 35:571, 1951.

Decreased Erythrocyte Production

Bomford, R. R.: Anaemia in Myxoedema. Quart. J. Med., 7:495, 1938.

———, and Rhoads, C. P.: Refractory Anaemia. Quart. J. Med., 10:175, 1941.

Callen, I. R., and Limarzi, L. R.: Blood and Bone Marrow Studies in Renal Disease. Am. J. Clin. Path., 20:3, 1950.

Cartwright, G. E., and others: The Anemia of Infection. J. Clin. Investigation, 25:65, 1946.

Castle, W. B.: Present Status of the Etiology of Pernicious Anemia. Ann. Int. Med., 34:1093, 1951.

Collins, D. H., and Rose, W. M.: The Nature of Anaemia in Leukaemia. J. Path. & Bact., 60:63, 1948.

Gairdner, D., Marks, J., and Roscoe, J. D.: Blood Formation in Infancy, Part II, Normal Erythropoiesis. Arch. Dis. Childhood, 27:214, 1952.

Girdwood, R. H.: Vitamin B_{12} and Related Factors: A Clinical and Experimental Review. Edinburgh M. J., 57:72, 1950.

Heath, C. W., and Patek, A. J., Jr.: The Anemia of Iron Deficiency. Medicine, 16:267, 1937.

Shen, S. C., and Homburger, F.: The Anemia of Cancer Patients and Its Relation to Metastases to the Bone Marrow. J. Lab. & Clin. Med., 37:182, 1951.

Singer, K., Motulsky, A. G., and Wile, S. A.: Aplastic Crisis in Sickle Cell Anemia: Study of Its Mechanism and Its Relation to Other Types of Hemolytic Crises. J. Lab. & Clin. Med., 35:721, 1950.

Thompson, R. B., and Ungley, C. C.: Megaloblastic Anaemia of Pregnancy and the Puerperium. Quart. J. Med., 20:187, 1951.

Wyatt, J. P., and Sommers, S. P.: Chronic Marrow Failure, Myelosclerosis, and Extramedullary Hematopoiesis. Blood, 5:329, 1950.

HEMORRHAGIC DISEASES

Definition. In these conditions in association with (1) vascular weakness, (2) defective numbers or function of blood platelets or (3) faulty coagulation of the blood, bleeding occurs either spontaneously or as a result of trauma ordinarily innocuous.

Pathologic Physiology. In the normal person when a small vessel is ruptured, the flow of blood is first diminished by local contraction of its smooth muscle. Blood platelets then become adherent to the edges of the vascular wound and either partially or completely close the orifice. Vasotonic substances are also released locally from the platelets. The retarded flow of blood allows substances derived from the damaged tissues to initiate processes leading to local conversion of the soluble fibrinogen of the blood to fibrin strands. The contraction of the fibrin strands at points of contact with platelets draws together the edges of the vascular wound, and a firm clot forms both within and without the vessel wall.

Figure 150 presents in schematic form modern modifications of the two-stage hypothesis of blood coagulation originally proposed by Morawitz. The production of thrombin from prothrombin, its first stage, is now regarded as involving at least two distinct autocatalytic reactions. The first of these, a "slow" phase, begins with the disintegration of platelets at the site of vascular injury. Then follows the formation of traces of plasma thromboplastin, and thereafter minute amounts of thrombin appear. Once thrombin is produced more platelets are rapidly "labilized" by it, and with quickened tempo and greater volume the cycle through thromboplastin repeats itself. Moreover, a second autocatalytic reaction is begun by thrombin and this "accelerated" phase also hastens the conversion of prothrombin to thrombin. Here labile plasma accelerators become even more active as serum accelerators of the prothrombin conversion process. These last as well as other stable serum accelerators interact with calcium and thromboplastin in what may be a stoichiometric conversion of prothrombin to thrombin. The final stage in which thrombin acting as an enzyme catalyzes the conversion of fibrinogen to fibrin remains essentially unchanged. This is the barest outline (see Fig. 150) of a vastly complicated and presently controversial subject concerning which the reader may well con-

formation of the clot that normally quickly supplements the primary mechanical action of the platelets in checking the flow of blood. These maladies include deficiency of prothrombin and its accelerators, hemophilia with its deficient plasma thromboplastinogen, fibrinogen deficiency and bleeding due to the presence of heparin or, rarely, spontaneously appearing anticoagulants. It is also perhaps necessary to take into account variations in the concentration of thromboplastin in the tissues, for example, in the hemophiliac.

Symptoms and Signs. Careful inquiry as to the extent of bleeding from cuts and abra-

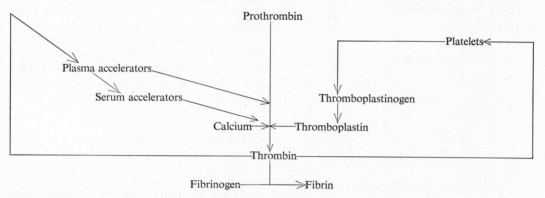

Fig. 150. Blood coagulation, the result of autocatalytic reactions. (Modified from Dr. W. H. Harrington.)

sult the articles included in the references cited.

The various types of hemorrhagic disorders are classified in the accompanying table. In vascular purpura the platelets appear to be normal in number and function, as is the coagulation of the blood. Hence, by exclusion, the ecchymoses and petechial hemorrhages, like those readily induced by raising the capillary pressure by means of a venous tourniquet, appear to be due to inherent vascular weakness. Purpura due to a diminished number of platelets may well result from defective mechanical function of the platelets in maintaining the competency of the vascular wall. Characteristic of this defect is the fact that bleeding continues from even a needle wound for an abnormally long time. To ordinary clinical tests the clotting time of the blood is often normal, but later the fibrin strands fail to contract to create a firm clot. Quick's test demonstrates that the conversion of prothrombin to thrombin is delayed. Finally there is the group of conditions in which typical large extravasation of blood or continuing hemorrhage is due to delay in the

sions, with menstruation and from minor or major dental or surgical procedures should be made. The bleeding may be insignificant or extensive enough to produce shock or later cause hypochromic anemia. When hemorrhage occurs in such areas as the larynx, pericardium or central nervous system, the local effects upon vital functions are serious. The small petechial hemorrhages in the skin, characteristic of thrombocytopenic purpura, cannot be obliterated by pressure (glass rod). They are often prominent in areas of greatest capillary pressure such as around the lower legs or forearms. When otherwise distributed, an embolic, vascular or allergic origin is suggested. The exposed position of the small blood vessels of the nasal septum and gingival margins is probably the reason that these areas are frequent sites of "spontaneous" bleeding in the purpuras. Slow oozing continues despite the presence of formed clots. The motility of the gastrointestinal and genitourinary tracts and the superficial location of the vasculature may account for the frequency of bleeding from these viscera. Coagulation defects, such as occur in prothrombin deficiency and in hemophilia, are likely to be associated with large extravasations of blood, and not with purpura. In further contrast to the purpuras, the bleeding is more clearly related to trauma. The peculiar tendency of

Functional Classification of Hemorrhagic Disorders

I. VASCULAR PURPURA
  A. Congenital
    1. Hereditary telangiectasia
    2. Pseudohemophilia (Willebrand)
    3. Thrombasthenia (Glanzmann)
  B. Defective vasoconstriction
    1. Hemorrhagic thrombocythemia
  C. Defective tissue support
    1. Senile purpura
  D. Infections
    1. Toxic
    2. Embolic
  E. Nutritional deficiency
    1. Scurvy
  F. Allergy

II. THROMBOCYTOPENIC PURPURA
  A. Secondary
    1. Menstruation, local infections, drug allergy
    2. Bone marrow disease: aplastic anemia, carcinomatosis, leukemia
  B. Primary
    1. Purpura hemorrhagica

III. COAGULATION DEFECTS
  A. Prothrombin deficiency
    1. Congenital: hypoprothrombinemia, hemophilia neonatorum
    2. Acquired: biliary obstruction, fatty diarrhea, liver disease, dicoumarins
  B. Prothrombin accelerator deficiencies
  C. Plasma thromboplastinogen deficiencies
    1. Hemophilia
  D. Fibrinogen deficiency
    1. Congenital
    2. Acquired: liver disease, fetal death
  E. Fibrinolysis
    1. Shock, placental separation
    2. Metastatic prostatic cancer
  F. Anticoagulants

hemorrhage to involve the joints in hemophilia may be due to lack of tissue thromboplastin. Hemorrhage into the central nervous system sometimes occurs in thrombocytopenic purpura, rarely in hemophilia. Unexplained are the long intervals between spontaneous bleedings in hemophilia or in congenital afibrinogenemia in which the blood is completely incoagulable.

Laboratory Studies. The multiple causes of the hemorrhagic disorders require that critical laboratory studies be carried out in order to identify the condition. In detecting and distinguishing vascular and thrombocytopenic purpura the tourniquet test, bleeding time, blood platelet count and inspection for clot retraction are well established procedures. The classic coagulation time of the blood in glass remains a standard procedure in detecting clotting defects. Long delay suggests hemophilia; resolution of the formed clot, fibrinolysis; and complete absence of clot, afibrinogenemia. Modern studies include determinations of the prothrombin concentration either by the one-stage or the more definitive two-stage method, and a test for prothrombin consumption. Careful use of these bedside and laboratory methods will permit recognition of the majority of the hemorrhagic disorders. For identification of the rare disturbances, including the detection of deficiencies of prothrombin accelerators or the presence of circulating anticoagulants, special methods are required, for the description of which space here is not available.

VASCULAR PURPURA

The various conditions listed as causing vascular purpura are shown in the table. *Hereditary telangiectasia* is a purely local vascular abnormality transmitted as a simple dominant by both sexes. The lesions may appear in childhood, but increase in number in adult life, characteristically appearing as 1- to 4-mm.-sized bright red or purplish, slightly elevated papules on the face, lips, tongue and tips of fingers. Pressure as with a glass slide causes them to disappear. Occasionally the lesions may be larger or may be associated with internal vascular nevi, rarely tumors of embryologically corresponding portions of the gastrointestinal, respiratory, genitourinary or central nervous systems. Unless hemorrhage develops, the condition is asymptomatic. However, because of the exposed nature of the lesions, which often have thin vascular walls, repeated bleeding may occur and produce all the characteristics of chronic hypochromic anemia, clinical and hematologic. Individual lesions can be obliterated by use of the thermocautery when accessible. Because premenstrual bleeding may occur from such lesions, it is interesting that estrogens have been reported to lessen bleeding in postmenstrual women and in elderly males, perhaps because of an effect on atrophied mucous membranes supporting the vascular anomalies.

Pseudohemophilia or constitutional thrombopathy is a hereditary hemorrhagic disorder that is more severe in females than in males and appears usually in childhood or youth. A prolonged bleeding time, except for an occasional positive tourniquet test, is the only hematologic abnormality and may be the result of defective contractility of the capillaries. Purpura is uncommon. The symptoms as described by von Willebrand are chiefly prolonged bleeding from wounds, ecchymoses and epistaxis. Menorrhagia and parturient bleeding are common. Fatal gastrointestinal or uterine bleeding occurs.

Thrombasthenia, as described by Glanzmann, differs clinically only in that purpura is more common. This rare hereditary syndrome is characterized by little or no prolongation of the bleeding time, but clot retraction is defective despite normal numbers of platelets. However, the platelets are of abnormal appearance: unusual variation in size, vacuolization and paucity of granules. Disturbances of either clot retraction or prothrombin consumption or both in patients with normal platelet levels have been described. No treatment is especially effective, but transfusion is indicated to replace blood lost by severe hemorrhage and to provide more effective platelets. In the early stages of polycythemia vera or of chronic myelogenous leukemia, platelet levels of a million or more may be associated with contrasting tendencies to thrombosis or to bleeding following small cuts or trauma. In explanation of the hemorrhages, the only relevant abnormality may be lack of the vasotonic principle (probably 5-hydroxy-tryptamine) normally evolved by disintegrating platelets.

Di Guglielmo first described an acquired hemorrhagic diathesis affecting middle-aged and older adults, associated with a markedly elevated platelet level, as piastrinemia or, translated, *thrombocythemia.*

The hemorrhagic lesions in *senile purpura* appear to result from trauma to inelastic skin or capillaries, and probably for this reason are especially common about the wrists and knees. The dark purple, slightly elevated, sharply circumscribed, irregular, round or oval lesions are characteristic. Petechiae are rare. Hemorrhage is never important.

The extensive purpura that is observed at the onset of certain *infectious diseases* such as meningococcal meningitis, measles or pneumonia, when not, as is frequently the case, associated with thrombocytopenia, is due to toxic injury to the vascular endothelium. In scarlet fever the erythrotoxin causes widespread capillary injury. In *septicemia* the scattered purpura is presumably due to local bacterial emboli as in typhoid fever, subacute bacterial endocarditis and meningococcal septicemia, for it is sometimes possible to demonstrate organisms in skin lesions. The fulminating purpura with vascular collapse and associated adrenal hemorrhage, known as the *Waterhouse-Friderichsen syndrome,* is usually due to meningococcal septicemia.

Deficiency of ascorbic acid results in disturbance of the laying down of intercellular collagen. This presumably explains the characteristic perifollicular hemorrhages in the dependent portions of the body in *scurvy.* Subperiosteal extravasations appear only in scorbutic children because the ununited epiphyseal junctions provide a point of origin for hemorrhage. In adults, usually elderly men, the most characteristic extravasation begins in the posterior aspect of the thigh and may involve the entire extremity. Some bleeding may occur also from the fungating gums, which appear only in apposition to teeth. Ascorbic acid is corrective of the bleeding tendency within 24 hours. The petechiae brought out by the positive tourniquet test appear chiefly in hair follicles and hence on the extensor side of the forearm. This, the only laboratory measure of the hemorrhagic diathesis, also disappears promptly.

Allergic purpura often develops a few days after an acute or recurrent infection or a few hours after the ingestion of food or drugs to which the patient has become sensitized. The platelets are not reduced significantly and blood loss is never great. The lesions, which involve skin, mucous membranes or viscera, result from the effusion of variable proportions of plasma and white and red cells. Associated with the purpura may be erythema multiforme, bullous lesions, urticaria, edema or even local tissue necrosis. Schoenlein described patients in whom joint manifestations were prominent; and Henoch recognized associated abdominal symptoms due to purpuric or edematous lesions of the bowel. In some patients the urine may contain red cells and albumin as in acute glomerular nephritis. Avoidance of unnecessary abdominal surgery is important. Relief from pain often promptly follows the injection of epinephrine. Antihistaminics or salicylates may also be useful, and cortisone should be tried if these are not successful against peripheral and joint manifestations.

THROMBOCYTOPENIC PURPURA

This condition occurs either as a secondary result of a primary process or as an idiopathic entity. A careful search for causative factors should always be made. Mild purpura, usually associated with "easy bruising" coincidental to a fall of platelets in the first day or two of the *menstrual cycle,* is a common phenomenon. With or without change in vascular permeability, a striking fall of platelets occurs at the onset of a variety of *infections,* including pneumonia, meningococcemia and some of the exanthemata. Thrombocytopenia also occurs in the period of convalescence from measles. Spontaneous recovery, as when purpura accompanies lymphocytosis, usually follows after a few days. In rare instances of meningococcemia the extravasation and injury to tissue may be extensive. Decreased numbers of platelets and recurrent purpura are frequent in *disseminated lupus.* A rare form of thrombocytopenia occurs, chiefly in women, accompanied by *multiple platelet thrombi* in capillaries. Suggestive relationships to the so-called collagen diseases have been noted. Bleeding is extensive and fever, hemolytic anemia, icterus, stupor, delirium and various neurologic signs herald a fatal outcome, usually within a few days or a week. Autopsy discloses widespread eosinophilic thrombi in arterioles, capillaries and venules of many organs which may in part represent accumulations of blood platelets.

Significant thrombocytopenia due to *allergy* to foods is rare. However, thrombocytopenia due to *drug sensitivity* is a well established clinical occurrence with the organic arsenobenzenes, occasionally the sulfonamides, quinine, quinidine and phenobarbital, but especially the drug Sedormid. Readministration of the last can cause a prompt fall of platelets in sensitized patients with reappearance of clinical purpura. Sedormid when applied to the skin may produce petechial hemorrhages at the site. *In vitro* Sedormid or quinidine produces specific agglutination of the patient's platelets or of normal platelets when suspended in the patient's, but not in normal plasma. If complement is present, lysis of platelets follows, presumably because the patient's plasma contains a specific antibody against a drug-platelet antigen. In pernicious and related macrocytic anemias *nutritional thrombocytopenia* and granulocytopenia are characteristic, but only in rare instances is purpura a prominent manifestation. A few retinal hemorrhages are common in any severe anemia. For these conditions treatment is directed against the underlying disease, involves discontinuance of the sensitizing drug, or is symptomatic, including the use of ACTH, cortisone and transfusions.

Toxic injury to the bone marrow may cause disturbance in platelet formation alone, more commonly associated with disturbances of red and white cell production. Injurious substances are benzol, gold salts and stilbestrol. External *irradiation,* when generalized and severe or when prolonged because of radium absorbed in the bone marrow, may produce thrombocytopenia in association with other hematologic disturbances. When the bone marrow becomes hypoplastic or even hyperplastic in the *"refractory macrocytic anemias"* or when it is extensively invaded by foreign cells such as those of *cancer* or *leukemia,* purpura is also due to the lowered platelet count. This often accompanies the onset of the acute or announces the final stages of the chronic leukemias. Thrombocytopenia is a late manifestation of miliary tuberculosis or of extensive fibrosis or osteosclerosis of the bone marrow. Significant bleeding is likely to occur when the platelets number less than 50,000 per cubic millimeter.

Idiopathic thrombocytopenic purpura is a primary condition of unknown etiology and variable severity. The plasma of some patients contains a globulin that, upon intravenous injection, promptly reduces the circulating platelet level of recipients of the same blood group. Rarely the patient's plasma agglutinates normal platelets *in vitro.* The chief clinical manifestations are petechial hemorrhages and traumatic ecchymoses in the skin and muscles, together with bleeding from the mucous membranes of the nose, mouth, gastrointestinal and genitourinary tracts. Hemorrhage into the central nervous system is to be feared, especially in adults over 40. The disease commonly begins in childhood, sometimes with severity at the time of the first menstruation. Measles or other infections occasionally appear to precipitate the onset. Frequently it is a mild chronic process with irregular exacerbations. Thrombocytopenic purpura is distinctly more common in female than in male children, and is almost wholly confined to women when the first symptoms appear in adults. In an adult male it is usually secondary to manifest or latent bone marrow disease. It may be the first sign of unsuspected disseminated lupus. Thrombocytopenic purpura may develop as a complication of pregnancy, and the newborn infant may exhibit thrombocytopenia with or without purpuric manifestations for a period of a few days or weeks.

Except for the signs of hemorrhage, the physical examination is usually normal. Rarely the spleen is slightly enlarged. Morphologic examination of the blood is normal except for the diminished number of platelets, which sometimes vary markedly in size, and except for the anemia secondary to blood loss. Occasionally eosinophilia of 5 to 10 per cent is found. Lymphocytosis suggests an association with infectious mononucleosis or related conditions. Bleeding may occur when the platelets in the peripheral blood are as numerous as 100,000, and is usually profuse if the platelets are less than 50,000 per cubic millimeter. However, such correlations are open to frequent exceptions such as little bleeding with less than 10,000 platelets. The bone marrow exhibits normal or perhaps somewhat increased numbers of megakaryocytes, which frequently do not appear to be forming platelets in normal numbers. With a history of chronic recurrent purpura, spontaneous cure is unlikely, but in a first attack some authorities believe that spontaneous recovery may occur at any time up to three or four months.

Splenectomy in normal persons, in instances of thrombocytopenia associated with splenomegaly, and in thrombocytopenic purpura, usually causes after a few days increases in the circulating platelets. Whether this is the result of the removal of an organ destroying excessive number of platelets or because of ablation of a humoral influence of the spleen upon the bone marrow remains unsettled. However, splenectomy is successful in producing clinical improvement in over two thirds of the patients. This is not necessarily accompanied by maintained normal platelet values. In general, the more acute the bleeding process, the less likely is splenectomy to be effective, despite its greater urgency in such patients. Splenectomy produces within the hour a decrease in the bleeding time, within a few hours an increase in capillary resistance, and only after a few days the maximal increase in platelet count. Qualitatively similar effects follow splenectomy in patients with thrombocytopenia secondary to other conditions. Final evaluation of its effectiveness may be impossible

until many weeks have elapsed. Recently ACTH or cortisone has been shown to be effective in controlling bleeding within a day or two, and with or without a subsequent rise of platelet level. Rarely this will be permanent. Cortisone therapy is probably a desirable preliminary to splenectomy and may be helpful subsequently if the platelet level again declines.

COAGULATION DEFECTS

The clinical manifestations of defective blood coagulation result from deficiencies of certain of the elements involved in the coagulation of normal blood (as shown in Fig. 150): prothrombin, plasma and platelet factors required for the rapid conversion of prothrombin to thrombin, and fibrinogen. Calcium deficiency is never responsible. In addition, fibrinolytic enzymes may appear in the blood stream. Finally, heparin, antibodies developed against the antihemophilic globulin, or, in rare instances, spontaneously developing anticoagulants of uncertain nature may cause defective clotting. The resulting clinical conditions are classified in the table on page 1198.

In general, bleeding follows definite trauma and is often extensive in tissues or prolonged externally. Capillary fragility, bleeding time, platelet number and retraction of the clot after it is eventually formed are normal unless fibrinolysis is active. Although the clotting time of the blood in hemophilia is grossly prolonged, or is infinite in the absence of fibrinogen, this test is not necessarily a satisfactory measure of other types of inefficiency of the clotting mechanism. This is because it detects the initiation of coagulation on the surface of the blood in the test tube rather than the rapid completion of the process that is required for effective hemostasis in the body. For this reason the one-stage prothrombin concentration test of Quick, which measures the sum of prothrombin and antiprothrombin factors, or the more precise two-stage method of Seegers is necessary to bring out quantitative deficiency in prothrombin. Quick's so-called prothrombin consumption test is invaluable in picking up the failure of the plasma prothrombin accelerators to effect quantitative conversion of prothrombin to thrombin. Unfortunately, the necessary experience with and precision in the performance of these tests are still beyond the capacity of many hospital laboratories.

PROTHROMBIN DEFICIENCY

Prothrombin is a glycoprotein formed in the normal liver when vitamin K is present. Significant bleeding does not occur unless the concentration of prothrombin by the one-stage method is less than 15 per cent of normal. Prothrombin deficiency as a congenital defect occurs in two forms: one, the so-called hemophilia neonatorum present only during the first few days of life, the other a rare, permanent, hereditary anomaly of the plasma proteins. Attention is drawn to the latter by various forms of spontaneous or operatively induced bleeding, often massive. Most of the patients are children or young adults. Reinvestigation of the precise nature of the coagulation defect would probably indicate deficiency of prothrombin accelerators rather than of prothrombin itself in some. In one patient only has vitamin K appeared to increase the prothrombin level of the blood.

Hemophilia neonatorum, or hemorrhagic disease of the newborn, not to be confused with various forms of hemorrhage due to birth trauma, appears to be an exaggeration of the processes normally producing low prothrombin levels in the blood of the newborn infant. Before the introduction of prophylaxis with vitamin K, the condition occurred in approximately one out of every 100 to 400 infants. Until an intestinal flora capable of synthesizing vitamin K becomes established, the prothrombin of the normal infant consists of the endowment originally derived from the maternal circulation. Probably for this reason, when conditioned by an inadequate prenatal storage of vitamin K or imperfect hepatic function, hemorrhagic disease of the newborn makes its appearance almost always before the fourth and never after the seventh day of life. Spontaneous bleeding is characteristic, usually not of large amounts, most commonly from the gastrointestinal tract, but also into the skin, mucous membranes and stump of the umbilical cord. Internal bleeding may occur with signs of circulatory collapse, but without the usual peripheral evidences of hemorrhage. Hemorrhage into the central nervous system produces drowsiness and convulsions. Petechiae are rare. The disease can be completely prevented by the oral or parenteral administration of synthetic vitamin K to the mother for a few days prior to delivery or by parenteral administration to the infant at birth. Bleeding can be controlled within a few hours by parenteral use of vitamin K or even more rapidly by transfusions of fresh whole blood which contains prothrombin. The blood should be Rh negative in order to obviate sensitization.

Acquired hypoprothrombinemia results either from defective assimilation of vitamin K or from defective formation of prothrombin in the liver. The tendency to surgical hemorrhage formerly encountered in patients with extrahepatic *biliary obstruction* or with biliary fistula was due to the failure of the bile salts to assist in the absorption of the fat-soluble vitamin K. Also due to *inadequate absorption* of vitamin K is the tendency to hemorrhage associated with hypoprothrombinemia observed in certain patients with sprue or idiopathic ulcerative colitis. A more common cause of hypoprothrombinemia in the adult is defective formation of prothrombin as a result of *liver disease,* for example, acute or chronic hepatitis or cirrhosis. Prothrombin deficiency due to exclusion of vitamin K responds readily to parenteral administration of the synthetic preparation. When hepatic cell dysfunction is responsible, this does not occur. *Dicumarol* administration interferes with the synthesis of prothrombin in the liver, perhaps because of the competition permitted by its structural resemblance to substances having vitamin K-like activity. Vitamin K_1 emulsion intravenously has been shown to be more effective in counteracting the effects of Dicumarol than the usual synthetic preparations. This also applies to the currently popular dicoumarin analogue Tromexan and to phenylindanedione. The administration of fresh plasma or whole blood will passively supply prothrombin.

PROTHROMBIN ACCELERATOR DEFICIENCIES

Deficiency of prothrombin accelerators was not distinguished from lack of prothrombin until Owren, in the study of a hemorrhagic condition in a young woman, defined it as a failure of a normal prothrombin concentration to be converted to thrombin. Normal plasma in small amounts supplied Owren's Factor V, which is probably identical with Quick's labile factor and Seeger's plasma (accelerator) Ac-globulin. Alexander has described a patient in whom the addition of normal plasma was not effective in promoting prothrombin conversion. However, serum was so effective, presumably because it supplied Owren's Factor VI or Alexander's SPCA, which is a component of Seeger's serum Ac-globulin. The rare persons affected exhibit the clinical manifestations of the hereditary deficiencies of prothrombin itself.

PLASMA THROMBOPLASTINOGEN DEFICIENCIES

Hemophilia is the classic example of prolonged blood coagulation. According to Quick, plasma thromboplastinogen is lacking for conversion to plasma thromboplastin by normally acting platelets. Plasma thromboplastinogen is presumably different from the plasma prothrombin accelerators just discussed, and is present in a globulin fraction of normal plasma free of platelets, prothrombin and fibrinogen. The blood is morphologically normal except for the secondary effects of hemorrhage. Bleeding time, capillary fragility, clot retraction and prothrombin concentration are normal. The coagulation time, which is more or less constant for a given individual, is usually greatly prolonged, but may in a few adults be almost normal. Prothrombin conversion to thrombin is much delayed. Modern laboratory studies indicate that clinically indistinguishable hemophilias comprise individuals with at least two distinct types of coagulation abnormality: the classic thromboplastinogen deficiency (hemophilia A) and plasma thromboplastin component deficiency (hemophilia B, Christmas disease). Each type of plasma corrects the clotting abnormality of the other. Normal plasma corrects both, as well as a coexisting deficiency of A and B responsible for a third laboratory variety of hemophilia.

Hemophilia is inherited as a sex-linked recessive character transmitted directly by unaffected females to male offspring. Though hemophilia in a female is genetically possible from the mating of a hemophilic male and a female carrier of the trait, very few such instances have been established. Most female bleeders reported in the earlier literature are probably examples of hypoprothrombinemia or of persons with spontaneous anticoagulants in the blood. Recently a nonhereditary hemophilia-like disease has been reported in two women in whom the greatly prolonged coagulation time in the blood was reduced by the addition of normal but not of hemophilic plasma.

Hemophilia is usually recognized in infancy or childhood either because of spontaneous bleeding or bleeding from slight trauma or minor surgery. In rare instances the condition is so mild that disability is slight, especially in adults; and this may be characteristic of entire family trees. Usually, however, persistent slow bleeding for days from trivial injuries greatly limits the activities of the person. Subcutaneous and intramuscular hemorrhages are frequent and often extensive. Purpura is rare. When the hemorrhage affects an area in which local swelling may interfere with vascular or respiratory functions, as in the extremities or the neck, it may result in gangrene or be immediately hazardous to life. Bleeding from the mucous membranes of the mouth is common and, like that from other insignificant wounds, difficult to control. Repeated hemorrhage into joints with the eventual production of a form of arthritis, deformity and limitation of motion is especially characteristic. Symptomless bleeding from the gastrointestinal tract is infrequent compared to that from the genitourinary tract. Bleeding into the colonic wall, mesentery or retroperitoneal tissues is not uncommon and can give rise to low abdominal pains and other symptoms that strongly suggest conditions requiring immediate surgical intervention. Fortunately, hemorrhage into the central nervous system is rare.

Treatment begins with the avoidance of injury and requires psychologic adjustment to the restrictions of the disease. The extent of hemorrhage into tissues can sometimes be limited by cold compresses. Conservative orthopedic and physiotherapeutic measures are best for the acute and chronic stages of hemarthroses. Pain requires relief by sedatives, including aspirin, codeine and Demerol. The control of external bleeding is best achieved by gentle cleansing and approximation of the edges of the wound without sutures. Then thrombin prepared from animal or human blood is applied directly to the site of bleeding on appropriate pressure dressings, which must sometimes be kept in place for days. Transfusions of 100 to 250 cc. of fresh citrated blood or preserved plasma at once reduce the coagulation time of the patient's blood nearly to normal. This effect persists from 6 to 12 hours. The intravenous injection of Cohn plasma Fraction I is effective only in hemophilia A. Moreover, this use of antihemophilic globulin has the distinct limitation that antibodies sometimes develop and render the patient refractory to subsequent administrations. The removal of a tooth requires both general and local hemostatic measures. Major surgery causes a 35 per cent mortality, but is probably less often required in this era of antibacterial chemotherapy.

FIBRINOGEN DEFICIENCY

Fibrinogen deficiency occurs as a rare complete or nearly complete congenital absence of plasma fibrinogen. The clinical manifestations resemble those of congenital hypoprothrombinemia. It is remarkable that, despite lack of fibrinogen, long periods may elapse without symptoms. Less severe reductions of fibrinogen occur on occasion in vitamin B deficiencies, myelogenous leukemia, polycythemia and liver disease. Hypoprothrombinemia is, however, more important than is fibrinogen deficiency in causing hemorrhage in patients with liver disease. In certain abnormalities of pregnancy, especially premature placental separation, the thromboplastin-rich placental and decidual tissues may be a source of circulating thromboplastin. This may cause progressive "defibrination" of the blood with deposition of the precipitated fibrin in various organs, especially the lungs. The resulting shock in turn may cause or be associated with fibrinolysis. In afibrinogenemia the blood completely fails to clot even with thrombin. Transfusions of whole blood are useful, but the intravenous injection of Cohn plasma Fraction I containing fibrinogen may be required for prompt control of bleeding.

FIBRINOLYSIS

Fibrinolysis due to enzymatic dissolution of fibrin strands may normally play an obscure but useful part in the metabolism of fibrin and the process of repair. When operative to an exaggerated degree, it may be a cause of serious hemorrhage from tissues already traumatized in surgery, especially of the lungs, and in obstetrics. Mild degrees of fibrinolysis in the plasma probably accompany the "alarm reaction" and are excited by the injection of epinephrine. Severe hemorrhage and shock, perhaps because of resulting anoxia and tissue autolysis, appear to release into the capillaries large amounts of the activator of the fibrinolytic enzyme precursor in the plasma, which may attack fibrinogen, prothrombin and its conversion accelerators. Fibrinolysis, due apparently to escape of such an enzyme from prostatic tissue, may occur in 10 per cent of patients with metastatic prostatic cancer. Cortisone and estrogens may diminish the prostatic fibrinolysin level in the blood. Premature separation of the placenta apparently provides natural perfusion of a mass of autolyzing tissue, and is the most common cause of this rare but potentially disastrous form of obstetrical hemorrhage. Treatment of this type of bleeding, always an acute emergency, is identical with that of fibrinogen deficiency: anti-shock therapy and enough fibrinogen to cause firm clotting at the site of bleeding.

ANTICOAGULANTS

The anticoagulant action of *heparin* derives from its mucoitin polysulfuric acid structure. It is useful therapeutically either when added to whole blood or when given intravenously because of its antithrombic action. This property is exhibited in plasma, but not in purified mixtures of thrombin and fibrinogen. Heparin is promptly neutralized by the strongly basic protamine salmine. *Dicumarol,* like its congeners and indanedione derivatives, also used for the prevention of intravascular thrombosis, is an anticoagulant only indirectly by inhibiting prothrombin formation in the liver.

In hemophilia the repeated injection of whole blood, plasma or probably especially plasma fractions containing antihemophilic globulin, appears to produce antibodies in the plasma of some patients. Thereupon, when antihemophilic globulin is therapeutically administered, these antibodies combine with and neutralize its action. In this refractory state the incoagulability of the blood may be difficult to overcome even with large amounts of whole blood or plasma derivatives. For this reason it is best not to use plasma fractions in the treatment of hemophilia if local measures and, when necessary, whole blood transfusions will suffice to control bleeding. Certain diseases, such as tuberculosis, chronic glomerular nephritis and lupus erythematosus, as well as pregnancy, appear to be able to cause similar sensitization. Different anticoagulants may oppose the formation of plasma thromboplastin or the conversion of prothrombin to thrombin. Spontaneous disappearance of the anticoagulant may occur. Small amounts of the plasma of these, as well as of other patients, prolong the clotting time of the blood. Hyperheparinemia may develop in patients given large amounts of roentgen irradiation or nitrogen mustard, and in rare instances there are reports of spontaneously developing anticoagulants of uncertain nature.

W. B. CASTLE

References

Ackroyd, J. F.: Allergic Purpura, Including Purpura Due to Foods, Drugs and Infections. Am. J. Med., 14:605, 1953.

Alexander, B., and Goldstein, R.: Parahemophilia in Three Siblings (Owren's Disease) with Studies on Certain Plasma Components Affecting Prothrombin Conversion. Am. J. Med., 13:255, 1952.

Barondess, J. A.: Thrombotic Thrombocytopenic Purpura. Am. J. Med., 13:294, 1952.

Bigelow, F. S.: Serotonin Activity in Blood: Measurements in Normal Subjects and in Patients with Thrombocythemia Hemorrhagica and Other Hemorrhagic States. J. Lab. & Clin. Med., 43:759, 1954.

Davidson, C. S., Epstein, R. D., Miller, G. F., and Taylor, F. H. L.: Hemophilia. A Clinical Study of Forty Patients. Blood, 4:97, 1949.

DeVries, A., Shafir, E., Efrati, P., and Shamis, Z.: Thrombocytopathic Purpura with Normal Prothrombin Consumption: Hemorrhagic Diathesis Due to Partial Platelet Dysfunction. Blood, 8: 1000, 1953.

Frick, P. G.: Hemophilia-like Disease Following Pregnancy: With Transplacental Transfer of an Acquired Circulating Anticoagulant. Blood, 8: 598, 1953.

Harrington, W. J., and others: Immunologic Mechanisms in Idiopathic and Neonatal Thrombocytopenic Purpura. Ann. Int. Med., 38:433, 1953.

Lawson, H. A.: Congenital Afibrinogenemia. New England J. Med., 248:552, 1953.

Moloney, W. C., Egan, W. J., and Gorman, A. J.: Acquired Afibrinogenemia in Pregnancy. New England J. Med., 240:596, 1949.

Mortensen, O.: Thrombocythemia Hemorrhagica. Acta med. Scandinav., 129:547, 1948.

Olwin, J. H.: The Significance of Different Methods for Prothrombin Estimation and Their Relative Values. Surg., Gynec. & Obst., 90:423, 1950.

Quick, A. J.: Studies on the Enigma of the Hemostatic Dysfunction of Hemophilia. Am. J. M. Sc., 214:272, 1947.

———, and Grossman, A. M.: The Nature of the Hemorrhagic Disease of the Newborn. Am. J. M. Sc., 199:1, 1940.

Robson, H. N.: Idiopathic Thrombocytopenic Purpura. Quart. J. Med., 18:279, 1949.

Soulier, J. P., and Larrieu, M. J.: Differentiation of Hemophilia into Two Groups: A Study of Thirtythree Cases. New England J. Med., 249:547, 1953.

Stefanini, M.: Mechanism of Blood Coagulation in Normal and Pathologic Conditions. Am. J. Med., 14:64, 1953.

Tagnon, H. J., Whitmore, W. F., Schulman, P., and Kravitz, S. C.: The Significance of Fibrinolysis Occurring in Patients with Metastatic Cancer of the Prostate. Cancer, 6:63, 1953.

Tocantins, L. M.: The Mechanism of Hemostasis. Ann. Surg., 125:292, 1947.

Weiner, A. E., Reid, D. E., and Rolsy, C. C.: Coagulation Defects Associated in Premature Separation of Normally Implanted Placenta. Am. J. Obst. & Gynec., 60:379, 1950.

Wintrobe, M. M.: Clinical Hematology. 3rd ed. Philadelphia, Lea & Febiger, 1951, Chaps. XV, XVI (bibliography).

POLYCYTHEMIA

Definition. An abnormal increase in hemoglobin concentration is invariably accompanied by an increase in red cells, although the converse is not always so. For this reason, and as the physiologic opposite of anemia, *polycythemia* is defined here as an increased concentration of hemoglobin rather than of red cells, as is the custom of most authors. Some writers use the term "erythrocytosis" for sustained polycythemias secondary to recognized causes, and use "erythremia" for the disease of unknown origin otherwise known as polycythemia (*rubra*) vera.

RELATIVE POLYCYTHEMIA

This temporary condition results from loss of plasma or its diffusible constituents relative to loss of red cells so that the latter become more concentrated. *Restricted fluid intake* alone may lead to restriction of plasma volume after several days, merely as a result of the irreducible losses of water from the lungs, skin and kidneys. More commonly in disease, with or without restricted fluid intake, *increased loss of water and electrolytes* occurs from increased sweating or from vomiting, diarrhea, hyposthenuria or adrenal insufficiency. In extensive skin burns or in traumatic shock, plasma escapes freely from the capillaries into dressings or tissues. The increased number of leukocytes usually accompanying dehydration is not simply the result of hemoconcentration, which indeed rarely gives rise to more than a 25 per cent increase in hematocrit, but is mainly due to an active leukocytosis. Restoration of fluid balance with appropriate amounts of water and electrolytes promptly abolishes the polycythemia. Release of red cells from storage areas such as the spleen is so slight in normal man as never to lead to significant polycythemia.

SECONDARY POLYCYTHEMIAS

These sustained elevations of red cells and hemoglobin result when some type of anoxia stimulates the cells controlling erythropoiesis in the bone marrow.

Pathologic Physiology. Secondary polycythemias of chronic duration often occur when the *amount* or *tension of the oxygen carried by the arterial blood is diminished.*

This directly, or indirectly through some humoral effect of the anoxic blood upon the metabolism of some other organ, presumably stimulates the bone marrow to morphologic and functional erythroid hyperplasia, as does the anoxia of anemia. At any rate, the plasma of anemic rabbits has been convincingly shown by Erslev to produce an erythropoietic response in normal rabbits. Whatever the mechanism, Hurtado has found that in groups of well persons residing at various altitudes in the Andes, there is a consistent inverse relation between the decreased oxygen tensions in the inspired air and arterial blood (anoxic anoxia) and the increased red cell and hemoglobin concentrations in the blood. Polycythemia secondary to the lowered oxygen tension of the fetal circulation as derived from the placental capillaries begins to diminish shortly after the establishment of pulmonary respiration. In patients with certain types of *cardiac or pulmonary disease,* polycythemia results from the passage of partially oxygenated blood into the aorta. This happens with two different sets of anatomic circumstances: first, when there is short circuiting of a normally functioning pulmonary capillary bed by passage of some venous blood from the right directly into the left side of the heart or into the aorta (e.g., defective atrial or ventricular septums, dextroposition of the aorta or pulmonary arteriovenous fistula); second, when restricted alveolar ventilation due to chronic pulmonary disease (e.g., emphysema or silicosis) or congestion of the alveolar membranes prevents normal aeration of the blood during its passage through the lung (e.g., mitral stenosis). It should be understood that the arterial anoxia of mitral stenosis or of *Ayerza's syndrome* is not directly due to a diminished rate of blood flow through the pulmonary capillaries (which would actually lead to increased aeration of the blood), but rather to changes in the lung itself. Chronic exposure to *aniline, nitrobenzol* or *phenacetin,* by producing methemoglobin or other abnormal forms of hemoglobin, decreases the capacity of the arterial blood for carrying oxygen quite as does anemia. Rarely, chronic exposure to carbon monoxide produces sufficient carboxyhemoglobin to lead also to polycythemia.

Stagnant anoxia of the bone marrow, or of some other tissue, perhaps as a result of diffuse vasoconstriction, conceivably results in the polycythemia noted in association with hypertension in *Cushing's syndrome* and in *subtentorial brain tumors. Cobalt* administration in animals and in man induces polycythemia theoretically as a result of the formation of oxygen-binding cobalt complexes possibly in the cytoplasm of the erythroid cells of the bone marrow (histotoxic anoxia). No abnormal forms of circulating hemoglobin have been detected after giving cobalt.

Except in polycythemia due to hemoconcentration, the blood volume is increased, chiefly as a result of the increment of circulating red cells. In polycythemia secondary to arterial anoxia, despite the increased oxygen capacity the oxygen tension of the arterial blood is still less than normal. This, together with the increased viscosity of the blood and the underlying circulatory burden imposed by the abnormalities in heart or lung, usually results in distinctly restricted delivery of oxygen to the tissue cells.

Clinical Symptoms. In contrast to the acute symptoms appearing upon ascent to an altitude of 10,000 feet or more is the satisfactory adjustment of most permanent residents to existence at such elevations. By virtue of the increased oxygen-carrying power of the blood, sufficient compensation for its lowered oxygen tension is achieved so that these persons are even able to carry on muscular work with comparative ease. However, Monge has described *chronic mountain sickness* in occasional persons living at such altitudes who presumably have chronic pulmonary disease as a superimposed additional cause of arterial anoxia. A long history of recurrent bronchitis and laryngitis develops into an incapacitating illness characterized by headache, tinnitus, dyspnea, anorexia, vomiting and lethargy. These symptoms are greatly enhanced by slight exertion. The chest is emphysematous, and the vital capacity is reduced. Cyanosis, clubbing of the fingers and congestion of the scleral capillaries are prominent. Examination of the blood reveals marked polycythemia relative to that of normal residents living at the same altitude. The blood volume is increased, and reticulocytosis, moderately increased bilirubinemia and sometimes leukocytosis are found. Return to sea level promptly relieves the symptoms, and the polycythemia gradually subsides.

Polycythemias secondary to cardiac and pulmonary disease are accompanied by pathognomonic symptoms and signs of disease of those organs: congenital anomalies, pulmonary hypertension or diffuse fibrosis and emphysema. The patients are invariably cyanotic and frequently exhibit clubbing of the fingers. Enlargement of the liver is common as a manifestation of cardiac failure. Splenomegaly may be due to this cause, but is more frequently associated with chronic pulmonary infection. An exaggerated degree of cyanosis and polycythemia resulting from chronic pulmonary insufficiency is sometimes called Ayerza's syndrome. In this condition signs of right-sided cardiac hypertrophy and failure eventually appear. Otherwise the symptoms closely resemble those of Monge's disease just described.

In these secondary forms of polycythemia the red cells often reach 8 million and sometimes 10 million per cubic millimeter, usually with somewhat less than normally corresponding hemoglobin and hematocrit values. Reticulocytosis and slight hyperbilirubinemia are characteristic. Leukocytosis is absent except when due to associated infection, which also seems in many instances to restrict the degree of the polycythemic response to the arterial unsaturation. The essential diagnostic criterion of secondary polycythemia of this type is an oxygen saturation of the arterial blood of less than 90 per cent. This is best demonstrated by blood gas analysis, but may be inferred in patients with diffuse pulmonary disease or congestion by the prompt disappearance of cyanosis when oxygen is breathed.

The **treatment** of secondary polycythemias is chiefly that of the underlying cardiac or pulmonary condition. Elimination of the offending drug or toxic exposure shortly relieves the polycythemias due to perverted forms of hemoglobin. In acute episodes of cyanosis, oxygen administration is indicated. The increased oxygen capacity of the blood of patients with heart or lung disease is presumably a useful physiologic response. However, in some patients occasional bleeding is of subjective benefit, perhaps because it decreases blood volume or viscosity.

PRIMARY POLYCYTHEMIA

This disease is manifested by a chronic and sustained elevation of the red cells and hemoglobin often accompanied by leukocytosis, and sometimes by great elevation of the platelet level. Splenomegaly is usual and may be massive.

Pathologic Physiology. The nature of the stimulus to the increased red cell and hemoglobin formation is unknown. Tenable theories regard the disease either as a neo-plastic condition of the erythropoietic tissues analogous to leukemia or as a response to diffuse stagnant anoxia of the bone marrow, for which there is no direct evidence. A frequent evolution into leukemia is the chief argument in favor of the former conception. In accord with the latter hypothesis is Reznikoff's observation of capillary wall fibrosis and thickening in the bone marrow. Also suggestive of local interference with or competition for the available oxygen in the bone marrow is the transient association of several different kinds of cellular hyperplasia of the bone marrow with polycythemia: early benzol and radium poisoning, myelogenous and monocytic leukemias and multiple myeloma. Moreover, in many patients with polycythemia vera, especially in those with splenomegaly, there is morphologic evidence of a chronic association with a leukemic or leukemoid process in the bone marrow. There, according to Zadek, the increased cellularity is due to white as well as to red cell proliferation. Megakaryocytes are also unusually prominent. Finally, the qualitatively normal hematologic responses of patients with polycythemia vera to such procedures as blood loss, hemolysis by phenylhydrazine and iron administration indicate that erythropoiesis is actually under usual physiologic controls, although adjusted for an abnormally high level of circulating hemoglobin.

In patients with polycythemia vera when at rest the cardiac and respiratory functions are normal unless there is coincidental heart failure, due usually to hypertension or arteriosclerosis. The slowing of the peripheral blood flow arising from the greatly increased viscosity of the blood does not result in inadequate delivery of oxygen to most tissues, because of the increased oxygen content and normal oxygen tension of the arterial blood. However, the increased blood viscosity produces a tendency to vascular thrombosis; and paradoxically, probably because of the congestion of the capillaries and veins required to accommodate the huge blood volume, these patients also tend to bleed freely from minor injuries or surgical procedures. In some, with high platelet levels, this may be related to a lack of the vasoconstrictor principle, serotonin. The frequently elevated basal metabolism and the increased amounts of uric acid in blood and urine are presumably reflections of the increased hematopoiesis and its accompanying enhanced nucleoprotein metabolism.

Clinical Symptoms. Polycythemia vera affects men more often than women and is usually of gradual onset, most frequently after 40 years of age. Its course is one of long duration, frequently ten, sometimes twenty years. Rarely, young adults or even children are affected. When this is the case, a familial incidence has been observed. The attention of the patient may be drawn to his ruddy color, or the frequently enlarged spleen or thrombotic or bleeding episodes may cause him to consult a physician. In most patients there are also complaints of fullness in the head, dizziness on arising, irritability, paresthesias, night sweats, lassitude or weakness. The red or purplish color is especially noticeable in the face, lips, oral cavity, neck, hands and feet. The veins of the sclerae and retina are engorged and conspicuous. In about half the cases systolic hypertension or cardiomegaly is found. Patients with hypertension, moderate polycythemia and no enlargement of the spleen were regarded as a distinct clinical category by Gaisböck. However, many of them eventually develop the large, firm spleen that can be felt in over three quarters of the entire group of patients. The organ may be so huge as to interfere with food intake. Some enlargement of the liver is also detectable in about half the patients.

Although even arterial blood samples appear dark red to purple in color, their oxygen saturation is normal. The red cells frequently number 8 million and not rarely 10 million per cubic millimeter. The hemoglobin and hematocrit values are also increased, but usually not proportionately. The red cells may be entirely normal in size, shape and hemoglobin content, but frequently are somewhat small and varied in size as well as slightly hypochromic. This is especially true if hemorrhages or therapeutic bleedings have taken place. The reticulocytes are usually increased, and stippled red cells and normoblasts are often noted on blood smears. Slightly increased bilirubinemia and stool pigments are usual. In perhaps half the patients, and especially in those with splenomegaly, there is a leukocytosis of from 10,000 to 15,000, not infrequently as high as 25,000, cells per cubic millimeter. The differential count demonstrates predominance and immaturity of the granulocytes; and metamelocytes and even occasional myelocytes are seen. Remarkable increases in thrombocytes sometimes occur, totaling well over a million per cubic millimeter. The bone marrow is usually hypercellular with active erythropoiesis

proceeding from the normoblast level. Myeloid hyperplasia is also present, and megakaryocytes are prominent, especially in the terminal stages of the disease when the bone marrow becomes fibrotic or even osteosclerotic in some patients and anemia develops. Other patients succumb with all the features of a terminal acute or chronic myelogenous leukemia.

Among the common complications of the long course of the disease are the vascular thromboses, which may be arterial or venous and may affect peripheral, mesenteric or cerebral vessels. Progressive thromboses of the portal vein radicles may lead to liver cirrhosis. Hemorrhage, from hemorrhoids, from varices of stomach or bowel or from duodenal ulcers that are said to occur in 8 per cent of the patients, is frequent and may be serious. In the patients with hypertension, chronic cardiac and renal disease frequently develops. Attacks of gout have been reported. Aside from the secondary effects of the greatly increased blood volume and viscosity, the course of the disease is best appreciated as an intimate association either with arteriosclerosis or more commonly with a chronic form of myelogenous leukemia.

The **treatment** of polycythemia vera is directed toward reduction of the increased viscosity and volume of the circulating blood, of which the hematocrit is the best single measure. Satisfactory means to this end depress the increased erythropoiesis: repeated venesections, irradiation of the bone marrow with x-rays or radioactive phosphorus or administration of nitrogen mustard conveniently used in the form of triethylene melamine as an oral medication. Phenylhydrazine should not be used, because it increases both red cell destruction and production and is a potentially toxic substance. Phlebotomy immediately reduces the blood volume by a corresponding amount and, when repeated, eventually produces sufficient iron deficiency to retard erythropoiesis. It is best begun with the removal of 500 cc. of blood one to three times a week until the hematocrit is in the vicinity of 50 per cent. Thereafter regular bleedings at biweekly and later monthly intervals wall usually suffice to maintain this level. Hypochromia of the red cells is a necessary consequence and indicator of an effective degree of inhibition of erythropoiesis. When the x-ray is used, exposures are made either to successive body quadrants or to the whole body as a "spray." The oral administration of P[32] or of triethylene melamine in doses of 5 mg. a week is carried out, much as in the treatment of chronic myelogenous leukemia. Leukopenia may soon appear, but, because of the 100-day average lifetime of the red cells, significant reduction in their number does not develop before one or two months have passed. The long latent period before neoplasia develops after experimental irradiation in animals indicates that the apprehension is unfounded, that irradiation, especially with P[32], causes leukemia to develop promptly in these patients. Conceivably, it may accelerate the overt clinical appearance of a latent process.

W. B. CASTLE

References

Altschule, M. D., Volk, M. C., and Henstell, H.: Cardiac and Respiratory Function at Rest in Patients with Uncomplicated Polycythemia Vera. Am. J. M. Sc., 200:478, 1940.

Erslev, A.: Humoral Regulation of Red Cell Production. Blood, 8:349, 1953.

Grant, W. C., and Root, W. S.: Fundamental Stimulus for Erythropoiesis. Physiol. Rev., 32:449, 1952.

Harrop, G. A., Jr.: Polycythemia. Medicine, 7:291, 1928 (bibliography).

Holmes, C. R., Kredel, F. E., and Hanna, C. B.: Polycythemia Secondary to Brain Tumor. Report of Two Cases. South. M. J., 45:967, 1952.

Hurtado, A., Merino, C., and Delgado, E.: Influence of Anoxemia on the Hemopoietic Activity. Arch. Int. Med., 75:284, 1945.

Lawrence, J. H.: The Control of Polycythemia by Marrow Inhibition. A Ten Year Study on 172 Patients. J.A.M.A., 141:13, 1949.

Minot, G. R., and Buckman, T. E.: Erythremia (Polycythemia Rubra Vera). Am. J. M. Sc., 166:469, 1923.

Reznikoff, P., Foot, N. C., and Bethea, J. M.: Etiologic and Pathologic Factors in Polycythemia Vera. Am. J. M. Sc., 189:753, 1935.

Richardson, W., and Robbins, L. L.: The Treatment of Polycythemia Vera by Spray Irradiation. New England J. Med., 238:78, 1948.

Rosenthal, N., and Bassen, F. A.: Course of Polycythemia. Arch. Int. Med., 62:903, 1938.

Wintrobe, M. M.: Clinical Hematology. 3d ed. Philadelphia, Lea & Febiger, 1951, Chap. XIV (bibliography).

HEMOGLOBINURIA AND MYOHEMO- GLOBINURIA

For discussion of hemoglobinuria and myohemoglobinuria, see under Diseases of the Kidneys, page 1091.

THE LEUKOPENIC STATE AND AGRANULOCYTOSIS

THE LEUKOPENIC STATE

Leukopenia exists whenever the white blood cell count falls below the normal range of values, i.e., lower than about 4000 cells per cubic millimeter. The decrease usually occurs predominantly in the granulocytic series but may involve lymphocytes and monocytes as well, particularly when the leukopenia becomes profound. If the differential count remains approximately normal, patients may tolerate leukopenias as low as 1500 cells per cubic millimeter for long periods of time without evident difficulty. When the total number of leukocytes is reduced below that level, however, or when the percentage of granulocytes is markedly decreased, resistance to infection is impaired so that microorganisms tend to invade the skin, mucous membranes and blood stream. Because leukocytes may exist in tissues as well as in the peripheral blood, and because there is no accurate method for measuring rates of white blood cell production or destruction, the pathogenesis of leukopenia is often obscure, even when its etiology can be identified.

Infections of various kinds are common causes of leukopenia: (*a*) bacterial (typhoid, paratyphoid, and sometimes tularemia and brucellosis); (*b*) viral (influenza, measles, rubella, psittacosis, dengue, infectious hepatitis, atypical pneumonia); (*c*) rickettsial (Rocky Mountain spotted fever, typhus, scrub typhus, rickettsialpox) and (*d*) protozoal (malaria, relapsing fever, kala-azar). In addition, septicemia or any overwhelming infection, particularly in elderly, debilitated or malnourished patients, may be associated with moderate to severe depression of the white blood cell count. Granulocytes under these circumstances may show vacuolization and toxic granulation as evidences of damage. Toxemia associated with the infection may depress the rate of leukocyte formation. In addition, white cells actively engaged in the process of trying to combat the invasion of microorganisms may be destroyed at an accelerated rate. Menkin has demonstrated both leukocytosis and leukopenia-promoting factors in exudates; he postulates that the leukocyte level in any infection depends on the over-all balance between these substances. In septicemias, the leukopenia, in part, may also result from the accumulation of leukocytes along the endothelial walls of capillaries, venules and arterioles where they can more readily trap and engulf bacteria within the blood stream.

The depressant effect of *drugs, chemical agents* and *ionizing irradiation* on leukopoiesis constitutes another major cause of leukopenia. The number of substances which may be listed under this heading is already legion and increases every year: benzol, dinitrophenol, antithyroid drugs, anticonvulsant drugs such as Tridione, sulfonamides, nitrogen mustard, triethylene melamine, folic acid antagonists, DDT, arsenic, gold, etc. The leukopenia produced by these chemical agents and by irradiation should be differentiated from the acute, explosive and fulminating disease, agranulocytic angina. The mechanism is one of direct depression or destruction of leukopoietic tissue rather than sensitization as in agranulocytic angina. The white blood cell count, for instance, may fall slowly in a patient taking sulfonamides, thiouracil, Tridione, gold, triethylene melamine, or other drugs to levels of 1500 or 2000 cells per cubic millimeter without producing any recognizable clinical manifestations. On the other hand, if the leukopenia is more severe, the signs and symptoms may be quite similar to those of acute agranulocytosis so that differentiation becomes more difficult. Treatment should be directed toward recognition and withdrawal of the offending agent, and antibiotic therapy either as prophylaxis against or treatment of infection. Because of the increasing use of radioactive substances and the threat of atomic warfare, many investigators are currently searching for ways to prevent and treat radiation-induced leukopenia and other evidences of bone marrow damage. No discoveries of practical importance, however, have yet been made.

Leukopenia may also develop during the course of any disease associated with *splenomegaly*: cirrhosis of the liver, splenic or portal vein thrombosis, conditions primarily affecting lymph nodes (the lymphomas), the leukemias, lupus erythematosus, rheumatoid arthritis, sarcoid, infectious granulomatous lesions of the spleen, kala-azar, Gaucher's disease and other disorders. Some observers believe that the abnormally functioning spleen is responsible for the low white cell count because it destroys the cells faster than they can be formed, while others insist that splenic inhibition of leukopoiesis must also occur. Granulocytic elements in the bone marrow are normal or hyperplastic, but the myelocytes may be immature. If treatment of the primary disorder fails to relieve the splenomegaly and leukopenia, then splenectomy should be done if the patient's clinical condition permits. Closely related, at least in terms of mechanism, is primary splenic neutropenia (see p. 1155).

A number of hematologic dyscrasias in addition to those listed are frequently associated with leukopenia: aplastic anemia, myelophthisic anemias, chronic hypochromic anemia and untreated pernicious anemia. The mechanisms here vary from aplasia of leukopoietic tissue, to replacement by cells invading the marrow, to deficiency of nutrients required for normal white blood cell production. In myelophthisic anemias, myelocytes and an occasional myeloblast are found in the peripheral blood.

Brief description should also be made of a rare disorder called *cyclic* or *periodic neutropenia*. The etiology and pathogenesis of this disease are obscure. It can occur at any age and is characterized by cyclic periods of moderately severe leukopenia during which neutrophils may almost disappear from the blood. The attacks may occur at intervals of weeks or months, and in the interim the peripheral blood is quite normal. Weakness, fatigue, stomatitis, arthralgia, infections of the skin and mucous membranes, and abscesses may occur. Splenectomy may lead to recovery or enough elevation of the white count so that the leukopenic episodes are less severe; in some instances, however, it has failed to give relief.

Because agranulocytic angina is such a fulminating disease, there is a tendency for many physicians to regard moderately severe leukopenic states with more alarm than is often justified. The cause should be identified and treated or removed as quickly as possible, of course, and antibiotic therapy should often be given prophylactically. But if the primary disease is one which cannot be corrected, or if splenectomy is not warranted when the spleen is enlarged, patients may tolerate the leukopenia for long periods of time without difficulty. The author has followed a number of patients with chronic splenomegaly (from chronic malaria, old splenic vein thrombosis, etc.) and leukocyte counts of 1000 to 2000 per cubic millimeter for more than ten years;

they are asymptomatic so that splenectomy has never seemed necessary.

AGRANULOCYTIC ANGINA
(Agranulocytosis)

Definition. Agranulocytosis is an acute disease in which the white blood cell count drops precipitously to low levels and neutropenia becomes extreme. Clinical manifestations usually appear in an explosive manner and are secondary to the bacterial invasion of tissues: high fever, prostration, ulcerations in the mouth, rectum or vagina, pyodermia, and septicemia. In all, or nearly all, instances the disease is caused by sensitization of granulocytic elements to drugs or other chemical substances. As more drugs have been recognized as causative agents, so-called idiopathic cases have almost vanished. Before sulfonamides and the antibiotics became available, patients succumbed to infection so that the mortality was very high. If the offending chemical is withdrawn and infection is prevented or controlled, recovery occurs after five to ten days.

History. Werner Schultz in 1922 described 6 patients with agranulocytosis. Detailed reports of similar cases had been published by Brown in 1902 and by Turk in 1907, but Schultz seems to deserve the credit for having recognized the disorder as a clinical entity. In 1931, Kracke suggested that the sudden increased incidence of agranulocytosis in Europe and America might possibly be correlated with the greater therapeutic use of certain coal-tar derivatives. In November, 1933, Madison and Squier presented evidence that amidopyrine had produced the disease and suggested that the reaction was allergic or anaphylactoid in nature. Since then, many other substances have been incriminated as causative agents.

Etiology and Pathogenesis. Agranulocytosis is caused by sensitization to drugs or other chemical substances to which the patient has been exposed. Because it takes time for sensitization to occur, the disease usually develops after repeated rather than initial contact with the offending agent or, in the case of continuous exposure, at any time after seven to fourteen days. For instance, the first time a patient takes amidopyrine or sulfapyridine he is not in much danger of agranulocytosis providing therapy is terminated after a few days. On the other hand, if the medication is continued for longer than seven to ten days, sensitization may occur at any time, even after weeks or months of treatment, and be followed by the explosive onset of the disease. Or, if the first or any subsequent short course of therapy has produced sensitization, agranulocytosis may develop after the first dose of the drug at any subsequent administration. Agranulocytosis occurs in only a small percentage of patients exposed even to those drugs which cause the greatest number of cases. The gravity of the complication, rather than its frequency, accounts for its great importance. Unfortunately, no one has been able to devise a method for detecting those persons who are most likely to become sensitized.

Drugs which have frequently been incriminated as causes of agranulocytosis include: amidopyrine, dinitrophenol, sulfonamide compounds, thiouracil, propylthiouracil, gold compounds, organic arsenical compounds, phenylbutazone and trimethadione (Tridione). In addition, many drugs have been reported to have caused the disease in a few instances: antipyrine, phenobarbital, amytal, allurate, Novaldin, pyribenzamine, Tapazole, Mesantoin, Apresoline, mercurial diuretics, Bismarsen, cinchophen, neocinchophen, quinine, Plasmochin, salol, Neostibosan, pyrithyldione (Presidon) and DDT.

In a few instances, after patients have recovered, small amounts of the offending drug given while the subjects were being carefully studied have been observed to reproduce the neutropenia. Attempts to demonstrate sensitization in other ways, i.e., by intradermal injection, patch tests, passive transfer tests, etc., have yielded negative results. Dameshek and Colmes, however, did obtain strongly positive skin tests by injecting intradermally a small amount of amidopyrine mixed with the blood serum of 3 patients who had recovered from amidopyrine-induced agranulocytosis. Recently, Moeschlin has reported a convincing series of experiments in which he first produced agranulocytosis in a sensitized patient by giving him 0.3 gm. amidopyrine orally. Three hours later, when the neutropenia was pronounced, 300 cc. of blood was withdrawn and administered to a normal recipient. The white cell count in the normal subject fell from 5000 to 800 per cubic millimeter within 40 minutes; recovery occurred after about 4 hours. Appropriate control studies were done. Similar results were obtained when the experiment was repeated on a second normal recipient. Plasma obtained from the patient 3 hours after the challenging dose of amidopyrine caused agglutination of leukocytes from both normal subjects and from the patient himself. From these observations, Moeschlin concluded that leukocyte agglutinins in agranulocytosis are responsible for the agglutination of white cells; the agglutinated leukocytes are subsequently phagocyted or lysed, possibly in large part in the lung.

A further comment should be made about the so-called idiopathic cases of agranulocytosis. It has been suggested that infection may at times be the cause rather than the result of agranulocytosis, possibly by a process of sensitization to bacterial or viral protein. Of interest, therefore, is the recent observation by Moeschlin that a patient with virus pneumonia, in whom the cold agglutinin titer reached 1:8000, developed a leukopenia of 230 cells per cubic millimeter along with a hemolytic anemia. One must be prepared for the demonstration that infectious agents and other substances may also possibly produce the kind of sensitization that results in agranulocytosis.

Incidence. Agranulocytic angina occurs, for some unknown reason, about three times more frequently in females than in males. Its incidence varies with the therapeutic popularity of the drugs which cause it.

Pathologic Anatomy. Except for the evidences of infection, pathologic changes are confined to the marrow. Granulocytic elements may be quantitatively normal, showing a shift to younger forms of myelocytes and a decrease in more mature cells; or in severe cases they may be markedly decreased in number as well. These changes have been variously interpreted as the result of maturation arrest, damage to the cells, or as exhaustion of the leukopoietic tissue produced by great peripheral demand.

Tissues contain numerous colonies of bacteria. The histopathology of ulcerative areas, pneumonia and other sites of infection is distinctive in that neutrophils are absent. The cellular reaction is made up principally of lymphocytes and plasma cells.

Signs and Symptoms. The onset of the disease is sudden with a chill, high fever and marked prostration. These symptoms were formerly regarded as due to bacterial invasion of tissues, but two observations indicate that they may result from the antigen-antibody re-action at the time white blood cells rapidly disappear from the circulation and are destroyed. When an amidopyrine-sensitized individual is given a test dose of the drug, a chill, fever and prostration occur within the first hour as the neutropenia is developing. Similar reactions were experienced by the two normal subjects in whom Moeschlin produced granulocytopenia by injecting 300 cc. of blood obtained from a sensitized patient 3 hours after a challenging dose of amidopyrine.

There then follows a period of brief but variable duration characterized by profound neutropenia, fatigue and continuing prostration in which no new symptoms appear.

The third stage begins when the tissues are invaded by bacteria. It is usually heralded by a return of fever, often to levels as high as 40° or 41° C., chills, headache, and the appearance of ulcerations most commonly in the pharynx, tonsils, gums or buccal mucous membranes, but also around the nose, rectum or vagina. The ulcers, in other words, tend to occur at those sites where bacteria are normally present in greatest numbers. These symptoms may be so severe that they dwarf those of the first two stages, and patients often regard them as the onset of the disease. The ulcers are frequently covered by a dirty gray or dark membrane, but the surrounding tissue shows little inflammatory change. Regional lymph nodes may become enlarged and tender. Pneumonitis and bacteremia may develop. Splenomegaly, jaundice and bone pain may appear as manifestations of septicemia. Swallowing may become difficult. Pain, with few physical signs of inflammation, may be present around the rectum or in other portions of the body, but when the patient recovers and has a return of white blood cells to his peripheral blood, abscesses often form at these sites, indicating that they had previously been infected. Ulcers in the gastrointestinal tract may be found at autopsy examination, but there usually are few symptoms which can be related to them. Dermatitis and pyodermia are not infrequent. When death occurs, it is almost always the result of infection.

Neutropenia dominates the changes in the peripheral blood. The total leukocyte count is often less than 1000 cells per cubic millimeter but may be as high as 2000 to 4000. Even with the higher levels, however, there are practically no granulocytes. The few that may be found show pyknotic nuclei with vacuolization of the cytoplasm and toxic granulation. Erythrocyte and platelet values are normal unless anemia or thrombocytopenia antedated the agranulocytosis.

The neutropenia usually persists for from five to ten or twelve days. In general, more rapid recovery can be correlated with the persistence of a large number of moderately immature granulocytes in the marrow, while the longer recovery times tend to be associated with those marrows in which leukopoietic tissue had initially all but disappeared. Recovery is probably delayed because more time is required for the regeneration and subsequent maturation of the myelocytes. The first signs of recovery in the peripheral blood are the appearance of a few myelocytes and often a transient monocytosis. Within a few days thereafter, the white cell count rises rapidly to normal or slightly elevated levels. The percentage of myelocytes may temporarily be as high as 10 to 15 per cent. If tissues have been infected so that localized abscesses are formed as the white cells return, leukocytosis of 30,000 to 40,000 or more cells per cubic millimeter may be observed.

Differential Diagnosis. When ulcerations are limited to the pharynx or tonsillar area, clinical manifestations of agranulocytosis may simulate those of acute ulcerative *pharyngitis* or *tonsillitis*. Differentiation becomes obvious, however, when the blood count is obtained and one finds a severe neutropenia rather than leukocytosis.

Aplastic anemia can be excluded by the absence of anemia and thrombocytopenia, and by the persistence of qualitatively normal erythroid and megakaryocytic elements in the bone marrow. Patients with *subleukemic leukemia* may resemble patients with agranulocytosis, particularly in the early stages of acute leukemia when severe leukopenia and ulcerations in the oral cavity may occur before anemia and thrombocytopenia develop. Aspirated bone marrow, however, reveals that normal cells have been replaced by leukemic leukocytes. In primary *splenic neutropenia,* the spleen is usually enlarged, the leukopenia is persistent, and the marrow is hyperplastic for granulocytic cells with or without evidences of immaturity.

Toxic depression of leukopoiesis and *irradiation damage* can be differentiated on the basis of history, longer course, and usu-ally the more gradual development of leukopenia.

It is common practice to have white blood cell counts done at intervals of several weeks or months in patients who for long periods of time take drugs capable of causing agranulocytosis, i.e., antithyroid drugs, Mesantoin, Tridione, phenylbutazone. While there may be medical-legal justification for this procedure, it can hardly, except under the most fortuitous circumstances, be expected to detect the onset of so fulminating a disease as agranulocytosis. Patients or their families should be told that the drug in question may rarely cause agranulocytosis, should be provided with a description of initial symptoms, and should be instructed to report to the physician promptly if the symptoms appear.

Prognosis. The mortality rate was very high before sulfonamides and antibiotics became available. There has been no extensive compilation of current mortality statistics, but at least 95 per cent of patients probably now recover. Those who succumb do so largely because the institution of antibiotic therapy is delayed too long or they are unfortunate enough to become infected with a resistant organism.

After recovery, the leukopoietic tissue seems to harbor no residual damage.

Treatment. Most patients with agranulocytosis will recover if the causative agent is withdrawn and infection is controlled. An attempt should be made immediately, therefore, to identify the responsible agent and to make certain that the patient has no further contact with it. If there are evidences of infection, appropriate cultures should be obtained from blood, spinal fluid, throat, sputum, ulcerated lesions or urine. Immediately thereafter, antibiotic therapy, designed to give broad coverage, should be started. Combinations of penicillin with dihydrostreptomycin or with tetracycline are satisfactory. Intramuscular injection of 200,000 to 400,000 units of penicillin G every 3 hours may be given plus 1 gm. of dihydrostreptomycin intramuscularly every 12 hours, or with 500 mg. of tetracycline orally every 6 hours. After the results of the cultures become known, antibiotic therapy should be altered according to the nature of the infecting agent. Therapy should be continued until the infection has been cured and the bone marrow has recovered. Unless streptomycin is the only effective antibiotic for the particular organisms involved, the dose of dihydrostrepto-mycin should be reduced within five to seven days to 1 gm. per day.

When the patient is seen before infection has begun, prophylactic therapy should be given in the form of 400,000 units of for-tified procaine penicillin and 0.5 gm. of di-hydrostreptomycin intramuscularly every 12 hours. Tetracycline, 1 gm. per day, may be substituted for the dihydrostreptomycin.

Cortisone and ACTH have been reported to hasten recovery from agranulocytosis in some instances. Their use is rational since a hypersensitivity reaction is involved in the pathogenesis of the disease. A satisfactory dose is 50 mg. of cortisone orally or intra-muscularly four times daily, or 20 to 30 mg. of adrenocorticotrophic hormone by slow in-travenous drip during an 8-hour period each day. They constitute a two-edged sword, how-ever, since they further depress resistance to infection. Antibiotic coverage as described above must be maintained while the patient is being treated with either hormone. The dan-ger of giving ACTH and cortisone must be weighed carefully in each case against the possible but not certain beneficial effect on the agranulocytic process.

Experimental evidence suggests that pent-nucleotides, yellow bone marrow extract, leukocytic creams, folic acid and liver ex-tracts may favorably influence white cell maturation under some circumstances. There is little reason to believe, however, that they contribute anything to the therapeutic meas-ures mentioned in the practical management of patients with agranulocytosis. Blood trans-fusions are usually not necessary, and should be given only as general supportive care for the very ill patient.

BAL (British anti-lewisite; 2,3-dimer-captopropanol) is of value when the agranulo-cytosis is due to gold salts or to arsenic. The dose should be 1.5 cc. of a 10 per cent solu-tion in oil, intramuscularly, every 4 hours. After the first two days, the interval between doses should be lengthened to 12 hours, and injections continued for an additional eight to ten days.

Precautions should be taken to keep the mouth clean. Frequent rinsing with warm physiologic salt solution or a mild alkaline mouth wash should be encouraged. Constipa-tion should be avoided because of the danger of perirectal abscess formation. Daily saline or soapsuds enemas, given carefully so as to avoid trauma, may be used for this purpose. Fluid balance should be maintained with parenteral fluids if necessary. Unless the pa-tient is debilitated at the onset of agranulocy-tosis, maintenance of nutrition is not a serious problem because of the short course of the disease.

CARL V. MOORE

References

Dameshek, W., and Colmes, A.: The Effect of Drugs in the Production of Agranulocytosis with Partic-ular Reference to Amidopyrine Sensitivity. J. Clin. Investigation, 15:85, 1936.

Kracke, R. R.: Recurrent Agranulocytosis. Am. J. Clin. Path., 1:385, 1931.

Madison, F. W., and Squier, T. L.: Etiology of Primary Granulocytopenia (Agranulocytic An-gina). J.A.M.A., 102:755, 1934.

Menkin, V.: The Determination of the Level of Leu-kocytes in the Bloodstream with Inflammation. Blood, 4:1323, 1949.

Moeschlin, S., and Wagner, K.: Agranulocytosis due to the Occurrence of Leucocyte Agglutinins (Pyramidon and Cold Agglutinins). Acta Haema-tologica, 8:29, 1952.

Reimann, H. A., and de Barardinis, C. T.: Periodic (Cyclic) Neutropenia. Blood, 4:1109, 1949.

Schultz, W.: Über eigenartige Halserkrankungen. Deutsch. Med. Wchnschr., 48:1495, 1922.

Wintrobe, M. M.: Clinical Hematology, 3rd Ed., Philadelphia, Lea and Febiger, 1951, pp. 211–214, 965–976.

Wiseman, B. K., and Doan, C. A.: A Newly Recog-nized Granulopenic Syndrome Caused by Exces-sive Splenic Leukolysis and Successfully Treated by Splenectomy. Ann. Int. Med., 16:1097, 1942.

Wood, W. B., Jr., Smith, M. R., Perry, W. D., and Berry, J. W.: Studies on the Cellular Immunology of Acute Bacteremia. I. Intravascular Leucocytic Reaction and Surface Phagocytosis. J. Exper. Med., 94:521, 1951.

THE LEUKEMIAS

Definition. Leukemia is a fatal disease, considered by many to be neoplastic in na-ture, which arises primarily in the blood-form-ing organs and is characterized by an exten-sive and abnormal proliferation of the white blood cells and their precursors, with cellular infiltrations into the various tissues of the body, especially the bone marrow, spleen, liver and lymph nodes. Almost invariably at some time during the disease, immature white corpuscles appear in the circulating blood, frequently in great numbers; in most cases there is an associated anemia, often of a severe degree.

Types of Leukemia and Allied States.

For practical purposes it is convenient to discuss the various types under the following divisions:

1. Lymphocytic
2. Granulocytic (Neutrophilic, Eosinophilic, Basophilic)
3. Monocytic
4. Plasmocytic
5. Megakaryocytic
6. Other varieties and allied pathologic states
   - (a) Lymphosarcoma cell leukemia
   - (b) Plasmocytic myeloma
   - (c) Hemocytoblastic leukemia
   - (d) Chloroma
   - (e) Mycosis fungoides
   - (f) Myeloid metaplasia of the spleen
   - (g) Leukemoid reactions.

Each variety of leukemia may be divided into the acute, subacute and chronic types, defined as follows: an *acute leukemia* is one which has a spontaneous course of three months or less; a *subacute leukemia* is one which has an expected duration, when untreated, of three months to one year from the appearance of the initial symptom; a *chronic leukemia* is one with an expected duration of one to twenty years or more, but averaging from three to five years from the first symptom.

Subleukemic and aleukemic aleukemia are discussed on page 1224.

A study of the incidence of the various types of leukemia by F. H. Bethell at the Simpson Memorial Institute of the University of Michigan showed that in a group of 495 patients with the disease, the percentage incidence of the various types was as follows: 48.3, granulocytic; 43.6, lymphocytic; 8.1, monocytic (histogenous or Schilling type). If the myelomonocytic group were removed from the classification of the granulocytic group, the percentage of cases in this subgroup would be 35.4, and if they were added to the monocytic variety, it would increase this division to 21 per cent.

A study of the incidence of the types of our cases of leukemia in recent years indicates a definite increase in the occurrence of acute leukemia and also of the combined chronic granulocytic and monocytic group.

History. Although the disease had been observed previously by Barth and others, and the initial examination of leukemic blood had been made by Donne in 1839, credit for first establishing the condition as a new clinical syndrome must be given to Hughes Bennett and Rudolf Virchow. In the autumn of 1845 these observers, independently and almost simultaneously, described in patients after death the greatly enlarged spleen and the increase in white corpuscles in the blood. Fuller in 1846 recognized the first case during life and confirmed the diagnosis by necropsy. The disease was called leukocythemia by Bennett and leukemia by Virchow. With the introduction of differential staining methods by Ehrlich in 1891, it became apparent that splenic and myelogenous leukemia were the same. The first case of acute leukemia was described by Friedreich in 1857. Lissaurer in 1865 was among the first to use arsenic in its treatment and observed symptomatic improvement, but it was not until 1878 that G. E. Cutler and E. H. Bradford made the first careful study of the effect of this drug on the blood. Pusey in 1902 introduced roentgen rays in the treatment of leukemia; this was followed in 1903 by the observations of Nicholas Senn and in 1904 by those of George Dock on the same subject. O. Naegeli in 1900 identified the myeloblast and emphasized its importance in relation to the leukemic states. Monocytic leukemia was first described by H. Reschard and Schilling-Torgau in 1913.

Etiology. There are two principal views concerning the nature of the leukemic process: one that the condition is an infection, the other that it is a malignant neoplasm. The latter is the more commonly accepted theory at present. Certainly the condition is an invariably fatal, invasive, pathologic process. Banti's conclusion in 1904 in regard to the cause of lymphatic leukemia epitomizes the most rational present-day tentative opinion concerning the etiology of leukemia in general. His statement is as follows: "A tissue with typical structure that has a tendency to spread locally from the involved to neighboring organs, that forms hematogenous metastases, cannot be called hyperplastic; it belongs, instead, in the group of new growths."

Those who argue for the infectious etiology are influenced to do so because some of the striking features, particularly in the acute leukemias, such as chills, fever and leukocytosis, are also present in diseases of a known infectious nature. Infection, especially about the mouth and throat, is commonly present, and septicemia may be observed. On the other hand, it has not been possible to produce leukemia in animals with any organism isolated from a patient; there is no evidence to indicate that the disease is transmissible from man to man; and it is not communicated to the fetus by a mother who has leukemia.

It is a more logical conclusion that the organisms which have been isolated from patients with leukemia are present in the role of secondary invaders rather than as primary etiologic agents.

Additional evidence is favor of the neoplastic theory other than that emphasized in Banti's statement is as follows: The disease, so far, has been produced in mice and guinea pigs only by the actual transference of malignant cells. Fowl leukemia is apparently a filterable form, but this is also true of certain types of neoplasms, such as sarcomas. Maude Slye maintained that spontaneous leukemia in mice follows the laws of heredity and is inherited as a simple mendelian recessive characteristic, as are other neoplasms.

The Hereditary Factor in the Etiology. The knowledge that the susceptibility to experimental leukemia, and the transmission of the spontaneous disease, follow definite genetic laws in experimental animals causes one to consider that in human beings the hereditary element might be of importance. Clinical experience gives some but not too convincing support to the idea. Ardashnikov concluded that, in some cases at least, hereditary factors play a role in the etiology of the disease in man. According to him the most probable explanation is a conditionally dominant type of inheritance, associated with the ordinary paired chromosomes, especially in the lymphatic form of leukemia, with great variation in the fully developed disease due to other genes or to external influences. It has been shown by Videback that the incidence of the condition in the blood relatives of patients with leukemia is 17 times as great as in a comparable control group.

Age and Sex Incidence. Leukemia of various types may be observed in either sex at any age. The greatest number of cases of chronic granulocytic leukemia is observed in the decade from 35 to 45 years, whereas the maximum incidence of chronic lymphocytic leukemia is between the ages of 45 and 54; some observers, however, place its greatest incidence somewhat later, namely, 50 to 69 years. Chronic leukemia of either type is less likely to occur in patients younger than 10 years, and it is not commonly observed before the age of 25 years. Acute leukemia is seen most frequently in persons younger than 25 years and has its greatest incidence in children under 5 years; it is relatively rare in patients older than 50 years, but may be present at any period of life and has been reported in old age.

Chronic granulocytic leukemia develops more frequently in men than in women in the ratio of 60:40 and chronic lymphocytic leukemia is three times as common in the male sex. Acute granulocytic leukemia of childhood appears to occur about equally in the two sexes. There is no evidence to indicate that leukemia of any type pursues a different course in either sex.

Pathology of Various Types of Leukemia. The fundamental pathologic change in any type of leukemia is an extensive proliferation of cells of the myeloid, lymphoid, monocytic group or primitive stem cells, which is usually associated with the presence of large numbers of these cells in various tissues of the body and the blood stream.

In chronic granulocytic leukemia, the bone marrow, most frequently of the sternum and other flat bones, is replaced by myeloid cells in which the myelocytes and metamyelocytes predominate, although a few myeloblasts may be present. A quantitative reduction of the red blood cell-forming marrow is the explanation of the commonly associated anemia of the disease. The spleen is usually grossly enlarged, and there may be a great increase in the myeloid cells of the splenic pulp, with often a fibrous thickening of the capsule; infarcts are commonly present. The liver is usually moderately increased in size, and myeloid metaplasia is frequently present in that organ.

In chronic lymphocytic leukemia the characteristic pathologic change consists in a replacement of the normal architecture of the lymph glands, spleen, liver, bone marrow and other tissues by lymphoid cells. Similar changes may be observed in the tonsils, lymphadenoid tissue of the pharynx, bronchi, esophagus, stomach, solitary lymph follicles, Peyer's patches, the bladder and urethra. The spleen is usually moderately enlarged because of the lymphocytic infiltration, and there may be infarction, perisplenitis, and thickening of the splenic capsule. The bone marrow is almost always involved with a similar lymphoid infiltration which eliminates most of the fat and normal marrow cells.

In the acute forms the leukemic infiltrations occur in various tissues throughout the body in a manner similar to that observed in the chronic leukemias. In the former, however, the abnormal collection of infiltrating cells consists almost entirely of myeloblasts, lymphoblasts, monoblasts, lymphosarcoma cells, hemocytoblasts or plasma cells. In addition, there is commonly a widespread and severe tendency to bleed, owing to the secondary thrombocytopenic purpura.

It is of interest to note, especially with reference to lymphocytic and monocytic leukemia, that Custer and Bernhard regard all lymphatic tumors as comprising a single neoplastic entity, with a number of variants. In this group are included follicular lymphoblastoma, lymphatic leukemia, lymphosarcoma, Hodgkin's granuloma, Hodgkin's paragranuloma and reticulum cell sarcoma. In the opinion of these authors, it is possible to have transitions from one form to any of the others of these lymphatic tumors.

CHRONIC GRANULOCYTIC LEUKEMIA

Symptoms and Signs. The onset is usually insidious; often the disease is well advanced when the patient is first examined. Definite and pronounced leukemic blood changes may be present for several years before the patient complains of symptoms.

Frequently the initial complaints are weakness, pallor, palpitation and dyspnea which are due to the associated myelophthisic type of anemia. In some cases there are no symptoms other than a dull dragging sensation in the left side of the abdomen or a bulging in the left upper quadrant which results from splenic enlargement. Fever of an intermittent or remittent type, rising as high as 101° or 102° F., is commonly observed, and this, sometimes associated with chills, may be an early complaint. As an increased basal metabolic rate is commonly encountered, the symptoms due to this, such as increased sweating, warmth, loss of weight and tachycardia, are frequently present.

During the acute exacerbations of the chronic form and as a terminal event, there may be an abnormal tendency to bleed which manifests itself as epistaxis, hemorrhages under the skin, from the uterus, kidneys, bowels or into the retinas or middle ear. Cerebral hemorrhage is an occasional complication. The hemorrhagic tendency is usually associated with a diminution of platelets in the circulating blood. Priapism, although always mentioned, is an exceedingly rare complication. Symptoms associated with an increasingly severe anemia, fever, and abnormal bleeding are likely to become more pronounced as the disease progresses.

The general appearance of the patient varies widely, depending largely on the degree of anemia which is present. When this is advanced, the patient has the aspects of a chronically ill persons with pronounced pallor and emaciation. In the earlier stages, when the red blood cell count and hemoglobin are within normal limits, the appearance may be that of a robust person in good health, although even then the white blood cell count may be several hundred thousand per cubic millimeter, and the spleen greatly enlarged.

Splenic enlargement, sometimes to a degree which causes this organ to occupy a large portion of the abdominal cavity, is characteristic of the disease. The lower edge commonly reaches below the umbilicus. The absence of a palpable spleen is strong evidence against the diagnosis of chronic granulocytic leukemia. The organ is firm and is not tender unless perisplenitis develops. The liver is usually palpable and may attain an enormous size.

Characteristically, the lymph nodes are not enlarged as they are in the lymphatic type, and this assists in differentiating the two types of the disease. Occasionally there may be a moderate increase in size of some of the lymph glands because of an infiltration with myeloid cells similar to that which occurs in other tissues of the body.

Skin lesions, other than the purpuric manifestations, are not commonly encountered. In some instances there is an infiltration of the skin with myelocytes and myeloblasts, which causes the formation of bluish-gray, elevated nodules, varying in size from a pin head to a walnut. They most frequently appear on the trunk, although they have been observed elsewhere on the body. Ordinarily they are not associated with itching or pain.

As leukemic infiltrations may be present in almost any tissue of the body, the possible complications are many. In addition to those already mentioned, the following may occur: the retinas may show hemorrhages and leukemic infiltrations; there may be destructive lesions of bone with pathologic fracture; deafness can occur, due either to hemorrhage or leukemic infiltrations in the inner or middle ears; various lesions of the nervous system may be observed due to hemorrhages, thromboses or tumor-like infiltrations; hematuria associated with infiltration of the kidneys may be encountered; myeloid changes may occur in the gastrointestinal tract resulting in hemorrhage, but this is more frequently observed in lymphocytic leukemia.

Blood Examination. The typical blood picture is an increase in the total number of leukocytes to 100,000 or more per cubic millimeter, of which 20 to 60 per cent are myelocytes, chiefly in the later stages of development, and 30 to 70 per cent are polymorphonuclear neutrophils with segmented nuclei. An occasional myeloblast may be seen. As the disease progresses, the proportion of myelocytes and myeloblasts increases, and in the advanced or terminal stages 70 per cent or more of the cells may be of the latter type. The total white blood cell count usually ranges between 100,000 and 500,000 per cubic millimeter, although as many as 1,000,000 or more leukocytes per cubic millimeter have been observed. It is not rare for the leukocyte count to become normal or for a leukopenia to develop, either spontaneously or after treatment. This is discussed in the section on Subleukemic Leukemia. An almost constant finding is an increase of 2 to 10 per cent of basophils, and occasionally these cells may comprise 50 per cent or more of all the leukocytes (basophilic leukemia). Likewise, the numbers of eosinophils and eosinophilic myelocytes are frequently increased to 5 or 6 per cent of the total leukocytes, and in some instances these types of cells are the predominating ones in the circulating blood (eosinophilic leukemia). Monocytes are usually present, but rarely exceed 3 per cent of the total number of leukocytes. There is characteristically a decrease in the percentage of lymphocytes, but their absolute number may be normal or actually increased. Care should be used in differentiating between lymphocytes and myeloblasts.

Most frequently there is a slight increase in the blood platelets above normal, but this may be excessive, or in some instances the numbers may be reduced, sometimes to a marked degree. The latter change usually prevails in the more acute and terminal, stages of the disease and is often associated with a hemorrhagic tendency. Occasionally an experienced observer may detect fragments of megakaryocytes in the blood.

An anemia is an almost constant finding at some stage during the course of every case of leukemia. It is usually normocytic and normochromic in nature, since almost always the mean corpuscular volume, mean corpuscular hemoglobin and mean corpuscular hemoglobin concentration are within normal limits. At the onset or after spontaneous or therapeutically induced remissions, it is often mild or may be absent. The general condition of the patient usually parallels the level of the red blood cell count and hemoglobin percentage. It is generally accepted that the anemia is of the myelophthisic type which results from the encroachment of the hyperplastic myeloid tissue in the bone marrow on the red blood cell-forming elements, causing a diminished rate of erythrocyte production. Occasionally, the anemia may be due in part to an increased destruction of erythrocytes and this has been attributed to a secondary hypersplenism. In the bone marrow there often remain areas of erythrocytic activity which as a compensatory mechanism may account for the presence of reticulocytes and nucleated red blood cells in the circulating blood.

Prognosis. Not a single well authenticated case of granulocytic leukemia has been observed in which a cure has actually been proved. It is known, however, that about 8 per cent of patients will undergo spontaneous remissions of a moderate degree, lasting for a few months to several years. Moffitt and Lawrence collected a group of 10 patients from the literature who have survived for intervals between nine and nineteen years. In a series of 129 patients treated with roentgen therapy and radioactive phosphorus (P^{32}) by Lawrence and his associates, there was an average survival period of 3.7 years from the onset of symptoms, and 33 patients, or 25.5 per cent of the total group, were still alive at the end of five years or longer. The longest survivor was living eleven years after the onset of the disease. These results are somewhat better than the previously accepted statement that the average length of life of patients with chronic granulocytic leukemia was between two and one half and three and one half years from the onset of the disease, and that treatment prolonged life only about six months.

It should be emphasized, however, that the benefit derived from treatment is not solely in increasing the length of life, although with the newer therapeutic agents the outlook for this is more encouraging. Undoubtedly it is of greatest benefit in the control of symptoms and the restoration of the patient to apparent health for considerable periods of time. It is fair to state that irradiation, either with roentgen ray or radioactive phosphorus, will improve markedly at least 75 to 85 per cent of patients with the chronic form of the disease. The benefit is such that it will permit them to live efficient and comfortable lives for 50 to 75 per cent of the period between the beginning of treatment and death from the disorder.

It is not possible to predict which patients will have the most favorable responses. The results attained are better when treatment is applied at a time when the earliest indications for it appear, although the effects when used later in the course of the disease are worth while. This uncertainty is because the degree of success depends on (1) the selective action of the therapeutic agent on the disordered cell growth, and (2) the ability of the individual patient to resume normal cell activity and differentiation when unrestrained growth has been checked by therapeutic measures.

Eventually there comes a time when irradiation produces little benefit. Emaciation develops, fever is often a prominent feature, the anemia becomes progressively worse, a hemorrhagic tendency frequently appears, and death usually ensues in a few weeks to several months after the onset of the period of decline. This stage of the disease is often associated with a striking increase in the myeloblasts of the circulating blood. The folic acid antagonists have been of little value in the treatment of patients with chronic leukemia, especially if they are 25 years of age or older. On the other hand, 6-mercaptopurine, when given in daily doses of 2.5 mg. per kilogram orally, may exert a favorable effect.

The unfavorable prognostic signs in myelogenous leukemia, as in any other form, are persistent high fever, continued loss of weight, a constantly and greatly elevated white blood cell count, progressive anemia, the presence of over 50 per cent of immature cells, and over 10 per cent of "blast" cells in the circulating blood, a decrease in blood platelets which is often associated with a hemorrhagic tendency, and failure to respond to roentgen therapy.

CHRONIC LYMPHOCYTIC LEUKEMIA

Symptoms and Signs. The onset is insidious, usually with one or two types of complaints. The patient observes a painless, nontender lymph node in the neck, axilla or groin, or the symptoms of an anemia develop, such as pallor, weakness, ease of fatigue, dyspnea and palpitation. Less frequently the initial symptom may be the occurrence of an abnormal tendency to bleed as indicated by hemorrhages from the mucous membranes or excessive bleeding following trauma. Occasionally an early symptom may be associated with a leukemic infiltration of the skin which causes itching and redness. In some instances the disease has been discovered as an incidental finding of a lymphocytosis when a routine blood examination has been done.

The commonly encountered findings on physical examination are associated with the anemia, the enlarged lymph glands and splenomegaly. Usually the patient appears pale and gives a history of recent increasing pallor and loss of weight. Evidences of abnormal bleeding are not ordinarily observed except during acute exacerbations of the disease and as a terminal event. The lymph nodes are most frequently enlarged in the cervical, axillary and inguinal regions. They vary in size from a pea to a hen's egg and are nontender, smooth, moderately firm and not adherent to each other. Usually they increase slowly in size unless reduced with radiation therapy; it is not uncommon to have them diminish in extent spontaneously, although it has been claimed that this may occur after an intercurrent infection. Roentgenograms may disclose an increase in the extent of the mediastinal lymph glands; rarely it is possible to palpate enlarged abdominal glands. Occasionally cases have been reported without enlargement of the lymph glands, but such a situation is exceedingly rare. The firm, nontender edge of the spleen is most often palpable 7 to 8 cm. below the left costal margin, but never is a huge size attained. The liver is usually moderately enlarged.

Blood Examination. It is ordinarily not difficult to conclude, from the blood examination alone, that a patient has chronic lymphocytic leukemia. This is because usually the total leukocyte count is increased to 30,000 to 100,000 per cubic millimeter and because 60 to 90 per cent of the cells resemble the normal small lymphocytes. In the early stages of lymphocytic leukemia the red blood cell count and hemoglobin percentage are normal, but eventually a normocytic normochromic anemia will develop, and it almost always reaches a severe degree as the disease advances. The number of blood platelets is characteristically decreased to a moderate extent, although they may at times show a slight increase. The difficulty in recognizing the disease arises when the total white blood cell count is normal or below normal, and the diagnosis from a study of the blood depends primarily on the recognition of the immature forms of lymphocytes. This is also puzzling in the acute phases when a large percentage of the cells are immature, since even experienced observers in hematology cannot always agree upon the criteria for differentiating immature lymphocytes from myeloblasts. Although the various stages of the myeloid cells are easily recognized, this is not true of the lymphocyte series. In general, the immature lymphocyte differs from the fully developed form in that the former is more commonly a large cell with a comparatively large nucleus; some believe that the nuclear pattern serves to differentiate it from the myeloblast. It is generally accepted that the degree of basophilia of the cytoplasm reflects the age of the lymphocyte series, and that young lymphocytes and lymphoblasts have a more basophilic cytoplasm.

There is a marked diminution or almost complete absence of monocytes, polymorphonuclear neutrophils, eosinophils and basophils in the circulating blood.

The Basal Metabolic Rate in Chronic Leukemia. The basal metabolic rate in untreated patients with either chronic granulocytic or lymphocytic leukemia may be elevated above normal limits, although the increase is moderate, usually varying between $+20$ and $+30$; occasionally the elevation may be more extreme, reaching levels as high as $+70$ or $+80$. It should be recognized that some of the important manifestations of the disease depend on an increased basal metabolic rate. These are dyspnea, tachycardia, sensation of increased body warmth, excessive sweating, intolerance to heat and loss of weight. These symptoms, however, are never as conspicuous as they are in patients with toxic goiter who have a similarly elevated basal metabolic rate. Often in leukemia the level of the basal metabolic rate is a more accurate index of the clinical condition of the patient than either the white blood cell count or the percentage of immature myeloid cells in the circulating blood. High estimations which persist despite irradiation suggest a poor prognosis.

The cause of the increased basal metabolic rate is not definitely known, but it is considered to be due in large part to the increased consumption of oxygen by the leukemic cells throughout the body. An accelerated rate of destruction of these cells may also be a factor of importance in this connection. The hypermetabolism differs from that observed in patients with hyperthyroidism, as in leukemia there is no associated increase in the protein-bound iodine, and the radioactive iodine uptake of the thyroid gland in leukemia is normal. When the basal metabolic rate is increased in leukemia, there is a decrease in the serum cholesterol.

Prognosis. Much which has been said in regard to the prognosis in chronic granulocytic leukemia may also be applied to the chronic lymphocytic form of the disease. The outlook in the latter variety is slightly better in my experience, especially in older persons, if care is taken to eliminate patients with chronic lymphosarcoma leukemia, which is sometimes erroneously regarded as the lymphocytic type, in whom the prognosis is relatively poor.

The average length of life in patients with chronic lymphocytic leukemia, from the onset of symptoms, is usually given as 3.5 years, and it is generally stated that roentgen therapy may prolong life for about six months. More recently, Lawrence and his associates have reported that in a group of 100 patients with this form of the disease, the average length of life was 3.69 years, *but 24 of the 100 patients were still living.* Hence the ultimate duration of life in this series will be even longer. Moreover, 35 per cent of the patients lived five years or longer, and 10 per cent eight years or more.

Undoubtedly a small percentage of patients with the disease may go into a spontaneous remission and live in comparatively good health for several months or years. Fifteen patients who have lived for periods varying from ten to twenty-five years have been collected from the literature by Moffitt and his associates. There can be no question, therefore, that some patients with or without treatment, may survive for a long time.

The unfavorable prognostic indications are essentially the same in chronic lymphocytic leukemia as those given for patients with chronic granulocytic leukemia.

Treatment of Chronic Leukemia. Since chronic leukemia, regardless of the type, invariably terminates fatally, any treatment now available must be discussed from the standpoints of its palliative value, the effect it may have on the prolongation of life, and the promise it provides for future therapeutic developments. The following therapeutic agents are now used: (1) roentgen ray therapy, (2) radioactive phosphorus (P^{32}), (3) urethane, (4) blood transfusions, (5) antibiotics. Folic acid antagonists are of value only in the treatment of acute leukemia in persons under the age of 25 or 30 years; likewise 6-mercaptopurine, although it may be of some benefit in patients with chronic leukemia, is of greater use in the acute leukemias. Nitrogen mustard, and also the similarly acting triethylene melamine (TEM), while somewhat helpful in the treatment of the leukemias, especially the lymphatic variety, are of greater use in Hodgkin's disease.

Roentgen Ray Therapy. This is the treatment of choice in most patients with chronic leukemia. The following conclusions in regard to it, in my opinion, are justified: (1) Roentgen therapy is valueless, in fact harmful, in patients with acute leukemia and most of those who have the subacute varieties. (2) In patients with chronic granulocytic leukemia total body irradiation ("spray") is the most satisfactory form of treatment, but localized therapy over the spleen may be used when gross splenomegaly is present, or if symptoms are referable to that organ. (3) In chronic lymphocytic leukemia the localized form of treatment is preferable. (4) Patients should usually be treated when symptoms appear or when the white blood cell count is elevated to 40,000 per cubic millimeter or higher. In general, the dosage should be regulated so that roentgen sickness does not appear. Usually this amounts to 50 to 100 roentgens when applied locally every other day. When total body irradiation is used, a dose of 15 to 20 roentgens is given daily or every other day.

Radioactive Phosphorus (P^{32}). This form of irradiation is of no value in the treatment of acute leukemia or lymphosarcoma. It is useful in chronic granulocytic leukemia, and is comparable in effect to total body irradiation with roentgen rays. It is much less useful in patients with lymphocytic leukemia but can be employed when the disease is present without demonstrable localized areas of involvement. It has wide tissue dispersion and a prolonged effect, and there is a high selective uptake of the element by the rapidly growing cells of the hematopoietic system.

The dosage of radioactive phosphorus is variable, and the hazards of overdosage, such as the risk of damage to normal tissue with resulting thrombopenia, leukopenia and anemia, should be kept in mind. A dosage of 1 to 2 millicuries intravenously a week until the desired effect has been attained has been suggested by Lawrence. It has been our custom to give 5 to 7 millicuries intravenously and repeat the dose in six to eight weeks if necessary. It has not been claimed that radioactive phosphorus produces better therapeutic results than roentgen irradiation, but, if the facilities are available, it is a convenient method of treatment, and no irradiation sickness results. The indications for its use are the same as with roentgen therapy.

Urethane. The use of urethane, or ethyl carbamate, is of value in the treatment of chronic granulocytic leukemia and plasmocytic myeloma but is of little benefit in the treatment of chronic lymphocytic leukemia or any of the acute types. It may be used in mild and early cases of the disease, and in the hope that it will prolong remissions induced by roentgen therapy. When given in enteric-coated tablets of 0.3 gm. three times daily, and the total dose increased 0.3 gm. a day until a total dosage of 3 gm. is reached, the leukocyte count will begin to fall within two to four weeks. The maintenance dose is variable, but in general it should be between 1 and 2 gm. daily, which is the amount to be given when the white blood cell count falls to approximately normal. Anorexia, nausea and vomiting may be troublesome symptoms and necessitate an adjustment of the dosage. It is possible to give the same amount by intravenous injection or by rectal suppositories as is given orally. Like all forms of treatment for this disease, its use is potentially hazardous, and patients should be kept under observation for evidence of overtreatment, especially leukopenia and thrombopenia.

Blood Transfusions. Blood transfusions should be given freely to patients with chronic leukemia in an attempt to maintain the hemoglobin level of the circulating blood at 11 to 12 gm. per 100 cc. of blood. Although effective treatment of the disease usually causes the anemia to disappear, this may require some time. Hence at the beginning of treatment, time may be saved by the use of one or more blood transfusions in order to bring the hemoglobin level rapidly to normal.

Antibiotics. In many patients, especially if the leukemia is of the acute or subacute variety, ulcerative lesions appear in the mucous membranes, especially of the mouth, but occasionally in the rectum and vagina. When this condition develops, it should be treated energetically and promptly with intramuscular injections of penicillin or other antibiotics, depending upon the nature of the infection.

ACUTE LEUKEMIA

Types of Acute Leukemia. In a fifteen-year period we observed 168 cases of acute leukemia at the Simpson Memorial Institute of the University of Michigan. In our opinion it has been possible to conclude with reasonable accuracy that at least six types of the condition have been observed: the myeloblastic, myelomonocytic, lymphosarcoma cell, lymphoblastic and histiomonocytic. Although there was not a great deal of difference in the incidence of each type, the myeloblastic was the most common, and the histiomonocytic the rarest. It should be admitted, however, that in some instances all of the white blood cells may be of such a primitive type that the acute leukemias can only be classified as the stem cell or hemocytoblastic type.

Symptoms and Signs. The onset of acute leukemia is usually abrupt with the development of symptoms often considered to be due to a "cold" or upper respiratory infection, an ulcerative stomatitis or acute tonsillitis. There is ordinarily no suspicion as to the serious basis for the complaints until attention is directed toward the rather sudden appearance of pallor indicative of a rapidly developing anemia or an unusual degree of prostration out of proportion to the minor nature of the initial symptoms. Fever, which may be associated with outspoken chills or chilly sensations, is almost invariably present in the advanced stages, but an increase in body temperature may also occur early.

A spontaneous hemorrhagic tendency is commonly present and is a manifestation of a secondary thrombocytopenic purpura with the characteristic decrease in blood platelets. It may be one of the early indications of the sinister nature of the patient's illness. Bleeding occurs into the skin and from the mucous membranes of the mouth, the gums or the nose, into the fundi of the eyes and the brain, from the gastrointestinal tract, and the uterus. The first evidence of the disease may be profuse hemorrhage following the extraction of a tooth, removal of the tonsils, or from minor injuries. Although a slight tendency to bleed may be noted early in the illness, the more extensive hemorrhagic manifestations occur late as a rule, and their appearance is usually an ominous sign.

Blood Examination. The characteristic change in the blood is the presence of a large number of mononuclear, nongranular cells which are usually either myeloblasts or lymphoblasts; rarely are they monoblasts. Frequently almost all the cells are of a uniform, immature type, and confusion arises as to their exact identity. Few, if any, intermediate cells representing stages between the mature and the primitive forms may be present, a fact which makes difficult the recognition of the predominant primitive cell type. It then becomes necessary to depend upon the cytologic characteristics of the myelocyte, lymphocyte and monocyte in order to classify the type of acute leukemia from which the patient is suffering. This is not possible in all instances even by experienced hematologists; in such cases, therefore, it is necessary to be content with the diagnosis of acute leukemia of hemocytoblastic or undetermined type. The total number of leukocytes, in the various types of the disease, is most frequently between 15,000 and 30,000 per cubic millimeter; rarely does the count exceed 100,000. At the onset it is commonly below 8000, and it may be 2000 to 3000 or less.

The characteristic alteration in the circulating blood in acute granulocytic leukemia is the presence of immature cells of the myeloid series. As previously mentioned, almost all the white corpuscles may be of the myeloblast type, which closely resembles both the lymphoblast and the monoblast. There is a parallelism between the number of myeloblasts and the acuteness of the disease. In the subacute granulocytic variety the intermediate cell stages, promyelocytes and myelocytes, are present, and classification can be made without difficulty. In acute lymphocytic leukemia some of the cells may be in the intermediate stage between the lymphoblast and the mature lymphocyte. As the large cells represent the more immature lymphocyte, it is this type that predominates in acute lymphatic leukemia, whereas the small lymphocyte is the commonly encountered cell in chronic lymphatic leukemia.

A severe anemia almost always develops in the acute leukemias in which the red blood cells may fall to 1,000,000 per cubic millimeter or less; in some cases there may be nucleated red blood cells, and an increase in reticulocytes in the circulating blood. The blood platelets are almost always reduced in number.

Prognosis. The disease frequently has a fulminating course and terminates fatally within a relatively brief interval. If untreated, more than three fourths of the patients succumb within eight weeks after the appearance of the initial symptoms, and about one fifth die after an illness of two or three weeks. There is no authentic record that a patient with true acute leukemia has ever recovered. Occasionally the disorder will change spontaneously from the acute to the subacute or chronic phase, but this is rare, and even then the duration of life is ordinarily not greater than six months.

Occasionally, a patient with acute leukemia may develop a spontaneous remission which may persist for variable periods of two to twenty-one months. At these times, such patients, without treatment of any kind, may become ambulatory and have few if any complaints. Furthermore, the splenomegaly and hepatomegaly may recede completely, and all evidence of the disease disappear from the peripheral blood.

Treatment. Treatment has had little to offer in this disease until recently. It should be emphasized that roentgen therapy, radioactive phosphorus and urethane are contraindicated since they may do more harm than good. There are five forms of treatment which are useful, namely: (1) blood transfusions, (2) antibiotics, (3) folic acid antagonists, (4) 6-mercaptopurine, (5) cortisone and ACTH.

Blood transfusions should be given repeatedly in an attempt to maintain the hemoglobin percentage and red blood cell count at normal levels. The antibiotic drugs should be used freely to control infection of the mucous membranes which invariably develops and combat secondary infection elsewhere.

In 1948 Farber and his associates introduced the folic acid antagonists in the treatment of the acute leukemias, and, more recently (1953), Burchenal and his associates have reported encouraging results from another anti-metabolite, 6-mercaptopurine. These preparations will cause a remission in 30 to 50 per cent of all cases of acute leukemia in children and adults under 25 years of age. The latter drug, 6-mercaptopurine, is of more value than folic acid antagonists in adults over 25 years of age but is much less effective in children.

The folic acid antagonist, 4-amino pteroylglutamic acid (Aminopterin), has been used most frequently. It is given intramuscularly or orally in doses of 1 or 2 mg. daily for three days, and then 1 mg. a day for ten to fourteen days, followed by an average maintenance dose of 1 mg. three times a week. Improvement is shown by control of many symptoms, regression of the enlarged lymph nodes, liver and spleen, a loss of the hemorrhagic tendency and a favorable change in the peripheral blood and the bone marrow. Similar results may be obtained by the use of A-Methopterin in an initial oral dosage of 5 to 10 mg. daily for three days, followed by 5 mg. a day for 10 to 14 days. The average maintenance dose is 5 mg. three times a week.

6-Mercaptopurine is useful in the treatment of acute leukemia and in some cases of the chronic granulocytic form of the disease. It is given orally in a daily dosage of 2.5 mg. per kilo of body weight, and after suitable improvement has occurred which is usually in one to three weeks, the drug may be continued in an oral maintenance dosage which varies from 50 mg. every other day to 100 mg. daily.

Two facts should be emphasized about 6-mercaptopurine and the folic antagonists. First, the patient may become refractory to one, and also to ACTH and cortisone, and not the other; and second, the effect of the drugs must be checked by repeated examinations of the peripheral blood, and in some instances the bone marrow, as they may cause a depressant action on the marrow with a resultant anemia, leukopenia and thrombocytopenia. Furthermore, ulcerative lesions of the mouth and bleeding from the gastrointestinal tract may follow the use of the folic acid antagonists.

Forty to 100 mg. of ACTH or 100 to 300 mg. of cortisone may be given in divided doses daily for two to three weeks during which time the patient should be placed on a low sodium diet. Frequently, a striking remission is induced with a favorable change in the bone marrow. Unfortunately, these remissions last on the average only about six weeks, and eventually the patient becomes resistant to this form of therapy.

MONOCYTIC LEUKEMIA

Within recent years it has been recognized that a leukemia may occur which differs from other types in that there is a significant increase in the cells of the monocyte series in the circulating blood. The characteristic pathologic change is an infiltration of the organs of the body, especially the spleen and the liver, with monocytic cells resembling those of the blood.

There is no agreement concerning the origin of the monocytes, but there is strong evidence that they are an independent strain of cells. Undoubtedly a leukemia does occur which has acute, subacute, chronic, aleukemic and subleukemic phases and in which the chief characteristic in common is the presence of an increased number of monocytes in the blood, some of which may be immature in type. A distinctive clinical feature is the occurrence of oral lesions such as gingivitis associated with swelling of the gums and a tendency of the teeth to become submerged in the gingivae. Purpura and bleeding from the mucous membranes with various other types of skin lesions occur in somewhat less than 20 per cent of the cases. Enlargement of the liver and spleen may be observed, but is uncommon and, when present, is usually of slight extent. The course is usually rapid, and a fatal termination commonly occurs within a period of months.

Downey recognizes two varieties of monocytic leukemia—the Schilling (histiomonocytic) type, and the Naegeli (myelomonocytic) type. In the former the monocytes are derived from the reticuloendothelial system; in the latter they develop presumably from the myeloblasts, thereby making this variety a variant of myelogenous leukemia.

Blood Examination. In the histiomonocytic type of leukemia the white blood cell count is usually between 25,000 and 100,000 per cubic millimeter, although extreme variations may be from 2000 or 3000 to several hundred thousand. The monocytes usually make up 50 per cent of all white blood cells, occasionally 90 per cent. In patients with the chronic form of the disease almost all the monocytes resemble the normal adult form. The monoblast is described as a cell having a nucleus with a density similar to that of the lymphoblast and myeloblast. As the cell develops, the bluish shade of the cytoplasm in films becomes less deeply stained and finally resembles the light blue mottled cytoplasm of the mature cell.

In the myelomonocytic type of the disease the distinctive feature is the presence of both immature cells of the myeloid series, that is, myeloblasts and myelocytes, in association with monoblasts and less immature cells of this series.

LESS COMMON VARIETIES OF LEUKEMIA AND ALLIED PATHOLOGIC STATES

SUBLEUKEMIC (ALEUKEMIC) LEUKEMIA

A subleukemic leukemia is defined as one in which the leukocyte count is below 15,000 per cubic millimeter yet the diagnosis can be made from the presence of abnormal cells in the circulating blood; an aleukemic leukemia is one with leukocyte count below 15,000 and often below 4000 per cubic millimeter, but the abnormal cell types are absent or present in such small numbers that the diagnosis cannot be made from an examination of the peripheral blood. The diagnosis of aleukemic leukemia must be made from a study of the marrow and this is usually also true in the case of the subleukemic leukemias.

The clinical picture in such patients depends to a certain extent upon the variety of subleukemic leukemia present. There are variable degrees of splenomegaly and lymphadenopathy, but in some cases these findings may be absent. The most common clinical features are as follows: (1) a progressive normocytic normochromic anemia, often reaching a severe grade, associated with which are the customary complaints of weakness, ease of fatigue, dyspnea, and palpitation on exertion. Aplastic anemia is the condition most commonly confused with subleukemic leukemia, but it is necessary also to distinguish from it pernicious anemia, Hodgkin's disease, myelophthisic anemia resulting from metastasis in bones, and achrestic anemia. (2) The anemia of this disease is refractory to all forms of treatment. Aside from the temporary improvement following blood transfusions, none is observed except that associated with rarely occurring spontaneous remissions. (3) The total white blood cell count is frequently below 4000 per cubic millimeter and may be as low as 1000 or 2000. In almost every instance there are immature white blood cells present in the circulating blood, but since they may be scarce, and the total white blood cell count is usually diminished, they are easily overlooked even by the expert hematologist. It is not uncommon for the less experienced to regard the myeloblasts, which may be present, as lymphocytes. It should be emphasized that careful examination in almost all instances will show that the differential formula of the white blood cells is abnormal. (4) Sternal puncture is exceedingly useful in establishing the diagnosis, for it may show the predominating cells of the marrow to be myeloblasts, lymphoblasts or monoblasts. In rare instances, however, the sternal marrow may not be infiltrated with abnormal cells. The examination, therefore, is of the greatest value in demonstrating positive evidence of the disease; it should be understood that a normal sternal marrow, as determined by sternal aspiration, does not necessarily eliminate the condition as a diagnostic possibility. (5) It is important to emphasize that there is commonly a decrease in the circulating blood platelets which may or may not be associated with purpuric manifestations such as bleeding from the mucous membranes, retinal hemorrhage and petechiae.

One should always consider the diagnosis of subleukemic leukemia in the presence of any one or a combination of the following: (1) a leukopenia with or without an associated normocytic or macrocytic anemia; (2) an unexplained lymphadenopathy or splenomegaly; (3) fever without obvious explanation; (4) tumefaction of the gums; (5) a hemorrhagic tendency; (6) certain characteristic skin lesions; (7) vague pain in the bones and about the joints; and (8) bone tenderness, especially if it involves the sternum.

LYMPHOSARCOMA CELL LEUKEMIA

Lymphosarcoma cell leukemia is a definite clinical entity characterized by the presence of lymphosarcoma cells in the blood stream. These vary in size from 12 to 14 microns in diameter, and have a sparse but deeply basophilic cytoplasm. The most striking identifying feature of the cell is the nucleolus, which is usually single, eccentrically placed and light blue in color. When stained with cresyl blue and Wright's stain, it is surrounded by an intensely staining, conspicuous blue-black rim.

Such a type of leukemia arises when lymph tissue undergoes sarcomatous change which at first is a localized new growth. Eventually the neoplastic cells escape from the confines of the surrounding tissue and appear in the blood stream. The earliest evidence of the disease is usually enlargement of the lymph glands or spleen, or symptoms referable to the anemia. Throughout the course of the disease, anemia, fever, hemorrhage and infection are the most conspicuous features. The disorder occurs most commonly in

males; it may appear at any age. Frequently the condition manifests itself at a time when the blood does not exhibit abnormal changes. It may be months or even several years before the lymphosarcoma cells invade the blood stream. When this occurs, the course is usually rapid, although beneficial effects may follow the cautious use of roentgen therapy. About one half of the patients die within one year after onset of symptoms or discovery of the tumor. Patients with this condition are usually regarded as suffering from lymphocytic leukemia; the careful exclusion of such cases will extend the average duration of life of patients with lymphocytic leukemia to four or five years, which is longer than usually stated.

In almost all instances the earliest evidence of the condition is a painless enlargement of the cervical lymph glands, although the initial change may be in the other superficial lymph glands of the body. In about one quarter of our cases, however, the first clinical manifestations were those associated with an anemia, namely, weakness, ease of fatigue, pallor, dyspnea and palpitation. Other less commonly occurring symptoms which may be present early in the course of the disease are evidences of infection of the oral cavity and throat, fever and a tendency to abnormal bleeding.

In a group of 70 patients with the malady the blood was found to be subleukemic in 63 per cent, and in about one half of these it was in this state when first observed. From 30 to 50 per cent of the white blood cells are usually of the lymphosarcoma type, but occasionally as many as 98 per cent are of this variety.

LEUKEMOID REACTIONS

It is now appreciated that there are a considerable number of conditions, in addition to true leukemia, in which immature white blood cells may appear in the circulating blood in association with a normal, increased or decreased leukocyte count. Such a blood picture is called a leukemoid reaction. This highly important differentiation can usually be accomplished by continued clinical observation, repeated blood examinations and a study of the sternal marrow.

As the hematopoietic tissues in infancy and childhood are more likely to react abnormally to various stimuli, especially infections, caution should be used before concluding that the hematologic changes in the blood of a young person are of a leukemic nature. Confusion is more likely to arise with the alterations observed in the acute leukemias. In this condition three important and almost constantly occurring changes are helpful in differentiating it from a leukemoid reaction; in leukemia (1) 60 to 70 per cent or more of the circulating white blood corpuscles are of the uniformly large, immature "blast" type; (2) a normocytic or slightly macrocytic anemia, often of severe grade, usually develops during the course of the disease; (3) the blood platelets are almost always reduced in number.

Lymphatic leukemoid reactions are observed in a number of diseases, including pertussis, typhoid fever and infectious mononucleosis. The last condition, which is characterized by complaints referable to the upper respiratory passages, fever, lymphadenopathy, a palpable spleen in 50 per cent of the cases, and atypical lymphocytes in the circulating blood, should receive most careful consideration in all young persons in whom the diagnosis of leukemia is a possibility. Of considerable assistance in the differential diagnosis is the heterophile antibody reaction, which is usually positive in infectious mononucleosis and is negative in leukemia.

Leukemoid reactions of the myeloid type are observed occasionally in almost any type of pyogenic infection. A pyonephrosis in which the infected kidney may be mistaken for the spleen when it is on the left side, if associated with a leukemic blood picture, may present a most puzzling diagnostic problem. Immature leukocytes may also be present in nonpyogenic infections such as subacute bacterial endocarditis and tuberculosis. Similar changes may be observed in various hemolytic anemias, of which congenital hemolytic icterus, sickle cell anemia, and acute hemolytic anemia are examples. Other blood dyscrasias, including pernicious anemia, especially at the beginning of a remission, polycythemia vera, erythroblastic anemia and anemia following hemorrhage, may be associated with such blood changes. A special group in which a leukemoid blood picture may be present consists of pathologic processes which involve the bones and bone marrow. Examples of such conditions are metastases from malignant processes, plasmocytic myeloma and osteosclerosis. Lastly, immature white blood cells may be noted in the blood stream of patients in diabetic coma, in poisoning with mustard gas, mercury and phenylhydrazine, and occasionally in cases in which the cause cannot be ascertained.

CHLOROMA

This disease is a rare variety of leukemia characterized by an invasive tumor-like growth of greenish color in various organs and tissues of the body, and by changes in the blood simulating closely those seen in acute granulocytic leukemia. Often many of the white blood cells are of the mononuclear nongranular type which commonly occur in acute leukemia, and the same difficulty arises in classifying these changes into the lymphocytic or granulocytic variety. Most present-day observers believe that they are myeloid cells.

The greenish tumors may be observed in any tissue in which leukemic infiltrations are known to occur. The bones of the skull are involved with relative frequency; a tumor of the orbital fossa causing exophthalmos was present in 11 of 18 cases collected by Dock and Warthin. Tumors may occur in the lymph nodes, spleen, kidneys and many other organs and tissues. The bone marrow may have a uniformly greenish color or circumscribed areas of pigmentation.

The condition is observed more frequently in males than in females and has its greatest incidence in childhood, adolescence or young adult life. It is similar to acute leukemia in that it has a brief course which usually terminates fatally in a few weeks or months. All types of therapy which have been used are ineffective.

PLASMACYTOMAS, PLASMA CELL LEUKEMIA AND MULTIPLE MYELOMA

A neoplasm in which the cell type is a plasma cell may occur in the body in three forms: (1) as a localized or metastasizing new growth which may be found in the bones, the upper respiratory passages, the conjunctivas, the cornea, the pleura and elsewhere; (2) one which is localized especially in the bones, causing destructive lesions, with the production of the syndrome of plasmocytic myeloma; (3) in some instances with a diffuse infiltration in the liver, spleen, lymph glands and bone marrow, associated with an anemia and an increase in the white blood cell count of the circulating blood to over 50,000 per cubic millimeter, a large percentage of the cells being of the plasma cell type. In some instances there may be osseous lesions, in others, extraosseous le sions, but in others only the diffuse infiltration of the various organs similar in all respects to the leukemic infiltrations observed in granulocytic and lymphocytic leukemias, except that the infiltrating cells are of the plasma cell type. Such a condition can properly be designated as a true plasma cell leukemia, such as reported by Patek and Castle, and others. In plasmocytic myeloma and patients with extraosseous plasmacytoma there may be a few plasma cells in the circulating blood; hence these conditions could properly be considered as subleukemic plasma cell leukemias. It appears logical to regard a plasma cell tumor as a pathologic entity, and the different forms as variants of the same disease process.

PLASMOCYTIC MYELOMA (MULTIPLE MYELOMA)

This disorder should be considered a variant of a plasmacytoma with osseous involvement. It may be defined as a malignant plasmacytoma arising in the bone marrow which tends to occur in persons after the fifth decade. It is usually characterized by pain in the back and weakness, destructive osseous lesions involving especially the bones of the trunk, pathologic fractures, a normocytic or macrocytic anemia of moderate degree, and the presence, in many cases, of a peculiar type of protein (Bence Jones) in the urine.

Symptoms and Signs. The condition is observed twice as commonly in males as in females. Almost all cases occur after the age of 40 years. Pain of a vague, intermittent, shifting type, often referable to the spine, is commonly the earliest evidence of the disease. As the condition progresses, this frequently is a severe and dominant symptom. Tumors and pathologic fractures, usually in bones containing red marrow, are common. Changes in the spine causing compression of the spinal cord with its resultant neurologic manifestations are not rare complications.

Blood. Although the anemia which is almost always present may be normocytic, it is slightly macrocytic in a majority of patients. The leukocyte count is ordinarily normal, slightly elevated or diminished, and the differential formula is usually not disturbed, or may reveal only an occasional abnormal white blood cell. In recent years it has been shown that small numbers of multiple myeloma or atypical plasma cells may be identified in the circulating blood by an expert hematologist in over half of the cases.

Their presence, therefore, is of some importance from a diagnostic standpoint.

A finding of great diagnostic importance is the presence of Bence Jones protein in the urine, which appears in about two thirds of the cases. It may occur occasionally in the urine of patients with leukemia and polycythemia. This protein precipitates at temperatures of 50° to 60° C.; further heating causes it to go into solution at about boiling, and on cooling it reappears. Its presence appears to be limited to pathologic conditions attacking the bone or bone marrow. Decreased renal function is present in about one fourth of the patients. There may be a pronounced hyperproteinemia, as indicated by plasma protein determinations, which are often found to be 10 gm. per 100 cc. of plasma, or above; figures twice as high as this have been reported. This may be due entirely to an increase in any one of the globulin fractions. Study of the blood serum and urine by paper electrophoresis is often of great help in establishing the diagnosis. Autohemagglutination, or spontaneous clumping of the erythrocytes, occurs in some cases. This accounts for the tendency to striking rouleau formation and an accelerated sedimentation rate. Serum calcium is frequently elevated to levels of 12 to 16 mg. per 100 cc., but the serum inorganic phosphates are usually normal.

In addition to those already mentioned, there are two diagnostic procedures which are of great importance: (1) sternal puncture, which usually reveals the presence of an excessive number of plasma cells, some of which are immature cells, and (2) roentgen ray examination, which demonstrates the characteristic punched-out areas, without evidence of bone regeneration, in the ribs, spine, clavicles, skull and the shoulder and pelvic girdles. It should be emphasized, however, that in about 15 per cent of the patients the only pathologic finding radiographically is a diffuse osteoporosis.

Prognosis and Treatment. The disease usually terminates fatally after an average length of time of two to three years. Occasionally the course is prolonged with periods of remission and exacerbation. Roentgen ray exposures over the areas of osseous involvement may give worthwhile relief from pain, and blood transfusions are indicated to combat the anemia. Loge and Rundles report that the administration of urethane (ethyl carbamate) will control the fever, skeletal pain and acute symptoms within two to four weeks. In addition, the blood values improve greatly toward normal. Though apparently the acute symptoms may be controlled to a certain extent, the long-term results are yet to be determined. These patients received from 4 to 6 gm. of urethane orally daily for the first three or four weeks of therapy. Then the dose was reduced to 2 gm. daily or completely suspended on account of the resultant leukopenia. My own observations on the use of urethane have been favorable. Certainly the drug merits a trial in all patients with the disorder, but the possibility should be kept in mind that a severe leukopenia makes necessary the observation of the patient's blood and regulation of the dosage accordingly. A fairly high proportion of patients experience nausea and vomiting from the medication. It may be given by suppositories or intravenously in the same amounts as orally, to avert this complication.

The use of ACTH in doses of 25 mg. four times daily, or cortisone, 75 mg. every 6 hours for ten days to two weeks, with a gradual reduction of dosage and elimination in several weeks, may give prompt temporary relief of pain, and some evidence of a reversion of the plasma protein levels toward normal limits.

MYELOID METAPLASIA OF THE SPLEEN

This condition simulates chronic granulocytic leukemia as there is a progressive gross enlargement of the spleen, a moderate anemia, a slight elevation or depression of the leukocyte count with immature white and nucleated red blood cells in the peripheral blood. The blood picture may be almost identical with that of chronic granulocytic leukemia; in some patients, however, there is leukopenia, thrombocytopenia and evidence of a hemolytic anemia probably associated with a superimposed hypersplenism.

The diagnosis of myeloid metaplasia is made during life by finding evidence of active hematopoiesis in material obtained by splenic aspiration, with cytologic evidence in the sternal aspirate that the marrow is normal, aplastic, hyperplastic or fibrotic, but not characteristic of leukemia. When these findings are present, along with leukemoid changes in the circulating blood, the diagnosis is suggested.

The etiology of the disorder is uncertain. Until recently the prevailing view has been that the initial change is a depression of bone marrow function from unknown causes and that the extramedullary blood formation is compensatory in nature. In recent years, however, it is more generally accepted that this condition is a proliferative one involving the primitive mesenchymal precursors from which the hematopoietic system arises.

Some patients survive eight to ten years or longer but occasionally one is said to have had a rapidly fatal course. Splenectomy, previously considered to be rigidly contraindicated, is now thought to be harmless, and in some patients with thrombocytopenia or hemolytic anemia or both, it may be followed by improvement. A much better course to follow, however, is to give cortisone or ACTH, along with repeated blood transfusions. If improvement does not follow, then the cautious application of the roentgen ray may be tried in order to diminish the size of the spleen, and possibly improve the patient's general condition.

MYCOSIS FUNGOIDES

This condition is usually associated with Hodgkin's disease but it may be observed in patients with lymphocytic leukemia. Usually in such patients there is a premycotic interval of several years during which the patient has a desquamative dermatitis with pruritus. At the end of this time, the typical mycotic lesions occur in the form of multiple cutaneous tumors which vary in size from a pea to a child's head.

CYRUS C. STURGIS

References

Ardashnikov, S. N.: Genetics of Leukemia in Man. J. Hyg., 37:286, 1937.
Best, W. R., and Limarzi, L. R.: Age, Sex, Race and Hematologic Classification of 916 Leukemia Cases. J. Lab. & Clin. Med. 40:778, 1952.
Bethell, F. H.: Leukemia; Relative Incidence of Its Various Forms and Their Response to Radiation Therapy. Ann. Int. Med., 18:757, 1943.
Bierman, H. R.: Chemical Agents in Neoplastic Diseases. California Med., 78:44, 1953.
Farber, S.: The Effect of Therapy on the Life History and Biologic Behavior of Leukemia. Proc. Inst. Med. Chicago, 18:311, 1951.
Furth, J.: Recent Studies on the Etiology and Nature of Leukemia. Blood, 6:964, 1951.
Green, T. W., Conley, G. L., Ashburn, L. L., and Peters, H. R.: Splenectomy for Myeloid Metaplasia of the Spleen. New England J. Med., 248:211, 1953.
Harris, L. J.: Leukemia and Pregnancy. Canad. M. A. J., 68:234, 1953.

Lawrence, J. H., Dobson, R. L., Low-Beer, B. V. A., and Brown, B. R.: Chronic Myelogenous Leukemia. J.A.M.A., *136*:672, 1948.

Lawrence, J. H., Low-Beer, B. V. A., and Carpenter, J. W. J.: Chronic Lymphatic Leukemia. J.A.M.A., *140*:585, 1949.

Mettier, S. R., and Purviance, K.: Aleukemic Myelosis (Aleukemic Leukemia) with Special Reference to the Clinical Significance of the Myeloblast. Analysis of Twenty Cases. California & West. Med., *49*:296, 1938.

Osgood, E. E.: Monocytic Leukemia, Report of Six Cases and Review of One Hundred and Twenty-seven Cases. Arch. Int. Med., *59*:931, 1937.

———, and Seaman, A. J.: Treatment of Chronic Leukemias. J.A.M.A., *150*:1372, 1952.

Patek, A. J., and Castle, W. B.: Plasma Cell Leukemia. A Consideration of the Literature with the Report of a Case. Am. J. M. Sc., *191*:788, 1936.

Poncher, H. G., Waisman, H. A., Richmond, J. B., Limarzi, L. R., and Horak, O. A.: Acute Leukemia in Children with and without Folic Acid Antagonist. J. Pediatrics, *41*:377, 1952.

Snapper, I., Turner, L. B., and Moscovitz, H. L.: Multiple Myeloma. New York, Grune & Stratton, 1953.

Sturgis, C. C.: Some Aspects of the Leukemia Problem. J.A.M.A. *150*:1551, 1952.

Videbaek, A.: Heredity in Human Leukemia and Its Relation to Cancer. Copenhagen, Denmark, Eljnra Munksgaard Forlag, 1947; London, H. K. Lewis & Co., Ltd.

Diseases of the Cardiovascular System

PATHOLOGIC PHYSIOLOGY OF GENERALIZED CIRCULATORY FAILURE

An adequate blood supply is essential for the proper function of every organ and tissue of the body. When the circulation as a whole fails, as in heart disease or shock, none of the organs of the body functions normally. The fact that the disturbance in circulation affects every organ and tissue is easily overlooked, because in many tissues a partial loss of function does not produce striking clinical symptoms. Interference with the function of the muscles produces a much less dramatic effect than does the same degree of disturbance in the function of the brain.

Failure of the circulation as a whole occurs whenever the heart is unable to pump out sufficient blood to meet the metabolic requirements of the body. This may result simply from the inability of the heart to pump out the blood returned to it by the great veins (heart failure), or it may result from an inadequate venous return to the heart (peripheral circulatory failure).

In the first instance—*heart failure*—symptoms and signs are produced by the following two mechanisms (*a*) diminished blood flow to the various tissues of the body (forward heart failure); (*b*) accumulation of an excess amount of blood in the various organs, because the venous drainage becomes inadequate when the heart is unable to pump out the blood returned to it (backward heart failure). Although backward and forward failure must of necessity occur together, since the circulation is a closed system, the distinction is useful because certain symptoms result primarily from congestion, while other symptoms are produced by poor tissue nutrition.

The amount of blood pumped normally by the heart varies considerably from person to person. In the same patient it varies greatly with various physiologic and pathologic states. Exercise, eating, apprehension and epineph-rine increase the cardiac output; motionless standing decreases it. In a person with a normal heart the resting cardiac output will be decreased if the subject has myxedema, and increased if he has anemia, thyrotoxicosis, beriberi or an arteriovenous fistula. There are no absolute levels of the circulation above which circulatory failure does not occur and below which it always occurs. The amount of blood pumped must be considered in terms of the immediate needs of the body rather than as an absolute value. These considerations apply equally to congestive heart failure and peripheral circulatory failure.

In the natural history of slowly progressive congestive heart failure it is the rule rather than the exception for congestion and edema to occur during periods when the cardiac output is above the resting level. Edema develops during the day when the subject is active. The output is increased above the resting value, but is below the level that is reached by a normal heart.

During sleep the cardiac output falls from a subnormal exercising level to a normal value for rest. The output is now sufficient for the resting needs, and diuresis occurs. As the heart becomes weaker, signs and symptoms of congestive failure persist at rest. In these patients the cardiac output is consistently below the resting value unless complicating physiologic or pathologic states are present.

Patients with advanced pulmonary disease, anemia, thyrotoxicosis, beriberi and arteriovenous fistula have a high resting cardiac output. Circulatory failure usually develops before the resting cardiac output falls below the value for normal subject. The significant fact is the fall in cardiac output to a value below that found in the diseased state in the absence of heart failure.

Stimuli which normally cause a rise in cardiac output frequently cause a fall in output in congestive failure. The reverse is also seen, and stimuli which cause a fall in the normal subject cause a rise in the patient with failure. Any stimulus, such as exercise or excitement, which normally increases the output may decrease the output in a fatigued heart. As fatigue increases, the ability of the heart to empty decreases. Anything which decreases the activity of the patient and normally decreases the output may increase the output of the fatigued heart.

In uncomplicated heart failure which persists at rest, blood flow has been reduced in all areas where it has been studied. The reduction in splanchnic blood flow and cerebral blood flow is proportionate to the decrease in cardiac output, the reduction in renal blood flow much greater. Fasting splanchnic oxygen consumption is maintained at normal level by widening of atrioventricular oxygen difference. Cerebral oxygen consumption is slightly decreased. Data are not available for the kidney. The reduction in blood flow to the various areas studied is related to the change in cardiac output and does not correlate with changes in venous pressure.

In the second type of generalized failure of the circulation—*peripheral circulatory failure*—symptoms are produced primarily by the inadequate blood supply to the tissues or by a precipitous fall in arterial pressure. In peripheral circulatory failure the reduction of renal blood flow is out of proportion to the reduction in output. Data for other organs in man are not available. It is presumed that they would show the changes which occur in congestive failure.

Symptoms of Heart Failure. *Dyspnea.* The patient's term for dyspnea is "breathlessness" or "shortness of breath." Dyspnea is said to be present when the patient becomes conscious of his breathing. It is to be differentiated from rapid breathing (tachypnea), in which the patient may have no feeling of respiratory distress, and from the deep breathing of acidosis (hyperpnea). Because dyspnea is a subjective complaint, it cannot be correlated closely with objective signs of circulatory failure. An anxious, apprehensive and introspective patient will complain of shortness of breath when there are few objective signs of circulatory failure. On the other hand, a phlegmatic person may have advanced congestive failure before he becomes conscious of shortness of breath. Hence, by study of the circulation one cannot determine the extent to which a given persons will experience dyspnea.

Normal persons have dyspnea on *unusual exertion.* In a given normal subject breath-

lessness will appear whenever the tidal air exceeds a given portion of the vital capacity. At this point the accessory muscles of respiration are brought into action and the subject becomes aware that breathing is an effort. Thus dyspnea in normal persons is primarily dependent on a large increase in pulmonary ventilation. In patients with diminished vital capacity less exertion will produce breathlessness because an increase in pulmonary ventilation more quickly causes the tidal air to approach the vital capacity. Failure of the heart produces a decreased vital capacity by causing the lungs to become engorged, inelastic and edematous. As the vital capacity becomes progressively diminished, smaller and smaller increases in pulmonary ventilation will cause dyspnea.

The *severity* of dyspnea will depend, not only on the extent of the pulmonary engorgement and the resulting encroachment on the vital capacity, but also on the volume of air respired per minute. A patient with a moderate degree of pulmonary engorgement may have no dyspnea at rest, but when the volume of air required is increased by exercise, dyspnea may occur. Thus the factors which control the rate and depth of respiration play an important part in the pathogenesis of dyspnea. In cardiac patients who complain of dyspnea at rest, the vital capacity is usually reduced and the ventilation is increased.

It was believed heretofore that this increase in ventilation rate was the result of stimulation of the respiratory center by anoxemia or by an increase in the hydrogen ion concentration in the region of the respiratory center because of slow cerebral blood flow. Studies of the oxygen content, the carbon dioxide content and the hydrogen ion concentration of the arterial blood and the blood from the internal jugular vein showed, however, that in cases with moderate dyspnea there are no arterial anoxemia and no measurable decrease in cerebral blood flow. These observations stimulated the study of the reflex control of respiration, and it was conclusively demonstrated that most of the changes in ventilation which occurred in normal subjects during the day were of reflex rather than chemical origin. Reflexes originating from moving muscles, from emotional stimuli, from the lungs, the great vessels and the auricles have all been shown to influence the respiratory rate. In cardiac failure the increased ventilation with the resulting tendency toward alkalosis is produced by the reflex stimulation of respiration from the congested lungs and great vessels.

PATHOGENESIS OF PULMONARY CONGESTION AND EDEMA. There are two main factors in the pathogenesis of pulmonary congestion and edema in heart failure: (a) increase in pulmonary venous pressure, and (b) failure of the kidneys to excrete salt and water normally. Catheterization of the right heart has shown that in man the dyspnea of heart failure is accompanied by a rise in pulmonary capillary and pulmonary arterial pressures. The initial rise in pulmonary arterial pressure is the reflection of the rise in the pulmonary venous and capillary pressures. When the capillary pressure exceeds the osmotic pressure of the plasma proteins, the pulmonary arterial pressure begins to rise out of proportion to the rise in capillary pressures. A stimulus such as exertion, which normally causes a rise in cardiac output without a rise in pulmonary arterial pressure, produces a further increase in pulmonary arterial pressure and pulmonary venous pressure without the expected rise in cardiac output. This elevated pressure within the pulmonary capillaries causes increased transudation of fluid and accounts for the occurrence of acute pulmonary edema as induced by exercise or apprehension. The increase in the amount of blood in the lungs, with its attendant rise in venous pressure, occurs whenever the right ventricle pumps more blood into the pulmonary vessels than the left ventricle is able to remove (left heart failure). Such difficulty in transferring blood from the lungs may result either from interference with the filling of the left ventricle, as in mitral stenosis, or from the inability of the left ventricle to empty itself adequately with each contraction, as in the heart failure produced by hypertension, coronary artery disease, aortic insufficiency and aortic stenosis. It is important to remember that excess blood may accumulate in the lungs even when the output of the left ventricle is normal or increased. With fever, exercise, anemia, beriberi and thyrotoxicosis, signs of pulmonary engorgement may appear when the output of the left ventricle is still above the normal basal level. The explanation is that in such cases the output of the left ventricle, though increased, is lagging behind that of the right ventricle.

In massive infarcts of the left ventricle in a patient without previous evidence of congestive failure, the increase in pulmonary venous pressure appears to be the only factor operative in producing the pulmonary engorgement and edema. The loss of fluid into the lungs causes a moderate degree of hemoconcentration. The right ventricle pumps blood into the pulmonary vessels which the infarcted left ventricle is unable to remove.

When heart failure develops more slowly, as usually happens, and when the left ventricle is more nearly capable of keeping up with the right ventricle, a second and important factor becomes operative in the development of the pulmonary congestion—namely, the tendency for a person with a failing heart to retain salt and water. The excess normal saline leaves the blood stream and is deposited in the tissues in areas where the tissue pressure is low or where the venous and capillary pressures are increased. This problem will be discussed in more detail under Edema (p. 1236). In these cases even a slight increase in pulmonary venous pressure because of heart failure is sufficient to cause a considerable portion of the retained water to accumulate in the lungs.

Dyspnea on *exertion* is the presenting symptom in most cases of congestive failure. The patient discovers that he becomes short of breath after an effort which formerly caused no discomfort. The first objective sign of this failure is usually a decrease in vital capacity, followed by an increase in the pulmonary circulation time. Moist rales at the bases are frequently present. It cannot be emphasized too strongly that, in the absence of the anxiety syndrome, dyspnea in heart disease always means pulmonary congestion and edema regardless of the physical findings in the lungs. In certain patients the edema is primarily pericapillary and not intra-alveolar. In these cases, intense dyspnea and pulmonary edema may be present even though auscultation of the lungs reveals no rales.

SUMMARY. Dyspnea in heart disease is produced by the changes in the lungs which result from interference with the venous drainage of the lungs and from the tendency of the cardiac patient to retain excess salt and water. Reflex stimulation from the congested lungs plays an important role in the mechanism of dyspnea. The pulmonary changes producing the dyspnea are the result of a combination of backward heart failure (increased venous pressure in the pulmonary veins because of mitral stenosis or failure of the left ventricle) and of failure of the kidneys to excrete salt and water normally. The backward failure in the lungs causes a large amount of the saline, retained by the kidneys, to be deposited in the lungs. It is obvious that anything which further decreases the vital capacity or which by reflex action increases the ventilation rate will increase the dyspnea. Hydrothorax, pulmonary infarcts and pneumonia all increase the dyspnea of cardiac failure through both these mechanisms. Fright, anxiety and pain precipitate attacks of dyspnea in cardiac patients, by increasing the pulmonary congestion and by a reflex increase in ventilation.

Orthopnea. Orthopnea is a more advanced stage of dyspnea in which the patient refuses to lie flat in bed because, when he assumes the horizontal position, his difficulty in breathing increases. In heart disease, dyspnea at rest is a relative state. With the trunk raised above a given angle, the patient may have no dyspnea. When the trunk is below that angle, dyspnea will occur. Orthopnea, like dyspnea, is a subjective sensation, and so, as in dyspnea, there is no close correlation between the degree of orthopnea and the objective signs of circulatory failure. The reflex sensitivity of the central nervous system of the individual patient determines at what level of pulmonary congestion and edema orthopnea first appears. In advanced heart failure with disturbance in consciousness, the patient may have less orthopnea despite increasing pulmonary edema. Because orthopnea is a subjective sensation, an unconscious patient cannot be orthopneic.

In many patients with orthopnea the venous pressure is normal, and marked elevation of the venous pressure in the brain in cases of superior mediastinal obstruction does not cause orthopnea. There is no constant change in arterial oxygen saturation when the orthopneic patient is lowered to a position where he complains of dyspnea. Estimation of the cerebral blood flow by determination of the oxygen content of arterial blood and of blood from the internal jugular vein reveals no constant change in cerebral blood flow with change in position. Thus there is no evidence that the circulation to the medullary centers is improved when the patient is upright.

Changes in posture do cause slight alterations in vital capacity. These are not marked even when the change is from the horizontal to the standing position. In many patients with orthopnea, lowering the trunk only a few degrees will cause dyspnea. It seems unlikely that this small change in position has caused a measurable change in vital capacity. In normal subjects the vital capacity is somewhat greater in the upright position than in the recumbent position. Hamilton and Morgan observed that the vital capacity of normal subjects in the recumbent position was increased when blood was pooled by the application of tourniquets to the four extremities. After the limbs were congested by tourniquets, change in posture caused little change in vital capacity. These data suggest that even in normal persons the blood volume in the lungs is appreciably increased when the subject lies down.

Clinical observation leaves little doubt that increased reflex activity with a rise in pulmonary ventilation as the body is lowered is the primary cause of orthopnea in cardiac failure. Whether this results from pulmonary congestion because of shift of blood from the lower part of the body as the effect of gravity becomes less marked, or from other reflex mechanisms, is not known. Any slight fall in the vital capacity would accentuate the dyspnea. The importance of the nervous system in orthopnea is emphasized by the common observation that the administration of morphine will allow a cardiac patient to rest comfortably in a position he had previously been unable to endure because of dyspnea. Reducing the sensitivity of the central nervous system in these patients relieves the dyspnea without producing any measurable change in the circulation.

Paroxysmal Dyspnea and Cardiac Asthma. Attacks of shortness of breath which come on suddenly—often while the patient is asleep —occur frequently in patients with cardiac failure from hypertension, coronary artery disease, aortic insufficiency and aortic stenosis, all diseases which cause strain or injury to the left ventricle. Although these attacks of dyspnea frequently occur in patients who are already incapacitated by chronic congestive failure, they may occur at night in patients who during the day seem to have a fairly good cardiac reserve and who are able to carry on their daily work. In many cases the liver is not palpable, and there is no pitting edema. Even though the peripheral circulation appears normal at rest, the lungs show signs of congestion. The mean velocity of pulmonary blood flow is usually decreased. On x-ray examination the hilar shadows are enlarged with a fanlike radiation toward the periphery. Moist rales are usually, though not always, present. The vital capacity is diminished, and the volume of the residual air is increased.

During the attack the patient sits up or stand up. The skin becomes ashen, the small veins are collapsed, and there is profuse sweating. The respiratory midposition of the thorax becomes elevated, and there is a tendency for the chest to become fixed in the forced inspiratory position. Both inspiratory and expiratory distress are usually present. Asthmatic wheezes and moist rales are frequently audible. In some cases only moist rales are heard. In certain patients, in spite of intense dyspnea, there are no rales. Tachycardia is invariably present. Embryocardia and gallop rhythm are common. The pulmonary second sound is accentuated. Though measurement of cardiac output has rarely been made during the acute spontaneous attacks, data on mild attacks produced by exertion have been studied in the laboratory. The cardiac output may be increased, unchanged or decreased. As the oxygen consumption is increased by struggling, the output per unit of oxygen consumption is always decreased, indicating progressive failure of output in terms of increased needs. The pulmonary arterial pressure is elevated. The systemic arterial pressure is usually increased above the resting level; the venous pressure either does not change or shows a moderate increase. The oxygen saturation of the arterial blood may show little or no decrease. If the bronchial constriction is marked or if severe pulmonary edema develops, the oxygen saturation may be markedly decreased. The mean velocity of blood flowing through the lungs is decreased. Diminished velocity without a decrease in volume of blood flowing through the lungs indicates that the cross-section area of the pulmonary vascular bed is increased and that the lungs contain more blood during the attack.

These data show that the paroxysm of dyspnea is caused by the sudden trapping of a few hundred cubic centimeters of blood in lungs which are already moderately congested. Because normal function has been impaired by disease, the left ventricle is unable to increase its output sharply enough to clear the lungs. This engorgement, then, is produced by a temporary imbalance between the outputs of the right and left ventricles, wherein the output of the right ventricle exceeds that of the left. In a short time the balance between the two ventricular outputs is restored, but the left ventricle is unable to do more than keep up with the right ventricle. It does not have enough reserve strength to remove the excess blood from the lungs. This excess blood reduces the efficiency of the lungs by decreasing the vital capacity and by decreasing the pulmonary elasticity. These changes in the lungs cause a reflex increase in pulmonary ventilation.

If the bronchi respond to the pulmonary congestion by spasm or if the lumina of the bronchi are narrowed by edema of the bronchial mucosa, asthmatic wheezes and groans will be present. Bronchial wheezes are more apt to develop if the patient has a history of repeated attacks of bronchitis or if he has chronic lung disease, such as emphysema or bronchiectasis. In some patients the edema that develops is pericapillary rather than intra-alveolar, in which case there are no rales. In any case the fundamental mechanism of the attack—namely, sudden pulmonary engorgement with a left ventricle incapable of removing the blood—is the same.

Paroxysmal attacks of dyspnea usually occur at night. In patients who have orthopnea the attack is frequently brought on by sliding into the horizontal position while asleep. In patients who are ambulatory the assumption of the horizontal position at rest tends to bring a redistribution of the blood and fluid in the body. When the patient lies down, blood is shifted from the abdomen and the upper and lower extremities to the lungs and to the great veins of the thorax. This redistribution of blood is one of the factors which cause the vital capacity of normal subjects to be less in the horizontal than in the upright position. Although there may be no pitting edema in many of these patients who have paroxysmal nocturnal dyspnea, the quantity of extracellular fluid is increased. During the day this fluid accumulates mainly in the lower part of the body because of the high venous and capillary pressures caused by the upright position. When the patient lies down, the venous pressure in the lower part of the body is decreased and excess fluid enters the blood stream, causing an increase in blood volume. If the pulmonary venous pressure is slightly elevated, much of the fluid is deposited in the lungs. The fall in pulmonary ventilation associated with sleep reduces the fluid loss from the lung by evaporation, and the decrease in lung motion tends to slow lymph flow. All these factors tend to increase pulmonary edema and decrease vital capacity. The stage is now set, and any stimulus which causes the patient to increase the output of the right ventricle for a short time will precipitate the paroxysms of dyspnea. Coughing, noise, nightmares and a distended bladder often act as the trigger mechanisms. The hyperpnea phase of Cheyne-Stokes breathing also frequently precipitates an attack.

Periodic Breathing (Cheyne-Stokes Respiration). In many patients with cardiac failure the regular sequence of respiratory movements is replaced by alternating periods of underbreathing and overbreathing. As the condition becomes more marked, apnea and hyperpnea occur. The periods of apnea may last 15 to 60 seconds. The apneic period is terminated by respirations of a gradually increasing depth until marked hyperpnea occurs. The depth of the respirations then gradually decreases until the next period of apnea begins. During the period of apnea the patient is frequently drowsy, sleepy or stuporous. As the hyperpnea begins, he frequently arouses, moves about restlessly, and not infrequently moans or cries out. He frequently complains of dyspnea, and if he has fallen back on the pillow he will sit upright. The hyperpnea of Cheyne-Stokes breathing is often the trigger mechanism which precipitates an attack of cardiac asthma.

Periodic breathing in heart failure is the result of incoordination of the nervous and chemical factors which normally control respiration. The exact nature of the incoordination has not been determined. This type of respiration may occur in normal sleeping babies. It may also be seen in patients after cerebral accidents or trauma to the central nervous system, or in patients with meningitis, uremia or other forms of coma. In all these conditions the sensitivity of the respiratory center is depressed. In sleep the depression is physiologic; in cardiac failure it is the result of the inability of the heart to maintain the normal cardiac output and to nourish the brain properly. That cerebral metabolism is disturbed in these patients is shown by their restlessness, the narrowing of the field of consciousness, and the difficulty in fixing attention.

The lowering of the blood flow to the brain because of decreased cardiac output is not the only factor responsible for depression of the respiratory center. Changes in cerebral blood flow because of local vascular disease play an important part. In addition, changes in the cerebral metabolism because of decreased blood supply to the liver, kidneys and all other tissues are probably important. The respiratory center becomes insensitive to the normal concentration of carbon dioxide, and apnea results. When respiration ceases, the carbon dioxide concentration of the arterial blood steadily increases until finally the sluglish respiratory center is stimulated and hyperpnea occurs. The carbon dioxide concentration continues to fluctuate, and the patient suffers alternately from apnea and hyperpnea.

Periodic breathing occurs in normal subjects at high altitudes. Both a decrease in oxygen tension and a decrease in carbon dioxide tension of the arterial blood appear to be operative. The fall in carbon dioxide tension is secondary to the stimulation of respiration resulting from the anoxemia. Whether the anoxemia affects the respiratory center directly or whether it works through peripheral receptors such as the carotid sinus is not clear. The administration of carbon dioxide invariably steps the periodic respiration. The administration of oxygen frequently makes the periodic breathing less marked, and occasionally stops it.

In cardiac failure there is usually a tendency for the carbon dioxide content of the arterial blood to be lowered because of the reflex stimulation of respiration from the engorged lungs. Both this tendency toward alkalosis and the depression of the respiratory center appear to be important in producing the periodic breathing. The interaction between these two factors probably accounts for the effect of sleep and morphine on Cheyne-Stokes breathing. In cardiac failure, periodic breathing frequently begins as the patient is going to sleep. Presumably the physiologic depression of the respiratory center, combined with the overbreathing produced by the reflexes from the congested lungs, initiates the periodic breathing. As sleep deepens, the ventilation decreases, the carbon dioxide content of the blood tends to increase, and the periodic breathing may cease. The effect of morphine is variable. In large doses it depresses the respiratory center and causes a marked prolongation of the periods of apnea and hyperpnea. In smaller doses it may cause the respirations to be more regular. This is probably due to the fact that smaller doses decrease the ventilation rate and reduce the tendency toward alkalosis, but are not powerful enough to cause any marked depression of the respiratory center.

When periodic breathing is marked and the heart is normal in size, the oxygen content of the arterial blood will be decreased during the apneic phase, and the carbon dioxide content of the arterial blood will be increased. These changes in the blood gases and corresponding changes in hydrogen ion concentration are the result rather than the cause of the periodic breathing. Once the periods of apnea and hyperpnea have begun, the changes in hydrogen ion concentration are probably important in explaining the variations in depth of respirations during the hyperpneic period. When the heart is very large, periodic breathing may occur without any disturbance in the respiratory center. The large bag of slowly moving blood interposed between the heart and brain prevents changes in pulmonary venous blood from being quickly reflected in cerebral arterial blood. In these patients the arterial blood is unsaturated with oxygen and high in CO_2 content during the height of the hyperpnea, and the reverse changes are present during apnea.

Periodic breathing in cardiac failure usually results from a combination of forward and backward failure of the left ventricle. The reflex overbreathing and pulmonary congestion (backward and forward failure) and the depression of the respiratory center (forward failure) are factors of importance.

Edema. Failure of the heart characteristically results in the retention of water and salt. The patient may retain 10 to 20 pounds of water before there is any objective sign of the increased extracellular fluid (subclinical edema). As the process continues, the patient notices that his shoes are tight and that his ankles are swollen in the evening. On arising in the morning the swelling has disappeared. In the more advanced stages pitting edema is present continually, and eventually the scrotum and abdominal wall become waterlogged. If the patient is confined to his bed, edema of the back and sacral regions may be more extensive than that of the lower extremities. Hydrothorax occurs, usually first on the right and later bilaterally. Ascites may develop.

Edema of the lower extremities produces a feeling of heaviness, but does not cause actual pain. The skin may become so tightly swollen that the body cannot nourish it. Therefore low grade cellulitis is not uncommon. At times the pressure of the extracellular fluid becomes so great that the skin ruptures and fluid drains freely from the part. Hydrothorax produces dyspnea by lowering the vital capacity. Less frequently, ascites is a factor in the production of dyspnea. It is possible that a portion of the anorexia and nausea occurring in congestive failure may be produced by the excess fluid in the tissues of the abdominal viscera. The generalized retention of water has already been discussed as an important factor in the production of dyspnea.

The *mechanism* of cardiac edema has never been completely explained. Formerly the edema was thought to be a manifestation of backward heart failure (failure of the right ventricle). The fact that elevation of the venous pressure produced edema was well known, and it was assumed that the edema in cardiac failure was secondary to the rise in venous pressure. Recent studies show that in patients with intractable chronic congestive failure, edema is present before there is a measurable rise in the resting venous pressure. The renal blood flow and glomerular filtration rate in patients with chronic failure are greatly reduced at rest. The greater the discrepancy between the cardiac output and the metabolic needs of the patient, the lower the renal blood flow. There is no correlation between the renal blood flow and the venous pressure.

The available data suggest that the retention of the sodium ion by the kidney is the fundamental cause of cardiac edema. The retention of water is secondary to the retention of the sodium ion. Everyone agrees that the retention of sodium is caused by some fault in the proper distribution of blood in the vascular system. Some believe that changes in blood flow or venous pressure cause the production of steroids which increase the reabsorption of sodium by the tubules. Others maintain that the decreased blood volume present in the arterial tree or the large blood volume present in the venous system causes increased renal reabsorption of sodium by hormonal or neurogenic mechanisms. In the author's opinion, this disturbance in renal function results from a decrease in renal blood flow because of the inability of the heart to maintain an adequate circulation while the patient is active. The low renal blood flow causes a reduction in glomerular filtrate. When the amount of sodium filtered falls below a critical level, the tubules reabsorb nearly the entire amount filtered, because the body is unable to depress the fundamental sodium-conserving function of the tubules below a certain level. As the salt and water retention becomes more marked, the plasma volume gradually increases and the quantity of circulating protein rises. The venous pressure may have already risen because of the vasoconstrictor response to a fall in cardiac output. The increase in blood volume causes a further rise. The retained salt and water are distributed throughout the body in areas where the capillary pressure is high or the tissue pressure is low. During the day, when the patient is upright, the high venous and capillary pressures produced by gravity cause most of the excess fluid to accumulate in the portion of the body below the level of the heart. When the patient lies down, the venous and capillary pressures throughout the body become more nearly equal. This results in a redistribution of the excess fluid over the body. If the pulmonary venous pressure is increased, owing to left ventricular failure, much of the excess fluid is deposited in the lungs. The remainder is lodged in areas where the tissue pressure is low.

In this discussion a distinction is made between the generalized rise in venous pressure which occurs in cardiac failure and the local rise in venous pressure which is produced by placing a part below the level of the heart. The rise in pressure throughout the venous system is produced by a large blood volume which distends the venous bed or by a redistribution of blood from vasoconstriction. At least in some patients, the elevated venous pressure is the *result,* rather than the cause, of the edema. The local increases in venous and capillary pressures produced by postural effects are of primary importance in determining the distribution of the excess saline retained by the kidney.

In chronic fixed congestive failure, changes in venous pressure are closely correlated with changes in blood volume; changes in venous tone secondary to changes in cardiac output are not observed, because the output is fixed at a subnormal level. In acute heart failure vasoconstriction secondary to the fall in cardiac output may increase the venous pressure. In these patients the venous pressure rises before the change in blood volume occurs. It is our opinion that in these patients the retention of salt and water and the rise in venous pressure both result from the fall in cardiac output and that the edema is not primarily due to the rise in venous pressure. In many patients with heart failure both the increase in blood volume and vasoconstriction occur. When the output is increased by digitalis, the venous pressure at first falls rapidly, but it may remain above the normal level until diuresis produces a decrease in blood volume.

The low protein content of cardiac edema fluid shows that neither increased capillary permeability nor lymphatic blockage plays a significant part in the mechanism of cardiac edema. Even in patients with marked lack of arterial oxygen saturation, capillary permeability seems to be normal. Lowering of the serum protein concentration always predisposes to the formation of edema. This is a secondary factor in certain patients with congestive failure.

Disturbances in Electrolyte Concentrations. In acute heart failure the plasma concentrations of sodium, chloride and potassium are normal. In any chronic long-lasting illness these values may drop strikingly and if the chronic illness in itself produces edema, one finds sodium retention, edema and low concentration of sodium in the plasma. Cardiac failure is no exception to this general rule. The characteristic finding of inability to increase the excretion of sodium and chloride in response to an increased sodium and chloride load persists. The fall in sodium and chloride values is an indication of the severity of the illness and its serious prognosis. It is not specific for heart failure.

As heart failure becomes more intractable and mercurial diuretics are relatively ineffective in reducing edema, the diuretic causes an increased loss of potassium and the syndrome of hypochloremic, hypokalemic alkalosis may develop. A fall in serum potassium potentiates the effect of digitalis on ventricular irritability and may cause extrasystoles.

Cough. Cough and expectoration are frequent complaints in patients with cardiac failure. The cough is produced by a reflex from the congested lungs and bronchi. Less commonly, it results from pressure of an aneurysm on the trachea, bronchi or recurrent laryngeal nerve. Rarerly, marked enlargement of the left atrium may produce cough by pressure on the bronchi. The cough produced by congestive failure may be severe enough to interfere with sleep, and is frequently the trigger mechanism which precipitates an acute attack of nocturnal dyspnea.

Hemoptysis. Bleeding from the lung or bronchial mucosa occurs frequently in heart failure. In mitral stenosis bleeding from the dilated pulmonary vessels or from dilated bronchial veins is common, and may occasionally be fatal. Bloody sputum is a frequent symptom of pulmonary infarction. In severe pulmonary edema caused by left ventricular failure, bloody froth may pour from the bronchial tree.

Weight Loss. Patients with chronic congestive failure suffer from a gradual loss of tissue which is frequently unnoticed because of the accumulation of edema. If failure persists for a long period of time, the cachexia may become as marked as that produced by advanced malignancy. The loss of weight is a manifestation primarily of forward heart failure. The heart does not pump enough blood to nourish the tissues properly. The observations of Gross on the nutritional state of children before and after ligation of a patent ductus are particularly significant. These studies show that physical development was retarded by poor peripheral blood flow even in the absence of the usual signs of congestive failure. When the peripheral blood flow was increased by obliteration of the patent ductus arteriosus, growth was accelerated.

Anorexia, Nausea and Vomiting. Gastrointestinal symptoms are common in congestive failure, and may originate in a number of ways. The reversible medullary-reflex interrelationship between the heart and stomach makes it possible for either stomach or heart to be the precipitating agent. Irritation of the gastric mucosa may produce reflex heart block or auricular standstill. Reflexes arising in the heart from myocardial infarction or from digitalis fixed in the heart may cause contractions of the stomach with reverse peristalsis, nausea and vomiting. Congestion of the abdominal viscera themselves may cause nausea and vomiting. Central stimulation of the reflex pathways producing vomiting may occur when the metabolism of the brain is disturbed. Hiccups is present at times in patients with myocardial infarction and is usually a symptom of serious prognostic significance.

Hepatomegaly and Abdominal Pain. The basal oxygen consumption of the area drained by the hepatic vein remains normal in heart failure in spite of a reduction in blood flow.

Thus there is an increased extraction of oxygen from blood in the splanchnic area which results in a lowered oxygen tension of venous blood. This happens most markedly in the hepatic sinusoids near the central veins. This anoxic state in the liver not only results in atrophy and necrosis of hepatic cells surrounding the central veins, but in edema and fatty changes in other parts of the lobule. Blood is pooled, particularly in conjunction with increases in venous pressure and blood volume, and in centro-lobular sinusoids which are now dilated as a result of the atrophy and necrosis of liver cells. Hepatomegaly is the consequence of. this train of events. It may be present with or without increase in venous pressure, and with or without detectable edema elsewhere.

Acute enlargement of the liver may occur with exercise or in rapidly developing congestive failure at rest. Palpation reveals an enlarged, tender liver. The sudden stretching of the liver capsule causes pain in the right upper quadrant which varies from a constant ache to, at times, colicky pain. Such pain is one of the most common symptoms of congestive failure. Once the hepatic capsule has been stretched, the liver may remain markedly enlarged and produce little discomfort. Over-all hepatic function usually remains good in hepatomegaly of heart failure, although mild elevation of serum bilirubin level is not uncommon.

Cerebral Symptoms. Symptoms of cerebral dysfunction are common in heart disease, although they do not usually appear until the patient has reached the stage when dyspnea is present at rest. Pulmonary congestion from poor venous drainage of the lungs and from retention of salt and water usually is present before the cardiac output decreases to a degree sufficient to produce a significant change in the metabolism of the brain. As the heart continues to fail, however, the cardiac output even at rest becomes inadequate to nourish the brain properly and irritability, restlessness and difficulty in fixing attention develop. The eventual sequence is that of stupor, coma and death. These symptoms of inadequate cerebral metabolism are often part of the clinical picture of congestive failure during the last few days or weeks of life. A change in personality, a mild delirium or mental depression is frequently the presenting symptom in the circulatory failure produced by myocardial infarction. It is probable that the changes in cerebral metabolism caused by heart failure have a mechanism more complicated than simple reduction of the blood supply to the brain. It seems evident that there must be widespread disorders of the intermediary metabolism produced by the decreased blood supply to the liver, endocrine glands, gastrointestinal tract and all other organs of the body. Such lack of proper function of other organs may well have a secondary effect on cerebral metabolism. The cerebral symptoms are accentuated if the oxygen saturation of the arterial blood is decreased because of severe pulmonary changes either secondary to or independent of the congestive failure.

Hypoglycemia. In severe congestive failure associated with reduction in cardiac output sufficient to give obvious disturbances in peripheral blood flow, profound hypoglycemia may occur. This is presumably the result of poor liver glycogen reserve and increased breakdown of glucose to lactic acid because of anoxia.

Palpitation. Persons—both sick and well—complain frequently of the fact that they are conscious of the beating of their hearts. On the one hand this may be due simply to increased awareness of normal physiologic variations in cardiac output (anxiety state). On the other hand, it may be the result either of changes in stroke volume or rate of the heart, or of cardiac enlargement. Anything which increases the stroke output of the heart will cause the patient to complain of palpitation unless his attention is centered elsewhere. For example, the beat after an extrasystole is noticed because a longer period of diastolic filling causes the stroke volume of this beat to increase. Exercise, excitement, thyrotoxicosis and anemia cause palpitation by increase in stroke volume and minute output of the heart. Increases in heart rate, without a rise in the minute volume output of the heart, are less apt to cause palpitation. Any change from the usual rhythm may cause awareness of the heart beat. When the heart is enlarged, palpitation is more likely to be experienced because the heart lies closer to the chest wall. Both normal subjects and patients with heart disease commonly complain of palpitation when lying quietly on the left side. This position causes the apex impulse to shift nearer the chest wall.

Anxiety State in Persons with Heart Disease. The layman knows that proper cardiac function is necessary to sustain life and that heart disease is a common cause of death.

The diagnosis of heart disease offers such a threat to security that it is safe for the physician to assume that anxiety is present whenever the patient knows or suspects that he has heart disease. The degree and manner in which this anxiety is expressed will depend on the personality structure of the individual person. Failure of the physician to differentiate between the symptoms of anxiety and those of heart failure frequently causes invalidism for years before the circulation actually becomes inadequate.

Persons who have real or imaginary heart disease without circulatory failure are apt to interpret many normal physiologic phenomena as evidence of heart failure. The slight feeling of giddiness which is produced by changing suddenly from the recumbent to the upright position and the palpitation which is produced by excitement, fear or exercise are frequently interpreted by the patient as signs of circulatory failure. Hyperventilation is easily produced by anxiety and may lead to the mistaken diagnosis of paroxysmal dyspnea due to early congestive failure. The following sequence of events is common. A patient with compensated heart disease is suddenly aroused from sleep by a noise or a nightmare. This produces an increase in pulmonary ventilation. At the same time the patient notices palpitation because of the increase in cardiac output from the sudden awakening. The palpitation is interpreted as a symptom of the circulatory failure, and the resulting anxiety causes a further increase in pulmonary ventilation. The rise in pulmonary ventilation without an increase in muscular activity produces alkalosis by lowering the carbon dioxide content of the arterial blood. The alkalosis alters the cerebral metabolism, and the patient feels giddy and uncertain. The hands and feet become cold and the extremities tingle. Rarely, tetany develops. These cerebral symptoms are interpreted as symptoms of heart failure, and sudden death is feared. The patient becomes conscious, also, of the increase in respiratory rate, and this, again, is interpreted as heart failure.

In taking the history, one should always ask whether the attacks of dyspnea, suspected of being caused by heart disease, are accompanied by faintness, giddiness, sense of unreality, loss of consciousness, coldness of the hands and feet, and tingling sensations around the mouth or down the extremities. Whenever the symptoms appear more severe than is compatible with the objective signs of heart disease, it is advisable to determine whether the sensations produced by voluntary hyperventilation are similar to those described by the patient as "shortness of breath."

Peripheral Circulatory Failure. The symptoms of peripheral circulatory failure are caused by (1) a marked decrease in cardiac output, which results from ineffective filling of the ventricles because of a decreased venous return; (2) a precipitous fall in arterial pressure because of arteriolar dilatation. The decreased venous return to the heart may result from a small blood volume from loss of blood, plasma or salt and water; it may result from increase in size of the circulatory bed so that the blood volume is inadequate to fill the distended bed, as in postural fainting. In the patients with circulatory failure from a small blood volume, the fall in arterial pressure is caused by the decrease in cardiac output, and arteriolar dilatation is not present. The pallor of the skin, coldness of the extremities, sweating, weak and thready pulse, narrowing of the field of consciousness and restlessness exhibited by the patients are also secondary to the diminished cardiac output. A precipitous fall in arterial pressure may be caused by arteriolar dilatation either reflexly or by the action of the products of infection on the arterioles directly. In these patients the cardiac output and venous return to the heart may be normal is spite of the low arterial pressure.

The signs and symptoms produced by a marked decrease in cardiac output are seen in varying degrees in patients with heart failure. In heart disease, however, the decrease in cardiac output is caused by cardiac weakness rather than by a decreased venous return to the heart. The clinical pictures of peripheral circulatory failure secondary to an inadequate venous return and of congestive failure are so different that at first glance it is difficult to believe that both result from the same cause, namely, a cardiac output below the needs of the body. The differences in the clinical picture result from the following factors: (1) The time relations are different. Chronic congestive failure usually occurs over a period of days, weeks or months. One must have time to ingest the 30 liters of edema fluid which may be present in chronic failure. Conditions leading to peripheral circulatory failure usually kill the patient, or recovery is complete. (2) The blood volume is frequently small in shock and usually large

in heart failure. A marked increase in venous tone in the presence of a small blood volume does not cause distention of the large veins; if the blood volume is normal or elevated, as in congestive failure, the venous pressure rises. (3) The reduction in cardiac output originally causes arteriolar constriction in both types of failure. The injured tissues and infection associated with many types of shock interfere with the maintenance of this normal constrictor response for long periods of time. (4) In most forms of heart failure there is a high capillary pressure in the lungs which causes pulmonary edema to develop early. Factors causing pulmonary edema are less likely to be present in the earlier stages of shock.

Syncope. Loss of consciousness from a transient decrease in cerebral blood flow is called *syncope.* The decrease in cerebral blood flow may result from cardiac standstill, from a fall in arterial pressure from reflex arteriolar dilatation or from a diminished cardiac output because of heart failure or peripheral circulatory failure. The *cardiac standstill* (Adams-Stokes syndrome) may be caused by heart block because of disease of the bundle of His, by ventricular fibrillation, or by overactivity of certain vagal reflexes whose afferent limb may originate in any organ of the body. Afferent impulses from the carotid sinus, the heart itself, any part of the gastrointestinal tract, the pleura, the peritoneum, the gallbladder, the uterus, the vagina or the prostate may produce sinoauricular standstill or auriculoventricular block by way of the vagus nerves.

The precipitous fall in arterial pressure may be due to reflex stimulation from the emotional content of thought, from the carotid sinus, from any sensory nerve or special sense organ. Syncope usually occurs while the subject is standing because the low arterial pressure is not able to pump blood to the brain against the force of gravity. This type of reaction is responsible for the usual benign faint. A fall in cardiac output rather than reflex arteriolar dilatation causes the sharp fall in arterial pressure in patients with hemorrhage, plasma loss, dehydration and pericardial tamponade. When widespread disease of the sympathetic nervous system is present, syncope may occur in the upright position because of failure of the normal reflex vasoconstrictor response to standing (postural hypotension). Less commonly, syncope occurs because of the decrease in cardiac output from marked tachycardia.

Reflex hyperventilation is a frequent cause of syncope. The alkalosis caused by the loss of carbon dioxide from the arterial blood either interferes with cerebral metabolism directly or produces its effect by a slowing of the cerebral blood flow. The combination of emotional hyperventilation and reflex arteriolar dilatation is responsible for many attacks of benign fainting.

Certain *afferent stimuli* apparently cause unconsciousness without affecting the circulation as a whole. Stimulation of the *carotid sinus* in certain persons causes unconsciousness without any slowing of the heart or fall in arterial pressure (central type of carotid sinus response). Engel and Romano have shown by the use of the electroencephalograph that slow waves of cortical origin are present in these patients, and they believe that they are caused either by local reflex vasoconstriction or by a direct cortical reflex mediated through the midbrain.

Any severe attack of *pulmonary congestion* from heart disease may be accompanied by unconsciousness. Syncope is seen most frequently with aortic stenosis, but has been described with pulmonary congestion resulting from coronary artery disease, mitral stenosis and aortic insufficiency. It appears that the suddenness and severity of the attack of failure are more important than the type of heart disease. The mechanism of these attacks of syncope has not been established. They may have a varied etiology. Reflex cardiac standstill, transient arrhythmia, cerebral anoxemia from a sudden inability of the heart to maintain an adequate cardiac output, and hyperventilation caused by the severe pulmonary congestion may each play an important role in certain cases.

Shock Syndrome in Heart Disease. A marked decrease in cardiac output causes a clinical syndrome resembling that described as peripheral circulatory failure or shock. Narrowing of the field of consciousness, restlessness, stupor, pallor, cold sweat, constricted veins in the extremities, low arterial pressure, narrow pulse pressure, weak and thready pulse are frequently seen in patients with heart disease. It is important to realize that though these signs are identical with those found in shock, they are the result of heart failure rather than peripheral circulatory failure. The picture may develop in a normal heart which is unable to pump blood

successfully because of marked tachycardia. In paroxysmal auricular tachycardia, auricular flutter or rapid auricular fibrillation the cardiac output may be markedly decreased because the period of diastole has been shortened until there is not sufficient time for proper ventricular filling. Interference with proper ventricular filling likewise causes the shock syndrome to develop in pericardial tamponade and to a lesser degree in constrictive pericarditis.

In the last few hours or days of life most patients with congestive failure exhibit the symptoms and signs of a marked decrease in cardiac output. These patients with chronic congestive failure usually have a large blood volume and high venous pressure, so that it is obvious that the decrease in cardiac output results, not from a decrease in venous return, but from the inability of the heart to pump blood in the presence of an adequate venous return. Patients with a massive myocardial infarct who have never had congestive failure have the clinical syndrome of shock without distention of the neck veins. They tend to show hemoconcentration rather than the increase in blood volume seen in chronic congestive failure. Roentgenograms of the lungs, however, show marked pulmonary congestion and edema. The pathologic findings in the heart help to explain the clinical picture. The area of infarction usually involves the left ventricle primarily. The right ventricle pumps blood into the lungs, but the infarcted left ventricle is not able to pump out the blood it receives. Sufficient fluid is lost into the lungs to cause some degree of hemoconcentration. The lungs become intensely engorged as the output of the left ventricle decreases. The decrease in output of the left ventricle causes the clinical syndrome of shock. The fall in arterial pressure adversely affects coronary blood flow. Attempts to raise the arterial pressure by transfusions of blood by artery or vein have been made. At present it must be determined by trial and error whether transfusion improves the circulation or increases the edema. The *slow* infusion of norepinephrine to maintain arterial pressure above levels of shock may prove of benefit in some cases.

In summary, heart disease may produce the *clinical* picture that is described as characteristic of peripheral circulatory failure or of shock. It is clear, however, that this failure is not peripheral in origin. It is caused by the inability of the heart to pump blood, and not by an inadequate venous return. The term "cardiac shock" is used only to describe the clinical appearance of the patient. It has no physiologic connotation.

EUGENE A. STEAD, JR.

References

Engel, G. L., Romano, J., and McLin, T. R.: Vaso-depressor and Carotid Sinus Syncope. Arch. Int. Med., 74:100, 1944.

Harrison, T. R.: Failure of the Circulation. 2d ed. Baltimore, Williams and Wilkins, 1939.

Merrill, A. J.: Edema and Decreased Renal Blood Flow in Patients with Chronic Congestive Heart Failure: Evidence of "Forward Failure" as the Primary Cause of Edema. J. Clin. Investigation, 25:389, 1946.

Stead, E. A., Jr., Warren, J. B., and Brannon, E. S.: Cardiac Output in Congestive Heart Failure. Am. Heart J., 35:529, 1948.

Warren, J. V., and Stead, E. A.: Fluid Dynamics in Chronic Congestive Heart Failure. Arch. Int. Med., 73:138, 1944.

Weiss, S.: Symptoms of Patients with Heart Disease and Their Interpretation. M. Clin. North America, 24:1295, 1940.

————, and Robb, G. P.: Cardiac Asthma (Paroxysmal Cardiac Dyspnea) and the Syndrome of Left Ventricular Failure. J.A.M.A., 100:1841, 1933.

CARDIAC DILATATION AND HYPERTROPHY

The heart may increase in size by enlargement of its cavities without an increase in muscle mass (dilatation), or by an increase in the size of the individual muscle fibers without an increase in the size of the cavities (hypertrophy). In many instances, dilatation and hypertrophy occur together.

Dilatation of the chambers of the heart is thought to occur when the muscle of the heart is injured by overwork, ischemia, chemical agents or bacterial toxins. The change may be reversible or irreversible.

Increased work of the heart without periods of rest is one of the stimuli for hypertrophy. In hypertension, aortic stenosis and insufficiency, and mitral regurgitation the left ventricle hypertrophies because of the added work. In mitral stenosis, hypertrophy and dilatation of the left atrium occur. In pulmonary hypertension from mitral stenosis or pulmonary arteriosclerosis the right ventricle hypertrophies. Failure of the left heart leads to right ventricular hypertrophy because of the rise in pulmonary arterial pressure

produced by the pulmonary congestion. Observations on patients with arteriovenous fistula demonstrate that an increased output of the heart without hypertension is an effective stimulus for hypertrophy. There is no good correlation between the amount of added work and the degree of hypertrophy. In a number of instances marked hypertrophy is found without any evidence that the work load has been abnormal. In these patients work may still be the stimulus to hypertrophy. Chemical or physiologic changes in the muscle of the heart may have occurred, which make normal work an overload for the damaged heart.

The evidence that heavy physical work causes hypertrophy of the heart is less convincing. The heart does not do extra work between the periods of exercise, and therein the situation differs from the pathologic overwork.

When the heart is enlarged, it is difficult to determine during life whether hypertrophy or dilatation, or a combination of both, has occurred. Marked reduction in the amplitude of pulsations of the chambers of an enlarged heart shows that dilatation is present. Hypertrophy may or may not be present in these dilated hearts.

Reversible changes in heart size are not uncommon. A reversible increase in heart size is seen in patients with acute infections, hypertension, arteriovenous fistulas, normal pregnancy, toxemia of pregnancy, acute glomerulonephritis, anemia, thyrotoxicosis, myxedema, beriberi and many other diseases. The relative importance of hypertrophy and dilatation in these changes is not known. A reversible decrease in heart size is seen in patients with Addison's disease and in starvation.

EUGENE A. STEAD, JR.

THE TREATMENT OF CONGESTIVE HEART FAILURE

General Considerations. Congestive heart failure occurs when the heart pumps less blood than is demanded by the body over a prolonged period. The objects of therapy are (1) to bring back into balance the demand for blood and the supply of blood, and (2) to remove and to prevent the reaccumulations of excess fluid and excess blood volume when the output of the heart cannot be made to meet the minimum requirements of the body. The means of accomplishing these ends are (1) reduction of the requirements of the body for blood; (2) increase in the output of the heart (*a*) by digitalis, and (*b*) by modifying the disease process responsible for the heart failure; (3) elimination of edema (*a*) by restriction of intake of sodium chloride, (*b*) by promoting the excretion of sodium chloride by the administration of diuretic drugs, and (*c*) by removal of fluid by aspiration.

Reduction of the Requirements of the Body for Blood. *Rest,* both physical and mental, is one of the most effective methods of reducing the cardiac output. Physical rest may be achieved by shorter working hours, regular midday periods of rest, longer hours in bed at night, walking more slowly, use of elevator and avoidance of hills and stairs. Bedroom and toilet should be on the ground floor. When orthopnea is present, a hospital bed with Gatch type of bedspring is a great asset. Rest at night is essential, and sedatives should be used as needed to obtain this. Constipation is to be avoided. *Reduction of weight* in obese persons and *reduction of weight by removal of edema* are important methods of decreasing the requirements for cardiac output. In patients with thyrotoxicosis, anemia, arteriovenous fistula, patent ductus arteriosus and beriberi the treatment of the underlying disease may reduce greatly the increased amount of blood pumped by the heart.

Mental rest is more difficult to achieve. This may be because the patient has a lifelong habit of expending large amounts of emotional energy in his daily activities or because the illness itself has caused family and financial difficulties. All the resources of a skillful and patient doctor plus the resources of the community and church may be needed.

Increase in the Output of the Heart. *Digitalis.* Digitalis preparations cause a sustained increase in cardiac output of the failing heart. The prime indication for digitalis is congestive heart failure. It is contraindicated in ventricular tachycardia. It can be given in the presence of heart block and ventricular extrasystoles. It is used with caution in the presence of myocardial infarction.

The tincture of digitalis was gradually replaced by the more stable powdered leaf, and in recent years the powdered leaf is being replaced by purified glycosides. These have the great advantages of prescription by weight rather than by biologic units, of causing less irritation to the gastrointestinal tract when given orally in large doses, and of availability for intravenous administration when indicated. The pharmacologic and toxic actions of the purified glycosides are the same as those of powdered digitalis leaf. They accomplish nothing therapeutically that cannot be done with the leaf.

Three cardioactive glycosides have been purified and are now in general use. Digitoxin is present in both *Digitalis purpurea* and *Digitalis lanata*. Lanatoside C is present only in *Digitalis lanata*. Digoxin is obtained from lanatoside C by hydrolytic removal of acetyl and glucose groups. Digitoxin is almost completely absorbed from the gastrointestinal tract, so that the oral and intravenous doses are the same. Digoxin is better absorbed than lanatoside C, but is less completely absorbed than digitoxin. Because of the variability of absorption of lanatoside C, digitoxin and digoxin are preferred for oral use. When toxic symptoms are produced by digitoxin, they persist for a longer time than when they are induced by lanatoside C or digoxin, probably because of the more rapid destruction of the latter substances.

Digitalis preparations are given until therapeutic effects occur or toxic symptoms develop. The more severe the heart failure, the closer the therapeutic approaches the toxic dose. The drug in therapeutic doses causes a rise in cardiac output, slight rise in arterial pressure, fall in peripheral resistance and venous pressure, fall in ventricular rate if auricular fibillation is present, and changes in the S segment and T wave of the electrocardiogram. The improvement in the circulation is manifested by diuresis and relief of signs and symptoms of congestive failure. The resting ventricular rate in persons with atrial fibrillation should be slowed to 70 to 80 beats per minute. If exercise causes a marked increase in rate, additional digitalis is needed. The toxic effects are loss of appetite, nausea and vomiting, diarrhea, disturbances in vision, mental confusion, ventricular premature beats, various degrees of heart block, atrial standstill, atrial fibrillation, and nodal and ventricular tachycardias.

The average total oral therapeutic dose of digoxin is around 4 mg. For moderately rapid digitalization, give an initial dose of 1.5 mg. and follow by 0.75 mg. at 6-hour intervals until the desired therapeutic effect is obtained or toxic symptoms develop. The oral maintenance dose ranges between 0.25 and 1.5 mg. with an average of 0.5 mg.

The average total oral digitalizing dose of digitoxin is around 2 mg. In patients who have not received digitalis, 1.2 mg. of digitoxin can be given orally as a single dose. As this will overdigitalize a small minority and underdigitalize a considerable number, most physicians prefer to give digitoxin in divided doses. An initial dose of 0.6 mg. is followed in 6 hours by an additional 0.6 mg. Subsequent doses of 0.2 mg. every 6 to 12 hours are given until therapeutic effects or minor toxic symptoms are obtained. The daily maintenance dose ranges from 0.05 to 0.3 mg. with most patients requiring about 0.15 mg.

Small doses of digitalis have a cumulative effect, and the usual maintenance dose is not disposed of within 24 hours until considerable quantities have accumulated in the body. For this reason, the average maintenance dose given over a long period of time will eventually produce a good digitalis effect.

All three glycosides can be given intravenously. Lanatoside C, in doses of 1.6 mg. intravenously, has been given many times as a single digitalizing dose without harmful effects. Digoxin in amounts of 0.75 to 1.5 mg., and digitoxin in doses of 1.2 mg., have also been used intravenously as single digitalizing doses, but fewer reports are available in the literature. Because of the more rapid disappearance from the body, lanatoside C or digoxin would appear to be the drugs of choice in the rare patient requiring intravenous medication.

Modification of the Disease Process Responsible for the Heart Failure. Treatment with thyroid gland extract may relieve dramatically the congestive heart failure caused by myxedema. Successful treatment of thyrotoxicosis, anemia and beriberi affects the metabolism of the heart muscle favorably and directly increases the reserve of the heart by reducing the demands for cardiac output. The course of congestive heart failure in acute rheumatic fever may be modified by therapy with cortisone or adrenocorticotrophic hormone. Congestive failure occurring in the course of subacute bacterial endocarditis may improve when the bacteria are killed, though recurrence is the rule because of the extensive damage of the valve. Congestive failure complicating coarctation of the aorta may be helped by surgical resection or by-pass procedures. Hypertension is a common cause of congestive heart failure. Rigid restriction of sodium chloride, the use of the rice diet of Kempner, antihypertensive drugs or sympathectomy, if successful in lowering blood pressure, lessens the load on the heart. When arterial blood is not normally saturated with oxygen, the administration of oxygen by tent, mask or catheter is beneficial.

Patients with organic heart disease may not have congestive failure until infection or pulmonary infarction occurs. Congestive failure may disappear when the infection is controlled or when further pulmonary infarcts are prevented by the use of anticoagulants or by ligation of femoral veins. When pulmonary infarction occurs in patients with congestive failure and atrial fibrillation, conversion to normal rhythm by the use of quinidine may cause improvement.

Prevention of Edema and Excess Blood Volume. *Restriction of Intake of Sodium Chloride.* Edema is composed largely of water and sodium chloride. When a patient is able to eat a normal diet without showing edema, he has a cardiac output that is approximately normal for his level of activity. When the patient has to have salt restriction to remain free of edema, the cardiac output, for long periods of time, is considerably below the normal volume for his level of activity. The degree of salt restriction will depend on the severity of failure. Restriction of the 24-hour intake to 2 gm. of sodium is sufficient in mild failure; restriction to 150 mg. of sodium is necessary in severe intractable failure. When sodium chloride is restricted, one does not have to limit the fluid intake. Thirst is not a problem unless salt is eaten. Large quantities of water are excreted without difficulty. The rice diet of Kempner causes a marked reduction in total solids excreted by the kidney and is compatible with a restricted intake of fluid. Patients on a larger electrolyte intake with similar fluid restriction may have cellular dehydration and for a short period may require a large intake of fluid.

Control of edema by restriction of sodium chloride in the diet gives the most satisfactory result in heart failure. It removes the need for restriction of water intake, it avoids the recurrent swelling which occurs when a mercurial diuretic is given once or twice weekly, and it escapes the danger of sodium depletion which may occur when a mercurial diuretic is given daily. The author prefers not to use salt substitutes and to avoid the use of ammonium chloride. If edema is not controlled on the prescribed diet, the 24-hour output of chloride in the urine is determined to decide whether the patient is breaking his diet or whether a more rigid restriction of sodium chloride is needed. This laboratory check on chloride excretion has proved a great boon both to patient and physician. It is as useful in following a patient with severe congestive failure as is the test for sugar in the urine in patients with diabetes.

When rigid restriction of salt is combined with the repeated use of mercurial diuretics, the levels of sodium and chloride in the blood may become depressed, even though considerable edema may still be present. The diuretic has caused an increased excretion of sodium chloride without an equal increase in output of water. We have seen many examples of the low salt syndrome from electrolyte loss in urine when patients with nephritis are placed on extremely low sodium intakes; this has not been seen in patients with congestive heart failure without renal disease unless diuretics have been given. Patients with severe heart failure do develop low concentrations of sodium and chloride in the plasma secondary to the severe disturbances in cell metabolism.

Use of Diuretics. The excretion of sodium chloride from the body can be greatly increased by the administration of diuretics. This is of great advantage when the patient is in acute distress from waterlogging. Once the acute situation is relieved, edema is best controlled by dietary limitation of sodium chloride. If complete cooperation of the patient in following a diet cannot be obtained, the prolonged use of diuretics to control edema becomes necessary. The organic mercurial diuretics are the most useful.

Meralluride sodium solution (Mercuhydrin) in 1 to 2 cc. doses intramuscularly has been very effective and is not painful. Mercurophylline injections (Mercuzanthin) and mersalyl and theophylline injection (Salyrgan-theophylline) are also effective in 1 to 2 cc. doses, but they cause more pain when given intramuscularly. As rare deaths, presumably from ventricular fibrillation, have been reported after the intravenous injections of mercurial diuretics, the intramuscular route is preferred. Muscular cramps, diarrhea and skin rash occur occasionally and may not recur when another mercurial preparation is tried. The signs of acute nephritis or an elevated nonprotein nitrogen are contraindications to the use of mercurial diuretics.

If the patient has chronic failure, the diuretic must be given routinely at least once or twice a week. Some authors recommend doses of 0.5 to 1 cc. daily and teach the patients to give the drug themselves. When salt restriction in the diet is combined with the continued use of a mercurial diuretic, salt depletion may occur even though edema persists. Replacement of salt may result in improvement.

Ammonium chloride in enteric-coated tablets may be given in daily doses of 6 to 10 gm. It is a mild diuretic by itself and often increases the diuresis produced by the mercurial preparations. For the latter purpose, it is usually given on the two days preceding and on the day of the injection of the mercurial diuretic. A rest period is then given until two days preceding the next mercurial injection. Ammonium chloride may cause marked acidosis in patients with renal failure.

Theophylline, theobromine calcium salicylate (Theocalcin), theobromine sodium salicylate (Diuretin), theophylline ethylene diamine (aminophylline) and urea are used occasionally as diuretics. They have the advantage that they can be taken by mouth, but they are so much less effective than the mercurial preparations that they are now little used.

Drainage of Edema by Needle. Hydrothorax and ascites are usually best treated by removal of fluid by paracentesis. These collections of fluid tend to disappear more slowly than subcutaneous edema. If massive subcutaneous edema cannot be controlled, the patient is allowed to sit in a chair with the feet and legs dependent. After local injection of procaine, No. 14 needles are inserted through the skin of the legs and left in place for a few minutes. They are then removed and edema fluid allowed to drain from the tracts made by the needles. The legs are wrapped lightly with alcohol sponges. Penicillin is given parenterally to prevent secondary infection.

Acute Pulmonary Edema. This is a medical emergency. If the patient is struggling and excited, morphine given hypodermically in doses of 15 to 30 mg. is a life-saving drug. If the patient is seen late in an attack and stupor is beginning, morphine should be withheld. The slow intravenous injection of 0.25 to 0.5 gm. of aminophylline may be effective in reducing bronchial spasm. If the patient is not digitalized, 1.2 mg. of digitoxin or 1.6 mg. of lanatoside C is given intravenously. If the patient is partially digitalized, smaller doses of these drugs can be given intravenously at hourly intervals. Oxygen by mask, tent or catheter is useful. The removal of 500 to 800 cc. of blood rapidly by venesection may cause a fall in blood pressure and increase in cardiac output. Tourniquets inflated to a pressure above the diastolic level may be applied to the four extremities. This bloodless venesection is frequently effective if the patient is thin and if the systemic venous pressure is not greatly elevated. If hypertension is present, lowering of the pressure by hexamethonium may be effective by reducing the load on the left ventricle.

Eugene A. Stead, Jr.

References

Batterman, R. C., and DeGraff, A. C.: Studies in the Rate of Dissipation of Digoxin in Man. Fed. Proc., 4:112, 1945.

————: Comparative Study on Use of Purified Digitalis Glycosides, Digoxin, Digitoxin and Lanatoside C for Management of Ambulatory Patients with Congestive Heart Failure. Am. Heart J., 34: 663, 1947.

Gold, H.: Pharmacologic Basis of Cardiac Therapy. J.A.M.A., 132:547, 1946.

Stead, E. A., Jr., Warren, J. V., and Brannon, E. S.: Cardiac Output in Congestive Heart Failure. Am. Heart J., 35:529, 1948.

————, Warren, J. V., and Brannon, E. S.: Effect of Lanatoside C on Circulation of Patients with Congestive Failure. Arch. Int. Med., 81:282, 1948.

Wheeler, E. O., Bridges, W. C., and White, P. D.: Diet Low in Salt (Sodium) in Congestive Heart Failure. J.A.M.A., 133:16, 1947.

VASCULAR HYPERTENSION

Definition. Hypertension may be defined as a pathologic elevation of the blood pressure. It is a physical sign reflecting an underlying disturbance of the heart or blood vessels. An elevated blood pressure can result from a variety of causes which may or may not be of clinical importance. Hypertensive disease, as opposed to a simple blood pressure elevation, is a disorder which is characterized by (1) a sustained elevation of blood pressure, and (2) the eventual appearance of cardiac, renal, retinal and cerebral vascular complications. Hypertensive disease is said to occur in about 5 per cent of the adult population.

Normal Variations. Blood pressure normally varies from moment to moment as a result of bodily movement, mental stress, pain and position. The degree of elevation depends upon the intensity of the stimulus and upon the individual response. At birth the blood pressure is about 75 mm. of mercury systolic and 40 mm. diastolic. There is a gradual rise of pressure to about 100/60 at adolescence and to about 120/80 between the ages of 20 and 40. There is a further rise of pressure to perhaps 140/90 at the age of 60; thereafter the diastolic pressure remains essentially unchanged, while the systolic pressure tends to become higher. It should be remembered, however, that these figures represent the mean average and that there is a normal scatter around this mean of about plus or minus 10 per cent or more. It is therefore difficult to assess normal values for blood pressure and impossible to define a truly normal level. The farther the blood pressure deviates from normal, the more likely is it to be pathologic. If it is consistently elevated over a number of examinations, with the patient considered to be relaxed, and if any of the hypertensive complications to be described are present, the elevated blood pressure may be considered pathologic.

Pathologic Physiology of Elevated Systolic and Diastolic Blood Pressures. The physiologically important blood pressure is the mean pressure. This is not the average value between systolic and diastolic, but is the average level throughout the cardiac cycle. It is usually about 40 per cent of the way between diastolic and systolic pressure, but may vary from 20 to 80 per cent in individual cases, depending on the pulse rate and other factors. Since mean pressure can be determined only by direct arterial puncture with a suitable recording device, it is measured only as a research procedure. Because mean pressure is usually nearer the diastolic than the systolic value, the diastolic blood pressure is of far greater clinical significance than the systolic.

Mean blood pressure may be defined as the product of cardiac output and the peripheral resistance. Cardiac output varies as a result of changes of blood volume, emotion and exercise and a number of disease conditions. The peripheral resistance is composed of several factors—pressure losses as the blood flows through arteries, arterioles, capillaries, venules and veins; blood viscosity; elasticity of the vessels; and many factors of minor importance. The resistance to blood flow through the arterioles makes up about three quarters of the total peripheral resistance, and at a given cardiac output the resistance varies inversely as the third to fifth power of the radius of these vessels. In other words, minor changes in the caliber of the arterioles have a profound effect on blood pressure. As with cardiac output, peripheral resistance may change as a result of emotion, exercise and a number of disease conditions and thus affect blood pressure. Apprehensive patients are frequently seen with elevated blood pressures due to an increased cardiac output or else to a temporary increase of peripheral resistance. Twenty minutes of quiet rest or two or three days in the hospital may result in a fall of blood pressure, even to normal levels, as cardiac output or the resistance decreases. Whether in any given person the elevated blood pressure at first was due to an elevation of cardiac output or to an increased peripheral resistance cannot be ascertained clinically with certainty. This is one of the main stumbling blocks in evaluating patients with high blood pressure. The decision as to the existence of hypertensive disease in contrast to a simple elevation of blood pressure depends in the last analysis on the recognition of hypertensive complications in the heart, brain, eyegrounds and kidneys.

The pulse pressure is the pressure which distends the aorta and its large branches each time the left ventricle discharges its volume of blood. Pulsatile flow from the heart becomes a steady flow in the capillaries, largely because of the reservoir function of the aorta and its branches which distend during systole to accommodate most of the blood expelled during ventricular systole. An increased cardiac output and decreased elasticity of the large arteries are therefore associated with a wide pulse pressure. A wide pulse pressure is observed in exercise, emotion, complete heart block, thyrotoxicosis, aortic insufficiency, patent ductus arteriosus and arteriovenous aneurysms, largely on the basis of an increased ventricular systolic output which results in greater changes of pressure. Decreased elasticity of the aorta and its main branches produces an elevation of systolic pressure only. When rigidity of these vessels is accompanied by an increased cardiac output from any cause, the systolic and, to a much less extent, the diastolic blood pressures become elevated and the pulse pressure remains wide. Rigidity of the large vessels from loss of elasticity is a common accompaniment of advancing years and is also seen in association with diabetes mellitus and hypertensive disease itself. Even when the ves-

sels and the volume of blood ejected by the left ventricle are normal, the distensibility of the aorta becomes less as blood pressure rises. When the diastolic pressure becomes elevated, the systolic pressure tends to rise to a greater extent with a resultant wide pulse pressure. In the older age group with inelastic arteries the pulse pressure is even wider. In patients with essential hypertension the pulse pressure is usually wider than in those with chronic nephritis. This is due to the difference in age incidence, essential hypertension being a disease of middle and old age and therefore accompanied by rigid vessels, and chronic nephritis being a disease of the young.

Pathogenesis of Hypertensive Disease. Hypertension due to a narrowing of the arterioles and characterized by a sustained elevation of diastolic pressure has long been suspected to be of renal origin, whether or not renal disease such as chronic nephritis can be demonstrated by the usual tests. The precise relation to the kidney has not yet been elucidated.

Two main types of hypertension have been produced experimentally in animals. A *neurogenic hypertension* is produced by section of the aortic and carotid sinuses, the so-called moderator nerves. This hypertension is characterized by wide swings of blood pressure from moment to moment, rapid heart rate, increased cardiac output and blood volume, and increased peripheral blood flow. The heart becomes greatly hypertrophied. Since it is neurogenic in origin, it is almost completely eradicated by complete sympathectomy. Though cardiac hypertrophy appears as a result of increased cardiac work, no consistent vascular lesions occur, even after many years of this type of hypertension. Because this experimental hypertension does not involve an alteration of the psychologic or emotional state, this type of experiment does not entirely exclude a neurogenic origin of human hypertension. Experimental neurogenic hypertension, however, bears little resemblance to the human disease, with the possible exception of that due to epinephrine- and norepinephrine-producing pheochromocytomas.

Renal hypertension was first produced in mammals by Goldblatt by constriction of the renal artery so as to reduce blood flow to the kidney. This is accompanied by a gradual rise of blood pressure which reaches its maximum in ten days to two weeks and, if the development of a collateral circulation through the capsule can be prevented, remains permanently elevated. This renal type of hypertension is similar in many respects to human hypertension. As in the human disease, the cardiac output, heart rate, blood volume and peripheral blood flow are normal. The peripheral arteriolar resistance is increased. The blood pressure is "set" at a higher level than normal, but behaves qualitatively the same, in that the blood pressure fluctuates in response to bodily activity and to emotion in an essentially normal fashion. By varying the degree of constriction of the renal artery in animals, either a benign or a malignant type of hypertension can be produced.

Complete sympathectomy neither prevents nor cures this type of experimental hypertension. It has been shown to be humoral in origin, but the precise mechanism by which the blood pressure rises has not been entirely elucidated. Many *pressor substances* have been described to be present in the blood of patients with hypertension. With few exceptions, other workers in the field have failed to confirm their presence. At this time it is not possible to evaluate the role played in hypertension by *pharentasin* (Schroeder), the long-sustained pressor principle (Helmer and Shipley), *norepinephrine* (Goldenberg and associates) or desoxycorticosterone and salt (Selye). Two humoral mechanisms—*renin* and *vaso-excitor material*—have been studied extensively and deserve comment.

In 1898 Tigerstedt and Bergman discovered renin, a renal enzyme. It has been studied extensively, especially by Braun-Menéndez and his co-workers in Houssay's laboratory in Argentina and by Page and his co-workers in the United States. Renin is an enzyme found only in the kidney which, in response to constricting the renal artery, is liberated directly into the blood stream. Here it acts upon its substrate, hypertensinogen, which is an alpha-2 globulin formed in the liver. From their interaction, the powerful pressor and constrictor substance, hypertensin, is produced. Hypertensin is thought to have a molecular weight of about 2700. It is rapidly destroyed by a group of enzymes generically called hypertensinase which are present in all tissues of the body. In the acute phase of experimental renal hypertension and in certain acute human hypertensions (acute glomerulonephritis and pre-eclampsia and eclampsia), sufficient amounts of renin are found in the circulating blood to account for the hypertension. Despite the persistence of the hypertension in the experimental animal and in human hypertensive disease, the concentration of renin gradually decreases until it is no longer recoverable by bio-assay techniques. Immunologic blocking of renin activity, however, results in a prompt fall of blood pressure to normal levels in experimental renal hypertension. Unfortunately, the immunologic blocking of renin in man has not been possible to date, so that the effect of neutralization of renin on human blood pressure remains to be determined. Evidence for the renal origin and renin origin of human essential hypertension is therefore suggestive but not convincing at this time.

Shorr and his co-workers have described a humoral mechanism in experimental renal and in human essential hypertension which consists of two substances, a vaso-excitor material (VEM) and a vasodepressor material (VDM), measured by the reactivity of mesenteric vessels to topically applied epinephrine as observed microscopically. Vaso-excitor material is produced by the anoxic kidney, vasodepressor material mainly by the anaerobic liver and skeletal muscles. Vasodepressor material has been identified as ferritin. Systems are present in the body for their inactivation. When renal hypertension is produced experimentally, the vasoexcitor material titer in the blood rises and then falls despite the persistence of the hypertension. The fall is only apparent, however, because it has been shown that in reality it remains elevated, its apparent fall being due to a concomitant rise of vasodepressor material.

The relation of this humoral system to experimental and human hypertension remains to be explained. Vaso-excitor material and vasodepressor material have not been demonstrated to have pressor or depressor activity in normal animals. Their site of action in the circulatory system is in the precapillaries. Indeed, present evidence seems to indicate that they play an important role in the regulation of the capillary circulation. Their site of action is distal to the point of the increased resistance in hypertensive disease, i.e., the arterioles. Whatever the relation to hypertension, it would seem necessary at this time to assume the existence of some other factor responsible for the rise of blood pressure. Whether vaso-excitor material stimulates the production of this other substance or whether the other substance stimulates the production of vaso-excitor material and vasodepressor material to control a resultant disturbance of the all-important capillary circulation, or whether the two are produced together as a result of a common stimulus, remains to be ascertained.

Present evidence indicates that the relation of the hypophysis to hypertension, as in Cushing's disease, is by way of the *adrenal cortex.* Hypertension produced by adrenocorticotrophic hormone (ACTH), especially when sodium chloride intake is not restricted, is due to an increased peripheral resistance. That there is a close tie-up cannot be denied, but the precise relationship requires more study.

The same is true of *sodium.* In acute hypertension—acute glomerulonephritis and toxemia of pregnancy—there is a direct relationship between the sodium chloride intake and the level of blood pressure. In chronic hypertension there is a relationship, but it is not so close, and how important it is also is not certain. An excellent summary of our knowledge of the relationship of the adrenal cortex and of sodium will be found in the article of Perera and Atchley. An attractive hypothesis, without factual basis, however, is that in human essential hypertension the adrenal cortex in some way stimulates the kidney to produce an elevation of blood pressure.

Etiology of Human Hypertension. *Predisposing Factors.* Although hypertensive disease is somewhat more common in women than in men, it is a more serious affliction in the male. There is a strong familial tendency, which is probably the most important of all predisposing factors. Ayman's studies indicated that if both parents had hypertension, 46 per cent of the children had hypertension, while if both parents were normotensive, there was only a 3 per cent incidence of hypertension in the children. Although no age is immune to hypertension, the vast majority of patients are first seen in the fourth decade or later in life. Until recently it was believed that the younger the age of onset, the more violent and rapid the course. There is an increasing body of evidence indicating that patients with benign hypertension in the fourth or fifth decade of life have had elevated blood pressures for many years. Hypertensive disease appearing after the age of 50 usually follows a benign course. The incidence of hypertensive disease is considerably higher in patients with diabetes mellitus and gout. Life insurance statistics have shown clearly that the death rate from hypertensive vascular disease is higher in the obese than in those whose weight is normal. Obesity is not apparently a genetic factor, because a loss of weight is often accompanied by a fall of blood pressure. Whether or not this is due to upper arm obesity producing a falsely high pressure as recorded by the cuff method has not been adequately studied. The European and North American white population have a somewhat higher blood pressure and a higher incidence of essential hypertension than certain Indian, Chinese, African, Philippine and North and South American people. The characteristic constitutional type is the stocky, thick-set, ruddy-complexioned person who is energetic, aggressive and a go-getter. Suppressed hostility, suppressed aggression and emotional lability are supposed to characterize the typical *hypertensive emotional pattern* and have been credited with specific etiologic significance. It seems more plausible to regard the emotional patterns in much the same light as constitutional factors; i.e., they are a frequent but not universal setting for hypertensive disease.

Acute Hypertension. There are two diseases associated with acute rises of blood pressure—acute glomerulonephritis and toxemia of pregnancy—to which the reader is referred on pages 1102 and 1125 for more detailed descriptions. The behavior of the elevated blood pressure in these two diseases is quite unlike that in chronic hypertension. In each there is a striking relationship between hypertension and salt and water retention. Once the hypertension appears, salt and water retention aggravates it, and with diuresis the blood pressure falls. In each the hypertension is transient, usually lasting one to two weeks in the case of acute glomerulonephritis; in pregnancy the hypertension may last for only a few days or may not disappear until delivery takes place. Occasionally in both diseases, however, the hypertensive process never disappears, but instead becomes chronic, in which case it is referred to as chronic glomerulonephritis and post-toxemic hypertension.

Chronic Hypertension. There are as many classifications of hypertension as there are authors, and by and large the common denominator of each classification is that it presents a list of those renal diseases with which hypertension is commonly associated. The author has found the classification shown in the accompanying table to be a convenient one. Most of the chronic renal diseases are sooner or later associated with hypertensive disease, although it is not rare to observe patients dying in uremia without any elevation of blood pressure. Certain renal diseases are seldom associated with hypertension; tuberculosis, hydronephrosis and pyonephrosis are conspicuous examples. Chronic glomerulonephritis and post-toxemic hypertension have already been mentioned. Chronic nephritis and the nephrotic syndrome are further examples of diffuse renal parenchymal disease commonly associated with hypertension. Chronic pyelonephritis is extremely important to recognize in all age groups because of its controllability with antibiotic agents and by surgical eradication of an underlying obstruction to urinary outflow. Congenital polycystic kidneys, though comparatively rare, are usually accompanied sooner or later by hypertension. Hypertension usually occurs in patients with coarctation of the aorta. In dogs, hypertension can be regularly produced by aortic constriction, provided that the aortic narrowing is above the origin of the renal arteries. The rare group of arteritides are usually associated with hypertension when the renal vessels are involved in the process. Pheochromocytomas of the adrenal medulla may produce a paroxysmal type of hypertension, since the adrenal sporadically discharges epinephrine and norepinephrine into the circulation. This type of hypertension is unique and does not fit well into any classification. Sometimes, however, these adrenal medullary tumors produce a sustained type of hypertension indistinguishable from other types of chronic hypertension. Chronic hypertension of this type has not yet been produced in the experimental animal by repeated injections of epinephrine, and its pathogenesis in man is not well understood. An interesting group are the tumors and hyperplasias of the adrenal cortex and of the basophile cells of the pituitary gland (Cushing's syndrome) in which diabetes, hirsuties, hypertension and other manifestations of adrenal cortical hyperactivity are present. The increased incidence of hypertension at the climacteric in both males and females is also a fact, but not well understood.

All these diseases account for only 20 or 25 per cent of hypertensive disease. The remaining 75 per cent are of unknown etiology; i.e., no constant underlying disease process can be identified. These are all combined under the time-honored name of *"essential hypertension"*—the hyperpiesia of All-

butt. Those hypertensive diseases associated with the underlying diseases just enumerated behave in a manner practically identical in all basic respects with essential hypertension with only one exception. If there is an associated renal disease, death is more likely to be due to renal insufficiency. As regards the severity of the vascular process and the complications that ensue, there is little in the behavior of the hypertensive disease to distinguish essential hypertension from those diastolic hypertensions due to other causes. The similarity in the behavior of all these hypertensions, essential or otherwise, has led many to suspect that they are all mediated through the kidney and that a disturbance in the function of some other organ may act upon the kidney to produce in turn essential hypertension. Proof of this hypothesis is still lacking.

Morbid Anatomy. The age-old controversy of which comes first, the elevated blood pressure or pathologic changes in the arterioles of the body, especially the kidney, is still unresolved. Renal biopsies in early hypertensive disease may show no clear-cut evidence of arteriolar nephrosclerosis. The significance of this observation is much debated. Later on in the disease, arteriolar sclerosis characterized by thickening of the media is found in scattered distribution throughout the body and almost constantly in the kidney—the arteriolar nephrosclerosis of the pathologist. This is the most important pathologic finding in benign hypertension. Prior to the stage of nitrogen retention, but when the clinical course has already taken on a rapid progression, intimal proliferation of the arterioles (the so-called onion-skin arteriole) is usually widespread pathologically. With the advent of nitrogen retention, necrotizing arteriolitis involving arterioles throughout the body, including the kidney (the malignant nephrosclerosis of the pathologist), often appears. Although there is a general relationship between the clinical course and the histologic appearance of the arterioles, there are many exceptions to this generalization.

The heart shows hypertrophy of the left ventricle, the hypertrophy being an increase in the size of the muscle cells. The kidney becomes decreased in size. The surface is granular, the cortex narrowed. The afferent arteriole particularly shows the changes just described. The glomeruli become ischemic and hyalinized, and the tubules degenerated. Replacement fibrosis becomes increasingly

Classification of Hypertension and Hypertensive Disease

I. HYPERTENSION (important only in reflecting the underlying disease)

    A. From increased stroke output:
        1. Complete heart block (R)
        2. Aortic insufficiency (C)
        3. Hyperthyroidism (NC)*
        4. Arteriovenous aneurysm (R)*
        5. Patent ductus arteriosus (R)*
        6. Anxiety state (VC)

    B. From rigid vessels:
        1. Generalized arteriosclerosis (VC)

    C. From neurogenic stimulation:
        1. Increased intracranial pressure (R)*
            (trauma, tumors, inflammation)
        2. Asphyxia: bulbar poliomyelitis (R)
        3. Anxiety state (VC)

II. HYPERTENSIVE DISEASE

    A. Acute
        1. Acute glomerulonephritis (NC)
        2. Toxemia of pregnancy (pre-eclampsia and eclampsia) (C)

    B. Chronic
        1. Affections of renal vessels
            (a) Coarctation of the aorta (R)*
            (b) Arteritis
                (1) Disseminated lupus erythematosus (R)
                (2) Polyarteritis nodosa (R)
                (3) Dermatomyositis (R)
                (4) Thrombo-angiitis obliterans (R)
            (c) Vascular anomalies and obstructions
                (embolism, venous and arterial; thrombosis; aneurysm; tumor; atherosclerotic plaques; hypogenesis of renal artery; dissecting aneurysm of aorta) (R)

        2. Affections of parenchyma
            (a) Chronic pyelonephritis (C)*
            (b) Chronic nephritis (C)
            (c) Post-toxemic hypertension (NC)
            (d) Nephrotic syndrome (R)
            (e) Congenital polycystic kidneys (R)
            (f) Congenital hypoplasia of kidneys (R)
            (g) Tumors (R)*

        3. Affections of perinephric structures
            (a) Perinephritis (x-ray, trauma, inflammation) (R)
            (b) Retroperitoneal masses causing pressure (tumor, hematoma) (R)*

        4. Endocrine
            (a) Adrenal cortical carcinoma, adenoma, or hyperplasia (R)
            (b) Cushing's syndrome (pituitary basophilism) (R)
            (c) Pheochromocytoma: adenoma or carcinoma (R)*
            (d) Menopause (C)

        5. Unknown: essential hypertension (benign or malignant) (VC)

The following abbreviations after the various diseases are designed to give an idea of the relative frequency of these lesions:

VC = very common
 C = common
NC = not common
 R = rare
  * = specifically remediable or potentially remediable

prominent as the nephrons are destroyed. In the retina, flame-shaped hemorrhages appear. Focal necroses in the superficial layers of the retina appear as exudates. Neuroretinal edema and papilledema are bad prognostic signs and may be accompanied by retinal detachment. Fatty star-shaped configurations around the macula may occur.

Clinical Course. The clinical course of hypertensive disease follows a rather set pattern, but varies enormously in the speed with which it progresses. When the course is one of slow progression over a period of many years, it is referred to as benign. When it progresses rapidly to cause death over a period of months, it is thought of as malignant. Current concepts of hypertensive disease indicate that the terms "mild" and "severe" could just as well be substituted for benign and malignant.

Benign Hypertension. The onset of hypertension is insidious. Periodic examination at the onset reveals a diastolic blood pressure that is sometimes somewhat elevated, at other times entirely normal, and sometimes borderline. Not too rarely, the blood pressure, after a period of days, weeks or months of elevation, becomes entirely normal and remains so. In maybe two thirds of the patients, however, the blood pressure eventually becomes constantly elevated. There is no way of making a correct diagnosis until the blood pressure becomes consistently high. In most cases the patient remains asymptomatic for years, and, were it not for the blood pressure cuff, there would be little or no evidence to suggest the presence of this disease. It is common experience that a patient first seeks medical advice in his forties or fifties because of some one of the complications of hypertension such as headaches, failing vision, cerebrovascular accident, exertional dyspnea, angina pectoris or coronary thrombosis. The diastolic blood pressure is usually in excess of 100 mm. of mercury, but rarely over 125 or 130 mm. The height of the blood pressure bears little relation to the severity of the process. It may vary markedly from visit to visit, such changes being of no clinical significance. *Indeed, it is only by evaluating the complications of the hypertension rather than the height of the blood pressure itself that insight may be gained in regard to the progression and severity of the hypertensive process.* Complications may appear ten or fifteen years after the onset, sometimes sooner and often later. The vulnerable organs are predominantly the heart, the eye, the brain and the kidneys.

The heart becomes enlarged and eventually may fail. Retinal examination usually reveals arterioles narrower than normal with an irregular caliber of their outline. Albuminuric retinitis is absent, although an associated diabetes mellitus or nephrotic syndrome may produce a similar retinal picture. Renal function is usually not significantly impaired unless there is some underlying renal disease. Urinalysis may be normal or show perhaps one-plus proteinuria and a few casts. Again, if there is an associated renal disease, these findings may be more pronounced. A variety of neurologic complaints may appear sooner or later, owing to cerebral vascular involvement. Such patients may live for many years without apparent change in their condition. Some may attain a ripe old age. Indeed, many patients with benign essential hypertension die from causes other than vascular. Their life expectancy, however, is less than normal, and death is the result of cardiac failure, a cerebrovascular accident or intercurrent disease. Death from uremia is not common in essential hypertension, and common if there is obvious underlying renal disease.

Malignant Hypertension. Classically, this occurs in young persons, often in their third decade. It may be the end result, however, of benign essential hypertension or hypertension due to any of the renal diseases enumerated in the table, and it may have its onset in the older age groups. The course of the hypertension until the present has been perfectly benign. For some reason not readily apparent, the progress of the disease becomes rapid, the evolution of the hypertensive life span becoming telescoped into a relatively few months instead of extending over a period of many years. Complications fall one upon the other in rapid succession. Cerebral symptoms, whether or not present previously, become severe. Cardiac function may deteriorate rapidly. Renal function decreases. Vision fails and blindness may ensue. Albuminuric retinitis appears, characterized by papilledema and retinal exudates and hemorrhages. The general condition of the patient is one of rapid degeneration. The character of the disease has changed from mildness to violence, from benign to malignant. Microscopic and occasionally gross hematuria, proteinuria and casts are found in the urine. The patient dies in uremia unless, as often happens, he has already succumbed as a result of congestive heart failure or a cerebral hemorrhage. The total duration of the illness from the onset of albuminuric retinitis and nitrogen retention is usually about six months and rarely exceeds a year.

Complications. *The Heart.* The heart gradually hypertrophies, owing, in part, to the high pressure required during systolic discharge and in part to intrinsic disease of the coronary vessels. The increased work involves only the left ventricle, since the pulmonary circuit does not partake in the hypertensive process. The electrocardiogram may show no changes for long periods other than those of left ventricular hypertrophy. Atrial fibrillation may appear sooner or later. As the left ventricle becomes incompetent, dyspnea appears on an amount of exertion previously well tolerated. This is followed by orthopnea. Paroxysmal nocturnal dyspnea, nightmares or apprehension are further manifestations of left ventricular failure. It is usually only a matter of a year or less after outright left ventricular failure that right ventricular failure with chronic passive congestion of the viscera, edema and distention of the neck veins becomes manifest. It should be remembered, however, that there is great individual variation in the rate at which heart failure progresses. This appears to depend particularly on two factors—the rate of progression of the hypertensive process, and the state of the coronary arteries. If angina pectoris is present or coronary thrombosis occurs, the outlook is much more gloomy. A considerable proportion of patients with hypertension die from cardiac failure.

The Eye. The one place in the body where arterioles are directly visible is the retina. Although many changes have been described, perhaps the easiest for those physicians who have had no special training in ophthalmology to see is the irregularity in the caliber of the vessels. Normally, the retinal arterioles have a smooth contour gradually becoming narrower as they extend out toward the periphery. In hypertensive patients the vessel becomes "puckered" with what appear to be short areas of narrowing, then widening, then narrowing. In more advanced cases the vessel "burrows;" i.e., it disappears for a short distance, only to reappear further along its path. An early change, but one requiring considerable ophthalmologic experience to evaluate, is narrowing of the retinal arteri-

oles. Arteriovenous nicking, the apparent pinching in of a vein where the arteriole crosses it, is commonly seen to some extent in normal eyegrounds. Unless accompanied by other manifestations of hypertensive disease, it is of no import. Tortuosity of the arterioles is likewise of no significance from the hypertensive viewpoint. "Albuminuric" retinitis is characterized by bilateral papilledema, retinal edema, cottonwool exudates, macular stars and hemorrhages. It is not seen in benign essential hypertension, but is often seen in chronic nephritis, the nephrotic syndrome and malignant hypertension. In the interpretation of the significance of retinal vascular lesions, the eye offers a glimpse of a generalized arteriolar disease. No two organs are involved to an identical extent in any given patient, and it is to be emphasized that retinal vascular changes reflect in general the condition of the arterioles in the body as a whole, but not specifically the condition of the vessels in the brain or the kidneys.

The Kidney. Renal function is, for many years, normal or only slightly impaired, as judged by concentration and phenolsulfonphthalein tests in patients with benign essential hypertension. Renal blood flow measured by Diodrast or para-aminohippurate clearance techniques is regularly reduced and the filtration fraction increased. Barring the complication of malignant hypertension, renal function seldom becomes seriously impaired in benign essential hypertension, and death from uremia is rare. When hypertension is associated with demonstrable renal disease (chronic nephritis, chronic pyelonephritis, polycystic kidneys, and the like), the kidney must be looked upon as suffering from two diseases—the primary renal disease producing destruction of the nephrons, and hypertension which, with its associated decrease in renal blood flow, leads to atrophy of the nephron. Because of this, renal function is reduced to a greater extent than either disorder alone would produce, and death in uremia is common.

The Brain. Many patients with hypertension suffer from a variety of complaints referable to the central nervous system. The typical hypertensive headaches are occipital in location, throbbing in character, and present in the morning on awakening. They characteristically wear off an hour or so after assuming the upright position. They may be predominantly frontal and parietal in location. It should be emphasized that many hypertensive patients complain of headaches not related to their hypertensive disease. Emotional instability and "nervousness" occur in patients with, as well as without, hypertension. Loss of concentrating ability and forgetfulness, especially of recent events, may occur in hypertensive patients and in those in the older age group with cerebral arteriosclerosis. Tinnitus may be bothersome. Transient episodes of weakness, tingling and numbness of hands or feet, partial aphasia, and a host of other neurologic symptoms and signs may appear for a few minutes, hours or days. At times, such fleeting neurologic manifestations may presage a more serious cerebrovascular accident. Cerebral hemorrhage can be one of the serious complications of hypertension. The more common cerebral thrombosis is a manifestation of cerebral atherosclerosis which is commonly associated with hypertensive disease.

Hypertensive encephalopathy refers to a symptom complex which resembles an epileptic seizure. Prodromata such as headache, vomiting, weakness, apathy or excitement, paresthesias and pallor may be present for hours or even several days. The blood pressure rises during this period. Convulsions may occur suddenly, with or without these prodromata. They are clonic or tonic and usually last only a few minutes. They frequently are repetitive. Coma may ensue. The patient may recover completely or be left with residual neurologic damage. This symptom complex covers a wide variety of underlying lesions. Identical manifestations are encountered in epilepsy and brain tumor, uremia, cerebral hemorrhage, thrombosis and embolism, encephalitis and lead poisoning. When convulsions appear in hypertensive patients, the cause is usually one of these conditions. In a small group, however, there is no obvious cause other than the hypertension, in which case it is permissible to make a diagnosis of hypertensive encephalopathy. It is to be emphasized, however, that this diagnosis should be made with caution, since serious and sometimes remediable underlying causes are usually found.

Atherosclerosis of Large Arteries. Atherosclerosis of large arteries is such a common accompaniment of hypertensive (arteriolar) disease that it may in a sense be considered a complication of the hypertensive process. It is more frequent in patients with hypertensive disease than in others. Its frequency parallels age, being rare in the young and common over 50. Evidence suggests that the atherosclerotic lesions arise at locations of stress, such as at vascular bifurcations, although metabolic factors may eventually turn out to be more important in their genesis.

Atherosclerosis usually produces no symptoms until thrombotic occlusion of a large artery occurs or impends. As a thrombotic disease, it leads to cerebral thrombosis, angina pectoris, and coronary thrombosis with myocardial infarction, intermittent claudication and gangrene of the legs, and infarction of various organs such as, for example, the kidney.

Physical signs of atherosclerosis are unreliable, because it has such a patchy distribution. If strategically located, one atherosclerotic plaque in a coronary artery may kill, the remainder of the larger arteries being essentially normal and free of disease. On the other hand, atherosclerosis is often diffuse and accompanied by a widespread loss of elasticity of the large arteries. The palpable large arteries, such as the radial or brachial, may feel rigid to the touch, and pulsations of the dorsalis pedis may no longer be detectable. As discussed earlier, the pulse pressure may widen, and this is often the only real clue to the existence of widespread arterial disease. Smithwick has devised a useful procedure for evaluating the pulse pressure in this regard. Patients with narrow pulse pressures which are less than one half the diastolic pressure have type I hypertension. Those with wider pulse pressures equal to or up to 19 mm. more than one half the diastolic pressure have type II hypertension. Those with the widest pulse pressures, 20 mm. or more greater than one half the diastolic pressure, have type III hypertension. Type I hypertension can in general be considered to be mainly arteriolar, type III mainly arterial and type II intermediate. This is a useful calculation to make in giving some idea as to the relative amounts of arterial and arteriolar disease present, but its limitations, as discussed before, are many. There are no laboratory tests for detecting the presence of atherosclerosis.

Thus, atherosclerosis is difficult to detect with any precision by any method as yet devised. Thrombosis and infarction of some organ may be the first definite clue of its presence. *Its importance cannot be overemphasized, because death from the atherosclerotic process is far more common than from the hypertensive disease (i.e., the arteriolar process) itself.*

Diagnosis and Evaluation. In advanced cases, diagnosis is easy. In early cases the diagnosis may be extremely difficult. Take, for example, a young person with a blood pressure at the first visit of 150/95. There are no retinal, cardiac or urinary abnormalities, and the patient is without symptoms. Is hypertensive disease present? There is no answer to this question. It is only by following the patient at intervals of six months or so for a period of a year or two that the diagnosis will be established. If, during this period, the physician's attitude makes the patient become conscious of blood pressure, the problem of diagnosis becomes even more difficult, since the blood pressure is liable to become elevated at the sight of a blood pressure cuff. If an elevated blood pressure is found repeatedly and consistently, and, more important, if there are vascular complications, it is fair to assume that the patient has hypertensive disease.

The next problem is to decide the cause of the elevated blood pressure, i.e., whether it is of the progressive arteriolar variety (early hypertensive disease), atherosclerotic in origin, particularly in the older age group, or incidental to one of the causes enumerated in the table on page 1251, such as aortic insufficiency or complete heart block. The elevated blood pressure associated with increased intracranial pressure from, for example, brain tumor may closely simulate primary hypertensive disease.

Assuming the existence of hypertensive disease itself, i.e., the progressive arteriolar type characterized by an elevation of diastolic blood pressure and ultimate damage to heart, brain or kidneys, search for evidence of cause and of complications must be made.

Coarctation of the aorta is recognized by the finding of a lower blood pressure in the legs than in the arms, using the standard blood pressure cuff. Intercostal pulsations, notching of the ribs by roentgenogram, and a systolic murmur which is as loud over the back as over the precordium, are salient points in diagnosis. Being curable surgically, it should never be overlooked.

Pheochromocytomas, producing epinephrine and norepinephrine, are rare. They may produce paroxysms of hypertension with a normal blood pressure between attacks or a sustained elevation of blood pressure indistinguishable clinically from essential hypertension. Their presence may be recognized by the response to such drugs as epinephrine, benzodioxane, histamine and others. Pyelography and perirenal air insufflation may reveal a tumor mass at the pole of one of the kidneys. The importance of these tumors is their surgical removability.

The presence of an underlying renal disease is usually suspected by the finding of abnormalities in the urine. On each visit the urine should be tested, and a concentration test or phenolsulfonphthalein test carried out at yearly intervals. In children and young adults up to the age of 35, retrograde pyelography with ureteral cultures should be routine as soon as hypertension is discovered, regardless of the presence or absence of symptoms referable to the urinary tract. Only in this way can congenital abnormalities of the urinary tract and chronic asymptomatic pyelonephritis be recognized. In the younger age group these two lesions are the commonest causes of hypertension, and both are potentially remediable. Over the age of about 35, pyelography should depend on urologic indications.

Azotemia in its early stages is often unaccompanied by symptoms, and yet its presence in heralding the approach of terminal uremia is important to recognize. It is rarely present in the absence of albuminuria. If albuminuria is present, it is wise to test the blood yearly for nitrogen retention—either a nonprotein nitrogen or a blood urea nitrogen.

The cerebral status is determined mainly by history. Inquiry is made for such symptoms as nervousness, insomnia, headaches, tinnitus, loss of concentrating ability, fatigue, weakness, dizziness, paresthesias, aphasia, hemiplegia, and the like. Objective findings are verified by neurologic examination.

The cardiac status is evaluated mainly in terms of function. Inquiry is made as to the existence of exertional dyspnea, orthopnea, paroxysmal nocturnal dyspnea, edema and angina. It is well to establish an objective baseline of heart size by roentgenogram, and electrical activity and rhythm by electrocardiogram, for comparison with subsequent films and tracings taken at yearly intervals. Some idea of the progress of the disease may then be obtained.

On each visit the eyegrounds should be examined for abnormalities of the optic disks, especially papilledema, and of the arterioles. Search for hemorrhages and exudates should be made.

Prognosis. It is difficult to render an accurate prognosis in any given patient. *There is little or no correlation between the height of the blood pressure and symptoms, rate of progression, and development of complications.* Complications may occur in a single organ, the function of the others remaining essentially normal, or several organ systems may become involved simultaneously with the same or different rates of progression.

Statistics are difficult to evaluate. The average duration of life exceeded sixteen years after its onset in the extensive studies by Perera and his associates. Survivals of twenty, thirty, and even more than forty years have been well documented. The prognosis is less favorable in men than in women and in patients with an underlying renal disease.

In malignant hypertension accompanied by papilledema and uremia the outlook for life is about six months and rarely exceeds one year. Fortunately, the incidence of these rapidly progressive hypertensions is only about 5 per cent.

More than half of the patients with hypertensive disease die from cardiac complications, less than a third from cerebrovascular accidents, and only about 10 per cent from renal insufficiency.

General Treatment. *Presymptomatic Stage.* If the patient is made overconscious of his blood pressure, his life becomes one of anxiety and even semi-invalidism. If, on the other hand, a fairly free rein is given to his activities, that period of his life before the onset of hypertensive complications remains full, enjoyable and useful. The author is aware of no evidence to indicate a prolongation of life by the application of any therapy at present available, since specific therapy for hypertensive disease is lacking. It is only reasonable, therefore, to emphasize that at the stage before symptoms or complications appear, the most important therapeutic principle is the prevention of anxiety on the part of the patient over his blood pressure. Prevention of anxiety is not believed to influence the hypertensive disease itself, but does make all the difference in the patient's outlook on life. Any anxiety exhibited by the physician is immediately transmitted to the patient. The patient should be told of his disease, referring to it as a blood pressure "tendency" or as high blood pressure, and immediate steps should be taken to explain what this means. The patient should be told in simple terms how pressure produces flow of blood through the body, how pressure rises and falls as a result of emotion, exercise and change of posture, and how, if it did not, the patient would faint every time he ran up stairs or got out of bed. He can be disabused of the general lay belief that a stroke will occur when pressure rises in this fashion, since strokes occur as often in bed as when the patient is ambulatory. One can emphasize that rises or falls of blood pressure from one visit to the next are of absolutely no significance to the physician. What the physician wishes to know is what the blood pressure is doing to the patient. To this end, questions will be asked, the eyes examined, the heart listened to, and the urine tested at periodic intervals. The chronicity of the process should be explained, with a statement that, although trouble will probably occur someday, it is impossible to tell whether it will be ten or fifteen or more years from now. Most patients do not inquire further as to the nature of this "trouble," and if they do, it has been projected so far into the future as to mean little to them. There is no need to mention the serious complications just to have it on the record. Finally, the physician can tell the patient, in light vein, that he should let him (the physician) do the worrying and that he will let the patient know when to become worried.

A full hypertensive work-up is indicated as described to establish a baseline, and after one or two visits at brief intervals to acquaint the patient with the results, again with the idea of reassurance, follow-up visits for check-up should not be more frequent than once or twice a year. Since, in the asymptomatic, well compensated hypertensive person with benign hypertension, complications do not ordinarily occur until some indeterminate time in the future, nothing is to be gained by more frequent ·visits except to make the patient worry about his blood pressure. If at any time any untoward or unforeseen complication appears, measures can immediately be introduced to handle the situation.

At this stage of the disease it is comforting to the patient to hear that there is no indication for dietary restriction (unless he is obese), surgery or radical change in his way of life. If the patient is young, he should follow the activity pattern of his more slow-moving companions, avoiding only the peak loads of exercise and avoiding intemperance. It is well for the patient to refrain from group competition in sports, such as basket-ball, football, soccer and crew, in which the desire not to let his teammates down may force him to excesses of exertion. On the other hand, tennis, swimming, baseball and the like should be permitted. More harm than good will result from imposing restrictions which make his pattern of life unnatural. In the middle and older age groups, their way of life need not change.

Excesses in general should be avoided. This includes tobacco, alcohol, coffee and tea, late hours, long working hours, overeating and no vacations. These are general measures which, after all, apply to all patients. In moderation or on occasion, none of these factors do harm.

A great deal has been written about therapy applied to the emotional aspects of the patient's life. This should be managed in the hypertensive as in the nonhypertensive person. Psychotherapy for the control of the hypertensive process has, with rare exceptions, been unrewarding. Psychotherapy should be reserved for psychiatric indications, but not with the idea of benefiting the hypertensive disease.

Considerable time has been spent in emphasizing that these patients not be pampered, restricted, dieted and overtreated in the asymptomatic phase of their disease. Watchful neglect, as advocated, makes life full and worth living for the patient. Overtreatment appears to do nothing except to produce an anxiety state and only too often semi-invalidism, all to no avail.

Symptomatic Stage. Headaches may yield to elevation of the head of the bed on 4- or 6-inch blocks, a cup of strong coffee or tea on arising, simple analgesics (aspirin, 0.6 gm.) or various commercial varieties of pills containing mixtures of aspirin, acetophenetidin and caffeine. Morphine and its derivatives should be avoided because of the danger of habit formation in those whose symptoms may persist for years. Intractable headaches sometimes respond to lumbar puncture and usually to sympathectomy. For giddiness, dizziness, irritability, easy fatigability, lack of energy, insomnia and the like, there is no specific therapy. These are often manifestations of frustration, maladjustment and neurosis, not of the hypertension, and occur about as frequently in patients without as with hypertensive disease. They respond to the sympathetic ear and the counsel of a wise physician better than to pills. For the

nervous, high-strung person, chloral hydrate, 0.3 gm., or elixir of sodium bromide, one teaspoonful three times a day after meals, is the preparation of choice. For insomnia, the choice of drug depends on the time of occurrence of the insomnia. For those having difficulty getting to sleep, chloral hydrate, 1 to 1.5 gm., should be taken about 30 minutes before bedtime. For those who go off to sleep, but awaken in the early morning hours, one of the slower-acting barbiturates, such as barbital (0.3 to 0.5 gm.) or phenobarbital (0.1 to 0.2 gm.), is preferable.

Treatment of the Blood Pressure. Various measures have been introduced from time to time with the purpose of lowering the blood pressure, since evidence seems to indicate that, if this can be accomplished, the underlying vascular disease with its complications improves accordingly. These measures can conveniently be grouped as medical and surgical.

Medical Therapy. ANTIHYPERTENSIVE AND DEPRESSOR AGENTS. Tissue extracts, vegetable extracts, vaccines, hormones, nitrites, sedatives, pyrogens, phlebotomies, thiocyanates and sympatholytic agents have all been administered for hypertensive disease, only to be abandoned.

Many new depressor drugs have recently been introduced and are being used in the treatment of hypertension. Their usage is based on the assumption that the underlying disease process will either become quiescent or recede if blood pressure falls to or toward normal. Whether such an assumption is justified remains to be proven. As Hoobler has stated, the ideal hypotensive agent should produce a prolonged fall of blood pressure in a large proportion of patients through generalized peripheral vasodilatation without serious side effects and without the development of tolerance. No such drug exists. Drugs which have received the widest study in the last few years are as follows:

1. Adrenergic blocking agents (Dibenzyline)
2. Ganglionic blocking agents (methonium compounds)
3. Centrally acting inhibitors (1-hydrazinophthalazine)
4. Activators of afferent reflex areas (veratrum compounds)
5. Drugs of unknown or mixed action (Rauwolfia serpentina)

Dibenzyline is an adrenergic blocker when

used in a dosage of 10 to 40 mg. three times a day by mouth. It produces tachycardia, drowsiness, nasal congestion and postural hypotension. The development of tolerance is only slight.

Methonium compounds are powerful ganglionic blockers and are difficult to administer orally because of irregular absorption. Various methonium derivatives are being studied, but hexamethonium has received the widest appraisal. The dosage varies from 125 to 250 mg. by mouth every 6 hours but because of its irregular absorption the dosage for any individual is unpredictable. Side reactions, which are very common, include constipation, collapse, urinary retention, postural hypotension and angina. In inexperienced hands, serious complications including death have been altogether too frequent as a result of this therapy. The dosage must be altered as tolerance develops.

1-Hydrazinophthalazine (Apresoline) is used in an oral dosage of 10 to 50 mg. every 6 hours. It produces a fall of blood pressure, tachycardia, increased cardiac output, headache, and at times angina pectoris. A disseminated lupus erythematosus-like syndrome has been increasingly reported to appear in as high as 10 per cent of patients on long-term treatment with Apresoline. Tolerance develops rapidly.

Veratrum compounds are powerful hypotensive agents. One of the most active principles is protoveratrine. The oral dose of protoveratrine is 0.75 to 1.5 mg. daily in divided dosage. Unfortunately, the effective dose usually produces nausea, vomiting, bradycardia, and a precipitate and often alarming fall of blood pressure. Tolerance develops within two to four weeks.

Rauwolfia serpentina is mildly hypotensive, has a relaxing type of sedative action and produces a mild bradycardia. The dosage of this drug varies from 25 to 100 mg. three times a day by mouth. One of the active principles is the purified alkaloid reserpine (Serpasil). Its initial dosage is 0.25 mg. three or four times a day, reduced after two to three weeks to 0.5 mg. daily according to the patient's response and needs.

For one reason or another, none of these various agents are entirely satisfactory. Toxic side reactions limit their usefulness. Hypotensive "cocktails," consisting of reduced dosage of two or three in combination, appear to be more promising than any single drug in their hypotensive effect and lack of toxic side reactions. One of the most serious side-effects in the usage of these drugs is the development of severe hypotension with syncope, collapse, renal shutdown or thrombosis of large vessels. The physician must have a thorough knowledge of the pharmacology and toxicology of these drugs. Since they are so powerful, since the initial dosage must be individualized, and since the patient must be almost as indoctrinated as is a diabetic with insulin, it is desirable to institute therapy under observation in the hospital until the precise dosage schedule is established.

DIETARY MEASURES. The use of a low salt diet (less than 1 gm. daily) for hypertension has recently been revived with considerable enthusiasm. The rice diet of Kempner is low in salt (0.2 gm. daily) and deficient in protein (20 gm. daily). The evaluation of low salt regimens is difficult because, although blood pressure may decrease in some cases, there is no convincing evidence as yet available that the progress of the disease is retarded or arrested. Whether the lowering of blood pressure from salt restriction is due to decreases in cardiac output, in peripheral resistance or in serum sodium has not been satisfactorily explained. One of the greatest obstacles to the implementation of a low salt diet is the lack of cooperation of almost all patients unless symptoms are alleviated by the diet. The use of a low salt diet before the occurrence of symptoms appears to be not only impractical, but of dubious benefit. After the appearance of symptoms, however, salt restriction may be highly beneficial. It may at times produce striking improvement in those with hypertensive headaches. It is time-honored in the therapy of cardiac insufficiency. In all but a few patients with renal insufficiency, dietary salt restriction is indicated.

Thus, before symptoms appear, extreme salt restriction is not practical, and there is no evidence that it slows down the progress of the hypertensive disease. Its main benefit is for the symptoms of hypertensive disease. During the heat of summer, it is well to add 1 or 2 gm. of salt to the diet in order to prevent sodium depletion—the so-called low salt syndrome, wherein the patient experiences cramps, weakness, nausea, vomiting, stupor, anuria and even death.

Surgical Therapy. There are in general

three operations on the sympathetic nervous system for hypertension: (1) splanchnicectomy and resection of the sympathetic chain from the ninth through the twelfth thoracic ganglia (Peet operation). This is performed supradiaphragmatically, both sides being done at one operation. Postoperative postural hypotension is rare. The patient can return to his usual activities in a month or six weeks. (2) Splanchnicectomy and resection of the sympathetic chain from the tenth thoracic ganglion or higher through the second lumbar ganglion (Smithwick operation). This is performed transdiaphragmatically in two stages. Postoperative hypotension is the rule. Postoperative disability lasts usually for at least six months and often more. (3) Complete sympathectomy (Grimson operation). The results of this operation have not been reported in a large enough series as yet for this author to render an evaluation.

Despite the fact that there are now about twenty years of experience with sympathectomy, its evaluation as a therapeutic procedure is still controversial. Many patients are not benefited. A few are dramatically improved, particularly those with rapidly progressing hypertensive disease before the stage of azotemia and without complicating atherosclerosis. Present evidence seems to indicate that in the reported results, only about 5 to 10 per cent of the patients have been sufficiently benefited by sympathectomy to have warranted the procedure. The problem of choosing those patients who will be helped is extremely difficult. At this time the most favorable candidates appear to be those under 45 or 50 years of age, with a narrow pulse pressure (Smithwick, type I) and a rapidly progressing course. Congestive heart failure, extensive retinal changes and associated renal disease (pyelonephritis, glomerulonephritis) are not contraindications to the operation. Cerebrovascular accidents should make one hesitate to suggest sympathectomy unless the patient is an ideal candidate in other respects. Definite contraindications are the presence of nitrogen retention, a wide pulse pressure (type III and usually type II of Smithwick), angina pectoris or a previous coronary thrombosis. If symptoms are not present, it is well to bear in mind that the patient will be made symptomatically much worse for many months. For this reason the writer considers the absence of symptoms to be a contraindication. In all reported series, relief of hyper-

tensive headaches has followed the operation in about 80 per cent of cases.

The after-effects of the operation depend on the extent of the procedure. Back pain usually persists for months. The choice of operation—Peet, Smithwick or Grimson—is likewise hard to evaluate. From the reported results, there appears to be little choice between the first two.

It seems probable that, in the future, sympathectomy will be relegated to a small group of patients with hypertensive disease. Though seldom if ever curative, the results when successful are indeed impressive.

LEWIS DEXTER

References

Ayman, D.: Arterial Hypertension. New York, Oxford University, 1948.
Braun-Menéndez, E., and others: Renal Hypertension, translated by L. Dexter. Springfield, Ill., Charles C Thomas, 1946.
Hoobler, S. W., and Dontas, A. S.: Drug Treatment of Hypertension. Pharmacol. Rev., 5:135, 1953.
Page, I. H., and Corcoran, A. C.: Arterial Hypertension. Its Diagnosis and Treatment. 2d ed. Chicago, Year Book Publishers, 1949.
Perera, G. A., and Atchley, D. W.: Hypertensive Vascular Disease, in Nelson's Loose-Leaf Medicine. New York, Thomas Nelson & Sons, 1949, Vol. 4, pp. 233–263.
Symposium on Hypertension by Various Authors. Am. J. Med., 4: January-June, 1948.

VASCULAR HYPOTENSION

Vascular hypotension has been arbitrarily defined as a systolic blood pressure below 110 mm. of mercury and a diastolic below 70 mm. in adults. Three groups of vascular hypotension are recognized: (a) primary hypotension, (b) secondary hypotension and (c) postural hypotension.

Primary Hypotension. Primary hypotension is extremely common, occurring in about 25 to 30 per cent of the population. It is found particularly in thin, flat-chested and slender members of each sex. It is not a disease in any way, but represents an ideal blood pressure level, since there are no symptoms attributable to it and life expectancy from life insurance statistics has demonstrated a lower mortality than in those with average pressures. Patients with low blood pressure have often been thought to have fatigability, loss of vitality and vigor, headaches, irritability and insomnia. These are symptoms which are more commonly found in hypertension and as frequently in patients with normal blood pressure. Obviously, the level of blood pressure is not the common denominator and it may be stated categorically that there are no symptoms ascribable to this type of low blood pressure. Medically speaking, the patient may be congratulated.

Secondary Hypotension. Hypotension may be secondary to serious disease processes, and usually there is no difficulty in recognizing the cause. Among such causes are (1) circulatory shock from hemorrhage, trauma, anesthesia, hyperinsulinism and a host of other causes; (2) Addison's disease; (3) Simmonds' disease; (4) cachexia and malnutrition; (5) acute and chronic infections. Secondary hypotension is of no significance except in the presence of circulatory collapse, i.e., shock or an Addison's crisis in which signs of an inadequate peripheral circulation occur, especially a cold and damp skin. The patient is weak and tired. On stooping over or assuming the upright position, vision becomes darkened (giddiness as opposed to vertigo), and syncope may occur. In the other conditions mentioned the level of blood pressure is apparently scaled to the metabolic needs of the patient, and the symptomatology present is due primarily to the underlying disease. The prognosis and treatment are those of the associated condition.

Postural Hypotension. In the standing position the amount of blood present in the upper part of the body is decreased, largely because of dilatation of blood vessels in the lower part of the body by a high hydrostatic pressure. This is normally compensated for by vasoconstriction and tachycardia mediated through the sympathetic nervous system so that the blood pressure is little affected. In postural hypotension the patient, on assuming the upright position, experiences blurred vision, weakness and syncope, the blood pressure having fallen to low levels. On lying down, consciousness returns. Postural hypotension occurs under two general sets of conditions, as follows:

Exaggerated Venous Pooling in the Presence of a Normally Functioning Sympathetic Nervous System. This is most commonly seen to a greater or lesser degree in many older people. It is one of the cardinal signs of circulatory collapse or shock. It is also seen at all ages in association with postinfectional states, immobile standing as in soldiers at attention, extensive varicose veins, large venous angiomas of the lower extremities, Addison's disease, and the squatting of cyanotic patients with low cardiac outputs who have congenital heart disease (tetralogy of Fallot, tricuspid atresia). Syncope usually occurs when the systolic blood pressure falls to a level of 70 or 80 mm. of mercury.

Failure of Sympathetic Nervous System Impulses in Response to the Normal Pooling of Blood on Assuming the Upright Position. There is a loss of reflex vasoconstriction in response to a fall of blood pressure. In certain patients only the postural vasoconstrictor reflexes are affected. If the lesion is more extensive, other signs of loss of sympathetic function may be present, such as loss of sweating and absence of an increase in heart rate when the blood pressure falls. In these persons there is no abnormally large pooling of blood in the lower extremities in the upright position. This type of postural hypotension has been reported in tabes dorsalis, multiple sclerosis, syringomyelia, amyotrophic lateral sclerosis and other types of neurologic disorders, and following extensive lumbodorsal sympathectomy for hypertension. In some cases there is no obvious associated disease. Syncope usually does not occur until the blood pressure falls to a level of about 50 mm. of mercury.

If there is a correctible underlying disorder, therapy should be directed at its removal. In the persistent cases, drug therapy may meet with variable success. Ephedrine, 25 to 50 mg., amphetamine sulfate, 10 to 40 gm., and paredrinol, 20 mg., at appropriate time intervals can be tried. When the severity of symptoms warrants, postural hypotension can usually be prevented by the use of snug elastic bandages or stockings to lower extremities applied with the legs horizontal or inclined upwards, and in the most severe cases by the addition of an abdominal binder.

LEWIS DEXTER

References

Robinson, S. C.: Hypotension: the Ideal Normal Blood Pressure. New England J. Med., 223:407, 1940.
Spingarn, C. L., and Hitzig, W. M.: Orthostatic Circulatory Insufficiency. Its Occurrence in Tabes Dorsalis and Addison's Disease. Arch. Int. Med., 69:23, 1942.
Stead, E. A., Jr., and Ebert, R. V.: Postural Hypotension, a Disease of the Sympathetic Nervous System. Arch. Int. Med., 67:546, 1941.

CIRCULATORY COLLAPSE AND SHOCK

The terms "circulatory collapse" and "shock" are used to describe the clinical appearance of patients with circulatory insufficiency in which the usual signs of congestive heart failure are absent. The patient appears ill and complains of weakness. The radial pulse is thready, the systolic arterial pressure is low and the pulse pressure is small. Pallor, sweating, tachycardia, nausea, restlessness, confusion or apathy may be present. The clinical picture of an inadequate circulation may be produced in many ways: (1) inability of the heart to pump the needed blood because of weakness of the heart itself; (2) failure of the heart to fill properly because of pericardial tamponade; (3) obstruction of the main arterial pathways as a massive pulmonary embolus; (4) failure of the heart to pump the needed blood not because of weakness of the heart, but because the venous inflow to the heart has failed; (5) widespread failure of cell metabolism; and (6) loss of vasoconstrictor tone.

Various authors have attempted to give a physiologic meaning to the word "shock." They would restrict its use to the circulatory failure resulting from a decreased venous return to the heart because of a small blood volume. Though this might be desirable from a theoretical point of view, it breaks down in practice, because frequently the mechanism responsible for the circulatory failure cannot be determined immediately. The physician sees a man with obvious circulatory failure. He wishes to describe in a word the appearance of this patient without committing himself to the cause of the inadequate circulation.

Shock Syndrome Produced by Failure of the Heart. The picture of shock may be produced by a marked decrease in the output of the heart from massive myocardial infarction. If the patient has had no evidence of congestive failure prior to the infarction, the venous pressure may be normal. The heart rate is frequently slow.

The circulation may become inadequate in patients with atrial and ventricular tachycardia, and atrial flutter. If the ventricles remain contracted too much of the time because of the tachycardia, they are not able to fill properly and the cardiac output decreases.

Patients with severe congestive heart failure frequently show the shock syndrome during the last few days or hours of life. The decrease in cardiac output has become so marked that the circulation to the tissues is obviously inadequate. The venous pressure is elevated because of the chronic congestive failure. The pallor, sweating, narrow pulse pressure and mental confusion result from the marked decrease in the output of the progressively failing heart.

Shock Syndrome from Pericardial Tamponade. Patients with pericardial tamponade from stab wound of the heart or effusion or empyema of the pericardium have an inadequate circulation when the pericardial pressure becomes sufficient to collapse the atria and interfere with cardiac filling. When the onset is acute, as in a stab wound of the heart, the circulatory failure may be profound. The venous pressure is elevated, though on casual inspection this point may be overlooked, especially when the neck veins are not dilated. The arterial pulse is paradoxical.

Shock Syndrome from Obstruction of the Main Arterial Pathways. Shock may be produced by blocking the flow of blood through the major arteries. Such a situation is seen in patients with a massive pulmonary embolus blocking both pulmonary arteries and in patients with the pulmonary capillaries plugged by neoplastic tissue.

Smaller pulmonary emboli may cause circulatory failure without blocking of a major portion of the pulmonary arterial tree. In these patients both reflex vasodilatation and the products of tissue breakdown may be responsible for the shock picture.

Shock Syndrome Produced by Failure of the Venous Return from a Small Blood Volume. The circulation will fail if the volume of fluid in the vascular bed is sufficiently decreased. The cardiac output falls, not because of inability of the heart muscle to pump blood, but because the ventricles do not receive the blood to pump. That the circulatory failure is the result of a small blood volume is easily demonstrated: when the blood volume is increased, the output of the heart immediately increases correspondingly.

The common causes of shock from a low blood volume are:

1. *Hemorrhage.* The blood may be lost externally. It may be lost internally into the body cavities, into the gastrointestinal tract or into the tissues from the rupture of numerous small blood vessels. All these forms of hemorrhage result in hemodilution.

2. *Plasma Loss.* This is a selective form of bleeding. The injury to the blood vessels is not sufficient to destroy the continuity of the capillaries, but the capillary damage is great enough to allow the blood pressure to force the plasma out of the vascular bed. This selective loss of plasma results in hemoconcentration as judged by the rising hemoglobin concentration and hematocrit reading. Circulatory failure from plasma loss is seen in burns, diffuse peritonitis and certain types of anaphylactic reactions. Loss of whole blood is more common than loss of plasma in most patients with trauma.

3. *Dehydration.* The blood volume may be strikingly decreased by the loss of water and electrolytes from the body. Circulatory failure from dehydration is seen in patients with vomiting, diarrhea, intestinal obstruction, diabetic acidosis and Addison's disease.

Many authors have attempted to differentiate between the circulatory failure caused by hemorrhage and that produced by loss of plasma or fluid from the blood stream. It is true that in one instance hemodilution occurs, while in the other hemoconcentration is present. Nevertheless, in both the circulatory failure is primarily the result of the inadequate venous return to the heart and in both the circulation can be restored to normal by increasing the blood volume. In patients with burns or extensive trauma the circulatory failure caused by the small blood volume may be accentuated by the effect on cell metabolism of the products of infection or tissue necrosis.

A considerable decrease in blood volume may occur before the signs of circulatory failure develop. This fact is best demonstrated by observations from the bleeding of blood donors. The blood volume may be decreased about 1 liter in an average-sized man without interfering with the cardiac output when the subject is prone. If fainting occurs, it is reflex in origin and not related to a fall in cardiac output.

Shock Syndrome from Failure of Cell Metabolism and Irreversible Shock. The circulation eventually fails in all patients who die. If the process of dying is slow and prolonged, signs of circulatory insufficiency will be present for days or hours before the breathing ceases. This type of circulatory failure is seen in patients with liver disease, renal failure, overwhelming infections and late burns. The blood volume is not at fault in these patients. The capillaries do not seem to be abnormally permeable to protein. The tone of the arterioles and veins is diminished. There is some evidence that the heart may not function normally. The disturbance in the circulation seems to be primarily related to the disturbance in the metabolic activities of all the cells of the body rather than to the failure of any particular portion of the circulation.

This type of circulatory failure may up to a certain point be reversible if the process causing the abnormality in cell metabolism can be controlled. In infectious diseases, control of the infection by the use of appropriate chemotherapy may result in striking improvement. If the patient is not dehydrated and is not anemic, plasma and whole blood are not effective.

Patients who have bled repeatedly will eventually exhibit this type of terminal circulatory failure. During the first few days, increasing the blood volume will improve the circulation, but after the circulation has been inadequate for a sufficient length of time the cells begin to die and transfusions no longer cause improvement. Any form of circulatory failure from a small blood volume will become irreversible once the metabolism of the cells of the body is sufficiently altered by prolonged circulatory insufficiency.

In dogs with irreversible shock from hemorrhage, irreversible changes occur first in the liver. It is doubtful if the death of any one organ will explain irreversible shock as it is seen in man. Preexisting pathology probably alters the susceptibility of the various organs to ischemia.

Shock Syndrome Produced by Changes in the Tone of the Small Blood Vessels. Acute circulatory collapse of reflex origin (primary shock, common faint), with or without loss of consciousness, produces the clinical picture of shock. If the circulatory collapse is of short duration and sweating is not excessive, the extremities remain warm. If it is more prolonged, the extremities may become as cold as in any other form of failure of the circulation. When the patient is first seen, it may be impossible to decide whether this is a benign state or whether the patient is *in extremis* from blood loss, pericardial tamponade or acute heart failure.

Observations have been made on the state of the circulation during the acute circulatory collapse which occurs in blood donors. As blood is removed, the right atrial pressure falls, but it does not fall further when the collapse occurs. The subject becomes pale, breaks out in a cold sweat, and complains of nausea. The arterial pressure falls precipitously, and the pulse usually slows. The cardiac output shows only a slight decrease or no decrease below the precollapse level.

The circulatory failure is caused by a sharp fall in peripheral resistance, presumably by arteriolar dilatation. It appears as if sensory stimuli from any efferent nerve or from the emotional control of thought may cause a sudden reflex arteriolar dilatation which results in a sharp fall in the arterial pressure. If the patient is upright, loss of consciousness will occur when the low arterial pressure is inadequate to maintain the cerebral blood flow against the force of gravity. This type of collapse is benign in the recumbent position because the overall tissue blood flow is not reduced.

The factors responsible for the circulatory failure which can be produced by motionless standing in normal subjects after the ingestion of sodium nitrite and in patients with acute infections and fatigue have never been completely determined. How much of the circulatory failure is caused by pooling in veins whose tone has been decreased by disease or drugs, and how much is the result of arteriolar vasodilatation secondary to reflex stimuli induced by the upright position, has never been demonstrated. It is possible that both mechanisms are important.

A marked decrease in arterial pressure without other evidences of circulatory insufficiency is seen after acute bouts of fever produced by malaria, or the intravenous injection of typhoid vaccine. Occasionally this occurs in other diseases, such as pneumonia. It would appear that the infection has caused a loss of arteriolar tone and a lowering of the arterial pressure. Certain drugs, such as alcohol, seem to have a similar action. Quantitative studies are needed in these patients before definite conclusions can be drawn.

Anaphylactic shock causes a marked fall in arterial pressure and the clinical picture of shock. It is not clear to what degree generalized interference with cell metabolism or hemoconcentration due to capillary damage produces the circulatory failure.

Multiple Factors in Shock. For clarity of presentation, the various mechanisms producing the picture of shock have been presented separately. In practice several factors are frequently responsible. Infection with its adverse effect on cell metabolism is a frequent complication in patients who have lost blood from trauma and in those who are dehydrated. Reflex arteriolar dilatation from pain occurs in patients with a diminished cardiac output resulting from a massive myocardial infarct. Both the loss of blood and reflex arteriolar dilatation are important in the circulatory failure caused by penetrating wounds of the chest.

Treatment. Correct treatment depends upon proper evaluation of the factors underlying circulatory failure. Often the frank development of shock can be anticipated and avoided by proper supportive therapy. Once circulatory failure has become manifest, the patient should be placed at rest, extremes in temperature avoided, and therapy begun. In general, the moderate application of heat may be recommended, although on certain theoretical grounds this alone might be deleterious. If combined with the other therapeutic measures, it appears to be advantageous. The patient's head should not be elevated, and in some instances improvement may follow elevation of the foot of the bed.

In those patients with the shock syndrome produced by failure of the heart, measures such as rapid digitalization and diuretics may be of value. Acute pericardial tamponade is relieved either by aspiration or, if resulting from a stab wound of the heart, by operation. Once pulmonary emboli have blocked the pulmonary circuit, little can be done to help except to prevent further emboli by means of anticoagulants and venous ligation.

Shock due to diminished blood volume is treated primarily by restoration of the volume of circulating blood to normal. If the problem is one of dehydration alone, simple physiologic saline solution is adequate. If the condition is of some duration, additional protein in the form of plasma may be required. In some conditions, such as peritonitis, in which the loss has been primarily plasma, plasma offers the best replacement fluid. In most conditions, however, the most rational replacement fluid is whole blood. Even in patients with severe burns and apparent hemoconcentration, there is enough red cell loss to make whole blood the best therapeutic fluid. In some patients the situation may be so critical that emergency therapy with plasma or even saline is life-saving while blood is being obtained. Although saline leaves the vascular system rapidly, an adequate increase in blood volume may be maintained for the duration of the infusion. As stated before, the patient is kept warm and extremes in temperature avoided. However, local cooling of an injured part may diminish the amount of local fluid loss. Morphine is of value in reducing pain, but it must be remembered that in patients with sluggish circulation it enters the blood stream slowly after hypodermic injection. Intravenous administration may be advisable. In general, pressor drugs are of little avail. If infection is already present, or felt to be likely, appropriate therapy should be instituted at once.

Shock caused by failure of cell metabolism does not respond to the administration of blood or plasma. Treatment of the underlying condition causing the shock is of major importance.

Circulatory failure due to changes in tone of the small blood vessels is usually benign and self-limited. Placing the patient in the horizontal position is usually adequate treatment. Drug therapy is not usually indicated because recovery is rapid.

Eugene A. Stead, Jr.

References

Blalock, A.: Principles of Surgical Care; Shock and Other Problems. St. Louis, C. V. Mosby Co., 1940.

Cannon, W. B.: Traumatic Shock. New York, D. Appleton & Co., 1923.

Stead, E. A., Jr., and Warren, J. V.: Orientation to the Mechanisms of Clinical Shock. Arch. Surg., 50:1, 1945.

Wiggers, C. J.: The Present Status of the Shock Problem. Physiol. Rev., 22:74, 1942.

DISEASES OF THE HEART

DISEASES OF THE PERICARDIUM*
ACUTE FIBRINOUS PERICARDITIS

Definition. Acute fibrinous pericarditis is an inflammation of the pericardium associated with the formation of a fibrinous exudate on the pericardial surfaces. The inflammatory process may subside or progress and be complicated by a serous, serosanguineous or purulent exudate (*pericarditis with effusion*).

Etiology. Acute pericarditis may be classified into the following eight groups: (1) Acute nonspecific pericarditis. Since this entity is receiving increasing recognition and since its clinical features sometimes closely simulate those of myocardial infarction, it is described separately in the next section. (2) Infectious pericarditis, which includes: (*a*) Pyogenic pericarditis. This is most commonly caused by the pneumococcus but may be produced by other organisms, especially the streptococcus and staphylococcus, as well as the gonococcus, meningococcus, influenza bacillus, colon bacillus and related bacteria. Pericarditis may occur in tularemia and brucellosis as well as in a variety of less common systemic infections. (*b*) Tuberculous pericarditis. (*c*) Mycotic pericarditis such as rarely occurs in actinomycosis and coccidioidomycosis. (*d*) Parasitic pericarditis as represented by the very rare echinococcal involvement of the pericardium. (3) Pericarditis occurring as a manifestation of the "collagen diseases": (*a*) Rheumatic pericarditis. (*b*) Pericarditis accompanying rheumatoid arthritis as reported by Bauer and Ropes. (*c*) Pericarditis of disseminated lupus erythematosus. (*d*) Pericarditis occurring in periarteritis nodosa. (4) Uremic pericarditis. (5) Pericarditis secondary to myocardial infarction. (6) Pericarditis due to neoplasm. (7) Traumatic pericarditis. (8) Rare forms of pericarditis of uncertain etiology. Pericarditis has been described in infectious mononucleosis. The extremely rare cholesterol pericarditis would

* Dr. Robert A. Helm has rendered invaluable assistance to the author in the revision of this section on pericarditis.

be included in this group, and also pericardial effusion due to myxedema.

Morbid Anatomy. Acute pericarditis is associated with an outpouring of fibrin. This may be exuded on the percardial surfaces without effusion of fluid (*dry pericarditis*), or serum may be admixed with the fibrin (*serofibrinous pericarditis*). In severe pericarditis the subjacent myocardium is involved, and this superficial myocarditis is probably the cause of the electrocardiographic abnormalities frequently found in pericarditis.

Symptoms. Since pericarditis is secondary to disease elsewhere in the body, the symptomatology is influenced by the character of the primary or underlying disorder. The visceral and the inner surface of the parietal pericardium apparently do not contain pain-sensitive nerve endings, and acute fibrinous pericarditis *per se* is often painless. The outer surface of the parietal pericardium below the fifth or sixth intercostal space is sensitive to painful stimuli. When this portion of the pericardium is involved, pain occurs and is frequently intensified during inspiration by a contiguous pleurisy. Agonizing pain of this character has been frequently observed in acute nonspecific pericarditis of unknown etiology, a disorder often complicated by pleurisy.

The pericarditis of uremia and other terminal conditions is usually painless, probably because complicating pleuropericarditis is infrequent.

Physical Examination. *Palpation* occasionally reveals a friction fremitus caused by the rubbing together of the roughened visceral and parietal layers of the pericardium. *Auscultation* yields the most important and, not infrequently, the sole evidence of fibrinous pericarditis. The friction rub is a to-and-fro sound, close to the ear, which corresponds to systole and diastole, and varies greatly in intensity in different cases and often in the same case. The timing of the sound differs from the timing of a to-and-fro valvular murmur, in that it does not begin immediately after the heart sounds and generally overlaps them. The rub may be only a slight, scratchy noise, perceptible with some difficulty and

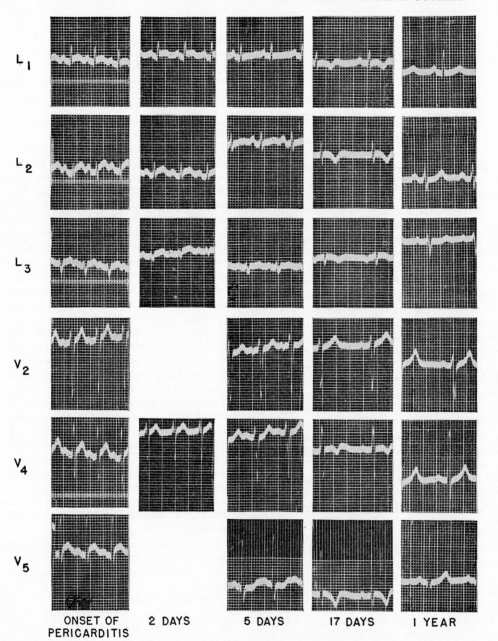

Fig. 151. Acute benign nonspecific pericarditis. Onset: acute stage, elevated S-T segments in leads I, II and V₅. Two days later: straightening of S-T segments in leads I and II. Five days later: subacute stage, S-T segments becoming isoelectric in limb leads. Seventeen days later: chronic stage, inversion of T waves in leads I, II, III, V₄ and V₅. One year later: return to normal.

easily overlooked, or an intense, grating sound. It may be heard at one examination and be absent at the next; not infrequently it persists only a few hours, but it may recur, with increased intensity. It disappears if a fluid exudate *completely separates* the layers of the pericardium. However, a pericardial friction rub frequently is audible in the pres-ence of large effusions, since adhesions may prevent separation of the entire visceral and parietal pericardial surfaces. The rub is most frequently heard over the right ventricle in the fourth and fifth spaces close to the sternum; it is, however, often encountered at the base of the heart or at the apex. In rare instances it may be heard posteriorly in the left thorax. At times the intensity of the friction can be augmented by precordial compression with the hand or stethoscope. Change of position of the patient may alter the intensity of the rub considerably.

Diagnosis. The friction rub is pathognomonic of the disease, but, since it is often present for only a few hours, repeated examination of the heart is necessary. Difficulty in diagnosis arises if there is intense pain without friction rub at the onset. A scratchy or crepitant quality of the heart sounds, particularly the first sound in the tricuspid and pulmonary areas, is encountered in a small percentage of normal hearts, and may be differentiated from a friction rub by its constancy, by its more definite timing with the heart sounds, by the fact that it does not change under pressure with the stethoscope, and by the absence of fever or other symptoms.

A *pleuropericardial friction rub* must be differentiated from a pure pericardial rub. The former has, in addition to the to-and-fro rhythm, definite intensifications associated with the respiratory cycle, which may be temporarily abolished by cessation of breathing. The bubbling, crunching sounds heard in mediastinal emphysema may be differentiated from a pericardial friction rub by their peculiar acoustics.

Electrocardiographic changes (Fig. 151) are usually but not invariably present in pericarditis and are believed to be due to subjacent myocarditis. The changes frequently show considerable variation from day to day.

Acute Pericarditis. Early in the course of acute pericarditis, elevation of the ST segment occurs in the limb and precordial leads in any of the following leads or combination of leads: (1) lead I, (2) leads I and II, (3) leads I and precordial leads, (4) leads I and II and the precordial leads. If the picture is typical, the S-T segment of lead III is isoelectric. In the unipolar extremity leads, RS-T segment elevation in the left arm lead or the left leg lead and depression of the RS-T segment in the right arm lead are the usual findings.

Subacute Pericarditis. As the inflammation of the subepicardial muscle subsides, the S-T segments return toward or to the isoelectric line, and the T waves decrease in size and usually become inverted.

Chronic Pericarditis. Low voltage of the QRS complexes and T waves is common. From this description it is apparent that the electrocardiographic changes may simulate those encountered in myocardial infarction; however, in acute and subacute pericarditis the QRS complex remains normal, reciprocal depression and elevation of the S-T segment in leads I and III is uncommon. Also, abnormally large Q waves do not occur with pericarditis in the limb or precordial leads.

Prognosis. The prognosis in acute fibrinous pericarditis is good, provided the underlying disease is not fatal. Adhesions of the layers of the pericardium by organized fibrinous exudate are a common sequel, and the patient should be followed carefully for the possible development of pericardial effusion or chronic constrictive pericarditis. The latter is most commonly due to tuberculosis.

Treatment. Specific therapy is directed toward the underlying disease as described in the section on Pericardial Effusion. Symptomatic treatment consists of combating pain with analgesic drugs. Application of an ice bag to the precordium often affords relief.

ACUTE NONSPECIFIC PERICARDITIS

Synonyms. Acute benign pericarditis, idiopathic pericarditis, acute primary pericarditis, acute serofibrinous pericarditis of benign type.

Incidence. This entity was described a century ago but has been well recognized only during the past decade. Although it is difficult to determine its relative incidence, it is evident that it rivals tuberculous and rheumatic pericarditis in frequency. The disease has been reported in all age groups through the seventh decade, but the average age is about 35. Approximately 75 per cent of the cases occur in males.

Etiology. The cause is unknown but either hypersensitivity to a preceding upper respiratory infection or invasion by an unidentified virus is considered the most likely possibility. An analogy to pleurisy with effusion has led to speculation concerning a tuberculous etiology, but the benign course of the disease strongly militates against such a concept.

Pathology. The serofibrinous inflammatory process involves both the visceral and parietal pericardium and the contiguous pleura. The visceral pericardium is insensitive, but the pleura and portions of the parietal pericardium are sensitive to painful stimuli. There is usually effusion which may be hemorrhagic. The relative importance of pericardial fluid and cardiac dilatation in the formation of an enlarged cardiac silhouette is controversial, but the presence of dilatation in certain cases is strongly suggested by failure to obtain more than relatively small amounts of fluid with pericardial paracentesis.

Symptoms. Approximately two thirds of all patients have an antecedent respiratory infection. This precedes the pericarditis by varying periods up to two months but averaging twelve days.

Pain is the most common presenting symptom and is characteristically intensified by deep breathing, coughing or rotation of the trunk. In about 60 per cent of reported cases the pain is sudden in onset. It may be sharply localized or may radiate widely over the chest and back as well as into the neck and upper extremities. Dyspnea, cough, malaise, anorexia, nausea and vomiting may be present.

Physical Signs. Fever is usually present and may range up to 105° F. It is usually present at onset and is often maximal on the first day. A pericardial friction rub is heard in at least 70 per cent of cases and may be noted within a few hours of the onset of chest pain. The duration of the friction rub is variable but may persist as long as two months. Gallop rhythm is rare. Arrhythmias occur occasionally. The heart sounds may or may not be distant. Shock develops infrequently, but signs of pericardial compression, rarely sufficiently severe to necessitate pericardial paracentesis, are more commonly found. Signs of pleural fluid, usually on the left or bilateral, and pneumonitis may be present.

Laboratory Findings. A polymorphonuclear leukocytosis with a white blood count exceeding 10,000 is found in the majority of cases. The sedimentation rate is increased early and parallels the course of the disease. Pericardial fluid may be straw-colored or hemorrhagic and no distinct cytologic pattern is characteristic. Pleural fluid may be similar to that present within the pericardial sac. Bacterial cultures are negative but adequate viral studies have not been reported.

Roentgenographic and Electrocardiographic Findings. These findings are similar to those described in the sections on pericarditis with effusion and acute fibrinous pericarditis respectively.

Prognosis. Complete recovery almost invariably occurs ultimately. The initial episode usually lasts several weeks but may persist for three months. Recurrences are common but are generally of less severity and of shorter duration than the initial illness. Rare in-

stances of failure of the electrocardiogram to return to normal have been reported. Constrictive pericarditis rarely, if ever, develops.

Differential Diagnosis. Nonspecific pericarditis is sometimes differentiated with difficulty from myocardial infarction, but the following findings suggest pericarditis: (1) pleuritic chest pain; (2) early development, frequently on the first day, of friction rub, fever, and elevation of the white blood count and sedimentation rate; (3) rapid change in size and configuration of the cardiac silhouette; (4) electrocardiographic findings typical of pericarditis; (5) an antecedent respiratory infection.

Since involvement of serosal surfaces which are sensitive to painful stimuli occurs less frequently in tuberculous and rheumatic pericarditis, the presence of pain increased by respiration and rotation of the trunk favors the diagnosis of nonspecific pericarditis. However, the ultimate differentiation from all other forms of pericarditis depends upon the demonstration in the latter of the specific underlying disease by clinical bacteriologic or serologic methods, or by microscopic examination of a pericardial biopsy. Other causes of chest pain, particularly pulmonary infarction, acute pleurisy of various types, spontaneous pneumothorax, mediastinal emphysema and less commonly angina pectoris, hiatus hernia, acute abdominal lesions and various causes of radicular pain, may simulate pericarditis.

Treatment. Sulfonamides and penicillin are ineffective and, in the majority of reported cases, streptomycin has produced no benefit. Chlortetracycline and oxytetracycline have been reported as producing dramatic improvement in some patients but have been used with indifferent results in others. One patient improved markedly when adrenocorticotrophic hormone was begun on the sixteenth day of illness. The specificity of these or other agents in a disease with variable course can be determined only in the future by well controlled studies. At the present time therapy may be considered to be symptomatic.

PERICARDIAL EFFUSION

Definition. The accumulation of fluid, either exudate or transudate, within the pericardial cavity is designated as pericardial effusion.

Etiology. Pericardial effusion may follow pericarditis due to any of the causative factors

Concretio Cordis). SYMPTOMS. Dy
dema, abdominal swelling, palpitat
he heart and cough are the usual sym
nd their onset is insidious. Orthop
are.

PHYSICAL SIGNS. Inspection reveal
picuous engorgement of the veins
eck (the venous pressure may be 20
m. of water, i.e., two to five times th
nal). The distention of the veins is
resent in the sitting as well as in t
umbent position. Cyanosis of the lip
ailbeds may be present. Inspiratory sv
f the veins of the neck is a commo
mportant sign. There is moderate or
xtreme enlargement of the abdomen, v
vith a fluid wave. Pitting edema of tl
nd ankles is often found. The liver is
arly enlarged and firm, but usually it
ender and does not pulsate. Splenor
ccasionally occurs. The pulse is smal
he systolic blood pressure and pulse pr
re characteristically low, or within the
imits of normal. A paradoxical pulse
liscussion under Pericardial Effusion
1269) may be observed. Pleural effu:
commonly absent. The fluid, like that
in the abdomen, usually has the cha
istics of a transudate.

The heart is usually small and quie
may be of normal size or moderate
larged. In most cases the rhythm is re
but irregularity arising from atrial f
tion or atrial flutter is found in abo
per cent. The sounds may be distan
otherwise are of normal quality. Mu
are extremely rare, but a distant third
sound at the apex is often audible. The
are usually remarkably free from rales.

The ELECTROCARDIOGRAM is help
the recognition of chronic constrictive
carditis. Usually there is low voltage o
complexes; and the T waves are freq
of low amplitude, or negative. If the h
immobilized by adhesions, the electri
may not alter with change of positi
the body, but fixation of the electric
by no means pathognomonic.

X-RAY FINDINGS. As mentioned l
the heart is usually normal in size, but
erate enlargement is not at all uncor
and even marked degrees of enlargeme
occasionally seen. The configuration
heart is sometimes normal, but there n
straightening of the waistline, poor vis
of the aortic knob and obliteration
cardiophrenic angles, giving the heart

Differentiation
cardial effusion a
cardiac enlargem
is usually not pea
instances the ap
cular shadow or
distinguishable ir
larged hearts t
normal unless ca
such cases, thou
markedly impair
invariably show

Angiocardiogra
by Williams and
method of establ
cardial effusion,
true in our expe
the dye-filled ri
ventricle lie wel
cardiopericardial
tween the two b

Diagnosis. T
effusion is often
effusion is not fu
examination is n
is examined from
lects, the physic
recognition of th
time. In doubtfu
tion may aid gre

The electroc
changes describ
Pericarditis in
pericardial effus
plexes of the ele
inish, probably
the electrical po

Diagnostic pu
the presence of
definitely demor
remembered tha
piration may le
ventricular wall
nary vessels tor
aspiration are t
tion for the relie
clinical and lab
edly elevated o
sure, and mark
ing arterial pres
relieving increa
(2) diagnostic
ing the etiologic
ulent pericardit
ally requiring s
case of pericard
best performed

described under Acute Fibrinous Pericarditis. Rheumatic pericarditis, tuberculous pericarditis, acute nonspecific pericarditis, bacterial pericarditis, malignant tumors invading the pericardium, and penetrating chest wounds are the commonest causes of pericardial effusion. In myxedema pericardial effusion frequently occurs.

Morbid Anatomy. The fluid exudate may be of several kinds—serous, serosanguineous, hemorrhagic, seropurulent or purulent. The quantity of fluid contained in the pericardial cavity varies greatly; in some cases only 100 to 200 cc. may be found, while in others 1.5 or 2 liters may distend the sac. In contrast to transudates, the inflammatory exudates have a relatively high specific gravity (1.017 +) and usually a total protein content of more than 30 gm. per liter. The fluid is clear, cloudy or hemorrhagic, according to the number and character of the cells and the amount of fibrin contained. Bacterial infections often produce creamy pus. Grossly hemorrhagic effusions usually are due to tuberculosis or malignant tumor, but have recently been observed in benign idiopathic pericarditis. Bloody effusions must be differentiated from hemorrhage into the pericardium due to ruptured myocardial infarct or a dissecting aneurysm. Chylopericardium may occur with obstruction or injury of the thoracic duct. Pericardial fluid of relatively high specific gravity and high protein content may develop in myxedema. Finally, it is not uncommon for a small amount of clear fluid (30 to 200 cc.) to collect in the pericardium especially in cardiac and renal disease (hydropericardium).

Pathologic Physiology. Pericardial effusion of sufficient magnitude to produce clinical manifestations does so primarily by causing cardiac tamponade, as follows: (1) Blood enters the heart with difficulty, since the pressure of the fluid between the distended pericardium and the heart impedes the entrance of blood from the great veins into the heart. This causes a rise of peripheral venous pressure from the normal 5 to 10 cm. of water to levels of 15 to 40 cm. of water. (2) The cardiac output per minute and per beat is decreased from the normal of 3.5 ± 0.3 liters per minute per square meter of body surface to approximately 2 liters. (3) The lowered cardiac output produces a decrease in systemic arterial blood pressure. Since the diastolic pressure is either slightly elevated or unchanged, the pulse pressure is markedly

reduced. (4) The pulse rate is increased, probably because of a compensatory reflex to aid the total blood flow per minute, since the output per beat is decreased. (5) The velocity of blood flow is diminished, as measured from arm to the tongue. (6) The movements of the heart are decreased, as seen fluoroscopically or in the roentgenkymograph. (7) The development of a weak or imperceptible pulse during inspiration is called pulsus paradoxus, a valuable, although not pathognomonic, sign of cardiac tamponade. There is disagreement concerning the precise cause of pulsus paradoxus but it is generally considered to be an accentuation of a normal mechanism. Normally during inspiration the sucking action of the thorax increases the systemic venous return, resulting in an increase of the stroke volume of the right ventricle in accordance with Starling's law. The increased inspiratory capacity of the pulmonary vascular bed is almost completely compensated by the increased right ventricular output during this phase of respiration. The net result is a slight inspiratory diminution of left ventricular inflow and stroke volume. Normally the intrapericardial structures are subjected to the same pressure changes during respiration as the intrathoracic extrapericardial structures. With the development of cardiac tamponade it is thought that the pressure variations within the right and left atria are less than those in the intrathoracic extrapericardial portions of the venae cavae and pulmonary veins. Therefore, during inspiration both the right and the left venoatrial pressure gradients are diminished. Consequently the right ventricular stroke volume is increased to a lesser degree and the left ventricular stroke volume is decreased to a greater degree than obtain normally. With expiration the opposite changes occur, resulting in an augmentation of left ventricular stroke volume. The pulsus paradoxus is, therefore, not actually paradoxical but is merely a marked accentuation of the rhythmic waxing and waning of the systemic pulse volume with respiration.

Symptoms. The onset of pericarditis with effusion is seldom abrupt, and often insidious. Because the disease is frequently secondary to serious trouble elsewhere in the body, it may not perceptibly alter the general condition of the patient. The fever is usually of the same type as that of the primary disease, although it may be somewhat aggravated.

The disease often causes little or no local

discon
ized (
cardit
there
disco
ting (

Dy
preser
rapidl

A
ity m
the v
lead
the p
cougl
tion,
and

Pl
ally s
of th
usua

P(
creas
and
palp
ante
A va
port
card
an i
The
by
this
note
The
spir
mm
larg
rapi

P
tive
spac
may
prec
ders
dull
tien
mer
and
assu
nes
lev(

me
the

ons

---

age must otherwise be ca
stillation of enzymes suc
and streptodornase to liqu
exudate has had a limited
but the status of this the
not well defined.

Tuberculous pericarditi
with streptomycin, 1 gr
twice weekly, in combina
oral administration of e
isonicotinic acid hydrazide
aminosalicylic acid. Loca
not used. Although a fa
frequently observed withir
present tendency is to con
for six months to one ye

The treatment of rhe
is that of the underlying
of adrenal steroids is co
present time. The peric
myxedema responds dran
therapy.

Evidence of extensive
carditis in the course of
infarction dictates caution
coagulants, since under
instances of pericardial l
ponade have been report

CHRONIC CONSTRICTI
FORMS OF ADHESIVE

(*Adherent Pericardium, Pick
Scar, Concretio Cordis,*

Definition. Adherent
condition usually resultin
hesions between the vis
layers of the pericardiu
between the parietal per
ous intrathoracic structu
the pericardial cavity ma
may be completely oblitei
tissue (*concretio cordis*).
adhesions extending from
the mediastinum, the pleu
and the chest wall (*accre*

Etiology. A history o
is usually not obtained
chronic constrictive peric
is demonstrated as the cau
15 per cent and probably
others in which the eti
Acute pyogenic pericard
pericarditis are responsib
Neoplastic involvement
sometimes produces the
Acute nonspecific pericar
pericarditis are rarely, if

---

various intrathoracic structures are sometimes
visualized by fluoroscopy or roentgenography.

Differential Diagnosis. Chronic constrictive pericarditis must be differentiated from
the following disorders:

*Arteriosclerotic Heart Disease with Con-
gestive Heart Failure.* The history, the electrocardiogram, and the persistence of an elevated venous pressure despite bed rest and
digitalization in constrictive pericarditis help
to differentiate the two conditions. Also careful roentgenographic and fluoroscopic studies
may demonstrate evidence of calcium deposits
within the pericardium itself.

Mitral and Tricuspid Valvular Disease.
Enlargement of the liver, edema, and dilatation of the cervical veins are commonly present with tricuspid stenosis and failure of the
right heart secondary to mitral stenosis. The
history, configuration of the heart, and the
presence of presystolic or diastolic murmur
are helpful differential findings.

Portal Cirrhosis of the Liver. The normal
level of venous pressure in the veins of the
arm in cirrhosis eliminates Pick's disease
from consideration.

Treatment. Chronic constrictive pericarditis may be cured by pericardial resection in
properly selected cases. The results in 60
per cent of cases are satisfactory, although
there is about a 10 to 20 per cent operative
mortality in various clinics. Medical treatment consists of the usual measures for combating the effects of venous congestion. Although digitalis has been thought to be without benefit except to slow the ventricular
rate when atrial fibrillation is present,
recent studies reported from Cournand's
laboratory indicate that some patients have
myocardial as well as mechanical factors contributing to their circulatory abnormalities.
Digitalis was demonstrated to be beneficial
in such instances. Restoration of the serum
protein to normal before operation has been
extremely important in reducing the operative mortality. The use of mercurial diuretics
preoperatively and postoperatively may be
lifesaving in the extremely edematous patient.

In adherent pericardium with external adhesions, Brauer has advocated the resection
of several ribs and costal cartilages overlying
the pericardium in order that the heart may
pull against yielding rather than rigid structures. This procedure is palliative rather than
curative.

PERICARDIAL DISEASES AS A CAUSE OF ACUTE CARDIAC COMPRESSION

Beck has described a "triad" which characterizes acute cardiac compression: "(1) A
rising venous pressure, (2) a falling arterial
pressure, (3) a small quiet heart" (see Fig.
152). The principal causes for acute cardiac
compression are penetrating wounds of the
chest causing laceration of the heart or
coronary vessels and extravasation of blood
into the pericardial cavity. Other causes are
rupture of a myocardial infarct, of an aortic
aneurysm, a dissecting aneurysm or rupture
of a contusion of the myocardium. Rapidly
developing effusions or the formation of gas
within the pericardial cavity also causes
acute cardiac compression.

The condition is characterized in its early
stage by weakness of the pulse, and often pulsus paradoxus. The skin is pale, cold and
clammy, and the heart sounds are weak. The
veins may not be conspicuously distended,
but measurement of venous pressure shows
definite elevation above the normal. Treatment depends upon the cause of the compression. In cases of cardiac laceration the
modern tendency is to aspirate the pericardium, simultaneously administering blood
or other plasma expander if shock is present. The patient is carefully observed and, if
tamponade rapidly reoccurs, suture of the
site of hemorrhage should be carried out immediately. If blood seeps slowly into the
pericardium, a second aspiration may sometimes be performed before resorting to surgery. Contusion of the heart following penetrating or nonpenetrating injuries to the
chest occasionally produces pericardial effusion and compression. Even in the absence
of effusion cardiac contusion resembles and
must be differentiated from cardiac tamponade. The diagnostic features of cardiac
contusion include thoracic trauma, precordial
pain, tachycardia, dyspnea and occasionally
cyanosis. Electrocardiographic changes in the
T waves and RS-T segments may occur in
either tamponade or myocardial contusion resembling the changes described under Acute
Fibrinous Pericarditis.

OTHER CONDITIONS AFFECTING THE PERICARDIUM

Pneumopericardium. Pneumopericardium, resulting from the presence of gases in
the pericardium, is a rare condition which may
follow penetrating wounds, an infection

dents and rupture of
excising the coarcted
the continuity of the a
of the hypertension in
operated on. Surgery
childhood years. Beyo
progressive sclerotic o
increase the surgical

BICUSPID AORTIC V
as an isolated anoma
associated with othe
acyanotic type. Bicus
prone to undergo th
scarring which may
petence, or become th
endocarditis.

SUBAORTIC STENOS
embryonic tissue may
the conus area of the
diately below the aorti
is no serious obstruct
cardiac strain; there is
infective endocarditis.
mur transmitted into
quently accompanied h
over the first and sec
Some post-stenotic dila
ing aorta is usually p
be evidence of some l
trophy.

PULMONARY STEN
forms. In *valvular ste*
form a dome-shaped p
tral opening. This type
by some to be the resul
and is most apt to occ
formation with closed
stances the foramen ov
by raised right atrial
II). In *infundibular ste*
ing of varying degree ar
or outflow area of the
is due to failure of ex
cordis which takes part
development of this ar
development of other
hence far more freque
stances of infundibular

There is wide variatic
and resultant physiolog
individual cases, as ha
n studies by cardiac ca
olic pressure in the pul
han in the right ventri
ween the two and the r
of right ventricular pr
narked are related to t

---

pulmonary arter
On this basis Bi
classification of
tion: (1) pulm
flow, and pulm
decreased; (2)
than systemic fl
pressure normal
flow equal to sy
exercise.

Conditions w
circulation, eith
development of
lead to hypertro
to such areas. T
the same type o
Pressure in the
force the blood
The severity of
sistance affect th
the additional
hypertrophy pre
Work of the ri
pulmonary valv
and also by and
creased resistanc
bed, as in certa
shunts. Right
results from ma
which partially
Since this chan
munication with
ing systole, righ
must be elevated
to maintain bloc
left ventricle m
sistance in the s
coarctation of t
stenosis. The
dominance as se
to the gross un
ventricle.

Enlargement
and the pulmon
communications
through which
higher pressure
side (*left to ri*
volume of bloo
recipient chamb
quires larger ca
of these areas.
part related to t
into the right si
cific chamber h
ent. The level at
accounts for the

---

caused by gas-forming organisms, rupture of
a hollow viscus, or rupture of the lung into
the pericardium.

When pneumopericardium is present, relative cardiac dullness is replaced by tympany,

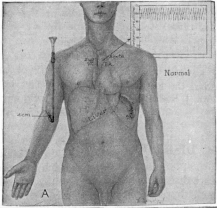

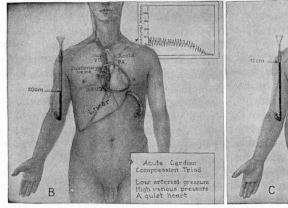

Fig. 152. Cardiac compression triads. For comparison, normal (A), acute (B) and chronic (C). The acute compression is produced by fluid in the pericardial cavity. Note collapse of the venous gateway and distention of the veins outside the pericardium. The ventricles are shrunken and the heart *per se* is smaller than normal. The parietal pericardium has not had time to dilate, nor has there been sufficient time for the liver to enlarge and for ascites to form. In the illustration for chronic compression of the heart the compression is produced by scar tissue. The heart is a small shrunken organ in contradistinction to cardiac dilatation. The veins dilate in response to the high venous pressure. The liver and spleen enlarge, and ascites develops. (C. S. Beck: J.A.M.A., Vol. 104.)

and if a fluid exudate collects, peculiar splash-
ing and churning sounds are audible. On
x-ray examination the air within the pericardium is apparent.

Tumors of the Pericardium. Benign
tumors arising in the pericardium include
lipoma, fibroma and angioma; sarcoma and
mesothelioma represent the only important
primary malignant neoplasms. However, in
contrast to primary neoplasms which are extremely rare, pericardial metastases have been
found at autopsy in 6 per cent of a large
group of patients dying of malignant disease.
The most common tumor types are carcinoma

---

and lymphoma. Lung and breast are the most
frequent primary sites of carcinomatous
metastases. The widespread metastases occurring with melanoma usually involve the
heart and pericardium.

Congenital Pericardial Defects. Rarely
the parietal pericardium is absent. This results in unusual mobility of the heart, and
pain and sudden death have been reported
with this condition, attributed to kinking of
the great vessels as a complication of excessive
cardiac mobility.

JOHNSON McGUIRE

References

Burchell, H. B.: Acute Nonspecific Pericarditis. Mod.
Concepts Cardiovas. Dis., *16*:[n.p.], March, 1947.
Freedman, E.: Inflammatory Diseases of the Pericar-
dium. Am. J. Roentgenol., *42*:38, 1939.

Harve
ard
My
car
Kotte,
tesi
Jul
McGu
Per
Paul,
Co
19
Willi
An
of
61

D

prise
norn
hear
reste
life.

Ir
cong
cal
age
in tl

E
men
of c
the
com
puln
from
proc
and
men
weel
have
of tl
prior
form
ceed
resu
anor
of t
are
and
caus
arte

T
card
infa
the
by

anomalous
pathic dila
(B) Ca
nosis possi
reversal o
ductus art
genital and
Valsalva,
atrial septa
Group I
venous art
stenosis wi
auricular s
Eisenmeng
derdevelop
position of
and trunci
Group
cardia the
chest with
frequently
inversus of
asymptoma
the heart
cardiac and
dextrocardi
the electroc
nomonic. L
mal; the tr
deflections
III those of
ANOMAL
ITS BRANCI
mally trans
aortic arch
occur. Anoi
double aort
right descer
crossing bel
the left sid
vessels from
origin and
occasionally
Many of
symptoms. I
ship and
trachea, res
swallowing
of these ani
study of tl
trachea and
symptoms a
to be of seric
lishment of
gical interve
"ring" and
plished by

pected when signs of heart failure occur. Usually there are no murmurs, arm and leg blood pressures are normal and the heart is found to be markedly enlarged. The electrocardiogram usually shows evidence of left ventricular enlargement with inversion of T waves. Intensive treatment for congestive failure should be tried. Definite diagnosis is established only by pathologic gross and microscopic findings.

ANOMALIES OF PULMONARY VENOUS RETURN vary in effect, depending on the number of pulmonary veins entering the right atrium or vena cava instead of the left atrium. The larger the number of such misplaced veins and the amount of pulmonary blood so returned, the greater is the strain on the right side of the heart and inadequacy of supply to the systemic circulation. When all four veins are involved, patency of the foramen ovale may maintain life for a time, but congestive failure and death usually occur in infancy. If this condition could be adequately diagnosed early, surgical transplantation of such pulmonary veins into the left auricle might be a life-saving procedure.

IDIOPATHIC DILATATION OF THE PULMONARY ARTERY, frequently associated with hypoplasia of the aorta, is probably due to maldivision of the embryonic truncus. There may be a systolic murmur over the pulmonic area due to swirling of blood in the dilated artery. The shadow of the main pulmonary artery and sometimes one or both branches is prominent, but does not show abnormally increased pulsations on fluoroscopic examination. This condition must be differentiated from other malformations which cause enlargement of the pulmonary artery on a dynamic basis, such as patent ductus arteriosus and septal defects, or poststenotic dilatation of the pulmonary artery beyond pulmonic stenosis. Cardiac catheterization may be necessary to clarify the diagnosis.

Group I-B. PATENT DUCTUS ARTERIOSUS. The ductus arteriosus is an essential passage during fetal life. The lung being unexpanded, most of the blood entering the pulmonary artery is shunted directly through the ductus into the aorta. With onset of respiratory function at birth the blood from the right ventricle is directed into the pulmonary vascular bed, and the lumen of the ductus arteriosus gradually becomes obliterated Normally this process is completed by the end of the second month. In some instances, for poorly understood reasons, closure fails to occur.

In persistent patency of the ductus arteriosus the direction of blood shunt is from the aorta into the pulmonary artery, because of the higher pressure in the systemic circulation after birth. The physiologic effects of this condition vary with the size of the ductus, its direction in relation to the aorta and pulmonary artery, as well as with the volume of blood shunted through the communication. Both sides of the heart are affected. The work of the right ventricle is increased by the additional volume of blood entering the pulmonary circulation. This increased blood flow returning from the lungs increases the size, output and work of the left side of the heart.

In cases with a small flow through the patent ductus arteriosus definite symptoms may be absent. When there is a large flow, such symptoms as easy fatigability, moderate exertional dyspnea and repeated pulmonary infections as well as signs of underdevelopment and pallor may be present. No clubbing of the digits occurs, and there is no cyanosis except with the occurrence of congestive failure or pulmonary disease.

The classic finding is a continuous systolic and diastolic murmur, frequently associated with a thrill, at the pulmonic area. The second pulmonic sound is accentuated. The murmur has a characteristic rasping to roaring quality often described as resembling a "train in a tunnel" or the "continuous running of a machine." It may be well localized or transmitted lower over the precordium as well as to the back. The blood pressure readings frequently show a low diastolic level and wide pulse pressure which become more pronounced after exercise. The diastolic phase of the murmur may be absent in infants and young children and in cases with development of high pulmonary pressure.

Fluoroscopic and x-ray findings vary considerably. Where the shunt is large, moderate cardiac enlargement is found with prominence and abnormally active pulsations of the pulmonary artery and hilar vessels ("hilar dance"). In instances with a small shunt the heart and pulmonary vessels may show relatively little deviation from normal. The electrocardiogram shows no axis deviation in the majority of cases.

Diagnosis is not difficult in the presence of a classic murmur. Problems of differential diagnosis arise when the auscultatory findings are atypical. Other conditions associated with a loud systolic murmur at the pulmonic area

instances, especially in infants, no d
murmur is audible. There is no diastoli
mur. Roentgenograms and fluoroscopy s
heart relatively normal in size, the
rounded and raised above the diaphragr
the presence of concavity without puls
instead of the normal convexity in the
left third or pulmonary segment of th
diac contour. In the left anterior obliqu
abnormal clarity of the pulmonary win
often demonstrated. Poststenotic dilatat
the pulmonary artery may fill out th
monary segment to some degree, b
fluoroscopic examination, pulsations i
area are either faint or absent. Because
creased pulmonary blood flow, the lung
show a rather striking clarity. The e
cardiogram in almost all instances sh
marked degree of right axis deviation.
to compensatory polycythemia, the red
cell count and hemoglobin value are ele
Arm-to-tongue circulation time is sho
because of overriding of the aorta.

Treatment for the tetralogy of Fallo
sists in a surgical procedure to increas
of blood to the lungs. In the Blalock-T
procedure a shunt is created by the ana
sis of a vessel from the aortic arch, usua
subclavian artery, to the pulmonary arte
the Potts procedure a side-to-side ana
sis between the aorta and pulmonary
is created. Instead of a shunt, direct su
relief of the pulmonary stenosis may be
These operations cause improved fun
capacity and decrease of cyanosis.

EISENMENGER COMPLEX. The featu
this condition are a high ventricular
dextroposition and overriding of the
and a normal or dilated pulmonary
Cyanosis is usually only moderate an
appear late. Radiologically, prominer
the pulmonary segment and increasec
shadows with vigorous pulsations serve
ferentiate this condition from the tetra
Fallot. As there is already excessive
nary blood flow in cases of Eisenr
complex, a surgical procedure desigi
increase flow of blood to the lungs
traindicated.

TRICUSPID ATRESIA OR HYPOPLASI
to underdevelopment of the right ver
including the pulmonary orifice. In po
circulation, blood from the right atriur
escape to the left atrium through an
ated interauricular septal defect or
tained patency of the foramen ovale.
ent patency of the ductus arterio:

are pulmonary stenosis, high ventricular
septal defect and atrial septal defect. In
the latter two conditions, when associated
with considerable enlargement of the pulmonary artery, there may be pulmonary regurgitation giving rise to a diastolic murmur.
This latter type of diastolic murmur is softer,
more blowing and usually heard somewhat
lower along the left sternal border than the
diastolic element of the murmur created by a
patent ductus arteriosus. In some cases in
which the diagnosis cannot be clearly established by standard methods and decision as to
possible surgery is important, resort to
catheterization of the heart or angiocardiography or aortography may be indicated.

Elimination of shunt by surgical ligation
or division of a patent ductus arteriosus in
the hands of surgeons familiar with the technique carries a low operative risk and restores
the circulatory dynamics to a normal state.
When the diagnosis is made in a child,
whether the flow through the ductus appears
to be large or small, operation at that age
should be recommended. This is advised both
for the relief or prevention of progressive cardiac strain and pulmonary vascular changes
and for providing optimum opportunity in
growth. In infants the diagnosis is frequently
less readily established, and, if there is not
serious difficulty, surgical intervention is
probably best deferred until after the age of
two years. When the diagnosis of a patent
ductus arteriosus is made in an adult, decision as to surgery must be balanced between the indications in the individual case
for the necessity of operation such as enlargement of the heart and decreased functional
capacity, and the greater risk in operation on
the ductus in older patients. With increasing
years a satisfactory surgical exposure of the
ductus is more difficult, and the vessels are
more rigid.

The presence of other congenital cardiac
abnormalities or acquired heart disease may
be found in certain cases with signs of a
patent ductus arteriosus. An associated ventricular or atrial septal defect does not
contraindicate surgical intervention. The
presence of pulmonary stenosis, however, is a
strong contraindication to elimination of a
ductus, which in this instance is acting as a
compensatory mechanism. Cyanosis or significant right axis deviation makes careful
investigation of the case imperative prior to
consideration of surgery. Superimposed rheumatic heart disease, provided all tests indicate

that the rheumatic process is inactive at the
time of surgery, does not contraindicate, but
rather enhances, the need for the elimination of the ductus.

A DEFECT OF THE AORTIC SEPTUM, due
to failure of the down-growing aorticopul-
monary septum to unite with the bulbar septum, occurs relatively rarely. An opening is
present in this disorder between the aorta and
pulmonary artery above the level of their
valves. In contrast to patent ductus arteriosus the continuous murmur is usually heard
lower along the left sternal border and cardiac
enlargement is apt to be greater. As the shunt
enters the pulmonary artery in both instances, cardiac catheterization may not
clarify the differential diagnosis between the
two conditions and exploratory thoracotomy
is indicated. In a few instances surgical
closure of an aortic septal defect has been
possible when there was adequate separation
of the two vessels proximal to the communication.

A communication between the aorta and
the conus of the right ventricle due to an
anomalous congenital channel or rupture of
a CONGENITAL ANEURYSM OF THE RIGHT
SINUS OF VALSALVA is also a rare condition
which may present signs suggestive of a
patent ductus. Again the murmurs are louder
over the midprecordium, and the diastolic
element is particularly prominent. Catheterization findings reveal an increased oxygen
content in the right ventricle similar to the
findings in a high ventricular defect.

VENTRICULAR SEPTAL DEFECTS. The
most common type of ventricular septal defect
is a perforation in the septal wall, usually
near the base of the septum and small in size.
The blood passing through this small opening
under high pressure from the left ventricle
creates a loud harsh murmur which is heard
with maximum intensity over the midsternal
or lower sternal area and is often widespread
both to the left and right in its transmission.
An accompanying systolic thrill is present in
many cases. As the volume of left to right
shunt is small, the size of the heart as confirmed by roentgenogram is usually normal.
Functional capacity is good. The striking intensity of the murmur has too frequently led
to unnecessary restrictions of activity.

A high septal defect, caused by the failure
of the ventricular septum to meet the aortic
septum, is less common than defects in the
septal wall. Because of the higher location of
this opening, blood shunted from the left ven-

tricle is ejected almost direc
monary artery. Such high s
usually larger than the defe
wall and may cause great
changes, owing both to la
shunt and possibly to more
nary vascular changes res
direct transmission of high
pressure. Pulmonary hyperte
In the presence of a large h
and marked increase in pres
ventricle, especially with the
sufficient reversal of flow th
may occur to cause cyanosis
ent. A systolic murmur is he
of the heart, and the second
is increased in intensity.
dilatation of the pulmonary
murmur of pulmonary insuf
be heard. The heart usuall
erate degree of enlargement,
nary artery and its branche
and pulsate actively. In som
ings are suggestive of those o
arteriosus and require speci
ing cardiac catheterization,
correct diagnosis.

ATRIAL SEPTAL DEFEC
logic development of the atri
plex and accounts for sever
of defects. Failure of compl
tum primum leaves a large
base of the atrial septum wh
associated with anomalous f
mitral valves and occasionall
valves. Incomplete developn
tum secundum leaves an ope
and posterior part of the s
natal life, because of norma
sure in the left atrium, the d
shunt through such defects
into the right atrium. A
foramen ovale may remain
pensatory escape mechanism
diac anomalies which cause
pressure in the right atrium.
nary stenosis or tricuspid d
atrial pressure here being
blood is shunted into the lef
the appearance of cyanosis.

An atrial septal defect
bined with congenital or
stenosis and marked enlarge
monary artery, and is know
bacher syndrome.

The presence of a large
fect allows a considerable

study are occasionally indicated to establish the diagnosis, especially in cases in which a decision is necessary as to the presence of a condition amenable to surgery. The procedures of cardiac catheterization and angiocardiography require special equipment and personnel trained to carry out and interpret the results of these tests.

Catheterization of the heart may give important information in several ways. In certain abnormal communications the route of the catheter as followed under fluoroscopic observation may be seen to take an unusual course. For instance, in the case of an interatrial septal defect it can be directed from the right into the left atrium; or, in the case of overriding of the aorta, the catheter may pass directly from the right ventricle into the aorta. Collection of individual blood samples is made successively from the venae cavae, right atrium, right ventricle and pulmonary artery. The oxygen content of these samples from the right side of the heart in normal circumstances shows no significant variation. In the presence of a left to right shunt the oxygen content will be higher in the blood sampled from the region receiving the shunt; e.g., in the presence of a patent ductus arteriosus the oxygen content of blood from the pulmonary artery is higher than that from the right ventricle. By the use of various formulas calculation can be made of the volume of blood shunted. Pressure recordings are taken at the various locations. From these, for example, the presence of pulmonary stenosis is demonstrated by the recording of a lower pressure in the pulmonary artery than in the right ventricle. Venous *angiocardiography* is helpful in demonstrating communications and areas of stenosis within the heart and also in delineating the pulmonary vascular tree. Aortography is most useful for visualizing coarctation of the aorta and patency of the ductus arteriosus.

Differential diagnosis between congenital and acquired heart disease is occasionally a problem. Significant points in the history are the age at which a murmur or other evidences of heart disease such as cyanosis were first noted, and the presence or absence of symptoms of rheumatic fever; the presence of other congenital anomalies is suggestive. On cardiac examination, physical findings in locations other than the mitral and aortic areas are immediately suggestive of a congenital lesion, although certain anomalies may also cause signs in these two areas. In children,

particularly, the frequent occurrence of relatively loud functional murmurs is often misleading. These functional murmurs are usually more musical and tend to be more variable in intensity than those caused by congenital lesions.

Prognosis. The prognosis in congenital heart disease varies widely and is dependent both on the type of anomaly and the degree of pathologic physiology created in the individual case. In many instances the prognosis is excellent. In certain conditions, because of grave disturbances of circulation, prognosis is poor.

The great advances in control of subacute bacterial endocarditis with antibiotics has radically changed the prognosis of this form of complication prone to develop in certain types of anomalies. The advent and continued developments in surgical treatment for certain cardiac malformations have greatly altered the prognosis in these conditions.

Treatment. Medical management of patients with a congenital heart lesion must vary according to the circulatory dysfunction or complications present in the individual case. When there is no cardiac enlargement and functional capacity is normal, as in many cases with a small ventricular defect, physical activities need not be restricted. In cases with lesions which cause considerable cardiac enlargement, or in the presence of significant hypertension due to coarctation of the aorta, strenuous exercise should be avoided. Children with cyanosis usually will limit the amount of their activity themselves with variations in the degree of hypoxia present. Individualization of limitation of activities is vital to avoid the occurrence of unwise strain in certain cases on the one hand and to avoid the more common error of unnecessary invalidism on the other.

The development of congestive heart failure in cases of congenital heart disease is not necessarily a terminal event and should be treated with digitalis and other standard methods of therapy. Congestive failure may occur as a transient complication due to the added strain imposed by an intercurrent infection, and specific therapy in these cases may be necessary only for a short time.

In infants and young children who suffer hypoxia due to lesions of the cyanotic group, episodes of severe dyspnea and cyanosis may occur. In such attacks the child should be placed on the abdomen with knees drawn up. If relief is not thus obtained, morphine

(1 mg. per 10 pounds of body weight) should be administered, as well as oxygen if available.

As a prophylactic measure against the development of subacute bacterial endocarditis, preventive measures against the development of foci of infection are important. Eradication of such foci, if present, is indicated with the use of antibiotic or chemotherapeutic treatment at the time of and for two days after dental extraction or tonsillectomy.

Treatment by the specific surgical procedures currently available has been discussed under the items on Anomalies of the Aortic Arch, Coarctation of the Aorta, Patent Ductus Arteriosus, Pulmonary Stenosis, the Tetralogy of Fallot and other anomalies causing inadequate flow of blood to the lungs. With further advances in cardiovascular surgery, other conditions will probably be added to the list of congenital cardiac anomalies amenable to surgical treatment.

JANET S. BALDWIN

References

Abbott, M. E.: Atlas of Congenital Heart Disease. New York, American Heart Association, 1936.
Bing, R. J.: Congenital Heart Disease. An Introduction and Classification. Am. J. Med., *12*:77, 1952.
Brock, R. C.: Congenital Pulmonary Stenosis. Am. J. Med., *12*:680, 1952.
Brown, J. W.: Congenital Heart Disease. 2nd ed. London, Staples Press, 1950.
Dotter, C. T., and Steinberg, I.: Angiocardiography in Congenital Heart Disease. Am. J. Med., *12*: 219, 1952.
Dow, J. W., and others: Studies of Congenital Heart Disease. IV. Uncomplicated Pulmonic Stenosis. Circulation, *1*:267, 1950.
Gross, R. E.: The Patent Ductus Arteriosus. Observations on Diagnosis and Therapy in 525 Surgically Treated Cases. Am. J. Med., *12*:472, 1952.
————: Coarctation of the Aorta. Circulation, 7: 757, 1953.
Holman, E., Gerbode, F., and Purdy, A.: The Patent Ductus. A Review of 75 Cases with Surgical Treatment Including an Aneurysm of the Ductus and One of the Pulmonary Artery. J. Thoracic Surg., 25:111, 1953.
Keith, J. D., Neill, C. A., Vlad, P., Rowe, R. D., and Chute, A. L.: Transposition of the Great Vessels. Circulation, 7:830, 1953.
Potts, W. J.: The Tetralogy of Fallot. Am. J. Med., *12*:596, 1952.
Taussig, H. B.: Congenital Malformations of the Heart. New York, Commonwealth Fund, 1947.
————, and Bauersfeld, S. R.: Follow-up Studies on the First 1000 Patients Operated on for Pulmonary Stenosis or Atresia (Results up to March, 1952). Ann. Int. Med., 38:1, 1953.

RHEUMATIC HEART DISEASE

Definition. Rheumatic heart disease includes inflammation of the endocardium, myocardium and pericardium, occurring in the course of acute rheumatic fever; also those sequelae which persist after the acute process has subsided.

Etiology (See section on Rheumatic Fever for complete consideration). Many economic, geographic, meteorologic and familial factors are apparently concerned, but one fact stands out above all others, namely, that hemolytic streptococcal infection (Lancefield Group A) is associated intimately with the onset of rheumatic fever and with its recurrence. Rheumatic recurrences can be prevented almost completely by preventing hemolytic streptococcal infections with sulfonamides or penicillin. Early and vigorous treatment of hemolytic streptococcal infections with penicillin reduces the incidence of rheumatic fever following such infections; but after rheumatic fever has begun, treatment with antimicrobial agents is ineffective.

Incidence. Average figures for the whole country vary from 1 to 8 per 1000. Large cities (London, New York) have shown an incidence of 10 to 20 per 1000 (Bland). Rheumatic heart disease was found in 31 of 3086 college students at the University of Pennsylvania (1932), a frequency of about 1 per cent. This incidence has been found by others in the study of similar groups. Rheumatic fever, hypertension and coronary artery disease are the three main causes of heart disease in America today. In the past, various statistics have placed one or the other of the three in the lead. However, preventive measures may soon put rheumatic heart disease in third place. Statistics published by the Metropolitan Life Insurance Company indicate that rheumatic heart disease now causes only half as many deaths as it did ten years ago, and only one-fifth as many deaths as it did forty years ago. Nevertheless, it has been estimated that a million people in the United States have rheumatic heart disease.

Morbid Anatomy. *Acute Stage.* At present, the primary lesion in the heart is thought to involve the collagen of the connective tissue. Involvement of the endocardium, the pericardium and the surfaces of the valves may be a secondary result. The myocardial fibers may be affected to some extent and occasionally myocardial damage is severe. Baggenstoss quotes Klinge as saying that typical Aschoff bodies are not present in the myocardium of patients dying within the first few weeks after onset of rheumatic fever, but that they develop later. However, they have been described in a 21-month-old infant who died five days after the onset of presumptive acute rheumatic fever. Their presence is thought to constitute evidence of active rheumatic heart disease. The atrioventricular rings may be dilated. The ventricles are often dilated. Characteristically, there are rows of small verrucae at the line of closure of certain valves, especially the mitral and aortic. The pericardium is often inflamed. Fibrinous or serofibrinous exudates are common. The valve leaflets may be thickened. Acute lesions of the coronary arteries have been described.

Late Stage. From the clinical point of view, the late stage of rheumatic heart disease is important chiefly because of lesions of the heart valves. These are discussed in the section on Chronic Valvular Heart Disease.

Pericardial adhesions are commonly found. There may be only a few or there may be enough to obliterate the pericardial cavity (*concretio pericardii*). Most observers do not believe that rheumatic heart disease produces the thick percardial scars which cause cardiac constriction, but there is some doubt on this point. Bland states that "constrictive pericarditis has not been observed in the follow-up of 3,000 cases of childhood rheumatism in 30 years experience at the House of the Good Samaritan in Boston."

Endocardial lesions, over surfaces other than valvular, occur and are well described by Baggenstoss. They usually occur in the left atrium, and may progress in rare instances to a thickening and whitening of the entire left atrial endocardium.

The myocardium of late rheumatic heart disease usually shows hypertrophy of the chambers, the work of which is increased by diseased valves. There are at times many scattered small scars. However, large areas of destruction of myocardial tissue are not usually seen, except occasionally in the atria, where they may give rise to aneurysmal dilatation, especially of the left atrium. Occasionally rheumatic lesions of coronary arteries are said to produce infarcts of the ventricular myocardium.

Pathologic Physiology. *Acute Rheumatic Carditis.* The major danger to the patient is cardiac failure. This development has been attributed by most observers to acute rheumatic myocarditis. That the myocardial lesion may be an important factor in the production of cardiac failure cannot be denied, yet extensive myocardial involvement is not the most striking histologic abnormality in the hearts of patients, dying of acute rheumatic carditis. It may be that the rheumatic lesion interferes with cardiac contraction by affecting the myocardial fibers in ways which are not obvious histologically, and in ways which do not lead to subsequent large-scale myocardial destruction. However, two other mechanisms should be considered: (1) The frequent, early and fairly marked dilatation of the atrioventricular rings, emphasized by Coombs, may be a major factor in producing cardiac failure. If the lesion in the connective tissue is the primary effect of acute rheumatic fever, dilatation of the atrioventricular rings may be an early result. Certainly a systolic murmur is present in almost all children seriously ill with rheumatic carditis. Furthermore, Powers has demonstrated experimentally that acutely developing mitral insufficiency may lead rapidly to cardiac failure. More recently the accidental production of acute regurgitation during mitral commissurotomy has provided further dramatic evidence of its seriousness. (2) Coombs has suggested that the bulk of the interstitial tissue of the heart is increased in acute rheumatic carditis, even before the development of obvious valvular lesions. If intermyocardial collagen swells, it might interfere with the blood supply of the myocardial fibers and also make it more difficult for them to shorten. Thus the cardiac failure which is the central clinical feature of acute rheumatic carditis may be due to a combination of factors: (*a*) myocarditis which is not very obvious histologically, (*b*) acute insufficiency of the atrioventricular valves, and (*c*) swelling of the collagen between the myocardial fibers.

Atrial fibrillation occurs occasionally during an attack of acute rheumatic carditis in a child. It occurs more commonly later in life as a result of chronic mitral valve disease or sometimes during a recurrence of rheumatic fever.

Late Stage. The pathologic physiology of the various valvular lesions is discussed in the section on Chronic Valvular Heart Disease.

The contribution which is made by pericardial adhesions to the unfavorable effects of late rheumatic heart disease has been the subject of much dispute. When pericardial and valvular lesions coexist, their relative importance has been particularly difficult to assess. It is now the general belief that pericardial scar tissue causes congestive heart failure only by producing constriction of the heart, not by the production of adhesions between the heart and its surroundings (see Wood and Krumbhaar for more complete discussion.)

Clinical Manifestations and Diagnostic Criteria. *Acute Stage.* The clinical evidences of acute rheumatic carditis are intimately intermingled with those of active rheumatic fever (see section on Rheumatic Fever).

The diagnosis of acute rheumatic fever is often missed because many patients fail to exhibit the so-called "textbook picture." The classic migratory joint pains are much less common in children than in adults; in fact, it is quite rare to see this clinical picture on a pediatric ward. What one does see is a pallid, sickly, listless child with anorexia, periodic fever and occasional mild discomfort in an extremity, as often in the thigh or calf as in a joint.

One should not wait for incontrovertible evidence to make the tentative diagnosis of active rheumatic fever in patients who are thought to be unusually susceptible; for example, in those with a known rheumatic valvular lesion, or with a history of a previous episode of typical rheumatic fever, or with a history of rheumatic heart disease in a parent or sibling, particularly if their illness follows a streptococcal pharyngitis. In such individuals, rheumatic fever should be suspected when the patient is ill in any way not clearly explained by some other diagnosis. Any fever, malaise, anorexia, muscle pain, anemia, leukocytosis or a rapid sedimentation rate otherwise unexplained may indicate rheumatic activity. Sometimes a sudden increase in the degree of cardiac disability may be the only manifestation. Almost certainly any patient with rheumatic heart disease, who develops congestive failure before the age of 20, has active rheumatic carditis and should be treated on that basis.

In patients with active rheumatic fever, congestive heart failure may cause the sedimentation rate to become normal. Under these circumstances, one of the best indications of the presence of rheumatic activity becomes unreliable as a guide to management.

The diagnosis of acute rheumatic heart disease is to be made by the inference that it is present to some degree during every attack of rheumatic fever. However, there are certain clinical findings which indicate its presence more definitely: (1) The heart may enlarge, causing the apex impulse to become diffuse and to be displaced to the left. (2) Various murmurs may appear. While systolic murmurs are most frequent, they are not always reliable evidence of carditis, since they occur so commonly in normal children, particularly during a febrile illness. Diastolic murmurs constitute more definite evidence, but are less frequent. These include a short apical, mid-diastolic murmur which does not indicate the presence of a true mitral stenosis since it often disappears when the active process subsides. Aortic diastolic murmurs may appear during active carditis. (3) Certain electrocardiographic abnormalities may occur. An increased or changing P-R interval can be demonstrated by serial tracings in many patients with acute rheumatic carditis. However, the P-R interval may also be affected in other febrile illnesses, so that such changes constitute suggestive rather than absolute diagnostic evidence. The QRS complex may become notched, slurred or widened; the Q-T interval may be prolonged; transient T wave changes are commonly seen in serial electrocardiograms. Atrial fibrillation usually indicates severe cardiac involvement.

Patients with severe carditis are usually acutely ill with fever, cough, dyspnea, tachycardia and gallop rhythm. These patients often have pericardial and pleural involvement with chest pain of a pleuritic type, and a pericardial friction rub. Congestive heart failure, when it appears, is a serious sign. It is usually of "right-sided" type with venous distention, liver enlargement and edema.

Chronic Stage. The clinical findings of the various rheumatic valvular lesions are discussed under Chronic Valvular Heart Disease.

The diagnosis of chronic rheumatic heart disease may be made by finding a form of chronic valvular disease known to be of rheumatic origin. For example, patients with mitral stenosis can be diagnosed as having rheumatic heart disease despite the absence of any history of rheumatic fever. This same principle should probably be applied to patients with acquired aortic stenosis, since pathologic studies seem to indicate that most, if not all, acquired aortic stenosis is of rheumatic origin. Degenerative vascular disease may contribute later to the progressive deformity of the valve. Similarly the presence of aortic insufficiency in a patient under 30 years of age, who has no history or findings of syphilis, is usually considered evidence of rheumatic heart disease.

Great care must be taken not to diagnose rheumatic valvular disease on the basis of invalid criteria. For example, a systolic apical murmur alone should not be considered as evidence of rheumatic heart disease. Approximately 50 per cent of school children have functional systolic murmurs, particularly during tachycardia caused by exercise or apprehension. Similarly, tachycardia is not uncommon in nervous, highstrung children and should not constitute a basis for restricting their activity in the absence of a rapid sedimentation rate or other significant evidence of active rheumatic heart disease. Finally extrasystoles in a child, unaccompanied by signs of active rheumatism, are not to be considered evidence of, or a harbinger of, rheumatic carditis.

When attempting to decide whether a murmur of questionable significance is due to rheumatic heart disease, the recognition of an earlier attack of rheumatic fever on the basis of the history may afford at least circumstantial evidence. The diagnosis of rheumatic fever in the past may be suggested, as a result of careful questioning, even in the absence of "typical" chorea or acute migratory joint pains, as indicated in the section on Rheumatic Fever.

Prognosis. Analysis of series of rheumatic subjects, collected before the introduction of current programs of prophylaxis and treatment of acute and chronic rheumatic heart disease and of bacterial endocarditis, revealed the following statistics: Less than 5 per cent of children with a first attack of rheumatic fever died within the first year. Of those who developed definite congestive heart failure, 70 per cent died. At the end of an attack of rheumatic fever, 65 per cent had evidence of heart disease. Thirty-five per cent showed no signs of cardiac injury. After ten years, 32 per cent showed no signs of cardiac disability, 48 per cent had heart disease and 20 per cent were dead. After twenty years, 32 per cent revealed no signs of heart disease, whereas 38 per cent had definite heart disease and 30 per cent had died. Approximately 5 per cent of patients with definite evidence of heart disease at the end of an attack of rheumatic fever lose those signs during the next ten years. In the past, about 2 to 5 per cent of patients with chronic rheumatic val-

vulitis died of subacute bacterial endocarditis. Without prophylaxis, rheumatic recurrences were to be expected in 50 to 75 per cent of children in the first five or ten years following the initial attack. Some statistics indicated a recurrence at the rate of one child in every four each year.

It is too early to give definite statistics concerning many aspects of the present-day prognosis in patients with rheumatic heart disease. However, it is already apparent that prophylaxis with sulfonamides or penicillin has sharply reduced the rate of recurrent attacks of rheumatic fever. Also, the prompt treatment of streptococcal pharyngitis and surgical treatment of valvular defects have improved the outlook. The recent improvement in the prognosis of bacterial endocarditis is demonstrated by the fact that the mortality rate has been reduced from approximately 100 per cent to less than 15 per cent in most clinics.

Treatment. *Treatment of the Patient with Active Rheumatic Carditis.* See section on Chronic Valvular Heart Disease for treatment of chronic rheumatic valvular disease.

Rest. It is of utmost importance to postulate the presence of active rheumatic carditis in all cases of active rheumatic fever, whether or not obvious cardiac symptoms or signs are present, and to keep the child at rest in bed until all evidence of activity subsides. The subsidence of active carditis usually takes months, not weeks. The last objective signs to return to normal are usually the weight chart and the erythrocyte sedimentation rate. A good rule of thumb is that when the child looks well, eats well, feels well and is gaining weight, the rheumatic fever is probably quiescent.

Salicylates. Although these drugs have been in use for many years, it is not yet known whether they have a favorable effect on the cardiac lesion. They are indicated for the relief of pain and to reduce fever. Amounts up to 0.065 gm. per pound of body weight may be used, usually divided into four to six doses. Adults may tolerate 10 gm. per day, but usually less is required. The drug is usually prescribed in the form of oral tablets of acetylsalicylic acid, but sodium salicylate may be used. Rectal administration of sodium salicylate in a starch retention enema is useful in patients who cannot take large doses by mouth. After fairly full doses for two to four days, if the pain and fever have subsided, the dose may be reduced by a third. A week later it may be cut to 50 per cent of the original amount. If well tolerated, it may be continued at this level for some months; premature withdrawal of salicylates is often associated with recrudescence of pain and fever. The practice of using sodium bicarbonate with salicylates reduces the blood level and is therefore equivalent to reducing the dose. Toxic signs include tinnitus, nausea, vomiting and headache. High doses, especially when used intravenously (a method we do not advise), may cause acidosis and hyperpnea. Salicyclates may in rare instances interfere with prothrombin formation and can cause a bleeding tendency. Some observers combine salicylate therapy with steroid therapy (see below).

Penicillin and Sulfonamides. These drugs exert no beneficial effect on the rheumatic fever itself. It has been suspected, but without clear evidence, that sulfonamides may do harm; however, there is no evidence that this is true in the case of penicillin. It is, therefore, customary to give penicillin in a dose of 300,000 units of procaine penicillin daily by injection for ten days (or 1 million units by mouth daily). After that, it is given in the prophylactic dose of 300,000 units once a day by mouth before breakfast. The object is to eradicate hemolytic streptococci and to keep them eradicated. This is especially indicated when steroid therapy is used (see below). Under these circumstances, the dose of penicillin should be doubled or tripled.

Steroid Therapy (ACTH, Cortisone and Hydrocortisone). There is considerable divergence of opinion concerning the value of steroid therapy in rheumatic fever. Some observers believe that it may be life-saving in certain instances. Others have almost given it up, believing that salicylate administration is less expensive and equally effective. It is of interest that preliminary reports of an attempt to decide, on a large-scale experience, whether steroid therapy prevents rheumatic heart disease, give no evidence that it does. The "control series" on salicylates alone is said to have shown the same subsequent incidence of heart disease as that shown by patients on steroid therapy. At the present time we are unsure of many things that should enable us to use steroid therapy unerringly in rheumatic heart disease. Nevertheless, an unofficial poll of several competent observers with a large experience in this field indicates that all would advise cortisone under certain circumstances, especially in the face of severe acute rheumatic fever and carditis of recent onset. The majority consider it relatively ineffective in smoldering rheumatic fever of long duration. Most use oral cortisone, starting with a fairly large dose, reducing it somewhat when signs and symptoms are controlled, maintaining this reduced level for approximately six weeks, and tapering off the last 75 mg. very slowly. The following regimen is suggested: 300 mg. daily, in three divided doses for the first few days; 200 mg. daily for the next ten days;100 mg. daily for the next four weeks; thereafter reduce the dose 25 mg. each week. Some continue the original 300 mg. dose for the full six weeks. The typical manifestations of hyperadrenalism induced by cortisone, hydrocortisone or ACTH may appear in the course of therapy. Limitation of the sodium intake and mercurial diuretics usually control fluid retention and pulmonary congestion. The administration of 2.0 to 3.0 gm. of potassium chloride daily will prevent potassium depletion. If the doses of ACTH or adrenal steroids required to control rheumatic activity produce cerebral or cardiac complications, they should be replaced by salicylate therapy.

Results to be hoped for include a decrease in "toxicity"; improvement in fever, joint pain and general condition; a return to normal of the erythrocyte sedimentation rate; a reduction in cardiac size; and, if salt is restricted sufficiently, a disappearance of signs of congestive heart failure.

When hormonal therapy is discontinued there is often a "rebound," i.e., a recrudescence of clinical and laboratory manifestations of the disease. This relapse may be severe and may require reinstitution of therapy. Usually a short period of salicylate therapy will suffice.

Diet and Other General Measures. The child should have a balanced diet insofar as possible. Most workers prescribe iron (ferrous sulfate, 0.3 gm. twice daily).

The Treatment of Congestive Heart Failure in the Presence of Acute Rheumatic Carditis. The rules are as follows: Use rest; cortisone as outlined above; strict salt restriction; and if needed, mercurial diuretics and xanthine diuretics (theobromine calcium salicylate, 1 gm. three times a day). Digitalis is not as helpful in this situation as it is in congestive failure without rheumatic activity. It may be used, but with caution. It may cause atrial fibrillation. In some cases it has been thought to predispose to sudden death. One should rarely exceed 0.1 gm. of the powdered leaf per 10 pounds of body weight as a "digitalizing" dose. If a child of 60 pounds has atrial fibrillation, not controlled with a dose of 0.6 gm. followed by 0.05 gm. daily thereafter, do not increase the dose without very careful consideration. A general rule of digitalis therapy is applicable here; do not try, by means of digitalis, to reduce the cardiac rate of a febrile patient with atrial fibrillation below the rate to be expected if the patient had normal sinus rhythm and was equally ill.

It is well to remember a point stressed by Coombs: During a severe attack of rheumatic carditis the time will often come when you find the cardiac dullness becoming larger, the heart sounds becoming muffled and the patient beginning to show circulatory embarrassment. At such a time you wonder if the patient is developing a functionally significant pericardial effusion. There may actually be a small amount of effusion, but these signs are usually the result of cardiac weakness and dilatation. If one will refrain from subjecting the patient to fatiguing studies to determine the presence or absence of pericardial effusion, and refrain from performing pericardial paracentesis, he will be justified in the vast majority of instances.

Prophylaxis. *Prevention of Recurrences of Rheumatic Fever.* This can now be achieved by preventing hemolytic streptococcal infections in persons who have had rheumatic fever. It is accomplished by administering penicillin or sulfonamides daily. The dose of penicillin is 300,000 units by mouth once daily 30 minutes before breakfast. Toxic effects are rare. Some patients experience urticaria and angioneurotic edema in the first two or three weeks. If these manifestations are not severe, they usually prove transient; penicillin is continued and antihistaminic drugs are given. The injection of 600,000 units of benzathine penicillin G twice a month in children or 1,200,000 units in adults is adequate to prevent recurrent streptococcal infections. The incidence of sensitization does not appear greater than with other penicillin preparations.

The dose of sulfadiazine is 0.5 gm. once daily by mouth for small children, and 1 gm. daily for larger children and adults. A certain proportion of patients develop toxic reactions, particularly leukopenia, and cannot continue. If undesired effects do not appear in the first four to six weeks, they are not likely to occur at all. Consequently, the daily observation and weekly blood count required during the first six weeks may give place to less frequent observation.

In the past, these preventive drugs were stopped during the summer. It is now the practice to continue them throughout the year. The question arises as to when to stop them. Those physicians with the most experience in this field do not necessarily stop prophylaxis even when the patient reaches age 20, as was the custom in the past. In fact, they do not like to stop prophylaxis at all. This is especially true when unusual exposure to streptococcal infection is to be anticipated as in the case of doctors, nurses or parents of school age children. One must think carefully about each individual and tend to advise continuation of prophylaxis almost indefinitely, unless there are good reasons to desist.

Tonsillectomy, once practiced as a prophylactic measure against rheumatic recurrence, has fallen into disrepute for this purpose. It should be done only if the condition of the tonsils requires it.

For the prevention of subacute bacterial endocarditis, any patient with rheumatic heart disease who is to have a tooth extraction or tonsillectomy should be protected by penicillin. An effective method is to use a combination of 100,000 units of aqueous penicillin and 300,000 units of procaine penicillin, one hour before operation and once daily for two days after the operation.

Control of the Child's Activity after the Rheumatic Attack Has Subsided. If there is no cardiac enlargement and no definite valvular lesion, it is usually safe to let the patient engage in normal activity. If such a patient develops "dyspnea," it is sometimes necessary to encourage him to undertake gradually increasing activity to prevent the development of a "cardiac neurosis." Rules are difficult to make for all cases, but exercise is not apt to hurt a person with a systolic murmur at the apex of slight to moderate intensity if the heart is of normal size and shape and if he does not have mitral stenosis or active rheumatism. Experience has taught us that when we advise the average child who likes athletics to give up competitive sports, he will do so only while he is being watched, or if he develops really uncomfortable symptoms as a result of indulging in sports.

A person with a definite cardiac lesion

and cardiac enlargement should be kept within his exercise tolerance. For reasons beyond our control we have watched a student with slight aortic regurgitation play football and take part in intercollegiate track (220 yard dash). We have seen another with a similar cardiac lesion play water polo. Neither suffered any harm that we could demonstrate.

Education. Since the child with rheumatic heart disease may well have to earn his living by brain rather than by brawn, his education is of particularly great importance. It may have to be interrupted temporarily by acute illness. However, all through the long convalescence it should be carried on at all costs.

F. C. WOOD AND H. F. ZINSSER, JR.

References

Baggenstoss, A. H.: Pathology of the Heart (edited by S. E. Gould). Springfield, Charles C Thomas, 1953, pp. 638–692.

Bland, Edward F.: In Levy, R. L.: Disorders of the Heart and Circulation. New York, Thomas Nelson and Sons, 1951, pp. 313–342.

Coombs, C. F.: Rheumatic Heart Disease. Bristol, John Wright and Sons, 1924.

Kuttner, Ann G.: Rheumatic Fever. In Nelson, W. E.: Textbook of Pediatrics, 6th ed., Philadelphia, W. B. Saunders Co., 1954.

Major, Ralph H.: Classic Descriptions of Disease. 3rd ed. Springfield, Ill., Charles C Thomas, 1948. William Charles Wells, p. 219; Jean Bouillard, p. 222.

Powers, John H.: Surgical Treatment of Mitral Stenosis, an Experimental Study. Arch. Surg., 25: 555, 1932.

Symposium on Rheumatic Fever and Rheumatic Heart Disease. Am. J. Med., 17:747, 1954.

Walsh, Benjamin J. and Sprague, Howard B.: The Treatment of Congestive Failure in Children with Active Rheumatic Fever. J.A.M.A., 116:560, 1941.

Wood, F. C. and Krumbhaar, E. B.: Diseases of the Pericardium. In Levy, R. L.: Disorders of the Heart and Circulation. New York, Thomas Nelson & Sons, 1951, pp. 49–95.

CHRONIC VALVULAR HEART DISEASE

Definition. The term "chronic valvular heart disease" includes any permanent organic deformity of one or more cardiac valves. By definition, the disease which produced the valvular deformity has become quiescent or chronic.

Etiology and Incidence. Most chronic valvular heart disease in America today is of rheumatic origin. Other causes include syphilis, congenital valvular anomaly, healed bacterial endocarditis, arteriosclerosis and trauma. The etiology and relative frequency of the various specific valvular lesions are presented in the appropriate subdivisions of this section. Changes in frequency of valvular heart disease should be expected in the future as a reflection of recent advances in treatment of contributing diseases such as syphilis and streptococcal infections.

Morbid Anatomy. The diseased valves become stenotic, insufficient or both. Further details of morbid anatomy may be found in standard textbooks of pathology.

Pathologic Physiology. The major difficulty results from mechanical interference with valvular function by valvular deformity. In general it can be said that stenosis of a valve increases the work of the chamber behind the obstruction, and that insufficiency of a valve tends to increase the work both of the chamber in front of and the one behind the insufficient valve. The way in which increasing cardiac work leads to congestive heart failure is considered in the section on Pathologic Physiology of Generalized Circulatory Failure.

Symptoms and Signs. The clinical picture associated with each lesion will be considered separately. With multiple valvular involvement, the findings become modified owing to summation or partial neutralization of various effects.

Treatment. Advances in cardiac surgery have revolutionized the treatment of chronic valvular defects. Furthermore, such surgery has stimulated clinical observation and research which has led to a better understanding of valvular disease. Simultaneously, great progress has been made toward the eradication of, or prophylaxis against such diseases as syphilis and rheumatic fever. These advances in prophylaxis and treatment may prove eventually of greater importance than the current dramatic treatment of valvular defects by surgery.

MITRAL VALVULAR DISEASE

Mitral disease is the most common form of chronic valvular heart disease. While its relative frequency varies somewhat, depending on the incidence of syphilis in certain series, mitral disease comprises well over half of all valvular heart disease. In several American series the mitral valve was involved in about 85 per cent of the cases. Isolated mitral involvement occurred in slightly over 50 per cent; mitral and aortic in 20 per cent; mitral, aortic and tricuspid in 11 per cent; mitral and tricuspid in 3 per cent; and all four valves in 1 per cent.

Mitral disease is of great economic importance because of its frequency and because it disables the individual at a time of life when familial obligations are greatest. Most adult patients with significant disability from mitral valve disease have mitral stenosis.

MITRAL STENOSIS

The normal mitral orifice will admit three fingers. The average patient who is treated surgically has an opening that will barely admit the index finger.

Etiology. Except for rare cases of congenital origin, mitral stenosis is practically always due to rheumatic heart disease.

Pathologic Physiology. The circulatory disturbances produced by mitral stenosis may be discussed in two stages.

In the *first stage,* the gradual narrowing of the mitral valve interferes with the flow of blood from the left atrium into the left ventricle during diastole. Pressure within the left atrium increases and this chamber enlarges. The increased pressure is transmitted backward through the pulmonary veins to the pulmonary capillaries producing pulmonary congestion and sometimes transudation into the alveoli. Early during this stage, the circulatory abnormalities may be insignificant while the patient is at rest, becoming apparent only at times when, for various reasons, blood flow or blood volume increases sufficiently to exaggerate the hemodynamic effect of the obstruction. During this stage, exertional dyspnea is the outstanding symptom. Other symptoms of pulmonary congestion may include orthopnea, paroxysmal nocturnal attacks, cough and hemoptysis. The duration of this first stage is extremely variable; it may persist for years in some patients, while in others it may be so brief that they do not recall this type of difficulty in their history.

In the *second stage,* a more advanced and chronic state of increased resistance to pulmonary blood flow develops. This must be compensated for by an increased pulmonary arterial pressure and the burden for producing this falls upon the right ventricle. Secondary pulmonary arteriolar changes may develop and increase the resistance to blood flow. Pulmonary hypertension may lead to the development of relative pulmonic valvular insufficiency which, if severe, may further handicap the right ventricle. Dilatation and failure of the right ventricle occasionally produces relative tricuspid valvular insufficiency which adds still another burden. The symptoms at this stage are those of so-called "right ventricular failure" and include an increase in venous pressure, distention of the neck veins, enlargement of the liver, ascites and peripheral edema. When these develop, dyspnea, orthopnea and pulmonary congestion sometimes disappear. Patients in stage two can occasionally be changed back to stage one by restoring the integrity of the right ventricle with digitalis and other measures; in such patients dyspnea, orthopnea and pulmonary congestion may reappear.

Symptoms. The history is of great importance in the evaluation of patients with mitral stenosis. The majority have had rheumatic fever during childhood or in early adult life. However, in approximately 35 per cent of patients, a history of such episodes cannot be obtained.

Onset. Some patients have no symptoms and the presence of mitral stenosis is discovered as an incidental finding on routine examination. Most patients, however, on careful questioning prove to have symptoms of varying degree. The usual story is one of slowly increasing difficulty which, because of its very gradual nature, is often not recognized by the patient until a considerable handicap has developed. Occasionally the onset is abrupt, owing to an attack of pulmonary edema, hemoptysis, arterial embolism or atrial fibrillation.

Stage of Pulmonary Congestion. Exertional dyspnea is common, but the degree of activity which produces dyspnea varies widely in different patients. Dyspnea may be more severe with certain activities requiring arm raising, which at first glance would appear less likely to cause trouble than seemingly heavier work. For example, a woman may be able to scrub floors or do a washing when she is unable to hang up clothes, sweep or arrange curtains. Sometimes dyspnea is more common with talking than with walking. At times these variations lead to an erroneous evaluation of the patient's capabilities.

Orthopnea is common, and patients often require from two to four pillows for comfort. Cough is frequent and often associated with exertion or recumbency; in these instances it represents the equivalent of exertional dyspnea or orthopnea. Hemoptysis of varying degrees may occur.

Cough or dyspnea may at times appear only in the form of paroxysmal nocturnal attacks. These vary in severity from mild episodes, which subside promptly when the patient sits up or gets out of bed, to severe episodes of pulmonary edema. Wheezing is not uncommon during these spells and the condition may be mistaken for bronchial asthma.

sionally, however, the patients present themselves initially in peripheral congestive failure and deny any antecedent pulmonary symptoms. Such patients may be able to lie absolutely flat in bed and may be capable of reasonable activity without significant dyspnea.

Edema of the feet or ankles may appear first as a transient phenomenon, perhaps only during the premenstrual period. Later, persistent and severe dependent edema may develop. Many patients complain of abdominal

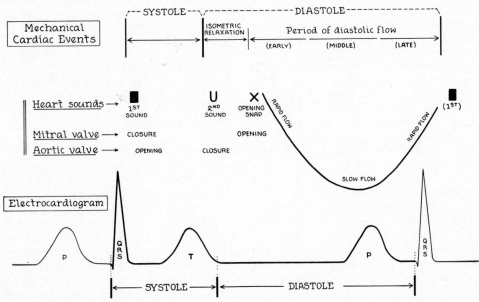

Fig. 153. Diagram indicating relations between cardiac ausculatory findings and physiologic phenomena. The diagram is intended to portray only left-sided events and has thus eliminated the contribution of the pulmonic and tricuspid valves.

The symptoms of pulmonary congestion may or may not be accompanied by peripheral evidence of congestive failure. Chest pain sometimes occurs and has been attributed to pulmonary arterial hypertension rather than to coronary insufficiency. Other symptoms associated with specific developments such as arterial embolism and arrhythmias will be considered later. The patient may complain of weakness and fatigability, which usually increase gradually, may become very severe, and at times are the chief difficulty. Some patients, however, do not recognize the presence of such symptoms except in retrospect after successful mitral commissurotomy.

Stage of Peripheral Congestive Failure. Most patients have had symptoms of the "pulmonary" type before they pass into the stage of so-called "right heart failure." Occa-

swelling or tightness together with symptoms of "indigestion." Occasionally, marked abdominal enlargement constitutes the only complaint and may be associated with ascites.

Physical Signs. The findings on physical examination may be divided into those signs produced directly by the narrowed valve orifice, and those occurring secondary to the development of associated conditions, including cardiac failure, arterial embolism and arrhythmias. The direct effects of the stenosed valve include the diastolic apical murmur and thrill, together with certain changes in the heart sound pattern.

The Diastolic Murmur. The characteristic murmur of mitral stenosis consists of sound vibrations produced because the narrowed orifice interferes with the flow of blood from the left atrium into the left ventricle during diastole. The time relationships of this murmur will be better understood by studying the normal curve of blood flow through the mitral valve as shown in Figure 153. The second heart sound in the diagram represents aortic semilunar valvular closure, and for a brief period following this there is normally no movement of blood into the left ventricle. Then the mitral valve opens and flow from the left atrium into the left ventricle takes place. Normally this flow is rapid during early diastole and subsequently slows through the middle of diastole. With contraction of the left atrium, the flow is again speeded up during the presystolic period (late ventricular diastole). Because the murmur results from an obstruction to this flow of blood, its intensity and timing will be correlated with the flow curve as diagrammed.

The murmur is characteristically low-pitched and of a coarse rumbling quality. A short gap representing the interval of isometric relaxation must be present between the second heart sound and the start of the murmur; the murmur cannot begin simultaneously with the aortic second heart sound because mitral valvular opening and aortic valvular closure are not simultaneous events. The early part of the murmur may be loud, but soon a decrescendo occurs so that the murmur becomes less intense through the middle of diastole. In patients with normal sinus rhythm, the murmur is again accentuated during late diastole, producing the so-called presystolic murmur. This presystolic crescendo murmur is simply one part of the complete murmur, although it may be the part most easily appreciated by untrained observers. This presystolic accentuation of the murmur disappears with the onset of atrial fibrillation. Consequently, recognition of the early part of the murmur is very important in such patients.

The murmur is usually best heard near the cardiac apex with the patient placed in the left lateral recumbent position. It may at times be sharply localized and thus require careful searching of the apical area for its discovery. It can be accentuated by increasing the heart rate, either by means of exercise or by having the patient inhale amyl nitrite. The murmur may at times be missed unless it is brought out by these maneuvers.

The murmur is often accompanied by a diastolic apical thrill. At times the thrill is more easily detected than the murmur, but when a thrill is present the murmur can be found by careful examination. Occasional patients with mitral stenosis have no diastolic murmur or thrill.

The Heart Sound Pattern. Mitral stenosis frequently produces changes in the heart sounds which strongly suggest the diagnosis, even in the absence of the characteristic murmur. The first heart sound at the apex becomes loud and sharp. In patients with isolated mitral insufficiency of marked degree, the loudness of the first heart sound tends to become diminished or the sound may even disappear. Thus, preservation of an accentuated first heart sound at the apex in patients with mitral disease points to mitral stenosis. The first heart sound in mitral stenosis may also be shown to be later than normal when timed against electrical systole as demonstrated by the electrocardiogram. In addition to these changes in the first heart sound, the second heart sound as heard at the pulmonic area may become quite loud and split.

The Mitral Opening Snap. In many patients with mitral stenosis an extra sound may be heard; the additional sound follows shortly after the second heart sound. The extra sound is short, and clicking or snapping in quality. It is higher pitched than the second heart sound and is usually heard best in the third or fourth intercostal space along the left sternal border. By referring again to the diagram in Figure 153, it can be seen that this extra sound occurs following isometric relaxation and at the time of the opening of the mitral valve. A normal mitral valve usually opens without producing any sound, whereas the opening of a stenotic valve may be accompanied by a clicking sound. One hears this sound at the beginning of the mitral diastolic murmur, although a well damped sound tracing shows that the sound occurs very slightly before the start of the murmur.

Diagnostically, this sound is second in importance only to the characteristic diastolic murmur. At times it will suggest the diagnosis in the absence of a murmur and should cause the examiner to resort to maneuvers designed to bring out the murmur. The sound must be differentiated from split second heart sounds, gallop rhythm and the physiologic third heart sound. By comparison with the opening snap sound, split second heart sounds are heard better over the base of the heart and the gap is shorter. Furthermore, the two components usually do not sound different, but produced as they are by asynchronous closure of the semilunar valves, they tend to have similar qualities. By comparison with the opening snap sound, gallop sounds and the physiologic third heart sound are better heard near the apex. The extra sound is lower pitched than the accompanying second heart sound, and the gap after the second sound is longer.

General Physical Findings. Patients with longstanding mitral stenosis tend to lose weight and often present the picture of chronic illness with emaciation and pallor. In patients with marked stenosis, the blood pressure will usually show a tendency to lowered systolic levels together with a narrowing of the pulse pressure. Readings in the range of 90/70 or 80/60 are not uncommon. Other findings include signs arising from associated conditions such as congestive heart failure, arrhythmias and embolism.

Roentgenologic Findings. With so-called "pure" mitral stenosis, changes in the cardiac silhouette involve chiefly the left atrium, right ventricle and pulmonary arteries. The left ventricle and aorta are not prominent. As viewed in the frontal projection, these changes combine to produce a straightening of the left border of the heart, sometimes referred to as "the mitral configuration" or "mitralization of the heart." A similar configuration may occur in other conditions, hence the diagnosis of mitral stenosis should not be based alone on the anteroposterior cardiac silhouette. Left atrial enlargement is best demonstrated by administering barium sulfate with the patient in the right anterior oblique or in the lateral position. The esophagus is displaced posteriorly and to the right by the enlarged left atrium. Calcification of the mitral valve can best be seen during fluoroscopy with the patient rotated into the right or left oblique position. The calcified mitral valve can be recognized fluoroscopically by its dancing movements, when it cannot be identified on an ordinary chest film. Angiocardiography may provide additional information in the study of patients with mitral stenosis. Its application to the selection of patients for cardiac surgery will be discussed subsequently.

Electrocardiogram. The tracing may be within normal limits. Atrial fibrillation is frequently present. Atrial flutter is less common. In patients with normal rhythm, the P wave may become broad, and notched or diphasic. Varying degrees of right ventricular predominance occur, ranging from simple right axis deviation to advanced right ventricular hypertrophy. Electrocardiographic changes resulting from digitalis administration are often present.

It is of interest that after successful mitral commissurotomy the R wave may increase in amplitude in lead I and in the lateral chest leads. This is believed to represent an increased contribution of the left ventricle to the electrocardiogram, subsequent to the operation.

Special Features. In patients with mitral stenosis certain events occur with a frequency that merits special attention. It is probably best to avoid calling them complications, since this term implies an untoward event of infrequent occurrence. For example, subacute bacterial endocarditis might properly be considered a true complication. It is relatively infrequent in patients with pure mitral stenosis and more likely to occur in patients with aortic or mitral valvular insufficiency. In contrast, however, the occurrence of arrhythmia or embolism is so common as to constitute part of the disease picture.

Arrhythmia. Most patients with mitral stenosis eventually develop atrial fibrillation. In some patients this may occur in paroxysmal form before becoming permanent. It may be preceded by the appearance of other atrial arrhythmias such as premature beats or flutter. The development of atrial fibrillation may produce sudden severe failure in a previously asymptomatic patient and give the first indication of heart disease. The onset may occasionally fail to cause any symptoms if the ventricular rate is slow (as in a digitalized patient). Atrial fibrillation developing in a young person constitutes strong presumptive evidence of mitral stenosis, provided hyperthyroidism, congenital heart disease or constrictive pericarditis can be excluded. The accentuated first heart sound and mitral opening snap are unaffected by the onset of atrial fibrillation, but the diastolic apical murmur may be altered or may become almost inaudible, as already noted.

Arterial Embolism. Arterial embolism is a relatively common manifestation of mitral stenosis. Narrowing of the mitral orifice together with enlargement of the left atrium and its atrial appendage produces a situation favorable to the formation of thrombi, and this tendency is increased by the presence of atrial fibrillation. It was previously thought that emboli broke off from mural thrombi, but many patients with a history of repeated embolic episodes have failed to show mural thrombi in the left atrium at the time of mitral commissurotomy. This observation suggests that most of the emboli represent recently formed clots rather than dislodgement of particles from fixed thrombi. In fact, old mural thrombi are found more commonly at operation in patients with no embolic history than in patients with previous embolism.

Emboli may lodge anywhere in the arterial tree, but most commonly in the brain, spleen, kidneys or extremities. The effects of cerebral embolism vary from mild, transient paresis or paresthesias, to severe attacks with residual hemiplegia and aphasia. The differential diagnosis of cerebral symptoms in a young person must include consideration of mitral stenosis with embolism. The diagnosis may be more obscure with intra-abdominal arterial embolism. Severe sudden abdominal pain is the rule. Renal infarction may be accompanied by hematuria. Splenic infarction occasionally produces a friction rub in the left upper quadrant or at the costal margin. The so-called "saddle embolism" deserves special mention because of the need for prompt recognition and surgical treatment. When sudden complete arterial occlusion occurs in an extremity, the underlying cause is usually recognized. Occasionally, however, lesser degrees of arterial insufficiency result and the correct etiology may not be recognized. Such patients may be thought to have some other peripheral vascular disease, such as thromboangiitis obliterans.

Pulmonary Infarction. Pulmonary infarction is common in patients with mitral stenosis and congestive failure. The patient is often mistakenly considered to have suffered an intercurrent infection with pneumonitis or pleurisy. Cough and hemoptysis may be attributed to the mitral stenosis itself rather than to an accompanying pulmonary infarction. The blood in hemoptysis due to mitral stenosis alone tends to be bright red, whereas that due to a superimposed pulmonary infarction tends to be darker in color. The diagnosis of pulmonary infarction should always be considered in any patient with mitral stenosis who develops acute pulmonary symptoms, or shows a sudden increase of "right-sided failure."

Common Diagnostic Errors. In eliciting the medical history of over 300 candidates for mitral commissurotomy, we have found that in many patients the presence of mitral stenosis remained unrecognized for long periods during which treatment was given for other conditions not really present. The following mistaken diagnoses were made frequently enough to be worthy of mention.

1. *Bronchial Asthma.* In certain patients with mitral stenosis, the stage of pulmonary congestion is accompanied by a prominent element of bronchial spasm with wheezing. In an astonishing number of such patients a diagnosis of bronchial asthma was made and the patients were referred for an allergic survey. Several had received prolonged treatment with pollen, dust or bacterial vaccines.

2. *Pulmonary Disease.* By causing a chronic cough, with or without hemoptysis and the presence of pulmonary rales, mitral stenosis can simulate pulmonary disease. The chest film may add to the deception by showing increased lung markings or occasionally a diffuse nodulation due to hemosiderosis. Thus, some of our patients had been considered to have tuberculosis and one had even been confined to a sanatorium for a year. Others of the group had been diagnosed as having bronchiectasis and several had undergone extensive studies, including bronchoscopy and bronchograms. Two older men with pleural effusions had been referred with diagnoses of bronchogenic carcinoma.

3. *Thyrotoxicosis.* Weight loss, nervousness, excessive sweating and tachycardia may occur in patients with mitral stenosis and strongly suggest the possibility of thyrotoxicosis. When such a patient coincidentally has a palpable thyroid gland, or nodule, the resemblance to thyroid disease may be remarkably close. Such patients have occasionally been referred for thyroidectomy. The presence of atrial fibrillation may lead to further difficulty in diagnosis since the diastolic murmur may escape detection more easily under such circumstances.

4. *Neurasthenia.* Certain patients with mitral stenosis complain chiefly of weakness, easy fatigue and other vague symptoms. Their only cardiovascular complaints may be those of palpitation or precordial discomfort, which commonly occur in "neurotic" patients. They may be thin, nervous and have cold hands. If the diastolic murmur is missed, the label of "neurasthenia" is frequently applied. Many patients have been treated for "nerves" for long periods before they were correctly diagnosed.

Treatment. Until recently, treatment of patients with mitral stenosis consisted chiefly of therapy for such associated conditions as congestive failure, arrhythmias and arterial embolism; the management of these is detailed elsewhere in this text. Now mitral commissurotomy has become established as a reasonably satisfactory procedure permitting direct surgical relief of the mitral valvular obstruction. Thus, the internist must concern himself not only with standard medical measures, but should select from among his patients those suitable for surgery, aid in their preoperative preparation and postoperative care, and supervise their long-term management.

The Choice of Patients for Surgery. Mitral commissurotomy now can offer to certain patients the prospect of considerable benefit at reasonably low risk. The results tend to be best in patients who have uncomplicated mitral stenosis, with symptoms of pulmonary engorgement. The presence of longstanding "right-sided failure" or of complicating valve lesions reduces the chance for marked improvement.

The risk varies widely among patients, and with the experience of the surgeon. Under the best circumstances the mortality is slightly less than 5 per cent in the "better risk" patients. This figure rises with the acceptance of "poor risk" patients.

In selecting patients for mitral surgery, it is the usual policy to choose only those who have significant, progressive disability, and to reject those with minimal or no symptoms. A minority holds the viewpoint that when a patient has mitral stenosis and left atrial enlargement, there is no advantage in waiting. In our opinion, however, asymptomatic patients should not be referred routinely for mitral surgery at the present time.

The difficulty of deciding whether or not a given patient should be subjected to mitral commissurotomy varies widely among patients. In some the decision may be quite easy. For example, one would not hesitate to recommend surgery to a 30-year-old patient whose physical signs were those of "pure" mitral stenosis and who was severely handicapped by exertional dyspnea, hemoptysis, orthopnea, cough, paroxysmal nocturnal attacks and pulmonary edema. On the other hand, in certain patients, the decision may be very difficult, and the following factors may require special consideration in the decision.

1. AGE. Most patients who develop difficulty due to "pure" mitral stenosis do so between the ages of 30 and 45. One rarely sees purely mechanical mitral obstruction in patients under 20 years of age. Most patients in their teens who develop serious rheumatic cardiac disability prove to have complicating rheumatic activity, severe mitral insufficiency, multiple valvular involvement, myocardial disease, marked cardiac enlargement or combinations of these. In patients over 50 the surgical risk is increased. Hence, one must be certain that in these older patients, their progressive cardiac disability cannot be managed effectively by medical measures. One should also attempt to exclude patients with other serious disease, so that a successful mitral commissurotomy could be expected to promise a reasonable addition to the life span. Despite these considerations, age is not an absolute contraindication to operation in patients under 20 or over 50 who are markedly handicapped by mitral obstruction. Extremely gratifying results were achieved in one patient aged 14 and in one aged 62.

2. RHEUMATIC ACTIVITY. Clinical evidence of active rheumatic fever or carditis is considered an absolute contraindication to mitral commissurotomy. The chief problem is the difficulty of recognizing such activity (see section on Rheumatic Heart Disease). Despite all efforts to exclude from operation those patients with active rheumatic carditis, surgical biopsy of the left atrial appendage has shown Aschoff bodies in as high a proportion as 45 per cent. This has led some to question whether Aschoff bodies in the left atrial appendage really indicate rheumatic activity. Most workers accept the finding as further evidence of the difficulty of recognizing rheumatic activity. However, operation should probably not be done when clinical and laboratory signs point to the probability of rheumatic activity.

3. PERSISTENT CONGESTIVE FAILURE. Patients who remain in severe "right-sided" congestive failure despite intensive medical therapy present a special problem. It has been suggested that such patients cannot be improved by surgery because of irreversible changes in the pulmonary circulation. Many of them have indeed failed to improve after surgery and the operative mortality in this group has been quite high. However, an occasional patient with this clinical picture has been improved remarkably by surgery, suggesting that in some instances the pulmonary

circulatory changes may be reversible. In view of the occasional dramatic results, one sometimes feels justified in recommending operation in an otherwise hopeless situation.

4. APICAL SYSTOLIC MURMURS. Cardiac auscultation has proved most reliable in those patients with so-called "pure" mitral stenosis who have loud apical diastolic murmurs but in whom apical systolic murmurs are either absent or faint. Auscultation, however, is particularly unreliable in evaluating the group of patients with prominent apical systolic murmurs. Formerly, such murmurs were thought to represent mitral insufficiency of a degree sufficient to contraindicate mitral commissurotomy. However, it has since been learned that this finding does not guarantee the presence of significant mitral regurgitation. Often, despite the presence of a systolic murmur the patient has proved to have severe mitral stenosis without significant insufficiency and has derived great benefit from mitral commissurotomy.

Since experience has emphasized the difficulty of diagnosing mitral insufficiency by ordinary methods of physical examination or by standard roentgenographic identification of left ventricular enlargement, various special tests have been used in an effort to recognize significant degrees of mitral regurgitation. Cardiac catheterization has been used to record "wedge" pressures (pulmonary capillary pressures) which are supposed by some to reflect actual pressure relationships within the left atrium. Combinations of phonocardiography, ballistocardiography and electrokymography have been used to provide data bearing on this problem. In our hands, angiocardiography has supplied additional helpful information by showing a characteristic pattern of opacification for pure mitral stenosis of severe degree, and a different angiocardiographic pattern for wide-open mitral insufficiency. In pure mitral stenosis the left atrium remains sharply outlined and densely opacified for a long period of time, whereas the left ventricle is poorly opacified and small. In severe mitral incompetence, on the other hand, the left atrium and left ventricle are opacified to equal degrees of density and the left ventricle is enlarged. Unfortunately, the angiocardiographic pattern occasionally lies somewhere between these two extremes and a decision may be difficulty. In no instance should a patient be rejected for operation merely because of the presence of an apical systolic murmur. Such patients deserve the benefit of special study including an angiocardiogram.

5. AORTIC VALVULAR DISEASE. Any significant disease of the aortic valve complicating mitral stenosis was previously considered an absolute contraindication to mitral commissurotomy. The presence of aortic stenosis was doubly feared because of its deleterious effect on the left ventricle postoperatively, and because its preoperative recognition was often difficult in the presence of mitral stenosis. Mitral obstruction can mask the presence of aortic stenosis by reducing the blood flow through the left ventricle and aortic valve, thus decreasing the intensity of the aortic systolic murmur; only after the mitral stenosis is treated surgically does the aortic murmur become prominent. An aortic stenosis so missed has occasionally led to the death of a patient following an otherwise successful mitral commissurotomy. This is no longer so serious a problem since the development of an instrument for dilating stenosed aortic valves. The aorta can now be palpated routinely after mitral commissurotomy, and if a significant systolic thrill appears the aortic valve can be dilated at the same operation. When the surgeon is not prepared to proceed with dilatation of the aortic valve, the presence of aortic stenosis still constitutes an absolute contraindication to mitral commissurotomy.

Aortic insufficiency, on the other hand, presents a more difficult problem. The methods proposed for treating this lesion surgically must await further development and evaluation before they can be considered satisfactory. Thus in patients with mitral stenosis, when aortic insufficiency is of major degree and accompanied by a wide pulse pressure and Corrigan pulse, mitral commissurotomy is clearly contraindicated. However, if the diastolic blood pressure is not lowered and the pulse pressure is not significantly widened, the presence of a basal diastolic murmur of semilunar valvular insufficiency should not necessarily contraindicate mitral commissurotomy. Under such circumstances a basal diastolic murmur may represent either an unimportant degree of aortic valvular insufficiency or else a Graham Steel murmur of relative pulmonic insufficiency. Many of the basal diastolic murmurs, which are unaccompanied by a widened pulse pressure, disappear after successful mitral commissurotomy, indicating their probable origin in the pulmonic valve.

6. PREGNANCY. With good medical management, many patients with mitral stenosis do well during pregnancy. Under such circumstances one would certainly avoid an elective operation. However, under special circumstances one might recommend valvulotomy in certain pregnant patients who develop severe failure before the seventh month, and in whom termination of pregnancy is not advisable.

7. VALVULAR CALCIFICATION. At times definite calcification of the mitral valve is visible fluoroscopically. In general this is an unfavorable finding which may well have an adverse influence on the success of the surgical procedure. It does not, however, constitute a contraindication to operation, since one can never be certain preoperatively that the presence of calcification will be an insurmountable difficulty to the surgeon.

8. SUBACUTE BACTERIAL ENDOCARDITIS. When active, this disease has generally been considered an absolute contraindication to operation. Although experience has been limited, it seems possible that mitral commissurotomy might be undertaken in these patients after bacterial endocarditis has been cured.

9. ATRIAL FIBRILLATION. The presence of this arrhythmia is no longer considered a contraindication to operation, and the majority of patients coming to operation have permanent fibrillation. These patients do very well provided the ventricular rate can be kept under good control by digitalization.

There are certain patients in whom the ventricular rate cannot be satisfactorily controlled despite extremely large doses of digitalis. Under such circumstances one must consider the possibility of overactivity of the thyroid gland, although there may be no clinical evidence of hyperthyroidism. Occasional patients have benefited from radioactive iodine therapy despite the fact that they appeared euthyroid. Following such treatment, the ventricular rate has been decreased with average doses of digitalis where control had previously been impossible. In general, control of the ventricular rate must be achieved prior to mitral commissurotomy. Otherwise, the rapid rate will be a hazard during surgery and the postoperative period.

10. ARTERIAL EMBOLISM. Previous embolism, if not too crippling, is no longer considered a contraindication to operation. In fact, repeated embolism actually may constitute an indication for mitral commissurotomy even in the absence of significant cardiac failure. Statistics are as yet not available to serve as a sound basis for this decision. However, there is hope and some evidence that removal of the left atrial appendage, together with successful opening of the stenosed mitral valve, will help reduce the tendency toward formation of thrombi.

Preoperative Preparation. In patients being prepared for mitral commissurotomy, certain points require special attention. Perhaps the most important of these is the proper *mental preparation* of the patient and his family. This preparation begins with the manner in which the physician proposes operation to the patient. In general, one must first assess and point out to the patient and family the prognosis to be expected with and without surgery; in doing this, prognosis must be pictured in its broader sense to include the prospect of useful living versus an invalid state, and not merely the question of survival. Then the patient and family must be permitted to make their own decision. This is usually easy for them when they realize the seriousness of the situation. It is harder when they do not recognize this, and under such circumstances, it is probably wiser not to insist on operation until they do. If possible, one should avoid frightening the patient; however, the family should be warned of the hazards common to any major surgical procedure plus certain unavoidable accidents incident to this specific operation, such as embolism which may result in hemiplegia, or even in death. When the patient has decided to accept the operation, it is wise to discuss its general nature, and the events which may occur during the postoperative period. Patients should be given the opportunity to ask whatever questions they wish. Above all, they should have a clear understanding of the results which may be expected; for example, a patient who has atrial fibrillation may not reasonably expect to omit his digitalis even after operation has produced its full benefit. If all these features are discussed prior to operation, the patient may be spared many misunderstandings and disappointments.

Before operation the patient should be freed, if possible, of excessive fluid. Those without obvious physical signs of congestive failure may still have fluid retention. This may be detected by weighing the patient daily and testing the effect of mercurial diuretic injections until a "dry weight" is established.

Patients with severe degrees of congestive failure may require a prolonged period of medical treatment prior to operation.

The question of digitalization requires special mention. Many patients have been adequately digitalized and merely require continuance of the daily maintenance dose. Those with atrial fibrillation must be digitalized so that the apical rate is well controlled. The chief problem arises in those with normal sinus rhythm, who have not received digitalis in the past. It may be wise to avoid digitalization of such patients immediately prior to operation. We have had the suspicion that under these circumstances, digitalis therapy may increase the risk of ventricular tachycardia or ventricular fibrillation during operation. It has been our experience that these patients usually do not develop atrial fibrillation until some time after the operation. They can be digitalized rapidly at that time if necessary.

The prothrombin level is frequently low and may require the preoperative institution of vitamin K therapy.

Postoperative Care. Certain of the problems in the immediate postoperative period are those attendant upon any thoracotomy. The tracheobronchial tree must be kept clear to avoid atelectasis. The patient is urged to cough and to use a "blow bottle," but intratracheal suction is often necessary. Oxygen is usually administered by nasal catheter for the first 24 hours after operation. *It is important to avoid excessive intravenous administration of blood or other fluids during the immediate postoperative period,* and the patient should be given oral fluids as soon as they are tolerated. Maintenance doses of digitalis can be given parenterally until the patient resumes eating. Anticoagulant therapy is usually started after 48 or 72 hours unless there is some special contraindication to its use. The average patient who does well is allowed to get out of bed into a chair on the fourth or fifth postoperative day. Once the patient is up, the weight is recorded daily and used as a guide to mercurial injections. In very sick patients, such injections may be necessary earlier in the postoperative period. There has been a tendency for some patients to develop salt depletion during the postoperative period. This may be prevented by relaxing the dietary salt restrictions rather than by parenteral administration of salt. Most patients are capable of gradually increased activity during the second week and are ready for discharge from the hospital in two weeks after the operation.

Throughout the postoperative period emergencies such as arrhythmias or embolic episodes must be carefully watched for and treated promptly. The possibility of pericardial effusion should be considered in those patients who do not progress as well as one might reasonably expect. Certain patients develop an acute depression which rarely may go on to a frank psychosis. This tendency to anxiety or depression is not uncommon. *All* these patients need reassurance. Sometimes it is necessary to get them out of bed sooner than usual in order to convince them that they are doing well. Anxious patients often are helped by sedation with phenobarbital (15 to 30 mg. four times a day). We have seen only one instance in which a psychotic episode failed to clear up.

For the first month following discharge from the hospital, patients are instructed to avoid all forms of exertion including stair climbing. During the following two or three months their activities are gradually increased. The principles during this period are similar to those applied to patients recovering from myocardial infarction. Certain patients with normal sinus rhythm may find that they require no cardiac medication throughout this period. Others are continued on their maintenance dose of digitalis, and are given mercurial injections to control any tendency to congestive failure. Many will improve gradually and require less and less diuresis. In a few patients, maximum improvement may not occur for a year after operation. Certain patients require continued medical treatment, but get along with less therapy than they could prior to operation.

Certain patients, at varying periods following operation, have developed peculiar febrile illnesses termed the "post-commissurotomy syndrome," associated with chest pain. At times this has been accompanied by fever, pleural friction rubs and even pleural effusions. Such illnesses developing after operation raise the question of possible reactivation of rheumatic fever, but the clinical picture has not been typical. Persistent chest pain has been less frequent in our experience than in that of others. Perhaps the lowered incidence may be explained in part by the fact that we have been routinely giving our patients acetylsalicylic acid 0.6 gm. four times a day for several months following operation.

It is important to realize that valvular surgery is merely one additional measure used in the treatment of rheumatic heart disease. The patients must understand that many of them have not been "cured" and will require further treatment. In some, it is obvious that the operation will simply grant a reprieve from invalidism or death. Furthermore, possible re-stenosis of the mitral valve must be kept in mind, although we have not as yet encountered a proven instance. Certainly the operation has proved of great value in properly selected patients. Its eventual place in the treatment of rheumatic heart disease has still to be determined.

MITRAL INSUFFICIENCY

Mitral regurgitation may be of organic type due to actual mitral valvular disease, or of functional type, the result of left ventricular dilatation secondary to other conditions, such as acute rheumatic carditis, hypertension or chronic aortic valvular disease. The majority of writers consider pure mitral regurgitation of severe grade less common but more serious than similar grades of mitral stenosis.

Etiology. Most cases of organic mitral insufficiency are of rheumatic origin. The condition is sometimes produced accidentally during mitral commissurotomy. Other causes include bacterial endocarditis, rupture of a papillary muscle secondary to myocardial infarction, and rarely trauma.

Pathologic Physiology. Pure mitral regurgitation places a stress on the left ventricle which leads to left ventricular dilatation and hypertrophy. In addition, when severe, it causes an increase of left atrial pressure which can lead to left atrial dilatation and a chain of events similar to those described in mitral stenosis. Acutely produced mitral insufficiency leads rapidly to severe congestive heart failure and often to death.

Symptoms. Minor grades of mitral regurgitation may be asymptomatic and are compatible with long and normal life. Severe insufficiency may give rise to either the pulmonary or peripheral congestive symptoms described under mitral stenosis.

Physical Signs. When significant mitral insufficiency is present, there is a loud apical systolic murmur. The first heart sound at the apex tends to be soft or may be entirely replaced by the murmur. The heart may be enlarged with the apex displaced downward and to the left. While mitral insufficiency is ac-companied by an apical systolic murmur, similar apical systolic murmurs may be heard in many patients with mitral stenosis who have no evidence of significant mitral insufficiency at operation. Thus, this sign is frequently an unreliable basis for diagnosing mitral insufficiency of sufficient degree to contraindicate commissurotomy, as pointed out in the section dealing with the selection of patients for surgery of the mitral valve.

Roentgenologic Findings. The left ventricle shows varying degrees of enlargement. The left atrium may also become enlarged and sometimes shows definite systolic pulsations. On the left cardiac border there may be a marked "see-saw" movement due to simultaneous inward movement of the left ventricle and outward movement of the "auriculo-pulmonic" segment.

Electrocardiogram. With major degrees of mitral insufficiency evidences of left axis deviation or left ventricular hypertrophy may appear. Atrial fibrillation may be present.

Diagnosis. In severe uncomplicated mitral insufficiency the diagnosis is usually easy. Difficulty arises in assessing the importance of an apical systolic murmur in a patient with a history of rheumatic fever but without obvious left ventricular enlargement or "see-saw" movement. One should remember that the vast majority of patients with apical systolic murmurs never develop cardiac failure; those that do first develop left ventricular enlargement.

As already pointed out, it is difficult to determine the degree of mitral insufficiency in patients with mitral stenosis. In such patients systolic apical murmurs may be present in the absence of significant insufficiency, and the determination of left ventricular enlargement by fluoroscopy or routine chest films may be unreliable. Additional data have been sought by using special techniques including cardiac catheterization, angiocardiography, ballistocardiography, phonocardiography and electrokymography. Of these, angiocardiography has proven most helpful to us as discussed in the section on mitral stenosis. Despite all these methods, the problem in certain instances remains a very difficult one.

Treatment. Medical treatment is similar to that outlined for mitral stenosis. Although several surgical techniques have been proposed for correcting mitral insufficiency, their mortality is high and the procedures are not yet ready for general use.

AORTIC VALVULAR DISEASE

Isolated aortic valvular disease occurs with one fourth to one third the frequency of isolated mitral disease. Furthermore, the mitral valve is also involved in approximately one half to two thirds of all patients with aortic valvular disease, depending on the incidence of syphilis in the particular series. Aortic valvular disease is three times more common in men than in women.

AORTIC STENOSIS

Aortic stenosis is chiefly a disease of older men, being three times more frequent in patients past 50 years of age than in younger persons. Calcification of the valve is an important feature of aortic stenosis, particularly in older individuals.

Etiology. Certain writers in the past have divided acquired aortic stenosis into two etiologic types; they considered calcific aortic stenosis in older patients to be of "sclerotic" origin as opposed to the rheumatic type found in younger patients. Extensive pathologic studies (Clawson; Karsner and Koletsky) have suggested that nearly all cases of aortic stenosis are initiated by inflammation due to rheumatic fever, and that the calcific or "sclerotic" changes develop later as a secondary process. In 200 cases, Karsner and Koletsky found definite evidence of other rheumatic cardiac stigmata in 196. Rarely, stenosis may be of congenital origin involving either the subaortic (infundibular, subvalvular) region, or less commonly the aortic valve itself.

Pathologic Physiology. In most cases aortic stenosis develops slowly; thus it may be compensated for, and tolerated well, for a long time. The left ventricle gradually undergoes hypertrophy without much dilatation. As the stenosis increases in severity, the coronary circulation becomes impaired; simultaneously the hypertrophied left ventricle requires more coronary blood flow. This combination of events can produce anginal pain, myocardial fibrosis or even infarction. When the left ventricle fails, the predominant effect may be one of pulmonary congestion, although peripheral congestion may also occur.

Symptoms. Many of the patients have a history of rheumatic fever or of a murmur heard earlier in life. Anginal pain is frequent and often severe. Patients with high grade stenosis may develop symptoms of deficient cerebral blood flow with faintness, dizziness, syncope or even epileptiform seizures. A carotid sinus mechanism may play a part in certain cases. Patients with anginal or cerebral episodes are notoriously subject to sudden death. Cardiac failure may occur and produce the symptoms of pulmonary congestion, or less often of peripheral congestive failure, as described under mitral stenosis.

Physical Signs. The classic signs of aortic stenosis include: (1) a harsh aortic systolic murmur which is transmitted up into the neck, especially on the right side, (2) an accompanying systolic thrill, (3) a reduced intensity of the second heart sound at the aortic area, (4) a narrow pulse pressure and (5) a small, slowly rising pulse (*pulsus parvus et tardus*). When these signs are present, the diagnosis may be considered certain. However, many patients with aortic stenosis lack certain of these findings; in fact, half of the patients found to have aortic stenosis at necropsy lacked all but the aortic systolic murmur. In general, however, it is better to reserve the diagnosis of aortic stenosis for patients in whom the obstruction to blood flow is functionally significant. The recognition of aortic stenosis may be particularly difficult in the presence of mitral stenosis, as discussed in that section.

Roentgenologic Findings. The heart shows varying degrees of enlargement particularly involving the left ventricle. The fluoroscopic recognition of calcification in the aortic valve is pathognomonic. In congenital subaortic stenosis the heart is frequently within normal limits of size and shape; however, the ascending aorta almost always shows increased prominence, sometimes approaching aneurysmal proportions (the so-called "post-stenotic dilatation").

Electrocardiogram. The changes may vary in degree from simple left ventricular predominance to advanced left ventricular hypertrophy.

Special Diagnostic Studies. Direct pressure measurements may be made from the aorta by means of small plastic catheters introduced retrograde through peripheral arterial puncture. Pulse curves obtained in this fashion or by means of the electrokymograph may be of aid in the diagnosis of aortic stenosis. Phonocardiography may show a "diamond-shaped" murmur.

Treatment. Medical treatment includes all the usual measures discussed elsewhere for combating congestive failure and angina.

Marked restriction of activity is recommended to reduce chances of sudden death in patients who have had anginal or syncopal episodes. Treatment with radioactive iodine to decrease thyroid function has been tried in certain of these patients with severe angina, but the results have not been impressive.

With the development of the Bailey dilator, a practical operation is now available for the surgical treatment of aortic stenosis. This has been particularly successful in correcting aortic stenosis present in combination with mitral stenosis; the mortality in this group has been approximately 11 per cent. However, in patients with isolated aortic stenosis, the surgical mortality has been at least double this figure, chiefly as a result of ventricular fibrillation. The reason for this difference in mortality between the two groups seems to stem from the fact that high grade mitral stenosis apparently "protects" the left ventricle from excessive hypertrophy. By contrast, in isolated aortic stenosis the left ventricle is greatly thickened and thus (1) seems more likely to fibrillate during surgery, (2) is more difficult to "pump" manually in maintaining the circulation during ventricular fibrillation, and (3) is more difficult to defibrillate electrically. Despite this increased risk, surgery should be considered in patients with severe isolated aortic stenosis, when life is threatened by episodes of cerebral ischemia, severe angina, or bouts of pulmonary edema. The chief problem in selecting patients is presented by the presence of complicating aortic insufficiency. This is not considered a contraindication to aortic valve dilatation so long as the diastolic blood pressure is well sustained and the pulse pressure not unduly widened.

AORTIC INSUFFICIENCY

Etiology. Aortic valvular insufficiency is most commonly of rheumatic or syphilitic origin. Occasionally, it may be due to subacute bacterial endocarditis, sometimes implanted on a congenitally bicuspid aortic valve. Rarely it appears suddenly, as a result of trauma or of dissecting aneurysm of the aorta with deformity or displacement of valve structures. Relative aortic regurgitation without actual valvular disease may occur in patients with marked hypertension.

Pathologic Physiology. In general, aortic regurgitation develops more rapidly than does stenosis, and is likely to produce left ventricular failure at an earlier age. The effects of this lesion are similar to those described for aortic stenosis, except that the left ventricle tends to become dilated as well as hypertrophied.

Symptoms. Cardiac failure usually produces symptoms of the pulmonary congestive type, but peripheral congestive phenomena may occur. Anginal pain is not uncommon. Patients with "wide-open" insufficiency may be extremely conscious of excessive pounding of the heart and throbbing of arteries in the neck and extremities.

Physical Signs. The findings depend upon the degree of aortic regurgitation and the associated hemodynamic effects. In some patients the only finding is the diastolic murmur of semilunar insufficiency type. Murmurs of semilunar insufficiency (pulmonic or aortic) characteristically tend to be soft, blowing and high-pitched. The quality is not unlike that of a breath sound. They may be heard over the base of the heart but are often best heard along the left sternal border in the third intercostal space. Semilunar diastolic murmurs characteristically begin with the second heart sound when it is present. Thus, even when transmitted down to the apex they may be differentiated from mitral diastolic murmurs since they "blow off" the second heart sound rather than beginning after a gap, as do mitral diastolic murmurs. The semilunar diastolic murmur is at times very difficult to hear. It may be heard best with the patient leaning forward and holding his breath in expiration.

If the regurgitation is of significant degree it may be accompanied by the well known peripheral signs associated with a widened pulse pressure. These include the "water-hammer" (Corrigan) pulse, Traube "pistol-shot" arterial sounds, Duroziez double arterial murmurs and Quincke capillary pulsations. The systolic blood pressure may be elevated; the diastolic blood pressure is lowered and sometimes is unobtainable because beats are audible down to zero.

Roentgenologic Findings. The heart may show varying degrees of left ventricular enlargement; the left ventricular and aortic pulsations may be markedly exaggerated.

Electrocardiogram. The changes are similar to those described for aortic stenosis.

Special Diagnostic Considerations. Pulmonic and aortic insufficiency are often very difficult to differentiate on the basis of the murmurs alone. In general, a semilunar diastolic murmur heard best to the right of the sternum is usually aortic. One heard over the base of the heart and again at the apex without being heard well at intervening positions is also probably aortic. Those semilunar diastolic murmurs which are heard well over the right ventricular area, but which fade out toward the apex, are probably pulmonic. However, decisions based on the distribution of the murmur are not sufficiently reliable for diagnosis when one is seeking maximum accuracy as in the selection of patients for valvular surgery. Occasionally the Valsalva maneuver is helpful as described in the section on pulmonic insufficiency. Differentiation usually depends on finding the hemodynamic effects of widened pulse pressure either in the peripheral or in the pulmonary arteries. Hemodynamic effects of pulmonic insufficiency may be demonstrated (1) fluoroscopically, or (2) by cardiac catheterization which can disclose a widened pulmonary pulse pressure and increased right ventricular diastolic pressure. Occasionally, angiocardiography may provide suggestive evidence of pulmonic insufficiency by demonstrating dilatation of the pulmonary artery and widening of the valvular region. Sometimes the diagnosis must remain that of "semilunar valve insufficiency" when more accurate clinical differentiation is impossible.

Treatment. Medical treatment includes the standard measures for managing congestive failure and anginal pain. In addition syphilitic patients should be treated with penicillin. Radioactive iodine to reduce thyroid function may occasionally prove of considerable benefit in patients with severe angina; the reason for this apparent difference in results between patients with aortic insufficiency and those with aortic stenosis (q. v.) is not clear.

Various surgical procedures have been tried, but operative treatment is generally less satisfactory than that for stenotic valvular lesions. The most promising method yet proposed involves the placement of a plastic valve in the descending aorta. This, at best, effects only partial correction of the situation. Further evidence must be awaited relative to this problem, including the durability of the plastic valve. For the present, surgical treatment of aortic insufficiency should be confined to those patients facing an otherwise hopeless prognosis.

PULMONIC VALVULAR DISEASE

Organic pulmonic valvular disease is relatively rare. The most important form is that of congenital pulmonic stenosis. Involvement of the pulmonic valve occurs in somewhat less than 2 per cent of patients with rheumatic heart disease and almost never appears as an isolated lesion.

PULMONIC STENOSIS

Etiology. Practically all instances of pulmonic stenosis are of congenital origin. Two forms are recognized—the valvular and the infundibular (subvalvular). These sometimes occur together.

Pathologic Physiology. Much confusion in the literature results from failure to distinguish between (1) isolated pulmonic stenosis with intact cardiac septums and (2) pulmonic stenosis in combination with septal defects (e.g., in the tetralogy of Fallot). *Isolated pulmonic stenosis* leads to right ventricular hypertrophy and may be well tolerated for long periods before the right ventricle fails. When not in failure such patients do not have cyanosis, and the arterial blood shows normal oxygen saturation because there is no shunt. When *pulmonic stenosis* is *combined with septal defects* (either interatrial or interventricular), right to left shunts commonly occur so that venous blood reaches the peripheral circulation. Arterial blood samples show oxygen unsaturation, and cyanosis of varying degree may appear. This situation is not tolerated so well as is isolated pulmonic stenosis, and with rare exceptions the prognosis is poor.

Symptoms. Patients with isolated pulmonic stenosis may be asymptomatic until right ventricular failure occurs. Such patients not uncommonly have normal exertional tolerance well into adult life. With combined (valvular and septal) lesions, however, the history is usually one of cyanosis and considerable cardiac handicap from birth; other symptoms include anorexia, deficient growth and poor exercise tolerance. Squatting by children may be an important feature in the tetralogy of Fallot. In these patients sudden "spells" may occur which the mother describes in various ways (e.g., rigidity, limpness, panting, syncope or convulsions).

Physical Signs. Characteristic findings include (1) a harsh systolic murmur best heard at the second or third left intercostal space, also usually audible in the left clavicular region and often posteriorly over the left chest, (2) a palpable systolic thrill in the second or third left interspace and (3) a decrease in intensity of the second heart sound at the pulmonic area. Rarely both the murmur and thrill may be absent. Those patients with associated right to left shunts usually show clubbing, cyanosis and polycythemia. Acneform lesions and severe dental caries frequently are present.

One must differentiate the systolic murmur of pulmonic stenosis from the rough systolic murmurs of functional type which may be heard at the pulmonic area. This type of murmur may be reproduced by light pressure on the pulmonary artery of an exposed dog's heart. By analogy, the ribs or sternum may indent the pulmonary outflow tract and produce this murmur in patients with a flat chest or dilated pulmonary artery. It will disappear if the patient takes a deep breath, thereby removing the compression from the pulmonary artery. This murmur is almost never accompanied by a thrill.

Roentgenologic Findings. The heart is frequently within normal limits of size but the configuration is that of right ventricular hypertrophy. With infundibular stenosis the pulmonary segment of the left cardiac border may appear hollow and the pulmonary arterial branches small. However, with valvular stenosis the pulmonary artery may be very large owing to "poststenotic" dilatation. On fluoroscopy one may observe a decrease of the pulmonary vascular pulsations which will aid in the diagnosis, but this may not always be easy to recognize.

Electrocardiogram. The changes are usually those of right ventricular hypertrophy with so-called right ventricular strain. The P waves may be large with abnormally pointed peaks.

Diagnosis. The diagnosis may be confirmed by cardiac catheterization which reveals an increase in systolic pressure recorded as the catheter is withdrawn from the pulmonary artery, past the obstruction, and back into the right ventricle. The character of the pressure tracing at various positions may help in deciding whether the stenosis is valvular, infundibular, or both. The site of a right to left shunt may also be discovered by cardiac catheterization if the catheter happens to pass through the defect. Angiocardiography may provide information relative to the nature of the stenosis, and the exact site of the right to left shunt if it exists.

Treatment. The medical treatment of pulmonic stenosis is nonspecific and involves various symptomatic measures described elsewhere. The surgical treatment has been of two types: (1) direct surgical relief of the pulmonic stenosis and (2) indirect methods designed to by-pass the obstruction by shunting blood from the aorta into the pulmonary artery. The choice of techniques depends on the type of pulmonic stenosis, and also on the site of any associated septal defect.

Surgery in patients *with isolated pulmonic stenosis* must relieve the pulmonic obstruction and shunting procedures are of no value. Even when asymptomatic, such patients should probably have cardiac catheterization to determine the right ventricular pressure; if the systolic pressure is over 100 mm. of mercury, operation should be considered despite the lack of symptoms.

In patients with the tetralogy of Fallot each type of operation has been used. At present we prefer a shunting operation of the Blalock type because it has a lower mortality than the direct Brock attack on the pulmonic obstruction (which is so frequently of the infundibular type). The optimum time for operation probably lies between the ages of 4 and 11.

In patients *with pulmonic stenosis and a right-to-left shunt through the atrial septum,* surgery *must* be directed toward relief of the pulmonic obstruction. Originally it was thought that a shunting procedure would improve these patients as it does those with the tetralogy of Fallot; actually the results were disastrous because right-sided heart failure occurred sooner or later in practically all patients. This is thought to be caused as follows: shunting operations transmit blood from the aorta into the pulmonary arterial circulation, producing an increased return of blood to the left atrium. The left atrial pressure rises and this tends to reduce, or close off entirely, the shunt from the right atrium into the left which formerly constituted the "safety valve" for the right heart. Since the shunting operation produces these changes without relieving the pulmonic obstruction, and *since the ventricular septum is intact,* the right ventricular work is increased beyond its tolerance and the right ventricle fails. For these reasons, surgery in such patients must correct the pulmonic obstruction.

PULMONIC INSUFFICIENCY

Etiology. Pulmonic insufficiency due to valvular disease is extremely rare but may occur with rheumatic heart disease or subacute bacterial endocarditis. Relative pulmonic regurgitation is apparently much more common than previously believed and occurs in association with pulmonary hypertension, most often secondary to mitral stenosis or to congenital cardiac disease such as atrioseptal defect or patent ductus arteriosus.

Pathologic Physiology. Pulmonary hypertension of itself places a stress on the right ventricle. When functional pulmonic insufficiency develops in association with pulmonary hypertension it may, if severe, add to the work load of the right ventricle. Among other things, it may increase the right ventricular diastolic pressure, thus interfering with the diastolic pressure gradient between the right atrium and ventricle. This may lead to increased venous pressure and eventually to "right-sided" failure with venous congestion and fluid collection.

Symptoms. The symptoms are chiefly those of the underlying disease causing pulmonary hypertension and of the cardiac failure which may ensue.

Physical Signs. The murmur of pulmonic insufficiency is similar to that of aortic insufficiency. The characteristics and differentiation of semilunar diastolic murmurs have been discussed previously. As noted, it is difficult to differentiate the two murmurs by auscultation alone. Occasionally by voluntary straining (Valsalva maneuver), we have been able to produce different responses in the two murmurs. Murmurs often become softer during the Valsalva maneuver, and following cessation of straining regain their former intensity. Right heart murmurs will recover promptly with the first or second beat after relaxation, whereas left heart murmurs return more slowly with the sixth or seventh beat.

Roentgenologic Findings. The changes are chiefly those of the underlying condition (e.g., mitral stenosis). The one important differential finding is the fluoroscopic demonstration of excessive pulmonary arterial pulsations in pulmonic insufficiency, as opposed to more active aortic pulsations in aortic insufficiency.

Electrocardiogram. The changes commonly include varying degrees of right ventricular predominance, right ventricular hypertrophy or so-called "right ventricular strain."

Special Diagnostic Studies. When contemplating mitral valvulotomy, it is especially important to differentiate pulmonic regurgitation from aortic insufficiency. Differentiation often requires special study which has been discussed in the section on aortic insufficiency.

Treatment. There is no specific treatment for pulmonic regurgitation. Frequently it will disappear following treatment of the underlying cause (e.g., after mitral commissurotomy, ligation of a patent ductus arteriosus or repair of an atrioseptal defect).

TRICUSPID VALVULAR DISEASE

Some degree of organic tricuspid disease can be demonstrated pathologically in 20 per cent to 30 per cent of patients with rheumatic heart disease, but significant involvement occurs in only about 10 per cent. Insufficiency of the valve is by far the predominant feature; marked degrees of stenosis are much less frequent. Dressler and Fischer found a "considerable degree of stenosis" in 6.5 per cent of 123 cases of endocarditis, which represented 21 per cent of their 38 cases with organic tricuspid disease. Tricuspid disease rarely occurs as an isolated lesion; mitral stenosis is practically always associated with it, and aortic involvement is found in about one third of the cases. Approximately 40 per cent of patients with combined mitral and aortic disease also have tricuspid involvement. Because of these associations tricuspid disease becomes a factor in considering for surgery patients with mitral or aortic disease.

TRICUSPID INSUFFICIENCY

Etiology. Organic tricuspid insufficiency is almost invariably of rheumatic origin. Very rarely it can be due to congenital displacement of the tricuspid valve (Ebstein's anomaly). Functional regurgitation in the absence of intrinsic valvular disease can occur as a result of right ventricular failure and dilatation secondary to various causes (most commonly mitral stenosis or atrioseptal defect).

Pathologic Physiology. Tricuspid insufficiency enlarges both the right ventricle and the right atrium. Right atrial and venous pressures are increased, and pressure curves from the right atrium and veins show an exaggerated wave at the time of ventricular systole. These changes lead to the clinical picture of "right heart" failure. The effects of tricuspid insufficiency are superimposed on those of the mitral and aortic lesions which usually coexist.

Signs and Symptoms. The clinical features are intermingled with those of the associated mitral or aortic valvular lesions. Nevertheless, there is a clinical picture made up of the following findings by which the diagnosis of tricuspid insufficiency can be made: (1) Marked cardiac enlargement, especially to the right. (2) Cardiac failure with some cyanosis, a high venous pressure, an enlarged liver, edema and ascites. (3) A systolic tricuspid murmur which, of itself, is practically never helpful, because it is difficult to be sure that it is not transmitted from other valve lesions. (4) *A palpable systolic venous pulse* in the neck and *a palpable pulse in the liver,* which are the *pathognomonic* signs of this condition.

In some patients one sees a lateral movement of the precordium in which the front of the chest moves rightward during systole and leftward during diastole as viewed from the foot of the bed.

Most of these patients can lie flat in bed without discomfort. Their exercise tolerance tends to be limited by muscular weakness and fatigue rather than by dyspnea. Severe intractable edema may develop. Their extremities often become mottled and cold. Frequent abdominal paracentesis may be required. Atrial fibrillation is usually present, sometimes accompanied by remarkably persistent bigeminal rhythm unrelated to digitalis administration. Pulmonary infarction with hemoptysis and jaundice is not uncommon. Despite a relatively miserable existence, these patients may continue to live for an astonishingly long time.

Roentgenologic Findings and Electrocardiogram. The only specific finding may be that of a pronounced systolic pulsation of the right atrium and vena cava visible fluoroscopically. Otherwise the changes are those of the associated valve lesions as previously described.

Diagnosis. When a patient has acute cardiac failure of the type described, *with a palpable venous and hepatic pulse,* one must be cautious about making an immediate diagnosis of *organic* tricuspid insufficiency. However, when these pulsations persist after the acute stage has subsided, the patient at ne-

cropsy usually shows organic rheumatic tricuspid disease. Whereas differentiation of the organic and functional forms is often difficult, clinical recognition of tricuspid insufficiency is generally easy.

Venous or right atrial pressure curves show prominent waves during ventricular systole. Angiocardiography may show irregular opacification of the right atrium due to the regurgitant jet.

Treatment. The problems are chiefly those of treatment of underlying rheumatic activity, congestive heart failure and of the associated mitral stenosis. No specific surgical operation has been devised for tricuspid insufficiency itself.

TRICUSPID STENOSIS

Etiology. Practically all cases of tricuspid stenosis are of rheumatic origin. Tricuspid atresia may occur as a congenital lesion.

Pathologic Physiology. Tricuspid stenosis of itself will impair the diastolic filling of the right ventricle and thus lead to right atrial enlargement with elevation of the right atrial and venous pressures. The association of tricuspid insufficiency, mitral stenosis or aortic valvular involvement will produce the changes previously described in those sections.

Symptoms and Signs. The clinical findings of tricuspid stenosis are intimately intermingled with those of the mitral stenosis which is practically always present. In addition, there is usually the characteristic picture of tricuspid disease as detailed in the section on tricuspid insufficiency. One can rarely diagnose tricuspid stenosis on the basis of physical signs for the following reasons: (1) The characteristic clinical picture described for tricuspid insufficiency is the same as that seen in tricuspid stenosis and is far more frequently caused by tricuspid insufficiency. (2) While tricuspid stenosis can produce, at the tricuspid area, a diastolic murmur and heart sound pattern similar to those described for mitral stenosis, these auscultatory signs are usually overshadowed by the mitral and aortic lesions. We have recognized such a murmur in only one of 30 patients. (3) Presystolic pulsations of veins and liver, presumably due to a reflux wave produced by contraction of the hypertrophied right atrium, have been described as pathognomonic. However, the value of this observation is questionable since most patients with tricuspid stenosis have atrial fibrillation and therefore have no atrial contraction to cause this presystolic pulse. Moreover, we have recorded classic presystolic pulses in a patient who had no tricuspid stenosis at necropsy.

Roentgenologic Findings and Electrocardiogram. The changes are those of the other associated valve lesions previously described. No specific changes attributable to tricuspid stenosis can be recognized.

Diagnosis. From pathologic data one can predict that 40 per cent of patients with both aortic and mitral disease will have tricuspid disease, that 50 per cent of patients with signs of tricuspid disease will have some degree of stenosis, and that 20 per cent will have stenosis of considerable degree. Despite recognition of these probabilities, the diagnosis can rarely be made with certainty on a clinical basis. Undiagnosed tricuspid stenosis was found at autopsy in two patients who developed progressive failure and died following mitral commissurotomy.

Preliminary work suggests the possibility that significant tricuspid stenosis might be recognized (1) when cardiac catheterization demonstrates a gradient in which the diastolic pressure of the right atrium exceeds that of the right ventricle, or (2) when angiocardiography in the right anterior oblique or anteroposterior position shows the right atrium to remain sharply opacified in contrast to the right ventricle (analogous to the findings described for mitral stenosis).

Treatment. Most patients with mitral stenosis and signs of tricuspid involvement will be managed adequately by treating the mitral stenosis. One may anticipate a certain number of patients in whom tricuspid disease will influence the outcome adversely; most of these will have tricuspid insufficiency while a few will have significant tricuspid stenosis.

Tricuspid commissurotomy would seem a logical treatment for tricuspid stenosis. However, the development of this operation has been delayed because: (1) significant tricuspid stenosis is rare, (2) its diagnosis is uncertain and (3) the valve anatomy makes commissurotomy difficult.

H. F. ZINSSER, JR.
F. C. WOOD

References

Bailey, C. P.: The Surgical Treatment of Mitral Stenosis (Mitral Commissurotomy). Dis. of Chest, 15:377, 1949.

———, Redondo, R., and Larzelere, H. B.: Surgical Treatment of Aortic Stenosis. J.A.M.A., 150: 1647, 1952.

Clawson, B. J., Noble, J. F., and Lufkin, N. H.: The Calcified Nodular Deformity of the Aortic Valve. Am. Heart J., 15:58, 1938.

Dressler, W., and Fischer, R.: Über Tricuspidalstenose. Klin. Wchnschr., 8:1267, 1316, 1929.

Ferrer, M. I., Harvey, R. M., Kuschner, M., Richards, D. W., and Cournand, A.: Hemodynamic Studies in Tricuspid Stenosis of Rheumatic Origin. Circulation Research, 1:49, 1953.

Harken, D. E., Ellis, L. B., Ware, P. F., and Norman, L. R.: The Surgical Treatment of Mitral Stenosis. I. Valvuloplasty. New England J. Med., 239:801, 1948.

Johnson, J., Kirby, C. K., and Zinsser, H. F.: The Present Status of the Surgery of Mitral and Aortic Stenosis. Surgery, 34:1090, 1953.

Karsner, H. T., and Koletsky, S.: Calcific Disease of the Aortic Valve. Philadelphia, J. B. Lippincott Co., 1947.

McNeely, W. F., Ellis, L. B., and Harken, D. E.: Rheumatic Activity as Judged by the Presence of Aschoff Bodies in Auricular Appendages of Patients with Mitral Stenosis II. Clinical Aspects. Circulation, 8:337, 1953.

Welch, K. J., Johnson, J., and Zinsser, H. F., Jr.: The Significance of Pulmonary Vascular Lesions in the Selection of Patients for Mitral Valve Surgery. Ann. Surg., 132:1027, 1950.

White, Paul D.: Heart Disease. 4th ed. New York, The Macmillan Co., 1951.

Zinsser, H. F., Jr.: The Selection of Patients for Mitral Commissurotomy. Am. J. Med., 17:804, 1954.

———, and Johnson, J.: The Use of Angiocardiography in the Selection of Patients for Mitral Valvular Surgery. Ann. Int. Med., 39:1200, 1953.

ENDOCARDITIS

Definition. Endocarditis is an inflammation of the endocardium, the membrane lining the cavities of the heart. The heart valves, which are specialized endocardial structures, are characteristically involved, and this fact is of particular significance, since a small valvular lesion may be responsible for widespread and dramatic clinical effects. Lesions of the mural endocardium occur less frequently and often go unrecognized. A simple classification of the various types of endocarditis is as follows:

1. *Nonbacterial*
    (a) Simple thrombotic (nonrheumatic)
    (b) Associated with disseminated lupus erythematosus
    (c) Rheumatic

(d) Calcific (calcareous)

2. *Bacterial*

   (a) Acute (malignant), due to pyogenic organisms

   (b) Subacute (endocarditis lenta), due to organisms of low virulence, especially the nonhemolytic streptococci.

Syphilitic damage to the aortic valve results primarily from a lesion of the aorta, and the valve is only secondarily involved. It is therefore not considered in this classification. The ventricular endocardium is often damaged, together with the myocardium in cardiac infarction resulting from coronary artery disease, but again this is not primarily an endocarditis.

Nonbacterial Endocarditis. 1. SIMPLE THROMBOTIC ENDOCARDITIS is the term applied to lesions of the heart valves consisting in aseptic ulcerations and thrombotic vegetations which are often found at autopsy in patients who die of chronic debilitating diseases. The valvular damage is rarely extensive; specific signs and symptoms are lacking; significant murmurs are usually absent; consequently the disease is seldom diagnosed ante mortem. This type of endocarditis is of unknown cause and has little clinical importance except that the thrombotic lesions may at times give rise to emboli, or may become infected and thus be transformed into the vegetations of bacterial endocarditis.

2. DISSEMINATED LUPUS ERYTHEMATOSUS. A type of verrucous endocarditis described by Libman and Sachs is now considered to be a manifestation of lupus erythematosus disseminatus. This disease, which is described fully elsewhere, is of importance in considering endocarditis because clinically it may closely simulate bacterial endocarditis or rheumatic fever.

3. RHEUMATIC ENDOCARDITIS is discussed in detail in the chapters on Rheumatic Fever and Chronic Valvular Cardiac Disease.

4. CALCAREOUS lesions of heart valves are considered in the chapter on Chronic Valvular Cardiac Disease. In the past this type of lesion was thought to result either from atheromatous changes or rheumatic valvulitis, but now healed bacterial endocarditis must be added as a cause of calcific valvular disease.

Bacterial Endocarditis. The usual classification of bacterial endocarditis as *acute* and *subacute,* based upon the rapidity of progress of the untreated disease, is a somewhat arbitrary one of no great importance. In general the acute, rapidly progressive form of the disease is caused by virulent, pyogenic bacteria; whereas the subacute type is associated with organisms of low virulence, typically the *Streptococcus viridans.* It is best whenever possible to characterize a case of bacterial endocarditis bacteriologically, viz., "bacterial endocarditis due to *Streptococcus viridans.*" Such classification is especially important because the type of therapy given and the prognosis are determined largely by the nature of the infecting organism.

Etiology. Although virulent bacteria may occasionally form vegetations on normal heart valves, the great majority of patients who have bacterial endocarditis have some pre-existing valvular abnormality. Rheumatic endocarditis is the most common predisposing lesion, and for some unknown reason bacterial implants occur most frequently on valves which are only slightly scarred. It is unusual to find bacterial infection of the valves when severe mitral stenosis and atrial fibrillation are present. Various congenital lesions of the heart and great vessels, particularly patent ductus arteriosus, ventricular septal defects and coarctation of the aorta, and rarely calcareous or syphilitic valvular damage, may also be the sites of bacterial vegetations.

Bacteria circulating in the blood stream lodge in a nidus of fibrin on the surface of one of these lesions, where they multiply, invade the substance of the endocardium and, with the deposition of further fibrin, produce the typical vegetations of the disease. The source of the original bacteremia is usually apparent in acute endocarditis, which generally develops as a complication of recognized infections such as pneumonia, osteomyelitis, furunculosis or gonorrhea. *Streptococcus viridans* infection often occurs after tooth extraction, but more frequently no obvious cause of bacteremia can be found. There is evidence, however, that transitory invasion of the blood stream by these organisms is common in the presence of minor oral infection. Although patients with predisposing valvular damage may suffer bacteremia many times without acquiring bacterial endocarditis, the disease occurs sooner or later in about 10 per cent of patients with chronic rheumatic or congenital heart disease. The exact conditions which lead to the inception of bacterial vegetations are unknown.

Almost every known bacterial pathogen has at one time or another been found the infecting agent in bacterial endocarditis, but the nonhemolytic streptococci account for about 90 per cent of all cases. The term "nonhemolytic" is here used to include both strains which produce greening on blood agar, otherwise known as Streptococcus viridans, and those which produce no hemolysis or pigment and are called Streptococcus anhemolyticus. These two types overlap considerably, and the distinction between them is of no great importance. Some of the organisms most frequently encountered in the remaining 10 per cent of cases are staphylococci, both aureus and albus, pneumococci, Neisseria, Hemophilus influenzae and members of the coliform group of bacteria.

Of the nonhemolytic streptococci approximately 90 per cent of strains are sensitive to penicillin; i.e., their growth is completely inhibited in suitable culture media by 0.1 unit per milliliter or less. The other strains show varying degrees of resistance to penicillin, some requiring up to 50 units per millimeter or more for inhibition. The enterococci deserve special mention because of their high degree of resistance to penicillin. This group of organisms, which is found particularly in the intestinal tract and in urinary tract infections, produces typical subacute bacterial endocarditis, except that therapy is unusually difficult. Serologically, the enterococci fall in Lancefield's group D, and are further characterized by heat resistance and the ability to grow in 6 per cent sodium chloride. Most of the organisms which are relatively resistant to penicillin are susceptible to the action of some of the other antibiotics, either singly or in combination with penicillin.

The reaction of different strains of bacteria to antibiotics is so variable that it becomes necessary to measure in vitro the activity of the appropriate antibiotics against the infecting organism in each individual case of bacterial endocarditis. With this information one is in a position to plan a rational course of therapy, and in general the correlation between the bactericidal activity of antibiotics against an organism in vitro and in the patient is good, although in some instances gross discrepancies may occur. The nonhemolytic streptococci rarely develop resistance to penicillin even when exposed to sublethal concentrations of the drug for long periods of time, but organisms may rapidly develop mutants which are highly resistant to streptomycin. Hence when blood cultures become positive again after a patient has received therapy, the sensitivity of the newly recovered organism should be redetermined.

Morbid Anatomy. The vegetations of bacterial endocarditis are typically large friable masses composed of fibrin, bacteria and necrotic valve substance. The cellular reaction in and around the vegetations is variable but rarely intense, and large areas are often virtually acellular. Fibrosis and a tendency to healing are usually present even in untreated cases, giving the picture of an indolent infection, except when pyogenic organisms are present. The healing process after successful therapy is extremely slow, consisting in gradual fibrosis, calcification of some areas, and finally after many months endothelialization of the surfaces. Serious valvular deformities may or may not occur, depending on the duration, extent and location of the vegetations. Focal myocarditis may further contribute to cardiac insufficiency. Embolic lesions are found throughout the body, particularly in the spleen, kidneys and brain. Emboli containing Streptococcus viridans rarely produce suppuration, but cause damage mainly by impairing blood supply to the area involved. In pyogenic infections, however, multiple abscesses, metastatic meningitis and septic arthritis may occur. In addition to the focal embolic nephritis regularly found, at times there is a diffuse renal lesion indistinguishable from chronic glomerulonephritis.

Emboli to the vasa vasorum of arteries may weaken the vessel wall and give rise to mycotic aneurysms. Once established, these may enlarge progressively and rupture in spite of antibiotic therapy. The resulting hemorrhage may be fatal, especially when it is intracranial.

If vegetations are present in the right heart or in association with abnormal shunts in which the flow of blood is from the left heart to the right, emboli breaking off lodge in pulmonary vessels and give rise to small pulmonary infarctions.

Symptoms and Signs. Bacterial endocarditis may occur at any age, but is rare in children under 5 years and most common in patients between 20 and 40 years of age. The onset in a typical case of subacute bacterial endocarditis is insidious. The patient often attributes his symptoms to "grippe" for several weeks or months, and the course of the disease may seem quite benign, with periods during which fever is absent and the patient continues about his business relatively free from symptoms, but gradually weakness, easy fatigability, anorexia, fever and malaise progress. Chills, sweats and arthralgias are often prominent, and sooner or later embolic phenomena are usually observed. Painful, tender, pea-sized nodules known as Osler nodes may appear on the pads of the fingers or toes, last for several days and disappear, as may crops of petechiae on the skin, or mucous membranes. Petechiae are commonly found in the conjunctivas, where they appear as small hemorrhagic spots a millimeter or so in diameter which do not fade on pressure. Fine linear hemorrhagic lesions under the fingernails or toenails and known as "splinter hemorrhages" may also occur. The term "Janeway lesion" is applied to erythematous, nontender, macular lesions a few millimeters in diameter characteristically found on the skin of the palms and soles. Lesions seen in the ocular fundi include various types of hemorrhages, but boat-shaped lesions with white centers are said to be particularly suggestive of bacterial endocarditis. Although petechiae and the other related lesions are usually assumed to be connected with embolization of small vessels, there is some doubt as to the exact pathogenesis of these phenomena. Some workers have described vascular changes in small vessels, including marked intimal thickening and perivascular infiltration which they felt did not clearly fit in with the embolic theory, and they have suggested an allergic etiology as a possibility. While petechiae and other hemorrhagic manifestations in the skin and mucous membranes are found in many diseases associated either with a bleeding tendency or with damage to small blood vessels, typical Osler lesions are practically pathognomonic of subacute bacterial endocarditis.

Sudden pain in the left flank aggravated by respiration or movements of the trunk, and perhaps associated with a friction rub, generally signifies a splenic infarct, although at times pulmonary or renal infarction may be difficult to distinguish from infarction of the spleen. All manner of neurologic signs, transitory or permanent, may result from cerebral emboli, but persistent severe headache, especially with signs of meningeal irritation, usually indicates bleeding from a mycotic aneurysm and probably a fatal outcome. The spleen is frequently palpable, but not greatly enlarged; and although splenomegaly often disappears during therapy, it may persist for years.

Significant heart murmurs are almost always present, although at times a soft systolic murmur may be the only sign of any cardiac abnormality, and early in the disease attention may not be directed particularly to the heart. Rapidly changing murmurs resulting from growth or breaking off of vegetations are particularly characteristic of bacterial endocarditis. The heart is usually overactive, but signs of myocardial damage are uncommon until late in the course of the disease. Many patients have been followed for several years after a successfully treated bout of bacterial endocarditis without showing any evidences of significant cardiac impairment, while others, even though the infection has been controlled, have gone on to progressive valvular damage, cardiac enlargement and heart failure. Occasionally heart failure may appear during the stage of active infection and then clear as the patient's general condition improves under therapy.

Signs and symptoms of renal insufficiency may be prominent, especially in elderly patients, usually as a late manifestation of the disease. Although severe renal damage is generally irreversible, in some cases kidney function returns to normal after cure of the infection. Clubbing of the fingers and toes appears only after several months of active disease and may regress completely after therapy.

The clinical picture in acute bacterial endocarditis is basically similar, with findings related to infection, embolization and cardiac damage. There may be no evidence of previous valvular disease, however, and the course of the illness is much more rapidly progressive and stormy, terminating fatally in one or two months unless therapy is instituted.

Laboratory Data. Positive blood cultures can be obtained eventually in nearly every untreated case of this disease, but cultures may remain sterile for weeks at a time even though active infection is present. It is particularly difficult to recover organisms from the blood after antibiotics have been administered, whether in adequate dosage or not. The nonhemolytic streptococci usually grow in culture after a few days, but in some instances incubation of cultures for three weeks may be necessary before growth is apparent. The white blood cell count is usually slightly elevated, but may be entirely normal or low. A leukocytosis greater than 15,000 cells per cubic millimeter is unusual except in acute bacterial endocarditis, or during the first few days after an embolic episode. In the well established disease a refractory normocytic anemia is almost a constant finding, but, as the infection clears, the anemia improves spontaneously. Although the erythrocyte sedimentation rate is almost invariably elevated, it is a poor index of activity, since it may not revert to normal for several months after cure of the disease. Albuminuria and microscopic hematuria are intermittently present in most cases, but gross hematuria usually signifies renal infarction. There are no diagnostic serologic tests for bacterial endocarditis, for antibodies against the non-hemolytic streptococci are commonly present in normal serums. Hyperglobulinemia of a moderate degree, together with positive cephalin-cholesterol flocculation and thymol turbidity tests, is often found, probably as a result both of increased antibody production and focal liver damage.

Diagnosis. Early recognition of bacterial endocarditis is of the utmost importance so that treatment can be started before irreparable valvular damage or serious embolization occurs. *The disease must therefore be suspected in any patient with valvular heart disease who has unexplained fever, even though other common signs and symptoms may be lacking.* The diagnosis can be established only by the finding of several positive blood cultures, although it may be unwise to withhold treatment until organisms are recovered if the clinical picture is strongly suggestive of the diagnosis and the condition of the patient precarious. In any event, every possible effort should be made to obtain the infecting organism, so that its sensitivity to antibiotics can be determined as a guide to therapy. Five or six blood cultures can be taken at hourly intervals if necessary, and some of the cultures should be kept anaerobically, under carbon dioxide, and at room temperature in order to facilitate the recovery of organisms with unusual growth characteristics.

The **differential diagnosis** of bacterial endocarditis includes a great variety of diseases associated with longstanding fever and involvement of multiple organ systems, including other chronic infections, such as brucellosis, tuberculosis and fungus diseases; some malignant disorders, especially the lymphomas; and the diffuse vascular or collagen diseases of the lupus erythematosus-periarteritis nodosa group. Most difficult of all is the differentiation of smouldering rheumatic fever, not only because the two diseases may resemble each other clinically, but also because the two may coexist in the same patient. A therapeutic trial of antibiotics may be helpful in distinguishing one from the other, and is indicated even though blood cultures are negative if there is a reasonable possibility that bacterial endocarditis may be present.

Treatment. Although there is some difference of opinion as to the details of therapy, certain broad principles appear to be well established. The primary objectives must be the *eradication* of bacteria from the vegetation. Experience has shown that treatment with bacteriostatic agents such as the sulfonamides or the broad spectrum antibiotics chloramphenicol and the tetracyclines is likely to produce only temporary remission of symptoms with a high relapse rate. On the other hand, experience with *bactericidal* agents such as penicillin, streptomycin and bacitracin alone or in combination has been more satisfactory. The aim of treatment should be to achieve blood levels several times as high as the concentration known to be bactericidal *in vitro*.

Patients with an infection caused by a penicillin-sensitive *Streptococcus viridans* can be cured bacteriologically in about 90 per cent of cases. Penicillin administered in doses of 2 to 5 million units daily for from four to six weeks has been the usually accepted regimen. Recent evidence indicates that equally good results can be obtained employing penicillin together with streptomycin for a period of only two weeks. These two agents have a synergistic effect on most strains of nonhemolytic streptococci, producing rapid and complete sterilization of large inocula *in vitro*. It should be emphasized that this short, two week course of therapy cannot be recommended for cases other than those caused by streptococci which are inhibited by 0.1 unit of penicillin or less.

In enterococcal endocarditis pencillin alone is usually unsuccessful, as are the broad spectrum antibiotics. The combination of large doses of penicillin, 10 to 20 million units, with streptomycin, 1 to 2 gm. daily, or occasionally with bacitracin, has proved to be the most effective therapy. These organisms are more slowly killed, however, and treatment must be continued for four to six weeks.

The response of staphylococci and the gram-negative organisms to various antibiotics is so variable that no specific recommendations can be made except to emphasize the principle already outlined. If no antibiotics can be shown to have a bactericidal effect on the organism, treatment with the best available bacteriostatic agent should be prolonged—at least two to three months.

The place of erythromycin in the treatment of bacterial endocarditis remains to be evaluated. Early reports on a small number of cases have not been too encouraging.

Anticoagulants are contraindicated, since they contribute nothing to the cure of the disease, and only add to the risk of hemorrhage. General supportive measures are important in maintaining the best possible nutrition and morale. Bed rest is indicated during the stage of active infection and when any signs of cardiac decompensation are present, but need not be prolonged if the patient's general condition is good. As a prophylactic measure it is wise, when possible, to remove any obvious foci of infection, such as abscessed teeth, during therapy with penicillin.

Under adequate treatment with antibiotics, organisms are cleared from the blood stream within a day or two. Further persistence of positive blood cultures is strong evidence that the therapeutic regimen is inadequate. Improvement in the patient's clinical condition may be much slower. Low grade fever often continues for several weeks, and fresh embolic lesions may appear many months after cure. Conversely, a regimen which proves inadequate to cure the disease may sterilize the blood stream temporarily, and produce such a striking clinical remission that the physician may have a false sense of security all during the course of therapy. There are, unfortunately, no reliable criteria by which to judge the success of a course of treatment while it is in progress, and it is sometimes difficult to decide when therapy should be stopped. It is rarely wise, however, to continue beyond six or eight weeks on a given dosage schedule, because, if the patient is not cured by that time, further prolongation of the same regimen will probably not meet with success. It is better to stop treatment altogether, observe the patient carefully for signs of relapse, and, if this occurs, to institute a new and more intensive course of treatment. Relapses, when they occur, are almost always evident within the first month after cessation of treatment.

Prophylaxis. Any patient with valvular heart disease, no matter how minimal, is in danger of contracting bacterial endocarditis every time bacteremia occurs. Although it is impossible to prevent bacteremia altogether by any known means, it seems wise to attempt to protect vulnerable patients at times when heavy bacteremia is known to occur. Any operation in an infected field, especially tooth extraction, tonsillectomy, and instrumentation of the genitourinary tract, presents a real hazard. At such times penicillin, 100,-000 to 200,000 units every 3 hours, or the equivalent in a long-acting preparation, should be started several hours before the procedure and continued for at least 48 hours. Although bacteremia is not eliminated by this measure, it is probable that any bacteria deposited on a damaged heart valve are prevented from multiplying and are killed *in situ* before a vegetation can be formed.

Prognosis. Untreated bacterial endocarditis is almost invariably fatal, although patients have survived as long as two years with only supportive therapy. It is now possible to eradicate the infection in over 90 per cent of cases. There is still an inevitable mortality from complications of the disease, which at present is between 10 and 20 per cent. Most deaths are due to cardiac failure, renal insufficiency or cerebral vascular accidents, either from emboli or ruptured mycotic aneurysms. The prognosis in an individual case is difficult to estimate, but depends primarily upon the degree of cardiac damage, and to a lesser degree upon the type of organism, the valves involved, and the duration of the disease. Patients with vegetations on the aortic valve are particularly prone to develop serious heart failure unless the infection is rapidly controlled.

THOMAS H. HUNTER

References

Cates, J. E., and Christie, R. V.: Subacute Bacterial Endocarditis. Quart. J. Med. (New Series), 20: 93, 1951.

Finland, M.: Clinical Uses of Currently Available Antibiotics. Brit. M. J., 2:1115, 1953.

Hunter, T. H.: Speculations on the Mechanism of Cure of Bacterial Endocarditis. J.A.M.A., 144: 524, 1950.

———: Bacterial Endocarditis. Am. Heart J., 42:427, 1951.

———: Treatment of Some Bacterial Infections of the Heart and Pericardium. Bull. N. Y. Acad. Med., 284:213, 1952.

Kelson, S. R., and White, P. D.: Notes on 250 Cases of Subacute Bacterial (Streptococcal) Endocarditis Studied and Treated between 1927 and 1939. Ann. Int. Med., 22:40, 1945.

Loewe, L., Cohen, C., Eiber, H. B.: Factors in the Proper Selection of Antibiotic Programs for the Cure of the Refractory Case of Subacute Bacterial Endocarditis. Antibiotics & Chemother. 3:681, 1953.

Parsons, W. B., Cooper, T., and Scheifley, C. H.: Anemia in Bacterial Endocarditis. J.A.M.A., 153:14, 1953.

Rosebury, T.: The Aerobic Nonhemolytic Streptococci. Medicine, 23:249, 1944.

DISEASES OF THE MYOCARDIUM

MYOCARDITIS

The heart is a muscular pump, the propulsive force of which is dependent upon the functional integrity of the myocardium. All other factors which contribute to the circulation of the blood (action of the valves of the heart and venous system, vasomotor regulation, blood volume regulation, and so forth) are secondary. Regardless of how efficiently the peripheral vascular system functions with its extraordinary mechanism for sustaining and storing the propulsive force given the blood by cardiac contraction, the myocardium is of the very essence in the maintenance of the circulation. The propulsive force supplied the blood by the myocardium is absolutely essential to its movement throughout the body. Therefore, disorders which affect the heart muscle affect the tissue which is of basic functional importance to the circulation.

Failure of the central circulation as a result of pericardial diseases, valvular defects, increased peripheral resistance to the flow of blood, arteriosclerosis, anemia, hypermetabolism, senescence, disturbances of cardiac rhythm or other factors is brought about through the effect of these conditions on the myocardium. In their presence the heart muscle undergoes physical and chemical changes which eventually result in impaired efficiency. Myocardial insufficiency secondary to the factors just enumerated is dealt with in other chapters under Diseases of the Cardiovascular System.

Alterations of the blood supply to the heart muscle, either abrupt or gradual, lead to structural and functional changes of the greatest importance. The myocardial ischemia resulting from insufficient coronary blood supply may produce clinical manifestations either of angina pectoris or myocardial infarction. These conditions represent the response of the heart muscle to impaired blood supply, which most commonly is caused by arteriosclerosis. At a time when knowledge of the coronary circulation was meager, many of the changes in the myocardium now known to be due either to the aging process or to be of vascular origin were interpreted as the end results of inflammation. "Chronic myocarditis" was a term frequently used to indicate the presence of myocardial fibrosis. As knowledge accumulated, it became apparent that almost all the changes formerly designated "chronic myocarditis" were in fact reflections either of involutional changes of senescence, or impaired coronary circulation, and the term fell into disrepute. At the same time clinical skepticism regarding acute myocarditis also increased, and a strong tendency developed among clinicians to recognize the presence of myocarditis only in acute rheumatic fever and diphtheria—diseases in which inflammation of the myocardium may be a most conspicuous clinical and pathologic feature.

With the development of electrocardiography and its widespread clinical application it became apparent that abnormalities of myocardial function are frequent in many infections and in some metabolic diseases. They are usually transient and are infrequently associated with significant evidence of disturbed circulation. However, exceptions occur. It is now apparent that the myocardium may be affected by a variety of noxious factors; that structural and functional changes may occur in the myocardium in the course of many diseases and also, apparently, as isolated phenomena; that, although in the vast majority of instances these changes are transient and unrelated to symptoms or signs of central circulatory disturbance, occasionally the latter may occur and the condition terminate in death or in subacute or chronic myocardial disease.

Incidence. As indicated, myocarditis is infrequently recognized except in the cardiac manifestations of acute rheumatic fever and diphtheria. Nevertheless, isolated clinical and autopsy reports continue to appear, and in recent years Saphir, Gore and others have accumulated incontestable evidence that it occurs far more frequently than is recognized at the bedside. Thus, in the autopsy material of the Army Institute of Pathology (World War II) acute rheumatic infection and diphtheria accounted for only 25 per cent of the cases of myocarditis.

In 1941 Saphir reported the occurrence of myocarditis 240 times in 5626 autopsies at the Michael Reese Hospital in Chicago. Contagious diseases were excluded from this material.

The following instances of myocarditis were noted: myocarditis in association with subacute bacterial endocarditis, 44; myocarditis in the form of abscesses in association with pyemia, 32, and in the form of an acute diffuse change, 12; rheumatic myocarditis with the presence of outspoken Aschoff bodies, 30; acute and subacute myocarditis without the presence of definite Aschoff bodies in association with acute endocarditis of the rheumatic type, 24; acute myocarditis associated with bronchopneumonia, 19, and with lobar pneumonia, 7; isolated (Fiedler's) myocarditis, 15; myocarditis in association with acute bacterial endocarditis, 14; myocarditis in chronic diseases such as chronic duodenal ulcers, ulcerative colitis and carcinoma, 12; myocarditis in the presence of bronchiectasis, 8; myocarditis in the presence of meningococcic meningitis, 2, and in the presence of streptococcic and of pneumococcic meningitis, 4; myocarditis in tuberculosis, 6 (in 3 of the instances miliary tubercles were seen and in 3 diffuse myocarditis); myocarditis in association with pyelitis, 4; myocarditis in the presence of acute glomerulonephritis, 3, and in that of chronic glomerulonephritis, 2; myocarditis in congenital cardiac anomalies, 1; myocarditis in postdiphtheritic disease, 1.

In the review (1946) of pathologic material accumulated at the Army Institute of Pathology during World War II, Gore and Saphir cite 1402 cases of myocarditis. Clinical recognition of these cases was infrequent, although it is stated that in the majority the cardiac complication "was instrumental in causing death." In this and in other material cited in the literature myocarditis followed acute pharyngitis and tonsillitis in a number of cases and occurred frequently in fatal cases of rickettsial infections. Myocarditis was present in every case of scrub typhus studied at the Army Institute of Pathology and in a large number of cases of epidemic typhus and Rocky Mountain spotted fever. In the viral diseases electrocardiographic changes are not uncommon, although clinical evidence of significant heart disease is rare. However, Finland presents strong evidence that the influenza A virus may produce severe myocarditis and a virus producing myo-

carditis in anthropoid apes and small animals has been described. Gore and Saphir found the incidence of myocarditis at autopsy to be relatively high in rickettsial disease, subacute bacterial endocarditis, rheumatic heart disease, diphtheria, meningococcemia, scarlet fever, Weil's disease, relapsing fever, coccidioidomycosis, streptococcal infections, sulfonamide hypersensitivity, heat stroke, burns and starvation. Among the 1402 cases of myocarditis there were 43 which were listed under disease unknown (so-called "idiopathic") by Gore and Saphir. These constituted the cases of "Fiedler's" or "isolated" myocarditis in the Army material. Myocardial changes are known to occur also in trichinosis, early syphilis, sarcoidosis, amyloid disease, scleroderma, infectious mononucleosis and muscular dystrophy.

From this it is apparent that the pathologist encounters acute and chronic myocarditis at autopsy a great deal more frequently than the clinician recognizes it during life. Death in many of the infections listed often follows peripheral circulatory failure with no signs of congestive heart failure. This point is emphasized by those who insist that much of the material cited here is of no clinical significance—that in such circumstances "myocarditis" at autopsy is part and parcel of general infection and intoxication and plays no significant role. This interpretation is based on the premise that in the absence of signs of congestive heart failure the myocarditis observed at autopsy could hardly have been of clinical importance during life or a factor leading to death. With regard to this point Rantz suggests that the sodium and water retention preceding the onset of congestive failure "requires time and the ingestion of considerable amounts of sodium chloride" and that, in certain infections associated with severe myocarditis, death may occur before congestive heart failure has time to develop. In these circumstances myocarditis could result in diminution of cardiac output and thus contribute to the peripheral circulatory failure and collapse which dominates the clinical picture.

Fiedler's "isolated myocarditis," also called "idiopathic myocarditis," is a term now restricted to instances of myocardial inflammation without associated endocarditis or pericarditis and apparently unrelated to infection or injury elsewhere in the body. Whether or not such an isolated myocarditis represents an etiologic and pathologic entity is unknown. It is interesting that in the Army Institute of Pathology material Gore and Saphir found only 43 instances of idiopathic myocarditis in 1402 cases. It is certain that many instances of Fiedler's myocarditis reported earlier in this century now would be classified "postinfectious." Acute tonsillitis and pharyngitis are implicated, as well as other more obviously serious infections which heretofore have been disregarded as likely etiologic factors in myocarditis. Encephalomyocarditis of virus origin is known to occur in apes, mice and hamsters and three possible instances in man have been described.

Symptoms and Signs. The clinical picture of myocarditis is dominated as a rule by the primary disease. Certainly this is true of the cases which are overlooked during life and recognized only at necropsy. It seems highly probable that the electrocardiographic changes frequently observed in the presence of acute infections, intoxications, drug reactions and allergic states represent structural as well as functional myocardial disorders. In the vast majority of instances they are transient. This fact is responsible for the generally accepted belief that electrocardiographic signs are never significant of actual myocarditis except in rheumatic fever and diphtheria. This is not true. As we have seen, clinically significant myocarditis may complicate many disorders. The fact that this is an unusual and infrequent phenomenon in no sense negates the statement. Moreover, "isolated" myocarditis unrelated to any other recognizable illness occurs.

There is no clear-cut *clinical picture* of nonrheumatic, nondiphtheritic myocarditis; indeed, except in acute rheumatic fever, diphtheria and rickettsial diseases, myocarditis is diagnosed so infrequently that a distinct clinical pattern is not recognized. In the author's experience the diagnosis is arrived at in most instances by a process of exclusion. The presence of a large heart and diminished cardiac reserve in the absence of signs of valvular, pericardial, hypertensive, arteriosclerotic, thyrotoxic disease or senile (involutional) heart disease strongly implicates the myocardium. Electrocardiographic changes indicating myocardial disease constitute strong confirmatory evidence. The history of a recent infection, which is known occasionally to be associated with or followed by myocarditis, is of course important. Streptococcal infection should be emphasized in this connection, because of its relation not only to rheumatic

fever, but also to upper respiratory tract infections. Experience of recent years indicates that the incidence of significant myocarditis may be considerably greater that is generally recognized.

In postinfectious myocarditis as in rheumatic carditis there may be an interval of one or more weeks between the time of the initial infection and the appearance of signs of myocardial involvement. This has been observed in a good many cases, especially those which follow upper respiratory tract infections, and suggests that sensitization may play a role. The first manifestation of postinfectious myocarditis may be sudden death. The possibility that myocarditis may contribute significantly to the peripheral circulatory collapse of certain acute infectious processes has been mentioned. The condition is recognized more readily when it produces diminished cardiac reserve or congestive heart failure.

The *physical signs* of myocardial insufficiency resulting from acute or chronic inflammation of the myocardium are not specific. Perhaps tachycardia disproportionate to fever, hypotension, diminished pulse pressure and pulse volume, arrhythmia and pulsus alternans occur more frequently here than in myocardial insufficiency due to other causes. Electrocardiographic changes not due to digitalis, quinidine or other factors are of the greatest importance. Q-T and T wave abnormalities are considered diagnostic of myocardial disease.

It is important to recognize postinfectious neurocirculatory asthenia and not to confuse it with myocarditis or other forms of organic heart disease. A careful history and an intimate knowledge of the patient concerned will help greatly in arriving at a correct diagnosis. The presence of a neurotic personality and unconvincing symptoms and the absence of significant cardiac and electrocardiographic changes are perhaps the most characteristic features of neurocirculatory asthenia. Treatment in such cases is directed toward the neurosis.

Prognosis. Little can be said regarding prognosis. Myocarditis is not infrequently encountered at autopsy, and in many instances in which it occurs it unquestionably plays an important role in producing death. It seems highly probable that inflammatory reactions in the myocardium are relatively common in many disorders and that they are usually reversible and heal without residual changes. If this be true, then we are concerned here with a common instead of a rare disorder, and one in which recovery is the rule rather than the exception.

Chronic inflammatory processes in the myocardium result in myocardial fibrosis which is productive of cardiac enlargement, diminished cardiac reserve and, eventually, congestive heart failure. The last may be associated with coronary pain, pulsus alternans, excessive tachycardia, gallop rhythm, hypotension and the characteristic electrocardiographic changes of myocarditis, As has been stated, myocarditis not infrequently terminates in death suddenly and unexpectedly.

Treatment. From a prophylactic and diagnostic point of view it is well to emphasize that signs or symptoms referable to the heart during or within one to three weeks following many acute infections, especially streptococcal disease, should be viewed critically and in the light of the possibility that myocarditis may be present. More commonly such signs, if due to organic disease of the heart, will point to pericardial or endocardial involvement with or without associated myocarditis. Conservative management and careful observation are in order until a diagnosis is established.

When myocarditis develops, prompt diagnosis and treatment may not only prevent sudden and unexpected death, but may greatly prolong life and also favor complete recovery. Energetic treatment of the primary infection is indicated if it can be recognized and if specific treatment is available. Complete bed rest and supportive treatment are mandatory until electrocardiographic and clinical manifestations indicate that the myocardial process has abated or has become stationary. The treatment of cardiac arrhythmia is discussed elsewhere. The development of congestive heart failure is indication for the usual therapeutic measures: bed rest, oxygen, regulation of sodium intake, diuretics and digitalization.

HUGH J. MORGAN

References

Fiedler, A.: Ueber akute interstitielle Myokarditis. Festchrift d. Stadtkrankenhauses Dresden-Friedrichstadt, 1899.

Finland, M., Parker, F., Jr., Barnes, M. W., and Jolliffe, L. S.: Acute Myocarditis in Influenza A Infections—Two Cases of Nonbacterial Myocarditis, with Isolation of Virus from the Lungs. Am. J. M. Sc., 209:455, 1945.

Gore, I., and Saphir, O.: Myocarditis—A Classification of 1402 Cases. Am. Heart J., 34:827, 1947.

Helwig, F. C., and Schmidt, E. C. H.: Filter-Passing Agent Producing Interstitial Myocarditis in Anthropoid Apes and Small Animals. Science, 102: 31, 1945.

House, R. K.: Diffuse Interstitial Myocarditis in Children. Am. J. Path., 24:1235, 1948.

Rantz, L. A.: Myocarditis in Infections, with a Selected Bibliography. Stanford Med. Bull., 7:12, 1949.

Saphir, O.: Myocarditis: A General Review, with an Analysis of Two Hundred and Forty Cases. Arch. Path., 32:1000, 1941; 33:88, 1942.

———: Virus Myocarditis. Mod. Concepts Cardiovas. Dis., 6:43, 1949.

———: Encephalomyocarditis. Circulation, 6:843, 1952.

SENILE HEART DISEASE

(Presbycardia)

Aging is a phenomenon of living which is continuous, inconspicuous and quite unimpressive as a rule, but it is as relentless in its development as is the passage of time itself and, barring termination of life by the accidents of disease and injury, it gradually but inevitably leads to disability and death. Because its role in health and its effect upon disease are usually not dramatic, it is often neglected and forgotten and is rarely accorded proper importance by physicians in appraisals of physical disabilities. There is a strong tendency to attribute all the invisible manifestations of aging to specific diseases, and amongst the latter arteriosclerosis is the one blamed most frequently. The longer man lives the greater the chance for the development, not only of the involutional changes of aging, but also the diseases which have their highest incidence in the aged, as atherosclerosis and cancer. The importance of heredity in predetermining the life span and biologic age of the various species is obvious and, of course, holds true for man.

Graying of the hair, atrophy and wrinkling of the skin, hyperpigmentation, bagginess beneath the eyes, baldness and keratoses are all manifestations of aging of the skin. The degree to which they occur and the time of their development vary greatly among both individuals and families. Involutional changes occur earlier in certain other body structures. The ductus arteriosus undergoes involution in the first two months after birth and the thymus at puberty. The time of onset of the menopause varies widely and so, too, must the involutionary changes in the ovaries which lead to amenorrhea. Senility itself may be greatly delayed in certain individuals. Achylia gastrica may be an early expression of aging and is almost always present in the eighth and ninth decades. The same is true of diminished gallbladder and small bowel function and associated mild digestive disturbances. The tottering gait, tremor and impaired motor and sensory functions of the aged, together with the emotional instability and memory lapses so characteristic of senility, are conspicuous and are well understood by the laity as being due to old age, whereas physicians very commonly attribute them to "cerebral arteriosclerosis." Medial sclerosis of blood vessels occurs as the body ages and this form of arteriosclerosis is believed often to be an expression of involutional change. In itself, medial sclerosis of whatever cause is not of great importance in significantly modifying blood supply. It is when atherosclerosis or intimal arterial disease is present that symptomatic circulatory disturbances occur.

Etiology. Senescence as an etiologic factor in cardiac arrhythmias and circulatory insufficiency is often either forgotten or interpreted as arteriosclerosis. Actually, senescence, alone and uncomplicated, is probably a very infrequent cause of congestive heart failure, just as "uncomplicated" old age is an infrequent cause of death. On the other hand, the aging process renders the heart increasingly susceptible to other factors adversely affecting cardiac efficiency. Thus, the ultimate development of congestive heart failure in chronic valvular disease, hypertension, atherosclerosis, chronic pulmonary disease, thyrotoxicosis and longstanding anemia is favored by the presence in the heart of the involutional changes of aging. The slow but steady diminution in circulatory efficiency which normally begins in the latter part of the third or early in the fourth decade is manifestly an expression of structural and functional changes incident to aging, plus the accumulated effects of previously experienced disease and injury. Actually, distinction between the two is very difficult, often impossible. Nevertheless, it is clear that an entirely stationary and nonprogressive rheumatic valvular defect well compensated during the younger years of life may eventually, with the passage of time and diminishing cardiac efficiency, result in congestive heart failure. The infrequency of "thyrotoxic heart disease" in the early decades of life and the frequency of serious cardiac manifestations in Graves' disease in individuals over 50 years old is well recognized. Severe anemia in the young is rarely associated with conges-

tive heart failure unless other complicating factors which reduce cardiac reserve exist, yet congestive heart failure was a common accompaniment of pernicious anemia in old people prior to the advent of liver therapy.

As has been said, the aging process operates most commonly as a cause of heart disease by reducing cardiac reserve, thus rendering the heart vulnerable to the effects of other factors which then precipitate congestive failure. It seems important to differentiate diagnostically the aging from the other factors. Occasionally these other conditions appear to be absent or insignificant in the aged but congestive failure or cardiac arrhythmia occurs, nevertheless. Under such circumstances it is appropriate to list aging as the primary etiologic factor, adopting the nomenclature proposed by Dock, "presbycardia," or Harrison, "senile heart disease."

Morbid Anatomy and Physiology. The chief anatomic and physiologic changes which are believed to be expressions of cardiovascular aging may be summarized as follows: atrophy and pigmentation of muscle cells; increased rigidity and diminished efficiency of the heart valves and thickening of the endocardium; fibrous tissue replacement of elastic tissue in the aorta and heart; disturbances of rhythm by ectopic beats and paroxysmal atrial fibrillation; medial fibrosis and calcinosis, elongation and tortuosity of the arteries with loss of elasticity and increase in systolic blood pressure; diminished skeletal muscle tone and activity with slowing of venous return from the periphery to the heart; diminution of the inspiratory suction of blood centralward to the great veins from the peripheral circulation as a result of poor muscle tone, obesity or emphysema. Most of these changes can be identified. Biochemical changes, poorly understood but probably of equal or greater importance, occur. It seems certain that both structural and biochemical changes are etiologically related to the steady encroachment upon the reserve capacity of the circulation which occurs with aging and expresses itself in diminished circulatory efficiency.

Symptoms and Signs. The manifestations of heart disease which may be due to the aging process are either extrasystolic arrhythmias, atrioventricular block, bundle branch block, atrial fibrillation or congestive heart failure. There is nothing distinctive about either the arrhythmias, conduction defects or the congestive heart failure to identify senescence as the underlying cause. Breathlessness first on exertion and later at rest, cough and orthopnea indicate the development of "left heart failure." At the same time or somewhat later "right heart failure" occurs with swelling and tenderness of the liver and edema of the ankles, sacrum and dependent portions of the body. On physical examination the usual manifestations of congestive heart failure with distended veins, dependent edema, moist lung bases and enlarged tender liver are encountered. Fluid may be present in pleural or peritoneal cavities. The heart is enlarged both to the right and left. Tachycardia is present. Arrhythmia due to ectopic beat or to atrial fibrillation may be present. If the lungs are very emphysematous the heart sounds may be quite distant. A gallop rhythm may be audible at the apex. The electrocardiogram is important in a negative fashion in the recognition of uncomplicated senile heart disease because the patterns usually associated with localized atherosclerotic heart disease are absent. The established presence of atherosclerotic heart disease in no wise negates the significance or importance of senescent changes. On the contrary, experience indicates that the older the patient, the graver the prognosis in thrombosis of a coronary artery.

Diagnosis. Age is important and should be recognized and evaluated in cardiovascular disease. When the changes of senescence reduce cardiac reserve sufficiently to produce either congestive heart failure or greatly increased susceptibility to congestive heart failure in the presence of other precipitating factors, then the aging process *per se* deserves a place in cardiac nosology. Unfortunately, this point of view is not as yet generally accepted.

The diagnosis of senile heart disease rests upon: (1) the fact that readily recognizable changes of senescence are present in the body, and (2) the absence of convincing evidence that other forms of heart disease, especially coronary atherosclerosis, are present and of significance. The history and electrocardiogram are very important in this regard. Thus, the absence of a history of angina pectoris or of myocardial infarction, and the absence of characteristic coronary disease patterns in the electrocardiogram, constitute strong evidence that congestive heart failure in old patients is due to senescence and not to atherosclerosis. Moreover,

senile changes in the heart exaggerate the effect of other factors which precipitate congestive heart failure.

Treatment. The management of congestive heart failure, cardiac arrhythmia and conduction disturbances due to aging is identical with the management of these disorders when due to other forms of heart disease. The response to treatment is usually very satisfactory and is impressively better than when coronary sclerosis is chiefly to blame.

HUGH J. MORGAN

References

Billings, F. T., Jr., Kalstone, B. M., Spencer, J. L., Ball, C. O. T., and Meneely, G. R.: Prognosis of Acute Myocardial Infarction. Am. J. Med., 7:356, 1949.

Burch, G. E., and Reaser, P.: A Primer of Cardiology. Philadelphia, Lea & Febiger, 1947.

Cowdry, E. V.: Problems of Ageing; Biological and Medical Aspects. 3rd ed. Ed. by A. I. Lansing. Baltimore, Williams and Wilkins Co., 1952.

Dock, W.: Presbycardia or Aging of the Myocardium. New York State J. Med., 45:983, 1945.

Harrison, T. R., Editor-in-Chief: The Principles of Internal Medicine. The Blakiston Co. Toronto, 1950.

Lansing, A. I., Alex, M., and Rosenthal, T. B.: Atheromatosis as a Sequel to Senescent Changes in the Arterial Wall. J. Gerontol., 5:314, 1950.

Morgan, H. J.: Senescence and Heart Disease. Tr. A. Am. Physicians, 44:54, 1951.

Shock, N. W., Editor: Conference on Problems of Aging. Josiah Macy, Jr. Foundation. New York, Feb. 5–6, 1951.

DISEASES OF THE CORONARY ARTERIES

The coronary arteries, the first peripheral branches given off by the aorta, are subject to the same lesions as other arteries. Atheromatosis leading to arteriosclerosis with narrowing and complete obstruction is the most prevalent lesion. Syphilitic aortitis distorting the coronary ostia, and rheumatic arteries, are next in frequency. Rarely, periarteritis nodosa, scleroderma, thromboangiitis obliterans, amyloid, hemorrhagic diseases, vegetations of bacterial endocarditis or tumors impinging on the ostia, emboli, and the arteritis associated with systemic infections may be responsible for significant clinical manifestations. Congenital malformations and trauma are sometimes encountered. The chief effect of these lesions is to interfere with coronary blood flow and prevent an adequate blood supply to the myocardium.

THE PATHOGENESIS OF CARDIAC PAIN, WITH PARTICULAR REFERENCE TO CORONARY ARTERIOSCLEROSIS

Cardiac pain is generally regarded as the result of an insufficient supply of blood to meet the requirements of the myocardium. The insufficiency may be in amount, as with sudden narrowing or occlusion of the coronary arteries, or in quality, as in asphyxia with anoxemia. Not infrequently, both deficiencies may be present. In a patient with sudden massive hemorrhage and shock, the coronary blood flow is reduced because of the lowered blood pressure; the oxygen supply to the myocardium is still further lowered because of the anemia.

It is of paramount importance to recognize that blood supply is deficient only in relation to the requirements of the myocardium to accomplish its work. The coronary blood flow may be adequate to meet the normal myocardial needs at rest, but insufficient for the increased requirements when the work of the heart is increased as in exercise, emotion, thyrotoxicosis, fever or rises in blood pressure. In such circumstances myocardial ischemia develops with its clinical representation of cardiac pain or discomfort. That this imbalance between supply and demand underlies cardiac pain is supported by the electrocardiographic evidence of ischemia; the induction of cardiac pain by inhalation of air with low oxygen tension; the prevention of attacks of pain by inhalation of high oxygen mixtures; the occurrence of angina pectoris on effort, emotion and in other states in which the work of the heart is increased; the relief of discomfort by rest, nitroglycerin and other vasodilators.

The pathologic basis for this discrepancy between supply and demand is revealed by the striking prevalence of arteriosclerotic coronary narrowings and occlusions in patients with the pain or discomfort of angina pectoris. Ninety per cent of the hearts of patients with angina pectoris studied by the writer and his associates have shown obstructive narrowings and occlusions of the main coronary arteries or their primary branches. Similar lesions occasionally were found in the hearts of patients who had no cardiac symptoms during life and who died of noncardiac causes, but the incidence and severity of such lesions were strikingly less. This apparent inconsistency between the presence of longstanding obstructive arterial lesions and the absence of pathologic or clinical evidence of myocardial infarction was dispelled by the demonstration of collateral channels which by-passed the obstructions or which supplied the myocardium distal to the areas of narrowing or occlusion from neighboring unoccluded coronary arteries.

In the normal heart, fine communications are present between the coronary arteries, but they are functionally inadequate to prevent the serious or fatal consequences of sudden occlusion. In the presence of marked narrowing and occlusion, collateral channels of larger than normal size are regularly demonstrable and safeguard the heart from the otherwise dire consequences of such obstructive lesions. Although serious damage is generally avoided by the development of such collateral circulation, the margin of safety or, as it may be termed, the "coronary reserve," is presumably reduced. The maximal blood supply originally available to the myocardium has been obviously reduced by arterial obstruction. Cardiac pain, evidently due to ischemia, develops under conditions which further reduce the available blood supply or increase the nutritional requirements of the heart. Sudden narrowing or occlusion due to a thrombus, subintimal hemorrhage or a ruptured atheromatous abscess results in immediate myocardial infarction, for there has been no adequate opportunity for the gradual development of sizable collateral channels.

Arterial hypertension with its arteriolar hypertrophy apparently predisposes to arteriosclerosis and is frequently associated with coronary narrowings and occlusions.

Conditions other than coronary arteriosclerosis are responsible for cardiac pain in approximately 10 per cent of patients. Arterial hypertension and valvular disease greatly increase cardiac work even under basal conditions and therefore limit the degree to which the work of the heart may be augmented, as on effort, without inducing relative ischemia and cardiac pain or distress. Syphilitic aortitis with aortic regurgitation or narrowing of the coronary ostia, periarteritis nodosa, thromboangiitis obliterans, rheumatic arteritis, scleroderma, amyloid, cor pulmonale with chronic pulmonary infection and anoxemia, and the arteries or myocarditis associated with systemic infections may be encountered.

Physicians often postulate "spasm" of the coronary arteries to explain episodes of angina pectoris and other types of cardiac pain. Spasm could result from a direct effect of epinephrine or other chemical circulating substances on the smooth muscle of the arteries, or it could be induced by vasomotor impulses. That important vasomotor effects on the coronary circulation are induced by emotion or exposure to cold is plainly evident from clinical observations and studies of Freedberg, Wilson, Gilbert and others. Such effects rarely, if ever, are the sole etiologic factor, for in the experience of the writer and his associates the heart of every patient with angina pectoris or myocardial infarction has disclosed unmistakable evidence of cardiovascular disease. But vasoconstriction, or absence of vasodilatation, is to be considered in the same category as anemia, tachycardia, arterial hypertension or the lowered blood pressure from any cause, as precipitating agents in the production of cardiac pain or distress in a heart already compromised by arterial obstruction.

ANGINA PECTORIS

Definition. Angina pectoris is a syndrome consisting in paroxysmal substernal or precordial pain or discomfort of short duration, frequently radiating to the shoulders and inner aspects of the arms, usually precipitated by exertion, emotion or other states in which the work of the heart is increased, and relieved by rest or nitroglycerin.

Etiology. The etiologic factors of angina pectoris may be considered as comprising three groups: (1) primary etiologic factors which set the stage for the appearance of angina pectoris, (2) the secondary predisposing influences which favor the development of the primary etiologic factors and (3) the immediate precipitating factors.

Primary Etiologic Factors. Coronary arteriosclerotic narrowings and occlusions are observed in approximately 90 per cent of cases. In the absence of such changes, arterial hypertension, valvular disease and the other causes mentioned before together account for probably less than 10 per cent. Aortic stenosis with its frequent distortion of the coronary ostia and the increased cardiac work likewise predisposes to angina pectoris.

Secondary Predisposing Factors. Men are affected approximately five times as often as women. Since arteriosclerosis increases generally with age, angina pectoris is most frequent in the sixth and seventh decades, but younger persons in the forties and thirties may be affected, even in the absence of arterial hypertension or other evident disorders. "The inherited quality of the vascular tubing," to quote Osler, apparently plays a decisive role in certain families in which angina pectoris appears in many members at a relatively early age and runs a rapidly progressive course.

Excessive emotional as well as physical strain promotes the appearance of angina pectoris; hence the sensitive, nervous, active, high-strung person is more prone to this disorder than the stolid or those who have achieved equanimity.

The incidence of angina pectoris is increased in patients with arterial hypertension, diabetes mellitus, polycythemia vera, thromboangiitis obliterans and periarteritis nodosa. In the presence of aortic regurgitation of syphilitic or rheumatic origin, angina pectoris is more frequent, doubtless because of the lowered diastolic pressure and consequently decreased coronary blood flow, as well as because of the increased work imposed on the heart.

Gallbladder disease, peptic ulcer or, indeed, any other pathologic state in the upper abdomen, chest, neck or extremities is believed by some observers to facilitate the appearance of pain or distress; not infrequently these lesions lead to reference of the anginal pain to the diseased part.

Immediate Precipitating Factors. These are factors which transiently increase the work of the heart or decrease the blood flow. Among the former are effort, emotion, large meals, the tachycardias and rises in blood pressure. Coronary flow may be decreased by the lowered blood pressure in shock and, at times, in dehydration, in hypoglycemia and in the tachycardias. Coronary blood flow may also be diminished because of increased resistance in the coronary system from the reflex vasomotor effects of emotions or exposure to cold. Drugs such as epinephrine, pitressin or thyroid may cause anginal pain.

Symptoms. *Usual Characteristics.* The cardinal characteristic of angina pectoris is the pain or discomfort. This is ordinarily substernal, or precordial, abrupt in onset, short in duration; it remains localized or radiates to the shoulders and arms, particularly the left, or to the neck or back.

The quality of the discomfort varies greatly in different patients, but in a given person is fairly constant and notably repetitive in its characteristics. It may be described as "vise-like," "heaviness," "tightness," "boring," "grinding," "crunching," "choking," "fullness," "aching," "pressure," "squeezing," and so on. Patients are usually unable to define the sensation more specifically; this difficulty in describing the symptom is indeed one of the characteristic features of the condition.

The onset is usually sudden and may strike without warning or mount within a few seconds or a minute to a crescendo until the patient stops or rests or takes nitroglycerin; it then rapidly disappears. Of great significance are the attendant circumstances of the attack. The onset on exertion, excitement, aggravation is characteristic.

In most persons, exertion is the precipitating factor, but occasionally emotion is the sole provocation. The attacks commonly are induced more readily after meals and also in cold weather by chilling or walking against the wind. Relatively slight exertion may induce an attack when first undertaken in the morning, after which much more exertion may be accomplished before an attack is experienced. In patients with advanced disease, slight exertion or eating may provoke attacks; episodes may occur while at rest, or may awaken the patient at night from sleep.

The duration of the pain, a most important feature, is usually estimated by the patient to be five minutes or less, but may be described as lasting fifteen minutes. Actual measurement by Riseman of attacks induced by exertion has revealed that they are practically always less than three minutes in duration. Also characteristic is the mode of relief of an attack of angina pectoris, i.e., by rest, or nitroglycerin.

Atypical Features. Approximately 75 per cent of patients exhibit the characteristics already described; in some 25 per cent, atypical features are displayed.

VARIATIONS IN THE LOCALIZATION AND RADIATION OF PAIN OR DISTRESS are not uncommon. The sites of origin other than the substernal area include the right anterior chest, the epigastrium and upper abdomen, various parts of one or both upper extremities, and, rarely, the upper back.

The aberrant sites of pain are sometimes related to disease elsewhere which, to use Mackenzie's concept, has given rise to an irritable focus which acts as a trigger or focal point of reference. Mackenzie cites a patient who suffered toothache whenever he exerted himself; the right molar tooth was the site of an abscess. Bursitis of the shoulder or the elbow, arthritis of the spine or the arms, gallbladder disease, diaphragmatic hernia, peptic ulcer may localize the anginal pain to such areas. In many instances the radiation from these aberrant sites is not to the substernal area, and the symptoms may be attributed to some other condition unless a detailed clinical history is obtained.

Although the pathway of radiation of substernal pain is characteristically along the inner, rather than the outer, aspects of the arm, and into the fourth and fifth fingers along the ulnar distribution, in some patients the pathway is not continuous. Substernal discomfort may be accompanied, immediately followed, or be replaced by localized discomfort about the elbows, wrist or in the fourth or fifth finger. Numbness and tingling of these areas during attacks may be experienced.

SENSE OF DISSOLUTION (ANGOR ANIMI). The patient's fear of sudden, impending death during an attack has been recognized as a hallmark of angina pectoris since the days of Heberden. The sense of dissolution may be strikingly out of proportion to the intensity of the discomfort produced by the pain itself. It occurs in only a small proportion of patients and is not to be confused with the anxiety constantly present in hypersensitive patients regarding their ailment.

GASTRO-INTESTINAL SYMPTOMS, particularly belching, are frequent accompaniments of the attacks. Substernal or epigastric distress, with relief after sodium bicarbonate or belching, may lead the patient to ascribe his symptomatology to "indigestion." Whenever a patient complains of thoracic or upper abdominal symptoms after meals, inquiry should always be made whether this occurs only on exertion after meals or whether it occurs on exertion alone.

OTHER SYMPTOMS. *Hyperesthesia* within the areas in which the pain or discomfort is experienced may linger, as noted by John Hunter, after the attack is ended. *Temporary breathlessness, palpitation and vasomotor phenomena,* including pallor, sweating and giddiness, are not infrequently described by patients; rarely, *syncope* occurs. By themselves these symptoms neither indicate nor exclude angina pectoris, but their presence is compatible with the syndrome.

Physical Examination. Physical examination does not reveal pathognomonic evidence.

If seen during an attack, the patient is immobile, his face pallid and anxious. Between attacks, in about one quarter of the patients with angina pectoris, cardiac study by physical examination, roentgenography and electrocardiography, including standard, unipolar limb and precordial leads, reveals normal findings; in them the only evidence of heart disease is the patient's clinical history. In the majority of patients, however, arterial hypertension, abnormal physical or electrocardiographic findings indicating cardiac enlargement, valvular or myocardial damage are observed. These evidences of cardiac damage frequently are no different than in other patients of advancing years who do not suffer from this disorder. Examination may reveal other conditions such as syphilis, anemia or thyrotoxicosis, which are not indicative of angina pectoris, but may be associated with it; when they are adequately treated, the intensity or frequency of attacks may decrease.

Diagnosis. "Listen to the patient's story; he is telling you the diagnosis." Nowhere in clinical medicine is the old adage more pertinent. The diagnosis is based on the patient's symptomatology reported between attacks or at the time of induced symptoms. The cardinal diagnostic feature is the pain or distress. *In general, any distress or sensation in the upper part of the body between the upper abdomen and the neck induced by effort or excitement and subsiding rapidly on rest should be suspected as possibly angina pectoris until ruled out by contrary considerations.*

Usually the diagnosis is readily made. The freedom from symptoms between attacks, and the characteristics of the symptomatology previously described, are diagnostic. The regularity of the amount of effort which induces an attack, and the uniformity of the symptoms from attack to attack in the individual patient, are helpful characteristics.

In some patients, inability to describe the distress or atypical localization and symptomatology may make it impossible to appraise the condition with assurance on the initial examination; further observation and close questioning may be necessary before a decision can be reached. Relief by nitroglycerin or amyl nitrite strongly suggests the diagnosis of angina pectoris, but is not pathognomonic, for they also relieve other spasmodic states. Moreover, in some patients with angina pectoris the drugs are not effective.

Various tests have been devised for the occasional instance in which, despite all one's effort, uncertainty remains. The proposed use of epinephrine to precipitate attacks is fallacious and dangerous; fatalities have resulted. Injection of posterior lobe pituitary extracts is likewise inadvisable. Various other procedures have been advocated, including study of the electrocardiographic changes and of the appearance of pain while the subject breathes a mixture of 10 per cent oxygen and 90 per cent nitrogen or undertakes standardized amounts of exercise. The most useful procedure in the writer's experience is the exercise test of Riseman and Stern which consists in walking over a two-step staircase at a standard rate of speed under constant conditions of temperature between 40 and 50° F. in a room especially devised for this purpose. This test is not without danger in severely affected patients, in whom attacks are readily provoked. In such cases the test is unnecessary, for the usual clinical examination almost always suffices. In those patients in whom attacks occur infrequently and in whom the symptomatology is vague, the exercise tolerance test may be considered safe, provided the patient is instructed to stop when the attack is induced. In actual practice, exercise at room temperature and, if necessary, with the subject holding an ice cube in his hand, as suggested by A. S. Freedberg, enables one to perform this test readily under the usual office or hospital conditions.

Ballistocardiography and its possible usefulness in the diagnosis and evaluation of coronary artery disease have evoked much interest. This technique yields a record of the movements imparted to the body by the forces associated with contraction of the heart, and acceleration and deceleration of blood as it is ejected and moved in the large vessels. Although the waves are clearly associated with specific events in the cardiac cycle, their qualitative and quantitative significance have not been precisely defined. In patients with angina pectoris, the ballistocardiogram is generally abnormal; however, similar abnormalities are encountered so frequently in other subjects of the same age without angina pectoris that the practical diagnostic value of this technique at its present stage of development is indeed minimal for this purpose.

Differential Diagnosis. Angina pectoris is to be differentiated from the prolonged precordial or substernal ache and discomfort which occur with *prolonged anxiety* or with the *nervous and physical debilitation* of long-continued illness. This type of distress is part of the constellation of signs and symptoms which has been denoted by the terms "neurocirculatory asthenia," "irritable heart," "effort syndrome" or "soldier's heart." It differs from angina pectoris in that the distress is an ache present for long periods of time and not constantly related to effort. It tends to be precordial rather than substernal and is attended by exhaustion, faintness and the presence, frequently, of the physical signs of anxiety, including tachycardia, cold moist hands, sighing respiration and the sensation of dyspnea on slight exertion in the absence of any organic disease. In addition to such phenomena, it is imperative to uncover positive psychologic evidence to support the diagnosis. It is to be remembered that the existence of a neurosis does not render the patient immune to angina pectoris.

Extrasystoles or *paroxysmal tachycardia* may cause discomfort or pain, but the nature of the symptoms and the lack of relation to effort permit clear differentiation. The sharp pain of *acute pericarditis* or *pleuritis* is occasionally mistaken for angina pectoris, but can be differentiated readily by analysis of the symptomatology, the physical signs and, in the instance of pericarditis, by serial electrocardiographic tracings.

Arthritis of the cervical or thoracic spine and *bursitis* are among the common causes of pain over the cardiac area and left upper chest and may be initially deceiving. *Ruptured intervertebral disks, intercostal neuritis, pulmonary hypertension, distention of the splenic flexure, lesions of the lungs and mediastinum,* particularly *acute interstitial mediastinal emphysema* (Hamman's syndrome) occasionally produce symptoms which bear some resemblance to angina pectoris, but can be differentiated without difficulty on careful study.

Hiatus hernia, gallbladder colic, peptic ulcers, esophageal ulcers, cardiospasm or *spasm of the esophagus* may give rise to severe substernal pain with radiation to the neck or to one or both arms, particularly on emotion or after eating a large meal. The symptoms may be dramatically relieved by nitroglycerin or amyl nitrite. The associated symptoms of these disorders, the longer duration of the discomfort and the lack of relation to effort usually permit the resolution of any diagnostic difficulties.

If the patient is first seen while experiencing an attack, the pain may be indistinguishable from that of *coronary failure* or *acute myocardial infarction.* The circumstances attending the onset, the duration and severity of the pain, and careful consideration of the respective clinical features almost invariably yield the correct diagnosis, but observation for several days for the signs of myocardial necrosis may be necessary.

Clinical Course. Mild attacks occurring at infrequent intervals may characterize an insidious onset. Over a period of years the attacks may be precipitated by lesser effort and the pain may become more severe. In patients with syphilitic aortitis or syphilitic aortic regurgitation the course is usually much more rapidly progressive.

Many patients, when closely questioned, vividly recall the precipitating circumstances, the exact date and, indeed, the hour of their first attack, which was intense, prolonged and not infrequently attended by cold sweat, followed by weakness lasting hours. Some of these patients, judging by the symptomatology and electrocardiographic evidence of old myocardial infarction, apparently suffered acute narrowing or complete occlusion of a major coronary artery which, though unrecognized, was responsible for the initial symptomatology and the ensuing attacks of angina pectoris.

In some patients the symptoms are not slowly progressive, but proceed in steplike gradation, remaining stationary for many months or years, abruptly becoming somewhat more intense and then again remaining stationary for a time. In practically all patients, for stretches of weeks or months, the attacks are induced with regularity by approximately the same amount of effort, if one excludes episodes of excitement, exposure to cold or overeating. With progression of the underlying cardiac pathology, some patients show increasing breathlessness on exertion between attacks. This eventually may lead to the frank evidence of congestive failure. With the limitation on effort imposed by congestive failure, the attacks of angina pectoris may be infrequent or disappear completely.

In some patients, especially those with arterial hypertension, attacks of paroxysmal nocturnal dyspnea complicate the clinical course with its attendant possibilities of pulmonary edema, ventricular fibrillation or cardiac standstill.

In a small proportion of patients marked temporary improvement may occur, evidently owing to the development of adequate collateral channels to regions of myocardial ischemia, or the correction of associated conditions such as thyrotoxicosis or anemia; an occasional patient may, indeed, be permanently relieved of the distress. Disappearance of the seizures occasionally occurs after acute myocardial infarction. In such instances the infarct evidently obliterates the portion of the myocardium which previously had been the site of relative anoxia, and the muscle fibers which had been the source of abnormal stimuli during attacks are replaced by insensitive fibrous tissue.

In all patients with angina pectoris the clinical course may be abruptly altered by the unpredictable catastrophic events which constantly hover over such persons. They may occur during the first or any subsequent attack. *There is no necessary relation between the mildness of the symptoms and the occurrence of serious complications such as acute myocardial infarction, cardiac standstill and sudden death.*

Prognosis. The wide variations in the clinical course and the unpredictable occurrence of serious complications, including sudden death, always render the prognosis uncertain. In a study by White, Bland and Miskall of 497 patients observed over a period of twenty-three years, 52 patients still survived with an average duration of eighteen years since the onset of the angina. It appears that the average duration of life after the onset for the entire group will approximate ten years; the average age of the group at the time of onset was 57 years. It is apparent that many patients with angina pectoris have a normal life span. General surveys of the prognosis of large groups of patients provide helpful guidance, but strict application to the individual patient is precarious and must be tempered by the findings in each instance. The tense, anxious patient rebellious against his disease, the presence of obesity, cardiac hypertrophy, arterial hypertension, previous cardiac infarctions, congestive failure and significant electrocardiographic abnormalities are clearly related to a higher mortality rate and a lower survival rate. Aortic stenosis, syphilitic aortitis and advanced rheumatic valvular disease are decidedly adverse factors.

Though one of the most serious cardiac disorders, angina pectoris must not be regarded as the equivalent of a death warrant. Many distinguished men in the professions and in public life continue active careers for many years and even decades by restricting their activities and adhering to the plan of management advised by their physician. In many of these, full expectation of life is achieved.

Treatment. Much can be achieved in the treatment of angina pectoris. It is of paramount importance to educate the patient to arrange his daily activities so that he may lead a comfortable and worthwhile existence within the confines of his malady. It is important to review in minute detail a daily program of the patient's life. He should be instructed to cease effort immediately on experiencing pain and to rest until the pain has gone for several minutes. The number of proposed remedies is legion, but nitroglycerin for the prevention as well as for the treatment of attacks, and long-acting vasodilators such as the xanthines, remain the most trustworthy of the medicinal agents. In exceptional circumstances, when all else has failed, surgical procedures may be considered.

Restriction of Effort. The guiding principle is that the patient live within the limits set by his pain. If the onset of the illness has been characterized by the sudden appearance of severe pain or frequent attacks of mild pain, a period of bed rest or marked restriction of activity for several weeks is usually indicated until it is clear that myocardial infarction has not occurred and that a new balance of coronary reserve is reached. Confinement to bed is also to be advised if, at any time, there is a sudden increase in the severity of the condition. In most patients the clinical course is stationary or only slightly progressive, and easy or moderate exercise, including walking or golf, is to be encouraged within the limits tolerated without anginal symptoms. Strenuous activity such as running, carrying heavy objects such as suitcases, walking fast upstairs or uphill in the cold or against strong winds should be forbidden. *It is the intensity of effort more than its duration which must be avoided.*

General Measures. During the cooler months of the year, patients should avoid chilling and should be instructed to dress too warmly rather than risk chilliness. Obese or overweight patients should lose 1 to 2 pounds weekly until they reach a proper weight. The use of desiccated thyroid to increase oxygen consumption or of amphetamine sulfate to diminish appetite is contraindicated. In the presence of moderate or severe angina pectoris, particularly when attacks are induced by eating or are prone to occur after meals, improvement frequently follows dividing the daily food intake into six small meals. In all patients, distribution of the daily food intake more evenly among the meals is desirable. There is divergence of opinion regarding the use of tobacco. In some patients, abstinence leads to increased nervousness and irritability or to increased weight; in others, alleviation of cardiac symptoms is noticeable. It is the writer's practice to advise a trial period of abstinence; for most patients who show no consequent improvement, tobacco in moderation is permitted. Alcohol in small amounts is usually well tolerated; especially in the elderly, brandy or whisky, 15 to 30 cc. for the prevention or relief of attacks, may be useful.

Medical Treatment. NITROGLYCERIN in tablets of 0.6 or 0.3 mg. remains the most effective agent for the relief of attacks. Only fresh hypodermic-type tablets which dissolve readily under the tongue should be used. Tablets older than six months had best be discarded. The patient is instructed to allow the tablet to dissolve completely in the mouth and to retain the saliva containing the nitroglycerin for at least a brief interval before swallowing. Some patients, particularly those with arterial hypertension, suffer severe throbbing with intense headache and flushing of the face, occasionally with nausea and vomiting lasting minutes to an hour or more. For such patients, and indeed for many others without such symptoms, smaller doses such as 0.3 mg. or even 0.12 mg. are equally effective therapeutically and entail no discomfort. It is well to administer tablets of various dosage to the patient at the time of visit and determine the optimum dosage. If a single dose is not effective, the patient should be instructed to take an additional one, two or even three doses at intervals of 5 minutes. If an attack is unusually long or severe, he should immediately rest and seek medical advice. All patients should be assured that nitroglycerin is not habit forming and that it will not lose its efficacy on continued use.

The prophylactic use of nitroglycerin emphasized by Murrell when he first introduced the drug in 1879 is frequently neglected. If attacks are induced by definite unavoidable activities, placing a tablet under the tongue a few minutes beforehand will prevent the attack. The duration of the prophylactic effect is frequently a half hour and may be as long as an hour. In patients with frequent attacks during the day, even at rest, regular use of the tablet every hour or two hours throughout the day may be advisable.

AMYL NITRITE, introduced by Brunton in 1867, is the most potent and rapidly acting of all nitrites. A liquid, it is dispensed in small glass perles or ampules which are crushed in a handkerchief or cloth at the time of attack. Two or three minims are contained in each perle. Amyl nitrite is rarely used, because nitroglycerin tablets are more convenient, less expensive and less likely to be attended by unpleasant symptoms. Octyl nitrite, which also is administered by inhalation, has no advantages over amyl nitrite. Erythrol tetranitrate and mannitol hexanitrate require approximately an hour to produce their full effect and have a duration of action of 6 hours. Their action is variable. In doses of 30 mg. erythrol tetranitrate is worthy of trial in patients with angina decubitus and in those with severe nocturnal attacks.

The XANTHINES are the preparations most commonly used for prolonged action to induce coronary vasodilatation and prevent attacks. Both theobromine and theophylline are relatively insoluble and are therefore prescribed in loose chemical combinations with the acetates, salicylates or ethylenediamine to increase solubility, absorption and effectiveness. The most commonly used preparations are theophylline with ethylenediamine (aminophylline), 0.1 to 0.2 gm.; theobromine sodium salicylate (Diuretin) in doses of 0.3 gm.; theobromine calcium salicylate, 0.5 gm.; and theobromine sodium acetate, 0.5 gm., three or four times daily. Drugs containing sodium should not be used for patients on markedly low sodium regimens. All these preparations induce nausea or even vomiting in some patients and in others may not lead to any discernible improvement. In some patients the clinical usefulness of these drugs is convincing. They therefore are worthy of trial over a period of weeks. Many of these preparations are available with enteric coating to obviate gastric distress; absorption is somewhat delayed and occasionally uncertain. In patients with nocturnal anginal attacks, diuretics may be useful.

QUINIDINE SULFATE, 0.3 gm. four times daily, also has been found useful. It occasionally causes toxic manifestations in these doses, but may be valuable in patients who experience no benefit from the purine derivatives. Its duration of action is approximately 6 hours.

Many other agents have been proposed for the treatment of angina pectoris: potassium iodide, testosterone propionate, papaverine, atropine sulfate, vitamin E. The writer has not found them of value.

DIGITALIS in the usual dosage should be given in the presence of congestive failure. In such patients, angina pectoris may be favorably influenced. Digitalis is not indicated, however, in uncomplicated angina pectoris; indeed, some patients experience aggravation of their symptoms.

Treatment of Special Conditions. SYPHILIS. When angina pectoris is due to syphilitic aortitis and the serologic tests are positive, treatment with procaine penicillin G in doses of 600,000 units daily for ten days is indicated. As a precautionary measure against a possible Herxheimer reaction, the administration of penicillin should be preceded by four intramuscular injections of 1.5 cc. of bismuth subsalicylate in oil at five- to seven-day intervals. Further long-term experience is necessary to appraise the efficacy of penicillin in this condition; antiluetic therapy occasionally yields gratifying improvement.

ANEMIA. In anemia, particularly when marked, the work of the heart is increased. In some patients with angina pectoris, correction of the anemia may be followed by amelioration or even disappearance of cardiac pain.

DIABETES MELLITUS. Hypoglycemia may be attended by greatly increased cardiac pain. Special care must be exercised in regulating the dosage of insulin to avoid hypoglycemia. It is frequently wise to be content with blood sugar levels somewhat higher than are usually considered optimal.

THYROTOXICOSIS. In some patients with thyrotoxicosis, particularly those of middle or advanced years, the attendant increased work of the heart and other cardiovascular derangements of the disease give rise to angina pectoris. Such patients probably have a moderate degree of coronary arteriosclerosis which by itself would not be sufficient to give rise to cardiac pain. They may show marked clinical improvement or even disappearance of angina after subtotal thyroidectomy or the use of antithyroid drugs.

MYXEDEMA. Myxedematous patients with angina pectoris must be given thyroid with great caution. The increased cardiac work attendant on the raising of the metabolic rate may aggravate angina pectoris or even result in death. The myxedematous patient is hypersensitive to thyroid; therefore 6 to 12 mg. daily may be sufficient to relieve the patient of the unpleasant symptoms of myxedema and cause a rise in the metabolic rate of 10 or 15 per cent, but still safeguard the heart from unnecessary work.

Surgical and Other Methods in the Treatment of Intractable Angina Pectoris. Under a program of medical therapy most patients are able to lead a comfortable existence. For those who remain incapacitated despite all medical measures, various special procedures have been proposed.

SURGICAL INTERRUPTION OF PAIN PATHWAYS FROM THE HEART is based on the fact that the pathways of cardiac pain are all concentrated in the upper thorax, and reach the upper four spinal nerves over the sympathetic *rami communicantes* to enter the spinal cord over the posterior roots. Consequently, these pain pathways may be interrupted by sympathectomy, posterior rhizotomy or paravertebral block with alcohol. Alcohol injection is the method of choice. In some patients comparative freedom from pain is achieved. Almost all such patients still experience slight residual symptoms on effort or excitement which, therefore, can be regarded as danger or warning signals, safeguarding the patients from undue risk of continuing with exercise. Not infrequently, alcohol injection is followed by severe intercostal neuritis, pleurisy or pneumothorax; toxic myelitis may occur. While this procedure is the simplest of all surgical methods, it requires high skill and extensive experience. J. C. White and Bland have advocated posterior rhizotomy as a comparatively safe and effective procedure when alcohol injection has failed or has caused severe neuralgia. This operation involves the risk of ischemic transverse myelitis and must be reserved for patients well able to withstand the stress of such a procedure.

OPERATIONS TO INCREASE CARDIAC BLOOD FLOW BY THE DEVELOPMENT OF ANASTOMOTIC COLLATERAL VESSELS. The pericardial implantation of subpectoral muscle or omentum, the establishment of pericardial adhesions by chemical or mechanical irritation of the pericardial sac, pericoronary neurectomy, ligation of the great cardiac vein and anastomosis of a systemic artery to the coronary sinus are methods still in the experimental stage and not to be recommended as acceptable forms of therapy.

ROENTGEN THERAPY of the upper six thoracic sympathetic rami communicantes and radiation applied to the suprarenal glands have been recommended, but in the writer's experience have not been successful.

INDUCTION OF THE HYPOMETABOLIC STATE. Surgical total thyroidectomy was proposed by the writer and associates to lessen the work of the heart and hence reduce relative myocardial ischemia. Significant clinical improvement in euthyroid patients was reported by various clinics, including the writer's. The rationale of the procedure was verified in that the degree of alleviation of angina pectoris was generally proportional to the degree of reduction in the metabolic rate. The magnitude of the operation, however, in these patients with advanced heart disease and the occurrence of complications and progression of the underlying disease, which prevented worth-while results in approximately half of the patients, precluded adoption of the procedure as a generally applicable practical measure.

The advent of RADIOACTIVE IODINE (I^{131}) offered the possibility of achieving the same result by medical rather than surgical means. The clinical results observed by the writer and his associates are most satisfactory and have been corroborated by the experience in many other clinics.

The THIOUREA DERIVATIVES, including propylthiouracil, also have been used to attain the hypometabolism of total thyroidectomy by medical instead of surgical means. These drugs are readily available, comparatively inexpensive and, like I^{131}, are administered by mouth. Unfortunately, however, hypothyroidism can be induced in only some patients. Moreover, to maintain hypothyroidism in the patients in whom it is effective, administration of the drug must be continued for the remainder of the patient's life. At any time during such administration, dangerous drug reactions, including granulocytopenia and agranulocytosis, and death may suddenly occur.

ACUTE MYOCARDIAL INFARCTION

(Coronary Occlusion, Coronary Thrombosis)

Definition. Acute myocardial infarction is the clinical syndrome characterized by prolonged substernal oppression or pain, a fall in blood pressure and other manifestations of shock, accompanied by characteristic progressive electrocardiographic changes, fever, leukocytosis and an increased sedimentation rate.

Etiology. Acute myocardial infarction is the most frequent cardiac emergency which confronts the physician. The primary cause is an inadequate coronary blood supply. Occlusion by thrombosis, subintimal hemorrhage, rupture of an atheromatous abscess or embolism is usually responsible. Prolonged effort or excitement in the presence of a previously compromised circulation may lead to infarction without the occurrence of fresh coronary arterial lesions. Since the myocardial infarct is the pathologic lesion responsible for the clinical syndrome, and since the presence, absence or exact character of the arterial occlusion cannot be diagnosed clinically, it is more accurate to use the term "acute myocardial infarction" rather than alternative designations such as coronary thrombosis, coronary occlusion, coronary insufficiency, and so on.

Arteriosclerosis is the most frequent etiology, but in a few cases arteritis due to syphilis, rheumatic fever, systemic infections or thromboangiitis obliterans may be responsible.

Acute myocardial infarction affects men approximately six times as often as women and occurs with increasing frequency with advancing years, particularly after 50 years of age. Occasionally it strikes in the forties, thirties or even twenties. Acute myocardial infarction may be the first clinical manifestation of coronary arteriosclerosis; in approximately half of the patients, however, angina pectoris, mild or severe, has been present. Other factors of etiologic importance have been discussed previously and will not be repeated here. In most instances acute myocardial infarction occurs without relation to effort or other discernible clinical event. In some persons, one or more of the following *precipitating factors* may be evident: unusual exertion, insulin hypoglycemia, concussion or trauma to the precordial area, or shock consequent to operation, paroxysmal tachycardia, hemorrhage or other cause.

Symptoms and Signs. The onset of acute myocardial infarction is signalled by the abrupt appearance of severe persistent pain. This is variously described as agonizing, sharp, viselike, tearing, cutting, gripping, burning, crushing or choking. In some patients it is described as a fullness, heaviness or pressure. Occasionally the pain initially is relatively mild, increasing progressively in severity and becoming intense only after 15 to 30 minutes. The pain is usually referred to the upper or middle third of the sternum, but may arise beneath the lower third, over the precordium, in the epigastrium or elsewhere in the upper abdomen. In the latter instances a substernal toris. They immediately recognize the difference in the pain, i.e., its greater severity and duration, its failure to respond to nitroglycerin, and occasionally its different quality. The pain almost always persists for at least a half hour and usually for several hours; after

Fig. 154

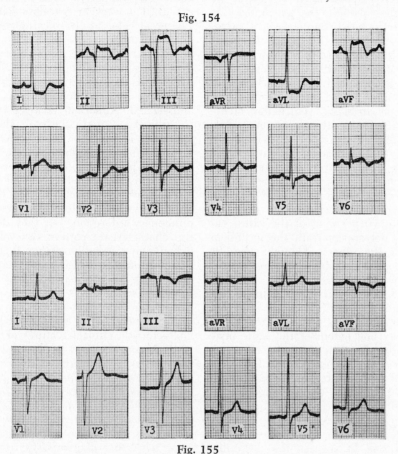

Fig. 155

Fig. 154. Acute posterior wall myocardial infarction. Deep Q in leads II, III and aVF indicates through and through, posterior wall infarction; Q in V6 indicates extension of infarct to lateral wall. S-T depression in leads I and aVL and elevation in leads II, III, aVF and V6, with late inversion of T waves, indicate an acute process.

Fig. 155. Old posterior wall myocardial infarction. Typical pattern of Q2, Q3, inverted T3, deep Q, and inverted T in aVF. No significant abnormality in precordial leads.

component may be disclosed by questioning the patient, a most important point in diagnosis. Radiation to the left and, at times, the right arm, into the left and right sides of the neck, and more rarely down into the abdomen, is observed. Patients occasionally complain of increased pain on swallowing. In contrast to the almost invariable immobility of patients with angina pectoris, some persons become restless or may even pace about the room.

Many patients have had prior angina pec-

it subsides a dull ache or heaviness remains. As Mackenzie pointed out, hyperesthesia frequently persists for hours or even days.

With the onset of the attack, the patient becomes cyanotic, pale or ashen gray, is frequently bathed in cold sweat, cannot get his breath, and in his anguish is apprehensive and feels that he is dying. Marked weakness is experienced and often helps distinguish the pain from angina pectoris. Physical examination discloses cold clammy skin and obvious dyspnea. Nausea is frequently present, and there may be repeated vomiting. The blood pressure may be at shock levels; in those with prior hypertension it may be profoundly lowered without reaching such low values. The pulse may not be detectable at the wrist and only barely palpable in the neck over the carotids. In most patients the ventricular rate is above 100, the heart sounds weak. Particularly in those who are in shock, the heart rate may be slow because of vagal inhibition or because of atrioventricular block. Gallop rhythm is frequently present. Ventricular extrasystoles, partial heart block, atrial fibrillation, or atrial or ventricular tachycardia is not infrequently encountered. Numerous medium moist rales may be heard over the chest, and in some patients expiration may be prolonged in the presence of musical ronchi and rales. In such patients the pulmonic second sound is usually accentuated. A pericardial friction rub is heard in approximately 10 per cent of the cases, but usually does not appear until the second or third day of the illness. Though generally transient or persisting for a day or two, it may last a week or more.

Fever and *leukocytosis* are commonly observed within the first 24 hours after the onset. The magnitude is roughly proportional to the severity and extent of the acute myocardial infarct. In some patients, fever appears only on the second or third day; in others the temperature may be normal throughout. Subnormal temperatures are often recorded in the presence of shock. The fever usually does not exceed 101°, but may reach 105° F. A high temperature should always lead one to suspect the possibility of complications such as pulmonary infarction, pneumonia or the concomitant presence of other infections.

Leukocytosis of 12,000 to 15,000 cells per cubic millimeter is commonly observed, and occasionally may reach 25,000 or more. Like the fever, the degree and duration of leukocytosis are a gauge of the extent of the infarction.

The *erythrocyte sedimentation rate* almost always becomes elevated within the first three or four days, even when the symptoms are mild and the temperature and white blood cell count remain normal. There is usually a lag of one or two days between the occurrence of infarction and the rise in the sedimentation rate.

The *electrocardiogram* is of paramount importance in establishing the diagnosis of acute myocardial infarction. The characteristic QRS changes, S-T segment displacements and T wave inversions are seen in practically every case (Figs. 154–158). These changes may appear immediately after the onset or may not develop for several days, in rare instances, not until a week or ten days have elapsed. The great value of electrocardiography in the diagnosis of acute myocardial infarction can be realized only if the meaning of the various deflections and their aberrations is understood and the limitations of electrocardiography are clearly defined and thoroughly appreciated. Abnormal changes in the electrocardiogram, particularly in the S-T segment and T wave, or the characteristic pattern of acute cor pulmonale, may be due to transient myocardial ischemia, nonischemic myocarditis, pericarditis, changes in position of the heart, or to noncardiac conditions such as cholecystitis, perforated peptic ulcer or pulmonary infarction, but they do not show the characteristic pattern of evolution seen in acute myocardial infarction. It is important, therefore, to take serial tracings every day or every few days to establish the progressive nature of the changes and to record the precordial and unipolar limb leads in addition to the standard limb leads. Contrariwise, the characteristic clinical features of acute myocardial infarction may be observed for days or even a week or more before electrocardiographic evidences appear. *In general, the greatest emphasis always should be placed on the clinical findings, and an unqualified diagnosis of acute myocardial infarction is hazardous unless the clinical features are in accordance with this diagnosis. Only rarely does one encounter unequivocal electrocardiographic evidence of acute myocardial infarction* in the absence of the clinical features.

Special Features, Complications and Sequelae. *Premonitory Symptoms and Signs.* The attack of acute myocardial infarction does not always appear unheralded. There may be forewarnings which, if heeded, permit the physician to suspect that an attack of acute myocardial infarction is impending, place the patient under close observation, diminish activities, and perhaps lessen the severity of the attack or even obviate its occurrence. Thus the appearance of angina pectoris in a previously well person, the abrupt, increased severity and frequency of attacks or the appearance of cardiac irregularities may signify the development of progressive narrowing or occlusion of a coronary artery.

Fig. 156

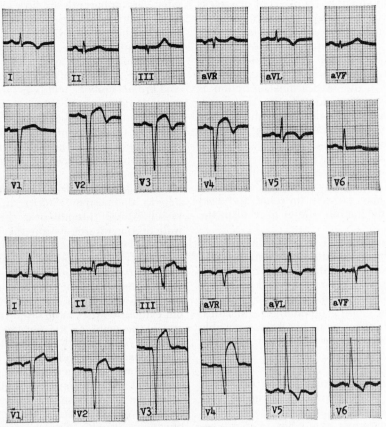

Fig. 157

Fig. 156. Recent anterior wall infarction and probable, old posterior wall infarction. Small Q in leads II, III and aVF suggests old posterior wall infarction. Deep QS in V4 indicates through and through apical infarction. Elevated S-T junction in V2 to V4 with coving and late, sharp inversion of T in leads I, aVL, and V2 to V5 indicate recent anterior wall process.

Fig. 157. Acute anteroseptal infarction plus left ventricular hypertrophy. Wide QRS, small Q, and inverted T in leads I, aVL, V5 and V6 indicate left ventricular hypertrophy. Deep QS and elevated S-T in V1 to V4 (most marked in V4) indicate acute anteroseptal infarction.

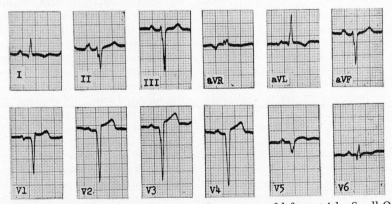

Fig. 158. Old anterior wall myocardial infarction with aneurysm of left ventricle. Small Q and inverted T in leads I and aVL, deep Q in V1, QS in V2 to V5, and Q in V6 indicate through and through, anterior wall infarction. Slightly elevated S-T junction in V1 to V4 persisted unchanged for months and is consistent with aneurysm of ventricular wall.

Painless Attacks with Dyspnea and Weakness. In approximately 10 per cent of attacks of acute myocardial infarction, pain is absent. Intense or moderate dyspnea, weakness and, occasionally, acute pulmonary edema occupy the foreground of the clinical picture. In some persons who experience no cardiac pain the onset of acute myocardial infarction is signalled by syncope and collapse. Acute myocardial infarction may develop without being evidenced by pain in any patient in whom the sensorium is clouded by diabetic coma, uremia, advanced congestive failure or hemiplegia. In such instances, unexplained fever, leukocytosis, the onset of dyspnea or cardiac irregularity may provide the clue and lead to electrocardiographic studies to confirm the diagnosis.

The Arrhythmias. Every known form of arrhythmia has been witnessed during attacks of acute myocardial infarction. Their recognition and treatment are described elsewhere (p. 1344). Atrial and ventricular extrasystoles are the most common irregularities; paroxysmal ventricular tachycardia, a possible precursor of ventricular fibrillation, is one of the most serious.

Rupture of the Heart. Rupture of the heart is responsible for approximately 10 per cent of all deaths occurring during the acute stage of myocardial infarction. It generally occurs without premonitory symptoms or signs between the fourth and fourteenth day after the onset of the attack. This fatal complication is particularly prone to occur in hypertensive patients with no previous history of old myocardial infarction or congestive failure. Sustained hypertension or excessive effort usually precedes rupture.

Rupture of the Interventricular Septum. This rare complication can be recognized clinically by the development of a loud systolic murmur, usually maximal in the fourth and fifth intercostal spaces to the left of the sternum. A palpable thrill may be present. This complication is not incompatible with survival of the patient even for several years.

Rupture of a papillary muscle is rare. Death usually occurs abruptly but acute and intractable pulmonary edema may be observed. A systolic murmur loudest over the cardiac apex may appear.

Aneurysm of the Ventricle. The scar tissue bulging out with each systolic contraction gives rise to paradoxical pulsation on fluoroscopy. Such aneurysms, while undoubtedly decreasing the efficiency of the heart somewhat, are apparently of little clinical importance and rarely rupture. Mural thrombi may form in the sac and give rise to embolic phenomena at any time, even years later. The most common site of aneurysm is in the region of the apex of the left ventricle.

Thromboembolic episodes are among the most dangerous and frequent complications. Central or peripheral extension of the original coronary thrombus may block important arterial branches and lead to necrosis of areas contiguous to the original infarct or of entirely different areas. A part of the thrombus may break off and lead to secondary infarction in the peripheral area supplied by the vessel. Mural thrombi over the endocardial wall of the infarct within the left ventricle may lead to embolization in the brain, extremities, spleen, kidneys or other organs. Pulmonary embolism is rather frequent; it may be due to emboli from mural thrombi on the right ventricular surface of the septum, but evidently arises more often from thromboses in the veins of the lower extremities or pelvis. The inactivity of the extremities, the reduced arterial blood pressure and systemic blood flow, and increased coagulability of the blood after the onset of acute myocardial infarction predispose the patient to these serious accidents. These thromboembolic complications usually develop within the first four weeks after the onset of the illness; their incidence is higher in the second week.

Pain in the Shoulder Girdle, Arm and Hand. Persistent pain in the left shoulder, and also at times the right arm and hand, within the first few months after acute myocardial infarction is not infrequent and may be severely painful and disabling. It was observed by Ernstene in approximately 15 per cent of patients. The symptoms and signs vary considerably. In approximately one third of the instances pain, swelling, tenderness and limitation of movement develop also in the joints of the fingers, hand and wrist of the affected side. Subsequent atrophy of the muscles may occur and often is more marked than that which would be anticipated on the basis of disuse only. The immobility of the shoulder and upper extremities during the period of enforced bed rest is undoubtedly an important factor in producing this *"shoulder-hand"* syndrome. The marked atrophy suggests that trophic disturbances, either primarily or secondarily induced by acute myocardial infarction, may play a prominent role. It is important to recognize the onset of this disability, since, to be effective, early treatment is urgently indicated.

Angina Pectoris. Antecedent angina pectoris is present in approximately one half of the patients prior to their attack of myocardial infarction. After acute myocardial infarction most patients experience an intensification of angina, and many who were free prior to the episode of infarction suffer mild or more severe attacks. Occasionally, but all too rarely, a patient who had angina pectoris prior to acute myocardial infarction experiences no further attacks. In some of these instances a concomitant fall of blood pressure from hypertensive to more normal levels occurs, but in other patients the mechanism is obscure; obliteration of a previously ischemic area may have occurred.

Differential Diagnosis. The diagnosis of acute myocardial infarction can be made with great accuracy. A mistaken diagnosis of its presence or the false diagnosis of other conditions will rarely be made if the cardinal criteria of acute myocardial infarction are kept clearly in mind and, in every instance, the other conditions with which it may be confused are briefly reviewed. Occasionally two conditions may be simultaneously encountered. Thus, the patient suffering from a bleeding or perforated peptic ulcer may go into shock, which in turn may lead to prolonged ischemia and acute myocardial infarction. Similarly, a patient with acute myocardial infarction with a mural thrombus on the septal wall of the right ventricle may suffer pulmonary embolism.

Acute abdominal disease must be clearly differentiated, lest a needless or even fatal operation be performed on a patient with acute myocardial infarction; or, conversely and equally disastrously, a false diagnosis of acute myocardial infarction be made and the patient allowed to die of an undiagnosed *ruptured gallbladder, acute appendicitis* or other acute abdominal condition. *Acute cholecystitis, penetrating* or *perforated peptic ulcer, acute pancreatitis, acute mesenteric thrombosis, renal colic* or *intestinal obstruction* also may simulate acute myocardial infarction. Such confusion is particularly likely when the pain of acute myocardial infarction is referred to the upper abdomen. Nausea, vomiting, slight distention, fever, muscle spasm and leukocytosis may be common to the two conditions. The presence of specific abdominal signs, such as localized pain, tenderness and spasm, or a palpable mass in the presence of a normal electrocardiogram and normal heart sounds, usually leads to the correct diagnosis.

Hiatus hernia and *cardiospasm* may give rise to severe substernal pain, but the absence of cardiac signs and, in the case of hiatus hernia, the tendency for the attacks to occur particularly on lying down after big meals, and the exacerbation of pain on deep inspiration serve to clarify the diagnosis.

It is a good rule to consider *pulmonary embolism* carefully whenever a diagnosis of acute myocardial infarction is made, but not firmly established. The character and localization of the pain, its relation to respiration, hemoptysis, the physical signs in the chest aided by x-ray studies and the clinical and electrocardiographic evidences of acute cor pulmonale will establish the presence of pulmonary embolism. As previously pointed out, both pulmonary embolism and acute myocardial infarction may be present.

Acute nonspecific idiopathic pericarditis, dissecting aneurysm, acute spontaneous pneumothorax, spontaneous mediastinal emphysema, herpes zoster or the prolonged precordial distress of *paroxysmal tachycardia* may simulate acute myocardial infarction; their recognition is discussed elsewhere under their respective headings.

Prognosis. Until fatal and unpredictable complications such as pulmonary embolism, rupture, syncope, cardiac standstill, ventricular paroxysmal tachycardia or fibrillation can be foretold, the prognosis of acute myocardial infarction always must remain uncertain, and our opinion must be expressed with reserve. These unpredictable complications occur largely within the first four weeks, but with decreasing frequency during this period. The first two weeks are the most dangerous. Patients who survive the third week generally recover, although the degree of residual disability because of congestive failure, angina pectoris or other complications and sequelae varies greatly from patient to patient. Patients with seemingly slight myocardial involvement and a smooth encouraging course may suddenly die; and, contrariwise, patients with a stormy, complicated course survive. Nevertheless, there are important general guideposts which are helpful in rendering an opinion as to the outlook in the individual patient.

The mortality of the acute attack varies

from 25 to 35 per cent in most reported series. The prognosis is somewhat better in younger persons than in those of advanced years and more favorable in men than in women.

The extent of cardiac damage greatly influences the outcome. Among the most important indices of widespread infarction are shock with conspicuous fall in blood pressure, cold clammy skin, tachycardia over 100, the presence of congestive failure, and fever, leukocytosis and elevated sedimentation rate. The degree and duration of such abnormalities weigh heavily in estimating the outlook. Fever of 102° F. or more, a leukocytosis of 20,000 cells per cubic millimeter or higher, and the appearance of pulmonary or hepatic engorgement with peripheral edema are ominous signs. Weak heart sounds, cardiac dilatation, gallop rhythm and the presence of irregular heart action are unfavorable. Electrocardiography, though of the greatest diagnostic importance and permitting localization of the infarct, is of little assistance in prognosis except in those instances in which the evidences of injury in many of the precordial leads suggest widespread involvement.

The probability of survival is enhanced by the absence of prior cardiac disease such as congestive failure, angina pectoris or previous attacks of myocardial infarction.

The mortality is increased by the presence of other diseases which add to the burden of the damaged heart. Thus diabetes mellitus with its tendency to progressive coronary arteriosclerosis, arterial hypertension demanding increased work of the heart, rheumatic and syphilitic heart disease affect the outcome adversely. Similarly, a family history of attacks in many other members of the family, particularly when they have occurred at a relatively early age, should lead to a more guarded prognosis.

Treatment. *The Immediate Management of the Acute Attack.* COMPLETE REST, PHYSICAL AND MENTAL, is essential. Superior nursing to spare the patient needless effort and to encourage equanimity is of utmost importance. In the presence of shock and profuse perspiration, the patient must be kept warm. The RELIEF OF PAIN should be prompt and complete. Morphine sulfate, 15 mg. subcutaneously, should be given at half-hour intervals until the desired effect is attained. The total dose should not exceed 0.065 gm. The effect of each dose should be carefully observed before administering the next dose. If the pain is intense, 30 mg. should be given at once, hypodermically; or if the pain is extreme or the situation critical, slow intravenous injection of 0.015 mg. is advisable. If an idiosyncrasy to morphine and related compounds is present, meperidine in doses of 75 to 100 mg. or one of the newer preparations such as methadone in doses of 5 to 15 mg. may be used by mouth or subcutaneously.

OXYGEN THERAPY is indicated in all moderate or severe cases, always when the pain is resistant to other measures, and whenever cyanosis is present. Dyspnea is relieved, pain is lessened, the heart rate is slowed, and not infrequently the patient soon lapses into quiet, restful sleep.

AMINOPHYLLINE (theophylline with ethylene diamine), 0.48 gm., or PAPAVERINE HYDROCHLORIDE, 30 to 90 mg., administered by *slow* intravenous injection, may be used if the relief of pain is not attained by the previously mentioned methods.

ATROPINE SULFATE, hypodermically, in an initial dose of 0.8 mg. and additional doses of 0.4 mg. every 8 hours during the first three or four days, has been strongly recommended in the hope of blocking adverse reflexes which occur after acute myocardial infarction. In patients with bradycardia it is occasionally useful, but its effect in causing an elevated heart rate in other patients, particularly in the presence of atrial fibrillation, is undesirable.

DIGITALIS should be administered to all patients with evidences of congestive failure or with rapid ventricular rate due to atrial fibrillation or atrial flutter. The rapid absorption of some of the purified glycosides such as digitoxin frequently obviates the necessity of parenteral administration. Rapid digitalization can be accomplished by 0.6 mg. of digitoxin followed by 0.2 mg. after 2 hours, and then by 0.2 mg. every 4 hours until the desired effect is attained. In the absence of these definite indications it is unwise to use digitalis. (For a discussion of the pharmacotherapeutics of digitalis and allied drugs, see the chapter on The Treatment of Congestive Heart Failure.)

QUINIDINE SULFATE has been advised routinely to minimize the possible development of paroxysmal tachycardia or fibrillation. The drug is not without occasional adverse effects, causing nausea, vomiting or diarrhea in some patients; in moderate dosage it may also cause a fall in blood pressure in some patients with acute myocardial infarction. In the presence of extrasystoles, however, its administration should be attempted in doses of 0.2 gm. every 3 or 4 hours. If gastrointestinal symptoms are induced, enteric-coated preparations or the administration of the drug parenterally is indicated.

NITROGLYCERIN is hazardous in the acute phase of acute myocardial infarction and should not be used. If the patient is first seen in his initial attack of cardiac pain, this drug should not be administered until the diagnosis of acute myocardial infarct has been excluded. In the presence of fresh coronary occlusion, administration of nitroglycerin may lead to a fall in blood pressure and precipitate massive infarction or death.

DIET. A low caloric intake of approximately 1000 calories and consisting of readily ingestible and digestible foods is indicated during the first two or three days. Fruit juices, milk, ginger ale, ice cream, custards, eggs and toast may be given. Fluids sufficient to produce a daily urinary output of 1500 cc. and restriction of salt to 2 gm. or less daily are indicated.

The BOWELS may be neglected at the onset, but one of the heavier mineral oils or emulsified preparations should be prescribed in 30 cc. doses once or twice daily to avoid the discomfort of constipation and abdominal distention. If constipation requires treatment, a retention enema of 90 cc. of plain mineral oil may be administered in the evening. If cathartics later prove necessary, one of the milder saline laxatives is preferable; straining at stool must be avoided.

Treatment of Certain Complications. SHOCK must be energetically combated. The patient must be kept warm. Continuous administration of oxygen in concentrations of 50 to 90 per cent, opiates and stimulants should be utilized. The slow intravenous infusion of 5 per cent glucose in physiologic saline solution is indicated especially in the presence of dehydration because of profuse perspiration or vomiting. Transfusions of plasma or blood in amounts of 200 to 250 cc. may be given in refractory situations, particularly in the presence of anemia, and repeated at 2- to 4-hour intervals to maintain the systolic pressure at or above 100 mm. Epinephrine is hazardous and is contraindicated.

The clinical usefulness of vasopressor drugs has become increasingly apparent. Neo-Synephrine 0.1 to 0.2 cc., Paredrine 8 to 15 mg., methoxamine or mephentermine (Wyamine) sulfate may be used at half-hour intervals intramuscularly as well as intravenously. The latter route should be used only in critical situations. The most potent agent is L-norepinephrine (arterenol) which may be effective when other preparations have failed. It cannot be given subcutaneously or intramuscularly. Extravascular administration produces severe necrosis and sloughing. Norepinephrine (arterenol) is best used by slow intravenous drip, each cubic centimeter containing 4 to 12 micrograms. Injection into leg veins is dangerous. The flow is maintained at a rate sufficient to elevate the systolic blood pressure to approximately 100 mm. Hg or to alleviate the clinical manifestations of shock. The use of pressor agents decreases the mortality of acute myocardial infarction to a significant though inevitably limited extent.

ACUTE PULMONARY EDEMA in the presence of cyanosis and engorged veins should be combated by adequate sedation, use of high concentrations of oxygen, and tourniquets applied to the legs and arms at pressures somewhat below diastolic. If the situation is critical and the patient plethoric, venesection should be considered. Ethyl alcohol inhalation may be useful with marked edema and frothy sputum.

Not infrequently the clinical characteristics of shock and of acute pulmonary edema are exhibited simultaneously. Opiates, oxygen therapy, and cautious administration of plasma and of vasopressor agents are indicated. Rapid digitalization may be employed to combat left ventricular failure.

PAROXYSMAL VENTRICULAR TACHYCARDIA must be treated vigorously, not only because of its inherently adverse effects, but also because it is often the immediate precursor of fatal ventricular fibrillation. Procaine amide hydrochloride (Pronestyl) and quinidine are the most effective agents. For the treatment of this disorder, as well as of the other arrhythmias which may complicate the clinical course, see the chapter on Cardiac Arrhythmias. Digitalis is almost always contraindicated in the presence of paroxysmal ventricular tachycardia. In the presence of cardiac standstill, intracardiac injection of 0.25 or 0.5 cc. of epinephrine may be tried. External electrical stimulation of the heart through electrodes applied to the chest wall has recently been shown by Zoll to be effective.

CONGESTIVE FAILURE is not uncommon and should be treated with digitalis, diuretics and the other measures usually employed, as outlined elsewhere.

Treatment of Subsequent Course of Acute Myocardial Infarction. After the pain of acute myocardial infarction has subsided, codeine sulfate, 30 mg. by mouth or subcutaneously, may be substituted together with relatively mild, quickly acting sedatives such as phenobarbital, 15 mg. four times a day, to promote rest. The xanthines, such as theobromine sodium acetate, 0.5 gm., or aminophylline, 0.1 to 0.2 gm. three or four times daily, are commonly used to promote vasodilatation and the healing process. The patient should be permitted to assume whatever position is most comfortable for him. A program of massage and passive movements of the arms and legs should be inaugurated after the acute phase of the illness to prevent venous thromboses and periarthritis of the shoulder girdle. Elastic stockings are frequently employed until the patient becomes ambulatory. Deep breathing should be encouraged to prevent atelectasis. The diet should be simple and not above caloric resting requirements; frequent small feedings may be desirable. A reduction regimen is to be used for obese patients. In the presence of diabetes mellitus requiring insulin, hypoglycemia is to be avoided. Management of the bowels as described during the acute phase is to be continued, and the use of a commode at the bedside may be permitted after a week or ten days to those who cannot use a bed pan without excessive straining.

ANTICOAGULANT THERAPY, consisting of Dicumarol or allied drugs, alone or in combination with heparin, has been shown by Wright, Allen and others to diminish the incidence of thromboembolic complications and to lower the mortality rate. In recent years strong evidence has been brought forward by Russek and his associates that anticoagulant therapy is unnecessary in "good risk" patients. Included in this group are patients who, when first seen, appear on the basis of history and symptoms to have a small and not severe lesion, and those who are having their first attack and do not manifest arrhythmias, congestive failure, thrombotic complications, or evidence of shock. Dicumarol is administered orally; no parenteral preparations are available. Three hundred milligrams are usually administered the first day if there are no contraindications. A single dose of Dicumarol requires 24 to 48 hours to attain its maximum effect; therefore subsequent dosage is gauged each day after the daily prothrombin report is available. Two hundred milligrams are usually given the second day, and 50 to 100 mg. on subsequent days to maintain the prothrombin time at approximately 30 seconds, corresponding to 10 per cent of normal. When the prothrombin time is 30 to 35 seconds, the drug is omitted. Anticoagulant therapy usually is maintained for twenty-one to twenty-eight days.

Heparin may be used in doses of 75 mg. every 4 hours or by constant intravenous drip during the first 24 to 48 hours until the action of Dicumarol becomes manifest, particularly if the patient is first seen several days after the onset.

Unless these drugs are given with a full knowledge of their pharmacologic characteristics, their contraindications and their inherent dangers, and unless absolutely reliable laboratory measurements are available, their use is hazardous and should be avoided.

The *duration of rest* after acute myocardial infarction is three months or longer. Complete rest for four to six weeks is usually indicated. After mild uncomplicated attacks the patient may be allowed to sit in a chair for increasing periods during the fifth and sixth weeks. After severe attacks, particularly when attended by congestive failure or prolonged weakness, longer periods of many months of bed rest may be necessary. In the exercise of clinical judgment, the sedimentation rate is helpful. Continued elevation should indicate caution, since, other conditions excluded, it bespeaks continued muscle necrosis. A return to normal or, if known, to the control value is a favorable sign.

CORONARY FAILURE: THE CLINICAL SYNDROME OF CARDIAC PAIN INTERMEDIATE BETWEEN ANGINA PECTORIS AND ACUTE MYOCARDIAL INFARCTION

Definition. Coronary failure denotes attacks of cardiac pain or distress too prolonged to be consistent with angina pectoris, but, on the other hand, not attended by the various recognized features of acute myocardial infarction such as sustained leukocytosis, fever, prolonged rise in sedimentation rate and progressive characteristic electrocardiographic changes.

Etiology and Pathologic Physiology. The pathologic physiology generally underlying all myocardial pain is relative ischemia; the clinical and pathologic consequences depend on its duration and degree, not on the particular mechanism of its production. In accordance with this concept, attacks of coronary failure are occasionally coincident with increased demands on the heart such as paroxysmal arrhythmia, emotion or effort; in other instances decreased coronary blood flow, consequent to the hypotension of shock due

underlying physiopathologic mechanism is prolonged but reversible myocardial ischemia. Correspondingly, on pathologic examination no resultant myocardial infarction or extensive fibrosis is found.

Symptoms and Signs. The attacks of pain or distress are infrequent compared to

Clinical Characteristics of Angina Pectoris, Coronary Failure and Acute Myocardial Infarction

	ANGINA PECTORIS	CORONARY FAILURE	ACUTE MYOCARDIAL INFARCTION
I. Clinical manifestations			
1. Pain			
Onset	Sudden	Sudden	Sudden
Location	Usually substernal with radiation to arms	Same	Same
Quality and intensity	Vague, pressure, squeezing, choking	Same as angina pectoris, but more intense; similar quality	More intense, viselike
Induced by	Effort, emotion, cold	Same, but may occur at rest	No necessary relation to effort, emotion or cold
Duration	Usually less than 15 minutes	Prolonged longer than 20 minutes	Usually more prolonged
Frequency	Usually frequent	Infrequent	Infrequent
Response to nitroglycerin	Usually striking	Unusual or temporary	None
2. Peripheral vascular collapse (hypotension, sweating, nausea)	Absent	Unusual	Frequent
3. Pulmonary edema	Absent or rare	Unusual	Frequent
4. Death	Uncommon	Uncommon	Frequent
II. Evidences of myocardial necrosis			
1. Fever	Absent	Absent	Frequent
2. Leukocytosis	Absent	Absent	Frequent
3. Erythrocyte sedimentation rate	Slightly elevated (0.75 to 1.38 mm./min. in over 60%)	Same; no progressive change, usually below 1.5 mm./minute	Progressive rise over 1.5 mm./min. in 2/3 of cases.
4. Pericardial friction rub	Absent	Absent	Diagnostic
5. Electrocardiograms	No change or transient changes in T waves and S-T segments	Same as angina pectoris; rarely marked changes, but temporary and nonprogressive	Progressive typical patterns; conduction defects, arrhythmias common

to hemorrhage, infection, dehydration, and so forth, is apparently responsible. When attacks of coronary failure occur without apparent precipitating factors or in circumstances which have not previously provoked pain, a recent reduction of coronary blood flow may be postulated. Such attacks may be due to the occurrence of acute coronary narrowing or occlusion. The exact pathologic mechanism of narrowing or occlusion, i.e., atherosclerosis, thrombosis, embolism, ulceration of an atheromatous plaque, subintimal hemorrhage or edema, is beyond determination by clinical means.

In all instances of coronary failure the

the oft-repeated episodes of angina pectoris. The distress is commonly more intense and prolonged than the patient's usual attacks of angina pectoris. The duration of pain is from one half hour to many hours. The pain is usually unresponsive to nitroglycerin and rest. The attacks may be provoked by exertion, emotion and other states in which the work of the heart is increased, but they may also occur during rest or sleep. The evidences of myocardial necrosis, such as sustained leukocytosis, progressive elevation of the sedimentation rate and fever, are absent. Electrocardiographic changes with the attacks are either absent or minor. Rarely, transient changes similar to those seen with myocardial infarction may be present for a period of hours with a return to the pattern present before the attack. Progressive electrocardiographic changes of the types characteristic of acute myocardial infarction do not occur. The blood pressure usually remains unchanged. Shock and pulmonary edema rarely occur.

Diagnosis. When a patient is first seen during or immediately after an attack of severe cardiac pain, the precise diagnosis often cannot be made. The evidences of acute myocardial infarction may appear only after hours or even days. When such manifestations are absent or are minor or transient during the ensuing days, the diagnosis of coronary failure becomes clear. The majority of instances occur in patients with angina pectoris; the fact that the pain is more prolonged and frequently of greater intensity and sometimes of different quality than that of angina pectoris is of diagnostic importance.

Differential Diagnosis. Coronary failure must be distinguished from the noncardiac conditions described under Angina Pectoris and Acute Myocardial Infarction, and also must be differentiated from these latter two types of cardiac pain (see table).

Treatment. The patients should be confined to bed for the first few days to observe the course of the symptoms and signs. Occasional instances of coronary failure are followed after an interval of hours or days by an attack of acute myocardial infarction, a sequence of events noted by Feil and by Sampson and Eliaser and designated by them as "preliminary pain" and "impending acute coronary artery occlusion." In the majority of cases this sequence does not occur and the patient is permitted to assume gradually increasing activity, sitting up in a chair after a week or ten days, and then becoming ambulatory. In' each case clinical judgment may modify the regimen, but in any event the episode will not be dismissed as an attack of angina pectoris, nor will the patient be bedridden for many weeks. Should the attack of coronary failure be the forerunner of myocardial infarction, the patient will be under favorable conditions permitting early diagnosis and immediate treatment. Anticoagulant therapy may be instituted as a prophylactic measure against the possible development of a coronary thrombus or its propagation if already present.

HERRMAN L. BLUMGART

References

Allen, E. V., Barker, N. W., and Waugh, J. M.: A Preparation from Spoiled Sweet Clover [3, 3′ Methylene-Bis-(4-Hydroxycoumarin)] Which Prolongs Coagulation and Prothrombin Time of the Blood: A Clinical Study. J.A.M.A., 120:1009, 1942.

Blumgart, H. L., Freedberg, A. S., and Kurland, G. S.: Hypothyroidism Produced by Radioactive Iodine (I^{131}) in the Treatment of Euthyroid Patients with Angina Pectoris and Congestive Heart Failure. Early Results in Various Types of Cardiovascular Diseases and Associated Pathologic States. Circulation, 1:1105, 1950.

Blumgart, H. L., Schlesinger, M. J., and Zoll, P. M.: Angina Pectoris, Coronary Failure and Acute Myocardial Infarction. J.A.M.A., 116:91, 1941.

Ernstene, A. C.: Coronary Heart Disease. Springfield, Ill., Charles C Thomas, 1948.

Freedberg, A. S., Blumgart, H. L., Zoll, P. M., and Schlesinger, M. J.: Coronary Failure—The Clinical Syndrome of Cardiac Pain Intermediate between Angina Pectoris and Acute Myocardial Infarction. J.A.M.A., 138:107, 1948.

Gubner, R. S., Rodstein, M., and Ungerleider H. E.: Ballistocardiography: An Appraisal of Technic, Physiologic Principles, and Clinical Values. Circulation, 7:268, 1953.

Kurland, G. S., and Malach, M.: The Clinical Use of Nor-Epinephrine in the Treatment of Shock Accompanying Myocardial Infarction and Other Conditions. New England J. Med., 247:383, 1952.

Russek, H. I., Zohman, B. L., White, L. G., and Doerner, A. A.: Indications for Bishydroxycoumarin (Dicumarol) in Acute Myocardial Infarction. J.A.M.A., 145:390, 1951.

Stewart, H. J.: Cardiac Therapy. New York, Paul B. Hoeber, Inc., 1952, p. 112.

White, P. D.: Heart Disease. 4th ed. New York, The Macmillan Co., 1951.

Wright, I. S., Marple, C. D., and Beck, D. F.: Anticoagulant Therapy of Coronary Thrombosis with Myocardial Infarction. J.A.M.A., 138:1074, 1948.

Zoll, P. M., Linenthal, A. J., Norman, L. R., with the assistance of Belgard, A. H.: Treatment of Stokes-Adams Disease by External Electric Stimulation of the Heart. Circulation, 9:482, 1954.

MISCELLANEOUS PATHOLOGIC CONDITIONS OF THE HEART

NEOPLASM OF THE HEART

Cardiac neoplasm is a rare and relatively unimportant cause of heart disease. Because of its rarity and the complex histopathology of the primary tumors, the number of reported cases is greatly out of proportion to the actual occurrence of the condition.

Incidence. Metastatic malignancies involving the heart and pericardium comprised

10.9 per cent of the 1082 cases of malignant disease discovered in 11,100 consecutive autopsies at the Cleveland City Hospital from 1919 to 1939. A total of 118 carcinomas of the bronchus and of the breast were found as the primary lesion in 48 per cent. The other primary sites may be the uterus, rectum, kidney, gallbladder and malignant melanoma.

Primary tumors of the heart and pericardium are less frequent than metastatic neoplasms. The total number of cases of primary neoplasm of the heart reported up to 1945 was 165. Any part of the heart may be involved, but the right chambers are the seat of the tumor much more frequently than the left, particularly the right atrium.

Morbid Anatomy. A review of the reported cases emphasizes the complex histopathology of cardiac tumors. However, they can, for clinical purposes, be grouped into the following basic types:

1. Sarcomas arising from any mesenchymal elements in the heart wall
2. Pseudomyomas, which are most likely organized thrombi, but not true neoplasms
3. Rhabdomyomas (congenital nodular glycogenic tumors of the heart, Batchelor-Mann 1945).

Diagnosis. Cardiac tumors are seldom suspected and less often diagnosed *ante mortem* because of the rarity of the disease and the lack of characteristic symptoms and physical signs. Occurrence of progressive signs of primary right heart failure not explained by valve lesions or pulmonary disease is suggestive of an intracardiac neoplasm involving the right atrium. Inconstant signs of mitral stenosis, changing rapidly and grossly with altered position, should make one suspicious of a pseudomyoma in the left atrium. If transient episodes of tamponade of the pulmonary circulation occur, owing to stoppage of the mitral orifice, the diagnosis is more *certain*. Neoplasm may be considered as a possible diagnosis when an otherwise inexplicable gross disturbance of rhythm is present in association with a bizarre cardiac silhouette. One may say that multiplicity and inconsistency of both symptoms and physical signs are admittedly the most helpful leads to a clinical diagnosis of cardiac neoplasm.

Hemorrhagic pericardial effusion is a frequent manifestation of metastatic malignancy to the heart and pericardium. Characteristically, the hemoglobin content of the aspirated fluid is high, 2 to 3 gm. per 100 cc., and the effusion invariably recurs promptly following aspiration. Following aspiration of the effusion, inflation of the pericardial sac with air and a restudy of the cardiac silhouette with x-rays and the fluoroscope frequently enables one to visualize tumor masses both in the pericardium and on the surface of the heart.

Prognosis of cardiac neoplasm is grave because neither surgery nor radiotherapy has as yet been developed sufficiently to justify optimism in their usage. It is conceivable that a pedunculated pseudomyoma of the auricle might be successfully removed by surgery.

WILLIAM B. PORTER

References

Batchelor, B. S., and Mann, M. E.: Congenital Glycogenic Tumors of the Heart. Arch. Path., 39:67, 1945.
Leach, W. B.: Primary Neoplasm of the Heart. Arch. Path., 22:198, 1947.
Pritchard, R. W.: Tumors of the Heart. Arch. Path., 51:98, 1951.
Ravid, J. M., and Sachs, J.: Tumors of the Heart. Am. Heart J., 26:385, 1943.
Wainwright, C. W.: Intracardiac Tumor Producing Signs of Valvular Heart Disease. Bull. Johns Hopkins Hosp., 48:187, 1938.
Weir, D. R., and Jones, B. C., Jr.: Primary Sarcoma of the Heart. Am. Heart J., 22:556, 1941.

SYPHILIS OF THE HEART

Occurrence of primary myocardial disease due to invasion of the heart muscle by the treponema of syphilis is extremely rare. The lesions which may be identified as syphilitic are localized gummas or diffusely scattered areas of interstitial myocardial infiltration with lymphocytic and plasma cells. The process is perivascular in location and is accompanied by varying degrees of muscle fiber degeneration. It is admittedly true that the latter condition is difficult, if not impossible, to differentiate from that caused by insufficiency of the coronary blood flow.

Symptoms and Diagnosis. There is no group of symptoms or physical signs peculiar to myocardial syphilis. Much emphasis has been given to the importance of syphilis in the causation of complete heart block; nevertheless, fibrosis of the bundle of His from coronary arteriosclerosis and occasionally from rheumatic myocarditis is the lesion usually found at necropsy in patients dying of Stokes-Adams syndrome.

Progressive and irreducible heart failure, unassociated with hypertension, valvular disease, coronary insufficiency or other obvious causes in a patient known to have syphilis, warrants a tentative yet conditional diagnosis of diffuse syphilitic myocarditis. Occurrence of ectopic ventricular rhythms from varying foci is suggestive of progressive myocardial disease which may be of syphilitic etiology, but is much more likely to be a result of severe coronary arteriosclerosis.

Sudden death may occur from syphilitic myocarditis, but certainly is much less frequent from that cause than from acute coronary insufficiency.

In view of its conceded rarity, the diagnosis of uncomplicated syphilis of the heart must be tentative and by exclusion. Because of the fact that symptoms are always delayed until widespread disease of the myocardium has occurred, the **prognosis** is grave.

Treatment. The care of patients who have heart failure is predicated on the basic principles established for such cases, with little primary concern for the specific etiology. With diminution of the symptoms and signs of cardiac insufficiency, appropriate antisyphilitic therapy should be instituted, as described in the chapter on Syphilis.

WILLIAM B. PORTER

References

Kobernick, S. D.: Gumma of the Coronary Artery, Myocardial Infarction, and Gumma of the Heart. Arch. Path., 44:490, 1947.
Magill, T. P.: Syphilitic Myocarditis. Bull. Johns Hopkins Hosp., 57:22, 1935.
Norris, J. C.: Syphilis of the Myocardium and Coronary Arteries. J.A.M.A., 108:169, 1937.
Steiger, H. P., and Edeiken, J.: EKG Changes in Early Syphilis. Am. Heart J., 34:674, 1947.

TRAUMA OF THE HEART

Penetrating wounds and contusions of the heart are common enough to constitute a problem of peculiar interest to the clinician and of real gravity to the patient.

The majority of wounds in civil practice are penetrating ones caused by sharp pointed objects such as ice picks, knives, daggers or swords. Less frequently the wounds are caused by pistol or rifle bullets, but such wounds usually cause prompt death.

Trauma to the heart from a blow on the anterior thorax, and crushing injuries may cause contusions of the myocardium and pericardial membranes; but because of the great mobility of the heart, such cases are relatively rare.

Wounds and contusions are, as a rule, problems of a different order. For that reason each can best be discussed separately.

WOUNDS

Three conditions must be instantly considered and differentiated when the physician is confronted by the problem of possible cardiac injury:

1. Injury of the internal mammary artery with intrapleural hemorrhage
2. Wound of the heart or great vessels and trapped hemopericardium with tamponade
3. Wound of the heart or great vessels with intrapleural escape of blood.

In any of these conditions the dynamics of the circulatory system are so speedily and seriously disturbed that partial or complete loss of consciousness may promptly occur; however, differentiation is as a rule possible.

Internal Mammary Artery Injury. The symptoms are those of a concealed hemorrhage, and the physical signs are those of hemothorax or hemopneumothorax. Unilateral (the wound side) distention of the neck veins may occur. All other surface veins are collapsed, as in other forms of hemorrhagic or traumatic shock.

Cardiac Tamponade. The symptoms and physical signs are those of circulatory collapse and hemorrhage, but with bilateral *distention of the neck veins*. Sinus tachycardia with a small and diminishing *pulse pressure* is present. The heart sounds are distant, and the area of absolute cardiac dullness is enlarged. In fluoroscopic examination there is slight increase in the size of the cardiac shadow, diminished amplitude of the contraction waves (dead heart), and elimination of the landmarks between the cardiac chambers. The electrocardiogram is significantly normal during the period immediately after the injury.

Escape of Blood. This is almost impossible to differentiate from an uncomplicated injury to the internal mammary artery. The fluoroscopic study may be helpful to determine whether the usual partial cardiac tamponade is present. The situation is urgent, and immediate surgical exploration is obligatory.

The *prognosis* of heart wounds, both early and late, is of interest. Regardless of the strides made in thoracic surgery, penetrating wounds of the heart, even when they receive appropriate treatment, have a high immediate mortality. In 141 cases reviewed by Bigger in 1939 the case fatality rate was 50 per cent. The late physical and physiologic status is invariably good. The writer reexamined a series of 21 patients one to eight years after surgical repair of heart wounds, in some of whom the coronary artery had been ligated. In all the patients the roentgenograms and electrocardiograms were normal. The latter were surprising, since all had previously shown RS-T and T wave changes after surgical treatment. One patient died from pneumonia two and a quarter years after surgical treatment of a penetrating wound of the apex of the left ventricle. The heart, at necropsy, weighed 260 gm. The pericardium was adherent over the entire heart, and the scar following the healing of the primary injury indicated that the wound had penetrated the left ventricle and extended through the interventricular septum into the apex of the right ventricle. It is reasonably certain that an adherent pericardium is a regular aftermath of hemopericardium, but this has no clinical significance.

It should be emphasized that the immediate mortality is dependent upon the clinical acumen of the physician who first sees the patient and on the skill of the surgeon. A satisfactory postoperative state is manifestly due in a considerable degree to the youth of the patients, for the majority of penetrating wounds occur in men aged 20 to 35 years.

WILLIAM B. PORTER

References

Beck, C. S.: Further Observations on Stab Wounds of the Heart. Am. Surg., 115:698, 1942.
Elkin, D. C.: The Diagnosis and Treatment of Wounds of the Heart, A Review of Twenty-two (22) Cases. J.A.M.A., 111:1750, 1938.
Kissane, R. W.: Traumatic Heart Disease: Nonpenetrating Injuries. Circulation, 6:421, 1952.
Porter, W. B., and Bigger, I. A.: Non-fatal Stab Wounds of the Ventricle. Am. J. M. Sc., 184:799, 1932.
———, and Bigger, I. A.: Stab Wounds of the Heart and Great Vessels. Tr. Am. Climat. & Clin. A., 54:96, 1938.

CONTUSION

Contusion of the heart may occur from trauma to the thorax, but its frequency is likely to be exaggerated. A "steering wheel" compression of the anterior thorax and other crushing injuries are frequent accidents in civil and industrial medicine; but just how often the heart and pericardium are contused by such accidents it is impossible to say. The only objective evidence clinically available is the electrocardiogram, which may show alterations indicating myocardial damage. If it shows varying changes, the evidence of muscle trauma is more convincing. Disturbance of rhythm may be produced by trauma to the thorax with or without definite evidence of heart trauma. Atrial fibrillation occasionally occurs, but as a rule the arrhythmia is transient and requires no therapy.

There is much convincing evidence that disturbances of cardiac rhythm are due, not to contusion of the heart, but to other factors, especially compression of the thorax. In this connection it is interesting how rarely arrhythmias are induced by penetrating wounds of the heart. This suggests that factors other than direct trauma to the heart are responsible for the arrhythmias occurring in compression injuries to the thorax. There is no evidence indicating that serious or permanent damage results from cardiac contusion. Rare instances of ruptured valves or laceration of the myocardium are the exceptions. But here again it is doubtful if trauma to the thorax ever produces such serious injury except in those patients who have either diseased hearts or congenital weakness of the involved tissues.

The medicolegal aspect of thoracic trauma with its implied dangers to the heart is likely to become a serious compensation problem. It emphasizes the importance of routine physical examinations of all industrial employees and the value of routine electrocardiograms in all cases of thoracic trauma.

WILLIAM B. PORTER

References

Arenberg, H.: Traumatic Heart Disease. A Clinical Study of 250 Cases of Non-penetrating Chest Injuries and Their Relation to Cardiac Disability. Ann. Int. Med., 19:326, 1943.
Barber, H.: Contusion of Myocardium. Brit. M. J., 2:520, 1940.
Bright, E. F., and Beck, C. S.: Non-penetrating Wounds of the Heart. A Clinical and Experimental Study. Am. Heart J., 10:293, 1935.
Kissane, R. W., Koons, R. A., and Fidler, R. S.: Traumatic Rupture of a Normal Aortic Valve. Am. Heart J., 12:231, 1936.

FOREIGN BODIES

A great variety of foreign bodies may enter the myocardium or heart chambers and remain there for long periods, producing few, if any, clinical symptoms. Occasionally those in the ventricles will migrate from the heart as emboli, blocking a major vessel. Fragments of projectiles, splinters of wood, fragments of bone, needles and tips of sharp-pointed objects have been found both in the heart chambers and in the myocardium. Some of them migrated to the heart by way of the great veins; others may migrate from the muscles of the thorax, esophagus or bronchi to the heart.

Removal of metal fragments lodged in the myocardium has become a feasible procedure, but is one which must remain in the domain of the highly specialized surgeon.

WILLIAM B. PORTER

References

Fair, G. L.: Foreign Bodies in the Heart. Report of a Case with Retention of Large Needle with Recovery. New York State J. Med., 35:453, 1935.
La Roque, G. P.: Penetrating Bullet Wounds of the Thoracic Aorta Followed by Lodgment of the Bullet in the Femoral Artery. Am. J. Surg., 33:827, 1926.
Shapiro, S.: Passage of a Hollow Needle into the Venous Stream to the Heart through the Cardiac Wall and into the Thorax. Am. Heart J., 22:835, 1941.
Silverman, J. J.: Shrapnel Wound of the Heart with Benign Manifestations. Am. Heart J., 34:419, 1947.

TUBERCULOSIS OF THE HEART

Except as a cause of pericarditis, tuberculosis is an unimportant etiologic factor in clinical heart disease.

Tuberculosis of the myocardium or of the endocardium is essentially not a clinical problem. It is an autopsy finding, rarely suspected during life. Miliary tubercles of the myocardium and endocardium do not modify the usual clinical signs or symptoms of miliary tuberculosis; nor is it likely that the prognosis of the case is altered.

Diffuse fibrosis with scarring of the myocardium, manifested clinically by irreducible congestive heart failure, may rarely result from extensive tuberculosis of the myocardium.

A solitary tubercle or a caseous abscess is occasionally found at autopsy, but such lesions rarely cause recognizable or specific symptoms. The rarity of myocardial tuberculosis is indicated by the autopsy studies by Raviart on 7683 cases of tuberculosis in which 49 showed myocardial tuberculosis (0.63 per cent).

Tuberculous endocarditis is invariably miliary. The tubercles are found on the endocardium of the valves and of the heart walls. Occasionally there are tuberculous ulcerations of the endocardium. Tubercle bacilli have been demonstrated in endocardial lesions. No case of chronic valvular disease has ever been reported as a sequel of tuberculous endocarditis.

WILLIAM B. PORTER

References

Bevans, M., and Wilkins, S. A., Jr.: Tuberculous Endocarditis. Am. Heart J., 24:843, 1942.
Horn, H., and Saphir, O.: The Involvement of the Myocardium in Tuberculosis—Review of the Literature and Report of Three Cases. Am. Rev. Tuberc., 321:492, 1935.
Rose, I.: Tuberculosis of the Myocardium. Am. Rev. Tuberc., 65:332, 1952.
Wilbur, E. L.: Myocardial Tuberculosis: Cause of Congestive Heart Failure. Am. Rev. Tuberc., 38:769, 1938.

PARASITES

It has been suspected for some time that in trichiniasis the myocardium may be involved along with other striated muscles. However, the number of larvae found in the myocardium is never great, and in many fatal cases the heart muscle may not show any parasites, even though there has been clinical evidence of cardiac disease before death.

Electrocardiographic studies have emphasized the effects of trichiniasis on the myocardium. In an outbreak studied by Reimann, 75 per cent of the severely infested cases showed abnormal electrocardiograms consisting in flattening or inversion of the T waves and minor changes in the QRS complex. It is interesting to note that the changes occurred five to seven weeks after the initial illness. With the encystation of the larvae the critical stage of intoxication ensues. The late development of the abnormal electrocardiograms strongly suggests that myocardial damage in trichiniasis results mainly from toxemia rather than from invasion of the heart muscle by the *Trichina spiralis*.

Respiratory symptoms suggesting heart

failure are in most instances due to the extensive involvement of the diaphragm and intercostal muscles rather than to heart failure of the congestive type. Circulatory failure resulting from severe toxemia is the usual mechanism of death in trichiniasis, and not primary myocardial insufficiency. Trichiniasis is not a cause of chronic heart disease.

Trypanosomiasis as a cause of heart disease has been reported from Brazil, but it has not yet been recognized in the United States or Europe. The parasites probably invade the myocardium during childhood, producing a focal and progressive type of inflammatory reaction which eventually results in focal fibrosis and muscle fiber degeneration. Clinically, congestive heart failure with arrhythmias occurs in middle life with no obvious signs of valve disease or hypertension. The prognosis is poor, regardless of adequate treatment.

The *Echinococcus* may involve the heart. Hydatid cysts are found attached to, or invading, the walls of the atria, ventricles or interventricular septum.

Calcified cysts of the heart are occasionally disclosed by roentgenogram, or the condition is suspected when a cyst discharges its contents into the circulation. This results in a peculiar syndrome, characterized by the phenomena of multiple embolization and anaphylactic shock.

WILLIAM B. PORTER

References

Beecher, C. H., and Amodon, E. G.: Electrocardiographic Findings in 44 Cases of Trichinosis. Am. Heart J., 16:219, 1938.

Chagas, E.: Foruma Cardiaca da Trypanosomiase Americana. Thesis, Rio de Janeiro, 1930.

Peters, J. H., Dexter, L., and Weiss, S.: Clinical and Theoretical Considerations of Involvement of the Left Side of the Heart with Echinococcal Cysts. Am. Heart J., 29:143, 1945.

Reimann, H.: Electrocardiograms in Trichiniasis. Deut. Militärarzt, 7: No. 7–4–48, 1942; abst. in Bull. War Medicine, 3: No. 6337, 1943.

HEART INVOLVEMENT IN SARCOIDOSIS

It is becoming increasingly obvious that sarcoidosis (Besnier-Boeck-Schaumann's disease) may manifest itself clinically in a variety of forms, owing to the involvement of any organ or tissue by the pathologic lesions of this interesting disease.

Invasion of the heart by sarcoids can no longer be recorded as a pathologic curiosity, for the presence of typical lesions, characteristic of Boeck's disease, are found in the myocardium or pericardium, or both areas, in the occasional fatal cases of sarcoidosis. When the heart is involved, the myocardium or pericardium is extensively infiltrated by characteristic granulomatous lesions, a finding which prompts the conclusion that the cardiac failure and fatal termination are the direct result of the involvement of the heart structures. No recorded fatal cases have been reported which showed involvement of the valves or endocardium.

The clinical syndrome resulting from sarcoidosis involving the heart is variable, and it is doubtful if one is justified in being dogmatic. A given patient's heart failure might be the result of sarcoidosis of the heart if the usual causes of heart failure are not obvious. Longcope and Fisher reviewed a series of 31 cases of sarcoidosis with special reference to heart involvement. Six patient showed some clinical evidence of myocardial insufficiency, type not specifically classified, during life, or sarcoids of the heart and pericardium were discovered at autopsy. Various degrees of heart failure with cardiac enlargement and electrocardiographic changes suggestive of nonspecific myocardial disease were noted in 5 of these 6 patients

Obviously, extensive diffuse myocardial lesions will result in heart failure of the congestive type. When failure occurs, it usually becomes progressively more severe, regardless of appropriate treatment. Focal lesions may be present in the heart without any clinical symptoms or arrhythmias, and conduction defects, including complete heart block may result. Scotti and McKeown recently reviewed 13 cases of sarcoidosis of the heart which resulted in death. It is interesting that 3 patients died suddenly. "Lymphogranulomatosis benigna" is generally a benign self-limiting disease. It does, however, have grave potentialities in a few patients.

At present no treatment is available which will modify the lesions of Boeck's sarcoid. It is too early to appraise the possible value of ACTH or cortisone or the nitrogen mustards, which are being evaluated currently.

WILLIAM B. PORTER

References

Johnson, J. B., and Jason, R. S.: Sarcoidosis of the Heart. Report of a Case and Review of the Literature. Am. Heart J., 27:246, 1944.

1344   DISEASES OF THE CARDIOVASCULAR SYSTEM

Kulka, W. E.: Sarcoidosis of the Heart: A Cause of
Sudden and Unexpected Death. Circulation, *1*:
772, 1950.

Longcope, W. T., and Fisher, A. M.: Involvement of
the Heart in Sarcoidosis or Besnier-Boeck-Schaumann's Disease. J. Mt. Sinai Hosp., 8:784, 1942.

Scotti, T. M., and McKeown, C. E.: Sarcoidosis Involving the Heart. Report of a Case with Sudden
Death. Arch. Path., *46*:289, 1948.

THE HEART IN HEMOCHROMATOSIS

In Sheldon's classic monograph on hemochromatosis, heart failure or other disturbances of myocardial function are mentioned
only as an incidental cause of death. It is
well known that the longer the life span of
a patient with hemochromatosis, the greater
the total amount of iron pigment found in
the body tissues. It is reasonable to assume,
therefore, that, with the prolongation of life
possible with the insulin control of bronze
diabetes, cardiac involvement may in the
future become more frequent.

In patients with bronze diabetes who die
with obvious symptoms of heart disease, the
heart at autopsy shows varying degrees of
dilatation, involving as a rule all the chambers, and the cut surface of the flabby myocardium has a peculiar coppery color. Histologically, the muscle cells contain much
iron pigment and show swelling with degeneration. There is some replacement of isolated
degenerated cells by connective tissue, but
extensive myocardial fibrosis is rare. The
coronary arteries are not primarily involved.

Obviously the clinical manifestations of
the heart disease as occasionally seen in patients with hemochromatosis are variable.
The occurrence of ectopic rhythms of varying types is suggestive, yet such disturbances
of rhythm cannot be classed as specific.
When heart failure of the congestive type
develops, its onset is usually rather sudden
and the course progressively more severe.
The over-all impression is one of a preponderance of right heart failure; however, the
syndrome is essentially total heart failure
similar to that seen in diffuse rheumatic myocarditis or beriberi.

In principle, the treatment of such patients should conform to that regimen established for congestive failure as it occurs in
other types of heart disease. The extensive
changes in the myocardium which were present before failure develops make the prognosis grave.

WILLIAM B. PORTER

References

Blumer, G., and Nesbit, R. R.: A Case of Hemochromatosis with Degeneration of the Heart Muscle
and Death from Congestive Heart Failure. New
England J. Med., *218*:295, 1938.

Shelden, J. H.: Haemochromatosis. London, Oxford
University Press, 1935.

Swan, W. G. A., and Dewar, H. A.: The Heart in
Hemochromatosis. Brit. Heart J., *14*:117, 1952.

Tucker, H. St. G., Jr., Moss, L. F., and Williams,
J. P.: Hemochromatosis with Death from Heart
Failure. Am. Heart J., *35*:993, 1948.

CARDIAC ARRHYTHMIAS

Cardiac rhythm connotes the sequence of
the heart beats. It may be regular or irregular. The irregularity may be perpetual, as in
atrial fibrillation, or may disturb the normal sequence occasionally or at regular intervals, and the cardiac rate may be rapid or
slow. The normal stimulus initiating the heart
beat arises in the sinus node, which lies in the
right atrium in the region of the opening of
the superior vena cava. It spreads in a radial
fashion over the atria and induces their contraction, and, arriving at the atrioventricular
node, which lies at the lower part of the
interatrial septum, proceeds rapidly down the
atrioventricular bundle and over the right
and left branches in the ventricular septum
simultaneously, and finally is distributed by
the Purkinje fibers to the ventricular muscle
and results in synchronous contraction of
the two ventricles.

The sinus discharge is usually more rapid
than the inherent rate of the atrioventricular node and the idioventricular center,
over which it takes precedence as the
pacemaker. Normally, conduction is forward
from atria to ventricles, but occasionally may
be retrograde. The activity of the sinus node
is affected by the vagus and the accelerator
nerves. Most of the fibers of the right vagus
are distributed to the sinus node, and most
of the fibers of the left vagus to the atrioventricular node, and a few to the bundle.
The heart beat is the expression of a physiologic mechanism and has no histologic counterpart that can be discovered at present
except in heart blocks.

The **physiologic properties** of heart muscle concerned with its rhythms are (1) *excitability* or *contractility*: it responds to a
stimulus by contracting; (2) *refractory period*: having contracted, a recovery period is
necessary before it can respond to the next

stimulus; (3) *automaticity* or *rhythmicity:* the property of initiating impulses; (4) *conductivity:* it conducts an impulse that it receives.

Method of Examination. Orderly examination facilitates the clinical recognition of arrhythmias. (1) The jugular bulbs and external jugular veins, which become distended if the patient lies flat, are observed for pulsations. The "a" (atrial contraction), "c" (ventricular contraction) and "v" (ventricular filling) waves can usually be identified by this technique when the heart is beating normally. (2) The sequence of beats in the radial pulse is analyzed. (3) The rhythm is analyzed on auscultation, correlating it with radial and carotid pulses; atrial contractions may be heard in complete heart block and in atrial flutter. (4) The apex and radial rates are counted simultaneously for one minute to estimate the pulse deficit. If careful clinical examinations are made and then checked with electrocardiograms whenever possible, a skill is acquired which permits proceeding without them when they are not available. Electrocardiograms record the electrical activity of the heart accompanying contraction. The normal cardiac cycle consists of a P wave, indicating atrial activity, followed by the QRS complex, recording the spread of the excitation wave through the ventricles, and in turn by the T wave, coinciding with the retreat of electrical activity associated with contraction, after which there is an isoelectric pause before the onset of the next P wave (Fig. 159).

SINUS NODE: NORMAL RHYTHM

The heart beat controlled by the sinoatrial node is called normal or regular (sinus) rhythm, or normal (sinus) mechanism. The discharge of impulses may be quite regular (Fig. 160, A) or may have the following variations.

SINUS IRREGULARITY OR SINUS ARRHYTHMIA

When the sinus discharge is irregular (Fig. 160, B, C), the length of the cycle varies. The rate may wax and wane in a repetitive pattern. When the irregularity is respiratory, the rate increases with inspiration and decreases with expiration (Fig. 160, B, C). It is a physiologic phenomenon. It is most common in children and young persons.

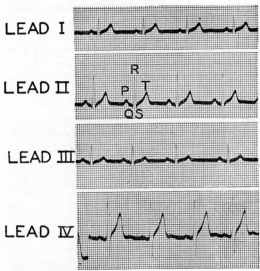

Fig. 159. The three standard leads and the chest lead of a *normal* electrocardiogram. The leads and waves are identified. The P waves, the major part of the QRS deflections, and the T waves are upright in all leads, and P-R_2 is 0.17 second, QRS_2, 0.06 second, rate 75 per minute. Lead I is derived from the electrodes placed on the right and left arms, lead II from the right arm and left leg, and lead III from the left leg and left arm. To obtain chest lead IV, the precordial electrode is placed 1 cm. outside the apex beat and the indifferent electrode on the left leg. Using lead III selector of the galvanometer control box, the left leg wire is attached to the precordial electrode and the left arm electrode to the left leg in order to secure upright T waves in normal curves. The P-R interval measures the time for passage of the excitation wave from the sinus node through the atria to the atrioventricular node, down the atrioventricular bundle to the beginning of ventricular activity, and normally does not exceed 0.20 second in adults. The QRS interval represents the time of spread of the excitation wave through the ventricles by way of the special conduction system and is normally not greater than 0.10 second. The Q-T time from the beginning of QRS to the end of T measures ventricular systole. The three standard leads of the electrocardiogram obey the laws of the Einthoven equilateral triangle, namely, that the amplitudes of any waves of the complexes in lead II equal the sum of those in leads I and III. Standardization in all records, unless specifically mentioned, is such that 1 millivolt produced 1 cm. deflection of the string. Divisions of the ordinates equal 10^{-4} volts. Divisions of the abscissae equal 0.04 second. Chest derivations over the base of the heart and esophageal leads may record P waves in paroxysmal tachycardia and flutter waves in atrial flutter. Unipolar limb and chest leads usually do not contribute to the diagnosis of cardiac arrhythmias.

It may disappear during rheumatic carditis. It may be confused with atrial fibrillation with a slow ventricular rate (Fig. 165, A);

however, in sinus irregularity there is no pulse deficit, and increasing the heart rate with exercise dispels the irregularity, but might elicit a pulse deficit in fibrillation. The sequence of P-QRS-T waves in the electrocardiogram is normal, but the P-P interval varies (Fig. 160, B, C).

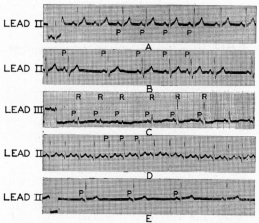

Fig. 160. Electrocardiograms showing variations in discharge from the sinus node. In A the discharge is regular and the complexes are equally spaced (lead II). In B there is sinus irregularity (lead II). In C there is sinus irregularity with marked respiratory variation in the amplitudes of the QRS complexes (lead III). D records sinus tachycardia (132 per minute) (lead II), and E, sinus bradycardia (37 per minute) (lead II). P = atrial complexes, R = ventricular complexes.

SINUS TACHYCARDIA

Sinus tachycardia occurs when the discharge of impulses from the sinus node is over 100 per minute. The rate may be 200, but the lower ranges above 100 are more common.

Etiology. Sinus tachycardia is normal in a few persons. It may result from depression of vagal activity or from stimulation of the accelerator nerves, and may be induced by atropine or epinephrine. It is a physiologic response to exercise, eating, excitement and fear. It occurs in neurasthenia, neurocirculatory asthenia, anemia, pulmonary tuberculosis, hyperthyroidism, infections (except typhoid fever), active rheumatic carditis, myocardial infarction, heart failure, and after hemorrhage.

Pathologic Physiology. The normal heart augments its output in response to exercise and increased oxygen consumption by increasing its rate.

Symptoms. There may be no symptoms,

or there may be palpitation or pounding of the heart.

Diagnosis. In sinus tachycardia the rate usually accelerates and retards gradually. In electrocardiograms the normal sequence of P-QRS-T is observed, but the P-P interval is short (Fig. 160, D).

Treatment. The heart rate accelerated by exercise retards on resting, as well as when other precipitating factors are alleviated. Sedatives may be effective.

SINUS BRADYCARDIA

Sinus bradycardia occurs when the sinus impulses are fewer than 60 per minute.

Etiology. Sinus bradycardia is not unusual in athletes and young adults. It occurs during sleep. It may be associated with mal-

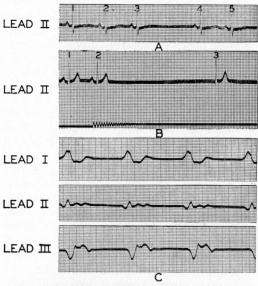

Fig. 161. A shows (lead II) sino-atrial block. The interval from 3 to 4 equals twice the interval from 1 to 2 or equals interval 1 to 3. B shows sinus arrest with cardiac standstill (asystole) for 3 seconds resulting from right carotid sinus pressure (lead II). Ventricular escape occurs at 3. The signal at the bottom indicates the onset of carotid sinus pressure. C records three standard leads showing atrial standstill with idioventricular rhythm and bundle branch block, which probably resulted from toxic effect of potassium chloride. The patient exhibited normal rhythm before the onset of this rhythm.

nutrition, jaundice and increased intracranial pressure. It may result from digitalis or from carotid sinus pressure.

Pathologic Physiology. In sinus bradycardia the cardiac output per minute may decrease; because of the slow rate the stroke volume, however, may be increased.

Symptoms. There are usually no symptoms.

Diagnosis. The diagnosis of sinus bradycardia is not difficult. It accelerates with exercise. If very slow, the atrioventricular node assumes pacemaking, or there may be ventricular escape. In electrocardiograms there is normal sequence of P-QRS-T, but the P-P interval is long (Fig. 160, *E*).

Treatment. Sinus bradycardia requires no specific treatment, except for the underlying condition which at times may be responsible. It is rarely necessary to use atropine.

SINO-ATRIAL PREMATURE CONTRACTIONS

It is unusual for the sinus node to initiate premature contractions. They cannot be differentiated clinically from other premature beats. In electrocardiograms the P waves are similar in form to the normal ones, but they occur early and are not followed by a compensatory pause.

SINO-ATRIAL BLOCK

Sino-atrial block, sinus pause or arrest, occurs when the discharge of impulses from the sinus node is interrupted. It may be occasional, frequent or in a recurrent pattern, or there may be longer periods of block.

Etiology. Sino-atrial block may result from increased vagal activity. It may be precipitated by quinidine, potassium salts or digitalis. When the sinus node is quiescent for a few seconds, syncope may result. It may follow carotid sinus stimulation. If this tissue is hypersensitive, attacks may be precipitated by sudden turning of the head, a tight collar, bending forward. One carotid sinus is usually more sensitive than the other.

Pathologic Physiology. Occasional sinoatrial block does not affect the functional capacity of the heart. When it is prolonged, the cardiac output and the blood pressure fall to zero until the ventricles escape.

Symptoms. Occasional sinus pause is usually without symptoms. If there are longer periods of block with asystole, Adams-Stokes-like attacks occur.

Diagnosis. Single sino-atrial block can occasionally be detected because the pause equals two usual intervals. It is to be differentiated from atrioventricular block. When the pause is of longer duration, as in carotid sinus hypersensitivity, the diagnosis should be suspected because of asystole. In testing for carotid sinus sensitivity (see p. 1350, point 4) pressure may be applied for 5 to 15 seconds (Fig. 161, *B*). In the electrocardiogram single sino-atrial block is recognized by the absence of atrial and ventricular activity, and the interval covering the block approximately equals two normal intervals (Fig. 161, A). Longer periods of sinus arrest may be recorded with ventricular escape (Figs. 161, *B;* 173, *B*).

Treatment. Occasional sino-atrial block requires no specific therapy. If it is due to carotid sinus hypersensitivity and associated with symptoms, atropine, 0.0006 gm. three times a day, tincture of belladonna, 0.6 to 1 cc. three times a day, ephedrine, 20 to 30 mg. three times a day, or phenobarbital, 0.015 gm. four times a day orally, may be used. Banthine, because of its atropine-like effects, in 100 mg. doses up to four times a day orally may be effective. If these measures are ineffective, one or both carotid sinuses may be denervated, or the ninth nerve sectioned intracranially. If block is due to digitalis and infrequent, digitalization may be continued if the drug is necessary.

ATRIAL STANDSTILL

In this rhythm the sinus node is quiescent, the atria fail to contract, and there is ventricular escape with idioventricular rhythm. It occurs transiently in carotid sinus hypersensitivity. As a persistent rhythm, only a few instances have been reported. Death results if the idioventricular center fails to initiate ventricular contractions. Atrial standstill may occur as a toxic effect of potassium salts, Pronestyl and quinidine on the sinus node and atrioventricular system. The administration of normal salt solution and 5 per cent glucose intravenously is the most effective therapy. In the electrocardiogram P waves are not seen, and there is idioventricular rhythm (Fig. 161, *C*).

PREMATURE CONTRACTION

Premature contraction is the best term for an irregularity resulting from contractions derived from abnormal stimuli arising in various parts of the heart. *Extrasystole* implies an extra beat of the heart; because of the pause following the premature contraction, the number of beats per minute is not increased. The term "extrasystole" applies only when the premature contraction is interpolated between two normal beats without disturbing the sequence (p. 1367). The terms "ectopic" and "aberrant" imply an unusual place of origin and manner of spread of the excitation wave, and would not include sino-atrial premature contractions. *Dropped beats* are seen in heart block. *Intermittent pulse* is vague. The occurrence and volume of the pulse accompanying a premature contraction depend on its time in the cardiac cycle. Premature contractions may arise from areas of increased irritability.

ATRIAL RHYTHMS

ATRIAL PREMATURE CONTRACTIONS

Atrial premature contractions are occasioned by abnormal stimuli arising in one of the atria which cause them to contract prematurely, and also, passing down the atrioventricular system, initiate ventricular contractions. Atrial premature contractions may occur occasionally (Fig. 162,

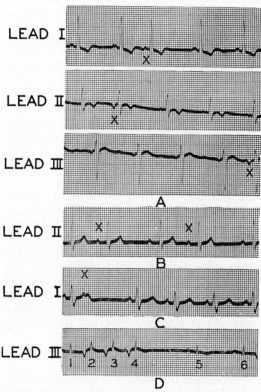

Fig. 162. *A* shows the three standard leads in which atrial premature contractions (X) are recorded in each lead. In *B* the atrial premature contractions (X) recur and give rise to coupling. In *C* there is an atrial premature contraction (X) superimposed on the T wave, and it occurs so early that it is blocked (ventricles refractory). In *D* the first complex (1) is normal followed by a run of 3 atrial premature contractions in succession (2, 3, 4), giving rise to a short run of atrial paroxysmal tachycardia, followed by reversion to normal rhythm in the fifth and sixth complexes.

A), several in a sequence (Fig. 162, *D*), or according to a pattern (Fig. 162, *B*).

Etiology. Atrial premature contractions occur more frequently in younger than in older persons and are not as common as ventricular ones. They may not be significant. They may be associated with active rheumatic fever and other infections, especially pneumonia; they occur in organic heart disease, especially mitral stenosis, coronary artery disease, and after myocardial infarction. They are frequent during periods of stress, and may result from coffee, alcohol, tobacco.

Pathologic Physiology. Occasional atrial premature contractions do not disturb the circulation significantly; when they cause coupling, the cardiac output decreases.

Symptoms. Patients may be unaware of the irregularity. They may complain of palpitation, the pause after the premature contraction, the prematurity, the "quick" beat, the forceful beat following the premature one, the heart "turning over," "fluttering in the heart," fullness of the neck veins, a catch in the throat and cough. Their persistency may cause fatigue.

Diagnosis. Atrial premature contractions are detected by their prematurity, both on auscultation of the heart and on palpation of the pulse. They cannot always be differentiated from ventricular or atrioventricular ones. The dominant rhythm is disturbed. The sounds accompanying the premature beat approach the usual ones. The premature complex in the electrocardiogram consists of a P wave of different contour, a P-R time exceeding 0.10 second, and a QRS complex of supraventricular form, which may differ from the usual ones (Fig. 162, *A*).

Prognosis. Their occurrence may be fleeting. They may occur for years without significance. They may precede the onset of atrial fibrillation in mitral stenosis and are common in patients subject to atrial paroxysmal tachycardia.

Treatment. Treatment is usually not necessary, for they may disappear when the precipitating factors are alleviated. Attention should not be directed to them, because it may induce symptoms. Patients are reassured. Cigarettes, coffee and alcohol are eliminated when implicated. When treatment is required, triple bromides, 1 gm. three times or twice a day orally, may dissipate them, and are usually more effective than phenobarbital, 0.015 gm. three times a day.

The patient is warned of drowsiness and drug rash. If effective, the drug is decreased and frequently may be discontinued. If sedation fails, digitalis in full therapeutic amounts (see Atrial Fibrillation) is the most effective drug. Quinidine, 0.2 gm. three times a day (see Atrial Fibrillation), is less effective than in the relief of ventricular ones. Occasionally, potassium chloride or phosphate, 2 gm. three times a day by mouth, is beneficial. Atrial standstill as a toxic effect of potassium must be kept in mind. Papaverine, 0.06 to 0.3 gm. three to four times a day at three to four hour intervals, may abolish them.

BLOCKED ATRIAL PREMATURE CONTRACTIONS

Occasionally, an atrial premature contraction may be blocked if it arises early in diastole, because the ventricles are still refractory. This irregularity is detected in electrocardiograms (Fig. 162, C).

ATRIAL PAROXYSMAL TACHYCARDIA

Atrial paroxysmal tachycardia is a rapid *regular* beating of the heart, controlled by stimuli arising from a focus in the atria, and characterized by sudden onset and sudden offset. It may be considered a succession of atrial premature contractions (see p. 1348). It may persist for a few beats only, or for days. The rate is usually rapid, around 150 per minute, but is frequently up to 250 per minute and rarely less than 100.

Etiology. It is more common in younger persons than the ventricular type. There may be a single attack, or recurrences at rare or frequent intervals. It occurs without organic heart disease. It may be precipitated by excessive alcohol intake, cigarettes or gastrointestinal upsets. It may be associated with acute infections, acute rheumatic fever being the most common. It occurs in mitral stenosis, thyrotoxicosis, myocardial infarction, and in patients with Wolff-Parkinson-White syndrome.

Pathologic Physiology. During atrial paroxysmal tachycardia the cardiac output per minute and per beat decreases. The heart dilates, and the circulation time increases. The vital capacity decreases. The oxygen saturation of both the arterial and venous blood decreases. If prolonged, heart failure may occur. *Transient* electrocardiographic changes have been reported, presumably due to the anoxemia of heart muscle from de-

creased coronary flow. There may be cyanosis. A few rales at the lung bases, fall in blood pressure, fever and leukocytosis are not unusual.

Symptoms. Patients are usually aware of the disturbed rhythm. They complain of fluttering of the heart starting suddenly, rapidity of the heart, palpitation, throbbing or fullness of the neck vessels. Common complaints are weakness, faintness, shortness of breath and sensation of the heart stretching. There may be apprehension and nervousness. Car-

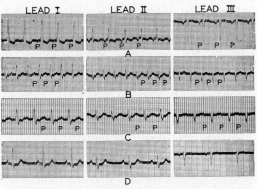

Fig. 163. *A* shows the three leads recording atrial paroxysmal tachycardia, rate 107 per minute (*P = P* waves). *B* shows another example of atrial paroxysmal tachycardia, rate 162 per minute. *C* shows the same paroxysm with the speed of the electrocardiographic film increased to spread out the complexes and aid in identifying the P waves. *D* shows the electrocardiogram after reversion to normal rhythm (rate, 61 per minute) from the atrial paroxysmal tachycardia recorded in *B* and *C*.

diac distress may simulate the symptoms of myocardial infarction. Nausea and vomiting, a sense of fullness, dizziness, fainting and loss of consciousness may be experienced. When the blood pressure falls, the picture may be one of shock.

Diagnosis. *Paroxysmal tachycardia* may be diagnosed from the *history* of sudden onset and offset, but the type cannot be decided unless the patient is examined during an attack, since atrial, nodal and ventricular tachycardia and atrial fibrillation and flutter may be paroxysmal. Awareness of an irregularity suggests fibrillation. The rapidity and regularity are apparent. The rate is not influenced by respiration or exercise, but may change in several hours. Pulsations in the jugular veins are rapid, and "c" waves may be identified. The pulse is rapid, of small volume and rarely alternating. If carotid sinus pressure or ocular pressure terminates the attack, it is likely to be supraventricular. In electrocardiograms P waves of abnormal form are detected with P-R exceeding 0.10 second, and usually a supraventricular form of the QRS complex (Fig. 163, A, B, C). There may be 2:1 block, which may be a toxic effect of digitalis.

Prognosis. Atrial paroxysmal tachycardia frequently indicates heart disease, but may recur for many years without other abnormalities; there may be a single attack. Its occurrence increases the hazards of the underlying disease.

Treatment. The first problem is to stop the attack and the second to prevent recurrence. The patient should be reassured and kept in bed, especially when mechanical stimuli or drugs are used. If possible, electrocardiograms should be taken before and during attempts to stop the paroxysm. Patients may report measures that have stopped previous attacks.

Attacks are usually terminated by inducing vagal or parasympathetic effects: (1) holding the breath as long as possible, or expiring against the closed glottis (*Valsalva*) or inspiring after closing the glottis (*Müller*); (2) bending forward, or (3) mechanical induction of *nausea* may terminate the attack. (4) *Carotid sinus pressure* is frequently effective. The patient should be recumbent during this maneuver and atropine, 0.0006 gm. for intravenous use, or epinephrine, 1 cc. 1:1000 (hypodermic), should be ready for immediate injection should asystole persist too long. The right and then the left carotid sinus is pressed, after which both may be stimulated. Pressure for 5 to 10 seconds is effective in suitable cases. The carotid bulb, which is easily identified in the bifurcation of the common carotid, is compressed against the cervical spine. This procedure should not be taught the patient. Auscultation warns of asystole.

(5) In the long run, the most effective drug is *digitalis*. With the patient in bed, digitalization is carried out rapidly in 24 hours (p. 1352); 1.8 gm. is the average digitalizing amount of the powdered leaf (U.S.P. XIV) if given orally in 24 hours and the subject has had no digitalis within three weeks. If reversion does not occur during the 24 hours of digitalization, as is common (Fig. 163, B, C, D), 0.2 gm. three times or twice a day is given the next day. If the clinical strength of the preparation is not known, smaller amounts are used. If more rapid action is required, lanatoside C, 1.6 mg., may be given intravenously in single or split amounts. (6) Acetyl-beta-methylcholine (*methacholine chloride*) subcutaneously is frequently effective; 10 to 20 mg. are given subcutaneously to those 10 to 20 years of age, 30 to 40 to 50 mg. to those more than 50 years, 30 mg. being the average dose. It should not be given without having atropine, 0.0006 gm., ready for intravenous use if asystole is prolonged, or if the side effects are marked. Gentle massage of the site of injection enhances the effect. The patient should be lying down in case fainting or asystole occurs. Because the drug induces increased bronchial secretions, profuse expectoration, asthmatic breathing due to bronchospasm, urticaria and involuntary stools, it should not be used without preparations beforehand to meet them. History of such allergic manifestations as asthma and hay fever, or of sensitivity to foods, are contraindications to its use. Methacholine chloride results in atrioventricular block, long periods of ventricular quiescence, or atrial standstill, before reversion to normal rhythm occurs. The synchronous use of methacholine chloride and carotid sinus pressure may be effective. (7) If these measures fail, *quinidine sulfate* orally is occasionally effective (p.1369). If there is nausea and vomiting, quinidine can be given intramuscularly (p. 1369). It should be used intravenously (p. 1369) only when other measures fail and persistence of the attack is hazardous. When electrocardiograms are not available and the diagnosis is not established, and therapy is required, it is better to use quinidine than digitalis, because of the danger of inducing ventricular fibrillation should the rhythm be ventricular paroxysmal tachycardia. (8) Unilateral ocular pressure is painful and is too rarely effective to use routinely. (9) Apomorphine, 5 mg. hypodermically, or syrup of ipecac, 4 to 8 cc. by mouth, which may be repeated, is used to induce vomiting, during which the attack may stop. They are not resorted to often. (10) Occasionally, triple bromide, 1 gm. three times a day by mouth, or morphine, 16 mg. hypodermically, may terminate the attack, although the latter is not recommended because paroxysmal tachycardia recurs. (11) Atabrine, 0.3 to 0.6 gm. dissolved in 10 cc. of 1 per cent procaine and administered intramuscularly, may be effective. Reversion to normal rhythm occurs in

Stanc
digitalis
The an
required
must th
shown t
can be
ventricu
digitaliz
is availa
establish
rapid v
tion to
is partia
or three
rate and
during
withheld
the rate
prematu
tion shou
Nausea,
contracti
failure a
The ver
guide to
aim shou
minute
slightly l
age amo
duced th
level by
is 0.2 gi
0.1 gm.
gm. alter
casionall
has shov
to 70 is
increase
Digita
complish
ing milli
average i
Toxic ef
the whol

a half hour. (12) Neostigmine methylsulfate, 1 mg. intramuscularly, may be effective within a few minutes. (13) Occasionally Pronestyl is effective in restoring normal rhythm (p. 1369). (14) Magnesium sulfate intravenously in 10 to 20 cc. amounts of the 25 per cent solution may be effective. Disturbance in conduction and ventricular premature contractions may result. (15) It is not safe to use Neo-Synephrine intravenously in 0.5 mg. amounts in the treatment of supraventricular paroxysmal tachycardia.

Prevention of attacks is more difficult. Elimination of the precipitating factors may be sufficient if attacks occur at wide intervals. If they occur at weekly or ten-day intervals, the most effective therapy is full digitalization followed by ration doses. In other instances quinidine, 0.2 gm. several times daily, is effective, although it is usually not desirable to give it over long periods. Electrocardiograms are taken occasionally to detect prolongation of P-R and of QRS conduction. The administration of propylthiouracil has been effective in preventing recurrent atrial paroxysmal tachycardia in a few patients refractory to other therapy.

ATRIAL FIBRILLATION

Atrial fibrillation is an irregularity in which the sinus node no longer controls the rhythm of the heart. It is characterized by absence of coordinated atrial contraction, tumultuous rapid twitching of atrial muscle fibers and total irregularity of the ventricular beats. Instead of the usual origin and spread of the sinus stimulus, an excitation wave courses continuously through the atrial muscle over a circular pathway about the opening of the great veins. The great speed of the excitation wave, 400 to 600 occurring per minute, and the continual variation in the length and course of the pathway account for the irregularity in the atrial action in the electrocardiogram. Not all these stimuli traverse the atrioventricular bundle, because of its refractoriness, nor can the ventricles respond to all arriving there because of their refractoriness; consequently, the ventricular rate before digitalization is usually rapid and irregular (Fig. 164, A), but slower than atrial activity. The validity of this circus motion theory has recently been questioned (p. 1356).

Etiology. Atrial fibrillation is the most common rhythm requiring therapy. Though commonly associated with organic heart dis-

ease, both transient and permanent types occur without it. It may follow excessive intake of alcohol, oversmoking, overeating, food poisoning, surgical operations. It occurs transiently in acute rheumatic fever, pneumonia, particularly in the later decades, myocardial infarction and pulmonary infarction. It is frequently associated with chronic rheumatic heart disease, especially mitral stenosis, less frequently with the arteriosclerotic and hypertensive types, infrequently with syphilitic and congenital forms, ex-

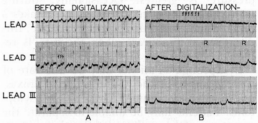

Fig. 164. A records three leads, showing atrial fibrillation before digitalization and showing the irregular fibrillation waves (fff), the rapid ventricular complexes (R, R) (ventricular rate approximately 175 per minute) which occur irregularly. B shows the effect of digitalization in this same patient: the slower ventricular rate (59 per minute), and the change in T waves.

tremely infrequently with subacute bacterial endocarditis, and occasionally with diphtheria and chronic constrictive pericarditis. After mitral stenosis its most frequent occurrence is in thyrotoxicosis.

Pathologic Physiology. On observation of the fibrillating heart the atria appear dilated and coordinated contraction is replaced by quivering of the atrial surfaces, while the ventricles beat at totally irregular intervals. There is decrease in cardiac output per minute and dilatation of the heart. Owing probably to the slow circulation rate permitting a longer time for oxygenation of the blood in the lungs, there is *increase* in the arterial oxygen saturation until heart failure supervenes, and decrease in venous oxygen saturation.

During tachycardia there is little blood in the ventricles when systole occurs, so that contraction fails either to open the aortic valve or to expel enough blood to form a radial pulse, accounting for the *pulse deficit;* at the next systole there will be a greater accumulation of blood, so that the radial pulse is barely palpable or will be larger, accounting for variations in pulse volume. The pulse deficit represents wasted cardiac

is warned of toxic symptoms. If the clinical potency of the preparation is not known, smaller amounts than those listed are recommended. Digitalization by 0.2 to 0.3 gm. daily takes too long to attain an adequate effect.

Occasionally, in terminal heart disease, digitalis fails to reduce the rate, or sufficient amounts cannot be given without inducing ventricular premature contractions. If there is heart failure, digitalization commonly results in diuresis, which may be sufficient to restore compensation.

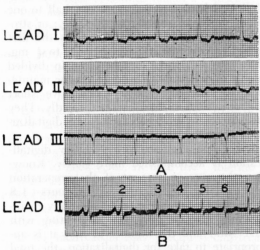

Fig. 165. *A* shows atrial fibrillation in which the ventricular sequences are regularly spaced, ventricular rate 60 per minute. *B* shows the transition from normal rhythm (88 per minute) to atrial fibrillation (ventricular rate 125 per minute). Complexes 1 and 2 are normal rhythm, and 3 to 7, inclusive, atrial fibrillation.

The reversion of *chronic* fibrillation to normal rhythm with *quinidine* is now undertaken infrequently. Reversion should not be attempted (1) if fibrillation has been present for a long time, because mural thrombi may be dislodged when the auricles begin contracting regularly; (2) if the heart is large; (3) during heart failure—compensation should be restored first; (4) if failure has been of long duration, because the formation of thrombi may have been encouraged; (5) without taking into consideration that some patients feel better and the heart rate is more easily controlled during fibrillation. The effectiveness of anticoagulants in the prevention of embolization in these circumstances is being explored. During attempts at restoration the patient should be in bed. The ven-

tricular rate is first reduced with digitalis and compensation is restored. Digitalis is then discontinued and test made for quinine idiosyncrasy with 0.2 gm. Two hours later the drug may be given as follows: 0.4 gm. four times a day at 4-hour intervals the first day; normal rhythm may recur at any time. If fibrillation persists, 0.4 gm. of quinidine is given five times a day the second day; and 0.4 gm. six times a day the third day. If reversion has not occurred, larger amounts should not be given at this time, but digitalis is resumed and the ventricular rate reduced again. If reversion is urgently desired, a second attempt may be made, attention being given to the occurrence of ventricular premature contractions. If normal rhythm is restored, maintenance doses of 0.2 gm. three times a day are given for a week longer. If normal rhythm is restored once, but fibrillation recurs while quinidine is being given, further attempts are not recommended. The use of larger amounts daily to restore normal rhythm is not recommended. Discontinuance of digitalis before giving quinidine avoids maximal concentrations of both drugs at the same time. If it recurs after being discontinued, another attempt may be made. It is not advisable to use quinidine daily over long periods to prevent recurrence. *Pronestyl* is occasionally effective in chronic atrial fibrillation, but amounts in the toxic range may be required (p. 1369).

PAROXYSMAL ATRIAL FIBRILLATION

Treatment. If paroxysms are infrequent and brief in an otherwise well subject, specific treatment is not required, beyond avoidance of precipitating factors (Fig. 165, *B*).

If, however, the attack has persisted for several hours or days, if tachycardia prevails, if the patient is uncomfortable, or if signs of failure are apparent, treatment is indicated. The patient should be in bed and the ventricular rate reduced with digitalis. There is no evidence clinically that digitalis fixes the rhythm and prevents reversion to normal, since (1) paroxysmal fibrillation may revert to normal rhythm on digitalization, (2) maintenance amounts of digitalis may prevent recurrent fibrillation and (3) normal rhythm recurs while digitalis is being given after thyroidectomy. If normal rhythm is not restored during preliminary digitalization, and if the signs of failure have not been present or have disappeared, quinidine may be given (*v. supra*). If the patient has been treated effectively with quinidine and has no idiosyncrasy, instructions may be given about taking the drug on recurrence. Ration doses of quinidine are usually not given daily over months or years; controlling the ventricular rate with digitalis is more satisfactory. Recurrent fibrillation is occasionally prevented by digitalization followed by maintenance doses, when quinidine has been ineffectual. In acute rheumatic fever it is transient and usually does not require therapy. In pneumonia and myocardial infarction prompt slowing of the ventricular rate is necessary; the use of quinidine is then considered. Occasionally, after quinidine, fibrillation changes to flutter, which persists in spite of large amounts of quinidine or digitalis. Pronestyl is frequently effective in paroxysmal atrial fibrillation (p. 1369).

The benefits of digitalis are more dramatic in atrial fibrillation than in normal rhythm because of marked slowing of the ventricular rate. Digitalis exerts certain other effects on the heart which can be recorded in patients. (1) An effect on heart muscle is observed objectively in changes in the form and amplitude of T waves of the electrocardiogram (Fig. 164, *A, B*). This effect, however, cannot be interpreted in terms of benefit, or degree of digitalization. (2) Digitalis increases the atrioventricular block and in adequate dosage prevents most of the fibrillation impulses from passing to the ventricles; those passing relatively infrequently find the ventricles containing more blood. The ventricular rate is retarded (Fig. 164, *A, B*) and the pulse deficit is decreased or abolished. The blocking effect of digitalis can be pushed to complete heart block. Atropine abolishes the vagal effects, so that the ventricular rate and pulse deficit increase. (3) Digitalis decreases the size of the dilated, fibrillating heart and increases its volume output. The failing and the digitalized heart as well as the normal heart appear to obey Starling's law of the heart. (4) The extent of ventricular contraction is also increased in roentgenkymograms. These effects contribute toward increase in cardiac output per minute and per beat, decrease of the circulation times toward normal and fall in venous pressure, if it has been elevated. When normal rhythm is restored spontaneously or by quinidine, still further increase in cardiac output may occur.

Quinidine brings about restoration of normal rhythm in fibrillation by increasing the refractory period of atrial muscle. As the excitation wave, moving in its circuit, reaches a certain point, it finds that tissue still refractory and unable to transmit it; the circus motion ends and the sinus node assumes control. Quinidine also slows the speed of conduction of the impulse and thereby tends to perpetuate the circus motion; thus, when the effect on the refractory period is greater than its contrary effect on conduction, normal rhythm supervenes.

Quinidine is to be discontinued should there occur ringing in the ears, deafness, diarrhea, nausea, vomiting, rash, fever, interventricular heart block, ventricular premature contractions, rapid regular rhythm or episodes of irregular rhythm suggesting ventricular fibrillation. Cerebral accidents or death occurring during quinidine therapy are in some instances due to embolism associated with dislodgment of mural thrombi on restoration of coordinated contraction of the atria. Other instances of death have been attributed to cardiac standstill resulting from depression of both the sinus and atrioventricular nodes, leaving no center available for pacemaking when the atria stop fibrillating.

When atrial fibrillation occurs in hyperthyroidism, the ventricular rate is reduced with digitalis. Larger than the average amounts may be required to attain adequate slowing. Maintenance doses are continued during treatment with iodine and propylthiouracil, or I^{131}, and after thyroidectomy. In most instances a few days to many weeks after operation the rhythm reverts to normal spontaneously. When this occurs, digitalis is discontinued, if heart failure does not require its continued use. If normal rhythm has not recurred after an adequate postoperative period, the use of quinidine is considered.

ATRIAL FLUTTER

Atrial flutter is a rhythm in which the atria contract regularly at a rate of 200 to 360 or more per minute, and in which the ventricles contract in response to some of these stimuli. Flutter is due to the passage of an excitation wave in a circus motion about the opening of the great veins in the right atrium. The passage is over a constant pathway, and only one impulse is given off from the circumference of the circular pathway with each circuit; the atrial impulses occur *regularly,* the rate ranging between 200 and 400 per minute, but commonly around 320 (Fig. 166), which is slower than in fibrillation. These impulses spread through the atrial muscle down the atrioventricular node and bundle to the ventricles, but are so rapid that the conducting system cannot readily transmit nor the ventricles respond to so many, and atrioventricu-

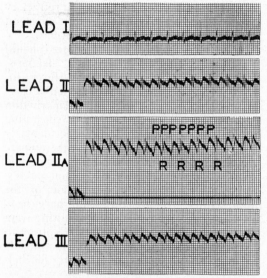

Fig. 166. The three standard leads recording 2:1 atrial flutter (ventricular rate 187, atrial rate 374). The flutter waves are poorly seen in lead I, but are easily identified in leads II and III (PPP) of which there are two to one ventricular complex (RRR). In lead IIA the galvanometer string was standardized for 2 cm. instead of 1 cm. in order to magnify the flutter waves.

lar block usually develops. The ventricular rate is usually regular and slower than the atrial rate and usually has a constant ratio to it; two atrial contractions to one ventricular, designated 2:1 atrial flutter, is common before treatment (Fig. 166). A 1:1 ratio is occasionally observed. The most frequent ventricular rate is 150 to 165 per minute. Ratios of 3:1, 4:1 or more occur after digitalization (Fig. 167, B, C) and occasionally before treatment. If the ratio fluctuates, the ventricular sequence is irregular (Fig. 167, A). Atrial flutter is more commonly paroxysmal than chronic. It may be transient (Fig. 167, E), but usually persists for hours, days or weeks, and rarely for many years. The validity of the circus motion theory has recently been questioned. According to recent observations, the excitation spreads in all directions from a focus. The mechanism in atrial

fibrillation, flutter and paroxysmal tachycardia is the same, but the rate and regularity of the discharge from the irritable focus differ, being fastest in fibrillation and slowest in paroxysmal tachycardia.

Etiology. Atrial flutter is commonly associated with heart disease. It occurs in chronic rheumatic heart disease, especially when mitral stenosis is present, in hyperthyroidism, pneumonia, active rheumatic infection, hypertensive and arteriosclerotic heart diseases, myocardial infarction, and less rarely in congenital heart disease. It is far less common than fibrillation and occurs more frequently in older than in younger persons.

Pathologic Physiology. When there is tachycardia, as in 2:1 block, the cardiac output per minute is markedly decreased, together with prolongation of the arm-to-tongue circulation time and cardiac dilatation. Rise in venous pressure may be recorded. Reversion to normal rhythm is accompanied by restoration of these functions toward normal levels. When the ventricular rate is moderately slow, the cardiac output may be normal.

Symptoms. The patient may complain of rapid heart beat or palpitation, which may be described as a "fluttering" sensation. Heart failure may be precipitated or aggravated by its onset.

Diagnosis. The ventricular rate is usually rapid, 150 to 160 per minute, and is not influenced by exercise or holding the breath. Block is increased transiently by carotid sinus pressure. If block varies, the ventricular sequence is irregular. When audible, approximately 300 atrial contractions may be counted per minute, and a ratio between the atrial and ventricular rates is detected. Occasionally, rapid atrial waves and slower larger ventricular waves are identified in the jugular pulse. During 4:1 block when the ventricular rate is around 75 per minute, the rhythm may escape recognition. The detection of regularly spaced flutter waves in the electrocardiogram establishes the diagnosis (Figs. 166; 167, A, B, C, and E). The atrial rate is greater than in atrial paroxysmal tachycardia, but the differentiation is difficult if there is 1:1 ratio.

Impure flutter is intermediate between fibrillation and flutter (Fig. 167, D). Clinically, it resembles fibrillation in irregularity of the ventricular sequence, but in the electrocardiogram there is a fairly but not absolutely regular spacing of flutter waves at a faster rate than in flutter, interspersed with runs of fibrillation waves.

Prognosis. Atrial flutter is usually associated with heart disease. It is commonly of short duration if treated, but may be chronic.

Treatment. Treatment is directed to restoration of normal rhythm. The patient should usually be in bed. Digitalis is the most effective drug. If the clinical strength of the preparation is known and the ventricular rate is rapid, digitalization may be accomplished in 24 hours by giving 1.8 gm., the average amount, in this time (p. 1352). As it becomes effective, the ventricular rate falls as block increases to 3:1 or 4:1 and may reach 75 per cent during the day. Reversion may occur during the first 24 hours. On the other hand, if the rate has not retarded sufficiently, 0.3 gm. twice during the second day may be required. Maintenance doses are given when satisfactory slowing results. It may be necessary to induce nausea and vomiting before reversion occurs. During digitalization the rhythm may become normal. When the ventricular sequence is irregular, it may be due to changing block or to the onset of fibrillation. After the onset of fibrillation, normal rhythm may follow. It may be restored directly from flutter, or often there is an intervening period of fibrillation. It is not necessary to discontinue digitalis at the onset of fibrillation to insure reversion to normal rhythm. Lanatoside C, 1.6 mg. intravenously, may restore normal rhythm earlier, if there is urgency.

After restoration of normal rhythm, digitalis is discontinued unless it is required because of heart failure. If normal rhythm is not occasioned by digitalis, or if the rhythm has changed to fibrillation which persists without giving way to normal rhythm, quinidine sulfate may be used orally, digitalis being used as required, to keep the ventricular rate slow. Fibrillation is more satisfactory as a chronic irregularity than flutter, because the ventricular rate is more easily controlled. If quinidine is effective, maintenance amounts are given for a few days. Occasionally these measures are not successful; it may be impossible even to retard the ventricles. Recurrent flutter may be prevented by digitalization followed by ration doses. If ration doses of quinidine are used for this purpose, which is not recommended, toxic effects should be foreseen. This drug should

not be used intravenously unless there is urgency.

Pronestyl (p. 1369) in large amounts occasionally restores normal rhythm in chronic atrial flutter, but is somewhat more effective in the paroxysmal type. When Pronestyl is used in atrial flutter and fibrillation

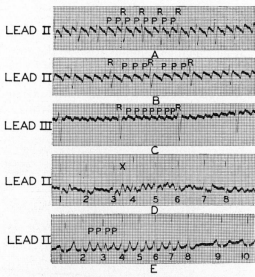

Fig. 167. A shows atrial flutter in lead II with the ratio of atrial waves (PPP) to ventricular ones (RRR) changing from 2:1 to 3:1 (ventricular rate 110, atrial rate 240). B, lead II, 4:1 atrial flutter is recorded (ventricular rate 57, atrial rate 228), and in C, lead III, the ratio is 7:1 (ventricular rate 42, atrial rate 294). D shows atrial fibrillation 1–2–3, changing at X to impure flutter for 4–5–6, and then atrial fibrillation again for 7 and 8. In E (lead II) the first complex 1 is normal rhythm followed by 7 complexes (2 to 8) of atrial flutter (PP), in which the position of the ventricular contraction changes, and is then followed by reversion to normal rhythm for complexes 9 and 10.

a toxic effect may be the onset of atrial flutter with 1:1 ratio.

The use of digitalis to restore normal rhythm is based on its vagal effects. Vagal stimulation by the drug shortens the refractory period of atrial muscle and increases the transmission rate. This action tends to maintain the gap in the circus and shortens the time to make a circuit, and the atrial rate increases. The direct action of the drug on the atrial muscle, on the other hand, lengthens its refractory period and slows conduction, which tends to close the gap and slow the atrial rate. Although the vagal and direct effects are opposite, the vagal effect overrides the direct action and converts flutter to fibrillation, from which normal rhythm may follow. The action of quinidine, effective in breaking up the circus motion, is the same as in fibrillation; it fails when the effect on conduction overbalances that on the refractory period.

ATRIOVENTRICULAR TISSUE

ATRIOVENTRICULAR, NODAL OR JUNCTIONAL PREMATURE CONTRACTIONS

If an abnormal stimulus arises in the atrioventricular node or bundle, a premature contraction results. In a large series of electrocardiograms they are frequently encountered. They may occur occasionally in a pattern.

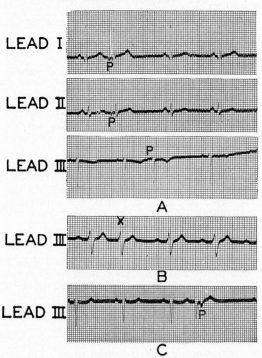

Fig. 168. *A* records the three standard leads of the electrocardiogram in which one atrioventricular premature contraction (*P*), arising high in the tissue, is recorded in each lead, so that the P wave is in front of the QRS complex and the P–R time of them 0.08 to 0.09 second. In *B* the atrioventricular premature contraction (*X*) arises near the middle of the tissue, and a P wave is not seen. In *C* the atrioventricular premature contraction (*P*) arises low in the atrioventricular bundle, and ventricular contraction precedes atrial activity, so that the P wave follows the QRS complex.

Etiology. Nodal premature contractions occur in normal as well as in diseased hearts, especially during active rheumatic carditis and myocardial infarction.

Pathologic Physiology. Occasional atrioventricular premature contractions do not embarrass the circulation appreciably.

Symptoms. There may be symptoms similar to those associated with atrial premature contractions.

Diagnosis. They cannot be differentiated clinically from atrial premature contrac-

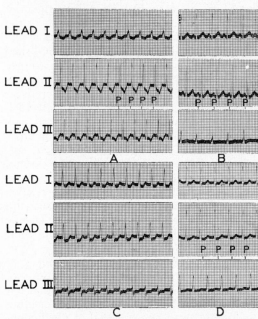

Fig. 169, *A* and *B* show the three standard leads, illustrating atrioventricular paroxysmal tachycardia (rate 206 and 150 per minute, respectively), in which the P waves (*PPP*) fall in front of the QRS. *C* shows the three standard leads, illustrating atrioventricular paroxysmal tachycardia (rate 176), in which the P waves are not seen and are presumably concealed in the QRS complexes, and in *D* the P waves (*PPP*) follow the QRS complexes (rate 172 per minute). Increasing the speed of the electrocardiograph film or loosening the galvanometer string may aid in identifying the P waves.

tions. The diagnosis is electrocardiographic. The impulse arising in the atrioventricular tissue passes backward by retrograde conduction to the atria and initiates their contraction, and simultaneously downward to the ventricles, stimulating them. If the stimulus arises high up in the junctional tissue, the atria contract first, followed in 0.10 second or less by the ventricles; if it arises in the middle of this tissue, it arrives simultaneously at the atria and ventricles, and they contract synchronously; if it arises at the lower part of the junctional tissue, the stimulus arrives at the ventricles first, causes them to contract, and, arriving later at the atria, results in their contraction; accordingly, in the electrocardiograms the P wave falls in front of (Fig. 168, *A*), during (Fig. 168, *B*), or after the QRS complex (Fig. 168, *C*).

One atrioventricular premature contraction occasionally initiates two ventricular contractions. The stimulus traverses the atrioventricular bundle and initiates the ventricular contraction and, in passing backward to the atria, stimulates their contraction; this atrial impulse spreads through the atrial muscle, and, arriving at the atrioventricular tissue, passes down the bundle if this tissue is no longer refractory, is distributed again to the ventricles and causes another ventricular systole, provided the ventricles have also recovered from their refractoriness.

Treatment. When treatment is required, it is similar to that given for atrial premature contractions.

ATRIOVENTRICULAR PAROXYSMAL TACHYCARDIA

This term designates a rapid, regular beating of the heart, controlled by stimuli arising in the junctional tissue and characterized by sudden onset and sudden offset. It may be looked upon as a succession of atrioventricular premature contractions. The excitation wave passes upward to the atria, initiating their contraction, and also downward to the ventricles, stimulating them. The rate is usually around 150 to 200 per minute, but may be slower or more rapid.

Etiology. It occurs in all age groups both in subjects with normal hearts and in those with organic disease. It occurs in acute rheumatic fever and myocardial infarction and in patients with Wolff-Parkinson-White syndrome. It may be transient or persist for days.

Pathologic Physiology. Atrioventricular paroxysmal tachycardia is associated with decreased cardiac output per minute and per beat. The circulation time may be prolonged, and the heart dilates. The blood pressure may fall and heart failure appear.

Symptoms. Symptoms are similar to those associated with atrial paroxysmal tachycardia.

Diagnosis. Clinically, this cannot be differentiated from atrial paroxysmal tachycardia, although the rate may be more rapid. The diagnosis is made in the electrocardiogram: the P wave falls before (0.10 second or less) (Fig. 169, *A, B*), during (Fig. 169, *C*), or after the QRS complex (Fig. 169,

D). Occasionally, supraventricular paroxysmal tachycardia is diagnosed if the origin cannot be more accurately localized.

Prognosis. Attacks may occur for many years without the appearance of signs of cardiac disease. Electrocardiographic changes may persist several weeks after an attack.

Treatment. Treatment is similar to that for atrial paroxysmal tachycardia. Digitalis is the most effective drug. Pronestyl either orally or intravenously is frequently effective even in small doses in restoring normal rhythm (see pp. 1369–1370).

ATRIOVENTRICULAR OR NODAL RHYTHM

Atrioventricular rhythm occurs when pacemaking is dislocated from the sinus node to the atrioventricular tissue, so that a focus in this tissue controls the beating of atria as well as ventricles. The rate is usually slower than the discharge from the sinus node. The sequence is usually regular.

Etiology. The dislocation of pacemaking to this node is precipitated either by factors depressing the sinus discharges by vagal

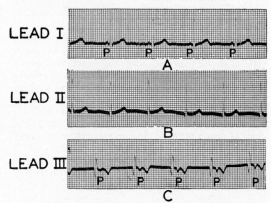

Fig. 170. *A* shows lead I, illustrating nodal rhythm (rate 66 per minute) in which the P waves (*PPP*) precede the QRS; the P-R time is 0.08 to 0.09 second. *B* shows lead II, illustrating nodal rhythm (rate 79 per minute) in which the P waves are not seen and it appears that the P and QRS occur simultaneously. *C* shows lead III of nodal rhythm in which the focus for pacemaking is low in the bundle so that the ventricular complexes (QRS) (65 per minute) occur first, followed by the atrial contractions (*PPP*).

stimulation, or those increasing the irritability of the atrioventricular tissue by sympathetic nerve stimulation. The rhythm occurs more commonly in subjects having heart disease. It may result from digitalis,

sometimes in doses less than the full therapeutic amount, and also after atropine. On
the other hand, atropine may restore sinus
pacemaking. It is encountered in acute infections.

Pathologic Physiology. Studies of the
circulation during this rhythm have not been
reported.

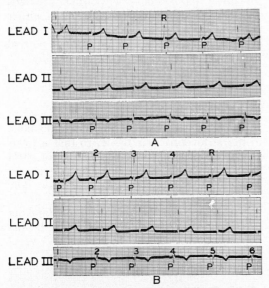

Fig. 171. A shows three leads of nodal rhythm
(rate 50 per minute) in which the focus for pacemaking shuttles up and down the junctional tissue,
indicated by the changing position of the P waves
(PPP) to the QRS complexes. B shows three leads of
wandering pacemaker. Complexes 1 and 2 arise in
the sinus node (58 per minute); 3 shifts to high up
in the junctional tissue (rate 48 per minute); the
place of origin of the excitation wave then gradually
moves down the bundle (shifting position of P
waves) in leads I and II, and in lead III the site is
again high up (complexes 2 and 3), then in 4–5–6
activity is restored to the sinus node.

Symptoms. The rhythm causes no symptoms unless the rate is very slow.

Diagnosis. The diagnosis should be suspected when large pulsations occur in the
jugular veins resulting from simultaneous
contraction of atria and ventricles. Electrocardiograms differentiate it from complete
block and sinus bradycardia. The stimuli may
arise in any part of the atrioventricular
tissue so that the P waves in the electrocardiogram precede (Fig. 170, A), occur simultaneously with (Fig. 170, B), follow the
QRS complex (Fig. 170, C), or shuttle up
and down (Fig. 171, A).

Prognosis. Normal rhythm is restored
when the precipitating factors are eliminated.

Treatment. Atrioventricular rhythm is
usually transient, but may persist for days.
It requires no special therapy. If digitalis is
implicated, normal rhythm follows its elimination. Heart failure, however, takes precedence in therapy.

WANDERING PACEMAKER

When pacemaking shifts back and forth
from the sinus to the atrioventricular node,
the rhythm is designated as *wandering
pacemaker*. It is commonly transient, but
may be persistent. It may follow digitalization. It is frequently observed in normal
persons, especially athletes with bradycardia,
and during deep breathing. It may be evidence of carotid sinus hyperactivity. In electrocardiograms the P waves shift location
with respect to the QRS complexes, indicating that the site of impulse formation shifts
from the sinus node to the upper part of the
atrioventricular node, then moves gradually down the atrioventricular tissues, after
which it retraces its course up the junctional tissue back to the sinus node (Fig.
171, B).

CONDUCTION DEFECTS
HEART BLOCK

Heart block refers to atrioventricular
heart block and occurs when stimuli arising
in the sinus node or atria are delayed or
obstructed in their passage down the atrioventricular bundle. Defect in the main bundle is more common than in its right and left
branches.

When there is delay in conducting the
sinus impulse, the interval from the beginning of atrial activity to the onset of ventricular activity in the electrocardiogram exceeds 0.20 second in adults. This is designated *prolonged P-R conduction time* or *first
degree heart block* (Fig. 172, A). When impulses are blocked from reaching the ventricles, so that ventricular contractions fail
to occur, there is *second degree, partial* or
incomplete heart block, which may assume
several patterns. In the *Wenckebach phenomenon* the delay in conduction increases
progressively until an impulse is blocked and
a *"dropped beat"* occurs; the bundle transmits
the next sinus impulse, after which the progressive increase in P-R time recurs (Fig.
172, B). Every third (3:2 heart block),
fourth, fifth, six, seventh or eighth stimulus
may be blocked. At other times, every second
or every second and third impulses are

blocked, giving rise to 2:1 (Fig. 172, C) and 3:1 (Fig. 172, D) block in which there are two and three atrial contractions to one ventricular beat, respectively. These are *high grade heart block*. Finally, when obstruction to the passage of sinus impulses is total, *complete heart block* or *complete atrioventricular dissociation* is present (Figs. 172, E, F; 173, A). When this occurs, the ventricles escape and contract at their own inherent rhythm, which is usually slow, 30 to 40 per minute, and rarely rapid: *idioventricular rhythm* prevails (Figs. 172, E, F; 173, A). The atria may beat regularly (Figs. 172, F; 173, A) or fibrillate (Fig. 172, E).

Etiology. Alterations in the conducting system resulting in heart block may be occasioned by (1) structural damage, (2) toxic effect of drugs, (3) nutritional changes and (4) vagal effects. Conduction changes are accepted as criteria of rheumatic activity which may cause all degrees of transient or permanent block. Any degree of block occurs in arteriosclerosis, and in myocardial infarction it may be transient or chronic. Likewise, diphtheria may cause any degree of block, especially complete block. Congenital heart block, especially when complete, may be associated with interventricular septal defect. Digitalis results in any grade of block. Methacholine chloride induces conduction defects through its stimulation of parasympathetic nerve effects. Nutritional or functional changes probably cause the alterations in uremia and in myxedema. Carotid sinus pressure may induce any grade block and cardiac standstill (Fig. 173, B, C).

Morbid Anatomy. In functional or nutritional block, pathologic lesions are not expected. In organic block, anatomic lesions are detected frequently, but may not be greater than in another heart in which defects are not recorded. The lack of correlation between the presence of block and the microscopic picture is not surprising, since the integrity of a few fibers may be sufficient to transmit the excitation wave. Inflammatory changes in rheumatic fever may involve the conduction system, although the changes are also attributed to vagal effects. Arteriosclerosis causes block either by myocardial fibrosis involving the bundle or by decrease in blood supply by narrowing or closure of coronary vessels supplying this tissue. There may be diffuse syphilitic involvement or gumma formation.

First degree heart block causes no symp-

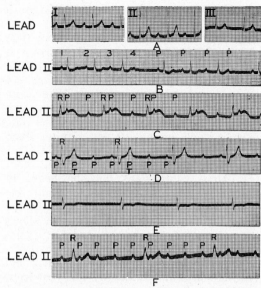

Fig. 172. *A* shows three standard leads with P-R conduction prolonged to 0.32 second in lead II. *B* shows in lead II gradual prolongation of P-R from 0.20 in 1st, to 0.27 in 2d, to 0.39 in the 3rd complex, and the fourth P wave is blocked; this pattern is then repeated (Wenckebach phenomenon). *C* shows lead II of 2:1 heart block (P = P waves, R = ventricular waves), with prolonged P-R time to 0.41 second (ventricular rate 48, atrial rate 96). The blocked P wave appears on the hump of the T waves. *D* shows lead I of 3:1 heart block (*PPP* = P waves and *R* = ventricular complexes) (ventricular rate 37, atrial rate 111). *E* shows atrial fibrillation with complete heart block and idioventricular rhythm, the ventricular rate 37 in lead II. *F* shows lead II of complete heart block with the atria (*PPP*) continuing to contract at the rate of the sinus node discharge (ventricular rate 30, atrial rate 120). Idioventricular rhythm with bundle branch block is present (QRS prolonged to 0.12 second).

toms. The P-R interval in the electrocardiogram exceeds 0.20 second (Fig. 172, A).

SECOND DEGREE HEART BLOCK

Pathologic Physiology. Occasional block is probably associated with no marked change in cardiac function; 2:1 block results in decrease in cardiac output per minute with prolongation of the circulation time.

Symptoms. Patients are usually unaware of occasional block; when occurring frequently, they may complain of the pause, of the forceful beat after the pause, or palpitation. In 2:1 block they may complain of the slow forceful beating and dyspnea, and rarely exhibit other signs of failure.

Diagnosis. During digitalis therapy or rheumatic fever the diagnosis is frequently possible. When there is occasional block, a sequence of regular beats followed by a pause will be detected on auscultation, then the regular sequence recurs. The pause is also apparent in the pulse. The irregularity differs from a premature contraction in not being preceded by an early beat. The pause may equal two regular cycles. When high grade block is present, the ventricular rate may be slow, around 40 per minute; when the ventricular rate suddenly halves, 2 : 1 heart block should be considered (Fig. 172, C). Atrial contractions may be heard in the middle of the long pauses, and one "c" to two "a" waves may be seen in the jugular pulse. The electrocardiogram shows the relationship between P and QRS complexes (Fig. 172, B, C, D).

In *interference dissociation* the atria and ventricles beat independently. The ventricles, under the direction of the atrioventricular node or the idioventricular center, contract slightly more rapidly than the atria, which are responding to the sinus node. This is in contrast to the common type of complete atrioventricular dissociation in which the ventricular rate is slower than the atrial rate and is very slow. Interference dissociation is seen in active rheumatic carditis and after digitalis.

Prognosis of First and Second Degree Heart Block. In rheumatic fever, block usually disappears with recovery; when resulting from digitalis, normal conduction is ́restored with its elimination. In syphilitic and arteriosclerotic heart diseases, or after myocardial infarction, block indicates myocardial damage and makes the prognosis more serious.

Treatment. Incomplete block usually requires no treatment. Digitalis, when implicated, is omitted for a few days or the dose diminished. If the patient complains of irregularity, atropine, 0.0006 gm., may abolish it. Digitalis can usually be given when necessary even though high grade organic block is present, without increasing the block.

COMPLETE HEART BLOCK

Etiology. Complete block is most common in arteriosclerotic heart disease, with or without myocardial infarction, less common in congenital heart disease, in rheumatic carditis, after diphtheria and digitalis intoxication.

Pathologic Physiology. Complete block is usually associated with marked decrease in the cardiac output *per minute,* but the stroke volume is usually increased. The circulation time may be prolonged. The heart rate cannot increase appreciably to provide increase in cardiac output. As a compensatory mechanism, the organism decreases its basal metabolic rate. The systolic blood pressure may be elevated.

Symptoms. When complete block has become established, patients may be without symptoms at rest, but experience dyspnea and dizziness on exertion. They may be unaware of the rhythm or may complain of the slow forceful beating of the heart. Other patients suffer the Adams-Stokes syndrome, characterized by syncope with convulsions, or milder symptoms of dizziness and faintness, because there may be several seconds of ventricular asystole at the onset of complete block before the idioventricular center becomes active. During this time the circulation is at a standstill. In recurrent complete block the Adams-Stokes syndrome may recur with each onset. When complete block has become established and adjustments have been made, the cardiac output is usually sufficient to supply the body needs, and the patient recovers from syncope and convulsions and may remain without symptoms. On further slowing of the rate, however, to 15 or 20 per minute, syncope will recur. Asystole and syncope may be transient or persist for several seconds. Heart failure may result.

Diagnosis. Complete heart block is to be suspected when the heart beats regularly around 35 per minute and the patient complains of syncopal attacks. It is to be differentiated from 2 : 1 heart block and sinus bradycardia. Exercise does not increase the rate appreciably. The cardiac and radial rates correspond. Atrial beats may be heard at a more rapid rate than the ventricular ones; "a" waves may be identified during the ventricular intervals, and a ratio is not apparent. Electrocardiograms confirm the diagnosis (Figs. 172, E, F; 173, A). When digitalis is being given in atrial fibrillation, the onset of a slow, *regular* ventricular sequence suggests complete block (Fig. 172, E). That paroxysmal tachycardia, ventricular flutter and transient ventricular fibrillation may also cause syncope must be kept in mind.

Prognosis. Complete block usually disappears with recovery from rheumatic carditis and diphtheria. Persistence after diphtheria is compatible with longevity. In syphilitic and arteriosclerotic heart disease and after myocardial infarction it indicates progressive damage to heart muscle and makes the prognosis more serious. Bundle branch block increases the hazards. Compensated patients tolerate surgical operations. Death follows prolonged ventricular asystole or too great

not known whether the patient will suffer another seizure shortly after recovery. If the attack is prolonged, intracardiac injection of epinephrine is indicated. In chronic complete block, patients may require epinephrine every 2 to 3 hours for many days, because of sudden decline in rate below that established. For more prolonged effect, ephedrine sulfate 20 to 30 mg. three times

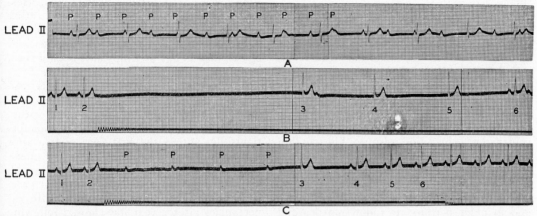

Fig. 173. A shows a long strip of lead II, showing complete heart block with idioventricular rhythm, atrial rate 75 and the ventricular rate 43 per minute. At times 3:1 or 4:1 heart block may be diagnosed unless a long enough strip is taken for the P waves and QRS complexes to get out of step. The P-P interval in which the QRS falls may be short. B shows in lead II asystole for 6 seconds, resulting from right carotid sinus pressure, ventricular escape finally occurring at 3 with three complexes of idioventricular rhythm, and reversion to normal sinus rhythm at 6, while pressure is still maintained. The signal at the bottom indicates the application of pressure. C shows in lead II complete heart block with ventricular asystole for 6 seconds on the application of pressure to the left carotid sinus. The atrial rate (PPP) is 43 per minute. There is ventricular escape at 3, followed by return to normal sinus rhythm at 4 while pressure is still maintained. The signal indicates onset and release of pressure.

ventricular slowing. Complete block occasionally disappears after being present for many months.

Treatment. When complete block has become established, treatment is usually not required. Patients lead active lives with restriction of overexertion. If heart failure occurs, digitalis is used. When block is due to digitalis, normal conduction follows its elimination.

When Adams-Stokes attacks occur frequently, 0.5 to 1 cc. of epinephrine, 1:1000, is given hypodermically. Its effect lasts 1 to 2 hours. It may be prolonged by using epinephrine in oil. It increases the irritability of the ventricular pacemaker and of ventricular muscle and may prevent long periods of asystole as well as increase the rate. Although it may be useless to give epinephrine during Adams-Stokes syncope, it is advisable to give it at once, nevertheless, because it is

a day orally, may be beneficial. *Isuprel hydrochloride* (isopropylarterenol hydrochloride) sublingually in 15 mg. doses may prevent attacks of syncope. In other instances, barium chloride, 30 to 40 mg. three or four times day orally, increases ventricular irritability. Thyroid extract, 0.1 gm. once to three times a day, may be tried. It is used cautiously, not only because it is inadvisable to increase the basal metabolic rate in patients with coronary artery disease, but also because fall in basal metabolic rate is one of the compensatory mechanisms in complete block. Atropine, 0.5 to 1 mg. orally or hypodermically several times daily, may decrease vagal block. Digitalis may prevent Adams-Stokes attacks, especially if heart failure is present. In other instances of complete heart block with syncope due to ventricular paroxysmal tachycardia or ventricular fibrillation, digitalis may abolish the attacks.

With the onset of complete heart block death results unless the idioventricular center or a focus in one of the ventricles takes over promptly. Recently, electrical impulses applied to the anterior chest wall within a few minutes after cardiac arrest in complete heart block have initiated cardiac contractions which have kept the heart beating until the intrinsic pacemakers revived and resumed activity.

BUNDLE BRANCH BLOCK

Bundle branch block or intraventricular block occurs when the excitation wave is impeded in its passage down the right or left branch of the atrioventricular bundle, an abnormality recorded in electrocardiograms. Excitation of the ventricle supplied by that branch is delayed, and asynchronism of ventricular contraction results. The rhythm is unaffected.

Etiology. It is usually chronic but may be transient. It occurs most commonly in arteriosclerotic and hypertensive heart diseases and in older persons. It follows myocardial infarction. Left bundle branch block is more common than right, probably because sclerotic changes are more common in the descending branch of the left coronary artery. It may be due to a congenital defect of the conduction system. It occurs occasionally in rheumatic carditis and in chronic valvular disease (aortic stenosis and insufficiency). Gumma and diffuse syphilitic involvement, as well as diphtheria, are less commonly implicated. Bundle branch block is occasionally functional in uremia, and a fatigue manifestation during tachycardia. It may be a toxic effect of quinidine or Pronestyl, and rarely has been attributed to digitalis. It occurs in association with a short P-R conduction (Wolff-Parkinson-White syndrome) (Fig. 174). It is seen in acute myocarditis of obscure origin associated with cardiac enlargement, heart failure and embolic phenomena (Fiedler's or isolated myocarditis).

Morbid Anatomy. Myocardial fibrosis involving the bundles has been found when bundle branch block was recorded electrocardiographically. It is, however, frequently impossible to differentiate microscopically the blocked from the unblocked side, or from the bundles in hearts not exhibiting this defect.

Pathologic Physiology. The lesion occurs most frequently in hearts subject to myocardial damage in which the functional capacity may be already reduced.

Symptoms. There are no symptoms attributable to bundle branch block.

Diagnosis. The clinical diagnosis cannot be made with certainty. Gallop rhythm, a bifid apex thrust, and reduplication of one or both heart sounds suggest its presence. Pulsus alternans may be present. The QRS time exceeds 0.1 second, usually 0.12 second or longer. Occasionally, every other beat shows block. There may be normal P-R conduction or any degree of atrioventricular block (Fig. 172, F). Unipolar limb and chest leads aid in the diagnosis.

Prognosis. Bundle branch block is usually associated with severe myocardial damage. The nature of the underlying disease determines its prognostic import. Many patients die within the first year or two after its recognition, the others may live many years. Patients with right bundle branch block of the S wave type have the best prognosis, and look forward to normal life expectancies after a year has elapsed following its recognition. If there are no other defects these patients may lead normal lives. Patients with the other types of bundle branch block with good functional capacities and without symptoms may also engage in activities commensurate with the underlying disease. If the functional capacity of the heart is unimpaired, patients sustain surgical procedures satisfactorily, but special care is given to anesthesia, avoidance of anoxia, and of overloading the circulation with fluids.

Treatment. In most instances specific treatment is not indicated. It may disappear in uremia when hypertonic glucose is given intravenously. It may also disappear with recovery from heart failure. Neither quinidine nor Pronestyl should be used in the presence of this lesion.

WOLFF-PARKINSON-WHITE SYNDROME

The Wolff-Parkinson-White syndrome is a conduction defect in the electrocardiogram characterized by a *short P-R interval* (0.10 second or less) and *prolonged QRS time* (0.11 second or more) (Fig. 173). It is a pre-excitation phenomenon. It is usually an accidental finding in subjects without evidence of organic heart disease. Patients are prone to attacks of paroxysmal rhythms, most commonly atrial or nodal and less frequently ventricular tachycardia, and rarely to atrial flutter and fibrillation. One explanation of this syndrome is the presence of a congenital accessory pathway of conduction, such as the bundle of Kent, bridging the atria and ventricles. The short P-R time would be accounted for if this accessory pathway offered a shorter and more rapid route for conduction from atria to ventricles; the long QRS would be explained by asynchronous contraction of the two ventricles, one ventricular contraction being initiated by the stimulus which has bridged the gap by the bundle of Kent, and the other contraction occurring at a later time by the excitation wave traversing the usual pathway down its bundle. Restoration of normal P-R and QRS intervals may take place with atropine and exercise, suggesting that vagal effects underlie this phenomenon. Both digitalis and quinidine have restored normal relationships in others.

Prognosis. This defect does not appear to carry a serious prognosis, except that it predisposes to paroxysmal rhythms which may be refractory to treatment. It may be associated with other congenital cardiac defects.

VENTRICULAR RHYTHMS

IDIOVENTRICULAR RHYTHM

With the onset of complete heart block or atrial standstill, the ventricles beat in response to stimuli from the idioventricular center, which is located in the atrioventricular bundle just before its bifurcation. It discharges impulses usually at a slow rate, around 35 per minute. The QRS complex in the electrocardiogram has a supraventricular form (Figs. 172, *E*; 173, *A*), unless there is a bundle branch defect (Fig. 172, *F*). Rarely when the site of origin is in the ventricular muscle below the bifurcation, the complexes resemble ventricular premature contractions. Because of the block, the impulses do not pass backward to the atria. Idioventricular rhythm differs from atrioventricular rhythm, in which stimuli arising in the atrioventricular tissue control both atrial and ventricular activity.

VENTRICULAR ESCAPE

Occasionally, when the sinus discharges are greatly retarded and the atrioventricular node is also depressed, there may be ventricular escape and one or more beats arise from the idioventricular center. It occurs in

normal persons and after carotid sinus stimulation. The QRS complex is usually of the supraventricular form without a preceding P wave (Figs. 161, *B*; 173, *B, C*) because of retrograde block; it may, however, be of aberrant form.

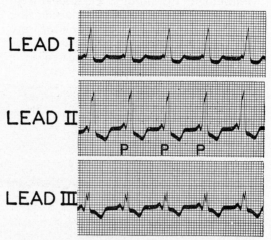

Fig. 174. An example of the short P-R (0.07 to 0.08 second) and the long QRS (0.12 second), or Wolff-Parkinson-White syndrome.

VENTRICULAR PREMATURE CONTRACTIONS

If an abnormal stimulus arises in the right or left ventricle or septum, a ventricular premature contraction results. The impulse spreads over the ventricles and up to the atrioventricular bundle and node, but *usually not* back to the atria, so that the dominant rhythm is uninterrupted; occasionally, however, retrograde conduction to the atria occurs. The normal impulse from the sinus node passing down the atrioventricular system usually finds the ventricles refractory, having just contracted prematurely.

Etiology. Stimuli causing ventricular premature contractions have been elicited in man *mechanically* and *electrically*. They occur more commonly in older persons. Forced respiration or excitement may incite them. They are common in organic heart disease, but more frequently no other cardiac signs are detected. They occur in acute infections, especially acute rheumatic fever, acute tonsillitis and pneumonia, in arteriosclerotic, hypertensive and chronic rheumatic valvular heart disease, and after coronary thrombosis. They may result from nervous tension, loss of sleep, coffee and cigarettes, and from overdigitalization, when coupled rhythm may appear (p. 1372). On the other hand, they may be a manifestation of heart failure and may disappear with digitalization. They may precede ventricular paroxysmal tachycardia.

Pathologic Physiology. Occasional ventricular premature contractions do not alter the functional capacity of the heart, but when they are frequent and persistent, the cardiac output is probably decreased.

the electrocardiogram when the QRS complex which is not preceded by or related to a P wave is wide and split, and the T wave usually opposite in direction to the main QRS deflection. Ventricular premature contractions may occur irregularly or in a recurrent pattern. Occasionally, retrograde conduction occurs and the excitation wave initiates an atrial premature contraction; the stimulus of this atrial premature contraction then passes downward through the atrioven-

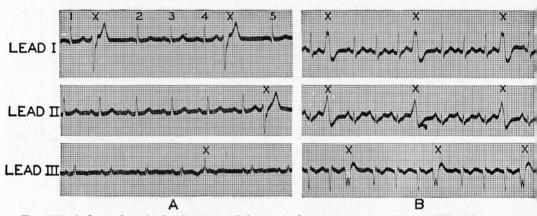

Fig. 175. A shows three leads, illustrating left ventricular premature contractions (X). There is compensatory pause. In lead I the interval 1 to 2 equals twice the regular intervals, 2–3, or equals 2 to 4. B shows three leads, illustrating right ventricular premature contractions (X) after every third normal contraction. The pause after the ventricular premature contractions is compensatory. If the main QRS deflection is upward in lead I, the premature contraction arises in the right ventricle (B); and if downward, in the left ventricle (A). The form of QRS in leads II and III is dependent upon the origin of the premature contractions in the apical, middle or basal part of the heart.

Symptoms. The symptoms do not differ significantly from those experienced with atrial premature contractions.

Diagnosis. Ventricular premature contractions can usually be diagnosed clinically. On ausculation the beat is premature; the radial pulse may be premature or may show a pulse deficit if the beat occurred so early that insufficient blood was available to form a radial pulse. There is an appreciable pause after the premature beat until the next regular one occurs. This *compensatory pause* may be too short, however, to make differentiation from supraventricular premature contraction certain. The interval from the last usual beat to the first one after the premature beat equals two normal cycles (Fig. 175, A, B). There may be a large wave in the jugular vein coinciding with the ventricular premature contraction, owing to the atria contracting while the ventricles are in systole. Ventricular premature contractions may disappear on exercise. The diagnosis is made in

tricular tissue and excites the ventricles to contract again; this one will be supraventricular in form (short QRS).

Prognosis depends upon the circumstances in which the premature contractions occur and upon other evidences of heart disease.

Treatment. When treatment is required, the general principles are the same as for atrial premature contractions: elimination of possible factors, and use of triple bromide or phenobarbital. Triple bromide, 1 gm. twice or three times a day, is frequently effective. If the premature contractions result from digitalis, the drug is stopped for a few days or the ration decreased. Except when the contractions are a manifestation of congestive failure, digitalis is not used, because it may increase their number. If they are numerous or multiple, digitalis may precipitate ventricular paroxysmal tachycardia or ventricular fibrillation. If other measures fail, *Pronestyl* is probably the most effective drug. It is given orally in 0.25 gm. amounts four times a day, but larger amounts may be required (p. 1370). It may be used in the presence of digitalis effect and when ventricular premature contractions are due to digitalis intoxication. Quinidine sulfate, 0.2 gm. three

the ventricles are capable of responding again. Auscultation reveals three rapid beats, the middle one being the *"extrasystole."* Interpolated premature contractions may arise from the atria (Fig. 176, C, D), atrioven-

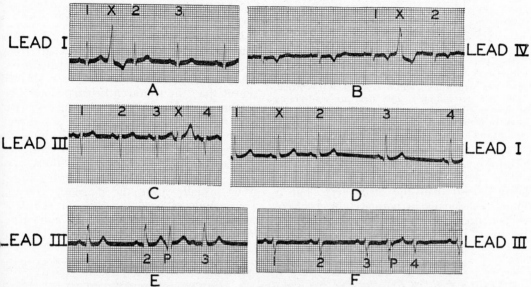

Fig. 176. A and B show leads I and IV, respectively, illustrating interpolated right ventricular premature contractions between normal complexes 1 and 2 (X) (see text). C shows in lead I an interpolated atrial premature contraction (X) between normal complexes 3 and 4, and, in D, in lead III interpolated atrial premature contraction (X) between normal complexes 1 and 2. QRS complexes of the premature beats are supraventricular in form. E reproduces lead III, showing an interpolated atrioventricular premature contraction in which the P wave (P) precedes the QRS between normal beats 2 and 3, and in F, lead III, the P wave (P) of the atrioventricular premature contraction falls after the QRS, between normal beats 3 and 4.

toxication. Quinidine sulfate, 0.2 gm. three times a day, may abolish the contractions. If successful, the drug may frequently be discontinued without their recurrence. If the drug is used over long periods, toxic effects must be avoided. Potassium phosphate or chloride or papaverine may abolish them (p. 1349).

INTERPOLATED PREMATURE CONTRACTIONS

Premature contractions are interpolated when they occur between two normal heart beats without disturbing the rhythm; they are true *extrasystoles*. In the electrocardiogram, if the premature stimulus occurs near the middle of the P-R interval and the ventricles are no longer refractory, a premature contraction will occur, and recovery will again take place, so that when the next normal atrial impulse arrives, the conduction tissue is receptive to transmit it and

tricular tissue (Fig. 176, E, F) or from the ventricles (Fig. 176, A, B).

VENTRICULAR PAROXYSMAL TACHYCARDIA

This is a fairly regular rhythm with a rapid rate caused by stimuli originating from an irritable focus in one of the ventricles, characterized by sudden onset and sudden offset. It may be considered a succession of premature contractions. If the preceding rhythm was normal, the sinus impulses continue and the atria contract at their usual rate (Fig. 177, A, B). Atrial fibrillation may, however, be present (Fig. 178, A, B). Ventricular paroxysmal tachycardia may result from a circus motion in the ventricles. The ventricular rate is commonly 150 to 200, rarely greater than 220. It may persist for a few beats (Fig. 179, B, C), several minutes, hours or many days and be resistant to treatment.

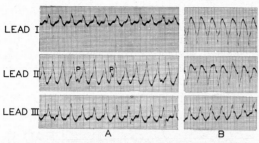

Fig. 177. A shows the three leads of ventricular paroxysmal tachycardia from the right ventricle (rate 182 per minute), and B, from the left ventricle (rate 206 per minute). The atria are contracting at their usual slower rate indicated by P in lead II of A. In B the standardization of the string is for 2 cm. instead of 1 cm. to magnify the waves.

Etiology. Ventricular paroxysmal tachycardia occurs more commonly in organic heart disease than the atrial type, but is found occasionally in normal subjects. Ventricular premature contractions may precede its onset. It is most common in the latter

crease in venous pressure unless heart failure supervenes. The heart dilates, and the blood pressure falls.

Symptoms. The patient experiences symptoms similar to those of atrial paroxysmal tachycardia. Since they occur more commonly as a complication of heart disease, however, patients appear more ill.

Diagnosis. Ventricular paroxysmal tachycardia is to be differentiated especially from atrial and nodal paroxysmal tachycardia. The rate is commonly 150 to 180, slightly slower than the supraventricular forms. The rhythm is slightly irregular as compared with atrial tachycardia. Frequently, "a" waves can be identified in the jugular vessels, and are especially large when the atria and ventricles contract simultaneously. Carotid sinus pressure is usually ineffectual. Electrocardiograms usually make the diagnosis certain. The complexes have the form of ventricular premature contractions and may arise from either ventricle (Fig. 177, A, B), or

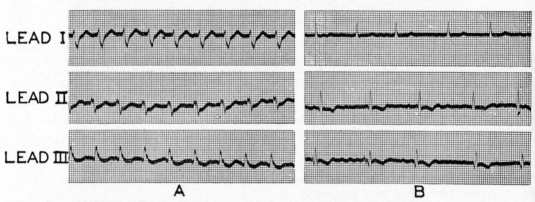

Fig. 178. A shows the three standard leads of ventricular paroxysmal tachycardia (rate 125 per minute) from the left ventricle during paroxysm, and B, after reversion to atrial fibrillation (ventricle rate approximately 75 per minute).

decades when arteriosclerotic and hypertensive heart diseases occur. It may follow myocardial infarction and at other times has been thought to lead to myocardial infarction due to the fall in blood pressure or decrease in coronary circulation. It occurs in acute rheumatic fever, in subjects with Wolff-Parkinson-White syndrome. It may be a toxic manifestation of digitalis, quinidine, or digitalis and quinidine given at the same time.

Pathologic Physiology. It is associated with marked decrease in the cardiac output per minute. There is prolongation of the arm to tongue circulation time, without in-

may be alternating (Fig. 179, A), or the QRS complexes may vary. If the preceding rhythm was normal, the atria continue to beat slowly and independent P waves appear (Fig. 177). The ventricular excitation waves are usually blocked from passing backward. Occasionally, however, *retrograde* conduction to the atria causes them to contract, the sinus node being superseded. If atrial paroxysmal tachycardia and bundle branch block occur together, the complexes will be similar to ventricular premature contractions. The detection of P waves may establish the rhythm as atrial, or the occurrence of ventricular premature contractions in other records of the patient may aid in the differentiation.

Prognosis. Ventricular paroxysmal tachycardia may be an alarming hazard when it occurs in the course of myocardial infarction. Impairment in the coronary circulation associated with marked decrease in cardiac output and fall in blood pressure is shown in the T wave changes, which may persist for days after reversion to normal rhythm. Heart failure may be precipitated.

Treatment. The patient should be in bed. If the paroxysm is brief, treatment is not required. More commonly it persists unless measures are taken to control it; most circumstances in which it occurs require its prompt abolition. Two drugs, namely quinidine and Pronestyl, are available for the treatment of this rhythm. Pronestyl has the advantage that it can be given intravenously more safely than quinidine when it is urgent to terminate the rhythm without delay. Quinidine is usually effective: 0.2 gm. is given; 2 hours later, if there have been no evidences of idiosyncrasy (see Atrial Fibrillation) and normal rhythm has not been restored, 0.4 gm. is given and repeated every 4 hours. Three to 4 gm. may be required in 24 hours before reversion occurs. If it is not urgent, 2 gm. may be given the first day, 3 gm. the next; but if myocardial infarction is present, restoration should be achieved promptly with the larger amounts without waiting to test for idiosyncrasy. When possible, electrocardiograms should be taken. Massive doses of quinidine may occasion ventricular fibrillation. After restoration of normal rhythm, 0.2 gm. three times a day is given for a few days. With therapy the ventricular rate declines, followed by reversion to normal rhythm or atrial fibrillation. It is rarely necessary to give quinidine hydrochloride in 0.2 to 0.3 gm. amounts *intravenously*. Great care must be exercised should quinidine lactate in 0.2 to 0.4 gm. amounts be used intravenously. A mixture of quinidine hydrochloride, 15 gm., antipyrine, 15 gm., urea, 20 gm., and distilled water to 100 cc. has been found to give a soluble quinidine preparation for intramuscular use with 0.45 to 0.6 gm. as the initial dose. Quinidine is not warranted routinely after myocardial infarction to prevent this rhythm. For recurrent attacks, quinidine sulfate, 0.2 gm. two or three times a day, is usually effective; patients should be instructed in its use. Digitalis is usually contraindicated, for it increases ventricular irritability and may precipitate ventricular fibrillation. If the rhythm is not susceptible to Pronestyl or quinidine and heart failure ensues, it may, however, be required and indeed, normal rhythm may be restored. Twenty cubic centimeters of magnesium sulfate, 20 per cent solution intravenously, may restore normal rhythm.

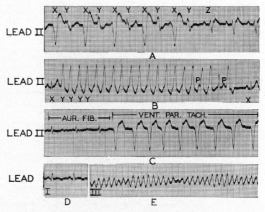

Fig. 179. *A* shows in lead II a run of ventricular paroxysmal tachycardia (134 per minute) with alternation of origin of the beats, XXX and YYY, followed by reversion to normal sinus rhythm at Z. *B* shows in lead II one normal complex (X) followed by a run of ventricular paroxysmal tachycardia, YYY (rate 230 per minute; the sequences are slightly irregular), with reversion to normal sinus rhythm at the end of the strip (X). The P waves of atrial contraction can be seen at intervals. *C*, in lead II are three ventricular complexes during atrial fibrillation (ventricular rate 80 per minute) with onset of ventricular paroxysmal tachycardia, in which the ventricular sequences are irregular (rate approximately 120 per minute). *D* shows lead I of electrocardiogram of a patient with normal rhythm which had changed to ventricular fibrillation (*E*) a few minutes later when lead III was being taken. The ventricular complexes are somewhat irregular and of bizarre and changing form.

Procaine amide hydrochloride (Pronestyl) is usually effective either intravenously, if it is urgent to restore normal rhythm or atrial fibrillation as soon as possible, or orally if the urgency is not so great. *Intravenously* it is given in 0.25 to 1.0 gm. doses not faster than 50 to 100 mg. per minute, and usually more slowly. It is diluted so that 1 cc. contains 20 mg. Normal rhythm is restored usually during its injection. The blood pressure should be determined and the rate of injection slowed or stopped if hypotension is marked. The drug should not be given intravenously unless electrocardiograms can be taken during injection because aberration of the ventricular complexes may occur and excessive dosage may cause toxic rhythms.

Orally Pronestyl is commonly effective in terminating ventricular paroxysmal tachycardia. The initial dose may be 1.25 gm. followed by 0.75 gm. in 2 hours, and if necessary 0.5 to 1.0 gm. every 2 hours. 1.25 gm. four times a day is the average maximal tolerated dose. Other schedules are 0.5 gm. three times a day or 1.0 gm. every 2 to 4 hours. After oral ad-

lent to quinidine 0.065 gm. in the treatment of arrhythmias.

Pronestyl may be effective in the treatment of ventricular paroxysmal tachycardia with alternation of the foci between the two ventricles due to digitalis intoxication, a rhythm which was uniformly fatal before the introduction of Pronestyl. In this case it should be used intravenously as the urgency is so great. Pronestyl is also effective orally in the treatment of angina pectoris due

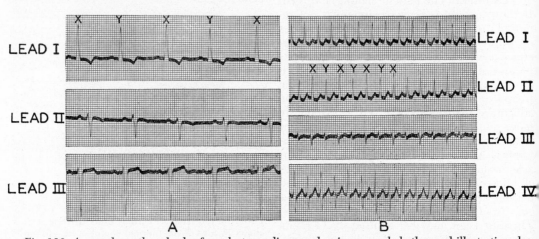

Fig. 180. *A* reproduces three leads of an electrocardiogram showing normal rhythm and illustrating electrical alternans. The QRS complexes marked X are taller than the alternate ones marked Y. *B* shows four leads of an electrocardiogram illustrating electrical alternans occurring in atrioventricular paroxysmal tachycardia (rate 214 per minute). The tall QRS complexes (X) alternate with the lower ones (Y).

ministration there may be delay of 1 hour or more for absorption and attaining an adequate blood level. After termination of the rhythm maintenance or prophylactic doses may be given, varying from 0.25 gm. every 4 hours to 0.5 to 1.0 gm. every 3 to 6 hours. Hypotension rarely occurs with its oral use. Pronestyl is also effective when given *intramuscularly*. Patients on maintenance doses should have occasional electrocardiograms to detect prolongation of QRS time or decrease in amplitude of QRS complexes. Toxic effects are not frequent, but nausea and vomiting, fever, chill, urticaria and agranulocytosis have been reported. Excessive dosage intravenously may lead to complete heart block, bundle branch block, ventricular fibrillation and death. The drug should not be used in the presence of known antecedent complete heart block, or antecedent bundle branch block. Pronestyl is about one quarter as strong as quinidine in prolonging the refractory period. Pronestyl 0.25 gm. is equiva-

to frequent ventricular premature contractions, or coupled rhythm due to ventricular premature contractions or runs of ventricular paroxysmal tachycardia.

VENTRICULAR FIBRILLATION

In this rhythm the coordinated contraction of the ventricles is replaced by rapid, irregular twitches of the ventricular muscle. Its persistence is incompatible with life, because the twitchings are ineffectual in expelling blood. The mechanism may be a circus motion in the ventricles. Brief paroxysms are not fatal. Ventricular fibrillation is a cause of sudden death, especially in patients with coronary artery disease. It has been observed in the electrocardiograms of dying patients and of subjects during electrocution. It may follow ventricular paroxysmal tachycardia and massive doses of Pronestyl, of quinidine or of quinidine and digitalis. Paroxysms which have been diagnosed were accompanied by Adams-Stokes-

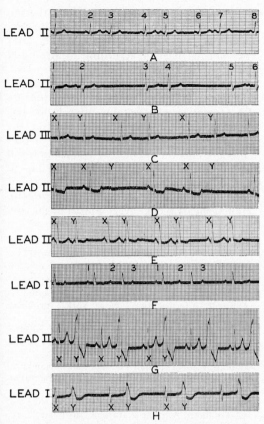

LEAD II
A
LEAD II
B
LEAD III
C
LEAD II
D
LEAD II
E
LEAD I
F
LEAD II
G
LEAD I
H

Fig. 181. A shows in lead II coupled rhythm due to recurrent sino-atrial block. Intervals 1 to 2, 3 to 4, 5 to 6 and 7 to 8 show sino-atrial block. The regular sequence is 2 to 3, 4 to 5 and 6 to 7, which was present in lead I with only an occasional sino-atrial block. B shows in lead II coupled rhythm due to normal sinus rhythm with recurrent sino-atrial block and ventricular escape. Complexes 2, 4, 6 are normal rhythm, and 1, 3, 5 are ventricular escape. Intervals 2 to 3, 4 to 5 are sino-atrial block. C shows lead III of coupled rhythm due to recurrent atrial premature contractions. X = normal rhythm complex, Y = atrial premature contractions. D shows in lead II coupled rhythm due to recurrent atrial premature contractions which are blocked. X = normal beat; Y = atrial premature contractions blocked; the form of these P waves is different from the normal P waves. E shows lead II of coupled rhythm due to recurrent atrioventricular premature contractions, the P waves in front of the QRS. X = normal beats, Y = atrioventricular premature contractions. F shows in lead I coupled rhythm due to incomplete heart block in which every third (3) P wave is blocked. P waves are indicated as 1, 2, 3. G shows lead II of basic normal rhythm with coupling due to recurrent ventricular premature contractions. X = normal beats, Y = ventricular premature contractions. H shows lead I of atrial fibrillation with coupled rhythm due to recurrent ventricular premature contractions. X = normal beats, Y = ventricular premature contractions.

like attacks and were characterized by the absence of pulse and of heart sounds. Quinidine or Pronestyl may be used to prevent attacks if complete heart block is not present. In a few instances digitalis has been effective in the treatment of syncope due to attacks of ventricular fibrillation and flutter in pa-

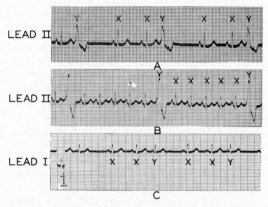

LEAD II
A
LEAD II
B
LEAD I
C

Fig. 182. A shows lead II, illustrating trigeminy due to ventricular premature contractions (Y) after every two normal beats (X), the compensatory pause after the ventricular premature contractions making the three beats fall in a group. B shows in lead II ventricular premature contractions (Y) recurring after every fifth normal beat (X). C shows trigeminy due to atrioventricular premature contractions (Y) occurring after every second normal beat (X). The short P-R (0.08 second) identifies the atrioventricular premature contractions.

tients with complete heart block. A rapidly acting and rapidly excreted preparation is recommended. In the electrocardiogram wide QRS complexes occur irregularly with bizarre and changing form (Fig. 179, D, E). Occasionally the QRS complexes resemble the vibrations of a tuning fork. Such rhythms are thought to be intermediate between ventricular paroxysmal tachycardia and fibrillation and may be called *ventricular flutter*.

PULSUS ALTERNANS

When the volume of the radial pulse alternates between a large and a small one, and the sequence is regular, *pulsus alternans* is present. It is found occasionally in syphilitic heart disease, but most commonly in the older age groups in which the arteriosclerotic and hypertensive forms and coronary thrombosis predominate. It occurs in marked heart failure.

Diagnosis is made by detection of alternation in volume of the radial pulse on palpation, which is easily observed while taking the blood pressure. *Alternation* may also appear in the electrocardiogram, tall QRS complexes coinciding with the larger radial pulse and lower ones with the smaller radial pulse (Fig. 180, *A, B*), or the reverse. Pulsus alternans should not be confused with coupled rhythm.

Treatment is directed to the underlying condition. It may disappear when digitalis is given. It carries a grave **prognosis.** It may be transient, but, if it persists or recurs, death may occur in a few months. Both pulsus alternans and *electrical alternans* may occur transiently in paroxysmal tachycardia or atrial flutter without a grave prognosis.

COUPLED RHYTHM

Coupled rhythm refers to recurrent grouping of the heart beats in pairs followed by a pause. The radial pulse may also show coupling. Coupled rhythm at the apex is most commonly caused by (1) ventricular premature contractions with the long compensatory pause regularly following each normal systole (Fig. 181, *G, H*). The radial pulse may be coupled also if the ventricular contractions occur late enough for sufficient ventricular filling; if the radial pulse is lacking, its rate is half the apical. The diagnosis of coupled rhythm due to ventricular premature contractions can usually be made clinically, especially if the patient is taking digitalis and atrial fibrillation is present (Fig. 181, *H*). Coupled rhythm at the apex and in the radial pulse may also be due to regularly recurring (2) atrial premature contractions (Fig. 181, *C*) after every normal beat, (3) blocked atrial premature contractions after every second beat (Fig. 181, *D*), (4) atrioventricular premature contractions after every normal beat (Fig. 181, *E*), (5) sino-atrial block, every third sinus impulse being blocked (Fig. 181, *A*), or sino-atrial block with ventricular escape (Fig. 181, *B*) and (6) block in atrial flutter alternating between 2:1 and 3:1 or 4:1. It may also be due to (7) incomplete heart block when every third atrial stimulus is blocked (Fig. 181, *F*). One motion of regularly recurring premature contractions is that of the *parasystole:* an ectopic pacemaker is constantly and regularly initiating stimuli in much the same fashion as the sinus or atrioventricular node; when the refractory state of the muscle is appropriate and does not interfere, the impulse from this new focus gives rise to premature contractions, which may be after every normal beat or according to any other fixed pattern (Figs. 181, *C, E, G, H;* 182, *A, B, C*).

Common causes of *trigeminal* rhythm are (1) premature contractions after every second normal beat, the long pause after the premature contraction making the two normal beats and the premature contraction fall together in a group of three (Fig. 181, *A, C*); (2) interpolated premature contractions (Fig. 176) and (3) regularly recurring incomplete heart block, every fourth atrial contraction being blocked (Fig. 172, *B*).

Harold J. Stewart

References

Barker, J. M.: The Unipolar Electrocardiogram. A Clinical Interpretation. New York, Appleton-Century-Crofts, Inc., 1952.

Burch, G., and Windsor, T.: A Primer of Electrocardiography. 2d ed. Philadelphia, Lea & Febiger, 1949.

Goodman, L., and Gilman, A.: The Pharmacological Basis of Therapeutics. New York, The Macmillan Co., 1955.

Hecht, H., Katz, L. N., Pick, A., Prinzmetal, M., and Rosenblueth, A.: The Nature of Auricular Fibrillation and Flutter: A Symposium. Circulation, 7: 591, 1953.

Levine, S. A.: Clinical Heart Disease. 4th ed. Philadelphia, W. B. Saunders Company, 1951.

Luisada, A. A.: The Heart Beat. Graphic Method in the Study of the Cardiac Patient. New York, Paul B. Hoeber, Inc., 1953.

Scherf, D., Schaffer, A. I., and Blumenfeld, S.: Mechanism of Flutter and Fibrillation. A.M.A. Arch. Int. Med., 91:333, 1953.

Stewart, H. J.: How to Use Digitalis. M. Clin. North America, 34:649, 1950.

————:Cardiac Therapy. New York, Paul B. Hoeber, Inc., 1952.

————, Deitrick, J. E., Crane, N. F., and Thompson, W. P.: Studies of the Circulation in the Presence of Abnormal Cardiac Rhythms. Observations Relating to (Part I) Rhythms Associated with Rapid Ventricular Rate and to (Part II) Rhythms Associated with Slow Ventricular Rate. J. Clin. Investigation, 17:449, 1938.

————, Deitrick, J. E., Crane, N. F., and Wheeler, C. H.: Action of Digitalis in Uncompensated Heart Disease. Arch. Int. Med., 62:569, 1938.

————, and Newman, A. A.: The Amount of Digitoxin (Digitaline nativelle) Required for Adequate Digitalization. Am. Heart J., 36:641, 1948.

Use of Digitalis. Conferences on Therapy. New York State Med. J., 42:2043, 1942.

Wolff, L.: Electrocardiography. Fundamentals and Clinical Application. Philadelphia, W. B. Saunders Company, 1950.

ANGINAL PAIN

Anginal pain is discussed in Angina Pectoris under Diseases of the Coronary Arteries.

NEUROCIRCULATORY ASTHENIA

(Psychoneurosis with Cardiovascular Symptoms, Soldier's Heart, Effort Syndrome)

Definition. Neurocirculatory asthenia is a functional disorder of the vasomotor system characterized by fatigue, dyspnea, palpitation and precordial pain on exertion.

Pathology. No definite pathologic changes can be ascribed to this condition. However, the slender, asthenic person with a low diaphragm, a small heart and inadequate personality is the type which may exhibit this syndrome under various forms of stress. There is also evidence that patients presenting this syndrome have a low cardiac output.

History. Because of the fact that neurocirculatory asthenia was first noted as a clinical entity in soldiers, it was originally termed "soldier's heart." DaCosta described it during the Civil War. Many cases were again reported in both World Wars. When civilians also were shown to exhibit this syndrome, the terms "effort syndrome" and "disordered action of the heart" were given to it. Neither term is quite so descriptive of the condition as the one suggested by Oppenheimer and now in common use, namely, "neurocirculatory asthenia."

Etiology. The precise mechanism by which this syndrome is brought about is still unknown. The disease is rare at the extremes of life, the greatest incidence being in young adults. In civilian life the age incidence is higher than in the army; Craig and White found the average to be 35 years. There seems to be little difference in the incidence as related to sex.

Symptoms. The chief symptoms are palpitation, shortness of breath, precordial pain or discomfort, and exhaustion, especially on mild exertion. The onset frequently occurs in anxiety or fear-producing situations. However, it may develop after other conditions such as pregnancy, prolonged bed rest or one of the infectious diseases. The symptom of palpitation usually consists in a consciousness of forceful pounding of the heart with little or no change in heart rate. Irregularities of the heart such as sinus tachycardia, paroxysmal tachycardia, ventricular premature contractions or transient atrial flutter and wandering pacemaker have been found. Shortness of breath on effort is the symptom which prompted some observers to name this condition the "effort syndrome." The dyspnea may vary from a simple awareness of ordinary respiratory effort to profound hyperventilation and symptoms of alkalosis. Occasionally there may be a marked increase in the rate of respiration. White mentions a frequent tendency to sigh as an important point in differentiating neurocirculatory asthenia from organic heart disease.

Precordial pain of a sharp, momentary, penetrating type occurs and may be related either to the forceful pounding of the heart or to the appearance of cardiac irregularities. There is also another type of precordial pain, dull, aching and persistent in character, which may or may not be related to exercise. This pain may last for many hours, days or weeks. According to Wood, this pain is associated with respiratory dysfunction and is in part due to fatigue of the chest muscles. Arteriolar constriction is often pronounced as indicated by cold, sometimes cyanotic, extremities. Giddiness which may be associated with peripheral arteriolar constriction or pooling of blood in the peripheral veins occurs. The exhaustion noted in nearly all cases not only is produced by slight effort, but is often unrelieved by rest.

Other symptoms are faintness, syncope, insomnia, headache, dizziness, increased perspiration, difficulty in swallowing, tremor, flushing and pallor.

Physical Signs. In a typical case the patient appears anxious, the face is flushed, and there is often profuse sweating at normal room temperature. The respirations may be rapid. Tremors are noted in pronounced cases. An examination of the heart is in the main negative. A forcible apex beat and some increase in the heart rate may be noted. The blood pressure is usually normal, but may be slightly elevated and slow to return to resting levels after exercise. Fluoroscopic examination is usually negative, but occasionally a small heart is found. Friedman found that if the tachypnea can be controlled, the exercise tolerance is within normal limits. The vital capacity, venous pressure, circulation time and electrocardiogram are also unchanged. In the group of asthenic subjects studied by Master there were electrocardiographic findings consisting in a tendency to right axis deviation, T wave changes and the changes indicative of a diminished exercise tolerance. There also appears to be a diminished tolerance to an atmosphere of 10 per cent oxygen in this group, but hot humid atmospheres and crowds may also be intolerable to these patients.

Ability to perform muscular work is definitely below normal. This may be due to a defect in aerobic metabolism, since a low oxygen consumption with high blood lactate during exercise is found. Abnormalities in the capillaries of the nailbed and an abnormal sensitivity to painful stimuli have also been noted. Ballistocardiographic studies indicate that most patients with neurocirculatory asthenia have an abnormal circulatory response. Starr suggests this test as of value in differentiating those with neurocirculatory asthenia from malingerers.

Diagnosis. The diagnosis of neurocirculatory asthenia should be suspected in a patient who has palpitation, respiratory distress, precordial pain and fatigue which develops in the presence of fear- or anxiety-producing situations. If, on further inquiry, historical evidence of a psychoneurotic personality (nail-biting, bed-wetting, hysterical episodes, nervous breakdowns) is obtained, and the patient presents signs of fear, anxiety or tension (pallor, sweating, tremor, wet cool hands, uneasiness), the diagnosis can usually be established.

Hyperthyroidism must be considered, but a normal basal metabolism together with the absence of the usual signs associated with an overactive thyroid gland would serve to exclude it as a possibility. Since, if anything, there is a tendency for a diastolic hypertension rather than hypotension, orthostatic hypotension can easily be ruled out.

Prognosis. No one ever dies of neurocirculatory asthenia. However, the course is usually protracted unless definite measures are taken early to remove the patient from the distressing situation or change his attitude toward it. Experience in the Armed Forces demonstrates that the latter is difficult to accomplish. Complete recovery can be expected in about 15 per cent, improvement in 17 per cent, and in the remainder the condition either remains stationary or gets progressively worse.

Treatment. Treatment consists in psychotherapy or removal of the patient from the situation in which the illness occurred. In mild cases, group activity in which the morale is high and leadership strong will often keep the symptoms in check. Some patients will be helped by reassurance, suggestive procedures and the sympathetic support of the physician. In special instances an intensive personality analysis may be helpful.

ARTHUR C. DEGRAFF

References

Cohen, M. E., White, P. D., and Johnson, R. E.: Neurocirculatory Asthenia, Anxiety Neurosis or the Effort Syndrome. Arch. Int. Med., 81:260, 1948.

Craig, H. R., and White, P. D.: Etiology and Symptoms of Neurocirculatory Asthenia: An Analysis of One Hundred Cases with Comments on Prognosis and Treatment. Arch. Int. Med., 53:633, 1934.

DaCosta, J. M.: On Irritable Heart; Clinical Study of a Functional Cardiac Disorder and Its Consequences. Am. J. M. Sc., 61:17, 1871.

Friedman, M.: Cardiovascular Manifestations of Neurocirculatory Asthenia. War Medicine, 6:221, 1944; Am. Heart J., 30:325, 478, 1945.

Starr, I.: Ballistocardiographic Studies of Draftees Rejected for Neurocirculatory Asthenia. War Medicine, 5:155, 1944.

CAROTID SINUS SYNCOPE

(Vasovagal Syncope)

At the point where the common carotid artery bifurcates to form the external and internal carotid arteries there is a slight bulging known as the carotid sinus. In the wall of the artery in this region there are specialized sensory end plates surrounded by a rich nerve plexus. By means of the carotid sinus nerve, which joins the glossopharyngeal nerve, connection is made with the central nervous system. Overactivity of the carotid sinus may cause attacks of dizziness, fainting and sometimes convulsions. The physical signs noted during the attack are a fall in arterial blood pressure and marked slowing of the heart rate. Attacks may come on without any apparent cause, follow an emotional upset, or be induced by pressure over the carotid sinus. Caution should be exercised in applying carotid sinus pressure, particularly in the aged, because paralysis may occur from the prolonged cerebral anoxemia resulting from cardiac asystole. The overactivity is usually functional without any pathologic change being noted. Occasionally some organic disturbance may be responsible, such as tumors in the neck pressing on the carotid sinus or a dilatation of aneurysmal proportion of the carotid artery. The carotid sinus may become hypersensitive reflexly, as has been found in gallbladder disease. In such cases the treatment is to correct the underlying condition responsible for the hypersensitivity When the primary condition appears to be in the carotid sinus, good results are often obtained by maintaining the patient on a dose of atropine (0.5 to 1 mg. two or three times a day) sufficient to prevent fainting, but not enough to cause dryness of the throat or visual disturbances. For the more serious cases surgical treatment may be necessary. Infiltration of the carotid sinus area with procaine will give some indication as to the possible success of surgical treatment. Best results are obtained if the carotid sinus nerve can be severed. Stripping of the nerve plexus from the carotid artery at the bifurcation may in some cases effect a cure, but in others gives only temporary relief.

ARTHUR C. DE GRAFF

References

Engel, E. L., and Engel, J. F.: The Significance of the Carotid Sinus Reflex in Biliary Tract Disease. New England J. Med., 227:470, 1945.

Ferris, E. B., Capps, R. B., and Weiss, S.: Carotid Sinus Syncope and Its Bearing on the Mechanism of the Unconscious State and Convulsions. Medicine, 14:377, 1935.

Heymans, C.: Le Sinus Carotidien et les Autres Zones Vasosensibles Reflexogenes. London, H. K. Lewis and Co., 1929.

Smith, H.: Attacks of Unconsciousness Resulting from Hyperactive Carotid Sinus Reflex. Am. Heart J., 33:711, 1947.

Weiss, S., and Baker, J. P.: The Carotid Sinus Reflex in Health and Disease. Its Role in the Causation of Fainting and Convulsions. Medicine, 12:297, 1933.

Zeman, F. D., and Siegal, S.: Monoplegia Following Carotid Sinus Pressure in the Aged. Am. J. Med. Sc., 213:603, 1947.

DISEASES OF THE PERIPHERAL VESSELS

GENERAL CONSIDERATIONS

By usage the term "peripheral vascular disease" is limited to conditions in which blood flow through the extremities is disturbed by structural or functional abnormality of the peripheral blood vessels. In many instances, however, the primary cause of the disorder is neither peripheral nor vascular, as illustrated by some cases of spasmodic cyanosis of the fingers, which, though closely resembling Raynaud's disease, may be caused by such distant lesions as spondylitis or cervical rib. Furthermore, a great variety of systemic disorders occasionally exert striking effects on peripheral blood flow. In this group are such unrelated conditions as the anemias, polycythemia vera, hyperthyroidism, myxedema and, of course, cardiac disease.

The extremities, particularly the digits, may be the first parts of the body to manifest a generalized vascular disease such as arteriosclerosis. This is not only because they are situated at the periphery of the vascular tree, "at the end of the line," as it were, but also because they are frequently exposed to varying temperature and to trauma. For correct diagnosis and efficient therapy, therefore, one must bear in mind the general, as well as the local, state of the circulation, and especially the influence of the sympathetic nervous system.

Physiology of the Peripheral Vascular System. The arterial pressure or, more accurately, the arteriovenous pressure gradient (arterial *minus* venous pressure), is the force that drives blood through the resistance of the peripheral blood vessels and produces blood flow. It is important to bear in mind that the terms "arterial pressure" and "venous pressure" in this connection refer to *local* pressures in the limb under study, and that these pressures may be, but usually are not, exactly the same as the *systemic* arterial or venous pressures measured centrally. For example the arterial pressure, or the venous pressure, may be altered locally in a limb by changing its position or by applying external constriction without affecting the systemic pressures at all.

If the caliber of all the blood vessels in a limb could be maintained constant, their resistance would remain constant, and blood flow through them could be altered only by changing the arteriovenous pressure gradient. Thus, if local arterial pressure were increased (and venous pressure were unchanged) blood flow would rise, and if arterial pressure were decreased, flow would fall. On the other hand, if local venous pressure were increased, flow would fall, and if venous pressure were decreased, flow would rise. But if the arterial and venous pressures were increased or decreased equally, flow would remain unchanged since the arteriovenous gradient would be the same. Incidentally, one should remember that venous pressure in the limbs cannot be decreased below zero (atmospheric) because the veins are collapsible and will not sustain negative pressures. Hence the principle of siphonage cannot be applied to blood flow in the limbs.

Although changes in peripheral blood flow do occur as a result of changes in arteriovenous pressure gradient, they are relatively small as compared with those that occur from changes in the caliber (resistance) of the peripheral blood vessels themselves. Changes in the caliber of blood vessels may be active, that is, may result from contraction or relaxation of the vascular smooth muscles, or they may be merely passive, that is, may result from changes in *effective* internal pressure (intravascular minus extravascular pressure). Of these two types, the active, i.e., muscular contraction (vasoconstriction) or relaxation (vasodilatation), is by far the more important.

Vasoconstriction and vasodilatation may be either reflex or local in nature. In the limbs reflex vasomotor activity is mediated over the sympathetic nervous system. However, sympathetic vasomotor activity in the hands and feet is much more important than that in the more proximal parts of the limbs (arms and legs). This is shown not only by the effects of sympathetic denervation, but also by the effects of applying reflex vasodilating or vasoconstricting stimuli (heating or cooling the trunk), all of which cause much more marked changes of blood flow in the hands and feet than in the arms and legs. Thus when the sympathetic nerves to an extremity are blocked, there is (acutely) a marked increase in blood flow in the digits, but slight if any increase in blood flow in the proximal muscular parts. Likewise sympathetic reflex vasospasm may be an important cause of ischemia in the hands and feet but is much less likely to be so in the arms or legs. It is interesting also that sympathetic reflex vasoconstriction is normally more pronounced in the *feet* than in the hands. Thus when a normal person is exposed in a cool room his feet will be cooler than his hands, and they warm up (undergo vasodilatation) more slowly than the hands when heat is applied to the trunk as a reflex vasodilating stimulus.

These several differences between the vasomotor "tone" in the hands, feet, arms and legs are related, in part at least, to the contrasting roles played by these parts in regulating body temperature or performing muscular work. Thus, the hands and feet are active radiators of body heat and are equipped with numerous arteriovenous anastomoses or shunts which open up during strong vasodilating procedures but close down during strong vasoconstrictor stimuli. The latter may cause circulation in the hands and feet virtually to cease while causing the circulation in the muscular parts, which are concerned primarily with body movement, to change little if at all.

Perhaps even more important than sympathetic reflex vasomotor responses in the limbs are vasodilator and vasoconstrictor reactions to local physicochemical factors. Among these are local temperature, local anoxia, local accumulation of metabolites and local humoral or drug actions. Local heat is a strong vasodilator and local cold (within limits) a strong vasoconstrictor influence. Another strong vasodilating mechanism is local anoxia and the accumulation of products of metabolism, demonstrable most easily by occluding the circulation for a few minutes, and then releasing it. This results in a marked vasodilation (reactive hyperemia). Finally, various other intrinsic or extrinsic substances such as histamine, epinephrine, nicotine or nitrites may have strong local vasodilating or vasoconstricting effects. It is worthy of special mention that epinephrine has effects in the hands and feet (skin) that are opposite to its effects in

the arms and legs (muscles), since epinephrine is a vasoconstrictor substance in skin but primarily a vasodilator substance in muscle.

Clinical Symptoms and Signs of Peripheral Ischemia. The vast majority of patients with peripheral vascular disease suffer from the effects of ischemia. (The opposite, namely excessive *hyperemia* due to abnormal dilatation of structurally normal vessels, does occur, but is rare and is known as *erythromelalgia*.) The symptoms and signs of patients with peripheral ischemia are usually classic and lead the thoughtful physician quickly to the diagnosis provided he understands their significance.

Coldness of the extremities signifies decreased blood flow but may be normal or abnormal, depending on the circumstances in which it occurs. Skin temperatures vary widely in health, and temporary coldness of the extremities particularly in a cool environment may be quite physiologic. However, severe coldness that persists even in a warm room usually is abnormal. Skin temperature measurements are of value only if they are made repeatedly under controlled conditions, especially during body warming. Consistent differences in the temperatures of corresponding parts of two symmetrical limbs, similarly treated and exposed, are highly significant. In the absence of disuse, atrophy and diseases of the nervous system, unilateral coldness is generally due to structural disease of the corresponding blood vessels. Exceptionally, however, the more grossly diseased limb will be warmer, apparently because the circulation in such a limb is largely maintained by superficially placed collateral channels which remain partially dilated all the time. However, if full vasodilation (reactive hyperemia) is produced in both limbs and the resultant "maximal" blood flow is measured, it will be found to be much less in the more diseased limb.

Intermittent claudication refers to aching or constricting pain which may arise during activity of any group of muscles, but typically affects the calf muscles. The pain appears gradually after a relatively constant amount of exercise and is promptly relieved by rest. If exercise is continued in spite of pain, the affected muscles become spastic and cramps may occur. In the absence of general anemia, intermittent claudication bespeaks structural arterial disease. Advance or quiescence of local vascular disease is reflected by gradual diminution or increase of exercise tolerance, which can be measured by controlled pacing or by some type of recording ergometer.

Rest pain accompanies (1) sudden arterial occlusion by thrombosis or embolism, (2) indolent ulceration, gangrene or other advanced trophic changes and (3) ischemic neuritis. In contrast to intermittent claudication, it is not relieved by rest and is usually worse at night. Patients often discover that they can relieve this agonizing pain somewhat by gently massaging the skin near lesions, or by hanging the extremity over the side of the bed.

Skin color depends, first, upon the number and fullness of the capillaries and subpapillary venules; second, upon the composition of the venous blood with reference to the number of erythrocytes and their oxygen saturation. Arterial blood normally enters the skin rapidly enough to prevent pallor of the digits even when the extremities of the recumbent patient are raised well above heart level. If general anemia is absent, *conspicuous blanching* of the elevated extremities, particularly in a warm room, strongly suggests, but does not prove, the presence of organic arterial occlusion. Delay in, or failure of, the natural pink color to return to such blanched extremities when the patient sits up and dangles them over the side of the bed is more significant in indicating organic arterial obstruction. Normally, such flushing should occur almost immediately, beginning in the toes and spreading proximally. If definite flushing requires more than 20 seconds (Smithwick) or does not occur at all, it denotes severe or virtually complete organic obstruction without adequate collateral circulation. If it does occur within 20 seconds, but not immediately, it denotes organic arterial obstruction, though with adequate collateral circulation. If on the other hand, flushing appears only in sites proximal to the digits, it suggests that these sites are the most dital part adequately supplied with arterial blood.

The speed of *filling of the veins* of the feet on dependency (after first emptying them by elevation) may also be of value in estimating the degree of arterial obstruction. If, in the absence of varicosities, these veins do not become visibly distended within 30 seconds after dependency, there is usually an "inadequate" arterial blood flow into the foot. Definite diffuse *cyanosis* limited to the extremities indicates that the capillaries, venules and veins are filled with excessively deoxygenated blood resulting from venous stasis or from slow arterial inflow. In a cold limb, pallor or cyanosis rarely may be due to vasospasm alone, the vessels still being capable of dilating widely under proper conditions. Such vasospasm can be abolished by warming the skin in a water bath at 37° to 40° C. for 20 minutes, after which either complete pallor on elevation, or failure to flush normally on dependency, provides practically conclusive evidence that both the main and collateral arterial channels are inadequate.

Rubor, a persistent dull red or reddish blue discoloration of the cold extremity, appears when the cutaneous capillaries and venules are persistently dilated owing to injury from anoxemia, cold or low grade inflammation. Moderate redness is normal in a naturally warm extremity. However, peripheral blood flow may be impaired though skin color is still normal, since blood flow and skin temperature depend chiefly upon the tone of the arterioles whereas skin color varies with the blood flow in the more minute vessels.

Trophic changes in the skin accompany nearly all slowly developing peripheral vascular conditions and indicate merely that ischemia is severe, or has been so at intervals. The subcutaneous tissues, ordinarily meager, may at first be puffy and thickened. Later the skin becomes dry, atrophic, shiny, tightly drawn and subject to indolent ulceration. The nails become hard, brittle, ridged and otherwise deformed. The severity of trophic manifestations corresponds so closely to fluctuations in the adequacy of peripheral circulation that there is no need to invoke the activity of so-called "trophic nerve impulses."

Diminished pulsation of the peripheral arteries is detected with the fingertip or with the oscillometer, the latter serving especially to determine the point at which pulsation ceases in the thigh or calf where the vessels are too deep to be palpated. The instrument is more reliable in demonstrating relative differences between the deep pulses of two symmetrical limbs than in measuring absolute deviations from normal. The stethoscope may also be used to detect the presence of obstructive bruits in the peripheral arteries, and occasionally may localize the site of a partial occlusion. A pulse not palpable in the cold extremity may reappear when vasoconstrictor tone is diminished by heat, since vasospasm occasionally abolishes pulsation in arteries still able to dilate. Peripheral pulses may be obliterated by aneurysm or coarctation of the aorta, whereas arterial anomalies may be responsible for failure to feel pulsations in their usual situations. A normal pulse is sometimes felt at the wrist or ankle, while the smaller, distal arteries and arterioles are occluded by advanced organic disease.

Indolent ulceration and gangrene indicate conspicuous or complete local ischemia. The vessels in and near the lesion are commonly thrombosed, whereas other vessels in the extremity usually show organic disease, but may be structurally normal if the underlying condition is essentially vasospastic. The occurrence of local gangrene and ulceration render it likely that widespread organic arterial occlusion is present, but does not justify this diagnosis unless other evidence of widely distributed structural disease is found.

Tests for Differentiating Vasospasm and Structural (Organic or Occlusive) Arterial Disease. The degree to which peripheral ischemia is due (1) to pure vasospasm or (2) to organic arterial disease can be determined by observing the rise of digital skin temperature which follows temporary abolition of vasoconstrictor tone in the extremities. The patient, thinly clad, lies with the extremities exposed to room air at a temperature between 20° and 22° C. When the digits have cooled sufficiently, vasoconstrictor tone in the extremities is abolished by one of the following procedures:

1. Injection of procaine around appropriate sympathetic ganglia.
2. Anesthetization by procaine of appropriate peripheral mixed nerves.
3. Spinal anesthesia (for lower limbs only).
4. General anesthesia.
5. Raising body temperature by (*a*) enclosing the body (excepting the limbs under observation) in an electric heat cabinet; (*b*) immersing two uninvolved limbs in water baths at 42° to 44° C. for 35 minutes. (As an alternative procedure, the entire room may be warmed to 29° C., but allowance must be made for this increase in environmental temperature in evaluating any rise in digital temperature.)
6. Autonomic blocking agents.

As soon as vasoconstrictor impulses fail to reach the extremity, normal vessels dilate, peripheral blood flow increases and digital skin temperature rises rapidly to the normal vasodilatation level, between 31° and 35° C. Such a normal vasodilator response indicates that the peripheral arteries are able to dilate fully and that significant organic arterial disease is absent. A partial vasodilator response, i.e., rise of digital skin temperature to between 27° and 29° C., indicates that moderate organic vascular disease is present in the area studied. If skin temperature fails to rise or actually diminishes during the procedure, the vasodilator response is absent, indicating advanced occlusive disease locally.

For studying the upper extremities, body warming is the simplest and most reliable method. For the lower extremities, body warming is generally satisfactory, but occasionally fails to release extreme vasospasm; under these conditions warming the entire room and/or anesthetization of the appropriate sympathetic ganglia or peripheral mixed nerves, or spinal anesthesia, may be necessary for reliable results. Autonomic blocking agents have also been advocated for testing vasodilator responses, although their effect may not be maximal.

To determine how far upward in the extremity organic occlusion extends, other procedures may be used, *viz.:* (1) the oscillometer, (2) histamine puncture, (3) reactive hyperemia and, in experienced hands, (4) arteriography. The limitations of the oscillometer have been mentioned. Histamine (1:1000), punctured into the skin of the warm, horizontally placed extremity, normally produces a wheal and hyperemic flare in 5 minutes or less (Starr). If a wheal fails to appear within 5 minutes, it can be concluded that blood flow is diminished in that skin area. Reactive hyperemia is produced by arresting blood flow completely for 5 minutes after the extremity has been warmed and emptied of blood. Sudden release of the circulation is followed by a brilliant hyperemic flush which normally reaches the tips of the digits in less than 5 seconds. If organic occlusion is present, the flush is delayed and faint. The actual increase in blood flow during reactive hyperemia may also be accurately measured with the venous occlusion plethysmograph for comparison with normal values. Compression and local arrest of circulation incur some risk of inducing thrombosis in diseased arteries.

Arteriography involves roentgenography after intra-arterial injection of radiopaque solutions. This procedure reveals the site and nature of anatomic changes in the peripheral vessels as well as the size and number of collateral channels. Arteriography is sometimes painful and is generally contraindicated in vascular disease in which there is danger of arterial thrombosis.

Vasodilator Drugs. Since, in treating peripheral vascular disease, prolonged vasodilatation is required, the evanescent effects of amyl nitrite, nitroglycerin and acetylcholine are generally of little therapeutic value. The efficacy of those drugs which have prolonged vasodilator action depends upon the grade of vasospasm to be overcome and the degree to which structural disease has rendered the peripheral arteries rigid and incapable of dilatation. In addition, vasodilator drugs often lower systemic blood pressure so that in many cases, particularly with structural disease, though vasodilatation is obtained, peripheral blood flow is increased but little. Nevertheless, appropriate vasodilator drugs should be tried in all cases because their action, though often feeble and capricious, is sometimes strikingly effective even under adverse conditions.

Ethyl alcohol, given in the form of acceptable beverages to provide 0.5 cc. of alcohol per kilogram of body weight, induces peripheral vasodilatation which lasts on the average for 4 hours. Acetyl-beta-methylcholine may be given orally in doses of 0.1 to 0.5 gm., and repeated as necessary. Undesirably intense side effects can be terminated promptly by injecting atropine. Prostigmine has been used in doses of 0.0075 to 0.030 gm. orally, three to four times daily. Papaverine hydrochloride may be given orally or subcutaneously (0.03 to 0.06 gm.), and intravenous administration (0.01 to 0.03 gm.) at intervals of 3 to 4 hours has been recommended for relaxing vasospasm in embolism. Aminophylline (theophylline ethylene diamine) (orally 0.1 to 0.3 gm., three times daily) and theobromine sodiosalicyclate (orally 0.1 to 1 gm., three times daily) are said to be helpful in certain vasospastic cases of thromboangiitis obliterans and arteriosclerosis, though useless in Raynaud's disease. Thyroid substance in dosage controlled by frequent estimations of basal metabolism is often used, especially if basal metabolism is low initially.

A number of newer sympatholytic, adrenolytic and ganglionic blocking drugs intended specifically to reduce adrenergic vasoconstriction are being tried in the treatment of peripheral vascular diseases associated with ischemia. These include tetraethylammonium chloride (TEA), hexamethonium chloride, 2-benzyl-4,5-imidazoline hydrochloride (Priscoline), phenoxybenzamine hydrochloride (Dibenzyline), N,N-dibenzyl beta-chloroethylamine hydrochloride (Dibenamine) and dihydroergocornine (DHO). Of these Priscoline, given orally in doses of 0.025 to 0.050 gm. every 3 or 4 hours, or Dibenzyline, given orally in doses of .005 to .020 gm. every 3 or 8 hours, appear to be the most practicable for prolonged clinical trial.

Anticoagulant Therapy. Anticoagulants have been demonstrated to be of great importance in the prevention and retardation of intravascular thrombosis, particularly after vascular surgery, in acute arterial or venous occlusions, and many other types of cases commonly complicated by thromboembolic disease, as well as in myocardial infarction and when mural thrombi are present in the heart. If an immediate anticoagulant effect is desired, heparin is the drug of choice, since its action is almost instantaneous after parenteral injection of a soluble preparation. The anticoagulant effect of heparin, measured by the clotting time of freshly shed unmodified whole blood, lasts but 3 to 6 hours when administered intravenously in the usual therapeutic dose. This brevity of action provides a safety-factor in cases in which hemorrhage may develop to contraindicate further anticoagulant therapy.

Dicumarol, which, after oral administration, inhibits prothrombin activity as measured by the Quick test, has similar prophylactic value. Although relatively inexpensive and easier to administer than heparin, the onset, degree and termination of its action are less predictable.

A variety of regimens have been recommended for the use of anticoagulants in the prevention and treatment of thromboembolic disorders. The following general program, which combines treatment with heparin and Dicumarol, has proved highly satisfactory in the majority of patients. It must be emphasized, however, that wide variations in response occur from patient to patient and in the same patient from time to time. Fifty milligrams of heparin are given subcutaneously, intramuscularly or intravenously at 6-hour intervals. The clotting time is determined 5 hours after the second dose, and then every 12 hours. The clotting time should be maintained at an elevated level, i.e., over 20 minutes, and the dosage raised or lowered to achieve this effect. An initial dose of 300 mg. of Dicumarol is given orally when heparin therapy is started. The next day a dose of 200 mg. is administered, and on the subsequent days a dose of 50 to 100 mg. is usually required to maintain the prothrombin time at 10 to 30 per cent of normal activity. If the prothrombin time exceeds 40 seconds, the dose is omitted on that day. The prothrombin time must be determined daily. If adequate laboratory facilities are not available, anticoagulants should not be used. Heparin is discontinued when the prothrombin time has reached 25 seconds. If the underlying clinical disorder permits, the patient is ambulated progressively after the fifth day, but treatment is continued for a total of about two weeks.

If bleeding occurs or the clotting time is excessively elevated in the course of heparin therapy, an injection of 50 to 100 mg. of protamine sulfate is given intravenously. This restores the clotting time to normal at once. Excessive effects of Dicumarol are controlled by the intravenous injection of 70 mg. of menadione, which may require about 12 hours for its effect, or by the transfusion of fresh whole blood or plasma, which has an immediate but temporary effect.

Dicumarol should not be administered to patients with severe liver disease or to those with advanced renal insufficiency or to patients exhibiting any hemorrhagic diathesis.

R. W. WILKINS

References

Allen, E. V., Barker, N. W., and Hines, W. A., Jr.: Peripheral Vascular Diseases. 2nd ed. Philadelphia, W. B. Saunders Company, 1955.

Buerger, L.: The Circulatory Disturbances of the Extremities. Including Gangrene, Vasomotor, and Trophic Disorders. Philadelphia, W. B. Saunders Company, 1924.

Cassirer, A.: Die vasomotorisch-tropischen Neurosen. 2d ed. Berlin, Karger, 1912.

LeFevre, F.: Management of Occlusive Arterial Diseases of the Extremities. J.A.M.A., 147:1401, 1951.

Lewis, T.: The Blood Vessels of the Human Skin and Their Responses. London, Shaw, 1927.

———: Vascular Disorders of the Limbs. New York, The Macmillan Co., 1936.

Montgomery, M., Naide, M., and Freeman, N. E.: The Significance of Diagnostic Tests in the Study of Peripheral Vascular Disease. Am. Heart J., 21: 780, 1941.

Smithwick, R. H.: Surgery of the Autonomic Nervous System. New England J. Med., 240:543, 1949.

Starr, I.: Physiologic Therapy for Obstructive Vascular Disease. New York, Grune & Stratton, 1953.

Van Dellen, T. R., Scupham, G. W., deTakats, G., and Fowler, E. F.: Vascular Diseases; Tenth Annual Review. Arch. Int. Med., 75:125, 197, 1945.

Wilkins, R. W., Halperin, M. H., and Litter, J. The Effects of Various Physical Procedures on the Circulation in Human Limbs. Ann. Int. Med., 33: 1232, 1950.

PERIPHERAL VASCULAR DISEASES DUE TO ORGANIC ARTERIAL OBSTRUCTION

THROMBOANGIITIS OBLITERANS

(Presenile Gangrene, Buerger's Disease)

Definition. Thromboangiitis obliterans is an inflammatory type of obliterative vascular disease affecting chiefly the peripheral arteries and veins, especially of males during early adult life. Identified first as endarteritis obliterans (von Winiwarter, 1879), it was described more fully and given its present name by Buerger (1908).

Etiology. Specific etiology is unknown, although infection or the activity of some toxic agent is generally taken to be responsible. Streptococci, trichophytons and *Rickettsia prowazekii* all have been suggested as possible etiologic agents. However, systemic reactions characteristic of infection are lacking, and infection alone certainly does not explain the sex incidence of the disease. Cigarettes are used moderately or excessively by many but not all patients with thromboangiitis obliterans. Since smoking produces transient vasoconstriction and probably favors extension of the disease, patients with Buerger's disease, or for that matter any type of occlusive arterial disease, should be prohibited from using tobacco in any form. Chronic ergotism and abnormalities of calcium or choline metabolism also have been mentioned as possible etiologic factors in Buerger's disease. Exposure to cold and repeated trauma favor reactivation and extension of the disease, but are not primary causes.

Incidence. All races are subject to thromboangiitis obliterans, but approximately half the patients are Jews. Men are affected far more frequently than women, in a ratio of 75 to 1. In women the disease is mild and may often escape diagnosis. Thromboangiitis obliterans has been observed at all ages from

17 to 73, but occurs most frequently between 20 and 45.

Pathology. The lesions are segmental, in that diseased sections of arteries or veins are separated by areas which are still normal. In the acute stage cellular proliferation of the intima is accompanied by the formation of red thrombi. Giant cells are found occasionally. Polymorphonuclear leukocytes and lymphocytes infiltrate all coats of the artery and extend into the thrombus, which is gradually organized. Finally, the occluded artery, the venae comites and contiguous nerves are bound inseparably into a bundle of hard fibrous cords. Additional segments of artery or vein are involved acutely at intervals varying from days to years; hence a single long artery commonly exhibits many stages of the cycle, ranging from earliest intimal proliferation to dense scar formation. Many partly organized thrombi are recanalized, thus aiding the conspicuously enlarged collateral vessels in restoring peripheral circulation.

Symptoms and Signs. Thromboangiitis obliterans follows a relapsing course in that periods of extending arterial involvement alternate with periods of quiescence during which developing collateral circulation gradually assumes, more or less efficiently, the function of the occluded vessels. Depending upon the relation between these two concurrent processes of occlusion and compensation, the onset and course vary from insidious to fulminant. Ordinarily, occlusion gradually outstrips the developing collateral circulation, and definite peripheral ischemia brings the patient to the physician within one to four years after the first mild symptoms appear. In fulminating or acute cases the whole course is condensed into a few months. The disease ordinarily runs an active course of six to twelve years and then advances much less rapidly.

The most frequent initial complaint is persistent coldness of one or both lower extremities and, less commonly, of the upper extremities. Aching pain in the digits, instep, ankle, calf (intermittent claudication), wrists or forearm follows exercise of the corresponding muscles. Migratory phlebitis may precede or accompany arterial involvement, and occasionally the veins alone are affected. Tender, red, elevated areas about 1 cm. in diameter appear suddenly in the skin near the valves of the small superficial veins of the foot or lower leg and gradually disappear during two or three weeks, to be followed after irregular intervals by new lesions. The patient may have observed cutaneous color changes such as cyanosis, rubor or even cyclic digital cyanosis and redness. Trivial trauma, ill advised minor surgery, excessive heat or irritant local medication may produce a small ulcer which, instead of healing rapidly, extends and becomes painful. Agonizing pain, sleeplessness and excessive smoking frequently form a vicious cycle as the ulcer extends and gangrene develops. Rest pain arising from thrombosis and ulceration is generally burning, gnawing or aching in type and tends to be constant, while the rest pain of ischemic neuritis, which may occur without cutaneous lesions, is paroxysmal and often lancinating. Gangrene is usually moist from the beginning, but local resistance to extending infection is much greater than in arteriosclerotic or diabetic gangrene.

Examination reveals coldness of the involved extremity, with reduced or absent arterial pulsations. Elevation of the extremity produces pallor, and dependency produces cyanosis. The grade of rubor, trophic changes and wasting of muscles depends upon the duration and severity of peripheral ischemia. Vasodilatation tests reveal definite organic vascular occlusion with coexisting vasospasm in one or more extremities. When the patient is first seen, the disease is usually well advanced in one extremity, while the opposite one presents at least vasospasm and frequently mild organic occlusion. Although the lower extremities are most frequently involved, the disease may begin in the small arteries of the hands. Moreover, *thrombosis of the mesenteric, coronary, cerebral or renal arteries is not uncommon.*

Roentgenograms usually reveal osteoporosis and, occasionally, osteomyelitis of the phalanges. In elderly patients roentgenographic or clinical evidence of arterial calcification does not exclude thromboangiitis obliterans, which may occur in association with arteriosclerosis.

Diagnosis. Typical thromboangiitis obliterans, when fully developed in the lower extremities of a young man, can hardly be confused with other conditions. Paroxysmal cyanosis of the digits sometimes leads to an erroneous diagnosis of Raynaud's disease, which, in contrast to thromboangiitis obliterans, is rare in men, affects the upper extremities more severely and does not obliterate arterial pulsation at the wrist and ankle.

Migratory thrombophlebitis, accompanied by normal arterial blood flow and a normal vasodilator response, may be the first sign of the disease. In the elderly patient with arteriosclerosis the certain diagnosis of thromboangiitis may require histologic study of an excised vein unless classic migratory phlebitis has been observed.

Failure to recognize early states of thromboangiitis obliterans is the common error. Patients frequently wear a succession of orthopedic appliances for "fallen arches" before it is recognized that the pain in the ankle or instep is due to organic vascular disease. Gangrene may be precipitated by excessive heat (baking), strong antiseptics or ill advised avulsion of a nail for pain or persisting paronychia. The rubor of longstanding ischemia will not be mistaken for inflammatory reaction if the coldness of the foot and the absence of arterial pulsation are observed and their significance appreciated.

Treatment. Early diagnosis is an important prerequisite for instituting preventive measures to avoid the more serious complications and eventual disability. Warm clothing should be worn routinely with fleece-lined gloves or shoes. Patients should avoid exposure to cold and, if possible, obtain sedentary indoor occupation. The potential dangers of trauma, minor surgery and dermatophytosis should be repeatedly explained. The skin should be kept scrupulously clean, dry and soft, with frequent inunctions of a bland oil. *Tobacco should never be used in any form.* In mild cases without lesions, diathermy, warm sitz baths, active postural exercises (Buerger, Allen) or passive oscillation of the limbs into and out of a dependent position (Sanders' bed), will often increase peripheral blood flow, at least temporarily. Reflex vasodilatation of those vessels still capable of expanding may be produced by applying electric heating pads to the body and unaffected extremities for a period of 45 minutes several times weekly. Local external heat should be used, if at all, only with greatest caution, because of the danger of blistering and burning.

A large fluid intake, 3 to 4 liters a day, with 5 to 10 gm. of sodium chloride, induces hydremia and may relieve distressing nocturnal cramps. Intravenous injections of sodium citrate, hypertonic sodium chloride solutions or sodium thiosulfate in repeated courses have been recommended. Insulin-free extracts of pancreas injected intramus-

cularly are said by some to diminish the severity of intermittent claudication, but do not affect ulcers or rest pain. If basal metabolism is low, thyroid substance or thyroxin may be of value. The administration of calcium has been recommended.

If rest pain is present, with or without lesions, absolute rest in bed is essential. The affected extremities should be kept horizontal or 20 to 30 degrees *below* (never *above*) horizontal. The dependent position aids peripheral blood flow and occasionally is the only one the patient can tolerate. Preferably it should be intermittent, and the development of edema and lesions arising from pressure or friction should be guarded against. External local warmth if used at all is best applied to the extremities by means of a thermoregulated cradle kept at the temperature at which the patient is most comfortable, usually between 30° and 34°, never above 38° C. (Starr). Infected lesions should be kept open, moist and clean by means of warm compresses. Strong antiseptics must be used with caution if at all because of the danger of injuring tissues already partially devitalized. Systemic chemotherapy, as well as topical application or irrigation of lesions, with antibiotic agents to which the infecting organisms are shown to be sensitive is the most effective method of decreasing infections (Howe).

Typhoid vaccine may be given intravenously in ascending doses every four to seven days in spaced courses of eight to sixteen injections. The smaller doses do not produce a chill, but may still be followed by vasodilatation, relief of pain and healing of ulcers. The usefulness of vasodilator drugs (see p. 1380) is limited by the degree of organic occlusion, but they should be tried because of the conspicuous relief occasionally obtained. The oscillating bed may be tried to increase blood flow temporarily in crises of ulceration and rest pain, but is useless with massive gangrene or osteomyelitis. Anticoagulant therapy may be advisable in sudden extensive occlusion, which may be followed by progressive thrombosis.

Rest pain may also be relieved by analgesic ointments applied directly to lesions and by the oral administration of acetylsalicylic acid, phenobarbital, codeine, meperidine (Demerol), methadone or morphine, with precautions against addiction. The alcoholic injection or the crushing of peripheral nerves produces anesthesia that persists for two to six months, after which the operation may, if necessary, be repeated. Chordotomy, though occasionally used, is rarely, if ever, justified.

Bilateral preganglionic sympathectomy has been advocated for the treatment of established, gradually advancing thromboangiitis obliterans with symptoms dating back two years or more, if organic occlusion is not pronounced and if vasospasm is prominent. This major operation is not indicated in mild cases responding well to medical treatment or in advanced cases with massive gangrene and gross organic vascular occlusion. The operation is said to have a certain prophylactic value in that the opposite extremity is involved less frequently and less severely. Opinion is still divided concerning the general usefulness of sympathectomy in the treatment of thromboangiitis obliterans. In skilled hands paravertebral injection of alcohol is an effective method of temporarily blocking sympathetic impulses and releasing vasospasm.

In thromboangiitis obliterans, resistance to systemic infection is fairly high and collateral circulation is usually good, so that minor amputations may be performed more safely than in arteriosclerotic gangrene. In the presence of ascending infection, advancing lymphangitis, fever and leukocytosis, prompt antibiotic chemotherapy is indicated. Delay in amputation may be hazardous, however, because the efficacy of the antibiotic agents may be limited by the ischemia of the affected tissues and by local necrosis. The color of the extremities on elevation and dependency, during reactive hyperemia, or after the intradermal injection of histamine will assist in deciding the safe level for amputation. High amputations are required in elderly patients and in those with progressive gangrene, rapidly ascending infection or extensive destruction of tissue.

R. W. WILKINS

References

Barker, N. W.: Results of Treatment of Thromboangiitis Obliterans by Foreign Protein. J.A.M.A., 97:841, 1931.

Brown, G. E., and others: Thrombo-angiitis Obliterans. Philadelphia, W. B. Saunders Company, 1928.

———, Craig, W. M., and Adson, A. W.: The Selection of Cases of Thrombo-angiitis Obliterans and Other Circulatory Diseases of the Extremities for Sympathetic Ganglionectomy. Am. Heart J., 10: 143, 1934.

Herrmann, L. G.: Passive Vascular Exercises. Philadelphia, J. B. Lippincott, 1936.

Howe, C. W., and Wigglesworth, W. C.: Control of Infections Associated with Obliterative Arterial Disease. Surg., Gynec. & Obst., 96:553, 1953.

Maddock, W. G., and Coller, F. A.: Peripheral Vasoconstriction by Tobacco and Its Relation to Thrombo-angiitis Obliterans. Ann. Surg., 98:70, 1933.

Naide, M.: The Causative Relationship of Dermatophytosis to Thrombo-angiitis Obliterans. Am. J. M. Sc., 202:822, 1941.

Samuels, S. S.: Management of Peripheral Arterial Diseases. New York, Oxford University Press, 1950.

PERIPHERAL ARTERIOSCLEROSIS

(Senile Gangrene, Diabetic Gangrene, Thromboarteriosclerosis Obliterans, Monckeberg's Sclerosis)

The etiology, pathology and general symptomatology of arteriosclerosis are discussed in the chapters on Atherosclerosis and Arteriosclerosis. It is unquestionably the leading cause of ischemic peripheral vascular disease in the extremities of elderly patients and should be considered whenever such a case appears. The diagnosis, localization and evaluation of the severity of the process are arrived at by utilizing the symptoms, signs and tests of peripheral ischemia detailed on pages 1377–1379. Treatment for practical purposes is identical with that outlined for Buerger's disease on page 1383, provided due allowance be made for the age of the patient, which on the average is two decades older in the arteriosclerotic. Surgical arterial grafting is being tried on an increasing scale. One must always remember that in elderly patients restorative and collateral vascular processes take place slowly if at all. (See also section on Arteriosclerosis, p. 1398.)

R. W. WILKINS

References

Howe, C. W., and Thompson, J. E. Management of Arteriosclerotic Vascular Disease of the Lower Extremities with Particular Reference to the Control of Infection. J. Am. Geriatrics Soc., 1:486, 1953.

ARTERIAL EMBOLISM

Dislodged fragments of centrally located thrombi may produce sudden occlusion of the peripheral arteries. Emboli usually originate from mural or valvular thrombi in the left side of the heart, and less commonly from an atheromatous ulcer in a large artery. Predisposing factors include (1) change from atrial fibrillation to normal rhythm, (2) bacterial endocarditis and (3) coronary occlusion with mural thrombosis. Large emboli lodge most commonly at branchings of the larger arteries, viz., at the origin of the iliac arteries (saddle or rider embolus), at the junction of the femoral artery with the profunda femoris and at the junction of the subscapular and axillary arteries. The embolus (1) stops blood flow through the vessel in which it lodges, (2) induces widespread secondary vasospasm in the affected extremity and (3) is followed within a few hours by secondary progressive arterial thrombosis below and sometimes above the point of obstruction.

Symptoms and Signs. The onset is usually sudden with severe pain in the region where the embolus lodges; the sensation may resemble that of a blow on the extremity. When large arteries are occluded, fainting, nausea, vomiting, abdominal pain and local tenderness may precede a shocklike state. The extremity is pallid and cold, and paresthesias, such as numbness or tingling, develop rapidly. Within one or two hours pain in the extremity is often agonizing, particularly if the patient has exercised it, sensation is absent, and muscular weakness or actual paralysis has developed. The initial pallor changes to blotchy cyanosis, and, if treatment is delayed, massive gangrene follows with mummification, bleb formation and spotty vermilion discoloration of the skin. Small emboli produce local cyanosis with or without pain.

On examination the extent of coldness and discoloration indicates roughly the size of the vessel affected, but it must be remembered that ischemia from secondary vasospasm is added to that from embolic obstruction per se. Arterial pulsation cannot be detected by finger or oscillometer, distal to the embolus. Anesthesia, paralysis and absence of reflexes are found if large arteries are occluded. The skin color on dependency or after injection of histamine, and the measurements of skin temperature and pulse oscillations, will indicate the boundary between normal and abnormal blood flow.

Treatment. If embolism is suspected, a vascular surgeon should be called immediately into consultation. Early diagnosis is essential and must be definitive, since the operation of embolectomy, to be successful, should be done within 8 or 10 hours after the embolus has lodged. Embolectomy is less often necessary in the upper extremity, where collateral circulation is good. If the patient is seen very early, it is best to abolish the widespread reflex vasospasm before deciding definitely whether embolectomy is advisable or not. The immediate results of embolectomy may be good, but new emboli are liable to appear, and the mortality after operation is usually due to the underlying condition that caused embolization.

In all cases in which surgical embolectomy has been decided *against,* vasoconstrictor tone should be relieved as soon as possible (1) by the paravertebral injection of procaine to block the sympathetic ganglia, (2) by administering alcohol by mouth, or papaverine hydrochloride intravenously and (3) by warming the body and the uninvolved extremities. The affected limb should be kept comfortably warm, as in a thermoregulated (30° to 34° C.) cradle. Every precaution should be taken to prevent burning and trauma which follow the indiscriminate use of uncontrolled heat. Anticoagulant therapy is indicated. Heparin is given at once intravenously or subcutaneously to prevent secondary thrombosis until the effect of orally administered Dicumarol achieves the desired prolongation of the prothrombin time. Suction and pressure therapy, applied early and carefully at frequent intervals, may be a useful adjuvant measure.

The advisability of amputation will depend upon the degree to which collateral circulation fails to compensate for sudden organic occlusion, the general condition of the patient, and the underlying condition responsible for embolism.

R. W. WILKINS

References

Linton, R. R.: Acute Peripheral Arterial Occlusion and Its Treatment. New England J. Med., *216:* 871, 1937.

Lund, C. C.: The Treatment of Embolism of the Greater Arteries. Ann. Surg., *106:*880, 1937.

McClure, R. D., and Harkins, H. N.: Recent Advances in the Treatment of Peripheral Arterial Embolism. Surgery, *14:*747, 1943.

Saland, G.: Acute Occlusions of the Peripheral Arteries; Clinical Analysis and Treatment. Ann. Int. Med., *14:*2027, 1941.

PERIPHERAL ARTERITIS AND GANGRENE IN SYSTEMIC INFECTIONS

Symptoms and signs of peripheral vascular disease, mild or severe, appear occasionally as complications in typhoid fever, typhus, pneumonia, influenza, cholera, bacterial endocarditis, septicemia, trichiniasis and scarlet fever. Mild focal degeneration of the media of the large arteries occurs frequently without producing vascular symptoms. Outspoken necrosis of the media and intimal hyperplasia may lead to thrombosis with signs of subacute or acute arrest of peripheral blood flow. Peripheral ischemia may be transitory and, in large part, vasospastic. On the other hand, thrombotic vascular occlusion affecting small arteries produces necrosis of the skin, while occlusion of large arteries leads to massive gangrene.

Tuberculosis of the peripheral arteries is rare, but occasionally metastatic infections or embolism produces panarteritis or endarteritis with fully developed tubercles in thrombosed vessels. Direct involvement by extension from adjacent tuberculous lesions, while common in centrally placed vessels, is rare in the extremities.

Syphilis may diminish peripheral circulation by producing periarteritis, obliterative intimal hyperplasia or panarteritis, but the media is much less affected than is the case in the large elastic arteries. True gummas have been found in the vessels of gangrenous limbs. Peripheral vascular complications of syphilis are more common in men than in women. Peripheral ischemia, vasospastic or organic, appears insidiously or suddenly, but gangrene is rare. Active antisyphilitic therapy ordinarily arrests the acute progress of the disease and relieves early vasospasm, but organic occlusion remains.

R. W. WILKINS

References

Bailly, L. A.: Occlusion of Arteries of Limbs in Diphtheria. Internat. Clin., 2:157, 1920.

Derick, C. L., and Hass, G. M.: Diffuse Arteritis of Syphilitic Origin. Am. J. Path., 11:291, 1934.

Learmonth, G. E.: Gangrene of the Lower Extremities Complicating Scarlet Fever. Canad. M. A. J., 15:69, 1925.

Slaughter, W. H.: Symmetrical Gangrene of Malarial Origin. J.A.M.A., 86:1607, 1926.

PERIARTERITIS NODOSA

See section on Diseases of Collagen.

PERIPHERAL VASCULAR DISEASES DUE TO ABNORMAL VASOCONSTRICTION OR VASODILATATION

RAYNAUD'S DISEASE

Raynaud's disease (Raynaud, 1862) is the primary or idiopathic form of paroxysmal, bilateral cyanosis of the digits, with or without local gangrene. The attacks of cyanosis are produced by cold or emotion and relieved by heat.

Etiology and Incidence. The etiology of Raynaud's disease is unknown, although constitutional predisposition may be a factor. Familial incidence has been described; nationality plays no role. Women who are underweight, asthenic and subject to mental stress are most frequently affected. Occurring at any age, it is less common before puberty and after 40, without relation to menopause or irregular menses. Men are affected but rarely, so that the essential diagnostic criteria should be considered carefully before making the diagnosis in a male.

Pathologic Physiology. The paroxysmal cyanosis of the digits is due to complete interruption of local blood flow by tight constriction of the digital and palmar, or plantar, arteries. Initial pallor, when it occurs spontaneously, indicates that the minute cutaneous vessels are sharing in the vasospasm. Later the digital capillaries become markedly dilated, but the intensely cyanotic blood in them remains stationary, and the skin is cold. Raynaud, in his original descriptions (1862, 1874), concluded that excessive vasoconstrictor tone of central origin must be responsible. In more advanced cases the involved vessels are also abnormally reactive to local cold (Lewis). Typical attacks of digital cyanosis can then be produced simply by immersing the affected extremities for 20 minutes in water at 15° to 18° C.

Pathology. In the early stages of the disease the arteries, large and small, are histologically normal. Later, in progressive cases, the intima is thickened and the muscular coat of the arteries hypertrophied. Eventually thrombosis of small arteries in the digits leads to focal gangrene, although elsewhere the arteries are still histologically normal or show only slight hypertrophy.

Symptoms and Signs. The onset is usually gradual, the first mild attacks appearing in winter or, less commonly, during a period of emotional stress. Initially, attacks may be unilateral, but they soon become bilateral and are induced regularly by emotion or by exposure of the body or digits, or both, to cold. Infections, fatigue and nervous exhaustion increase their frequency and severity. In a typical well developed attack from one to four digits (thumb often excepted) on each hand become deeply blue or initially white, then blue. The digits are affected to different levels, and the terminal phalanges most severely. The fingers are cold, more or less numb, and may be covered with perspiration. Prolonged cyanosis is accompanied by aching pain and awkwardness in fine movements. The attacks end spontaneously or can be terminated at any time by immersing the hands in warm water or by going into a very warm room. During recovery the cyanotic areas are gradually invaded by tongues of reactive hyperemia which extend slowly or rapidly until the affected digits are brilliantly red throughout. If recovery is slow, pallor, cyanosis and hyperemia may coexist in adjacent patches of skin. Tingling, throbbing, slight swelling and rising skin temperature accompany the rapid return of arterial blood flow. Depending on the severity of the condition, attacks may be rare, or they may occur many times a day; between attacks the digits appear normal or, in severe cases, remain mildly cyanotic. The attacks may disappear entirely during pregnancy.

The hands alone are affected in half the cases, hands and feet in the remainder; nose, cheeks, ears and chin are involved much more rarely. The course of the disease varies; after onset it may persist indefinitely in mild form or improve spontaneously. Approximately one third of the cases are progressive; the attacks become more numerous, persist during summer, last longer and disappear less completely until mild cyanosis is more or less constantly present. The vasodilator response is usually still normal or slightly reduced.

Trophic changes appear in progressive cases usually one to four years after onset. The fingers become thin and tapering, their skin smooth, shiny, less mobile, and eventually tightly stretched (sclerodactyly). The nails grow slowly and are ridged or curved. Recurrent infections, blisters and small areas of local cutaneous gangrene appear on the fingertips, but gangrene of a whole digit is rare. Minute scales of necrotic tissue separate slowly and painfully, leaving tiny depressed scars or pits. At this stage the abolition of vasoconstrictor tone produces a vasodilator response which is slow and incomplete in the more involved digits, but usually normal in the others.

Prognosis. Mild grades of Raynaud's disease improve slowly or remain stationary for years, and the attacks, being few and avoidable, are merely an inconvenience. The progressive form, with recurring infection and local gangrene, becomes increasingly painful and disabling, though only rarely is more than the distal phalanx lost. Generalized scleroderma and rheumatoid arthritis, which are not infrequently associated with progressive Raynaud's disease, may produce extreme deformity and disability.

Diagnosis. The essential diagnostic criteria are (1) digital pallor or cyanosis occurring in intermittent attacks, induced by cold or emotion, and followed by recovery with the redness of reactive hyperemia; (2) symmetric or bilateral involvement of digits; (3) absence of occlusive arterial disease or, at most, in progressive cases, mild involvement of the digital arteries; (4) gangrene, if present, usually limited to small areas of skin; (5) conspicuously greater incidence in women than in men (10 to 1); (6) absence of any disease or anatomic abnormality to which paroxysmal digital cyanosis might be secondary.

Paroxysmal digital cyanosis, or *Raynaud's phenomenon* of the secondary type, which is to be distinguished from primary Raynaud's disease, occurs with thromboangiitis obliterans, arteriosclerosis ("dead finger"), crutch trauma, pneumatic hammer disease, cervical rib, disseminated lupus erythematosus and after recovery from severe cold injury. More or less typical Raynaud's phenomenon may occur secondarily in diseases of the central nervous system, osteoarthritis of the spine, traumatic arthritis, with painful osteoporosis, spina bifida, neuritis, causalgia and poisoning by arsenic or certain heavy metals. Raynaud's phenomenon also occurs in certain patients exhibiting cold agglutinins and cryoglobulinemia. Spasmodic digital cyanosis, hemoglobulinuria and urticaria from cold occasionally occur together in congenital syphilis.

Sudden "bilateral gangrene of the digits" (Lewis) rarely may appear in children or young adults without previous attacks of discoloration and without exposure to cold. The fingers, toes, nose and ears become permanently cyanotic, and within a few days gangrene develops in the distal phalanges of one or more fingers, often symmetrically and bilaterally. Cyclic color changes of the Raynaud type first appear during the stage of healing. This syndrome should not be termed fulminant Raynaud's disease, since gangrene is extensive and due to sudden thrombotic occlusion of the final end branches of the digital arteries. Raynaud's phenomenon has also been observed *after* massive gangrene occurring in malnutrition and during certain infections, e. g., typhoid fever, typhus, pneumonia, influenza and streptococcal sore throat.

Simple disuse of an extremity, paralysis and section of mixed nerves eventually produce coldness of the affected parts with vasoconstriction, but not the cyclic color changes of Raynaud's disease. Some normal subjects, at or before puberty, have incomplete cyanosis or pallor of one or two digits ("dead finger") after exposure to cold, or rarely after emotional disturbance. No necrosis or trophic changes are observed, and the attacks disappear within a few years. There is no reason to regard this mild form of vasospasm as a prodromal stage of Raynaud's disease.

Treatment. Mild cases, with infrequent, slight attacks limited to the winter months, and without trophic changes or gangrene, may be relieved by taking high caloric diets, relaxing mental stress, wearing heavier clothing, protecting the extremities whenever exposure to cold cannot be avoided, and moving to a warm climate. Smoking has been shown to produce vasoconstriction, and the use of tobacco should, therefore, be avoided. Psychotherapy and even simple reassurance concerning the nature of the condition may reduce its severity by allaying excessive fear. If there is evidence of hypothyroidism, thyroid substance should be tried. Vasodilator drugs (see p. 1380) taken immediately before the extremities are exposed to cold will abort some mild attacks. Repeated reactive hyperemia and contrast baths have been used. At best, however, medical measures provide only partial relief.

Vasoconstrictor tone is an important factor in bringing on and maintaining attacks of vasospasm, whether or not the local arteries are abnormally reactive to cold. Removal of vasoconstrictor impulses by regional sympathectomy is the treatment of choice for the progressive type of Raynaud's disease with increasing distress, indolent ulcers, local gangrene or early diminution of vasodilator response in the digits. If trophic changes or complications are well advanced, the useful-

ness of the operation will depend upon the degree to which the normal capacity for vasodilatation is preserved as shown by the vasodilator response.

In early Raynaud's disease of the lower extremities lumbar sympathetic ganglionectomy, which is essentially a preganglionic sympathectomy of the limbs, gives complete relief of symptoms. For the upper extremity preganglionic cervicodorsal sympathectomy is the operation of choice (Smithwick, Telford). After successful sympathectomy, sweating is absent in those areas of skin which have been deprived of sympathetic impulses, and the extremities will be warmer to a degree that can be gauged roughly before operation by vasodilatation tests. In late Raynaud's disease, when the digital vessels are hypersensitive to local cold, exposure may still produce color changes after sympathectomy, but the attacks are less severe and, in general, less persistent. In patients with complications such as scleroderma or arthritis, vasospasm may be relieved with or without improvement of the associated disease.

R. W. WILKINS

References

Allen, E. V., and Brown, G. E.: Raynaud's Disease. J.A.M.A., 99:1472, 1932.
Lewis, T.: Raynaud's Disease, with Special Reference to the Nature of the Malady. Brit. M. J., 2: 136, 1932.
———, and Pickering, G. W.: Observations upon Maladies in Which the Blood Supply to Digits Ceases Intermittently or Permanently, and upon Bilateral Gangrene of Digits; Observations Relevant to So-called "Raynaud's Disease." Clin. Sc., 1:327, 1934.
Raynaud, A. G. M.: De l'asphyxie locale et de la gangrène symétrique des extrémités. Paris, Leclerc, 1862.
Smithwick, R. H.: The Value of Sympathectomy in the Treatment of Vascular Disease. New England J. Med., 216:141, 1937.
Telford, E. D.: Sympathetic Denervation of the Upper Extremities. Lancet, 1:70, 1938.
White, J. C., and Smithwick, R. H.: The Autonomic Nervous System. 2d ed. New York, Macmillan Co., 1941.

ACROCYANOSIS

Acrocyanosis (Crocq, 1896; chronic acroasphyxia, Cassirer, 1900) is a symmetrical cyanosis of the hands and feet which causes few or no symptoms and no serious consequences. Of unknown etiology, it is primarily a vasospastic disturbance of the smaller arterioles of the skin with secondary dilatation of the capillary beds and the subpapillary venous plexuses. It occurs in men or women without special age incidence, and may be associated with asthenia and various endocrine disorders as well as with certain anxiety states.

Acrocyanosis is characterized by an unevenly mottled blue and red discoloration of the skin extending from a line above the wrists and ankles to the digits, and increasing in degree distally. The cyanosis is intensified by cold or emotion and relieved by warmth. The digits are habitually cold and sweat profusely, but the soft tissues are normal or at most puffy. Hypesthesia of mild grade may be present. It is easily differentiated from various types of generalized cyanosis because the discoloration is limited to the hands or feet and disappears when the extremities are warmed. It can be distinguished from Raynaud's disease by the type of discoloration and by the absence of even slight pain. In acrocyanosis, histamine puncture produces a brilliant flare and conspicuous wheal in the cyanotic digits. In Raynaud's disease histamine produces neither hyperemic flare nor wheal in the digits *during a paroxysm of cyanosis*.

Except for reassurance, treatment is usually unnecessary. Possible endocrine abnormalities should be investigated. For cosmetic reasons the condition may be made less conspicuous by local protection from cold, wearing of warm clothing, vasodilator drugs (see p. 1380), contrast baths and lotions for hyperhidrosis. The trivial nature of the condition rarely, if ever, warrants surgical treatment.

R. W. WILKINS

References

Elliott, A. H., Evans, R. D., and Stone, C. S.: Acrocyanosis: A Study of the Circulatory Fault. Am. Heart J., *11:*431, 1936.
Lewis, T., and Landis, E. M.: Observations upon the Vascular Mechanism in Acrocyanosis. Heart, 15:229, 1930.
Stern, E. S.: Acrocyanosis. J. Ment. Sc., 83:408, 1937.

ERGOTISM

Ergotism is an acute or chronic intoxication arising from the ingestion of bread made from rye or wheat infected with ergot fungus (*Claviceps purpurae*), or the chronic use of drugs derived from this source. Diarrhea, colic and vomiting are followed by headache, vertigo, paresthesias, convulsive seizures and, occasionally, gangrene of the digits, nose or ears. It occurred during the past in epidemic form, but is now seen only sporadically, or after the repeated administration of ergot in abortion and of ergotamine (Gynergen) in pruritus or migraine. Peripheral gangrene is due to long-continued arteriolar spasm and slow blood flow with secondary intimal hyperplasia and thrombosis. In chronic intoxications the nonocclusive form is said to affect especially women, children and the aged, while the gangrenous form is more frequent in men during early adult life.

R. W. WILKINS

References

Gould, S. E., Price, A. E., and Ginsberg, H. L.: Gangrene and Death Following Ergotamine Tartrate (Gynergen) Therapy. J.A.M.A., *106:*1631, 1936.
Perlow, S., and Bloch, L.: Impending Gangrene of the Feet Due to Ergotamine Tartrate. J.A.M.A., *109:*27, 1937.

ERYTHROMELALGIA

Erythromelalgia (Weir Mitchell, 1872) is a primary or idiopathic form of paroxysmal, bilateral vasodilatation associated with burning pain, increased skin temperature and more or less redness of the skin, particularly in the feet. The etiology is unknown, and no uniform pathology has been found thus far. It occurs with equal frequency in men and women without special age incidence.

Symptoms and Signs. The onset is gradual, and symptoms may remain mild for years or may become so severe and continuous that total disability results. Attacks of bilateral, burning pain, superficial or deep, first involve circumscribed areas on the soles or palms, but later may spread over the whole extremity. The attacks follow stimuli which normally induce only physiologic peripheral vasodilatation or engorgement, *viz.*, local heat, a warm environment, exercise, standing or simple dependency of the extremity. Arterial pulsation is increased locally and the affected skin is hot and often sweats profusely, but trophic changes, gangrene and ulceration are absent. Rest, elevation of the extremity and local application of cold will relieve the congestion, hyperthermia and pain.

Differential Diagnosis. Polycythemia vera and arteriosclerosis may produce localized and often unilateral burning pain and redness, but, unlike erythromelalgia, rarely cause a rise in skin temperature. Many chronic inflammatory states produce in the skin a "susceptible state" (Lewis) with diminished capillary and arteriolar tone. Burning pain (erythralgia, Lewis) is then induced by mild grades of heat, cold, friction and congestion which leaves normal skin unaffected. Neuritis, infectious ganglionitis and poisoning by thallium, lead or arsenic occasionally produce painful peripheral hyperemia. A temporary reactive vasodilatation of the cutaneous vessels normally occurs after prolonged exposure to cold in response to a histamine-like substance liberated by local tissue damage (Lewis). This is easily distinguished from erythromelalgia by the history. Glomus tumor and arteriovenous fistula produce venous engorgement, local pulsation and increased skin temperature, but not the type of pain observed in erythromelalgia.

Treatment. The therapy of true erythromelalgia is in general unsatisfactory. Attacks can be avoided or aborted by rest, elevation of the extremity and cold applications. Contrast baths, using heat below the threshold for pain, and local irradiation often afford considerable relief, at least temporarily. Severe attacks require liberal doses of sedative. Acetylsalicylic acid (0.3 to 0.6 gm.) relieves pain in some cases. Occasionally section or alcohol injection of peripheral nerves is required; sympathectomy has been advocated.

R. W. WILKINS

References

Lewis, T.: Clinical Observations and Experiments Relating to Burning Pain in Extremities, and to So-called "Erythromelalgia" in Particular. Clin. Sc., 1:175, 1933.

Mitchell, S. W.: On a Rare Vasomotor Neurosis of the Extremities, and on the Maladies with Which It May be Confounded. Am. J. M. Sc., 76:17, 1878.

Smith, L. A., and Allen, E. V.: Erythermalgia (Erythromelalgia) of the Extremities. Am. Heart J., 13:483, 1937.

Telford, E. D., and Simmons, H. T.: Erythromelalgia. Brit. M. J., 2:782, 1940.

PERIPHERAL VASCULAR DISEASES DUE TO EXPOSURE TO COLD

Exposure to cold stimulates vasoconstriction and, if severe, results in definite tissue damage that varies directly with the degree and duration of the exposure and the suscep-tibility of the patient. Even brief exposure to nonfreezing cold is followed in susceptible persons by an exaggerated and prolonged type of reactive vasodilatation, characterized by persistent local redness, low grade edema and tingling pain. Similar exposure in more susceptible patients produces pronounced edema of the angioneurotic or urticarial type, with increased skin temperature persisting for 12 to 24 hours. In still more susceptible subjects such exposure may be followed by an even greater local vasodilatation, and also by systemic effects, similar to those produced by injecting histamine intravenously, viz., flushing of the face, tachycardia, decreased arterial pressure, faintness and syncope.

TRENCH FOOT AND IMMERSION FOOT

Prolonged exposure to low but not freezing temperatures, combined with persistent dampness or, more usually, actual immersion in water, can damage severely the skin, peripheral vessels, nerves and muscles of the lower and, more rarely, the upper extremities. This form of injury, recognized by Larrey during the Napoleonic wars, was an important cause of disability in both the Crimean War and World War I. In the latter this syndrome was fully described under the name of "trench foot." The maritime and "home front" hazards of World War II added subvarieties of this syndrome under the titles of "immersion foot," "immersion hand" and "shelter foot."

Though prolonged exposure to cold is always an important factor, it is by no means the sole or, in some cases, even the predominant cause of immersion foot. In fact, several contributory factors seem almost equally important, viz., prolonged dampness or actual immersion in cold or cool water, immobility and dependency of the lower extremities, chilling of the body, exhaustion or dehydration and, in some instances, semistarvation with deficient intake of proteins and vitamins. It may be noted that most of these factors tend singly or together to reduce blood flow to the extremities. Persistent local tissue anoxia, combined with mild or severe cold, injures the capillary wall. Plasma passes freely into the tissue spaces, leaving packed red cells in the minute vessels. The tense edema, increased further by immobility, constricting garments and sometimes hypoproteinemia or vitamin deficiency, embarrasses peripheral circulation still more and is finally accompanied by Wallerian degeneration of the nerves in the affected area. In the more severe cases the brawny edema is associated with organic vascular occlusion, desquamation of the skin, deep fibrosis and superficial gangrene even as the injured nerve tracts regenerate. The nerves may be embedded in contracting fibrous tissue; the walls of arterioles and venules also show fibrosis. Practically all the characteristic lesions have been reproduced in laboratory animals by prolonged immersion of extremities in cold water.

The condition may develop insidiously with only numbness, "cotton wool sensation" and slight swelling as long as the tissues are supported by shoes or boots. When the tissues are not supported, or as soon as boots are removed, rapid transudation appears with marked edema, tingling, itching and severe pain. The skin is red at first, particularly at low temperatures, but later becomes a mottled "sickly yellow," blue or black in color.

Symptoms and Signs. At the time of rescue at sea, or when first seen by medical officers in trench warfare, severely injured extremities are often pulseless and cold with a sock or glove type of hypesthesia or anesthesia with respect to touch, pin prick, temperature, vibration and deep pressure, though joint sense is usually retained.

Within the first few hours or days of hospitalization at normal environmental temperatures the "hyperemic stage" appears and lasts for one to ten weeks, depending upon the grade of initial injury. In areas still free of organic vascular occlusion the skin becomes hot, red and dry, the areas of anhidrosis coinciding with those showing sensory loss. Pulses are bounding, the minute vessels are widely dilated and skin temperatures are high, as though a complete vasomotor paralysis had been produced. Tissue swelling increases as blisters form, weep serous fluid and then slowly heal. Muscle weakness and wasting appear in severe cases.

In areas of skin with thrombosed vessels the color remains mottled and the skin itself becomes gangrenous. Fortunately, gangrene is often superficial, and the necrotic skin is sometimes shed like a glove, leaving healthy skin beneath. Even in the absence of gangrene, extensive exfoliation is common. Meanwhile the areas of hypesthesia and anesthesia diminish and give way, early in this period of hyperemia, to throbbing or burning pain, tingling, pins and needles sensations and sudden intermittent lancinating pain.

These are worse at night, increased by dependency or warmth and decreased by elevation or mild cooling. Pain reaches maximum intensity in seven to ten days and then decreases during the next two to six weeks. The vessels become hypersensitive to epinephrine as in any injury to postganglionic fibers.

The next stage, blending indistinguishably with the preceding stage, is characterized by return of vascular tone, with restoration of normal skin color and temperature. Recovery may be complete in mild cases within two to five weeks, but severe cases often require three to twelve months. At the end of one or even two years a few show sequelae such as sensitivity to cold with Raynaud's phenomenon; general or marginal hyperhidrosis; persistent indurated swelling progressing to fibrosis, limited joint motion and deformity; painful indolent ulcers of the digits or their stumps, and tingling or burning which is increased by warmth, dependency or exertion.

Prophylaxis. The exigencies of warfare make preventive measures difficult, but the value of meticulous foot hygiene in the trenches and at sea is well established. In life rafts it is helpful to move the feet frequently and to avoid dependency by placing them whenever possible on the sides of the raft.

Treatment. For developed trench or immersion foot, treatment of the hyperemic stage consists of rest in bed, correction of dietary deficiencies, cleansing and moderate elevation of the extremities, accompanied by cooling of the hyperemic tissues to reduce local metabolism and to control pain and edema. Hydrous wool fat should be applied to the skin with light massage. Infected abrasions and epidermophytosis may require special applications. For cooling it may be sufficient merely to expose the extremities to room air at 20° C. (70° F.) or less. For more severe pain and swelling it is sometimes necessary to expose the limb in a cool room or to use a blast of air from an electric fan cooled further by water sprayed into the blast from a nebulizer. With sufficient cooling, pain should be relieved in a few hours, but in some instances it is necessary to discover an optimum temperature, since too low a temperature may again produce pain.

Sympathetic block and ganglionectomy have not been helpful in the stage of hyperemia, but appear to improve certain late sequelae such as chronic painful ulcers, persistent vasospasm with Raynaud's phenomenon and hyperhidrosis.

R. W. WILKINS

References

Lange, K., Weiner, D., and Boyd, L. J.: The Functional Pathology of Experimental Immersion Foot. Am. Heart J., 35:238, 1948.

Ungley, C. C., and Blackwood, W.: Peripheral Vasoneuropathy after Chilling. Immersion Foot and Immersion Hand. Lancet, 2:447, 1942.

Webster, D. R., Woolhouse, F. M., and Johnston, J. L.: Immersion Foot. J. Bone & Joint Surg., 24:785, 1942.

White, J. C.: Vascular and Neurologic Lesions in Survivors of Shipwreck. I. Immersion Foot Syndrome Following Exposure to Cold. II. Painful Swollen Feet Secondary to Prolonged Dehydration and Malnutrition. New England J. Med., 228:211, 1943.

CHILBLAIN AND PERNIO

Chilblain and *pernio* (erythrocyanosis) occur commonly in patients with a history of cool limbs in summer as well as in winter. This suggests that they are liable to occur on the basis of a preexisting circulatory disturbance in the limbs.

Chilblain occurs on the dorsum of the fingers, hands or feet as a localized, warm, red, pruritic swelling that may disappear in a few days, but more often becomes an indolent lesion, dull red or violaceous, proceeding to painful bleb formation or ulceration. It is due to repeated or prolonged exposure to cold insufficient to freeze the tissues and appears (in temperate zones) at the onset of cold weather, recurring each year in the same exposed areas of the body.

Pernio, an essentially similar lesion involving the lower parts of the legs, occurs especially in women because their mode of dress affords inadequate protection for their legs against cool weather.

R. W. WILKINS

References

Lewis, T.: Observations on Some Normal and Injurious Effects of Cold upon Skin and Underlying Tissues. II. Chilblain and Allied Conditions. Brit. M. J., 2:837, 1941.

McGovern, T., Wright, I. S., and Kruger, E.: Pernio: A Vascular Disease. Am. Heart J., 22:583, 1941.

FROSTBITE

Strictly speaking, frostbite, in contradistinction to immersion foot, chilblain and pernio, is due to freezing of the tissues, with mechanical disruption of cell structure. Actually, however, it frequently occurs in association with one of the other syndromes. When the freezing is superficial, thawing is followed by the typical cutaneous response to injury, namely, local reddening, wheal and flare; but, when the skin is frozen more extensively, or when the subcutaneous tissues are involved, it is accompanied by bleb formation or by necrosis and ulceration.

Frostbite results from exposure to cold air usually at temperatures below $-13°$ C. ($10°$ F.). Theoretically, the freezing point of the skin cannot be far from $-1°$ C. ($30°$ F.), but, when dry and oily, the skin's property of supercooling without freezing affords considerable protection. High winds, dampness and general chilling of the body make freezing more likely at less rigorous temperatures, e.g., $-5°$ C. ($23°$ F.). Once started, freezing progresses rapidly, and the tissues of the cheeks, nose, ears or digits are injured to increasing depth by the formation of minute ice crystals.

Symptoms and Signs. Predisposing factors are bodily weakness, insufficient or improper clothing, general chilliness, and any peripheral vascular disturbance of the ischemic type. The first indication of actual frostbite is often a sharp, pricking sensation which draws attention to a yellowish white, numb area of hard skin. However, cold itself produces numbness and anesthesia which may permit serious freezing to develop without the helpful warning of acute discomfort. The local injury found in frostbite ranges from simple erythema, transient anesthesia and superficial bullae to persisting ischemia, secondary thrombosis, livid cyanosis, deep tissue destruction and gangrene.

Prophylaxis. Frostbite is preventable and occurs rarely among those who have been trained properly to protect themselves against the effects of cold. Prophylactic measures include the wearing of abundant warm, dry clothing with windbreakers and gloves or preferably mittens; only brief periods of exposure to cold, particularly if vigorous exercise is not possible; and the avoidance of smoking before and during exposure. Feet and socks should be kept scrupulously dry, and all exposed skin should be greased liberally.

Treatment. When patches of frostbite appear on the face, irreversible damage may be prevented by placing the bare, warm hand immediately over the area. Frostbitten skin should not be rubbed with snow or warmed too vigorously. Affected extremities should be warmed immediately between the layers of one's own or a companion's clothing.

After rescue, it is best to rewarm the frozen tissues as rapidly as possible (in warm water up to 42° C.) until thawing has occurred. They should then be exposed to room air (70° C.). Massage, too vigorous warming (water temperatures above 45° C.) and reactive hyperemia should be avoided because they tend to increase pain and edema. To control severe pain, cooling may be required as described under Trench Foot (p. 1391). Early and continuous heparinization to combat thrombosis and gangrene has been stressed.

If vasodilatation is slow and incomplete, vasodilator drugs (alcohol, papaverine) and exposure in a room at a moderate temperature will be helpful. For late and prolonged ischemia resulting from widespread arterial thrombosis, suction and pressure therapy in brief repeated periods may be helpful, and sympathetic ganglionectomy may be considered for residual spasm. Eventual recovery is usually surprisingly good, though sensitivity to cold and predilection to repeated frostbite often persist. For this reason, and because of the difficulty in judging accurately the extent of eventual injury, initial therapy should always be very conservative. In deep frostbite, sepsis and gangrene may develop, and these complications must be treated according to the general precautions and surgical principles applying to ischemic and vulnerable tissue. Amputation may be required at levels to be determined by the line of demarcation and the amount of secondary thrombosis.

R. W. WILKINS

References

Gottschalk, C. W.: Frostbite. Mod. Concepts Cardiovasc. Dis., 22:202, 1953.

Greene, R.: Frost-Bite and Kindred Ills. Lancet, 2: 689, 1941.

Lewis, T.: Observations on Some Normal and Injurious Effects of Cold upon the Skin and Underlying Tissues. Brit. M. J., 2:837, 1941.

Lange, K., Boyd, L. J., and Weiner, D.: Prerequisites of Successful Heparinization to Prevent Gangrene after Frostbite. Proc. Soc. Exper. Biol. & Med., 74: 1, 1950.

Frostbite. Editorial. J.A.M.A., 148:940, 1952.

PERIPHERAL VASCULAR DISEASES DUE TO ABNORMAL COMMUNICATIONS BETWEEN ARTERIES AND VEINS

ARTERIOVENOUS FISTULA

Arteriovenous fistula refers to abnormal communications, single or multiple, between arteries and veins by which arterial blood enters the vein directly without traversing a capillary network. These fistulas are classified as (1) congenital, usually multiple and present from birth, and (2) acquired, usually single and saccular, arising after bullet or stab wounds involving an artery and a contiguous vein.

Arterial blood, following the path of least resistance, rushes directly into the vein instead of through the corresponding capillary bed. The thin-walled veins are distended by the pressure transmitted from the artery through the fistulous opening and eventually become prominent and cirsoid. Increased blood flow makes the tissues near the fistula abnormally warm, while diminished flow distal to the fistula may produce peripheral coldness and trophic changes. Large fistulas impose a burden on the heart, the output of which must be increased above normal by an amount proportional to the size of the fistula in order to maintain an efficient general circulation. The low peripheral resistance tends to decrease diastolic blood pressure and increase systolic and pulse pressures. Men and women are affected equally, and any part of the body may be involved.

Symptoms and Signs. Patients complain of aching pain, edema, disfigurement from dilated veins or hypertrophied extremities and, occasionally, cardiac symptoms such as palpitation, substernal pain and dyspnea on exertion.

On inspection the superficial veins are prominent under spongy subcutaneous tissue, and venous pulsation can be felt unless the fistula is small or deeply placed. Arterial pulsation is also increased and skin temperature often elevated. Local bruit and thrill occur frequently, but not uniformly. The tissues near the fistula may be tender, more or less edematous, and either red or slightly cyanotic. The circumference of the extremity is increased by edema or true hypertrophy, but bony structures are hypertrophied only if the fistula had been present before epiphyseal ossification occurred. Distal to the fistula, decreased capillary flow may lead to the formation of shallow, indolent ulcers, rarefaction of bone and occasionally to unilateral arthritic changes. Temporary compression of the artery leading to a large fistula diminishes the heart rate (Branham's sign), but no effects are observed if the fistula is small.

The oxygen saturation of blood removed from distended veins is greater than that of blood removed from corresponding veins in the opposite extremity. Deeply placed fistulas require comparisons between blood samples from deeper veins. Arteriography reveals the exact location, number and size of the communications.

Treatment. Single fistulas can be eradicated by ligating the involved artery and vein, both above and below the fistula, if adequate collateral circulation is available. Multiple fistulas are much less amenable to surgical treatment. If the arterial supply depends upon one large anomalous artery, ligation of this vessel, followed by stenosing injections of the dilated veins, may be effective. Ulcers, edema and pain are relieved by applying supporting elastic bandages or stockings. Amputation is required for large, inoperable fistulas producing cardiac decompensation or gross deformity.

R. W. Wilkins

References

Horton, B. T.: Hemihypertrophy of Extremities Associated with Congenital Arteriovenous Fistula. J.A.M.A., 98:373, 1932.

Nickerson, J. L., Elkin, D. C., and Warren, J. V.: The Effect of Temporary Occlusion of Arteriovenous Fistulas on Heart Rate, Stroke Volume, and Cardiac Output. J. Clin. Investigation, 30:215, 1951.

Reid, M.: Abnormal Arteriovenous Communications, Acquired and Congenital. Arch. Surg., 11:237, 1925.

Veal, J. R., and McCord, W. M.: Congenital Abnormal Arteriovenous Anastomoses of the Extremities, with Special Reference to Diagnosis by Arteriography and by the Oxygen Saturation Test. Arch. Surg., 33:848, 1936.

Warren, J. V., Nickerson, J. L., and Elkin, D. C.: The Cardiac Output in Patients with Arteriovenous Fistulas. J. Clin. Investigation, 30:210, 1951.

———, Elkin, D. C., and Nickerson, J. L.: The Blood Volume in Patients with Arteriovenous Fistulas. J. Clin. Investigation, 30:220, 1951.

GLOMANGIOMA OR GLOMUS TUMOR

(Painful Subcutaneous Nodule, Angioneuroma or Angiomyoneuroma)

Glomangioma or glomus tumor designates painful, benign hypertrophy of an arteriovenous anastomosis with its associated smooth muscle coat, nonmyelinated nerve fibers and connective tissue (collectively termed a "glomus"). Histologically, the lesion is encapsulated, occasionally diffuse but never invasive, and contains numerous "glomus" cells without inflammatory reaction. These extremely tender but inconspicuous subcutaneous tumors develop slowly during adult life, often following slight trauma. They are found in various parts of the upper and lower extremities, but most frequently (30 per cent) beneath the fingernail. The diameter of the tumor is 1 cm. or less. The intact skin or nail over the lesion is flat or slightly raised with discoloration ranging from red to blue, usually the latter. Excruciating burning or shooting pain, both local and referred up the extremity, occurs spontaneously or is produced by pressure on the tumor. Heat, excessive cold, and even contact with clothing become intolerable so that protection is required continuously day and night. The tumor may pulsate slightly, and skin temperature may be elevated locally.

In **treatment,** radium has proved useless. Surgical excision brings complete and immediate relief without recurrence.

R. W. Wilkins

References

Bailey, O. T.: The Cutaneous Glomus and Its Tumors—Glomangioma. Am. J. Path., 11:915, 1935.

Bergstrand, H.: Multiple Glomic Tumors. Am. J. Cancer, 29:470, 1937.

Stabins, S. J., Thornton, J. J., and Scott, W. J. M.: Changes in Vasomotor Reaction, Associated with Glomus Tumors. J. Clin. Investigation, 16:685, 1937.

DISEASES OF THE PERIPHERAL VEINS

The conditions affecting venous blood flow in the extremities may be divided into two categories: (1) intrinsic disorders produced primarily by disease of the walls of the veins or by abnormality of their contained blood and (2) extrinsic disorders resulting secondarily from invasion or external pressure. These various maladies are disabling in proportion to the grade of venous stasis produced (1) by anatomic blockage as in thrombosis and external pressure or (2) by hydrostatic forces as in varicose veins.

VARICOSE VEINS

Varicose veins are caused (1) by constitutionally defective valves in association with postural strain, usually of occupational type, or (2) by any condition which obstructs venous blood flow and distends collateral veins over long periods of time, especially pregnancy and pelvic or abdominal neoplasm. The veins are distended and tortuous, while chronic venous stasis produces local edema, stabbing or aching pain, indolent ulceration, overgrowth of connective tissue and, occasionally, hemorrhage or ecchymosis.

The extremities are warm and the arterial pulses normal. Elevation of the foot produces no blanching, but empties the veins rapidly unless obstruction is present, when emptying is slow and incomplete. Retrograde flow of blood past incompetent valves in the long saphenous vein is demonstrated by the Trendelenburg test. The leg of the recumbent patient is elevated to empty the varices, and then, while firm pressure with the thumb or a tourniquet closes the proximal end of the long saphenous vein, the patient quickly assumes the standing position. Sudden release of the saphenous vein will make the varices prominent and turgid within a few seconds if back-flow is present. If pressure is maintained for a longer time in the standing position, dilated communications with incompetent deep veins can be identified. In advanced stages the vein responsible for brawny induration and ulceration may be invisible under the deformity it has produced, but careful palpation will usually detect the dilated vein. Venography has been advocated for doubtful cases. Phlebosclerosis is common in chronic cases.

Therapeutic measures include bed rest with elevation of the extremity, elastic stockings or bandages, sponge rubber dressings, the gelatin boot, injection of sclerosing solutions and high ligation or excision. Acetyl-beta-methylcholine by iontophoresis, excision and skin grafting have been used successfully for treating chronic ulcers resisting other therapy.

R. W. WILKINS

References

Ferguson, L. K.: Ligation of Varicose Veins; Ambulatory Treatment Preliminary to Sclerosing Injections. Ann. Surg., *102*:304, 1935.

McPheeters, H. O., and Anderson, J. K.: Injection Treatments of Varicose Veins and Hemorrhoids. Philadelphia, F. A. Davis Co., 1938.

Saylor, L., Kovacs, J., Duryee, A. W., and Wright, I. S.: The Treatment of Chronic Varicose Ulcers by Means of Acetyl Beta Methylcholine Chloride Iontophoresis. J.A.M.A., *107*:114, 1937.

PHLEBOTHROMBOSIS AND THROMBOPHLEBITIS

Venous obstruction by thrombosis may be either a primary, simple, noninflammatory process (*phlebothrombosis*) or a secondary reaction to local or distant inflammatory agents with active inflammation of the wall of the affected vein (*thrombophlebitis*). Sometimes it is difficult to distinguish clinically between the two, though characteristically *phlebothrombosis,* being accompanied by little or no local reaction, produces no symptoms, while *thrombophlebitis* is associated with the classic symptoms and signs of inflammation both locally and systematically. *Pylephlebitis* is described on page 930.

Etiology of intravenous clotting consists of one or more predisposing factors: (1) venous stasis associated with prolonged bed rest or external pressure, (2) local injury of the endothelium by stretching, contusion, chemicals or bacteria, and (3) thrombophilia or changes in the circulating blood which favor coagulation.

A number of different clinical conditions predispose to the development of *phlebothrombosis,* including myocardial failure, malignancy, obesity, debility, senility, varicosities, trauma and surgery. While these conditions probably operate in a variety of ways, a factor common to them all is their tendency to slow the circulation, particularly in the veins of the limbs. Saccular dilatations of the calf veins in patients over the age of 40 may explain the greater incidence of phlebothrombosis in the elderly. Greater vein length in tall persons may predispose to stasis and cause venous thrombosis, especially after effort (Naide). Slowing of the peripheral circulation postoperatively is said to be maximal at the time when phlebothrombosis and pulmonary embolism most commonly develop. Other changes suggested as possibly important in predisposing to phlebothrombosis include an increase in clot-promoting factors and a decrease in clot-inhibiting factors after operation, and the development of cold agglutinins and other auto-agglutinins after certain infections. Polycythemia vera and certain forms of anemia in which the coagulability of the blood is increased are frequently complicated by phlebothrombosis.

True *thrombophlebitis* occurs during prolonged bed rest with associated infection, e.g., after operations, intravenous therapy, in the puerperium and during convalescence from pneumonia, influenza or typhoid fever. It may be produced by direct extension from local suppurative foci, e.g., mastoiditis and osteomyelitis. So-called "resting phlebitis" in varicose veins may be reactivated periodically by trauma, exercise or minor infection elsewhere.

Symptoms and Signs. Noninflammatory *phlebothrombosis* may occur suddenly or gradually without pain, local tenderness or systemic symptoms. Edema and cyanosis may appear rapidly, but unfortunately are often overlooked until the symptoms of pulmonary embolism call attention to the limbs. A sudden increase in the circumference of the limb, pain in the calf and/or popliteal space on dorsiflexion of the foot (Homans's sign) or diminished pulsation in the femoral artery on the ipsilateral side may be found if looked for.

The onset of true *thrombophlebitis* is usually sudden with mild or severe symptoms, depending on the size of the vein involved. Pain may be absent, mild and localized, or severe and throbbing through the whole extremity. When the pelvic veins are obstructed, abdominal pain, faintness, nausea or vomiting may appear suddenly and persist for some hours. When a peripheral and superficial vein is affected, the thrombosed vessel can usually be felt beneath the skin as a tender cord. Local tenderness in the calf and pain on forced dorsiflexion of the foot suggest involvement of the deeper branches of the popliteal vein. Edema and mottled cyanosis are present if collateral venous drainage is poor, but are absent when small veins are obstructed and the collateral channels are adequate. Arterial pulsation usually is normal and the extremity is not persistently cold. Occasionally, however, in sudden extensive venous thrombosis, vasospasm is so conspicuous that arterial embolism may be suspected and even gangrene may appear imminent. However, the oscillometer may detect arterial pulsation even when it is too feeble to be palpated. Elevation of the extremity does not produce abnormal pallor; on the contrary, cyanosis may persist during elevation. General malaise, anorexia, fever and leukocytosis appear shortly after onset and, barring extension of thrombosis, gradually disappear. In "migrating thrombophlebitis," however, several widely separated veins may be involved in succession, with healing in one location occurring simultaneously with fresh thrombosis in a totally different region.

The most serious complication of *phlebothrombosis* or *thrombophlebitis* is pulmonary embolism which follows dislodgement of a thrombus shortly after it has formed and before organization has fixed it firmly in the vein of origin. In general, the greater the local tenderness and pain in the extremity, the less is the danger of embolism, since thrombi usually loosen before pronounced inflammatory reaction develops. Large thrombi dislodged from the femoral, iliac or pelvic veins commonly produce fatal pulmonary embolism, a frequent cause of sudden death after operation or deep pelvic irradiation. Smaller emboli produce pulmonary infarction, pleuritis, bronchopneumonia or abscess.

Repeated attacks of thrombophlebitis and continued venous stasis, with more or less lymphangitis, cause edema, fibrosis, pigmentation and trophic ulceration in the limbs, and the eventual deformity in untreated cases may be extreme.

Prophylaxis. Frequent turning, deep breathing, bicycle exercises, and flexion and extension of the extremities are useful in speeding the circulation and lessening the danger of venous thrombosis. Unfortunately, in debilitated and especially in cardiac patients, it is not always practicable to carry out these procedures. However, elastic compression of the legs and prophylactic anticoagulant drugs (p. 1380) may be used in almost every case in which venous thrombosis is liable to occur. Excessive dehydration should be avoided.

Treatment. Once thrombosis has developed, the objects of therapy are (1) to prevent pulmonary embolism by loosened thrombus, and (2) to relieve the edema before connective tissue overgrowth in the protein-rich edema fluid produces permanent brawny organization. Pulmonary embolism may occur suddenly before symptoms and signs of peripheral thrombosis appear. Just as soon as it seems probable that thrombosis has occurred, active or passive motion of the limbs is contraindicated. Phlebotomy and removal of the thrombus (thrombectomy) have been advocated, especially for simple, noninflammatory thrombosis of large veins. Such surgical treatment is contraindicated if diagnosis is late and if there is local inflammatory reaction. However, when the distal segments of superficial veins, e. g., the long or short saphenous, or the deep veins of the calf are thrombosed, proximal ligation is a minor procedure which reduces the danger of pulmonary embolism. It has been emphasized that unilateral ligation may not be sufficient, since the predisposing factors to phlebothrombosis operate generally, and often thrombosis is present in both legs. Furthermore, embolization is more liable to occur from the less obviously involved (less symptomatic) limb. Finally, ligation should be performed high enough to preclude the possibility of embolization from proximal extension of the clot. In some cases it has seemed advisable to ligate even as high as the inferior vena cava.

As soon as *thrombophlebitis* is suspected, the patient should be kept at rest in bed with the affected extremity slightly elevated to diminish edema. Blocking the sympathetic ganglia by the paravertebral injection of procaine abolishes reflex vasospasm, relieves pain and diminishes edema. Anticoagulants, as mentioned before, can have little effect on existing thrombi, but should be used to prevent propagation, as described under Anticoagulant Therapy (p. 1380). Local heat should be applied by means of a thermoregulated cradle. Proximal venous ligation should be considered if the thrombus is extending into the thigh, is suppurating, or if a history of pulmonary embolism is obtained. There is increasing tendency to shorten greatly the period of absolute bed rest for all types of patients, because sluggish blood flow predisposes to development of thrombi or propagation of an existing thrombus.

After temperature and pulse are normal, the patient may sit up in bed unless activity is followed by return of symptoms or a rise in temperature. Passive, and later active, movements of the affected extremity are started gradually to help recovery of muscle

tone and to assist the function of collateral venous channels. If edema still forms, the limbs should be elevated nightly. When normal activity is resumed, an elastic stocking should be worn until measurement of the extremity reveals no accumulation of edema fluid while the tissues are unsupported. Brawny swelling and induration may be somewhat relieved by vigorous massage and heat if there has been no recent phlebitis. Gross deformity, ulceration and infection rarely may require amputation.

R. W. WILKINS

References

Allen, A. W., Linton, R. R., and Donaldson, G. A.: Venous Thrombosis and Pulmonary Embolism. J.A.M.A., *128*:397, 1945.

D'Alessandro, A. J.: An Early Clinical Sign of Venous Thrombosis. J.A.M.A., *147*:1759, 1951.

Homans, J.: Venous Thrombosis in the Lower Limbs; Its Relation to Pulmonary Embolism. Am. J. Surg., 38:316, 1937.

Murray, W. D. G.: Heparin in Thrombosis and Embolism. Brit. J. Surg., 27:567, 1940.

Naide, M.: Spontaneous Venous Thrombosis in the Legs of Tall Men. J.A.M.A., *148*:1202, 1952.

Ochsner, A., and DeBakey, M.: Therapeutic Considerations of Thrombophlebitis and Phlebothrombosis. New England J. Med., 225:207, 1941.

Roe, B. B., and Goldthwait, J. C.: Pulmonary Embolism. New England J. Med., *241*:679, 1949.

Wilkins, R. W., and Stanton, J. R.: Elastic Stockings in the Prevention of Pulmonary Embolism. II. A Progress Report. New England J. Med., *248*:1087, 1953.

Thromboembolism. Combined Staff Clinic. Am. J. Med., 3:753, 1947.

DISEASES OF THE PERIPHERAL LYMPHATIC VESSELS

The lymphatic capillaries form a rich intercellular network and collect excess tissue fluid which, as lymph, is conducted by valved channels of increasing size to regional lymph nodes and thence through trunk lymphatics to the subclavian veins. The flow of lymph depends on muscular contraction, respiratory movements and, to a certain extent, on gravity.

LYMPHANGITIS

Lymphangitis refers to acute or chronic inflammation, usually streptococcal in origin, affecting the lymphatic vessels and the immediately adjacent tissues. Advancing lymphangitis indicates that infection is spreading and is therefore a danger signal of special importance. The path by which bacteria penetrate the skin cannot be discovered in some cases, but usually local trauma, trichophytosis or chronic ulcers are obvious portals of entry. Slightly indurated, red, tender streaks appear in the skin of the leg or forearm, and the regional lymph nodes in the knees, groin or axilla rapidly become swollen and tender. Malaise, chills, fever, increased pulse rate and leukocytosis indicate systemic reaction and possible blood stream infection. Lymphangitis may be of grave import and is especially dangerous in the ischemic tissues of patients with peripheral vascular disease. Only under these unfavorable conditions is prompt high amputation often required. When circulation is normal, drainage of the original focus, rest, hot wet dressings and antibiotic therapy will usually produce rapid recovery.

LYMPHEDEMA

Lymphedema is a form of chronic bilateral or unilateral edema of the extremities due, in its primary form, probably to congenital hypoplasia of the lymphatic vessels and, in its secondary form, to obstruction by external pressure or repeated low grade inflammation.

Primary lymphedema occurs more commonly in women. Three forms are described: (1) congenital lymphedema, present at birth or developing shortly thereafter; (2) lymphedema (praecox), appearing at or near puberty; and (3) Milroy's disease (hereditary tropho-edema), or lymphedema of familial type. The onset is gradual and symptomless except for the increasing size of the limb. The edema pits easily at first and disappears when the limb is elevated, but later, owing to fibrosis, pits with difficulty and is not relieved by elevation. Low grade lymphangitis and cellulitis, absent in the early stages, often appear later and add to the original deformity.

Secondary lymphedema may be noninflammatory or inflammatory. The former is due to compression of main lymphatic trunks by neoplasm or scar, surgical removal of lymph nodes, fibrosis following irradiation, or direct invasion of lymph vessels or nodes by neoplasm.

Secondary lymphedema of the inflammatory type follows recurrent low grade lymphangitis. In tropic and subtropic regions, filari-

asis must be considered. Each attack of lymphangitis produces additional edema, which disappears only partially after acute inflammation subsides. Recurrences at irregular intervals are due to reinfection from the exterior or to intermittent activity of foci in the extremity itself. The edema fluid contains considerable protein and offers an excellent medium, not only for recurrent bacterial invasion, but also for overgrowth of connective tissue. The skin finally becomes thick, coarse, folded and hard, and the extremities are subject to indolent ulceration, erysipeloid infection and excoriation, so that the eventual deformity may be extreme, well deserving the name "elephantiasis."

Treatment. Painstaking care in keeping the tissues free of edematous fluid will do much to avoid fibrosis and recurrent infection of the extremity. In the early stages, frequent elevation of the extremity and assiduous use of elastic bandages or stockings will suffice. Local infection and obvious lesions, such as epidermophytosis, in the extremity should be eradicated. Recurrent lymphangitis is best treated by rest, antibiotic therapy, elevation of the extremity and hot, moist dressings for comfort, with resumed elastic compression after the patient is again active. In advanced cases with fibrosis and resistant edema the Kondoleon operation and its modifications produce some relief.

R. W. WILKINS

References

Allen, E. V.: Lymphedema of the Extremities. Arch. Int. Med., 54:606, 1934.
Homans, J.: The Treatment of Elephantiasis of the Legs. New England J. Med., 215:1099, 1936.
Matas, R.: The Surgical Treatment of Elephantiasis and Elephantoid States Dependent upon Chronic Obstruction of the Lymphatic and Venous Channels. Am. J. Trop. Dis., 1:60, 1913.
Milroy, W. F.: Chronic Hereditary Edema; Milroy's Disease J.A.M.A., 91:1172, 1928.

ARTERIOSCLEROSIS

A simplified classification of arteriosclerosis appears justified on clinical grounds. (1) *Medial* (hyperplastic) *sclerosis* of blood vessels, resulting in widening and lengthening but in no significant diminution in blood carrying capacity. This is an inevitable manifestation of the involutional changes of aging. When calcification occurs in the media it is called Mönckeberg's arteriosclerosis. Involvement of arterioles (arteriolar sclerosis) is a constant occurrence in sustained hypertension. Medial sclerosis is thought by many to predispose to (2) *intimal sclerosis* (atherosclerosis). It is this form of arteriosclerosis which, by narrowing the lumina of arteries, leads to diminution or failure of blood supply. The latter results in a wide variety of clinical manifestations.

There is a great deal of experimental and clinical evidence that atherosclerosis is intimately related to lipid metabolism, and there is little doubt that manifestations of the disease "arteriosclerosis" encountered in patients are almost exclusively the expression of atherosclerosis. Nevertheless, until additional knowledge becomes available it seems best to continue to consider the clinical problems under the general heading arteriosclerosis, recognizing that medial sclerosis appears to be a manifestation chiefly of either aging or of elevated blood pressure and is in the main asymptomatic; that medial sclerosis appears to predispose to the development of intimal sclerosis; and that intimal sclerosis (atherosclerosis) is chiefly responsible for the interference with blood supply and, therefore, the symptoms and signs attributable to arterosclerosis. (See also discussions under Peripheral Arteriosclerosis and under Atherosclerosis.)

Morbid Anatomy and Physiology. Although medial sclerosis probably causes no significant reduction in the amount of blood delivered to the parts, vasomotor responsiveness is doubtless affected. The loss of elasticity of the larger vessels reduces their capacity as reservoirs, since the ability of the arteries to store the peak-work of cardiac systole and to release it during diastole is reduced. As a result, the systolic blood pressure tends to rise. Thus, in medial sclerosis, more work may be required of the heart for the preservation of normal blood flow, and a corresponding reduction in cardiac reserve may ensue. Demonstrable loss of elasticity of vessels occurs as early as the third decade (Winternitz). This emphasizes the importance of the "vital rubber" at an early stage in the aging process.

In the aorta and larger vessels the earliest macroscopic evidence of atherosclerosis occurs in the form of yellow streaks in the intima. These are produced by the presence of newly formed connective tissue and fat-ladened wandering cells. As these lesions increase in size, they lead to excrescences on the intima which project into the lumen of the vessel. Hyaline changes or necrosis occurs. Injection specimens indicate a rich network of blood vessels, vasa vasorum, about these lesions. Thus is formed the atheroma—so-called because of the soft, fatty, porridge-like material contained in the depth of the lesion. Well marked intimal lesions are generally associated with less conspicuous changes in the media. The atheroma eventually exhibits varying degrees of calcium deposition, even bone formation. Ulceration of the surface of an atheroma with discharge of its fatty contents into the blood stream commonly occurs. The presence of such "ulcers" in the intima favors thrombosis, especially in the smaller vessels.

It has been emphasized that the usual location of the major arteriosclerotic changes in the aorta is the intima. In the arteries of the extremities the media is frequently the site of maximum involvement (Mönckeberg's sclerosis). Degeneration here frequently leads to the development of localized and sometimes encircling calcium plaques which result in palpable beads or rings along the course of the arteries. Thus, the brachial or femoral artery may feel like the trachea. When the process is confined to the media, no encroachment upon the lumen occurs and the amount of blood delivered by the vessel is affected but little, if at all. However, in association with these characteristic changes in the media in Mönckeberg's sclerosis, thickening of the intima frequently occurs and results in reduction in or even obliteration of the vessel lumen. Arteriosclerosis of this type is common in the peripheral vessels of the aged and in diabetes and produces profound disturbances in the circulation of the extremities, often terminating in gangrene.

Clinical Manifestations. The frequency with which arteriosclerosis is associated with hypertension produces confusion and difficulty in distinguishing between the clinical manifestations of the two conditions. It may prove useful to summarize briefly certain alterations in physiology and structure induced by arteriosclerosis: (1) The reduction in elasticity of the walls of the aorta and great vessels (medial sclerosis) diminishes their capacity as reservoirs; vasomotor regulation is less effective; the systolic blood pressure tends to rise, and additional work is required of the heart. (2) Involvement of the intima (atherosclerosis) narrows the vessel lumen, and this narrowing may progress to occlusion. Structures supplied by vessels thus affected respond clinically with the development of manifestations of ischemia. Thus, reduction in the blood supply to an area of the myocardium may result in angina pectoris; if the blood supply is completely destroyed, in myocardial infarction. Reduction of blood supply to the kidney has been shown to produce hypertension. Indeed, it appears that renal artery sclerosis may be a common etiologic factor in so-called essential hypertension. These are but isolated examples of the importance of atherosclerosis in the production of structural and functional changes in all parts of the body, changes due to interference with the normal blood supply. (3) Destruction of the elastic and muscular coats produces weakness of the vessel wall, thus predisposing to rupture and hemorrhage. The greater the blood pressure in such vessels, the more prone the vessel is to rupture.

When the blood supply to various parts of the body is reduced sufficiently by atherosclerosis, symptoms and signs appear. This being the case, it follows that manifestations may be absent or confined to one or more areas or systems, or generalized. From the clinical point of view, the organs more commonly affected are heart, brain and kidneys. Atherosclerosis of the vessels of the extremities also produces typical clinical syndromes.

Well marked peripheral and retinal arteriosclerosis may be demonstrable by physical examination, in the absence of any symptoms or signs of impairment of function of either these parts or of internal organs. It is a common observation that generalized arteriosclerosis may be present for long periods of time without giving rise to symptoms.

Treatment of Arteriosclerosis. Perhaps more important at the present time than attempts to treat arteriosclerosis specifically is the management of the aging process which is invariably associated with medial sclerosis of blood vessels and commonly mistaken for atherosclerosis. There is no specific treatment for the medial sclerosis of arteries which is associated with senescence. A graceful, sane mental and physical adjustment to the aging process is certainly the most desirable and practical measure to be hoped for, and the physician can often do much to encourage this. The tactful suggestion that the demands of the third and fourth decades cannot be met easily by the body in its fifth and sixth decades, together with the definition of a manner of living compatible with the patient's age, is often helpful. Encouragement is more important than drugs. Indeed, the latter are effective chiefly through suggestion. Bromides and the barbiturates are useful when nervousness and apprehension are present, but should be administered with care to old patients. The time-honored iodides provide medicine which is usually administered by drops and taken thrice daily, good attributes for a placebo. The judicious use of simple analgesics and hypnotics, when indicated, is in order, and constipation should be corrected. The problem usually resolves itself into symptomatic treatment with due attention to the psyche. Resourcefulness and optimism characterize the successful therapeutist.

For a discussion of the treatment of hypertension and atherosclerosis, see the appropriate chapters. The use of low cholesterol, low fat diets, estrogens, heparin, choline and inositol to influence favorably lipid metabolism in atherosclerosis is controversial.

Heart. *Atherosclerotic* disease of the heart is one of the commonest causes of death. It is responsible for 25 to 40 per cent of cases of chronic heart disease. It has been observed at all ages, but is commonest after 50 and increases in frequency with advancing years. Men are more frequently affected than women. The classic symptoms and signs are those of angina pectoris and myocardial infarction with either diminished cardiac reserve or heart failure. Myocardial degeneration and fibrosis and cardiac arrhythmias occurring in the elderly in the absence of either angina pectoris or myocardial infarction are much more likely due to the involutional changes of aging than to coronary atherosclerosis. Aortic insufficiency secondary to arteriosclerosis of the aorta and dilatation of the aortic ring is rare, but does occur, especially when hypertension is present. The reader is referred to the chapters on Angina Pectoris, Diseases of the Coronary Arteries, Senile Heart Disease, Cardiac Arrhythmias, Diseases of the Myocardium and the Treatment of Congestive Heart Failure.

The Aorta. As stated elsewhere, arteriosclerosis of the root of the aorta, hypertension and dilatation of the aortic ring may lead to aortic valve incompetency. However, syphilitic disease of the root of the aorta is common and arteriosclerotic disease relatively rare, a point of importance in the etiologic diagnosis of aortic valve incompetency. Saccular aneurysm of the thoracic aorta are almost always syphilitic in origin, although arteriosclerosis may coexist.

Dissecting Aneurysm. In the presence of hypertension the intima of the aorta may rupture. When this occurs, blood extravasates between the coats of the aorta, and a dissecting aneurysm is formed. Sudden agonizing thoracic or abdominal pain developing, often, during great physical exertion and followed by shock is characteristic. The pain may radiate to the head, back, pelvic region and lower extremities and rarely to the arms. In spite of varying degrees of shock, even with loss of consciousness, the blood pressure tends to remain elevated. Evidence of arterial obstruction in branches of the aorta supplying various parts of the body, especially the legs or head, may develop. Moderate fever and leukocytosis occur. Death usually occurs within a few hours or days from rupture of the aneurysm into the mediastinal, pleural, pericardial or peritoneal cavities. Clinically, the condition is usually confused with coronary and peripheral artery occlusion. The absence of electrocardiographic changes is helpful in differentiating the condition from coronary occlusion. Arteriosclerosis of the aorta with atheromatous degeneration of the intima was formerly considered the cause of dissecting aneurysms. However, Erdheim in 1930 described a rare form of cystic degeneration of the media which is generally accepted now as the commonest etiologic factor. Hypertension is almost invariably present. Atheromatous ulcers may be important factors, especially in dissecting aneurysms which originate in the descending aorta.

Thrombotic obliteration of the aortic bifurcation first described by Leriche (1940) is being recognized more frequently in recent years. Intermittent claudication, hip pains and weakness of the legs occur. Obstructive lesions in the aorta can be diagnosed and accurately localized by angiography. Surgical resection of certain thoracic and abdominal aneurysms and thrombotic lesions with restoration of continuity by grafts can now be accomplished.

The Brain. The manifestations of cerebral arteriosclerosis may be general or focal. Alterations in the blood supply to the brain are brought about by arteriosclerosis through interference with normal vasomotor control of the cerebral vessels, or by a general narrowing of the vascular bed as a result of athero-

sclerosis, or by actual thrombosis or hemorrhage of cerebral vessels. Hypertension greatly favors the occurrence of cerebral hemorrhage in a person with cerebral arteriosclerosis. It seems probable that in the absence of evidence of focal vascular disease the involutional changes of aging of the central nervous system are responsible for the commonly designated "cerebral arteriosclerosis" symptom complex. This consists of irritability, forgetfulness, emotional instability, tremor and muscular weakness. The reader is referred to the chapter on Affections of the Blood Vessels of the Brain.

Kidneys. The classic experiments of Goldblatt have focused attention on the significance of renal ischemia in the etiology of hypertension. Atherosclerosis of the large renal vessels leads to atrophy of the parenchyma with fibrous tissue replacement (benign nephrosclerosis). Renal function usually is not impaired greatly. This is in striking contrast to arteriosclerosis of the kidney wherein the arterioles become involved apparently as a result of hypertension. Here serious impairment of function may occur and lead to uremia, although death from cardiac failure is much more common.

The Extremities. Atherosclerosis is by far the commonest cause of arterial disease of the extremities. It is rare before the age of 55 years except in diabetes mellitus, when it may appear early in life. Clinical manifestations practically never occur in the upper extremities. In the lower extremities obliterative lesions in the terminal branches of the posterior tibial and dorsalis pedis arteries commonly produce the earliest symptoms of the disease: numbness, and tingling and burning sensations in the toes. A sense of heaviness and pain, nocturnal cramps, and weakness of the legs and feet are common complaints. The foot is colder than normal, and the skin may appear shiny and atrophic. Faint discoloration of the toe tips may be present. The pulse is feeble or absent in the posterior tibial and dorsalis pedis arteries. If the process is of slow development, dry gangrene may ensue; if rapid, moist gangrene occurs.

Intermittent claudication may develop before the signs of complete arterial occlusion are apparent. This symptom is characterized by the occurrence of severe cramping pain in the calf muscles during walking, which subsides with rest. The degree of exercise tolerance is determined to a nicety by the patient, and continuous walking beyond this critical point is avoided. The symptom is due to narrowing of the vascular bed supplying the muscles and loss of capacity to increase vascularity adequately during periods of muscular activity.

Although peripheral atherosclerosis is bilateral, clinical manifestations are practically always confined to the lower extremities and commonly begin on one side only. The lack of pulsation in the posterior tibial and dorsalis pedis arteries is the most important diagnostic sign. When the extremity is elevated, it blanches promptly; when placed in a dependent position, color returns slowly and the veins remain collapsed for some time. Atherosclerosis must be differentiated from thromboangiitis obliterans and from vasomotor disturbances (Raynaud's disease, erythromelalgia). Atherosclerosis rarely occurs before the fifth decade, and the clinical manifestations are usually of short duration, unilateral and confined to a lower extremity; the vessel pulsations are faint or absent; gangrene develops early; the vessels can be visualized by the roentgenogram. Thromboangiitis obliterans rarely develops after 50, occurs almost exclusively in the male and especially in the Jewish race. The clinical manifestations extend over a period of years, gangrene is late in development, and the vessels are not demonstrable by roentgenogram. As in atherosclerosis, the lower extremities are affected, symptoms at first are unilateral commonly, and the superficial arteries are usually pulseless. Phlebitis and evidence of sluggish circulation may be present in superficial veins. Patients with vasomotor disturbances are relatively young, predominantly female; the disturbance is characteristically chronic; and gangrene develops late. The vessels pulsate and are not demonstrable by roentgenogram. The upper extremities are predominantly affected. The process is usually bilateral and manifests its presence by paroxysmal attacks.

The *treatment of peripheral atherosclerosis* is unsatisfactory. The early recognition and proper management of diabetes should delay the development of atherosclerosis in this condition. High carbohydrate, low fat diets are given. It should be emphasized that the control of the diabetes rather than the type of diet used appears to be the important factor. Actual proof is lacking that cholesterol-poor diets are of value. Patients with arteriosclerotic disease of the extremities should take every precaution against trauma, cold, dampness and infections. Prophylactic care of the feet is of the greatest importance, and lists of instructions should be provided. Poorly fitting shoes, improper care of corns and calluses and exposure to cold and dampness are especially hazardous and predispose to infection. Measures favoring the development of collateral circulation are used. Of these, Buerger's postural exercises, contrast baths, passive vascular exercise and the use of heat cradles and typhoid vaccine intravenously are of established value. If definite gangrene develops, amputation must be performed.

When sclerotic changes have progressed to the point where the arteries are incapable of dilating, little is to be expected from the use of vasodilator drugs. However, an element of vasospasm may be and commonly is present in the circulatory disturbance of advanced arteriosclerosis. In such circumstances ethyl alcohol, neostigmine, papaverine, theobromine, aminophylline and intra-arterial Priscoline have been given but with indifferent results. A good temperature response to paravertebral or spinal anesthesia encourages the trial of lumbar sympathectomy with the hope of improving collateral circulation. Sympathectomy rarely helps intermittent claudication and results are poor when calcification of vessels is demonstrable by x-ray.

Anticoagulants. Theoretically, the use of anticoagulants in occlusive arteriosclerotic lesions should help prevent the extension of thrombosis and thus favor the prevention of gangrene. Experience does not indicate clearly that this is the case.

The Abdomen. Many of the digestive disturbances which occur in the aged doubtless are related directly to the involutional changes of senescence rather than to the effects of arteriosclerosis upon the blood supply of the digestive organs. The mild diabetes mellitus of the aged, and the achlorhydria, intestinal atony and obstipation which commonly appear late in life, doubtless are due in small part if at all to impairment of the circulation.

Mesenteric Thrombosis. The syndrome which develops with occlusive lesions in the mesenteric arteries, resulting in infarction of the bowel, is by far the most definite clinical expression of atherosclerosis of the abdominal vessels. This is characterized by the sudden occurrence of agonizing abdominal pain, usually accompanied by nausea and vomiting. Exquisite tenderness and boardlike rigidity of the abdominal wall rapidly develop. The blood pressure and frequently the body temperature fall. Abdominal distention with constipation becomes marked. If bowel movements occur, the stools are usually bloody. In the absence of melena the clinical picture strongly suggests intestinal perforation. Gangrene of the infarcted segment of bowel, peritonitis and death rapidly ensue, unless the affected portion of gut can be resected.

HUGH J. MORGAN

References

Allen, E. V., Guest Editor, Katz, L. N., Keys, A., Gofman, J. W., et al.: Atherosclerosis. A Symposium. Circulation, 5:98, 1952.

Barr, D. P.: Some Chemical Factors in the Pathogenesis of Atherosclerosis. Circulation, 8:641, 1953.

Best, C. H., and Taylor, N. B.: Physiological Basis of Medcial Practice. 5th ed. Baltimore, Williams and Wilkins, 1950.

Cowdry, E. V.: Arteriosclerosis, a Survey of the Problem. New York, The Macmillan Company, 1933.

DeBakey, M. E., and Cooley, D. A.: Surgical Treatment of Aneurysms of Abdominal Aorta by Resection and Restoration of Continuity with Homograft. Surg., Gynec. & Obst., 97:257, 1953.

Gofman, J. W., and others: Blood Lipids and Human Atherosclerosis. Circulation, 2:161, 1950.

Harrison, T. R.: Failure of the Circulation. Baltimore, Williams and Wilkins Company, 1939.

Ivins, J. C., and others: Symposium on Recent Advances in the Surgical Treatment of Aneurysms. Proc. Staff Meet., Mayo Clin., 28:705, 1953.

Lansing, A. I., Alex, M., and Rosenthal, T. B.: Atheromatosis as a Sequel to Senescent Changes in the Arterial Wall. J. Gerontol., 5:315, 1950.

Leriche, R., and Morel, A.: The Syndrome of Thrombotic Obliteration of the Aortic Bifurcation. Ann. Surg., 127:193, 1948.

Winternitz, M. C., Thomas, R. M., and LeCompte, P. M.: The Biology of Arteriosclerosis. Baltimore, Charles C Thomas, 1938.

SYPHILITIC AORTITIS AND ANEURYSM

A discussion of these topics will be found in the section on Spirochetal Infections (p. 357).

Diseases of the Locomotor System

DISEASES OF THE MUSCLES

INTRODUCTION

In the minds of many, diseases of muscle represent a collection of odd, infrequent, dimly understood and therapeutically gloomy mishaps, which occur so rarely that they are of little moment in comparison to most other diseases. If disease of muscle were limited to such peculiar defects then this view might be tenable, but in fact clinical disorders of muscle function are ubiquitous. For, if one considers that weakness and pain in muscles indicate disordered function, then it becomes evident that, in a larger sense, disease of muscle accompanies almost every pattern of disease. Indeed, most physicians make use of this phenomenon when they inquire into and make rough assessment of muscular strength in attempting to gauge the extent and severity of many diseases which are not primarily muscular in origin.

Muscle makes up some 45 per cent of total body weight in man and constitutes thereby a large portion of certain carbohydrate, protein, mineral and water stores of the body. These depots are not stagnant backwaters but rather participate vigorously in the ebb and flow of metabolic tides which sweep through the body in disease. It is not surprising, therefore, that a host of diseases, which disturb circulation and metabolism in direct or indirect fashion, are prone also to result in disorders of muscular function. In addition to the muscular disorders which accompany constitutional disease, as does malfunction in many other organs and tissues not involved in the primary process, there are certain well recognized but little understood diseases which appear to arise primarily within the muscle fiber itself.

It is worth emphasis that it may prove difficult to distinguish by the usual clinical means the primary diseases of the muscle cell from those disorders in which muscular malfunction is only part of disease arising in other tissues. Perhaps the main reason for this difficulty lies in the fact that the clinical manifestations of disease of muscle are extraordinarily unvaried and may be so extensive as to mask the underlying process.

In the main, muscular disease of any sort is evidenced by these phenomena: *weakness, atrophy, limitation of motion* and *pain,* either spontaneous or evoked by movement or pressure. In certain circumstances there may be observed extraordinarily involuntary phenomena such as myotonic contractions, myoidema of various bizarre forms, cramps and coarse fasciculations. Unfortunately, the certain diagnosis of specific disease of muscle frequently cannot be established by histopathologic techniques because the structural alterations demonstrable by generally available methods are equally stereotyped in many diseases which appear to differ widely in origin.

Weakness is a very common symptom and may be generalized, be noticeable in a group of muscles, or occasionally appear in one muscle alone. Its cause may reside in the highest levels of the nervous system as in the forms of weakness which accompany certain neurotic or hysterical behavior, it may follow disease at any other level of the nervous system out to and including the motor nerve endings, or it may arise as a result of injury restricted to the muscle cell itself. Thus weakness may be either an expression of change in the contractile mechanism of the muscle fiber or a failure somewhere in the system responsible for evoking contraction.

Atrophy of muscle, which may develop with explosive speed, occurs in three different situations: following interruption of direct innervation, with disuse, and when the muscle cells themselves disintegrate because of their primary disease. The first instance is a special case in that muscular atrophy is secondary to neural disease. The atrophy of disuse is the commonest form and may be seen as a regrettable sequel to injudicious, as well as unavoidable, immobilization of the patient or any of his joints. The loss of muscle bulk which follows primary disease of the fibers may masquerade as one of the other secondary forms, and in certain circumstances biopsy and histologic study may be required to arrive at a decision, although it must be emphasized again that even this kind of examination may yield information of little differentiating value.

Pain in muscles occurs so commonly that few persons are unaware of its characteristic qualities. These vary from the dull ache which follows unaccustomed heavy exercise or accompanies the prodromal period of a febrile infection, through the more severe, unpleasant pain which follows an acute strain or occurs during muscular cramps, to the agonizing bright pain experienced briefly at the moment of sprain or in more prolonged fashion during acute myositis. The processes within muscle which produce pain are not understood with much clarity but appear to be related to swelling, circumscribed arterial supply and venous drainage with accompanying metabolic disturbances, trauma or inflammation. Not infrequently pain and even exquisite tenderness arise as phenomena referred from lesions existing in skeleton, central nervous system or viscera.

The lack of much certain knowledge about muscular diseases has resulted in descriptions which vary widely in their bases. Some diseases are defined by genetic characteristics, by anatomic distributions, by temporal evolution and by the pathologic changes noted in microscopic section. Some diseases are accompanied by a clinically distinct functional disturbance, such as myotonia, or by some chemically recognized anomaly, such as alterations in the concentration of potassium in serum or the appearance of myoglobin in the urine. Under certain circumstances the primary process, which leads to a clinical state suggesting primary disease of muscle, may be extramuscular in origin, as, for example, in the extensive myopathy which accompanies apathetic variants of hyperthyroidism. Conversely patients in the early stages of dystrophy have been thought on occasions to represent examples of behavioral disturbance or outright malingering. It would seem judicious, therefore, to bear in mind that the muscles may be the site of symptoms which arise either primarily in the muscle fibers themselves or represent the response of muscle to disease much wider in distribution and originating in other tissues.

In order to provide some framework to consider the extraordinarily varied processes which produce disturbances in muscle function, a classification is provided below. Any classification, and particularly in a field so ill understood, properly should evoke question and disagreement, but in this case a valuable function may be served in addition if it but reminds the reader of the numerous diseases which result so often in disorders of muscle. Indeed, it may be noted that by far the greater number of the diseases listed below appear for discussion in other sections of this book.

Classification of Diseases of Muscle

I. "PRIMARY" MYOPATHIES, limited to or predominant in muscle.
  (a) Progressive muscular dystrophies
  (b) Myotonias (dystrophic, congenital, acquired)
  (c) Periodic paralyses
  (d) Myositides, including poly- or dermatomyositis
  (e) Metabolic defects (glycolytic, myoglobinuric)
  (f) Miscellaneous (amyoplasias, contractures, degenerations)

II. "SECONDARY" MYOPATHIES, representing muscular reaction to primarily extramuscular disease.
  (a) Atrophy
    1. Denervation (traumatic, neuropathic secondary to metabolic, vascular, nutritional, infectious and toxic processes)
    2. Disuse and fixation
    3. Aging and cachexia
  (b) Endocrine (pituitary, thyroid, parathyroid, adrenal, pancreas, gonad)
  (c) Internal environment
    1. Chemical milieu
    2. Vascular supply
  (d) Infection
    1. "Specific" (Trichinella, Toxoplasma, Coxsackie viruses)
    2. General (rickettsial, typhoid, pneumococcal pneumonia)
    3. Postinfectious asthenia

The "primary" myopathies are remarkable for the high incidence of genetic factors which determine their appearance, and for the related fact that in many of them suspicion runs high that the underlying defect or defects are metabolic in nature. But even in those instances in which some biochemical disturbance has been demonstrated, we are no closer to any substantial understanding of how the defect produces the disease. It may well transpire eventually that our concept of these diseases as being restricted to muscle is too limited; perhaps a warning may be seen in the case of myotonic dystrophy, in which there occurs a dystrophic process in muscle fiber which also exhibits a myotonic reaction. These phenomena are held to be characteristic of primary disturbances of muscle, yet these patients display baldness, cataracts, hyperostosis of the frontal bones and gonadal insufficiency with associated hormonal changes, all indications of some very general process. It is curious that despite the wealth of available information concerning many physiologic and biochemical aspects of the muscle fiber, not an inkling has been gained of how these primary disturbances arise.

The "secondary" myopathies are better understood in a few instances, to the extent that the disturbances produced by the underlying disease interfere with the normal environment required by muscle to perform its usual functions. Perhaps the clearest examples are furnished by the many disease processes which lead to deficit or accumulation of several electrolytes in the interstitial and intracellular waters of the body. Sodium chloride depletion during exposure to heat results in weakness and cramps; accumulation of potassium during renal insufficiency leads to flaccid paralysis, as may potassium depletion. Invasions of muscle cells by Trichinella or Coxsackie virus evoke reactions which are related readily to the symptoms which develop. Much more obscure is the extraordinary wasting of muscle which characterizes some forms of hyperthyroidism, or the profound and protracted asthenia which may follow hepatitis or atypical pneumonia. Although etiology is little understood, it is encouraging that so many of these disorders of muscle are improved if the basic process is amenable to treatment.

JOSEPH L. LILIENTHAL, JR.

References

Adams, R. D., Denny-Brown, D. and Pearson, C. M.: Diseases of Muscle. A Study in Pathology. New York, Paul B. Hoeber, 1953.

Denny-Brown, D.: The Nature of Muscular Diseases. Canad. M. A. J., 67:1, 1952.

———: Clinical Problems in Neuromuscular Physiology. Am. J. Med., 15:368, 1953.

Fenn, W. O., Editor: Muscle. Lancaster, Pa., Jaques Cattell Press, 1941.

Gerard, R. W., and Taylor, R. E.: Muscle and Nerve —Physiologic Orientation. Am. J. Med., 15:83, 1953.

Hoagland, C. L.: Some Biochemical Problems Posed by a Disease of Muscle, in Green, D. E.: Currents in Biochemical Research. New York, Interscience Publishers, 1946.

Lewis, T.: Pain. New York, The Macmillan Co., 1942.

Schapira, G., Editor: The Muscle. A Study in Biology and Pathology. Paris, L'Expansion Scientifique Française, 1952.

Stephens, F. E.: Inheritance of Diseases Primary in the Muscle. Am. J. Med., 15:558, 1953.

Zierler, K. L., and Lilienthal, J. L., Jr.: The Myopathies: Including Their Appearance in Constitutional Disease. Am. J. Med., 15:829, 1953.

THE DYSTROPHIES

PROGRESSIVE MUSCULAR DYSTROPHY

This is a hereditary disease characterized by progressive muscular wasting and weakness. The condition is found in three or more recognized forms, but the main clinical and pathologic features are similar in all. About 45 per cent of the patients give a history of at least one other member of the family affected with the disease. Heredity in the pseudohypertrophic form usually is by a recessive factor, often sex-linked. In the facio-scapulohumeral form, heredity usually is by a dominant factor. The disease affects males about three times as frequently as females.

The onset usually is during early or late childhood, at the age of puberty or in adolescence, and more rarely later in life. The muscles earliest affected are those of the proximal groups, although, as the disease progresses, practically all the muscles of the body become involved. The hands are not affected, and, except in the Landouzy-Déjerine form, the face is spared. Pseudohypertrophy is prominent in many patients. Frequently the onset is so insidious that considerable time elapses before the seriousness of the symptoms is recognized. The course usually is steadily and slowly progressive, although in some instances rapid increase in weakness can occur, especially during periods of prolonged physical inactivity. As a general rule, however, disability develops much faster in patients in whom the disease appears early in life than in those in whom the first symptoms appear at a later age. Contractures develop sooner or later in most patients; not only do they interfere seriously with muscular function, but they hasten muscular wasting by restricting activity. Pain is not a prominent feature. No signs of structural disease of the nervous system are present. The tendon reflexes are diminished or absent. Fasciculations and a reaction of degeneration are lacking. Defects in the metabolism of creatine usually are present; large amounts are eliminated in the urine, and the ability of the muscles to retain ingested creatine is impaired (low creatine tolerance). However, in the Landouzy-Déjerine form of the disease, creatinuria can be only moderate in the early stages of the disease.

The early age of onset, the sparing of the hands and feet even in instances of advanced wasting of the proximal groups of muscles, the presence of pseudohypertrophy, the impairment of creatine metabolism, the absence of fasciculations and the lack of a reaction of degeneration clearly distinguish this disease from forms of progressive muscular atrophy subsequent to disease of the nervous system.

The *pseudohypertrophic form* commences in childhood. The child has increasing difficulty in climbing stairs and in running, falls easily and has more and more difficulty in erecting the body. In getting up from the supine position, the patient first turns over on the abdomen, uses the arms to assume a kneeling position, extends the knees while supporting himself with the hands on the floor and then places the hands on the knees and by alternately moving the hands higher on the thighs, gradually "climbs up" to the erect position. Lordosis develops, and the gait becomes waddling. Pseudohypertrophy of various muscle groups is a prominent feature, and the contrast between the size and power of the calves is often striking. In the later stages of the disease the pseudohypertrophy frequently disappears. Contractures of the calf muscles can produce pes equinus so pronounced that the patient walks on his toes. Later, the soles of the feet turn inward; development of talipes equinovarus may thereafter confine the patient to wheel chair or bed. Involvement of the upper arms and shoulder girdle results in increasing disability in raising the arms; the upper extremities appear to be loosely attached to the trunk, and the scapulae become winged. Disability develops steadily to complete infirmity.

The *juvenile form* has its onset in childhood or a little later. The muscles earliest affected are those of the shoulder girdle; the muscles of the upper arms, thighs and back become wasted; those of the forearms and calves are usually spared for a long time. Hypertrophy of certain muscle groups can occur.

In the *Landouzy-Déjerine form* the muscles earliest involved are those of the face, shoulder girdle and upper arms. The facial expression is characteristic; the face is weak, the eyes cannot be closed completely, the lips are prominent and the patient is unable to whistle. Lordosis and scoliosis often become pronounced.

Though classification according to these forms serves a useful purpose in some instances, progressive muscular dystrophy may be considered a clinical and pathologic unit in which the various types are distinguished by no fundamental differences.

At the present time there is no suitable treatment. Some workers have postulated a defect in the utilization of vitamin E as the cause of the muscular changes. In some patients, physical therapy may be of limited value, especially in the management of contractures.

MYOTONIA CONGENITA

(Thomsen's Disease)

This is a hereditary condition in which the defect is an inability to relax the muscles promptly after an initial forceful contraction. Thus, in initiating a movement the muscles remain contracted for several seconds, but on continued repetition of the movements the defect disappears. The delay in relaxation can be shown also by mechanical stimulation of the muscles (myotonic reaction). The syndrome usually has its onset during childhood and persists for life. Evidence of muscular wasting or other structural disease is absent. In fact, most patients show excellent muscular development. Prolonged rest, exposure to low temperatures and emotional excitement aggravate the symptoms. Quinine (0.3 to 0.6 gm. two or three times daily) affords relief in many instances. However, most patients consider the side effects of the drug (tinnitus, blurring of vision and nausea) more bothersome than the muscular symptoms and reserve the use of the drug for occasions when improvement in myotonia is of special importance.

AMYOTONIA CONGENITA

(Oppenheim's Disease)

This disease is characterized by pronounced flaccidity and weakness of the muscles, noted either at the time of birth or during the first few months of life. In some instances the cry of the newborn baby is weak and the child is too feeble to nurse. Often, however, no abnormality is suspected until the patient reaches the age at which more advanced physical performances may be expected. The child is unable to turn over, sit up or hold up the head. Extreme weakness and almost complete flaccidity of most of the muscles are noted. The extremities are slack, and the joints can be extended to an abnormal degree. The reflexes are absent, and on palpation no muscle groups can be distinguished. About one third of the patients die within the first year. Others show suggestive improvement for a time, with subsequent relapse. Most patients die within five years, usually from pneumonia. A few patients are said to have improved, but instances of this unusual course have not been adequately studied. The underlying defect appears to be an absence of muscular development; degenerative changes are generally considered to be lacking. The condition is often familial. The clinical features resemble those of Werdnig-Hoffmann disease so closely that in some instances it is almost impossible to distinguish the two conditions, although the latter usually has its onset during the second half of the first year and is associated with alterations in the anterior horn cells of the spinal cord. Often the distinction can be made only on the basis of the pathologic changes.

MYOTONIA ATROPHICA

This is a hereditary disease characterized by myotonia (delayed relaxation of muscles after an initial contraction), muscular wasting and weakness, lens opacities and, in males, testicular atrophy. The basal metabolic rate usually is decreased. The muscles earliest and most severely affected by wasting are those of the face (myasthenic facies, nasal speech and poor enunciation), the sternocleidomastoids, those of the forearms, the quadriceps and the dorsiflexors of the feet (tendency to trip and fall). Many patients complain of increased need for sleep. The onset usually is during the third decade of life, and the course is insidiously progressive. In the later stages of the disease, muscular wasting and weakness can be generalized, the myotonia usually disappears, and occasionally the lens opacities, when sufficiently dense, require cataract extraction. Not infrequently, other members of the family show only lens opacities; these are subcapsular in type. The etiology is not known, and there is no effective therapy. Thyroid administration usually is of no value. Quinine for control of myotonia sometimes is useful. In a few cases, adrenocorticotrophic hormone appears to have had mild beneficial effects.

A. T. MILHORAT

References

Abramson, A. S.: An Approach to the Rehabilitation of Children with Muscular Dystrophy. Proc. Second Med. Conf. Muscular Dystrophy Associations of America, Inc., 1953.

Anderson, L. R., and Reeves, D. L.: Amyotonia Congenita (Oppenheim's Disease). Report of a Case with Autopsy Findings. Bull. Los Angeles Neurol. Soc., 5:210, 1940.

Burdick, W. F., Whipple, D. V., and Freeman, W.: Amyotonia Congenita (Oppenheim). Report of Five Cases with Necropsy; Discussion of the Relationship between Amyotonia Congenita, Werdnig-Hoffman Disease, Neonatal Poliomyelitis and Muscular Dystrophy. Am. J. Dis. Children, 69: 295, 1945.

Milhorat, A. T.: Creatine and Creatinine Metabolism and Diseases of the Neuro-Muscular System. In Metabolic and Toxic Diseases of the Nervous System. Association for Research in Nervous and Mental Disease, New York, 1953, pp. 400–421.

———, and Wolff, H. G.: Studies in Diseases of Muscle. XII. Heredity of Progressive Muscular Dystrophy; Relationship between Age at Onset of Symptoms and Clinical Course. Arch. Neurol. & Psychiat., 49:641, 1943.

Tyler, F. H., and Perkoff, G. T.: Studies in Disorders of Muscle. VI. Is Progressive Muscular Dystrophy an Endocrine or Metabolic Disorder? Arch. Int. Med., 88:175, 1951.

Waring, J. J., Ravin, A., and Walker, C. E., Jr.: Studies in Dystrophia Myotonica. II. Clinical Features and Treatment. Arch. Int. Med., 65:763, 1940.

MYOSITIS

PARENCHYMATOUS MYOSITIS

Parenchymatous myositis is a disease of the muscles which simultaneously affects the muscle cells and the intramuscular fibrous supporting tissue. It may be suppurative or nonsuppurative. It may appear without localized infection elsewhere, but in most cases it is part of a systemic infection or pyemia, or it results from extension from an infected viscus, bone, joint or wound.

SUPPURATIVE MYOSITIS

PRIMARY SUPPURATIVE MYOSITIS

Primary suppurative myositis may affect one or more muscular regions. It is of bacterial origin, and its course may be acute or chronic. It has been called a primary disease because the mode of entry of the infection has not been found. Certain special forms are observed in the tropics (Miyake, Sayers and others).

Etiology. Trauma, bruising, strain and exposure to cold or dampness have been regarded as predisposing causes of primary suppurative myositis. *Staphylococcus aureus* is the organism most frequently found in the abscesses in the muscles; however, other organisms have also been found. Either sex and any age group may be affected, although in most cases the patients are young men.

Morbid Anatomy. There may be one or multiple abscesses, or there may be diffuse infiltration in the muscles. When the abscess is close to the surface, the skin and subcutaneous tissue may also be inflamed. The affected muscle is edematous and friable, and appears red or gray. Microscopic examination of the walls of the abscess during the acute stage reveals bacteria and evidences of acute serous, serofibrinous or purulent inflammation. The abscess contains pus, fragments of necrotic tissue, and blood. During the chronic stage, granulation tissue is present. Healing takes place by scar formation.

Symptoms. The onset of symptoms is usually sudden. Headache, fever, chills and sweating are soon followed by localization of pain and swelling in the affected muscles. Fluctuation occurs in four to ten days, and the abscess rarely resolves without evacuation of pus. A single abscess well drained may heal in a few weeks. When multiple abscesses occur, the patient may be confined to bed for months.

Diagnosis. The localized painful fluctuant swelling in a muscle usually makes an early diagnosis relatively easy; but if the affected region is juxta-articular, a diagnosis of pyoarthrosis is sometimes entertained.

Prognosis. The prognosis is good if the abscesses are drained early. Miyake reported 1 death in 33 cases, and Sayers reported 2 deaths in 26 cases. After the abscess heals, the muscle usually recovers good function. In severe cases there is much destruction of muscle, with replacement by scar tissue which may lead to deformity when it contracts.

Treatment. Hot applications may be applied during the early stage of the infection to hasten localization. As soon as fluctuation

is present the abscess should be freely drained by a broad incision. It is better to err by opening an indurated region than to allow an unrecognized collection of pus from suppurative myositis to infiltrate the surrounding tissue. Penicillin should be administered parenterally if the infection is produced by staphylococcus or other penicillin-sensitive bacteria.

If there is not a prompt reaction to incision of the abscess and the administration of penicillin, the sensitivity of the causative organism to other antibiotic agents should be determined.

SECONDARY SUPPURATIVE MYOSITIS

Secondary suppurative myositis is associated with other dominant infection elsewhere in the body. The infection may reach the muscle because of a pyemia, or by extension from an adjacent infected viscus, bone, joint or wound. The most common causative organisms are the staphylococcus, streptococcus, tubercle bacillus and *Treponema pallidum*. The disease may be associated with actinomycosis, gas gangrene and erysipelas. If contractures ensue, massage and orthopedic correction should be given.

NONSUPPURATIVE MYOSITIS

DERMATOMYOSITIS

For a discussion of dermatomyositis, the reader is referred to the section on Collagen Diseases.

PROGRESSIVE MYOSITIS FIBROSA

Progressive myositis fibrosa is a localized or generalized, subacute or chronic inflammation of a muscle and its fibrous tissue. The muscles that are involved atrophy and are eventually almost completely replaced by fibrous tissue.

Etiology. The etiology is unknown. The incidence of the disease bears no apparent relation to sex.

Morbid Anatomy. Muscle most recently affected may appear swollen. Later, the muscles atrophy, feel firm and, when cut, grate on the knife. The muscles chiefly involved appear white; those which are less severely affected are reddish yellow. On microscopic examination some muscle fibers are seen to be larger than normal, others are atrophied. Hyaline and hydropic degenerations occur, and there is a loss of transverse striations.

There are local increases in fibroblasts and lymphocytes with a few plasma cells and neutrophilic polymorphonuclear leukocytes. Fibrous tissue eventually replaces the diseased muscles.

Symptoms. The onset usually is insidious. A voluntary muscle or a group of muscles, usually in the lower extremities, is first involved. Clinical features are weakness of involved muscles, clumsiness and absence of fever. Pain usually is minimal or absent, except when muscle spasms occur. Subjective stiffness of muscles may be present, but usually is minimal. At first, there is a doughy feel to the muscles; later, an increased firmness is felt.

Finally, the muscles atrophy and are replaced by fibrous tissue. Severe contractures may occur. Pain and tenderness are not prominent features. In reported cases, the ages of the patients have varied from 9 months to 48 years. Until the disease is well advanced, the diagnosis cannot be made definitely without biopsy.

A small group of patients have a condition that is being reported as menopausal dystrophy, polymyositis, "atypical progressive muscular atrophy," and this condition is indistinguishable from myositis fibrosis. Results of electromyographic studies and biopsy of muscles indicate a similar inflammatory reaction and similar symptoms.

Prognosis. The course of generalized myositis may be rapid and last only a few months, or it may be slowly progressive, as in the case reported by Burton, Cowan and Fleming, in which the patient was still physically active after having had the disease ten years.

Treatment. Specific treatment is unknown. Massage and electric treatment may relieve symptoms somewhat. Drugs are of little help.

TRICHINOUS MYOSITIS

(Trichiniasis)

This is a myositis resulting from the invasion of voluntary muscles by *Trichinella*. Trichinellae have been recovered from the diaphragm in from 3.5 to 27.6 per cent of cases at necropsy. The condition is only recognized in cases in which the infestation is severe and associated with diarrhea, acutely painful muscles, edema of the muscles and subcutaneous tissues, and eosinophilia. Fur-

ther details will be found in the chapter on Trichinosis.

CHARLES H. SLOCUMB

References

Burton, J. A. G., Cowan, J., and Fleming, J.: Generalized Myositis Fibrosa. Quart. J. Med., 24:369, 1931.

Dowling, H. F.: The Acute Bacterial Diseases; Their Diagnosis and Treatment. Philadelphia, W. B. Saunders Company, 1948, p. 188.

Leedham-Green, J. C., and Evans, W.: Myositis Tropica. Tr. Roy. Soc. Trop. Med. & Hyg., 36: 359, 1943.

Schwab, E. H., Brindley, P., Bodansky, M., and Harris, T. H.: Generalized Myositis Fibrosa. Ann. Int. Med., 6:422, 1932.

Stewart, A. M., and MacGregor, A. R.: Myositis Fibrosa Generalisata. A.M.A. Arch. Dis. Child., 26: 215, 1951.

INTERSTITIAL MYOSITIS

MYOSITIS OSSIFICANS

There are three types of myositis ossificans: namely, progressive, circumscribed and traumatic. The traumatic type is associated with the formation of bone in a traumatized region. Myositis ossificans circumscripta is usuallay associated with the formation of bone in a scar. The progressive form will be considered more in detail.

PROGRESSIVE MYOSITIS OSSIFICANS

Progressive myositis ossificans is a disease of unknown etiology which is characterized by proliferative inflammation in portions of the fibrous tissue of muscles, tendons, aponeuroses, fasciae and ligaments. It progresses to the formation of bone which eventually leads to destruction of the involved muscles and ankyloses of adjacent joints.

Etiology and Incidence. The etiology is unknown. In 102 of 112 cases collected by Nutt the disease started before the age of 10 years. It can start later in life, however. Males are more frequently affected than females. Microdactylia of the thumbs or great toes, and occasionally of other toes or fingers, is an accompaniment in most cases.

Morbid Anatomy. Three stages have been recognized. Swelling, edema and hemorrhage in the fibrous tissue in and around the involved muscles, and proliferation of fibrous tissue are present in the first stage. The skin and subcutaneous tissue may appear normal, or may be swollen and red. In the second stage the newly formed fibrous tissue contracts and forms a firm mass. Bundles of muscle fibers are caught in the fibrous tissue and undergo degeneration. In the fibrous tissue there appear cells, resembling cartilage, and clefts which resemble osteoid trabeculae and contain cells which later become osteoblasts and bone corpuscles. When calcification occurs, the parts enclosed by trabeculae form bone marrow. In the third stage, ossification occurs. The new bone has been regarded as chemically and structurally the same as normal bone. *No abnormalities have been found in studies of the chemical constituents of the blood.*

Symptoms. Progressive myositis ossificans may be present for years before it is recognized that limitations in the movements of certain muscles or joints are the result of bony deposits in muscle. It may start as a soft doughy swelling in a muscle, usually of the neck or back. There may or may not have been an antecedent trauma. Fever, local tenderness and pain, and edema and redness of the overlying skin and subcutaneous tissues may or may not be present. After a few days the edema disappears, leaving a firm nodule. Other similar nodules may develop in adjacent muscles and fibrous tissues. These firm nodules usually increase in size for a variable period and then regress, but they seldom disappear completely. Within about two to eight months deposits of bone in the involved regions can often be demonstrated by roentgenograms or by palpating a hard bony mass. When the disease is extensive, the deformities that develop usually stiffen the spinal column in the position of kyphosis; the scapulae are attached to the thorax by bony ridges, which limit movements of the shoulders; the neck is rigidly anteflexed; and the arms, legs and jaws may become ankylosed. Amenorrhea and atrophy of the testes and scrotum have been noted in some cases.

Diagnosis. The diagnosis is not difficult in advanced cases. In early cases the early onset of swelling in the muscles, gradual progression of the disease, microdactylia, and formation of hard masses in muscles and fibrous tissue should make one suspect the diagnosis, which may be confirmed by roentgenographic examination or by microscopic evidence of the bone deposited in muscles. Myositis ossificans traumatica and myositis ossificans circumscripta are distinguished from the progressive form by the absence of progression to other regions, the presence of the ossification in injured regions or in regions in which a scar is present or an incision has been made. Spondylitis deformans can be readily distinguished from progressive myositis ossificans; in cases of spondylitis there is generally early roentgenographic evidence of arthritis of the sacro-iliac joints, and there is an absence of the formation of bone in muscles.

Prognosis. The disease may progress with remissions and exacerbations, but the tendency is for the inflammation to spread progressively and irregularly into surrounding muscles, fibrous tissue and bones, producing destruction of muscles, limitation of movements of joints, and ankyloses. Exostoses develop, especially over fibrous and tendinous attachments to bones. Death usually results from intercurrent infection, from edema of the glottis or from suffocation as a result of limitation of costal breathing.

Treatment. No medical treatment has been of help. Excision of the bony deposits is sometimes advised in cases in which localized ossification interferes with function of the joints, but this procedure is useless in cases of generalized myositis ossificans. Surgical removal of new bone may be followed by the formation of more bone in the same region. Protection against cold and dampness may prevent some exacerbations.

MYOPATHIES

Myopathies include the diseases which are regarded as primary diseases of muscles, but which are associated with secondary changes in the somatic nervous system. The relation between the myopathies and the autonomic nervous system is not understood. A consideration of the myopathies will be found elsewhere.

CHARLES H. SLOCUMB

THE FIBROSITIS SYNDROME

The name fibrositis was first introduced by Sir William Gowers in 1904, when he used the term to denote the inflammatory changes in fibrous tissue which he felt were responsible for lumbago. Stockman (1920) was the first to describe what he felt was the underlying pathology, and he defined fibrositis as a condition of chronic inflammation of the white fibrous tissue, occurring in all parts of the body, and giving rise to pain, aching and stiffness, the result of preceding general infection or local inflammation or injuries. This plausible theory was at first eagerly accepted as the cause of the many aches and pains in nonarticular tissues, but subsequent histologic studies failed to confirm the presence of chronic inflammation. Lacking a firm pathologic background and a definite diagnostic boundary, fibrositis has become the most controversial condition in the field of rheumatism. Attempts are therefore being made to limit the use of the term to a well recognized symptom complex which is best called the fibrositis syndrome.

Etiology. The cause continues to be a controversial subject, but it is probable that the fibrositis syndrome represents a yet unknown soft tissue reaction to a variety of different stimuli. Most agree that the syndrome may be initiated by many factors, and such agents as trauma, infection, exposure, fatigue or vascular, metabolic, postural, occupational and psychogenic conditions have all been put forward.

The theory of direct infection now has little support, although the fibrositis syndrome does occur in association with influenza, malaria and other general infections. The relevance of septic foci, once strongly supported, is rapidly losing ground. Trauma, either as a single incident or recurring over a long period, is considered a common cause. There would seem to be no doubt that exposure to cold, wet, drafts, chilling and sudden changes in temperature can initiate an attack. The syndrome is believed by some to result from the abnormal retention of fluid by fat confined in indistensible fibrous tissue, the origin of the selective swelling being probably endocrine in nature (Copeman). Sir Thomas Lewis (1938) thought that the pain of fibrositis is of the same quality as that experienced in intermittent claudication. Elliot (1944) postulates that the myalgia arises from an irritated nerve root and that tender spots are due to local muscle spasm. Others favor a nutritional basis with particular reference to vitamin E. (Steinberg). Many agree that emotional factors play an important role. There would seem to be no doubt that the syndrome may be initiated or profoundly

affected by the emotional state of the individual which is manifested by aching, pain and stiffness.

It is probable that in most cases the fibrositis syndrome is precipitated by a psychosomatic disorder, and this view is supported by the fact that the symptoms disappear when the life situation improves. Such a mechanism has long been accepted as a basis for cardiac and gastric complaints, and the failure of its acceptance in the field of rheumatism can only lead to misfortune in treatment. It is necessary to accept the basic concept that people can become physically sore and stiff from mental as well as physical trouble. Such patients are not necessarily psychoneurotics, but they are emotionally unstable, oversensitive physically and mentally and complain of symptoms that the average person would consider insignificant. When they meet what most people would consider ordinary trials of life, they become tense, "keyed-up," "tied in knots," and are seldom able to relax. The resulting clinical picture may duplicate the so-called fibrositis syndrome: aching muscles, soreness and stiffness, local tenderness and trigger points. The pain and discomfort, however, must not be considered as something imaginary in the patient's mind. Although a psychologic factor is uniformly present in such patients, the local stiffness, pain and tenderness are due to a related peripheral physical factor, the exact nature of which is still unknown.

In view of the multiplicity of etiologic factors outlined above, it is obvious that fibrositis is not a disease entity but a syndrome brought about by a variety of widely separate conditions and, if considered in this light, much confusion will be avoided.

Incidence. Fibrositis is considered by many to be the most common form of acute and chronic rheumatism, but a true analysis of its incidence is rendered impossible by the elastic limits which define the syndrome in various countries. For example during World War II, the incidence of fibrositis in the British forces was many times that seen in American troops subject to the same conditions. The discrepancy is due to the fact that patients with psychogenic rheumatism were included by the British in the fibrositis group, whereas in the American series, patients with psychogenic rheumatism were listed separately. Such conflicting figures illustrate the fact that the composite term fibrositis is too broad a label and must be subdivided into its etiologic components in order to obtain diagnostic uniformity.

Morbid Anatomy. Pathologic studies have not yet revealed the fundamental nature of the syndrome. Fibrositic nodules and thickenings, varying in size, shape and location, have been described by many authors, but in spite of biopsy studies there is as yet no typical microscopic appearance whereby they can be identified histologically. Authors have pictured the outpouring of serofibrinous exudate, the proliferation of fibroblasts and laying down of fresh fibrous tissue as the pathologic basis for the symptomatology, but such theories still lack microscopic support. A pathologic basis for pain and local tenderness in certain cases has been adequately established in the herniated fat nodule (Copeman), and many nodules, tender or nontender, formerly referred to as fibrositic nodules undoubtedly represent such fat herniations.

Classified according to location, fibrositis has been separated on an anatomic basis (Slocumb) into (1) intramuscular (myositis, muscular rheumatism), (2) periarticular, (3) tendinous or fascial, (4) perineural, (5) bursal, (6) panniculitis. Classified on clinical grounds fibrositis has been considered as (1) primary—without demonstrable cause or sign of systemic disease; and (2) secondary—a manifestation of diseases such as infection, or associated with various forms of arthritis such as rheumatoid, rheumatic fever, osteoarthritis and gout, or the result of strain, or postural and structural abnormalities. However, recent studies suggest that if the patient is adequately studied not only physically but psychologically, a cause for the symptoms will not be lacking and the use of the term primary or idiopathic fibrositis will seldom be necessary.

Symptoms. The chief symptoms are pain, stiffness and soreness, and the usual signs are tenderness and perhaps some limitation of movement. The most frequent sites are in the neck, shoulder, lower back and chest areas. The onset may be sudden or slow and insidious, and the course may be acute, subacute or chronic with remissions and exacerbations, the patient being relatively free of symptoms for varying periods. There is little or no effect upon the general health except that most patients complain of an unusual degree of tiredness and easy fatigue which is not relieved by the night's rest. The distress is most often a dull ache, sometimes a burning sensation. The patient is worse after rest, worse in the morning and worse after sitting. The muscles seem to gel with rest but the discomfort is relieved by activity. The patient can to some extent "work it off" by exercise, but with the onset of fatigue the discomfort tends to return. The symptoms may be precipitated or augmented by cold, dampness, drafts and emotional upsets. Relief is often obtained, at least temporarily, by heat such as a hot bath, salicylates, alcohol, and mental and physical relaxation. No constitutional disturbance is found and, apart from local tenderness, physical examination is notoriously negative. Palpation may disclose a localized tender area or myalgic spot, the so-called "trigger point" of fibrositis, and it would seem that these tender areas may be largely responsible for the symptoms. Any discussion about the so-called fibrositis nodule is still entirely speculative. Many claim to have felt them but biopsies have not revealed a specific lesion. For this reason it is probable that nodules have been overstressed as a diagnostic aid.

Differential Diagnosis. It is important that the pain and stiffness of fibrositis be differentiated from that of diseases which carry a more unfavorable prognosis. Early rheumatoid arthritis may be suspected, but the onset of the intra-articular, extra-articular and systemic features of rheumatoid disease will soon readily separate them. An adequate history will distinguish between chest pain due to fibrositis and that of angina pectoris. Low back pain is more often due to a skeletal lesion, and rheumatoid spondylitis, spondylolisthesis, disk lesions, carcinoma and osteoarthritis must be considered. In general those suffering from fibrositis are better with activity whereas those with structural lesions are sometimes worse. Pain in the region of the shoulder is most often due to bursitis or tendonitis. Limitation of shoulder movement will distinguish it from fibrositis. The shoulder-hand syndrome may begin with pain and stiffness but the swelling of the hand and palmar fascial changes are not seen in fibrositis. In the cervical area a roentgenogram may be necessary to rule out referred pain from a disk or osteoarthritic lesion.

Prognosis. The fibrositis syndrome may result from many different conditions so that prognosis will naturally depend upon the

joint or may develop as a secondary complication in a patient with bacteremia. Occasionally the arthritis is secondary to an adjacent osteomyelitis which involves one of the bones entering into the formation of the joint. By far the largest number are secondary to some form of bacteremia, the original focus being a furuncle, an infected wound, a mastoid infection or some other localized inflammatory focus.

Like most joint infections, suppurative arthritis starts in the synovial membrane. This rapidly becomes swollen and inflamed, and an exudate rich in polymorphonuclear leukocytes forms in the joint cavity. Many of the patients give a history of trauma to the affected joint, a day or two after which there is sudden pain and swelling in the joint and excessive pain on movement. There may be an initial chill and a rise in temperature to 38° or 39°. The joint is hot, swollen and tender, and in a short time fluctuation is present.

Aspiration of the joint reveals purulent fluid, cultures from which usually show streptococci or staphylococci.

The treatment consists in sulfonamide or penicillin therapy and surgical drainage if necessary.

Syphilitic Arthritis. Syphilis may manifest itself in the joints during either the secondary or the tertiary stages of the disease.

The arthritis of *secondary syphilis* is associated with the other symptoms of secondary lues and is characterized by swelling, tenderness and limitation of motion of several of the larger joints.

The arthritis of *tertiary syphilis* is usually monarticular. It develops late in the disease and is characterized by gummatous thickening of the synovial membrane and capsule. Clinically, this form of arthritis runs a chronic course similar in many respects to that of tuberculous arthritis. There is considerable swelling, but no redness, and fluctuation is usually demonstrable. The knee is particularly prone to involvement. Hydrops of the knee joint associated with periostitis immediately adjacent to the joint is strongly suggestive of syphilis, especially when the patient gives no history of trauma.

The treatment of luetic arthritis is that of syphilis elsewhere in the body. In a case which has not been too long neglected, penicillin therapy usually yields excellent results.

Tuberculous Arthritis. Tuberculous arthritis occurs most frequently in children. It is usually monarticular. Almost any joint in the body may be involved, but tuberculosis of the hip joint and of the spine are the two most common forms.

The treatment of tuberculous arthritis is largely surgical and orthopedic. Favorable results have been obtained with streptomycin in some cases, but a final evaluation of the drug cannot be made at this time. For a full discussion of tuberculous arthritis, the reader is referred to any standard treatise on surgery or orthopedics.

Other Forms of Infectional Arthritis. In addition to the common forms of infectional arthritis already described, other bacteria occasionally localize in the joints and set up inflammation. Among these may be mentioned:

The Arthritis of Scarlet Fever. This occurs in two types: (*a*) so-called "scarlatinal rheumatism"; (*b*) septic arthritis caused by the *Streptococcus hemolyticus* and differing in no respect from the ordinary surgical joint.

The arthritis of cerebrospinal fever also occurs in two forms, one resembling rheumatic fever and usually running a transitory course; the other a true meningococcal infection of the joint and characterized by the formation of a seropurulent exudate, rich in pus cells and meningococci.

The Arthritis of H. Influenzae. Several cases of influenzal arthritis, monarticular in type, have been reported. Most cases have occurred in children. The affected joint contains a seropurulent fluid, cultures from which yield *Hemophilus influenzae*.

The Arthritis of Brucellosis. Arthritis is a frequent and characteristic symptom of brucellosis. Several of the large joints are usually affected, and the acute manifestations migrate from joint to joint. Eventually the joints clear up spontaneously.

The Arthritis of Subacute Bacterial Endocarditis. In the course of this disease the patient may complain of pain and stiffness in some of the joints. This may be fleeting and mild, or the joints may be swollen and red and the symptoms persist for some time. The symptoms suggest a mild form of rheumatic fever. The treatment is that of bacterial endocarditis.

The Arthritis of Typhoid Fever. Typhoid arthritis is a rare condition; it is described in the chapter on Typhoid Fever (p. 224).

The Arthritis of Bacillary Dysentery. Arthritis is one of the commonest complications of bacillary dysentery and usually affects the knee, though other joints may be involved. It develops after the acute stage of dysentery is over and is accompanied by a recrudescence of fever and serous effusion into the joint.

The Arthritis of Lymphogranuloma Venereum. The arthritis which occurs in this disease may be either acute or chronic. In a series of 24 cases reported by Dawson and Boots, the arthritis was of an indolent serous type, usually polyarticular, and with a tendency to relapse. Joint fluid was sterile on culture.

ARTHRITIS OF RHEUMATIC FEVER

Rheumatic fever is a generalized affection characterized in most instances by acute inflammation of the joints. Rheumatic fever is described in detail on page 167.

RHEUMATOID ARTHRITIS

(Atrophic Arthritis, Arthritis Deformans)

Definition. Rheumatoid arthritis is a chronic systemic disease characterized by inflammatory changes in the joints, and by atrophy and rarefaction of the bones. In the earlier stages the disease manifests itself as a migratory swelling and stiffness of the joints, in the later stages by more or less deformity and ankylosis. Rheumatoid arthritis affects chiefly the collagen substance of connective tissue, and is now generally looked upon as one of the "collagen diseases."

Incidence. Unfortunately we have no accurate figures concerning the incidence of rheumatoid arthritis. It is known, however, to be prevalent in the temperate zone and rare in the tropics. It is fairly common in the southern portion of the United States. A large proportion of cases observed in New York City have their onset in the spring months, particularly in March. Rheumatoid arthritis is three times as common in females as in males. It is essentially a disease of young people, the average age at onset being 35 years.

Etiology. The etiology of rheumatoid arthritis has not been finally determined. In spite, however, of the lack of knowledge concerning the exact cause of the disease, certain precipitating factors are generally accepted as being conducive to its development.

Precipitating Causes. Among the more important precipitating factors may be mentioned:

SHOCK. A severe physical or emotional shock often precedes the onset of rheumatoid arthritis. A death in the family, a difficult labor, a surgical operation or some business calamity is often mentioned as having occurred just before arthritis developed.

FATIGUE. Fatigue, either mental or physical, especially if prolonged, is another important precipitating cause.

TRAUMA. Rheumatoid arthritis sometimes makes its first appearance in a joint which has previously been the seat of trauma. A sprained ankle, a fracture or a gunshot wound lowers the local resistance, and the rheumatoid process is initiated at this particular point. The disease may for a time remain localized in one joint, but other joints soon become involved.

INFECTIONS. Rheumatoid arthritis occasionally makes its first appearance shortly after an acute infection, particularly the more common ones, such as coryza, tonsillitis, sinus infection, influenza or pneumonia.

EXPOSURE. Sudden or repeated exposure to dampness, rain and cold is one of the predisposing causes of rheumatoid arthritis. This was shown by Pemberton in his statistical study of arthritis in soldiers. A high percentage of the men who acquired arthritis gave a definite history of standing in water, marching or sleeping in the rain, or of prolonged exposure to cold weather.

CONSTITUTIONAL INFERIORITY. Osgood has stressed the high incidence of rheumatoid arthritis in the thin, visceroptotic type of person. The muscles are poor, the thoracic cage is narrow, the chest expansion small, the weight-bearing lines of the joints are not true, and because of poor muscle tone the patient is easily fatigued.

HEREDITY. Rheumatoid arthritis is said to run in families. The writer has been rather impressed with the tendency of the disease to develop in the offspring of arthritic patients.

CLIMATE. Rheumatoid arthritis is a disease of the temperate zones. It is rarely encountered in the tropics.

Exciting Cause. The exciting cause of rheumatoid arthritis is still very much under debate. Many students of the disease have looked upon it as a chronic infection. The clinical course is suggestive of an infectious disease, and the lesions in the joints are essentially inflammatory, similar in many respects to those in other well known infections of the joints.

In 1912 Billings and his co-workers first

called attention to focal infection as an etiologic factor in chronic arthritis. These foci were found most frequently in the tonsils or sinuses or at the roots of devitalized teeth. The theory of focal infection was widely accepted for a number of years, but has very few supporters at the present time. One thing seems to be quite certain, and that is that foci of infection are not any more frequently encountered in rheumatoid arthritis than they are in other diseases or in healthy persons.

ALLERGIC FACTORS. Certain similarities between rheumatoid arthritis and rheumatic fever, periarteritis nodosa and other collagen disorders give some weight to the theory that they all are expressions of tissue hypersensitivity to some protein. Rich and others have produced clinical and experimental evidence in support of this concept. Further investigations along this line are indicated.

ENDOCRINE FACTORS. Students of arthritis have long suspected that rheumatoid arthritis might be due to some disturbance in the hormones. Selye was able to produce an experimental arthritis in rats by the injection of desoxycorticosterone. The arthritis was even more striking when an adrenalectomy was performed on the rats before desoxycorticosterone was injected. Hench and others have stressed the beneficent effect of jaundice and pregnancy on the course of rheumatoid arthritis.

The remarkable effect (to be discussed later) which is produced on the rheumatoid joint by cortisone or ACTH should not be interpreted as evidence that rheumatoid arthritis is caused by adrenal cortical deficiency. Many other conditions which are obviously unrelated etiologically to rheumatoid arthritis are greatly benefited by treatment with cortisone or ACTH, at least temporarily. Ragen has shown that cortisone and ACTH tend to retard the formation of granulation tissue in mesenchymal tissue. This fact alone might explain in part the relief of symptoms which are caused by an inflammatory exudate.

AGGLUTINATION REACTIONS. In approximately 70 per cent of cases of rheumatoid arthritis the serum of the patient will agglutinate group A hemolytic streptococci. More recently it has been found that rheumatoid serum will also agglutinate sensitized sheep red blood cells. The significance of these reactions is not clear.

EXPERIMENTAL ARTHRITIS. When various strains of streptococci are injected into rabbits, arthritis in one or more joints develops in a large proportion of the animals. The condition roughly resembles the rheumatoid arthritis of man. Sabin has produced a subacute proliferative polyarthritis in mice by the intravenous injection of a microorganism of the pleuropneumonia-like group.

In conclusion, it must be admitted that the etiology of rheumatoid arthritis has not yet been determined. Though the disease presents some of the characteristics of a chronic low grade infection, it seems quite likely that the pathogenesis of this disease will not yield to such a simple explanation. It would seem more plausible to assume that rheumatoid arthritis is the result of tissue reaction to some noxious product, possibly nonspecific in nature. It would then be somewhat analogous to asthma, a disease in which the tissue changes can be induced indirectly by bacterial infection or result from hypersensitivity to various heterologous proteins.

Morbid Anatomy. In the early stages, swelling of the joint is the most characteristic feature. This swelling is due to active inflammation in the various parts of the joint, particularly in the synovial membrane, the capsule and the surrounding soft tissue. The synovial membrane is swollen and deep red in color, and the villous processes show marked hypertrophy. In advanced cases, granulation tissue extends over the articular surfaces of the joint in the form of a pannus which eventually is converted into dense fibrous tissue. This binds the two contiguous articulating surfaces together in fibrous ankylosis. In other instances, ankylosis does not occur, but the cartilage ulcerates and there is an increase of fluid in the joint cavity. Finally, subluxation and distortions of the affected joints lead to deformities characteristic of the disease.

In addition to the destructive changes in the joint itself, a certain amount of atrophy occurs in the long bones, in the muscles and in the skin. In an advanced case of rheumatoid arthritis the bones are smaller and more brittle than normal, the muscles show marked wasting, and the skin over the affected parts is thin, tight and glossy.

Microscopically, the histologic changes in the joints are those of a chronic granulomatous process. In a section taken through the synovial membrane, the surface is often found covered with a thin layer of necrotic material densely infiltrated with leukocytes, beneath which there is vascular granulation tissue rich in fibroblasts, monocytes and leukocytes of various kinds.

Perhaps the most interesting pathologic lesion in rheumatoid arthritis is the subcutaneous nodule which occurs in about 15 per cent of the cases. Microscopic sections of these nodules show small granulomatous foci somewhat suggestive of miliary tubercles, which consist of an area of central necrosis surrounded by a zone of large mononuclear

tabolism in rheumatoid arthritis is close to the average normal level.

Symptoms. The patient with rheumatoid arthritis can often date the onset of symptoms from some disturbance of his physical equilibrium such as an acute infection, exposure to cold, a surgical operation, fatigue from overwork or an emotional strain. Certain prodromal symptoms may first be noted, the more common of which are weakness and fatigue, loss of weight, anemia and vasomotor

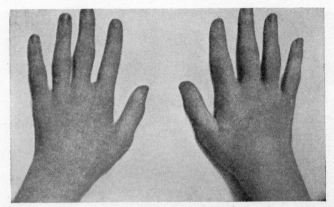

Fig. 183. Hands of a young woman with early rheumatoid arthritis, showing typical fusiform swelling of the proximal interphalangeal joints. Notice the symmetric distribution of the joint swelling. (From Oxford Monograph, Cecil's Diagnosis and Treatment of Arthritis, courtesy of the Editor, Dr. Henry A. Christian, and Oxford University Press.)

cells arranged in characteristic radial fashion, and an enveloping area of dense fibrous connective tissue. The changes in the heart are usually insignificant except in those cases of rheumatoid arthritis in which there is a history of rheumatic fever. In such cases the various lesions characteristic of rheumatic fever may be found on the valves or in the heart muscle. In cases not associated with rheumatic fever, perivascular collections of lymphoid and plasma cells have been described in the heart muscle; however, similar collections of cells have been noted in conditions other than rheumatoid arthritis. Focal collections of cells also occur in the skeletal muscles and in the connective tissue sheaths of the peripheral nerves. These too are not limited to rheumatoid arthritis.

Physiology. There are surprisingly few chemical changes in the blood of rheumatoid patients. The blood urea and the nonprotein nitrogen are well within normal figures. The carbon dioxide-combining power for blood, the calcium of the circulating blood and the total fat and cholesterol of the fasting blood are all within normal limits. The basal me-

disturbances, particularly tingling and numbness in the hands and feet. The onset may be sudden, but is usually gradual. When the onset is acute, the pain and swelling of the joints come on rapidly and are associated with chills, fever, prostration and other features of an acute illness, but in a great majority of cases the disease makes its appearance insidiously.

When the onset is gradual, symptoms usually appear first in only one joint. Often there is pain and stiffness in this particular joint for weeks or even months before other joints are affected. Gradually the joint begins to swell. The temperature is normal or only slightly elevated, often running for weeks from 37° to 38°C. The pulse is somewhat accelerated, and even early in the disease there may be some anemia.

Regardless of whether the symptoms develop suddenly or gradually, the disease eventually assumes a chronic course. The characteristic clinical features of rheumatoid arthritis are the swelling of the joints, particularly those of the fingers, hands and knees; the symmetrical distribution of the arthritic manifestations; the migratory character of the joint symptoms, especially in the early stages; the tendency of the disease to progress into a chronic state; and the eventual ankylosis and deformity of the joints if the disease is not arrested.

The degree of pain in the affected joints varies considerably and is not entirely proportional to the amount of swelling in the joint. With many of these patients there is comparatively little pain except with exercise.

in rheumatoid arthritis than in any other form of joint disease, and causes the patient considerable pain and discomfort when the jaw is exercised.

As the disease progresses, flexion deformities take place in the elbows and knees, as well as in the fingers and wrists. At first these muscle spasms can be overcome by traction or splints, but as time goes on the joints often become fixed in this position and extension becomes more and more difficult.

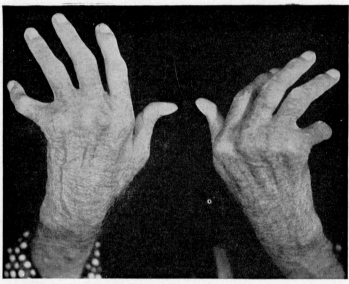

Fig. 184. Hands of an elderly man with advanced rheumatoid arthritis, showing the characteristic deformities and ulnar deviation of fingers. Most of the swelling has disappeared from the joints.

In the majority of patients the hands are sooner or later involved and present a characteristic appearance. In the fingers one sees the badge of the disease, a pod-shaped swelling of the proximal interphalangeal joint, the so-called fusiform or sausage finger. The distal interphalangeal joints are rarely involved. As the disease progresses, many or all of the fingers may be implicated, and swelling appears in the knuckles and wrists. The knees are nearly always affected, usually early in the disease. The joint becomes swollen and warm, and contains a moderate excess of fluid. There is considerable tenderness on pressure, and flexion is painful and limited. The ankles are frequently affected, but the toes are often spared, possibly because they are subject to little exercise. The metatarsophalangeal joints of the feet are often exquisitely tender on deep pressure; this finding may be of diagnostic value in doubtful cases. The temporomandibular joint is more frequently involved

Marked muscular atrophy and wasting leads to still more deformities and subluxations. In the hands, lateral deflection and subluxation at the metacarpophalangeal joint produce the characteristic ulnar deviation which is one of the earmarks of the disease.

The heart is rarely affected in rheumatoid arthritis. In those cases in which valvular disease is present the patient usually gives a history of a preceding rheumatic fever. The pulse rate may be accelerated, running between 90 and 100.

Among the most remarkable accompaniments of rheumatoid arthritis are the so-called "subcutaneous nodules" which occur in 15 per cent or more of all cases. They are usually found about the elbows, wrists or fingers, occasionally over the ankles, and appear as hard, usually movable nodules which vary in size from that of a pea to that of a walnut. They may disappear in a short time or persist for years. Iritis is a rare complication.

Physical Signs. The typical arthritic presents certain constitutional signs that are striking. These patients are usually anemic; many of them appear chronically ill and undernourished; some are markedly emaciated, particularly those in whom the disease has lasted for some time. A few patients, however, show excellent nutrition and no anemia.

Examination of the tonsils may occasionally show chronic infection. The gums may be the seat of various grades of gingivitis or pyorrhea. Transillumination of sinuses may reveal a chronic sinusitis. In the experience of the writer, however, the existence of frank focal infection is unusual in these patients and certainly no more prevalent than in patients suffering from other ailments.

In the early stages the joints affected usually present a characteristic appearance. There is more or less swelling of the soft parts, and the overlying skin is warm and sometimes reddened. In some cases there is an increase in synovial fluid. The swelling is due for the most part to the outpouring of inflammatory exudate into the periarticular structures. Tenderness is usually present and is most marked on the lateral aspects of the joints. Motion, either active or passive, is painful. In the early stages of the disease there is no crepitation.

The hands are cold and clammy. Several or all of the fingers are apt to show the characteristic fusiform enlargement of the proximal interphalangeal joint. Flushing of the thenar and hyperthenar eminences (the so-called "liver palm") is nearly always noted. The patient is unable to make a completely closed fist.

In the later stages some of the swelling may disappear, but a certain amount of thickening persists about the joint, owing to a new growth of fibrous tissue in this region. In the joint itself the granulation tissue may become converted into adhesions which eventually lead to partial or complete fibrous ankylosis. In those cases in which proliferation of the perichondrium predominates, bony ankylosis is apt to occur. Ankylosis is usually associated with considerable atrophy of the neighboring muscles. Muscular atrophy appears to be an integral part of the disease and is not solely attributable to disuse or muscular malnutrition. The skin of the extremities becomes smooth, glossy and atrophic, and in a few cases a secondary sclerodactyly makes its appearance.

The longer the duration of the disease, the more frequently bony changes can be demonstrated in the joints. In patients who are seen very early there may be no swelling or bony changes present and the disease is manifested solely by subjective sensations of pain. In these cases, examination of the joint reveals nothing abnormal except possibly slight tenderness on pressure.

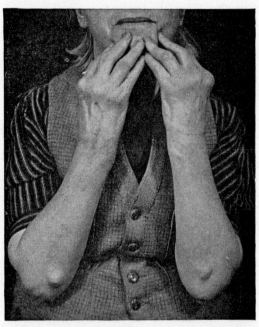

Fig. 185. Rheumatoid arthritis in an elderly woman, showing swelling and deformity of the hands and large subcutaneous nodules near the elbows.

Constitutional Manifestations. The general nutrition usually suffers in rheumatoid arthritis, and in severe cases profound cachexia may occur. The spleen is enlarged in 5 to 10 per cent of cases, and a general glandular enlargement may also be observed. As mentioned before, the cardiac changes are usually histologic rather than clinical. The patient rarely shows evidence of clinical heart disease unless there has been a history of previous rheumatic fever.

Clinical Course. When the onset of rheumatoid arthritis is acute, the disease may run a comparatively short course with complete disappearance of symptoms. The patient may then be entirely free from joint trouble for several months or even years. In a majority of cases, however, the condition returns after a lapse of time and with each recurring attack it takes on a more chronic course.

In those cases in which the onset is gradual the disease may run a chronic progressive course extending over years. There may be periods of comparative comfort alternating with periods of active advance. With each exacerbation the joints become progressively stiffer and more permanently injured. With loss of function, muscular atrophy becomes more and more pronounced, and flexion deformities, especially in the fingers, elbows and knees, make their appearance.

If the process is checked in its early stages, all the symptoms of arthritis may disappear, with complete return of normal function in the affected joints. Even in well established cases, remission sometimes occurs either spontaneously or as a result of treatment. In such cases the patient recovers partial or complete use of the affected joints, even when swelling and deformity do not entirely disappear. If the disease is not checked, the patient may eventually become a bedridden cripple, presenting a pitiful picture with his contracted, deformed limbs and markedly wasted muscles.

Roentgenographic Findings. In the early stages of rheumatoid arthritis, radiographs of the affected joints may be entirely negative. Later on, as the process advances, there is haziness and narrrowing of the interarticular space, as well as moderate osteoporosis of the bones adjacent to the affected joints. Still later in the disease, as the inflammatory tissue destroys the cartilage, the adjacent articular surfaces come into actual contact, so that the two bones appear to be fused together. At this stage there is considerable atrophy and rarefaction of the cancellous bone due to the diminished calcium content, and small areas of bone destruction, frequently referred to as "punched-out areas," are often demonstrable. These areas of erosion are smaller than those which occur in gout. In the last stages of the disease, when the bone itself is partially destroyed and ankylosis has occurred, the markings of the joint are replaced completely by a diffuse shadow which merges with the adjacent bone.

Laboratory Findings. Secondary microcytic anemia, sometimes of fairly severe grade, is present in the majority of patients with rheumatoid arthritis.

A moderate leukocytosis is found in a considerable number of cases, and the Schilling hemogram frequently shows increase of the immature cells, particularly in active cases.

The sedimentation rate of the red blood cells is increased in approximately 95 per cent of cases. In active cases it may be three or four times the normal rate.

In 70 per cent of well established cases the patient's serum will give a positive agglutination reaction to the hemolytic streptococcus, and in an almost equally high percentage of cases to sensitized sheep red blood cells.

The urine shows no characteristic changes.

The *synovial fluid* in rheumatoid arthritis ranges from normally clear to frankly turbid. Clot formation is frequent. In mild cases the cell count may be as low as 600 per cubic millimeter, but the average is 14,000, and it may be as high as 50,000 or 60,000. The polymorphonuclear count varies from 5 to 95 per cent. Protein concentration is above normal, averaging 5 gm. per 100 cc. of fluid. The sugar content is reduced, and hyaluronate is increased in rheumatoid joint fluids.

Diagnosis. The diagnosis of a typical case of rheumatoid arthritis presents little difficulty. The important features in diagnosis are:

1. Its tendency to occur in young adults, though it may occur at any age.

2. The migratory character of the joint symptoms is characteristic, particularly in the early stages. Later on the changes in the joints become chronic and persistent, and tend to a symmetrical distribution.

3. The affected joints usually are swollen and tender. In mild cases there may be an entire absence of swelling, but as a rule some degree of infiltration is present, and one should hesitate to make a diagnosis of rheumatoid arthritis is no swollen joints are demonstrable.

4. Rheumatoid arthritis is prone to attack the metacarpophalangeal and proximal interphalangeal joints, with the production of fusiform fingers.

5. In severe cases which are not checked, more or less deformity and ankylosis eventually take place.

6. Laboratory findings are helpful. The high sedimentation rate is important, and the x-ray findings, while not absolutely specific, are quite characteristic. The positive agglutination reactions would be more valuable if they appeared earlier in the disease. Changes in the joint fluid may settle the diagnosis in doubtful cases.

Differential Diagnosis. The most important differential diagnosis is that between rheumatoid arthritis and hypertrophic or so-called "degenerative arthritis." In the latter type there is an absence of inflammatory swelling. The disease does not spread, but remains localized in a few joints. In rheumatoid arthritis there is a loss of calcium in the bone which shows up in the roentgenogram, the bone being much more transparent than normal. In hypertrophic arthritis there is an increased amount of calcium deposit around the joint, which in the roentgenogram appears as a condensation of the bone

tiated from subacute rheumatic fever, a distinction which is not always easy to make. In both conditions the patient may give a history of a preceding tonsillitis or sore throat, followed by an acute arthritis with fever and swelling of the joints. In rheumatic fever, however, the temperature is higher, the sweating is more profuse and cardiac complications are frequent. The patient's serum yields a positive antistreptolysin reaction in rheumatic fever. In rheumatoid arthritis this reaction is negative. The therapeutic test is

Differential Diagnosis of Rheumatoid Arthritis

	RHEUMATOID ARTHRITIS	DEGENERATIVE ARTHRITIS
Average age of onset.......	Third and fourth decades	Fifth and sixth decades
Weight...................	Normal or underweight	Usually overweight
Condition of bones........	Osteoporosis	Condensation of articular margins
Joints involved............	Any joint in body	Chiefly knees, spine and fingers
Type.....................	Migratory	Not migratory
Appearance of joints.......	Periarticular swelling	No swelling
Special signs.............	Fusiform finger joints	Heberden's nodes
Subcutaneous nodules......	Present in 10 per cent of cases	Never present
Roentgen ray.............	Narrowing and clouding of joint space	Lipping of bony margins of joint
Joint fluid................	Turbid. Increased cells and protein.	Clear. Few cells. Low protein.
Streptococcal or sheep cell agglutinins..............	Usually present	Never present
Blood count..............	Secondary anemia and slight leukocyosis	Normal blood count
Sedimentation of R.B.C....	Considerably accelerated	Normal or slightly accelerated
Course...................	Usually progressive	Stationary or slightly progressive
Termination..............	Ankylosis and deformity	No ankylosis; usually no deformity

adjacent to the articular surface, and an actual new formation of bone around the margins of the joint. The distinction between rheumatoid arthritis and hypertrophic arthritis is important, since the line of treatment to be instituted is quite different for the two groups.

It must not be forgotten that in a middle-aged patient, rheumatoid arthritis may be superimposed on a degenerative arthritis, and that both processes may attack the same joint.

It is easy to mistake gonococcal arthritis for rheumatoid arthritis, especially in women who have no vaginal discharge. Gonorrheal arthritis is polyarticular, and the swollen, painful joints may bear a close resemblance to those of rheumatoid arthritis. In this differentiation the history is of great importance, as well as the examination of the genitourinary tract. The sedimentation rate is increased in both diseases. Penicillin and the sulfonamides are so specific for gonococcal arthritis that these drugs may be used for therapeutic tests in doubtful cases.

Rheumatoid arthritis must be differen-

valuable. Adequate treatment with sodium salicylate or aspirin (6 to 8 gm. a day) usually gives instant and permanent relief in rheumatic fever. In rheumatoid arthritis these drugs produce only a temporary improvement.

Tuberculous arthritis possibly might be mistaken for rheumatoid arthritis. The former, however, is nearly monarticular; the latter is polyarticular. X-ray examination will be of great assistance in making the disinction, but in some cases it may be necessary to resort to biopsy and animal inoculation.

Gouty arthritis may easily be confused with rheumatoid arthritis. In acute gout the therapeutic response to colchicine is so sharp that it constitutes a valuable method of differentiation. In chronic gout, tophi in the helix of the ear or in other parts of the body, when combined with an elevated blood uric acid and the characteristic x-ray changes, serve to differentiate the two conditions. It should be noted, however, that punched-out areas in the bone are found in the roentgenograms of both rheumatoid and gouty patients.

Prognosis. The prognosis in rheumatoid

arthritis is dependent on many factors. Perhaps the most important of these is the application of rational treatment early in the disease. The prognosis is affected by the morale of the patient and by his constitutional make-up. Robust, well developed patients respond to treatment more readily than those with inferior physiques. The actual number of patients who make a complete and permanent recovery is not accurately known. However, it must be quite small. Often the disease becomes arrested or quiescent, only to flare up again later on when for some reason the patient's resistance has been lowered. In rough figures, 10 to 15 per cent recover and remain well, 35 per cent improve, and the remaining 50 per cent exhibit persistent or progressive symptoms. These figures are of course modified by the newer forms of therapy. Patients who are running an acute febrile course appear to respond more quickly to treatment than those who present a chronic indolent type of arthritis.

Rheumatoid arthritis alone is never a menace to life. In advanced cases, however, when the patient's general health has undergone marked deterioration, the danger of death from some intercurrent infection is quite real.

Prophylaxis. As long as the etiology of rheumatoid arthritis remains in doubt, the prophylaxis of the disease will continue to present a difficult problem.

One of the most striking features of rheumatoid arthritis is its tendency to relapse. Many patients recover completely from the first attack of the disease and remain free from symptoms for several years. The second or third attack is nearly always more stubborn in its course and often goes on into the chronic progressive form. In view of this characteristic of the disease, every effort should be made to prevent a subsequent attack. The patient's life and personal hygiene must be carefully regulated to a point well within his capacity to function without fatigue.

Treatment. Rheumatoid arthritis is a chronic systemic disease, and the physician should approach the patient with this idea constantly in mind. Local treatment to painful joints often gives symptomatic relief, but much more than this is needed for successful results. The physician must also bear in mind that rheumatoid arthritis is subject to spontaneous remissions and exacerbations, a fact which often leads one to attribute therapeutic efficacy to agents which have no value as such.

Active incipient cases with fever can often be greatly benefited by four to six weeks' intensive treatment in a hospital. This will rarely be sufficient to produce a remission, but the patient comes out feeling better and stronger and often afebrile. He can then be treated at home or at the physician's office as seems desirable. Even those patients with more advanced arthritis will often benefit considerably from a few weeks of hospital care. A well equipped hospital not only provides complete rest and good nursing, but offers facilities for laboratory study, blood transfusions, physical therapy, orthopedic treatment, and so forth, which are difficult to obtain at home.

Rest. All students of rheumatoid arthritis are agreed that complete and prolonged rest is the keynote to successful treatment of this disease. This can best be obtained in a hospital or sanatorium, particularly in the earlier stages of treatment. It should be pointed out, however, that patients who receive hospital care, unless febrile, should not be allowed to remain in bed 24 hours a day. Such "overrest" encourages ankylosis of the affected joints and further atrophy of the muscles in the back and legs. In many ambulant cases complete rest is a difficult form of therapy to enforce, chiefly because the patient is anxious to keep up his daily duties. However, if patients in the early stages of rheumatoid arthritis can be persuaded to give up work and take a rest cure for six months or a year, a much higher percentage of them will make a complete recovery. As it is, and chiefly for economic reasons, the physician must usually compromise on the rest issue, and the patient is advised to take from one to two hours' rest in bed every day after lunch. If a real rest cure can be taken, it is far preferable, because the patient gets a mental and emotional rest as well as a physical one. In well established cases, rest in bed for a considerable part of the day is absolutely essential. There should also be long sleeping hours at night, induced by some mild hypnotic if necessary.

Dietary and Vitamin Regimen. No special diet is indicated in the treatment of rheumatoid arthritis. Most rheumatoid patients are undernourished and underweight, and one of the duties of the physician is to try to restore the lost weight by means of a nutritious, well balanced diet. In order to achieve this, a high calorie, high vitamin diet, rich in vegetables and fruits, is indicated. There may be occasional instances of overweight patients who need a low calorie diet, but these are exceptions to the rule.

The use of vitamins in the treatment of arthritis is purely empiric. However, some patients feel better while taking vitamins, and some such schedule as the following may be tried:

Cod liver oil and viosterol, one capsule twice a day (vitamins A and D). The highly concentrated preparations of vitamin D (Ertron and others), which some writers have hailed as a cure for rheumatoid arthritis, have no advantage over the less concentrated preparations. There are several reports in the medical literature of hypercalcemia, sometimes associated with renal failure, which has resulted from long-sustained doses of concentrated vitamin D. Some of these cases with vitamin D intoxication have terminated fatally.

Orange juice and tomato juice, one glass of each a day (vitamin C).

Wheat germ or brewers' yeast once or twice a day (vitamin B).

Many physicians prefer to maintain an adequate vitamin balance by the administration once or twice a day of one of the "shotgun" vitamin capsules now being manufactured by various pharmaceutical houses.

Foreign protein therapy has been advocated as a method of treating arthritis, but is not very popular at the present time. Various substances such as milk, horse serum, peptone and proteoses, and typhoid vaccine have been injected intramuscularly or intravenously with the idea of mobilizing the patient's immune bodies or producing a febrile reaction. Of the various agents used, typhoid vaccine is the most popular.

Fever Therapy. In the writer's opinion, fever therapy has a very limited place in the treatment of rheumatoid arthritis. It is not recommended for the chronic, well established cases. In the initial stages of the disease, particularly in acute febrile patients, fever therapy will sometimes bring about a rapid cessation of symptoms. Unfortunately, a considerable number of patients who are relieved by fever therapy will suffer a relapse after a few weeks of comfort.

There are two methods of inducing fever: (1) typhoid vaccine intravenously; (2) artificial hyperthermia by some form of hot box.

TYPHOID VACCINE administered intravenously is the simpler and, in the author's opinion, the safer method of fever therapy. The first dose should be 25,000,000 bacteria. It is usually desirable to double the dose with each subsequent injection in order to obtain good febrile reactions of 103° to 105° F. The maximum benefit is obtained by the first three or four injections. Typhoid vaccine therapy is contraindicated in patients with chronic cardiac disease, in elderly patients and in those who give a history of tuberculosis.

ARTIFICIAL HYPERTHERMIA. Artificial fever is produced by several methods: (1) the hot bath, (2) high frequency diathermy currents, (3) radiothermy, (4) electrically heated cabinets. In the writer's opinion, hyperthermia by induced heat has more disadvantages than typhoid vaccine. The production of heat by radiant energy seems to be the preferable method because of its cheapness, simplicity and freedom from danger.

Transfusions. Transfusions of blood have been advocated by Copeman, Holbrook and others. Holbrook treated 70 patients in this manner, and found that in the subacute or early phases of rheumatoid arthritis, with or without anemia, they responded well and in a few instances dramatically. The amount usually given is 500 cc. of blood, and it may be repeated a few days later if desirable. In recent years, transfusions have become less popular because of the danger of transmitting infectious hepatitis.

Drugs. Drugs play a small but important part in the treatment of rheumatoid arthritis.

IRON in the form of ferrous sulfate, 0.2 gm. four times a day, or reduced iron, 0.6 gm. three times a day, may be tried for the anemia which is common with this disease, though too often the results are disappointing.

SALICYLATES. For the control of pain there is no drug that stands up as well month after month as acetylsalicylic acid. The dose should be 0.6 gm. three to four times a day, and in some patients even larger doses are well tolerated. There is less danger of gastric disturbance if the drug is combined with sodium bicarbonate or taken in the form of enteric-coated tablets. In severe cases the writer sometimes combines aspirin with aminopyrine and phenacetin in a formula such as the following:

Acetylsalicylic acid	0.3 gm.
Aminopyrine	0.1 gm.
Phenacetin	0.1 gm.

When the pain is not controlled by these drugs, codeine, 0.03 gm., may be necessary. Codeine seems to work particularly well in combination with aspirin.

The analgesic effect of alcohol should not be forgotten. A small drink of whisky or some other alcoholic beverage will do much to brighten the end of the day for the arthritic patient and usually gives definite relief from pain. Many physicians are in the habit of prohibiting alcoholic beverages for patients with arthritis. The writer, however, has rarely seen any ill effects from the moderate use of spirits.

GOLD SALTS. Since 1932 various salts of gold have been tried with considerable success in the treatment of rheumatoid arthritis. This form of therapy was originally introduced by Forestier, and has received support from various clinics in England and America. The mechanism by which gold acts in rheumatoid arthritis is not understood. It has been shown, however, that gold salts have chemotherapeutic properties against hemolytic streptococci and certain other pathogenic bacteria.

Freyberg and his co-workers have studied the rate of absorption and excretion of various gold salts injected into human subjects. These writers found that about 75 per cent of gold is retained in the body during a course of gold therapy, while the other 25 per cent is excreted, for the most part through the urine and a small part through the feces. The gold salt continues to be excreted for months after the injections have been concluded. This slow excretion of gold products probably explains the toxic effects which are sometimes produced.

The most popular forms of gold now in use are sodium gold thiosulfate, the aurothiomalate of sodium (Myochrysine) and aurothioglucose (Solganal-B). The sodium gold thiosulfate is usually administered intravenously, while Myochrysine and Solganal-B are injected deep into the gluteal muscles. The dosage of gold salts has been a matter of considerable controversy. In the beginning of gold therapy the dosage varied from 100 to 500 mg. It was soon discovered, however, that such doses were extremely dangerous. Freyberg has shown that a dose of even 100 mg. is unnecessarily large and that smaller doses will produce almost equally good clinical results. At the present time the doses advocated by most authorities in America are as follows:

First dose	10 mg. intramuscularly
Second dose	25 mg. intramuscularly
Third and succeeding doses	50 mg. intramuscularly

The total amount administered in the course should be 750 to 1000 mg. It is customary to administer gold therapy in several series or courses with intervals of four to eight weeks between. The reason for these intervals is to permit the body to excrete some of the accumulated gold.

Gold salts are most efficacious when administered early in the course of rheumatoid arthritis. In a study made by the writer in collaboration with Chester Adams, it was found that, in 106 patients with rheumatoid arthritis treated during the first year of their illness by chrysotherapy, remissions occurred in 66 per cent of the gold-treated patients; in 83 control cases treated by conventional methods during the first year of the disease, only 24 per cent had remissions. On the average, remissions were noted ten months sooner in the gold-treated cases than in the controls (7.1 months versus 17.1 months).

Unfortunately, gold therapy is attended by certain dangers which militate against its general acceptance. Approximately 25 per cent of the patients on gold therapy exhibit a rash or some other form of gold intoxication such as stomatitis or gastroenteritis. Depression of the bone marrow has been observed in a small number of cases with a consequent development of hemorrhage, purpura, aplastic anemia or agranulocytosis. Because of this tendency toward gold intoxication, which is occasionally fatal, patients who are subjected to gold therapy must be watched carefully for reactions. A blood count and urinalysis should be made at least once a month and the skin carefully watched for drug rashes. In spite of careful watching, however, an occasional patient will acquire an unpleasant and persistent exfoliative dermatitis.

BAL (British anti-lewisite) was developed by the British to combat the toxic effects of lewisite, an arsenical poison. Its effectiveness against arsenic, mercury and other heavy metal intoxications led to its trial in cases of gold intoxication. Toxic reactions occur when gold is in combination with tissue protein. BAL competes successfully with the tissues for gold, and the inert gold-BAL complex is rendered nontoxic.

There is an increase in the urinary excretion of gold for a short while after treatment with BAL. BAL is prepared in a 10 per cent solution of benzyl-benzoate in peanut oil for intramuscular use. The dose is 2.5 mg. per kilogram of body weight every 4 hours during the first and second days, then twice daily for five to eight days. BAL may produce nausea, vomiting and abdominal pain.

BAL, if given promptly, mitigates gold intoxication. Cortisone in doses of 50 to 75 mg. a day may be quite valuable in relieving gold dermatitis.

Another disappointing feature of gold therapy is the comparatively high percentage of relapses, 40 per cent or higher in several reported series. The relapse may come a few weeks or months after cessation of gold therapy, or it may be postponed for several years.

Patients on gold therapy should have determination of the sedimentation rate of the red blood cells about every two or three months. Those who react well to gold therapy usually have a rapid drop in the sedimentation rate during the first course of treatment. If a patient shows no improvement after two or three months of gold therapy, further administration of the agent is contraindicated.

Because of the toxic reactions and because of the high percentage of relapses, some authors (Short, Beckman and Bauer) seriously question the advisability of gold therapy, believing that in the end, results with rest, physiotherapy and other conservative measures equal or surpass those obtained with gold salts.

The majority of rheumatologists endorse the use of gold therapy in spite of its drawbacks. Many advise the administration of maintenance doses of gold salts after the regular course of chrysotherapy has been completed. The maintenance dose consists of 25 to 50 mg. of gold salt administered intramuscularly every two to four weeks. The incidence of relapse appears to be considerably reduced by this procedure, but adequate data are lacking.

Cortisone and Corticotropin Therapy. Cortisone is a crystalline hormone derived originally from the adrenal cortex. It is a pure compound of definite chemical structure and has been produced by chemical synthesis from bile and other substances. Cortisone (Compound E) has a rather complicated chemical structure, 17-hydroxy-11-dehydrocorticosterone.

Cortocotropin (ACTH) is the pituitary corticotrophic hormone which stimulates responsive adrenal glands to the production of cortisone and possibly other steroids.

Hench, Kendall, Slocumb and Polley have shown that, when cortisone or corticotropin is injected intramuscularly into a patient with rheumatoid arthritis, there is a marked and rapid amelioration in the patient's symptoms. The response to these agents usually begins within 24 to 48 hours after the first injection and is characterized by a rapid decrease in subjective stiffness, diminution in articular tenderness and decrease of pain on motion. This immediate effect is usually followed by decrease in swelling of the joints, improvement in appetite and replacement of malaise with euphoria.

Unfortunately, when either of these agents is discontinued, signs and symptoms of arthritis usually begin to reappear within 24 to 48 hours, and within a short time the patient's condition returns to its previous state. In a few exceptional cases remission has persisted for as long as several weeks or months. When cortisone or corticotropin is readministered, prompt remission is usually again induced.

OTHER EFFECTS OF CORTISONE. In addition to the marked antirheumatic effect of cortisone, this hormone produces other noteworthy effects.

1. Fever usually disappears when cortisone is administered.

2. There is a marked increase in appetite which may result in more or less increase in weight.

3. Retention of salt and water. As a rule this produces no problem, but if the patient has a rapid increase in weight and edema of the ankles, cortisone should be discontinued temporarily.

4. Excess excretion of potassium.

5. Rapid drop in the sedimentation rate to normal, or almost normal. When cortisone is discontinued, the rate rises again to approximately its previous level.

6. Cortisone produces a drop in the total eosinophil count.

7. Large doses of cortisone may produce hyperglycemia and glycosuria. However, in the routine treatment of rheumatoid patients, glycosuria is not often observed. The coexistence of diabetes mellitus and rheumatoid arthritis, though not a rigid contraindication to cortisone therapy, makes the handling of both the diabetes and the arthritis difficult

and should be undertaken only when the arthritis is severe.

8. Effect of cortisone on excretion of steroids. Urinary 17-ketosteroids are normal in rheumatoid arthritis. Hench found that, when 100 mg. of cortisone were given daily, there was moderate increase in the excretion of 17-ketosteroids in the urine.

CORTICOTROPIN (ACTH). In general, the response of the rheumatoid patient to corticotropin is the same as that to cortisone. There is a marked diminution in stiffness, pain and swelling. The euphoria is more marked, and the general improvement is striking, but there is the same tendency to relapse when the hormone is withdrawn. The effect on various physiologic and biochemical functions of the body is similar to that of cortisone.

COMPARISON OF CORTISONE AND CORTICOTROPIN. Cortisone and corticotropin should not be looked upon as competing therapeutic agents. Both produce striking effects on the patient with rheumatoid arthritis, though they act in different ways. Cortisone is a substitution product, actually replacing or supplementing the natural cortisone excreted by the adrenal cortex. Corticotropin stimulates the adrenal cortex to the production of more cortisone. Both agents, therefore, induce a state of hyperadrenalism in the patient. Long-continued use of cortisone may result in adrenal atrophy, at least while the cortisone is being given. Corticotropin, on the other hand, may produce hypertrophy of the adrenal cortex if continued over a long period of time or, if used in too large doses, may actually exhaust the adrenal from overstimulation. Corticotropin, if used immediately after a course of cortisone, may prove temporarily disappointing. The adrenal becomes lazy after long-continued use of cortisone and does not respond to stimulation from corticotropin until after a certain amount of time. Fortunately the adrenal atrophy which accompanies long-continued use of cortisone is temporary. The gland soon returns to normal after cortisone therapy has been discontinued.

SIDE EFFECTS OF CORTISONE AND CORTICOTROPIN. Certain side effects are observed in connection with both cortisone and corticotropin therapy. These side effects are more frequently observed when large doses (200 mg. of cortisone or 100 mg. of corticotropin daily) are given, or when smaller doses are continued for a long period, and indicate hyperadrenalism, or so-called Cushing's syndrome. Among such manifestations are:

1. "Moon facies" and "buffalo hump," resulting from deposition of fat in the neck and upper dorsal spine.

2. Retention of salt associated with weight gain, edema and some elevation of blood pressure.

3. Hypopotassemia with resulting muscular weakness.

4. Osteoporosis, purple striae over abdomen and buttocks, and diabetes.

5. Hirsutism, acne, amenorrhea.

No definite effect on libido or potentia has been reported.

Side Effects on the Nervous System. Though euphoria and increased cerebral activity are desirable effects, cortisone and corticotropin occasionally produce undesirable effects such as nervousness, variation in mood or psyche, paresthesias, and occasionally psychotic states. In some cases the psychosis may be of such severe degree that resort to shock therapy is necessary. This is one of the major danger signals and can lead to much trouble. In these patients there is usually some evidence of an abnormal personality previous to hormone therapy. A mild restlessness or nervousness is not an infrequent symptom, and may be accompanied by insomnia. Several observers have noted changes in the electro-encephalogram.

DOSAGE OF CORTISONE. Cortisone is usually prepared in the form of an acetate salt. In its original form the salt was suspended in an aqueous medium for intramuscular injection. Cortisone is now available in tablet form for oral administration. The tablets, supplied in 5, 10 and 25 mg. sizes, have largely supplanted the suspension because of their obvious practical advantages. The dosage is essentially the same for either tablets or suspension and varies with circumstances. In the treatment of active rheumatoid arthritis, it is customary to start with four or five 25 mg. tablets every 24 hours. If for any reason the cortisone suspension must be used, 100 mg. should be the initial dose in a single intramuscular injection. In either case, after two or three days, dosage is reduced by 25 mg., and again after a few days more to a maintenance dose of approximately 50 mg. a day. In divided doses this would be equivalent to two 25 mg. tablets a day, or four half tablets (12.5 mg.). At this dosage cortisone can be maintained for weeks or months in most cases without much danger of unpleasant side effects. Men as a rule tolerate cortisone better than women and can take somewhat larger doses.

DOSAGE OF CORTICOTROPIN. The dosage of corticotropin is roughly about half that of cortisone. In its original form the crystals are suspended in water or saline for intramuscular injection. Because of its rapid action and elimination, this hormone must be injected every 6 to 12 hours. Such a schedule becomes burdensome to both patient and physician, and because of this disadvantage, corticotropin has not enjoyed so wide a usage as cortisone. Its popularity has recently been increased by the introduction of corticotropin in a gel suspension, which is much more slowly absorbed than the aqueous product, and reduces the number of injections to one or two every 24 hours. The usual initial dose of corticotropin is 40 to 60 mg. a day in single or divided injections.

Some authorities believe that for theoretical reasons, courses of cortisone and corticotropin should be alternated in the treatment of the rheumatoid, and practically this procedure seems to work very well in some cases.

HYDROCORTISONE or Compound F is another hormone which is now being widely used, not only orally but as an intra-articular agent in the treatment of rheumatoid arthritis. Hydrocortisone tablets are reported to be more potent as an anti-inflammatory agent than cortisone itself. A 20 mg. tablet is approximately the equivalent of a 25 mg. tablet of cortisone. The general effect of the two agents is the same.

Hydrocortisone acetate has been prepared as an aqueous suspension for intra-articular injection. When this agent in doses of 25 to 50 mg. is introduced into an inflamed joint, the result is often spectacular, both subjectively and objectively. Unfortunately, the benefit is usually temporary; after a week or ten days of relief, the swelling and pain return and the injection must be repeated. In spite of this disadvantage hydrocortisone is a useful therapeutic agent, and sometimes two or three injections of this hormone will induce a permanent remission in a rheumatoid joint.

Is cortisone or corticotropin indicated for every case of rheumatoid arthritis? By no means. Certain mild cases will recover with rest and physiotherapy. Others will respond promptly to gold salts and will remain in remission often for months or even years. None of the new hormones *cure* rheumatoid arthritis. The value of these agents lasts only so long as they are being administered. Cortisone does not repair damaged tissue, hence it will not restore deformed or ankylosed joints. The physician should employ cortisone therapy with some reluctance, realizing that once started the patient will usually wish to continue it indefinitely. However, cortisone should be considered in the acute inflammatory progressive form of rheumatoid arthritis, especially if other forms of treatment have proved unavailing. In chronic cases, some improvement can be expected, and in a significant percentage of cases this improvement is so great that the drug is a godsend to the patient. Even in this group disillusionment may come when because of some side effect, or because of lessening effectiveness, cortisone has to be discontinued, and the patient relapses to a state often more severe than that which existed before cortisone was started.

The contraindications to the use of cortisone or corticotropin are cardiac decompensation or advanced cardiorenal disease, malignant vascular hypertension, osteoporosis, severe diabetes mellitus, active tuberculosis and other infections. Active peptic ulcer and various mental disturbances are contraindications.

Treatment with Other Steroids. The dramatic effect of cortisone and ACTH in the treatment of rheumatoid arthritis has spurred efforts toward the isolation of other steroid agents which might prove effective in this condition. Thus testosterone propionate and pregnenolone (the 3-hydroxy analogue of progesterone) have both been reported as highly efficacious in the treatment of rheumatoid arthritis. However, in the hands of most observers, including the writer, these agents have been disappointing.

METACORTANDRACIN. A new synthetic steroid, the chemical structure of which differs only slightly from that of cortisone, has recently been isolated by Herzog et al., and subjected to clinical trial by Bunim and co-workers. This agent is known as metacortandracin (Meticorten). Its adrenocortical activity, measured by eosinopenic response, is three to four times that of cortisone. Bunim found that in a series of 15 rheumatoid patients treated with this steroid, the clinical improvement was more marked than with cortisone or corticotropin, and that this enhanced potency was not accompanied by a proportionate increase in the frequency or severity of undesirable side effects. The writer has had an opportunity to try metacortandracin on some 50 patients with rheumatoid arthritis and the results have confirmed the observations of Bunim. In every case the clinical improvement has been striking, even in those patients in whom cortisone had failed to give satisfactory relief. One gratifying feature of this new steroid is that, with ordinary therapeutic doses, it does not cause retention of sodium or loss of potassium.

The optimal dosage has not yet been finally determined, but varies with the severity of the arthritis. Most of our patients have been started on 10 mg. three times a day. After a week or ten days the suppressive dose is gradually reduced every four or five days until symptoms of recurrence appear. The maintenance dose is kept at the lowest level necessary to give the patient maximal comfort and disappearance of objective signs; it ranges from 5 to 20 mg. daily. Metacortandracin (at this writing) has been in use for approximately six months—too short a period to allow of any final conclusion as to its safety or its lasting therapeutic value. However, it does appear to mark a distinct advance in the development of hormone therapy for rheumatoid arthritis. Most of the well recognized symptoms of Cushing's syndrome may appear after prolonged use of this agent, but do not appear to be as conspicuous a feature as in cortisone or ACTH therapy.

Phenylbutazone (Butazolidin). This new drug has received favorable comment from a number of writers as an analgesic in the treatment of rheumatoid arthritis. Some have gone so far as to claim real antirheumatic qualities for phenylbutazone, but this seems unlikely.

Phenylbutazone is available in 100 mg. tablets for oral administration. It can also be given intramuscularly. The dose is 100 mg. three or four times a day by mouth, or 2.5 cc. of a 20 per cent solution (500 mg.) intramuscularly every two or three days.

The great drawback to phenylbutazone therapy is the rather high incidence of toxic reactions following its use. Like cortisone it may cause sodium retention with edema in elderly patients or in those with cardiac or renal disease. Other toxic manifestations are abdominal pain and nausea, skin rashes, dizziness and anemia. Leukopenia, thrombocytopenia and even agranulocytosis are occasionally encountered, and a few fatalities

have been reported. Patients on phenylbutazone must be kept under medical supervision and should have frequent blood counts.

Physical Therapy. The more common types of physical therapy, such as dry heat, diathermy, massage and exercises, all have a place in the treatment of rheumatoid arthritis. Their chief function is to increase circulation in the affected joints and to preserve as far as possible the tone of the skeletal muscles.

Heat is perhaps the most important form of physical therapy and can be applied either locally to the joint or to the entire body. The local application of heat to one joint is carried out by means of the ordinary electric baker or by diathermy. Some prefer moist heat in the form of hot towels or submersion of the joint in hot water. In the experience of the writer, diathermy is usually disappointing in the treatment of rheumatoid arthritis. From a theoretical standpoint, diathermy should be ideal, since it heats the tissues as well as the skin, but practically, a good many rheumatoid patients, especially those in the active stage, complain that diathermy actually increases the pain. One of the simplest ways of applying heat to the joint is by means of infra-red light. Generalized heat is best applied by means of the hot tub bath, the hot pack or the electric light bridge. The advantage of generalized heat is that, in addition to stimulating the circulation, copious perspiration is induced in the patient.

Hydrotherapy has come to have an important place in the modern treatment of arthritis. The rheumatism cures of Europe date back to the Roman Empire and are still popular, both on the Continent and in Great Britain. The European spas which make a specialty of arthritis are Bath and Harrogate in England, Aix-les-Bains and Dax in France, Wiesbaden and Baden-Baden in Germany, Bad-Gastein in Austria and Pistiany in Czechoslovakia. Alternating hot and cold baths, or contrast baths as they are usually called, have the advantage of stimulating the sympathetic system as well as the local circulation in the joint.

Massage complements heat in that both have more or less the same object—the improvement of blood and lymph flow through the joints. Successful results in the use of massage depend on the qualifications of the masseur and the proper selection of cases for massage therapy. Massage is contraindicated in any patient whose joints are in a highly active, painful stage. However, in many chronic cases there is little tenderness on pressure over the joints, and in such cases massage can be used with advantage, not only to the joints themselves, but to the adjacent muscles as well.

Exercises. The object of exercises and calisthenics is, first, to preserve the function of the joint by preventing ankylosis; second, to maintain the tone of the muscles; and third, to prevent and overcome contractions and deformities. Every arthritic should have some exercise, and one of the most important factors in the treatment of arthritis is to determine just the right balance between rest and exercise in the patient's routine. In the average case with several swollen fingers or knuckles and a certain amount of swelling and cartilaginous injury in the knees and feet, ordinary calisthenics taken lying down will usually serve the purpose. The reason for the recumbent posture is to prevent strain and fatigue.

Perhaps the most important of the exercises are those that have to do with maintaining posture, and of these the most useful is the quadriceps drill. The patient, lying supine in bed, is instructed to contract and relax the quadriceps muscles forty to fifty times at least three times a day, in order to prevent atrophy and weakness in this important group of muscles. In advanced arthritics passive exercises may be necessary, or a combination of passive with active exercises. At the New York Hospital we have found active and passive exercises in the warm pool a valuable procedure in the rehabilitation of the arthritic patient. If a warm pool is not available, the Hubbard tub provides facilities for exercising the patient under water. The optimum temperature for exercise under water is 98° to 100° F. Higher temperatures are not desirable.

Climatotherapy. Some rheumatoid patients respond well to a change of climate, particularly when they are transferred to a dry warm climate, such as that of Arizona, New Mexico or the West Indies. Holbrook believes that the various forms of heliotherapy contribute the main benefit in climatotherapy. A physician who advises a patient to go to Arizona should stress the importance of his remaining there for at least six months or even a year. Patients who, for financial or other reasons, cannot make the pilgrimage to the Southwest should be exposed as much as possible to sunlight and dry heat at home.

Orthopedic Treatment. If every patient with rheumatoid arthritis could receive prompt and efficient medical treatment, comparatively few of them would need orthopedic measures. There are certain simple orthopedic measures with which every physician should be familiar. The arthritic should sleep on a flat bed with only one pillow. Many patients will require a board at the foot of the bed to prevent foot-drop. If the patient shows a tendency to rapid ankylosis, it is important for the physician to be familiar with the optimum position for ankylosed joints, particularly those of the knees, elbows, wrists and fingers. Unfortunately there are a good many patients who for one reason or another do not receive prompt medical treatment, or perhaps are lacking in resistance to the disease and advance rapidly to ankylosis and deformity. For such patients, orthopedic procedures of various kinds are of great importance for both prophylaxis and treatment. Some of these measures can be applied to ambulant cases. Others can be used only in institutions. The amount of rehabilitation which may be achieved, even in an advanced case of rheumatoid arthritis, is remarkable, but such improvement requires months or even years of patient care and supervision. In patients who are badly disabled from a previously active arthritis, cortisone or corticotropin may prove helpful in relieving pain and stiffness and thereby allowing a somewhat more aggressive attack on joint deformities by the physiotherapist.

Surgical Treatment. Great strides have been made in recent years in the surgical treatment of advanced arthritic conditions. Manipulation under an anesthetic, synovectomy, osteotomy, arthrodesis and various reconstruction and arthroplastic operations all have an important place in modern orthopedic surgery. Synovectomy is particularly useful in the correction of rheumatoid knees or elbows which have developed villous arthritis. This operation involves the removal almost *en masse* of the proliferative synovial membrane. A new synovial membrane may be expected to re-form, and a good but not complete range of motion is to be anticipated.

Sympathectomy of the cervical or lumbar ganglia has been tried, but rarely gives permanent benefit.

Psychotherapy. Most patients with rheumatoid arthritis suffer a great deal from mental depression and consequently need an abundant measure of psychotherapy. On the other hand, there are some patients, usually men, who do not take their affliction seriously enough, and the physician, in all fairness to the patient, should make clear to him the serious potentialities of the disease. The small, slender type of neurotic woman is particularly susceptible to rheumatoid arthritis and often responds poorly to treatment. It is this type of patient that needs the greatest amount of moral encouragement. Unless the physician makes earnest efforts along this line, he will fail to get the full cooperation and confidence of the patient, factors that mean much in the stubborn fight against the disease.

Other forms of treatment for rheumatoid arthritis which have been tried from time to time and found of little or no value are (1) vaccine therapy, (2) massive doses of vitamin D, (3) low carbohydrate diet, (4) sulfur therapy, (5) bee venom therapy, (6) sulfonamide derivatives, (7) penicillin, (8) antireticular-cytotoxic serum, and (9) prostigmine therapy. The author can recommend none of these forms of therapy.

CLINICAL VARIANTS OF RHEUMATOID ARTHRITIS

Arthritis Associated with Infections. Certain cases of arthritis are definitely associated with localized infections. So-called subacute infectious polyarthritis usually follows some form of acute respiratory infection, though it may occur after infections in other parts of the body, notably those of the genitourinary tract. It is occasionally seen following cholecystitis, ulcerative colitis or some gastrointestinal infection. Some writers believe that this type of arthritis should be classified either as rheumatic fever or rheumatoid arthritis, but it does not conform strictly to either. It differs from rheumatic fever in absence of heart lesions and failure to respond to salicylates; it differs from rheumatoid arthritis in running an active febrile course, with hot, swollen, painful joints, in contrast to the sluggish, inactive swelling characteristic of rheumatoid arthritis. Furthermore, the prognosis in subacute infectious polyarthritis is excellent; most of these patients make a complete recovery after the condition has run a course of several weeks or months. This type of arthritis was prevalent in military hospitals during World War II.

Still's Disease. In 1897 Still described a form of polyarthritis in children and reported 12 cases of the disease. This syndrome is now looked upon as a juvenile form of rheumatoid arthritis.

So far as the morbid anatomy of the disease is concerned, the findings in the joints are similar to those of rheumatoid arthritis. In the later stages, ankylosis and deformity occur with marked atrophy of the muscles. Lipping and spurring of the articular surfaces almost never occur, but considerable rarefaction of the bone is shown by roentgenograms. In addition to the changes in the joints, hyperplasia of the lymph nodes and enlargement of the liver and spleen frequently occur. Amyloid degeneration has been noted in the liver, spleen, lymph nodes and kidneys.

Rheumatoid Spondylitis. Most patients with rheumatoid arthritis sooner or later exhibit symptoms in some part of the spine, usually the cervical portion. However, there is a special form of arthritis in which the entire spine may become implicated. This may exist with or without involvement of peripheral joints, and is known as ankylosing, rheumatoid or Marie-Strümpell spondylitis (poker spine). Many students believe that this disease is distinct from rheumatoid arthritis. Certainly it differs fundamentally in one respect from rheumatoid arthritis in being a disease mostly of young men. Typical Marie-Strümpell spines are unusual in the female.

Ankylosing spondylitis makes its first appearance in the lower back, affecting primarily the sacro-iliac joints. The small articulations of the apophyseal and costovertebral joints are involved early in the disease. The pathologic changes are similar to those which occur in rheumatoid arthritis, but, in addition, the longitudinal ligaments show a marked tendency to become calcified. As the disease progresses upward, more and more of the vertebrae are involved, until, in advanced cases, complete ankylosis of the entire spine may occur.

These young men present a characteristic appearance. The lumbar curve is flattened and the dorsal curve exaggerated. The chest is flat and rigid, and there is spasm of the deep back muscles. The body is flexed at the hips, the entire spine held rigid, and chest expansion is markedly curtailed. The patient is usually poorly nourished, and there is marked atrophy of the trunk muscles. In advanced cases the spinal column becomes fused into one piece which admits of no motion in any direction, and there is a tendency for the disease to extend into the shoulder and hip joints, with eventual ankylosis in these joints also.

The fact that more than 30 per cent of these patients sooner or later show arthritic changes in the peripheral joints, as well as the spine, and that these changes are indistinguishable from those seen in typical rheumatoid arthritis, lends support to the theory that ankylosing spondylitis is merely a special form of rheumatoid arthritis. However, there are differences. The sex incidence is quite different from that in rheumatoid arthritis. Response to gold therapy is not satisfactory. The agglutination reaction against the hemolytic streptococcus is nearly always negative in rheumatoid spondylitis.

Radiographs are characteristic and establish the diagnosis. Even in early cases there are destructive changes in the sacro-iliac joints. In advanced cases there is demineralization of the bones, obliteration of the small intervertebral articulations, and calcification of the intervertebral ligaments (bamboo spine). The sacro-iliac joints are affected in almost 100 per cent of the cases and are usually the first joints to be involved by the disease.

Treatment of rheumatoid spondylitis is similar to that for rheumatoid arthritis. In both conditions it is highly important that the physician recognize the condition early, in order that proper treatment be instituted before irreversible changes in the joints take place. Early recognition of Marie-Strümpell disease is more difficult that that of rheumatoid arthritis, chiefly because the affected joints show no demonstrable swelling. However, changes in the sacro-iliac joints can be demonstrated roentgenographically early in the disease, and these changes make the diagnosis. In the early stages the treatment is largely medical, and consists in rest, high calorie, high vitamin diet, the use of boards under the mattress, sleeping without a pillow, and special postural and deep-breathing exercises.

Cortisone and corticotropin produce the same striking benefit in rheumatoid spondylitis that they produce in rheumatoid arthritis (see Treatment of Rheumatoid Arthritis). However, there is the same tendency to relapse when treatment with these agents is discontinued.

This form of joint disease often responds well, particularly in the early stages, to deep x-ray therapy. In the more advanced cases a certain amount of pain and ankylosis persists, but the pain may disappear, and, as time goes on, often the stiffness becomes less marked.

In advanced cases, when there is a tendency to flexion deformity of the spine, orthopedic treatment is essential in order to support the spine adequately and prevent

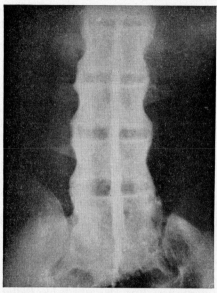

Fig. 186. Radiograph of spine of a young man with advanced ankylosing spondylitis (Marie-Strümpell spine). Notice how the bodies of the vertebrae are fused together by membrane of calcifying fibrous tissue. The sacro-iliac joint markings have been obliterated.

even more marked deformities. Excellent results have been reported from the use of plaster and leather jackets. In both the early and the late cases of Marie-Strümpell disease, active and passive exercises are extremely important, and should be supplemented by breathing exercises to increase the capacity of the thorax.

Psoriatic Arthritis. Psoriatic arthritis, or *psoriasis arthropathica,* is frequently referred to in the literature on arthritis and is considered by some clinicians as a separate disease entity. However, the majority of these patients present a fairly characteristic picture of rheumatoid arthritis. Five to 10 per cent of patients with rheumatoid arthritis are also the victims of psoriasis. Psoriasis usually precedes the arthritis, but the reverse may be true. It is also interesting to note that remissions and exacerbations of arthritis are usually accompanied by remissions and exacerbations of the psoriasis.

The treatment is the same as that for rheumatoid arthritis.

Felty's Syndrome. In 1924 Felty reported what he considered to be a specific type of chronic arthritis, characterized by fever, swollen joints, leukopenia and splenomegaly. In a certain percentage of these cases a palpable liver and general adenopathy were also noted. The clinical picture was much like that of an active Still's disease, except that it occurred in adults. In 60 per cent of the patients Felty noted a pigmentation of the exposed surfaces. In a review of the literature on this subject, Bauer and his co-worker conclude that this condition is essentially a rheumatoid arthritis with associated splenomegaly and leukopenia, and advise that the term "Felty's syndrome" be dropped from the medical literature. At the present time the general trend is to accept the conclusions of Bauer and to consider Felty's syndrome as an atypical form of rheumatoid arthritis.

Reiter's Disease. This syndrome is characterized by subacute or chronic polyarthritis associated with urethritis and conjunctivitis. A low grade fever is usually present, and there may be gastrointestinal symptoms. The condition was first described by Reiter in 1916 under the title of *spirochetosis arthritica*. The urethritis usually precedes the other features of the triad and is characterized by purulent discharge which is free from gonococci. The condition is not related to sexual exposure. Several reports on this syndrome have appeared in the literature based on cases seen in the U. S. Army. The etiology of the condition is unknown, though a certain number of cases have occurred in association with bacillary dysentery. Organisms of the pleuropneumonia-like group have been isolated from the urethra by Dienes and others.

The joint infiltration is usually multiple, affecting chiefly the fingers, knees, feet and ankles. The conjunctivitis is accompanied by abundant pus and may be followed by keratitis or iritis. A certain number of cases are associated with cutaneous lesions, resembling keratodermia blenorrhagica. In recent reports it has been pointed out that the triad of polyarthritis, urethritis and conjunctivitis is not always complete. The disease tends to run in cycles with one or more recurrences. The affected joints may be permanently injured, but this is unusual.

Reiter's syndrome does not respond to penicillin or sulfonamides. Gold salts appear to have been helpful in some cases and good results have been claimed for streptomycin. There are also favorable reports on the effect of cortisone in this disease.

Palindromic Rheumatism. Hench and Rosenberg reported an unusual and oft-recurring form of arthritis to which they gave the name of palindromic rheumatism. In 1944 they reported 34 cases of this syndrome which had been observed in the Mayo Clinic since 1928. The outstanding features are multiple afebrile attacks of acute arthritis and periarthritis with pain, swelling, redness and disability of one or more joints. The attacks appear suddenly and develop rapidly, last a few hours or at most a few days, then disappear completely, to recur repeatedly at long or short irregularly spaced intervals. In spite of the frequent recurrences and the transitory presence of acute or subacute inflammatory exudate in the articular tissues, little or no constitutional reaction or abnormality has been revealed by physical examination or laboratory tests, and no significant functional pathologic or roentgenologic residue occurs, even after years of the disease or scores of attacks.

The *etiology* of palindromic rheumatism has not been determined. Repeated cultures from the joints are sterile. The clinical picture is highly suggestive of some type of allergic reaction, but no definite hypersensitive state has been demonstrated in any of the cases. Biopsies of acutely inflamed joints reveal exudation of polymorphonuclear leukocytes and thickening of the synovial villi. The blood count is essentially normal, and the sedimentation rate is not elevated. Roentgenograms reveal no definite abnormalities.

The *prognosis* with respect to recovery is not good. The great majority of these patients continue to have frequent recurrences of general pain and swelling in spite of all therapeutic measures. Some observers look upon palindromic rheumatism as an atypical form of rheumatoid arthritis.

The treatment is symptomatic. Some of these patients have responded well to gold therapy. The value of hormone treatment has not yet been determined.

RUSSELL L. CECIL

References

Adams, C. H., and Cecil, R. L.: Gold Therapy in Early Rheumatoid Arthritis. Ann. Int. Med., 33: 163, 1950.

Bauer, W.: Rheumatoid Arthritis: The Importance of a Comprehensive Approach in Treatment. J.A.M.A., 138:397, 1948.

———, Bennett, G. A., and Zeller, J. W.: Pathology of Joint Lesions in Patients with Psoriasis and Arthritis. Tr. A. Am. Physicians, 56:349, 1941.

Boland, E. W., and Headley, N. E.: Management of Rheumatoid Arthritis with Smaller (Maintenance) Doses of Cortisone Acetate. J.A.M.A., 144:365, 1950.

Brown, E. M., Frain, J. B., Udell, L., and Hollander, J. L.: Locally Administered Hydrocortisone in the Rheumatic Diseases. A Summary of Its Use in 547 Patients. Am. J. Med., 15:656, 1953.

Brown, R., Bunim, J. J., and McEwen, C.: Differential Sheep-Cell Agglutination Test in Rheumatoid Arthritis. Ann. Rheumat. Dis., 8:299, 1949.

Bunim, J. J., Pechet, M. M., and Bollet, A. J.: Studies on Metacortandralone and Metacortandracin in Rheumatoid Arthritis. J.A.M.A., 157: 311, 1955.

Cecil, R. L., and DeGara, P. F.: The Agglutination Reaction for Hemolytic Streptococci in Rheumatoid Arthritis: Its Significance in Diagnosis and Treatment. Am. J. M. Sc., 211:472, 1946.

———, Kammerer, W. H., and DePrume, F. J.: Gold Salts in the Treatment of Rheumatoid Arthritis; Study of 245 Cases. Ann. Int. Med., 16:811, 1942.

Copeman, W. S. C., and others: A Study of Cortisone and Other Steroids in Rheumatoid Arthritis. Brit. M. J., 2:849, 1950.

Coss, J. A., Jr., and Roots, R. H.: Juvenile Rheumatoid Arthritis; Study of 56 Cases with Note on Skeletal Changes. J. Pediat., 29:143, 1946.

Dienes, L., Ropes, M. W., Smith, W. E., Madoff, S., and Bauer, W.: The Role of Pleuropneumonia-like Organisms in Genito-urinary and Joint Diseases. New England J. Med., 238:509, 563, 1948.

Freyberg, R. H., Block, W. D., and Wells, G. S.: Gold Therapy for Rheumatoid Arthritis; Considerations Based upon Studies of the Metabolism of Gold. Internat. Clin., 1:537, 1942.

Hench, P. S., and Rosenberg, E. F.: Palindromic Rheumatism. Arch. Int. Med., 73:293, 1944.

———, Kendall, E. C., Slocumb, C. H., and Polley, H. F.: Effects of Cortisone Acetate and Pituitary ACTH on Rheumatoid Arthritis, Rheumatic Fever and Certain Other Conditions: Study in Clinical Physiology. Arch. Int. Med., 85:545, 1950.

Hollander, J. L.: Diagnosis and Treatment of Reiter's Syndrome. M. Clin. North America, 30:716, 1946.

———: Comroe's Arthritis and Allied Conditions. Philadelphia, Lea & Febiger, 1953.

Ragan, C., and Tyson, T. L.: Chrysotherapy in Rheumatoid Arthritis; 3-year Study of 142 Cases. Am. J. Med., 1:252, 1946.

Rheumatism and Arthritis: Review of American and English Literature of Recent Years (Tenth Rheumatism Review). Part I. Ann. Int. Med., 39:498, 1953. Part II. Ann. Int. Med., 39:757, 1953.

Ward, L. E., Polley, H. F., Slocumb, C. H., and Hench, P. S.: Cortisone in Treatment of Rheumatoid Arthritis. J.A.M.A., 152:119, 1953.

DEGENERATIVE JOINT DISEASE

(Osteoarthritis, Hypertrophic or Degenerative Arthritis)

Definition. Degenerative joint disease, or osteoarthritis as it is usually called, is a chronic arthropathy occurring usually in elderly people and characterized by hypertrophic and degenerative changes in the bone and cartilage. In some cases there is considerable thickening of the synovial membrane.

Degenerative arthritis occurs in both a generalized and localized form. The generalized form is polyarticular and affects both the large and small joints. It is a senescent process, occurring in middle-aged and elderly people. Its etiology is unknown.

The localized form occurs in one or several joints and may be secondary to trauma, structural abnormalities or previous infections in the joint. It occurs most frequently in the hips, knees or lumbar spine.

Morbid Anatomy. One of the first changes seen is a slight roughening of the cartilaginous surfaces. At the edges of the surface there is more or less lipping and spur formation, the latter consisting in spongy bone covered with cartilage. As these irregularities become more prominent, the cartilage is worn away and the underlying bone is finally laid bare. The exposed bone becomes dense and hard, and takes on a highly polished, eburnated surface. These changes take place gradually and irregularly and in some cases may lead to considerable bony deformity. Ossification may occur in the fibrous tissue about the joints, and even in the ligaments, the tendon insertions and the bursae. The synovial membrane in the beginning is altered little or not at all, but later on it may show thickening and hypertrophy of the villous processes. These changes in the synovial membrane apparently are due to trauma from the bony deformities, to which they are secondary. Small, cartilaginous tumors sometimes form in these hypertrophied villi and, when they become free in the joint cavity, constitute the so-called "joint mice."

In this form of arthritis the joint cavity is

never obliterated. The joint may be partially dislocated, but the synovial membrane does not form adhesions and ankylosis does not occur.

Etiology. Degenerative arthritis is sometimes called senescent arthritis, since it occurs almost exclusively in middle-aged and elderly people. It is particularly common in women at the time of menopause. As the years advance, the wearing quality of the joint is diminished, depending possibly upon some disturbance in the local circulation. Just as the teeth wear down in many old people, so the joints, particularly the weight-bearing joints, are prone to wear out in the middle-aged and elderly.

It is generally supposed that degenerative arthritis has no specific etiology. It is more prevalent in some families than in others; Stecker has shown that heredity is a factor.

Perhaps the most important single etiologic factor is trauma. The trauma may be in the nature of a mild and long-continued irritation or an acute rather violent form, such as might result from an accident or fracture. The trauma to the weight-bearing joints which results from overweight is one of the most frequent causes of degenerative arthritis. In such cases the knees, hips and lumbar spine are the joints which suffer most.

Physical defects, such as curvature of the spine or abnormalities of the vertebrae, predispose to hypertrophic changes in the spine of middle-aged patients.

Faulty posture predisposes to hypertrophic arthritis by putting an unnatural strain on the joint, or by bringing about unequal pressure on the joint surfaces. Incorrect sitting or standing places a strain on the lower spine, and an improper gait puts an unnatural tension on the joints of the leg, particularly on the knee and ankle joints. Obese patients nearly all have a bad posture. The lower abdomen is abnormally prominent, the upper back is rounded, and the shoulders pushed forward. The feet are abducted, producing a distinct tendency toward knock-knee. This posture leads to a strain on the lumbar spine, as well as on the knees and feet, a condition which, of course, is accentuated by the overweight of the patient.

Occupation has an important bearing on the etiology of degenerative arthritis. Laborers and mechanics are affected most often. Any joint which has been subjected to constant strenuous usage is apt to develop osteoarthritic changes as the patient advances to middle age. This is seen frequently in sportsmen, particularly those who have engaged in the more active sports, such as football, baseball, tennis and high jumping.

Exposure is possibly a predisposing factor in degenerative arthritis, though certainly to a less extent than in rheumatoid arthritis. Elderly people who lead hard and exposed lives appear to be more prone to degenerative arthritis than those whose circumstances are more fortunate.

Symptoms and Physical Signs. The onset of hypertrophic arthritis is insidious. The patient, usually middle-aged or elderly, first notices a slight stiffness in the affected joint which gradually becomes more uncomfortable, especially during exercise. The disease progresses more slowly than rheumatoid arthritis. As time goes on, however, the symptoms become more marked and there may be constant pain in the joints involved. The joints most frequently affected are the hips, knees, fingers and vertebrae, although, under certain conditions, any joint in the body may undergo hypertrophic changes.

On physical examination the patient is usually middle-aged and often overweight, and the weight-bearing joints are the ones generally affected. The posture is often bad, and there may be some degree of flatfoot. The affected joints are rarely swollen and never ankylosed. On movement, some crepitation is usually noted. Occasionally there may be an increase of fluid in the joint cavity. When the affected joint is palpated, it may be possible, if the joint is superficial, to feel the hypertrophied bony outgrowths around the margins of the joint.

Diagnosis. The diagnosis of primary osteoarthritis can usually be made without much difficulty. The age of the patient and the gradual onset of pain and stiffness in one or more joints without soft tissue swelling are almost sufficient evidence on which to make a presumptive diagnosis. The presence of crepitation in the joint gives additional support, and the finding of the characteristic bony changes in the roentgenogram confirms the diagnosis. The sedimentation rate should be normal or only slightly elevated. If symptoms are limited to one joint, the history of trauma should make one suspicious of an osteoarthritis even before roentgenograms have been examined. An experienced internist will always suspect an osteoarthritis of the knees when an obese middle-aged woman limps into the consultation room!

Some confusion may arise in those cases which are often labeled "mixed arthritis," in which osteoarthritis is superimposed on a preceding rheumatoid arthritis. It is a fact that the two great types of chronic arthritis, the rheumatoid and the degenerative, can be present in the same joint, one form being superimposed on the other. It is also important to remember that a mild osteoarthritis can be present in a joint without causing symptoms, and that in many cases of osteoarthritis of the lumbar spine the pain is due, not so much to the osteoarthritis, as to bad posture, developmental abnormalities, spinal curvature, and so on.

Laboratory Findings. The sedimentation rate of the red blood cells is normal or only slightly accelerated. The patient's serum reveals no agglutinins for the hemolytic streptococcus or for sensitized sheep cells.

Roentgenographic Examination. In hypertrophic arthritis, characteristic findings can be made out in the radiographs fairly early in the disease. In incipient cases these changes take the form of bony lipping and spur formation along the articular margins of the bone. In the later stages the joint interspace is narrowed and there is erosion of the articular bone and alteration in the shape of the articulating surfaces. The surface itself, however, remains well defined, and there is some condensation of bone immediately below the articular surface. The periarticular lipping becomes more marked as the disease progresses.

Differential Diagnosis. The differential diagnosis of osteoarthritis from rheumatoid arthritis has been discussed in the chapter on Rheumatoid Arthritis. Osteoarthritis is occasionally confused with gout, though this should rarely happen. The clinical course of gout is very characteristic, with its paroxysmal and intermittent attacks; the presence of tophi and an elevated uric acid level in the blood should serve to identify it. Secondary osteoarthritis is frequently seen in patients with chronic tophaceous gout. Osteoarthritis should never be confused with a Charcot joint, which develops suddenly with a large effusion and is usually free from pain, tenderness and heat. The x-ray findings are quite different in the two conditions, and positive Wassermann and spinal fluid reactions should identify the Charcot joint.

The physician should never forget the possibility of metastatic malignant disease as a cause of pain in the cervical or lumbar spine or in the hips or pelvis. Routine roentgenograms will prevent such an unfortunate error.

Prognosis. There is no "cure" for an osteoarthritic joint; that is to say, the destruction of cartilage and the hypertrophic changes in the bone are permanent. However, the progress in osteoarthritis is usually slow, and the prognosis is much better than in rheumatoid arthritis. In many cases the patient's discomfort can be completely relieved by proper treatment, even though the pathologic changes in the joint persist. This is particularly true of the knees and back, where weight reduction, physiotherapy and orthopedic measures often give marked relief.

Treatment. The successful treatment of osteoarthritis depends upon a correct evaluation of the etiologic factors. Perhaps the most important feature of the treatment is rest for the affected joints. In obese patients, weight reduction is best accomplished by a low calorie diet. Diet itself plays no part in the treatment of osteoarthritis except in relation to obesity. Physiotherapy and other forms of heat give much relief, but care must be taken in massaging affected joints lest trauma be induced over the hypertrophied margins of bone. Moist heat appears to be more efficacious than dry heat. Deep x-ray therapy has been recommended by some writers, but in the author's experience is rarely effective except in some cases of osteospondylitis.

Moderate *exercises* are helpful and should be repeated two or three times daily. Several short walks are preferable to one long one. Analgesics are most useful, especially aspirin either alone or in combination with acetophenetidin. Narcotics are rarely necessary, though one may encounter an occasional osteoarthritis of the hip which occasions excessive pain.

Cortisone and *corticotropin* may give some temporary relief in osteoarthritis, but their use is not recommended. In this type of joint disease the pain can usually be relieved by less drastic measures such as rest, heat and aspirin.

Intra-articular injection of *hydrocortisone* is worth trial in joints that fail to respond to simpler measures. Painful knees are particularly amenable to this treatment. Sometimes the discomfort will disappear for several weeks after such treatment. (See Treatment of Rheumatoid Arthritis.)

Phenylbutazone (Butazolidin), 100 mg. tablet four times a day, will sometimes control pain when aspirin has failed. However, the incidence of toxic reactions is too high to justify its prolonged administration.

SPECIAL FORMS

Hypertrophic arthritis occurs in a number of well recognized clinical forms.

OSTEOARTHRITIS OF THE HIP

(*Morbus Coxae Senilis*)

This form of osteoarthritis occurs in the hip. It usually develops in middle age, in patients well past 50, though occasionally it is encountered in the forties.

Etiology. Osteoarthritis of the hip is often referable to trauma in the form of either an actual injury or repeated minor injuries, such as might result from constant overuse of a joint. Congenital malformations account for some cases. The condition, as the title indicates, is usually monarticular, though occasionally one sees both hips affected.

Symptoms. The patient is middle-aged or elderly. In the early stages the patient with osteoarthritis of the hip complains of pain in the distribution of the sciatic, obturator or anterior crural nerve. At this stage it may be mistaken for neuritis. In the later stages the pain is related more definitely to the hip joint, with radiating pain to the groin and to the knee joint. In some cases the symptoms in the knee joint are so pronounced that the physician is led to a mistaken diagnosis of disease in the knee, while the affected hip joint entirely escapes attention.

The patient walks with a limp, with his weight on the unaffected side. On palpation of the joint in a well developed case, crepitation is readily made out. On passive movement of the hip joint, rotation, abduction and other movements may be much limited.

Diagnosis. The diagnosis of osteoarthritis of the hip can be made without much trouble from the symptoms and physical signs. A middle-aged or elderly man complaints of increasing pain and stiffness in one hip. He may give a history of a fall or some other trauma affecting the hip joint. If, on examination, crepitation is made out, the presumptive diagnosis is morbus coxae senilis. As in other forms of degenerative arthritis, the final diagnosis is made by roentgenogram. Radiographs disclose the characteristic lipping and spur formation, with thinning of the joint space. Later on, degenerative

changes occur in the bone. In longstanding cases there may be some deformity resulting from absorption of the head and shortening of the neck of the femur.

Treatment. The treatment of osteoarthritis of the hip is difficult and unsatisfactory. As long as the pain is not too severe, rest and other conservative measures are all that should be attempted. Extension traction to the lower leg is an effective method of relieving pain and correcting deformity. Relief of pain is proportional to the amount of protection from weight-bearing, hence the benefit from rest, crutches and cane. When the pain and disability are severe, surgery may become necessary. In such cases, arthrodesis gives complete relief, but leaves the patient with a stiff hip joint. Plastic operations, particularly the vitallium cup operation, are popular with some surgeons. Obturator neurectomy will often relieve the patient, at least partially, of severe pain.

HEBERDEN'S NODES

One of the mildest and commonest forms of osteoarthritis is the so-called "Heberden's node." These nodes begin to make their appearance in middle life, particularly in the female sex, and manifest themselves as bony outgrowths around the bases of the terminal phalanges of the fingers. They are more prone to develop in people who work hard with their hands.

Symptoms. The development of Heberden's nodes, like that of other forms of osteoarthritis, is slow and insidious and causes little inconvenience; usually it does not even interfere with the normal movements of the joints. Many times they are free from tenderness and pain. Sometimes, however, particularly in the early stages, they may occasion a good deal of pain and some limitation of movement. At times the nodes undergo exacerbations and become swollen and tender. The lesion may appear on only one finger, but as a rule several or all of the distal phalangeal joints are involved.

Treatment. Painful Heberden's nodes are often relieved by resting the hand as much as possible, and by the local use of heat. In this connection the paraffin bath is often helpful. The method of applying paraffin is as follows:

Equipment. A candy or fat thermometer
2 to 4 pounds of parawax
1 piece of oil silk, 12 x 14 inches

1 square of absorbent cotton and piece of wool.

Melt parawax over slow fire, then remove from stove and allow it to cool until the thermometer registers 110° to 120° F. Having soaked the hand for about three minutes in hot water, and while still wet, dip in and out of the parawax twelve to fifteen times. Quickly wrap oil silk about parawax which has accumulated on hand, then around that the cotton, and a piece of wool about the whole so that the heat may be retained. Let hand rest quietly in the paraffin pack for about an hour. Then remove the wax, which may be used for the next application.

MENOPAUSAL ARTHRITIS OR ARTHROSIS

This type of arthritis occurs in two forms: (1) in women who have been subject to artificial menopause by hysterectomy or deep x-ray therapy. In such patients, the disease may appear even in the early thirties. (2) In women during or immediately after normal menopause. The age of onset in these cases is usually between 45 and 55.

In most cases the symptoms of discomfort are most noticeable in the knees, fingers and lumbar spine, and x-ray examination will show, particularly in the middle-aged patient, the usual hypertrophic changes in the bones. Many students object to the term "menopausal arthritis" and believe that all these cases should be classified as degenerative arthritis. There are some cases, however, particularly those seen in younger women, in which careful examination reveals no signs of osteoarthritis. For such cases the term "menopausal arthrosis" has been suggested.

Symptoms develop insidiously, the first signs of discomfort usually being in the knees. A large percentage of these patients show Heberden's nodes on the distal phalangeal joints. The progress of the disease is slow, and there is little tendency toward involvement of other joints.

Treatment. Menopausal arthralgia, when unaccompanied by osteoarthritic changes, is often relieved by estrogenic therapy, 2000 to 10,000 rat units twice a week, administered every three to five days. As the patient improves, oral treatment can be substituted for the parenteral injections. Stilbestrol, 0.5 to 1 mg. in tablet form, sometimes gives good results. It is much cheaper than the natural hormone, but is more likely to cause gastrointestinal symptoms. When menopausal arthralgia is accompanied by osteoarthritis, the therapeutic measures already described should be instituted in addition to the hormone therapy.

HYPERTROPHIC SPONDYLITIS

The vertebrae of most people past 50 years of age will show some evidence of this condition. The bodies of the vertebrae undergo more or less hypertrophy and lipping at their bases, and there may be some ossification of the ligaments. The articular processes of the vertebrae may be enlarged, eburnated and marked by bony outgrowths. Actual ankylosis does not occur, but there may be considerable limitation of movement due to the marked bony changes.

This condition develops slowly, usually without much pain. The bony outgrowths may press on spinal nerve roots, however, and produce pain and paresthesias. Other joints may show bony changes, particularly the hips and knees.

Treatment. The treatment of hypertrophic spondylitis should be that of osteoarthritis in general; but if the discomfort persists in spite of physiotherapy and other symptomatic remedies, traction and other orthopedic measures may be necessary. Many of these patients become dependent on a strong back brace for the relief of pain.

Osteospondylitis of the cervical spine is often associated with attacks of severe radicular pain. In such cases, cervical immobilization and traction are indicated. Roentgen therapy is worth the trial if other measures fail.

RUSSELL L. CECIL

References

Bennett, G. A., and Bauer, W.: Joint Changes Resulting from Patellar Displacement and Their Relation to Degenerative Joint Disease. J. Bone & Joint Surg., 19:667, 1937.

Cecil, R. L., and Archer, B. H.: Arthritis of Menopause. J.A.M.A., 84:75, 1925.

Heberden, W.: Commentaries on History and Cure of Diseases. London, T. Payne, 1802.

Stockman, R.: Rheumatism and Arthritis. Edinburgh, W. Green and Son, Ltd., 9:113, 1930.

ARTHRITIS ASSOCIATED WITH DISTURBANCES OF METABOLISM

The arthritic manifestations associated with gout and other diseases of metabolism are discussed in the chapters which deal with these diseases.

NEUROGENIC ARTHROPATHY

(Charcot Joint)

The Charcot joint occurs most frequently as a complication of tabes dorsalis, though it is also seen in association with syringomyelia and other conditions which compress or injure the spinal cord. The Charcot joint is commoner in men than in women and develops usually after the age of 40. Trauma appears to be the most important contributing cause, loss of deep sensation the essential etiologic factor.

The pathology of Charcot joint consists primarily of decalcification of bone with gradual destruction of the joint surfaces. This is followed by hypertrophic overgrowth of bone about the margins of the joint.

The characteristic features of the Charcot joint are the absence of pain (though there are exceptions) and the remarkable hypermotility of the affected joint. The knees and the spine are most frequently affected. Roentgenograms reveal marked destruction of the articular surface and of the underlying bone with compensatory hypertrophy of the bone and cartilage.

Diagnosis is made from the marked hypermotility of the joint, the absence of pain and the x-ray findings. When the Charcot joint is secondary to tabes, the presence of rigid pupils, absent knee jerks and positive findings in the blood and spinal fluid will corroborate the diagnosis. Charcot joint is sometimes confused with osteoarthritis, but the differentiation should not be difficult.

Treatment is not very satisfactory. Penicillin has no value. In early cases, a fusion operation may be successful. Braces and splints are necessary for protecting the joint against further damage.

NEOPLASMS OF THE JOINTS

Benign or malignant new growths involving any of the structures of a joint produce symptoms which may simulate those of arthritis. Benign soft tissue tumors, such as lipoma, hemangioma or cystic degeneration of the external semilunar cartilage of the knee, excite mechanical disorders such as limitation of motion, locking, and synovial effusion.

Single or multiple xanthomas arising in the synovium (usually in the knee) produce symptoms similar to those of any low grade synovitis. The synovial fluid, which is often yellowish-brown, is sterile. The blood cholesterol is usually elevated. Synovioma is a similar but definitely malignant tumor.

Bone tumors occurring near joints, such as giant-cell tumors, multiple or single bone cysts, osteogenetic sarcoma and metastatic carcinoma, cause stiffness, swelling, pain, limitation of motion, and even deformity if destruction of bone has been sufficient to produce a pathologic fracture.

Although the disability may be great, there is usually little local heat or redness. With malignant tumors the general condition of the patient rapidly deteriorates.

The **treatment** of joint neoplasms is surgical and orthopedic.

RUSSELL L. CECIL

MECHANICAL DERANGEMENTS OF JOINTS

Traumatic Arthritis. Any injury to the cartilage, bone or ligaments of a joint is apt to produce persistent or transient pain, swelling and limitation of motion. When the joint is badly sprained, temporary effusion of fluid may take place in the joint cavity. Traumatic arthritis is often an important predisposing factor in the development of a localized osteoarthritis.

The *treatment* of traumatic arthritis consists in rest, physiotherapy and orthopedic measures if necessary.

Joint Disturbances Secondary to Abnormal Postural Strain. Pronation of the feet, poor posture and congenital or acquired deformities produce undue strain on the weight-bearing joints and, if not corrected, may in the course of time lead to the development of secondary osteoarthritis. Deformities, such as congenitally flat feet, knock-knees and spinal scoliosis, are particularly important predisposing factors. Obesity is another common cause of joint disturbance secondary to postural strain.

The *treatment* consists in correction of the postural strain.

RUSSELL L. CECIL

MISCELLANEOUS FORMS OF ARTHRITIS

Arthritis of Serum Sickness. This form of arthritis is described in detail in the chapter on Serum Sickness (p. 487).

Intermittent Hydrarthrosis. This is a rare and peculiar condition of the joints characterized by acute, regularly recurring effusions of fluid into the joint cavity. The etiology of this disease is still obscure. There is some evidence to support the theory that it is an allergic manifestation. Schlesinger has pointed out the similarity between intermittent hydrarthrosis and angioneurotic edema. Féré and Garrod have each reported a case of intermittent hydrarthrosis in which the disease was associated with generalized urticaria, and Burchard refers to a case in which hydrops occurred in an asthmatic.

The striking features of intermittent hydrops are its periodic recurrence and its tendency to affect the knee joint. The exact regularity of the recurrences is the most interesting feature, the usual interval being ten or eleven days. When several joints are involved, the swelling may appear in all simultaneously or in one earlier than in the others. The average duration of each attack is four to five days. During the attack the joint is distended with fluid, and the patient is rarely able to use the extremity because of the resulting pain. In the interval between attacks the joint in most cases is practically normal, although in some patients there may be a residual stiffness. A slight rise in temperature and a leukocytosis have been reported in some cases. According to Miller and Lewin, one or both knees have been involved in every case reported in the literature. Occasionally, additional joints are implicated, such as the wrist or hip. Some cases progress into typical rheumatoid arthritis.

The *diagnosis* is comparatively easy and is based on the following criteria:

1. Acute attacks of effusion of fluid into the joint (usually a knee) occur at regular intervals of ten to eleven days.

2. After a period of four to five days, fluid disappears from the joint almost as rapidly as it forms, leaving the joint practically normal.

3. Puncture of the joint reveals clear and practically normal joint fluid.

The *treatment* of intermittent hydrops is rather unsatisfactory. Fortunately a certain number of patients recover spontaneously. During the acute attack the patient should rest in bed or in an easy chair. Local discomfort may be relieved by hot applications and acetylsalicylic acid. In view of its close similarity to rheumatoid arthritis, gold therapy or one of the steroids should be given a trial in every case. Krida has reported complete and permanent cure by synovectomy.

Pulmonary Osteoarthropathy. The arthritic manifestations of pulmonary osteoarthropathy are discussed in the chapter on this disease (p. 1467).

Hysterical Joints. Joint symptoms can occur without any organic basis. Partial or complete fixation of a knee in full extension or a foot in equinovarus may be a purely hysterical phenomenon. Other patients, especially compensation cases, may present many of the features of arthritis of the spine or those of an internal derangement of the knee. Subjective complaints overshadow physical findings. Swelling and local heat are absent. Tenderness is often too acute to be genuine. Typically hysterical conditions, such as paralysis or paresthesias, may occur in the same patient.

The *treatment* is that for hysteria (p. 1662).

Psychogenic rheumatism is closely related to the hysterical joint. During World War II psychogenic rheumatism was an extremely common finding in many hospitals and field areas. Various emotional stresses, particularly in a psychoneurotic person, can induce psychogenic rheumatism. It is characterized by arthralgia, stiffness and aching in the muscles and tendons, and other rheumatic symptoms which resemble those of either arthritis or fibrositis. Absence of joint changes on clinical and x-ray examination, with normal laboratory findings and good general health in a psychoneurotic patient, makes the diagnosis probable. More difficult is the differentiation from fibrositis. However, lack of consistent localization of symptoms, lack of relief from analgesics, and failure to improve in spite of all therapy are useful points in differentiation. The treatment should be directed toward relieving the emotional conflict, rationalization of problems and correction of the psychoneurosis.

RUSSELL L. CECIL

References

Berger, H.: Intermittent Hydrarthrosis with an Allergic Basis. J.A.M.A., *112*:2402, 1939.

Boland, E. W.: Psychogenic Rheumatism; The Musculoskeletal Expression of Psychoneurosis. Ann. Rheumat. Dis., *6*:195, 1947; also, California Med., *68*:273, 1948.

Hench, P. S.: Differentiation Between "Psychogenic Rheumatism" and True Rheumatic Disease. Postgrad. Med., *1*:460, 1947.

Krida, A.: Intermittent Hydrarthrosis of the Knee Joint. J. Bone & Joint Surg., *15*:449, 1933.

THE PAINFUL SHOULDER

One of the most prevalent ailments in the field of rheumatic disease is the painful shoulder. Though pain in the shoulder can be caused by a wide variety of factors, the great majority of cases will fall into one of four groups:

1. Calcific tendinitis (subacromial bursitis).
2. Adhesive peritendinitis (frozen shoulder).
3. Arthritis of the shoulder.
4. Shoulder-hand syndrome.

CALCIFIC TENDINITIS
(*Subacromial Bursitis*)

Calcific tendinitis of the shoulder is a fairly common condition, manifesting itself as a sudden and intense pain over the acromial region of the shoulder joint. Less frequently it occurs in a chronic form.

The calcareous deposit takes place primarily in the tendon tissue. Following certain degenerative changes in the fibers, calcific granules accumulate in the injured tissue and eventually form a deposit large enough to be readily demonstrable by x-ray. The tendons of insertion of the supraspinatus and the infraspinatus muscles are most frequently involved. When exposed, this deposit has the appearance of a cyst or "sterile furuncle" in the floor of the subdeltoid bursa.

Trauma and the aging process are important etiologic factors. Cultures from the pasty contents of the cyst are invariably sterile.

Symptoms. When the calcific deposit produces sufficient tension, pain results and may be very intense. The shoulder is immobilized and there is marked tenderness over the great tuberosity. X-rays reveal the opaque rounded shadow of the deposit overlying the head of the humerus.

Diagnosis is based on the local symptoms, with corroboration from the x-ray findings.

Treatment. Calcific bursitis in the acute form tends to be self-limiting, the pain being relieved when the calcareous sac ruptures into the bursa. Once the contents of the sac have been discharged, the foreign material is quickly absorbed by the wall of the bursa. This explians why roentgenograms taken weeks or months later fail to reveal any residual chalk.

During the painful stage local heat and other palliative measures are indicated. Roentgen therapy is popular and, when administered in divided doses not exceeding a total of 600 roentgen units, is often accompanied by rapid and spectacular disappearance of pain. However, control cases which have received no roentgen therapy do just about as well. In either case the end results are usually excellent, with complete restoration of function in the affected shoulder.

When conservative therapy fails, irrigation of the bursal cavity by needle may be tried or, better still, incision and drainage.

Chronic Type of Calcareous Bursitis. In some instances, calcific bursitis takes a mild chronic form. In McLaughlin's series, this represented only 5 per cent of all cases of calcific deposit.

The prognosis, however, is excellent, even in subacute and chronic cases. Palliative measures and maintenance of shoulder function are indicated. Roentgen therapy provides no beneficial effect. In rare instances surgery may have to be instituted in order to restore complete range of motion.

ADHESIVE PERITENDINITIS
(*Frozen Shoulder, Adhesive Capsulitis, Periarthritis of Shoulder, Adhesive Bursitis*)

Adhesive peritendinitis or "frozen shoulder" is quite distinct from calcific bursitis. The pathologic change is one of obliteration of the subdeltoid bursa by adhesions, and of adhesive inflammation between the joint capsule and the peripheral articular cartilage. It may originate from inflammatory changes in the long head of the biceps in the bicipital groove. These chronic inflammatory changes result in loss of the normal gliding function of the constituents of the shoulder girdle. The cause of this condition is not always clear. Some cases undoubtedly result from trauma, others from prolonged rest or immobilization of the shoulder joint. A considerable number follow an attack of coronary thrombosis.

Symptoms. The onset is gradual, with slowly increasing pain and stiffness in the affected joint. Occasionally the condition is bilateral, or the involvement of one is followed weeks or months later by implication of the other shoulder. The pain may be quite severe and persistent, and it is not unusual for it to extend up into the neck or down the arm to the hand. There is marked loss of function, particularly noticeable with lateral abduction and external rotation of the arm. Increasing atrophy of the muscles of the shoulder girdle is an almost constant finding. Roentgen ray examination reveals atrophy of the greater tuberosity and occasionally a calcific deposit in cases which have followed an attack of acute bursitis.

Diagnosis is usually easy, but the examiner must keep in mind other possibilities, such as calcific bursitis and the shoulder-hand syndrome. Various writers have pointed out the occurrence of occasional cases where accurate classification is impossible.

Treatment. The treatment of frozen shoulder is not entirely satisfactory. It requires great patience on the part of both the physician and the patient. Rest and sedatives are indicated to relieve pain and muscle spasm. As the pain eases, a gradually increasing program of exercises is introduced. Manipulation of the shoulder under anesthesia may be tried in stubborn cases, but is rarely necessary. X-ray therapy can be employed, but is rarely so helpful as it is in the acute calcific deposits. In the writer's experience cortisone has been disappointing. Hydrocortisone, when injected directly into the shoulder joint, may be of real value and the same is true of intramuscular or oral use of phenylbutazone.

ARTHRITIS OF THE SHOULDER

Arthritis of various types may occur in the shoulder in both the acute or chronic form. Specific infectious arthritis is usually acute, and the exciting micro-organism can be recovered from the joint exudate. Chronic arthritis of the shoulder may be either a typical monarticular osteoarthritis secondary to trauma or the initial manifestation of rheumatoid disease. When rheumatoid arthritis shows itself primarily in the shoulder, it may easily be mistaken for peritendinitis

until roentgen studies and other laboratory procedures reveal the true nature of the condition.

Osteoarthritis of the shoulder is not an uncommon finding in elderly patients. The writer recalls a case in an aging street car conductor, the result of ringing up fares for thirty years!

THE SHOULDER-HAND SYNDROME

(Reflex Dystrophy of the Upper Extremity, Post-infarctional Sclerodactylia)

Definition. The shoulder-hand syndrome is a clinical disorder of the upper extremity, characterized by pain and stiffness in the shoulder girdle, and puffy swelling and pain in the homolateral hand. In chronic cases the puffiness in the hand is often followed by digital contractures.

Etiology. This syndrome appears to be one of a group of shoulder ailments which may or may not be associated with pain, swelling and deformity in the hand. Other related conditions are causalgia, Sudeck's atrophy, postinfarctional shoulder, posthemiplegic and postherpetic syndromes, shoulder-hand pain secondary to cervical osteoarthritis, and a few others. Students of these conditions are now disposed to look upon all of them as mediated by similar neurovascular mechanisms. The group as a whole are spoken of as reflex dystrophies. The symptoms appear to result from vasomotor trophic disturbances arising from reflex stimulation of the sympathetic nerve supply. Any one of a number of etiologic agents may act as the stimulus. In the so-called idiopathic type of shoulder-hand syndrome no causative factor is apparent. In Steinbrocker's study of 42 cases, 11 were idiopathic and 9 followed myocardial infarction. Other common precursors were trauma and hemiplegia.

Steinbrocker divides the reflex dystrophies of the upper extremity into incomplete and complete forms. Under *incomplete* or abortive forms there are contractures of the palmar fascia, painful vasospasm or vasodilatation of the hand, swelling and atrophy of the hand, and painful disability of the shoulder. Under the *complete* form comes the typical shoulder-hand syndrome.

Symptoms. The first manifestations of the condition are usually pain and stiffness in the shoulder. Soon the pain and stiffness spread to the homolateral hand and fingers, usually without implication of the elbow. In some cases the shoulder and hand are affected simultaneously. The pain and limitation of motion in the shoulder joint are quite marked and similar to that observed in bursitis. The hand and fingers are diffusely puffy, brawny and sometimes of a dusky red hue. The fingers are moderately flexed and closure of the hand is painful and incomplete. The syndrome usually runs a rather chronic course, with gradual abatement of the disability in the shoulder and decrease of swelling in the hand. However, as the swelling subsides there is a tendency toward progression of the stiffness and deformity in the fingers, with atrophy of the muscles and subcutaneous tissue of the hand. Eventually the picture may resemble Dupuytren's contracture. At this stage the skin of the hand is tight, smooth and glossy, and the interossei show marked atrophy.

Fortunately, all cases do not progress to deformity. Either spontaneously or as the result of treatment, the symptoms and signs gradually disappear, leaving behind no evidence of ankylosis or deformity. In the early stages, roentgenograms are negative, but as time goes on, diffuse or patchy osteoporosis of the bones is demonstrable.

Diagnosis of the shoulder-hand syndrome in the complete form is simple enough. In the incomplete form, this condition resembles frozen shoulder or subacromial bursitis. The latter is readily spotted if roentgenograms reveal a calcareous deposit. Shoulder-hand syndrome is more probable if there is history or other evidence of cardiac or pulmonary disease. Other conditions which may simulate the shoulder-hand syndrome are localized rheumatoid arthritis, scalenus anticus syndrome and scleroderma.

Treatment is difficult and often disappointing. The usual forms of physiotherapy such as heat, massage and manipulative procedures are not recommended. Spontaneous and complete recovery does occur in some cases but only after the lapse of several months. Local procaine injections give only temporary relief. Cortisone in large doses (200 mg. daily) is a fairly satisfactory method of therapy but has to be continued for months. The dosage, of course, must be reduced to the minimal maintenance amount after the first ten or twelve days of high level administration. Steinbrocker has found that block of the stellate ganglion with procaine gives very satisfactory results. If sympathetic blocks fail to give relief, periarterial sympathectomy or ganglionectomy may be necessary. Complete recovery follows either of these surgical procedures in a majority of cases.

RUSSELL L. CECIL

References

Bayles, T. B., Judson, W. E., and Potter, T. A.: Reflex Sympathetic Dystrophy of the Upper Extremity (Hand-Shoulder Syndrome). J.A.M.A., 144: 537, 1950.
Bosworth, B. M.: Calcium Deposits in Shoulder and Subacromial Bursitis: Survey of 12,122 Shoulders. J.A.M.A., 166:2477, 1941.
Codman, E. A.: The Shoulder: Rupture of the Supraspinatus Tendon and Other Lesions in or about the Subacromial Bursa. Boston, Thomas Todd Co., 1934.
Howorth, M. B.: Calcification of the Tendon Cuff of the Shoulder. Surg., Gynec. & Obst., 80:337, 1945.
Jesperson, K.: Cervical Sympathetic Block in Periarthrosis of Shoulder Joint with Secondary Reflex Dystrophy. Ann. Rheumat. Dis., 8:220, 1949.
Key, J. A.: Calcium Deposits in the Vicinity of the Shoulder and Other Joints. Ann. Surg., 129:737, 1949.
McLaughlin, H. L.: Lesions of the Musculo-tendinous Cuff of the Shoulder. I. The Exposure and Treatment of Tears with Retraction. J. Bone & Joint Surg., 26:31, 1944.
———: Lesions of the Musculo-tendinous Cuff of the Shoulder: II. Differential Diagnosis of Rupture. J.A.M.A., 128:563, 1945.
———: Lesions of the Musculo-tendinous Cuff of the Shoulder: III. Observations on the Pathology, Course and Treatment of Calcified Deposits. Ann. Surg., 124:354, 1946.
Patterson, R. L., and Darrach, W.: Treatment of Acute Bursitis by Needle Irrigation. J. Bone & Joint Surg., 19:993, 1937.
Steinbrocker, O.: Shoulder-Hand Syndrome: Associated Painful Hemolateral Disability of Shoulder and Hand with Swelling and Atrophy of Hand. Am. J. Med., 3:402, (Oct.) 1947.
———, Spitzer, N., and Friedman, H. H.: The Shoulder-Hand Syndrome in Reflex Dystrophy of the Upper Extremity. Ann. Int. Med., 29:22, 1948
Steindler, A.: The Traumatic Deformities and Disabilities of the Upper Extremity. Springfield, Ill., Charles C Thomas, 1946.

DISEASES OF THE BONES

OSTEOPOROSIS

Definition. Osteoporosis is a condition wherein the bone mass is decreased as the result of a decrease in the rate of bone matrix formation. Since bone matrix is composed in part of nitrogenous tissues, osteoporosis is rather a disorder of protein than of calcium and phosphorus metabolism. Osteoporosis is clearly separable from the other metabolic bone diseases in that there is no failure of matrix to calcify (as in osteomalacia), nor is there increased bone destruction (as in osteitis fibrosa cystica).

The authors designate as "metabolic" bone diseases those in which all the bone tissue is involved (to a greater or lesser degree) and humoral factors are thought to play a part. These include osteoporosis, fragilitas ossium, osteomalacia, and osteitis fibrosa cystica generalisata.

Classification. The accompanying table, modified from that of Albright and Reifenstein, presents a classification of the causes of osteoporosis. The various categories will be considered *seriatim* under Etiology.

Causes of Osteoporosis

I. DEFECT IN OSTEOBLASTS
    A. Loss of strains on skeleton: atrophy of disuse
    B. Lack of estrogen
        1. Postmenopausal state
        2. Congenital hypoestrinism: ovarian agenesis

II. DEFECT IN MATRIX
    A. Absolute or relative inadequacy of nitrogenous components
        1. Malnutrition
        2. Hyperthyroidism
        3. Diabetes
    B. Inability to retain or form matrix from nitrogenous components
        1. Hypovitaminosis C
        2. Cushing's syndrome
        3. "Alarm reaction"
        4. Cortisone and ACTH therapy
        5. Androgen lack
            (a) Eunuchoidism
            (b) Senility
    D. DEFECT UNKNOWN
        1. Congenital: osteogenesis imperfecta
        2. Acromegaly
        3. "Idiopathic" osteoporosis

Etiology. A deficiency of bone matrix formation may result from deficient osteoblastic activity, or from a lack of, or inability to retain, the essential nitrogenous components of which the matrix is composed. In most cases of osteoporosis, one or the other of these factors appears to be at fault; in some the mechanism of the disorder is entirely obscure. The normal strains on the skeleton provide an essential stimulus to osteoblastic activity, and their diminution by immobilization leads to disuse atrophy of bone. This form of osteoporosis may be localized to the immobilized parts of the skeleton; all other forms have a generalized distribution. Estrogenic hormones likewise stimulate osteoblastic activity, and cessation of their secretion is associated with postmenopausal osteoporosis, the most common form of osteoporosis. In ovarian agenesis, in which estrogenic hormones are never present, osteoporosis appears at an early age.

When the structural materials essential for matrix formation are present in inadequate amounts (as in starvation) or are diverted towards caloric requirements (as in hyperthyroidism or in uncontrolled diabetes), osteoporosis may appear. It is likely that other factors contribute to the production of the osteoporosis of hyperthyroidism.

In hypovitaminosis C, there is a generalized defect in the formation of cement substances, the counterpart of which in the bones is poor matrix formation, and hence osteoporosis. The "carbohydrate-active" steroids of the adrenal cortex have the property of blocking anabolism (or causing catabolism) of protein tissues. This property helps to explain the osteoporosis seen when such steroids are present in excess, as in Cushing's syndrome, the "alarm reaction" or prolonged ACTH and cortisone therapy.

Androgenic steroids, on the other hand, have the property of producing anabolism of protein tissues, and lack of such steroids largely accounts for the osteoporosis seen in males with eunuchoidism and possibly also that of senility.

There remains a group of patients with osteoporosis for which no adequate explanation has been found. The first of these is a congenital disorder, fragilitas ossium, or "brittle bone disease." It is dealt with in a following chapter. In acromegaly, overproduction of thyroid or adrenal cortical hormones, and, in some cases, the associated hypogonadism, may cause the osteoporosis which is commonly present. However, the action of growth

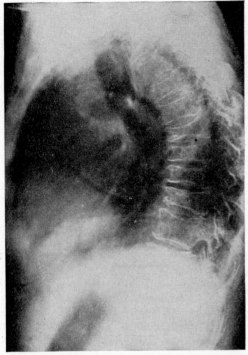

Fig. 187. Postmenopausal osteoporosis. Note "codfish" vertebrae, bulging of intervertebral disks, collapse of thoracic vertebrae and generalized radiolucency.

hormone or of other factors not yet elucidated cannot be ruled out.

Finally, in an interesting group of patients with "idiopathic" osteoporosis, none of the mechanisms discussed above can be implicated. In men the condition may follow a mild accident; in women it frequently follows a normal pregnancy.

Incidence. Osteoporosis is the most widespread of the metabolic bone diseases. As it is an almost "physiologic" accompaniment of old age in either sex and occurs with great frequency even in comparatively young women after the menopause, no exact figures as to its incidence are available.

Morbid Anatomy. Grossly, osteoporosis is characterized by thinning of the long bones, often with spontaneous fractures, and thinning of the bodies of vertebrae, with con-

cave deformities or rupture of the end-plates or collapse.

Microscopically, a decrease in the number and size of the bony trabeculae is found. The bone that remains is normal in histologic appearance, showing minimal evidence of bone formation (osteoblasts and osteoid "seams") and bone destruction (osteoclasts). In some cases of hyperthyroidism, there is evidence of both increased formation and destruction of bone.

Pathologic Physiology and Chemistry. In osteoporosis, the primary disorder is an inability to produce bone matrix. Therefore, as bone destruction proceeds at a normal (or, indeed, a decreased) rate, the bone mass diminishes, and strains on the skeleton increase. This stimulus does not result in increased bone matrix formation because of the basic defect. If, however, the sole cause of the disease is the loss of such strains (as with immobilization), it will be cured when mobilization is reinstituted.

The characteristic findings in the serum of patients with osteoporosis serve clearly to differentiate osteoporosis from the other metabolic bone diseases. Thus, in osteoporosis the serum calcium, phosphorus ("serum inorganic phosphate") and alkaline phosphatase are normal; in osteomalacia the phosphorus is low and the alkaline phosphatase high; and in osteitis fibrosa cystica generalisata the calcium is high and the phosphorus low when it results from primary hyperparathyroidism, the calcium is low and the phosphorus high when it results from chronic nephritis, and the alkaline phosphatase is high in both forms.

Symptoms. Osteoporosis tends to be more marked in the spine and pelvis than in the remainder of the skeleton, except in those cases due to partial immobilization (as by a plaster cast). For this reason, low back pain is the most common of all symptoms. Loss of height may follow extensive collapse of vertebrae. With the exception of the spine, osteoporotic bones are generally neither painful nor tender, in contrast to those involved by osteomalacia or osteitis fibrosa cystica generalisata.

By roentgenogram, the spine (Fig. 187) may show generalized radiolucency, with loss of finer trabeculations and increased prominence of those remaining, which often stand out as parallel vertical striations. In addition, there may be concave deformities of the end-plates due to pressure from the nucleus pulposus ("codfish" vertebrae), rupture of the end-plates (Schmorl's nodes) or collapse of the bodies. The lamina dura about the teeth is preserved—an important point in differentiating osteoporosis from osteomalacia or osteitis fibrosa cystica, in which it is absent. The skull is characteristically normal by roentgenography. The remaining bones may show varying degrees of demineralization, with decrease in number and increase in clarity of trabeculae. Pathologic fractures may appear, the neck of the femur being the favorite site.

Diagnosis. The chemical findings, which should rule out the other metabolic bone diseases, have been discussed. The diagnosis of osteoporosis *cannot be made on the basis of roentgenographic changes,* since osteomalacia, osteitis fibrosa cystica and metastatic malignancy may present an identical picture. Multiple myeloma presents special difficulties in differential diagnosis, in that it usually does not produce a rise in alkaline phosphatase, even with extensive bone involvement. With other types of widespread malignant disease in bone, an elevated alkaline phosphatase is commonly found. Although this, the presence of areas of destruction, and the discovery of a primary site will, in most cases, lead to the correct diagnosis, bone biopsy will be required in some to establish it with certainty.

Treatment. The treatment of osteoporosis should be directed, when possible, toward its cause. Disuse atrophy is, of course, best treated by mobilization. Indeed, all types of osteoporosis tend to heal faster with activity than with bed rest. In all forms, a diet adequate in protein is essential. When there is estrogen lack, replacement therapy is indicated. For example, stilbestrol, 1 to 3 mg. a day orally, will produce symptomatic relief far sooner than roentgenologic change. It must be discontinued for seven to ten days after every forty to allow withdrawal bleeding.

When there is evidence of malnutrition, hyperthyroidism, diabetes, vitamin C deficiency or excessive adrenal cortical hormones, the appropriate treatment should be instituted. When there is androgen lack, testosterone therapy is indicated. For example, methyl testosterone, 10 mg. a day by linguet, is often effective. For "senile" osteoporosis a combination of estrogens and androgens is the therapy of choice, as indeed is often the case in the postmenopausal form. In women the dosage of testosterone should be re-

duced after the first forty days to avoid masculinization. Excessive doses of calcium and vitamin D should *not* be used in the treatment of osteoporosis, as they do no good and are not without danger.

WALTER BAUER
FREDERIC C. BARTTER

References

Albright, F., and Reifenstein, E. C., Jr.: Parathyroid Glands and Metabolic Bone Disease. Baltimore, Williams and Wilkins Company, 1948.
Albright, F., Smith, P. H., and Richardson, A. M.: Postmenopausal Osteoporosis. Its Clinical Features. J.A.M.A., 116:2465, 1941.
Black, J. R., Ghormley, R. K., and Camp, J. D.: Senile Osteoporosis of the Spinal Column. J.A.M.A., 117:2144, 1941.
Bogdanoff, M. D., Shock, N. W., and Nichols, M. P.: Calcium, Phosphorus, Nitrogen and Potassium Balance Studies in the Aged Male. J. Gerontol., 8:272, 1953.
Schmorl, G.: Über die an den Wirbelbandscheiben vorkommenden Ausdehnungs- und Zerreissungsvorgänge und die dadurch an ihnen und der Wirbelspongiosa hervorgerufenen Veränderungen. Verhandl. d. deutsch. path. Gesellsch., 22:50, 1927.

FRAGILITAS OSSIUM

Definition. Fragilitas ossium is a rare congenial disease of the skeleton in which the bone mass is subnormal for the size and activity of the individual, and the bones are hard and brittle. It is characterized by pathologic fractures and may be part of a syndrome involving blue sclerae, hypermobility of the joints and otosclerosis.

Classification and Terminology. As the bone disease is thought to result primarily from a generalized failure of bone matrix formation, it is essentially a form of osteoporosis. The underlying biochemical abnormality is not known. Although the bone disease appears to be identical in all cases, past attempts to differentiate clinical entities of which fragilitas ossium forms a part have given rise to a confusing number of terms describing them. The recorded clinical terms and eponyms are reviewed briefly in the following outline:

I. *Osteogenesis imperfecta, Vrolik's disease, osteopsathyrosis congenita (Looser).* In this group the first fractures occur *in utero,* skull changes are generally present, short stature and early death are the rule, and both parents frequently have normal bones and sclerae.

II. *Osteopsathyrosis, idiopathic osteopsathyrosis, Lobstein's disease, osteopsathyrosis tarda (Looser).* In this group the first fractures occur after delivery, generally in childhood, the sclerae may or may not be blue, and both parents have normal bones and sclerae. It is familial but probably not hereditary, but cases with blue sclerae may show all the other characteristics of group III.

III. *Brittle bones and blue sclerae, Spurway's disease, hereditary hypoplasia of the mesenchyme (Key).* In this group the first fractures occur after delivery, generally in childhood, the sclerae are always blue, one parent always has blue sclerae (with or without the bone disease) which may be traced as a Mendelian dominant, the joints show hypermobility, and fractures tend to become less frequent after puberty, when otosclerosis often appears.

Etiology. When the disorder is hereditary, a genetic defect is clearly indicated. In many, perhaps all cases, there are associated defects in tendons, ligaments and blood vessels, tissues which share a mesenchymal origin with the bones and sclerae. As has been stated, the bone disease is esentially one of decreased matrix formation, and thus a form of congenital osteoporosis. Nothing further is known of the etiology of fragilitas ossium.

Incidence. Fragilitas ossium is a rare disease, the incidence of which in the general population cannot be accurately evaluated. Among families with the hereditary form, however, the incidence of blue sclerae (and thus, presumably, of hypoplasia of the mesenchyme) can be predicted by Mendelian law. With one parent affected, the disease may be anticipated in 50 per cent of the children; with both parents affected, in 75 per cent. Among the children with blue sclerae, about 40 per cent will suffer multiple fractures. In families in which one child has the nonhereditary form, there is a definitely increased probability that a second will be afflicted.

Morbid Anatomy. Grossly, fragilitas ossium is characterized by deformities of the skeleton resulting from fractures. The long bones may be unusually slender, increasing in diameter abruptly towards the epiphysis. They may, on occasion, be normal or even increased in diameter (Fairbank). The cortex, which is brittle and very hard, may or may not be thin. The skull may show a characteristic decrease in supero-inferior diameter, with occipital and bitemporal protuberances—a defect most often noted in Group I cases. Bone tissue in the skull and rarely in the long bones may be present only in isolated islands. The periosteum strips with ease and is friable; blood vessels, tendons and ligaments are thin, as are the sclerae.

Microscopically, the bone shows wide "canals" containing vascular fibrous tissue, coursing more or less irregularly through the cortex, with canal volume often equal to bone volume. The bone lamellae are irregularly arranged. Osteoclasts and osteoblasts are usually present in normal numbers. In some studies the osteoblasts have been found to be increased in number relative to the amount of matrix they have produced. The walls of the smaller blood vessels may show defects in the medial coats and a tendency to form varicosities.

Pathologic Physiology and Chemistry. As in other forms of osteoporosis, the primary disorder is an inability to form bone matrix. In addition, such bone as is formed has a structure (see above) not as ideally adapted to function as that of normal bone. The serum calcium and phosphorus are normal. The serum alkaline phosphatase may be slightly elevated, suggesting that the basic defect is not a paucity of osteoblasts but rather their inability to produce adequate matrix.

Signs and Symptoms. Patients with fragilitas ossium are often shorter than normal, not only as a result of deformities from fractures but also, apparently, as a manifestation of the mesenchymal defect. The deformity of the head has been mentioned. It may be so marked as to direct the ears partially downward. The sclerae, when they are affected, vary in color from a robin's egg blue to a deep slate color. The bones are not tender, but fracture with minimal trauma. They often show old deformities. Characteristically, fractures may be almost painless. The femoral neck—a favorite site of fracture in other forms of osteoporosis—is rarely fractured in fragilitas ossium. Incomplete fractures are common, but complete ones tend to be "clean," owing to the brittleness of the bones.

The ligaments are often abnormally relaxed, with hypermobility of the joints. Perhaps as a manifestation of this abnormality, scoliosis is relatively common. In a number of cases arcus senilis appears prematurely. Otosclerosis rarely appears before the third decade.

Roentgenographically, the long bones may show slender shafts with cortices *thick* but radiolucent, or normal shafts with thin cortices. A rare form has been described in which the cortices appear cystic. The "canals" described above may be reflected in prominent trabeculations by roentgenogram. The calvarium is thin. In Group I cases, it may show islands of ossification.

Prognosis. Patients in group I, if not born dead, often die at an early age. Any patient who survives through puberty is likely to show a decreasing tendency to fractures. Fractures which do occur heal readily at any age. The hereditary aspects of the disorder should be seriously considered by patients in group III who plan to become parents.

Diagnosis. A typical case of fragilitas ossium rarely presents any serious diagnostic problem. The generalized radiolucency of the bones may suggest rickets. It can be ruled out by the normal epiphyseal plates, the normal serum calcium and phosphorus, and the normal or only slightly elevated serum alkaline phosphatase. Renal osteitis fibrosa cystica can be excluded by the normal chemical findings in the blood and the absence of signs of renal disease. Although scurvy may cause a form of osteoporosis, it produces characteristic changes in the epiphyses and hemorrhages, with pain and tenderness and subsequent ossification—alterations which are not found in fragilitas ossium.

Treatment. Administration of estrogens and androgens will cause deposition of calcium and phosphorus in fragilitas ossium, although a definite preventive effect of such therapy upon fractures has not been demonstrated. It is obvious that measures should be taken to avoid fractures. However, immobilization should be avoided if possible, as it may be expected to increase the degree of osteoporosis. The treatment of fractures as they occur is that of fractures in general. There is no treatment known for otosclerosis.

FREDERIC C. BARTTER
WALTER BAUER

References

Fairbank, H. A. T.: Generalized Diseases of the Skeleton. Proc. Roy. Soc. Med., 28:1611, 1935.

Key, J. A.: Brittle Bones and Blue Sclera. Hereditary Hypoplasia of the Mesenchyme. Arch. Surg., *13:* 523, 1926.

Lobstein, J. F.: Lehrbuch der pathologischen Anatomie. Stuttgart, vol. 2, p. 179, 1835.

Looser, E.: Zur Kentniss der Osteogenesis imperfecta congenita et tarda. Mitt. a. d. genzb. d. Med. u. Chir., *15:*161, 1906.

Ropes, M. W., Rossmeisl, E. C., and Bauer, W.: The Effect of Estrin Medication in Osteogenesis Imperfecta. Conference on Metabolic Aspects of Convalescence. Tr. 14th Meeting, Josiah Macy, Jr. Foundation, New York, 1946, p. 87.

Spurway, J.: Hereditary Tendency to Fracture. Brit. M. J., 2:845, 1896.

OSTEOMALACIA

Definition. Osteomalacia is a condition wherein the mass of calcified bone is decreased as the result of a failure of calcium salts to be deposited in the newly formed bone matrix (osteoid tissue). This failure of bone matrix calcification is attributable to inadequate concentrations of phosphorus or calcium in the body fluids. The pathologic physiology and the histologic picture of osteomalacia are the same as those found in rickets, the essential difference being that rickets develops before epiphyseal closure. Osteomalacia is clearly separable from the other metabolic bone diseases in that there is no failure of matrix production (as in osteoporosis) nor is there an increase of bone destruction (as in osteitis fibrosa cystica).

Etiology. Osteomalacia is always due to inadequate concentrations of calcium or phosphorus in the body fluids. In man this may be the result of decreased intestinal absorption of calcium, increased urinary excretion of calcium, or, rarely, of abnormally rapid deposition of calcium and phosphorus in the skeleton following removal of a parathyroid adenoma. Loss of calcium and phosphorus from the body during pregnancy and lactation has not been shown to produce osteomalacia in man but may accentuate symptoms in predisposed subjects. It has been postulated, but not conclusively demonstrated, that urinary phosphate loss alone may give rise to osteomalacia.

Decreased intestinal absorption of calcium may be due to inadequate amounts of calcium or vitamin D in the diet, excessive loss of calcium and vitamin D in the feces, or, rarely, resistance to vitamin D. Clinically, osteomalacia resulting from dietary deficiency of calcium and vitamin D, although relatively common in northern India and China, has not been found in the United States. Increased fecal loss of calcium and vitamin D is commonly seen in steatorrhea resulting from chronic pancreatitis and the sprue syndrome. "Resistance to vitamin D" is a rare condition in which rickets (in children) or osteomalacia (in adults) is present in spite of a normal intake of vitamin D, whether this be given orally or parenterally or supplied by ultraviolet irradiation of the skin. It can be alleviated with very large doses of vitamin D.

Increased urinary excretion of calcium is found in "renal tubular insufficiency" and in essential hypercalcuria. In the former condition calcium is lost together with other cations as required to "cover" urinary anions in the face of an impairment of the ability of the renal tubules to secrete hydrogen ions. This may appear as an isolated renal disorder or may be accompanied by other renal tubular defects as in the "Fanconi syndrome." In the condition known as essential hypercalcuria, inadequate reabsorption of calcium appears to be an isolated renal tubular defect. It is observed occasionally in pyelonephritis resulting from coccal infections.

Abnormally rapid deposition of calcium and phosphorus in the skeleton may be seen following surgical removal of a parathyroid adenoma which has caused osteitis fibrosa cystica. Following operation, bone destruction abruptly ceases and rapid matrix formation continues. The amount of calcium and phosphorus in the extracellular fluid is no longer adequate to allow normal calcification of the newly formed matrix. Consequently, the serum calcium and phosphorus fall, and the bone presents histologically the wide osteoid seams characteristic of osteomalacia.

Incidence. Osteomalacia is endemic over wide areas in northern India and China, where it occurs chiefly in women and may be more severe in each succeeding pregnancy. In these regions, the underlying cause is dietary lack. In other parts of the world, osteomalacia is a rare disease resulting from gastro-intestinal, renal or preexisting bone disorders, as already indicated.

Morbid Anatomy. Grossly, osteomalacia is characterized by a softening of the bones, with the result that incomplete fractures and bending occur much more frequently than do complete fractures. When the disease is severe and of long duration, gross deformities of all the bones may appear, especially those of the spine, thorax and pelvis. The bones are easily cut, although they may not otherwise appear abnormal on gross examination. When the disease is mild, alterations in bone structure are detectable only by histologic examination.

Microscopically, there is found an increase in the width of the osteoid seams, together with a decrease in the amount of calcified bone. The total amount of bone, calcified and uncalcified, may be greater than normal. Osteoblasts are present in greatly increased numbers, osteoclasts virtually absent. These striking features serve to distinguish osteomalacia from osteoporosis and osteitis fibrosa cystica.

Pathologic Physiology and Chemistry. It is apparent that the various factors leading to osteomalacia (decreased absorption, increased excretion or increased deposition of calcium) have as a "final common pathway" a decrease in the circulating calcium. This in turn may act as a stimulus to parathyroid activity, resulting in (1) hyperplasia of the parathyroids, (2) increased secretion of parathyroid hormone, (3) increased urinary excretion of phosphorus (in the osteomalacia following parathyroidectomy, the "compensatory" hyperparathyroidism so produced is less than that initially present, and urinary phosphorus excretion actually falls), (4) fall of serum phosphorus, (5) increased resorption of bone (in osteomalacia due to increased urinary loss of calcium, there may also be increased absorption of calcium from the gastro-intestinal tract at this time), (6) rise of serum calcium.

The biochemical abnormalities of osteomalacia are a low or normal serum calcium, a low serum phosphorus and a high serum alkaline phosphatase (a reflection of increased osteoblastic activity). These findings serve to distinguish osteomalacia from the other metabolic bone diseases. Thus, the serum calcium is high in primary hyperparathyroidism, the serum phosphorus is high in renal osteitis, and the serum calcium, phosphorus and alkaline phosphatase are normal in osteoporosis. The urinary calcium is of cardinal importance in establishing the etiology, since it is decreased (and may be negligible) when osteomalacia results from decreased intestinal absorption or the rapid deposition of calcium, and is, of course, increased when it results from abnormal renal loss of calcium.

Symptoms. Albright divides clinical osteomalacia into four degrees of severity, as follows: (1) chemical osteomalacia with a normal serum alkaline phosphatase, (2) chemical osteomalacia with a high serum alkaline phosphatase, (3) Milkman's syndrome and (4) advanced osteomalacia. In the first, the tendency to hypocalcemia has been met by compensatory hyperparathyroidism, but bone disease has not developed. In the second, osteoblastic activity is increased, but there is no clinical or roentgenographic evidence of bone disease. The diagnosis in these two categories may be made only by determining the serum calcium, phosphorus and alkaline phosphatase. In the third (Milkman's syndrome) there are bone pain and tenderness, and roentgenographic examination reveals incomplete fractures (pseudofractures) which have a tendency to be bilateral and symmetrically placed. LeMay and Blunt have shown that they frequently occur at the point where arteries impinge on bony structures; the lateral margin of the scapula is a favorite site (Fig. 188). In the fourth (advanced osteomalacia) there is generalized radiolucency of the bones, and gross skeletal deformities.

The most striking symptoms in osteomalacia are bone pain and tenderness, which are frequently much more severe in relation to the degree of radiolucency than they are in the other metabolic bone diseases. Back pain, with or without collapse of vertebrae, is especially prominent and may keep the patient virtually immobilized. Muscular weakness is a striking symptom in osteomalacia, even when there is not an associated hypokalemia. When hypocalcemia is present, spontaneous tetany may occur and both Chvostek's and Trousseau's signs may be elicited.

Other symptoms will depend on, and give a clue to, the fundamental cause of the disorder. When the defect is of gastrointestinal origin, diarrhea, steatorrhea and signs of deficiency of fat-soluble vitamins other than D may be present. When it is of renal origin, there may be kidney stones, pyuria, hematuria, amino-aciduria and a metabolic acidosis.

Diagnosis. Osteomalacia is to be distinguished from two other groups of generalized bone diseases which result in increased radiolucency, namely, osteoporosis and osteitis fibrosa cystica. The chemical findings, which should rule out the other metabolic bone diseases, have been discussed.

Radiologically, osteomalacia is distinguished from osteoporosis (but not from osteitis fibrosa cystica) by the absence of lamina dura. The skull may be involved in osteomalacia (and in osteitis fibrosa cystica),

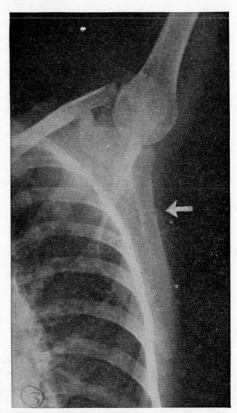

Fig. 188. Osteomalacia secondary to renal acidosis. Arrow points to a typical pseudofracture of the scapula.

but does not show roentgenographic changes in osteoporosis.

Treatment. Osteomalacia responds promptly to adequate therapy. Treatment should be directed towards both the osteomalacia *per se* and the underlying disorder. For the osteomalacia, a very high intake of calcium (calcium lactate, 30 gm. a day) and vitamin D (50,000 units a day orally) provide effective specific therapy. In osteomalacia due to vitamin D resistance, however, doses of vitamin D as high as 1,000,000 units a day may be required; in osteomalacia following removal of a parathyroid adenoma, calcium may be required intravenously (10 to 30 cc. of 10 per cent calcium gluconate). If the underlying disorder is chronic pancreatitis or the sprue syndrome, the appropriate therapeutic regimen must of course be instituted; if it is renal tubular acidosis, this should be controlled with adequate alkali.

WALTER BAUER
FREDERIC C. BARTTER

References

Albright, F., and Reifenstein, E. C., Jr.: Parathyroid Glands and Metabolic Bone Disease. Baltimore, Williams and Wilkins Company, 1948.
——, and others: Osteomalacia and Late Rickets. Medicine, 25:399, 1946.
LeMay, M., and Blunt, J. W., Jr.: A Factor Determining the Location of Pseudo Fractures in Osteomalacia. J. Clin. Investigation, 28:521, 1949.
Liu, S. H., and others: Calcium and Phosphorus Metabolism in Osteomalacia. Chinese M. J., 49:1, 1935.
Maxwell, J. P.: The Modern Conception of Osteomalacia and Its Importance to China. Chinese M. J., 49:47, 1935.
McCune, D. J., Nathan, H. H., and Clarke, H. D.: Intractable Hypophosphatemic Rickets with Renal Glycosuria and Acidosis (the Fanconi Syndrome). Am. J. Dis. Child., 65:81, 1943.
Milkman, L. A.: Multiple Spontaneous Idiopathic Symmetrical Fractures. Am. J. Roentgenol., 32:622, 1934.

OSTEITIS FIBROSA CYSTICA GENERALISATA

Definition. Osteitis fibrosa cystica generalisata is a condition in which the bone mass is decreased as the result of an increase in the rate of bone destruction. It is clearly separable from the other metabolic bone diseases, in that there is no failure of matrix formation (as in osteoporosis) or of matrix calcification (as in osteomalacia). It is separable from osteitis fibrosa cystica disseminata (fibrous dysplasia of bone) in that no bone is spared, at least histologically, and the serum alkaline phosphatase is invariably elevated.

Etiology. The two conditions in which osteitis fibrosa generalisata is found are primary hyperparathyroidism and chronic nephritis. In the former disease, excess of parathyroid hormone is clearly responsible (see below for discussion of mechanism); in the latter, although there is virtually always hyperplasia of the parathyroids, the bone disease is generally attributed to the disordered metabolism produced by the renal failure rather than to the parathyroid hormone excess.

Incidence. Primary hyperparathyroidism is a relatively rare disease. Renal failure is of course extremely common, but the frequency with which it is associated with osteitis fibrosa has not been established. It is relatively rare for the bone disease to become clinically significant after epiphyseal closure, but relatively common for the serum alkaline phosphatase to rise, indicating that histologic bone disease is present.

Morbid Anatomy. Grossly, osteitis fibrosa cystica generalisata is characterized by generalized rarefaction of the skeleton, cysts of the skull and long bones and by the appearance of pathologic fractures. Gross cysts within the cortices of long bones occur rarely, if at all, in renal osteitis. All the bones may become thinned and softened as the disease progresses. The teeth are never decalcified, but they may be loosened in their sockets. The jaw may be the site of the "epulis" tumor.

Microscopically, there is an increase in the number of osteoclasts and of osteoblasts, with fibrosis of the marrow. The osteoid seams are slightly increased in width (as in rapidly growing bone generally) but not to the extent seen in osteomalacia. The "cysts" are found to be true cysts, or to contain fibrous tissue or to be highly vascular areas containing osteoblasts and osteoclasts (brown tumors). The epulis is likewise a "brown tumor."

Pathologic Physiology and Chemistry. In osteitis fibrosa, the primary disorder is an increase in the rate of bone destruction. As bone destruction proceeds, the bone mass diminishes, and strains on the skeleton increase. This provides a stimulus to increased bone matrix formation. The matrix which is formed calcifies readily. The cause of the bone destruction that originates this sequence is a matter of controversy.

Some workers hold that the primary action of the parathyroid hormone is to decrease renal tubular reabsorption of phosphorus, resulting in (1) increased excretion of phosphorus, (2) decreased serum phosphorus, (3) undersaturation of the serum and extracellular fluid with respect to calcium phosphate and (4) resorption of bone. Adherents of this view believe the osteitis fibrosa of renal failure results from the metabolic abnormalities of the renal disease, and not from the associated parathyroid hyperplasia. Other workers are of the opinion that the primary action of the hormone is to increase bone destruction. This theory does not explain the cases of hyperparathyroidism with normal bones (see chapter on Hyperparathyroidism) or the lowered serum phosphorus in primary hyperparathyroidism.

The chemical findings serve clearly to differentiate osteitis fibrosa cystica generalisata from the other metabolic bone diseases. Thus, the serum calcium is high and the serum phosphorus low in primary hyperparathyroidism, the serum calcium low or normal and the serum phosphorus high in chronic nephritis. The serum alkaline phosphatase is elevated with osteitis fibrosa in both conditions. In contrast, all these values are normal in osteoporosis, whereas the serum calcium is never high and the serum phosphorus is virtually always low in osteomalacia. The urinary calcium is high with the hypercalcemia of primary hyperparathyroidism, and is often low with glomerular insufficiency.

Symptoms and Signs. Osteitis fibrosa cystica generalisata may be entirely asymptomatic. In advanced cases, bone tenderness appears. Cysts or brown tumors may distort the cortex of bones, and appear as swellings, tender areas or the sites of pathologic fractures. The "epulis" of the jaw, previously mentioned, may lead to detection of the disease.

Symptoms which are a result of the underlying condition rather than the bone disease itself include those due to hypercalcemia, to hypercalciuria, and to renal failure. Chief among the first are anorexia, constipation, nausea and vomiting, polyuria, polydipsia and weakness; chief among the second are renal stones; in the third are included, of course, all the symptoms that characterize renal failure.

By roentgenogram, the bones may show generalized radiolucency, with loss of trabecular markings. The involvement is characteristically uneven, the most markedly affected areas appearing as "cysts" which may expand the cortex over them, and are frequently the sites of pathologic fractures. Cysts within the cortices of long bones are common in primary hyperparathyroidism, but are rarely if ever seen in the osteitis fibrosa secondary to chronic nephritis. Subperiosteal resorption of cortical bone, giving a jagged or feathery appearance, is almost pathognomonic of osteitis fibrosa cystica generalisata. The skull often shows a characteristic mottled or ground-glass appearance; the lamina dura about the teeth is absent.

Before epiphyseal closure, the osteitis of prolonged renal insufficiency produces characteristic irregular deformities of the epiphyses. The term "renal rickets" has unfortunately been applied to this condition, which is in fact "renal osteitis fibrosa." There may be slipping, tilting, and fragmentation of epiphyses, especially that of the femoral head. Longstanding involvement of the epiphyses of the knee joint leads to the characteristic genu valgum.

Diagnosis. Osteitis fibrosa cystica generalisata resembles osteoporosis and osteomalacia in showing generalized radiolucency of the bones. The chemical findings, which should rule out the other metabolic bone diseases, have been discussed. It differs from osteoporosis by the loss of lamina dura about the teeth, and from both osteoporosis and osteomalacia by the presence of "cysts" and of subperiosteal resorption of bone. Osteitis fibrosa cystica disseminata (fibrous dysplasia) may present a strikingly similar radiologic picture, but without absence of lamina dura, or abnormalities of the serum calcium and phosphorus. The noninvolved bone is histologically normal in the disseminated variety, in which may also be found brown spots in the skin and precocious puberty in females. Paget's disease seldom presents a serious problem in differential diagnosis, as the roentgenographic pattern of involved bone is generally distinctive, with some normal bone always present. Furthermore, the serum calcium and phosphorus are normal.

Prognosis. The bone disease in primary hyperparathyroidism heals rapidly upon surgical removal of the cause. In chronic nephritis, control of the acidosis often leads to control of the bone disease. (This therapy, however, does not materially alter the course of the renal disease.) The use of Amphojel to lower the serum phosphorus, on the other hand, has been reported to *increase* bone destruction.

Treatment. The treatment of primary hyperparathyroidism is surgical removal of the parathyroid tumor. When extensive bone disease is present, the immediate result may be a fall of serum calcium and a further fall of serum phosphorus, with the development of tetany. This may require vigorous treatment with calcium by vein (10 to 30 cc. of 10 per cent calcium gluconate) and calcium (calcium lactate, 5 gm. six times daily) and vitamin D (50,000 units daily) by mouth.

The treatment of renal osteitis fibrosa is that of the renal disease, especially of the acidosis.

WALTER BAUER
FREDERIC C. BARTTER

References

Albright, F., Drake, T. G., and Sulkowitch, H. W.: Renal Osteitis Fibrosa Cystica; Report of a Case with Discussion of Metabolic Aspects. Bull. Johns Hopkins Hosp., 60:377, 1937.

———, and Reifenstein, E. C., Jr.: Parathyroid Glands and Metabolic Bone Disease. Baltimore, Williams and Wilkins Co., 1948.

Ginzler, A. M., and Jaffe, H. L.: Osseous Findings in Chronic Renal Insufficiency in Adults. Am. J. Path., 17:293, 1941.

von Recklinghausen, F. D.: Die fibrose oder deformirende Ostitis, die Osteomalacie und die osteoplastische Carcinose in ihren gegenseitigen Beziehungen. Festschrift f. Rudolf Virchow, Berlin, 1891.

Snapper, I.: Medical Clinics on Bone Diseases. 2nd ed. New York, Interscience Publishers, 1949.

Sussman, M. L., and Poppel, M. H.: Renal Osteitis. Am. J. Roentgenol., 48:726, 1942.

FIBROUS DYSPLASIA OF BONE

(Osteitis Fibrosa Cystica Disseminata)

Definition. Fibrous dysplasia of bone is a condition in which the architecture of one or more bones is distorted, with characteristic fibrous changes in the marrow spaces. When multiple bones are involved, it is termed polyostotic fibrous dysplasia or osteitis fibrosa cystica disseminata; it may form a part of a syndrome (Albright) involving brownish pigmentation of the skin and precocious puberty in females.

Etiology. Nothing is known of the etiology of fibrous dysplasia of bone. The tendency for the polyostotic variety to show unilateral involvement of the skeleton has suggested a neurologic or an embryologic disorder. The former possibility is suggested, perhaps, by the finding of early secretion of gonadotrophin in affected females.

Incidence. Albright's syndrome involving bone changes, areas of pigmentation of the skin and precocious puberty in the female is a relatively rare condition. The combination of skin and bone changes, without endocrine abnormality, is seen much less infrequently. The bone changes alone are relatively common. As they are often asymp-

tomatic and an incidental roentgenologic finding, it is clear that the true incidence cannot be evaluated.

Morbid Anatomy. Grossly, fibrous dysplasia is characterized by expansion and distortion of involved bones, especially the cranium and femurs, often with evidence of old and new pathologic fractures.

Microscopically, there is found an increase in the number of osteoclasts and of osteoblasts, with fibrosis of the marrow spaces. The lesion differs from that of osteitis fibrosa cystica generalisata in the occasional inclusion of areas of cartilage in the involved areas and in the normal histologic appearance of noninvolved bones.

Pathologic Physiology and Chemistry. Inasmuch as some normal bone tissue always remains, it is clear that fibrous dysplasia is not a generalized "metabolic" bone disease. The pathogenesis is not understood. Although histologically the lesions are virtually the same as those of osteitis fibrosa cystica generalisata, their progress appears clinically to be much slower. The inclusion of islands of cartilage in the diaphysis of long bones suggests a relationship with Ollier's disease, but does not illuminate the fundamental mechanism. When fractures occur, healing is normal in rate and in architectural features.

Biochemically, fibrous dysplasia of bone is characterized by a normal serum calcium and phosphorus. These findings serve to differentiate it clearly from the osteitis fibrosa of primary hyperparathyroidism, in which the calcium is high and the phosphorus low. The serum alkaline phosphatase may be normal when the total amount of involved bone is small, or increased with greater involvement or during the healing of fractures.

Symptoms. Single, or even multiple and quite extensive bone lesions may be present without producing symptoms. Swelling and deformity of involved bones or a pathologic fracture may first call attention to the presence of the disease. Pain, which may result from lesions in certain sites such as the spine, is rare in the syndrome as a whole. The femoral necks are favorite sites for the disorder (Fig. 189). The femurs may become bowed, with upward displacement of the trochanters, shortening of the legs and increasing difficulty in walking. As the hips assume the varus position, the gait may become "waddling."

Areas of brownish pigmentation of the

skin, non-raised and with a characteristically jagged outline, are found in some cases. When involvement of bone has a tendency to unilateral distribution, the same is often true of the skin lesions. In a few girls with the disorder, precocious puberty occurs as well. The triad of bone, skin and menarchal disorders is known as Albright's syndrome.

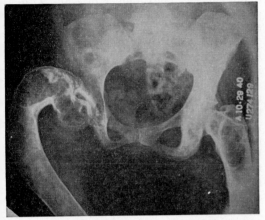

Fig. 189. Note cystic lesions in both femurs, in one of which they have produced the characteristic "shepherd's crook" deformity.

Roentgenograms fail to show generalized radiolucency, subperiosteal resorption or loss of lamina dura. Otherwise, the involved bones may resemble closely those found in osteitis fibrosa cystica generalisata. They differ from the latter in the presence of areas of increased density, especially at the base of the skull, and in a predilection for certain sites—notably the femoral necks and the occiput (see Fig. 189 and 190). Islands of cartilage in the long bones may produce striking radiolucent areas of irregular outline superficially resembling cysts. A "torn paper" appearance in the bone roentgenogram has been considered almost pathognomonic of the disease. The lesions of fibrous dysplasia may show very slow advance over a span of years.

Diagnosis. The diagnosis of extensive fibrous dysplasia seldom presents difficulties. The x-ray picture suggests that of primary hyperparathyroidism, not that of renal osteitis. Its chemical differentiation from osteitis fibrosa cystica generalisata has been mentioned. The lamina dura about the teeth, which is preserved, also serves to rule out the latter condition. When there is little bone involvement, biopsy may be necessary to distinguish the lesions from those of other

diseases, such as eosinophilic granuloma, enchondroma or hypernephroma. In none of these are there regions of increased bone density. Neurofibromatosis may resemble fibrous dysplasia in showing both bone and skin lesions. The former, however, tend to occur at foramina where nerves enter bone, and rarely show increased density; the areas of skin pigmentation have a characteristically smooth outline, may be raised and are often associated with subcutaneous nodules.

Prognosis. The lesions of fibrous dysplasia may show slow progression, and undergo partial or complete fracture, with bending and deformity of the involved bone and consequent mechanical difficulties. The fractures heal readily, as do the sites of operative intervention.

Treatment. The treatment is that of the complications, the fractures and deformities. The "shepherd's crook" deformity of the femurs may require excision with attachment of the femoral shaft to the head. A cortex so thinned as to be almost certainly a future

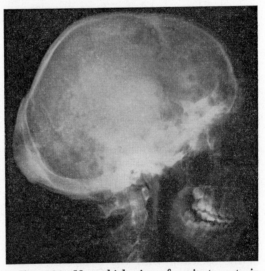

Fig. 190. Note thickening of occiput, cysts in frontal region and increased density of the bones of the base.

fracture site may be strengthened by scraping and filling with bone chips.

WALTER BAUER
FREDERIC C. BARTTER

References

Albright, F.: Polyostotic Fibrous Dysplasia: A Defense of the Entity. J. Clin. Endocrinol., 7:307, 1947.

Albright, F., Butler, A. M., Hampton, A. O., and Smith, P.: Syndrome Characterized by Osteitis Fibrosa Disseminata, Areas of Pigmentation, and Endocrine Dysfunction, with Precocious Puberty in Females. New England J. Med., 216:727, 1937.

Lichtenstein, L.: Polyostotic Fibrous Dysplasia. Arch. Surg., 36:874, 1938.

———, and Jaffe, H. L.: Fibrous Dysplasia of Bone. Arch. Path., 33:777, 1942.

Snapper, I.: Medical Clinics on Bone Diseases. 2nd ed. New York, Interscience Publishers, 1949.

OSTEITIS DEFORMANS

(Paget's Disease of Bone)

Definition. Osteitis deformans is a chronic disease of the adult skeleton characterized by increased bone destruction, increased bone formation and an abnormal architecture in the newly formed bone. Although hypertrophy, bowing and deformation of the bones may be widespread, the disease never involves all the bones. Thus, it is a "localized" and not a generalized or "metabolic" bone disorder.

Etiology. Virtually nothing is known of the etiology of osteitis deformans. Sir James Paget considered it to be a form of chronic inflammation of the bones, as is implied by the term "osteitis." Although this term persists in descriptions of this and other bone disorders in which fibrosis of the marrow spaces is found, the absence of cellular infiltration or of the usual clinical signs of inflammation suggests that the term is inappropriate. A relationship of osteitis deformans to weight-bearing and trauma is suggested by a predilection for those bones or parts of bones most frequently subjected to strain. Thus, there is a high incidence of the disease in the sacrum, femur and lower spine, and a relatively low incidence in those bones higher in the skeleton, with the exception of the skull. Albright has suggested that the semi-lunar distribution frequently seen in the initial lateral skull films (osteoporosis circumscripta) may be related to the pull of the temporal muscles, whose attachments describe a similar pattern. It has been shown that blood flow through bone affected with Paget's disease is greatly in excess of that through normal bone, but it is not known whether the vascular abnormality is primary, or secondary to the bone disease.

Incidence. Paget's disease is rare before the age of 35. (Cases of "juvenile Paget's disease" have been reported, but many or all of these appear in retrospect to be cases of polyostotic fibrous dysplasia.) After the age of 35, the incidence of Paget's disease increases rapidly. Schmorl reported an incidence of 3 per cent among autopsied subjects over 40. As many small lesions must never be detected, the true incidence is undoubtedly higher. Males are more commonly affected than females. The number of cases with a positive family history is significantly greater than that predictable as random distribution.

Morbid Anatomy. Grossly, bones affected with Paget's disease show characteristically: an increase in size, with loss of normal contour, the most characteristic deformities being the bowed tibias and femurs, and the enlarged skull; areas of softening, often with incomplete, occasionally with complete pathologic fractures, the most characteristic lesions being the incomplete anterior tibial fractures; areas of sclerosis, where the new-formed bone is abnormally hard and dense; and increased vascularity. Portions of involved bones may remain completely normal, and the line of transition is often apparent grossly, normal cortex giving way abruptly to thick, rough, periosteal new bone which may be cut easily, revealing a very vascular thick cortex, often coarsely trabeculated, usually with a widened marrow cavity. With extensive involvement of the pelvis, the acetabulums may be thrust upward by the femoral heads, with "heart-shaped" or triradiate deformity of the pelvic outlet. Similarly, the occipital bone may be bent inward by the spine (convexobasia).

Microscopically, the initial lesion consists of bone destruction, with numerous osteoclasts, and fibrosis of the marrow. In more mature lesions bone formation is prominent, the new bone characteristically lacking the structural orientation of normal bone. The resulting pattern of fragments of newer bone deposited on partially destroyed segments of older bone (which may in turn contain fragments of yet older bone partially destroyed), all without recognizable orientation, constitutes the "mosaic" described by Schmorl. Periosteal new bone lacking mosaic structure is deposited over involved areas in the long bones, and is rapidly replaced by "Paget's" bone. The histologic picture is further characterized by the presence of abrupt transitions from normal to diseased bone.

Pathologic Physiology and Chemistry. The initial lesion in Paget's disease is one of bone destruction. If this were the only defect, one would expect to find hypercalciuria, with a tendency to renal stone formation, and, in rapidly developing cases, hypercalcemia. Kidney stones are, indeed, frequently found in early cases. There is a greater tendency for these complications to develop when for any reason an increase of new bone formation does not ensue. Thus, in patients who are senile or in the postmenopausal state and in those subjected to extensive immobilization, these complications are not uncommon. When, however, new bone formation, as well as bone destruction, is increased—as generally occurs—the tendency towards calcium loss is diminished. The serum alkaline phosphatase, index of osteoblastic activity, is increased, often to values so high as to require dilution techniques for accurate evaluation.

When the disease is widespread, the increase of blood flow to involved bone may result in a condition akin to an arteriovenous fistula, with cardiac hypertrophy and congestive failure.

Symptoms. The best known clinical manifestations of osteitis deformans are the bowing of the tibias and the enlargement of the skull first clearly described by Sir James Paget. Any bone may be affected, however, with the exception of the bones of the hands and feet, where osteitis deformans is virtually never found. In Schmorl's extensive autopsy series, the most commonly affected bones were, in descending order of frequency, the sacrum, the spine, the right femur, the skull, the sternum, the pelvis, the left femur, the clavicle and the tibia. Depending on the site and extent of the lesion, the involved bone may show no change except as revealed by x-ray and be asymptomatic, or it may be enlarged and deformed. Pain in the involved bones is relatively uncommon save when pathologic fractures occur. The healing of repeated incomplete fractures may account for much of the deformity—a phenomenon seen most clearly in the tibia and femur, which are not only bowed but elongated as a result. The advanced case may present a clinical picture so characteristic as to establish the diagnosis upon inspection (Fig. 191). The whole calvarium is enlarged and the temporal arteries are prominent and tortuous, the head is carried forward with the chin resting almost on the sternum, the clavicles are prominent and distorted, there is a marked dorsal kyphosis, the thorax is deformed, with the lower ribs approaching the

pelvic brim, and the legs are held in outward rotation and show curved, massive bone structures describing an arc from hip to ankle.

Radiologically, Paget's disease is characterized by expansion of the bony cortex, with

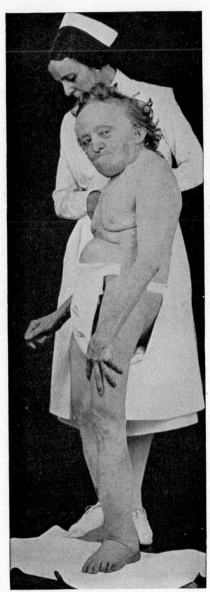

Fig. 191. Advanced Paget's disease. The head is characteristically enlarged, the chin rests on the sternum, there is scoliosis of the spine, and the femurs and tibiae are bowed anteriorly.

marked exaggeration and distortion of trabecular pattern. Whereas the initial destructive edge of a lesion shows increased radiolucency, areas involved for a longer time may be more or less dense than the surrounding bone, depending upon the extent of new bone formation. Figure 192 shows a skull in which Paget's disease has produced bone destruction and new bone formation, with widening of the bone and areas of sclerosis. It has resulted in the characteristic "cotton wool" appearance in the frontal region. The involved tibia and femur frequently show radiolucent bands (incomplete cortical fractures), extending part way into

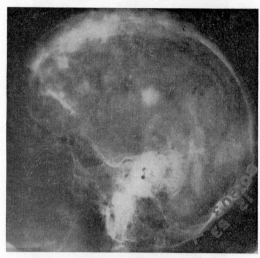

Fig. 192. Lateral view of the skull shows typical thickening of both tables involving primarily the frontal and parietal bones in a patchy fashion.

the cortex from the margin of greatest curvature. The teeth may show thickening of the cementum (hypercementosis), and the roots may be partially destroyed and replaced by Paget's bone.

The skin over an involved bone may be perceptibly warmer than the surrounding tissue. Arteriosclerosis of a greater degree than would be expected for the patient's age is quite constantly found with extensive Paget's disease. Deafness occurs commonly, both as a result of involvement of the ossicles and auditory canal and as a result of otosclerosis, the histologic picture of which suggests a close relationship to Paget's disease. Examination of the eyegrounds may reveal the presence of "angioid streaks" around the optic disk.

The course of Paget's disease is extremely variable. It may remain stationary for long periods of time, or may spread gradually to produce extensive deformity and crippling. Aside from pain, it has only three serious complications. Pathologic fractures have been

mentioned. They heal readily enough with the usual orthopedic measures (save that screws and pins hold poorly in affected bone). Osteogenic sarcoma after the age of 40 is much more frequent in patients with Paget's disease than in the populace at large. It not infrequently develops in two sites simultaneously. Finally, congestive failure may occur, as discussed above.

Diagnosis. The serum chemical values in osteitis deformans (normal serum calcium and phosphorus, elevated serum alkaline phosphatase) serve to differentiate it from osteitis fibrosa cystica generalisata. Osteitis fibrosa cystica localisata (fibrous dysplasia) may present similar serum chemical values, although the alkaline phosphatase is rarely markedly elevated in this condition. However, the radiographic pattern (see chapter on Fibrous Dysplasia), the characteristic lesions of occiput and femur, the frequent involvement of hands and feet, and the frequent association of "brown spots" in the skin should serve to establish the diagnosis of fibrous dysplasia without difficulty. Metastatic carcinoma from the prostate produces lesions closely resembling those of osteitis deformans. They do not, however, expand the cortex or bend the long bones, nor do they produce the coarsening of trabeculae that characterizes Paget's disease. They do produce elevations in the serum acid phosphatase, which is not elevated in Paget's disease.

Treatment. There is no specific treatment for osteitis deformans. If a sarcoma develops, it should be treated early and radically in the hope of avoiding metastases. We have administered high calcium diets, with added vitamin D, to allow rapid calcification of newly formed matrix. When patients must be immobilized or confined to bed, it is essential that a low calcium diet be given and fluids forced to prevent hypercalcemia and renal damage.

WALTER BAUER
FREDERIC C. BARTTER

References

Edholm, O. G., Howarth, S., and McMichael, J.: Heart Failure and Bone Blood Flow in Osteitis Deformans. Clin. Sc., 5:249, 1945.

Freund, E.: Zur Frage der Ostitis deformans Paget. Virchows Arch. f. path. Anat., 274:1, 1929–30.

Gutman, A. B., and Kasabach, H. H.: Paget's Disease (Osteitis Deformans). Analysis of 116 Cases. Am. J. M. Sc., 191:361, 1936.

Marie, P., Leri, A., and Chatelin, C.: Déformation de la base du crane dans la maladie de Paget. Bull.

méd. d. hôp. de Paris, 34:89, 1912; 43:901, 1919.

Paget, J.: On a Form of Chronic Inflammation of Bones (Osteitis Deformans). Medico-Chirurg. Trans., 60:37, 1877.

Reifenstein, E. C., Jr., and Albright, F.: Paget's Disease: Its Pathologic Physiology and the Importance of This in the Complications Arising from Fracture and Immobilization. New England J. Med., 231:343, 1944.

Schmorl, G.: Über Osteitis Deformans Paget. Virchows Arch. f. path. Anat., 283:694, 1932.

Snapper, I.: Medical Clinics on Bone Disease. 2nd ed. New York, Interscience Publishers, 1949.

Thoma, K. H.: Oral Pathology. 3rd ed. St. Louis, C. V. Mosby Co., 1950.

LEONTIASIS OSSEA

Leontiasis ossea is a term introduced by Virchow to describe the "leonine" appearance of the face imparted by deforming overgrowth of the facial bones.

As the term is a descriptive one, it is not surprising that it has been applied clinically to a number of pathologic entities. In many reported cases the nature of the lesion can only be guessed at from roentgenograms; in others, biopsy has been inconclusive. Rarely have biochemical data been reported. Whereas in a few cases the underlying disorder may have been periostitis, Paget's disease, and even osteopetrosis, it appears likely that, in most instances, the condition is a manifestation of polyostotic fibrous dysplasia. Indeed, moderate asymmetric deformity of the face is a common finding in the latter disorder—often the presenting sign. A few cases show associated metaphyseal dysplasia, a finding which suggests that the skull changes are developmental in origin. Microscopically, the majority of reported biopsies show the fibrosis of the marrow, with osteoclasts and osteoblasts, characteristic of fibrous dysplasia. In a few cases the "mosaic" of Paget's disease has been observed. Finally, there are a few cases in which histologic examination has shown great overgrowths of normal-appearing bone, with wide vascular channels, and has given no clue as to the pathogenesis.

Radiologically, expansion of the bony cortex of facial bones is seen, with cyst-like lesions often containing "spicules" of bone. A number of cases show marked "cystic" enlargement of the occiput. Other bones, especially those of the base of the skull, often show greatly increased radio-opacity. These are, of course, findings typical of fibrous dysplasia of bone.

Clinically, the deformities, often grotesque, are generally painless. They often come to medical observation for cosmetic reasons, or because pressure symptoms develop, including exophthalmos, visual and auditory difficulties, obstruction to nares or lacrimal ducts, and paresthesias, neuralgias and paralyses. Convulsions and coma are rare complications of the disorder.

Treatment is confined to surgical measures for the relief of pressure symptoms.

Walter Bauer
Frederic C. Bartter

References

Falconer, M. A., and Cope, C. L.: Fibrous Dysplasia of Bone with Endocrine Disorders and Cutaneous Pigmentation (Albright's Disease). Quart. J. Med., N. S. 11:121, 1942.

Freedman, E.: Leontiasis Ossea. Radiology, 20:8, 1933.

Knaggs, R. L.: Leontiasis Ossea. Brit. J. Surg., 11: 347, 1923–4.

Pugh, D. G.: Fibrous Dysplasia of the Skull: A Probable Explanation for Leontiasis Ossea. Radiology, 44:548, 1945.

Windholz, F.: Cranial Manifestations of Fibrous Dysplasia of Bone. Their Relation to Leontiasis Ossea and to Simple Bone Cysts of the Vault. Am. J. Roentgenol., 58:51, 1947.

DYSCHONDROPLASIA

(A. Hereditary Deforming Chondrodysplasia; B. Ollier's Disease)

The terms dyschondroplasia and chondrodysplasia have been used to describe two clinical syndromes which, although superficially resembling each other, are probably remotely if at all related. The first, hereditary deforming chondrodysplasia, an inherited disease, has also been termed multiple cartilaginous exostoses, diaphysial aclasis, multiple congenital osteochondromas, multiple cancellous exostoses, hereditary multiple exostoses and familial chondrodystrophy.

The second, Ollier's disease, a nonhereditary disease, has also been termed multiple cartilaginous enchondroses and enchondromatosis. When multiple hemangiomas are also present, it is part of Maffucci's syndrome.

HEREDITARY DEFORMING CHONDRODYSPLASIA

This is a fairly common disorder, in which bony protuberances, often with a cartilaginous cap, are found arising from the cortex of the bones. Müller has produced strong evidence to show that they arise within the periosteum. By far the commonest sites are the long bones, in which they are usually found in the metaphysial region, although they may appear more centrally in regions which constituted the metaphyses at an earlier date. The metaphyses are commonly broad, showing various degrees of failure of remodeling to the normal "trumpet shape." The exostoses join the bone with an obtuse angle distally, and an acute angle centrally, thus virtually always pointing towards the center of the bone. In a single radiographic view, an osteochondroma may be indistinguishable from an enchondroma. A second picture taken at 90 degrees from the first seldom fails to distinguish them. The disorder is generally bilaterally, albeit asymmetrically, distributed. In decreasing order of frequency, the most commonly affected regions are the tibia, femur, humerus, hand, radius, fibula, ulna, scapula and ribs. It is noteworthy that the hands are relatively infrequently involved. In Stock's series, they showed changes in 8 per cent of cases. Frequently the ulna is shorter than the radius, which may show bowing, dislocation of the head or incurving at the distal end, with or without ulnar deviation of the hand. The distal end of the ulna may end in a point, which, together with the broadened metaphysis, constitutes the characteristic "arrow head" deformity. The fibula is often foreshortened at the distal end, allowing valgus deformity of the ankle. There is characteristically some shortening of all the long bones (even those not otherwise involved), and subjects with the disease are generally below normal height.

With the onset of puberty and epiphysial closure, the lesions cease to enlarge, and some may partially regress. They may become completely ossified.

Aside from the strong hereditary tendency, nothing is known of the etiology of the disorder. Keith has attempted to explain the exostoses as a manifestation of partial failure of resorption analogous to the complete failure (aclasis) which produces the broadened epiphyses. As the exostoses are often much larger than the initial metaphysis, this phenomenon could not explain all the findings. Although tendons are not found attached to the exostoses, their attachment thereto at an earlier date may have played a part in their formation. Jacobsen attributes the condition to an inherited tendency of areas of the periosteum to initiate chondrogenesis, which is followed by normal transformation to bone.

Although the condition is most frequently asymptomatic, the exostoses may interfere mechanically with normal activity, alter the direction of tendon pull or cause pressure on nerves or, rarely, erosion of blood vessels. In addition, the deformities of wrists and ankles may produce symptoms for mechanical reasons. Pathologic fractures do not occur. Sarcomatous degeneration is rare. When treatment is necessary, it consists of simple excision of the growths.

OLLIER'S DISEASE

This is a rare disorder in which irregular fragments of cartilage are found persisting in the substance of endochondral bone. Speiser has produced strong evidence to show that they represent portions of the epiphysial plate which have failed to undergo normal bony replacement and become incorporated in the mature bone. The commonest sites are the long bones, in which they, like the exostoses described above, are usually found in the metaphysial region, but may appear in regions which were formerly metaphysial. In bones with but one metaphysis, like the metatarsals, metacarpals and phalanges, they are rarely seen in the end which lacked an epiphysis. In this disorder there is no failure of remodelling of metaphyses. The enchondromas may, however, expand, producing gross deformities of the part. The usefulness of the hands may be completely destroyed by such a process. Occasional exostoses are found in the disease, but they lack the characteristic shape of the hereditary osteochondromas described above. Expanding enchondromas may, in distorting the bony cortex, superficially resemble osteochondromas. Examination of the base, of the shape of the tumor and of the remaining bones should easily establish the true nature of the lesion. The disorder was thought by Ollier to be characteristically unilateral in distribution, but most cases show lesions on both sides, albeit often markedly asymmetrical in extent. In decreasing order of frequency the most commonly affected regions are the hand (but rarely the carpal bones), the foot, the femur, the ribs, the fibula and the pelvis. It is noteworthy that the hands are most frequently involved. In Stock's series, they showed changes in 74 per cent of cases. As in hereditary deforming chondrodysplasia, the distal end of the ulna may be abnormally short, and this, together with involvement of the distal end of the radius, may give rise to curvature of the radius and ulnar deviation of the hand. An involved bone is characteristically shorter than its uninvolved counterpart. When, as often happens, the lesions are present in only one side of a metaphysis linear growth may be more rapid on the healthy side, with resultant curvature of the bone. With the onset of puberty the lesions often cease to enlarge and may calcify. They often begin to calcify in highly irregular fashion much earlier, the calcified regions often appearing more dense radiographically than the normal bone. The resultant picture of bones distorted by irregular radiolucent masses which are in turn mottled with radio-opaque flecks is almost pathognomonic.

Nothing is known of the etiology of the disorder. When few bones are involved, there may be no symptoms. Symptoms may result from the disturbance of function as a result of bending, shortening and expansion of involved bones. Pathologic fractures are not uncommon and may lead to discovery of the condition. Sarcomatous degeneration is rare. When treatment is attempted, it consists of osteotomies to correct curvature and removal of cartilaginous tumors with replacement by bone chips to prevent further growth of, or fracture through, a lesion.

WALTER BAUER
FREDERIC C. BARTTER

References

Carleton, A., Elkington, J. St. C., Greenfield, J. G., and Robb-Smith, A. H. T.: Maffucci's Syndrome (Dyschondroplasia with Haemangiomata). Quart. J. Med., N. S., 11:203, 1942.
Ehrenfried, A.: Multiple Cartilaginous Exostoses— Hereditary Deforming Dyschondroplasia. J.A. M.A., 64:1642, 1915; 68:502, 1917.
Jacobsen, S. A.: Critique on the Inter-relationships of the Osteogenic Tumors. Am. J. Cancer, 40:375, 1940.
Keith, A.: Studies on the Anatomical Changes which Accompany Certain Growth Disorders of the Human Body. I. The Nature of the Structural Alterations in the Disorder Known as Multiple Exostoses. J. Anat., 54:101, 1919.
Ollier, L.: De la dyschondroplasia. Bull. d. l. Soc. d. Chir. de Lyon, 3:22, 1899.
Speiser, F.: Ein Fall von Systematisierter Enchondromatosis des Skeletts. Virchows Arch. f. path. Anat., 258:126, 1925.
Stocks, P.: Diaphyseal Aclasis (Multiple Exostoses), Multiple Enchondromatoma, Cheido-cranial Dysostosis. London University Eugenics Lab. Memorial No. 22, Treasury of Human Inheritance III. Hereditary Disorders of Bone Development. 1:48, 1925.

ACHONDROPLASIA

(Chondrodystrophia Foetalis, "Fetal Rickets")

Definition. Achondroplasia is a disease of the skeleton which begins in fetal life and is characterized by shortness of stature with the extremities relatively shorter than the trunk, a large brachycephalic head with the nose bridge sunken, "square" stubby hands, and a dorsal kyphosis terminating abruptly in a backward-tilted sacrum. Although Kaufman classified cases on the basis of differences in the (always abnormal) cartilage growth, they are probably all variations of the same disease process.

Incidence. Moerch's data suggest that the sporadic occurrence of achondroplasia in the populace at large is approximately one in 10,000. A child of an achondroplastic parent has a 50 per cent chance of showing the disorder, however. Caffey found it to be the commonest of the congenital bone dystrophies among patients seen at a children's hospital.

Etiology. Although the pathologic physiology of achondroplasia is not fully understood, it is clear that it is essentially a disorder of cartilage growth and of endochondral bone formation. It is also clear that it is frequently or always hereditary. In animals, hereditary achondroplasia is not uncommon, and the mode of inheritance, not the same in all species, has been well established, Thus, examples of achondroplasia are found in Ancon sheep, Telemark and Dexter-Kerry cattle, creeper fowl and a cross-breed of rabbits (Brown and Pearce). In some of these the trait is recessive, in some dominant; the phenotype may be heterozygous or homozygous; when it is heterozygous, the homozygous condition is sometimes lethal. Moerch has shown that human achondroplasia is probably always inherited as a dominant trait. Jansen has presented an ingenious study attempting to explain all the manifestations as results of abnormal amnion pressure between the second and sixth weeks of gestation. Even if this is the immediate mechanism, it is clear that a defect in the germ plasm can or must be ultimately responsible. The age of the parents of sporadic cases of achondroplasia is significantly greater than that of normal children.

Morbid Anatomy. All bony structures formed in cartilage are affected to a greater or less degree. As the membranous bones of the skull show secondary changes, the dis-

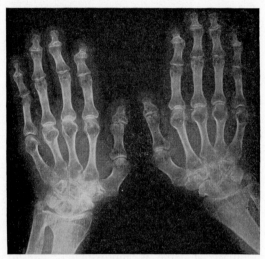

Fig. 193. Hands of a patient with achondroplasia. Note short metacarpals, thickened in epiphysial region.

ease can be said to affect the entire skeleton. Jansen has shown that many of the abnormalities represent persistence of fetal relationships, and that those structures that are formed latest are most affected. In the skull, the osseous centers for the basilar part of the occipital bone, the presphenoid and the postsphenoid are crowded together and fuse early, resulting in a shortened basis cranii, brachycephaly, and, occasionally, in a rudimentary or absent sella. The hard palate is thrust inward and its posterior end elevated, resulting in a narrowing of the nasal pharynx and a relative prognathism of the mandible; the bridge of the nose is depressed; the bones of the vault show a relative increase in size to accommodate the brain; the base of the occipital squama may be displaced forward, with narrowing of the foramen magnum. The last-named deformity probably accounts for many fetal deaths.

The spine is affected to a comparatively minor extent. The vertebrae are thinner than

normal (the lower ones being more affected than the upper), the intervertebral disks wider. There may be wedged vertebrae. The bodies do not show the "tongues," "beaks" or biconvexity characteristic of the other osteochondrodystrophies. A dorsal kyphosis is frequently present. The long bones are short and relatively thick for their length; the humerus and femur are characteristically relatively shorter than the bones of the forearm and lower leg. The femoral necks may be barely apparent. The radii are occasionally longer than the ulnas, resulting in dislocation of the head of the radius; the fibulas are quite regularly elongated relative to the tibias, even reaching the knee joint above, and presenting an abnormally low external malleolus below. Varus deformity of the knees may be in part a result of this disproportion. Muscular attachments on the long bones are often thickened, distorting the cortex. The long bones of the hands and feet are often short, and the epiphyses thick (Fig. 193). The sternum is sometimes short, sloping outward from above downward; the ribs, abnormally short, may be "beaded" anteriorly. The scapulas may show "squared" angles. The pelvis is often poorly developed, the ischia relatively infantile, the outlet narrowed.

The lips may be thick, the tongue protruding. The fingers are short and thick, diverging from their bases like the prongs of a trident (Marie). The skin, especially in fetal and early postnatal life, is redundant for the short limbs, hanging in folds like knickerbockers (Jansen) about the knees.

The histologic picture always shows a failure of pre-osseous cartilage cells to assume the orderly columnar structure, and little or no endochondral bone formation. Fibrous bands may appear between the metaphysial bone and the cartilaginous endplates. The periosteal bone may extend beyond, and "embrace" the epiphysial plate. In addition, some cases show distortion (chondrodystrophia malacica) and abnormal proliferation (chondrodystrophia hyperplastica), with "slipping" of the epiphyseal cartilage.

Pathologic Physiology. There is no known biochemical abnormality characteristic of achondroplasia. The available evidence is against the existence of pituitary or other glandular disease.

Symptoms. Many of the objective changes have been described. The shortening of the extremities produces a striking dwarfism, wherein the central point of the body is in the region of the xiphoid rather than the symphysis pubis, and the hands may barely reach the hips. The majority of the infants with this disease are stillborn. Those who survive often enjoy a normal life span, and, indeed, unusual strength and vigor. The narrowing of the nasal pharynx may result in stertorous respiration. Limitation of extension of the elbows is almost a constant feature. The commonly present dorsal kyphosis is compensated for by a sharp backward rotation of the sacrum, with resulting characteristic prominence of the buttocks. The acetabulums are thus displaced backward, and a "rolling" gait may result. The promontory of the sacrum is thrust forward into the pelvic inlet. This, and the pelvic deformity already alluded to, may make it impossible for the achondroplastic to bear children without cesarean section.

Achondroplastics may be unusually well developed muscularly, and possess a strength relatively much greater than that of normal persons. They are not abnormal mentally. They are reputed to have abnormally great potencia and libido. The sexual organs of male subjects, normal relative to the size of the trunk, often appear large relative to total body size.

Roentgenologic studies, while seldom necessary to establish the diagnosis, reveal striking and characteristic changes. The epiphyses, which may close early or late, reveal a pathognomonic "cupping" of the metaphysis around the ossification center of the epiphysis, which is placed nearer the shaft than normally. The joint spaces, like the intervertebral spaces, may be abnormally wide; the glenoid fossae and acetabulums are often incompletely formed. The shafts of the long bones may show, in addition to their shortening, thickening of the cortex and abrupt flaring at the metaphyses, terminating, when the epiphyses are closed, in blunt, poorly formed, club-like ends (Fig. 193).

As Pierre Marie pointed out, the apparent bowing of long bones in this condition is generally due to distortions at or immediately below the epiphyses, and is thus unlike that seen in rickets or Paget's disease.

Diagnosis. The features of achondroplasia are so unique that a typical case presents little difficulty in differential diagnosis. In the other osteochondrodystrophies (Morquio's disease, gargoylism) which produce dwarfism, the spine is abnormally short, rather than the limbs, and thus the abnormality is not apparent at birth, as it is in achondroplasia. Rickets is easily distinguished both by its radiologic and by its biochemical characteristics. Osteogenesis imperfecta may resemble achondroplasia superficially at the time of delivery, but x-ray studies readily establish its true nature.

Prognosis. The majority of achondroplastics die *in utero*. Those who survive the first year may reach extreme old age. They seldom exceed 140 cm. in height. Of importance to the normal mother of an achondroplastic child is the extreme improbability that a succeeding child will be affected.

Treatment. No known treatment affects the disease. Surgical measures to correct deformities are seldom necessary.

WALTER BAUER
FREDERIC C. BARTTER

References

Brown, W. H., and Pearce, L.: Hereditary Achondroplasia in Rabbits. J. Exper. Med., 82:241, 1945.
Caffey, J.: Achondroplasia. Brenneman's Practice of Pediatrics. Vol. IV, Ch. 28. Hagerstown, Md., W. F. Prior Co., 1945.
Fairbank, H. A. T.: Atlas of General Affections of the Skeleton. Baltimore, Williams and Wilkins Co., 1951.
Jansen, M.: Achondroplasia: Its Nature and Cause. Leiden, E. J. Brill, Ltd., 1912.
Kaufmann, E.: Untersuchungen über die sogenannte foetale Rachitis (Chondrodystrophia Foetalis). Berlin, 1892.
Marie, P.: L'achondroplasie dans l'adolescence et l'age adulte. Presse Méd., 8, ii, 17, 1900.
Moerch, E. T.: Achondroplasia Is Always Hereditary and Is Inherited Dominantly. J. Heredity, 31:439, 1940.
———: Chondrodystrophic Dwarfs in Denmark. Opera ex Domo Biologiae Hereditariae Humanae Universitatis Hafniensis, v. III. Copenhagen, Munksgaard, 1941.

OXYCEPHALY

(Acrocephaly, Acrocephalosyndactyly)

Definition. Oxycephaly refers strictly to a condition in which the cranium is elongated from base to apex (height/length greater than .77), and is essentially synonymous with the terms acrocephaly, turricephaly and steeple head. The term is often used, however, in a generic sense, to include other disorders of the cranium which have a common pathogenesis—namely, premature synostosis. Such disorders include scaphocephaly, keel- or boat-shaped head, where the cranium is elongated from before backward (width/length less than .76) and low (height/length less than .58), and plagiocephaly, where the cranium is distorted asymmetrically. Crouzon's disease, or craniofacial dysostosis, once mistakenly set apart because of its hereditary tendency, is another name for oxycephaly. In all of these disorders, there is aplasia of the bones of the cranial vault and the maxilla, with premature synostoses and resulting deformity of the skull. Exophthalmos is common, and partial or complete blindness is the complication most frequently observed. In many cases there are associated symmetrical deformities of the extremities.

Incidence. The incidence of premature synostosis has not been established. The later the closure occurs, the less need there is for later expansion of the brain, and hence the less deformity will occur and the fewer complications will appear. Thus, many mild cases, in which roentgenography alone would establish the diagnosis, doubtless go unrecognized.

Etiology. There is strong evidence that oxycephaly and acrocephalosyndactyly can be inherited as a dominant feature, so that a mutation is presumably the remote cause of the condition. A similar, clearly hereditary syndrome is found in rabbits. The immediate pathogenesis was ascribed by Park and Power to abnormality in, or partial absence of, the specialized mesenchymal tissue which is destined to separate the primordial (mesenchymal) anlage of the skeleton into individual bones. In the vault of the skull, the result is a premature fusion as bone arising from one ossification center meets that arising from a contiguous one. In the extremities, the result is a partial failure of the normal separation of long bones both transversely and longitudinally. This ingenious theory thus offers an explanation not only for the cranial synostoses, but also for the malformations of joints and the failure of separation of the bones and soft tissues of the digits which are so frequently present. Many secondary changes, including the characteristic shapes of the skull, are clearly the result of continued brain growth after synostosis has occurred. (When brain growth ceases as the primary event and premature synostosis occurs as a result, as in microcephaly, none of these secondary changes are found.)

Morbid Anatomy. Although all the bones of the skull show premature synostosis in oxycephaly, the earliest fusions largely determine the ultimate shape of the head. In this section we shall consider, first, those changes attributable to the primary mesenchymal defects, second, the shapes of the skull that may result, and third, the pressure changes which follow in all forms when expansion of the cranial contents is seriously interfered with.

When synostosis occurs, a more or less prominent ridge marks the line of fusion (this feature, indeed, gave rise to the name scaphocephaly). The ossification centers are displaced toward the ridge, and appear to blend into one across it. In part because these centers help form the frontal, occipital and parietal bosses, and in part because of the flattening of the bones of the vault towards the vertical, these eminences are lost— the first two in acrocephaly, the third in scaphocephaly.

There may be hypoplasia of the basioccipital and premature fusion (or failure of separation) of the pre- and postsphenoid and of the sphenoid with the occipital bones, but this is not a constant finding. Hypoplasia of the maxilla is a fairly constant feature, resulting in a narrow upper alveolar arch, with malocclusion, a high arched palate, deviation of the nasal septum, a curving of the nose into the "bec de perroquet" and a relative prognathism of the mandible. The optic foramina may be smaller or more elliptical than normal, a feature contributing to the visual impairment.

As mentioned above, premature synostosis produces three characteristic skull shapes— acrocephaly, scaphocephaly and plagiocephaly. In acrocephaly, the coronal suture, the the lambdoidal suture, or both are replaced (in whole or in part) by synostoses, and any further expansion of the vault must take place by depression of the base, and by expansion at the sagittal, and, to a lesser extent, at the metopic suture lines. The skull becomes elongated vertically, with deep fossae, and may be expanded laterally and thus brachycephalic. Whereas the parietal and occipital bosses are characteristically absent (see above), the superciliary ridges often appear prominent. The frontal and occipital bones may rise vertically from the neck and orbits. The apex of the elongated skull tends to be located posteriorly when the frontal and parietal bones fuse first, anteriorly when the parietals and occipitals fuse first, and centrally when all fuse simultaneously. In scaphocephaly, the sagittal suture is replaced by a synostosis, and any further expansion of the vault must take place by depression of the base and by expansion at the metopic, coronal and lambdoidal suture lines. The skull becomes elongated anteroposteriorly, with deep fossae, and fails to attain normal height. The parietal bosses are characteristically absent. Secondary changes (see below) tend to be less marked with scaphocephaly than with acrocephaly. In plagiocephaly, synostoses occur asymmetrically, with resulting asymmetric distortion of the head. Secondary changes, with one exception, all result from pressure imparted by the expanding brain in the restricted cranial cavity. The exception is the occasional direct damage to the optic nerves whose growth is restricted by narrowed optic foramina.

The posterior fossa is depressed, occasionally to such an extent as to cause the odontoid process of the axis to enter and narrow the foramen magnum. The middle fossa is pressed downward and anteriorly, with increase of the sphenoidal angle (basilar lordosis) and anterior displacement of the great sphenoid wings. The anterior fossa is deepened by downward displacement of the orbital plates of the frontal bones; the frontal sinus is usually absent. These changes combine to produce orbits that are shallower than normal, slant downward and outward, and are sometimes farther apart than normal (hypertelorism). Exophthalmos is a very common result.

All the bones facing the cranial cavity may show convolutional markings, and, histologically, a lack of inner table and diploë; in severe cases, the outer table as well may be perforated. The cerebrospinal fluid presure may be high, albeit rarely to an extreme degree. The brain has been observed, upon decompression, to lack its normal pulsations. Bone changes and pressure phenomena prevent normal drainage, and the venous channels of the vault are often distended. Foramina for emissary veins, normally small, may be greatly enlarged, and new ones may appear; venous distention about the scalp and face may be striking.

Syndactyly has been mentioned as a commonly associated phenomenon (about one fourth of cases reviewed by Ferriman). It involves bones and soft parts, and is strikingly symmetrical. Associated joint defects are common, ranging from minor deformities with limitation of motion especially in hands, elbows, and shoulders, to an occasional complete ankylosis.

Symptoms. The objective signs have been covered in large part under morbid anatomy. Severe degrees of acrocephalic and scaphocephalic deformity are recognizable on sight, the one revealing an unnaturally high head, narrowed from before backward, face and forehead parallel, surmounted by a "cap" of

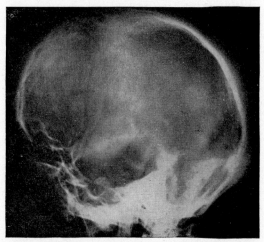

Fig. 194. The calvarium is abnormally short and the frontal fossa particularly shows foreshortening and a steeply sloping floor. The middle fossa is unusually deep. The posterior fossa is shallow. The coronal and lambdoid sutures are completely fused and obliterated.

hair high above the ears; the other an unnaturally low head, elongated from before backward, forehead and occiput protruding.

Headaches, nausea and vomiting and convulsions are not uncommon. They are undoubtedly a result of increased intracranial pressure, and are relieved by decompression. Visual impairment is extremely common. It may result from secondary optic atrophy following prolonged elevation of intracranial pressure with papilledema, or from primary atrophy due to damage to the optic nerve. The latter has been attributed to narrowing of the foramina, to tipping of the lesser wings of the sphenoid, or to impingement of the carotoid arteries upon the nerves at the foramina.

Mouth breathing may be a prominent feature, and anosmia has been reported in a number of cases. Mentality is generally normal. The exophthalmos is a cardinal feature, and may be so severe as to result in corneal ulcerations, or even dislocation of the orbit. Divergent squint may be present.

Prognosis. Beyond the age of 5 (when 90 per cent of brain growth is completed) serious complications seldom appear *de novo*. Before 5, the prognosis may well depend upon the promptness and adequacy with which therapy is instituted. Once the diagnosis is made, the patient must be watched with extreme care. Infants related to the patient should also be carefully watched.

Treatment. Treatment may be instigated to relieve pressure in general, to protect the optic nerves and to enlarge the orbits. It is surgical in all cases. In general, it must be performed before the age of 5 to be of benefit. For relief of pressure, "cruciectomy" of the vault (Faber and Towne) may be performed, or the more extensive "mosaic" operation of King. An operation such as these, performed early, may prevent the development of all the serious complications. In older cases, exophthalmos may be treated directly by unroofing the orbit, provided there is no longer any increased pressure. In those cases in which the optic foramina are narrow as a part of the original hypoplasia of bone, relief may be obtained by unroofing the foramina.

WALTER BAUER
FREDERIC C. BARTTER

References

Faber, H. K., and Towne, E. B.: Early Cruciectomy as Preventive Measure in Oxycephaly and Allied Conditions, with Special Reference to Prevention of Blindness. Am. J. M. Sc., *173*:701, 1927.

Ferriman, D.: Acrocephaly and Acrocephalosyndactyly. New York, Oxford University Press, 1941.

Greene, H. S. N.: Oxycephaly and Allied Conditions in Man and in the Rabbit. J. Exper. Med., 57:967, 1933.

Grieg, D. M.: Oxycephaly. Edinburgh M. J., N.S., 33:189, 280, 357, 1926.

King, J. E. J.: Oxycephaly. Ann. Surg., *115*:488, 1942.

Park, E. A., and Powers, G. F.: Acrocephaly and Scaphocephaly with Symmetrically Distributed Malformations of the Extremities. Am. J. Dis. Child., 20:235, 1920.

Reeves, D. L.: Craniofacial Dysostosis of Crouzon. The Surgical Treatment of Oxycephaly. Brennenman's Practice of Pediatrics. Hagerstown, Md., W. F. Prior Co., 1945, Vol. 4.

HYPEROSTOSIS FRONTALIS INTERNA

(L'hyperostose frontale interne, metabolic craniopathy, enostoses of the calvarium, calvarial hyperostosis, Stewart-Morel syndrome)

Definition. Hyperostosis frontalis interna is a condition almost exclusively of women, in which newly formed bone is deposited on the inner aspect of the frontal bones. As the outer table is not affected, the diagnosis depends essentially upon radiologic or postmortem evidence. There are a number of clinical reports in which it is suggested that it forms part of a *syndrome* involving also metabolic and psychiatric abnormalities. None of these reports is convincing, and no single associated abnormality is found in all or even the majority of cases.

The condition was clearly described by Morel, who reviewed the literature and reported 17 new cases. It consists of essentially symmetrical inward thickenings of the squama frontalis on either side of the midline, where the floor of the superior sagittal sinus is always spared. The enostoses may arise abruptly or gradually from the surrounding bone, and may be smooth or nodular. They frequently show a roughly radiate arrangement, the "spokes" descending from the highest central region to the level of the old inner table. The new bone may be cancellous bone indistinguishable from the old, or show areas of compact bone of ivory hardness. The dura mater is characteristically closely adherent, shredded and "literally absorbed" (Canavan) in the region of the enostoses—a finding which suggested to Morel his theory of the etiology. The enostoses do not involve the parietal bones or the orbital plates of the frontal bones. Moore has suggested that this condition is related to three others (nebula frontalis, hyperostosis calvariae diffusa and hyperostosis frontoparietalis) in which there is condensation of diploic bone without displacement of the tables. There are no established criteria by which such a relationship can be affirmed or denied.

Incidence. Hyperostosis frontalis interna has been reported in all age groups. The incidence among reported cases is greatest after the age of 40, but few series are available in which the population sample does not have a strong age bias. The commonly associated advanced arteriosclerosis is probably not beyond that expected in the general population of corresponding age. The incidence of hyperostosis has been reported as between 1 and 1.5 per cent in most large series, generally based on roentgenographic findings. Canavan, who studied autopsy protocols, found an incidence of "enostoses" of some 7 per cent in a mental institution, but the exact criteria for establishing the diagnosis are not stated. A corresponding autopsy study from a general hospital is not available.

Etiology. Nothing is known of the etiology of the condition. Morel attributed it to the pull of the attached dura in patients who spend considerable periods in dorsal decubitus. He was impressed by degenerative changes in the nerve cells in the walls of the third ventricle. A number of cases have had pituitary tumors, some with associated acromegaly. Stewart found partial pituitary fibrosis in 3 of his cases, whereas Canavan reported no typical lesion in the pituitary gland in 20 cases. Some authors have found underlying atrophy of brain, and interpreted the bone changes as secondary thereto. Any satisfactory explanation will have to account for the incidence almost exclusively in women. There is no known biochemical abnormality in the condition.

Obesity (favoring the upper arms and thighs, hence "rhizomélique") was thought by Morel to form a part of the syndrome mentioned above, although half of his subjects were apparently not obese. Less than half of the cases subsequently reported have been obese (Fig. 195), and it is not clear that this association is other than a chance one.

Mental disease has been commonly thought to be a part of a syndrome involving hyperostosis frontalis interna. As many of the studies, including Morel's, were done in mental institutions, there are few "control" data available. Even here, however, all types of mental disease are represented. Moore's series from a general hospital shows a scatter of asociated complaints typical of those for which skull roentgenograms are ordinarily ordered in a general hospital, and does not give support to the concept of a "syndrome."

WALTER BAUER
FREDERIC C. BARTTER

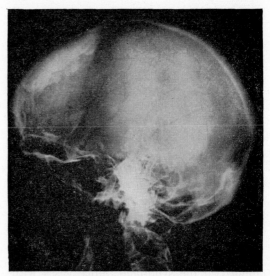

Fig. 195. Hyperostosis frontalis interna. The patient (who was normal mentally and not obese) had myotonia dystrophica.

References

Canavan, M. M.: Enostoses of Calvarium. Arch. Neurol. & Psychiat., 39:41, 1938.
Grieg, D. M.: On Intracranial Osteophytes. Edinburgh M. J., 35:165, 237, 1928.
Moore, S.: Hyperostosis Frontalis Interna. Surg., Gynec. & Obst., 61:345, 1935.
———: Metabolic Craniopathy. Am. J. Roentgenol., 35:30, 1936.
Morel, F.: L'Hyperostose frontale interne. Thèse, Genève, Chapaloy and Montier, 1929.
Stewart, R. M.: Localized Cranial Hyperostosis in the Insane. J. Neurol. & Psychiat., 8:321, 1927–8.

HYPERTROPHIC OSTEO-ARTHROPATHY

(Hippocratic or Clubbed Fingers, Secondary Hypertrophic Osteoarthropathy, Hypertrophic Pulmonary Osteoarthropathy, Marie-Bamberger Syndrome, Osteoarthropathie Hypertrophiante Pneumique, Familial Idiopathic Hypertrophic Osteoarthropathy, Touraine-Solente-Golé Syndrome)

Definition. Hypertrophic osteoarthropathy is a syndrome characterized by (1) clubbing of the fingers, (2) periosteal new bone formation involving especially the long bones, (3) swelling and pains of the joints, generally of moderate degree, and (4) signs of autonomic disorder, flushing and blanching, and profuse sweating—confined to or most marked in the hands and feet. The complete tetrad is not found in every case, but the bone and joint changes without the clubbing are extremely rare. Although the majority of cases are secondary to intrathoracic disease, there are a number which are not.

Etiology. There is little question that the pathogenesis of clubbing of the fingers is the same as that of hypertrophic osteoarthropathy, the latter representing a more advanced stage of the disorder. In many cases thought to show simple clubbing, a review of the roentgenograms will reveal early periosteal new bone formation.

Although the mechanism of their mediation is not known, it is certain that diseases elsewhere in the body are responsible for most cases—hence the term "secondary" often applied to the syndrome. Since cases without a remote "cause" exist, "secondary," like the term "pulmonary," becomes a misnomer when applied to the syndrome as a whole.

In roughly decreasing order of frequency, the conditions in which secondary hypertrophic osteoarthropathy is found are (1) lesions in the lungs, mediastinum and pleura, including benign and malignant tumors, chronic infections and, rarely, aneurysms, (2) diseases of the cardiovascular system, especially cyanotic congenital heart disease and subacute bacterial endocarditis, (3) diseases of the liver, especially hypertrophic biliary cirrhosis, but including cirrhosis of other cause, amyloidosis and liver abscess, and (4) diseases of the gastrointestinal tract, generally in association with chronic diarrhea, including ulcerative colitis, regional enteritis, chronic dysentery, neoplasm and steatorrhea. It may occur with the polycythemia of high altitudes, and has been reported in a few cases of hypothyroidism. It may occur in the absence of any "primary" disease, as an hereditary dominant trait (hereditary clubbing) or as a familial disease of young men (Touraine-Solente-Golé Syndrome). It may be unilateral, as with aneurysmal dilatation of a subclavian or innominate artery, or even unidigital.

No satisfactory explanation for the osteoarthropathy has been found. Many have ascribed it to "toxins," and one author produced similar lesions in guinea pigs treated with an extract of a bronchiolar carcinoma. This theory is supported by the common observation that osteoarthropathy often regresses promptly when the "primary" lesion is removed. It does not explain the pathogenesis in cyanotic heart disease or in the "idiopathic" varieties. Other authors have ascribed it to anoxia, as a result of venous stasis from back pressure, or arterial undersaturation, a view that fails to explain the numerous cases with no increase in venous pressure and normal arterial oxygen saturation. Still other authors, struck with certain similarities between osteoarthropathy and acromegaly, have invoked anterior pituitary overactivity (itself secondary to the underlying disease) to explain the syndrome. This view is perhaps strengthened by the frequent finding of an elevated serum phosphorus with osteoarthropathy, but is weakened by frequent findings of normal carbohydrate tolerance curves, and by the absence of most of the classic signs of growth hormone activity. Mendlowitz has shown that the digital blood flow is generally increased, and the brachiodigital pressure gradient decreased, with acquired clubbing but not with the hereditary form, and that both may return to normal with removal of the remote cause in the lungs. These findings, taken together with the frequently associated vasomotor and sudomotor instability, suggest that the autonomic nervous system may play a role in the disorder.

Incidence. The "idiopathic" varieties of osteoarthropathy are rare, but the "secondary" varieties are relatively common, their incidence being correlated, of course, with that of the primary disease. With improvement in surgical and chemotherapeutic measures for elimination of intrathoracic disease, the incidence is steadily declining. Males are affected more frequently than females, a datum which presumably merely reflects the sex distribution of the underlying disorders.

Morbid Anatomy. Grossly, the involved bones show periosteal new growth which ranges in extent from scattered "osteophytes" to complete sheaths of new bone surrounding and distorting the old bone. Although this may result first in a bone denser as well as larger than the original, resorption of the old cortex soon ensues, and the ultimate structure is often thinner and weaker than normal. The extremities are affected earliest and generally show the most advanced lesions. In the long bones of the lower legs and arms, the distal ends are involved first, the process often starting at the attachment of the interosseous membrane, and spreading upward but sparing the region of the epiphysis until late. In the bones of the hands, "collars" may form about the distal third of the metacarpals and first and second phalanges, often thickening the cortex in this region until this is the widest part of the bone. The terminal phalanx, the site of the clubbing, seldom shows periosteal proliferation, although subungual osteophytes have been described. The progress is roughly centripetal

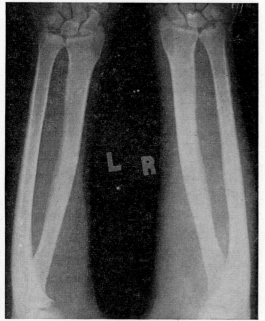

Fig. 196. A roentgenogram depicting the subperiosteal overgrowth of the long bones of the forearm of a patient with generalized osteoarthropathy.

and any bone of the body may be involved in the process, which tends to be symmetrical, although it may, curiously, be more marked on the same side as a lung lesion. The skull is least involved.

Microscopically, the earliest change is round cell infiltration in periosteum, followed by proliferation of the cambial layer and new formation of fibrous bone therefrom. The old compact bone soon shows widening of haversian canals, and may proceed to disappear almost completely. The new bone may be replaced by lamellar haversian systems, and may itself be the subject of considerable resorption.

The clubbed terminal phalanges show edema of the soft parts, with proliferation of fibrous tissue and thickening of blood vessel walls. The bone may show increased tufting, or, with prolonged clubbing, resorption of the normal distal flare.

The joints show thickening of synovium with round cell infiltration and hydrarthrosis, or may develop fibrinoid degeneration of cartilage, and loss of structure by resorption from above by pannus and from below by ad-

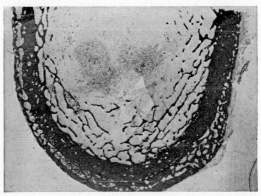

Fig. 197. A cross section of a tibia of the same patient (Figure 196) obtained at post mortem. There is no evidence of osteogenic activity at this time. The new bone has formed a cancellous sheath about the old cortex which now shows foci of lacunar resorption. The radial appearance of the trabeculae has disappeared and a well defined pseudocortex has formed.

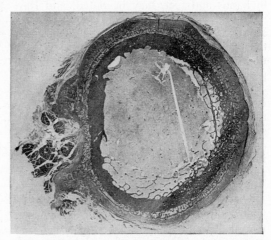

Fig. 198. A cross section through a metatarsal of the same patient (Figure 196). The periosteum is thickened and divided into an outer fibrous and an inner cambial layer. There is an irregular deposit of new bone on the cortex. The latter shows some osteoporosis.

vancing fibrous marrow. The skin and soft tissues of the ankles, wrists, hands and feet may show marked nonpitting swelling ("elephant foot"), a constant finding in familial osteoarthropathy.

Pathologic Physiology and Chemistry. New bone formation is the most prominent abnormality, and it is not surprising that the serum alkaline phosphatase is often moderately elevated. Osteoporosis of the old bone may progress *pari passu,* and the net effect may be to decrease the bone mass. Thus, the urinary calcium may be elevated. The serum phosphorus is often moderately elevated, a finding which has not been explained. The sedimentation rate is generally elevated when arthropathy is present.

Symptoms. The onset is insidious, the patient often failing to note the clubbing of the fingers that is usually the earliest sign. This may be grossly apparent, with "watch glass" or "parrot-beak" nails, or consist only of "floating" of the nail beds, with loss of the normal angle of inclination of nail toward bone. As the bone lesions progress, gross deformities may be noted. Though the pain is usually mild, it can on occasion be severe, unremitting and difficult to control. Discomfort, swelling and, less commonly, severe pain in joints may occur, the knees, ankles, wrists, elbows and metacarpophalangeal joints being most frequently involved.

Bouts of profuse sweating, often confined to hands and feet, may be noted, and Raynaud's phenomena with cold sensation may alternate with episodes of distal flushing of the extremities, with heat and burning. In a number of cases gynecomastia has been reported.

In the idiopathic familial syndrome there is generally marked thickening of the skin of the forehead, which, together with the coarse swelling of the extremities mentioned above, and the clubbing, may allow diagnosis upon inspection. The sella turcica is not enlarged, nor the lower jaw prognathic.

The course is extremely variable, the osteoarthropathy often fluctuating with the underlying primary disease. If this disease is removed the joint and autonomic disorders may disappear rapidly, and the clubbing and, finally, the bone deformity may in turn regress. Mere exploration of the chest has on occasion relieved the pain in the bones and joints resulting from osteoarthropathy secondary to bronchiogenic carcinoma.

Diagnosis. The features of the complete syndrome are so distinctive as to present no problem in diagnosis. Cases are rarely seen in which joint changes and the autonomic disorder precede detectable clubbing or bone changes. Diagnosis is difficult or impossible at this stage unless a primary disease is discovered. In all cases in which it is not apparent, a diligent search for a primary condition, notably bronchogenic carcinoma, should be instituted.

Treatment. The therapy is clearly that of the primary disease when this is possible. The joint pains and swelling may respond rapidly to cortisone therapy.

WALTER BAUER
FREDERIC C. BARTTER

References

Bamberger, E.: Ueber Knochenveranderungen bei chronischer Lungen und Herzkrankheiten. Ztschr. f.°klin. Med., *18:*193, 1890.

Bariety, M., and Croury, Ch.: L'ostéo-arthropathie hypertrophiante pneumique et les dysacromélies d'origine thoracique. Semaine hôp. Paris, *26:* 1681, 1950.

Crump, C.: Histologie der allgemeinen Osteophytose (Osteoarthropathie Hypertrophiante Pneumique). Virchows Arch. f. path. Anat., *271:*467, 1929.

Gall, E. A., Bennett, G. A., and Bauer, W.: Generalized Hypertrophic Osteoarthropathy. Am. J. Path., *27:*349, 1950.

Marie, P.: De l'ostéo-arthropathie hypertrophiante pneumique. Rev. de méd., *10:*1, 1890.

Mendlowitz, M.: Clubbing and Hypertrophic Osteoarthropathy. Medicine, *21:*269, 1942.

Touraine, A., Solente, A., and Golé, L.: Un syndrome ostéodermopathique. La pachydermie plicaturee avec pachypériostose des extrémités. Presse méd., *43:*1820, 1935.

TUMORS OF BONE

Tumors of bone are new growths which derive from the cellular elements of bone or arise in bone or spread to bone from some other primary source. They are encountered not infrequently by those engaged in the practice of internal medicine or in general medicine. Some are of rare occurrence and are often overlooked or mistaken for other diseases which may affect the musculoskeletal system. Early diagnosis is essential for prompt and effective treatment; unfortunately, early diagnosis is not usually made. In this brief chapter on neoplasms of bone, emphasis will be placed on measures which will assist in their prompt recognition, and only the more important types will be discussed.

At the outset it is imperative to have a workable classification of bone tumors. The accompanying classification, chiefly the concept of the late Dr. James Ewing, is the one widely used (Table 1).

Clinical Features of Benign Tumors of Bone. In general, benign tumors of bone are associated with little or no pain and only slight discomfort. They are nearly always of relatively slow growth. The lesions are usually circumscribed and orderly, and present characteristic roentgenographic features which differ from those usually associated with bone cancer. They may be present for many years before discovery, which often is accidental. Chondromas, osteochondromas

pear soon after the first complaint of pain, but often is not detected for weeks or months later. Its rate of growth may be the index of its degree of malignancy, since, as a rule, the more rapid the growth, the more malignant the tumor. Disability may appear as an early symptom, but is sometimes a late manifestation. It is often referred to the contiguous joint, e.g., knee, shoulder, hip, and the like. Neglected cases of bone sarcoma may show evidence of weight loss, anemia, cachexia and marked local swelling of the primary area. The majority of cases, when

Table 1. Classification of Bone Tumors

MALIGNANT	BENIGN
Fibrosarcoma of bone...	{ Nonosteogenic fibroma of bone { Fibrous dysplasia of bone
Osteogenic sarcoma..	{ Osteoma { Osteoid osteoma { Exostosis
Primary chondrosarcoma Secondary chondromyxosarcoma }	{ Chondroma { Benign chondroblastoma (Codman's epiphyseal giant cell tumor)
Malignant giant cell tumor..	Benign giant cell tumor
Endothelioma (diffuse, Ewing's sarcoma)	
Angiosarcoma...	{ Cavernous angioma { Plexiform angioma
Myeloma (plasma cell)	
Reticulum cell sarcoma	
Metastatic cancer in bone	

This table does not include several other entities that may be encountered, such as adamantinoma of the jaws (rarely of the tibia), chordoma, and so forth.

and occasionally angiomas of bone may undergo malignant transformation, the former to chondrosarcoma, and the latter to angiosarcoma. The advent of pain or increase in size of a preexisting benign tumor is strong presumptive evidence of such malignant alteration.

Some benign bone tumors require no treatment; others, by causing pressure on overlying soft tissues, nerves or blood vessels, or by mechanical interference with function, may require resection or excision. This is sometimes done in the absence of symptoms as a prophylactic measure against malignant degeneration.

Clinical Features of Malignant Tumors of Bone. Pain is the earliest, most constant and most significant symptom. It is usually insidious and intermittent at first, but becomes progressively severe and is followed by swelling and disability. Swelling may ap-

first seen, show none of these characteristics. Unexplained pain in a long bone calls for the *suspicion* of a tumor and an immediate roentgenographic examination. Deeply seated pain in the ribs, pelvis, spine or extremities which is found in a patient who is known to have had a cancer of the lung, prostate, breast, kidney or thyroid or, in fact, in any organ, should arouse suspicion of skeletal metastases. It is a sound principle that major or mutilating operations or roentgen therapy should not be proposed until a microscopic diagnosis has been made.

Benign Giant Cell Tumor. This well established entity is a benign tumor occurring near the ends of long bones of subjects in early adult life. Actually, the lesion is seldom found prior to epiphysial closure—a feature which serves to distinguish it from solitary bone cyst, which roentgenographically it may otherwise closely resemble. It is seen

Table 2. Differential Diagnosis by Exclusion

TUMOR

Benign
- Central
  - Benign chondroblastoma (Jaffe)
  - Chondroma
  - Chondromyxoid fibroma
  - Nonosteogenic fibroma
  - Bone cyst
  - Fibrous dysplasia
  - Giant cell tumor, benign
- Central and cortical
  - Angioma of bone
  - Osteoid osteoma
- Cortical (osteoma)
  - Exostosis
  - Osteochondroma
  - Multiple osteochondroma

Malignant
- Primary
  - Monostotic
    - Osteogenic sarcoma
    - Fibrosarcoma of bone
    - Chondrosarcoma—primary (chondroblastic)
    - " —secondary
    - Ewing's sarcoma (endothelioma)
    - Reticulum cell sarcoma
    - Angiosarcoma of bone
    - Sarcoma arising in irradiated bone
    - Malignant giant cell tumor
  - Polyostotic: Plasma cell myeloma
- Metastatic
  - Breast
  - Kidney
  - Thyroid
  - Prostate
  - Lung, etc.

NOT A TUMOR

- Inflammatory
  - Pyogenic
  - Syphilitic
  - Tubercular
  - Chronic sclerosing osteitis

Posttraumatic–Myositis ossificans
Parasitic–Hydatid disease of bone

- Mycotic infections
  - Actinomycosis
  - Sporotrichosis
  - Coccidioidomycosis
  - Blastomycosis, etc.

- Metabolic
  - Gaucher's disease
  - Niemann-Pick's disease

- Granulomas of uncertain etiology
  - Letterer-Siwe's disease
  - Hand-Schüller-Christian's disease
  - Eosinophilic granuloma

- Circulatory
  - Aseptic necrosis (Caisson disease)
  - Calcinosis

- Osteoporosis
  - Endocrine
    - Hyperparathyroidism (von Recklinghausen's disease)
    - Postmenopausal and senile
  - Nutritional

- Uncertain etiology
  - Paget's disease (Osteitis deformans)
  - Melorrheostosis
  - Osteopetrosis
  - Spontaneous absorption of bone (Phantom bone)
  - Fibrous dysplasia

most often in those between 21 and 35 years of age, and is unusual after the age of 40. It is a purely osteolytic process which destroys the cancellous ends of the long bones, but only occasionally involves the shaft. It may expand and ultimately destroy the cortex. It has a slow and insidious onset, and pain is the presenting symptom. Until expansion has occurred there may be little evidence of its presence on physical examination.

Owing to its proximity to the joint it is often confused with a sprain, ligamentous tear, rheumatic process or a traumatic synovitis. Fortunately the practice of taking roentgenograms promptly in all cases of pain in an extremity has resulted in establishing a correct diagnosis earlier than was possible a few decades ago. The appearance of giant cell tumor on the films is usually quite specific and easily interpreted, so that there is a high percentage of accurate roentgenographic diagnoses.

The clinical course of most cases treated either by roentgen therapy or by surgery is one of eventual healing of the process by ingrowth of new bone which fills the cavity more or less completely, and from then on the situation is a quiescent one. Treatment by either method is acceptable; both have their proponents. Most orthopedic surgeons prefer to curet the tumor tissue from the cavity and then pack it with cancellous bone chips. On the other hand, most roentgen therapists administer x-rays. Both methods have given excellent results in experienced hands, but combined therapy is considered inadvisable.

Despite thorough surgical measures or competent roentgen therapy some cases will present recurrences; some of these will undergo transformation into a malignant tumor (usually termed malignant giant cell tumor) and terminate fatally with lung metastases. This metamorphosis probably does not occur in more than 10 per cent of the cases. When, after treatment, recurrence is detected and biopsy material reveals a more aggressive histologic appearance of the stroma, one should be on guard, and, in the event of further recurrences, proceed to amputate the limb without further delay.

Fibrosarcoma. Often this tumor is included with osteogenic sarcoma, but it has seemed advisable to place it in a separate category. It may present itself as a periosteal fibrosarcoma or as a central lesion, medullary fibrosarcoma. There may be considerable variation in the histologic appearance; some may present all the criteria of highly malignant tumors, while others may be of extremely low grade and be locally invasive with but little tendency to metastasize. The prognosis for fibrosarcoma of bone as a whole is poor since pulmonary metastasis usually supervenes.

Chondrosarcoma. This tumor also is often grouped with osteogenic sarcoma and fibrosarcoma of bone. It is possible to separate chondrosarcoma into two subdivisions. The first, which we have called *primary chondrosarcoma,* resembles osteogenic sarcoma in its location, age and sex incidence, as well as in its roentgenographic appearance. Moreover, it requires the same treatment and has an equally unfavorable prognosis.

The second type we have called *secondary chondrosarcoma* because it arises in a preexisting osteochondroma or in a central chondroma. This variety has a slow, insidious onset, it occurs later in life, has a much slower course, tends to metastasize later and offers a considerably better prognosis for five-year survival. It also has a higher incidence in the scapula and pelvic bones than has osteogenic sarcoma. Because it arises in a preexisting benign cartilage tumor, one must appreciate the fact that pathologic reports of *benign chondroma,* in cases in which clinical and roentgenographic studies suggest a malignant tumor, are not always dependable.

Osteogenic Sarcoma. This highly malignant tumor derives from bone, and has a predilection for the metaphysial portion of a long bone, especially the proximal end of the humerus and tibia, and distal end of the femur. It is the most frequently encountered primary malignant tumor of bone, and affects chiefly children and young adults; males are slightly more subject to it than are females. It occurs in several forms, some of which are characterized by bone production as well as destruction, while others are almost entirely osteolytic. Some authorities include fibrosarcoma of bone and chondrosarcoma as subdivisions of osteogenic sarcoma. None of these types is radiosensitive. Surgery is the method of choice, and in long bones this usually means amputation of the extremity. Recent revival of interest in the operation known as hemipelvectomy has resulted in extending the field of operability to include some tumors arising in the proximal end of the femur and in the innominate bone. Occasional opportunities are encountered where conservative procedures, such as segmental resection, are justified. Roentgen therapy, though not curative, may have its place as a palliative method of treatment, particularly in cases beyond the scope of any amputation, or for those who refuse amputation.

The **prognosis** varies with the histologic type of tumor, its location in the skeleton and the age of the patient. The outlook in children under 12 is most unfavorable. The disease is characterized by early metastasis to the lung which, unfortunately, in the majority of cases has already occurred at the time amputation is performed.

Ewing's Sarcoma (Endothelioma of Bone). This neoplasm is characterized by a rapidly growing destructive process usually affecting the shafts of long bones, but at times the flat bones as well. It is found in children and adolescents, but rarely in patients past the age of 30 years. Since it may be associated with fever and leukocytosis, and the roentgenograms may closely resemble those in osteomyelitis, the differential diagnosis has proved difficult at times.

Ewing's sarcoma of bone is radiosensitive; the primary tumor can usually be subjected to long-term control by high-voltage x-rays. However, the disease metastasizes both to the lungs and to other bones with amazing constancy, so that five-year survivals in microscopically unquestioned cases are extremely rare (less than 5 per cent in our series at Memorial Hospital). Since amputation is consistently followed by metastasis and death, and since in the primary lesion long-term control by radiation can be maintained, the latter appears to be the method of choice.

Reticulum Cell Sarcoma of Bone. This is now widely accepted as a primary tumor of bone which, while microscopically similar to Ewing's sarcoma and sometimes closely resembling metastatic neuroblastoma, is nevertheless a distinct entity. It has a rather slow onset with periods of apparent quiescence, and its roentgenographic appearance is quite variable. It occurs at any age, but is most often seen in young and middle-aged adults. It is radiosensitive, perhaps more so than any malignant bone tumor. Moreover, it has by far the best prognosis. In our experience, about one half of the cases have had a five-year survival, while one third have been free of disease for a period of ten years after treatment. In addition to roentgen therapy the use of Coley's toxins is recommended. Attention is called to the great difference in prognosis of reticulum cell sarcoma as compared to Ewing's sarcoma despite their histologic similarity.

Plasma Cell Myeloma. (See chapter on Multiple Myeloma, page 1227.)

Metastatic Cancer in Bone. Any malignant tumor may metastasize to the skeletal system, but the majority do so only infrequently. Cancers of the breast, prostate, kidney, lung and thyroid, however, have a decided tendency to spread to bone. Whereas a malignant process in bone in childhood or adolescence is most apt to be a primary bone sarcoma, when it occurs after the age of 40 it is much more likely to be metastatic cancer.

Most bone metastases begin in the spongiosa and hence are marrow metastases. In patients with metastatic tumors of bone, pain may be the most constant and even the only symptom. The lesions being chiefly destructive and usually medullary in origin, swelling is often a late complaint or may be entirely absent. It is worthy of note that not infrequently the first indications of the presence of a cancer of the thyroid, lung, kidney or prostate are the symptoms and signs referable to a metastatic focus in bone. When the presence of a primary cancer is known, the diagnosis of metastatic bone involvement is usually not difficult.

Plasma cell myeloma may closely simulate multiple metastases to bone if reliance is placed solely on the roentgenographic examination.

The **treatment** of bone metastasis is palliative. Hormone therapy may be applicable to cases in which the primary tumor is prostatic or mammary. A small proportion of cases of thyroid cancer with bone metastases may be benefited by radioactive iodine. Roentgen therapy is generally worthy of trial for solitary lesions which may respond by a lessening of pain. Unfortunately, the majority of bone metastases are not radiosensitive. Relief or amelioration of suffering is the essential responsibility of the medical attendant, whose ingenuity is often sorely taxed in caring for these patients.

BRADLEY L. COLEY

References

Coley, B. L.: Neoplasms of Bone. New York, Paul B. Hoeber, Inc., 1949.

———, and Harrold, C. C.: An Analysis of Fifty-nine Cases of Osteogenic Sarcoma with Survival for Five Years or More. J. Bone & Joint Surg., 32: 307, 1950.

———, Higinbotham, N. L., and Bowden, L.: Endothelioma of Bone. Ann. Surg., 128:533, 1948.

———, Higinbotham, N. L., and Groesbeck, H. P.: Primary Reticulum-cell Sarcoma of Bone. Radiology, 55:641, 1950.

———, and Higinbotham, N. L.: Tumors of Bone. Annals of Roentgenology, Vol. XXI. New York, Paul B. Hoeber, Inc., 1953.

Ewing, J.: Diffuse Endothelioma of Bone. Proc. New York Pathol. Soc., n.s. 21:17, 1921.

Jaffe, H. L.: "Osteoid-osteoma": Benign Osteoblastic Tumor Composed of Osteoid and Atypical Bone. Arch. Surg., 31:709, 1936.

———, and Lichtenstein, L.: Benign Chondroblastoma of Bone. Am. J. Path., 18:969, 1942.

Parker, F., Jr., and Jackson, H., Jr.: Primary Reticulum-cell Sarcoma of Bone. Surg., Gynec. & Obst., 68:45, 1939.

Phemister, D. B.: Chondrosarcoma of Bone. Surg., Gynec. & Obst., 50:216, 1930.

Sherman, R. S., and Snyder, R. E.: The Roentgenological Appearance of Primary Reticulum-cell Sarcoma of Bone. Am. J. Roentgenol., 58:291, 1947.

Diseases of the Nervous System

IMPORTANT SYMPTOMS AND SIGNS

HEADACHE

Though pain always means "something wrong," with headache it most often means "wrong direction" or "wrong pace," a biologic reprimand rather than a threat. Thus the vast majority of discomforts and pains of the head stem from readily reversible bodily changes and are accompaniments of resentments and dissatisfactions. Headache may be equally intense whether its complications are malignant or benign, and though there are few instances in human experience in which so much pain may mean so little in terms of tissue injury, failure to separate the ominous from the trivial may cost life or create paralyzing fear.

Categories of Headache. The most frequently encountered headaches are vascular headaches of the migraine type and the headaches associated with sustained contraction of skeletal muscle about the face, scalp and neck ("tension headache"). Many daily recurrent ("chronic") headaches following head injury are in one or both of these categories and perhaps rank next in frequency along with certain headaches associated with sustained arterial hypertension. Next in order of frequency are the vascular headaches which accompany pyrexia, bacteremia and sepsis, as in typhoid fever, influenza, typhus fever and malaria. Headache from acute or chronic disease of the nose, paranasal spaces, ears, teeth or eyes is relatively infrequent. Even less frequent are the headaches due to intracranial disease—brain tumor, brain abscess, meningitis, arteritis, subdural and subarachnoid hemorrhage. These fortunately constitute but a small proportion of the total —less than 5 per cent. A final small group includes the head and face pain of the major neuralgias and neuritides, and the vascular headaches associated with acute or chronic hypoxic states, carbon monoxide inhalation, polycythemia vera, nitrite or nitrate administration and methemoglobinemia from any cause.

Disease involving structures below the diaphragm rarely induces headache except indirectly through fever, sepsis or bacteremia. Headache is almost invariably associated with disturbances of function and/or structure in tissues within or adjacent to the cranium. With few exceptions, pain in the head is not referred pain from other remote parts of the body. Uncommonly, referred pain in the jaw or upper neck is experienced during episodes of coronary insufficiency. Pain may also be referred to the neck and shoulder when disease involves the diaphragm or phrenic nerve.

HEADACHE MECHANISMS

Pain-Sensitive Structures of the Head. The principal pain-sensitive tissues and structures within and covering the cranium have been identified during surgical procedures on the head.

1. Of the tissues covering the cranium, all are more or less sensitive to pain, especially the arteries.

2. Of the intracranial structures, the great venous sinuses and their venous tributaries from the surface of the brain, parts of the dura at the base, the dural arteries and the cerebral arteries at the base of the brain, the fifth, seventh, ninth and tenth cranial nerves, and the upper three cervical nerves are sensitive to pain.

3. The cranium (including the diploic and emissary veins), the parenchyma of the brain, most of the dura, most of the pia-arachnoid, the ependymal lining of the ventricles and the choroid plexuses are not sensitive to pain.

The pathways for pain from pain-sensitive intracranial structures on or above the superior surface of the tentorium cerebelli are contained in the fifth cranial nerve. Pain from these structures is experienced in various regions in front of a line drawn vertically joining the ears across the top of the head, i.e., in the frontotemporoparietal region, and within and behind the eyes.

The pathways for pain from pain-sensitive

structures on or below the inferior surface of the tentorium cerebelli are contained chiefly in the ninth and tenth cranial nerves and the upper two or possible three cervical nerves. Pain from these structures is experienced in various regions behind the line just described, i.e., in the auricular, postauricular and occipital portions of the head.

MECHANISMS OF HEADACHE FROM INTERCRANIAL SOURCES

Six basic mechanisms of headache from intracranial sources have been formulated: (1) traction on and displacement of the veins that pass to the venous sinuses from the surface of the brain, and of the great venous sinuses; (2) traction on and displacement of the middle meningeal arteries; (3) traction on and displacement of the large arteries at the base of the brain and their main branches; (4) dilatation and distention of intracranial arteries; (5) inflammation in or about any of the pain-sensitive structures of the head and portions of the pia and dura at the base of the skull; and (6) direct pressure by tumors on the cranial and cervical nerves which contain many pain afferent fibers for the head.

Intracranial diseases commonly cause headache through more than one of these mechanisms and by involvement of more than one pain-sensitive structure. Traction, displacement, distention and inflammation involving cranial vascular structures are chiefly responsible for headache from intracranial sources. Traction-displacement, an important mechanism, is further discussed in connection with the headache of brain tumor.

The head pain associated with fever ("pyrexial headache"), bacteremia, sepsis, nitrite and foreign protein administration, carbon monoxide inhalation, hypoxia and asphyxia is due principally to dilatation and distention of intracranial arterial structures. A similar mechanism is the probable basis for the headaches following epileptic seizures (with or without convulsions), certain "hangover headaches," and, in some instances, migraine headache, the vascular headaches associated with arterial hypertension and Menière's disease, and headaches occurring with certain emotional states. Painful distention of intracranial arteries is likewise responsible for the headaches induced by procedures which evoke sudden, brisk elevation of the arterial blood pressure. Examples

are the headaches associated with: (a) distention of the rectum or urinary bladder in paraplegics with transection of the spinal cord above the eighth thoracic segment, (b) intravenous infusion of epinephrine, (c) the "hypertensive crises" occurring spontaneously or following abdominal massage in a patient with pheochromocytoma. There is no evidence of inflammation within or about the dilated and distended vessels during any of the aforementioned headaches.

In contrast, the headache of meningitis is primarily related to the lowered pain threshold of inflamed tissues and structures within or adjacent to the coverings of the brain. Though generalized, the inflammatory changes are usually most marked in the basal dura and pia and adjacent blood vessels and nerves at the base of the brain. Under these circumstances, the slight, usually painless arterial dilatation and distention during each cardiac systole becomes painful,—thus the characteristic throbbing headache. In addition, sepsis and bacteremia may have headache-inducing effects on arteries.

The mechanism of the headaches so frequently associated with abnormally high or low cerebrospinal fluid pressure has long been the subject of contradictory speculations. Headache can be induced in normal erect human subjects by the free drainage of approximately 20 cc. of cerebrospinal fluid, or about 10 per cent of the total amount. The intensity of such drainage headaches is reduced by the intrathecal injection of a volume of saline equal to that of spinal fluid removed or lost, by flexion or extension of the head, or by tilting the subject toward the horizontal. The intensity of drainage headache is not directly related to the estimated intracranial pressure. Significantly, however, the headache is usually intensified during intracranial venous distention secondary to bilateral jugular compression. This type of headache is primarily due to dilatation of and traction upon pain-sensitive intracranial venous structures. Its clinical analogue is the variety of headache following lumbar puncture and usually secondary to prolonged leakage of fluid through the needle hole in the slowly healing spinal dura.

When headache is associated with increased intracranial pressure, the abnormal cerebrospinal fluid pressure, *per se,* has generally been considered the cause of the head pain. However, headache due to intracranial tumor masses occurs with normal pressure, and conversely some patients may be free of headache despite a considerably elevated pressure. Further, repeated experimental elevation of the cerebrospinal fluid pressure to more than 500 mm. of water by saline infusions into the lumbar subarachnoid space consistently failed to induce headache in healthy subjects. These and other observations indicate that increased intracranial pressure is neither a prime nor an essential factor in such headaches. Instead, headaches associated with such tumor masses result from traction and displacement, by the mass, of the aforementioned pain-sensitive structures, regardless of the level of intracranial pressure.

Headache due to intracranial disease may be secondarily associated with extracranial muscle contraction headache, usually at the occiput, but often elsewhere. The mechanism of this muscle component of the head pain is discussed below.

MECHANISMS OF HEADACHE FROM EXTRACRANIAL SOURCES

As already mentioned, all of the tissues covering the cranium, especially the arteries, are more or less sensitive to pain. Six main categories of head and face pain from these tissues and related structures can be distinguished: (1) vascular headaches; (2) muscle contraction headaches; (3) headache from disease of the nose, paranasal spaces, eyes, ears and teeth; (4) craniofacial pain of the major neuralgias and the postinfectious neuritides; (5) headache due to nonspecific inflammation of cranial arteries ("Cranial Arteritis," "Temporal Arteritis"); (6) the head pain due to trauma, infection, new growth, involving extracranial tissues (see respective topics).

The Vascular Headaches. Vascular headaches are principally due to painful dilatation and distention and edema of one or more of the extracranial and probably dural branches of the external carotid artery. However, other vascular beds both within and outside the cranium may be involved.

Vascular headaches of the migraine type are most frequently associated with dilatation and distention of one or both frontal, supraorbital and superficial temporal arteries, and the usual site of the head pain is the temple or the forehead. Certain headaches associated with arterial hypertension and Menière's disease are in this category.

The lower half of the head and the face,

the upper jaw in the vicinity of the back teeth, the neck and even the shoulder, may all be the site of head pain of vascular origin. Such headaches may be accompanied by the awareness of unusually forceful throbbing in the neck. "Atypical facial neuralgia" is but one of many designations applied to headaches in this region, depending mainly upon the location of the pain. These head and face pains very probably result from dilatation and distention of the extracranial portion of the middle meningeal artery, of the internal maxillary artery, and of the other branches and the trunks of the external and the common carotid arteries.

Finally, certain headaches at the back of the head and the neck are associated with painful dilatation and distention of the postauricular and/or occipital arteries and comprise one type of "occipital neuralgia." Ergotamine tartrate, an agent which constricts cranial arteries, eliminates these headaches as effectively as it does the headache of migraine.

The Muscle Contraction Headaches. Muscle contraction headaches are due to long sustained contraction of skeletal muscle about the face, scalp and neck. Concurrent vasoconstriction of relevant nutrient cranial arteries is a very frequent finding, and the resultant ischemia contributes to the irritability of the involved muscle and the head pain.

Sustained muscle contraction and related headache are often secondarily associated with noxious stimuli arising from other cranial tissues and structures, e.g., with distended arteries from vascular headache, inflammation or other disease in the eye, ear, nose, paranasal spaces, teeth, scalp, from brain tumor, etc. Painful, sustained muscle contraction is also the primary source of many headaches associated with emotional tension states.

HEADACHES ARISING CHIEFLY FROM INTRACRANIAL STRUCTURES

Lumbar Puncture Headache and Its Management. Following lumbar puncture, headache is least likely if there is minimal loss of cerebrospinal fluid by leakage through the needle hole in the slowly healing spinal dura. This headache can be prevented by inserting a small caliber needle only once into the subarachnoid space of the immobile patient. It is uncertain whether 24 hours of bed rest, following the tap, reduces the incidence of these headaches; but if headache ensues, the recumbent position with the foot of the bed slightly elevated is usually most comfortable. The headache usually subsides spontaneously within seven to ten days and during this time useful measures are vigorous reassurance and use of suitable analgesics. Secondary muscle contraction headache may require treatment as described below.

BRAIN TUMOR HEADACHE WITH OR WITHOUT INCREASED INTRACRANIAL PRESSURE

The Quality and Intensity of Brain Tumor Headache. The headache of space-occupying intracranial lesions is deep, aching, steady, dull rather than sharp, and seldom rhythmic or throbbing. Intermittent headache is usual, but the pain is continuous in one tenth of the patients. The headache may be more intense during the acute phase of minor infections. Occasionally there is a history of headache which commences during, but persists after, the subsidence of an acute upper respiratory infection. Coughing or straining at stool may aggravate the headache. Some patients prefer the recumbent to the erect position. If there is any variation during the 24-hour cycle, headache intensity is generally worse in the morning.

Acetylsalicylic acid in 0.3 gm. amounts and local application of cold packs usually diminish the intensity of the head pain. Rarely is the headache as intense as that associated with migraine, ruptured cerebral aneurysm or meningitis, and interference with sleep is uncommon. Even when there is direct compression and extensive traction-displacement of pain-sensitive cranial nerves by slowly growing tumors, headache may be absent or slight, and rarely as intense as the pain of tic douloureux.

One less common form of intense headache is encountered in patients in the terminal phase of brain tumor. This headache is generalized, paroxysmal and agonizing, and often ends in stupor. The pain may last 30 seconds to a half hour, and then disappear as quickly as it commenced, leaving the patient exhausted. During an attack the patient may become comatose and expire.

Tumor headache, when severe, is associated with nausea, and vomiting may result from such painful stimulation. However, vomiting due to new growth may occur with slight or no nausea, even in the absence of headache, and is then the result of compression of the medulla. Such vomiting may be projectile, at least in part, because when nausea is slight or absent, vomiting is unexpected.

When the headache is occipital or suboccipital in location, it is sometimes associated with "stiffness" or aching of the muscles of the neck and tilting of the head toward the side of the lesion.

The Mechanism of Brain Tumor Headache. As already indicated, increased intracranial pressure, *per se,* is not necessarily associated with headache. Brain tumor headache results from traction-displacement of intracranial pain-sensitive structures, chiefly the large arteries, veins, venous sinuses and certain cranial nerves.

"Local traction" may be exerted by the tumor upon adjacent structures. *"Distant traction"* is consequent upon extensive displacement of the brain, effected either directly by the enlarging tumor mass, or indirectly by ventricular obstruction (internal hydrocephalus). These two types of traction may operate singly or in combination to evoke pain from structures adjacent to, as well as remote from the tumor. Hence tenderness of the scalp in a given location, a manifestation of irritation of pain-sensitive intracranial tissues, may result from disease of widely separated intracranial structures. Accordingly, since the headache of brain tumor is usually *referred pain,* the site thereof has limited value in the localization of the lesion. Not only may the headache be remote from the site inducing it, but this site itself (e.g., through distant traction) may be remote from the tumor.

Despite these limitations, knowledge of the site of brain tumor headache may aid significantly in the diagnosis and localization of the lesion, when interpreted in terms of the known principles of intracranial pain production and pain reference.

1. About one third of all brain tumor headaches approximately overlie the tumor.

2. In the absence of papilledema, headache can be of value in localizing a brain tumor. In these circumstances two thirds of headaches are near or overlying the tumor. When unilateral, the headache is on the same side as the tumor.

3. Headache is almost always present with posterior fossa tumor and is the first symptom of such tumors, excepting cerebellopontine angle tumors. The headache is almost always over the back of the head. When headache occurs

with cerebellopontine angle tumors it is frequently and sometimes solely postauricular.

4. Headache may be absent but is a first symptom in about one third of supratentorial tumors, and is usually in the front of the head. With such tumors headache rarely occurs in the back of the head as well, unless associated with papilledema.

5. When headache is both frontal and occipital, the symptom signifies extensive displacement of the brain and has little localizing value.

6. Brain tumor headache is usually intermittent. Of greater localizing value, however, is continuous headache occupying one predictable site.

In other words, when patients with brain tumors and evidence of increased intracranial pressure have headache, it is usually generalized, and hence is of little localizing significance. On the other hand, when patients with brain tumors, without papilledema or evidence of increase in intracranial pressure, have headache, its site may indicate where the intracranial tumor is. Thus, when solely unilateral and frontal, the tumor may be above the tentorium on the same side. When solely occipital, the tumor may be infratentorial, and when unilateral, on the same side. When headache is predictably localized behind one ear, acoustic neuromas and pontine angle tumors are suggested. Also, when headache is generalized, a history of its onset on the left or right, in front or in back may indicate the site of the lesion.

Management of Headache Associated with Increased Intracranial Pressure and Brain Tumor. Decompression procedures may, for short periods, diminish the pain intensity or eliminate the headaches resulting from traction-displacement of pain-sensitive structures associated with increased cerebrospinal fluid pressure, with or without an intracranial mass. Effective, though transient, decompression results from the intravenous infusion of 50 cc. of 50 per cent dextrose or sucrose. Lumbar drainage is contraindicated for the relief of headache associated with increased intracranial pressure from brain tumor and has no predictable effect on the headache of meningitis or subarachnoid hemorrhage. Rarely, ventricular puncture may reduce the intensity of the headache associated with brain tumor. Sudden changes in position from recumbent to sitting should be avoided since headache intensity may be thereby augmented. The rare headaches attributable to tumors obstructing the acqueduct of Sylvius and the posterior portion of the third ventricle may be reduced in intensity by continuous ventricular drainage through a catheter.

More lasting results are achieved by surgical removal of tumor masses. If an irremovable tumor causing headache is above the tentorium, transection of the right middle meningeal artery and the removal of a portion of the temporal bone with a stellate opening of the dura diminish the intensity of the headache. If such a tumor is in the posterior fossa, removal of a portion of the occipital bone with a stellate opening of the dura similarly reduces the headache intensity. The subsequent herniation of the brain through the defect seldom causes more than slight pain until massive displacement occurs, shortly followed by death. Sometimes surgical exploratory procedures are justified in attempts to reduce headache due to clearly defined metastatic disease, especially when the primary tumor is a known hypernephroma.

Headache resulting from craniopharyngioma or pituitary tumors does not, in itself, constitute an indication for surgical procedures. Indeed, only failing vision is a justifiable reason for such intervention. Not only are such tumors difficult to remove, but removal is no assurance that headache will be eliminated. Furthermore, such headache is not predictably reduced by creating a bony defect.

HEADACHES ARISING CHIEFLY FROM EXTRACRANIAL STRUCTURES

More than 90 per cent of the extracranial headaches are due to painful dilatation and distention of cranial arteries (e.g., migraine syndrome), and sustained contraction of skeletal muscle about the face, scalp, neck (muscle contraction headache). These headaches very commonly occur in a life setting of sustained anxiety and emotional tension. The headaches caused by inflammation or disease in the eye, ear, nose, paranasal structures, teeth and scalp are much less common.

MIGRAINE SYNDROME

Formulation of the Mechanism of the Migraine Syndrome. The migraine syndrome is a pattern of dysfunction integrated within the central nervous system and manifested as mood and widespread bodily disturbances both nonpainful and painful. The attacks may vary in duration from a few hours to several days, and in severity from trifling symptoms to prolonged disabling illness. The outstanding feature is periodic headache, usually unilateral in onset, but at times becoming bilateral or generalized. The headaches are associated with "'irritability," nausea and often photophobia, vomiting, constipation or diarrhea. Although most commonly in the temple, headaches may be experienced anywhere in the head, and in some patients there is pain in the face and neck.

For a period of several hours to several days preceding the headache, there is increased variability of the contractile state of the cranial arteries. Facial flushing, pallor and other transient cranial vasomotor phenomena may be noted. In the hour preceding the headache there is commonly constriction of the extracranial arteries as well as local constriction of the cerebral arteries or, sometimes, of retinal vessels, producing visual and other nonpainful sensory preheadache phenomena. These may take the form of scintillating scotomas or visual field defects, such as unilateral or homonymous hemianopsia. Vertigo may also appear as a forerunner of the migraine attack. As the vasoconstrictor preheadache phenomena recede, vasodilator headache manifestations commence. Sometimes these vasodilator manifestations overlap the last traces of preheadache phenomena, and sometimes the headache begins after a short symptom-free interval. The headache is characterized as a throbbing, aching pain, appreciably reduced by pressure on the common carotid artery, sometimes by pressure on a superficial artery, and by the action of ergotamine tartrate.

Painful vasodilatation sustained for several hours is often associated with a thickening or edema of the affected vascular and perivascular tissues. The soft, easily compressed arteries become rigid and relatively noncompressible. Further, the pulsatile pain becomes a nonpulsatile ache and the involved artery is usually tender to palpation. Redness and swelling of the nasal mucosa, with or without epistaxis, may occur with the headache attacks. The scalp may become more edematous and tender, at first locally and then diffusely.

Secondary to the vascular head pain, in half the cases, there is prolonged and ultimately painful contraction of the skeletal muscle of the head and neck. This muscle contraction component of the headache may outlast the vascular pain.

The migraine attack is but one aspect of a diffuse disturbance in function occurring episodically during or shortly after a stressful period in which resentment, fatigue and prolonged tension are features. In certain circumstances, even during intervals of stress, the migraine headache or preheadache phenomena may diminish, or actually fail to recur. However, other bodily or mood disturbances may be accentuated and become the basis of the dominant complaint. These other phenomena, referred to as "migraine equivalents," include a variety of abdominal, chest or extremity pains, and nonpainful attacks of vomiting, diarrhea, diffuse edema, transient mood disorder and fever.

Management and Prevention of Migraine Headache. Headaches of low intensity are usually eliminated by the oral administration of 0.3 gm. to 0.6 gm. of acetylsalicylic acid; 60 mg. of codeine phosphate may be required to reduce the intensity of moderate or severe headache.

For severe vascular headache the restoration of the painfully dilated vessels to a nonpainful constricted state is accomplished best by the intramuscular administration of 0.25 mg. to 0.5 mg. of ergotamine tartrate. Nausea and vomiting may accompany the use of this agent, and the total dose should not exceed 0.5 mg. in any one week. Although a less effective method, ergotamine tartrate may also be given by mouth in 3 mg. amounts, to be swallowed or absorbed sublingually. This first dose may be repeated in 30 minutes and a third in another 30 minutes if the headache persists. The amount so administered should not exceed 10 mg. in any one week.

Norepinephrine can terminate vascular headache without inducing nausea. It is administered by *infusion* of a 0.0008% solution in 5% dextrose in water (one 4 cc. ampule of 0.2% norepinephrine/1000 cc. solute) at a rate sufficient to raise systolic blood pressure 10–20 mm. Hg until headache is terminated, usually in 20 to 60 minutes. This rate varies from 30 to 60 drops per minute.

Resection of the superficial vessels involved in vascular headache has not been successful in eliminating the headaches except for short periods. At present there is no suitable surgical treatment for migraine headaches.

Much more important, although more difficult, is the *prevention* of attacks. Any procedure that enlists the interest or enthusiasm of the physician, and imparts to the patient the conviction that he is receiving adequate care, will diminish the frequency and intensity of the attacks for a time. Hence the large variety of recommended therapies. From this fact, it is apparent that procedures aimed at a better understanding of the patient, his life situation and the factors that constitute a threat to him can be of basic therapeutic importance.

Patients with migraine headaches are anxious, striving, perfectionistic, order-loving, rigid persons who, during periods of threat or conflict, become progressively more tense, resentful and fatigued. The elaboration of a pattern of inflexibility and perfectionism to deal with feelings of insecurity begins early in childhood. The person with migraine attempts to gain approval by doing more and better than his fellows, by "application" and "hard work," and to gain security by holding to a stable environment and a given system of excellent performance, even at a high cost of energy. This pattern brings the person increasing responsibility and admiration with but little love, so that he feels greater and greater resentment at the pace he feels obliged to maintain. During late adolescence or perhaps shortly thereafter, the increasing complexity of his life situation may lead the patient to further increase his demands upon himself despite progressively diminishing energy resources. The rigidity and inflexibility of the patient do not permit him to modify his established performance pattern. Then tension associated with repeated frustration, sustained resentment and anxiety, often followed by fatigue and prostration, become the setting in which the migraine attack occurs.

Comprehensive therapy in this area is directed toward enabling the patient to recognize and understand the basis of his anxiety and tension, the precipitating factors in his life situation that aggravate these feeling states, and to aid him in resolving his conflicts. About two out of three patients can be appreciably helped by such aid.

MUSCLES OF THE HEAD AND NECK AS SOURCES OF HEAD PAIN

The pain of muscle contraction headache is a steady nonpulsatile ache, unilateral or bilateral, in the temporal, occipital, parietal or frontal regions, or all, and in any combination. Additional descriptive terms include "tightness" bitemporally or at the occiput, bandlike sensations about the head which may become caplike in distribution, viselike ache, weight, pressure, drawing or soreness. "Cramplike" head pains are described by some patients and "feeling as if the neck and upper back were in a cast."

With prolonged sustained contraction, the muscle tissues of the head, neck and upper back become tender to palpation and there may be one or many painful, palpable, sharply localized areas or "nodules." Commonly there is pain on combing or brushing the hair, or on placing a hat upon the head. Exposure to cold and shivering may precipitate or aggravate the headache.

The patient may limit the motion of the head, neck and jaws. Pressure on the contracted, tender muscles may augment headache intensity and may elicit tinnitus, vertigo and lacrimation—features which also occur spontaneously. This procedure may also cause spread of the pain to adjacent portions of the head.

Although muscle contraction headaches may be fleeting, with frequent changes in the site and pain intensity of recurrences, this is also the type of headache which, localized in one region, may be sustained for weeks, months or even years.

Sustained painful muscle contraction may be secondary to noxious stimuli from any part of the head, and is the primary source of the headache associated with the adverse life situations of tense, aggressive, frustrated or anxious persons.

Management of Muscle Contraction Headache. Removal of the primary stimulation may eliminate the headaches secondary to noxious stimuli from disease of the eye, ear, nose and paranasal structures, or teeth. Perhaps a majority of persons with painful disease in any structure of the head may have secondary muscle contraction headache; but tense persons subject to sustained contraction of cranial skeletal muscle are especially susceptible.

Reassurance, rest, heat, massage, manipulation and manual stretching of the nuchal and occipital muscles, acetylsalicylic acid (0.3 gm. to 0.6 gm. every 2 to 3 hours for short periods) and phenobarbital (30 mg. three times a day) reduce the intensity of such headaches or completely eliminate them. Headaches resulting from trauma or infection with resultant painful sustained contraction of the involved muscles may be similarly managed. Bed rest or chair rest, local heat, submersion in warm tubs of water for 20 to 30-minute periods, and the passage of time are important adjuvants. Headaches due to sustained muscle contraction associated with life stress and emotional tension are only temporarily modified by sedative or analgesic medicaments. Treatment is best directed at an improvement in the relation of the patient to his environment, by allowing him free and repeated expression of his conflicts, resentments and dissatisfactions; by enabling him to recognize the nature of his dilemma and its relationship to the physiologic basis of his pain; by guiding him toward the acceptance of a more realistic appraisal of his needs; by encouraging appropriate modification of his environment and the establishment of a more efficient regimen compatible with his individual equipment; and especially by aiding the patient to accept the consequences of his past decisions, and the irreversibility of certain events.

RECURRENT ("CHRONIC") POST-TRAUMATIC HEADACHE

Head injury may be followed by headache from intracranial as well as extracranial sources. The intracranial headaches associated with post-traumatic subdural hematomas or subarachnoid hemorrhages are relatively infrequent. Recurrent extracranial headaches are much more common and three varieties may be distinguished: (1) Severe pain or circumscribed tenderness due to local tissue damage in a scar or at a site of impact; such tenderness may persist for years. (2) Muscle contraction headaches. (3) Attacks of throbbing and aching pain, usually unilateral in the temporal or frontal region, and due to painful dilatation and distention of certain branches of the external carotid artery, and probably other cranial arteries as well. Fleeting vertigo with sudden movement or rotation of the head often accompanies the headache.

Recurrent ("chronic") post-traumatic headache is due principally to sustained contraction of cranial skeletal muscle. Patients with such headache usually also have periodic vascular headaches. Many of these patients harbor resentment related to the circumstances of their accident, or fear that they have sustained permanent brain injury. These emotional reactions and attitudes are inti-

mately related to the mechanism and "chronicity" of post-traumatic headaches.

The *management* of post-traumatic headaches is as described for other vascular and muscle contraction headaches.

HEADACHES ASSOCIATED WITH ARTERIAL HYPERTENSION

When otherwise symptom-free, and in the absence of hypertensive encephalopathy with renal failure, or pheochromocytoma, persons with arterial hypertension may experience severe, even disabling headaches. Recent studies show that these headaches are principally of two types: (1) vascular headaches, and (2) muscle contraction headaches.

It seems clear that the contractile state of the cranial arteries is relevant to the headaches associated with sustained arterial hypertension. However, the following observations indicate that the elevated blood pressure, *per se,* is not the direct cause of the headaches, nor is the extent of this elevation directly related to the frequency or severity of the attacks. (1) Half of the patients with arterial hypertension do not have headaches, and the half that have headaches have blood pressure levels no higher than the half that do not. (2) During headache in any given person, the blood pressure level is not higher and may be lower than preheadache levels. (3) From daily records of the blood pressure level and headache incidence in such patients, headache attacks were not less frequent when the blood pressure was least elevated. Paradoxically, some of these patients did not have headaches when their blood pressure elevation was maximal. (4) Certain individuals with sustained arterial hypertension were headache-free for many years, whereas others who had headaches lost them as the blood pressure was further elevated with time. The onset or cessation of headaches in such patients was not associated with any detectable change in the blood pressure levels.

Management of Headache Associated with Arterial Hypertension. The headache associated with arterial hypertension often regresses spontaneously with reassurance, bed rest, sedative medication and the passage of time, especially when the patient is hospitalized. These headaches resemble the vascular headaches of migraine, and of sustained contraction of cranial skeletal muscle, in the mechanism of the pain, and the relation to life stress, fatigue and emotional tension. The management is also similar except that ergotamine tartrate is not used.

The headache associated with hypertensive encephalopathy with renal failure, high intracranial pressure and the distortion of pain-sensitive structures is occasionally reduced in intensity by lumbar spinal drainage. However, this procedure is not often effective, since increased cerebrospinal fluid pressure, *per se,* is not the cause of the headache.

NASAL AND PARANASAL STRUCTURES AS SOURCES OF HEADACHE AND OTHER HEAD PAIN

During experimental stimulation of various sites within the nasal and paranasal structures, the ostia of the maxillary and frontal sinuses were found to be most pain-sensitive and many times more sensitive than the sinus walls, which are relatively insensitive to pain. Numerous sites of stimulation evoked pain similarly referred: over the zygoma, into the upper teeth, and the temporal and frontal regions. Stimulation of structures near the midline results in the same area of referred pain as does stimulation of the ostium and the more lateral wall of the maxillary sinus. It is therefore likely that most of the discomfort from infection in this region stems from the nasal rather than the paranasal structures.

The location of "sinus" headache is diffusely frontal (frontal sinuses), zygomatic and nasal (antral disease), or occasionally (sphenoid and ethmoid disease) behind the eyes and over the vertex. Pain at the back of the head and the neck is usually due to secondary sustained skeletal muscle contraction. Typically, "sinus" headache commences in the morning (frontal), or early afternoon (maxillary) and subsides in the early or late evening.

The pain of "sinus" disease is dull and aching and seldom if ever associated with nausea or vomiting. Pain intensity is increased by shaking the head or holding it dependent. Measures that increase the venous pressure, e.g., straining, coughing or a tight collar, aggravate the headache. The pain intensity is also augmented by states that increase the engorgement of the mucosa, such as anxiety and resentment, menstruation, cold air, sexual excitement or the effects of alcohol.

Low intensity headache accompanies chronic sinus disease, but even though increased with acute disease, the pain intensity is not as great as in some instances of migraine, meningitis or certain febrile diseases.

Pain from disease of the nose and paranasal sinuses is due to mucosal inflammation and engorgement of the turbinates, ostia, nasofrontal ducts and superior nasal spaces. Headache not associated with turbinate engorgement and inflammation is probably not due to nose or sinus disease. Nor is disease of these structures commonly the cause of frontal, temporal, zygomatic or vertex headache, if the pain intensity is not greatly reduced or eliminated by intranasal application of vasoconstrictor agents or topical anesthetics, especially about the ostia to the sinuses.

Mucosal engorgement of the superior nasal spaces, and related headache, are frequently encountered as part of the life adjustment of certain resentful and anxious individuals. An infectious basis for such engorgement is by no means universal.

Suppurative disease in the frontal, ethmoid and sphenoid sinuses, or the mastoid air cells, may result in osteomyelitis and inflammation of adjacent cranial tissues. The development or persistence of headache following surgical drainage of the diseased sinus is evidence for extradural and possibly subdural infection.

HEAD PAIN AND DISEASE OF THE TEETH

The second and third divisions of the fifth cranial nerve contain afferent fibers for sensation in the teeth. Noxious stimuli arising in a tooth usually evoke local toothache. Tissues remote from the source of such stimuli may also exhibit surface hyperalgesia, tenderness and vasomotor reactions—such as tender eyeballs, reddening of the conjunctivas and tenderness of the auricular and temporal tissues. Other tender sites may be noted in the occiput, behind the ears, behind the lower border of the mastoid process, and in the muscles about the lower neck and shoulders.

Rarely, prolonged intense toothache is associated with headache at a distance from the involved tooth, in areas supplied by the first as well as the second and third divisions of the trigeminal nerve. Secondary muscle contraction headache in the occiput is usual.

The teeth in the upper jaw are frequently the site of tenderness and pain in association with disease of the nasal and paranasal structures. Occasionally, in coronary insufficiency, pain is experienced in the lower jaw because of the close approximation of the